# *Current*
# Medical
# Diagnosis &
# Treatment 1988

*From inability to let well alone; from too much zeal for the new and contempt for what is old; from putting knowledge before wisdom, science before art and cleverness before common sense; from treating patients as cases; and from making the cure of the disease more grievous than the endurance of the same, Good Lord, deliver us.*

—Sir Robert Hutchison

# *Current* Medical Diagnosis & Treatment 1988

Edited By

**STEVEN A. SCHROEDER, MD**
Professor of Medicine and Chief
Division of General Internal Medicine
University of California, San Francisco

**MARCUS A. KRUPP, MD**
Clinical Professor of Medicine Emeritus
Stanford University School of Medicine, Stanford
Director (Emeritus) of Research Institute
Palo Alto Medical Foundation, Palo Alto

**LAWRENCE M. TIERNEY, JR., MD**
Professor of Medicine
University of California, San Francisco
Assistant Chief of Medical Services
Veterans Administration Medical Center, San Francisco

with Associate Authors

**APPLETON & LANGE**
Norwalk, Connecticut/San Mateo, California

0-8385-1344-1

**Spanish Edition:** Editorial El Manual Moderno, S.A. de C.V.,
   Av. Sonora 206, Col. Hipodromo, 06100-Mexico, D.F.
**Italian Edition:** Piccin Nuova Libraria, S.p.A., Via Altinate, 107,
   35121 Padua, Italy
**German Edition:** Springer-Verlag GmbH & Co. KG, Postfach 10 52 80,
   6900 Heidelberg 1, West Germany
**Serbo-Croatian Edition:** Savremena Administracija, Crnotravska 7-9,
   11100 Belgrade, Yugoslavia
**Portuguese Edition:** Atheneu Editora São Paulo Ltda.,
   Rua Marconi, 131 – 2.o andar, 01047 São Paulo, Brazil
**Greek Edition:** Gregory Parisianos, 20, Navarinou Street,
   GR-106 80 Athens, Greece
**Dutch Edition:** Kooyker Scientific Publications B.V., Postbus 24,
   2300 AA Leiden, The Netherlands

88 / 5 4 3 2 1

Prentice-Hall of Australia, Pty. Ltd., Sydney
Prentice-Hall Canada, Inc.
Prentice-Hall Hispanoamericana, S.A., Mexico
Prentice-Hall of India Private Limited, New Delhi
Prentice-Hall International (UK) Limited, London
Prentice-Hall of Japan, Inc., Tokyo
Prentice-Hall of Southeast Asia (Pte.) Ltd., Singapore
Whitehall Books Ltd., Wellington, New Zealand
Editora Prentice-Hall do Brasil Ltda., Rio de Janeiro

ISSN: 0092–8682
ISBN: 0–8385–1344–1

Cover: M. Chandler Martylewski

PRINTED IN THE UNITED STATES OF AMERICA

# Table of Contents

# The Authors

**Michael J. Aminoff, MD, FRCP**
Professor of Neurology, University of California, San Francisco.

**Robert B. Baron, MD**
Assistant Clinical Professor of Medicine, University of California, San Francisco.

**R. Laurence Berkowitz, MD**
Clinical Assistant Professor of Plastic & Reconstructive Surgery, Stanford University School of Medicine, Stanford, California.

**James J. Brophy, MD**
Associate Clinical Professor of Psychiatry, University of California School of Medicine, San Diego, California.

**Carlos A. Camargo, MD**
Associate Clinical Professor of Medicine, Stanford University School of Medicine, Stanford, California.

**Milton J. Chatton, MD**
Clinical Professor of Medicine Emeritus, Stanford University School of Medicine, Stanford, California; and Senior Attending Physician, Santa Clara Valley Medicine Center, San Jose, California.

**Richard Cohen, MD, MPH**
Assistant Clinical Professor, Division of Occupational Medicine, University of California, San Francisco.

**Robert H. Dreisbach, MD, PhD**
Clinical Professor of Environmental Health, School of Public Health and Community Medicine, University of Washington, Seattle.

**Lawrence Z. Feigenbaum, MD**
Clinical Professor of Medicine, University of California, San Francisco; and Director of Professional Services and Medical Education and Director of Institute on Aging, Mount Zion Hospital and Medical Center, San Francisco.

**Armando E. Giuliano, MD**
Associate Professor of Surgery, University of California, Los Angeles.

**Robert S. Goldsmith, MD, MPH, DTM&H**
Professor of Tropical Medicine and Epidemiology, University of California, San Francisco.

**Sadja Greenwood, MD, MPH**
Assistant Clinical Professor of Obstetrics, Gynecology, and Reproductive Sciences, University of California, San Francisco.

**Moses Grossman, MD**
Professor of Pediatrics, University of California, San Francisco; and Chief of Pediatrics, San Francisco General Hospital.

**Carlyn Halde, PhD**
Professor of Microbiology and Immunology and Professor of Dermatology, University of California (San Francisco).

**Richard A. Jacobs, MD, PhD**
Assistant Clinical Professor of Medicine and Co-Director, Outpatient Infectious Disease Service, University of California (San Francisco).

**Robert K. Jackler, MD**
Assistant Professor of Otolaryngology, University of California (San Francisco).

**Ernest Jawetz, MD, PhD**
Professor of Microbiology and Medicine Emeritus, University of California, San Francisco.

**Michael J. Kaplan, MD**
Assistant Professor, Department of Otolaryngology-Head and Neck Surgery, University of California (San Francisco); and Chief, Otolaryngology-Head and Neck Surgery, San Francisco Veterans Administration Medical Center.

**C. Michael Knauer, MD**
Chief of Division of Gastroenterology, Santa Clara Valley Medical Center, San Jose, California; and Clinical Professor of Medicine, Stanford University School of Medicine, Stanford, California.

**Felix O. Kolb, MD**
Clinical Professor of Medicine, University of California, San Francisco.

**Margaret S. Kosek, MD**
Staff Physician, Palo Alto Medical Foundation, Palo Alto, California.

**Marcus A. Krupp, MD**
Clinical Professor of Medicine Emeritus, Stanford University School of Medicine, Stanford, California; and Director (Emeritus) of Research Institute, Palo Alto Medical Foundation, Palo Alto, California.

**Joseph LaDou, MD**
Associate Clinical Professor of Medicine and Acting Chief, Division of Occupational Medicine, University of California, San Francisco.

**Charles A. Linker, MD**
Associate Clinical Professor of Medicine, University of California (San Francisco).

**Alan J. Margolis, MD**
Professor of Obstetrics, Gynecology, and Reproductive Sciences, University of California, San Francisco.

**Barry Massie, MD**
Associate Professor of Medicine, University of California (San Francisco); Associate Staff Member, Cardiovascular Research Institute; and Chief, Hypertension Unit, and Director, Coronary Care Unit, San Francisco Veterans Administration Medical Center.

**Richard B. Odom, MD**
Clinical Professor of Dermatology, University of California (San Francisco).

**Kent R. Olson, MD**
Assistant Clinical Professor of Medicine and Adjunct Lecturer in Pharmacy, University of California, San Francisco; and Director of San Francisco Bay Area Regional Poison Control Center.

**Rees B. Rees, Jr., MD**
Clinical Professor of Dermatology Emeritus, University of California, San Francisco.

**Sydney E. Salmon, MD**
Professor of Internal Medicine and of Hematology and Oncology, University of Arizona College of Medicine, Tucson, Arizona; and Director of Arizona Cancer Center, Tucson.

**Steven A. Schroeder, MD**
Professor of Medicine and Chief, Division of General Internal Medicine, University of California, San Francisco.

**Martin A. Shearn, MD**
Clinical Professor of Medicine, University of California, San Francisco.

**Sol Silverman, Jr., DDS**
Professor of Oral Medicine and Chairman of the Division, University of California, San Francisco.

**Maurice Sokolow, MD**
Professor of Medicine Emeritus and Senior Staff Member, Cardiovascular Research Institute, University of California, San Francisco.

**John L. Stauffer, MD**
Associate Professor of Medicine, Milton S. Hershey Medical Center, Pennsylvania State University, Hershey, Pennsylvania.

**Daniel P. Stites, MD**
Professor of Laboratory Medicine and Director of Section on Immunology and Blood Banking, University of California (San Francisco).

**Lawrence M. Tierney, Jr., MD**
Professor of Medicine, University of California, San Francisco; and Assistant Chief of Medical Services, San Francisco Veterans Administration Medical Center.

**Daniel Vaughan, MD**
Clinical Professor of Ophthalmology, University of California, San Francisco; and Member, Francis I. Proctor Foundation for Research in Ophthalmology, San Francisco.

**Susan D. Wall, MD**
Assistant Professor of Radiology, University of California (San Francisco); and Assistant Chief of Radiology, San Francisco Veterans Administration Medical Center.

**Ralph O. Wallerstein, MD**
Clinical Professor of Medicine, University of California, San Francisco.

# Preface

*Current Medical Diagnosis & Treatment 1988* is the twenty-seventh annual revision of a general medical text designed to function as the complete physician's single most useful source of information about adult medicine. The practical features of patient management are emphasized. Appropriate background information is provided as necessary to facilitate understanding of concepts.

## OUTSTANDING FEATURES

- Reissued annually in Jan/Feb to incorporate current advances.
- Over 1000 diseases and disorders.
- All aspects of internal medicine *plus* obstetrics/gynecology, dermatology, ophthalmology, neurology, and other topics of concern to the office practitioner.
- Consistent readable format, permitting efficient use in various practice settings.
- Selected references.

## INTENDED AUDIENCE

*House officers and students* will find the concise descriptions of diagnostic and therapeutic procedures, with access to the current literature, of daily usefulness in the immediate management of patients.

*Internists, family physicians, and other specialists* will find *CMDT* useful as a ready reference and refresher text.

*Physicians in other specialties, surgeons, and dentists* will find the book useful as a basic treatise on internal medicine,

*Nurses and other health practitioners* will find that the concise format and broad scope of the book facilitate their understanding of diagnostic principles and therapeutic procedures.

## ORGANIZATION

*CMDT* is developed chiefly by organ system. Chapters 1–3 present general information on patient care,

including disease prevention, pain management, special problems of the elderly patient, and fluid/electrolyte therapy. Chapters 4–19 describe diseases and disorders and their treatment. Chapter 20 sets forth the basic concepts of nutrition in modern medical practice. Chapters 21–28 cover infectious diseases and antimicrobial therapy. Chapters 29–33 cover special topics: physical agents, poisoning, genetics, malignant disorders, and immunologic disorders. The appendix provides data on normal values of daily relevance to medical practice as well as sections on MRI, CPR, and the emergency treatment of airway obstruction.

## NEW TO THIS EDITION

- Revised, expanded, and updated section on AIDS.
- Complete revision of chapters on Blood, ENT, and the Heart and Great Vessels.
- Extensive revision of the chapters on Pulmonary Diseases, Nutrition, and Poisoning.
- Drug information and bibliographies updated through July 1987.
- New section in Appendix on MRI.
- Increased emphasis on costs of medical care and on prevention.

## ACKNOWLEDGEMENTS

We wish to thank our associate authors for participating once again in the annual effort of updating this important book. Many students and physicians have contributed useful suggestions to this and previous editions, and we are grateful. We continue to solicit comments and recommendations for future editions. Please address correspondence to us at Lange Medical Publications, 2755 Campus Drive, Suite 205, San Mateo, CA 94403.

Steven A. Schroeder
Marcus A. Krupp
Lawrence M. Tierney, Jr.

*January, 1988*

# *Current* Medical Diagnosis & Treatment 1988

# General Care—Symptoms & Disease Prevention

**1**

*Steven A. Schroeder, MD, & Milton J. Chatton, MD*

## DISEASE PREVENTION

Preventing disease is more important than treating it. Preventive medicine is categorized as primary, secondary, or tertiary. Examples in the case of cancer are giving up or not starting smoking, thereby reducing the incidence of lung carcinoma (primary prevention); routine periodic surveillance by cervical Papanicolaou smear (secondary prevention); and mastectomy to remove localized breast cancer (tertiary prevention). Primary prevention is by far the most effective and economical of all methods of disease control.

## INFECTIOUS DISEASES

**Immunization** remains the best means of preventing many infectious diseases, including tetanus, diphtheria, poliomyelitis, measles, mumps, hepatitis B, yellow fever, influenza, and pneumococcal pneumonia. Recommended immunization schedules for children and adults are set forth in Chapter 21.

**Skin testing for tuberculosis** and then treating selected skin-positive patients with prophylactic isoniazid reduces the risk of reactivation tuberculosis. Treatment is recommended for high-risk reactors regardless of age. These patients include recent tuberculin converters, postgastrectomy patients, persons taking immunosuppressive drugs, and patients with silicosis. For tuberculin-positive patients without these risk factors, treatment with isoniazid is recommended only for those under the age of 35 in order to minimize the risk of hepatitis. It now appears that prophylaxis for only 6 months (300 mg daily) is as effective as 12 months. BCG vaccine should be reserved for use in selected cases, such as protection of health workers in areas where tuberculosis is endemic.

The impressive 20th century accomplishments in immunization and antibiotic therapy notwithstanding, much of the decline in the incidence and fatality rates of infectious diseases is attributable to public health measures—especially improved sanitation, better nutrition, and greater prosperity.

**AIDS** is now the major infectious disease problem in the Western world. Until a vaccine or cure is found, prevention will be the only weapon against this disease. Since sexual contact is the usual mode of transmission, prevention must rely on safe sexual practices. These include abstinence, prudent selection of partners, avoidance of promiscuity, the use of condoms, and the limiting or avoidance of anal and oral sex except with partners known to be uninfected.

## CARDIOVASCULAR & CEREBROVASCULAR DISEASES

Impressive declines in age-specific mortality rates from heart disease and stroke have been achieved in all age groups in North America during the past 2 decades. The chief reason for this favorable trend appears to be a reduction in risk factors, especially cigarette smoking, hypercholesterolemia, and hypertension.

### Cigarette Smoking

Cigarette smoking remains the most important cause of preventable morbidity and early demise in developed countries. Smokers die 5–8 years earlier than nonsmokers; have twice the risk of fatal heart disease; 10 times the risk of lung cancer; several times the risk of cancers of the mouth, throat, esophagus, pancreas, kidney, bladder, and cervix; a 2- to 3-fold greater incidence of peptic ulcers (which heal less well than in nonsmokers); and about a 2- to 4-fold greater risk of fractures of the hip, wrist, and vertebrae.

The children of parents who smoke have lower birth weights, more frequent respiratory infections, less efficient pulmonary function, and a higher incidence of chronic ear infections than the children of nonsmokers and are more likely to become smokers themselves.

Recently there has been an encouraging national trend in North America away from smoking, so that now less than a third of all Americans smoke. To the clinician, the established smoker is a vexing problem, since many people who stop smoking do so without a doctor's help, leaving the clinician to deal with the recalcitrant heavily addicted smokers who need help but won't accept it.

The clinician should adopt a 3-step smoking cessation strategy with smoking patients: (1) Ask the patient about smoking and interest in quitting. (2) Motivate the patient to stop smoking. (3) Set a date to stop entirely, and follow up to find out what happens.

Pharmacologic aids have not been effective. Nicotine gum may be useful for some patients, but it is expensive and maintains the addiction. Clinicians should avoid appearing to disapprove of patients who are unable to stop smoking. Concerned exhortation, family or social pressures, or the opportunity presented by an intercurrent illness may eventually enable even the most addicted chronic smoker to give up the habit.

## Hypercholesterolemia

A National Institutes of Health Consensus Panel has recently concluded that lowering definitely elevated LDL cholesterol concentrations will reduce the risk from coronary heart disease. It is estimated that each 1% reduction in blood cholesterol yields about a 2% reduction in coronary heart disease. The data in Table 1–1 can be used as a guide to when dietary and other measures to lower blood cholesterol should be instituted. A recent model for assessing the benefits of lowering blood cholesterol levels, however, indicates that the calculated gain in life expectancy is low, especially in patients without other risk factors such as cigarette smoking and hypertension. Surprisingly, treatment of hypercholesterolemia conveys more benefit in women than in men.

Specific methods of therapy, which include diet, weight reduction, exercise, and drugs, are discussed in Chapter 19.

## Hypertension

Over 60 million adults in the USA have hypertension. It is well recognized that hypertension is a continuous and not a dichotomous risk factor. In every adult age group, higher values of systolic and diastolic blood pressure carry greater risks of stroke and congestive heart failure. Even so, clinicians must be able to apply specific blood pressure criteria as a means of deciding at what levels treatment should be considered in individual cases. Table 1–2 presents a classification of hypertension based on blood pressures that was developed in 1984 by the United States National High Blood Pressure Coordinating Committee of the National Institutes of Health. During the past 15 years, there have been great improvements in detection and control of hypertension, so that now about 65% of hypertensive patients in the United States are adequately controlled, compared with only 16% in 1972.

**Table 1–1.** NIH guidelines for treatment of hypercholesterolemia.

| Age (years) | Moderate Risk (mg/dL) | High Risk (mg/dL) |
|---|---|---|
| 20–29 | >200 | >220 |
| 30–39 | >220 | >240 |
| >40 | >240 | >260 |

**Table 1–2.** Classification of blood pressure in individuals aged 18 years or older.

| | Category* |
|---|---|
| **Diastolic blood pressure (DBP) (mm Hg)** | |
| <85 | Normal blood pressure |
| 85–89 | High normal blood pressure |
| 90–104 | Mild hypertension |
| 105–114 | Moderate hypertension |
| ≥115 | Severe hypertension |
| **Systolic blood pressure (SBP) (mm Hg) when DBP <90 mm Hg** | |
| <140 | Normal blood pressure |
| 140–159 | Borderline isolated systolic hypertension |
| ≥160 | Isolated systolic hypertension |

* A classification of borderline isolated systolic hypertension (SBP 140–159 mm Hg) or isolated systolic hypertension (SBP ≥160 mm Hg) takes precedence over a classification of high normal blood pressure (DBP 85–89 mm Hg) when both occur in the same individual. A classification of high normal blood pressure (DBP 85–89 mm Hg) takes precedence over a classification of normal blood pressure (SBP <140 mm Hg) when both occur in the same person.

**A. Indications for Starting Treatment:** Before specific therapy is recommended, the diagnosis of hypertension should be confirmed on at least 2 additional office visits. Controversy continues over at just what blood pressure level treatment should be started. All agree that treatment is indicated for sustained diastolic blood pressure readings over 100 mm Hg and not indicated for diastolic pressures under 90 mm Hg. In the case of patients with diastolic readings between 90 and 100 mm Hg and those with isolated high systolic readings, clinicians must decide on an individual basis whether to begin treatment or continue to observe the patient.

**B. Treatment:** Treatment strategies include nonpharmacologic interventions (most effective for mild hypertension) such as dietary salt and alcohol restriction, weight reduction, exercise programs, and relaxation techniques as well as specific antihypertensive drug therapy as set forth in detail in Chapter 8.

## CANCER

### Primary Prevention

Cigarette smoking is the most important preventable cause of cancer. Primary prevention of skin cancer consists of restricting exposure to ultraviolet light by wearing appropriate clothing and use of sunscreens. Prevention of occupationally induced cancers involves minimizing exposure to carcinogenic substances such as asbestos, ionizing radiation, and benzene compounds.

## Secondary Prevention

Generally recognized and used techniques exist for secondary prevention of cancers of the breast, colon, and cervix through cancer screening procedures (Table 1–3). Screening for other cancers in normal asymptomatic or even high-risk segments of the population is not generally recommended. There is even some controversy about the cost effectiveness, frequency, and age categories flagged for screening in Table 1–3.

## ACCIDENTS & VIOLENCE

Accidents remain the most important cause of loss of potential years of life before age 65, followed by cancer, heart disease, and suicide and homicide. Despite incontrovertible evidence that seat belt use protects against serious injury and death in motor vehicle accidents, fewer than 30% of all adults use seat belts routinely. As part of routine medical care, physicians should try to educate their patients about seat belts, drinking and driving, and gun safety in the home. Males age 16–35 are at especially high risk for serious injury and death from accidents and violence.

## THE PHYSICIAN-PATIENT RELATIONSHIP

One of the most effective therapeutic tools available to the clinician is a confident and trusting relationship with the patient. Good communication is essential to maximize the effects of therapy by ensuring patient compliance, helping patients to understand and choose among therapeutic options, and enabling them to bear the burden of serious illness and death. The old French folk saying, "To cure sometimes, to relieve often, to comfort always" is as apt today as it was 5 centuries ago.

**Table 1–3.** American Cancer Society (1983) guidelines for the early detection of cancer in people without symptoms.

| Test or Procedure | Sex | Age | Frequency |
|---|---|---|---|
| Sigmoidoscopy | M&F | Over 50 | Every 3–5 years after 2 negative examinations 1 year apart. |
| Stool guaiac slide test | M&F | Over 50 | Every year. |
| Digital rectal examination | M&F | Over 40 | Every year. |
| Papanicolaou test | F | 20–65; under 20 if sexually active. | At least every 3 years after 2 negative examinations 1 year apart. |
| Pelvic examination | F | 20–40 | Every 3 years. |
| | | Over 40 | Every year. |
| Endometrial tissue sample | F | At menopause; women at high risk.[*] | At menopause. |
| Breast self-examination | F | Over 20 | Every month. |
| Breast physical examination | F | 20–40 | Every 3 years. |
| | | Over 40 | Every year. |
| Mammography | F | 35–39 | Baseline. |
| | | 40–49 | Every 1–2 years. |
| | | 50+ | Every year. |
| Chest x-ray | | | Not recommended. |
| Sputum cytologic examination | | | Not recommended. |
| Health counseling and cancer checkup[†] | M&F | Over 20 | Every 3 years. |
| | | Over 40 | Every year. |

[*] History of infertility, obesity, failure of ovulation, abnormal uterine bleeding, or estrogen therapy.
[†] To include examination for cancers of the thyroid, testicles, prostate, ovaries, lymph nodes, oral region, and skin.

American Cancer Society: *1985 Cancer Facts and Figures.* American Cancer Society, 1985.

Centers for Disease Control: Advancements in meeting the 1990 hypertensive objectives. *MMWR* (March 20) 1987; **36**:144.

Centers for Disease Control: General recommendations on immunization. *Ann Intern Med* 1983;**98**:615.

Consensus Conference: Lower blood cholesterol to prevent heart disease. *JAMA* 1985;**253**:2080.

Fielding JE: Smoking: Health effects and control. (2 parts.) *N Engl J Med* 1985;**313**:491, 555.

National Committee on Detection, Evaluation, and Treatment of High Blood Pressure: The 1984 Report of the Joint National Committee on Detection, Evaluation, and Treatment of High Blood Pressure: *Arch Intern Med* 1984;**144**:1045.

Taylor WC et al: Cholesterol reduction and life expectancy: A model incorporating multiple risk factors. *Ann Intern Med* 1987;**106**:605.

## GENERAL SYMPTOMS

### PAIN

#### Approach to the Patient

Pain is the most common symptom causing patients to seek medical attention. It can provide the clinician with important diagnostic information. Because pain is a highly subjective phenomenon, the patient's description may be difficult to interpret. Information about the timing, nature, location, and radiation is crucial for proper treatment; the same is true for aggravating or alleviating factors.

Many emotional and cultural factors influence the perception of pain. The primary cause (eg, trauma, infection), pathogenesis (eg, inflammation, ischemia), and contributory factors (eg, recent changes in life situation, symbolic attributes of pain) must all be sought for.

Administration of a systemic analgesic is the usual method of pain management, but many other nonpharmacologic methods are useful. Examples include graded physical activity, simple reassurance, support groups, biofeedback training, and transcutaneous electrical nerve stimulation.

## 1. DRUGS FOR SEVERE PAIN

The addicting analgesics—narcotics, opioids—are indicated for severe pain that cannot be relieved with less effective agents. Examples are the pain of severe trauma, myocardial infarction, ureteral stone, and postoperative pain. Table 1–4 lists the addicting analgesics with some of their characteristics.

These drugs have pharmacologic similarities to opium. They are employed principally for the control of severe pain, but they also act to suppress severe cough and gastrointestinal motility. All can produce **physical dependence,** but to varying degrees and after varying periods of use. The risk of addiction or habituation should not prevent their appropriate use, especially in the management of terminal illness.

*A common error in management of pain from cancer is to prescribe insufficient doses "prn" rather than adequate doses around-the-clock at stated intervals.* In such cases, the major goal of management should be patient comfort.

The "Brompton cocktail," a mixture of heroin or morphine, cocaine, a phenothiazine, alcohol, and chloroform water for oral administration, was widely publicized as an effective analgesic in British hospices. Subsequent studies have shown that morphine alone is just as effective. The effects of all narcotics are reversed by naloxone. Continued use produces tolerance, so that increasing doses are needed to produce the same analgesic effect.

### Contraindications

The narcotic drugs are contraindicated in some acute illnesses. In acute abdomen, for example, the pattern of pain may provide important diagnostic clues; and in acute head injuries these drugs interfere with clinical interpretation of neurologic changes.

### Adverse Effects

The drugs in this category have the potential adverse effects listed below. Patients with hypothyroidism, adrenal insufficiency, hypopituitarism, reduced blood volume, and severe debility are particularly apt to suffer adverse effects from the addicting analgesics.

(1) Opioid narcotics should be given with great caution to patients with pulmonary insufficiency, because of dose-dependent respiratory depression.

(2) Central nervous system effects include sedation, euphoria, nausea, and vomiting. Antidepres-

**Table 1–4.** Useful narcotic analgesics.[*]

| | Approximate Equivalent Dose (mg) | Oral:Parenteral Potency Ratio | Duration of Analgesia (hours) | Maximum Efficacy | Addiction/Abuse Liability |
|---|---|---|---|---|---|
| Morphine | 10 | Low | 4–5 | High | High |
| Hydromorphone (Dilaudid) | 1.5 | Low | 4–5 | High | High |
| Oxymorphone (Numorphan) | 1.5 | Low | 3–4 | High | High |
| Methadone (Dolophine) | 10 | High | 4–6 | High | High |
| Meperidine (Demerol) | 60–100 | Low | 2–4 | High | High |
| Codeine | 30–60[†] | High | 3–4 | Low | Medium |
| Oxycodone[‡] (Percodan) | 4.5[†] | Medium | 3–4 | Moderate | Medium |
| Propoxyphene (Darvon) | 60–120[†] | Oral use only | 4–5 | Very low | Low/medium |
| Pentazocine (Talwin) | 30–50[†] | Medium | 3–4 | Moderate | Low/medium |

[*] Modified and reproduced, with permission, from Katzung BG (editor): *Basic & Clinical Pharmacology,* 3rd ed. Appleton-Lange, 1987.
[†] Analgesic efficacy at this dose not equivalent to 10 mg of morphine. See text for explanation.
[‡] Available only in tablets containing aspirin (Percodan) or acetaminophen (Percocet).

sants, antihistamines, phenothiazines, and hypnotics can potentiate these effects.

(3) Cardiovascular effects of particular importance are hypotension and circulatory collapse, though this is less common than hypoventilation.

(4) Gastrointestinal effects are chiefly decreased bowel motility and consequent constipation.

(5) Genitourinary effects include bladder spasm and urinary retention.

(6) Enhanced sensitivity to the drugs occurs in patients with hepatic insufficiency; biliary spasm may cause severe biliary colic.

(7) Allergic manifestations also occur, but rarely.

## Frequently Used Addictive Analgesics

**A. Morphine sulfate,** 8–15 mg subcutaneously or intramuscularly, is the most effective drug for control of severe pain. The effects last 4–5 hours. In acute anterior myocardial infarction or in acute pulmonary edema due to left ventricular failure, 2–6 mg may be injected slowly intravenously in 5 mL of saline solution.

**B. Morphine congeners** give effects equivalent to 10 mg of morphine sulfate but have no specific advantages—eg, hydromorphone or oxymorphone, 2–4 mg of either orally every 4 hours, or 1–3 mg of either subcutaneously every 4 hours.

**C. Meperidine (Demerol),** 50–150 mg orally or intramuscularly every 3–4 hours, provides analgesia similar to that achieved with morphine. Its indications and side effects are similar to those of morphine. Some clinicians prefer its use in inferior wall myocardial infarction, as it is less vagotonic.

**D. Methadone,** 10 mg orally, is most often used for treatment of addiction. Its side effects are similar to those of morphine, but tolerance and physical dependence are slower to develop.

**E. Codeine** (sulfate or phosphate), 15–65 mg orally or subcutaneously every 4–6 hours, is somewhat less effective than morphine but also less habit-forming. It is often given together with aspirin or acetaminophen for enhanced analgesic effect. Codeine is a powerful cough suppressant in a dose of 15–30 mg orally every 4 hours but is constipating.

**F. Oxycodone** is given orally and prescribed with another analgesic. The dosage is 5 mg every 4–6 hours in tablets that contain aspirin (Percodan) or acetaminophen (Percocet).

**G. Propoxyphene (Darvon),** 65 mg orally every 4–6 hours, has an analgesic effect little better than that of aspirin, but the side effects are minimal. When the drug is combined with aspirin or acetaminophen, the analgesic action is enhanced but is still similar to optimal doses of aspirin. Compared with other drugs in this category, it has a low potential for addiction.

**H. Pentazocine (Talwin),** 50 mg orally or 30 mg intramuscularly every 3–4 hours, is one of a group of agonist–antagonist opioids—ie, it can induce withdrawal symptoms in addicts while also having a morphinelike action. It has moderate analgesic action. Pentazocine offers little advantage, can cause addiction, and is less effective than morphine.

## 2. DRUGS FOR MODERATE OR MILD PAIN

Most people can manage their minor aches and pains with OTC analgesics available at the drug store or food store. Drugs such as codeine, oxycodone, and pentazocine, listed above as ''addictive narcotics,'' are sometimes used for moderate pain, but salicylates or acetaminophen in higher doses or the highly visible class of NSAIDs are often better for this purpose. (See Table 1–5.)

The activity—both anti-inflammatory and analgesic—of aspirin and other NSAIDs is mediated through inhibition of the biosynthesis of prostaglandins. All of these drugs to varying degrees inhibit prothrombin synthesis and platelet aggregation and may cause gastric irritation and kidney damage. All NSAIDs are analgesic, antipyretic, and anti-inflammatory in dose-dependent fashion. Their principal uses are in the control of moderate pain of arthritis (rheumatoid, degenerative, etc), other musculoskeletal disorders, menstrual cramps, and other—mainly self-limited—conditions, including moderate postoperative discomfort. Suicide attempts with overdoses of NSAIDs are less serious and less often successful than attempts with aspirin.

Table 1–5 lists the most commonly used NSAIDs along with dosages and pertinent comments.

The ability to tolerate minor degrees of discomfort varies greatly in different individuals. The most widely used agents for these purposes are aspirin and acetaminophen.

**Aspirin** is the drug of first choice for management of mild to moderate pain and is an effective antipyretic and anti-inflammatory agent. Analgesia is achieved with much lower doses and blood levels than are needed for anti-inflammatory action. Aspirin is available in many forms for oral administration in a single 325-mg unit dose, as well as smaller (eg, 60 mg) and larger (eg, 500 mg) doses. The usual dose is 2 tablets (650 mg) every 4 hours as needed, taken with fluid. Gastrointestinal irritation can be reduced by ingestion with food or with an antacid. Enteric-coated aspirin, which is more expensive (Ecotrin; many others), can be used to avoid gastric irritation, but absorption is delayed.

The main untoward effect of aspirin—especially in large doses or when taken chronically—is gastric irritation and microscopic blood loss from the gut. Rarely, there may be massive gastrointestinal hemorrhage, most commonly in heavy drinkers or patients with a history of peptic ulcer disease.

Aspirin allergy occurs infrequently and may be manifested as rhinorrhea, the growth of nasal polyps, asthma attacks, and—very rarely—anaphylactic shock. The incidence of true aspirin allergy is less than 0.1% in the general population.

**Table 1–5.** Useful nonsteroidal anti-inflammatory drugs.

| Generic Name | Proprietary Name | Dosage Range | Costs (AWP/100)* | Comments† |
|---|---|---|---|---|
| Fenoprofen | Nalfon | 300–600 mg 3–4 times daily | $44 for 600-mg pill | |
| Ibuprofen pill | Advil (OTC), Motrin, etc | 200–600 mg 3–4 times daily | $11.50 for 600-mg | Now available without prescription; relatively well tolerated. |
| Indomethacin | Indameth, Indocin, etc | 25–50 mg 2–4 times daily | $16 for 25-mg pill | Prototype untoward effects: headache, tinnitus, dizziness, confusion, rashes, anorexia, nausea, vomiting, gastrointestinal bleeding, diarrhea, nephrotoxicity, visual disturbances, etc. |
| Meclofenamate sodium | Meclomen | 100 mg 2–4 times daily | $50 for 100-mg pill | Diarrhea relatively more common. |
| Naproxen | Anaprox, Naprosyn | 250–500 mg twice daily | $78 for 500-mg pill | Useful for menstrual cramps. |
| Piroxicam | Feldene | 20 mg daily | $128 for 20-mg pill | Single dosage convenient; relatively expensive; may have higher rate of gastrointestinal bleeding. |
| Sulindac | Clinoril | 150–200 mg twice daily | $78 for 200-mg pill | Adverse effects similar to those of indomethacin; relatively expensive. |
| Tolmetin | Tolectin | 200–600 mg 4 times daily | $49 for 400-mg pill | |
| Aspirin | | 325–625 mg 2–4 times daily | $1.10 for 325-mg pill | |

* AWP/100 = average wholesale cost per pill. When estimating daily costs for medications, dosage frequency should be taken into account.
† The adverse effects listed for indomethacin and others can occur with any of the drugs that have been available for shorter periods. Tolerance and efficacy are subject to great individual variations among patients.

Aspirin in high doses may produce a vitamin K-responsive prolongation of the prothrombin time.

Because of a reported association with Reye's syndrome, the FDA has advised against use of salicylates by children and teenagers with febrile viral illnesses such as influenza and chickenpox.

**Acetaminophen** in the same dosage as aspirin (650 mg orally every 4 hours) has comparable analgesic and antipyretic effects but lacks the anti-inflammatory property of aspirin. It is useful for people who cannot tolerate aspirin and for those with bleeding disorders. In very large doses (eg, > 4 mg/d chronically, > 7 g/d acutely), acetaminophen can be hepatotoxic, manifested by appreciable hepatic necrosis with very high serum transaminase levels. Toxicity may occur at considerably lower doses in the chronic alcoholic.

See Chapter 30 for further details on salicylate and acetaminophen overdosage.

### 3. MANAGEMENT OF CHRONIC PAIN

The patient with chronic pain is one of the most difficult problems the clinician must deal with. Once pain becomes chronic, a number of self-perpetuating factors encourage its persistence, including sleep loss, muscle weakness, loss of control, feelings of depression and hopelessness, anger, narcotics addiction, and often secondary gain. Narcotics are much less effective in chronic than in acute pain. Their use is accompanied by tolerance and often by addiction or dependence, depression, sleep disorders, constipation, and depressed mentation.

In treating patients with chronic pain, the following approaches are important:

(1) The physician must acknowledge that the patient is suffering with "real pain"; chronic pain is rarely fictitious.

(2) Diagnostic workups should be circumscribed and avoid redundancy.

(3) If the patient is heavily addicted to narcotics, detoxification should be the first treatment goal. Moderate addiction may respond to withdrawal from narcotics according to a specified schedule.

(4) Patients should be directed to the goals of improved function and control rather than cure. Thus, increased activity and stress reduction are important.

In addition to analgesic drugs, a variety of alternative strategies may be offered, including antidepressant drugs, psychologic techniques such as hypnosis and biofeedback training, physical therapy, transcutaneous electrical nerve stimulation, and acupuncture. For severe intractable cases, neurosurgical procedures such as cordotomy or epidural morphine sometimes must be considered.

Clifford DB: Treatment of pain with antidepressants. *Am Fam Physician* (Feb) 1985;**31**:181.
Clive DM, Stoff JS: Renal syndromes associated with nonsteroidal anti-inflammatory drugs. *N Engl J Med* 1984;**310**:563.
Drug combinations for pain. (Editorial.) *Lancet* 1984;**2**:793.

Fields HL, Levine JD: Pain: Mechanisms and management. *West J Med* 1984;**141**:347.

Foley KM: The treatment of cancer pain. *N Engl J Med* 1985;**313**:84.

Fordyce WE, Roberts AH, Sternbach KA: The behavioral management of chronic pain: A response to critics. *Pain* 1985;**22**:113.

Kanner R: Pain management. *JAMA* 1986;**256**:2112.

Levine J: Pain and analgesia: The outlook for more rational treatment. *Ann Intern Med* 1984;**100**:269.

Sriwatanakul K et al: Analysis of narcotic analgesic usage in the treatment of postoperative pain. *JAMA* 1983;**250**:926.

Way WL, Way EL: Opioid analgesics and antagonists. Chapter 29 in: *Basic & Clinical Pharmacology*, 3rd ed. Katzung BG (editor). Appleton & Lange, 1987.

Wolf RE: Nonsteroidal anti-inflammatory drugs. *Arch Int Med* 1984;**144**:1658.

## FEVER & HYPERTHERMIA
## (Table 1-6)

Body temperature varies slightly in different individuals and according to physiologic factors such as exercise, digestion, or sudden changes in environmental temperature. The normal diurnal variation may be as much as 1 °C, being lowest in the early morning and highest in the late afternoon. There is a slight sustained temperature rise following ovulation during the menstrual cycle and in the first trimester of pregnancy.

The average normal oral body temperature is 36.7 °C (range 36–37.4 °C), or 98°F (range 96.8–99.3 °F). These ranges include 2 standard deviations and thus encompass 95% of a normal population, measured in mid-morning. The normal rectal or vaginal temperature is 0.5 °C (1 °F) higher than the oral temperature, and the normal axillary temperature is correspondingly lower. Rectal temperature measurement is more reliable than oral temperature, particu-larly in the case of patients who are mouth-breathers or who are tachypneic.

Fever is a regulated rise to a new "set point" of body temperature. When bacterial toxins or other stimuli act on the body's bone marrow-derived mono-cyte-macrophages, they produce a polypeptide, inter-leukin I, that causes elevation of the set point. This rarely exceeds 41.1 °C (106 °F). The elevation may result from either increased heat production (eg, shiv-ering) or decreased heat loss (eg, peripheral vasocon-striction).

Hyperthermia—not mediated by interleukin I—oc-curs when body metabolic heat production or environ-mental heat load exceeds normal heat loss capacity or when there is impaired heat loss; heat stroke is an example. Body temperature may rise to potentially lethal levels (> 106 °F), and no diurnal variation is observed. Prolonged elevation of temperature over 40.5 °C orally or 41 °C rectally may cause permanent brain damage. Oral temperatures over 42.5 °C (108.4 °F) or rectal temperatures over 43 °C (109.4 °F) are seen in heat stroke, with a high mortality rate.

**Malignant hyperthermia** that may follow certain types of anesthesia (succinylcholine and potent inhala-tion anesthetics) may occasionally be prevented by identifying patients with a personal or family history of difficult anesthesia or previous muscle abnormali-ties and then choosing the proper anesthetic agent, with temperature monitoring during the entire course of anesthesia. As soon as the syndrome is detected, emergency treatment is required.

### Effect of Fever

While fever as a symptom should generally be regarded with appropriate concern, in some circum-stances it may play a beneficial role. Markedly ele-vated body temperature may result in profound meta-bolic disturbances. High temperature during the first trimester of pregnancy may cause birth defects, such

**Table 1–6.** Pathophysiology, clinical findings, and treatment of fever and hyperthermia.[*]

| Pathophysiologic Basic for Fever | Clinical Findings | Treatment |
|---|---|---|
| Interleukin 1 on hypothalamus to induce fever (eg, infection, collagen disease, allergy). | Patient complains of feeling cold. Shivering. "Gooseflesh." | Antipyretic drugs: aspirin or acetaminophen, 300–600 mg 4 times daily. |
| Agent or illness acts on hypothalamus to induce hyperthermia (eg, central nervous system lesions, radiation). | Cold extremities. Minimal sweating. | Supply clothing and covers just sufficient for maximal comfort. *Avoid* measures for physical removal of heat (eg, sponging, ice bags). |
| Heat production exceeds normal heat loss mechanisms (eg, malignant hyperthermia, thyroid storm). | Patient complains of feeling hot. Hot extremities. Active sweating (except in cases where there is defective heat loss mechanism). | Remove excessive clothing or covers. Eliminate excess environmental heat source. Employ measures for physical removal of heat (eg, sponging, ice bags, ice-water enemas). *Avoid* antipyretic drugs. |
| Environmental heat load exceeds normal heat loss mechanisms (eg, exposure to industrial heat, overuse of sauna). | | |
| Defective heat loss mechanisms cannot cope with normal heat load (eg, heat stroke, burns, sweat gland disorders). | | |

[*] Modified and reproduced, with permission, from Stern RC: Pathophysiologic basis for symptomatic treatment of fever. *Pediatrics* 1977;**59**:92.

as anencephaly. Fewer may increase insulin requirements and also alter the metabolism and disposition of drugs used for the treatment of the diverse diseases associated with fever.

The body temperature may provide important information about the presence of illness and about changes in the clinical status of the patient. The fever pattern, however, is of rather limited use for specific diagnosis. Furthermore, the degree of temperature elevation does not necessarily correspond to the severity of the illness. In general, the febrile response tends to be greater in children than in adults; in elderly persons, the febrile response is less marked than in younger adults. A sudden fall in temperature in the febrile patient is not necessarily a favorable sign unless there is a corresponding clinical improvement.

### Diagnostic Considerations

The outline below illustrates the wide variety of clinical disorders that may cause fever. Most febrile illnesses are due to common infections, are shortlived, and are relatively easy to diagnose. In certain instances, however, the origin of the fever may remain obscure ("fever of undetermined origin," FUO) after careful diagnostic examination. The term FUO is reserved for patients with sustained fever of over 38.3 °C (101 °F) for 3 weeks and in whom the diagnosis is not apparent after 1 week or more of diagnostic studies.

In about 40% of cases, the cause of FUO is infectious disease. About 20% of cases of FUO are due to neoplasms, 25% to immunologic disorders, and the remainder to miscellaneous causes. In 5–10% of cases, the diagnosis is never established.

Hasty, empiric use of polypharmaceutic measures (eg, multiple antimicrobials, corticosteroids, antipyretics, analgesics) may seriously interfere with rational diagnosis and therapy and may be hazardous.

### Important Causes of Fever & Hyperthermia (With Examples)

**A. Infections:** Viral, rickettsial, bacterial, fungal, and parasitic infections.

**B. Autoimmune Diseases:** Systemic lupus erythematosus, polyarteritis nodosa, rheumatic fever, Still's disease; less prominent in dermatomyositis, adult rheumatoid arthritis.

**C. Central Nervous System Disease:** Cerebral hemorrhage, head injuries, brain and spinal cord tumors, degenerative central nervous system disease (eg, multiple sclerosis), spinal cord injuries. (This category represents interference with the thermal regulatory process rather than true "fever.")

**D. Malignant Neoplastic Disease:** Primary neoplasms (eg, of lung, liver, pancreas, and kidney), tumors metastatic to the liver.

**E. Hematologic Disease:** Lymphomas, leukemias, hemolytic anemias, hemorrhage (gastrointestinal tract or soft tissue).

**F. Cardiovascular Disease:** Myocardial infarction, pulmonary embolism.

**G. Gastrointestinal Disease:** Inflammatory bowel disease, liver abscess.

**H. Endocrine Disease:** Hyperthyroidism, pheochromocytoma may raise temperature because of impaired thermoregulaton.

**I. Diseases Due to Chemical Agents:** Drug reactions (including serum sickness), anesthesia (malignant hyperthermia; see below), anaphylactic reactions, chemical poisoning, pyrogen reactions (following intravenous fluids).

**J. Miscellaneous Diseases:** Sarcoidosis, familial Mediterranean fever, chronic fatigue syndrome.

**K. Psychogenic fever.**

**L. Factitious, or "false," fever.**

### Treatment

**A. Removal of the Specific Cause of the Fever:** Measures directed solely toward depression of elevated body temperature are indicated except for temperatures above 40.5 °C (105 °F) or to relieve symptoms. Prompt and vigorous body cooling (see below), hyperventilation with 100% oxygen, diuresis, intravenous dantrolene, and measures to correct metabolic acidosis and renal failure are instituted.

**B. Reduction of Fever by Nonspecific Means:** Most fever is well tolerated. When the temperature is greater than 40 °C (104 °F), particularly if prolonged, symptomatic treatment may be required (Table 1–6). *Temperature over 41°C (105.8°F)—is a medical emergency.* (See Heat Stroke, p. 998.)

**1. Measures for removal of heat**–Alcohol sponges, cold sponges, ice bags, ice-water enemas, and ice baths will lower body temperature and provide physical comfort for patients who complain of feeling *hot.*

**2. Antipyretic drugs**–Aspirin or acetaminophen, 0.3–0.6 g every 4 hours as needed, is quite effective in reducing fever.

**3. Fluid replacement**–Oral or parenteral fluids must be administered to compensate for increased insensible fluid and electrolyte losses as well as those from perspiration.

Atkins E: Fever: New perspectives on an old problem. (Editorial.) *N Engl J Med* 1983;**308**:958.

Kauffman CA et al: Diagnosing fever of unknown origin in older patients. *Geriatrics* (Feb) 1984;**39**:46.

Larson EB, Featherstone HJ, Petersdorf RG: Fever of undetermined origin: Diagnosis and follow-up of 105 cases, 1970–1980. *Medicine* 1982;**61**:269.

Rosenberg H: Malignant hyperthermia. *Hosp Pract* (March 15) 1985;**20**:139.

### WEIGHT LOSS

Marked unexplained weight loss is often an indication of serious physical or psychologic illness. If the weight loss appears evident from the patient's physical appearance, the clinician should proceed with appropriate diagnostic studies based upon the findings of a history, physical examination, and routine laboratory studies.

Weight loss may be due to a wide variety of disease processes of any organ system, as well as to psychiatric disorders. In the initial evaluation, many of the physical causes of weight loss can be quickly uncovered. It is important to correlate weight change with appetite, dietary intake, physical activity, and psychosocial factors.

When the patient complains of weight loss but appears to be adequately nourished, inquiry should be made about exact weight changes (with approximate dates) and about changes in clothing size. Family members may provide confirmation of weight loss, as may old documents such as driver's licenses.

Once it has been established that the patient has marked weight loss, further methodical laboratory and radiologic investigation may be indicated. Involuntary weight loss is rarely due to "occult disease." Almost all physical causes are clinically evident during the initial evaluation of the patient. Marked weight loss can sometimes occur in the absence of serious physical illness. Psychiatric consultation should be considered when there is evidence of depression, anorexia nervosa, or other psychologic problems (see Chapter 20).

Health and Public Policy Committee, American College of Physicians: Eating disorders: Anorexia nervosa and bulimia. *Ann Intern Med* 1986;**105**:790.
Marton KI, Sox HC JR, Krupp JR: Involuntary weight loss: Diagnostic and prognostic significance. *Ann Intern Med* 1981;**95**:568.

# FATIGUE

Fatigue, or lassitude, and the closely related complaints of weakness, tiredness, and lethargy are most often readily explained by apparent common factors such as overexertion, poor physical conditioning, inadequate rest, obesity, inadequate nutrition, and emotional problems. A history of the patient's daily living habits and working environment may obviate the need for extensive and unproductive medical studies. The presence of fatigue on arising in the morning (that clears as the day progresses) and a history of emotional stress or recurrent episodes of anxiety or depression lend support to a diagnosis of fatigue caused by psychologic illness.

The possibility that excessive fatigue may be due to nonpsychologic physical illness, particularly in its incipient phase, sometimes makes it necessary to search for a wide variety of organic causes, including the following:

**A. Endocrine Disorders:** Addison's disease, hypothyroidism, hyperthyroidism, diabetes mellitus.

**B. Neurologic Disorders:** Myasthenia gravis.

**C. Infectious Disease:** Hepatitis, infectious mononucleosis, tuberculosis, brucellosis, infective endocarditis, intestinal parasites.

**D. Respiratory Disorders:** Emphysema.

**E. Hematologic Disorders:** Anemia.

**F. Autoimmune Disorders:** Rheumatoid arthritis, systemic lupus erythematosus.

**G. Neoplastic Disease.**

**H. Drugs and Toxins:** Alcohol, sedative-hypnotics, environmental toxins.

Havad CWH: Lassitude. *Br Med J* 1985;**290**:1161.
Strauss SE et al: Persisting illness and fatigue in adults with evidence of Epstein-Barr virus infection. *Ann Intern Med* 1985;**102**:7.

# SHOCK SYNDROME

Shock occurs when the circulation of arterial blood is inadequate to meet tissue metabolic needs. Without proper treatment, shock can progress to cellular dysfunction, organ damage, and death. Treatment must be directed both at the manifestations of shock and at its cause.

## Classification

See Table 1–7.

**A. Hypovolemic Shock:** Decreased intravascular volume resulting from loss of blood or plasma may be obvious (eg, external hemorrhage) or subtle (eg, sequestration in a "third space," as in pancreatitis). Compensatory vasoconstriction temporarily reduces the size of the vascular bed and may temporarily maintain the blood pressure, but if fluid is not replaced, hypotension occurs, peripheral resistance increases, capillary and venous beds collapse, and the tissues become progressively more hypoxic. Even a moderate sudden loss of circulating fluids can result in severe damage to vital centers.

**B. Cardiogenic Shock:** (See Chapter 8.) Inadequate cardiac function may result from disorders of the heart muscle, valves, or the electrical pacing system. Shock associated with myocardial infarction or other serious cardiac disease carries a very high mortality rate (75–80%) despite therapy. Clinical findings are of limited value in predicting the course or assessing the prognosis of shock due to myocardial infarction.

**C. Obstructive Shock:** (See Chapter 8.) Obstruction of the systemic or pulmonary circulation, the aortic and mitral valves, or venous inflow, as in pericardial disease, may reduce cardiac output sufficiently to cause shock. Cardiac tamponade and massive pulmonary embolism are medical emergencies requiring prompt diagnosis and treatment. Tamponade

**Table 1–7.** Classification of shock.[*]

**Hypovolemic shock**
  Loss of blood (hemorrhagic shock):
    External hemorrhage:
      Trauma
      Gastrointestinal tract bleeding
    Internal hemorrhage:
      Hematoma
  Loss of plasma:
    Burns
  Loss of fluid and electrolytes:
    External:
      Vomiting
      Diarrhea
      Excessive sweating
      Hyperosmolar states (diabetic ketoacidosis)
    Internal ("third-spacing"):
      Pancreatitis
      Ascites
      Bowel obstruction
**Cardiogenic shock**
  Dysrhythmia
  Tachyarrhythmia (nearly always ventricular tachycardia)
  Bradyarrhythmia
  "Pump failure" (secondary to myocardial infarction or other cardiomyopathy)
  Acute valvular dysfunction (especially regurgitant lesions)
  Rupture of ventricular septum or free ventricular wall
**Obstructive shock**
  Pericardial disease (tamponade, constriction)
  Disease of pulmonary vasculature (massive pulmonary emboli, pulmonary hypertension)
  Cardiac tumor (atrial myxoma)
  Obstructive valvular disease (aortic or mitral stenosis)
**Distributive shock**
  Septic shock
  Anaphylactic shock
  Neurogenic shock
  Vasodilator drugs
  Acute adrenal insufficiency

[*] Adapted from Trunkey DD, Salber PR, Mills J: Shock. In: *Current Emergency Diagnosis & Treatment,* 2nd ed. Mills J et al (editors). Lange, 1985.

calls for immediate echocardiography and pericardiocentesis. The prognosis for patients with massive pulmonary embolism is guarded despite therapy with anticoagulants or thrombolytics; surgical embolectomy adds little. The success or failure of treatment undertaken for less common causes of obstructive shock such as atrial myxoma with pulmonary hypertension depends upon early diagnosis, relying especially on echocardiography.

**D. Distributive Shock:** Changes in vascular resistance or permeability from such diverse causes as sepsis, anaphylaxis, or acute adrenal insufficiency may result in inadequate cardiac output despite normal circulatory volume.

**1. Septic shock–**(See Chapter 21.) Most commonly, vascular shock is due to gram-negative bacteremia (so-called septic shock). In overwhelming infection, there is an initial short period of vasoconstriction followed by vasodilatation, with venous pooling of blood in the microcirculation. There may be a direct toxic action on the heart and adrenals. The mortality rate is high (40–80%). Responsible organisms include *Escherichia coli, Klebsiella, Proteus,* and *Pseudomonas* but also gram-negative anaerobes (eg, *Bacteroides*). Septic shock occurs more often in the very young and the very old; in diabetes, hematologic cancers, and diseases of the genitourinary, hepatobiliary, and intestinal tracts; in meningitis or pneumonia; and in association with corticosteroid, immunosuppressive, or radiation therapy. Immediate precipitating factors may be urinary, biliary, or gynecologic manipulations.

Septic shock is suspected when a febrile patient has chills associated with hypotension. Early, the skin may be warm and the pulse full ("warm shock"). Hyperventilation results in respiratory alkalosis. The sensorium and urinary output are often initially normal, with classic signs of shock becoming manifest later. The symptoms and signs of the inciting infection are not invariably present.

**2. Neurogenic shock–**Neurogenic or psychogenic factors, eg, spinal cord injury, pain, trauma, fright, gastric dilatation, or vasodilator drugs, may also cause distributive shock. Sudden autonomic overactivity results in vasodilatation and rapid peripheral and splanchnic pooling of blood. Following a period of anxiety (tachycardia, tremors, and pallor), there is a sudden reflex vagal stimulation with decreased cardiac output, hypotension, and decreased cerebral blood flow. Simple fainting in response to strong emotion is the most common example of neurogenic shock. This **vasovagal syncope** is not true shock because it seldom continues long enough to result in tissue ischemia and the clinical hallmarks of shock. In the absence of other complicating factors, the patient usually revives promptly in the recumbent position or following the administration of simple forms of treatment (eg, spirits of ammonia, physical stimuli), but further observation may be required.

**3. Distributive shock–**Distributive shock may also be due to anaphylaxis (see below), histamine response, ganglionic blockade, and hypnotic drug intoxication.

### Diagnosis of Shock & Impending Shock

Shock may be impending if the following signs are present.

**A. Hypotension:** Hypotension in adults is traditionally defined as a systolic blood pressure of 90 mm Hg or less. However, some normal adults may have levels that low without ill effects, and some hypertensive persons may go into shock with what would ordinarily be considered normal blood pressures.

**B. Orthostatic Changes in Vital Signs:** Patients who are not clearly hypotensive when tested in the supine position should have blood pressures measured and pulses counted while sitting up with the legs dangling. If no change occurs when this is done, repeat the measurements with the patient standing. Three to 5 minutes between measurements are allowed to permit the pulse and blood pressure to stabilize. A drop in systolic pressure of 10–20 mm Hg or more associated with an increase in pulse rate of more than 15 beats/min suggests depleted intravascular volume. Some normovolemic patients with peripheral neuropathies or those taking certain medications (eg, some antihypertensive drugs) may demonstrate an orthostatic fall in blood pressure, but without associated increase in pulse rate.

**C. Peripheral Hypoperfusion:** Patients in shock have cool or mottled extremities and weak or absent peripheral pulses.

**D. Altered Mental Status:** Patients may demonstrate normal mental status or may be restless, agitated, confused, lethargic, or comatose as a result of inadequate perfusion of the brain.

## Treatment

Treatment depends upon prompt assessment of the cause, type, severity, and duration of shock as well as an accurate appraisal of underlying conditions that may influence the onset or maintenance of shock.

**1. Position–**The patient is placed in the supine position to maximize cerebral blood flow.

**2. Oxygenation–**A patent airway is established or maintained and 100% oxygen is given initially at a rate of 5–10 L/min by mask or nasal prongs. If blood gas measurements show an arterial oxygen partial pressure ($P_{a_{O_2}}$) below 60 mm Hg or if dyspnea or cyanosis is present, the oxygen flow rate should be increased. If $P_{a_{O_2}}$ fails to show a prompt rise, pulmonary shunting with or without shock may be present. Artificial ventilation with positive end-expiratory pressure (PEEP) may be used to treat the latter; it requires constant monitoring of cardiopulmonary function, because although PEEP can increase $P_{a_{O_2}}$, it may reduce cardiac output. In addition, PEEP may cause pneumothorax and pneumomediastinum (especially at higher levels (eg, $> 10$ cm $H_2O$).

**3. Temperature–**The patient is kept comfortably warm. A blanket may be used to prevent heat loss. Excessive external heat should be avoided because it further dilates the peripheral vessels and increases metabolic requirements.

**4. Control bleeding–**External hemorrhage is controlled by direct compression by any available means.

**5. Analgesics–**Severe pain is treated promptly with analgesic drugs. Morphine sulfate, 8–15 mg subcutaneously, is appropriate for severe pain; since subcutaneous absorption is poor in patients in shock, 4–8 mg slowly intravenously may be used as an alternative. **Caution:** Morphine should not be given to unconscious patients, to those who have head injuries, or to those with respiratory depression.

**6. Laboratory studies–**Hemoglobin, hematocrit, and red cell count are determined immediately for baseline and follow-up values, and a specimen is sent for typing and cross-matching. Laboratory studies for rapid serial determination of serum electrolytes, pH, $P_{a_{O_2}}$, and $P_{a_{CO_2}}$ may be invaluable.

**7. Urine flow–**In the patient without preexisting renal disease, urine output is a reliable indication of vital organ perfusion. An indwelling catheter to monitor urine flow (which should be kept above 0.5 mL/kg/h) is indicated. Urine flow of less than 25 mL/h indicates inadequate renal circulation, which, if not corrected, can result in renal tubular necrosis.

**8. Monitor cardiac rhythm–**Periodic electrocardiography or continuous automated monitoring will permit early detection and prompt treatment of myocardial ischemia from hypoperfusion, and arrhythmias from similar causes or from electrolyte and acid-base disturbances.

**9. Central venous pressure (CVP) or pulmonary artery wedge pressure (PAWP)–**Monitoring of central venous pressure or pulmonary artery wedge pressure may be helpful in evaluating and treating the patient in shock. Central venous pressure determination is relatively simple and may be useful when serial measurements are made and are correlated with simultaneous clinical and laboratory observations. Central venous pressure is not as reliable, however, as determinations of the pulmonary artery wedge pressure by the Swan-Ganz catheter technique, which provides a better index of left ventricular function.

In central venous pressure determination, a catheter is inserted percutaneously (or by cutdown) through the antecubital vein or through a major vein (eg, external jugular) and is connected to a saline manometer. Normal values range from 5 to 8 cm of water. A low central venous pressure in the presence of intense peripheral vasospasm (pale, clammy skin) suggests a low blood volume and need for fluid replacement. A high central venous pressure (about 15 cm of water) suggests fluid overload or insufficient cardiac output.

The central venous pressure, however, may be normal in left ventricular failure and neurogenic shock. Spuriously high central venous pressure readings may occur with chronic obstructive pulmonary disease; low readings may be found in aortic stenosis and acute left ventricular failure. Pressure changes in response to cautious administration of small amounts of intravenous fluids may increase the value of central venous pressure as an indicator of blood volume and cardiac efficiency.

Pulmonary artery wedge pressure determinations using a Swan-Ganz flotation catheter are more reliable than central venous pressure for assessing adequacy of restoration of fluid volume. A mean pressure of 12 mm Hg is considered to be the upper limit of normal. An elevated pulmonary artery wedge pressure ($> 14$ mm Hg) may serve as a warning of impending pulmonary edema and of the hazard of fluid overload. Catheter insertion requires a skilled and experienced physician and is expensive. Surveillance for the catheter-induced complications of hemorrhage, sepsis, pneumothorax, arrhythmias, and pulmonary infarction should be considered an important part of catheter care.

**10. Volume replacement–**Initial or emergency needs may be determined by the history, general appearance, vital signs, and hematocrit. There is no simple technique by which to accurately judge the fluid requirements. An estimate of total fluid losses is an essential first step. Response to therapy—particularly the effect of carefully administered, gradually increasing amounts of intravenous fluids on the central venous pressure or pulmonary artery wedge pressure—is a valuable index.

Selection of the proper fluid for restoration and maintenance of hemodynamic stability is often difficult and controversial. It will depend upon the type of fluid that has been lost (whole blood, plasma, water, electrolytes), associated medical problems, availability of the various replacement solutions, clinical and laboratory monitoring facilities, and, in some circumstances, expense.

The most effective replacement fluid in case of gross hemorrhage is usually packed red cells with saline, but other available fluids should be given immediately pending the results of preliminary laboratory work and the procurement of blood. Rapid volume replacement in the case of blood loss will often prevent shock. If central venous or pulmonary artery wedge pressure is low and the hematocrit greater than 35%—and if there is no clinical evidence to suggest occult blood loss—blood volume should be supported with crystalloid solutions or colloids.

**a. Crystalloid solutions–**Crystalloid fluids include sodium chloride (physiologic saline, 0.9%) or lactated Ringer's injection. Five hundred to 2000 mL of the selected solution is given rapidly intravenously—ideally under central venous pressure or pulmonary artery wedge pressure monitoring. The crystalloids are readily available for emergencies and mass casualties. They may obviate the need for blood or colloids. They are often effective, at least temporarily, when given in adequate doses. When large volumes of crystalloids are given, patients should be monitored for evidence of volume overload and pulmonary complications. If shock persists after prompt fusion of 2 L of crystalloids, it is necessary to give blood or other colloids.

**b. Colloids–**Colloids are high-molecular-weight substances that do not diffuse readily across normal capillary membranes. Colloidal solutions increase the plasma oncotic pressure and thus can draw fluid from the interstitial space into the intravascular space to cause additional fluid volume expansion. Capillary membranes in the lungs are often damaged in the patient in shock, so that larger molecules may leak from the intravascular space into the interstitium and have an adverse effect on pulmonary function.

**(1) ·Blood–**Blood is used for patients requiring increased blood oxygen-carrying capacity, as in hemorrhagic shock. Packed or frozen red cells are preferred to whole blood. Remaining blood products may be used for other purposes. The amount of blood given depends on the clinical course, the hematocrit, and hemodynamic findings.

Screening of blood donors for hepatitis B infection and for AIDS virus antibodies has reduced the frequency of those infections following transfusion. Non-A, non-B hepatitis remains the commonest complication of transfusion.

**(2) Plasma fractions–**Group-specific frozen plasma is a satisfactory colloidal volume expander and occasionally can correct specific coagulation defects. Because of its expense, risk, and relative ineffectiveness, however, its use should be limited. Unit-bagged plasma is preferable to pooled plasma. Albumin 5% in saline, albumin 25% concentrate, or plasma protein fraction (containing 80–85% albumin) may be rapidly set up for emergencies, and blood typing is not required. These substances have been heat-treated to minimize the risk of infectious hepatitis.

**(3) Dextrans–**Dextrans are high-molecular-weight polysaccharide colloids that are fairly effective plasma expanders. Because they can impair blood coagulation and interfere with blood typing and because they may cause anaphylactoid reactions, dextrans are used very infrequently now.

**11. Vasoactive drugs–**Some adrenergic drugs can be useful in the adjunctive therapy of shock. *The adrenergic drugs should not be considered a primary form of therapy in shock.* Simple blood pressure elevation produced by the vasopressor drugs has little beneficial effect on the underlying disturbance, and in many instances, the effect may be detrimental. Correction of hypovolemia and a search for treatable causes deserve first consideration. Continuous clinical monitoring is essential to determine if, when, for how long, and in what quantity adrenergic drugs are to be used.

**a. Dopamine hydrochloride** (Intropin) has an advantage over other adrenergic drugs because it has a beneficial effect on renal blood flow and also increases cardiac output and blood pressure. Dopamine hydrochloride, 200 mg in 500 mL of sodium chloride injection USP (400 μg/mL), is given initially at a rate of 2.5 μg/kg/min. This dosage stimulates both the dopaminergic receptors, which increase the renal blood flow and urinary output, and the beta-adrenergic cardiac receptors, which increase the cardiac output. If shock is profound, gradually increasing doses of dopamine in excess of 20 μg/kg/min may be required. At these levels, however, the effect is nearly all alpha-adrenergic. After an effective dosage level has been reached, the infusion rate should be adjusted periodically to the lowest point necessary to maintain adequate organ perfusion. Dopamine alone may fail to maintain adequate perfusion pressure or to relieve intense vasoconstriction, and it may sometimes be necessary to use it in combination with another appropriate adrenergic drug.

Adverse reactions include ventricular arrhythmias, anginal pain, nausea and vomiting, headache, hypotension, azotemia, and rare cases of peripheral gangrene. Special care should be exercised when dopamine is used in the treatment of shock following myocardial infarction, because the drug's inotropic effect may increase myocardial oxygen demand. Dopamine should not be used in patients with pheochromocytoma or uncorrected tachyarrhythmias or in those who are receiving monoamine oxidase inhibitors.

**b. Dobutamine,** a synthetic catecholamine similar to dopamine but with greater inotropic effect, may be useful when filling pressures are high because of fluid overload or heart failure, as in some cases of septic shock or acute myocardial infarction with heart failure.

**c. Isoproterenol,** a beta-adrenergic stimulator, increases cardiac output by its action on myocardial contraction. Since it produces peripheral vasodilatation, it should not be given if central venous pressure is low. Because of its inotropic effect, an increased incidence of cardiac arrhythmias precludes its use if the cardiac rate is greater than 120/min.

**12. Corticosteroids**–The use of corticosteroids for the treatment of the many types of shock is controversial. Cortisol is, of course, lifesaving in the treatment of shock associated with acute adrenal insufficiency (see Acute Adrenal Insufficiency, p. 723). The value of corticosteroids for other forms of shock is questionable and is not approved by the FDA. In septic shock, a condition with extremely high mortality rates with current treatment methods, a set of recent studies indicates that steroid use conveys no benefit and may even be harmful.

**13. Diuretics**–The cautious early administration of mannitol as a 10–25% solution in 500–1000 mL of normal saline or Ringer's injection has been recommended in selected patients in whom oliguria is present or impending. Furosemide, 20 mg intravenously, has also been recommended. Urine flow and central venous pressure must be carefully monitored. The effectiveness of these agents in shock is still unknown; their use is controversial; and they are not without risk. Prior to the use of diuretics, it may be helpful to determine the urinary sodium; values greater than 30 meq/L suggests acute tubular necrosis and the possible advantage of diuretic therapy in converting oliguric to nonoliguric expression of the disorder.

**14. Heparin**–(See Disseminated Intravascular Coagulation, p. 335.)

**15. Fluid and electrolyte balance**–Abnormalities of fluid, electrolyte, and acid-base balance are addressed. There is growing evidence that vigorous treatment with sodium bicarbonate should not be used as standard therapy. It should probably be reserved for use when acidosis fails to respond to adequate fluid resuscitation.

**16. Cardiac disorders**–Digitalis glycosides are indicated only for those patients with preexisting or presenting evidence of cardiac failure or digitalis-responsive arrhythmias. Atropine may be of value in treating selected postmyocardial infarction bradycardias. The use of vasopressor drugs in myocardial infarction is controversial and is reserved for patients with hypotension and elevated left ventricular filling pressure. Continuous cardiac monitoring is required. The hemodynamic effectiveness of vasodilator drugs in reducing preload and outflow resistance in patients with left ventricular failure has been established,

but the mortality rate of cardiogenic shock is unchanged.

Following myocardial infarction, mechanical circulatory assistance that reduces myocardial work and increases coronary perfusion—utilizing intra-aortic balloon counterpulsation on an emergency basis—may be temporarily helpful; it is used only if cardiac surgery is contemplated. Emergency coronary bypass operations; infarctectomies; and repair of ventricular aneurysms, chordae tendineae rupture, and septal defects following myocardial infarctions offer hope for some patients.

Cullen DJ et al: Objective, quantitative measurement of severity of illness in critically ill patients. *Crit Care Med* 1984;**12:**155.

Heineman HS et al: Corticosteroids for septic shock. [Letters in response to Sprung article-see below]. *N Engl J Med* 1985;**312:**509.

Jacobson MA, Young CS: New developments in the treatment of gram-negative bacteremia. *West J Med* 1986;**144:**185.

Leier CV, Unverferth DV: Drugs five years later: Dobutamine. *Ann Intern Med* 1983;**99:**490.

MacLean LD: Shock: A century of progress. *Ann Surg* 1985;**201:**407.

Parker MM et al: Profound but reversible myocardial depression in patients with septic shock. *Ann Intern Med* 1984;**100:**483.

Pierson DJ, Hudson LD: Monitoring hemodynamics in the critically ill. *Med Clin North Am* 1983;**67:**1343.

Robin ED: The cult of the Swan-Ganz catheter: Overuse and abuse of pulmonary flow catheters. *Ann Intern Med* 1985;**103:**445.

Sprung CL et al: The effects of high-dose corticosteroids in patients with septic shock: A prospective controlled study. *N Engl J Med* 1984;**311:**1137.

Stacpoole PW: Lactic acidosis: The case against bicarbonate therapy. *Ann Int Med* 1986;**105:**276.

Trunkey DD, Salber PR, Mills J: Shock. Chap 2, pp 25–40, in: *Current Emergency Diagnosis & Treatment*, 2nd ed. Mills J et al (editors). Lange, 1985.

## SYSTEMIC ALLERGIC REACTIONS (Table 1–8)

Allergic, or hypersensitivity, disorders present as generalized systemic reactions as well as with localized reactions in any organ system of the body. The reactions may be acute, subacute, or chronic, immediate or delayed, and may be caused by an endless variety of offending agents (antigens)—pollens, molds, dusts, feathers, fur, venoms, food, drugs, etc. Many hypersensitive patients have a positive family history of allergy.

### Immunologic Factors (See Chapter 33.)

Some of the immunologic factors underlying hypersensitivity reactions are known. IgE is a humoral immunoglobulin that contains the reaginic antibody that plays a primary role in mediating many allergic reactions of the "immediate" hypersensitivity type (eg, asthma, acute urticaria, hay fever, anaphylaxis).

**Table 1–8.** Classification of allergic diseases (after Coombs and Gell).

| Type | Mechanism | Principal Antibody | Examples |
|------|-----------|--------------------|----------|
| I | Anaphylactic (immediate, homocytotropic, antigen-induced, antibody-mediated) | IgE | Anaphylaxis (drugs, insect venom, antisera), atopic bronchial asthma, allergic rhinitis, urticaria, angio-edema |
| II | Cytotoxic (antimembrane) | IgG, IgM (activate complement, causing cell lysis) | Transfusion reactions, Goodpasture's syndrome, autoimmune hemolysis, hemolytic anemia, certain drug reactions |
| III | Immune complex (serum sickness-like) | IgG, IgM (form complexes with complement, injuring vessels and basement membranes) | Serum sickness, lupus nephritis, occupational allergic alveolitis, allergic contact dermatitis |
| IV | Cell-mediated (delayed) or tuberculin type response | | Allergic contact dermatitis, infectious granulomas (tuberculosis, mycoses), tissue graft rejection |

When IgE antibody fixed to mast cells combines with antigen, the resulting complex disrupts the mast cell or basophil membranes, releasing histamine, slow-reacting substances of anaphylaxis (SRS-A; leukotrienes C and $D_5$), eosinophilic chemotactic factor of anaphylaxis (ECF-A), kinins, and prostaglandins. These chemical mediators act on target organs (eg, skin, bronchioles) and are responsible for the clinical manifestations of the immediate type of allergy.

## Atopic Allergies

Atopic, "spontaneous," allergies occur in about 10% of the population, often with a family history of similar disorders. Determination of the allergens in the atopic patient is difficult. Positive skin tests to multiple antigens are found frequently in atopic individuals. Eosinophilia and increased serum IgE levels are characteristic but not pathognomonic of atopic disorders. The atopic disorders include hay fever (allergic rhinitis), atopic dermatitis, allergic eczema, allergic asthma, and anaphylactic reactions.

## Delayed Allergies

"Delayed" hypersensitivity reactions—based upon a longer interval for the reaction to occur following a challenging antigen dose—are due largely to cell-mediated immunity and not dependent upon circulating immune globulins. Sensitized T lymphocytes react directly with antigen, producing inflammation through the action of soluble lymphokines. The tuberculin response and the various types of contact dermatitis are examples of delayed reactions, which usually take hours or days to occur. Anergy, primarily a deficiency in the lymphocyte-mediated response, is present in viral infections, Hodgkin's disease, organ transplantation, immunosuppressive therapy, and debility.

Naclero RM et al: Inflammatory mediators in late antigen-induced rhinitis. *N Engl J Med* 1985;**313**:165.

Salvaggio JE (editor): Primer on allergic and immunologic diseases. *JAMA* 1982;**248**:2579. [Entire issue.]

Stites DP et al (editors): *Basic & Clinical Immunology*, 6th ed. Lange, 1986.

## 1. ANAPHYLACTIC & ANAPHYLACTOID REACTIONS

Anaphylactic reactions are the immediate shock-like and frequently fatal reactions that can occur within minutes following the injection of sera, penicillin and other antibiotics, and practically all repeatedly administered parenteral diagnostic and therapeutic agents. Emergency drugs should be available whenever injections are given.

Anaphylactoid reactions are idiosyncratic reactions that occur generally when the patient is first exposed to a particular agent. Their emergency management is the same.

Symptoms and signs of anaphylaxis include apprehension, paresthesias, generalized urticaria, cyanosis, wheezing, cough, incontinence, shock, fever, dilatation of pupils, loss of consciousness, and convulsions. Death may occur within 5–10 minutes.

## Emergency Treatment

(1) Epinephrine, 0.4–1 mL of 1:1000 solution (0.4–1 mg), is given intramuscularly, repeated in 5–10 minutes and later as needed. If the patient does not respond, give 0.1–0.2 mL of 1:1000 solution diluted in 10 mL saline *slowly* intravenously.

(2) The patient is placed in the recumbent position.

(3) An adequate oral airway or endotracheal tube is essential. Emergency tracheostomy may be necessary on rare occasions for laryngeal edema.

(4) Antihistamines are not usually helpful in reversing acute anaphylaxis, but they may shorten its duration and prevent relapse. Diphenhydramine hydrochloride, aqueous, 5–20 mg intravenously, may be tried.

(5) Oxygen, 4–6 L/min, may be useful.

(6) Intravenous fluids to correct hypovolemia are essential, because hypotension due to profoundly decreased vascular resistance. Not surprisingly, large amounts of fluid are required. If arterial hypotension is severe, vasopressor agents (eg, dopamine, 200 mg in 500 mL of dextrose in water) may be given slowly by intravenous infusion. Hypotension is a major contributor to death in anaphylaxis.

(7) Hydrocortisone, 100–250 mg in water or saline intravenously over a period of 30 seconds, after epinephrine or diphenhydramine, may prevent prolonged reactions.

## Prevention

**A. Precautions:** Clinicians must be prepared for the occurrence of anaphylaxis when administering drugs likely to produce it, must identify the early manifestations of the syndrome, and must have epinephrine and other resuscitative aids available. Special precautions are observed in giving drugs to patients with a history of hay fever, asthma, or other allergic disorders. If there is a report of any allergic reaction in the past, the hazard of giving the drug, *either orally or by injection,* must be weighed. Scratch, intradermal, or conjunctival tests with dilute solutions of the test substance are unreliable and not without hazard. Individuals with known sensitivity to drugs and stings should wear a medical identification bracelet or tag (Medic-Alert) or carry an identification card.

**1. Drug anaphylaxis**—One of the most common forms of drug anaphylaxis is due to penicillin. Avoidance of penicillins is the only sure method of avoiding allergic reactions. All penicillins and related compounds are in varying degrees cross-allergenic. Oral administration of penicillin seems to be safer than parenteral but is not without risk. Specific penicillin antigen tests can be done with ''major'' and ''minor'' determinants, but these are not routinely available. A negative history does not always assure safety, but a history of penicillin reaction or a positive skin test should warn the physician not to use penicillin if another effective drug can be safely substituted. In rare instances where penicillin alone or in combination is the only effective regimen, progressive desensitization may be cautiously attempted. Since this involves risks, desensitization must be done under close supervision in a hospital with adequate resuscitation measures at hand.

Among other drugs that are likely to induce anaphylaxis are immune antisera (eg, tetanus, snake antivenin), protein drugs (eg, chymotrypsin), dehydrocholate sodium, nitrofurantoin, water-soluble iodine radiographic contrast media for parenteral use, and, rarely, vaccines.

**2. Insect stings**—Hymenoptera (honey bees, hornets, yellow jackets, and wasps) are the most common causes of allergic emergencies due to stinging in the USA, although there has been an increasing menace from stings of fire ants (*Solenopsis*). Sensitized patients should always carry an insect-sting first aid kit containing a preloaded syringe of epinephrine, 1:1000 (the solution should not be more than 1 year old); ephedrine sulfate tablets (25 mg); antihistamine tablets; and a tourniquet and should be familar with the use of these items.

**3. Dietary allergies**—Allergies to such foods as nuts, strawberries, and shellfish commonly cause anaphylaxis. Patients with a history of these allergies should take the same types of preventive and precautionary measures as described for insect stings. In addition, they must be instructed to inquire about the possible presence of the offending foods when dining out.

**B. Prior Administration of Antihistamines and Corticosteroids:** Antihistamines and corticosteroids may be given before cautious administration of important drugs to which the individual is sensitive in an attempt to anticipate hypersensitivity reactions, but the results are unpredictable.

**C. Desensitization:** (See p 833.) Hypersensitivity to insect allergens may be extreme, and desensitization is best performed by an experienced allergist. Patients with a history of bee sting anaphylaxis should be desensitized with venom immunotherapy.

Beall GN, Casaburi R, Singer A: Anaphylaxis—Everyone's problem. *West J Med* 1986;**144:**329.

Beeley L: Allergy to penicillin. *Br Med J* 1984;**288:**511.

Perkins RM, Anas NG: Mechanisms and management of anaphylactic shock not responding to traditional therapy. *Ann Allergy* 1985;**54:**202.

Schwartz HJ: Appropriate evaluation and therapy of stinging insect hypersensitivity. (Editorial.) *Arch Intern Med* 1984;**144:**1580.

## 2. SERUM SICKNESS-LIKE REACTIONS

''Serum sickness'' is a systemic allergic reaction that can occur within 1–2 weeks after administration of any foreign serum or drug. It may also appear as a disease prodrome, most notably in hepatitis B. The vasculitic type of response in the serum sickness syndrome is due primarily to circulating immune complexes induced by the offending agent. It is characterized by malaise, fever, urticaria, patchy or generalized rash, lymphadenopathy, musculoskeletal aches and pains, nausea and vomiting, and abdominal pain. Neuropathy and glomerulonephritis occur very rarely. In previously sensitized individuals, the reaction may be severe or even fatal; the onset may occur immediately or after a latent period of hours to days.

## Prevention & Treatment

Recognition of individual hypersensitivity depends upon a history of allergic diathesis or previous drug or serum reactions. It warrants careful precautions in administering immunizing sera and drugs.

Antihistamines or salicylates may be given as needed for mild reactions. Epinephrine, ephedrine, or the corticosteroids may also be required for moderate or prolonged reactions. Severe reactions should be treated as for anaphylaxis.

Lawley TJ et al: A prospective clinical and immunological analysis of patients with serum sickness. *N Engl J Med* 1984;**311:**1407.

## OTHER DRUGS USED IN ALLERGIC DISORDERS

Many manifestations of allergic reactions are due to the liberation of histamine and other chemical mediators of the hypersensitivity reactions from storage sites in the body-tissue mast cells and circulating blood basophils. The treatment of allergies consists of the following drugs:

**A. Antihistamines:** These block some of the effects of histamine. (See below).

**B. Beta-adrenergic Drugs:** These inhibit the release of histamine by increasing intracellular levels of cyclic nucleotides.

**C. Theophyllines:** These inhibit the release of histamine by blocking the enzyme that inactivates intracellular cAMP (see p 137).

**D. Cromolyn:** This agent prophylactically inhibits the release of histamine by an unknown mechanism. It has been used successfully in the prevention of allergic (often seasonal) conjunctivitis as a 4% ophthalmic solution (Opticrom) and for allergic rhinitis (Nasalcrom). In a minority of patients with allergic asthma, prophylactic use of inhaled cromolyn may reduce the frequency of attacks.

**E. Corticosteroids:** These suppress the allergic inflammatory reaction. They are available as nasal spray for allergic rhinitis (beclomethasone [Beconase, Vancenase], flunisolide [Nasalide]), as an inhalant for bronchial asthma (beclomethasone [Beclovent, Vanceril], flunisolide [Aerobid]), and systemically.

### The Antihistamines

These drugs, besides blocking the effects of histamine, also have sedative and atropinelike effects. The several dozen available antihistamine drugs differ from each other principally in potency, duration of action, degree of sedation, and incidence of side effects. It may be necessary to try different types of antihistamines to determine optimal effectiveness for a given patient.

The antihistamines are most useful in the symptomatic treatment of seasonal allergic rhinitis, urticaria, angioneurotic edema, insect stings, and serum sickness. They are less predictably useful in vasomotor or perennial rhinitis and least effective in atopic dermatitis and bronchial asthma. By themselves, even when used intravenously, they fail to protect against severe allergic reactions (eg, anaphylaxis).

Some commonly used antihistaminic drugs and their usual oral dosages are listed below. All are available as parenteral preparations. (AWP/100 = average wholesale price per hundred pills or capsules.)

**A. Sedation Rare:**

1. Terfenadine (Seldane), 60 mg twice daily. (AWP/100 = approximately $48.00.)

**B. Sedation Infrequent:**

1. Chlorpheniramine (Chlor-Trimeton), 4 mg 3–4 times daily. (AWP/100 = approximately $1.60.)

2. Brompheniramine (Dimetane), 4 mg 3–4 times daily. (AWP/100 = approximately $1.50.)

**C. Sedation Often Prominent:**

1. Diphenhydramine (Benadryl), 25–50 mg 3–4 times daily. (AWP/100 = 50 mg approximately $3.00.)

2. Hydroxyzine (Atarax, Vistaril), 25–100 mg 3–4 times daily. (AWP/100 = 25 mg approximately $9.50.)

3. Tripelennamine (Pyribenzamine), 25 mg 3–4 times daily. (AWP/100 = approximately $1.80.)

4. Promethazine (Phenergan), 12.5–25 mg twice daily. (AWP/100 = approximately $2.40.)

Antiallergic, antiviral and immunologic agents. Chapter 9 in: *AMA Drug Evaluations*, 5th ed. American Medical Association, 1983.

Norman FS: Role of immunotherapy in asthma. *Chest* 1985;**87(Suppl):**623.

# Geriatric Medicine & the Elderly Patient

**2**

*Lawrence Z. Feigenbaum, MD*

The biologic changes associated with aging are influenced by hereditary and environmental factors. A distinction should be made between physiologic aging—the normal wear and tear that occurs with the passage of time—and pathologic phenomena occurring in old people that are the result of disease or adverse features of the individual's life-style. The long-term effects of disuse and physical deconditioning are other factors that should logically be distinguished from the physiologic aging process.

Aging ordinarily occurs gradually throughout life, but quite unevenly from individual to individual; some persons age more rapidly than others. Specific chronologic age criteria for designating older individuals as a group are unavoidably arbitrary and may be harmful. The terms "elderly" and "senior citizen" are better defined in terms of functional status rather than by chronologic age, though for purposes of administrative convenience, age 65, age 75, etc, are often used. Some writers now subclassify the elderly into the "young-old" (ages 65–74) and the most rapidly growing group, the "old-old" (over 80 or 85).

Some of the consequences of aging that determine the nature and degree of functional impairment are listed below:

(1) Decreased function of one or more organ systems. Table 2–1 lists changes that occur as a result of "normal" aging.

(2) Decreased stress tolerance. A major characteristic of aging is a diminution or slowing of homeostatic mechanisms required to meet stress. Thus, accidental hypothermia and heat stroke are more common in the elderly, and mortality rates associated with burns, trauma, and disease increase significantly with age.

(3) Increased psychologic stress due to personal losses, eg, loss of physical vigor, deaths of friends and family members, retirement, reduced income, loss of sense of identity and self-worth.

(4) Impaired immunity, eg, greater susceptibility to infection, neoplastic disease.

(5) Increased susceptibility to disease, often to multiple diseases.

(6) Altered pharmacokinetics, eg, adverse drug reactions.

(7) Decreased physical conditioning, eg, loss of muscle tone.

This list of age-related psychophysiologic changes is intended only to emphasize the variety of problems

**Table 2–1.** Changes frequently associated with aging.

| Organ or System | Age-Related Change |
|---|---|
| Skin | Decrease in subcutaneous fat; atrophy of sweat glands; wrinkling and dryness. |
| Eyes | Presbyopia with marked decrease in accommodation; lens opacification and discoloration; decrease in pupil size; increase in drusen. |
| Ears | Decrease in hearing high frequencies; increase in sensitivity to loud noise. |
| Nose | Decrease in sense of smell. |
| Respiratory system | Decrease in bronchial ciliary activity; less lung elasticity; decrease in maximal breathing capacity; decrease in maximal oxygen uptake; decrease in sensitivity of cough reflex. |
| Cardiovascular system | Decrease in elasticity and compliance of arteries; sclerotic changes in aorta and valves; decrease in cardiac output and heart rate response to stress; decrease in baroreceptor response. |
| Gastrointestinal system | Decrease in salivary flow; decreased sense of taste; lower gastric acidity; decrease in absorption of calcium; decrease in colonic motility. |
| Genitourinary system | Atrophy and drying of vaginal mucous membrane; slower sexual response; enlargement of prostate; decrease in number of glomeruli; decrease in renal blood flow; decrease in maximal urine osmolality. |
| Nervous system | Decrease in size and weight of brain; slower psychomotor performance; decrease in "righting" reflexes; fewer nighttime hours of stage 4 and rapid eye movement (REM) sleep. |
| Musculoskeletal system | Decrease in bone mass; decrease in lean body mass. |
| Endocrine system | Glucose intolerance; increase in ADH response; decrease in estrogen secretion; decrease in aldosterone and renin response to upright posture and sodium restriction. |
| Immunologic system | Absent thymic hormone secretion; decrease in T cell function; increase in autoantibodies. |
| General | Decrease in total body water; decrease in lean body mass; increase in percentage of total body fat; decrease in height and weight; graying of hair. |

that may require special consideration in the medical management of elderly patients. It is important to recognize that there is immense variation in these changes within the elderly population and from organ system to organ system. Stereotypic concepts of hopelessness or progressive physical and mental deterioration must be avoided, since most older patients do enjoy good health and respond well to proper medical care.

An awareness of special problems of the elderly, a willingness to listen, a realistic and understanding attitude in dealing with older patients, and a knowledge of community support services can help the elderly function independently and actively as long as possible.

## HISTORY TAKING WITH ELDERLY PATIENTS

It must not be assumed that an older patient is unable to provide a reliable medical history. At the initial interview, the examiner should note any impairment of hearing or speech, mood disturbance, or apparent difficulty with thought processes, any of which may interfere with the history-taking process. If the patient has a hearing aid, be sure that it is used and is working properly. The elderly patient, just as any other patient, should be interviewed in an unhurried, reassuring manner in quiet, pleasant surroundings. If the patient is unable to comprehend or communicate, data should be sought from family and friends. The history should include pertinent information about daily living activities, presence or absence of stairs or elevator, availability of family and friends, and socioeconomic circumstances.

### Drug History

It is essential to review *all* drugs the patient has been taking. Have the patient or family bring in both prescription and over-the-counter drugs. Review them one by one by name, inquiring about the reason for taking the drug, its dosage and frequency of administration, and any adverse side effects the patient may attribute to the drug. Repeat this important exercise as often as necessary to make certain the patient's drug intake is both rational and minimal.

### Dietary History

Many elderly patients have limited nutritional intake. It is important to inquire about the diet, asking specifically about adequacy of income, problems with shopping or preparing meals, eating habits, impaired senses of taste and smell, and difficulties with dentures.

### Psychiatric History

Depression and anxiety resulting from severe psychologic stress or organic disease are common in the elderly. (The highest incidence of suicide in the USA is in white men over age 75.) Depression is a treatable condition that may be overlooked unless one is alert to its possibility. Depression can easily be mistaken for early dementia, since decreased attention span, loss of sense of humor, irritability, and poor performance on mental status testing may occur in both conditions. Loss of appetite, change in sleep patterns, and constipation are common in the well elderly but may also be signs of depression. Ask openly about suicidal thoughts and crying spells and any past history of mental illness. Psychiatric illness in old people can often be successfully treated, and psychiatric consultation should be recommended without hesitation if the history arouses concern about the patient's emotional status.

Do not avoid questions about sexual feelings or problems, since elderly patients may welcome an opportunity to discuss such matters. Many elderly people worry that it is abnormal for them to still have sexual feelings. Impotence or unreliable erections may be a significant problem for elderly men, and dryness of the vagina with a history of dyspareunia for elderly women.

Be aware of the possibility of drug abuse and alcoholism; they are more common in the elderly than is generally recognized.

## PHYSICAL EXAMINATION

A complete physical examination, including pelvic examination in women and rectal examination in both sexes, is essential. Note abnormalities of gait and steadiness on standing. Examine the patient completely undressed (with gown) so that the skin can be carefully inspected. Check for postural blood pressure changes. Test and record hearing and vision. Remove excess cerumen from the external auditory canals, look for cataracts, test ability to read, and check visual fields. Note redness or tenderness over the temporal artery. Look to see if dentures fit well, and inspect the oral cavity carefully with dentures removed, remembering that malignant lesions of the mouth are more often red than white. In auscultating the chest, bear in mind that the presence of an $S_4$ in an elderly patient does not imply clinically significant cardiac disease. Be sure to check for fecal impaction in inactive patients and those with fecal or urinary incontinence. Check muscle strength and range of motion of joints, and observe for neurologic deficit. Diminished or absent vibratory sense in the lower extremities may be found in elderly patients with no evidence of neurologic disease. Careful examination of the feet, including how well the shoes are fitted, is important in the patient with gait disturbance. If the patient uses a cane, be sure it is the correct length (ie, equal to the distance from the wrist crease to the ground) and has a good grip. If the patient is chair-bound or bed-bound, great care must be taken to examine the skin for reddening or evidence of early ulceration over pressure points.

## MENTAL STATUS EXAMINATION

Some form of cognitive testing is desirable with all elderly patients. Remember that patients with mild degrees of dementia may mask intellectual impairment by a cheerful and cooperative manner. If the patient appears mentally competent, the physician should explain that a mental status evaluation is part of every complete examination, so that the patient will not feel singled out and insulted. An examination that tests only orientation as to person, place, and time is not sufficient to detect mild or moderate intellectual impairment. Many practical mental status tests are available (eg, Jacobs Cognitive Capacity Screening Test, the Short Portable Mental Status Questionnaire [SPMSQ], Mini-Mental Status Examination of Folstein) and provide a numerical score that can be of great value as a baseline test.

## EVALUATION OF FUNCTIONAL CAPACITY IN THE ELDERLY

Simply taking a history, performing a physical examination, and listing medical diagnoses are not sufficient for elderly patients, particularly those who are frail and at high risk, for institutional care. A clear description of the patient's degree of fitness or functional incapacity based on both medical and psychosocial problems is essential. Before nursing home placement is recommended, a thorough multidisciplinary geriatric functional assessment should be done in most instances. In addition to the physician, the assessment team usually includes the following:

(1) A social worker who assesses the ability of the family, friends, and community agencies to provide those supports which will allow the patient to remain in his or her home.

(2) An occupational therapist who assesses the patient's ability to perform the activities of daily living. The Katz Index of Activities of Daily Living is a commonly used instrument (Katz S et al: *JAMA* 1963;**185**:94), as are the Barthel Index and Barthel Self-Care Ratings. These tests classify patients according to their functional independence or dependence in the following areas: bathing, dressing, feeding, transferring, using the toilet, and continence. For those patients who are less incapacitated, testing of more complex functions requiring both physical and cognitive ability should be done. These instrumental activities of daily living include reading, writing, cooking, shopping, using the telephone, and managing money and medications. Assessment of these functions and careful consideration of what steps can be taken to help the patient become more independent are often the most important contributions the health team can make in improving the patient's quality of life and preventing or delaying institutionalization. The occupational therapist is also helpful in detecting perceptual disorders, swallowing problems, and apraxias.

(3) A speech pathologist who may detect speech, hearing, and communication problems that might otherwise be overlooked.

(4) A psychiatrist or psychologist who may help differentiate depression (''pseudodementia'') from dementia, as well as organic from psychogenic symptoms.

Other consultants may be required—physiatrist, neurologist, urologist, gynecologist, dentist, and nutritionist being the most frequent.

A home visit is of great value in assessing the patient's ability to function in his or her own environment. Practical advice can be given to the patient or family on how to decrease risks of accidents in the home.

About 25% of patients on waiting lists for nursing home care can remain in their homes if a multidisciplinary functional assessment is carried out and appropriate recommendations implemented.

## LABORATORY EXAMINATIONS

Standard normal laboratory values are essentially the same for the elderly as for younger adults. (There is, for example, no ''anemia of old age.'') An elevated sedimentation rate should arouse a suspicion of polymyalgia rheumatica, cranial arteritis, infection, or cancer. The fasting blood glucose is not significantly altered by age, but the postprandial blood glucose may be higher than normal. Serum creatinine is not a good index of renal sufficiency in the elderly, since creatinine levels may be low because of the decrease in lean body mass. An age-corrected creatinine clearance can be used as a guide for dosage of ototoxic and nephrotoxic antibiotics. Since ''apathetic'' hyperthyroidism is commoner in the aged, thyroid function tests (including plasma TSH measurement) may be indicated. In the confused elderly patient, the following may be of diagnostic value: urinalysis; serum electrolytes; renal, thyroid, and hepatic function tests; blood gases; serum vitamin $B_{12}$ and red blood cell folate levels; and toxicology screening tests.

## SPECIAL CLINICAL CONSIDERATIONS

The following clinical characteristics of the elderly differ from those of the young or middle-aged and must be kept in mind when evaluating and treating elderly patients:

(1) Multiple diseases commonly present.

(2) Atypical presentations of disease.

(3) Frequent adverse drug reactions.

(4) More disability and dependence.

(5) Serious consequences from relatively minor insults.

(6) High frequency of associated social and psychologic problems.

(7) Higher mortality rates.

Diseases more common in the elderly are listed

**Table 2–2.** Diseases more common with aging.

Atherosclerotic cardiovascular and cerebrovascular diseases with resultant myocardial infarction, strokes, multi-infarction dementia, and abdominal aneurysms (see Chapters 8, 9, and 16).
Senile dementia of the Alzheimer type (see below).
Polymyalgia rheumatica (see Chapter 14).
Type II diabetes mellitus and nonketotic hyperglycemic coma (see Chapter 19).
Cancer—especially of the colon, prostate, and lung (see Chapter 32).
Tuberculosis (see Chapter 7).
Cataracts (see Chapter 5).
Osteoarthritis, osteoporosis, and hip fracture (see Chapters 14 and 18).
Parkinson's disease (see Chapter 16).
Depression and suicide (the latter is most common in elderly white men) (see Chapter 17).
Benign prostatic hypertrophy (see Chapter 15).
Diverticulitis (see Chapter 11).
Herpes zoster (see Chapters 4 and 22).

in Table 2–2. Geriatric medicine, although concerned with each of these many disorders, deals most frequently with a number of medical problems that do not usually present as clear-cut organ-specific diagnoses. These problems are most common in the frail elderly, especially those over 80 years of age, and are referred to as the "five *I*'s."

# THE FRAIL ELDERLY & THE FIVE *I*'S

Frail elderly patients are subject to certain problems that are referred to as the "five *I*'s" of geriatrics: (1) intellectual impairment, (2) immobility, (3) instability, (4) incontinence, and (5) iatrogenic drug reactions.

## INTELLECTUAL IMPAIRMENT (Dementia)

Dementia is probably the most feared condition among the aging population. It is important to reassure elderly patients who may have some degree of benign forgetfulness that senile dementia is not inevitable. Clinically significant intellectual impairment affects an estimated 5% of people over age 65 and only 20% of people over age 80. About 60–70% of cases of senile dementia are of the Alzheimer type, and 15–20% are what is called multi-infarction dementia. Another 15–20% of patients show evidence of both forms of the disorder.

## Clinical Features

Early manifestations of dementia include decrease in attention span, impaired powers of concentration, some personality change, and forgetfulness. These changes will often be noted by the family during periods of physical or emotional stress. Many patients with dementia maintain their social graces even in the face of significant cognitive impairment; thus, a clinical impression without mental status testing may miss the diagnosis. As the disease progresses, there is loss of computational ability, word-finding problems, difficulty with ordinary activities such as dressing, cooking, and balancing the checkbook, then severe memory loss and, ultimately, complete disorientation and social withdrawal. Senile dementia of the Alzheimer type has an insidious onset and is steadily progressive. Multi-infarction dementia is more common in men, associated with hypertension with or without a history of transient ischemic attacks or strokes, and is more likely to progress in a series of recognizably distinct steps. Its progression may be slowed by antihypertensive therapy.

## Diagnosis

Diagnosis is based on the history and the physical, laboratory, and mental status examinations. CT scanning is useful only to rule out structural brain disorders, such as hematomas, tumors, hemorrhage, hydrocephalus, and infarction. The scan may show minimal or no cerebral atrophy or ventricular enlargement in patients with severe dementia; conversely, these abnormalities may be incidental findings of no clinical significance in the normal elderly. At present, magnetic resonance imaging (MRI) offers no advantage except perhaps in chronic subdural hematoma. MRI may be impractical for the demented patient who is restless, since the test requires that the patient lie still for a relatively long period.

## Differential Diagnosis

One of the most important tasks of the physician dealing with older people is to rule out treatable causes of confusional states that may mimic dementia. These treatable causes are uncommon, however. The following common causes of confusional states may be missed if not specifically looked for:

**A. Drugs:** A wide variety of agents may cause confusion in the elderly. The most common are sedatives, hypnotics, neuroleptics, antidepressants, anticholinergics, antihypertensives, and nonsteroidal antiinflammatory drugs. If, as sometimes happens, the patient is receiving the same drug under different brand names, there is an increased likelihood of drug-induced confusion. Chronic alcoholism is not rare in the elderly.

**B. Depression:** Depression in the elderly often mimics dementia ("pseudodementia") or may be superimposed on mild dementia. Differentiation may be difficult and may warrant a therapeutic trial of antidepressant drugs.

**C. Other Psychiatric Problems:** Confusion may result from the anxiety and disorienting effect of being in a hospital or other unfamiliar surroundings. Severe anxiety over normal forgetfulness or psychotic behavior may be misdiagnosed as dementia.

**D. Sensory Loss:** Hearing loss not only leads to social isolation but results in inappropriate answers that may be misinterpreted as evidence of dementia. Behavior resulting from abnormalities of perception in patients with lesions of the nondominant parietal lobe may be mistaken for dementia.

**E. Metabolic Disturbances:** Hyponatremia is a common cause of confusional state in hospitalized elderly people because of the age-related increase in antidiuretic hormone (ADH) responsiveness to stress (eg, hypovolemia, morphine, trauma) and the syndrome of inappropriate antidiuretic hormone (SIADH) secretion, many of whose causes are common in the elderly (eg, tuberculosis, carcinoma of the lung and prostate, head injury, brain tumor). Other metabolic derangements such as liver failure, renal failure, and cardiopulmonary failure can also cause metabolic confusional states. Confusion due to hypercalcemia is particularly apt to occur in bone disorders that are more often seen in elderly patients (eg, Paget's disease, multiple myeloma, metastatic carcinoma).

**F. Endocrine Abnormalities:** Hypothyroidism and hyperparathyroidism (even in the absence of hypercalcemia) may cause confusion and be interpreted as senile dementia.

**G. Nutritional Deficiencies:** Cognitive impairment can be produced by folate, niacin, riboflavin, and thiamine deficiencies. Many factors including poor appetite, loss of taste and smell, poorly fitting dentures, and difficulty in shopping for and preparing meals increase the likelihood of nutritional problems.

**H. Trauma:** Subdural hematoma must always be considered as a possible cause of confusion. Falls with head injury may be forgotten or not reported by the patient and unknown to the family.

**I. Brain Tumor:** Metastatic lesions and gliomas are the most common brain tumors in old people, but in published reports they are rare as a cause of dementia.

**J. Infections:** Acute infection in the elderly may cause confusion. Suspect acute infection (eg, pneumonia, pyelonephritis) when an older patient without fever or neurologic deficit suddenly becomes confused. Chronic infections of lung, bone, kidneys, skin (associated with pressure sores), and the central nervous system may also present as dementia.

**K. Cardiovascular or Cerebrovascular Accidents:** Acute myocardial infarction, acute congestive heart failure, or pulmonary embolism may present as an acute confusional state. Strokes that result in fluent or receptive aphasias are often mistaken for dementia.

## Treatment

**A. General Measures:** The important first step in management of a "demented" elderly patient is the search for treatable factors contributing to the confusional state (see above). Patients with these treatable conditions should receive appropriate treatment, which may result in dramatic improvement. However, the patient and family should be advised that treatment often does not result in full recovery.

1. Discontinue nonessential medications, particularly sedatives, and hypnotics.

2. Provide for the patient's comfort and safety. Whenever possible, allow patients to remain in their own living quarters to minimize confusion and disorientation. Remember that the patient who becomes confused for the first time during a hospital stay is likely to recover at home. The adverse consequences of isolation must be balanced against the normal desire for an appropriate degree of privacy.

3. Provide adequate nutrition and hydration, and treat associated medical problems.

4. Remember that no drug treatment has consistently been shown to alter the course of dementia.

5. Help the patient's family cope with this devastating condition. Urge the family to read *The Thirty-Six Hour Day,* by Mace and Rabins (Johns Hopkins University Press, 1981). Support groups such as the Alzheimer's Disease and Related Disorders Association (ARDRA) often are of great value to the family and help to anticipate problems.

6. Ethical decisions about such issues as life support, treatment of acute conditions in a severely demented patient, tube feeding, etc, should be anticipated and, when appropriate, discussed with the patient or family.

**B. Management of Depression:** The elderly patient with early dementia deserves evaluation for possible depression. Since early dementia and depression may be indistinguishable, a cautious therapeutic trial of antidepressant medication may be required.

There is no ideal antidepressant drug. All of the tricyclic antidepressants seem about equally effective, but there are significant differences in side effects (see Chapter 17) that must be considered. Initial dosage should be low, and drug increases should be made slowly to avoid serious side effects; in addition, tricyclics in low doses (eg, doxepin, 10–20 mg daily) may be effective in the elderly. Careful follow-up supervision is required in order to anticipate and minimize anticholinergic side effects, orthostatic hypotension, sedating effects, confusion, bizarre mental symptoms, cardiovascular complications, and drug overdose with suicidal intent. Provide the patient and family with all of the necessary information and warnings, so that adverse drug reactions are not assumed to be due to the aging process.

Experience in the elderly with the tetracyclic agents and other new antidepressants has been limited. The monoamine oxidase inhibitors, used cautiously, are sometimes of benefit when other antidepressants are ineffective. Monoamine oxidase inhibitors should not be used in combination with the cyclic compounds. Electroconvulsive therapy has been successfully used and is usually well tolerated by elderly patients who remain severely depressed despite drug treatment.

## IMMOBILITY
## (Chair- or Bed-bound)

The main causes of immobility in the elderly are weakness, stiffness, pain, imbalance, and psychologic problems. Weakness may result from disuse of muscles, malnutrition, electrolyte disturbances, anemia, neurologic disorders, or myopathies. The commonest cause of stiffness in the elderly is osteoarthritis, but rheumatoid arthritis, gout, and pseudogout also occur in this age group. Polymyalgia rheumatica should not be overlooked in the elderly patient with pain and stiffness, particularly of the pelvic and shoulder girdle, and with associated systemic symptoms (see Chapter 14).

Pain, whether from bone (eg, osteoporosis, osteomalacia, Paget's disease, metastatic bone cancer, trauma), joints (eg, osteoarthritis, rheumatoid arthritis, gout), or muscle (eg, polymyalgia rheumatica, intermittent claudication), may immobilize the patient. Foot problems are common and include plantar warts, ulceration, bunions, corns, and ingrown toenails. Poorly fitting shoes are a frequent cause of these disorders.

Imbalance and fear of falling are major causes of immobilization. Imbalance may result from general debility, neurologic causes (eg, stroke; loss of postural reflexes; peripheral neuropathy due to diabetes, alcohol, or malnutrition; vestibulocerebellar abnormalities), anxiety, or drugs or may occur following prolonged bed rest (see Instability, below).

Psychologic conditions such as severe anxiety, depression, or catatonia may produce or contribute to immobilization.

Iatrogenic factors, particularly excessive bed rest and drugs (eg, haloperidol), may immobilize the patient.

### Treatment

**A. General Measures:** Treatment should be directed toward correction of malnutrition, anemia, and electrolyte disturbances that may be responsible for the patient's immobilized status. Installing handrails, lowering the bed, and providing chairs of proper height with arms and rubber skid guards may allow the patient to be safely mobile in the home. A properly fitted cane or walker may be necessary for getting the patient out for walks. (These aids should not be encouraged if the patient can manage without them.) Podiatric care, including proper footwear, is often essential.

In treating arthritis in the elderly, it must be remembered that nonsteroidal anti-inflammatory drugs, especially indomethacin, may cause central nervous system side effects with resultant confusion.

The hazards of bed rest must be recognized and avoided. Prevention is the best means of dealing with the serious and sometimes life-threatening complications of immobilization. Appropriate active exercises, no matter how limited the patient's capacity, should be encouraged on a regular basis when the patient is chair- or bed-bound.

**B. Management of Specific Complications:**

**1. Bedsores (decubitus ulcers)**—Prevention requires frequent and careful observation of the skin, particularly over pressure points. Keep the skin clean and dry. A special mattress (eg, foam-rubber eggcrate mattress) or water bed may be required for the very debilitated patient. If the patient is chair-bound, the skin over the coccyx and ischial tuberosities must be inspected daily. Correction of malnutrition and anemia is essential (see Chapter 4).

**2. Muscle weakness and wasting and osteoporosis**—Graded exercises and early ambulation are important.

**3. Contractures**—These may be avoided by early institution of range-of-motion exercises. Getting the immobile patient out of bed and into the chair is not enough; unless leg exercises are done regularly, 90-degree knee contractures may result.

**4. Venous thrombosis**—(See Chapter 9.) Frequent ankle flexion while in bed, elastic stockings, correction of dehydration, and early ambulation are important.

**5. Incontinence**—Spurious urinary incontinence is a common problem in immobilized elderly patients who cannot get to the bathroom if the bedpan or urinal is not made easily available. Such functional incontinence must be avoided because of its devastating psychologic effect as well as the potential for skin maceration, bedsores, and secondary skin infections. The patient should be toileted frequently, preferably in the bathroom or on a bedside commode rather than a bedpan. Avoid restraints and side rails whenever possible. (See Urinary Incontinence, below.)

## INSTABILITY (Physical Instability, Falls, Unstable Gait)

Falls are a major problem for elderly people, especially women, and are often the major cause of loss of independence. It is often difficult to tell from the history what caused a fall. The patient who is uncertain about what happened will often say, "I must have tripped."

### Causes of Falls

Causes of falls in the elderly are often classified as intrinsic (host) or extrinsic (environmental). General physiologic impairments associated with aging that may increase the risk of falling include reduced vision, general debility and excessive bed rest, impaired "righting" reflexes, and increased body sway when the patient assumes the upright posture. The older, more debilitated or demented the patient, the more likely it is that a fall will occur. Some specific factors that cause old people to fall are the following:

**A. Environmental:** The home environment often poses hazards, especially for a patient with poor vision, weakness, confusion, or problems of mobility.

These consist of slippery floors or loose or worn carpeting, loose appliance and telephone cords, poor lighting, steep stairs, and absence of handrails in halls and bathrooms and on stairways. All of these are an even greater hazard if the patient wears loose-fitting slippers or walks in stocking feet. Accidental falls are far more common than those associated with specific disease.

**B. "Drop Attacks":** These occur without warning and without loss of consciousness, possibly as a result of sudden loss of antigravity reflexes. The patient usually falls backward. Pressure on the soles of the feet is one stimulus that often helps the patient to get up again.

**C. Loss of Consciousness, Syncope, Vertigo:** (See Chapters 6 and 16.) Such episodes may be due to cerebrovascular or cardiovascular disease (eg, arrhythmias, aortic stenosis, postural hypotension). Leading questions should be avoided, since many patients will say they were "dizzy," if asked.

**D. Spasticity and Rigidity:** These may be due to pyramidal or extrapyramidal disease. Patients with Parkinson's disease may fall because of their spasticity as well as their abnormal center of gravity with festinating gait.

**E. Alcohol:** Excessive alcohol consumption is often overlooked as a cause of falls in old people. Falls occurring while the patient is intoxicated may be forgotten or denied, and a resulting subdural hematoma may be overlooked.

**F. Drugs:** Any drug that causes postural hypotension (eg, neuroleptics, antihypertensives, antidepressants), arrhythmias (eg, antidepressants), dizziness or vertigo, rigidity (eg, neuroleptics), or confusion can affect balance and result in falls. Sedatives and hypnotics should be avoided whenever possible.

**G. Genitourinary Factors:** Urgency (especially at night), straining, and micturition syncope may be unrecognized factors in falls in elderly people.

### Complications of Falls

Fear of falling again is a serious complication and is a major factor in the elderly person's loss of confidence and independence. The most common fractures resulting from falls are of the wrist, hip, and vertebrae. These are more likely to occur in thin white women. There is a high mortality rate (approximately 25% in 1 year) in elderly women with hip fractures, particularly if they were debilitated prior to the time of the fracture.

Subdural hematoma is a treatable but easily overlooked complication of falls that must be considered in any elderly patient presenting with new neurologic signs, including confusion.

Dehydration, electrolyte imbalance, and hypothermia may all occur and endanger the patient's life following a fall.

### Prevention & Management

A home visit by the physician, nurse, or physical therapist is often helpful to correct environmental factors. Cataract surgery or correction of refractive errors may be necessary. Leg muscles can sometimes be strengthened by graded exercises. Instructing patients to change position slowly (from lying to sitting, from sitting to standing) may prevent light-headedness and falls.

Teaching the patient how to get up after a fall if alone can have an important effect on the patient's confidence. Lightweight radio call systems are available that patients can wear to obtain help when out of reach of a telephone.

Estrogen therapy (eg, conjugated estrogens, 0.625 mg daily) for prevention or retardation of bone loss reduces the risk of fractures in women.

Medication and bed rest should be used judiciously.

## URINARY INCONTINENCE

### Classification

**A. Spurious (Functional) Incontinence:** Inability of the patient to get to the toilet without a long delay is probably the most common cause of incontinence in a hospitalized patient. Do not assume the patient will need nursing home care if urinary incontinence occurs for the first time in the hospital, since the problem may disappear at home. The delay in toileting may be related to an inaccessible call light, restraints, side rails, immobility, communication problems, or debility. Medications (eg, hypnotics, sedatives, diuretics) are apt to aggravate the problem.

**B. Detrusor Instability (Spastic or Uninhibited Bladder):** Neuropathic bladder is the commonest cause of chronic incontinence in patients with senile dementia of the Alzheimer type. Bladder volume is small, and uninhibited detrusor contractions result in urinary incontinence.

**C. Overflow Incontinence:** This may occur in elderly men with benign prostatic hypertrophy and partial bladder outlet obstruction. In addition, the large neuropathic bladders seen in diabetes and tabes dorsalis may result in overflow incontinence. Drugs with anticholinergic effects (eg, atropine, antidepressants, antihistamines) may cause urinary retention and overflow incontinence.

**D. Stress Incontinence:** This is a common problem in postmenopausal women and may be due to estrogen deficiency, urethral and vaginal atrophy, or pelvic floor relaxation. If the latter is severe, it may result in persistent incontinence.

**E. Fecal Impaction:** Fecal impaction in immobilized elderly patients is a common cause of urinary incontinence. The mechanism may be local irritative factors, change in urethrovesical angle, or other neurogenic stimuli. Whatever the cause, this is an easily treatable type of urinary incontinence.

### Treatment

Proper diagnosis is essential, since many disorders associated with urinary incontinence are treatable.

**A. Spurious Incontinence:** It is essential that the nursing staff be encouraged to toilet the patient frequently. A bedside commode is often preferable to a bedpan or enclosed toilet at a distance from the bed. Restriction of fluids, especially coffee and tea in the evening, may help. To prevent nocturia, avoid administration of rapidly acting diuretics at night, if possible. Avoid heavy sedation.

**B. Detrusor Instability:** The general measures noted for treatment of spurious incontinence are important here also. Anticholinergic drugs (eg, oxybutinin, 5 mg 2 or 3 times daily, or flavoxate, 200 mg 3 times daily) have been used and may help; however, they are likely to produce serious side effects in elderly people. Imipramine, 25 mg at bedtime, may be helpful but should be used cautiously. Calcium channel blockers (eg, nifedipine, 10–20 mg twice daily) may decrease incontinence in some patients. If senile vaginitis is also present, estrogen therapy (conjugated estrogens, 0.3–0.625 mg daily) may help.

**C. Overflow Incontinence:** Benign prostatic hypertrophy should be corrected surgically. Discontinue or decrease the dosage of anticholinergic drugs. Encourage frequent toileting. Bethanechol chloride, 5 mg cautiously 2 or 3 times daily, may be helpful.

**D. Stress Incontinence and Pelvic Floor Relaxation:** Give estrogen as ethinyl estradiol, 0.02–0.05 mg orally every other day. For pelvic floor relaxation, exercises to strengthen the pelvic floor musculature should be tried. Cystocele and severe pelvic floor relaxation may require surgery. A pessary may be of help if the patient is a poor surgical risk or refuses surgery.

**E. Fecal Impaction:** The impaction must be broken up digitally or dislodged with a sigmoidoscope. Recurrence should be avoided by regular toileting; by increasing the amounts of fluids, fiber, and stewed fruit in the diet; and by using mild laxatives (eg, milk of magnesia, 15–30 mL at bedtime or as necessary), bowel softeners (eg, docusate [Colace]), and bulk-forming agents (eg, psyllium hydrophilic mucilloid [Metamucil], 15 g in a glass of water or fruit juice 2 or 3 times daily). Frequent oil retention enemas or rectal suppositories (glycerin, bisacodyl [Dulcolax]) may be necessary. It is equally important to increase the patient's physical activity if possible.

## General Comments

Make the diagnosis of the type of incontinence first. Urinary tract infection is less often a cause than a consequence of urinary incontinence.

Avoid catheterization, since it imposes a risk of urinary tract infection. If essential, a condom catheter may be used in men with proper hygienic care. Absorbent underpants may simplify management.

Frequent toileting is often the single most important feature of treatment.

Sedatives, hypnotics, and diuretics should be discontinued whenever possible.

## "IATROGENIC" DRUG REACTIONS

Older patients are more likely than young to middle-aged adults to have adverse drug reactions, for a number of reasons. Changes in absorption, even with achlorhydria, are usually not of clinical significance, but drug clearance is often markedly reduced. This is due to a decrease in renal plasma flow and glomerular filtration rate as well as reduced hepatic clearance. The latter is due to a decrease in activity of the drug-metabolizing microsomal enzymes as well as an overall decrease in blood flow to the liver with aging. The volume of distribution of drugs also is affected, since the elderly have a decrease in total body water and a relative increase in body fat. Thus, water-soluble drugs become more concentrated, and fat-soluble drugs have longer half-lives. In addition, serum albumin levels decrease, so that there is some decrease in protein binding of some drugs (eg, warfarin, phenytoin), leaving more free (active) drug available.

In addition, the older patient with multiple chronic conditions is likely to be receiving many drugs. Thus, dosage errors are more likely to occur, especially if the patient has visual, hearing, or memory deficits.

## Precautions in Administering Drugs

To avoid drug toxicity in the elderly, the following should be kept in mind:

**A. Drug Selection and Administration:**

1. Use drug therapy only when the benefit clearly outweighs the risk.

2. Start with less than the usual adult dosage, and increase the dosage slowly.

3. Keep the dosage schedule as simple as possible.

4. Keep the number of tablets or capsules to a minimum, but try to avoid combination drugs. Combinations may be used only after the benefit of and tolerance to each drug, given separately in the same dose as in the combination preparation, have been established.

5. Have the patient or a family member bring in all medications at frequent intervals for reinforcing instructions regarding reasons for drug use, dosage, frequency of administration, and possible adverse effects.

6. As long as the special problems of drug therapy in the elderly are kept in mind, the physician should not withhold essential drugs from older patients.

7. Instruct the pharmacist not to use safety cap containers unless the patient is confused or at high risk for suicide, since it may be difficult or impossible for the patient to open them.

**B. Over-the-Counter Drugs:** Adverse drug reactions may result from taking over-the-counter drugs or drugs prescribed for others in the household in addition to those prescribed for the patient. Have the patient or a family member bring in for review all over-the-counter drugs as well as prescription drugs the patient may be taking.

**C. Sedative-Hypnotics:** Remember that the effects of sedative-hypnotics persist much longer in the elderly and may produce confusional states. Avoid this class of drugs whenever possible.

**D. Antibiotics:** Serum creatinine is not a good index of renal function in old people. An age-corrected creatinine clearance determination should be used to calculate drug doses of ototoxic and nephrotoxic antibiotics.

**E. Cardiac Drugs:** Both digitalis and quinidine have prolonged half-lives in older patients, so toxicity is common at the usual dosages.

**F. Cimetidine:** Cimetidine lowers hepatic blood flow, which reduces drug metabolism and thus results in a higher incidence of toxicity of drugs metabolized mainly in the liver (eg, propranolol). In addition, cimetidine often produces confusion in the elderly.

**G. Antidepressants:** Antidepressants are very likely to produce anticholinergic side effects in old people (eg, confusion, urinary retention, constipation, dry mouth). A period of cautious drug withdrawal should be attempted before assuming that such symptoms are age-related or due to other diseases.

# SUMMARY

## Special Considerations in Treating the Elderly

**A. Encourage Hopeful Attitude:** Remember that 80% of patients over age 80 function well and relatively independently in the community and should not be assumed to be demented, helpless, or hopeless. Remember also that the average 75-year-old man can expect to live to age 84 and the average 77-year-old women to age 87.

**B. Provide Prompt Medical Care:** Impaired homeostasis or even mild changes in physical status in the frail elderly dictate *prompt* medical attention.

**C. Assess Psychosocial Problems:** Early attention to social and psychologic problems may be critical factors in the patient's ability to remain independent.

**D. Utilize Other Health Professionals:** It is essential to be familiar with the roles of other health professionals and to use them as necessary. Inappropriate or unnecessary utilization of hospitals and nursing homes should be avoided and often can be avoided by appropriate "case management," ie, coordination of community social and health services.

**E. Encourage Home Care:** Every attempt should be made to allow the patient to stay at home. A thorough assessment of the patient medically, psychologically, and socially may prevent unnecessary nursing home placement. Some community resources that may be of value include the following: Home

Health Care, Day Health Care, Respite Beds (families who care for elderly relatives at home often require periods of relief from that burden if they are to be able to continue to keep the patient at home), Meals on Wheels, Home Health Aides, Transportation Services for the Disabled, and Visiting Nurses. Daily telephone contact, emergency radio systems, and communal and sheltered living arrangements all have obvious advantages in overall management of old people needing care and attention. Keep in mind the burden that maintaining the patient at home may impose on the family's primary caregiver. This person will need a great deal of support.

**F. Monitor Drug Therapy:** Allow enough time for the patient to respond to treatment before switching to different medications or other forms of treatment.

**G. Assess Feasibility of Surgery:** Age alone should not be the criterion for deciding whether a surgical procedure should be done. Survival following surgery in the elderly has increased dramatically in recent years. Premorbid health status and the patient's wishes are far more important in making this decision.

**H. Assist the Family:** If the patient has dementia, the family often needs the physician's support even more than the patient.

## Identification of the "High-Risk" Elderly

The following patients are at greater risk of rapid deterioration than others and should be monitored more closely:

(1) Those over age 80.
(2) Those who live alone.
(3) Those who are bereaved or depressed.
(4) Those who are intellectually impaired.
(5) Those who have fallen several times.
(6) Those with incontinence.
(7) Those who have not coped well in the past.

## General Instructions to the Elderly Patient

The elderly patient should be given some general practical instructions for maintaining health, dignity, and independence. The following is a partial list of subjects that can be introduced as the occasion arises:

**A. Outside Interests:** Maintain an active interest in others and the outside world (eg, by doing volunteer work such as with foster grandparents, reading daily newspapers, taking educational courses, traveling (there are now many tours specifically arranged for the elderly), and participating in recreational activities).

**B. Nutrition:** Eat nourishing food with adequate protein, fruit, vegetables, and fiber content. Avoid excess calories and salt intake. This sometimes requires smaller and more frequent meals.

**C. Exercise:** Exercise briskly by walking outside of the house at least 3–4 times weekly if possible. A patient who is unable to walk should be taught how to do muscle and movement exercises in a chair or in bed at least 4 times daily, accepting the use of a cane or walker when necessary.

**D. Fluids:** Drink 3–4 glasses of water daily to avoid dehydration.

**E. Skin Hygiene:** Devote proper attention to the skin, with adequate hygiene, but avoid overdrying of the skin by too frequent bathing.

**F. Eyeglasses:** Make sure eyeglasses are properly fitted and checked periodically.

**G. Foot Care:** Make sure that shoes are properly fitted and that feet are examined periodically.

**H. Hearing Aid:** Accept the use of a hearing aid when needed, and talk to a physician for advice in obtaining one. They are less visible now and, even if noticed, are evidence that the wearer is interested in communicating.

**I. Dentures:** Obtain dental services as needed, including being sure dentures fit properly.

**J. Unnecessary Drugs:** Avoid all types of nonessential medicines, especially sleeping pills and tranquilizers. Remember that with age, it is normal for sleep patterns and sleep requirements to change.

**K. Misuse of Alcohol:** Avoid intemperate use of alcoholic beverages.

**L. Physical Safety:** Take appropriate measures to prevent home accidents and injuries. Install handrails, provide adequate lighting, resurface or replace slippery floors, and keep loose appliance and telephone cords off the floor. Night lighting in the bedroom and bathroom is very useful. Avoid hypothermia by means of adequate clothing, heating, and physical activity. Care is needed in preventing burns (eg, when using hot water or electric heating pads).

**M. Medical Care:** Seek prompt medical attention and openly discuss symptoms of dread diseases such as cancer or dementia. The physician should be contacted even when symptoms are equivocal.

**N. Natural Limitations:** Recognize the natural limitations imposed by aging, but be certain that medical and other problems are given proper consideration and are not ascribed to "old age" without suitable diagnostic evaluation.

## REFERENCES

Avorn J: Benefit and cost analysis in geriatric care: Turning age discrimination into health policy. *N Engl J Med* 1984;**310:**1294.

Bortz W: Disuse and aging. *JAMA* 1982;**248:**1203.

Cutler NR et al: Brain imaging: Aging and dementia. *Ann Intern Med* 1984;**101:**355.

Eslinger PJ et al: Neuropsychologic detection of abnormal mental decline in older persons. *JAMA* 1985;**253:**670.

Friedland RP et al: The diagnosis of Alzheimer-type dementia. *JAMA* 1984;**252:**2750.

Greenblatt DJ, Sellers EM, Shader RI: Drug therapy: Drug disposition in old age. *N Engl J Med* 1982;**306:**1081.

Hazzard WR: Preventive gerontology: Strategies for healthy aging. *Postgrad Med* (Aug) 1983;**74:**279.

Health and Public Policy Committee, American College of Physicians: Long-term care of the elderly. *Ann Intern Med* 1984;**100:**760.

Kane R, Ouslander J, Abrass I: *Essentials of Clinical Geriatrics.* McGraw-Hill, 1984.

Kelsey J, Hoffman S: Risk factors for hip fracture. (Editorial.) *New England J Med* 1987;**316:**404.

Kennie DC: Good health care for the aged. *JAMA* 1983;**249:**770.

Lakshmanan M, Mion LC, Frengley JD: Effective low dose tricyclic antidepressant treatment for depressed geriatric rehabilitation patients: A double-blind study. *J Am Geriatr Soc* 1986;**34:**421.

Larson EB et al: Diagnostic tests in the evaluation of dementia: A prospective study of 200 elderly outpatients. *Ann Intern Med* 1986;**146:**1917.

Leaf A: Dehydration in the elderly. (Editorial.) *N Engl J Med* 1984;**311:**791.

Lipschitz DA et al: Cancer in the elderly: Basic science and clinical aspects. *Ann Intern Med* 1985;**102:**218.

Lipsitz LA: Syncope in the elderly. *Ann Intern Med* 1983;**99:**92.

Michel SL et al: Surgical procedures in nonagenarians. *West J Med* 1984;**141:**61.

Nickens H: Intrinsic factors in falling among the elderly. *Arch Int Med* 1985;**145:**1089.

Palmore E, Nowlin J, Wang M: Predictors of function among the old-old: A 10-year follow-up. *J Gerontol* 1985;**40:**244.

Rango N: The nursing home resident with dementia: Clinical care, ethics and policy implications. *Ann Intern Med* 1985;**102:**835.

Resnick NM, Yalla SV: Management of urinary incontinence in the elderly. *N Engl J Med* 1985;**313:**800.

Reuler JB, Cooney TG: The pressure sore: Pathophysiology and principles of management. *Ann Intern Med* 1981;**94:**661.

Rivlin RS: Nutrition and the health of the elderly: A growing concern for all ages. *Arch Intern Med* 1983;**143:**1200.

Rossman I: The pathology of normal aging. *Geriatric Med Today* (April) 1984;**3:**37.

Rowe JW: Health care of the elderly. *N Engl J Med* 1985;**312:**827.

Salzman C: Geriatric psychopharmacology. *Ann Rev Med* 1985;**36:**217.

Schneider E: Infectious diseases in the elderly. *Ann Intern Med* 1983;**98:**395.

Schneider E, Reed JD Jr: Life extension. *N Engl J Med* 1985;**312:**1159.

Schrier RW (editor): Musculoskeletal problems in the elderly. Chapter 11 in: *Clinical Internal Medicine in the Aged.* Saunders, 1982.

Setia U, Serventi I, Lorenz P: Bacteremia in a long-term care facility: Spectrum and mortality. *Arch Intern Med* 1984;**144:**1633.

Terry RD, Katzman R: Senile dementia of the Alzheimer type. *Ann Neurol* 1983;**14:**497.

Thompson TL II, Moran MG, Nies AS: Drug therapy: Psychotropic drug use in the elderly. (2 parts.) *N Engl J Med* 1983;**308:**134, 194.

Tyler KL, Tyler HR: Differentiating organic dementia. *Geriatrics* (March) 1984;**39:**38.

Williams ME, Pannill FC III: Urinary incontinence in the elderly: Physiology, pathophysiology, diagnosis, and treatment. *Ann Intern Med* 1982;**97:**895.

# Fluid & Electrolyte Disorders    3

*Marcus A. Krupp, MD*

Normally, the body fluids have a specific chemical composition and are distributed in discrete anatomic compartments of relatively fixed volumes. Disease can produce abnormalities in the amounts, distribution, and solute concentrations of the body fluids. Correct diagnosis and treatment of fluid and electrolyte disorders depend upon an understanding of the processes that control volume, distribution, and composition. In addition, the pharmacologic or physiologic action of some components of body fluids must be considered.

## BASIC FACTS & TERMS

### VOLUME & DISTRIBUTION OF BODY WATER

The volume of body water in a healthy normal individual is quite constant. Body water content differs inversely with obesity. Fat cells contain very little water, and lean tissue is rich in water. Thus, bodies heavy with fat will contain a smaller ratio of water to body weight than lean bodies. After childhood, women usually have a higher ratio of fat to lean tissue. As humans age, they tend to gain proportionately more fat. In the average well-nourished population of the USA, the total body water varies as shown in Table 3–1.

The distribution of water among the body fluid compartments is dependent upon the distribution and content of solute. Membranes and cells restrict movement of solute into and from capillaries, interstitial fluid, and cells. This results in compartmentalization of solute with resultant distribution of water by osmo-sis to sustain (1) equal osmolal concentrations of solute in compartments and (2) equal concentrations of water in compartments.

Solute concentration is expressed in terms of osmoles. The term osmole (osm) refers to the relationship between molar concentration and osmotic activity of a substance in solution. The osmolality of a substance in solution is calculated by multiplying the molar concentration by the number of particles per mole (mol) provided by ionization. Glucose in solution provides 1 particle per molecule; NaCl in solution—for all practical purposes—totally dissociates into $Na^+$ and $Cl^-$, yielding 2 particles per molecule. One mole of glucose in solution thus yields 1 osmole; 1 mole of NaCl, 2 osmoles. The milliunit (mosm) is more convenient. Osmole-per-kilogram-of-water is termed osmolal; osmole-per-liter-of-solution is termed osmolar. The normal osmolality of body fluids is 285–295 mosm/L.

In all problems of altered osmolality, the alteration exists in all body compartments, and the excess or deficit of solute or of water must be calculated on the basis of total body water (TBW).

### ELECTROLYTES
### (Table 3–2)

In clinical medicine, the measurement of concentrations of electrolyte in body fluids is expressed in milliequivalents per liter of the fluid. Salts in solution dissociate into ions with positive charges (cations) and with negative charges (anions). The numbers of

**Table 3–1.** Total body water (as percentage of body weight) in relation to age and sex.[*]

| Age | Male | Female |
|---|---|---|
| 10–18 | 59% | 57% |
| 18–40 | 61% | 51% |
| 40–60 | 55% | 47% |
| Over 60 | 52% | 46% |

[*] Modified and reproduced, with permission, from Edelman & Liebman: Anatomy of body water and electrolytes. *Am J Med* 1959;**27**:256.

**Table 3–2.** Molar and milliequivalent weights.

| | Valence | Molar Weights (g) | Milliequivalent Weights (mg) |
|---|---|---|---|
| **Cations** | | | |
| $Na^+$ | 1 | 23 | 23 |
| $K^+$ | 1 | 39 | 39 |
| $Ca^{2+}$ | 2 | 40 | 20 |
| $Mg^{2+}$ | 2 | 24 | 12 |
| **Anions** | | | |
| $Cl^-$ | 1 | 35.5 | 35.5 |
| $HCO_3^-$ | 1 | 61 | 61 |
| $H_2PO_4^-$ | $\begin{Bmatrix}1\\2\end{Bmatrix}$ | 31 (as P) | |
| $HPO_4^{2-}$ | | | |
| $SO_4^{2-}$ | 2 | 96 | 48 |

27

positive and negative charges are equal, ie, a divalent cation $(2^+)$ will be balanced by 2 monovalent anions or 1 divalent anion $(2^-)$.

One mole (gram-molecule) of a substance is the molecular weight of the substance expressed in grams. One mole of a substance contains $6.023 \times 10^{23}$ molecules of that substance. If the substance can exist in ionized form, its combining capacity with a substance of opposite charge will be determined by its valence, ie, the number of charges per atom or molecule. One mole of a monovalent ion is defined as an equivalent. Thus, 1 mole of a divalent ion will yield 2 equivalents. The term equivalent, therefore, is an expression of concentration in terms of electrical charge. The concentrations of ions in body fluids are small and better expressed in terms of $10^{-3}$ equivalents (milliequivalents) per liter. Dissociation of some complex ions such as phosphate and protein varies with pH. Thus, at pH 7.4, the normal pH of plasma, phosphate exists as a buffer mixture of $H_2PO_4^-$ and $HPO_4^{2-}$ to yield an effective valence of 1.8.

## BODY FLUID COMPARTMENTS
(Table 3–3)

The principal fluid compartments include plasma and interstitial fluid, which comprise the extracellular fluid, and intracellular fluid. Body fluids also are distributed to dense connective tissue, bone, and "transcellular" spaces (gut lumen, cerebrospinal fluid, intraocular fluid), but these are usually of little clinical significance in body fluid abnormalities except in a few situations (eg, burns, bowel obstruction).

Sodium salts constitute the bulk of osmotically active solute in extracellular water (ECW), whereas potassium salts constitute the bulk of osmotically active solute in intracellular water (ICW). Almost all other solutes present in body water can be considered to be either freely diffusible between ICW and ECW (such as urea) or osmotically inactive (such as intracellular magnesium, which is largely bound to protein) and consequently are not osmotically active in either compartment. The electrolyte concentrations within the compartments are shown in Table 3–4.

Interstitial fluids are not readily available for assay. One relies on determinations on plasma or serum to assess water and electrolyte derangements in the clinical setting.

# PHYSIOLOGY OF WATER & ELECTROLYTE & TREATMENT OF ABNORMAL STATES

In the subsequent discussion, the homeostatic mechanisms and their disturbances are listed under the headings of volume, concentration, and physiologic effects.

## WATER VOLUME

The volume of body water is maintained by a balance between intake and excretion. Water as such, in foods and as a product of combustion, is excreted by the kidneys, skin, and lungs. Electrolytes important in maintaining volume and distribution include the cations sodium for extracellular fluid and potassium and magnesium for intracellular fluid, and the anions chloride and bicarbonate for extracellular fluid and organic phosphate and protein for intracellular fluid.

In response to changes in volume, appropriate feedback mechanisms come into play. The principal elements in regulation are antidiuretic hormone (water); aldosterone and other corticosteroids (sodium and potassium); vascular responses affecting glomerular filtration rate (water and sodium); atrial natriuretic peptide, a hormone from the right atrium (sodium); and renal prostaglandins $PGA_2$ and $PGE_2$ (intrarenal circulation and tubule function).

The average adult requires at least 800–1300 mL of water per day to cover obligatory losses. A normal adult on an ordinary diet requires 500 mL of water for renal excretion of solute in a maximally concentrated urine plus additional water to replace that lost via the skin and respiratory tract.

Fluid losses most often include electrolytes as well as water. Sweat, gastrointestinal fluids, urine, and fluid escaping from wounds contain significant quantities of electrolytes. In order to ascertain deficits of water and electrolytes, one must consider the history, change in body weight, clinical state, and appropriate determinations in plasma of concentration of each of the electrolytes, osmolality, protein, and pH. Assessment of renal function is required before repair and maintenance requirements can be determined and prescribed. The capacity of the kidney to excrete a

**Table 3–3.** Body water distribution in an average normal young adult male.[*]

|  | mL/kg[†] Body Weight | % of Total Body Water |
|---|---|---|
| Total extracellular fluid | 270 | 45 |
| Plasma | 45 | 7.5 |
| Interstitial fluid | 120 | 20 |
| Connective tissue and bone | 90 | 15 |
| Transcellular fluid | 15 | 2.5 |
| Total intracellular fluid | 330 | 55 |
| Total body water | 600 | 100 |

[*] Modified from Edelman & Liebman: Anatomy of body water and electrolytes. *Am J Med* 1959;**27**:256.

[†] $\dfrac{mL/kg}{10}$ = %, eg, 45 mL/kg = 4.5% body weight.

**Table 3–4.** Concentrations of cations and anions present in plasma, interstitial water (ISW), and intracellular water (ICW). (n.d. = Not determined.)

| | Plasma meq/L | | Plasma meq/kg H$_2$O | ISW meq/kg H$_2$O$^*$ | ICW meq/kg H$_2$O |
|---|---|---|---|---|---|
| | Average | Range | Average | Average | Average |
| Na$^+$ | 140 | 138–145 | 150 | 144 | 5–10 |
| K$^+$ | 4 | 3.5–5 | 4 | 4 | 155 |
| Ca$^{2+}$ | 5 | 4.8–5.65 | 5 | 3 | 3 |
| MG$^{2+}$ | 2 | 1.8–2.3 | 2 | 2 | 30 |
| Total | 151 | | 161 | 153 | |
| Cl$^-$ | 103 | 97–105 | 110 | 114 | 5–10 |
| HCO$_3^-$ | 26 | 26–30 | 27 | 28 | 10 |
| Protein | 16 | 14–18 | 2 | 2 ⎫ | |
| HPO$_4^{2-}$; H$_2$PO$_4^-$ | 2 | 1.2–2.3 | 1 | 1 ⎬ | 180$^†$ |
| SO$_4^{2-}$ | 1 | n.d. | 17 | 4 ⎭ | |
| Organic acids | 3 | n.d. | 4 | 4 | |
| Total | 151 | | 161 | 153 | |

$^*$ Concentrations derived by converting plasma concentrations to meq/L of plasma water, accounting for nonwater volume of plasma and applying Donnan factors of 0.96 for monovalent ions and 0.92 for divalent ions.
$^†$ Protein, organic phosphates, other organic compounds.

concentrated or a dilute urine sets the limits of water requirement.

## 1. WATER DEFICIT (Volume Depletion)

Water deficit results in a decrease in volume of both ECW and ICW, with an increase in solute concentration. With decreased blood volume, perfusion of the kidneys and other tissues diminishes and antidiuretic hormone (ADH) release is stimulated, resulting in some conservation of water.

Water deficit results from reduced intake or unusual losses. Reduced intake is likely if the patient is (1) obtunded, unconscious, or disabled; (2) unable to ingest water because of interference with swallowing or esophageal obstruction; (3) given inadequate volumes of fluid to provide for maintenance (insensible loss and urine) and replacement of fluid lost via the gastrointestinal tract (vomiting, diarrhea, ileostomy); (4) has sequestration of fluids (burns, bowel obstruction, peritonitis); or (5) suffers fluid loss due to kidney disorders (diabetes insipidus, osmotic diuresis). Fever or a hot environment increases water loss from the lungs and skin.

### Clinical Findings

**A. Symptoms and Signs:** Early signs are thirst; flushed and loose skin; ''dehydrated'' appearance, with sunken eyes and dry mucous membranes; hypotension; blood pressure; tachycardia; and oliguria. Later, if dehydration progresses, hallucinations, delirium, and coma may ensue.

**B. Laboratory Findings:** The decrease in ICW and ECW results in an increase in solute concentration. Serum sodium and protein concentrations are increased. Serum urea nitrogen and, at times, creatinine are elevated, as a result of reduced renal blood flow. Serum osmolality is increased. Urine specific gravity and osmolality are elevated unless the kidney is the primary source of water loss.

### Treatment

An essential guideline for treatment is acute change in weight, which is directly related to change in fluid volume.

Water may be provided with or without electrolyte. If water alone is needed, 2.5% or 5% dextrose solution may be given intravenously; the dextrose is rapidly metabolized, leaving free water. Electrolyte (Na$^+$) is often required to replenish losses and to sustain adequate circulation and urine output; indeed, 0.9% NaCl should be administered first in patients with volume depletion severe enough to cause hypotension.

In the presence of normal renal function, 2000–3000 mL of water per day (1500 mL/m$^2$ of body surface) will provide a liberal maintenance ration. If dehydration is present with increased serum sodium concentration and osmolality, extra water replacement can be estimated on the basis of restoring normal osmolality for the total body fluid volume. The need for intracellular water is reflected in the extracellular fluid with which it is in osmotic equilibrium; therefore, any correction of deviation in osmolality must be considered on the basis of the total volume of body water.

The water requirement is increased in the presence of fever as a result of increased loss via the skin and lungs.

## 2. WATER EXCESS

Water excess (**dilution syndrome**) produces an expansion of both ECW and ICW, with a corresponding decrease in solute concentration. Both of these effects operate to reduce secretion of antidiuretic hormone (ADH).

Decreased excretion of water can produce an excess of body water, particularly when coupled with increased intake. Decreased renal perfusion results in water retention in the presence of such states as (1) acute or chronic renal failure, (2) nephrotic syndrome, (3) congestive heart failure, or (4) liver disease with ascites. Renal retention of water also occurs in the presence of secretion of vasopressin (ADH) or in the syndrome of inappropriate ADH secretion (SIADH). SIADH is associated with the stress of surgery or anesthesia; pulmonary disease (pneumonia, lung abscess, tuberculosis, mycoses); central nervous system disease (encephalitis, trauma, tumor, hemorrhage); malignant tumors (small cell carcinoma of the lung, prostate, or pancreas; thymoma); hypothyroidism; and a wide variety of drugs (narcotics, chlorpropamide, barbiturates, clofibrate, indomethacin, cyclophosphamide, vincristine, acetaminophen, psychotropic drugs, and diuretics). (See Hyponatremia, below.)

### Clinical Findings

**A. Symptoms and Signs:** Clinical evidence of water excess depends on the cause. If it occurs acutely or is severe, "water intoxication" is manifested by headache, nausea, vomiting, abdominal cramps, weakness, stupor, convulsions, and coma.

**B. Laboratory Findings:** The increased volume of body water produces a dilution of solute. Serum $Na^+$ and protein concentrations are reduced, and serum urea nitrogen concentrations are often low. Plasma osmolality is low. Tests for vasopressin in plasma are available in some laboratories; levels are increased.

### Treatment

The basic treatment consists of water restriction. If a real deficit of sodium exists as well, saline solutions should be employed. In the presence of severe water intoxication, administration of hypertonic saline solution may be useful to move excess intracellular water to the extracellular space, ie, to increase ECF osmolality and diminish intracellular water volume. Overexpansion of extracellular volume, which may precipitate acute congestive heart failure and pulmonary edema, may be prevented by use of a loop diuretic and replacement of urinary sodium loss with 0.9% sodium chloride supplemented with potassium and magnesium as required.

### CONCENTRATION

The total concentration of solute (osmolality) is apparently the same in intracellular and extracellular water. In the intracellular compartment, protein concentration plays a more important osmolar role than in the plasma. The protein content of interstitial fluid is small, and osmolar effects are therefore negligible. The most accessible and best index of osmolality is the measurement of the solute concentration in the plasma or serum by ascertaining the depression of the freezing point or by measurement of vapor pressure. The normal range is 285–295 mosm/L. Serum osmolality can be calculated from the following formula:

$$Osmolarity = 2(Na^+ \text{ mmol/L}) + Glucose \text{ mmol/L} + BUN \text{ mmol/L}$$

$$or = 2(Na^+ \text{ meq/L}) + \frac{Glucose \text{ mg/dL}}{18} + \frac{BUN \text{ mg/dL}}{2.8}$$

(1 mosm of glucose = 180 mg/L and 1 mosm of urea nitrogen = 28 mg/L.)

Measurement of serum sodium by flame photometry may yield an artifactually low result when there is an increased concentration of protein or lipid in the serum. These displace water in which electrolyte is dissolved. Measurement with ion-sensitive electrodes is not so affected.

### HYPEROSMOLAR STATES

Hyperosmolar concentrations of solute in body fluids are harmful when increased concentration of solute confined to the extracellular fluid results in loss of water from cells. Hyperosmolarity may be asymptomatic or give rise to the manifestations listed below.

### Hyperosmolarity With Only Transient or No Symptomatic Shift in Water

Urea and alcohol are 2 substances that readily cross cell membranes and can produce hyperosmolarity. Urea may be administered acutely in large doses to "draw" water from cells, but the effect is transient, as is the diuresis, and urea soon equilibrates throughout body water. Alcohol quickly equilibrates between intracellular and extracellular water, adding 22 mosm/L for every 1000 mg/L. The hyperosmolarity does not produce significant difficulty, but in any condition of stupor or coma in which measured osmolarity exceeds that calculated from values of serum $Na^+$, glucose, and urea nitrogen, alcohol should be considered to explain the discrepancy (osmolar gap). Methanol ingestion is another cause of osmolar gap; it is characterized by severe metabolic acidosis (see p 1020).

### Hyperosmolarity Associated With Significant Shifts in Water

Increased concentrations of solutes that do not readily enter cells produce a shift of water from the intracellular space to effect a true intracellular dehydration. Sodium and glucose are the solutes commonly involved.

# 1. HYPERNATREMIA

Hypernatremia almost always follows loss of water when an excess of $Na^+$ occurs (eg, diabetes insipidus or the osmotic diuresis associated with high-protein feedings coupled with inadequate water intake).

## Clinical Findings

**A. Symptoms and Signs:** Usually there is thirst (except if hypothalamic lesions are the cause), weight loss, flushed loose skin, tachycardia and hypotension, and oliguria. Fever, delirium, hyperpnea, and coma may be seen with severe hyperosmolality.

**B. Laboratory Findings:** Elevated serum $Na^+$ and osmolality are essential findings. Increased concentrations of serum urea nitrogen reflect decreased renal perfusion. Urine osmolality is elevated.

## Treatment

Treatment is directed to correct the cause of the fluid loss and to replace water and, as needed, electrolyte. Water deficit is calculated to restore normal osmolality for total body water. The volume of water required can be determined as follows: Calculate total body water (TBW). (TBW = 0.5–0.6 of body weight for well-nourished to lean adults.) Then,

$$\text{Volume (in liters) to be replaced} = \text{TBW} \frac{[Na^+] - 140}{140}$$

Initially, dextrose 5% in water may be employed. As correction of water deficit progresses, therapy should continue with 0.45% NaCl with dextrose or, if $Na^+$ depletion has also been significant, 0.9% saline. Potassium and phosphate may be added as indicated by serum levels. As soon as possible, oral intake should be resumed.

Replacement should be slow (over 24–72 hours) to permit readjustments through diffusion among fluid compartments. Maintenance requirements should be added to each 24-hour replacement ration.

**A. Hypernatremia With No Change in Total Body $Na^+$:** This rare occurrence may be associated with a hypothalamic malfunction and requires no treatment besides urging the patient to consume an adequate amount of water.

**B. Hypernatremia With an Increase in Total Body $Na^+$:** Accidental intravascular injection of hypertonic saline used for induction of abortion may be responsible. The use of large doses of $NaHCO_3$ in treating cardiac arrest may be a cause, particularly when renal function is impaired. The increase in $Na^+$ produces expansion of extracellular volume at the expense of intracellular water, ie, extracellular overload and intracellular dehydration.

Treatment consists of providing water as 5% glucose at a rate that will expand extracellular fluid volume and reduce hyperosmolarity but not induce congestive heart failure. Simultaneously, loop diuretics such as furosemide should be administered intravenously to remove the excess $Na^+$ and water.

# 2. HYPERGLYCEMIA (Hyperglycemic Hyperosmolar Syndrome)

Hyperglycemia, usually without ketosis, occurs in patients with non-insulin-dependent diabetes mellitus. When hyperglycemia is severe enough to produce significant hyperosmolarity in the extracellular fluid, the loss of water from cells and the loss of total body water consequent to the osmotic diuresis (glycosuria) result in severe dehydration and loss of $Na^+$, $K^+$, and phosphate.

## Clinical Findings

**A. Symptoms and Signs:** The common symptoms and signs are obtundation; severe dehydration with loose, dry skin, sunken eyes, and dry mucous membranes; and hypotension with tachycardia and fall in blood pressure that are more severe when the patient is upright. Impaired consciousness and coma are late manifestations.

**B. Laboratory Findings:** Extreme elevation of serum glucose is seen (usually > 800 mg/dL), as are elevated serum urea nitrogen, creatinine, and, at times, $K^+$. Serum $Na^+$ values may be high or low; in either event, the value should be corrected for the shift of water from the cells to the extracellular fluid as follows: For every 100 mg of serum glucose greater than 180 mg/dL, add 1.6 meq to the measured value of $Na^+$ to obtain the concentration of $Na^+$ that would exist in the absence of hyperglycemia.

## Treatment
(See also p 772.)

Treatment of the hyperosmolar state due to hyperglycemia requires an estimation of the state of total body sodium, for if $Na^+$ deficit is severe, prompt replacement of both $Na^+$ and water is essential. The presence of clinical evidence of low blood (plasma) volume is the best immediate indicator of $Na^+$ deficit. The serum $Na^+$ level is not a reliable index. Initially, it is essential to expand the extracellular fluid volume until blood pressure and urine volume are stable, employing isotonic saline. Low doses of insulin will reduce hyperglycemia. Once circulation is improved, water losses can be calculated on the basis of the degree of hyperosmolarity (see calculation for water replacement for hypernatremia, above) and hyposmolar solutions such as 0.45% saline introduced. Correction of deficit should not be rapid to allow for diffusion and equilibration of water and osmolarity. Serum electrolyte and urea nitrogen levels should be monitored closely. Potassium and phosphate may be required, as their concentration falls routinely with correction of blood glucose. If correction with hyposmolar solutions is too rapid, cerebral edema may result.

## HYPOSMOLAR STATES

### 1. HYPONATREMIA WITH DECREASED EXTRACELLULAR FLUID VOLUME

Hyponatremia with decreased extracellular fluid volume is caused by excessive use of diuretics, chronic renal disease, adrenocorticoid deficiency, and fluid sequestration with burns, peritonitis, and pancreatitis.

#### Clinical Findings

**A. Symptoms and Signs:** Diminished plasma volume and dehydration occur, with thirst, faintness, and dizziness on standing. There is dry mucosa, loss of skin turgor, tachycardia and orthostatic hypotension, and oliguria. Rarely, shock and coma result.

**B. Laboratory Findings:** Low serum $Na^+$ and $Cl^-$ are present. Serum urea and creatinine may be elevated. Serum $K^+$ may be low or high, depending on the cause.

#### Treatment

Treatment consists of replacement of volume loss with isotonic saline and treatment of the underlying disorder. Empiric use of corticosteroids is indicated if hypocortisonism is considered in the differential diagnosis.

### 2. HYPONATREMIA WITH INCREASED EXTRACELLULAR FLUID VOLUME

Hyponatremia with increased extracellular fluid volume occurs when decreased effective circulating blood volume with decreased renal perfusion results in retention of sodium and water. Total body sodium is increased. Secretion of antidiuretic hormone results in a greater retention of water.

#### Clinical Findings

**A. Symptoms and Signs:** Edema occurs in congestive heart failure, hepatic cirrhosis, nephrotic syndrome, and hypoproteinemia.

**B. Laboratory Findings:** Low serum $Na^+$ is present. Serum urea nitrogen and creatinine may be increased.

#### Treatment

Diuretics should be given and the underlying disorder treated. Do not attempt to correct hyponatremia with saline solutions.

### 3. HYPONATREMIA WITHOUT DEHYDRATION OR EDEMA (Normal Extracellular Fluid Volume)

Most commonly, the syndrome of inappropriate secretion of antidiuretic hormone (SIADH) produces retention of water with a dilution of electrolyte. See Water Excess, above, for a list of causes of SIADH.

#### Clinical Findings

**A. Symptoms and Signs:** This disorder is asymptomatic, with no signs of hyponatremia.

**B. Laboratory Findings:** There is low serum $Na^+$ and, often, low serum uric acid. There is increased loss in the urine of sodium, urate, and phosphate.

#### Treatment

Water should be restricted to 800 or 500 mL/d until serum $Na^+$ approaches normal. Demeclocycline (300–600 mg twice daily) is useful in the chronic state. In cases of severe hyponatremia, furosemide or ethacrynic acid may be used to promote diuresis simultaneously with administration of saline 0.9–3% supplemented with $K^+$ replacement.

Hyponatremia must not be corrected rapidly, but osmotic equilibration must be attained gradually to avoid acute volume overload or central pontine myelinolysis. If hyponatremia (water excess) is life-threatening, rapid correction of serum $Na^+$ to 120 meq/L can be accomplished, followed by slower correction thereafter.

The cause of SIADH must be treated. Vasopressin antagonists are under development.

### 4. ARTIFACTUAL HYPONATREMIA

When plasma water per unit volume of plasma is diminished (displaced) by lipids of lipidemia or by protein of hyperproteinemia, sodium concentration will be low when measured by flame photometry. With hyperglycemia, plasma water is increased (shift from cells), and sodium concentration is reduced by 1.6 mmol/L for each 100-mg/dL increase over 180 mg of glucose.

---

## ELECTROLYTES ASSOCIATED WITH PHYSIOLOGIC EFFECTS

---

Hydrogen ion, $K^+$, $Ca^{2+}$, $Mg^{2+}$, and phosphate ion are included in this category. An abnormality of concentration of any one of these is often accompanied by alteration of concentration and effects of others.

### HYDROGEN ION CONCENTRATION

The hydrogen ion concentration ($H^+$) of body fluids is closely regulated with intracellular concentrations of $10^{-7}$ mol/L (pH 7.0) and extracellular fluid concentrations of $4 \times 10^{-8}$ mol/L (pH 7.4). These concentrations are maintained at nearly normal levels by buffer substances that remove or release $H^+$. The capacity of buffers is limited, however, and regulation is accomplished mostly by the lungs and kidneys. The principal buffers include proteins, the oxyhemoglobin-reduced hemoglobin system, primary and secondary phosphate ions, some intracellular phosphate esters, and the carbonic acid-sodium bicarbonate system.

Most of the food used for energy is completely utilized, with production of water, $CO_2$, and urea. Sulfate and phosphate end products are strong acid anions that must be ''neutralized'' by cation such as sodium. In the utilization of fat and carbohydrate, intermediate products include the strong acids acetoacetic acid and lactic acid. Buffers provide cation and remove $H^+$, which is ultimately excreted by the kidneys as acid or as ammonium ion and by the lungs as $CO_2$ and $H_2O$, equivalent to carbonic acid. The anions of strong acids with cations such as sodium and ammonium are eliminated by the kidney.

The role of the lung and kidney in removal of $H^+$ and in regulation of $H^+$ concentration can be viewed as follows:

$$\frac{[H^+]\ [HCO_3^-]}{[B^+]\ [HCO_3^-]} \rightleftharpoons P_{CO_2} \qquad \frac{\text{lung}}{\text{kidney}}$$

Respiratory control of the partial pressure of $CO_2$ ($P_{CO_2}$) in pulmonary alveoli and therefore in the arterial plasma determines the $H_2CO_3$ concentration in body fluids:

$$CO_2 + H_2O \rightleftharpoons H_2CO_3$$

The elimination of $CO_2$ via the lung in effect removes carbonic acid. The kidney is responsible for $BHCO_3$ concentration in body fluids, which, with $H_2CO_3$, constitutes one of the buffer systems for regulation of pH.

In kidney tubule cells, carbonic anhydrase catalyzes the conversion of metabolic $CO_2$ and water to carbonic acid. The carbonic acid serves as a source of $H^+$ that can be exchanged for $Na^+$ in the tubular urine so that $H^+$ is excreted and $Na^+$ reabsorbed.

Although the pH of urine cannot be lowered below pH 4.5, additional $H^+$ ion can be excreted by combination with $NH_3$, generated principally from glutamine within the tubule cell. $NH_3$ diffuses from the tubule cell into the urine, where it combines with $H^+ \rightarrow NH_4^+$, providing cation for excretion with anions of strong acids with no increase in $H^+$ concentration (no lowering of pH). These exchanges in the renal tubule involve active transport systems capable of maintaining a gradient in concentration of extracellular fluid $H^+$ of $4 \times 10^{-8}$ mol/L (pH 7.4) against a tubular urine $H^+$ of $32 \times 10^{-6}$ mol/L (pH 4.5), an 800-fold increase in $H^+$ concentration.

## CLINICAL STATES OF ALTERED $H^+$ CONCENTRATION

The clinical term acidosis signifies a decrease in pH (increase in $H^+$) of extracellular fluid; alkalosis signifies an increase in pH (decrease in $H^+$) of extracellular fluid. The change in $H^+$ concentration may be the result of metabolic or respiratory abnormalities. Mixed abnormal states are common.

## 1. RESPIRATORY ACIDOSIS

Respiratory acidosis follows ventilatory abnormalities resulting in $CO_2$ retention and elevation of $P_{CO_2}$ in alveoli and arterial blood (hypercapnia), with increased $H_2CO_3$ and lowered pH. $CO_2$ retention follows inadequate ventilation during anesthesia, following suppression of the respiratory center by central nervous system disease or drugs, or results from respiratory muscle weakness or paralysis. Structural changes in the lung (emphysema, chronic obstructive disease) or pulmonary circulation and abnormal thoracic structure (kyphoscoliosis) may alter alveolocapillary blood exchange or diminish effective ventilation to prevent $CO_2$ excretion. In association with impaired $CO_2$ excretion ($P_{a_{CO_2}}$), there usually is impaired $O_2$ exchange with low alveolar and arterial $P_{O_2}$ (hypoxemia). In the presence of $CO_2$ retention and the resultant increase in $H_2CO_3$ concentration, compensatory reabsorption of $HCO_3^-$ by the kidney provides buffer to reduce $H^+$ concentration, but this protection cannot be accomplished rapidly and is effective only in chronic situations.

The hazard of acute hypercapnia cannot be overemphasized. Buffer protection is severely limited, and renal response is very slow. Thus, an increase in $P_{a_{CO_2}}$ can quickly produce sharp increases in $H^+$ concentration (decrease in pH) to levels incompatible with life. Respiratory inadequacy or acute, severe reduction of pulmonary circulation resulting in sudden increase in $P_{a_{CO_2}}$ will usually result in a severe decrease in $P_{a_{O_2}}$, compounding the threat to life. It is apparent that periods of hypoventilation constitute a serious and often lethal complication in the immediate postoperative state, following injury of the thoracic cage, in severe illness or shock accompanied by obtunded consciousness, in trauma to the central nervous system, and in the presence of heart failure, cardiac arrhythmias or arrest, and myocardial infarction.

### Clinical Findings

**A. Symptoms and Signs:** With acute onset, there is somnolence, confusion, and asterixis. Coma from $CO_2$ narcosis ensues. In chronic disease, shortness of breath and cyanosis occur.

**B. Laboratory Findings:** Arterial blood pH is low; $P_{CO_2}$ is elevated. Serum bicarbonate is elevated but not enough to compensate completely for the hypercapnia. In chronic respiratory acidosis, arterial $P_{O_2}$ is low and polycythemia may be present.

## Treatment

Treatment is directed toward improvement of ventilation by maintaining an open airway, use of mechanical aids, treatment with bronchodilators, restoration of circulation, correction of heart failure, and antidotes for anesthetics or drugs suppressing the respiratory center. Tracheal intubation is often required. Close monitoring of arterial blood pH, $P_{CO_2}$, and $P_{O_2}$ is essential. The respiratory center is readily rendered unresponsive by high $P_{aCO_2}$ (hypercapnia), and recovery may be slow. In the presence of hypercapnia, relief of hypoxemia with oxygen therapy may deprive the patient of the only remaining stimulus to the respiratory center and produce more severe hypoventilation with resultant $CO_2$ narcosis. However, hypoxemia also has serious consequences, and it cannot be allowed to exist untreated for fear of $CO_2$ narcosis. Thus, careful clinical observation is required while judicious amounts of oxygen are given. Endotracheal intubation should be performed if the patient becomes exhausted or if adequate oxygenation cannot be maintained.

## 2. RESPIRATORY ALKALOSIS

Respiratory alkalosis is a result of hyperventilation, which produces lowered $P_{aCO_2}$ and elevated pH of extracellular fluid. Anxiety is the usual cause. Hyperventilation may also occur during anesthesia or when mechanical ventilatory devices are incorrectly used. Renal compensation by excretion of $HCO_3^-$ (with $Na^+$ predominantly) is too slow a response to be effective, and elevation of pH may reach a point at which asterixis, tetany, and increased neuromuscular irritability appear (probably as a result of a decrease in ionized calcium). Respiratory alkalosis often results from the hyperventilation associated with asthma, congestive heart failure, pulmonary embolism, and pneumonia. Chronic hypocapnia is associated with advanced liver disease and pregnancy.

## Clinical Findings

**A. Symptoms and Signs:** In acute cases (hyperventilation), there is light-headedness, anxiety, paresthesias, numbness about the mouth, and a tingling sensation in the hands and feet. Tetany occurs in more severe alkalosis. In chronic cases, asymptomatic findings are those of the primary disease.

**B. Laboratory Findings:** Arterial blood pH is elevated, and $P_{CO_2}$ is low. Serum bicarbonate is decreased in chronic alkalosis.

## Treatment

Treatment of spontaneous hyperventilation consists of reducing anxiety by drugs or psychotherapy. Tetany may be alleviated by rebreathing exhaled air, which will increase $P_{aCO_2}$ and lower blood pH. Regulation of devices used in assisting with ventilation should be guided by measurement of the $P_{CO_2}$ and pH of arterial blood.

## 3. METABOLIC ACIDOSIS

Metabolic acidosis (lowered blood pH and bicarbonate) occurs with starvation; in uncontrolled diabetes with ketoacidosis and in lactic acidosis; with electrolyte (including bicarbonate) and water loss from diarrhea or enteric fistulas; and with renal insufficiency or tubular defect producing inadequate $H^+$ excretion. Cation loss ($Na^+$, $K^+$, $Ca^{2+}$) and organic acid anion retention occur with starvation and uncontrolled diabetes mellitus. In the presence of renal insufficiency, phosphate and sulfate are retained and cation (especially $Na^+$) is lost because of limited $H^+$ secretion for exchange with cation in the renal tubule. Respiratory compensation for metabolic acidosis by hyperventilation reduces $P_{CO_2}$ and thereby reduces $H_2CO_3$ concentration in extracellular fluid.

When acidosis is evident, it is important to distinguish between bicarbonate loss and the accumulation or retention of strong acid by calculating the "anion gap," or the amount of anion not identified by the usual serum electrolyte determination (Table 3–5).

$$\text{Anion gap} = [Na^+] - ([HCO_3^-] + [Cl^-]) = 8-12 \text{ meq}$$

When bicarbonate is lost (diarrhea, ileostomy, ileal loop bladder, renal tubular acidosis), chloride is usually retained to keep the "gap" normal. When chloride is taken in as $NH_4Cl$ or amino acid-chloride (total parenteral nutrition), bicarbonate is lost and the gap remains normal. An anion gap greater than

**Table 3–5.** Anion gap.

**Normal (8–12 meq)**
Loss of $HCO_3^-$
    Diarrhea
    Pancreatic fluid loss
    Ileostomy (unadapted)
    Carbonic anhydrase inhibitors
Chloride retention
    Renal tubular acidosis
    Ileal loop bladder
    Administration of HCl equivalent
        $NH_4Cl$
        Arginine and lysine in parenteral nutrition
**Increased (>12 meq)**
Metabolic anion
    Diabetic ketoacidosis
    Alcoholic ketoacidosis
    Lactic acidosis
    Renal insufficiency ($PO_4^{3-}$, $SO_4^{2-}$)
    Starvation
    Metabolic alkalosis (increased number of negative
        charges on protein)
Drug or chemical anion
    Salicylate intoxication
    Sodium carbenicillin therapy
    Methanol (formic acid)
    Ethylene glycol (oxalic acid)
**Decreased (<8 meq)**
Plasma cell dyscrasias
    Monoclonal protein (cationic paraprotein) (accompanied
        by chloride and bicarbonate)
Hypoalbuminemia (decreased unmeasured anion)

12 meq indicates accumulation of organic acids such as acetoacetate, β-hydroxybutyrate, and lactate. In the case of renal insufficiency, an anion gap exists because of retention of phosphate, sulfate, and other ions, but the increased hydrogen ion concentration results from inability to excrete hydrogen ion. A smaller than normal anion gap occurs when there is elevation of monoclonal immunoglobulins (with isoelectric point higher than serum pH), particularly IgG, in plasma cell dyscrasias and lymphoproliferative disorders, or with hypoalbuminemia (about 2.5 meq/g of albumin at normal blood pH).

## Clinical Findings

**A. Symptoms and Signs:** Symptoms include thirst, shortness of breath, weakness, and those of the primary disease (eg, polyuria in diabetic ketoacidosis). Signs include dehydration, tachypnea, restlessness, impaired consciousness, and coma, plus those of the primary disease (eg, fruity breath odor in diabetic ketoacidosis).

**B. Laboratory Findings:** Blood pH and $P_{aCO_2}$ and serum $HCO_3^-$ are low. The anion gap may be elevated or normal (see above). Elevated serum urea nitrogen, creatinine, and potassium reflect the degree of renal impairment due to dehydration or renal disease. With diabetic or alcoholic ketoacidosis and with starvation, tests for ketone bodies are positive in urine and serum.

## Treatment

Treatment is directed toward correcting the metabolic defect (eg, insulin for control of diabetes) and replenishment of water and of deficits of $Na^+$, $K^+$, $HCO_3^-$, and other electrolytes. If arterial blood pH is less than 7.1, anion replacement may include bicarbonate, but quantities of bicarbonate should not exceed 50–100 mmol. Renal insufficiency requires careful replacement of water and electrolyte deficit and closely controlled rations of water, sodium, potassium, chloride, and bicarbonate to maintain normal extracellular fluid concentrations; the elevated serum phosphate may be lowered by interfering with phosphate absorption from the gut by oral administration of aluminum hydroxide preparations. In the presence of renal insufficiency, elevated extracellular $K^+$ concentrations may be reduced by either oral or rectal administration of ion exchange resins that bind $K^+$ and prevent absorption in the intestine (see Hyperkalemia, below), or by hemodialysis or peritoneal dialysis. (See Diabetic Ketoacidosis in Chapter 19.)

## Lactic Acidosis

Lactic acidosis is a serious form of metabolic acidosis characterized by reduced serum bicarbonate concentration, a high anion gap, and usually a normal serum chloride. Two general causes are poor tissue perfusion (anoxia; cardiogenic, septic, or hemorrhagic shock; carbon monoxide poisoning) and metabolic abnormalities (diabetes mellitus, liver disease, renal failure, leukemia; toxicity from phenformin, ethanol, methanol, salicylates, isoniazid; ketoacidosis from any cause). Acidosis usually develops abruptly and is manifested by hyperventilation and often by abdominal pain. Blood chemical changes include low pH (< 7.20) of arterial blood, low bicarbonate, and occasionally high serum phosphate. Arterial blood lactate exceeds 5 mmol/L and may reach 10–15 mmol/L or more. The mortality rate is high (60–70%).

Treatment of severe lactic acidosis is that of the underlying disease: restoring tissue blood flow; correcting hypoxia, ketoacidosis, and liver failure, and removing toxic causative agents. Oxygen, intravenous fluids, avoidance of vasoconstrictors, and general supportive measures are required. Until recently, large doses of sodium bicarbonate were given to elevate blood pH and relieve acidosis, but the use of bicarbonate is now controversial. Administration of large amounts of bicarbonate may have deleterious effects by reducing cardiac output and blood pressure and perfusion of tissues and by reducing oxygen release from hemoglobin. The metabolism of lactate will yield bicarbonate to restore bicarbonate buffer and pH toward normal. Small doses of sodium bicarbonate (50–100 mmol) may be indicated for severe acidosis with arterial blood pH < 7.00. (See also p 773.)

## 4. METABOLIC ALKALOSIS

Metabolic alkalosis results from either acid loss or bicarbonate gain (Table 3–6). In both cases, serum bicarbonate is increased, chloride concentration is diminished, and pH is elevated. Moderate or severe metabolic alkalosis (alkalemia) is frequently associated with an increased anion gap because of (1) loss of $H^+$ and resultant increase in negative charge of plasma proteins, and (2) extracellular fluid volume deficit that results in increased concentration of the plasma proteins.

In defense of plasma pH, a decrease in ventilation permits retention of $CO_2$ to provide more of the $H_2CO_3$ fraction of the bicarbonate buffer system. With meta-

**Table 3–6.** Causes of metabolic alkalosis.

**Acid loss**
　Acid gastric juice (vomiting, suction)
　Chloride excretion with increased reabsorption of $HCO_3^-$ from potent diuretics (furosemide, thiazide, ethacrynic acid)
　Renal acid excretion from excess mineralocorticoid (especially aldosterone)
　$K^+$ deficiency with $H^+$ secretion in distal nephron
　Chloride-losing diarrhea (rare)
**Bicarbonate gain**
　Excessive intake of bicarbonate or precursors (alkalinizing salts). Usually requires some degree of renal insufficiency.
　Milk-alkali syndrome
　Metabolism of acetoacetic acid, β-hydroxybutyric acid, ketones, and lactic acid to bicarbonate
　Abrupt decrease of arterial $P_{CO_2}$ during treatment of chronic hypercapnia (compensated respiratory acidosis)
　Contraction alkalosis (body fluid volume depletion)

bolic alkalosis, $K^+$ and $H^+$ are excreted by the kidney, and $K^+$ depletion commonly results.

## Clinical Findings

**A. Symptoms and Signs:** There are no characteristic symptoms or signs. Weakness and hyporeflexia occur if serum $K^+$ is low. Tetany and neuromuscular irritability occur rarely.

**B. Laboratory Findings:** The arterial blood pH and bicarbonate are elevated. The arterial $P_{CO_2}$ is increased. Serum potassium and chloride are decreased. There may be an increased anion gap.

## Treatment

Treatment includes restoration of normal body water volume, $K^+$, $Cl^-$, and $Na^+$. The anion should be exclusively $Cl^-$ until correction is achieved. Alkalosis resulting from mineralocorticoid excess is often resistant to treatment, as the kidney is unable to retain $Cl^-$.

## POTASSIUM

Potassium is the major intracellular cation, parallel to that of sodium in extracellular fluid. Potassium plays an important role in muscular contraction, conduction of nerve impulses, enzyme action, and cell membrane function.

Cardiac muscle excitability, conduction, and rhythm are markedly affected by changes in concentration of $K^+$, $Mg^{2+}$, and $Ca^{2+}$ in extracellular fluid. Both an increase and a decrease of extracellular $K^+$ concentration diminish excitability and conduction rate. Higher than normal concentrations produce a marked depression of conductivity with cardiac arrest in diastole; in the presence of very low concentrations, cardiac arrest occurs in systole. The effects of abnormal $K^+$ concentrations upon the cell membrane potential of cardiac muscle and upon depolarization and repolarization are manifested in the ECG.

At both extremes of abnormal concentration of $K^+$ in extracellular fluid, skeletal and smooth muscle contractility is impaired and flaccid paralysis ensues.

Potassium concentration of extracellular fluid is closely regulated between 3.5 and 5 meq/L. Excretion of the 35–100 meq of potassium contained in the daily diet of the average adult is predominantly via the kidney. Loss or retention of $K^+$ by the kidney depends on many factors: renin-angiotensin-aldosterone effects, blood pH, serum $K^+$ concentration, glomerular filtration rate, and renal prostaglandins.

### 1. HYPERKALEMIA

The usual basis for hyperkalemia ($K^+$ concentration > 5 meq/L) is reduced excretion by the kidney. Table 3–7 lists the common causes.

## Clinical Findings

**A. Symptoms and Signs:** The elevated $K^+$ con-

**Table 3–7.** Causes of hyperkalemia.

**Diminished excretion**
  Renal failure, acute and chronic
  Severe oliguria due to severe dehydration or shock
**Increased supply of $K^+$**
  Overtreatment with $K^+$, orally or parenterally
  Massive release of intracellular $K^+$ in burns, rhabdomyolysis or crush injury, or severe infection
**Endocrine disease**
Adrenocortical insufficiency
  Hyporeninemic-hypoaldosteronism (often with long-term diabetes mellitus)
**Physiologic causes**
  Metabolic acidosis
**Artifacts**
  Leakage from erythrocytes if separation of serum from clot is delayed
  Thrombocytosis, with release of $K^+$ from platelets (plasma $K^+$ not affected)

centration interferes with normal neuromuscular function to produce weakness and flaccid paralysis; abdominal distention and diarrhea may occur. As extracellular concentration of $K^+$ increases, the ECG reflects impaired conduction by peaked T waves of increased amplitude, atrial arrest, spread in the QRS, and biphasic QRS–T complexes. The heart rate may be slow; ventricular fibrillation and cardiac arrest are terminal events.

**B. Laboratory Findings:** The serum $K^+$ is elevated. There is evidence of renal impairment (eg, elevated serum urea nitrogen, creatinine, phosphate, and urate; decreased $HCO_3^-$). With metabolic acidosis, the shift of $K^+$ from cells into the extracellular fluid produces an increase in serum potassium of approximately 0.6 meq/L per 0.1 unit decrease in pH from 7.4.

## Treatment

First confirm that the elevated level of serum or plasma $K^+$ is genuine (see p 1100). Treatment consists of withholding potassium and employing cation exchange resins by mouth or enema. Kayexalate, a sodium cycle sulfonic polystyrene exchange resin, 40–80 g/d in divided doses, is usually effective. In an emergency, insulin plus 10–50% glucose may be employed to deposit $K^+$ with glycogen in the liver, and $Ca^{2+}$ may be given intravenously as an antagonist ion. Sodium bicarbonate can be given intravenously as an emergency measure in severe hyperkalemia; the increase in blood pH results in a shift of $K^+$ into cells. Hemodialysis or peritoneal dialysis may be required to remove $K^+$ in the presence of protracted renal insufficiency. Therapy of the precipitating even proceeds concurrently.

### 2. HYPOKALEMIA

Hypokalemia is caused by decreased intake or absorption and increased loss (Table 3–8). Potassium

**Table 3–8.** Causes of hypokalemia.

**Poor intake**
  Starvation, alcoholism
  Prolonged use of intravenous fluids lacking potassium
**Reduced absorption**
  Malabsorption
  Small bowel bypass; short bowel
**Increased loss**
  Gastrointestinal: Vomiting, gastrointestinal suction, obstruction, small bowel fistula, diarrhea, villous adenoma, laxative abuse
  Renal: Congenital tubular defects (renal tubular acidosis, Fanconi's syndrome); renal failure; diuresis (diuretics, osmolar); acidosis (especially diabetes); metabolic alkalosis; corticotropin or glucocorticoid excess (Cushing's syndrome); mineralocorticoid excess (aldosterone-renin); licorice abuse; Bartter's syndrome; some antibiotics (amphotericin B, aminoglycosides, sodium load with carbenicillin or ticarcillin)
  Skin: Burns; excessive sweating
**Hypokalemia with no deficit (shift into cells)**
  Insulin; beta-adrenergic agonists
  Athletic training; testosterone (anabolic agent) therapy
  Respiratory alkalosis
  Familial periodic paralysis

deficit may or may not be accompanied by lowered extracellular fluid $K^+$ concentration ($< 3.5$ meq/L); however, when hypokalemia is present, total potassium deficit is usually profound. Exceptions to this common circumstance include the hypokalemia of alkalosis and that following administration of insulin.

## Clinical Findings

**A. Symptoms and Signs:** Weakness, paresthesias, and nocturia are frequent complaints. Skeletal muscle weakness, hyporeflexia, and even flaccid paralysis are characteristic. Smooth muscle involvement results in paralytic ileus. The diurnal pattern of urine excretion may be reversed.

**B. Laboratory Findings:** The serum $K^+$ is low ($< 3.5$ meq/L). Depending on the cause, serum $Na^+$, $Ca^{2+}$, or $Mg^{2+}$ may be low. The serum $HCO_3^-$ is usually elevated.

The ECG shows decreased amplitude and broadening of T waves, prominent U waves, sagging ST segments, and in more severe deficit, atrioventricular block and finally cardiac arrest. (Hypokalemia increases the likelihood of digitalis toxicity; see p 250).

## Treatment

Treatment requires replacement of potassium orally or parenterally. Because of the toxicity of potassium, it must be administered slowly and cautiously to prevent hyperkalemia. Confirmation of adequate renal function is important when potassium is administered, since the principal route of excretion is via the kidney. KCl in a total dose of 1–3 mmol/kg/d may be given parenterally in glucose or saline solutions (or both) at a rate that will not produce hyperkalemia. Except in an emergency in which serum $K^+$ is extremely low and cardiac muscle and respiratory muscle activity seriously impaired, the administration

of $K^+$ should be at a rate of 10–20 meq per hour or less. $Cl^-$ is always needed to relieve the hypochloremia of the accompanying metabolic alkalosis. The $K^+$ depletion of renal tubular acidosis requires $K^+$ and $HCO_3^-$ replacement. (See Renal Tubular Acidosis, p 552.) The hypokalemia of Bartter's syndrome responds to potassium replacement. If serum $Mg^{2+}$ or $Ca^{2+}$ is low, treatment should include these cations (see below).

## CALCIUM

Calcium constitutes about 2% of body weight, but only about 1% of the total body calcium is in solution in body fluid. In the plasma, calcium is present as a nondiffusible complex with protein (33%); as a diffusible but undissociated complex with anions such as citrate, bicarbonate, and phosphate (12%); and as $Ca^{2+}$ (55%). The normal total plasma (or serum) calcium concentration is 2.25–2.6 mmol/L (9–10.3 mg/dL). The serum calcium level is responsive to 2 hormones: parathyroid hormone elevates and calcitonin lowers the concentration. Vitamin D, particularly its active form 1,25-dihydroxycholecalciferol, and serum $PO_4^{3-}$ also influence $Ca^{2+}$ regulation. Bone serves as a reservoir of calcium available to body fluids. Excretion of $Ca^{2+}$ is via the kidney.

Calcium functions as an essential ion for many enzymes. Along with other cations (especially $K^+$ and $Mg^{2+}$), calcium exerts an important effect on cell membrane potential and permeability manifested prominently in neuromuscular function. It plays a central role in muscle contraction. At the synapse, the synaptic knobs release acetylcholine. The action potential opens gated $Ca^{2+}$ channels to increase the discharge of acetylcholine commensurate with $Ca^{2+}$ influx.

In cardiac muscle, augmentation of intracellular $Ca^{2+}$ with $Ca^{2+}$ from the extracellular fluid via the slow channels of the muscle cell membrane contributes significantly to contraction. Cardiac muscle responds to elevated $Ca^{2+}$ concentration with increased contractility, ventricular extrasystoles, and idioventricular rhythm. These responses are accentuated in the presence of digitalis. With severe calcium toxicity, cardiac arrest in systole may occur. Low concentration of $Ca^{2+}$ produces diminished contractility of the heart and a lengthening of the QT interval of the ECG by prolonging the ST segment.

## 1. HYPERCALCEMIA

Important causes of hypercalcemia are listed in Table 3–9.

## Clinical Findings

**A. Symptoms and Signs:** Anorexia, nausea and vomiting, constipation, polyuria, muscle weakness

**Table 3–9.** Causes of hypercalcemia.

**Increased intake or absorption**
  Milk-alkali syndrome
  Vitamin D and/or vitamin A excess
**Endocrine disorders**
  Primary hyperparathyroidism (adenoma, hyperplasia,
    carcinoma)
  Secondary hyperparathyroidism (renal insufficiency, malab-
    sorption)
  Acromegaly
  Adrenal insufficiency
**Neoplastic disease**
  Tumors producing PTH-like peptides (ovary, kidney, lung)
  Metastases to bone
  Lymphoproliferative disease, including multiple myeloma
  Secretion of prostaglandins and osteolytic factors
**Miscellaneous causes**
  Thiazide diuretic-induced
  Sarcoidosis
  Paget's disease of bone
  Hypophosphatasia
  Immobilization
  Familial hypocalciuric hypercalcemia
  Complications of renal transplantation
  Iatrogenic

with hyporeflexia, tremor, lethargy, and confusion are common. Stupor, coma, and azotemia ensue. Death is usually due to cardiac arrhythmia or asystole.

**B. Laboratory Findings:** A significant elevation of serum $Ca^{2+}$ is seen; the level must be interpreted in relation to the serum albumin level (see Hypocalcemia). Serum phosphate may or may not be low, depending on the cause. The ECG shows a shortened QT interval.

### Treatment

Treatment consists of control of the primary disease. Symptomatic hypercalcemia is associated with a high mortality rate; treatment must be promptly instituted. Until the primary disease can be brought under control, renal excretion of calcium with resultant decrease in serum $Ca^{2+}$ concentration should be promoted. Excretion of $Na^+$ is accompanied by excretion of $Ca^{2+}$; therefore, inducing natriuresis by giving $Na^+$ salts intravenously and by adjunctive use of diuretics, this is the emergency treatment of choice. Sodium in large quantities (50–80 mmol/h), as chloride or sulfate, with or without diuretics (furosemide) for 12–48 hours may be required. Replacement of water and of $K^+$ and $Mg^{2+}$ is usually necessary. Calcitonin may be a useful adjunct, but tachyphylaxis develops in 24–48 hours. The use of phosphate is hazardous and should be reserved for unusual cases refractory to saline therapy. When elevated $Ca^{2+}$ concentrations result from sarcoidosis or neoplasm, corticosteroids such as prednisone may be effective. Mithramycin is useful if elevated $Ca^{2+}$ is the result of neoplasm metastatic to bone (see p 1063). Recent experience with diphosphonates indicates that they may play a central role in treatment of hypercalcemia; toxicity appears minimal.

## 2. HYPOCALCEMIA

Important causes of hypocalcemia are listed in Table 3–10.

### Clinical Findings

**A. Symptoms and Signs:** Hypocalcemia affects neuromuscular function to produce muscle cramps and tetany, convulsions, stridor and dyspnea, diplopia, abdominal cramps, and urinary frequency. Cataracts may appear and calcification of basal ganglia of the brain may occur in chronic hypoparathyroidism. Mental retardation and stunted growth are common in childhood. (See Hypoparathyroidism, p 708).

**B. Laboratory Findings:** Serum $Ca^{2+}$ is low. The level of serum $Ca^{2+}$ must be correlated with the simultaneous concentration of serum albumin: When albumin concentration is depressed, serum $Ca^{2+}$ concentration is also depressed in a ratio of 0.8–1 mg of $Ca^{2+}$ to 1 g of albumin. Serum phosphate is usually elevated. Serum $Mg^{2+}$ is commonly low, and hypomagnesemia reduces tissue responsiveness to parathyroid hormone. Other findings are those of the primary disease. The ECG shows a prolonged QT interval.

### Treatment

Treatment depends on the primary disease. Treatment of hypoparathyroidism with vitamin D and calcium is discussed in Chapter 18. For tetany due to hypocalcemia, calcium gluconate, 1–2 g, may be given intravenously. A continuous infusion to sustain plasma calcium concentration may be required. Oral medication with the chloride, gluconate, levulinate, lactate, or carbonate salts of calcium will usually control milder symptoms or latent tetany. Vitamin D may be required to ensure adequate absorption of calcium. (See Vitamin D, p 804.) The low serum $Ca^{2+}$ associated with low serum albumin concentration does not require replacement therapy. Treatment of low serum $Mg^{2+}$ may normalize serum calcium.

**Table 3–10.** Causes of hypocalcemia.

**Decreased intake or absorption**
  Malabsorption
  Small bowel bypass, short bowel
  Vitamin D deficit (decreased absorption, decreased
    production of 25-hydroxyvitamin D or 1,25-
    dihydroxyvitamin D)
**Increased loss**
  Chronic renal insufficiency
  Diuretic therapy
**Endocrine disease**
  Hypoparathyroidism (genetic, acquired)
  Pseudohypoparathyroidism
  Calcitonin secretion with medullary carcinoma of the thyroid
**Physiologic causes**
  Associated with decreased serum albumin
  Decreased end organ response to vitamin D
  Hyperphosphatemia
  Induced by aminoglycoside antibiotics, mithramycin, loop
    diuretics

# MAGNESIUM

About 50% of total body magnesium exists in the insoluble state in bone. Only 5% is present as extracellular cation; the remaining 45% is contained in cells as intracellular cation. The normal plasma concentration is 1.5–2.5 meq/L, with about one-third bound to protein and two-thirds as free cation. Excretion of magnesium ion is via the kidney.

Magnesium is an important activator ion, participating in the function of many enzymes involved in phosphate transfer reactions. Magnesium exerts physiologic effects on the nervous system resembling those of calcium. Magnesium acts directly upon the myoneural junction.

## 1. HYPERMAGNESEMIA

Magnesium excess is almost always the result of renal insufficiency and the inability to excrete what has been taken in from food or drugs, especially antacids.

### Clinical Findings

**A. Symptoms and Signs:** Muscle weakness, mental obtundation, and confusion are characteristic manifestations. Weakness, even flaccid paralysis, and fall in blood pressure are evident on examination. There may be respiratory muscle paralysis or cardiac arrest.

**B. Laboratory Findings:** Serum $Mg^{2+}$ is elevated. In the common setting of renal insufficiency, concentrations of serum creatinine, urea nitrogen, phosphate, and uric acid are elevated; serum $K^+$ may be elevated. Serum $Ca^{2+}$ is often low. The ECG shows increased PR interval, broadened QRS complexes, and elevated T waves.

### Treatment

Treatment is directed toward alleviating renal insufficiency. Calcium acts as an antagonist to $Mg^{2+}$ and may be given intravenously as calcium chloride, 500 mg or more at a rate of 100 mg (4.5 mmol)/min. Hemodialysis or peritoneal dialysis may be indicated.

## 2. HYPOMAGNESEMIA

Relatively common causes of hypomagnesemia are given in Table 3–11.

### Clinical Findings

**A. Symptoms and Signs:** Common symptoms are weakness, muscle cramps, and tremor. There is marked neuromuscular and central nervous system hyperirritability, with tremors, athetoid movements, jerking, nystagmus, and a positive Babinski response. There may be hypertension, tachycardia, and ventricular arrhythmias. Confusion and disorientation may be prominent.

**Table 3–11.** Causes of hypomagnesemia.

| |
|---|
| **Diminished absorption or intake** |
|   Malabsorption, chronic diarrhea, laxative abuse |
|   Prolonged gastrointestinal suction |
|   Small bowel bypass |
|   Malnutrition |
|   Alcoholism |
|   Parenteral alimentation with inadequate $Mg^{2+}$ content |
| **Increased loss** |
|   Diabetic ketoacidosis |
|   Diuretic therapy |
|   Diarrhea |
|   Hyperaldosteronism, Bartter's syndrome |
|   Associated with hypercalciuria |
|   Renal magnesium wasting |
| **Unexplained** |
|   Hyperparathyroidism |
|   Postparathyroidectomy |
|   Vitamin D therapy |
|   Induced by aminoglycoside antibiotics, cisplatin |

**B. Laboratory Findings:** The serum $Mg^{2+}$ is low. Hypocalcemia and hypokalemia are often present. The ECG shows a prolonged QT interval particularly due to lengthening of the ST segment.

### Treatment

Treatment consists of the use of intravenous fluids containing magnesium as chloride or sulfate, 10–50 mmol/d during the period of severe deficit followed by 5 mmol/d for maintenance. Magnesium sulfate may also be given intramuscularly, 8–33 mmol/d in 4 divided doses. Serum levels must be monitored to prevent the concentration from rising above 2.5 mmol/L. $K^+$ and $Ca^{2+}$ may be required as well. Magnesium oxide, 250–500 mg by mouth 2–4 times daily, is useful for repleting stores in those with chronic hypomagnesemia.

# PHOSPHORUS

Eighty percent of the phosphorus in the body is combined with calcium in bones and teeth. Only 10% is incorporated in a variety of organic compounds, and 10% is combined with proteins, lipids, carbohydrates, and other compounds in muscle and blood. Organic phosphate is the principal intracellular anion; inorganic phosphate comprises only a small fraction of intracellular phosphorus.

Phosphate compounds are integral agents in energy transfer and in the metabolism of carbohydrate, protein, and fat. Phosphate serves as the principal urinary buffer ($HPO_4^{2-}$, $H_2PO_4^{-}$), constituting most of titratable acidity.

Renal tubular reabsorption of filtered phosphate is reduced (phosphate excretion increased) by parathyroid hormone, expansion of extracellular fluid volume, increased intake of sodium, hypercalcemia, calcitonin, glucocorticoids, and growth hormone.

Phosphorus metabolism and homeostasis are intimately related to calcium metabolism. See sections on calcium metabolism and bone disease.

# 1. HYPERPHOSPHATEMIA

Causes of hyperphosphatemia are given in Table 3–12. Growing children normally have serum phosphate levels higher than those of adults.

## Clinical Findings

**A. Symptoms and Signs:** The clinical manifestations are those of the underlying disorders (eg, chronic renal failure, hypoparathyroidism).

**B. Laboratory Findings:** Serum phosphate is increased. Other blood chemistry values are those characteristic of the underlying disease.

## Treatment

Treatment is that of the underlying disease and of acute onset of hypocalcemia. In acute and chronic renal failure, dialysis will reduce serum phosphate. Absorption of phosphate can be reduced by administration of aluminum hydroxide gel, 30 mL or (as tablets) 4–5 g 3–4 times daily.

# 2. HYPOPHOSPHATEMIA & PHOSPHORUS DEFICIENCY

Hypophosphatemia may occur in the presence of normal phosphate stores. Serious depletion of body phosphate stores may exist with low, normal, or high concentrations of phosphorus in serum. Leading causes of hypophosphatemia are listed in Table 3–13.

## Clinical Findings

**A. Symptoms and Signs:** Acute, severe hypophosphatemia (0.1–0.2 mg/dL) can lead to acute hemolytic anemia with increased erythrocyte fragility; impaired oxygen delivery to tissues, increased susceptibility to infection from impaired chemotaxis of leukocytes, and platelet dysfunction with petechial hemorrhages. Rhabdomyolysis, encephalopathy (irritability, confusion, dysarthria, convulsive seizures, and coma), and heart failure are uncommon but serious manifestations.

Chronic severe depletion may be manifested by

**Table 3–12.** Causes of hyperphosphatemia.

**Endocrine disease**
  Excessive growth hormone (acromegaly)
  Hypoparathyroidism associated with low calcium
  Pseudohypoparathyroidism associated with low calcium
**Renal disease**
  Chronic renal insufficiency
  Acute renal failure
**Catabolic states; tissue destruction**
  Stress or injury, particularly if renal insufficiency exists
  Chemotherapy of malignant disease, particularly lymphoproliferative
**Excessive intake or absorption**
  Laxatives or enemas containing phosphate
  Hypervitaminosis D

**Table 3–13.** Causes of phosphate depletion and hypophosphatemia.

| Causes of Phosphate Depletion |
| --- |

**Diminished supply or absorption**
  Starvation
  Parenteral alimentation with inadequate phosphate content
  Malabsorption syndrome, small bowel bypass
  Absorption blocked by aluminum hydroxide or bicarbonate
  Vitamin D-deficient and vitamin D-resistant osteomalacia
**Increased loss**
  Hyperparathyroidism (primary or secondary)
  Hyperthyroidism
  Renal tubular defects permitting excessive phosphaturia (congenital, induced by monoclonal gammopathy, heavy metal poisoning)
  Hypokalemic nephropathy (potassium depletion)
  Inadequately controlled diabetes mellitus

| Causes of Hypophosphatemia |
| --- |

**All of the conditions listed above**
**Intracellular shift of phosphorus**
  Administration of glucose, fructose (transient)
  Administration of insulin (transient)
  Anabolic steroids, estrogen, oral contraceptives
  Respiratory alkalosis
  Salicylate poisoning
**Electrolyte abnormalities**
  Hypercalcemia
  Hypomagnesemia
  Metabolic alkalosis
**Causes of clinically significant hypophosphatemia** (losses followed by inadequate repletion)
  Diabetes mellitus with acidosis, particularly during aggressive therapy
  Recovery from starvation or prolonged catabolic state
  Total parenteral nutrition with inadequate ration of phosphate
  Chronic alcoholism, particularly during restoration of nutrition; associated with hypomagnesemia (magnesium deficit)
  Respiratory alkalosis
  Recovery from severe burns

anorexia, pain in muscles and bones, and fractures.

**B. Laboratory Findings:** In acute symptomatic hypophosphatemia, serum phosphorus is less than 1 mg/dL. Evidence of anemia due to hemolysis may be present (eg, elevated serum lactate dehydrogenase). Rhabdomyolysis results in elevated serum creatine kinase (which contains mostly MM fraction but also some MB fraction) and, often, in myoglobin in the urine. Other values vary according to the cause. In chronic depletion, radiographs and biopsies of bones show changes resembling those of osteomalacia.

## Treatment

Treatment is best directed toward prophylaxis by including phosphate in repletion and maintenance fluids. For parenteral alimentation, 20 mmol of phosphorus is required for 1000 nonprotein kcal to maintain phosphate balance and to ensure anabolic function. A daily ration for prolonged parenteral fluid maintenance is 20–40 mmol phosphorus. A commercially available $KH_2PO_4/K_2HPO_4$ mixture (pH 6.5) provides potassium, 4.4 mmol/L, and phosphate, 3 mmol/mL; 5 mL added to each of 2 L of fluid would provide potassium, 44 mmol, and phosphate, 30 mmol (= 930 mg phosphorus). For asymptomatic hypophosphatemia (serum phosphorus 0.7–1 mg/dL), the infusion should provide 9–10 mmol/12 h until the serum phosphorus exceeds 1 mg/dL. A magnesium deficit often coexists and should be treated simultaneously. In administering phosphate-containing solutions, renal function must be assessed and serum calcium must be monitored to guard against production of hypocalcemia. For oral use, phosphate salts are available in skim milk (approximately 33 mmol/L). Tablets or capsules of mixtures of sodium and potassium phosphate may be given to provide 16–32 mmol of phosphorus (0.5–1 g of phosphate) per day.

Contraindications to therapy with phosphate salts include hypoparathyroidism, renal insufficiency, tissue damage and necrosis, and hypercalcemia.

# THE APPROACH TO DIAGNOSIS & TREATMENT OF WATER, ELECTROLYTE, & ACID-BASE DISTURBANCES

In the diagnosis and treatment of water and electrolyte derangements, one must rely upon clinical appraisal of the patient, including details of the history, the presenting disease and its complications, recent and abrupt change in weight, the physical examination, and the laboratory data bearing upon altered volume, osmolarity, distribution, and physiologic manifestations. Although a thorough knowledge of the physiologic principles of water and electrolyte metabolism and of renal function is essential for sound management, the physician must always consider and be grateful for the homeostatic resources of the patient. If renal function is reasonably good, the range between acceptable lower and upper limits of amounts of water and electrolytes is broad and the achievement of "balance" not difficult. In the presence of renal insufficiency, some endocrinopathies influencing water and electrolyte metabolism, shock, heart failure, hepatic insufficiency, severe gastrointestinal fluid loss, pulmonary insufficiency, and some rarer diseases, the patient is deprived of homeostatic resources, and the physician is called upon to substitute meticulous quantitative therapy.

## MAINTENANCE

Most of those who require water and electrolyte intravenously are relatively normal people who cannot take orally what they require for maintenance. Table 3–14 shows that the range of tolerance for water and electrolytes (homeostatic limits) permits reasonable latitude in therapy provided normal renal function

**Table 3–14.** Daily maintenance rations for patients requiring parenteral fluids.

|  | Per m² Body Surface | Average Adult (60–100 kg) |
|---|---|---|
| Glucose | 60–75 g | 100–200 g |
| Na⁺ | 50–70 meq | 80–120 meq |
| K⁺ | 50–70 meq | 80–120 meq |
| Water | 1500 mL | 2500 mL |

exists to accomplish the final regulation of volume and concentration.

An average adult whose entire intake is parenteral would require for maintenance 2500–3000 mL of 5% or 10% dextrose in 0.2% saline solution (34 meq $Na^+ + Cl^-$/L). To each liter, 30 meq of KCl could be added. In 3 L, the total chloride intake would be 192 meq, which is easily tolerated. An alternative would be to eliminate the KCl if parenteral fluids would be required for only 2–3 days. Other solutions available for maintenance therapy contain electrolyte mixtures designed to meet average adult requirements: in one example, each liter contains dextrose, 50 g; $Na^+$, 40 meq; $K^+$, 35 meq; $Cl^-$, 40 meq; $HCO_3^-$ equivalent, 20 meq; and $PO_4^{3-}$, 15 meq. The daily administration of 2500–3000 mL satisfies the needs listed in Table 3–14.

In situations requiring maintenance or maintenance plus replacement of fluid and electrolyte by parenteral infusion, the total daily ration should be administered continuously over the 24-hour period in order to ensure the best utilization by the patient. Periodic large infusions result in responsive excretion by the kidney. With modern techniques for continuous infusion, around-the-clock administration imposes little discomfort or hardship on the patient.

If parenteral fluids are the only source of water, electrolyte, and calories for longer than a week, more complex fluids containing amino acids, lipid, trace metals, and vitamins should be used under carefully controlled conditions. (See Total Parenteral Nutrition, p 812.)

## DEFICITS

To the maintenance ration one must add water and appropriate electrolyte for replacement of losses previously incurred and to replace current losses. The amounts of water and electrolytes are dictated by clinical evaluation of deficits of each, and a further choice of anion would be dictated by the presence of metabolic acidosis or alkalosis and in some instances of respiratory acidosis.

The severity of dehydration (volume depletion) is assessed by means of the history, the magnitude of acute weight loss, and, on physical examination, the loss of elasticity of the skin and subcutaneous tissues, dry mucous membranes, tachycardia and hypotension, lethargy, and weakness. As dehydration becomes more severe, the decrease in plasma volume results in progression of hypotension and shock. An increase in blood urea nitrogen reflects the decreases in glomerular filtration rate associated with low blood volume.

Changes in effective extracellular fluid volume and circulating blood volume accompany the acute redistribution of fluid following burns, bowel obstruction, peritonitis, venous obstruction, and, rarely, lymphatic obstruction.

Treatment consists of replacement of water deficit with appropriate electrolyte according to serum osmolarity ($Na^+$ concentration), blood pH, and serum $K^+$ concentration. In the presence of hyperosmolarity (hypernatremia), electrolyte-free or hypotonic solutions should be employed; if serum $Na^+$ concentration is normal, repletion can be accomplished with isotonic solutions. If hyposmolarity (hyponatremia) exists due to sodium loss, hypertonic (3%) NaCl solutions or hypertonic $NaHCO_3$ solutions may be required, but only if the serum sodium is less than 120 mg/dL. In addition to replacement needs, maintenance requirements must be met, requiring correlation of volume, electrolyte concentration, and rate of administration to effect a normal state.

One should aim for total replacement in 48–72 hours. Time is required for circulation, diffusion, equilibration, renal response, and restoration of normal homeostatic mechanisms; a general rule is to provide daily maintenance needs plus half the deficit in the first 24 hours and a quarter of the deficit daily for 2 days thereafter to complete restitution in 72 hours. To this must be added the equivalent of continuing losses.

Common situations in which deficits may be large are discussed below. Other less common derange-

ments are beyond the scope of this chapter. For guidance on therapy, consult more detailed texts and specific treatises.

### Gastrointestinal Disease

Gastrointestinal disease is often accompanied by large losses of water, sodium, and potassium. Loss of chloride or bicarbonate is related to site of the disease or obstruction, eg, pyloric obstruction with loss of HCl; small bowel fluid losses with loss of bicarbonate. (See Table 3–15.) Following intubation, the collected secretions should be assayed to determine the volume and losses of electrolyte that must be replaced.

### Diabetic Ketosis

Diabetic ketosis is characterized by significant losses of water, sodium, and potassium in addition to retention of ketone body acids and a decrease in bicarbonate and pH in the extracellular fluid. Therapy is outlined on p 768.

### Ascites

The association of liver disease with ascites and the consequences of therapy with diuretics may produce complex alterations of fluid distribution and electrolyte concentrations. (See Chapter 11.)

### Peritonitis

Inflammation may produce a large collection of fluid in the peritoneal cavity. Prompt restoration of plasma volume and extracellular fluid is essential.

### Burns

Edema accompanying the trauma to tissue results in sequestration of fluids in tissues beneath the burns with consequent decrease in circulating plasma vol-

**Table 3–15.** Volume and electrolyte content of gastrointestinal fluid losses.[*]

|  | $Na^+$ (meq/L) | $K^+$ (meq/L) | $Cl^-$ (meq/L) | $HCO_3^-$ (meq/L) | Volume (mL) |
|---|---|---|---|---|---|
| Gastric juice, high in acid | 20 (10–30) | 10 (5–40) | 120 (80–150) | 0 | 1000–9000 |
| Gastric juice, no acid | 80 (70–140) | 15 (5–40) | 90 (40–120) | 5–25 | 1000–2500 |
| Pancreatic juice | 140 (115–180) | 5 (3–8) | 75 (55–95) | 80 (60–110) | 500–1000 |
| Bile | 148 (130–160) | 5 (3–12) | 100 (90–120) | 35 (30–40) | 300–1000 |
| Small bowel drainage | 110 (80–150) | 5 (2–8) | 105 (60–125) | 30 (20–40) | 1000–3000 |
| Distal ileum and cecum drainage | 80 (40–135) | 8 (5–30) | 45 (20–90) | 30 (20–40) | 1000–3000 |
| Diarrheal stools | 120 (20–160) | 25 (10–40) | 90 (30–120) | 45 (30–50) | 500–17,000 |

[*] Average values per 24 hours with range in parentheses.

ume and circulatory collapse. Therapy is described in Chapter 29.

• • •

## SUMMARY OF CLINICAL APPROACH

The following outline summarizes an approach to therapy with water and electrolytes. Listed are factors essential to an assessment of the state of the patient, of the urgency for treatment, and of the choice of the therapeutic agents and the quantities to be administered. This outline has been useful in planning the therapeutic attack and averting the omission of essential elements of treatment.

### Problems
1. Simple maintenance.
2. Repair of deficit plus maintenance.
3. Repair plus replacement of continuing losses plus maintenance.
4. Replacement of continuing losses plus maintenance.

### Situations: Acute or Chronic
**A. Acute:**
1. Respiratory–$P_{CO_2}$ and pH. Often overlooked. $H^+$ concentration can change rapidly to life-threatening levels.
2. Organic ion acidosis (lactate, ketones), "anion gap." Normally, $Cl^- + HCO_3^- + 12 = Na^+$ in meq/L.
3. Plasma $K^+$, $Mg^{2+}$, $Ca^{2+}$, and $PO_4^{3-}$ deficit or excess.
4. Hyper- or hyposmolality, often iatrogenic.
5. Explosive gastrointestinal loss; Addison's disease in crisis.
6. Acute renal failure.
**B. Chronic:**
1. Renal insufficiency.
2. Pulmonary insufficiency.
3. Chronic gastrointestinal disease (gut, liver).
4. Endocrine abnormality, especially myxedema.

### Determinants in Establishing Therapy
Sex: Females have proportionately more body fat than males.

Size: Fat or lean; more fat means lower ratios of total body water/kg.

Renal and pulmonary function.

Cause of abnormal state, ie, shock, gastrointestinal obstruction, third space sequestration, diabetes or other endocrine abnormality, malnutrition, drug effect, or therapeutic error.

### Observations
Weight.

Intake, output, and loss record.

Serum electrolytes, osmolarity, urea, creatinine, protein, glucose.

Arterial blood $P_{CO_2}$, pH, $P_{O_2}$ as indicated.

Urine specific gravity, osmolarity, volume.

• • •

Tables 3–16, 3–17, 3–18, and 3–19 show examples of the wide choices available for planning the restoration of water and electrolyte in the variety of clinical problems that may occur. A sound understanding of the physiologic mechanisms discussed above enables the physician to direct therapy rationally and with considerable skill. If renal and pulmonary function are compromised, the task becomes difficult and hazardous for even the best-informed clinicians.

**Table 3–16.** Equivalent values of salts used for therapy.[*]

| Salt | g | mmol of Cation per Amount Stated |
|---|---|---|
| **IV or oral** | | |
| NaCl | 9 | 155 |
| NaCl | 5.8 | 100 |
| NaCl | 1 | 17 |
| NaHCO₃ | 8.4 | 100 |
| Na lactate | 11.2 | 100 |
| KCl | 1.8 | 25 |
| K acetate | 2.5 | 25 |
| K₂HPO₄ | 1.35 | 25 |
| KH₂PO₄ | 1.27 | |
| CaCl₂ | 0.55 | 5 |
| Ca gluconate | 2.2 | 5 |
| MgCl₂ | 0.57 | 5 |
| **Oral** | | |
| K citrate | 3 | 25 |
| K tartrate | 5 | 27 |

[*] Reproduced, with permission, from Krupp MA et al: *Physician's Handbook,* 21st ed. Lange, 1985.

**Table 3–17.** Examples of solutions for parenteral infusion.

| | Electrolyte Content in meq/L | | | | | | | Glucose (g/L) |
|---|---|---|---|---|---|---|---|---|
| | Na$^+$ | K$^+$ | Ca$^{2+}$ | NH$_4^+$ | Cl$^-$ | HCO$_3^-$ Equiv[*] | PO$_4^{3-}$ | |
| 5% glucose in water | | | | | | | | 50 |
| 10% glucose in water | | | | | | | | 100 |
| Isotonic saline (0.9%) | 155 | | | | 155 | | | |
| Ringer's injection | 147 | 4 | 4 | | 155 | | | |
| Ringer's lactate (Hartmann's) | 130 | 4 | 3 | | 109 | 28 | | |
| Potassium chloride<br>  0.2% in dextrose 5% | | 27 | | | 27 | | | 50 |
|   0.3% in dextrose 5% | | 40 | | | 40 | | | 50 |
| Ammonium chloride, 0.9% | | | | 170 | 170 | | | |
| Sodium lactate, ⅙ molar | 167 | | | | | 167 | | |
| Sodium bicarbonate, ⅙ molar | 167 | | | | | 167 | | |
| Examples of "maintenance solutions":<br>Maintenance electrolyte "No. 75" with dextrose 5% | 40 | 35 | | | 40 | 20 | 15 | 50 |
| 5% dextrose in 0.2% saline | 34 | | | | 34 | | | 50 |
| 10% dextrose in 0.45% saline | 77 | | | | 77 | | | 100 |

[*] HCO$_3^-$ equivalent may be bicarbonate, lactate, acetate, gluconate, or citrate, or combinations of these.
*Note:* A variety of modifications of multiple electrolyte solutions are commercially available.

**Table 3–18.** Examples of electrolyte concentrates.

| | Ampule Volume | Electrolyte Content in mmol per Ampule | | | | | | | | PO$_4^{3-}$ (mmol) |
|---|---|---|---|---|---|---|---|---|---|---|
| | | Na$^+$ | K$^+$ | Ca$^{2+}$ | Mg$^{2+}$ | NH$_4^+$ | Cl$^-$ | HCO$_3^-$ | Other Anion | |
| Potassium chloride[*] | 10 mL | | 20 | | | | 20 | | | |
| Potassium acetate[*] | 20 mL | | 40 | | | | | | 40 (acetate) | |
| Potassium phosphate[*] | 15 mL | | 65 | | | | | | | 45 |
| Calcium gluconate, 10% | 10 mL | | | 2.25 | | | | | 4.5 (gluconate) | |
| Sodium bicarbonate, 1 mmol/mL | 50 mL | 50 | | | | | | 50 | | |
| Sodium lactate, molar † | 40 mL | 40 | | | | | | | 40 (lactate) | |
| Ammonium chloride[*] | 30 mL | | | | | 120 | 120 | | | |
| Magnesium sulfate, 50% | — | | | | 4‡ | | | | | |

*Note:* The physician should always check the contents of the ampule as listed by the manufacturer.
[*] Dilute to 1 L or more.
† Dilute as indicated by the manufacturer.
‡ 2 mmol/mL.

**Table 3–19.** Examples of oral electrolyte preparations.

| Preparation | Supplied As | Electrolyte Content* | | | | | |
|---|---|---|---|---|---|---|---|
| | | Na$^+$ | K$^+$ | NH$_4^+$ | Ca$^{2+}$ | Cl$^-$ | HCO$_3^-$ |
| NaCl | Salt | 17 | | | | 17 | |
| NaHCO$_3$ | Salt | 12 | | | | | 12 |
| KCl | Salt | | 14 | | | 14 | |
| K-triplex | Elixir | | 15 meq/5 mL | | | | |
| K gluconate (Kaon) | Elixir | | 7 meq/5 mL | | | | |
| Ca gluconate | Salt | | | | 2.25 | | |
| Ca lactate | Salt | | | | 3.25 | | |
| NH$_4$Cl (acidifying salt) | Salt | | | 19† | | 19 | |
| Keyexalate | Salt | 1‡ | ‡ | | | | |

* mmol/g unless otherwise specified.
† NH$_4^+$ is converted to H$^+$ in the body, mmol for mmol.
‡ 1 g resin removes 1 mmol K$^+$ and contributes 3 mmol Na$^+$ to patient.

# REFERENCES

## General

Brenner BM, Rector FC Jr (editors): *The Kidney,* 3rd ed. Vol 1. Saunders, 1986.

Knochel JP: Neuromuscular manifestations of electrolyte disorders. *Am J Med* 1982;**72:**521.

Maxwell M, Kleeman CR (editors): *Clinical Disorders of Fluid and Electrolyte Metabolism,* 4th ed. McGraw-Hill, 1987.

Mitch WE, Wilcox CS: Disorders of body fluids, sodium and potassium in chronic renal failure. *Am J Med* 1982;**72:**536.

Narins RG, Emmett M: Simple and mixed acid-base disorders: A practical approach. *Medicine* 1980;**59:**161.

Narins RG et al: Diagnostic strategies in disorders of fluid, electrolyte and acid-base homeostasis. *Am J Med* 1982;**72:**496.

Skorecki KL, Brenner BM: Body fluid homeostasis in congestive heart failure and cirrhosis with ascites. *Am J Med* 1982;**72:**323.

## Fluid Volume & Sodium

Anderson RJ: Hospital-associated hyponatremia. *Kidney Int* 1986;**29:**1237.

Anderson RJ et al: Hyponatremia: A prospective analysis of its epidemiology and the pathogenetic role of vasopressin. *Ann Intern Med* 1985;**102:**164.

Decaux G et al: Treatment of the syndrome of inappropriate secretion of antidiuretic hormone with furosemide. *N Engl J Med* 1981;**304:**329.

DeFronzo RA, Thier SO: Pathophysiologic approach to hyponatremia. *Arch Intern Med* 1980;**140:**897.

Dzau VJ, Hollenberg NK: Renal response to captopril in severe heart failure: Role of furosemide in natriuresis and reversal of hyponatremia. *Ann Intern Med* 1984; **100:**777.

Gardenswartz MH, Berl T: Drug-induced changes in water excretion. *The Kidney* (May) 1981;**14:**19.

Gennari FJ: Serum osmolality: Uses and limitations. *N Engl J Med* 1984;**310:**102.

Jamison RL, Kriz W: *Urinary Concentrating Mechanism.* Oxford Univ Press, 1982.

Jamison RL, Oliver RE: Disorders of urinary concentration and dilution. *Am J Med* 1982;**72:**308.

Manning PT et al: Vasopressin-stimulated release of atriopeptin: Endocrine antagonists in fluid hemostasis. *Science* 1985;**229:**395.

Moran SM et al: The variable hyponatremic response to hyperglycemia. *West J Med* 1985;**142:**49.

Moses AM, Notman DD: Diabetes insipidus and syndrome of inappropriate antidiuretic hormone secretion (SIADH). *Adv Intern Med* 1982;**27:**73.

Narins RG et al: Diagnostic strategies in disorders of fluid, electrolyte and acid-base homeostasis. *Am J Med* 1982;**72:**496.

Packer M, Medina N, Yushak M: Correction of dilutional hyponatremia in severe chronic heart failure by converting-enzyme inhibition. *Ann Intern Med* 1984;**100:**782.

Robertson GL, Aycinena P, Zerbe RL: Neurogenic disorders of osmoregulation. *Am J Med* 1982;**72:**339.

Rose BD: A physiologic approach to solute and water balance in hyponatremia. *Kidney* (Jan) 1984;**17:**1.

Schrier RW: Treatment of hyponatremia: Editorial retrospective. *N Engl J Med* 1985;**312:**1121.

## Hydrogen Ion

Cogan MG et al: Metabolic alkalosis. *Med Clin North Am* 1983,**67:**903.

Cohen RD, Woods HF: Lactic acidosis revisited. *Diabetes* 1983;**32:**181.

Harrington JT: Metabolic alkalosis. (Clinical conference.) *Kidney Int* 1984;**26:**88.

Kassirer JP: Life-threatening acid-base disorders. *Adv Nephrol* 1985;**14:**67.

Kreisberg RA: Lactate homeostasis and lactic acidosis. *Ann Intern Med* 1980;**92:**227.

Kurtzman NA, Batlle DC (editor): Symposium on acid-base disorders. *Med Clin North Am* 1983;**67:**751.

Lever E, Jaspan JB: Sodium bicarbonate therapy in severe diabetic ketoacidosis. *Am J Med* 1983;**75:**263.

Narins RG, Cohen JJ: Bicarbonate therapy for organic acidosis: The case for its continued use. *Ann Intern Med* 1987;**106:**615.

Oster JR, Epstein M: Acid-base aspects of ketoacidosis. *Am J Nephrol* 1984;**4**:137.

Relman AS: "Blood gases": Arterial or venous? (Editorial.) *N Engl J Med* 1986;**315**:188.

Schade DS (editor): Metabolic acidosis. *Clin Endocrinol Metab* 1983;**12**:265. [Entire issue.]

Stacpoole PW: Lactic acidosis: The case against bicarbonate therapy. *Ann Intern Med* 1986;**105**:276.

Weil MH et al: Difference in acid-base state between venous and arterial blood during cardiopulmonary resuscitation. *N Engl J Med* 1986;**315**:153.

Williams HE: Alcoholic hypoglycemia and ketoacidosis. *Med Clin North Am* 1984;**68**:33.

## Potassium

Cannon-Babb ML, Schwartz AB: Drug-induced hyperkalemia. *Hosp Pract* 1986;**21**:99.

DeFronzo RA, Bia M, Smith D: Clinical disorders of hyperkalemia. *Annu Rev Med* 1982;**33**:521.

Hollenberg NK (editor): Potassium, magnesium and cardiovascular morbidity. *Am J Med* 1986;**80(Suppl 4A)**:1.

Hollenberg NK, Hollifield JW (editors): Potassium/Magnesium depletion: Is your patient at risk of sudden death. *Am J Med* 1987;**82(Suppl 3A)**:1.

Kaplan NM: Our appropriate concern about hypokalemia. (Editorial.) *Am J Med* 1984;**77**:1.

Knochel JP: Etiologies and management of potassium deficiency. *Hosp Pract* 1987;**22**:153.

Knochel JP: Hypokalemia. *Adv Intern Med* 1984;**30**:317.

Narins RG et al: Diagnostic strategies in disorders of fluid, electrolyte and acid-base homeostasis. *Am J Med* 1982;**72**:496.

Williams ME, Rosa RM, Epstein FH: Hyperkalemia. *Adv Intern Med* 1986;**31**:265.

## Calcium

Agus ZS, Wasserstein A, Goldfarb S: Disorders of calcium and magnesium homeostasis. *Am J Med* 1982;**72**:473.

Alveoli LV, Haddad JG: The vitamin D family revisited. (Editorial.) *N Engl J Med* 1984;**311**:47.

Body J-J et al: Dose/response study of aminohydroxypropylidene biphosphonate in tumor-associated hypercalcemia. *Am J Med* 1987;**82**:957.

Harinck HIJ et al: Role of bone and kidney in tumor-induced hypercalcemia and its treatment with bisphosphonate and sodium chloride. *Am J Med* 1987;**82**:1133.

Mundy GR et al: The hypercalcemia of cancer: Clinical implications and pathogenic mechanisms. *N Engl J Med* 1984;**310**:1718.

Rabin D, McKenna TJ: Calcium and phosphate homeostasis. Pages 324–371 in: *Clinical Endocrinology and Metabolism.* Vol 9 in: *The Science and Practice of Medicine.* Grune & Stratton, 1982.

Sutton RA: Disorders of renal calcium excretion. *Kidney Int* 1983;**23**:665.

Zaloga GP et al: Hypocalcemia in critical illness. *JAMA* 1986;**256**:1924.

## Magnesium

Agus ZS, Wasserstein A, Goldfarb S: Disorders of calcium and magnesium homeostasis. *Am J Med* 1982;**72**:473.

Cronin RE, Knochel JP: Magnesium deficiency. *Adv Intern Med* 1983;**28**:509.

Hollenberg NK (editor): Potassium, magnesium and cardiovascular morbidity. *Am J Med* 1986;**80(Suppl 4A)**:1.

Hollenberg NK, Hollifield JW (editors): Potassium/magnesium depletion: Is your patient at risk of sudden death. *Am J Med* 1987;**82(Suppl 3A)**:1.

Levine BS, Coburn JW: Magnesium, the mimic/antagonist of calcium. *N Engl J Med* 1984;**310**:1253.

Rude RK, Singer FR: Magnesium deficiency and excess. *Annu Rev Med* 1981;**32**:245.

Whang R et al: Frequency of hypomagnesemia in hospitalized patients receiving digitalis. *Arch Intern Med* 1985;**145**:655.

Whang R et al: Predictors of clinical hypomagnesemia: Hypokalemia, hypophosphatemia, hyponatremia, and hypocalcemia. *Arch Intern Med* 1984;**144**:1794.

Zaloga GP et al: Hypomagnesemia is a common complication of aminoglycoside therapy. *Surg Gynecol Obstet* 1984;**159**:561.

## Phosphorus

Fisher JN, Kitabichi AE: A randomized study of phosphate therapy in the treatment of diabetic ketoacidosis. *J Clin Endocrinol Metab* 1983;**57**:177.

Knochel JP: The clinical status of hypophosphatemia: An update. (Editorial.) *N Engl J Med* 1985;**313**:447.

Stoff JS: Phosphate homeostasis and hypophosphatemia. *Am J Med* 1982;**72**:489.

Vannatta JB, Whang R, Papper S: Efficacy of intravenous phosphorus therapy in the severely hypophosphatemic patient. *Arch Intern Med* 1981;**141**:885.

# Skin & Appendages

# 4

*Rees B. Rees, Jr., MD, & Richard B. Odom, MD*

## Diagnosis of Skin Disorders

Take a thorough history. Do not neglect the role of systemic disorders. Inquire about systemic and topical medications. Question about recent or unusual exposure to physical factors and chemical agents in the home and work environment. Examine the entire body surface in good (preferably natural) light.

## Planning Topical Treatment

Many topical agents are available for the treatment of dermatologic disorders. In general, it is better to be thoroughly familiar with a few drugs and treatment methods than to attempt to use a great many.

Consider the individual character of the patient's skin. Dry skins usually require lubricating or softening agents; moist or oily skins, greaseless drying agents.

Begin treatment with mild, simple remedies. In general, acute, inflamed lesions are best treated with soothing, nonirritating agents; chronic, thickened lesions with stimulating or keratolytic agents. When appropriate, apply a small amount of drug to a small area and observe for several hours for skin sensitivity.

Instruct the patient carefully on how to apply medicaments. Do not change remedies before the agent has had time to demonstrate its effectiveness. However, discontinue the drug immediately if an untoward reaction develops. When in doubt about the proper method of treatment, *undertreat* rather than overtreat.

## General Rules Governing Choice of Topical Treatment of Various Stages of Dermatoses

*Note:* The choice of treatment will vary with the individual case, depending upon the characteristics of the dermatosis, the extent of the lesions, the general character of the patient's skin, previous medication and drug allergies, environment, and other factors.

**A. Acute Lesions:** (Recent onset; red, burning, swollen, itching, stinging, blistering, or oozing lesions.) Use wet preparations, such as soaks, for lesions localized to extremities; cool, wet dressings or compresses for localized lesions of the head, neck, trunk, or extremities; or baths for generalized lesions (see below under Pruritus). Lotions or powders may be used in intertriginous areas (axillas, groin, between toes, beneath breasts).

**B. Subacute Lesions:** (Intermediate duration; subsiding lesions or lesions that are less inflamed in appearance.) Use wet preparations as outlined above, shake lotions, or both. Emulsions and water-soluble creams may also be used for soothing and drying effects and to apply medication.

**C. Chronic Lesions:** (Longer duration; quiescent, thickened, crusted, fissured, scaly lesions.) Use wet preparations or compresses for crusted lesions and emulsions, hydrophilic ointments, pastes (high powder content), water-soluble (vanishing) creams, or greasy ointments, especially for thickened, scaly lesions. Special medications can be incorporated in these preparations.

## Prevention of Complications

**A. Pyoderma:** Infected, inflamed, or denuded areas of skin are receptive environments for pyogenic organisms introduced by scratching, rubbing, or squeezing of skin lesions. Patients should be instructed to wash their hands frequently and to avoid manipulation of infected areas. Medications should be kept in closed containers. Crusts (scabs) should be removed by repeated soaks or compresses. If an infection occurs in a hairy portion of the body, special care should be taken in cleansing and shaving the area.

**B. Local or Systemic Spread of Infection:** Almost any skin infection may spread by extension or through vascular or lymphatic channels. In most cases, this complication is a much greater threat to the patient's health and life than the primary skin infection. A most striking and serious example is the extension of staphylococcal infections of the face to the cavernous sinuses. Lymphangitis, lymphadenitis, septicemia, and glomerulonephritis may occur as sequelae to primary skin infection. For these reasons, it is important to institute vigorous local and systemic measures for the control of skin infections. Systemic antibiotics, selected on the basis of bacteriologic studies if time permits, should be used promptly for potentially serious infections or those associated with systemic reactions.

**C. Overtreatment Dermatitis:** This may be avoided if the physician and the patient are aware that undertreatment is preferable to overtreatment and if the patient is warned to avoid overenthusiastic application of topical remedies (either too much or too long). Injudicious use of topical corticosteroids in large amounts or over prolonged periods, especially with occlusive plastic wrapping, can result in significant systemic absorption of steroids. Fluorinated topical corticosteroids may induce acnelike processes on the face (steroid rosacea) and atrophic striae in body folds and in cirrhotic patients may induce acute adrenocortical insufficiency and aseptic bone necrosis.

**D. Exfoliative Dermatitis:** This complication cannot always be anticipated or avoided, but it may be minimized if a careful history of drug sensitivity is obtained before institution of drug therapy. In allergic individuals, it is important to apply a small amount of topical medication in order to determine hypersensitivity. Drugs that may be required for systemic use (eg, sulfonamides, antibiotics, or antihistamines) should preferably not be used in topical preparations. Sodium sulfacetamide and erythromycin appear to be safe for topical use. Neomycin, because of its high sensitizing potential, is not the antibiotic of first choice for topical use.

**E. Cosmetic Disfiguration:** Disfiguration due to skin disorders may be avoided by early, careful treatment of skin lesions and by appropriate dermatologic operative techniques. Self-manipulation of skin lesions, especially on the face and exposed skin areas, should be avoided.

# PRURITUS
## (Itching)

Pruritus is a disagreeable sensation that provokes a desire to scratch. It is a primary sensory impulse carried on unmyelinated C fibers in the spinothalamic tract. It is modulated by central factors, including cortical ones. Not all cases of pruritus are mediated by histamine, although several mediators—bradykinin, neurotensin, secretin, and substance P—release histamine.

Although most cases of generalized pruritus can be attributed to dry skin—whether naturally occurring and precipitated or aggravated by climatic conditions or arising from disease states—there are many other causes: scabies, dermatitis herpetiformis, atopic dermatitis, pruritus vulvae et ani, miliaria, insect bites, pediculosis, contact dermatitis, drug reactions, urticaria, urticarial eruptions of pregnancy, psoriasis, lichen planus, lichen simplex chronicus, folliculitis, sunburn, bullous pemphigoid, fiberglass dermatitis, trichinosis, onchocerciasis, and echinococcosis.

Perhaps the commonest cause of pruritus associated with systemic disease at present is uremia in conjunction with hemodialysis. Both this condition and the pruritus of obstructive biliary disease may be helped by irradiation with ultraviolet B. Endocrine disorders, psychiatric disturbances, myeloproliferative disorders, visceral cancers, iron deficiency anemia, and certain neurologic disorders may also be manifested by pruritus.

Burning or itching involving the face, scalp, and genitalia may be "depressive equivalents," treatable with antidepressant heterocyclic drugs such as amitriptyline, imipramine, doxepin, and others.

## Treatment

**A. General Measures:** External irritants (eg, rough clothing, occupational contactants) should be avoided. Soaps and detergents should not be used by persons with dry or irritated skin. Baths containing a small amount of bath oil may be used. Nails should be kept trimmed and clean (see below). Prevent scratching, if possible. Unnecessary medication should be discontinued, since medication itself often produces pruritus.

**B. Specific Measures:** Remove or treat specific causes whenever possible.

**C. Local Measures:**

**1. Corticosteroids–**Representative topical corticosteroid creams, lotions, ointments, gels, and sprays are presented in the following list:

Least potency: hydrocortisone and desonide. Best for chronic use and for the face.

Mid potency: flurandrenolide, fluocinolone, triamcinolone, hydrocortisone valerate, and clocortolone pivalate.

Higher potency: desoximetasone, diflorasone, amcinonide, halcinonide, and fluocinonide.

Highest potency: betamethasone and clobetasol. Should be used for brief periods only, on limited areas, and not on the face or genitalia or in body folds.

**2. Petrolatum–**If the skin is too dry, wet it, as in a bath (to hydrate the keratin), and then apply petrolatum to the wet skin to trap the moisture.

**3. Drying agents–**If the skin is too moist, drying agents may afford relief, eg, wet dressings, soaks, shake lotions (eg, starch or calamine lotions), and powders (especially if the process is acute).

**4. Tub baths–**Generalized pruritus may often be effectively controlled by lukewarm baths, 15 minutes 2–3 times daily. Elderly patients with dry skin should bathe as infrequently as possible, however. After bathing, the skin should be blotted (not rubbed) dry. (*Caution:* Avoid excessive drying of skin by overbathing, prolonged bathing periods, and exposure to drafts after bathing.) Useful bath formulations are as follows: (1) Tar bath: Dissolve 50–100 mL of coal tar solution USP in 1 tubful (50 gallons) of warm water. (Watch for sensitivity.) (2) Bath oils: 5–25 mL in 1 tubful (50 gallons) of warm water (eg, Alpha-Keri, DOB, Domol Lubath). Bubble baths should be avoided. Preferably, oils, creams, lotions, and ointments should be applied to hydrated skin immediately after the shower or bath.

**5. Five percent lactic acid in petrolatum or a lotion vehicle** may relieve the pruritus and the appearance of dry skin and ichthyosis. A 12% lactate lotion is useful (LacHydrin).

**D. Potentiation of Topical Corticosteroid Creams:** By covering selected lesions of psoriasis, lichen planus, and localized eczemas each night, first with the corticosteroid, then with a thin plastic pliable film (eg, Saran Wrap), an appreciable amount of the medicament may be systemically absorbed. Complications include miliaria, striae, pyoderma, local skin atrophy, malodor, fungal infections, urticarial erythema, and, rarely, adrenocortical suppression when extensive areas of body surface are occluded.

**E. Systemic Antipruritic Drugs:**

**1. Antihistaminic and "antiserotonin" drugs**–In general, $H_1$ blockers are the agents of choice for pruritus, because $H_2$ receptors are not involved in itching. Hydroxyzine and doxepin are useful, as are all other agents that act as antihistamines. Cyproheptadine or chlorpheniramine may be useful when sedation is to be avoided. The newer nonsedating antihistamines—specifically terfenadine—may be beneficial and appear to be well tolerated (see Chapter 1).

**2. Diazepam** may provide useful sedation in agitated or distracted patients. Barbiturates may rarely produce dermatitis.

**3. Corticotropin or the corticosteroids**–(See Chapter 18.) The role of corticosteroids in controlling the endogenous mediators of inflammation is not known. Histamine, kinins, lysosomal enzymes, and prostaglandins have been examined, but experimental clarification of modes of action is lacking. The antimitotic effects of corticosteroids on human skin may account for some benefit in psoriasis and in other diseases associated with increased cell turnover.

**4. Psychotropic drugs**–The analgesic properties of some antidepressants, such as doxepin and imipramine (see Chapter 17), may alleviate intractable pruritus, since pain and pruritus share the same central nervous system pathways.

**Prognosis**

Elimination of external factors and irritating agents is often successful in giving complete relief from pruritus. Pruritus accompanying specific skin disease will subside when the disease is controlled. Idiopathic pruritus and that accompanying serious internal disease may not respond to any type of therapy.

Gupta M et al: Psychotropic drugs in dermatology: A review and guidelines for use. *J Am Acad Dermatol* 1986;**14:**633.

Denman ST: A review of pruritus. *J Am Acad Dermatol* 1986;**14:**375.

---

# COMMON DERMATOSES

---

## CONTACT DERMATITIS
## (Dermatitis Venenata)

### Essentials of Diagnosis

- Erythema and edema, often followed by vesicles and bullae in area of contact with suspected agent.
- Later, weeping, crusting, and secondary infection.
- Often a history of previous reaction to suspected contactant.

- Patch test with agent usually positive in the allergic form.

**General Considerations**

Contact dermatitis is an acute or chronic dermatitis that results from direct skin contact with chemicals or allergens. Lesions are most often on exposed parts. Four-fifths of such disturbances are due to excessive exposure to or additive effects of primary or universal irritants (eg, soaps, detergents, organic solvents). Others are due to actual contact allergy. The most common allergies to dermatologic agents include antimicrobials (especially neomycin), topical antihistamines, anesthetics, and preservatives.

**Clinical Findings**

**A. Symptoms and Signs:** Itching, burning, and stinging are often extremely severe, distributed on exposed parts or in bizarre asymmetric patterns. The lesions consist of erythematous macules, papules, and vesicles. The affected area is often hot and swollen, with exudation, crusting, and secondary infection. The pattern of the eruption may be diagnostic (eg, typical linear streaked vesicles on the extremities and erythema and swelling of the genitalia in poison oak dermatitis). The location will often suggest the cause: Scalp involvement suggests hair tints, lacquer, shampoos, or tonics; face involvement, creams, cosmetics, soaps, shaving materials; neck involvement, jewelry, fingernail polish, etc.

**B. Laboratory Findings:** The patch test may be useful but has limitations. In the event of a positive reaction, the clinical relevance of the chemical agent and the dermatitis must be determined. Photopatch tests (exposing the traditional patch test site to ultraviolet light after 24 hours) may be necessary in the case of suspected photosensitivity contact dermatitis.

**Differential Diagnosis**

Asymmetric distribution and a history of contact help distinguish contact dermatitis from other skin lesions. Eruptions may be due to primary irritation from chemicals or allergic sensitization to contactants. The commonest sensitizers are poison oak and ivy, rubber antioxidants and accelerators, nickel and chromium salts, paraphenylenediamine, formalin, ethylenediamine, turpentine, benzocaine, and neomycin. Differentiation may be difficult if the area of involvement is consistent with that seen in other types of skin disorders such as scabies, dermatophytid, atopic dermatitis, dishidrotic eczema, and other eczemas.

**Prevention**

Prevent reexposure to irritants. Avoid soaps and detergents. Use unscented cosmetics or eliminate cosmetics entirely. Protective gloves may be used; in such cases, a cotton glove liner must be used. Protective (barrier) creams are almost useless. It may be necessary to change occupation or duties if occupational exposure is otherwise unavoidable.

Prompt and thorough removal of irritants by prolonged washing or by removal with solvents or other chemical agents may be effective if done very shortly after exposure.

Most well-controlled studies indicate that injection or ingestion of *Rhus* antigen is of no practical clinical value for the prevention of *Rhus* (*Toxicodendron*) dermatitis.

### Treatment

**A. General Measures:** For acute severe cases, one may give prednisone, 30–40 mg/d orally for 10 days. Triamcinolone acetonide (Kenalog-40), 40 mg once intragluteally, may be used instead. (See Chapter 18.) An age-old remedy for itching disorders is repeated exposure to hot water, as in a shower, without soap; this treatment may have the effect of prolonging and aggravating the underlying disorder (eg, atopic or nummular dermatitis).

**B. Local Measures:** Treat the stage and type of dermatitis (see above).

**1. Acute weeping dermatitis–**Do not scrub lesions with soap and water. Apply solutions. Calamine or starch shake lotions may be indicated instead of wet dressings or in intervals between wet dressings, especially for involvement of intertriginous areas or when oozing is not marked. Lesions on the extremities may be bandaged with wet dressings. Potent topical corticosteroids, in ointment or cream form, may help suppress acute contact dermatitis and relieve itching. A soothing formulation is 0.1% triamcinolone acetonide in SARNA (0.5% camphor, 0.5% menthol, 0.5% phenol) lotion. Frequent continued use may induce tachyphylaxis (acute tolerance).

**2. Subacute dermatitis (subsiding)–**Use shake lotions or antipruritic-steroid lotion.

**3. Chronic dermatitis (dry and lichenified)–**Treat with hydrophilic, greasy ointments or creams. Tars, often combined with moderate-strength corticosteroid (eg, 0.1% triamcinolone) are useful.

### Prognosis

Contact dermatitis is self-limited if reexposure is prevented. Spontaneous desensitization may occur. Increasing sensitivity to industrial irritants may necessitate a change of occupation. Contact allergen alternatives are available.

Adams RM, Fisher AA: Contact allergen alternatives: 1986. *J Am Acad Dermatol* 1986;**14**:951.
Fisher AA: *Contact Dermatitis*, 3rd ed. Lea & Febiger, 1986.

### ERYTHEMA NODOSUM

### Essentials of Diagnosis

- Painful red nodules on anterior aspects of legs.
- No ulceration seen.
- Slow regression over several weeks to resemble contusions.

- Some cases associated with infection or drug sensitivity.
- Women are predominantly affected.

### General Considerations

Erythema nodosum is a symptom complex characterized by tender, erythematous nodules that appear most commonly on the extensor surfaces of the legs. It usually lasts about 6 weeks and may recur. The disease may be associated with various infections (streptococcosis, primary coccidioidomycosis, other deep fungal infections, primary tuberculosis, rheumatic fever, or syphilis) or may be due to drug sensitivity (penicillin, progestins). It may accompany leukemia, sarcoidosis, and ulcerative colitis. Infections with unusual organisms such as *Pasteurella* (*Yersinia*) *pseudotuberculosis* may be responsible. Erythema nodosum may be associated with pregnancy.

Keep in mind the possibility of a hepatitis B virus when seeing a patient with erythema nodosum or erythema multiforme or even chronic urticaria if there is accompanying hepatomegaly.

### Clinical Findings

**A. Symptoms and Signs:** The swellings are exquisitely tender and are usually preceded by fever, malaise, and arthralgia. The nodules are most often located on the anterior surfaces of the legs below the knees but may occur (rarely) on the arms, trunk, and face. The lesions, 1–10 cm in diameter, are at first pink to red; with regression, all the various hues seen in a contusion can be observed. The nodules occasionally become fluctuant, but they do not suppurate.

**B. Laboratory Findings:** The histologic finding of septal panniculitis is strongly suggestive of erythema nodosum. Hilar adenopathy is often seen on chest x-ray. Antistreptolysin titer may be elevated, and the throat smear and culture may be positive in cases caused by streptococci.

### Differential Diagnosis

Erythema induratum is seen on the posterior surfaces of the legs and shows ulceration. Nodular vasculitis is usually on the calves and is associated with phlebitis. Erythema multiforme occurs in generalized distribution. In the late stages, erythema nodosum must be distinguished from simple bruises and contusions.

### Treatment

**A. General Measures:** Eliminate or treat the underlying cause, eg, systemic infection and exogenous toxins. Saturated solution of potassium iodide, 5–15 drops 3 times daily, may result in prompt involution in many cases. Side effects of potassium iodide include salivation, swelling of salivary glands, and headache. Complete bed rest may be advisable. Focal infections should be treated, although this does not appear to influence the course of the disease. Systemic therapy directed against the lesions themselves may include corticosteroid therapy (see Chapter 18) unless it is contraindicated (tuberculosis must be ruled out) and salicylates for several days during the acute painful stage.

**B. Local Treatment:** This is usually not necessary. Hot or cold compresses may help.

## Prognosis

The lesions usually disappear after about 6 weeks, but they may recur.

Horio T et al: Potassium iodide in the treatment of erythema nodosum and nodular vasculitis. *Arch Dermatol* 1978; **117:**29.

Maggiore G, Grifeo S, Marzani MD: Erythema nodosum and hepatitis B virus (HBV) infection. (Letter.) *J Am Acad Dermatol* 1983;**9:**602.

## ERYTHEMA MULTIFORME

### Essentials of Diagnosis

- Sudden onset of symmetric erythematous skin lesions with history of recurrence.
- May be macular, papular, urticarial, bullous, or purpuric.
- "Target" lesions with clear centers and concentric erythematous rings may be noted.
- Mostly on extensor surfaces; may be on palms, soles, or mucous membranes.
- Herpes simplex, systemic infection or disease, and drug reactions may be associated.

### General Considerations

Erythema multiforme is an acute inflammatory, polymorphic skin disease due to multiple causes or of undetermined origin. In one study of erythema multiforme, 4 out of 5 cases followed outbreaks of herpes simplex. Of the remaining 20%, half were associated with administration of a sulfonamide drug and half with miscellaneous causes—drug, viral, fungal, and bacterial. The most serious cases (Stevens-Johnson syndrome) by far followed sulfonamide exposure, with possible renal damage and death. Those associated with herpes simplex were not serious. Deposition of C3 and fibrin along the dermoepidermal junction and of IgM, C3, and fibrin around dermal blood vessels appears to occur in all cases. Little is known about the pathogenesis.

*Mycoplasma pneumoniae* may be causative in the more severe cases (erythema multiforme major).

### Clinical Findings

**A. Symptoms and Signs:** Erythema multiforme is characterized by fixed erythematous papules and wheals, some of which evolve into blisters or target lesions. It has rather characteristic histologic features. Stevens-Johnson syndrome and some cases of toxic epidermal necrolysis are major forms of erythema multiforme. More than 50% of ordinary cases of erythema multiforme follow attacks of recurrent herpes simplex infection. A host of other etiologic factors

play a role in other cases. Major forms of the disease occur as complications of drug therapy or of recent *Mycoplasma pneumoniae* infection. Mucous membrane ulcerations are frequent. The tracheobronchial mucosa may be involved in severe cases (Stevens-Johnson variant), causing bronchitis and atelectasis. A rare type, erythema perstans, may exist for months or years. Chronic low-grade stomatitis may be an erythema multiforme variant.

Erythema multiforme-like eruptions may follow topical contact with medications, including ophthalmologic and intravaginal agents. Such topicals include balsam of Peru, chloramphenicol, econazole, ethylenediamine, furazolidone, mafenide acetate, neomycin, nifuroxime, promethazine, scopolamine, sulfonamides, and vitamin E.

**B. Laboratory Findings:** There are no characteristic laboratory findings. Histologic changes may be suggestive but are not pathognomonic.

### Differential Diagnosis

Secondary syphilis, urticaria, drug eruptions, and toxic epidermal necrolysis must be ruled out. The bullous variety of erythema multiforme is more severe and should be differentiated from dermatitis herpetiformis, pemphigus, pemphigoid, and bullous drug eruptions. In erythema multiforme there is usually some constitutional reaction, including fever.

### Complications

Visceral lesions are a complication (eg, pneumonitis, myocarditis, nephritis).

### Prevention

Avoid all unnecessary medications in patients with a history of erythema multiforme.

### Treatment

**A. General Measures:** When fever is present, the patient should be at bed rest and good nursing care should be provided. **Erythema multiforme major (Stevens-Johnson syndrome)** may resemble toxic epidermal necrolysis, with extensive denudation of skin, and is best treated in a burn unit.

**B. Specific Measures:** Eliminate causative factors such as chronic systemic infections, focal infections, and sensitizing drugs. Corticosteroids may be tried in more severe cases, although their use is controversial. Oral acyclovir, 200 mg 5 times daily or 800 mg twice daily for 5 days, is effective in preventing herpes-associated erythema multiforme. Antibacterial preparations are used for secondary infection.

**C. Local Measures:** Treat the stage and type of dermatitis (see above). For acute lesions, employ simple wet dressings and soaks or soothing lotions. Zinc sulfate solution, 0.01–0.025%, may be used as a mouth rinse several times daily. Subacute lesions require soothing lotions.

### Prognosis

The illness usually lasts 2–6 weeks and may recur.

Stevens-Johnson syndrome, in which visceral involvement may occur, may be serious or even fatal. The prognosis depends in part on that of the primary disease.

Fisher AA: Erythema multiforme-like eruptions due to topical medications: Part II. *Cutis* 1986;**37**:158.

Lemak MA, Duvic M, Ben SF: Oral acyclovir for the prevention of herpes-associated erythemia multiforme. *J Am Acad Dermatol* 1986;**15**:50.

Schosser RH: The erythema multiforme spectrum: Diagnosis and treatment. *Curr Concepts Skin Dis* (Summer) 1985;**6**:6.

## PEMPHIGUS

### Essentials of Diagnosis

- Relapsing crops of bullae appearing on normal skin.
- Often preceded by mucous membrane bullae, erosions, and ulcerations.
- Superficial detachment of the skin after pressure or trauma variably present (Nikolsky's sign).
- Acantholysis on biopsy.
- Immunofluorescence studies are confirmatory.

### General Considerations

Pemphigus is an uncommon intraepidermal blistering disease occurring on skin and mucous membranes. The cause is unknown, and the condition, if untreated, is always fatal within 2 months to 5 years. The bullae appear spontaneously and are relatively asymptomatic, but the lesions become extensive and the complications of the disease lead to great toxicity and debility. There is a surprising lack of pathologic findings; no primary lesions are found in internal organs at biopsy. The disease occurs almost exclusively in middle-aged or older adults and in all races and ethnic groups. Studies have demonstrated the presence of circulating autoantibodies to intercellular substances. Drug-induced autoimmune pemphigus from penicillamine and captopril has been reported. The pathogenetic role of IgG antibodies has been proved by passive transfer of antibodies to neonatal mice, reproducing the disease. There is an association with HLA-A10 antigen. Pemphigus may present with atypical features, and repeated reevaluation of clinical findings and changes shown by immunofluorescence and histopathologic studies may be necessary.

There are 2 forms of pemphigus: **pemphigus vulgaris** and its variant, **pemphigus vegetans;** and **pemphigus foliaceus** and its variant, **pemphigus erythematosus.** Both forms may occur at any age. The vulgaris form begins in the mouth in over 50% of cases. The foliaceus form, particularly, may be associated with other autoimmune diseases or may be drug-induced, eg, by exposure to penicillamine.

### Clinical Findings

**A. Symptoms and Signs:** Pemphigus is characterized by an insidious onset of flaccid bullae in crops or waves. The lesions often appear first on the oral mucous membranes, and these rapidly become erosive. Toxemia and a "mousy" odor may occur soon. Rubbing the thumb laterally on the surface of uninvolved skin may cause easy separation of the epidermis **(Nikolsky's sign).**

**B. Laboratory Findings:** On a smear taken from the base of a bulla and stained with Giemsa's stain **(Tzanck test),** one may see an almost unique histologic picture of disruption of the epidermal intercellular connections called **acantholysis.** There may be leukocytosis and eosinophilia. As the disease progresses, low serum protein levels may be found, as well as serum electrolyte changes. The sedimentation rate may be elevated, and anemia may be present. Intercellular antibody may be detected by the indirect immunofluorescence test on the patient's serum.

Microscopically, acantholysis is the hallmark of pemphigus, but in some patients, there may be eosinophilic spongiosis initially. Immunoelectron microscopy shows deposits of IgG intercellularly in the epidermis. These IgG antibodies may have titers corresponding with disease activity. C3 and other immunoglobulins and complement components may be present on occasion. Acantholysis can develop in a culture of normal human skin tissue when pemphigus serum is added.

### Differential Diagnosis

Acantholysis is not seen in other bullous eruptions such as erythema multiforme, drug eruptions, contact dermatitis, or bullous impetigo, or in the less common dermatitis herpetiformis and pemphigoid. All of these diseases have gross clinical characteristics and different immunofluorescence test results that distinguish them from pemphigus. Transient acantholytic dermatosis (harmless) may be a source of confusion.

### Complications

Secondary infection commonly occurs, often causing extreme debility. Terminally there may be shock, septicemia, disturbances of electrolyte balance, cachexia, toxemia, and pneumonia.

### Treatment

**A. General Measures:** Hospitalize the patient at bed rest and provide antibiotics, blood transfusions, and intravenous feedings as indicated. Anesthetic troches used before eating ease painful oral lesions.

**B. Specific Measures:** High dosages of prednisone, 200–400 mg/d for 6–10 weeks, may be lifesaving in pemphigus when given in time. Intermediate dosages, between 40 mg every other day and 200 mg daily, should be avoided. After initial control is achieved, azathioprine, 100 mg/d, is given concurrently with prednisone, which is gradually reduced to 40 mg/d for the first week, 30 mg/d for the second week, and 25 mg/d for the third week. Thereafter, 40 mg is given every other day, as a single morning dose, together with 100 mg/d orally of azathioprine, for years if necessary. This regimen reduces the incidence of death due to therapy. Gold sodium thiomalate, given as for rheumatoid arthritis, is said to be effective following initial prednisone. Many investigators feel that by initiating and carefully monitoring treatment with concomitant use of methotrexate, azathioprine, gold, and corticosteroids, it is possible to reduce the dosage of steroids gradually with fewer of the hazards of long-term steroid therapy. Dapsone, 100 mg daily or less, controls some cases of pemphigus.

**C. Local Measures:** Skin and mucous membrane lesions should be treated as for vesicular, bullous, and ulcerative lesions due to any cause. Complicating infection requires appropriate systemic and local antibiotic therapy.

### Prognosis

Infection is the most frequent cause of death, usually from *Staphylococcus aureus* septicemia. Signs and symptoms are often masked by high-dose corticosteroids, suggesting caution in their use. One-half of all deaths are now related to the complications of therapy.

Anhalt GJ, Patel H, Diaz LA: Mechanisms of immunologic injury: Pemphigus and bullous pemphigoid. *Arch Dermatol* 1983;**119**:711.

Bean SF, Fritz KA, Jordon RE: Bullous dermatoses: Pemphigus. *J Am Acad Dermatol* 1984;**11**:1151.

Lever WF, Schaumberg-Lever G: Treatment of pemphigus vulgaris. *Arch Dermatol* 1983;**120**:44.

Tuffanelli DL et al: Pemphigus. (Medical Staff Conference, University of California, San Francisco.) *West J Med* 1983;**138**:699.

## OTHER BLISTERING DISEASES

There is a wide variety of other skin disorders characterized by formation of bullae, or blisters. These include bullous pemphigoid, cicatricial pemphigoid, dermatitis herpetiformis, herpes gestationis, and other less common bullous disorders.

### Bullous Pemphigoid

Bullous pemphigoid is relatively benign, usually remitting in 5 or 6 years, with a course characterized by exacerbations and remissions. Oral lesions are present in about one-third of affected persons. The disease may occur in various forms, including localized, vesicular, vegetating, erythematous, erythrodermic, and nodular. There is no statistical association with internal malignant disease. The subepidermal bullae that characterize pemphigoid may closely resemble those of dermatitis herpetiformis.

With immunoelectron microscopy, deposits of IgG and C3 are found in the lamina lucida of the basement membrane. Circulating basement membrane antibodies can be found in the sera of patients in about 70% of cases. With direct immunofluorescence, IgG and C3 are commonly found, but other immunoglobulins and complement components may be found. Complement activation plus the presence of proteinases may be the cause of the blisters.

Corticosteroids are the treatment of choice. Some authorities add methotrexate, azathioprine, or cyclophosphamide. In a few cases, sulfapyridine or dapsone may be adequate.

### Cicatricial Pemphigoid

Cicatricial pemphigoid occurs most commonly in the mouth. The eyes are the second most common site. The nasal mucosa, larynx, pharynx, genitalia, anus, and esophagus may be involved. Desquamative gingivitis is a common presenting sign. The skin is involved in about one-third of cases. The **Brunsting-Perry** variant involves only the skin of the head and neck, sparing the mucous membranes. A subepidermal blister is seen microscopically. With immunologic techniques, C3, IgG, and other immunoglobulins and complement components are seen at the basement membrane zone.

The differential diagnosis includes acquired epidermolysis bullosa, but in that disorder clinical lesions of trauma-induced bullae are seen over the joints of the hands, feet, elbows, and knees as well as atrophic scars, milia, and nail dystrophy.

Dapsone, alone or with prednisone, may be tried initially, but prednisone in combination with azathioprine or cyclophosphamide may be necessary.

### Dermatitis Herpetiformis

Dermatitis herpetiformis occurs most commonly on the scalp, the sacral area, elbows, and knees. The clinical lesions are tense, very pruritic vesicles. Excoriations and hyperpigmentation or hypopigmentation may be seen.

There are 3 different forms of the disease, each having a different pattern of immunoreactants in the lamina lucida and the sub-lamina densa zone. The commonest form has a granular pattern and a high prevalence of HLA-B8/Dw3 immunogens. This form is associated with a gluten-sensitive enteropathy and slowly responds to a gluten-free diet. The other 2 forms each have different linear patterns of IgA deposits localized in the lamina lucida or below the lamina densa. The pathophysiology of these 2 types differs from that of the first type. Sulfapyridine or dapsone is the drug of choice. Dapsone may cause profound methemoglobinemia in persons with glucose-6-phosphate dehydrogenase deficiency.

Serologic studies for IgA-class antiendomysial antibodies, when positive, are specific in 70% of cases of dermatitis herpetiformis.

### Herpes Gestationis

Herpes gestationis occurs in about one in 50,000–60,000 deliveries. The bullae often appear first in periumbilical distribution, and there may be erythematous papules and plaques, vesicles, and large bullae. It usually begins in the fifth or sixth month of pregnancy or the onset may be delayed to the post-partum period. The disease is self-limited, but it may recur in subsequent pregnancies. Use of estrogens or progesterone or the onset of menses may trigger flareups. The risks to mother and fetus appear to be less significant than was formerly thought. Blisters are subepidermal, with eosinophils present. Direct immunofluorescence shows C3 at the basement membrane zone in most cases. IgG is found less often. Although C3 is found in the lamina lucida, as in pemphigoid, the antigen is in a different part of the stratum lucidum. Herpes gestationis factor is an avid complement-fixing IgG antibody found in the serum but rarely in the basement membrane zone.

Corticosteroids are the treatment of choice and are sometimes effective when used topically only.

Accetta P et al: Anti-endomysial antibodies: A serologic marker of dermatitis herpetiformis. *Arch Dermatol* 1986;**122**:459.

Bean SF, Fritz KA, Jordon RE: Bullous pemphigoid. *J Am Acad Dermatol* 1984;**11**:1152.

Bean SF, Fritz KA, Jordon RE: Cicatricial pemphigoid. *J Am Acad Dermatol* 1984;**11**:1153.

Bean SF, Fritz KA, Jordon RE: Herpes gestationis. *J Am Acad Dermatol* 1984;**11**:1154.

Beutner EH, Chorzelski TP, Jablonska S: Immunofluorescence tests: Clinical significance of sera and skin in bullous diseases. *Int J Dermatol* 1985;**24**:405.

## ATOPIC DERMATITIS
## (Eczema)

### Essentials of Diagnosis

- Pruritic, exudative, or lichenified eruption on face, neck, upper trunk, wrists, and hands and in the folds of knees and elbows.
- Personal or family history of allergic manifestations (eg, asthma, allergic rhinitis, eczema).
- Tendency to recur, with remission from age 2 to early youth and beyond.

### General Considerations

Diagnostic criteria for atopic dermatitis must include pruritus, typical morphology and distribution (flexural lichenification in adults; facial and extensor involvement in infancy), and a tendency toward chronic or chronically relapsing dermatitis. In addition, there should be 2 or more of the following features: (1) personal or family history of atopic disease (asthma, allergic rhinitis, atopic dermatitis), (2) immediate skin test reactivity, (3) white dermographism or delayed blanch to cholinergic agents, and (4) anterior or posterior subcapsular cataracts; plus 4 or more of the following features: (1) xerosis/ichthyosis/hyperlinear palms, (2) pityriasis alba, (3) keratosis pilaris, (4) facial pallor/infraorbital darkening, (5) Dennie-Morgan infraorbital fold, (6) elevated serum IgE, (7) keratoconus, (8) tendency toward nonspecific hand dermatitis, and (9) tendency toward repeated cutaneous infections.

### Clinical Findings

**A. Symptoms and Signs:** Itching may be extremely severe and prolonged, leading often to emotional disturbances, which have been erroneously interpreted by some as being causative. The distribution of the lesions is characteristic, with involvement of the face, neck, and upper trunk ("monk's cowl"). The bends of the elbows and knees are involved. An abortive form may involve the hands alone (in which case the history of atopy is all-important). In infants, the eruption usually begins on the cheeks and is often vesicular and exudative. In children (and later) it is dry, leathery, and lichenified, although intraepidermal vesicles are occasionally present histologically. Adults generally have dry, leathery, hyperpigmented or hypopigmented lesions in typical distribution.

The role of food allergy in atopic dermatitis is debatable. Several studies have implicated eggs, cow's milk, and peanuts in flare-ups of dermatitis, especially in younger children.

**B. Laboratory Findings:** Laboratory findings in general, including scratch and intradermal tests, are disappointing. Eosinophilia may be present. The delayed-blanch reaction to methacholine may help in diagnosing atypical atopic dermatitis.

There is increased IgE binding to *Staphylococcus aureus*. Interaction of staphylococcal antigen and specific antistaphylococcal antibodies may induce mast cell release, causing itching and aggravation of the dermatitis. Painful fissures indicate staphylococcal infection clinically. Therefore, treatment of severe flareups, such as with erythromycin or dicloxacillin, is helpful.

In children and adults with atopic dermatitis alone and no coexisting asthma or allergic rhinitis, circulating reagins against common allergens can be demonstrated with the radioimmunologic allergen-specific IgE in vitro assay technique (RAST), but this is not of great practical value ("the rich man's scratch test").

### Differential Diagnosis

Distinguish from seborrheic dermatitis (frequent scalp and face involvement, greasy and scaly lesions, and quick response to therapy), contact dermatitis (especially that due to weeds), and lichen simplex chronicus (flat, more circumscribed, less extensive lesions).

### Treatment

**A. General Measures:** Hospitalization is infrequently necessary today. Systemic corticosteroids are indicated in extensive and more severe cases. Oral prednisone dosages should be high enough to suppress the dermatitis quickly. The dosage is then reduced over a period of 2–5 weeks. Triamcinolone acetonide suspension, 20–30 mg intramuscularly every 4–6 weeks (or less often), may exert control **(caution)**. In mild cases, topical corticosteroid therapy may be adequate. The antihistamines may be used to aid in the relief of severe pruritus. Hydroxyzine or doxepin may be useful, but the dosage must be increased gradually to avoid extreme drowsiness. Warm temperate climates and exposure to ultraviolet rays are helpful for atopic dermatitis, reducing the need for topical corticosteroids. The skin in atopic dermatitis is usually colonized by large numbers of *Staphylococcus aureus,* which may aggravate the dermatitis or prevent resolution. *S aureus* may have a direct biologic action, or the deleterious effect may be due to indirect damage mediated by the immune (IgE) and inflammatory systems. Antibiotics given systemically, such as erythromycin or dicloxacillin, may be helpful in management.

**Eczema herpeticum,** a generalized herpes simplex infection superimposed on atopic dermatitis or other extensive eczematous processes, may sometimes be treated successfully with intravenous acyclovir in a dose of 1500 mg/m$^2$/d, administered over a 1-hour period 3 times a day. Renal impairment due to precipitation of the drug in the kidneys may be minimized by giving adequate fluids. Phlebitis may be a problem at the infusion site.

**B. Specific Measures:** Avoidance of temperature changes and stress may help to minimize abnormal cutaneous vascular and sweat responses.

The dry skin of atopic patients should be hydrated with hydrophilic creams and lotions.

The diet should be adequate and well-balanced. There is no evidence that standardized or routine dietary restrictions are of value, especially in adults.

Attempts at desensitization to various allergens by graded injections are disappointing and may cause severe flare-ups.

An attempt should be made to identify and treat emotional disturbances, but this is of little practical value in the management of the dermatitis.

**C. Local Treatment:** Avoid all unnecessary local irritations to the skin, such as may occur from excessive bathing or as a result of exposure to irritating drugs, chemicals, greases, and soaps. Soapless detergents are not advisable. Clear up skin infections promptly (particularly those with exudates) by appropriate measures (see Chapter 28). Corticosteroids in lotion, cream, or ointment form have almost completely supplanted all other topical medications because of greater efficacy. They should be applied sparingly twice daily.

Treat the clinical type and stage of the dermatitis:

1. For acute weeping lesions use saline, bicarbonate, or aluminum subacetate solutions as soothing or astringent soaks, baths, or wet dressings for 30 minutes 3 or 4 times daily. Calamine or starch shake lotions may be employed at night or when wet dressings are not desirable. Lesions on extremities, particularly, may be bandaged for protection at night. Apply steroid lotions or creams for this stage.

2. Subacute or subsiding lesions may be treated with shake lotions, which may incorporate mild antipruritic or mild stimulating agents. Shake lotions are usually preferred for lesions that are widespread.

Creams or ointments containing a steroid or mild tar should also be used.

3. Chronic, dry, lichenified lesions are best treated with ointments, creams, and pastes containing lubricating, keratolytic, antipruritic, and mild keratoplastic agents as indicated. Topical corticosteroids and tars are the most popular agents in chronic eczema. Useful corticosteroids are hydrocortisone valerate, hydrocortisone butyrate, alclometasone dipropionate, triamcinolone acetonide, fluocinolone acetonide, fluocinonide, desoximetasone, betamethasone valerate, betamethasone dipropionate, and clobetasol propionate—in creams, ointments, lotions, solutions, and sprays. **Tachyphylaxis,** the rapid onset of tolerance to the action of a drug after too-frequent application, may be overcome by applying a potent corticosteroid twice daily for 2 days, alternating with 2 days without treatment. Fluorinated topical steroids may cause rosacea, striae, and skin atrophy. Coal tar is available as 2–5% ointment, creams, and pastes. The least irritating soaps are Alpha Keri, Basis, Neutrogena, Purpose, and Emulave. The skin may be cleansed with a lipid-free lotion, Cetaphil.

### Prognosis

The disease runs a chronic course, often with a tendency to disappear and recur. Poor prognostic factors for eventual complete remission in atopic dermatitis include onset early in childhood, early generalized disease, and asthma. Only 40–60% of these patients have lasting remissions.

Dahl MV: *Staphylococcus aureus* and atopic dermatitis. *Arch Dermatol* 1983;**119:**840.

Hanifin JM: Atopic dermatitis. *J Am Acad Dermatol* 1982;**6:**1.

Hannuksela M et al: Ultraviolet light therapy in atopic dermatitis. *Acta Derm Venereol* (Stockh) 1985;**114(Suppl):**137.

Rystedt I: Long term follow-up in atopic dermatitis. *Acta Derm Venereol* (Stockh) 1985;**114:**117.

## LICHEN SIMPLEX CHRONICUS (Circumscribed Neurodermatitis)

### Essentials of Diagnosis

- Chronic itching associated with pigmented lichenified skin lesions.
- Exaggerated skin lines overlying a thickened, well-circumscribed scaly plaque.
- Predilection for nape of neck, wrists, external surfaces of forearms, inner thighs, genitalia, postpopliteal and antecubital areas.

### General Considerations

A traditional explanation for lichen simplex chronicus (circumscribed neurodermatitis) is that it represents a self-perpetuating scratch-itch cycle. Hypertrophic nerve fibers have been found in lichenified, thickened lesions of long standing. Definite personality patterns seem to be associated with the disorder, including inability to be aggressive. In some instances, the disease may be a well-compensated equivalent of a psychosis. Some patients are better off having the itching disorder than having knowledge of its cause. In rare instances, total abstinence from stimulants such as caffeine may result in severe withdrawal symptoms, followed by cure.

## Clinical Findings

Intermittent itching incites the patient to manipulate the lesions. Itching may be so intense as to interfere with sleep. Dry, leathery, hypertrophic, lichenified plaques appear on the neck, wrist, perineum, thigh, or almost anywhere. The patches are well-localized and rectangular, with sharp borders, and are thickened and pigmented. The lines of the skin are exaggerated and divide the lesion into rectangular plaques.

## Differential Diagnosis

Differentiate from other plaquelike lesions such as psoriasis, lichen planus, seborrheic dermatitis, and nummular dermatitis.

## Treatment

The area should be protected and the patient encouraged to avoid stressful and emotionally charged situations if possible. Topical corticosteroids give relief. The injection of dilute triamcinolone acetonide suspension into the lesion may occasionally be curative. Application of triamcinolone acetonide 0.1%, fluocinolone 0.025%, betamethasone valerate 0.1%, or fluocinonide 0.05% cream nightly with occlusive plastic wrap (eg, Saran Wrap) covering may be helpful. Betamethasone dipropionate 0.05% and clobetasol propionate 0.05% are effective creams and ointments without occlusion when applied twice daily. Stimulants (caffeine, etc) should be avoided. The mechanism of the itch-scratch cycle should be explained to the patient in hope of breaking the pattern.

## Prognosis

The disease tends to persist despite treatment.

Arnold HL Jr: Paroxysmal pruritus: Its clinical characterization and a hypothesis of its pathogenesis. *J Am Acad Dermatol* 1984;**11**:322.

## DERMATITIS MEDICAMENTOSA
## (Drug Eruption)

### Essentials of Diagnosis

- Usually, abrupt onset of widespread, symmetric erythematous eruption.
- May mimic any inflammatory skin condition.
- Constitutional symptoms (malaise, arthralgia, headache, and fever) may be present.

### General Considerations

As is well recognized, only a minority of cutaneous drug reactions result from allergy. Such factors as overdose, toxic side effects, neoplastic disease, super-infection, drug interaction, impaired degradation or excretion, conditions mimicking allergic reactions (eg, Jarisch-Herxheimer reaction), ampicillin reactions with infectious mononucleosis, Stevens-Johnson syndrome, intolerance with low doses, and idiosyncrasy may be operative. True allergic drug reactions involve prior exposure, an "incubation" period, reactions to doses far below the therapeutic range, manifestations different from the usual pharmacologic effects of the drug, involvement of only a small portion of the population at risk, restriction to a limited number of syndromes (anaphylactic and anaphylactoid, urticarial, vasculitic, etc), occasional identification of antibodies or T lymphocytes that react specifically with the drug or a metabolite, and reproducibility.

Rashes are among the most common adverse reactions to drugs and occur in 2–3% of hospitalized patients. Amoxicillin, trimethoprim-sulfamethoxazole, and ampicillin or penicillin are the commonest causes, followed by phenazones. Toxic epidermal necrolysis and Stevens-Johnson syndrome were most commonly produced by sulfonamides. Phenazones and barbiturates were the major causes of fixed drug eruptions.

## Clinical Findings

**A. Symptoms and Signs:** The onset is usually abrupt, with bright erythema and often severe itching, but may be delayed (penicillin, serum). Fever and other constitutional symptoms may be present. The skin reaction usually occurs in symmetric distribution. In a given situation, the physician may suspect one specific drug (or one of several) and must therefore inquire specifically whether it has been used or not.

**1. Toxic erythema–**(Commonest skin reaction to drugs; causes many patterns of erythema.) Often more pronounced on the trunk than on the extremities. In previously exposed patients, the rash may start in 2–3 days. In the first course of treatment, the eruption often appears about the ninth day. Fever may be present. Common offenders include antibiotics (especially ampicillin), sulfonamides and related compounds (including thiazide diuretics, furosemide, and sulfonylurea hypoglycemics), barbiturates, phenylbutazone, and aminosalicylic acid.

**2. Erythema multiforme–**Targetlike lesions mainly on the extensor aspect of the limbs. Bullae may occur. The commonest offenders are the sulfonamides, barbiturates, phenylbutazone, sulindac, and fenoprofen.

**3. Erythema nodosum–**Oral contraceptives.

**4. Allergic vasculitis–**Inflammatory changes most severe around veins and venules. Lesions may present as urticaria, hemorrhagic papules ("palpable purpura"), vesicles, bullae, or necrotic ulcers. Common offenders include sulfonamides, phenylbutazone, indomethacin, phenytoin, and ibuprofen.

**5. Purpura–**(Results from thrombocytopenia, by damaging blood vessel or by affecting blood coagulation.) Itchy, brownish, petechial macular rash on dependent areas. Common offenders include thiazides, sulfonamides, phenylbutazone, sulfonylureas, barbiturates, quinine, and sulindac.

**6. Eczema**–Rare epidermal reaction similar to contact dermatitis in patients previously sensitized by external exposure who are given the same or a related substance systemically. The commonest offenders include penicillin, neomycin, phenothiazines, and local anesthetics.

**7. Exfoliative dermatitis and erythroderma**–(Entire skin surface is red and scaly.) Common offenders include allopurinol, sulfonamides, phenylbutazone, aminosalicylic acid, isoniazid, gold, carbamazepine.

**8. Photosensitivity**–(An exaggerated response to ultraviolet light.) Affects the exposed skin of the face, neck, and backs of the hands, and also, in women, the lower legs. On occasion, the ultraviolet emission from fluorescent lighting may be sufficient. Common offenders are sulfonamides and sulfonamide-related compounds (thiazide diuretics, furosemide, sulfonylurea hypoglycemics), tetracyclines (especially demeclocycline), phenothiazines, nalidixic acid, sulindac, amiodarone, and indomethacin.

**9. Drug-related lupus erythematosus**–May present with a photosensitive rash accompanied by fever, polyarthritis, myalgia, and serositis. Less severe than systemic lupus erythematosus, and recovery often follows drug withdrawal. Common offenders are hydralazine, isoniazid, procainamide, and phenytoin, as well as many other drugs.

**10. Lichenoid and lichen planus-like eruptions**–Amiphenazole, benzthiazides, bismuth, carbamazepine, chlordiazepoxide, chloroquine, chlorpropamide, dapsone, ethambutol, furosemide, gold salts, hydroxychloroquine, levamisole, quinacrine, meprobamate, methyldopa, aminosalicylic acid, paraphenylenediamine salts, penicillamine, phenothiazines, pindolol, propranolol, quinidine, quinine, streptomycin, sulfonylureas, tetracyclines, thiazides, triprolidine.

**11. Fixed eruptions**–Demarcated, round, erythematous plaques that recur at the same site when the drug is repeated. Pigmentation remains after healing. Fixed drug eruptions have been described with at least 69 drugs, including antimicrobials, analgesics, barbiturates, cardiovascular drugs, heavy metals, antiparasitics, antihistamines, ibuprofen, and naproxen. Immunologic studies strongly indicate that the immune system plays a major role in pathogenesis.

**12. Toxic epidermal necrolysis**–(Rare.) Large sheets of erythema develop, followed by separation, which looks like scalded skin. In adults, the eruption has occurred after administration of practically all classes of drugs, particularly barbiturates, phenytoin, sulfonamides, and nonsteroidal anti-inflammatory drugs.

**13. Urticaria**–(Rare in chronic form.) The penicillins and salicylates may be responsible.

**14. Pruritus**–Itchy skin without rash may be due to a wide variety of drug reactions. Pruritus ani may

be due to overgrowth of *Candida* after systemic antibiotic treatment. The following drugs may produce this symptom during biliary stasis: contraceptive pills, phenothiazines, and rifampin.

**15. Hair loss**–Predictable side effect of cytotoxic agents and oral contraceptives. Diffuse hair loss also occurs unpredictably with a wide variety of other drugs, including anticoagulants, antithyroid drugs, newer antimicrobials, cholesterol-lowering agents, heavy metals, corticosteroids, androgens, nonsteroidal anti-inflammatory drugs, and nadolol.

**16. Pigmentation**–Drugs can cause many types of pigmentary disturbances.

a. Flat hyperpigmented areas on the forehead and cheeks (chloasma or melasma) are the most common pigmentary disorder associated with drug ingestion. Improvement is slow despite stopping the drug. Oral contraceptives are the usual cause.

b. A blue-gray discoloration on light-exposed areas may occur with chlorpromazine and related phenothiazines.

c. A generalized brown or blue-gray pigmentation may occur with heavy metals (silver, gold, bismuth, and arsenic).

d. A generalized yellow color is usually due to quinacrine (Atabrine).

e. Blue-black patches on the shins, pigmentation of the nails and palate, and depigmentation of the hair may be due to chloroquine or minocycline.

f. A slate gray color with amiodarone.

**17. Psoriasiform eruptions**–Amodiaquine, chloroquine, debrisoquin, lithium, oxprenolol, pindolol, propranolol, quinacrine, sulfonamides.

**18. Pityriasis rosea-like eruptions**–Arsenic trioxide, barbiturates, bismuth, clonidine, gold salts, methopromazine, metoprolol, metronidazole, tripelennamine.

**19. Seborrheic dermatitis-like eruptions**–Arsenic, cimetidine, gold salts, methyldopa.

**20. Bullous eruptions**–Aspirin, barbiturates, bromides, chlorpromazine, warfarin, phenytoin, sulfonamides and related compounds, and promethazine.

**B. Laboratory Findings:** The complete blood count may show leukopenia, eosinophilia, agranulocytosis, or evidence of aplastic anemia. Patch tests performed with the suspect drug, although not routinely useful, may detect an offending drug when contact sensitivity is also present.

Direct immunofluorescence studies may help distinguish drug eruptions from other skin conditions in patients with a histologic pattern of lichenoid dermatitis, vasculitis, perivascular lymphocytic infiltrate, nonspecific inflammation, and mild dermatitis. Blood vessel fluorescence with IgM, C3, or fibrin deposition may be found in nearly half such patients, and others may have basement membrane zone fluorescence that suggests bullous pemphigoid. Common drugs that may be associated with such changes include nonsteroidal anti-inflammatory drugs and antibiotics, as well as triamterene, trimethoprim-sulfamethoxazole, and quinidine. Antibody studies for certain drugs, such as triamterene and quinidine, may be possible in the future.

## Differential Diagnosis

Distinguish from other eruptions, usually by history and subsidence after drug withdrawal, although fading may be slow.

## Complications

Blood dyscrasias, anaphylaxis, laryngeal edema, photosensitivity, and hepatic, renal, ocular, central nervous system, and other complications may occur with dermatitis medicamentosa.

## Prevention

People who have had dermatitis medicamentosa should avoid analogs of known chemical "allergens" as well as known offenders. The physician should pay careful attention to a history of drug reaction.

## Treatment

**A. General Measures:** Treat systemic manifestations as they arise (eg, anemia, icterus, purpura). Antihistamines may be of value in urticarial and angioneurotic reactions, but epinephrine, 1:1000, 0.5–1 mL intravenously or intramuscularly, should be used as an emergency measure. Corticosteroids may be used as for acute contact dermatitis in severe cases. Dialysis may speed drug elimination.

**B. Specific Measures:** Stop all drugs, if possible, and hasten elimination from the body by increasing fluid intake. Dimercaprol (BAL) or other chelating agents such as calcium disodium edetate may be tried in cases due to heavy metals (eg, arsenic, mercury, gold). Sodium chloride, 5–10 g/d orally, may hasten elimination of bromides and iodides in cases due to those drugs.

**C. Local Measures:** Treat the varieties and stages of dermatitis according to the major dermatitis simulated. Watch for sensitivity. Extensive blistering eruptions resulting in erosions and superficial ulcerations demand hospitalization and nursing care as for burn patients.

## Prognosis

Drug rash usually disappears upon withdrawal of the drug and proper treatment. If systemic involvement is severe, the outcome may be fatal.

Bigby M, Stern R: Cutaneous reactions to nonsteroidal anti-inflammatory drugs: A review. *J Am Acad Dermatol* 1985;**12**:866.

Bigby M et al: Drug-induced cutaneous reactions. *JAMA* 1986;**256**:3358.

Bruinsma W: *A Guide to Drug Eruptions.* Excerpta Medica, 1982.

Kauppinen K, Stubb S: Drug eruptions: Causative agents and clinical types. *Acta Derm Venereol* (Stockh) 1984;**64**:320.

Millikan LE: Cutaneous adverse drug reactions. *Curr Concepts Skin Disorders* (Spring) 1984;**5**:5.

Westly ED, Wechsler HL: Toxic epidermal necrolysis. *Arch Dermatol* 1984;**120**:721.

Wintroub BU, Stern R: Cutaneous drug reactions: Pathogenesis and clinical classification. *J Am Acad Dermatol* 1985;**13**:167.

# EXFOLIATIVE DERMATITIS (Generalized Erythroderma)

## Essentials of Diagnosis

- Scaling and erythema over large area of body.
- Itching, malaise, fever, weight loss.
- Primary disease or exposure to toxic agent (contact, oral, parenteral) may be evident.

## General Considerations

As a causative factor, a preexisting dermatosis may be found in half of cases, including psoriasis, atopic dermatitis, contact dermatitis, pityriasis rubra pilaris, seborrheic dermatitis, photosensitivity, nummular eczema, and ichthyosis. Reactions to external and internal drugs account for perhaps one-fourth of cases, and cancer for 4–8%. Causation of the remainder is undeterminable.

## Clinical Findings

**A. Symptoms and Signs:** Symptoms include itching, weakness, malaise, fever, and weight loss. Exfoliation may be generalized or universal and sometimes includes loss of hair and nails. Generalized lymphadenopathy may be due to lymphoma or leukemia or may be part of the clinical picture of the skin disease (dermatopathic lymphadenitis). There may be mucosal sloughs. Skin biopsy is mandatory and may show changes of a specific inflammatory dermatitis or cutaneous T cell lymphoma or leukemia.

**B. Laboratory Findings:** Blood and bone marrow studies and lymph node biopsies may show evidence of lymphoma or leukemia. There may be pathologic serum electrophoresis, elevated erythrocyte sedimentation rate, eosinophilia, elevated serum IgE, elevated white blood count, anemia, and peripheral blood lymphocytosis.

## Differential Diagnosis

It is often impossible to delineate exfoliative dermatitis early in the course of the disease, so careful follow-up is necessary. Differentiate from other scaling eruptions such as psoriasis, lichen planus, severe seborrheic dermatitis, and dermatitis medicamentosa, which may themselves develop into exfoliative dermatitis.

## Complications

Septicemia, debility (protein loss), pneumonia, high-output cardiac failure, masking of fever, hypermetabolism, thermoregulatory disorders, and anemia.

## Prevention

Patients receiving sensitizing drugs should be watched carefully for the development of skin reactions of all types. The drug should be withheld until the nature of the skin reaction is determined. Proved sensitization should be considered an absolute contraindication to further administration of the drug. Dermatitis or dermatoses should not be overtreated.

## Treatment

**A. General Measures:** Hospitalize the patient at bed rest with talc on bed sheets. Keep the room at a warm, constant temperature and avoid drafts. Transfusions of blood or plasma may be required. Avoid all unnecessary medication.

Systemic corticosteroids may provide spectacular improvement in severe or fulminant exfoliative dermatitis, but long-term therapy should be avoided if possible (see Chapter 18). For recalcitrant cases of psoriatic erythroderma and pityriasis rubra pilaris, either isotretinoin, etretinate, or methotrexate—or isotretinoin and methotrexate in combination—may be indicated. Erythroderma secondary to lymphoma or leukemia requires specific topical or systemic chemotherapy combined with radiation therapy. Suitable antibiotic drugs should be given when there is evidence of bacterial infection; pyoderma is a common complication of exfoliative dermatitis.

**B. Specific Measures:** Stop all drugs, if possible, and hasten elimination of the offending drug by all means, eg, by increasing fluid intake. Dimercaprol (BAL) may lessen the severity or duration of reactions due to arsenic or gold (see Chapter 30).

**C. Local Measures:** Observe careful skin hygiene and avoid irritating local applications. Treat skin as for acute extensive dermatitis first with midpotency topical steroids under wet dressings or plastic suit occlusion and soothing baths; and later with soothing oily steroid lotions and ointments. Topical antiinfective drugs may be used when necessary.

## Prognosis

Most patients recover completely or improve greatly over time. Deaths have been reported but are rare unless there is underlying cancer. A minority will suffer from undiminished erythroderma for indefinite periods of time.

Hasan T, Jansen CT: Erythroderma: A follow-up of fifty cases. *J Am Acad Dermatol* 1983;**8**:836.

## PHOTODERMATITIS
## (Dermatitis Actinica, Erythema Solare or Sunburn, Polymorphous Light Sensitivity, Contact Photodermatitis)

## Essentials of Diagnosis

- Painful erythema, edema, and vesiculation on sun-exposed surfaces.
- Fever, gastrointestinal symptoms, malaise, or prostration may occur.
- Proteinuria, casts, and hematuria may occur.

## General Considerations

Photodermatitis is an acute or chronic inflammatory skin reaction due to overexposure or hypersensitivity to sunlight or other sources of actinic rays, photosensitization of the skin by certain drugs, or idiosyncrasy to actinic light as seen in some constitutional disorders including the porphyrias and many hereditary disorders (phenylketonuria, xeroderma pigmentosum, and others). Contact photosensitivity may occur with perfumes, antiseptics, and other chemicals.

## Clinical Findings

**A. Symptoms and Signs:** The acute inflammatory skin reaction is accompanied by pain, fever, gastrointestinal symptoms, malaise, and even prostration. Signs include erythema, edema, and possibly vesiculation and oozing on exposed surfaces. Exfoliation and pigmentary changes often result.

**B. Laboratory Findings:** Proteinuria, casts, hematuria, and hemoconcentration may be present. Look for porphyrins in urine and stool, protoporphyrins in blood, and findings in other inborn errors of metabolism. Elaborate testing for photosensitivity may be performed by experts.

## Differential Diagnosis

Differentiate from contact dermatitis that may develop from one of the many substances in suntan lotions and oils. Sensitivity to actinic rays may also be part of a more serious condition such as porphyria, erythropoietic protoporphyria, lupus erythematosus, or pellagra. Phenothiazines, sulfones, chlorothiazides, griseofulvin, oral antidiabetic agents, and antibiotics may photosensitize the skin. Polymorphous light eruption appears to be an idiopathic photodermatosis that affects both sexes equally.

In a 7-year follow-up evaluation of 114 patients with polymorphous light eruption, the condition was found to be chronic in nature but with diminishing sunlight sensitivity over the long term. Transitory periods of spontaneous remission do occur, and the risk of developing systemic lupus erythematosus and possibly other autoimmune collagen disorders is negligible or nonexistent. The action spectrum often lies in both long (320–400 nm) and short (below 320 nm) ultraviolet wavelengths. Contact photodermatitis may be caused by halogenated salicylanilides (weak antiseptics in soaps, creams, etc).

## Complications

Delayed cumulative effects in fair-skinned people include keratoses and epitheliomas. Some individuals become chronic light-reactors even when they apparently are no longer exposed to photosensitizing or phototoxic drugs.

## Prevention

Persons with very fair, sensitive skins should avoid prolonged exposure to strong sun or ultraviolet radiation. Preliminary conditioning by graded exposure and protective clothing is advisable.

Protective sunscreening agents (eg, those containing PABA and oxy- or dioxybenzone) may be applied before exposure, although PABA itself may cause photosensitivity dermatitis.

The use of psoralens orally is controversial.

In those photodermatoses in which the action spectrum involves wavelengths beyond the short ultraviolet range (320 nm), sunshades that contain titanium dioxide (Maxafil) must be used. RVPaque, which contains zinc oxide, may also be used.

## Treatment

**A. General Measures:** Treat constitutional symptoms by appropriate supportive measures. Control pain, fever, and gastrointestinal and other symptoms as they arise. Aspirin may have some specific value. Corticosteroids, both systemically and topically, may be required for severe reactions. Beta-carotene (Solatene), 60 mg/d orally, is effective treatment for erythropoietic protoporphyria. Beta-carotene, 90–300 mg/d orally, may be tried in adults with photosensitive eczema, polymorphous light eruptions, or solar urticaria, although double-blind studies have not been done because of unavoidable skin staining. Chloroquine, 125 mg orally twice weekly for 3–9 months, is effective in treating porphyria cutanea tarda. Patients must be followed clinically and ophthalmologically and with laboratory uroporphyrin determinations. This is not suitable if the patient has hepatitis or cirrhosis. Phlebotomy, letting 500 mL of blood every 2 weeks, is an alternative mode of therapy but is often complicated by anemia, other hematologic disorders, hypoproteinemia, or vasomotor dysfunction. Liver toxins, including alcohol, should be interdicted.

Triamcinolone acetonide suspension, 30–40 mg, may be given deep in the gluteal muscle once yearly for flare-ups of polymorphous light eruption.

Trioxsalen (Trisoralen), 25–30 mg orally, followed by sunlight exposure 2 hours later, may control polymorphous light eruption. Treatment may be given for 4 days each month if needed. Initial flare-ups may occur.

**B. Local Measures:** Treat as for any acute dermatitis. First use cooling and soothing wet dressings with saline, bicarbonate, or aluminum subacetate solutions and follow with calamine or starch lotions. Greases must be avoided because of the occlusive effect.

For maximum protection, sunscreens with a sun protective factor (SPF) of 15 or greater should be used. These aid in delaying sun damage and aging of fair skin and in the management of photodermatoses. Unfortunately, contact or photoallergy may be caused by sunscreens themselves, in which case sunshades containing titanium dioxide, zinc oxide, or talc may be used instead.

## Prognosis

Dermatitis actinica is usually benign and self-limiting unless the burn is severe or when it occurs as an associated finding in a more serious disorder.

Frain-Bell W (guest editor): Photodermatoses. *Semin Dermatol* 1982;**1**:153. [Entire issue.]

Jansen CT, Karvonen J: Polymorphous light eruption: A seven-year follow-up evaluation of 114 patients. *Arch Dermatol* 1984;**120**:862.

Rapaport M: Sunlight and sunscreens. *Dermatology and Allergy* 1982;**5**:34.

## LICHEN PLANUS

### Essentials of Diagnosis

- Pruritic, violaceous, flat-topped papules with fine white streaks and symmetric distribution.
- Commonly seen along linear scratch mark (Koebner phenomenon).
- Anterior wrists, sacral region, penis, legs, mucous membranes.
- Usually occurs in an otherwise healthy but emotionally tense person.
- Histopathology is diagnostic.

### General Considerations

Lichen planus is an inflammatory pruritic disease of the skin and mucous membranes, characterized by distinctive papules with a predilection for the flexor surfaces and trunk. It may be an "allergic" reaction pattern, particularly following exposure to dyes, color film developers, and gold. The 3 cardinal findings are typical skin lesions, histopathologic features of band infiltration of T cells in the dermis, and fluorescence with IgG and C3 at the basement membrane. Links have been seen with bullous pemphigoid, alopecia areata, vitiligo, chronic ulcerative colitis, hypogammaglobulinemia, and graft-versus-host reactions. Drugs associated with lichen planus include gold, demeclocycline, streptomycin, tetracycline, arsenic, iodides, chloroquine, quinacrine, quinidine, and paraphenylenediamine. Antimony, phenothiazine, aminosalicylic acid, chlorothiazide, hydrochlorothiazide, and amiphenazole have also been incriminated. Colloid bodies appear in the upper dermis and may contain IgM as well as small amounts of IgG. Fibrin may be found in the upper dermis. These findings are not highly specific.

### Clinical Findings

Itching is mild to severe. The lesions are violaceous, flat-topped, angulated papules, discrete or in clusters, on the flexor surfaces of the wrists and on the penis, lips, tongue, and buccal and vaginal mucous membranes. Mucosal lichen planus has been reported in the genital and anorectal areas, the gastrointestinal tract, the bladder, the larynx, and the conjunctiva. The papules may become bullous or ulcerated. The disease may be generalized. Mucous membrane lesions have a lacy white network overlying them that is often confused with leukoplakia. Papules are 1–4 mm in diameter, with white streaks on the surface (Wickham's striae).

A special form of lichen planus is the erosive variety. On palms and soles, it can be disabling. It is a major problem in the mouth, since squamous cell carcinoma may develop. The disease must be distinguished from systemic lupus erythematosus, both clinically and by laboratory findings.

### Differential Diagnosis

Distinguish from similar lesions produced by quinacrine or bismuth sensitivity and other papular lesions such as psoriasis, papular eczema, and syphiloderm. Lichen planus on the mucous membranes must be differentiated from leukoplakia. Certain photodeveloping or duplicating solutions may produce eruptions that mimic lichen planus.

### Treatment

**A. General Measures:** Patients with lichen planus are sometimes tense and nervous, and episodes of dermatitis may be temporally related to emotional crises. Measures should be directed at relieving anxiety, and judicious use of sedatives or hydroxyzine may be helpful. Corticosteroids (see Chapter 18) may be required in severe cases.

Psoralens plus long-wave ultraviolet light (PUVA) is effective for most cases of lichen planus, and maintenance therapy apparently is not required.

Isotretinoin by mouth may be effective for oral and cutaneous lichen planus, although this is not a listed indication for this drug, and precautions must be observed (see Acne Vulgaris).

After testing for the presence of glucose-6-phosphate dehydrogenase, treat erosive lichen planus with dapsone, 50 mg/d; this may be given over a period of many weeks, if necessary, with appropriate clinical and laboratory monitoring.

**B. Local Measures:** Use shake lotions containing tar. X-ray or grenz ray therapy (by a specialist) may rarely be used when involvement is particularly severe. Intralesional injection of triamcinolone acetonide is useful for localized forms. Corticosteroid cream or ointment may be used nightly under thin pliable plastic film. Betamethasone dipropionate or clobetasol propionate creams or ointments applied twice daily are helpful.

Application of tretinoin cream (retinoic acid; vitamin A acid), 0.05%, to mucosal lichen planus, followed by a corticosteroid ointment, may be helpful. For disabling hypertrophic lichen planus of the soles, tretinoin cream applied and covered with thin, pliable polyethylene film nightly is said to be effective.

### Prognosis

Lichen planus is a benign disease, but it may persist for months or years and may be recurrent. Oral lesions tend to be especially persistent, and neoplastic degeneration has been described.

Falk DK, Latour DL, King LE Jr: Dapsone in the treatment of erosive lichen planus. *J Am Acad Dermatol* 1985;**12:**567.

Fox B, Odom R: Papulosquamous diseases: A review. *J Am Acad Dermatol* 1985;**12:**597.

Gonzalez E, Momtaz-T K, Freedman S: Bilateral comparison

of generalized lichen planus treated with psoralens and ultraviolet A. *J Am Acad Dermatol* 1984;**10:**958.

Woo TY: Systemic isotretinoin treatment of oral and cutaneous lichen planus. *Cutis* 1985;**35:**385.

## PSORIASIS

### Essentials of Diagnosis

- Silvery scales on bright red plaques, usually on the knees, elbows, and scalp.
- Stippled nails.
- Mild itching unless psoriasis is eruptive or occurs in body folds.
- Possible associated psoriatic arthritis.
- Specific histopathologic features.

### General Considerations

Psoriasis is a common benign, acute or chronic inflammatory skin disease that apparently is based upon genetic predisposition. A genetic error in the epidermal mitotic control system has been postulated. For the relationship of psoriasis to histocompatibility (HLA) antigens, see Chapter 33. The decreased responsiveness of the cAMP system in psoriatic epidermis to prostaglandin $E_1$ suggests that altered response of the epidermis to prostaglandins may be one of the factors in the pathophysiology of psoriasis. Injury or irritation of psoriatic skin tends to provoke lesions of psoriasis in the site. Psoriasis occasionally is eruptive, particularly in periods of stress or after streptococcal pharyngitis. Grave, life-threatening forms may occur. There is some evidence that immunologic factors may play a part in the pathogenesis of psoriasis, but this is inadequately confirmed. Extensive erythrodermic psoriasis with abrupt onset may accompany AIDS.

### Clinical Findings

There are usually no symptoms. Eruptive psoriasis may itch, and psoriasis in body folds itches severely ("inverse psoriasis"). The lesions are dull red, sharply outlined plaques covered with silvery scales. The elbows, knees, and scalp are the most common sites. Nail involvement may resemble onychomycosis. Fine stippling ("pitting") in the nails is highly suggestive of psoriasis. There may be associated arthritis that resembles the rheumatoid variety but with a negative latex fixation test.

### Differential Diagnosis

Differentiate in the scalp from seborrheic dermatitis; in body folds from intertrigo and candidiasis; and in the nails from onychomycosis.

### Treatment

**A. General Measures:** Desert climates seem to exert a favorable effect. Severe psoriasis calls for treatment in the hospital or a day-care center with the Goeckerman regimen.

Corticotropin or corticosteroids may be necessary

to give relief in fulminating cases. Parenteral corticosteroids should not be used except in the most severe cases, because of the possibility of changing plaques to pustular lesions. Methotrexate is available for severe psoriasis. FDA guidelines must be followed.

Reassurance is important, since these patients are apt to be discouraged by the difficulties of treatment. An attempt should be made to relieve anxieties.

**B. Local Measures:**

**1. Acute psoriasis**—Avoid irritating or stimulating drugs. Begin with a calamine or starch lotion or bland ointment containing 10% solution of coal tar. As the lesions become less acute, gradually incorporate mild keratoplastic agents into lotions and hydrophilic ointments. Betamethasone dipropionate, 0.05% in a glycol formulation (Diprolene ointment), rubbed into the skin once daily so that 45 g lasts 1 week, is sometimes highly effective in treating resistant psoriasis and other dermatoses; adrenal function remains relatively unaffected. It is best to restrict the ointment to 3 weeks' use until more is known about topical and systemic side effects.

**2. Subacute psoriasis**—Give warm baths daily, scrubbing the lesions thoroughly with a brush, soap, and water. Apply increasing concentrations of keratoplastic or stimulating agents incorporated in lotions and hydrophilic ointments. Solar or ultraviolet irradiations may be applied in gradually increasing doses.

**3. Chronic psoriasis**—The Goeckerman regimen in psoriasis day-care centers is highly effective and cost-effective and has high patient compliance. With treatment for 6 days a week for 6 or 7 hours daily, a remission rate of 90% clearing of the skin occurs in an average of 18 days. Long remissions occur. Intensive exposure to 2–5% crude coal tar in petrolatum to which 2.5% polysorbate 80 is added, coupled with exposure to ultraviolet light in the B range (UVB) in 290- to 320-nm wavelength range), with the addition of 2% or 5% salicylic acid to the tar ointment for thick plaques, are the essentials of the treatment; mild corticosteroid creams are added, plus a 10% solution of coal tar USP in a skin oil for the scalp. The Mayo Clinic Goeckerman treatment is the standard with which other forms of psoriasis treatment must be compared.

Estar gel, psoriGel, Aquatar, and Fototar are elegant substitutes for crude coal tar. Anthralin ointment 0.1% may be helpful. It tends to be irritating, however, and it discolors white or gray hair. It should not be used near the eyes. Short-contact anthralin therapy (SCAT)—anthralin 1% applied for 15–30 minutes—is an effective and safe method of treatment.

Exposure to sunlamps or blacklight lamps, without systemic or topical therapy, may benefit chronic psoriasis.

PUVA (psoralen plus ultraviolet-A, ie, ultraviolet light in the 320- to 400-nm wavelength range; same as black light) tends to be a long-term form of treatment, as maintenance therapy is usually required. The ultraviolet dose is cumulative, and the relapse rate is about 63% in 1–6 months. The total safe dose is unknown, and the incidence of skin cancer is 9 times the normal incidence, with a reversal of the usual basal cell to squamous cell carcinoma ratio. Epidermal dystrophy by light microscopy is seen in 50% of patients treated with PUVA, and there is rapid aging of the skin. Cataracts are a potential threat, and there may be immunologic changes.

The simple application twice daily of commercial tar plus topical corticosteroids may be helpful.

For recalcitrant scalp lesions, one may rub in, nightly, a cream or ointment containing 0.5% anthralin, followed at once by Neutrogena T/Derm oil. This treatment stains pillowcases and may irritate the eyes.

Etretinate (aromatic retinoid), 0.3–1 mg/kg/d, appears to be the first choice in the treatment of severe pustular psoriasis. It is also useful for psoriatic erythroderma, psoriasis vulgaris, and psoriatic arthritis. Liver enzymes must be checked periodically. The drug has a prolonged half-life. An ominous finding is that of diffuse idiopathic skeletal hyperostosis (DISH syndrome) from long-term, high-dose therapy (eg, 4 mg/kg/d orally for many months).

Isotretinoin works on occasion. (See below for side effects and cautions.)

Clobetasol propionate, 0.05% ointment, is the newest member of the class of highly potent topical corticosteroid agents. It is the most effective of all the topical corticosteroids available in the USA for suppression of lesions of psoriasis. Caution is advised, as extensive use for prolonged periods may lead to suppression of the hypothalamic-pituitary-adrenocortical axis. Pseudoatrophy, striations, "steroid acne," and other complications may occur.

## Prognosis

The course tends to be chronic and unpredictable, and the disease may be refractory to treatment.

Gip L, Hamfelt A: Studies on the efficacy and adrenal effects of Diprolene ointment 0.05% and Dermolate ointment 0.05% in patients with psoriasis or other resistant dermatoses. *Cutis* 1984;**33:**215.

Jacobson C, Cornell RC, Savin RC: A comparison of clobetasol propionate 0.05% ointment and an optimized betamethasone dipropionate 0.05% ointment in the treatment of psoriasis. *Cutis* 1986;**37:**213.

Johnson TM et al: AIDS exacerbates psoriasis. *N Engl J Med* 1985;**313:**1415.

Menter A, Cram DL: The Goeckerman regimen in two psoriasis day care centers. *J Am Acad Dermatol* 1983;**9:**59.

Moy RL, Kingston TP, Lowe NJ: Isotretinoin vs etretinate therapy in generalized pustular and chronic psoriasis. *Arch Dermatol* 1985;**121:**1297.

Muller SA, Perry HO: The Goeckerman treatment in psoriasis: Six decades of experience at the Mayo Clinic. *Cutis* 1984;**34:**265.

Roenigk HH Jr, Maibach HI (editors): *Psoriasis.* Marcel Dekker, 1985.

## PITYRIASIS ROSEA

### Essentials of Diagnosis

- Oval, fawn-colored, scaly eruption following cleavage lines of trunk.
- Herald patch commonly precedes eruption by 1–2 weeks.
- Occasional pruritus.

### General Considerations

This is a common, mild, acute inflammatory disease which is 50% more common in females. Young adults are principally affected, mostly in the spring or fall. Concurrent household cases have been reported, and recurrences may take place over a period of years. The cause is unknown, but it is speculated that a picornavirus may be causative.

### Clinical Findings

Occasionally, there is severe itching. The lesions consist of oval, fawn-colored macules 4–5 mm in diameter following cleavage lines on the trunk. Exfoliation of the lesions causes a crinkly scale that begins in the center. The proximal portions of the extremities are involved. An initial lesion (''herald patch'') usually precedes the later efflorescence by 1–2 weeks. Attacks usually last 4–8 weeks.

### Differential Diagnosis

Differentiate from secondary syphilis, especially when lesions are numerous or smaller than usual. Tinea corporis, seborrheic dermatitis, tinea versicolor, viral exanthems, and drug eruptions may simulate pityriasis rosea.

### Treatment

Acute irritated lesions (uncommon) should be treated as for acute dermatitis with wet dressings or shake lotions. Apply coal tar solution, 5% in starch lotion, twice daily. Ultraviolet light is helpful.

### Prognosis

Pityriasis rosea is usually an acute self-limiting illness that disappears in about 6 weeks.

Arndt KA et al: Treatment of pityriasis rosea with UV radiation. *Arch Dermatol* 1983;**119**:381.

Chuang T-Y et al: Pityriasis rosea in Rochester, Minnesota, 1969 to 1978: A 10-year epidemiologic study. *J Am Acad Dermatol* 1982;**7**:80.

## SEBORRHEIC DERMATITIS & DANDRUFF

### Essentials of Diagnosis

- Dry scales or dry yellowish dandruff with or without underlying erythema.
- Scalp, central face, presternal, interscapular areas, umbilicus, and body folds.

### General Considerations

Seborrheic dermatitis is an acute or chronic papulosquamous dermatitis. It is based upon a genetic predisposition mediated by an interplay of such factors as hormones, nutrition, infection, and emotional stress. The possibility exists that *Pityrosporon orbiculare* (*Malassezia furfur*) or *P ovale* plays a central role in the pathogenesis of seborrheic dermatitis. Dandruff per se is merely an intensification of the physiologic process of desquamation. Induction or aggravation of seborrheic dermatitis has been described from overgrowth of *Pityrosporon ovale* (*Malassezia ovalis*) in AIDS patients, with clinical response to application of 2% ketoconazole cream.

It is difficult to distinguish between seborrheic dermatitis, simple dandruff, and scalp psoriasis on clinical or histologic grounds. The etiology and pathogenesis of seborrheic dermatitis and dandruff are poorly understood. Numerous disparate agents are useful in controlling dandruff, including selenium sulfide, zinc pyrithione, and antifungals (against yeasts) such as nystatin and the imidazoles. There is a reawakening of interest in *Pityrosporon* yeasts as possible agents of seborrheic dermatitis, but opinion is divided about whether imidazoles help these conditions because of their antifungal activity or because they have a nonspecific cytostatic effect.

### Clinical Findings

Pruritus may be present but is an inconstant finding. The scalp, face, chest, back, umbilicus, and body folds may be oily or dry, with dry scales or oily yellowish scurf. Eyelid margins (seborrheic blepharitis) may be involved in the process. Erythema, fissuring, and secondary infection may be present.

### Differential Diagnosis

Distinguish from other skin diseases of the same areas such as intertrigo and fungal infections; and from psoriasis (location).

### Treatment

**A. General Measures:** Hygienic habits of living, with an adequate diet, regular working hours, recreation, sleep, and simple cleanliness are recommended. Treat aggravating systemic factors such as infections and emotional stress.

*Pityrosporon ovale* folliculitis of the scalp, previously resistant to treatment, responds to a brief course of ketoconazole by mouth (200 mg/d for 1 week).

Two percent ketoconazole cream appears to benefit most patients with seborrheic dermatitis.

**B. Local Measures:**

**1. Acute, subacute, or chronic eczematous lesions**–Treat as for dermatitis or eczema (see p 54). An emulsion base containing 0.5% hydrocortisone and 10% sodium sulfacetamide is useful. Corticosteroid creams, lotions, or solution may be used in all stages. Potent fluorinated corticosteroids used regularly on the face may produce steroid rosacea. Therefore, nonfluorinated steroids are recommended for the face and intertriginous areas.

**2. Seborrhea of the scalp**–Use one of the following: (1) Selsun (selenium sulfide) suspension or Exsel once a week after shampoo. Fostex cream (containing soapless cleansers, wetting agents, sulfur, and salicylic acid) or Sebulex may be used as a weekly shampoo for oily seborrhea. The patient should be instructed to shampoo vigorously once and then shampoo again, leaving the shampoo on for 5–10 minutes to loosen the scales. (2) Neutrogena T/Gel shampoo, containing tar, may succeed where others fail. (3) Shampoos and soaps containing zinc pyrithione may be helpful. (4) Betamethasone valerate (Valisone), 0.1% lotion, is excellent.

An alcoholic solution of aluminum chloride plus an antibiotic topical lotion rubbed in once or twice daily, may work where other measures fail.

Newer antifungal lotions (miconazole, clotrimazole, econazole) may help.

**3. Seborrhea of nonhairy areas**–Mild stimulating coal tar lotion, mild sulfur-salicylic acid ointment, or 3–5% sulfur in hydrophilic ointment may be used. (The addition of 1% salicylic acid to these preparations aids in removing scales.)

**4. Seborrhea of intertriginous areas**–Avoid greasy ointments. Apply astringent aluminum subacetate wet dressings followed by 3% iodochlorhydroxyquin and 1% hydrocortisone in an emulsion base.

## Prognosis

The tendency is to lifelong recurrences. Individual outbreaks may last weeks, months, or years.

Editorial: Scales in the balance: Dandruff reconsidered. *Lancet* 1985;**2**:703.

Ford GP et al: The response of seborrheic dermatitis to ketoconazole. *Br J Dermatol* 1984;**111**:603.

Skinner RB et al: Seborrheic dermatitis and acquired immunodeficiency syndrome. (Correspondence.) *J Am Acad Dermatol* 1986;**14**:147.

## ACNE VULGARIS

### Essentials of Diagnosis

- Pimples (papules or pustules) over the face, back, and shoulders occurring at puberty.
- Open and closed comedones.
- Cyst formation, slow resolution, scarring.
- The most common of all skin conditions.

### General Considerations

Acne vulgaris is a common inflammatory disease of unknown cause that is apparently activated by androgens in those who are genetically predisposed. It may occur from puberty through the period of sex hormone activity. Eunuchs are spared. Similar involvement may occur in identical twins.

The disease is more common and more severe in males. Contrary to popular belief, it does not always clear spontaneously when maturity is reached. If untreated, it may persist into the fourth and even sixth decade of life. The skin lesions follow sebaceous overactivity, plugging of the infundibulum of the follicles, retention of sebum, overgrowth of the acne bacillus (*Propionibacterium acnes*) in incarcerated sebum, irritation by accumulated fatty acids, and foreign body reaction to extrafollicular sebum. The role of antibiotics in controlling acne is not clearly understood, but they may work because of their antianabolic effect on the sebaceous gland. (Topical occlusive corticosteroids may produce acne.)

When a resistant case of acne is encountered in a woman, hyperandrogenism may be suspected. Look for hirsutism, irregular menses, or other signs of virilism. Dexamethasone, 0.5 mg nightly, may help.

### Clinical Findings

There may be mild soreness, pain, or itching; inflammatory papules, pustules, ectatic pores, acne cysts, and scarring. The lesions occur mainly over the face, neck, upper chest, back, and shoulders. Comedones are common.

Self-consciousness and embarrassment may be the most disturbing symptoms.

### Differential Diagnosis

Distinguish from acneiform lesions caused by bromides, iodides, steroids, and contact with chlorinated naphthalenes and diphenyls.

### Complications

Cyst formation, severe scarring, and psychic trauma.

### Treatment

**A. General Measures:**

**1. Education of the patient**–It should be explained that treatment is essential not only to produce an acceptable cosmetic result while the condition is active but also to prevent permanent scarring.

**2. Diet**–Specific dietary factors are less important than formerly thought in causing acne.

**3.** Avoid exposure to oils and greases.

**4.** Aggravating or complicating emotional disturbances must be taken into consideration and treated appropriately.

**5. Antibiotics**–Tetracycline may discolor growing teeth.

Blood counts, blood chemistries, and urinalyses give essentially normal findings in persons on long-term low-dose tetracycline or erythromycin therapy for acne. Gram-negative folliculitis developing from acne during broad-spectrum antibiotic therapy will respond to oral isotretinoin (*caution*). Chloramphenicol should not be used. A number of commercial topical antibiotic lotions are available. The most effective are erythromycin or clindamycin, in hydroalcoholic or other special vehicles. Clindamycin phosphate should be used topically instead of the hydrochloride.

**6. Isotretinoin** (Accutane; 13-*cis*-retinoic acid), a vitamin A analog, is approved for treatment of severe cystic acne in the USA. A dosage of 0.5–1 mg/kg/d for 4–5 months is usually adequate for severe cystic acne. The drug is *absolutely contraindicated during pregnancy,* because of teratogenicity, and therapeutic abortion must be considered if the patient takes the drug during pregnancy. Side effects occur in most patients, usually related to dry skin and mucous membranes (dry lips, nosebleed, and dry eyes). If headache occurs, pseudotumor cerebri must be ruled out. At the higher dosage level, about 25% of patients will develop hypertriglyceridemia, 15% hypercholesterolemia, and 5% lowering of high-density lipoproteins. Miscellaneous adverse reactions, usually not seen with doses of 0.5 mg/kg/d, include musculoskeletal or bowel symptoms, rash, thinning of hair, exuberant granulation tissue in lesions, and bony hyperostosis (seen only with very high doses). No serious liver or hematologic disturbances have been reported.

Isotretinoin, in contrast to its prototype, vitamin A (retinol), is not stored in the liver, and few significant laboratory abnormalities have been reported. At doses of 1 mg/kg/d or less in teenage patients, even elevations of serum triglycerides have rarely been high enough to be of concern. Elevations of liver enzymes and triglycerides return to normal once the drug is stopped.

Serious adverse effects with isotretinoin include fetal abnormalities in women taking the drug during pregnancy, pseudotumor cerebri, hyperuricemia, regional ileitis, and reversible corneal opacities.

**B. Local Measures:** Desquam-X wash or Benzac W wash may be used. Avoid greasy cleansing creams and other cosmetics. Shampoo the scalp 1–2 times a week. Extract blackheads with a comedo extractor. Incise and drain fluctuant cystic lesions with a small sharp scalpel.

**1. Keratoplastic and keratolytic agents–**A sulfur-zinc acne lotion may be applied locally to the skin at bedtime and washed off in the morning. Tretinoin (Retin-A) cream or gel is recommended for comedo acne, but it may be irritating, in which case a lower concentration may be necessary.

**2. Commercial preparations** for acne include Fostex cream and cake; Acne-Dome cleanser, cream, and lotion; Benzac W gel and wash; Desquam-X gel and wash; Benzagel; and Xerac BP. All of these gels contain benzoyl peroxide. Benzoyl peroxide products are available in concentrations of 2.5%, 5%, and 10%.

**3. Dermabrasion–**Cosmetic improvement may be achieved by abrasion of inactive acne lesions, particularly flat, superficial scars. The skin is first frozen and anesthetized with ethyl chloride or Freon and then carefully abraded with fine sandpaper, special motor-driven abrasive brushes, or diamond fraises. The technique is not without untoward effects, since hyperpigmentation, hypopigmentation, grooving, and scarring have been known to occur. Dark-skinned individuals do poorly.

**4. Irradiation–**Simple exposure to sunlight in graded doses is often beneficial. Ultraviolet irradiation

may be used as an adjunct to other treatment measures. Use suberythema doses in graded intervals up to the point of mild erythema and scaling.

**5. Intralesional triamcinolone acetonide suspension,** 3 mg/mL, is helpful for acutely inflamed acne cysts.

**6. Topical antibiotics–**If dryness occurs with benzoyl peroxide-containing agents or topical antibiotics in hydroalcoholic vehicles, 2% erythromycin ointment (Akne-mycin) is an alternative.

**7. Azelaic acid,** 15% cream (investigational), is beneficial.

### Prognosis

Untreated acne vulgaris often remits spontaneously, but the condition may persist throughout adulthood and may lead to severe scarring. The disease is chronic and tends to recur in spite of treatment. Remissions following systemic treatment with isotretinoin tend to be lasting.

Dicken CH: Retinoids: A review. *J Am Acad Dermatol* 1984;**11:**541.

Lesher JL et al: An evaluation of a 2% erythromycin ointment in the topical therapy of acne vulgaris. *J Am Acad Dermatol* 1985;**12:**526.

Nader S et al: Acne and hyperandrogenism: Impact of lowering androgen levels with glucocorticoid treatment. *J Am Acad Dermatol* 1984;**11:**256.

Nazzaro-Porro M et al: Beneficial effect of 15% azelaic acid cream on acne vulgaris. *Br J Dermatol* 1983;**109:**45.

Strauss JS et al: Isotretinoin therapy for acne: Results of a multicenter dose-response study. *J Am Acad Dermatol* 1984;**10:**490.

## ROSACEA

### Essentials of Diagnosis

- A chronic face disorder of middle-aged and older people.
- There is a large vascular component (erythema and telangiectasis).
- An acneiform component (papules, pustules, and seborrhea) is present.
- There is a glandular component accompanied by hyperplasia of the soft tissue of the nose (rhinophyma).

### General Considerations

Aside from obvious genetic overtones, no single factor adequately explains the pathogenesis of this disorder. Emotional disturbances, chronic alcoholism, a seborrheic diathesis, and a dysfunction of the gastrointestinal tract may be significant associated factors. A statistically significant incidence of migraine headaches accompanying rosacea has been reported.

A variant of rosacea is so-called **demodex acne (demodicidosis),** in which large numbers of the mite *Demodex folliculorum* are found in pores. These may be demonstrated under the microscope when squeezings from pores are examined in glycerin on a microscope slide.

Strong topical steroids can change trivial dermatoses of the face into a recognizable entity called **perioral dermatitis.** This occurs predominantly in young women and may be confused with acne rosacea. It yields to 1% hydrocortisone cream topically, plus tetracycline by mouth.

### Clinical Findings

These are described above. The entire face may have a rosy hue. One sees few or no comedones. Inflammatory papules are prominent, and there may be pustules. Associated seborrhea may be found. The patient often complains of burning or stinging with episodes of flushing.

### Differential Diagnosis

Distinguish from acne, bromoderma, iododerma, and demodicidosis, as described above. The rosy hue of rosacea generally will pinpoint the diagnosis.

### Treatment

**A. General Measures:** Tetracycline, 250 or 500 mg orally daily on an empty stomach, when used in conjunction with the topical treatment described below, may be very effective.

Isotretinoin (13-*cis*-retinoic acid; Accutane) may succeed where other measures fail. A large-scale cooperative study in West Germany has shown an excellent response to isotretinoin, 0.5–1 mg/kd/d orally for 12–28 weeks, with minimal side effects. Pregnancy must be avoided during treatment.

Metronidazole, 250 mg twice daily for 3 weeks, may be worth trying for rosacea. Side effects appear to be minimal. It has a disulfiramlike effect when the patient uses alcohol.

**B. Local Measures:** Hydrocortisone cream 0.5–1%, desonide cream 0.05%, hydrocortisone valerate (Westcort) 0.1%, hydrocortisone butyrate (Locoid), or alclometasone dipropionate 0.05% (Aclovate), used morning and night, along with tetracycline orally, is a very effective regimen. Topical antibiotics in special vehicles may be helpful (see Acne Vulgaris). Benzoyl peroxide, 5–10% in an acetone gel, apparently will clear erythema, papules, pustules, and nodules but not telangiectasia of rosacea. Five to 8 weeks of treatment are needed for significant response. About one person in 6 or 7 experiences irritation, burning, edema, and erythema from the applications.

### Prognosis

Rosacea tends to be a stubborn and persistent process. With the regimens described above, it can usually be controlled adequately. Complicating rhinophyma may require surgical correction.

Kürkçüoglu N, Atakan N: Metronidazole in the treatment of rosacea. (Letter.) *Arch Dermatol* 1984;**120:**837.

Plewig G, Nikolowski J, Wolff HH: Action of isotretinoin in acne rosacea and gram-negative folliculitis. *J Am Acad Dermatol* 1982;**6:**766.

## URTICARIA & ANGIOEDEMA

### Essentials of Diagnosis

- Eruptions of evanescent wheals or hives.
- Itching is usually intense but may on rare occasions be absent.
- Special forms of urticaria have special features (hereditary angioedema, dermographism, cholinergic urticaria, solar urticaria, or cold urticaria).
- Most incidents are acute and self-limited over a period of 1–2 weeks.
- Chronic urticaria may defy the best efforts of the clinician to find and eliminate the cause.

### General Considerations

Urticaria can result from many different stimuli. The pathogenetic mechanism may be either immunologic or nonimmunologic. The most common immunologic mechanism is the type I hypersensitivity state mediated by IgE. Another immunologic mechanism involves the activation of the complement cascade, which produces anaphylatoxins. These in turn can release histamine. Whether the pathogenesis is allergic or nonallergic, modulating factors affect mast cells and basophils to release mediators capable of producing urticarial lesions. These mediators include histamine, serotonin, kinins, leukotrienes, prostaglandins, acetylcholine, degradation products of fibrin, and anaphylatoxins that increase vascular permeability, producing wheals. Intracellular levels of cAMP have a modulating role in the secretory release of histamine from mast cells and basophils.

### Clinical Findings

**A. Symptoms and Signs:** Itching is the classic presenting symptom but (paradoxically) may be absent in rare cases. Lesions are acute, with pseudopods and intense swelling. The morphology of the lesions may vary over a period of minutes to hours. There may be involvement of the lips, tongue, eyelids, larynx, palms, soles, and genitalia. Papular urticaria resulting from insect bites may persist for long periods and may occasionally be mistaken for lymphoma or leukemia cutis on the basis of histologic findings. A central punctum can usually be seen as with flea or gnat bites. Streaked urticarial lesions may be seen in acute allergic plant dermatitis, eg, poison ivy, oak, or sumac.

In familial angioedema, there is generally a positive family history, and the urticarial lesions may be massive. Death may occur from laryngeal obstruction.

Contact urticaria may be caused by a host of substances varying from chemicals to foods to medications on a nonimmunologic basis, or it may be due to allergy.

**B. Laboratory Findings:** Laboratory studies are

not likely to be helpful in the evaluation of chronic urticaria unless there are suggestive findings in the history and physical examination. Sinus x-rays may be an exception.

### Differential Diagnosis

Distinguish from contact dermatitis and from dermographism, which are different diseases.

### Treatment

**A. Systemic Treatment:** Look for and eliminate the cause if possible. The chief nonallergic causes are drugs, eg, atropine, pilocarpine, morphine, codeine; arthropod bites, eg, insect bites and bee stings (although the latter may cause anaphylaxis as well as angioedema); physical factors such as heat, cold, sunlight, injury, and pressure; and, presumably, neurogenic factors such as tension states and cholinergic urticaria induced by physical exercise, excitement, hot showers, etc.

Allergic causes may include penicillin reactions, inhalants such as feathers and animal danders, ingestion of shellfish or strawberries, injections of sera and vaccines as well as penicillin, external contactants including various chemicals and cosmetics, and infections such as viral hepatitis.

A few patients with chronic urticaria may respond to a salicylate- and tartrazine-free diet. Although salicylates are ubiquitous in nature, drugs and food are the most obvious sources.

Systemic treatment includes antihistamines orally. Hydroxyzine, 10 mg twice daily to 25 mg 3 times daily, may be very useful. Cyproheptadine, 4 mg 4 times daily, may work where hydroxyzine fails and is especially useful for cold urticaria.

Doxepin, a tricyclic antidepressant, 25–50 mg 3 times daily, appears to be effective in some cases of chronic urticaria, whether it be of the simplex, lymphocytic, or vasculitic type. It is given orally.

Enthusiasm for antihistamines has lessened. Clinicians no longer claim 95% symptomatic relief; 35% may be closer to the mark. It may be necessary to give a burst of oral prednisone in a dose of 40 mg daily for 10 days. Terfenadine (Seldane), a new nonsedating antihistamine, has been reported to be effective in chronic idiopathic urticaria. The dosage is 60 mg twice daily. The drug is considerably more expensive than other antihistamines. It use is not recommended during pregnancy and lactation.

For generalized cases, it may be necessary to give a course of oral prednisone in a dose of 40 mg/d for 10 days. Epinephrine 1:1000, a few minims given subcutaneously sequentially, may be useful.

For hereditary angioedema, methyltestosterone buccal tablets, 10 mg once or twice daily, may reduce the episodes. Danazol is effective for hereditary angioedema but is expensive. Stanozolol is a cheaper anabolic agent and is effective. Lyophilized, partially purified C1-inhibitor concentrate, in 5% dextrose, given intravenously in 10–45 minutes, may be lifesaving during an acute attack.

There is a continuing search for effective treatment for chronic idiopathic urticaria. The combined use of $H_1$ and $H_2$ receptor blockers, such as chlorpheniramine and cimetidine or ranitidine, has given inconsistent results. Agents are needed to counteract the kinins, the slow-reacting substance of anaphylaxis leukotrienes, the prostaglandins, the components of complement, and the potent factor that activates platelets.

When urticarial lesions persist indefinitely, biopsy is necessary to rule out vasculitis, and it may be desirable to determine the erythrocyte sedimentation rate, quantitative immunoglobulins, cryoglobulins, cryofibrinogens, antinuclear antibodies, total hemolytic complement, and circulating immune complexes. Hepatitis B is one factor that may cause persisting lesions.

**B. Local Treatment:** Starch baths twice daily or Aveeno baths may be very useful. One cupful of finely refined cornstarch or a packet of Aveeno may be used in a comfortably warm bath. Alternatively, one may use a lotion containing 0.5% camphor, 0.5% menthol, and 0.5% phenol (SARNA) topically or in addition to the bathing.

Solar urticaria is treated by graded exposure to sunlight or with cyproheptadine, 4 mg 4 times daily.

### Prognosis

Acute urticaria usually lasts only a few days. The chronic form may persist for years.

Greene SL, Reed CE, Schroeter AL: Double-blind crossover study comparing doxepin with diphenhydramine for the treatment of chronic urticaria. *J Am Acad Dermatol* 1985;**12:**669.

Monroe EW et al: Vasculitis in chronic urticaria: An immunopathologic study. *J Invest Dermatol* 1981;**76:**103.

Shelley WB: Commentary: Antihistamines and the treatment of urticaria. *Arch Dermatol* 1983;**119:**442.

Winton GB, Lewis CW: Contact urticaria. *Int J Dermatol* 1982;**21:**573.

## INTERTRIGO

Intertrigo is caused by the macerating effect of heat, moisture, and friction. It is especially likely to occur in obese persons and in humid climates. Poor hygiene is an important etiologic factor. There is often a history of seborrheic dermatitis. The symptoms are itching, stinging, and burning. The body folds develop fissures, erythema, and sodden epidermis, with superficial denudation. Urine and blood examination may reveal diabetes mellitus, and the skin examination may reveal candidiasis. A direct smear may show abundant cocci. "Inverse psoriasis," tinea cruris, erythrasma, and candidiasis must be ruled out.

Maintain hygiene in the area and apply talc powder. If there is evidence of colonization of yeasts or bacteria, apply a topical antifungal or antibacterial solution, lotion, or powder. Recurrences are common.

## MILIARIA
## (Heat Rash)

### Essentials of Diagnosis

- Burning, itching, superficial aggregated small vesicles, papules, or pustules on covered areas of the skin.
- Hot, moist climate.
- May have fever and even heat prostration.

### General Considerations

Miliaria is an acute dermatitis that occurs most commonly on the upper extremities, trunk, and intertriginous areas. A hot, moist environment is the most frequent cause, but individual susceptibility is important, and obese persons are most often affected. Bedridden febrile patients are also susceptible. Plugging of the ostia of sweat ducts occurs, with consequent ballooning and ultimate rupture of the sweat duct, producing an irritating, stinging reaction. Increase in numbers of resident aerobes, notably cocci, apparently plays a role.

### Clinical Findings

The usual symptoms are burning and itching. In severe cases, fever, heat prostration, and even death may result. The lesions consist of small, superficial, reddened, thin-walled, discrete but closely aggregated vesicles, papules, vesicopapules, or pustules. The reaction occurs most commonly on covered areas of the skin.

### Differential Diagnosis

Distinguish from similar skin manifestations occurring in drug rash and folliculitis.

### Prevention

Provide favorable working conditions when possible, ie, controlled temperature, ventilation, and humidity. Avoid overbathing and the use of strong, irritating soaps. Graded exposure to sunlight or ultraviolet light may benefit persons who will later be subjected to a hot, moist atmosphere. Susceptible persons should avoid exposure to adverse atmospheric conditions.

### Treatment

Triamcinolone acetonide, 0.1% in SARNA lotion, should be applied 2–4 times daily. Alternative measures that have been employed with varying success are drying shake lotions and antipruritic powders or other dusting powders. Treat secondary infections (superficial pyoderma) with erythromycin or cloxacillin, 1 g daily by mouth. Tannic acid, 10% in 70% alcohol, applied locally twice daily, serves to toughen the skin. Anticholinergic drugs given by mouth may be very helpful in severe cases, eg, glycopyrrolate, 1 mg twice daily.

### Prognosis

Miliaria is usually a mild disorder, but death may

occur with the severe forms (tropical anhidrosis and asthenia) as a result of interference with the heat-regulating mechanism. The process may also be irreversible to some extent, requiring permanent removal of the individual from the humid or hot climate.

## ANOGENITAL PRURITUS

### Essentials of Diagnosis

- Itching, chiefly nocturnal, of the anogenital area.
- There may be no skin reactions, or excoriations and inflammation of any degree may occur up to lichenification.

### General Considerations

Most cases have no obvious cause, but multiple specific causes have been identified. Anogenital pruritus may have the same causes as intertrigo, lichen simplex chronicus, or seborrheic or contact dermatitis (from soaps, colognes, douches, contraceptives) or may be due to irritating secretions, as in diarrhea, leukorrhea, or trichomoniasis, or local disease (candidiasis, dermatophytosis, erythrasma). Diabetes mellitus must be ruled out. Psoriasis or seborrheic dermatitis may be present. Uncleanliness may be at fault. It has been postulated that fecal bacterial endopeptidases play a causative role in pruritus ani.

Up to 10% of gynecologic patients may present with pruritus vulvae. In women, pruritus ani by itself is rare, and pruritus vulvae does not usually involve the anal area, although anal itching will usually spread to the vulva. In men, pruritus of the scrotum is less common than pruritus ani. When all possible known causes have been ruled out, the condition is diagnosed as idiopathic or essential pruritus—by no means rare.

Proctosigmoidoscopic examination is seldom helpful. Oxyuriasis (pinworm) is almost nonexistent in adults. Psychoneurosis is not a common cause. Lichen sclerosus et atrophicus may at times be the cause, but gross pathologic changes are evident in this disorder. Erythrasma is easily diagnosed by demonstration of coral-red fluorescence with Wood's light; it is easily cured with erythromycin, orally and topically.

### Clinical Findings

**A. Symptoms and Signs:** The only symptom is itching, which is chiefly nocturnal. Physical findings are usually not present, but there may be erythema, fissuring, maceration, lichenification, excoriations, or changes suggestive of candidiasis or tinea.

**B. Laboratory Findings:** Urinalysis and blood glucose determination may lead to a diagnosis of diabetes mellitus. Microscopic examination or culture of tissue scrapings may reveal yeasts, fungi, or parasites. Stool examination may show intestinal parasites.

### Differential Diagnosis

The etiologic differential diagnosis consists of *Candida* infection, parasitosis, local irritation from contact with drugs and irritants, and other primary skin disorders of the genital area such as psoriasis, seborrhea, intertrigo, or lichen sclerosus et atrophicus.

### Prevention
Treat all possible systemic or local causes. Instruct the patient in proper anogenital hygiene.

### Treatment
### (See also Pruritus)
**A. General Measures:** Avoid "hot" (spicy) foods, and drugs that can irritate the anal mucosa. Treat constipation if present. Instruct the patient to use very soft or moistened tissue or cotton after a bowel movement and to clean the perianal area thoroughly. Women should use similar precautions after urinating. Anal douching is the best cleansing method for all types of pruritus ani. Instruct the patient regarding the harmful and pruritus-inducing effects of scratching.

**B. Local Measures:** Hydrocortisone or iodochlorhydroxyquin-hydrocortisone creams are quite useful. Potent fluorinated topical corticosteroids may lead to atrophy and striae. Sitz baths twice daily using silver nitrate, 1:10,000–1:200; potassium permanganate, 1:10,000; or aluminum subacetate solution, 1:20, are of value if the area is acutely inflamed and oozing. Underclothing should be changed daily. Paint affected areas with Castellani's solution. Balneol Perianal Cleansing Lotion or Tucks premoistened pads, ointment, or cream (all Tucks preparations contain witch hazel) may be very useful for pruritus ani.

### Prognosis
Although usually benign, anogenital pruritus may be persistent and recurrent.

Jillson OF: Pruritus ani: Disputing the passage. *Cutis* 1984;**33**:537.

## CALLOSITIES & CORNS
## (OF FEET OR TOES)

Callosities and corns are caused by pressure and friction due to faulty weight-bearing, orthopedic deformities, improperly fitting shoes, or neuropathies such as occur in diabetes mellitus. Some persons are hereditarily predisposed to excessive and abnormal callus formation. It is crucial to provide optimal foot care for diabetics and those with insensitive extremities.

Tenderness on pressure and "after-pain" are the only symptoms. The hyperkeratotic well-localized overgrowths always occur at pressure points. On paring, a glassy core is found (which differentiates these disorders from plantar warts, which have multiple capillary bleeding points when cut). A soft corn often occurs laterally on the proximal portion of the fourth toe as a result of pressure against the bony structure of the interphalangeal joint of the fifth toe.

Treatment consists of correcting mechanical abnormalities that cause friction and pressure. Shoes must be properly fitted and orthopedic deformities corrected. Callosities may be removed by careful paring of the callus after a warm water soak or with keratolytic agents, eg, Keralyt gel, which contains 6% salicylic acid. Apply locally to the callus every night and cover with a polyethylene plastic film (Saran Wrap); remove in the morning. Repeat until the corn or callus is removed.

Extensive and severe palmar and plantar hyperkeratosis can be treated successfully by applying equal parts of propylene glycol and water nightly and covering with thin polyethylene plastic film (Baggies), or by soaking in 3% acetic acid solution.

A metatarsal leather bar, 1.25 cm (½ inch) wide and 0.65 cm (¼ inch) high, may be placed on the outside of the shoe just behind the weight-bearing surface of the sole.

Women who tend to form calluses and corns should not wear confining footgear and high-heeled shoes.

Gibbs RC, Boxer MC: Abnormal biomechanics of feet and their cause of hyperkeratoses. *J Am Acad Dermatol* 1982;**6**:1061.

## CHRONIC DISCOID
## LUPUS ERYTHEMATOSUS

### Essentials of Diagnosis
- Red, asymptomatic, localized plaques, usually on the face, often in butterfly distribution.
- Scaling, follicular plugging, atrophy, and telangiectasia of involved areas.
- Histology distinctive.

### General Considerations
Lupus erythematosus is a superficial, localized discoid inflammation of the skin occurring most frequently in areas exposed to solar or ultraviolet irradiation. The cause is not known. The disseminated type is discussed in Chapter 14.

### Clinical Findings
**A. Symptoms and Signs:** There are usually no symptoms. The lesions consist of dusky red, well-localized, single or multiple plaques, 5–20 mm in diameter, usually on the face and often in a "butterfly pattern" over the nose and cheeks. The scalp, external ears, and oral mucous membranes may be involved. There is atrophy, telangiectasia, and follicular plugging. The lesion is usually covered by dry, horny, adherent scales.

Where indicated, a complete medical study should be made to rule out systemic lupus erythematosus.

**B. Laboratory Findings:** There are usually no significant routine laboratory findings in the chronic discoid type. If there is leukopenia or proteinuria, with or without casts, one must suspect the disseminated or systemic form of the disease. Histologic changes are distinctive. The antinuclear antibody test is perhaps best for ruling out systemic lupus erythematosus. A direct immunofluorescence microscopy test reveals basement membrane antibody. "Uninvolved" skin adjacent to a lesion tends to be negative to direct immunofluorescence testing in discoid lupus erythematosus but positive in the systemic form of the disease.

One may also obtain a complete blood count, sedimentation rate, urinalysis, and anti-DNA, CH50, and C3 tests.

In patients with marked photosensitivity and negative antinuclear antibody tests, tests of other cellular—and organ—tissues may be required.

### Differential Diagnosis

The scales are dry and "tacklike" and can thus be distinguished from those of seborrheic dermatitis and psoriasis. Differentiate also from the morphea type of basal cell epithelioma and, by absence of nodules and ulceration, from lupus vulgaris.

### Complications

Dissemination may occur. There may be scarring.

### Treatment

**A. General Measures:** Provide protection from sunlight and all other powerful radiation. *Caution:* Do not use any form of radiation therapy. Avoid using drugs that are potentially photosensitizing.

**B. Medical Treatment:** (For discoid type only.) *Caution:* The following drugs may cause serious eye changes. If the medication is continued, ophthalmologic examination should be done every 3 months. Chloroquine, 250 mg/d, or hydroxychloroquine, no more than 400 mg/d, is unlikely to cause retinopathy or other eye damage. Wherever possible, chronic discoid lupus erythematosus should be considered a cosmetic defect only and treated topically or with camouflaging agents.

1. Chloroquine phosphate, 0.25 g daily for 1 week, then 0.25 g twice weekly. Watch for signs of toxicity.

2. Hydroxychloroquine sulfate, 0.2 g orally daily and then twice weekly, may occasionally be effective when chloroquine is not tolerated.

3. Quinacrine (Atabrine), 100 mg daily, may be the safest of the antimalarials, since eye damage has not been reported. It colors the skin yellow.

**C. Local Infiltration:** Triamcinolone acetonide suspension, 2.5 mg/mL, may be injected into the lesions once a week or once a month. This should be tried before internal treatment (see above).

**D. Corticosteroids:** Corticosteroid creams applied each night and covered with airtight, thin, pliable plastic film may be useful. Clobetasol propionate (Tenovate) cream or ointment applied twice daily without occlusion should be attempted before systemic therapy.

**E. Dapsone:** Dapsone, 50 mg/d orally, may be helpful.

**F. Isotretinoin:** In a limited open study, isotretinoin, 80 mg/d, was effective in returning the skin and laboratory findings to normal in chronic or subacute cutaneous lupus erythematosus. Because of teratogenicity, the drug cannot be used if there is any possibility of pregnancy.

### Prognosis

The disease is persistent but not life-endangering, unless it turns into the disseminated variety.

McCormack LS, Elgart ML, Turner MLC: Annular subacute cutaneous lupus erythematosus responsive to dapsone. *J Am Acad Dermatol* 1984;**11**:397.

Newton RC et al: Mechanism-oriented assessment of isotretinoin in chronic or subacute cutaneous lupus erythematosus. *Arch Dermatol* 1986;**122**:170.

Olansky AJ: Antimalarials and ophthalmologic safety. *J Am Acad Dermatol* 1982;**6**:19.

# VIRAL INFECTIONS OF THE SKIN

## HERPES SIMPLEX (Cold or Fever Sore)

### Essentials of Diagnosis

- Recurrent small grouped vesicles on an erythematous base, especially around oral and genital areas.
- May follow minor infections, trauma, stress, or sun exposure.
- Regional lymph nodes may be swollen and tender.
- Tzanck smear is positive for large multinucleated epithelial giant cells surrounded by acantholytic balloon cells.

### General Considerations

Although approximately 90% of the population acquire herpes simplex infection before the age of 4 or 5 years based on antibody studies, it is generally type 1 infection, following which the virus may remain in some form in the regional ganglia for life. No present means of treatment can eliminate the hidden foci of infection. The disease may manifest itself as severe gingiovostomatitis in small children, or the initial infection may be subclinical. Thereafter, the subject may have recurrent attacks, provoked by fever, a cold, fatigue, menstruation, and other triggering factors such as sun and wind. *Herpes simplex virus type 1 and the AIDS virus are the most important causes of fatal sporadic encephalitis in the USA.*

The incidence of genital herpes in the USA in patients treated in private clinics increased about 10-fold from 1966 to 1981.

In addition to mucocutaneous lesions, the virus may cause encephalitis, with a high morbidity and fatality rate, ophthalmitis, and a virulent infection in neonates.

Herpes simplex virus antibodies are found in 85% of young adults in lower economic classes.

## Clinical Findings

The principal symptoms are burning and stinging. Neuralgia may precede and accompany attacks. The lesions consist of small, grouped vesicles which can occur anywhere but which most often occur on the lips, mouth, and genitals. Regional lymph nodes may be swollen and tender.

## Differential Diagnosis

Lesions clinically diagnosed as chancroid, syphilis, pyoderma, or trauma have been found to be herpes simplex virus infections on culture. Viral culture, although not completely sensitive, is most helpful in confirming the clinical diagnosis and for showing viral shedding in asymptomatic patients. Other methods rely on detection of viral particles by electron microscopy, detection of viral antigen by immunologic methods (immunoperoxidase or immunofluorescence), or demonstration of multinucleated cells or intranuclear inclusion cells. The latter (Tzanck test) is the least sensitive but is readily available and easy to perform.

## Complications

Complications include pyoderma, eczema herpeticum, whitlow, esophagitis, transplacental fetal infection, keratitis, and a severe encephalitis.

## Treatment

For persistent or severe, recurrent herpes:

**A. General Measures:** Eliminate precipitating agents when possible.

Acyclovir is effective systemically (intravenously, subcutaneously, intramuscularly, or orally) and is practically nontoxic, but experience remains relatively limited. With first episodes of primary genital herpes simplex, the period of viral shedding, pain, crusting, and other symptoms can be shortened and healing can be hastened by giving acyclovir, 200 mg orally 5 times daily—or 800 mg twice daily—for 10 days. Acyclovir is effective in preventing subsequent genital recurrences if suppressive dosages of 200 mg 3 times daily are maintained. If recurrences are infrequent (every 3–6 months), episodic treatment employing 200 mg orally 5 times daily or 800 mg twice daily is effective if initiated at the first sign or symptom of recurrence. Long-term acyclovir therapy appears to be effective and safe. Intravenous acyclovir is nephrotoxic and is reserved for patients with severe and life-threatening infections.

Recurrences and symptoms may be reduced by giving L-lysine by mouth for several months. Two grams daily are needed.

**B. Local Measures:** Apply a moistened styptic pencil several times daily to abort lesions. Zinc sulfate solution, 0.025–0.05%, may be used as a warm com-press, 10 minutes twice daily. Or one may apply epinephrine, 1:100 solution, frequently. Applied topically, toluidine blue has an anesthetic effect and appears to hasten drying of vesicles.

If there is associated cellulitis and lymphadenitis, apply cool compresses. Treat stomatitis with water and milk of magnesia mouthwashes.

There is no really safe and effective systemic approach to cure recurrent herpes simplex infections of the skin. It is strongly urged that topical use of 5% acyclovir ointment (Zovirax) be limited to the restricted indications for which it has been approved, namely, initial herpes genitalis and mucocutaneous herpes simplex infections in immunocompromised patients, because of promotion of resistant strains of the virus and the mild mutagenicity of the drug.

## Prognosis

Aside from the dread complications described above, recurrent attacks last 1–2 weeks. A retrospective study indicated that 50% of those with genital herpes were found to be essentially free of frequently recurring episodes 7 years after onset.

Becker TM, Blount JH, Guinan ME: Genital herpes infections in private practice in the United States, 1966 to 1981. *JAMA* 1985;**253**:1601.

Bierman SM: A retrospective study of 375 patients with genital herpes simplex infections seen between 1973 and 1980. *Cutis* 1983;**31**:548.

Friedman-Kien AE: Herpes zoster: A possible early clinical sign for development of acquired immunodeficiency syndrome in high-risk individuals. *J Am Acad Dermatol* 1986;**14**:1023.

Guinan ME: Oral acyclovir for treatment and suppression of genital herpes simplex virus infection: A review. *JAMA* 1986;**255**:1747.

## HERPES ZOSTER
## (Shingles)

## Essentials of Diagnosis

- Pain along course of a nerve followed by painful grouped vesicular lesions.
- Involvement is unilateral. Lesions are usually on face and trunk.
- Swelling of regional lymph nodes (inconstant).
- Tzanck smear is positive.

## General Considerations

Herpes zoster is an acute vesicular eruption due to a virus that is morphologically identical with the virus of varicella. It usually occurs in adults. With rare exceptions, one attack of zoster confers lifelong immunity. Persons in anergic states (Hodgkin's disease, lymphomas, or those taking immunosuppressive drugs) are at greater risk, and generalized, life-threatening dissemination (varicella) may occur.

Zoster is the response to the varicella-zoster virus of a partially immune person. In patients at risk for AIDS, development of zoster may be one sign that precedes marked depression of cellular immunity associated with AIDS or ARC.

## Clinical Findings

Pain usually precedes the eruption by 48 hours or more and may persist and actually increase in intensity after the lesions have disappeared. The lesions consist of grouped, tense, deep-seated vesicles distributed unilaterally along the neural pathways of the trunk. The commonest distributions are on the trunk or face. Regional lymph glands may be tender and swollen.

It used to be felt that herpes zoster appearing in an older adult was a sign of occult malignant neoplastic disease. This suspicion has not been verified by controlled studies.

## Differential Diagnosis

Since poison oak and poison ivy dermatitis may be produced unilaterally and in a streak by a single brush with the plant, it must be differentiated at times from herpes zoster. Differentiate also from similar lesions of herpes simplex, which is usually less painful.

## Complications

Persistent neuralgia, anesthesia of the affected area following healing, facial or other nerve paralysis, and encephalitis may occur.

## Treatment

**A. General Measures:** Sedatives may be required to control tension and nervousness associated with neuralgia. Aspirin with or without codeine phosphate, 30 mg, usually controls pain. A single intragluteal injection of 40 mg of triamcinolone acetonide suspension may give prompt relief. Prednisone, 60 mg orally for 10 days, may be the treatment of choice. Steroid therapy may decrease the incidence of postherpetic neuralgia. Ophthalmologic consultation should be considered for supraorbital involvement to avoid serious ocular complications. Hospitalization may be necessary in serious cases. Zoster has developed despite normal varicella-zoster antibody levels, indicating that cell-mediated immunity is more important in preventing zoster than are circulating antibodies. (See Chapters 21, 22, and 28.)

The supply of varicella-zoster immune globulin is limited, and its use is restricted to susceptible children under 15 years of age who have underlying immunosuppression or immunodeficiency diseases and have had intimate exposure to chickenpox; the globulin must be given within 72 hours after exposure. It is not effective in established zoster. Zoster immune plasma is ineffective in established zoster.

The goal of herpes zoster therapy for immunocompromised patients is prevention of possibly life-threatening viral spread. Both intravenous acyclovir and vidarabine will prevent progression in this patient population. The advantages of using intravenous acyclovir for herpes zoster, especially in the immuno-

compromised patient, probably outweigh the disadvantages. Adverse effects include decreased renal function from crystallization, and nausea, vomiting, and abdominal pain. One may give acyclovir sodium, 7.5 mg/kg of ideal body weight, 3 times daily for 7 days. Acyclovir has not been shown to prevent postherpetic neuralgia.

**B. Local Measures:** Calamine or starch shake lotions are often of value. Apply lotion liberally and cover with a layer of cotton. Do not use greases.

**C. Postzoster Neuralgia:** Infiltration of skin with triamcinolone acetonide and lidocaine has been disappointing. High doses of systemic corticosteroids and oral acyclovir, 400–800 mg 5 times daily, early in the disease may reduce the incidence of post-herpetic neuralgia. Vitamin E (d-alpha tocopheryl acetate), 800 units daily, should be tried. Chronic postherpetic neuralgia is usually not relieved by regional blocks (stellate ganglion, epidural, local infiltration, or peripheral nerve) with bupivacaine hydrochloride, with or without corticosteroids added to the injections. Severe initial pain—or age over 60 years—tends to increase the likelihood of postherpetic neuralgia. Amitriptyline, 25 mg orally 3 times daily, and perphenazine, 4 mg orally 3 times daily, or fluphenazine, 1 mg 4 times daily, has also been suggested. Doxepin, 25–50 mg 3 times daily, has also been reported to be helpful. Somnolence may occur with either type of drug.

## Prognosis

The eruption persists 2–3 weeks and does not recur. Motor involvement may lead to temporary palsy. No age group is exempt from the possibility of postzoster neuralgia persisting for a year or more, but the likelihood is greater in the 60- to 69-year age group (20%) and in those over 70 (30%). Ocular involvement may lead to blindness.

Balfour HH Jr: Acyclovir therapy for herpes zoster: Advantages and adverse effects. *JAMA* 1986;**255**:387.

Keczkes K, Basheer AM: Do corticosteroids prevent post-herpetic neuralgia? *Br J Dermatol* 1980;**102**:551.

Liesegang TJ: The varicella-zoster virus: Systemic and ocular features. *J Am Acad Dermatol* 1984;**11**:165.

Riopelle JM, Naraghi M, Grush KP: Chronic neuralgia incidence following local anesthetic therapy for herpes zoster. *Arch Dermatol* 1984;**120**:747.

## WARTS

### Essentials of Diagnosis

- Warty elevation anywhere on skin or mucous membranes, usually no larger than 0.5 cm in diameter.
- Prolonged incubation period (average 2–18 months).
- Spontaneous ''cures'' are frequent (50%), but warts are often unresponsive to any form of treatment.
- ''Recurrences'' (new lesions) are frequent.

## General Considerations

Nearly a million visits to physicians for warts took place in 1981, nearly triple the incidence for genital herpes. Over 30 different subtypes of human papilloma viruses have been identified by serologic typing of viral proteins, molecular hybridization of viral DNA, and monoclonal antibody assays, using immunoperoxidase staining. About 25% of abnormal Papanicolaou smears are associated with the presence of human papilloma viruses, and 80% of cases of carcinoma of the cervix have similar associations, indicating that wart viruses may be more important than herpes simplex virus.

Six human papilloma virus types are associated with malignant neoplasms: types 5, 8, and 14 with squamous cell carcinomas occurring in the rare **epidermodysplasia verruciformis;** and types 6, 16, and 18 with uterine cervical carcinomas. Type 6 has also been implicated in giant condylomas of Buschke-Löwenstein and type 16 with bowenoid papulosis.

Cervical warts may be transmitted to the newborn via passage through the infected birth canal. Colposcopy with application of 3% acetic acid to suspicious lesions on the cervix may detect premalignant flat warts. A number of children with laryngeal papillomas (types 11 and 6) treated with x-rays have developed squamous cell carcinoma of the larynx.

## Clinical Findings

There are usually no symptoms. Tenderness on pressure occurs with plantar warts; itching occurs with anogenital warts. Occasionally a wart will produce mechanical obstruction (eg, nostril, ear canal).

Warts vary widely in shape, size, and appearance. Flat warts are most evident under oblique illumination. Subungual warts may be dry, fissured, and hyperkeratotic and may resemble hangnails or other nonspecific changes. Plantar warts resemble plantar corns or calluses.

## Prevention

Avoid contact with warts. A person with flat warts should be admonished not to scratch the areas. Using an electric shaver will in occasional cases prevent the spread of warts in razor scratches. Anogenital warts may be transmitted sexually.

## Treatment

**A. Removal:** Remove the warts whenever possible by one of the following means:

**1. Surgical excision–**Inject a small amount of local anesthetic into the base and then remove the wart with a dermal curet or scissors or by shaving off at the base of the wart with a scalpel. Trichloroacetic acid or Monsel's solution on a tightly wound cotton-tipped applicator may be painted on the wound, or electrocautery may be applied.

**2. Liquid nitrogen** applied for a few seconds may be used every 2 weeks for a period of 3 months if necessary.

**3. Keratolytic agents–**Either of the following may be used:

| ℞ | Salicylic acid | 2.5 |
|---|---|---|
| | Lactic acid | 2.5 |
| | Flexible collodion, qs ad | 15.0 |
| | (Duofilm, Verukan-20, Viranol) | |

Sig: Paint on warts each night with glass rod.

| ℞ | Salicylic acid | 3.6 |
|---|---|---|
| | Alcohol, 40% qs ad | 120.0 |

Sig: Paint on *flat* warts with cotton swab daily.

**4. Anogenital warts** are best treated by painting them weekly with 25% podophyllum resin in compound tincture of benzoin if they are moist and occluded by apposing skin surfaces. Dry genital warts are best treated with applications of liquid nitrogen. Intralesional recombinant interferon alfa-2a is more effective than placebo in clearing a single condyloma, but plantar warts do not respond.

**5. Plantar warts** may be treated by applying a 40% salicylic acid plaster after paring. The plaster may be left on for 5–6 days, then removed, pared down, and reapplied. Although with this method it may take weeks to months to eradicate the wart, it is safe and effective with almost no side effects.

Application of cantharidin (Cantharone) is also effective in managing plantar warts. It is applied to the wart after it is pared, allowed to dry, and covered by tape. The area may be sensitive or slightly painful for 2 or 3 days. It should be debrided in 10–14 days and the treatment repeated.

Bleomycin diluted to 0.1% with physiologic saline may be injected under warts, not exceeding 0.1 mL per puncture; with multiple punctures, it has been shown to have a high cure rate for plantar and common warts. It may cause loss of nails and symptoms similar to those of Raynaud's syndrome when used for periungual warts.

**B. Immunotherapy:** Dinitrochlorobenzene (DNCB) is useful for resistant warts. Initially, 400 μg of freshly prepared dinitrochlorobenzene is applied as a sensitizing dose to 2 or 3 sites on the forearm. Then the warts are painted with an Eppendorf pipette with precisely 20 μL of dinitrochlorobenzene at 2-week intervals until they recede. DNCB gives positive results with the Ames test.

Persistent conservative application of topical irritants may cure warts by nonspecific boosting of wart antibodies. Specific wart antibodies (especially IgG) have been found in the serum of individuals with regressing warts.

**C. Laser Therapy:** The carbon dioxide laser is particularly effective for treating recurrent warts, plantar warts, and condylomata acuminata. The wart tissue is vaporized under magnified vision in a bloodless procedure without damage to surrounding areas.

**D. Retinoids:** Extensive warts have been reported to disappear when etretinate was given by mouth for a month. This drug is now available for use in the USA. Oral isotretinoin may cure some warts (see Acne Vulgaris).

## Prognosis

There is a striking tendency to the development of new lesions. Warts may disappear spontaneously or may be unresponsive to treatment.

Bailin PL: Lasers in dermatology: 1983. (Editorial.) *Cleve Clin Q* 1983;**50**:53.

Bender ME: Papillomavirus infection of the urogenital tract: Implications for the dermatologist. *Curr Concepts Skin Disorders* (Spring) 1985;**6**:16.

Donagin WG, Millikan LE: Dinitrochlorobenzene immunotherapy for verrucae resistant to standard treatment modalities. *J Am Acad Dermatol* 1982;**6**:40.

Jablonska S, Orth G (editors): Warts/human papilloma viruses. *Clin Dermatol* 1985;**3**:No. 4. [Entire issue.]

Mackie RM: Extensive warts treated with etretinate. *Br J Dermatol* 1982;**107(Suppl 22)**:97.

Rees RB: The treatment of warts. *Clin Dermatol* 1985;**3**:179.

Vance JC et al: Intralesional recombinant alpha-2 interferon for the treatment of patients with condyloma acuminatum or verruca plantaris. *Arch Dermatol* 1986;**122**:272.

# BACTERIAL INFECTIONS OF THE SKIN

## IMPETIGO

Impetigo is a contagious and autoinoculable infection of the skin caused by staphylococci or streptococci or both. The infected material may be transmitted to the skin by dirty fingernails. In children, the source of infection is often another infected child.

Itching is the only symptom. The lesions consist of macules, vesicles, bullae, pustules, and honey-colored gummy crusts (streptococcal) that when removed leave denuded red areas. The face and other exposed parts are most often involved.

Ecthyma is a deeper form of impetigo caused by streptococci, with ulceration and scarring. It occurs frequently on the legs and other covered areas, often as a complication of debility and infestations.

Impetigo neonatorum is a highly contagious, potentially serious form of staphylococcal impetigo occurring in infants. It requires prompt systemic treatment and protection of other infants (isolation, exclusion from the nursery of personnel with pyoderma, etc). The lesions are bullous and massive and accompanied by systemic toxicity. Death may occur.

Impetigo must be distinguished from other vesicular and pustular lesions such as herpes simplex, varicella, and contact dermatitis (dermatitis venenata). A Gram stain and a Tzanck smear may be useful in differentiating the organisms.

Treatment is as for folliculitis. Some question has

been raised about the efficacy of topical antibiotics. If there is fever or toxicity or any concern over the possibility of a nephritogenic strain of *Streptococcus* being causative, systemic antibiotics may be given. Either erythromycin or dicloxacillin, 1 g daily, is usually effective, or one may use cephalexin, 50 mg/kg/24 h. For ping-ponging furunculosis in the family setting or in a live-in group of people, a course of vancomycin may be necessary.

Feingold DS, Wagner RF Jr: Antibacterial therapy. *J Am Acad Dermatol* 1986;**14**:535.

## FOLLICULITIS
## (Including Sycosis Vulgaris or Barber's Itch; Pseudofolliculitis)

### Essentials of Diagnosis
- Itching and burning in hairy areas.
- Pustules in the hair follicles.
- In sycosis, inflammation of surrounding skin area.

### General Considerations

Folliculitis is caused by staphylococcal infection of a hair follicle. When the lesion is deep-seated, chronic, and recalcitrant, it is called sycosis. Sycosis is usually propagated by the autoinoculation and trauma of shaving. The upper lip is particularly susceptible to involvement in men who suffer with chronic nasal discharge from sinusitis or hay fever.

Bockhart's impetigo is a staphylococcal infection that produces painful, tense, globular pustules at the follicular orifices. It is a form of folliculitis.

Gram-negative folliculitis, which may develop from antibiotic-treated acne, may be best treated with isotretinoin given orally, although this is not a listed indication for the drug. A range of gram-negative organisms has been implicated as the cause. An absolute contraindication to use of isotretinoin is pregnancy.

Pseudofolliculitis is caused by ingrowing hairs in the beard area and on the nape. It may be treated by growing a beard or by using the PFB shaving system, American Safety Razor Co., Staunton, VA 24401.

### Clinical Findings

The symptoms are slight burning and itching, and pain on manipulation of the hair. The lesions consist of pustules of the hair follicles. In sycosis, the surrounding skin becomes involved also and so resembles eczema, with redness and crusting.

### Differential Diagnosis

Differentiate from acne vulgaris or pustular miliaria and infections of the skin such as impetigo or fungal infections.

### Complications

Abscess formation.

## Prevention

Correct any precipitating or aggravating factors: systemic (eg, diabetes mellitus) or local causes (eg, irritations of a mechanical or chemical nature, discharges).

## Treatment

**A. Specific Measures:** Systemic anti-infectives may be tried if the skin infection is resistant to local treatment; if it is extensive or severe and accompanied by a febrile reaction; if it is complicated; or if it involves the so-called danger areas (upper lip, nose, and eyes).

Local anti-infective agents should be tried in sequence until a favorable response is obtained (allowing 3–4 days for evaluation in each case). These include polymyxin B in combination with bacitracin or oxytetracycline. They should be applied initially at night and protected by dressings; soaks should be applied during the day. After the area has cleared, any of the following preparations may be applied 2–4 times daily: (1) Iodochlorhydroxyquin, 3% in cream or ointment form, locally twice daily. (2) Antibiotics, alone or in combination, as ointments locally 2–4 times daily.

Penicillin and sulfonamides should not be used topically.

**B. Local Measures:** Cleanse the area gently with a weak soap solution and apply saline or aluminum subacetate soaks or compresses to the involved area for 15 minutes twice daily. When skin is softened, gently open the larger pustules and trim away necrotic tissue.

Anhydrous ethyl alcohol containing 6.25% aluminum chloride (Xerac AC), applied to lesions and environs and followed by an antibiotic ointment (see above), may be very helpful. It is especially useful for chronic folliculitis of the buttocks.

## Prognosis

Folliculitis is often stubborn and persistent, lasting for months and even years.

James WD, Leyden JJ: Treatment of gram-negative folliculitis with isotretinoin: Positive clinical and microbiologic response. *J Am Acad Dermatol* 1985;**12**:319.

## FURUNCULOSIS (BOILS) & CARBUNCLES

## Essentials of Diagnosis

- Extremely painful inflammatory swelling of a hair follicle that forms an abscess.
- Primary predisposing debilitating disease sometimes present.
- Coagulase-positive *Staphylococcus aureus* is the causative organism.

## General Considerations

A furuncle (boil) is a deep-seated infection (abscess) involving the entire hair follicle and adjacent subcutaneous tissue. The most common sites of occurrence are the hairy parts exposed to irritation and friction, pressure, or moisture or to the plugging action of petroleum products. Because the lesions are autoinoculable, they are often multiple. Thorough investigation usually fails to uncover a predisposing cause, although an occasional patient may have uncontrolled diabetes mellitus, nephritis, or other debilitating disease. Groups may be subject to epidemics.

A carbuncle is several furuncles developing in adjoining hair follicles and coalescing to form a conglomerate, deeply situated mass with multiple drainage points.

## Clinical Findings

**A. Symptoms and Signs:** The extreme tenderness and pain are due to pressure on nerve endings, particularly in areas where there is little room for swelling of underlying structures. The pain, fever, and malaise are more severe with carbuncles than with furuncles. The follicular abscess is either rounded or conical. It gradually enlarges, becomes fluctuant, and then softens and opens spontaneously after a few days to 1–2 weeks to discharge a core of necrotic tissue and pus. The inflammation occasionally subsides before necrosis occurs.

Infection of the soft tissue around the nails (paronychia) is usually due to staphylococci when it is acute. This is a variant of furuncle. Other organisms may be involved.

**B. Laboratory Findings:** There may be slight leukocytosis.

## Differential Diagnosis

Differentiate from deep mycotic infections such as sporotrichosis and blastomycosis; from other bacterial infections such as anthrax and tularemia; and from acne cysts and infected epidermoid or pilar cysts.

## Complications

Serious and sometimes fatal cerebral thrombophlebitis may occur as a complication of a manipulated furuncle on the central portion of the upper lip or near the nasolabial folds. Perinephric abscess, osteomyelitis, and other hematogenous staphylococcal infections may also occur.

## Treatment

**A. Specific Measures:** Systemic anti-infective agents are indicated (chosen on the basis of cultures and sensitivity tests if possible). Sodium cloxacillin or erythromycin, 1 g daily in divided doses by mouth for 10 days, is usually effective. Cephalexin is an effective alternative drug. Minocycline may be effective against strains of staphylococci resistant to other antibiotics.

Recurrent furunculosis may be effectively treated with a combination of dicloxacillin, 250–500 mg 4 times daily, and rifampin, 300 mg twice daily. Family members and intimate contacts may need evaluation for staphylococcal carrier state and perhaps concomitant treatment.

Strains of pathogenic staphylococci may carry a plasmid, or episome, causing resistance to antibiotics such as erythromycin.

**B. Local Measures:** Immobilize the part and avoid overmanipulation of inflamed areas. Use moist heat to help larger lesions "localize." Use surgical incision and debridement *after* the lesions are "mature." Do not incise deeply. Apply anti-infective ointment and bandage the area loosely during drainage. It is not necessary to incise and drain an acute staphylococcal paronychia. Inserting a flat metal spatula or sharpened hardwood stick into the nail fold where it adjoins the nail will release pus from a mature lesion.

### Prognosis

Recurrent crops may harass the patient for months or years. Carbunculosis is more severe and more hazardous than furunculosis.

An alcoholic aluminum chloride solution (see above) may be very useful in controlling repeated attacks of furuncles.

Gorbach SL (guest editor): Antibacterial therapy update: 1985: Skin and soft tissue infections. *Cutis* 1985;**36:**No. 5A:1. [Special issue.]

## ERYSIPELAS

### Essentials of Diagnosis

- Edematous, spreading, circumscribed, hot, erythematous area, with or without vesicle or bulla formation.
- Pain, malaise, chills and fever.
- Leukocytosis, increased sedimentation rate.

### General Considerations

Erysipelas is an acute inflammation of the skin and subcutaneous tissue caused by infection with beta-hemolytic streptococci. It occurs classically on the cheek.

### Clinical Findings

**A. Symptoms and Signs:** The symptoms are pain, malaise, chills, and moderate fever. A bright red spot appears first, very often near a fissure at the angle of the nose. This spreads to form a tense, sharply demarcated, glistening, smooth, hot area. The margin characteristically makes noticeable advances from day to day. The patch is somewhat edematous and can be pitted slightly with the finger. Vesicles or bullae occasionally develop on the surface. The patch does not usually become pustular or gangrenous and heals without scar formation. The disease may complicate any break in the skin that provides a portal of entry for the organism.

**B. Laboratory Findings:** Leukocytosis and increased sedimentation rate almost invariably occur.

### Differential Diagnosis

Distinguish from cellulitis, with its less definite margin and involvement of deeper tissues; and from erysipeloid, a benign bacillary infection producing redness of the skin of the fingers or the backs of the hands in fishermen and meat handlers.

### Complications

Unless erysipelas is promptly treated, death may result from extension of the process and systemic toxicity, particularly in the very young and in the aged.

### Treatment

Place the patient at bed rest with the head of the bed elevated, apply hot packs, and give aspirin for pain and fever. Penicillin is specific for beta-hemolytic streptococcal infections. Erythromycin is a good alternative.

### Prognosis

Erysipelas formerly was very dangerous to life, particularly in the very young and in the aged. It can now usually be quickly controlled with systemic penicillin or erythromycin therapy. Prompt and adequate treatment usually will limit it to one attack.

## CELLULITIS

Cellulitis, a diffuse spreading infection of the skin, must be differentiated from erysipelas (a superficial form of cellulitis) because the 2 conditions are quite similar. Cellulitis involves deeper tissues and may be due to one of several organisms, usually cocci. The lesion is hot and red but has a more diffuse border than does erysipelas. Cellulitis usually occurs after a break in the skin. Recurrent attacks may sometimes affect lymphatic vessels, producing a permanent swelling called "solid edema."

The response to systemic anti-infective measures (penicillin or broad-spectrum antibiotics) is usually prompt and satisfactory.

## ERYSIPELOID

*Erysipelothrix insidiosa* infection must be differentiated from erysipelas and cellulitis. It is usually a benign infection commonly seen in fishermen and meat handlers and characterized by purplish erythema of the skin, most often of a finger or the back of the hand, which gradually extends over a period of several days. Systemic involvement occurs rarely and is manifested by reversal of the albumin/globulin ratio and other serious changes. Endocarditis may occur.

Penicillin is usually promptly curative. Broad-spectrum antibiotics may be used instead.

## DECUBITUS ULCERS
### (Bedsores, Pressure Sores)

Bedsores (pressure sores) are a special type of ulcer caused by impaired blood supply and tissue nutrition due to prolonged pressure over bony or cartilaginous prominences. The skin overlying the sacrum and hips is most commonly involved, but bedsores may also be seen over the occiput, ears, elbows, heels, and ankles. They occur most readily in aged, paralyzed, debilitated, and unconscious patients. Low-grade infection may occur.

Good nursing care and nutrition and maintenance of skin hygiene are important preventive measures. The skin and the bed linens should be kept clean and dry. Bedfast, paralyzed, moribund, or listless patients who are candidates for the development of decubiti must be turned *frequently* (at least every hour) and must be examined at pressure points for the appearance of small areas of redness and tenderness. Water-filled mattresses, rubber pillows, alternating pressure mattresses, and thick papillated foam pads are useful in prevention and in the treatment of early lesions.

Early lesions should also be treated with topical antibiotic powders and adhesive absorbent bandage (Gelfoam). Established lesions require surgical consultation and care. A spongy foam pad placed under the patient may work best in some cases. It may be laundered often. A continuous dressing of 1% iodochlorhydroxyquin (Vioform) in Lassar's paste may be effective.

Deep infections are usually present in pressure sores, often requiring systemic antibiotics.

Parish LC, Witkowski JA, Crissey JT: *The Decubitus Ulcer.* Masson, 1983.
Sugarman B: Infection and pressure sores. *Arch Phys Med Rehabil* 1985;**66**:177.

# FUNGAL INFECTIONS OF THE SKIN

Mycotic infections are traditionally divided into 2 principal groups: superficial and deep. In this chapter we will discuss only the superficial infections: tinea capitis, tinea corporis, and tinea cruris; dermatophytosis of the feet and dermatophytid of the hands; tinea unguium (onychomycosis, or fungal infection of the nails); and tinea versicolor. Candidiasis belongs in an intermediate group but will be considered here as well as with the deep mycoses.

The diagnosis of fungal infections of the skin is usually based on the location and characteristics of the lesions and on the following laboratory examinations: (1) Direct demonstration of fungi in 15% potassium hydroxide preparations of scrapings from suspected lesions. (2) Cultures of organisms. Dermatophytes responsive to griseofulvin are easily detectable, with color change from yellow to red on dermatophyte test medium (DTM); or one may use a microculture slide that produces color change and allows for direct microscopic identification. (3) Skin tests, eg, trichophytin (not reliable) for superficial mycoses. (This test has exclusion value in suspected dermatophytid.) (4) Examination with Wood's light (an ultraviolet light with a special filter), which causes hairs to fluoresce a brilliant green when they are infected by *Microsporum* organisms. The lamp is also invaluable in following the progress of treatment. Ringworm of the scalp may be totally unsuspected yet discovered easily with Wood's light in mass surveys of schoolchildren. *Trichophyton*-infected hairs do not fluoresce. (5) Histologic sections stained with periodic acid-Schiff (Hotchkiss-McManus) technique. Fungal elements stain red and are easily found.

Serologic tests are of no value in the diagnosis of superficial fungal infections.

Delayed sensitivity to intradermal trichophytin appears to be a correlate of immunity, whereas immediate trichophytin reactivity is associated with chronic tinea infections.

### Principles of Treatment

Treat acute active fungal infections initially as for any acute dermatitis. *Note:* It may be necessary to treat the dermatitis before applying topical fungistatic medication.

Many topical fungistatic agents are strong skin irritants. *It is easy to overtreat.*

In 1981, ketoconazole was approved in the USA for treatment of candidiasis, chronic mucocutaneous candidiasis, oral thrush, candiduria, coccidioidomycosis, histoplasmosis, chromoblastomycosis, and paracoccidioidomycosis. It is also indicated for the treatment of patients with severe recalcitrant cutaneous dermatophyte infections who have not responded to topical therapy or oral griseofulvin or who are unable to take griseofulvin. Chief concerns are abnormal levels of liver enzymes, gynecomastia, nausea, and urticaria.

One person in 10,000–15,000 may have liver damage. It is critical to warn patients to stop the drug at the first onset of nausea, indigestion, dark urine, clay-colored stools, or jaundice. Of those who developed jaundice, 82% did so within 11–168 days of treatment (average, 49 days). Liver function tests rapidly return to normal when the drug is stopped. Tests may be done every 2–4 weeks, though clinical signs and symptoms are more reliable. Gynecomastia can be avoided by giving the total dose once daily. It is best to avoid giving more than 200 mg/d (one tablet) if possible.

Antifungal agents are now being designed and tested like antibacterial drugs instead of being discovered by chance, as was the case until recently.

### General Measures & Prevention

Keep the skin dry, since moist skin favors the growth of fungi. A cool climate is preferred. Reduce exercise and activities to prevent excessive perspiration. Dry the skin carefully after bathing or after perspiring heavily. Loose-fitting underwear is advisable. Socks and other clothing should be changed often. Sandals or open-toed shoes should be worn. Skin secretions should be controlled with talc or other drying powders or with drying soaks. Sedatives (eg, phenobarbital) may be effective in reducing skin secretions in tense, nervous people. Graded daily sunbaths or quartz lamp exposure may be helpful.

Duarte PA et al: Fatal hepatitis associated with ketoconazole therapy. *Arch Intern Med* 1984;**144:**1069.

Rippon JW: A new era in antimycotic agents. (Editorial.) *Arch Dermatol* 1986;**122:**399.

### TINEA CAPITIS (Ringworm of Scalp)

### Essentials of Diagnosis

- Round, gray, scaly "bald" patches on the scalp.
- Usually in prepubertal children.
- Occasionally fluorescent under Wood's lamp.
- Microscopic examination or culture identifies the fungus.

### General Considerations

This persistent, contagious, and sometimes epidemic infection occurs almost exclusively in children and disappears spontaneously at puberty. Two general species (*Microsporum* and *Trichophyton*) cause ringworm infections of the scalp. *Microsporum* accounts for many of the infections, and hairs infected with this genus fluoresce brilliantly under Wood's light. *Trichophyton tonsurans* is the most common cause of tinea capitis in the USA today. *Trichophyton* species account for some of the very resistant infections, which may persist into adulthood.

### Clinical Findings

**A. Symptoms and Signs:** There are usually no symptoms with noninflammatory tinea capitis, although there may be slight itching. The lesions are round, gray, scaly, apparently bald patches on the scalp. (The hairs are broken off, and the patches are not actually bald.) "Black-dot" ringworm caused primarily by *T tonsurans* presents as multiple areas of alopecia studded with black dots representing infected hairs broken off at or below the surface of the scalp. At times, scalp ringworm presents as a localized spot accompanied by pronounced swelling and develops into boggy and indurated areas exuding pus known as kerion celsi. Scalp ringworm may be undetectable with the naked eye, becoming visible only under Wood's light, in which case the hairs exhibit a brilliant green fluorescence extending down into the hair follicle.

**B. Laboratory Findings:** Microscopic or culture demonstration of the organisms in the hairs may be necessary.

### Differential Diagnosis

Differentiate from other diseases of scalp hair such as pediculosis capitis, pyoderma, alopecia areata, and trichotillomania (voluntary pulling out of one's own hair).

### Prevention

Exchange of headgear must be avoided, and infected individuals or household pets must be vigorously treated and scrupulously reexamined for determination of cure. The scalp should be washed after haircuts.

### Complications

Kerion (a nodular, exudative pustule), possibly followed by scarring, is the only complication. It responds dramatically to saturated solution of potassium iodide orally and prednisone, 1 mg/kg daily for 10–14 days.

### Treatment

Microcrystalline griseofulvin, 0.125–0.25 g/d for children weighing 3–50 lb, 0.2–0.5 g/d for children weighing 50–90 lb, and 0.5–1 g/d for children and adolescents over 90 lb and for adults, may be given by mouth for 8 weeks or more. The drug is best taken with the midday meal. Selenium sulfide shampoo is recommended to reduce spore shedding.

### Prognosis

Tinea capitis may be very persistent but usually clears spontaneously at puberty, except for infections caused by certain resistant organisms such as *Trichophyton tonsurans*. Kerion responds promptly to saturated solution of potassium iodide by mouth or short-term prednisone therapy.

Allen HB et al: Selenium sulfide: Adjunctive therapy for tinea capitis. *Pediatrics* 1982;**69:**81.

Rudolph AH: The diagnosis and treatment of tinea capitis due to *Trichophyton tonsurans*. *Int J Dermatol* 1985;**24:**426.

### TINEA CORPORIS OR TINEA CIRCINATA (Body Ringworm)

### Essentials of Diagnosis

- Pruritic, ringed, scaling, centrally clearing lesions; small vesicles in a peripherally advancing border.
- On exposed skin surfaces.
- History of exposure to infected domestic animal.
- Laboratory examination by microscope or culture confirms diagnosis.

### General Considerations

The lesions are often on exposed areas of the body such as the face and arms. A history of exposure to an infected cat may be obtained. All species of dermatophytes may cause this disease, but some are more common than others.

## Clinical Findings

**A. Symptoms and Signs:** Itching is usually intense; this distinguishes the disease from other ringed lesions. Rings, erythema, or vesicles with central clearing are grouped in clusters and distributed asymmetrically, usually on an exposed surface.

**B. Laboratory Findings:** Hyphae can be demonstrated by removing scale or the cap of a vesicle and examining it microscopically in a drop of 15% potassium hydroxide. The diagnosis may be confirmed by culture.

Material can be obtained for culture on Sabouraud's medium by thoroughly rubbing a cotton swab over the lesion and then rotating the swab while thoroughly rubbing it on the medium; this technique is just as accurate as scraping the lesions with a scalpel or curet.

## Differential Diagnosis

Itching distinguishes tinea corporis from other skin lesions with annular configuration, such as the annular lesions of psoriasis, syphilis, erythema multiforme, and pityriasis rosea.

## Complications

Complications include extension of the disease to the scalp hair or nails (in which case it becomes much more difficult to cure), overtreatment dermatitis, pyoderma, and dermatophytid.

## Prevention

Avoid contact with infected household pets and exchange of clothing without adequate laundering.

## Treatment

**A. Specific Measures:** Griseofulvin (microcrystalline), 0.5 g orally daily for children and 1 g orally daily for adults. Dermatophytosis is an unlisted indication for ketoconazole, but griseofulvin and topical antifungals are preferred therapy.

**B. Local Measures:** One percent salicylic acid and 3% precipitated sulfur in hydrophilic ointment may be rubbed into lesions twice daily. *Caution:* Do not overtreat.

Compound undecylenic acid ointment may be used in the less chronic and nonthickened lesions.

The following applied topically are effective against dermatophyte infections other than those of the nails: tolnaftate, 1% solution or cream; haloprogin, 1% solution or cream; miconazole, 2% cream; clotrimazole, 1% liquid, cream, or lotion; ketoconazole, 2% cream; sulconazole, 1% cream; and ciclopirox, 1% cream. Betamethasone dipropionate with clotrimazole (Lotrisone) applied twice daily for 3–5 days is beneficial for acutely inflamed tinea lesions. After the inflammation subsides, switch to a topical antifungal without a steroid component.

## Prognosis

Body ringworm usually responds promptly to griseofulvin by mouth or to conservative topical therapy.

Conti-Diaz IA, Civila E, Asconegui F: Treatment of superficial and deep-seated mycoses with oral ketoconazole. *Int J Dermatol* 1984;**23:**207.

Head ES, Henry J, MacDonald EM: The cotton swab technic for the culture of dermatophyte infections: Its efficacy and merit. *J Am Acad Dermatol* 1984;**11:**797.

## TINEA CRURIS
## (Jock Itch)

### Essentials of Diagnosis

- Marked itching in intertriginous areas.
- Peripherally spreading, sharply demarcated, centrally clearing erythematous macular lesions, with or without vesicle formation.
- May have associated tinea infection of feet.
- Laboratory examination with microscope or culture confirms diagnosis.

### General Considerations

Tinea cruris lesions are confined to the groin and gluteal cleft and are as a rule more indolent than those of tinea corporis and tinea circinata. The disease often occurs in athletes as well as in persons who are obese or who perspire a great deal. Any of the dermatophytes may cause tinea cruris, and it may be transmitted to the groin from active dermatophytosis of the foot. Intractable pruritus ani may occasionally be caused by tineal infection.

### Clinical Findings

**A. Symptoms and Signs:** Itching is usually more severe than that which occurs in seborrheic dermatitis or intertrigo. Inverse psoriasis, however, may itch even more than tinea cruris. The lesions consist of erythematous macules with sharp margins, cleared centers, and active, spreading peripheries in intertriginous areas. There may be vesicle formation at the borders, and satellite vesicular lesions are sometimes present. Follicular pustules are sometimes encountered.

**B. Laboratory Findings:** Hyphae can be demonstrated microscopically in 15% potassium hydroxide preparations. The organism may be cultured readily.

### Differential Diagnosis

Differentiate from other lesions involving the intertriginous areas, such as candidiasis, seborrheic dermatitis, intertrigo, psoriasis of body folds ("inverse psoriasis"), and erythrasma.

### Treatment

**A. General Measures:** Drying powder should be dusted into the involved area 2–3 times a day, especially when perspiration is excessive. Keep the area clean and dry but avoid overbathing. Prevent intertrigo or chafing by avoiding overtreatment, which predisposes to further infection and complications. Underwear should be loose-fitting. Rough-textured clothing should be avoided.

**B. Specific Measures:** Griseofulvin is indicated for severe cases. Give 1 g orally daily for 1–2 weeks.

**C. Local Measures:** Treat the stage of dermatosis. Secondarily infected or inflamed lesions are best treated with soothing and drying solutions, with the patient at bed rest. Use wet compresses of potassium permanganate, 1:10,000 (or 1:20 aluminum acetate solution), or, in case of anogenital infection, sitz baths.

**Fungistatic preparations.** Any of the following may be used: (1) Weak solutions of iodine (not more than 1% tincture) twice daily. (2) Carbolfuchsin solution (Castellani's paint), one-third strength, once a day. (3) Compound undecylenic acid ointment twice daily. (4) Sulfur-salicylic acid ointment. (5) Tolnaftate (Tinactin) solution or cream. (6) Haloprogin (Halotex), 1% cream or solution. (7) Miconazole, 2% cream. (8) Clotrimazole, 1% liquid or cream. (9) ketoconazole, 2% cream. (10) Sulconazole, 1% cream. (11) Ciclopirox, 1% cream.

Initial control of symptoms of tinea cruris and tinea corporis can be achieved with use of an antifungal-corticosteroid combination (clotrimazole plus betamethasone dipropionate [Lotrisone cream]). After 2 weeks' use, results with clotrimazole alone are as good as with the combination.

### Prognosis

Tinea cruris usually responds promptly to topical or systemic treatment.

Katz HI et al: SCH 370 (clotrimazole-betamethasone dipropionate) cream in patients with tinea cruris or tinea corporis. *Cutis* 1984;**34**:183

### TINEA MANUUM & TINEA PEDIS (Dermatophytosis, Tinea of Palms & Soles, "Athlete's Foot")

### Essentials of Diagnosis

- Itching, burning, and stinging of interdigital webs, palms, and soles.
- Deep vesicles in acute stage.
- Exfoliation, fissuring, and maceration in subacute or chronic stages.
- Skin scrapings examined microscopically or by culture may reveal fungus.

### General Considerations

Tinea of the feet is an extremely common acute or chronic dermatosis. It is possible that some causative organisms are present on the feet of most adults at all times. Certain individuals appear to be more susceptible than others. Most infections are caused by *Trichophyton* and *Epidermophyton* species.

### Clinical Findings

**A. Symptoms and Signs:** The presenting symptom is usually itching. However, there may be burning, stinging, and other sensations, or frank pain from secondary infection with complicating cellulitis, lymphangitis, and lymphadenitis. Tinea pedis often appears as a fissuring of the toe webs, perhaps with denudation and sodden maceration. Toe web "tinea" may not be tinea at all but rather an intertrigo that may be called "athlete's foot." It may respond better to 30% aqueous aluminum chloride or to carbolfuchsin paint or a keratolytic agent (Keralyt gel) than to antifungal agents. However, there may also be grouped vesicles distributed anywhere on the soles or the palms, a generalized exfoliation of the skin of the soles, or destructive nail involvement in the form of discoloration and hypertrophy of the nail substance with pithy changes. Acute reddened, weeping vesicular lesions are seen on the skin in the acute stages.

**B. Laboratory Findings:** Hyphae can often be demonstrated microscopically in skin scales treated with 15% potassium hydroxide. Culture with Sabouraud's medium is simple and often informative but does not always demonstrate pathogenic fungi.

### Differential Diagnosis

Differentiate from other skin conditions involving the same areas such as interdigital intertrigo, candidiasis, gram-negative toe web infection, psoriasis, contact dermatitis (from shoes, powders, nail polish), atopic eczema, and scabies.

### Prevention

The essential factor in prevention is personal hygiene. Rubber or wooden sandals should be used in community showers and bathing places. Careful drying between the toes after showering is recommended. Socks should be changed frequently. Apply dusting and drying powders as necessary.

### Treatment

**A. Specific Measures:** Griseofulvin has been disappointing in the treatment of dermatophytosis of the feet and should be used only for severe cases or those that are recalcitrant to topical therapy.

Ketoconazole, 200 mg daily by mouth, is an effective agent for griseofulvin-resistant dermatophytosis, although relapse may occur after discontinuing therapy. The drug is well tolerated; hepatotoxicity has been reported from its use. Dermatophytosis is not a listed indication for ketoconazole.

**B. Local Measures:** *Caution:* Do not overtreat.

**1. Acute stage (lasts 1–10 days)**—Give aluminum subacetate solution soaks for 20 minutes 2–3 times daily. If secondary infection is present, use soaks of 1:10,000 potassium permanganate. If secondary infection is severe or complicated, treat as described on p 48.

**2. Subacute stage**—Any of the following may be used: (1) Miconazole cream, 2%. (2) Clotrimazole cream or lotion, 1%. (3) Ketoconazole cream, 2%.

(4) Solution of coal tar, 5% in starch lotion. (5) Coal tar, 1–2% in Lassar's paste.

**3. Chronic stage—**Use any of the following: (1) Sulfur-salicylic acid ointment or cream. (2) Whitfield's ointment, one-fourth to one-half strength. (3) Compound undecylenic acid ointment twice daily. (4) Alcoholic Whitfield's solution. (5) Carbolfuchsin solution (Castellani's paint). (6) Tolnaftate (Tinactin) solution or cream. (7) Haloprogin, 1% cream or solution. (8) Miconazole, 2% cream. (9) Clotrimazole (Lotrimin or Mycelex), 1% cream or lotion. (10) Ketoconazole cream (Nizoral), 2%. (11) Sulconazole, 1% cream. (12) Ciclopirox (Loprox), 1% cream.

**C. Mechanical Measures:** Carefully remove or debride dead or thickened tissues after soaks or baths.

### Prognosis

Tinea of the hands and feet usually responds well to treatment, but recurrences are common in strongly predisposed persons.

Robertson MH et al: Ketoconazole in griseofulvin-resistant dermatophytosis. *J Am Acad Dermatol* 1982;**6**:224.

## DERMATOPHYTID
## (Allergy or Sensitivity to Fungi)

### Essentials of Diagnosis

- Pruritic, grouped vesicular lesions involving the sides and flexor aspects of the fingers and the palms.
- Fungal infection elsewhere on body, usually the feet.
- Trichophytin skin test positive. No fungus demonstrable in lesions.

### General Considerations

Dermatophytid is a sensitivity reaction to an active focus of dermatophytosis elsewhere on the body, usually the feet. Fungi are present in the primary lesions but are not present in the lesions of dermatophytid. The hands are most often affected, but dermatophytid may occur on other areas also.

### Clinical Findings

**A. Symptoms and Signs:** Itching is the only symptom. The lesions consist of grouped vesicles, often involving the thenar and hypothenar eminences. Lesions are round, up to 15 mm in diameter, and may be present on the side and flexor aspects of the fingers. Lesions occasionally involve the backs of the hands or may even be generalized.

**B. Laboratory Findings:** The trichophytin skin test is positive, but it may also be positive with other disorders. A negative trichophytin test rules out dermatophytid. Repeated negative microscopic examination of material taken from the lesions is necessary before the diagnosis of dermatophytid can be established. Culture from the primary site tends to reveal *Trichophyton mentagrophytes* organisms rather than *Trichophyton rubrum*. There appears to be selective anergy in patients with chronic *T rubrum* infections.

### Differential Diagnosis

Differentiate from all diseases causing vesicular eruptions of the hands, especially contact dermatitis, dyshidrosis, and localized forms of atopic dermatitis.

### Prevention

Treat fungal infections early and adequately, and prevent recurrences.

### Treatment

General measures are as outlined on p 48. The lesions should be treated according to type of dermatitis. The primary focus should be treated with griseofulvin or by local measures as described for dermatophytosis (see above). A single injection of triamcinolone acetonide suspension, 40 mg intragluteally, may suppress the eruption until the causative focus is controlled.

### Prognosis

Dermatophytid may occur in an explosive series of episodes, and recurrences are not uncommon; however, it clears with adequate treatment of the primary infection elsewhere on the body.

## TINEA UNGUIUM & CANDIDAL ONYCHOMYCOSIS

### Essentials of Diagnosis

- Lusterless, brittle, hypertrophic, friable nails.
- Fungus demonstrated in nail section or nail dust by microscope or culture.

### General Considerations

Tinea unguium is a destructive *Trichophyton* infection of one or more (but rarely all) fingernails or toenails. The species most commonly found are *Trichophyton mentagrophytes* and *Trichophyton rubrum*. *Candida albicans* causes candidal onychomycosis. "Saprophytic" fungi may cause onychomycosis.

### Clinical Findings

**A. Symptoms and Signs:** There are usually no symptoms. The nails are lusterless, brittle, and hypertrophic, and the substance of the nail is friable and even pithy. Irregular segments of the diseased nail may be broken.

**B. Laboratory Findings:** Laboratory diagnosis is mandatory. Portions of the nail should be cleared with 15% potassium hydroxide and examined under the microscope for branching hyphae or collections of spores. Fungi may also be cultured, using Sabouraud's medium. Periodic acid-Schiff stain of a histologic section will also demonstrate the fungus readily.

## Differential Diagnosis

Distinguish from nail changes caused by contact with strong alkalies and certain other chemicals and from those due to psoriasis, lichen planus, candidiasis, and trauma.

## Treatment

**A. General Measures:** See p 48.

**B. Specific Measures:** Onychomycosis is an unlisted indication for ketoconazole. Griseofulvin ultramicrosize, 1000 mg/d, is about as effective as ketoconazole, 200 mg/d. Increasing ketoconazole to 400 mg/d will substantially increase the cure rate of onychomycosis, but the side effects of ketoconazole (liver abnormalities, effects on the adrenal cortex, and antiandrogenic activity) must be taken into account.

**C. Local Measures:** Sandpaper or file the nails daily (down to nail bed if necessary). Ciclopirox (Loprox) is a topical fungicidal cream that contains a pyridone-ethanolamine salt and seems to penetrate nails better than other topical agents. Early reports indicate this might be the most effective topical agent in the treatment of dermatophyte infections of the fingernails and toenails (onychomycosis).

## Prognosis

Cure is difficult, even with microcrystalline griseofulvin by mouth in a dose of 1–2 g daily for months, or with ketoconazole, miconazole, or clotrimazole topically. Even when the nails clear after months of treatment, recurrences can be expected shortly after discontinuation of systemic therapy.

Scher RK: Differential diagnosis and treatment of onychomycosis. *Curr Concepts Skin Dis* 1985;**6**:4.

Zaias N, Drachman D: A method for the determination of drug effectiveness in onychomycosis: Trials with ketoconazole and griseofulvin ultramicrosize. *J Am Acad Dermatol* 1983;**9**:912.

## TINEA VERSICOLOR
## (Pityriasis Versicolor)

## Essentials of Diagnosis

- Pale macules that will not tan.
- Velvety, chamois-colored macules that scale with scraping.
- Trunk distribution the most frequent site.
- Fungus observed on microscopic examination of scales.

## General Considerations

Tinea versicolor is a mild, superficial *Pityrosporon orbiculare (Malassezia furfur)* infection of the skin (usually of the trunk). The eruption is called to the patient's attention by the fact that the involved areas will not tan, and the resulting pseudoachromia may be mistaken for vitiligo. A hyperpigmented form is not uncommon. The disease is not particularly contagious and is apt to occur more frequently in those who wear heavy clothing and who perspire a great deal. Epidemics may occur in athletes.

Pityrosporon folliculitis is common. Stubborn scalp folliculitis may occur.

## Clinical Findings

**A. Symptoms and Signs:** There may be mild itching. The lesions are velvety, chamois-colored macules that vary from 4 to 5 mm in diameter to large confluent areas. Scales may be readily obtained by scraping the area. Lesions may appear on the trunk, upper arms, neck, face, and groin.

**B. Laboratory Findings:** Large, blunt hyphae and thick-walled budding spores (''spaghetti and meatballs'') may be seen under the low-power objective when skin scales have been cleared in 15% potassium hydroxide. *P orbiculare* or *P ovale* is difficult to culture.

## Differential Diagnosis

Distinguish from vitiligo on basis of appearance. Differentiate also from seborrheic dermatitis of the same areas.

## Treatment & Prognosis

Encourage good skin hygiene. Topical treatments include Selsun suspension or Exsel lotion (both contain selenium sulfide), which may be applied daily and left on for 5 minutes; or one may use equal parts of propylene glycol and water topically, diluting with water if there is irritation. Other choices are 3% salicylic acid in rubbing alcohol and Tinver lotion (contains sodium thiosulfate). Relapses are common.

Sulfur-salicylic acid soap or shampoo (Sebulex) used on a continuing basis may be effective.

Ketoconazole, 200 mg daily orally for 1 week, apparently results in cure of 90% of cases. (Use caution because of possible hepatotoxicity.)

Newer antifungal creams, solutions, and lotions are also available (see p 79).

Bäck O, Faergemann J, Hörnqvist R: *Pityrosporum* folliculitis: A common disease of the young and middle-aged. *J Am Acad Dermatol* 1985;**12**:56.

Faergemann J, Fredriksson T: Propylene glycol in the treatment of tinea versicolor. *Acta Derm Venereol (Stockh)* 1980;**60**:92.

Savin RC: Systemic ketoconazole in tinea versicolor: A double-blind evaluation and 1-year follow-up. *J Am Acad Dermatol* 1984;**10**:824.

## CUTANEOUS CANDIDIASIS
## (Moniliasis)

## Essentials of Diagnosis

- Severe pruritus of vulva, anus, or body folds.
- Superficial denuded, beefy-red areas with or without satellite vesicopustules.
- Whitish curdlike concretions on the surface.
- Fungus on microscopic examination of scales or curd.

## General Considerations

Cutaneous candidiasis is a superficial fungal infection that may involve almost any cutaneous or mucous surface of the body. It is particularly likely to occur in diabetics, during pregnancy, and in obese persons who perspire freely. Antibiotics and oral contraceptive agents may be contributory. When the patient presents with chronic mucocutaneous candidiasis, baseline and yearly follow-up tests will screen for development of endocrinopathy. Tests for diabetes include glycosylated hemoglobin (hemoglobin A1c) and fasting and 2-hour postprandial glucose; for thyroid function, TSH, T4, resin T3 uptake, thyroglobulin, and microsomal antibody tests; for parathyroid function, calcium, phosphorus, and alkaline phosphatase tests; for adrenal function, electrolyte, blood glucose, and adrenal antibody tests and ACTH and cortisol levels. Oral candidiasis may be the first sign of AIDS or AIDS-related complex (ARC). Esophageal candidiasis can be detected by endoscopy in all patients with AIDS and oral candidiasis.

## Clinical Findings

**A. Symptoms and Signs:** Itching may be intense. Burning sensations are sometimes reported, particularly around the vulva and anus. The lesions consist of superficially denuded, beefy-red areas in the depths of the body folds such as in the groin and the intergluteal cleft, beneath the breasts, at the angles of the mouth, and in the umbilicus. The peripheries of these denuded lesions are superficially undermined, and there may be satellite vesicopustules. Whitish, curdlike concretions may be present on the surface of the lesions (particularly in the oral and vaginal mucous membranes). Paronychia and interdigital erosions may occur.

**B. Laboratory Findings:** Clusters of budding cells and short hyphae can be seen under the high-power lens when skin scales or curdlike lesions have been cleared in 15% potassium hydroxide. The organism may be isolated on Sabouraud's medium. In the more severe forms of mucocutaneous candidiasis, there may be negative skin tests to all common antigens including *Candida,* as well as inability to be sensitized to dinitrochlorobenzene.

## Differential Diagnosis

Differentiate from intertrigo, seborrheic dermatitis, tinea cruris, and erythrasma involving the same areas.

## Complications

In the debilitated or immunosuppressed patient, candidiasis may spread from the skin or mucous membranes to the bladder, lungs, and other internal organs.

## Treatment

**A. General Measures:** Treat associated diabetes, obesity, or hyperhidrosis. Keep the parts dry and exposed to air as much as possible. If possible, discontinue systemic antibiotics; if not, give nystatin by mouth concomitantly in a dose of 1.5 million units 3 times daily. Ketoconazole, 200 mg daily by mouth, will eradicate lesions with minimal side effects except for rare instances of liver damage. Liver function must be monitored. Recurrences follow discontinuation of therapy. Immune enhancers such as thymosin, transfer factor, levamisole, and cimetidine may play a role in maintaining control, as may supplemental iron.

**B. Local Measures:**

**1. Nails and skin–**Apply 1% ciclopirox cream, nystatin cream, 100,000 units/g, or miconazole, ketoconazole, or clotrimazole cream or lotion, 3–4 times daily. Gentian violet, 1%, or carbolfuchsin paint (Castellani's paint) may be applied 1–2 times weekly as an alternative.

**2. Vulva, anal mucous membranes–**For vaginal candidiasis, use miconazole cream (Monistat 7), one applicatorful vaginally at bedtime for 7 days; or clotrimazole (Gyne-Lotrimin, Mycelex-G), one suppository vaginally per day for 7 days; or nystatin, one tablet (100,000 units) vaginally twice daily for 7 days. Gentian violet or carbolfuchsin (see above) can also be used. Clotrimazole troches have proved effective in controlling chronic oral candidiasis. Ketoconazole, 200 mg daily for 10 days, is quite effective for chronic, recurrent, or recalcitrant vulvovaginal candidiasis.

## Prognosis

Cutaneous candidiasis may be intractable and prolonged, particularly in children, in whom the disturbance may take the form of a granuloma that resists all attempts at treatment.

Dolen J, Varma SK, South MA: Chronic mucocutaneous candidiasis: Endocrinopathies. *Cutis* 1981;**28:**592.

Jorizzo JL: Chronic mucocutaneous candidiasis: An update. *Arch Dermatol* 1982;**18:**963.

Tavitian A, Raufman J-P, Rosenthal LE: Oral candidiasis as a marker for esophageal candidiasis in the acquired immunodeficiency syndrome. *Ann Intern Med* 1986;**104:**54.

Tkach JR, Rinaldi MG: Severe hepatitis associated with ketoconazole therapy for chronic mucocutaneous candidiasis. *Cutis* 1982;**29:**482.

# PARASITIC INFESTATIONS OF THE SKIN

## SCABIES

### Essentials of Diagnosis

- Nocturnal itching.
- Pruritic vesicles and pustules in "runs" or "galleries," especially on the sides of the fingers and the heels of the palms.

- Mites, ova, and brown dots of feces visible microscopically.

## General Considerations

Scabies is a common dermatitis caused by infestation with *Sarcoptes scabiei*. An entire family may be affected. The infestation usually spares the head and neck (although even these areas may be involved in infants). The mite is barely visible with the naked eye as a white dot. Scabies is usually acquired by sleeping with an infested individual or by other close contact. This infestation is on the increase worldwide.

## Clinical Findings

**A. Symptoms and Signs:** Itching occurs almost exclusively at night. The lesions consist of more or less generalized excoriations with small pruritic vesicles, pustules, and "runs" or "galleries" on the sides of the fingers and the heels of the palms. The run or gallery appears as a short irregular mark (perhaps 2–3 mm long), as if made by a sharp pencil. Characteristic lesions may occur on the nipples in females and as pruritic papules on the scrotum or penis in males. Pruritic papules may be seen over the buttocks. Pyoderma is often the presenting sign.

**B. Laboratory Findings:** The adult female mite may be demonstrated by probing the fresh end of a run or gallery with a pointed scalpel. The mite tends to cling to the tip of the blade. One may shave off the entire run or gallery (or, in the scrotum, a papule) and demonstrate the female mite, her ova, and small brown dots of feces. A sharp bone or dermal curet yields an excellent specimen. The diagnosis should be confirmed by microscopic demonstration of the organism, ova, or feces in a mounted specimen in glycerin, mineral oil, or 15% sodium or potassium hydroxide. The diagnosis can be confirmed in most cases with the burrow ink test. Apply ink to the burrow and then do a superficial shave biopsy by sawing off the burrow with a No. 15 blade, painlessly and bloodlessly. The mite, ova, and feces can be seen under the light microscope.

## Differential Diagnosis

Distinguish from the various forms of pediculosis and from other causes of pruritus.

## Treatment & Prognosis

Unless the lesions are complicated by severe secondary pyoderma, treatment consists primarily of disinfestation. If secondary pyoderma is present, it should be treated with systemic and topical antibiotics.

Disinfestation with lindane (gamma benzene hexachloride), 1% in cream or lotion base, applied from the neck down overnight, is a popular treatment. A warning has been issued by the FDA regarding potential neurotoxicity, and any use in infants and pregnant women, as well as overuse in adults, is discouraged. Bedding and clothing should be laundered or cleaned. This preparation can be used before secondary infection is controlled. An alternative drug is crotamiton (Eurax) cream or lotion, which may be applied in the same way as gamma benzene hexachloride. The old-fashioned medication consisting of 5% or 6% sulfur in petrolatum may still be used, applying it nightly from the collarbones down, for 3 nights, but one must be prepared to treat irritant dermatitis. Benzyl benzoate may be compounded as a lotion or emulsion in strengths from 20% to 35% and used as generalized (from collarbones down) applications overnight for 2 treatments 1 week apart. The NF XIV formula is 275 mL benzyl benzoate (containing 5 g of triethanolamine and 20 g of oleic acid) in water to make 1000 mL. It is cosmetically acceptable, clean, and not overly irritating. Persistent pruritic postscabietic papules may be painted with undiluted crude coal tar or Estargel.

Unless treatment is aimed at all infected persons in a family or institutionalized group, reinfestations will probably occur.

Resistant forms requiring multiple forms of treatment are appearing.

Davies JH et al: Lindane poisonings. *Arch Dermatol* 1983;**119:**142.

Felman YM, Nikitas JA: Scabies. *Cutis* 1984;**33:**266.

Orkin M, Maibach HI (editors): *Cutaneous Infestations and Insect Bites.* Marcel Dekker, 1985.

Rees RB: Earlier treatments for scabies. Pages 101–102 in: *Cutaneous Infestations and Insect Bites.* Orkin M, Maibach HI (eds). Marcel Dekker, 1985.

# PEDICULOSIS

## Essentials of Diagnosis

- Pruritus with excoriation.
- Nits on hair shafts; lice on skin or clothes.
- Occasionally, sky-blue macules (maculae caeruleae) on the inner thighs or lower abdomen in pubic louse infestation.

## General Considerations

Pediculosis is a parasitic infestation of the skin of the scalp, trunk, or pubic areas. It usually occurs among people who live in overcrowded dwellings with inadequate hygiene facilities, although pubic lice may be acquired by anyone sitting on an infested toilet seat—and, more commonly, by sexual transmission. There are 3 different varieties: (1) pediculosis pubis, caused by *Pthirus pubis* (pubic louse, "crabs"); (2) pediculosis corporis, by *Pediculus humanus* var *corporis* (body louse); (3) pediculosis capitis, by *Pediculus humanus* var *capitis* (head louse).

Head and body lice are similar in appearance and are 3–4 mm long. Head louse infestations may be transmitted by shared use of hats or combs. The body louse can seldom be found on the body, because the insect comes onto the skin only to feed and must be looked for in the seams of the underclothing.

Trench fever, relapsing fever, and typhus may be transmitted by the body louse.

## Clinical Findings

Itching may be very intense in body louse infestations, and scratching may result in deep excoriations over the affected area. The clinical appearance is of gross excoriation. Pyoderma may be present and may be the presenting sign in any of these infestations. Head lice can be found on the scalp or may be manifested as small nits resembling pussy-willow buds on the scalp hairs close to the skin. They are easiest to see above the ears and at the nape of the neck. Body lice may deposit visible nits on the vellus hair of the body. Pubic louse infestations are occasionally generalized, particularly in a hairy individual; the lice may even be found on the eyelashes and in the scalp.

## Differential Diagnosis

Distinguish head louse infestation from seborrheic dermatitis, body louse infestation from scabies, and pubic louse infestation from anogenital pruritus and eczema.

## Treatment

For all types of pediculosis, lindane lotion (Kwell, Scabene) is used extensively. A thin layer is applied to the infested and adjacent hairy areas. It is removed after 12 hours by thorough washing. Remaining nits may be removed with a fine-toothed comb or forceps. Sexual contacts should be treated. Synergized pyrethrins (A-200 Pyrinate, Pyrinyl, Rid) are over-the-counter products that are applied undiluted until the infested areas are entirely wet. After 10 minutes, the areas are washed thoroughly with warm water and soap and then dried. Nits may be treated as indicated above. For involvement of eyelashes, petrolatum is applied thickly twice daily for 8 days, and remaining nits are then plucked off. There is controversy about whether lice and the acarus of scabies can develop resistance to lindane.

Malathion lotion, 0.5% (Prioderm), compared with A-200 Pyrinate shampoo, R&C shampoo, Rid, Kwell shampoo (lindane), and A-200 Pyrinate liquid, is the only product for pediculosis capitis that shows excellent ovicidal activity. Hatching of eggs following treatment with the other agents leads to recurrence of the infestation.

## Prognosis

Pediculosis responds to topical treatment.

Meinking TL et al: Comparative efficacy of treatments for pediculosis capitis infestations. *Arch Dermatol* 1986;**122**:267.
Parish LC, Witkowoski JA, Kucirka SA: Lindane resistance and pediculosis capitis. *Int J Trop Dermatol* 1983;**22**:572.

## SKIN LESIONS DUE TO OTHER ARTHROPODS

## Essentials of Diagnosis

- Localized rash with pruritus.
- Furunclelike lesions containing live arthropods.
- Tender erythematous patches that migrate ("larva migrans").
- Generalized urticaria or erythema multiforme.

## General Considerations

Some arthropods (eg, most pest mosquitoes and biting flies) are readily detected as they bite. Many others are not, eg, because they are too small, because there is no immediate reaction, or because they bite during sleep. Reactions may be delayed for many hours; many severe reactions are allergic. Patients are most apt to consult a physician when the lesions are multiple and pruritus is intense. Severe attacks may be accompanied by insomnia, restlessness, fever, and faintness or even collapse. Rashes may sometimes cover the body.

Many persons will react severely only to their earliest contacts with an arthropod, thus presenting pruritic lesions when traveling, moving into new quarters, etc. Body lice, fleas, bedbugs, and local mosquitoes should be borne in mind. Spiders are often incorrectly believed to be the source of bites; they rarely attack humans, although the brown spider (*Loxosceles laeta, Loxosceles reclusa*) may cause severe necrotic reactions and death due to intravascular hemolysis, and the black widow spider (*Latrodectus mactans*) may cause severe systemic symptoms and death.

In addition to arthropod bites, the most common lesions are venomous stings (wasps, hornets, bees, ants, scorpions) or bites (centipedes), dermatitis due to vesicating furunclelike lesions due to fly maggots or sand fleas in the skin, and a linear creeping eruption due to a migrating larva.

## Clinical Findings

The diagnosis may be difficult when the patient has not noticed the initial attack but suffers a delayed reaction. Individual bites are frequently in clusters and tend to occur either on exposed parts (eg, midges and gnats) or under clothing, especially around the waist or at flexures (eg, small mites or insects in bedding or clothing). The reaction is often delayed for 1–24 hours or more. Pruritus is almost always present and may be all but intolerable once the patient starts to scratch. Secondary infection, sometimes with serious consequences, may follow scratching. Allergic manifestations, including urticarial wheals, are common. Papules may become vesicular. The diagnosis is aided by searching for exposure to arthropods and by considering the patient's occupation and recent activities. The principal arthropods are as follows:

**(1) Bedbugs:** In crevices of beds or furniture; bites tend to occur in lines or clusters. Pustular urticaria is a characteristic lesion of bedbug bites. It is thought that *Cimex lectularius* (bedbug) may play a significant role in the transmission of hepatitis B. The closely related kissing bug has been reported with increasing frequency as attacking humans.

**(2) Fleas:** Fleas are bloodsucking ectoparasites that feed on dogs, cats, humans, and other species. Flea saliva produces papular urticaria in sensitized individuals. *Ctenocephalides felis* and *Ctenocephalides canis* are the most common species found on cats and dogs, and both species attack humans. The human flea, *Pulex irritans,* is not commonly recognized by veterinarians as a pet animal problem.

To break the life cycle of the flea, one must treat the home, pets, and outside environment, using quick-kill insecticides, residual insecticides, and a growth regulator. Obviously, this is a repetitive job for the exterminator. Home foggers and flea collars are not adequate. Birds and fish are especially sensitive and must be protected during disinfestation.

**(3) Ticks:** Usually picked up by brushing against low vegetation. Larval ticks may attack in large numbers and cause much distress; in Africa and India they have been confused with chiggers. Ascending paralysis may occasionally be traced to a tick bite, and removal of the embedded tick is essential. Ticks may transmit Rocky Mountain spotted fever and Lyme disease.

**(4) Chiggers or redbugs** are larvae of trombiculid mites. A few species confined to particular countries and usually to restricted and locally recognized habitats (eg, berry patches, woodland edges, lawns, brush turkey mounds in Australia, poultry farms) attack humans, often around the waist, on the ankles, or in flexures, raising intensely itching erythematous papules after a delay of many hours. The red chiggers may sometimes be seen in the center of papules that have not yet been scratched. Chiggers are the commonest cause of distressing multiple lesions associated with arthropods.

**(5) Bird mites:** Larger than chiggers, infesting chicken houses, pigeon lofts, or nests of birds in eaves. Bites are multiple anywhere on the body, although poultry handlers are most often attacked on the hands and forearms. Room air conditioning units may suck in bird mites and infest the inhabitants of the room. Rodent mites from mice or rats may cause similar effects.

The diagnosis of bird mites, rodent mites, or carpet mites may readily be overlooked and the patient treated for other dermatoses or for psychogenic dermatosis. Intractable "acarophobia" (delusions of parasitosis) may result from early neglect or misdiagnosis.

**(6) Mites in stored products:** These are white and almost invisible and infest products such as copra ("copra itch"), vanilla pods ("vanillism"), sugar, straw, cottonseeds, and cereals. Persons who handle these products may be attacked, especially on the hands and forearms and sometimes on the feet. Infested bedding may occasionally lead to generalized dermatitis.

**(7) Caterpillars of moths with urticating hairs:** The hairs are blown from cocoons or carried by emergent moths, causing severe and often seasonally recurrent outbreaks after mass emergence, eg, in some southern states of the USA.

**(8) Tungiasis** is due to the burrowing flea known as *Tunga penetrans* (also known as chigoe, jigger; not the same as chigger), found in Africa, the West Indies, and South America. The female burrows under the skin, sucks blood, swells to 0.5 cm, and then ejects her eggs onto the ground. Ulceration, lymphangitis, gangrene, and septicemia may result, possibly with fatality. Ethyl chloride spray will kill the insect when applied to the lesion, and disinfestation may be accomplished with insecticide applied to the terrain.

### Differential Diagnosis

Arthropods should be considered in the differential diagnosis of skin lesions showing any of the above symptoms.

### Prevention

Arthropod infestations are best prevented by avoidance of contaminated areas, personal cleanliness, and disinfection of clothing, bedclothes, and furniture as indicated. Lice, chiggers, red bugs, and mites can be killed by lindane (gamma benzene hexachloride; Gammexane, Kwell, Scabene) applied to the head and clothing. (It is not necessary to remove clothing.) Benzyl benzoate and dimethylphthalate are excellent acaricides; clothing should be impregnated by spray or by dipping in a soapy emulsion.

### Treatment

*Caution:* Avoid local overtreatment.

Living arthropods should be removed carefully with tweezers after application of alcohol. Preserve in alcohol for identification. (*Caution:* In endemic Rocky Mountain spotted fever areas, do not remove ticks with the bare fingers, because infection may occur.) Children in particular should be prevented from scratching.

Apply corticosteroid lotions or creams. Crotamiton (Eurax) cream or lotion may be used; it is a miticide as well as an antipruritic. Calamine lotion or a cool wet dressing is always appropriate. Antibiotic creams, lotions, or powders may be applied if secondary infection is suspected.

Localized persistent lesions may be treated with intralesional corticosteroids. Avoid exercise and excessive warmth. Codeine may be given for pain. Creams containing local anesthetics are not very effective and may be sensitizing.

Stings produced by many arthropods may be alleviated by applying papain powder (Adolph's Meat Tenderizer) mixed with water, or Xerac AC.

Extracts (expensive) from venom sacs of bees, wasps, yellow jackets, and hornets are now available for immunotherapy of patients at risk for anaphylaxis. Approximately 5% of patients fail to respond.

Chipps BE et al: Diagnosis and treatment of anaphylactic reactions to Hymenoptera stings in children. *J Pediatr* 1980;**97**:177.

Crissey JT: Bedbugs: An old problem with a new dimension. *Int J Dermatol* 1981;**20**:411.

Medleau L, Miller WH Jr: Flea infestation and its control. *Int J Dermatol* 1983;**22**:378.

Pien FD, Grekin JL: Common ectoparasites. *West J Med* 1983;**139**:382.

# TUMORS OF THE SKIN

Excessive exposure of fair skin to sun radiation is a cancer risk of major degree. Inculcation of new attitudes about sunbathing and development of measures to counteract the adverse effects of sun damage are important public health objectives. Sunlight on sandy complexions can induce actinic (solar) keratoses, nevi, basal and squamous cell carcinoma, and melanoma. The best protection is shelter, but protective clothing, avoidance of direct sun exposure during the 4 peak hours of the day, and the assiduous use of commercially available chemical sunscreens or sunshades are helpful.

A number of highly effective sunscreens are available. Fair-complexioned persons should not use a sunscreen with a rating less than SPF 15 (sun protective factor 15). For those who are sensitive to PABA (*p*-aminobenzoic acid), Neutrogena PABA-Free sunscreen SPF 15 Solbar SPF 15 PAPA-free cream or Presun 29 may be used.

The sunshades include those containing opaque materials such as titanium dioxide or zinc oxide.

## Classification

The following classification is admittedly oversimplified; almost any tumor arising from embryonal tissues in the various stages of their development can be found in the skin.

**A. Benign:** Seborrheic keratoses, considered by some to be nevoid, consist of benign overgrowths of epithelium that have a pigmented velvety or warty surface. They are relatively common, especially in the elderly, both on exposed and covered parts, and are commonly mistaken for melanomas or other types of cutaneous neoplasms. Skin tags frequently develop on the eyelids, around the neck, and in the axillae and groins.

Keratoacanthomas are rapidly growing tumors resembling squamous cell carcinomas.

**B. Nevi:** Any of the following (except freckles) may be excised if there are suspicious features.

**1. Junctional nevi,** which consist of clear nevus cells and usually some melanin, have nevus cells on both sides of the epidermal junction. They are possible forerunners of malignant melanoma, although most melanomas arise de novo. If a nevus grows rapidly, darkens, or bleeds, the possibility of melanomatous degeneration should be considered.

**2. Compound nevi,** composed of junctional elements as well as clear nevus cells in the dermis, also may develop into malignant melanoma.

**3. Dermal nevi** are almost always benign, and almost everyone has at least a few of these lesions. They usually appear in childhood and tend to undergo spontaneous fibrosis in old age. Pigmented nevi that are present at birth show a greater tendency toward the development of melanoma than those developing in later years and should be excised wherever possible. This is especially true of bathing trunk nevi, which should be excised in decrements if possible.

**4. Dysplastic nevi** range from 6 to 12 mm in diameter. They may be pebbly, papular, nodular, or plaquelike. They may be tan to dark brown, perhaps with a pink component, and may have an inflamed appearance. They may occur anywhere on the body but are usually on exposed areas. An individual may have more than 100 lesions—instead of about 25, as is the case with common melanocytic nevi ("moles"). They usually appear in adolescence, may continue developing throughout life (ordinary moles tend to disappear with aging), and may be familial, in which case the rate of development of malignant melanoma may be much higher than in sporadic cases. Dysplastic nevi have an overall lifetime risk for malignant melanoma of between 5 and 10%, with the rate approaching 100% in familial cases—especially if there is a history of malignant melanoma in close relatives. Several lesions should be biopsied and the rest followed carefully.

**5. Blue nevi** are benign, although in some instances they behave in an invasive manner requiring multiple excisions. These lesions in the pristine state are small, slightly elevated, and blue-black.

**6. Epithelial nevi** include several types of verrucous epithelial overgrowths, usually in linear distribution. Microscopically, cells found normally in the epidermis are present. Such lesions rarely degenerate into squamous or basal cell carcinomas. The nevus sebaceus of Jadassohn, which occurs commonly in the scalp, is composed of a number of embryonal elements and is considered to be particularly likely to give rise to carcinomas.

**7. Freckles,** which in the juvenile form are called ephelides and in the adult delayed form are called lentigines, consist of excess amounts of melanin in the melanocytes in the basal layer of the epidermis. Juvenile freckles tend to disappear with time, whereas lentigines come on in later life and are more persistent.

**C. Premalignant:** Actinic or solar keratoses are flesh-colored and feel like little patches of sandpaper when the finger is pulled over them. When they degenerate, they become squamous cell carcinomas. They occur on exposed parts of the body in persons of fair complexion. Nonactinic keratoses may be provoked by exposure to arsenic systemically or occupational irritants such as tars. In keratoses, the cells are atypical and similar to those seen in squamous cell epitheliomas, but these changes are well contained by an intact dermoepidermal junction. Application of liquid nitrogen is a rapid and effective method of eradication. The lesions are frozen for a few seconds with a cotton-tipped applicator that has been dipped in liquid nitrogen or with a spraying unit containing liquid nitrogen. The lesions disappear in a few days. They may be excised or removed superficially with a scalpel followed by cautery or fulguration. An alternative treatment is the use of 1–5% fluorouracil in propylene glycol or in a cream base. This agent may be rubbed into the lesions morning and night until they become briskly sore (usually 1–3 weeks); the treatment should then be continued for several days longer and then stopped. The eyes and the mouth should be avoided. Any lesions that persist may then be excised for histologic examination.

### D. Malignant:

**1. Squamous cell carcinoma** usually occurs on exposed parts in fair-skinned individuals who sunburn easily and tan poorly. They may arise out of actinic or solar keratoses. They tend to develop very rapidly, attaining a diameter of 1 cm within 2 weeks. These lesions appear as small red, conical, hard nodules that quickly ulcerate. Squamous cell carcinomas of the lip, oral cavity, tongue, and genitalia are serious cancers and deserve special care and management. Metastases may occur early, although they are said to be less likely with squamous cell carcinoma arising out of actinic keratoses than in those that arise de novo. Keratoacanthomas are benign growths that resemble squamous cell carcinoma but which for all practical purposes should be treated as though they were skin cancers. The preferred treatment of squamous cell carcinoma is excision. X-ray radiation may be used instead, and Mohs' fresh tissue microscopically controlled excision, where available, is excellent treatment also.

**2. Basal cell carcinoma** occurs mostly on exposed parts. These lesions grow slowly, attaining a size of 1–2 cm in diameter only after a year's growth. There is a waxy appearance, with telangiectatic vessels easily visible. Metastases almost never occur. Neglected lesions may ulcerate and produce great destruction, ultimately invading vital structures. It is important to widely excise basal cell carcinomas where possible. Excision and suturing may be used, or one may carve out the entire growth (called a ''shave biopsy'' by some physicians), following which the base of the wound is treated with curettage and electrodesiccation. If the growth is in areas such as the inner canthers of the eye or the nasolabial fold, where pockets of extension may occur, fresh tissue microscopically controlled extirpation may be done (modified Mohs' technique). X-ray therapy and cryosurgery are alternative methods of treatment.

**3. Bowen's disease** (intraepidermal squamous cell epithelioma) is relatively uncommon and resembles a plaque of psoriasis. The course is relatively benign, but malignant progression may occur, and it is best to excise the lesion widely if possible.

**4. Paget's disease,** considered by some to be a manifestation of apocrine sweat gland carcinoma, may occur around the nipple, resembling chronic eczema, or may involve apocrine areas such as the genitalia. There seems to be less likelihood of an underlying sweat gland carcinoma if the lesions are on the vulva than if they are on the nipple or perianal area.

**5. Malignant melanoma–**Malignant melanoma is the leading cause of death from skin disease. It is estimated, based on rates from the NCI SEER program 1977–1981, that there will be 25,800 new cases of melanoma in the USA in 1987, with the sex incidence nearly equal. Furthermore, 5800 deaths from melanoma are projected. Five-year survival rates for whites in 1977–1982 were 96% for localized disease, 83% for all stages, and 71% for melanomas that had spread. Insufficient data are available for blacks. Deaths from malignant melanoma are increasing at a faster rate than death from any other malignant neoplastic disease except lung cancer. Melanomas cause most of the deaths from skin cancer. The mean age of those dying from melanomas is less than that of those dying from other skin cancers. There is a trend toward a younger age incidence each year. Primary malignant melanomas may be classified into 6 clinicohistologic types, including lentigo maligna melanoma; superficial spreading malignant melanoma (the most common type, occurring in two-thirds of individuals developing melanoma); nodular malignant melanoma; acral-lentiginous melanomas; malignant melanomas on mucous membranes; and miscellaneous forms such as those arising from blue nevi and congenital and giant nevocytic nevi.

True melanomas vary from macules to nodules, with a surprising play of colors from flesh tints to pitch black and a frequent admixture of white, blue, purple, and red. The border tends to be irregular, and growth may be rapid.

Treatment of melanoma consists of wide excision, with lymph node dissection varying with the depth and location of the lesions and the background of the surgeon. Deaths from melanoma are increasing at a rate of 2% per year for females and 3% for males. Depth of invasion is the single most important prognostic factor (according to Breslow; see Balch reference, below).

**6. Kaposi's sarcoma–**Until recently in the USA, this rare malignant skin lesion was seen mostly in elderly white men, had a chronic clinical course, and was rarely fatal. Kaposi's sarcoma occurs endemically in an often aggressive form in young black men of equatorial Africa, but it is rare in American blacks. Within the past few years, epidemic clusters of Kaposi's sarcoma, predominantly in homosexual men, have been found in various large cities of the USA. Disseminated Kaposi's sarcoma in the homosexual population recurs as one feature of the only partially explained acquired immunodeficiency syndrome (AIDS). The disease has also been described in intravenous drug abusers, patients who have received multiple blood transfusions, and very infrequently in others (see Chapter 22).

The putative cause of AIDS is the AIDS retrovirus (HTLV-III, LAV, ARV; now called HIV [human immunodeficiency virus]). Fever, adenopathy, and gastrointestinal complaints associated with red, purple, or dark plaques or nodules on cutaneous or mucosal surfaces should alert the clinician to the possibility of the disease. Both T and B cell deficiencies have been found.

Management of AIDS-associated Kaposi's sarcoma consists of observation and supportive care for slowly progressive disease; vinblastine, 0.1–0.5 mg/mL intralesionally for cosmetically objectionable lesions; radiation therapy for accessible and space-occupying lesions; and, for progressive disease, intravenous vinblastine or etoposide.

Successful treatment and remission of Kaposi's sarcoma unfortunately do not affect patient survival. In New York City (1984), the median cumulative survival for patients with Kaposi's sarcoma alone was 125 weeks; length of survival was reduced to about half that when there was associated opportunistic infection.

There is no therapy for the underlying immunodeficiency of AIDS (see Chapter 22).

Balch CM: Measuring melanomas: A tribute to Alexander Breslow. *J Am Acad Dermatol* 1981;**5**:96.

Brooks NA: Curettage and shave excision: A tissue-sparing technic for primary cutaneous carcinoma worthy of inclusion in graduate training programs. *J Am Acad Dermatol* 1984;**10**:279.

Dixon SL: Dysplastic nevus syndrome: A clinical review. *Curr Concepts Skin Disorders* (Spring) 1985;**6**:5.

Fauci AS et al: The acquired immunodeficiency syndrome: An update. (NIH Conference) *Ann Intern Med* 1985;**102**:800.

Friedman RJ, Rigel DS, Kopf AW: Early detection of malignant melanoma: The role of physician examination and self-examination of the skin. *CA* (May-June) 1985;**35**:130

Lane HC, Fauci AS: Immunologic reconstitution in the acquired immunodeficiency syndrome. *Ann Intern Med* 1985;**103**:714.

Quinn TC: Perspectives on the future of AIDS. (Editorial.) *JAMA* 1985;**253**:247.

Rivin BE et al: AIDS outcome: A first follow-up. (Letter.) *N Engl J Med* 1984;**311**:857.

Silverberg E, Lubera J: Cancer statistics, 1986. *CA: A Cancer Journal for Clinicians* 1986;**36(Jan/Feb)**:9.

Volberding P et al: Vinblastine therapy for Kaposi's sarcoma in the acquired immunodeficiency syndrome. *Ann Intern Med* 1985;**103**:335.

---

# MISCELLANEOUS SKIN, HAIR, & NAIL DISORDERS

---

## PIGMENTARY DISORDERS

Melanin is formed in the melanocytes in the basal layer of the epidermis. Its precursor, the amino acid tyrosine, is slowly converted to dihydroxyphenylala-nine (dopa) by tyrosinase, and there are many further chemical steps to the ultimate formation of melanin. This system may be affected by external influences such as exposure to sun, heat, trauma, ionizing radiation, heavy metals, and changes in oxygen potential. These influences may result in hyperpigmentation, hypopigmentation, or both. Local trauma may destroy melanocytes temporarily or permanently, causing hypopigmentation, sometimes with surrounding hyperpigmentation as in eczema and dermatitis. Hypermelanosis appears to be associated with increased plasma immunoreactive $\beta$-MSH (melanocyte-stimulating hormone from the pituitary) only in Addison's disease. Melatonin, a pineal hormone, regulates pigment dispersion and aggregation.

Other pigmentary disorders include those resulting from exposure to exogenous pigments such as carotenemia, argyria, deposition of other metals, and tattooing. Other endogenous pigmentary disorders are attributable to metabolic substances, including hemosiderin (iron), in purpuric processes and in hemochromatosis; mercaptans, homogentisic acid (ochronosis), bile pigments, and carotenes.

### Classification

Pigmentary disorders may be classified as primary or secondary and as hyperpigmentary or hypopigmentary.

**A. Primary Pigmentary Disorders:** These are nevoid or congenital, and include pigmented nevi, Mongolian spots, and incontinentia pigmenti, vitiligo, albinism, and piebaldism. In vitiligo, pigment cells (melanocytes) are destroyed. The greater the pigment loss, the fewer the number of melanocytes. At the borders of lesions, the melanocytes are often large and have long dendritic processes, and they resemble pigment cells in tissue cultures that are blocked in the G phase of the cell cycle. Loss of pigment surrounding nevi, and in melanomas, may represent immune responses. Vitiligo, found in approximately 1% of the population, may be associated with hyperthyroidism and hypothyroidism, pernicious anemia, diabetes mellitus, addisonism, and carcinoma of the stomach. Albinism, partial or total, occurs as a genetically determined recessive trait. Piebaldism, a localized hypomelanosis, is an autosomal dominant trait.

**B. Secondary Pigmentary Disorders:** Hyper or hypopigmentation may occur following overexposure to sunlight or heat or as a result of excoriation or direct physical injury. Hyperpigmentation occurs in arsenical melanosis or in association with Addison's disease (due to lack of the inhibitory influence of hydrocortisone on the production of MSH by the pituitary gland). Several disorders of clinical importance are as follows:

**1. Melasma–**This occurs as patterned hyperpigmentation of the face. The localized pigmentation of chloasma may be a direct effect of certain steroid hormones, estrogens, and progesterones in predisposed clones of melanocytes. It occurs not only during pregnancy but also in 30–50% of women taking oral contraceptives.

**2. Berloque hyperpigmentation** can be provoked by phototoxicity from essential oils in perfumes, and these should be excluded wherever possible.

**3. Leukoderma,** or secondary depigmentation, may complicate atopic dermatitis, lichen planus, psoriasis, alopecia areata, lichen simplex chronicus, and such systemic conditions as myxedema, thyrotoxicosis, syphilis, and toxemias. It may follow local skin trauma of various sorts or may complicate dermatitis due to exposure to gold or arsenic. Antioxidants in rubber goods, such as monobenzyl ether of hydroquinone, cause leukoderma from the wearing of gauntlet gloves, rubber pads in brassieres, etc. This is most likely to occur in blacks.

**4. Ephelides** (juvenile freckles) and **lentigines** (senile freckles)–The number of functioning melanocytes decreases by about 10% per decade. The loss is often blotchy, particularly in areas of solar degeneration. Compensatory hypertrophy of some melanocytes gives rise to lentigines.

**5. Drugs**–Pigmentation may be produced by chloroquine, chlorpromazine, minocycline, and amiodarone.

### Differential Diagnosis

One must distinguish true lack of pigment from pseudoachromia, such as occurs in tinea versicolor, pityriasis simplex, and seborrheic dermatitis. It may be difficult to differentiate true vitiligo from leukoderma and even from partial albinism.

### Complications

Solar keratoses and epitheliomas are more likely to develop in persons with vitiligo and albinism. Vitiligo tends to cause pruritus in anogenital folds. There may be severe emotional trauma in extensive vitiligo and other types of hypo- and hyperpigmentations, particularly when they occur in naturally dark-skinned persons.

### Treatment & Prognosis

There is no increase of pigment in partial or total albinism; return of pigment is rare in vitiligo; in leukoderma, repigmentation may occur spontaneously. Therapy of vitiligo is long and tedious. The patient must be strongly motivated. If less than 20% of the skin is involved (most cases), topical methoxsalen, 0.1% in ethanol and propylene glycol or in Acid Mantle cream or Unibase, is used, with cautious exposure to long-wavelength ultraviolet light (UVA), followed by thorough washing, application of an SPF 15 sunscreen, and wearing of UVA-protective goggles for 48 hours. With 20–25% involvement, oral methoxsalen, 0.6 mg/kg 2 hours before UVA exposure, is best. Severe phototoxic response may occur with topical or oral psoralens plus UVA. For more than 50% skin involvement, the use of 20% monobenzone cream to totally depigment the skin has been reported.

Potent topical corticosteroids have been advocated for the treatment of vitiligo. Betamethasone dipropionate ointment may be rubbed thoroughly into the moistened skin once daily for 10 days, followed by 10 days' rest, then repetition, over a period of time. Caution must be exercised, especially on the face and on thin skin, to avoid pseudoatrophy and other changes.

Localized ephelides and lentigines may be destroyed by careful application of a saturated solution of liquid phenol on a tightly wound cotton applicator, or by brief application of liquid nitrogen. Chloasma and other forms of hyperpigmentation may be treated by protecting the skin from the sun and with cosmetics such as Covermark or Maxafil. Cosmetics containing perfumes should not be used.

Bleaching preparations generally contain hydroquinone or its derivatives. This is not without hazard, and it is best to start with the weakest preparation offered by the manufacturer. The use of this kind of bleach may result in unexpected hypopigmentation, hyperpigmentation, and even ochronosis and pigmented milia, particularly with prolonged use.

Treatment of other pigmentary disorders should be directed toward avoidance of the causative agent if possible (as in carotenemia) or treatment of the underlying disorder. Melasma, ephelides, and postinflammatory hyperpigmentation may be treated with 3–4% hydroquinone solution or cream and a sunscreen with an SPF of 15. Tretinoin cream, 0.05%, may be added. The superficial melasma responds well, but if there is predominantly dermal deposition of pigment, the prognosis is poor. Senile lentigines are resistant.

Azelaic acid, 15% cream, is described as beneficial for melasma and postinflammatory hyperpigmentation. This is investigational.

Breathnach AS, Nazzaro-Porro M, Passi S: Azelaic acid. (Comment.) *Br J Dermatol* 1984;**111**:115.

Fisher AA: Hydroquinone uses and abnormal reactions. *Cutis* 1983;**31**:240.

Kenney JA Jr., Grimes P: How we treat vitiligo. *Cutis* 1983;**32**:347.

## BALDNESS (Alopecia)

### Baldness Due to Scarring

Cicatricial baldness may occur following chemical or physical trauma, lichen planopilaris, severe bacterial or fungal infections, severe herpes zoster, chronic discoid lupus erythematosus, scleroderma, and excessive ionizing radiation. The specific cause is often suggested by the history, the distribution of hair loss, and the appearance of the skin, as in lupus erythematosus and other infections. Biopsy may be necessary to differentiate lupus from the others.

Scarring alopecias are irreversible and permanent. There is no treatment, except for surgical hair transplants.

## Baldness Not Due to Scarring

Noncicatricial baldness may be classified according to distribution as alopecia universalis (generalized total hair loss), alopecia totalis (complete scalp hair loss), and alopecia areata (patchy baldness).

Nonscarring alopecia may occur in association with various **systemic diseases** such as systemic disseminated lupus erythematosus, cachexia, lymphomas, uncontrolled diabetes, severe thyroid or pituitary hypofunction, and dermatomyositis. The only treatment necessary is prompt and adequate control of the underlying disorder, in which case hair loss may be reversible.

**Male pattern baldness,** the most common form of alopecia, is of genetic predetermination. The earliest changes occur at the anterior portions of the calvarium on either side of the "widow's peak." Associated seborrhea is evident as excessive oiliness and erythema of the scalp, with scaling. Premature loss of hair in a young adult male may give rise to a severe neurotic reaction. The extent of hair loss is variable and unpredictable. Investigative studies are under way regarding topical use of minoxidil in 1–5% concentrations or less for alopecia areata and androgenetic alopecia. Results are encouraging, and the commercial product, Rogaine, should be available in late 1987. Response takes several months. Clinical use is unwarranted at this time. Seborrhea may be treated as described on p 63.

Hair loss or thinning of the hair in women results from the same common baldness that affects men (androgenic alopecia). Treatment is aimed at antagonizing the follicular effects of androgens. Cyproterone acetate is the only widely available antiandrogen in Europe; it is not available in the USA. Spironolactone, a synthetic steroidal aldosterone antagonist, has been used successfully for the treatment of diffuse hair loss in women (androgenetic alopecia) in a dose of 25 mg daily by mouth. This is not a listed indication for the drug, which has been shown to be a tumorigen in long-term toxicity studies in rats. Oral corticosteroids have been recommended to suppress adrenal androgen production; give prednisolone, 2.5–7.5 mg/d plus oral antiandrogens. There are no well-documented studies to prove the efficacy of these approaches. Topical estrogens are of occasional value.

Women who complain of thin hair but show little evidence of alopecia may have unrelated psychiatric difficulties that would explain this disproportionate anxiety.

**Telogen effluvium** may be the cause of temporary hair loss in some women. A transitory increase occurs in the number of hairs in the telogen (resting) phase of the hair growth cycle. This may occur spontaneously, may appear at the termination of pregnancy, may be precipitated by "crash dieting" or malnutrition, or may be provoked by hormonal contraceptives, especially the monophasic contraceptives. Whatever the cause, telogen effluvium usually has a latent period of 2–4 months. The prognosis is generally good. If an abnormally high proportion of telogen hairs is present before taking the contraceptive, lasting improvement in hair growth may be expected. In one study, the only cause of telogen effluvium was found to be iron deficiency, and the hair counts bore a clear relationship to serum iron levels.

**Alopecia areata** is of unknown cause. Histopathologically, there are numerous small anagen hairs and a lymphocytic infiltrate. The bare patches may be perfectly smooth, or a few hairs may remain. Severe forms may be treated by systemic corticosteroid therapy, although systemic therapy is rarely justified unless the disease is of serious emotional or economic significance.

Anthralin, 0.5% ointment applied daily, may provoke hair growth (*caution*). Intralesional corticosteroids are frequently effective. Triamcinolone acetonide, in a concentration of 5 mg/mL, is injected in aliquots of 0.1 mL at approximately 1- to 2-cm intervals, not exceeding a total dose of 50 mg per month for adults. Alopecia areata is usually self-limiting, with complete regrowth of hair, but some mild cases are permanent and the extensive forms are usually permanent, as are the totalis and universalis types. Both topical dinitrochlorobenzene (DNCB) and an experimental topical allergen, squaric acid dibutyl ester, have been used to treat persistent alopecia areata. The principle is to sensitize the skin, then intermittently apply weaker concentrations to produce and maintain a slight dermatitis. Hair regrowth in 3–6 months in some patients has been reported to be remarkable. Long-term safety and efficacy have not been established.

New contact allergens are being sought to replace DNCB for the treatment of alopecia areata, because of the positive Ames test, which has shown that the substance is carcinogenic in laboratory animals. Squaric acid dibutyl ester and diphencyprone apparently are as effective as DNCB.

Minoxidil, a peripheral vasodilator given orally for hypertension, causes hypertrichosis in 80% of users. Trials with topical minoxidil in a water, ethanol, and propylene glycol vehicle have been performed with 1%, 3%, and 5% solutions applied twice daily to the scalp. Benefit is slow, and some hair regrowth occurs in a minority of patients treated for alopecia areata or androgenetic hair loss. The treatment is experimental but looks promising. It is expected that the FDA will approve minoxidil for the topical treatment of alopecia in late 1987.

Cataracts may complicate extensive alopecia areata.

In **trichotillomania** (the pulling out of one's own hair), the patches of hair loss are irregular, and growing hairs are always present, since they cannot be pulled out until they are long enough.

**Drug-induced alopecia** is becoming increasingly important. Such drugs include thallium, excessive and prolonged use of vitamin A, antimitotic agents, anticoagulants, clofibrate (rarely), antithyroid drugs, oral contraceptives, trimethadione, allopurinol, propranolol, indomethacin, amphetamines, salicylates, gentamicin, and levodopa.

Fiedler-Weiss VC et al: Topical minoxidil dose-response effect in alopecia areata. *Arch Dermatol* 1986;**122**:180.

Nelson DA, Spielvogel RL: Alopecia areata: A review. *Int J Dermatol* 1985;**24**:26.

Unapproved use of minoxidil: *FDA Drug Bulletin* (December) 1985;**15**:38.

## HIRSUTISM

Hirsutism is not curable except in rare surgically treatable Cushing's syndrome, prolactinoma, or androgen-secreting tumors of ovary or adrenal glands. Androgen levels can be reduced by a low-dose corticosteroid, eg, prednisolone, 5 mg nightly and 2.5 mg in the morning, or dexamethasone (not as good for suppression). A combined estrogen and nonandrogenic progestogen may help. However, these chemical treatments do not often suppress terminal hair growth enough to justify the long-term side effects. Dark facial and abdominal hair may be bleached with 5% hydrogen peroxide solution or commercial preparations, and hair removal may be done with chemical depilatories (*caution*) or by electrolysis.

Spironolactone, which is tumorigenic in rats, is effective in treating hirsutism in women in a dose of 200 mg/d. Hirsutism is not a listed indication for spironolactone, and the dose is relatively high.

Screening tests for hirsutism include levels of serum testosterone, androstenedione (peripheral conversion of which accounts for 40–60% of circulating testosterone levels), luteinizing and follicle-stimulating hormones, and prolactin. Second-line tests might include dexamethasone suppression, ovarian ultrasound scan, adrenal CT scan, pituitary fossa x-ray, and visual field tests.

Rentoul J: Management of the hirsute woman. *Int J Dermatol* 1983;**22**:265.

## KELOIDS & HYPERTROPHIC SCARS

Keloids are tumors consisting of actively growing fibrous tissue and occur as a result of trauma or irritation in predisposed persons, especially those of dark-skinned races. The trauma may be relatively trivial, such as an acne lesion. Keloids behave as neoplasms, although they are not malignant. Spontaneous digitations may project from the central growth, and the tumors may become large and disfiguring. There may be itching and burning sensations with both types of tumor.

Hypertrophic scars, usually seen following surgery or accidental trauma, tend to be raised, red, and indurated. After a few months or longer, they lose their redness and become soft and flat. Removal should not be attempted until all induration has subsided.

Intralesional injection of a corticosteroid suspension is effective against hypertrophic scars. The treatment of keloids is less satisfactory; surgical excision, x-ray therapy, and freezing with liquid nitrogen are used, as well as injection of corticosteroid suspensions into the lesions. They tend to involute in older age groups.

Keloids can be removed with carbon dioxide laser excision. Ring block anesthesia is accomplished with 1% lidocaine with epinephrine 1:200,000. The bulk of keloidal tissue is removed, using the focused mode to perform a shave excision. The base of the wound is palpated to remove residual areas of firmness, and the base is injected with triamcinolone acetonide suspension, 40 mg/mL. The wound is allowed to heal by granulation.

Wheeland RG, Bailin PL: Dermatologic application of the argon and carbon dioxide lasers. *Curr Concepts Skin Disorders* (Summer) 1984;**5**:5.

## NAIL DISORDERS
## (See also Candidal Onychomycosis, above.)

Nail changes are generally not diagnostic of a specific systemic or cutaneous disease. All of the nail manifestations of systemic disorders may be seen also in the absence of any systemic illness.

Nail dystrophies cannot usually be related to changes in thyroid function, hypovitaminosis, nutritional disturbances, or generalized allergic reactions.

### Classification

Nail disorders may be classified as (1) local, (2) congenital or genetic, and (3) those associated with systemic or generalized skin diseases.

**A. Local Nail Disorders:**

**1. Onycholysis** (distal separation of the nail plate from the nail bed, usually of the fingers) is caused by excess exposure to water, soaps, detergents, alkalies, and industrial keratolytic agents. Nail hardeners and demeclocycline may cause onycholysis. Hyper- and hypothyroidism are said to play a part.

**2. Distortion of the nail** occurs as a result of chronic inflammation of the nail matrix underlying the eponychial fold.

**3. Discoloration and pithy changes,** accompanied by a musty odor, are seen in ringworm infection.

**4. Grooving** and other changes may be caused by warts, nevi, synovial cysts, etc, impinging on the nail matrix.

**5. Allergic reactions** (to formaldehyde and resins in undercoats and polishes) involving the nail bed or matrix formerly caused hemorrhagic streaking of the nails, accumulation of keratin under the free margins of the nails, and great tenderness of the nail beds.

**6. Beau's lines** (transverse furrows) may be due to faulty manicuring.

**7. Onychogryphosis,** usually involving the nails of the great toes, is characterized by grossly distorted, hypertrophic, and misshapen nails. The disorder may respond to correction of chronic edema associated with stasis dermatitis, stasis ulcers, and other conditions of the lower extremities that are adversely affected by gravitational factors.

**B. Congenital and Genetic Nail Disorders:**

**1. A longitudinal single nail groove** may occur as a result of a genetic or traumatic defect in the nail matrix underlying the eponychial fold.

**2. Nail atrophy** may be congenital.

**3. Clubbed fingers** may be congenital.

**C. Nail Changes Associated With Systemic or Generalized Skin Diseases:**

**1. Beau's lines** (transverse furrows) may follow any serious systemic illness.

**2. Atrophy of the nails** may be related to trauma or vascular or neurologic disease.

**3. Clubbed fingers** may be due to the prolonged hypoxemia associated with cardiopulmonary disorders.

**4. Spoon nails** may be seen in anemic patients.

**5. Stippling or pitting of the nails** is seen in psoriasis.

**6. Nail changes** may be seen also with alopecia areata, lichen planus, and keratosis follicularis.

## Differential Diagnosis

It is important to distinguish congenital and genetic disorders from those caused by trauma and environmental disorders. Nail changes due to dermatophyte fungi may be difficult to differentiate from onychia due to *Candida* infections. Direct microscopic examination of a specimen cleared with 15% potassium hydroxide, or culture on Sabouraud's medium, may be diagnostic. Onychomycosis may be closely similar to the changes seen in psoriasis and lichen planus, in which case careful observation of more characteristic lesions elsewhere on the body is essential to the diagnosis of the nail disorders. Suspect malignancy with any persistent solitary subungual or periungual lesion.

## Complications

Secondary bacterial infection occasionally occurs in onychodystrophies and leads to considerable pain and disability and possibly more serious consequences if circulation or innervation is impaired. Toenail changes may lead to an ingrown nail, in turn often complicated by bacterial infection and occasionally by exuberant granulation tissue. Poor manicuring and poorly fitting shoes may contribute to this complication. Cellulitis may result.

## Treatment & Prognosis

Treatment consists usually of careful debridement and manicuring and, above all, reduction of exposure to irritants (soaps, detergents, alkali, bleaches, solvents, etc). Antifungal measures may be used in the case of onychomycosis and candidal onychia; antibacterial measures may be used for bacterial complications. Congenital or genetic nail disorders are usually uncorrectable. Longitudinal grooving due to temporary lesions of the matrix, such as warts, synovial cysts, and other impingements, may be cured by removal of the offending lesion. Intradermal triamcinolone acetonide suspension, 2.5 mg/mL, may be injected in the area of the nail matrix at intervals of 2–4 weeks for the successful management of various types of nail dystrophies (psoriasis, lichen planus, onycholysis, longitudinal splitting, grooving from synovial cysts, and others).

If it is necessary to remove nails for any reason (eg, fungal nails or severe psoriasis), one may apply urea 40%, anhydrous lanolin 20%, white wax 5%, white petrolatum 25%, and silica gel type H. The nail folds are painted with compound tincture of benzoin and then covered with cloth adhesive tape. Apply the urea ointment generously to the nail surface, and cover with plastic film and then adhesive tape. Avoid water. Leave the ointment on for 5–10 days; then lift off the nail plate. Medication can then be applied that is appropriate for the condition being treated.

South DA, Farber EM: Urea ointment in the nonsurgical avulsion of nail dystrophies. *Cutis* 1980;**25**:609.

Stone OJ: Resolution of onychogryphosis. *Cutis* 1984;**34**:480.

## REFERENCES

Arndt KA: *Manual of Dermatologic Therapeutics With Essentials of Diagnosis,* 3rd ed. Little, Brown, 1983.

Braverman IM: *Skin Signs of Systemic Disease,* 2nd ed. Saunders, 1981.

Burgdorf WHC et al: *Dermatopathology.* Springer-Verlag, 1984.

Domonkos AN, Arnold HL Jr, Odom RB: *Andrews' Diseases of the Skin.* Saunders, 1982.

Fitzpatrick TB et al: *Dermatology in General Medicine.* 3rd ed. McGraw-Hill, 1987.

Landow RK: *Handbook of Dermatologic Treatment.* Jones Medical Publications, 1983.

Lever WF, Schaumberg-Lever G: *Histopathology of the Skin,* 6th ed. Lippincott, 1983.

Moschella SL, Hurley HJ: *Dermatology,* 2nd ed. 2 vols. Saunders, 1985.

Pinkus H, Mehregan AH: *A Guide to Dermatohistopathology,* 3rd ed. Appleton-Century-Crofts, 1981.

Sherertz EF, Flowers FP: Rational use of topical corticosteroids. *Am Fam Physician* (Jan) 1984;**29**:262.

Taylor JS et al: Environmental reactions to chemical, physical, and biologic agents. *J Am Acad Dermatol* 1984;**11(5–Part 2):**1007.

# 5

# Eye

*Daniel Vaughan, MD*

## NONSPECIFIC MANIFESTATIONS OF EYE DISEASES

### Redness

Redness is the most frequently encountered symptom in ocular disorders. It is due to hyperemia of the conjunctival, episcleral, or ciliary vessels. Redness is caused by irritation, infection, inflammation, trauma, tumors, dryness, or increased intraocular pressure (Table 5–1).

### Dryness

Scratchiness, itching, and burning due to dryness of the eye are common complaints of older people, but they may occur as any age. These symptoms may be due to many causes, including dry environment, local ocular disease, systemic disorders, and drugs that lead to a deficiency of any of the tear film components. (See p 99.)

### Pain

Ocular pain may be caused by trauma (chemical, mechanical, or physical), infection, inflammation, or sudden increase in intraocular pressure. Common eye disorders that cause pain include corneal injuries, foreign bodies, infections, iritis, and acute glaucoma.

### Conjunctival Discharge

Discharge is usually caused by bacterial or viral conjunctivitis. A purulent discharge usually indicates bacterial infection. If the discharge is watery and is accompanied by photophobia or burning, viral conjunctivitis or keratoconjunctivitis may be present.

Obstruction of the lacrimal drainage system may also cause tearing, and infections of the lacrimal sac may lead to purulent discharge. Allergic conjunctivitis usually causes tearing and ropy discharge associated with itching. Any disruption of the corneal surface causes tearing.

### Visual Impairment & Blindness

An individual may be considered to be visually impaired if the best corrected distant visual acuity in the better eye is less than 20/70 (6/21) or if visual fields are significantly restricted. Legal blindness (partial) in the USA is defined for practical purposes as visual acuity for distant vision of 20/200 (6/60) or less in the better eye with best correction, or widest diameter of the visual field subtending an angle of less than 20 degrees. WHO estimates that at least 10 million of the world's population are totally blind, and millions more have loss of sight sufficient to interfere with normal living.

A wide variety of causative factors, including infection, malnutrition, toxins, degenerative changes, immunologic reactions, neoplasms, hereditary factors, and trauma that may involve any portion of the visual apparatus, can result in visual impairment. The most frequent causes of preventable blindness in the world are trachoma, leprosy, onchocerciasis, and xerophthalmia. Glaucoma, diabetic retinopathy, and other retinal disorders (many of which are related to the aging process) are leading causes of blindness in the USA and Western world. There are approximately 500,000 legally blind persons in the USA; about half are over age 65.

### Blurred Vision

The most important causes of blurred vision are refractive error, corneal opacities, cataract, vitreous clouding, hemorrhage, retinal detachment, macular degeneration, central retinal vein thrombosis, central retinal artery occlusion, optic neuritis, and optic atrophy.

### "Eyestrain"

This is a common ocular complaint that usually means eye discomfort associated with prolonged reading or close work. Significant refractive error, early presbyopia, inadequate illumination, or phoria (usually exophoria with poor convergence) should be ruled out.

### Photophobia

Photophobia is commonly due to corneal inflammation, aphakia, iritis, and albinism. A less common cause is fever associated with viral infections (eg, influenza, dengue, pneumonia), which characteristically produces aching of the eyes along with photophobia.

### "Spots Before the Eyes"

"Spots" are vitreous opacities that usually have no clinical significance though in some cases they signify impending retinal detachment or posterior uveitis.

**Table 5–1.** Differential diagnosis of common causes of inflamed eye.

| | Acute Conjunctivitis | Acute Iritis* | Acute Glaucoma† | Corneal Trauma or Infection |
|---|---|---|---|---|
| Incidence | Extremely common | Common | Uncommon | Common |
| Discharge | Moderate to copious | None | None | Watery or purulent |
| Vision | No effect on vision | Slightly blurred | Markedly blurred | Usually blurred |
| Pain | None | Moderate | Severe | Moderate to severe |
| Conjunctival injection | Diffuse; more toward fornices | Mainly circumcorneal | Diffuse | Diffuse |
| Cornea | Clear | Usually clear | Steamy | Clarity change related to cause |
| Pupil size | Normal | Small | Moderately dilated and fixed | Normal |
| Pupillary light response | Normal | Poor | None | Normal |
| Intraocular pressure | Normal | Normal | Elevated | Normal |
| Smear | Causative organisms | No organisms | No organisms | Organisms found only in corneal ulcers due to infection |

\* Acute anterior uveitis.
† Angle-closure glaucoma.

## Headache

Headache is only occasionally due to ocular disorders. The causes of ocular headache are in general the same as those of "eyestrain" (above).

## Diplopia

Double vision results from extraocular muscle imbalance. This may be caused by involvement of the third, fourth, or sixth cranial nerve by head injury, vascular disturbance, intracranial tumor, meningitis, or demyelination. Direct involvement of muscle, as in thyroid myopathy, or entrapment, as a result of orbital blow-out fracture, also results in diplopia.

## Proptosis (Exophthalmos)

The most frequent cause of proptosis in the adult is thyroid disease. Other causes of (usually unilateral) proptosis include orbital tumors and inflammatory disorders, hemorrhage, cysts, and cavernous sinus syndrome.

## OCULAR EMERGENCIES*

## SUDDEN LOSS OF VISION

Sudden loss of vision is a serious symptom requiring emergency ophthalmologic consultation. Some of the most important causes include occlusion of the central retinal artery or central retinal vein, vascular occlusion associated with giant cell arteritis, retinal detachment, and retinal or vitreous hemorrhage from any cause, especially if the macula is involved. Optic

\* Ophthalmologic consultation should be considered for all patients with ocular emergencies.

neuritis may also cause sudden and alarming visual loss. Many of these disorders are treatable and require immediate consultation.

## ACUTE (ANGLE-CLOSURE) GLAUCOMA

Acute glaucoma can occur only with the closure of a preexisting narrow anterior chamber angle. If the pupil dilates spontaneously or is dilated with a mydriatic or cycloplegic, the angle will close and an attack of acute glaucoma is precipitated; for this reason, it is a wise precaution to examine the anterior chamber angle before instilling these drugs. Dilation of the pupil should be avoided if the anterior chamber is shallow (readily determined by oblique illumination of the anterior segment of the eye). About 1% of people over age 35 have narrow anterior chamber angles, but many of these never develop acute glaucoma; thus, the condition is very uncommon.

A quiet eye with a narrow anterior chamber angle may convert spontaneously to angle-closure glaucoma. The process can be precipitated by anything that will dilate the pupil, eg, indiscriminate use of mydriatics or cycloplegics by the patient or the physician. The cycloplegic can be administered in the form of eye drops or systemically, eg, by an anesthetist ordering scopolamine or atropine in preparation for general anesthesia, or by a physician prescribing an atropinelike drug for any disorder. Increased circulating epinephrine in times of stress can also dilate the pupil and cause acute glaucoma. Sitting in a darkened movie theater can have the same effect.

Patients with acute glaucoma seek treatment immediately because of extreme pain and blurred vision. The eye is red, the cornea steamy, and the pupil is moderately dilated and nonreactive to light. Tonometry reveals elevated intraocular pressure.

Acute glaucoma must be differentiated from conjunctivitis, acute iritis, and corneal abrasion.

Laser or surgical peripheral iridectomy within 12–48 hours after onset of symptoms will usually result in a permanent cure. The fellow eye should have prophylactic laser iridectomy. Untreated acute glaucoma results in complete and permanent blindness within 2–5 days after onset of symptoms. Before surgery, the intraocular pressure must be lowered by miotics (pilocarpine, 4%) instilled locally and osmotic agents and carbonic anhydrase inhibitors administered systemically.

Three different osmotic agents (urea, mannitol, and glycerol) are available for lowering intraocular pressure preoperatively in angle-closure glaucoma. Urea and mannitol are administered intravenously, and glycerol is given orally. The usual dosage of all 3 of these osmotic drugs is 1.5 g/kg. Intravenous acetazolamide (Diamox), 500 mg, may also be used.

Behrendt T: Eye emergencies: Treatment. *Fam Pract Recertification* (July) 1982;**4**:23.

Keltner J: Giant cell arteritis. *Ophthalmology* 1982;**89**:1101.

Kolker AE, Hetherington J: *Becker-Shaffer's Diagnosis and Therapy of the Glaucomas,* 5th ed. Mosby, 1983.

McDonnell PJ et al: Temporal arteritis: A clinicopathologic study. *Ophthalmology* 1986;**93**:518.

## FOREIGN BODIES

If a patient complains of "something in my eye" and gives a consistent history, a foreign body is usually present on the cornea or under the upper lid even though it may not be readily visible. Almost all foreign bodies can be seen under oblique illumination with the aid of a hand flashlight and loupe.

Note the time, place, and other circumstances of the accident. Test visual acuity before treatment is instituted as a basis for comparison in the event of complications.

### Conjunctival Foreign Body

Foreign body of the upper tarsal conjunctiva is suggested by pain and blepharospasm of sudden onset in the presence of a clear cornea and by less pain on blinking when the eye is turned (right or left) so that the cornea is away from the foreign body location. After instilling a local anesthetic, evert the lid by grasping the lashes gently and exerting pressure on the mid portion of the outer surface of the upper lid with an applicator. If a foreign body is present, it can be easily removed by passing a sterile wet cotton applicator across the conjunctival surface.

### Corneal Foreign Body

When a corneal foreign body is suspected but is not apparent on simple inspection, instill fluorescein into the conjunctival sac and examine the cornea with the aid of a magnifying device and strong illumination. The foreign body may then be removed with a sterile wet cotton applicator. An antibiotic should be instilled, eg, gentamicin ointment. It is not necessary to patch the eye, but the patient must be examined 24 hours later for secondary infection of the crater. If a corneal foreign body cannot be removed in this manner, it should be removed by an ophthalmologist. Steel foreign bodies usually leave a diffuse rust ring. This requires excision of the affected tissue and is best done under local anesthesia using a slit lamp. *Caution:* Anesthetic drops should not be given to the patient for self-administration. If there is no infection, a layer of corneal epithelial cells will line the crater within 24 hours. It should be emphasized that the intact corneal epithelium forms an effective barrier to infection. Once the corneal epithelium is disturbed, the cornea becomes extremely susceptible to infection.

Early infection is manifested by a white necrotic area around the crater and a small amount of gray exudate. These patients should be referred immediately to an ophthalmologist.

Untreated corneal infection may lead to severe corneal ulceration, panophthalmitis, and loss of the eye.

### Intraocular Foreign Body

A patient with an intraocular foreign body should be referred immediately to an ophthalmologist. With delay, the ocular media become progressively more cloudy, and a foreign body visible shortly after the injury may not be visible several hours later. The foreign body can often be removed with a magnet through the point of entry or through an incision in the sclera near its site of lodgment.

Brinton GS et al: Posttraumatic endophthalmitis. *Arch Ophthalmol* 1984;**102**:68.

Holt JE, Holt GR, Blodgett JM: Ocular injuries sustained during blunt facial trauma. *Ophthalmology* 1983;**90**:14.

Penna EP, Tabbara KF: Oxybuprocaine keratopathy: A preventable disease. *Br J Ophthalmol* 1986;**70**:202.

## CORNEAL ABRASIONS

A patient with a corneal abrasion complains of severe pain and photophobia.

Record the history and visual acuity. Examine the cornea and conjunctiva with a light and loupe to rule out a foreign body. If an abrasion is suspected but cannot be seen, instill sterile fluorescein into the conjunctival sac; the area of corneal abrasion will stain a deeper green than the surrounding cornea.

Instill gentamicin ophthalmic ointment and apply a bandage with firm pressure to prevent movement of the lid. The patient should rest at home, keeping the fellow eye closed, and should be observed on the following day to be certain that the cornea has healed. Recurrent corneal erosion may follow corneal abrasions, and all such cases should be referred to an ophthalmologist.

## CONTUSIONS

Contusion injuries of the eye and surrounding structures may cause ecchymosis (''black eye''), subconjunctival hemorrhage, edema or rupture of the cornea, hemorrhage into the anterior chamber (hyphema), rupture of the root of the iris (iridodialysis), paralysis of the pupillary sphincter, paralysis of the muscles of accommodation, cataract, subluxation or luxation of the lens, vitreous hemorrhage, retinal hemorrhage and edema (most common in the macular area), detachment of the retina, rupture of the choroid, fracture of the orbital floor (''blowout fracture''), and optic nerve injury. Many of these injuries are immediately apparent; others may not become apparent for days or weeks. Patients with moderate to severe contusions should be seen by an ophthalmologist.

Any injury severe enough to cause hyphema involves the danger of secondary hemorrhage, which may cause intractable glaucoma with permanent visual loss. Any patient with traumatic hyphema should be put at bed rest for 6–7 days with both eyes bandaged to lessen the chance of secondary hemorrhage. Secondary hemorrhage rarely occurs after this time. Aminocaproic acid given orally may reduce the incidence of secondary hemorrhage.

Archer DB: Injuries of the posterior segment of the eye. *Trans Ophthalmol Soc UK* 1985;**104:**597.

Hutton WL: Factors influencing final visual results in severely injured eyes. *Am J Ophthalmol* 1984;**97:**715.

Palmer DJ et al: A comparison of two dose regimens of epsilon aminocaproic acid in the prevention and management of secondary traumatic hyphema. *Ophthalmology* 1986;**93:**102.

Vinger PF: Sports eye injuries: A preventable disease. *Ophthalmology* 1981;**88:**108.

## ULTRAVIOLET KERATITIS
### (Actinic Keratitis)

Ultraviolet burns of the cornea are usually caused by use of an ultraviolet sunlamp without proper eye protection, exposure to a welding arc, or exposure to the sun when skiing (''snow blindness''). There are no immediate symptoms, but about 6–12 hours later the patient complains of agonizing pain and severe photophobia. Slit lamp examination after instillation of sterile fluorescein shows diffuse punctate staining of both corneas.

Treatment consists of binocular patching, instillation of cycloplegic agents, systemic analgesics, and sedatives as indicated. All patients recover within 24–48 hours without complications. Local anesthetics should not be prescribed.

## CORNEAL ULCER

Corneal ulcers constitute a medical emergency. The typical gray, necrotic corneal ulcer may be pre-

ceded by trauma, usually a corneal foreign body. A modern cause of corneal ulceration is the soft continuous-wear contact lens. Some of these lenses tend to harbor organisms (like a sponge) and prevent proper corneal oxygenation. The eye is red, with lacrimation and conjunctival discharge, and the patient complains of blurred vision, pain, and photophobia.

Prompt treatment is essential to help prevent complications. Visual impairment may occur as a result of corneal scarring or intraocular infection.

Corneal ulcers have many causes, including bacterial, viral, and fungal infections and allergic disorders. Only the most common types will be discussed here.

### Pneumococcal ("Acute Serpiginous") Ulcer

*Streptococcus pneumoniae* is a common bacterial cause of corneal ulcer. The early ulcer is gray and fairly well circumscribed; hypopyon is often present.

Since the pneumococcus is sensitive both to sulfonamides and to several antibiotics, local therapy is usually effective. However, the commonly used broad-spectrum aminoglycosides gentamicin and tobramycin are not generally effective against *S pneumoniae*. If untreated, the cornea may perforate. Concurrent dacryocystitis, if present, should also be treated; later, dacryocystorhinostomy must be considered to prevent recurrence of the ulcer.

### *Pseudomonas* Ulcer

A common and devastating cause of corneal ulcer is *Pseudomonas aeruginosa*. The ulceration characteristically starts in a traumatized area and spreads rapidly, often causing perforation of the cornea and loss of the eye within 48 hours. *P aeruginosa* usually produces a pathognomonic bluish-green pigment.

Early diagnosis and vigorous treatment with local application and subconjunctival injection of antibiotics (tobramycin, gentamicin, carbenicillin, colistin) are essential to save the eye.

### Herpes Simplex (Dendritic) Keratitis

Corneal ulceration caused by herpes simplex virus is more common than any bacterial ulcer. It is almost always unilateral and may affect any age group of either sex. It is often preceded by upper respiratory tract infection with fever.

The commonest finding is of one or more dendritic ulcers (superficial branching gray areas) on the corneal surface. These are composed of clear vesicles in the corneal epithelium; when the vesicles rupture, the area stains green with fluorescein. Although the dendritic figure is its most characteristic manifestation, herpes simplex keratitis may appear in a number of other configurations.

Treatment consists of removing the virus-containing corneal epithelium without disturbing Bowman's membrane or the corneal stroma. This is best done by an ophthalmologist. *Caution:* Do not give local corticosteroids, as they enhance the activity of the virus by suppressing the local immune mechanisms. This may lead to perforation of the cornea and loss of the eye. (See also Chapter 21.)

Idoxuridine (IUDR; 5-iodo-2'-deoxyuridine) is commonly used against herpes simplex keratitis. It is instilled locally as 0.1% solution.

Trifluridine (Viroptic) and vidarabine (Vira-A) are generally effective in superficial epithelial herpetic infection and have less local toxicity than idoxuridine. Acyclovir (Zovirax), a new agent that is more specific in action, is sometimes effective. A number of ophthalmologists still prefer to remove the affected corneal epithelium mechanically and apply a pressure bandage for a few days until the epithelium regenerates.

Alfonso E et al: *Pseudomonas* corneoscleritis. *Am J Ophthalmol* 1987;**103**:90.

Darougar S, Wishart MS, Viswalingam ND: Epidemiological and clinical features of primary herpes simplex virus ocular infection. *Br J Ophthalmol* 1985;**69**:2.

Holden BA et al: Effects of long-term extended contact lens wear on the human cornea. *Invest Ophthalmol Vis Sci* 1985;**26**:1489.

Hung SO et al: Oral acyclovir in the management of dendritic herpetic corneal ulceration. *Br J Ophthalmol* 1984;**68**:398.

Roberts DStC: Steroids, the eye, and general practitioners. (Editorial.) *Br Med J* 1986;**292**:1414.

Sanitato JJ et al: Acyclovir in the treatment of herpetic stromal disease. *Am J Ophthalmol* 1984;**98**:537.

Smolin G, Tabbara K, Whitcher J: *Infectious Diseases of the Eye.* Williams & Wilkins, 1984.

## CHEMICAL CONJUNCTIVITIS & KERATITIS

Chemical burns are treated by irrigation of the eyes with saline solution or plain water as soon as possible after exposure. Do *not* neutralize an acid with an alkali or vice versa, as the heat generated by the reaction may cause further damage. Alkali injuries are more serious and require prolonged irrigation, since alkalies are not precipitated by the proteins of the eye as are acids. The pupil should be dilated with 0.2% scopolamine or 2% atropine. Complications include mucus deficiency, scarring of the cornea or conjunctiva (or both), symblepharon, tear duct obstruction, and secondary infection. Alkali burns have a poorer prognosis than acid burns.

Pfister RW: Chemical injuries of the eye. *Ophthalmology* 1983;**90**:1246.

## GONOCOCCAL CONJUNCTIVITIS

Gonococcal conjunctivitis, which may cause corneal ulceration, is manifested by a copious purulent discharge. The diagnosis may be confirmed by a stained smear and culture of the discharge. Prompt treatment with both local and systemic penicillin is required (see p 880).

## SYMPATHETIC OPHTHALMIA (Sympathetic Uveitis)

Sympathetic ophthalmia is a rare type of severe bilateral granulomatous uveitis. The cause is not known, but the disease may occur at any time from 1 week to many years after a penetrating injury through the ciliary body. The injured (exciting) eye becomes inflamed first and the fellow (sympathizing) eye second. Symptoms and signs include blurred vision, light sensitivity, and redness.

The best treatment of sympathetic ophthalmia is prevention by enucleating the injured eye. Any severely injured eye (eg, one with perforation of the sclera and ciliary body, with loss of vitreous) can incite sympathetic uveitis. Early enucleation may prevent this. The decision about whether or not enucleation should be performed—and, if so, when—is controversial and requires the most careful consideration. In established cases of sympathetic ophthalmia, systemic corticosteroid therapy may be helpful. Without treatment, the disease progresses gradually to bilateral blindness.

Chan C-C et al: Sympathetic ophthalmia: Immunopathologic findings. *Ophthalmology* 1986;**93**:690.

Sharp DC et al: Sympathetic ophthalmia. *Arch Ophthalmol* 1984;**102**:232.

## LACERATIONS

### Lids

If the lid margin is lacerated, the patient should be referred for specialized care, since permanent notching may result. Lacerations of the lower eyelid near the inner canthus often sever the lower canaliculus. These require treatment by an ophthalmologist to attempt to restore the function of the torn canaliculus. Lid lacerations not involving the margin may be sutured just as any other skin laceration.

### Conjunctiva

In superficial lacerations of the conjunctiva, sutures are not necessary. In order to prevent infection, instill a broad-spectrum antibiotic or sulfonamide into the eye until the laceration is healed.

### Cornea or Sclera

Keep examination and manipulation at an absolute minimum, since pressure may result in extrusion of the intraocular contents. Bandage the eye lightly and cover with a metal shield that rests on the orbital bones above and below. The patient should be instructed not to squeeze the eyes shut and to remain as quiet as possible and should be transferred to an ophthalmologist. Always examine the eye by radiography to exclude the presence of foreign bodies.

de Juan E Jr, Sternberg P Jr, Michels RG: Penetrating ocular injuries: Types of injuries and visual results. *Ophthalmology* 1983;**90:**1318.

## ORBITAL CELLULITIS

Orbital cellulitis is manifested by an abrupt onset of fever, proptosis, and swelling and redness of the lids. It is usually caused by a pyogenic organism. Immediate treatment with systemic antibiotics is indicated to prevent brain abscess. The response to antibiotics is usually excellent. Patients with orbital cellulitis may need to be admitted to the hospital.

Bargin DJ, Wright JE: Orbital cellulitis. *Br J Ophthalmol* 1986;**70:**174.
Check WA: Many misjudge severity of orbital cellulitis. *JAMA* 1982;**247:**1236.
Hornblass A et al: Orbital abscess. *Surv Ophthalmol* 1985;**29:**169.
Weiss A et al: Bacterial periorbital and orbital cellulitis in childhood. *Ophthalmology* 1983;**90:**195.

## VITREOUS HEMORRHAGE

Hemorrhage into the vitreous body may obscure a retinal detachment. Treatment by an ophthalmologist is indicated. The commonest causes of vitreous hemorrhage are diabetic retinopathy, retinal tears, severe hypertension, blood dyscrasias, and trauma.

O'Malley C: Vitreous. Chap 13, pp 151–162, in: Vaughan D, Asbury T: *General Ophthalmology,* Appleton-Lange, 1986.

# COMMON OCULAR DISORDERS

## CONJUNCTIVITIS

Conjunctivitis is the most common eye disease. It may be acute or chronic. Most cases are exogenous and due to bacterial, viral, or chlamydial infection, although endogenous inflammation may occur (eg, phlyctenular conjunctivitis, a delayed hypersensitivity response to circulating tuberculoprotein). Other causes are allergy, chemical irritations, and fungal or parasitic infection. The mode of transmission of infectious conjunctivitis is usually direct contact via fingers, towels, handkerchiefs, etc, to the fellow eye or to other persons.

Conjunctivitis must be differentiated from iritis, glaucoma, corneal trauma, and keratitis.

### Bacterial Conjunctivitis

The organisms found most commonly in bacterial conjunctivitis are *Streptococcus pneumoniae, Staphylococcus aureus,* Koch-Weeks bacillus, and Morax-Axenfeld bacillus. All may produce a copious purulent discharge. Examination of stained conjunctival scrapings for white blood cells and bacteria is helpful; if the disease is purulent or membranous, culture studies are recommended. There is no pain or blurring of vision. The disease is usually self-limited, lasting about 10–14 days if untreated. A sulfonamide (eg, sulfacetamide, 10% ophthalmic solution or ointment) instilled locally 3 times daily will usually clear the infection in 2–3 days. Topical antibiotics are usually to be avoided for minimal infections and limited to those unlikely to be used systemically (see p 106).

### Viral Conjunctivitis

One of the commonest causes of viral conjunctivitis is adenovirus type 3, which is usually associated with pharyngitis, fever, malaise, and preauricular adenopathy. Locally, the palpebral conjunctiva is red, and there is a copious watery discharge and scanty exudate. Children are more often affected than adults, and contaminated swimming pools are sometimes the source of infection. Epidemic keratoconjunctivitis (EKC) is caused by adenovirus types 8 and 19. There is no specific treatment, although local sulfonamide therapy may prevent secondary bacterial infection. The disease usually lasts at least 2 weeks. (See p 852.)

### Keratoconjunctivitis Sicca (Dry Eye Syndrome)

This is a common disorder, particularly in elderly women. The patient complains of dryness, redness, or a scratchy feeling of the eyes. A wide range of conditions predispose to or are characterized by dry eyes. Hypofunction of the lacrimal glands may be due to aging, hereditary disorders, systemic disease (eg, rheumatoid arthritis and other connective tissue disorders), and systemic and topical drugs. Excessive evaporation of tears may be due to environmental exposure (eg, a hot, dry, or windy climate). Mucin deficiency may be due to malnutrition, infection, burns, or drugs.

Treatment depends upon the cause. In most early cases, the corneal and conjunctival epithelial changes are reversible.

Aqueous deficiency can be treated by replacement of the aqueous with various types of artificial tears. Mucin deficiency can be partially compensated for by the use of ophthalmic vehicles of high molecular weight—eg, water-soluble polymers—or by the use of the patient's own serum as local eye drops. Serum used for this purpose must be kept refrigerated at all times. It acts by lowering the surface tension of the tears, assisting in the spreading of the tears, and wetting the epithelium. If the mucus is tenacious, as in Sjögren's syndrome, mucolytic agents (eg, acetylcysteine, 20%) may provide some relief.

Limberg MB et al: Topical application of hyaluronic acid and chondroitin sulfate in the treatment of dry eyes. *Am J Ophthalmol* 1987;**103**:194.

## Chlamydial Keratoconjunctivitis

**A. Trachoma:** Trachoma is a major cause of blindness worldwide. In endemic areas, it is contracted in childhood. In children, trachoma is usually insidious, with minimal symptoms. In adults, the disease is acute and is manifested by redness, itching, tearing, and slight discharge. The clinical picture consists of bilateral follicular conjunctivitis, epithelial keratitis, and corneal vascularization (pannus). Cicatrization of the conjunctiva occurs in the later stages of trachoma and usually follows necrosis of the conjunctival follicles. Scarring of the tarsal conjunctiva may result in entropion and trichiasis. Scarring of the limbal follicles results in round peripheral depressions with a clear central epithelium known as Herbert's pits. Superficial vascularization and scarring of the cornea cause decrease in vision. In endemic areas, superimposed bacterial conjunctivitis may aggravate the process.

The specific diagnosis can be made in Giemsa-stained conjunctival scrapings by the presence of typical cytoplasmic inclusions in epithelial cells. In active trachoma, the smear may also include polymorphonuclear leukocytes, plasma cells, and debris-filled macrophages (Leber cells).

Trachoma is transmitted from eye to eye by contact with contaminated fingers, towels, eye cosmetics, or other objects.

Treatment should be started on the basis of clinical findings without waiting for laboratory confirmation. Medical treatment consists of oral tetracycline given in full doses for 3–5 weeks. Local treatment is not necessary. *Caution:* Do not give tetracyclines during pregnancy or to young children, and do not use old preparations.

Hygienic measures are of great importance both in prevention and in treatment.

Corneal scarring may require corneal transplantation. Entropion and trichiasis require plastic surgery to evert the lids. Dacryocystorhinostomy may be required in nasolacrimal duct obstruction.

**B. Inclusion Conjunctivitis:** The agent of inclusion conjunctivitis is a common cause of genital tract disease in adults. The eye is usually involved following accidental contact with genital secretions. The newborn contracts the disease by passage through the infected birth canal. In the past, the disease had been transmitted by exposure of the eyes to contaminated water in swimming pools, and for this reason it was referred to as "swimming pool conjunctivitis."

Adequate chlorination of swimming pools has eliminated this mode of transmission.

Inclusion conjunctivitis (blennorrhea) of the newborn usually occurs about 5–12 days after birth. The disease is characterized by bilateral redness, a mucopurulent exudate, papillary hypertrophy, and, in some cases, a diffuse punctate keratitis. If pseudomembranes occur, the disease may result in conjunctival scars. Corneal scars occur rarely and never lead to blindness, as in trachoma.

In babies, treatment with a systemic antibiotic (eg, erythromycin) is recommended, since there is often associated pharyngitis and occasionally pneumonitis.

Adult inclusion conjunctivitis occurs most frequently in sexually active young adults. The disease starts with acute redness, discharge, and irritation. The eye findings consist of follicular conjunctivitis with mild keratitis. A nontender preauricular lymph node can often be palpated. Healing leaves no sequelae. The cytology of the conjunctival scrapings is similar to that of trachoma, but cytoplasmic inclusions are found more frequently.

In adults, treatment is with tetracycline, 1–2 g daily orally for 2–3 weeks.

Vaughan D, Asbury, T: *General Ophthalmology*, 11th ed. Lange, 1986.

## Ophthalmia Neonatorum

Any infection of the newborn conjunctiva is referred to as ophthalmia neonatorum. The eyes of the newborn are usually inoculated with the causative agent during passage through the birth canal. The causes of ophthalmia neonatorum include *Neisseria gonorrhoeae,* the agent of inclusion conjunctivitis, herpesvirus hominis type 2 (genital herpes), and certain opportunistic bacteria. The etiologic agent should be identified in Giemsa- and Gram-stained scrapings of the conjunctiva and smears of exudates and by conjunctival cultures for bacteria and viruses.

The Credé 1% silver nitrate prophylaxis is effective for the prevention of gonorrheal ophthalmia but does not protect against herpesvirus infection or inclusion blennorrhea. In many institutions, erythromycin (0.5%) or tetracycline (1%) ointment is now used for prophylaxis. Appropriate topical antibiotics should be instilled to treat bacterial infections.

Rapoza PA et al: Epidemiology of neonatal conjunctivitis. *Ophthalmology* 1986;**93**:456.

## Allergic Conjunctivitis

Allergic conjunctivitis is a common disorder that is most often associated with hay fever. It causes bilateral tearing, itching, and redness and a minimal stringy discharge. It is usually chronic and recurrent. Short-term local corticosteroid therapy is often effective. Allergy is the usual cause of the alarming sudden painless chemosis seen in children.

Vernal conjunctivitis is a seasonal condition often associated with keratitis. In atopic individuals, it may be quite serious. Sodium cromoglycate drops are generally effective in reducing the severity and frequency of episodes.

Feducowicz HB, Stetson S: *External Infections of the Eye: Bacterial, Viral, and Mycotic, With Noninfections and Immunologic Diseases,* 3rd ed. Appleton-Century-Crofts, 1985.

Ormerod LD et al: Microbial keratitis in children. *Ophthalmology* 1986;**93**:449.

Symposium on bacterial infection and the eye. *Trans Ophthalmol Soc UK* 1986;**105**:18.

Vaughan D, Asbury T: Conjunctiva. Chap 7 in: *General Ophthalmology,* 11th ed. Appleton-Lange, 1986.

## PINGUECULA

Pinguecula is a yellow elevated nodule on either side of the cornea (more commonly on the nasal side) in the area of the palpebral fissure. Histologically, pinguecula is an elastoid degeneration of the conjunctival substantia propria. The nodules rarely grow, but inflammation (pingueculitis) may occur. No treatment is indicated. Pinguecula is common in persons over age 35.

## PTERYGIUM

Pterygium is a fleshy, triangular encroachment of the conjunctiva onto the nasal side of the cornea and is usually associated with constant exposure to wind, sun, sand, and dust. Pterygium may be either unilateral or bilateral. There may be a genetic predisposition, but no hereditary pattern has been described. Pterygium is fairly common in the southwestern USA. Excision is indicated if the growth threatens to interfere with vision by approaching the pupillary area. Recurrences are frequent.

Pinkerton OD, Hokama Y, Shigemura LA: Immunologic basis for the pathogenesis of pterygium. *Am J Ophthalmol* 1984;**98**:225.

## UVEITIS
### (Iritis, Iridocyclitis, Choroiditis)

Uveitis is any inflammation of the uveal tract (iris, ciliary body, and choroid). Inflammation primarily of the iris is called anterior uveitis, iridocyclitis, or iritis; inflammation of the choroid (and usually the retina as well) is called posterior uveitis or chorioretinitis.

Uveitis may be either granulomatous (exogenous) or nongranulomatous (endogenous); the latter is more common. The disease is usually unilateral, and signs and symptoms are similar in both types, varying only in intensity. Early diagnosis and treatment are important to prevent the formation of posterior synechiae.

All patients with uveitis should have a thorough history, systems review, and physical examination.

Pertinent laboratory studies should include at least an erythrocyte sedimentation rate, VDRL, FTA-ABS, and serologic tests for toxoplasmosis. PPD and anergy skin tests should be performed. Obtain x-rays of the chest and (if symptomatic) the sacroiliac joint.

Uveitis must be differentiated from conjunctivitis, acute glaucoma, and corneal ulcer.

### Nongranulomatous Uveitis (Endogenous)

Nongranulomatous uveitis is primarily an anterior noninfectious disease, and it is occasionally associated with ankylosing spondylitis or Crohn's disease. The iris and ciliary body are primarily affected, but occasional foci are found in the choroid.

The onset is acute, with marked pain, redness, photophobia, and blurred vision. A circumcorneal flush, caused by dilated limbal blood vessels, is present. Fine white keratic precipitates on the posterior surface of the cornea can be seen with the slit lamp or with a loupe. The pupil is small, and there may be a collection of fibrin with cells in the anterior chamber. If posterior synechiae are present, the pupil will be irregular and the light reflex will be absent.

Local corticosteroid therapy tends to shorten the course. Warm compresses will decrease pain. Atropine, 1%, 2 drops in the affected eye twice daily, will prevent posterior synechia formation and alleviate photophobia. Recurrences are common, but the prognosis is good.

### Granulomatous Uveitis (Exogenous)

Granulomatous uveitis usually follows invasion by the causative organism, eg, *Mycobacterium tuberculosis* or *Toxoplasma gondii,* although these pathogens are rarely recovered. Other common causes are sarcoidosis, syphilis, and leprosy. Any or all parts of the uveal tract may be affected, but there is a predilection for the choroid.

Granulomatous uveitis is more subtle than nongranulomatous uveitis in that there is usually less pain and redness, but the permanent eye damage is relatively devastating. The onset is usually slow, and the affected eye may be only slightly and diffusely red. Because of vitreous haze and retinal involvement, vision may be more blurred than would be expected in view of the apparent mildness of the process. Pain is minimal or absent, and photophobia is slight. The pupil may be normal or, if posterior synechiae are present, irregular and slightly smaller than normal. Large gray "mutton fat" keratic precipitates on the posterior surface of the cornea may be seen with the slit lamp or loupe. The anterior chamber may be cloudy. Iris nodules are commonly present, and there may be vitreous haze. Fresh lesions of the choroid appear yellow when viewed with the ophthalmoscope.

Treatment depends on the causative agent. The pupil should be kept dilated with atropine and associated systemic disease treated as indicated. The visual prognosis is fair.

Henderly DE et al: Changing patterns of uveitis. *Am J Ophthalmol* 1987;**103**:131.

Lowder CY, Char DH: Uveitis: A review. *West J Med* 1984;**140**:421.

Vaughan D, Asbury T: The uveal tract. Chap 11, pp 132–150, in: Vaughan D, Asbury T: *General Ophthalmology*, 11th ed. Appleton-Lange, 1986.

## DISORDERS OF THE LIDS & LACRIMAL APPARATUS

### Hordeolum

Hordeolum is a common staphylococcal abscess that is characterized by a localized red, swollen, acutely tender area on the upper or lower lid. Internal hordeolum is a meibomian gland abscess that points to the skin or to the conjunctival side of the lid; external hordeolum or sty (infection of the glands of Moll or Zeis) is smaller and on the margin.

The chief symptom is pain of an intensity directly related to the amount of swelling.

Warm compresses are helpful. Incision is indicated if resolution does not begin within 48 hours. An antibiotic or sulfonamide instilled into the conjunctival sac every 3 hours may be beneficial during the acute stage. Internal hordeolum may lead to generalized cellulitis of the lid.

### Chalazion

Chalazion is a common granulomatous inflammation of a meibomian gland characterized by a hard, nontender swelling on the upper or lower lid. It may be preceded by a sty. Most chalazions point toward the conjunctival side.

If the chalazion is large enough to impress the cornea, vision will be distorted. The conjunctiva in the region of the chalazion is red and elevated.

Excision is done by an ophthalmologist.

### Tumors

Verrucae and papillomas of the skin of the lids can often be excised by the general physician if they do not involve the lid margin. Cancer should be ruled out by microscopic examination of the excised material.

### Blepharitis

Blepharitis is a common chronic, bilateral inflammation of the lid margins. It may be ulcerative (*Staphylococcus aureus*) or nonulcerative (seborrheic). Both types are usually present. Seborrhea of the scalp, brows, and frequently of the ears is almost always associated with seborrheic blepharitis.

Symptoms are irritation, burning, and itching. The eyes are "red-rimmed," and scales or "granulations" can be seen clinging to the lashes. In the staphylococcal type, the scales are dry, the lid margins are red and ulcerated, and the lashes tend to fall out; in the seborrheic type the scales are greasy, ulceration is absent, and the lid margins are less red. In the more common mixed type, both dry and greasy scales are present, and the lid margins are red and may be ulcerated.

Cleanliness of the scalp, eyebrows, and lid margins is essential to effective local therapy. Scales must be removed from the lids daily with a damp cotton applicator.

An antistaphylococcal antibiotic or sulfonamide eye ointment is applied with a cotton applicator daily to the lid margins. The treatment of both types is similar except that in severe staphylococcal blepharitis, antibiotic sensitivity studies may be required.

### Entropion & Ectropion

Entropion (inward turning of the lid, usually the lower) occurs occasionally in older people as a result of degeneration of the lid fascia and may follow extensive scarring of the conjunctiva and tarsus. Surgery is indicated if the lashes rub on the cornea.

Ectropion (outward turning of the lower lid) is fairly common in elderly people. Surgery is indicated if ectropion causes excessive tearing, exposure keratitis, or a cosmetic problem.

### Dacryocystitis

Dacryocystitis is a common infection of the lacrimal sac. It may be acute or chronic and occurs most often in infants and in persons over 40. It is usually unilateral.

The cause of obstruction is usually unknown, but a history of trauma to the nose may be obtained. In acute dacryocystitis, the usual infectious organisms are *Staphylococcus aureus* and beta-hemolytic streptococci; in chronic dacryocystitis, *Streptococcus pneumoniae* (rarely, *Candida albicans*). Mixed infections do not occur.

Acute dacryocystitis is characterized by pain, swelling, tenderness, and redness in the tear sac area; purulent material may be expressed. In chronic dacryocystitis, tearing and discharge are the principal signs. Mucus or pus may be expressed from the tear sac.

Acute dacryocystitis responds well to systemic antibiotic therapy, but recurrences are common if the obstruction is not surgically removed. The chronic form may be kept latent by using antibiotic eye drops, but relief of the obstruction is the only cure.

## OPEN-ANGLE (CHRONIC) GLAUCOMA

### Essentials of Diagnosis

- Insidious onset in older age groups.
- No symptoms in early stages.
- Gradual loss of peripheral vision over a period of years, resulting in tunnel vision.
- Persistent elevation of intraocular pressure associated with pathologic cupping of the optic disks.

● *Note:* "Halos around lights" are not present unless the intraocular tension is markedly elevated.

## General Considerations

In open-angle glaucoma, the intraocular pressure is consistently elevated. Over a period of months or years, this results in optic atrophy with loss of vision varying from a slight constriction of the upper nasal peripheral visual fields to complete blindness.

The cause of the decreased rate of aqueous outflow in open-angle glaucoma has not been clearly demonstrated. The disease is bilateral and is genetically determined. Development is multifactorial, with no clear inheritance pattern. Most cases of congenital glaucoma are sporadic. Glaucoma occurs at an earlier age and more frequently in blacks and may result in more severe optic nerve damage.

In the USA it is estimated that 1–2% of people over 40 have glaucoma; about 25% of these cases are undetected. About 90% of all cases of glaucoma are of the open-angle type.

## Clinical Findings

Patients with open-angle glaucoma have no symptoms initially. On examination, there may be slight cupping of the optic disk. Changes in the retinal nerve fiber layer may be observed as an earlier finding in some patients. The visual fields gradually constrict, but central vision remains good until late in the disease.

Tonometry, ophthalmoscopic visualization of the optic nerve, and central visual field testing are the 3 prime tests for the diagnosis and continued clinical evaluation of glaucoma. The normal intraocular pressure is about 10–25 mm Hg. Except in acute glaucoma, however, the diagnosis is never made on the basis of one tonometric measurement, since various factors can influence the pressure (eg, diurnal variation). Transient elevations of intraocular pressure do not constitute glaucoma (for the same reason that periodic or intermittent elevations of blood pressure do not constitute hypertensive disease). Field testing may prove unreliable in some patients.

## Prevention

All persons over age 20 should have tonometric and ophthalmoscopic examinations every 3–5 years. The examination may be performed by the general physician, internist, or ophthalmologist. If there is a family history of glaucoma, annual examination is indicated. Mydriatic and cycloplegic drugs should not be used in any patient with a shallow anterior chamber angle.

## Treatment

Timolol, a beta-adrenergic blocking agent, is an effective antiglaucoma agent in a dosage of 1 drop every 12 hours of 0.25% or 0.5% solution. It is used alone (every 12 hours) or in combination with other intraocular pressure-lowering agents. It should not be used in patients with reactive airway disease or cardiovascular abnormalities. In those situations, betaxolol may be a safer alternative. Timolol is often used in combination with epinephrine eye drops, 0.5–1%. Pilocarpine, the standard drug for a century, is still very useful and may be used along with timolol and epinephrine. Carbonic anhydrase inhibitors (eg, acetazolamide) are used less commonly since the advent of timolol. When local eye drops are ineffective, laser treatment (trabeculoplasty) has been shown to be an effective method of reducing intraocular pressure. Surgery (trabeculectomy) is necessary for patients whose intraocular pressure remains elevated despite medical and laser therapy. Therapeutic ultrasound treatment of glaucoma is presently under study.

## Prognosis

Untreated chronic glaucoma that begins at age 40–45 will probably cause complete blindness by age 60–65. Early diagnosis and treatment will preserve useful vision throughout life in most cases.

Allen RC et al: A double-masked comparison of betaxolol vs timolol in the treatment of open-angle glaucoma. *Am J Ophthalmol* 1986;**101**:535.

Glaucoma. *Ophthalmology* 1981;**88**:175. [Entire issue.]

Hitchings RA: Screening for glaucoma. (Editorial.) *Br Med J* 1986;**292**:505.

Kolker AE, Hetherington J: *Becker-Shaffer's Diagnosis and Therapy of the Glaucomas,* 5th ed. Mosby, 1983.

Martin MJ et al: Race and primary open-angle glaucoma. *Am J Ophthalmol* 1985;**99**:383.

Quigley ITA: Better methods of glaucoma diagnosis. (Editorial.) *Arch Ophthalmol* 1985;**103**:186.

Sharpe ED, Simmons RJ: Argon laser trabeculoplasty as a means of decreasing intraocular pressure from "normal" levels in glaucomatous eyes. *Am J Ophthalmol* 1985;**99**:704.

Transactions of the New Orleans Academy of Ophthalmology: *Symposium on the Laser in Ophthalmology and Glaucoma Update.* Mosby, 1985.

Van Buskirk EM, Fraunfelder FT: Ocular beta-blockers and systemic effects. *Am J Ophthalmol* 1984;**98**:623.

Watson PG et al: Argon laser trabeculoplasty or trabeculectomy: A prospective randomised block study. *Trans Ophthalmol Soc UK* 1985;**104**:55.

## RETINAL DISORDERS ASSOCIATED WITH SYSTEMIC DISEASES

Many systemic diseases are associated with retinal manifestations. Some of the more common ones include essential hypertension, diabetes mellitus, preeclampsia-eclampsia of pregnancy, blood dyscrasias, sarcoidosis, syphilis, and toxoplasmosis. The retinal damage caused by these disorders can be easily observed with the aid of the ophthalmoscope.

**Hypertensive retinopathy.** One method of classifying hypertensive retinopathy (modified after Keith and Wagener) is shown in Table 5–2.

**Diabetic retinopathy** is the leading cause of new blindness among American adults aged 20–65. In

**Table 5–2.** A classification of hypertensive retinopathy. (Modified after Keith and Wagener.)

| Stage | Ophthalmoscopic Appearance | Clinical Classification |
|---|---|---|
| I | Minimal narrowing or sclerosis of arterioles. | "Essential" hypertension (chronic, benign, "arteriosclerotic"). |
| II | Thickening and dulling of vessel reflection (copper wire appearance). Localized and generalized narrowing of arterioles. Changes at arteriovenous crossings (A-V nicking). Scattered tiny round or flame-shaped hemorrhages. Vascular occlusion may be present. | |
| III | Sclerotic changes may not be marked. "Angiospastic retinopathy": localized arteriolar spasm, hemorrhages, exudates, "cotton wool patches," retinal edema. | Malignant hypertensive retinopathy. |
| IV | Same as III, plus papilledema. | |

recent years, it has been broadly classified as proliferative or nonproliferative.

**Nonproliferative retinopathy** is characterized by dilatation of veins, microaneurysms, and retinal hemorrhages plus retinal edema and hard and soft exudates. **Proliferative retinopathy** is more devastating and is characterized by neovascularization and hemorrhage that result in fibrovascular proliferation into the vitreous, a forerunner of virtually untreatable total retinal detachment. Without treatment, the visual prognosis with proliferative retinopathy is generally much worse than with nonproliferative retinopathy.

It is essential that proliferative retinopathy be recognized early and treated with laser photocoagulation to prevent devastating blindness. Early recognition of collections of hard exudates in the region of the macula is also important. This maculopathy is the most common cause of legal blindness in maturity-onset diabetics. It can often be adequately treated with laser photocoagulation in its early stages. Patients with diabetes mellitus should have a careful yearly ophthalmoscopic examination through dilated pupils. Examination by an ophthalmologist is usually advisable if the diabetes is of more than 10 years' duration, or earlier if ocular symptoms are present or if there are suspicious findings of retinopathy on ophthalmoscopic examination. Failure to diagnose nonproliferative retinopathy by ophthalmoscopic examination is common (see Sussman reference below). Fluorescein angiography may be required to allow a detailed assessment of the retinal vasculature. There is adequate evidence now to show that the risk of diabetic retinopathy can be lessened by careful control of blood glucose levels.

**Age-related macular degeneration** is the leading cause of permanent blindness in the elderly. The exact cause is unknown, but the incidence increases with each decade over age 50. Other associations besides age include race (usually white), sex (slight female predominance), family history, and a history of cigarette smoking. Age-related macular degeneration includes a broad spectrum of clinical and pathologic findings, which can be classified into 2 groups: nonexudative ("dry") and exudative ("wet"). Although both types are progressive and usually bilateral, they differ in terms of their manifestations, prognosis, and management. The more severe exudative form accounts for approximately 90% of all cases of legal blindness due to age-related macular degeneration.

**Preeclampsia-eclampsia** is manifested in the retina as rapidly progressive hypertensive retinopathy, and extensive permanent retinal damage may occur if the pregnancy is not terminated. Occasionally, the choroidal circulation is mainly affected, leading to infarction of the retinal pigment epithelium.

In **blood dyscrasias,** various types of hemorrhages are present in both the retina and choroid and may lead to blindness. If the underlying dyscrasia is successfully treated and macular hemorrhages have not occurred, it is possible to regain normal vision.

The chorioretinitis associated with **syphilis** is striking. There are many small yellow dots and pigment clumps in the peripheral fundus, giving a typical "salt and pepper" appearance.

**Toxoplasmosis** produces necrotizing lesions of retinochoroiditis that may involve the posterior pole and the macular area. The active lesion appears as a white elevated granuloma with inflammatory cells in the vitreous. The vitreous appears hazy and may sometimes obscure the lesion. In the healed stage, a punched-out pigmented chorioretinal lesion develops through which the sclera is clearly visible. Treatment consists of the administration of sulfadiazine and pyrimethamine and, in severe cases, systemic corticosteroids.

### Retinal Vasculitis

Inflammation of the retinal veins (retinal periphlebitis) may occur as an isolated phenomenon or as part of a multisystem disorder such as sarcoidosis or Behçet's disease. Fluffy white thickening of the vein wall with associated venous occlusion may occur.

Patients with retinal vasculitis may need systemic steroids or cytotoxic therapy.

### Acquired Immunodeficiency Syndrome (AIDS)

Patients with AIDS commonly develop retinal cotton wool spots and hemorrhages indistinguishable from those seen in systemic hypertension. There may also be opportunistic infections of the retina and choroid, including cytomegalovirus retinitis that may lead to rapid loss of vision and is especially difficult to treat. Patients have low white cell counts and a marked reversal of normal helper/suppressor T lymphocyte ratios. Overwhelming opportunistic infection may be apparent on ocular examination before other clinical features of AIDS appear.

Callen JP, Eifferman RA (editors): Oculocutaneous diseases. *Int Ophthalmol Clin* 1985;**25**. [Entire issue.]

Diabetic Retinopathy Study Research Group: Photocoagulation treatment of proliferative diabetic retinopathy. *Ophthalmology* 1981;**88**:583.

Early Treatment Diabetic Retinopathy Study Research Group: Photocoagulation for diabetic macular edema. *Arch Ophthalmol* 1985;**103**:1796.

Ferris FL III: Senile macular degeneration: Review of epidemiologic features. *Am J Epidemiol* 1983;**118**:132.

Freeman WR, O'Connor GR: Acquired immune deficiency syndrome retinopathy, *Pneumocystis*, and cotton-wool spots. (Editorial.) *Am J Ophthalmol* 1984;**98**:235.

Friberg TR et al: The effect of long-term near normal glycemic control on mild diabetic retinopathy. *Ophthalmology* 1985;**92**:1051.

Graham EM: Retinal vasculitis. Chap 18, pp 380–394, in: *The Eye in General Medicine*. Rose FC (editor). University Park Press, 1983.

Henderly DE et al: Cytomegalovirus retinitis as the initial manifestation of the acquired immunodeficiency syndrome. *Am J Ophthalmol* 1987;**103**:316.

Holland GN et al: Treatment of cytomegalovirus retinopathy in patients with acquired immunodeficiency syndrome. Use of the experimental drug 9-[2-hydroxy-1-(hydroxymethyl)-ethoxymethyl]guanine. *Arch Ophthalmol* 1986;**104**:1794.

Howard-Williams J et al: Retinopathy is associated with higher glycaemia in maturity-onset type diabetics. *Diabetologia* 1984;**27**:198.

Macular Photocoagulation Study Group: Argon laser photocoagulation for senile macular degeneration. *Arch Ophthalmol* 1983;**100**:912.

Phelps RL et al: Changes in diabetic retinopathy during pregnancy. Correlations with regulation of hyperglycemia. *Arch Ophthalmol* 1986;**104**:1806.

Sigelman J: *Retinal Diseases*. Little, Brown, 1984.

Smith RE, Nozik RM: Toxoplasmic retinochoroiditis. Chap 26, p 120, in: *Uveitis: A Clinical Approach to Diagnosis and Management*. Williams & Wilkins, 1983.

Witkin SR, Klein R: Ophthalmologic care for persons with diabetes. *JAMA* 1984;**251**:2534.

## RETINAL DETACHMENT

### Essentials of Diagnosis

- Blurred vision in one eye becoming progressively worse. ("A curtain came down over my eye.")
- No pain or redness.
- Detachment seen by ophthalmoscopy.

### General Considerations

Detachment of the retina is usually spontaneous but may be secondary to trauma. Spontaneous detachment occurs most frequently in persons over 50 years of age. Aphakia and myopia are the 2 commonest predisposing causes.

### Clinical Findings

As soon as the retina is torn, fluid vitreous is able to pass through the tear and behind the sensory retina. This, combined with vitreous traction and the pull of gravity, results in progressive detachment. The superior temporal area is the most common site of detachment. The area of detachment rapidly increases, causing corresponding progressive visual loss. Central vision remains intact until the macula becomes detached.

On ophthalmoscopic examination, the retina is seen hanging in the vitreous like a gray cloud. One or more retinal tears, usually crescent-shaped and red or orange, are always present and can be seen by an experienced examiner.

### Differential Diagnosis

Sudden partial loss of vision in one eye may also be due to retinal or vitreous hemorrhage and central retinal vessel (artery or vein) occlusion.

### Treatment

All cases of retinal detachment should be referred immediately to an ophthalmologist. During transportation over a long distance, the patient's head should be positioned so that the detached portion of the retina will fall back with the aid of gravity. For example, a patient with a superior temporal retinal detachment in the right eye should lie supine, head turned to the right. Head position is less important during transportation for a short distance.

Treatment is aimed at closing retinal breaks to reattach the retina. This can often be achieved without draining subretinal fluid. A cryoprobe is applied to the sclera in the region of the tear, and an indentation is made in the sclera with a silicone sponge or buckle. More complicated cases may require drainage of subretinal fluid. Occasionally, removal of vitreous and internal tamponade of the retina with air, special gas, or even silicone oil is necessary.

Retinal tears without detachment may be successfully sealed by cryotherapy or photocoagulation either with xenon light or the argon laser.

### Prognosis

About 80% of uncomplicated cases can be cured with one operation; an additional 10% will need repeated operations; the remainder never reattach. The prognosis is worse if the macula is detached, if there are many vitreous strands, or if the detachment is of long duration. Without treatment, retinal detachment almost always becomes total in 1–6 months. Spontaneous detachments are ultimately bilateral in 20–25% of cases.

Kanski JJ: *Retinal Detachments*. Butterworths, 1986.

Michels RG: Scleral buckling methods for retinal detachment. *Retina* 1986;**6**:1.

Ratner CM et al: Pars plana vitrectomy for complicated retinal detachments. *Ophthalmology* 1983;**90**:1323.

## CATARACT

### Essentials of Diagnosis

- Blurred vision, progressive over months or years.

- No pain or redness.
- Lens opacities (may be grossly visible).

## General Considerations

A cataract is a lens opacity. Cataracts are usually bilateral. They may be congenital or may occur as a result of trauma or, less commonly, systemic disease. Senile cataract is by far the most common type; most persons over 60 have some degree of lens opacity.

## Clinical Findings

Even in its early stages, a cataract can be seen through a dilated pupil with an ophthalmoscope, a slit lamp, or an ordinary hand illuminator. As the cataract matures, the retina will become increasingly more difficult to visualize, until finally the fundus reflection is absent. At this point, the pupil is white and the cataract is mature.

The degree of visual loss corresponds to the density of the cataract.

## Treatment

Functional visual impairment is the prime criterion for surgery. The cataract is removed either with its entire capsule (intracapsular) or by a technique in which the delicate posterior lens capsule remains (extracapsular).

Over recent years, it has become common practice to implant an intraocular lens at the time of surgery. This dispenses with the need for heavy cataract glasses or contact lenses. With modern techniques and improved intraocular lenses, the success rate is high. Intraocular lens implants are generally not suitable for patients with uveitic cataract or those with significant diabetic retinopathy.

An alternative to the intraocular lens is the continuous-wear soft contact lens that can be worn day and night for weeks to months at a time.

In the USA, the most significant innovation in cataract surgery has been the change to outpatient ambulatory surgery. This change was prompted by financial concerns. Whether it benefits patients is doubtful.

## Prognosis

If surgery is indicated, lens extraction improves visual acuity in 95% of cases. The remainder either have preexisting retinal damage or develop postoperative complications such as glaucoma, hemorrhage, retinal detachment, or infection.

Apple DJ: Complications of intraocular lenses: A historical and histopathological review. *Surv Ophthalmol* 1984;**29**:1.

Dowling JL, Bahr RL: A survey of cataract surgical techniques. *Am J Ophthalmol* 1985;**99**:35.

Oxford Cataract Treatment and Evaluation Team (OCTET): I. Cataract surgery: Interim results and complications of a randomised controlled trial. *Br J Ophthalmol* 1986;**70**: 402.

Trevor-Roper PD: Who should have an intraocular lens? *Br Med J* 1985;**290**:581.

# PRINCIPLES OF TREATMENT OF OCULAR INFECTIONS

## Identification of Pathogen

Before one can determine the drug of choice, the causative organism must be identified. For example, a pneumococcal corneal ulcer will respond to treatment with a sulfonamide, penicillin, and several broad-spectrum antibiotics, but this is not true in the case of corneal ulcer due to *Pseudomonas aeruginosa*, which requires vigorous treatment with tobramycin, gentamicin, or polymyxin. Another example is staphylococcal dacryocystitis, which, if it does not respond to penicillin, is most likely to respond to erythromycin.

## Choice of Alternative Drugs

In the treatment of infectious eye disease, eg, conjunctivitis, one should always use the drug that is the most effective, the least likely to cause complications, and the least expensive. It is also preferable to use a drug that is not usually given systemically, eg, sulfacetamide or bacitracin. Of the available antibacterial agents, the sulfonamides come closest to meeting these specifications. Two reliable sulfonamides for ophthalmic use are sulfisoxazole and sodium sulfacetamide. The sulfonamides have the added advantages of low allergenicity and effectiveness against the chlamydial group of organisms. They are available in ointment or solution form.

Among the most effective broad-spectrum antibiotics for ophthalmic use are gentamicin, tobramycin, and neomycin. These drugs have some effect against gram-negative as well as gram-positive organisms but are not generally effective against the pneumococcus. Allergic reactions to neomycin are common. Other antibiotics frequently used are erythromycin, the tetracyclines, the cephalosporins, bacitracin, and polymyxin. Combined bacitracin-polymyxin ointment is often used prophylactically after corneal foreign body removal for the protection it affords against both gram-positive and gram-negative organisms.

## Method of Administration

Most ocular anti-infective drugs are administered locally. Systemic administration as well is required for all intraocular infections, corneal ulcer, orbital cellulitis, dacryocystitis, and any severe external infection that does not respond to local treatment.

## Ointment Versus Liquid Medications

Ointments have greater therapeutic effectiveness than solutions, since contact can be maintained longer. However, they do cause blurring of vision; if this must be avoided, solutions should be used.

Barza M, Baum J: Ocular infections. *Med Clin North Am* 1983;**67**:131.

**Table 5–3.** Adverse ocular effects of systemic drugs.

| Drug | Possible Side Effects |
|---|---|
| **Respiratory agents** | |
| Oxygen | Retrolental fibroplasia (in premature infants). Blurring of vision, constriction of visual fields. |
| **Cardiovascular system drugs** | |
| Cardiac glycosides (digitalis, etc) | Disturbances of color vision, blurring of vision, scotomas. |
| Quinidine | Toxic amblyopia. |
| Thiazides (Diuril, etc) | Xanthopsia (yellow vision), myopia. |
| Carbonic anhydrase inhibitors (acetazolamide) | Ocular hypotony, transient myopia. |
| Amiodarone | Corneal deposits. |
| Oxyprenolol | Photophobia, ocular irritation. |
| **Gastrointestinal drugs** | |
| Anticholinergic agents (eg, atropine) | Risk of angle-closure glaucoma due to mydriasis. Blurring of vision due to cycloplegia (occasional). |
| **Central nervous system drugs** | |
| Barbiturates | Extraocular muscle palsies with diplopia, ptosis, cortical blindness. |
| Chloral hydrate | Diplopia, ptosis, miosis. |
| Phenothiazines (eg, chlorpromazine) | Toxic amblyopia, deposits of pigment in conjunctiva, cornea, lens, and retina. Oculogyric crises. |
| Amphetamines | Widening of palpebral fissure. Dilatation of pupil, paralysis of ciliary muscle with loss of accommodation. |
| Monoamine oxidase inhibitors | Nystagmus, extraocular muscle palsies, amblyopia (toxic). |
| Tricyclic agents | Dilatation of pupil (risk of angle-closure glaucoma), cycloplegia. |
| Phenytoin | Nystagmus, diplopia, ptosis, slight blurring of vision (rare). |
| Neostigmine | Nystagmus, miosis. |
| Morphine | Miosis. |
| Haloperidol | Capsular cataract. |
| Lithium carbonate | Exophthalmos, oculogyric crisis. |
| Diazepam | Nystagmus, allergic conjunctivitis. |
| **Hormones** | |
| Corticosteroids | Cataract (posterior subcapsular), local immunologic suppression causing susceptibility to viral (herpesvirus hominis), bacterial, and fungal infections; steriod-induced glaucoma. |
| Female sex hormones | Retinal artery thrombosis, retinal vein thrombosis, papilledema, ocular palsies with diplopia, nystagmus, optic neuritis and atrophy, retinal vasculitis, scotomas, migraine, mydriasis and cycloplegia, and macular edema. |
| **Antibiotics** | |
| Chloramphenicol | Optic neuritis and atrophy and aplastic anemia. Toxic amblyopia (rare). |
| Streptomycin | Toxic amblyopia (rare). |
| Tetracycline | Pseudotumor cerebri, transient myopia. |
| **Antimalarial agents** | |
| Eg, chloroquine | Macular changes, central scotomas, pigmentary degeneration of the retina, chloroquine keratopathy, ocular palsies, ptosis, ERG depression. |
| **Amebicides** | |
| Iodochlorhydroxyquin | Optic atrophy. |
| **Chemotherapeutic agents** | |
| Sulfonamides | Conjunctivitis in Stevens-Johnson syndrome causing cicatrization of the conjunctiva. Toxic amblyopia (rare). |
| Ethambutol | Toxic amblyopia, optic neuritis and atrophy. |
| Isoniazid | Toxic amblyopia, optic neuritis and atrophy. |
| Aminosalicylic acid | Toxic amblyopia. |
| **Heavy metals** | |
| Gold salts | Deposits in the cornea and conjunctiva. |
| Lead compounds | Toxic amblyopia, papilledema, ocular palsies. |
| **Chelating agents** | |
| Penicillamine | Ocular pemphigoid, optic neuritis, ocular myasthenia. |
| **Oral hypoglycemic agents** | |
| Chlorpropamide | Transient change in refractive error, toxic amblyopia, diplopia. |
| **Vitamins** | |
| Vitamin A | Papilledema, retinal hemorrhages, loss of eyebrows and eyelashes, nystagmus, diplopia, blurring of vision. |
| Vitamin D | Band-shaped keratopathy. |
| **Antirheumatic agents** | |
| Salicylates | Toxic amblyopia, cortical blindness (rare). |
| Indomethacin | Corneal deposits, toxic amblyopia, diplopia, retinal changes. |
| Phenylbutazone | Toxic amblyopia, retinal hemorrhages. |

Baum J, Barza M: Topical versus subconjunctival treatment of bacterial corneal ulcers. *Ophthalmology* 1983;**90**:162.

Havener WH: *Ocular Pharmacology,* 5th ed. Mosby, 1983.

Shell JW: Ophthalmic drug delivery systems. *Surv Ophthalmol* 1984;**29**:117.

Vaughan D, Asbury T: *General Ophthalmology,* 11th ed. Appleton-Lange, 1986.

## TECHNIQUES USED IN THE TREATMENT OF OCULAR DISORDERS

### Instilling Medications

Place the patient in a chair with head tilted back, both eyes open, and looking up. Retract the lower lid slightly and instill 2 drops of liquid into the lower cul-de-sac. Have the patient look down while finger contact on the lower lid is maintained. Do not let the patient squeeze the eyes shut.

Ointments are instilled in the same general manner.

### Self-Medication

The same techniques are used as described above, except that drops are usually better instilled with the patient lying down.

### Eye Bandage

Most eye bandages should be applied firmly enough to hold the lid securely against the cornea. An ordinary patch consisting of gauze-covered cotton is usually sufficient. Tape is applied from the cheek to the forehead. If more pressure is desired, use 2 or 3 bandages. The black eye patch is difficult to sterilize and therefore is seldom used.

### Warm Compresses

A clean towel or washcloth soaked in warm tap water is applied to the affected eye for 10–15 minutes 2–4 times a day.

### Removal of a Superficial Corneal Foreign Body

Record the patient's visual acuity, if possible, and instill sterile local anesthetic drops. With the patient sitting or lying down, an assistant should direct a strong light into the eye so that the rays strike the cornea obliquely. Using either a loupe or a slit lamp, the physician locates the foreign body on the corneal surface. It may then be removed with a sterile wet cotton applicator or, if this fails, with a spud, with the lids held apart with the other hand to prevent blinking. An antibacterial ointment (gentamicin) is instilled after the foreign body has been removed. It is preferable not to patch the eye, but the patient must be seen on the following day to make certain healing is under way.

## PRECAUTIONS IN MANAGEMENT OF OCULAR DISORDERS

### Use of Local Anesthetics

Unsupervised self-administration of local anesthetics is dangerous because the patient may further injure an anesthetized eye without knowing it. The drug may also prevent the normal healing process.

### Pupillary Dilation

Use cycloplegics and mydriatics with caution. Dilating the pupil can precipitate an acute glaucoma attack if the patient has a narrow anterior chamber angle.

### Local Corticosteroid Therapy

Repeated use of local corticosteroids presents several serious hazards: herpes simplex (dendritic) keratitis, fungal overgrowth, open-angle glaucoma, and cataract formation. Furthermore, perforation of the cornea may occur when the corticosteroids are used for herpes simplex keratitis.

### Contaminated Eye Medications

Ophthalmic solutions must be prepared with the same degree of care as fluids intended for intravenous administration.

Tetracaine, proparacaine, and fluorescein are most likely to become contaminated. The most dangerous is fluorescein, as this solution is frequently contaminated with *Pseudomonas aeruginosa,* an organism that can rapidly destroy the eye. Sterile fluorescein filter paper strips are now available and are recommended in place of fluorescein solutions.

The following rules should be observed in handling eye medications for use in the diagnostic examination of uninjured eyes: (1) Obtain solutions in small amounts from the pharmacy. (2) Be certain that the solution is sterile as prepared and that it contains an effective antibacterial agent. (3) Date the bottle at the time it is procured.

Plastic dropper bottles are in widespread use; solutions from these bottles are safe to use in uninjured eyes. Whether in plastic or glass containers, eye solutions should not remain in use for long periods after the bottle is opened. Two weeks after opening is a reasonable maximal time to use a solution before discarding.

If the eye has been injured accidentally or by surgical trauma, it is of the greatest importance to use sterile medications supplied in sterile disposable single-use eyedropper units.

### Ocular Irritation

Patients receiving long-term topical therapy may develop local toxic reactions to preservatives, especially if there is inadequate tear secretion. Burning and soreness are exacerbated by drop instillation; occasionally, fibrosis and scarring of the conjunctiva and cornea may occur.

## Fungal Overgrowth

Since antibiotics, like corticosteroids, when used over a prolonged period of time in bacterial corneal ulcers, favor the development of secondary fungal corneal infection, the sulfonamides should be used whenever they are adequate for the purpose.

## Systemic Effects of Ocular Drugs

The systemic absorption of certain topical drugs (through the lacrimal drainage system) must be considered when there is a systemic medical contraindication to the use of the drug. Exercise caution, for example, when using ophthalmic solutions of the beta-blocker timolol (Timoptic) in patients with cardiac disease, asthma, or diabetes mellitus. Atropine oint-

ment should be prescribed for children rather than the drops, since absorption of the 1% topical solution may be toxic. Phenylephrine eye drops can precipitate hypertensive crises. Also to be considered are adverse interactions between systemically administered and ocular drugs. Patients who have used echothiophate drops to manage glaucoma are at risk of prolonged apnea from succinylcholine used in anesthesia. On the other hand, oral levodopa administration has been shown to reduce the mydriasis following topical phenylephrine. A few minutes of nasolacrimal occlusion or eyelid closure improves efficacy and decreases systemic side effects of topical agents.

## Sensitization

An antibiotic instilled into the eye can sensitize the patient to that drug and cause a hypersensitivity reaction upon subsequent systemic administration.

## REFERENCES

Beard C: *Ptosis,* 3rd ed. Mosby, 1981.

Ellis PP: *Ocular Therapeutics and Pharmacology,* 7th ed. Mosby, 1985.

Ellis PP: Commonly used eye medications. Chap 28, pp 372–383, in: Vaughan D, Asbury T: *General Ophthalmology,* 11th ed. Appleton-Lange, 1986.

Ernest JT (editor): *Year Book of Ophthalmology.* Year Book, 1985.

Fraunfelder FT, Mayer SM: Ocular and systemic side effects of drugs. Pages 379–382 in: Vaughan D, Asbury T: *General Ophthalmology,* 11th ed. Appleton-Lange, 1986.

Fraunfelder FT, Hampton RF: *Current Ocular Therapy 2,* 2nd ed. Saunders, 1985.

Hansten PD: *Drug Interactions,* 5th ed. Lea & Febiger, 1985.

Harrington DO: *The Visual Fields: A Textbook and Atlas of Clinical Perimetry,* 5th ed. Mosby, 1981.

Havener WH: *Ocular Pharmacology,* 5th ed. Mosby, 1983.

Henkind P et al (editorial consultants): *Physicians' Desk Reference (PDR) for Ophthalmology.* Medical Economics, 1986.

Kolker AE, Hetherington J: *Becker-Shaffer's Diagnosis and Therapy of the Glaucomas,* 5th ed. Mosby, 1983.

Little HL et al: *Diabetic Retinopathy.* Thieme-Stratton, 1983.

March WF (editor): *Ophthalmic Lasers: Current Clinical Uses.* Slack, 1984.

Melamed MA: A generalist's guide to eye emergencies. *Emergency Med* (Feb 15) 1984;**16**:99.

Miller NR: *Walsh & Hoyt's Clinical Neuro-Ophthalmology,* 4th ed. Vol 1. Williams & Wilkins, 1982.

Newell FW: *Ophthalmology: Principles and Concepts,* 6th ed. Mosby, 1986.

Scheie HG, Albert DM: *Textbook of Ophthalmology,* 9th ed. Saunders, 1977.

Smolin G, Thoft RA (editors): *The Cornea: Scientific Foundation and Clinical Practice.* Little, Brown, 1983.

Spalton DJ, Hitchings RA, Hunter PA: *Atlas of Clinical Ophthalmology.* Gower, 1984.

Spencer WH: *Ophthalmologic Pathology: An Atlas and Textbook,* 3rd ed. 3 vols. Saunders, 1985.

Trevor-Roper PD: *Lecture Notes on Ophthalmology,* 6th ed. Blackwell, 1980.

Van Buskirk EM, Fraunfelder FT: Ocular beta-blockers and systemic effects. *Am J Ophthalmol* 1984;**98**:623.

Vaughan D, Asbury T: *General Ophthalmology,* 11th ed. Appleton-Lange, 1986.

Von Noorden GK: *Atlas of Strabismus,* 4th ed. Mosby, 1983.

Wilson FM Jr: Adverse external ocular effects of topical ophthalmic therapy: An epidemiologic, laboratory, and clinical study. *Trans Am Ophthalmol Soc* 1983;**81**:854.

Zimmerman TJ et al: Improving the therapeutic index of topically applied ocular drugs. *Arch Ophthalmol* 1984;**102**:55.

# 6

# Ear, Nose, & Throat

*Robert K. Jackler, MD, & Michael J. Kaplan, MD*

## DISEASES OF THE EAR

### HEARING LOSS

#### Classification

**A. Conductive Hearing Loss:** Conductive hearing loss results from dysfunction of the external or middle ear. There are 4 mechanisms, each resulting in impairment of the passage of sound vibrations to the inner ear: (1) obstruction (eg, cerumen impaction), (2) mass loading (eg, middle ear effusion), (3) stiffness effect (eg, otosclerosis), and (4) discontinuity (eg, ossicular disruption). Conductive hearing loss is generally correctable with medical or surgical therapy—or in some cases both.

**B. Sensory Hearing Loss:** Sensory hearing loss results from deterioration of the cochlea, usually due to loss of hair cells from the organ of Corti. Among the many common causes are noise trauma, ototoxicity, and aging (presbycusis). Sensory hearing loss is not correctable with medical or surgical therapy but often may be prevented or stabilized.

**C. Neural Hearing Loss:** Neural hearing loss occurs with lesions involving the eighth nerve, auditory nuclei, ascending tracts, or auditory cortex. It is the least common clinically recognized cause of hearing loss. Examples include acoustic neuroma, multiple sclerosis, and cerebrovascular disease.

#### Epidemiology of Hearing Loss

**A. Children:** Conductive losses in children are very common, especially before age 6. Most are due to middle ear effusion resulting from immaturity of the auditory tube (eustachian tube). Significant conductive losses during this critical period of speech and language acquisition are especially deleterious. Uncorrected hearing loss during this time may lead to a lasting deficit in communication skills.

Sensorineural loss in children may be congenital (eg, familial, teratogenic) or acquired (eg, meningitis, viral infection). Profound congenital deafness is usually not recognized by parents until age 12–18 months. For this reason, careful screening of high-risk infants is indicated in order to implement auditory rehabilitation at the earliest possible time. Some criteria for

high risk include prematurity, congenital malformation involving the head and neck region or urinary tract, hyperbilirubinemia, meningitis, exposure to teratogens, and a familial history of deafness.

**B. Adults:** Conductive losses in adults are most commonly due to cerumen impaction or transient auditory tube dysfunction associated with upper respiratory tract infection. Persistent conductive losses usually result from chronic ear infection, trauma, or otosclerosis.

Sensorineural losses in adults are common. A gradually progressive, predominantly high-frequency loss with advancing age is typical though not invariable. Other than aging effects, common causes of sensorineural loss include excessive noise exposure, head trauma, ototoxicity, and systemic diseases such as diabetes mellitus.

#### Evaluation of Hearing (Audiology)

In a quiet room, the hearing level may be estimated by having the patient repeat aloud words presented in a soft whisper, a normal spoken voice, or a shout. Tuning forks are useful in differentiating conductive from sensorineural losses. A 512-Hz tuning fork is employed, since frequencies below this level elicit a tactile response. In the **Weber test,** the tuning fork is placed on the forehead or front teeth. In conductive losses, the sound appears louder in the poorer-hearing ear, whereas in sensorineural losses it radiates to the better side. In the **Rhine test,** the tuning fork is placed alternately on the mastoid bone and in front of the ear canal. In conductive losses, bone conduction exceeds air conduction; in sensorineural losses, the opposite is true.

Formal audiometric studies are performed by an audiologist in a soundproofed room. Pure-tone thresholds in decibels (dB) are obtained over the range of 250–8000 Hz (the main speech frequencies are between 500 and 3000 Hz) for both air and bone conduction. Conductive losses create a gap between the air and bone thresholds, whereas in sensorineural losses both air and bone conduction are equally diminished. The threshold of normal hearing is from 0 to 20 dB, which corresponds to the loudness of a soft whisper. Mild hearing loss is indicated by a threshold of 20–40 dB (soft spoken voice), moderate loss by a threshold of 40–60 dB (normal spoken voice), severe loss by a threshold of 60–80 dB (loud spoken voice), and profound loss by a threshold of 80 dB (shout).

The clarity of hearing is often impaired in sensorineural hearing loss. This is evaluated by speech discrimination testing, which is reported as percentage correct (90–100% is normal). The site of the lesion responsible for sensorineural loss—whether it lies in the cochlea or in the central auditory system—may be determined with auditory brain stem-evoked responses.

### Hearing Rehabilitation

Patients with hearing loss not correctable by medical therapy may benefit from hearing amplification. Contemporary hearing aids are comparatively free from distortion and have been miniaturized to the point where they often may be contained entirely within the ear canal. To optimize the benefit, a hearing aid must be carefully selected to conform to the nature of the hearing loss.

Aside from hearing aids, many assistive devices are available to improve comprehension in individual and group settings, to help with hearing television and radio programs, and for telephone communication. In individuals with profound sensory deafness, the cochlear implant—an electronic device that is surgically implanted to stimulate the auditory nerve—offers socially beneficial auditory rehabilitation to most adults with acquired deafness.

Rupp RR, Vaughn GR, Lightfoot RK: Nontraditional "aids" to hearing: Assistive listening devices. *Geriatrics* 1984; **39**:55.

Schindler RA et al: The UCSF/Storz multichannel cochlear implant: Patient results. *Laryngoscope* 1986;**96**:597.

## DISEASES OF THE AURICLE

Disorders of the external ear are for the most part dermatologic. Skin cancers due to actinic exposure are common and may be treated with standard techniques. Traumatic auricular hematoma must be recognized and drained to prevent significant cosmetic deformity (cauliflower ear) resulting from dissolution of supporting cartilage. Similarly, cellulitis of the auricle must be treated promptly to prevent development of perichondritis and its resultant deformity.

Senturia BH, Marcus MD, Lucente F: *Diseases of the External Ear: An Otologic-Dermatologic Manual.* Grune & Stratton, 1980.

## DISEASES OF THE EAR CANAL

### 1. CERUMEN IMPACTION

Cerumen is a protective secretion produced by the outer portion of the ear canal. In most individuals, the ear canal is self-cleansing. Recommended hygiene consists of cleaning the external opening with a washcloth over the index finger without entering the canal itself. In most cases, cerumen impaction is self-induced through ill-advised attempts at cleaning the ear. It may be relieved with detergent ear drops (eg, 3% hydrogen peroxide; 6.5% carbamide peroxide [Debrox]), mechanical removal, suction, or irrigation. Irrigation is performed with water at body temperature to avoid a vestibular caloric response. The stream should be directed at the ear canal wall adjacent to the cerumen plug. Irrigation should be performed only when the tympanic membrane is known to be intact.

### 2. FOREIGN BODIES

Foreign bodies in the ear canal are more frequent in children than in adults. Firm materials may be removed with a loop or a hook, taking care not to displace the object medially toward the tympanic membrane. Aqueous irrigation should not be performed for organic foreign bodies (eg, beans, insects), because water may cause them to swell. Living insects are best immobilized before removal by filling the ear canal with lidocaine.

### 3. EXTERNAL OTITIS

External otitis, commonly known as swimmer's ear, presents with otalgia, frequently accompanied by pruritus and purulent discharge. There is often a history of recent water exposure or mechanical trauma (eg, scratching, cotton applicators). External otitis is usually caused by gram-negative rods (eg, *Pseudomonas, Proteus*) or fungi (eg, *Aspergillus*), which grow in the presence of excessive moisture.

Examination reveals erythema and edema of the ear canal skin, often with a purulent exudate. Manipulation of the auricle often elicits pain. Because the lateral surface of the tympanic membrane is ear canal skin, it is often erythematous. However, in contrast to acute otitis media, it moves normally with pneumatic otoscopy. When the canal skin is very edematous, it may be impossible to visualize the tympanic membrane. Fundamental to the treatment of external otitis is protection of the ear from additional moisture and avoidance of further mechanical injury by scratching. Otic drops containing a mixture of aminoglycoside antibiotic and anti-inflammatory corticosteroid in an acid vehicle are generally very effective (eg, Cortisporin Otic). Purulent debris filling the ear canal should be gently removed to permit entry of the topical medication. Drops should be used abundantly (5 or more drops), since too much is harmless and too little will fail to penetrate the depths of the canal. When substantial edema of the canal wall prevents entry of drops into the ear canal, a wick is placed to facilitate entry of the medication.

Persistent external otitis in the diabetic or immunocompromised patient may evolve into osteomyelitis of the skull base, often referred to as **malignant exter-**

**nal otitis.** Usually caused by *Pseudomonas aeruginosa,* osteomyelitis begins in the floor of the ear canal and may extend into the middle fossa floor, the clivus, and even the contralateral skull base. The patient usually presents with persistent foul aural discharge, granulations in the ear canal, deep otalgia, and progressive cranial nerve palsies involving nerves VI, VII, IX, X, XI, or XII. Diagnosis is confirmed by the demonstration of osseous erosion on CT and radionuclide scanning.

Treatment is chiefly medical, requiring prolonged intravenous administration of antibiotics, often for several months. Surgical debridement is reserved for cases of deterioration despite medical therapy.

Bell DN: Otitis externa: A common, often self-inflicted condition. *Postgrad Med* (Sept) 1985;**78:**101.

Chandler JR et al: Osteomyelitis of the base of the skull. *Laryngoscope* 1986;**96:**245.

## 4. EXOSTOSES & OSTEOMAS

Bony overgrowths of the ear canal are a frequent incidental finding and occasionally have clinical significance. Clinically, they present as skin-covered mounds in the medial ear canal obscuring the tympanic membrane to a variable degree. Solitary osteomas are of no significance as long as they do not cause obstruction or infection. Multiple exostoses, which are generally acquired from repeated exposure to cold water, often progress and require surgical removal.

## 5. NEOPLASIA

The most common neoplasm of the ear canal is squamous cell carcinoma. Clinically, this tumor may simulate persistent external otitis. When an apparent otitis externa does not resolve on therapy, early biopsy is warranted. This disease carries a very high 5-year mortality rate and must be treated with wide surgical resection and radiation therapy. Adenomatous tumors, originating from the ceruminous glands, generally follow a more indolent course.

## DISEASES OF THE AUDITORY (EUSTACHIAN) TUBE

### 1. AUDITORY TUBE DYSFUNCTION

The tube that connects the middle ear to the nasopharynx—the auditory tube, or eustachian tube—provides ventilation and drainage for the middle ear cleft. It is normally closed, opening only during the act of swallowing or yawning. When auditory tube function is compromised, air trapped within the middle ear becomes absorbed and negative pressure results. The most common causes of auditory tube dysfunction are diseases associated with edema of the tubal lining, such as viral upper respiratory tract infections and allergy. The patient usually reports a sense of fullness in the ear and mild to moderate impairment of hearing. When the tube is only partially blocked, swallowing or yawning may elicit a popping or crackling sound. Examination reveals retraction of the tympanic membrane and decreased mobility on pneumatic otoscopy. Following a viral illness, this disorder is usually transient, lasting days to weeks. Treatment with systemic and intranasal decongestants combined with autoinflation by forced exhalation against closed nostrils may hasten relief. Air travel should be avoided. Autoinflation should not be recommended to patients with active intranasal infection, since this maneuver may precipitate middle ear infection. Allergic patients may also benefit from desensitization or intranasal corticosteroids.

### 2. SEROUS OTITIS MEDIA

When the auditory tube remains blocked for a prolonged period, the resultant negative pressure will result in transudation of fluid. This condition, known as serous otitis media, is especially common in children because their auditory tubes are narrower and more horizontal in orientation than adults. It is less common in adults, in whom it usually follows an upper respiratory tract infection or barotrauma. In an adult with persistent unilateral serous otitis media, nasopharyngeal carcinoma must be excluded. The tympanic membrane in serous otitis media is dull and hypomobile, occasionally accompanied by air bubbles in the middle ear and conductive hearing loss. The treatment of serous otitis media is similar to that for auditory tube dysfunction. When medication fails to bring relief after several months, a ventilating tube placed through the tympanic membrane may restore hearing and alleviate the sense of aural fullness.

Sade J (editor): *Secretory Otitis Media and Its Sequelae.* Churchill Livingstone, 1979.

### 3. BAROTRAUMA

Individuals with auditory tube dysfunction due either to congenital narrowness or to acquired mucosal edema may be unable to equalize the barometric stress exerted on the middle ear by air travel or underwater diving. The problem is generally most acute during airplane descent, since the negative middle ear pressure tends to collapse and lock the auditory tube. Several measures are useful to enhance auditory tube function and avoid otic barotrauma. The patient should be advised to swallow, yawn, and autoinflate frequently during descent. Systemic decongestants (eg, pseudoephedrine, 30–60 mg) should be taken several hours before anticipated arrival time so that they will be maximally effective during descent. Topical decongestants such as 1% phenylephrine nasal spray should be administered 1 hour before arrival. It is important that the susceptible individual not sleep during the descent phase, since one may awaken with severe pain and markedly negative pressure from a collapsed auditory tube. Infants are especially prone to barotrauma and should be given a bottle to suck during descent.

The treatment of acute negative middle ear pressure that persists on the ground is with decongestants and attempts at autoinflation. Myringotomy provides immediate relief and is appropriate in the setting of severe otalgia and hearing loss. Repeated episodes of barotrauma in persons who must fly frequently may be alleviated by insertion of ventilating tubes.

## DISEASES OF THE MIDDLE EAR

### 1. ACUTE OTITIS MEDIA

Acute otitis media is a bacterial infection of the mucosally lined air-containing spaces of the temporal bone. Purulent material forms not only within the middle ear cleft but also within the mastoid air cells and petrous apex when they are pneumatized. Acute otitis media is usually precipitated by a viral upper respiratory tract infection that causes auditory tube edema. This results in accumulation of fluid and mucus, which becomes secondarily infected by bacteria. The most common pathogens both in adults and in children are *Streptococcus pneumoniae, Haemophilus influenzae,* and *Streptococcus pyogenes.* In newborn infants, gram-negative enteric bacilli predominate.

Acute otitis media is most common in infants and children, though it may occur at any age. The patient presents with otalgia, aural pressure, decreased hearing, and often fever. The typical physical findings are erythema and decreased mobility of the tympanic membrane. Occasionally, bullae will be seen on the tympanic membrane. Although it is commonly taught that this represents infection with *Mycoplasma pneumoniae,* most cases involve more common pathogens.

Rarely, when middle ear empyema is severe, the tympanic membrane can be seen to bulge outward. In such cases, tympanic membrane rupture is imminent. Rupture is accompanied by a sudden decrease in pain, followed by the onset of otorrhea. With appropriate therapy, spontaneous healing of the tympanic membrane occurs in most cases. When perforation persists, chronic otitis media frequently evolves. Mastoid tenderness often accompanies acute otitis media and is due to the presence of pus within the mastoid air cells. At this stage, this does not indicate suppurative (surgical) mastoiditis.

The treatment of acute otitis media is specific antibiotic therapy, often combined with nasal decongestants. Surgical drainage of the middle ear (myrin-gotomy) is reserved for patients with severe otalgia or when complications of otitis (eg, mastoiditis, meningitis) have occurred.

Tympanocentesis for culture may be performed with a 20-gauge spinal needle bent 90 degrees to the hub of a 3-mL syringe. Tympanocentesis is useful for otitis media in immunocompromised patients; in neonates, in whom gram-negative organisms are common; and in cases of persistent infection despite multiple courses of antibiotics.

The first-choice antibiotic treatment is either amoxicillin (20–40 mg/kg/d) or erythromycin (50 mg/kg/d) plus sulfonamide (150 mg/kg/d). Alternatives useful in resistant cases are cefaclor (20–40 mg/kg/d) or amoxicillin-clavulanate (20–40 mg/kg/d) combinations.

Recurrent acute otitis media may be managed with long-term antibiotic prophylaxis. Single daily doses of sulfamethoxazole (500 mg) or amoxicillin (250 or 500 mg) are given over a period of 1–3 months. Failure of this regimen to control infection is an indication for insertion of ventilating tubes. In children with recurrent nasopharyngitis and nasal obstruction, adenoidectomy may be a useful adjunct to tympanostomy tubes.

Eichenwald H: Developments in diagnosing and treating otitis media. *Am Fam Physician* 1985;**31:**155.

Kaleida PH et al: Amoxicillin-clavulanate potassium compared with cefaclor for acute otitis media in infants and children. *Pediatr Infect Dis* 1987;**6:**265.

### 2. CHRONIC OTITIS MEDIA & CHOLESTEATOMA

Chronic infection of the middle ear and mastoid generally develops as a consequence of recurrent acute otitis media, although it may follow other diseases and trauma. Perforation of the tympanic membrane is usually present. This may be accompanied by mucosal changes such as polypoid degeneration and granulation tissue and osseous changes such as osteitis and sclerosis. The bacteriology of chronic otitis media differs from that of acute otitis media. Common organisms include *P aeruginosa, Proteus* sp, *Staphylococcus aureus,* and mixed anaerobic infections. The clinical hallmark of chronic otitis media is purulent aural discharge. Drainage may be continuous or intermittent, with increased severity during upper respiratory tract infection or following water exposure. Pain is uncommon except during acute exacerbations. Conductive hearing loss results from destruction of the tympanic membrane and ossicular chain. The medical treatment of chronic otitis media includes regular removal of infected debris, use of earplugs to protect against water exposure, and topical antibiotic drops for exacerbations.

The definitive management of chronic otitis media is surgical in most cases. Tympanic membrane repair may be accomplished with temporalis muscle fascia or with homograft middle ear structures. Successful reconstruction of the tympanic membrane may be achieved in about 90% of cases, often with elimination of infection and significant improvement in hearing. When the mastoid air cells are involved by irreversible infection, they should be exenterated through mastoidectomy.

Cholesteatoma is a special variety of chronic otitis media. The most common cause is prolonged auditory tube dysfunction, with resultant chronic negative middle ear pressure that draws inward the upper flaccid portion of the tympanic membrane. This creates a squamous epithelium-lined sac, which—when its neck becomes obstructed—fills with desquamated keratin and becomes chronically infected. Cholesteatomas typically erode bone, with early penetration of the mastoid and destruction of the ossicular chain. Over time, they may erode the inner ear or facial nerve and on rare occasions may spread intracranially. Physical examination reveals an epitympanic retraction pocket or marginal tympanic membrane perforation that exudes keratin debris. The treatment of cholesteatoma is surgical marsupialization of the sac or its complete removal. This often requires creation of a ''mastoid bowl'' in which the ear canal and mastoid are joined into a large common cavity that must be periodically cleaned.

Farrior JB: Management of the chronically draining ear. *South Med J* 1985;**78:**271.

## 3. COMPLICATIONS OF OTITIS MEDIA

### Mastoiditis

Acute suppurative mastoiditis usually evolves following several weeks of inadequately treated acute otitis media. It is characterized by postauricular pain and erythema accompanied by a spiking fever. Radiography reveals coalescence of the mastoid air cells due to destruction of their bony septa. Initial treatment consists of intravenous antibiotics and myringotomy for culture and drainage. Failure of medical therapy indicates the need for surgical drainage (mastoidectomy).

### Petrous Apicitis

The medial portion of the petrous bone between the inner ear and clivus may become a site of persistent infection when the drainage of its pneumatic cell tracts becomes blocked. This may cause foul discharge, deep ear and retro-orbital pain, and sixth nerve palsy (Gradenigo's syndrome). Treatment is with prolonged antibiotic therapy and surgical drainage via petrous apicectomy.

### Otogenic Skull Base Osteomyelitis

Infections originating in the external or middle ear may result in osteomyelitis of the skull base, usually due to *P aeruginosa*. The diagnosis and management of this disease is discussed in the section on external otitis.

### Facial Paralysis

Facial palsy may be associated with either acute or chronic otitis media. In the acute setting, it results from inflammation of the nerve in its middle ear segment, perhaps mediated through bacterially secreted neurotoxins. Treatment consists of myringotomy for drainage and culture, followed by intravenous antibiotics. The use of corticosteroids is controversial. The prognosis is excellent, with complete recovery in the vast majority of cases.

Facial palsy associated with chronic otitis media usually evolves slowly due to chronic pressure on the nerve in the middle ear or mastoid by cholesteatoma. Treatment requires surgical correction of the underlying disease. The prognosis is less favorable than for facial palsy associated with acute otitis media.

### Sigmoid Sinus Thrombosis

Trapped infection within the mastoid air cells adjacent to the sigmoid sinus may cause septic thrombophlebitis. This is heralded by signs of systemic sepsis (spiking fevers, chills), at times accompanied by signs of increased intracranial pressure (headache, lethargy, nausea and vomiting, papilledema). If not recognized early, it may lead to widespread septic embolization and death. Treatment is with intravenous antibiotics, surgical drainage, and—when emboli are suspected—ligation of the internal jugular vein in the neck.

### Central Nervous System Infection

Otogenic meningitis is by far the most common intracranial complication of ear infection. In the setting of acute suppurative otitis media, it arises from hematogenous spread of bacteria, most commonly *H influenzae* and *S pneumoniae*. In chronic otitis media, it results either from passage of infections along preformed pathways such as the petrosquamous suture line or from direct extension of disease through the dural plates of the petrous pyramid.

Epidural abscesses arise from direct extension of disease in the setting of chronic infection. They are usually asymptomatic but may present with deep local pain, headache, and low-grade fever. They are usually discovered as an incidental finding at surgery. Intraparenchymal brain abscesses may arise in the temporal lobe or cerebellum. They most commonly evolve from retrograde thrombophlebitis adjacent to an epidural abscess. The predominant causative organisms are *Staphylococcus aureus, S pyogenes,* and *S pneumoniae*. Rupture into the subarachnoid space results in catastrophic meningitis and often sudden death.

Gower D, McGuirt WF: Intracranial complications of acute and chronic infectious ear disease: A problem still with us. *Laryngoscope* 1983;**93:**1028.

Olsen KD: Facial nerve paralysis. 2. ''All that palsies is not Bell's.'' *Postgrad Med* ( July) 1984;**76:**95.

## 4. OTOSCLEROSIS

Otosclerosis is a progressive disease with a marked familial tendency that affects bone surrounding the inner ear. Lesions involving the footplate of the stapes result in increased impedance to the passage of sound through the ossicular chain, producing conductive hearing loss. This may be corrected through surgical replacement of the stapes with a prosthesis (stapedectomy). When otosclerotic lesions impinge on the cochlea, permanent sensory hearing loss occurs. Some evidence suggests that this level of hearing loss may be stabilized by treatment with oral sodium fluoride over prolonged periods of time (Florical—8.3 mg sodium fluoride and 364 mg calcium carbonate—2 tablets orally each morning).

## 5. TRAUMA TO THE MIDDLE EAR

Tympanic membrane perforation may result from impact injury or explosive acoustic trauma. Spontaneous healing occurs in the great majority of cases. Persistent perforation may result from secondary infection brought on by exposure to water. Patients should be advised to wear earplugs while swimming or bathing during the healing period. Hemorrhage behind an intact tympanic membrane (hemotympanum) may follow blunt trauma or extreme barotrauma. Spontaneous resolution over several weeks is the usual course. When a conductive hearing loss greater than 30 dB persists for more than 3 months following trauma, disruption of the ossicular chain should be suspected. Middle ear exploration with reconstruction of the ossicular chain, combined with repair of the tympanic membrane when required, will usually restore hearing.

## 6. MIDDLE EAR NEOPLASIA

Primary middle ear tumors are rare. Glomus tumors arise either in the middle ear (glomus tympanicum) or in the jugular bulb with upward erosion into the hypotympanum (glomus jugulare). They present clinically with pulsatile tinnitus and hearing loss. A vascular mass may be visible behind an intact tympanic membrane. Large glomus jugulare tumors are often associated with multiple cranial neuropathies, especially involving nerves VII, IX, X, XI, and XII. Treatment may require surgery, radiotherapy, or both.

## DISEASES OF THE INNER EAR

## 1. SENSORY HEARING LOSS

Diseases of the cochlea result in sensory hearing loss, usually irreversible. The primary goals of management are prevention of further losses and func-

tional improvement with amplification and auditory rehabilitation. Most cochlear diseases result in bilateral symmetric hearing loss. The most common example is presbycusis, the progressive, predominantly high-frequency hearing loss of advancing age. Approximately 25% of people between the ages of 65 and 74 years and almost 50% of those over 75 experience hearing difficulties.

Noise trauma is the second most common cause of sensory hearing loss. Sounds exceeding 85 dB are potentially injurious to the cochlea, especially with prolonged exposures. The loss typically begins in the high frequencies (especially 4000 Hz) and progresses to involve the speech frequencies with continuing exposure. Among the more common sources of injurious noise are industrial machinery, weapons, and excessively loud music. In recent years, monitoring of noise levels in the workplace by regulatory agencies has led to preventive programs that have reduced the frequency of occupational losses. Individuals of all ages—especially those with existing hearing losses—should wear earplugs when exposed to moderately loud noises and specially designed earmuffs when exposed to explosive noises such as gunfire.

Head trauma has effects on the inner ear similar to those of severe acoustic trauma. Some degree of sensory hearing loss may occur following simple concussion and is frequent after skull fracture.

Ototoxic substances may affect both the auditory and vestibular systems. The most common ototoxic medications are salicylates, aminoglycosides, loop diuretics, and several antineoplastic agents, notably cisplatin. The latter 3 categories of ototoxic agents may cause irreversible hearing loss even when administered in therapeutic doses. When using these medications, it is important to identify high-risk patients, such as those with preexisting hearing losses or renal insufficiency. Patients simultaneously receiving multiple ototoxic agents are at particular risk due to ototoxic synergy. Useful measures to reduce the risk of ototoxic injury include serial audiometry and monitoring of serum peak and trough levels to ensure use of the lowest dose compatible with therapeutic efficacy, and substitution of equivalent (monototoxic) drugs whenever possible.

There are numerous less common causes of sensory hearing loss. Metabolic derangements (eg, diabetes, hypothyroidism, renal failure), infections (eg, measles, mumps, syphilis), autoimmune disorders (eg, polyarteritis, lupus), and hereditary syndromes are some of the chief examples.

Unilateral or asymmetric sensorineural hearing loss raises the question of a lesion proximal to the cochlea. Lesions affecting the eighth nerve and central auditory system are discussed in the section on neural hearing loss. A notable cause of unilateral cochlear dysfunction is the syndrome of sudden sensory hearing loss. This may occur at any age but is more common in the elderly. It most probably is the result of sudden vascular occlusion of the internal auditory artery or of a viral inner ear infection. Prognosis is mixed, with many patients suffering permanent deafness in the involved ear while others enjoy complete recovery. Oral corticosteroids are felt by many to improve the odds of recovery. A common regimen is prednisone, 80 mg/d, followed by a tapering dose over a 10-day period.

Anderson RG, Meyerhoff WL: Otologic manifestations of aging. *Otolaryngol Clin North Am* 1982;**15:**353.

Byl FM Jr: Sudden hearing loss: Eight years' experience and suggested prognostic table. *Laryngoscope* 1984;**94:**647.

D'Alonzo BJ, Cantor AB: Ototoxicity: Etiology and issues. *J Fam Pract* 1983;**16:**489.

Glorig A: Noise: Past, present, and future. *Ear Hear* 1980;**1:**4.

Miller JJ: *CRC Handbook of Ototoxicity.* CRC Press, 1985.

## 2. TINNITUS

Tinnitus is the perception of abnormal ear or head noises. Persistent tinnitus usually indicates the presence of sensory hearing loss. Intermittent periods of mild, high-pitched tinnitus lasting for several minutes are common in normal-hearing persons. When severe and persistent, tinnitus may interfere with sleep and the ability to concentrate, resulting in considerable psychologic distress.

The most important treatment of tinnitus is avoidance of exposure to excessive noise, ototoxic agents, and other factors that may cause cochlear damage. Masking the tinnitus with music or through amplification of normal sounds with a hearing aid may also bring some relief. Although pharmacologic treatment with antiarrhythmic drugs has been advocated, recent evidence suggests no benefit with available oral regimens.

Pulsatile tinnitus should be distinguished from tonal tinnitus. Pulsations most often result from conductive hearing loss, which renders transmitted carotid pulsations more apparent. However, it may also indicate a vascular abnormality such as glomus tumor, carotid vaso-occlusive disease, arteriovenous malformation, or aneurysm. CT scan and vascular studies are often necessary to establish a definitive diagnosis.

Meyerhoff WL, Shrewsbury D: Rational approaches to tinnitus. *Geriatrics* 1980;**35:**90.

## 3. VERTIGO
### (Table 6–1)

Vertigo is the cardinal symptom of vestibular disease. It is either a sensation of motion when there is no motion or an exaggerated sense of motion in response to a given bodily movement. Thus, vertigo is not just "spinning" but may present, for example, as a sense of tumbling, of falling forward or backward, or "earthquakelike" ground rolling beneath one's feet. It should be distinguished from imbalance and light-headedness, both of which are usually nonvestibular in origin.

A minimal physical examination of the patient with vertigo includes the Romberg test, an evaluation of gait, and observation for the presence of nystagmus. The Fukuda test, in which the patient marches in place with eyes closed, is useful for detecting subtle defects. A positive response is when the patient rotates, usually toward the side of the diseases labyrinth.

Electronystagmography consists of objective recording of the nystagmus induced by head and body movement, gaze, and caloric stimulation. It is helpful in quantifying the degree of vestibular hypofunction and may help with the differentiation between peripheral and central lesions. Computer-driven rotatory chairs and posturography platforms offer improved diagnostic abilities but are not widely available.

Dix MR, Hood JD: *Vertigo.* Wiley, 1984.

Hotson JR: Clinical detection of acute vestibulocerebellar disorders. *West J Med* 1984;**140:**910.

Hybels RL: History taking in dizziness: The most important diagnostic step. *Postgrad Med* (Feb) 1984;**75:**41.

### Endolymphatic Hydrops (Meniere's Syndrome)

Meniere's syndrome results from distention of the endolymphatic compartment of the inner ear. The primary lesion appears to be in the endolymphatic

**Table 6–1.** Differential diagnosis of some common vestibular disorders based on their classic presentations.

| Duration of Typical Vertiginous Episodes | Auditory Symptoms Present | Auditory Symptoms Absent |
|---|---|---|
| Seconds | Perilymphatic fistula | Positioning vertigo (cupulolithiasis), vertebrobasilar insufficiency, cervical vertigo |
| Hours | Endolymphatic hydrops (Meniere's syndrome), syphilis | Recurrent vestibulopathy, vestibular migraine |
| Days | Labyrinthitis, labyrinthine concussion | Vestibular neuronitis |
| Months | Acoustic neuroma, ototoxicity | Multiple sclerosis, cerebellar degeneration |

sac, which is thought to be responsible for endolymph filtration and excretion. Although a precise cause of hydrops cannot be established in most cases, 2 known causes are syphilis and head trauma. The classic syndrome consists of episodic vertigo, usually lasting 1–8 hours; low-frequency sensorineural hearing loss, often fluctuating; tinnitus, usually low-tone and "blowing" in quality; and a sensation of aural pressure. Symptoms wax and wane as the endolymphatic pressure rises and falls.

Specific treatment is intended to lower endolymphatic pressure. A low-salt diet, at times supplemented by diuretics, adequately controls symptoms in the great majority of patients. In those who have failed medical therapy and remain disabled by their vertigo, surgical decompression of the endolymphatic sac may bring relief.

Episodic vertigo resembling that of Meniere's syndrome but without accompanying auditory symptoms is known as recurrent vestibulopathy. The pathogenic mechanism of this symptom complex is unknown in most cases, though a few patients suffer from a variant of migraine whereas others go on to develop the classic syndrome of endolymphatic hydrops.

Thomsen J: Defining valid approaches to therapy for Meniere's disease. *Ear Nose Throat J* 1986;**65:**396.

## Labyrinthitis

Patients with labyrinthitis suffer from continuous, usually severe vertigo lasting several days to a week, accompanied by hearing loss and tinnitus. During a recovery period that lasts for several weeks, rapid head movements may bring on transient vertigo. Hearing may return to normal or remain permanently impaired in the involved ear. The cause of labyrinthitis is unknown, although it frequently follows an upper respiratory tract infection. For this reason, it is generally known as "viral" or "infectious" labyrinthitis.

## Vestibular Neuronitis

This disorder is distinguished from labyrinthitis by the absence of auditory symptoms. The vertigo of vestibular neuronitis is disabling and usually lasts several days to a week. Viral mononeuritis has been suggested as the cause.

## Traumatic Vertigo

The most common cause of vertigo following head injury is labyrinthine concussion. Symptoms generally diminish within several days but may linger for a month or more. Basilar skull fractures that traverse the inner ear usually result in severe vertigo lasting several days to a week and deafness in the involved ear. Chronic posttraumatic vertigo may result from cupulolithiasis. This occurs when traumatically detached statoconia (otoconia) settle on the ampulla of the posterior semicircular canal and cause an excessive degree of cupular deflection in response to head motion. Clinically, this presents as episodic positioning vertigo. A less common source of posttraumatic

vertigo is disruption of the oval or round window with leakage of perilymph into the middle ear. Perilymphatic fistulization may follow physical or barometric trauma or may result from erosion of the inner ear by cholesteatoma or neoplasm. Symptomatic fistulas are usually associated with both vertigo and hearing loss. Surgical repair may be necessary.

## Positioning Vertigo

Transient vertigo following changes in head position is a frequent complaint. The term "positioning vertigo" is more accurate than "positional vertigo" because it is provoked by changes in head position rather than by the maintenance of a particular posture. Use of the term "benign positional vertigo" is discouraged except for cases known to be unassociated with central nervous system disorders. True positional vertigo suggests either vertebrobasilar insufficiency or dysfunction of the cervical spine.

The typical symptoms of positioning vertigo last up to 30 seconds and occur in clusters that persist for several days. During these periods, vertigo is provoked by most head movements, especially vigorous ones.

This syndrome often evolves several months after an episode of acute vestibular disease such as labyrinthitis or vestibular neuronitis. Head trauma is also a frequent cause.

Mohr DN: The syndrome of paroxysmal positional vertigo: A review. *West J Med* 1986;**145:**645.

## Management of the Patient With Vertigo

Unfortunately, few specific treatments for labyrinthine disorders have been designed to reverse a known pathogenic mechanism. Examples include low-salt diet and diuretics in Meniere's disease, antibiotic treatment of infectious diseases, and surgical repair of perilymphatic fistulas.

Symptomatic treatment is useful in the vertiginous patient to lessen the abnormal sensation and to alleviate vegetative symptoms such as nausea and vomiting. The most common drug classes employed are the antihistamines, anticholinergics, and sedative-hypnotics. Ample evidence exists that vestibular suppressant medications adversely affect the process of central compensation following acute vestibular disease. For this reason, these drugs should be used only for brief periods. Generally, they are best administered to patients with prominent vegetative symptoms and are best tapered and halted when symptoms are resolved.

In acute severe vertigo, diazepam, 2.5–5 mg intravenously, may abate an attack. Relief from nausea and vomiting usually requires antiemetic delivered intramuscularly or by rectal suppository (eg, prochlorperazine, 10 mg intramuscularly, or 25 mg rectally every 6 hours). Less severe vertigo may often be successfully alleviated with antihistamines such as meclizine, 25 mg, or dimenhydrinate, 50 mg, orally every 6 hours. Scopolamine, administered in low dosage transdermally, has proved beneficial to many patients with recurrent vertigo, although side effects (dry mouth, blurred vision) often limits its utility.

In chronic or recurrent vertigo, one of the most important therapies is exercise. Physical activity substantially enhances the central nervous system's ability to compensate for labyrinthine dysfunction and should be encouraged once nausea and vomiting have resolved. In general, the patient should be instructed to repeatedly perform maneuvers that provoke vertigo—up to the point of nausea or fatigue—in an effort to habituate them.

Surgical remedies are reserved for those who remain substantially disabled despite a prolonged and varied trial of medical therapy and exercises. Selective section of the vestibular portion of the eighth nerve brings relief of vertigo in over 90% of such patients. Surgical removal of the semicircular canals (labyrinthectomy) is also highly effective but is appropriate only for patients with little or no hearing in the involved ear.

Baloh RW: The dizzy patient: Symptomatic treatment of vertigo. *Postgrad Med* (May) 1983;**73**:317.

Hughes GB, Hahn JF: Surgery for vertigo: Update 1985. *Am J Otol* 1985;**6**:423.

Peppard SB: Effect of drug therapy on compensation from vestibular injury. *Laryngoscope* 1986;**96**:878.

Zee DS: Perspectives on the pharmacotherapy of vertigo. *Arch Otolaryngol* 1985;**111**:609.

## DISEASES OF THE CENTRAL AUDITORY & VESTIBULAR SYSTEMS
### (Table 6–1)

Lesions of the eighth cranial nerve and central audiovestibular pathways produce neural hearing loss and vertigo. One characteristic of neural hearing loss is deterioration of speech discrimination out of proportion to the decrease in pure tone thresholds. Another is auditory adaptation, wherein a steady tone appears to the listener to decay and eventually disappear. Auditory evoked responses are useful in distinguishing cochlear from neural losses and may give insight into the site of lesion within the central pathways.

Vertigo arising from central lesions tends to be more chronic and debilitating than that seen in labyrinthine disease. The associated nystagmus is nonfatigable, vertical rather than horizontal in orientation, without latency, and unsuppressed by visual fixation. Electronystagmography is useful in documenting these characteristics. The evaluation of central audiovestibular dysfunction usually requires imaging of the brain with CT or MRI scans.

### 1. ACOUSTIC NEUROMA

Tumors of the cerebellopontine angle, most notably acoustic neuroma, cause central audiovestibular symptoms. Acoustic neuromas are among the most common intracranial neoplasms. These schwannomas generally arise from the vestibular division of the eighth nerve. When small, they may occasionally be excised, with preservation of hearing. Large tumors can also be safely removed in most cases, but cranial nerve palsies—especially facial paralysis—are common sequelae.

Brackmann DE: A review of acoustic tumors: 1979–1982. *Am J Otol* 1984;**5**:233.

### 2. VASCULAR COMPROMISE

Vertebrobasilar insufficiency is a common cause of vertigo in the elderly. It is often triggered by changes in posture or extension of the neck. Empirical treatment is with vasodilators and exercise.

Migraine may cause vertiginous attacks. The diagnosis is obvious when vertigo accompanies a typical headache pattern, but this is not always the case. In patients with a history of both migraine headaches and recurrent vertigo, a therapeutic trial of $\beta$-adrenergic blocking drugs and ergots is reasonable.

Vascular loops that impinge upon the brain stem root entry zone of cranial nerves have been shown to cause dysfunction. Widely recognized examples are hemifacial spasm and tic douloureux. It has been suggested that hearing loss, tinnitus, and disabling positioning vertigo may result from such a loop abutting the eighth nerve.

Ausman JI et al: Vertebrobasilar insufficiency: A review. *Arch Neurol* 1985;**42**:803.

### 3. MULTIPLE SCLEROSIS

Most patients with multiple sclerosis suffer from episodic vertigo and chronic imbalance. Hearing loss in this disease is most commonly unilateral and of rapid onset. Spontaneous recovery may occur.

## DISEASES OF THE NOSE & PARANASAL SINUSES

## INFECTIONS OF THE NOSE & PARANASAL SINUSES

### 1. VIRAL RHINITIS
### (Common Cold)

The nonspecific symptoms of the ubiquitous common cold are present in the early phases of many diseases that affect the upper aerodigestive tract. Because there are numerous serologic types of rhinoviruses, adenoviruses, and other viruses, patients remain susceptible throughout life. Headache, nasal congestion, watery rhinorrhea, sneezing, and a scratchy throat accompanied by general malaise are typical in viral infections. Nasal examination usually shows reddened, edematous mucosa and a watery discharge. The presence of purulent nasal discharge suggests bacterial infection.

There is no proved specific treatment for a cold, but supportive measures such as decongestants (pseudoephedrine, 30 mg every 4 hours, or 120 mg twice daily) may provide some relief of rhinorrhea and nasal obstruction. Nasal sprays such as oxymetazolone or phenylephrine are rapidly effective. They should not be used for more than a few days at a time, since chronic use leads to a rebound congestion that is often worse than the original symptoms. This chronic nasal stuffiness is known as rhinitis medicamentosa. Treatment requires complete cessation of the sprays. This triggers a period of severe nasal congestion that usually lasts 1–2 weeks. Topical intranasal corticosteroids (flunisolide [Nasalide], 2 sprays in each nostril twice daily) or a short tapering course of oral prednisone may help during the process of withdrawal.

Other than transient middle ear effusion, complications of viral rhinitis are unusual. Secondary bacterial infection may occur and is suggested by a change in color of the rhinorrhea from clear and watery to mucoid and yellow or green. The most common pathogens are the same as those responsible for acute otitis media. Nasal cultures may help guide treatment.

## 2. ACUTE SINUSITIS

Acute sinus infections are uncommon compared to viral rhinitis. Because sinusitis usually has followed an acute respiratory infection and because media advertisements often use the term "sinusitis" when "rhinitis" would be more accurate, it is understandable that patients and physicians alike sometimes confuse these entities. In addition to the symptoms of rhinitis, the diagnosis of sinusitis requires clinical signs and symptoms that indicate involvement of the affected sinus or sinuses such as pain and tenderness over the involved sinus.

Sinusitis occurs when an undrained collection of pus accumulates in a sinus. Diseases that swell the nasal mucous membrane, such as viral or allergic rhinitis, are usually the underlying cause. Edematous mucosa causes obstruction of a sinus drainage tract, resulting in the accumulation of mucous secretion in the sinus cavity that becomes secondarily infected by bacteria. The typical pathogens of bacterial sinusitis are the same as those that cause acute otitis media: *S pneumoniae,* other streptococci, *H influenzae,* and, less commonly, *S aureus* and *Branhamella catarrhalis.*

## Clinical Findings

**A. Symptoms and Signs:** Because the maxillary sinus is the largest of the paranasal sinuses and its drainage into the nose is not fully dependent, it is the most commonly affected sinus. Pain and pressure over the cheek are the usual symptoms. Pain may refer to the upper incisor and canine teeth via branches of the trigeminal nerve, which traverse the floor of the sinus. It is not uncommon for maxillary sinusitis to result from dental infection, and teeth that are tender should be carefully examined for signs of abscess.

Acute ethmoiditis in adults is usually accompanied by maxillary sinusitis. In such cases, the symptoms of maxillary sinusitis generally predominate. Ethmoidal infection presents with pain and pressure over the high lateral wall of the nose that may radiate to the orbit. In children, however, because the maxillary sinus is poorly developed, isolated ethmoiditis is not rare. It usually presents as periorbital cellulitis, with the most common pathogen being *H influenzae.*

Sphenoid sinusitis is usually seen in the setting of pansinusitis. The patient may complain of a headache "in the middle of the head" and often points to the vertex. Sixth nerve palsy may occur as the abducens nerve courses just lateral to the sinus.

Acute frontal sinusitis usually causes pain and tenderness of the forehead. This is most easily elicited by palpation of the orbital roof just below the medial end of the eyebrow. Palpation here is more accurate than percussion of the supraorbital area or forehead.

**B. Imaging:** Although it is often possible to make the diagnosis of sinusitis on clinical grounds alone, radiologic confirmation allows a more definitive diagnosis and is an objective monitor of the course of infection. The standard set of sinus films and the sinus best seen in each view are Caldwell (frontal), Waters (maxillary), lateral (sphenoid), and submentovertical (ethmoid). Opacification without bone destruction is a typical feature of sinusitis. An air-fluid level may be seen if the films are taken with the patient upright rather than supine. The frontal sinus may occasionally appear normal even in the face of clinically compelling evidence of sinusitis.

## Treatment

In uncomplicated sinusitis with mild symptoms, outpatient management is usually successful. Oral decongestants, nasal decongestant sprays, and oral antibiotics are recommended. If purulent discharge is seen in the nose, it should be cultured. Because amoxicillin has better sinus penetration that ampicillin, it is an appropriate first choice. Alternatives are discussed in the section on acute otitis media. Antibiotic treatment for sinusitis should be continued for 2 weeks, with longer courses sometimes required to prevent relapses.

Failure of sinusitis to resolve after an adequate course of oral antibiotics may necessitate hospital admission for intravenous antibiotics and possible surgical drainage. Frontal sinusitis that does not promptly respond to outpatient care should be managed aggressively, because the posterior sinus wall is adjacent to the dura and because undertreated infection may lead to intracranial extension. If intravenous antibiotics fail to ameliorate symptoms, a frontal sinus trephine may be necessary to drain and irrigate the sinus. Persistent maxillary empyema may be cultured and relieved with a needle inserted through the lateral or anterior wall of the nose.

### Complications

Local complications of sinusitis include osteomyelitis and mucocele. Mucoceles, a consequence of long-standing ductal obstruction, are more common in the supraorbital ethmoids and frontal sinuses and may become secondarily infected. They appear radiologically as a smoothly expanded sinus filled with homogeneous soft tissue density. Treatment is surgical, requiring either drainage of the mucocele intranasally or its complete excision with fat ablation of the sinus cavity.

Osteomyelitis requires prolonged antibiotics as well as removal of necrotic bone. The frontal sinus is most commonly affected, with bone involvement suggested by a tender puffy swelling of the forehead. Following treatment, secondary cosmetic reconstructive procedures may be necessary.

Intracranial complications of sinusitis occur either through hematogenous spread, as in cavernous sinus thrombosis and meningitis, or by direct extension, as in epidural and intraparenchymal brain abscesses. Fortunately, they are rare today. Cavernous sinus thrombosis is heralded by opthalmoplegia, chemosis, and visual loss. Frontal epidural abscess is usually quiescent. It may be detected on CT scan, a study recommended in all cases of atypical or complicated sinusitis.

It should always be kept in mind that paranasal sinus cancer is in the differential diagnosis of sinusitis. The presence of bone destruction radiologically, cranial neuropathies (especially $V_2$), persistent pain, epistaxis, or a prolonged clinical course should raise the suspicion of possible cancer.

Bluestone CD: Medical and surgical therapy of sinusitis. *Pediatr Infect Dis* 1984;**3(Suppl 3)**:S13.

Goodman A, Cleary JG, Pickering LK: Is it a "cold"—or a mimic that mandates treatment? *J Respir Dis* 1985;**6**:21.

Stool SE: Diagnosis and treatment of sinusitis. *Am Fam Physician* 1985;**32**:101.

### 3. NASAL VESTIBULITIS

Inflammation at the nasal vestibule commonly results from folliculitis of the hairs that line this orifice. Systemic antibiotics effective against *S aureus* and streptococci—in addition to local antimicrobial ointments—are indicated. If a furuncle exists, it should be incised and drained, preferably intranasally. Adequate treatment of these infections is important to prevent retrograde spread of infection through valveless veins into the cavernous sinus and intracranial contents.

### 4. RHINOCEREBRAL MUCORMYCOSIS

Although mucormycosis is rare, any physician seeing patients in a primary care setting must be aware of its presenting signs and symptoms. The fungus (*Mucor, Absidia, Rhizopus*) spreads rapidly through vascular channels and may be lethal if not detected early. Patients with mucormycosis almost invariably have an underlying disease, often diabetes mellitus or uremia. The initial symptoms may be similar to those of bacterial sinusitis, although facial pain is often more severe. Examination of the nasal mucosa is likely to show black, necrotic eschar adherent to the inferior turbinate. Cranial neuropathies and black necrotic skin overlying the ethmoid sinuses are advanced signs. Diagnosis requires biopsy, which reveals broad nonseptate hyphae within tissues.

Mucormycosis represents a medical and surgical emergency. Once recognized, prompt wide surgical debridement and amphotericin B by intravenous infusion are indicated. Close management of the underlying disease is also of great importance. Even with early diagnosis and immediate appropriate intervention, the prognosis is guarded. In diabetics, the mortality rate is about 20%; in patients with renal failure, the mortality rate is over 50%.

Abedi E et al: Twenty-five years' experience treating cerebro-rhino-orbital mucormycosis. *Laryngoscope* 1984;**94**:1060.

Oakley LA, Fisher JF, Dennison JH: Bread mold infection in diabetes: The life-threatening condition of rhinocerebral zygomycosis. *Postgrad Med* (Aug) 1986;**80**:93.

Parfrey NA: Improved diagnosis and prognosis of mucormycosis: A clinicopathologic study of 33 cases. *Medicine* 1986;**65**:113.

### ALLERGIC RHINITIS

The symptoms of "hay fever" are similar to those of viral rhinitis but are usually more persistent and show seasonal variation. Nasal symptoms are often accompanied by eye irritation, which causes pruritus, erythema, and excessive tearing. Numerous allergens may cause these symptoms: pollens are most common in the spring, grasses in the summer, and ragweed in the fall. Dust and household mites may produce year-round symptoms.

On physical examination, the mucosa of the turbinates is usually pale or violaceous because of venous engorgement—in contrast to the erythema of viral rhinitis. Nasal polyps, which are yellowish boggy masses of hypertrophic mucosa, may be seen.

Treatment is symptomatic in most cases. Oral decongestants alone are usually helpful, although antihistamines more specifically counteract allergic mechanisms. Numerous over-the-counter preparations are available. Nasal corticosteroid sprays such as beclomethasone and flunisolide (Nasalide), are remarkably effective if used appropriately. These sprays should be administered as 2 activations into each nostril twice daily for 1 month. Compliance is poor unless patients know that improvement usually does not begin until 1–2 weeks after starting therapy. Intranasal steroids are especially helpful in shrinking nasal polyps, often eliminating the need for surgery. Intranasal cromolyn (Nasalcrom) may be useful, especially when administered before expected contact with an offending allergen.

Maintaining an allergen-free environment by covering pillows and mattresses with plastic covers, substituting synthetic materials (foam mattress, acrylics) for animal products (wool, horsehair), and removing dust-collecting household fixtures (carpets, drapes, bedspreads, wicker) is worth the attempt to help more troubled patients. When symptoms are extremely bothersome, a search for offending allergens may prove helpful. This can either be done by skin testing or by serum RAST testing. Desensitization by gradually increasing subdermal exposure to identified allergens may be tried in selected patients, with variable results.

Broide D, Schatz M, Zeigler R: Current status of pharmacotherapy in the treatment of rhinitis. *Ear Nose Throat J* 1986;**65**:222.

Buesse WW: Chronic rhinitis: A systematic approach to diagnosis and treatment. *Postgrad Med* 1983;**73**:325.

Frazer JP: Allergic rhinitis and nasal polyps. *Ear Nose Throat J* 1984;**63**:172.

Leffert FH: Nasal and paranasal allergy. *J Asthma* 1984;**21**:131.

Norman PS: Allergic rhinitis. *J Allergy Clin Immunol* 1985;**75**:531.

Parkin JL: Topical steroids in nasal disease. *Otolaryngol Head Neck Surg* 1983;**91**:713.

Toohill RJ et al: Rhinitis medicamentosa. *Laryngoscope* 1981;**91**:1614.

## EPISTAXIS

Bleeding from Kiesselbach's plexus, a vascular plexus on the anterior nasal septum, is by far the most common type of epistaxis encountered. Predisposing factors include nasal trauma (nose picking, foreign bodies, forceful nose blowing), rhinitis, drying of the nasal mucosa from low humidity, and deviation of the nasal septum. Most cases of anterior epistaxis may be successfully treated by direct pressure on the bleeding site. The nasal alae should be firmly compressed for at least 10 minutes. Venous pressure is reduced in the sitting position, and leaning forward lessens the swallowing of blood. Nasal decongestant sprays, which act as vasoconstrictors, may also be helpful. When the bleeding does not readily subside, the nose should be examined, using good illumination and suction, in an attempt to locate the bleeding site. Topical 4% cocaine applied either as a spray or on a cotton strip serves both as an anesthetic and as a vasoconstricting agent. When visible, the bleeding

site may be cauterized with silver nitrate, diathermy, or electrocautery. A supplemental patch of Surgicel or Gelfoam may be helpful.

Occasionally, a site of bleeding may be inaccessible to direct control, or attempts at direct control may be unsuccessful. In such cases, nasal packing is necessary. A properly placed anterior pack requires several feet of half-inch iodoform packing lubricated with bacitracin or petroleum ointment. The packing is carefully and systematically placed along the floor and then the vault of the nose. If the equipment necessary to place a pack is not available, various manufactured nasal balloons may serve as either a temporizing or definitive solution.

About 5% of nasal bleeding originates in the posterior nasal cavity. This requires placement of a pack to occlude the choana before placement of a pack anteriorly. Because this is uncomfortable for the patient and because it requires oxygen supplementation to prevent hypoxia, hospitalization for several days is indicated. Narcotic analgesics are needed to reduce the considerable discomfort and elevated blood pressure caused by a posterior pack. Immediate ligation of the nasal arterial supply (internal maxillary artery and ethmoid arteries) is a reasonable alternative to posterior nasal packing. This surgery is certainly necessary when packing fails to control life-threatening hemorrhage. On rare occasions, selective arterial embolization or ligation of the external carotid artery may be necessary.

After control of epistaxis, the patient is advised to avoid vigorous exercise for several days. Avoidance of hot or spicy foods and tobacco is also advisable, as they may cause vasodilation. Avoiding nasal trauma is an obvious necessity and may require trimming children's nails. Lubrication with petroleum jelly or bacitracin ointment and increasing home humidity may be useful ancillary measures.

It is important in all patients with epistaxis, especially if recurrent, to consider underlying causes of the bleeding. A check of the PT, PTT, and platelet count is prudent. Similarly, once the acute episode has passed, careful examination of the nose and paranasal sinuses to rule out neoplasia is wise.

Johnson JT, Rood SR: Epistaxis management. *Postgrad Med* (Nov) 1981;**70**:231.

Kirchner JA: Current concepts in otolaryngology. *N Engl J Med* 1982;**307**:1126.

Okafor BC: Epistaxis: A clinical study of 540 cases. *Ear Nose Throat J* 1984;**63**:153.

## NASAL TRAUMA

The nasal pyramid is the most frequently fractured bone in the body. Fracture is suggested by crepitance or palpably mobile bony segments. Epistaxis and pain are common, as are soft tissue hematomas ("black eye"). It is important to make certain that there is no palpable step-off of the infraorbital rim, which would indicate the presence of a zygomatic complex fracture. Radiologic confirmation may at times be helpful but is not necessary in complicated nasal fractures.

Treatment is aimed at maintaining long-term nasal airway patency and nasal aesthetics. Closed reduction, using topical 4% cocaine and locally injected 1% lidocaine, should be attempted within a week of injury. In the presence of marked nasal swelling, it is best to wait several days for the edema to subside before undertaking reduction. Persistent functional or cosmetic defects may be repaired by delayed reconstructive nasal surgery.

Intranasal examination should be performed in all cases to rule out septal hematoma, which appears as a widening of the anterior septum, visible just posterior to the columella. The septal cartilage receives its only nutrition from its closely adherent mucoperichondrium. An untreated subperichondrial hematoma will result in loss of the nasal cartilage with resultant saddle-nose deformity. Undrained septal hematomas may become infected, with *S aureus* the predominant organism. Treatment consists of incision and drainage via an intranasal septal mucosal incision. It is important to be sure that both sides of the septal cartilage are adequately drained. A small Penrose drain sutured in place is helpful. Antibiotics should be given and the drained fluid sent for culture.

Ambrus PS et al: Management of nasal septal abscess. *Laryngoscope* 1981;**91**:575.
Harrison DH: Nasal injuries: Their pathogenesis and treatment. *Br J Plast Surg* 1979;**32**:57.

## TUMORS & GRANULOMATOUS DISEASE

## 1. BENIGN NASAL TUMORS

### Nasal Polyps

Nasal polyps are pale, edematous, mucosally covered masses commonly seen in patients with allergic rhinitis. They may result in chronic nasal obstruction and a diminished sense of smell. In patients with nasal polyps and a history of asthma, aspirin should be avoided, as it may precipitate a severe episode of bronchospasm. The presence of polyps in children should alert the physician to the possibility of cystic fibrosis.

Medical treatment with topical nasal steroid sprays (such as beclomethasone) is usually successful for small polyps. A short course of oral corticosteroids (eg, prednisone) may also be of benefit. When medical management is unsuccessful, polyps should be removed surgically. In healthy persons, this is a minor outpatient procedure, but a higher level of cure is advisable for those with asthma. In recurrent polyposis it may be necessary to remove polyps from the ethmoid, sphenoid, and maxillary sinuses to provide longer-lasting relief. This may be done intranasally,

endoscopically, via a Caldwell-Luc approach, or through external incision depending on the extent of disease.

Small P, Frenkiel S, Black M: Multifactorial etiology of nasal polyps. *Ann Allergy* 1981;**46**:317.

### Inverted Papilloma

Inverted papillomas are benign tumors that usually arise from the lateral wall of the nose. They present with unilateral nasal obstruction and occasionally hemorrhage. Because squamous cell carcinomas are seen in 5–10% of inverted papillomas, complete excision is necessary. Lateral rhinotomy and medial maxillectomy, with all tissue carefully processed for the pathology laboratory, is usually the procedure of choice.

Suh KW et al: Inverting papilloma of the nose and paranasal sinuses. *Laryngoscope* 1977;**87**:35.

### Juvenile Angiofibroma

These highly vascular tumors arise in the nasopharynx, typically in adolescent males. Initially, they cause nasal obstruction and hemorrhage. Any adolescent male with recurrent epistaxis should be checked to be sure he is not harboring an angiofibroma. Though benign, these tumors expand locally from the nasopharynx to involve the nasal cavity, the sphenoid and other paranasal sinuses, the clivus, and the intracranial structures.

## 2. MALIGNANT NASAL TUMORS

Unfortunately, malignant tumors of the nose, nasopharynx, and paranasal sinuses tend to remain asymptomatic until late in their course. In general, the prognosis is poor. Early symptoms are nonspecific, mimicking those of rhinitis or sinusitis. Unilateral nasal obstruction and discharge are common, with pain and recurrent hemorrhage often clues to the diagnosis of cancer. Any patient with unilateral or persistent nasal symptoms should be thoroughly evaluated. A high index of suspicion remains a key to the earlier diagnosis of these tumors. Patients often present with advanced symptoms such as proptosis, expansion of a cheek, or ill-fitting maxillary dentures. Malar hypesthesia, due to involvement of the infraorbital nerve, is common in maxillary sinus tumors. Biopsy is necessary for definitive diagnosis, and MRI or CT scan will usually delineate the extent of disease.

Squamous cell carcinoma is the most common cancer seen in this anatomic region. It is especially common in the nasopharynx, where it obstructs the auditory tube and results in serous otitis media. Any adult with persistent serous otitis media, especially when unilateral, requires careful evaluation of the nasopharynx. Adenocarcinoma, mucosal melanomas, sarcomas, and non-Hodgkin's lymphomas are less commonly encountered neoplasia of this area.

Treatment depends on the tumor type and the extent of disease. Nasopharyngeal carcinoma may be treated, with considerable success, by radiotherapy alone. Other squamous cell carciomas are best treated—when resectable—with a combination of surgery and irradiation. Numerous protocols investigating the role of chemotherapy are under evaluation.

Johns ME, Kaplan MJ: Advances in the management of paranasal sinus tumors. Page 53 in: *Head and Neck Oncology.* Wolf GT (editor). Martinus Nijhoff, 1984.

## 3. WEGENER'S GRANULOMATOSIS, POLYMORPHIC RETICULOSIS, SARCOIDOSIS

The nose and paranasal sinuses are involved in Wegener's granulomatosis more commonly than either the lungs or the kidneys. Nasal crusting, obstruction, and vague pain are common. Examination shows bloodstained crusts and friable mucosa. Biopsy classically shows necrotizing granulomas and vasculitis, but in practice the differential diagnosis may be more difficult. Sarcoidosis also commonly presents in the paranasal sinuses and is clinically similar. Biopsy shows nonnecrotic granulomas. Polymorphic reticulosis (also known as lethal midline granuloma) is clinically similar to Wegener's granulomatosis, but there is often more bone destruction in the midface. Histologically, there is a dense infiltrate of mature lymphocytes, histiocytes, and immunoblasts. Differentiation from lymphoma may be difficult.

Fauci AS et al: Wegener's granulomatosis: Prospective clinical and therapeutic experience with 85 patients for 21 years. *Ann Intern Med* 1983;**98**:76.
Hall SL et al: Wegener granulomatosis in pediatric patients. *J Pediatr* 1985;**106**:739.
McDonald TJ, DeRemee RA: Wegener's granulomatosis. *Laryngoscope* 1983;**93**:220.

# DISEASES OF THE ORAL CAVITY & PHARYNX

## STOMATITIS

**Aphthous stomatitis** (canker sore) is the most common form of ulcerative stomatitis. Its cause remains uncertain. Lesions are usually 1–2 mm in diameter but may be up to 10 times larger. They are commonly buccal or gingival in location. Lesions typically present as gray vesicles that ulcerate, developing intensely painful yellow fibrinoid centers with a red halo. This painful stage lasts 48–96 hours. While no treatment has proved successful, topical anesthetics may offer symptomatic relief.

The lesions of herpetic stomatitis are similar in size to those of aphthous stomatitis but are multiple and often occur in proximity to the mucocutaneous junction. They are caused by herpes simplex type 1 and are self-limited. Topical or systemic acyclovir has been suggested to prevent recurrences, decrease postherpetic pain, and shorten the clinical course.

**Acute necrotizing ulcerative gingivitis** (Vincent's angina) is caused by infection with a synergistic combination of fusiform bacilli and oral spirochetes. It is common in young adults, often occurring at times of stress. There is superficial mucosal necrosis, resulting in a gray pseudomembrane on the tonsils, gingiva, and elsewhere in the mouth. Halitosis is a prominent feature. Treatment includes penicillin and hydrogen peroxide rinses.

**Oral candidiasis** is common in patients receiving broad-spectrum antibiotics and in those undergoing radiation therapy or chemotherapy. It is increasingly being seen early in the course of AIDS and ARC. Angular cheilitis is often seen in candidiasis, but it is also frequent in nutritional deficiency. The intraoral lesions are usually painful and have a shaggy white surface over a hemorrhagic base. The white membrane is easily scraped off with a tongue depressor—unlike lichen planus or leukoplakia. It may be stained with potassium hydroxide to reveal the hyphae. Oral ketaconazole (200 mg daily for 10–14 days) is the treatment of choice. Nystatin troches 5 times a day are an alternative.

In children, several additional causes of vesicular stomatitis are seen. **Herpes zoster** (varicella) vesicles and ulcers are seen on the palate in association with chickenpox on the trunk and face. Varicella is more common in the winter months and in children under 10. Acute herpetic gingivostomatitis is seen in 1- to 3-year-olds and is characterized by yellow-gray gingival ulcers 2–10 mm in diameter accompanied by fever and submandibular adenopathy. Because of the severe pain, toddlers do not eat, and intravenous hydration may be needed for the 4- to 10-day self-limited course.

**Herpangina** is caused by coxsackieviruses types A and B. It affects children under 6 years old, usually in summer. Abrupt onset of fever and dysphagia is accompanied by white-gray vesicular and ulcerative lesions 1–2 mm in diameter with surrounding bright red halos limited to the tonsillar fossae and soft palate.

**Hand-foot-and-mouth disease,** also caused by one or more coxsackieviruses and also occurring in young children usually in summer, is characterized by vesicular-ulcerative lesions on the lips and buccal mucosa. It is distinguished from herpangina by the presence of lesions on the soles and palms, accompanied by a transient erythematous rash.

Armstrong RB: Cutaneous aids in the diagnosis of oral ulcers. *Laryngoscope* 1981;**91**:31.
Greenberg MS: Ulcerative, vesicular and bullous lesions. Page 163 in: *Burket's Oral Medicine: Diagnosis and Treatment,* 8th ed. Lynch MA (editor). Lippincott, 1983.
Guy JT: Oral manifestations of systemic disease. Page 1231

in: *Otolaryngology: Head and Neck Surgery.* Cummings CW, Frederickson J (editors). Mosby, 1986.

## LEUKOPLAKIA & ERYTHROPLAKIA

Leukoplakia is any white mucosal lesion that cannot be removed by simply rubbing the surface. It may consist of simple hyperkeratosis resulting from chronic irritation (eg, dentures, chronic alcohol exposure, chewing tobacco) or may represent histologic dysplasia. In about 2–6% of cases, leukoplakia represents early squamous cell carcinoma. Erythroplakia is similar except that there is an erythematous component to it. About 90% of erythroplakia is early squamous cell carinoma. Any leukoplakic area that enlarges or contains an erythematous component should be managed by incisional biopsy or scraping for cytologic examination.

A systematic and thorough intraoral examination, including the lateral tongue, the floor of the mouth, the gingiva, the buccal region, the palate, and the tonsillar fossa, should be part of any general physical examination, especially in patients over the age of 45 who smoke or who drink immoderately. Numerous benign lesions may mimic carcinoma, including necrotizing sialometaplasia, pseudoepitheliomatous hyperplasia, median rhomboid glossitis, oral epithelial residues, and the juxtaoral organ of Chievitz. The threshold for specialty referral should be low.

Brightman VJ: Red and white lesions of the oral mucosa. Page 209 in: *Burket's Oral Medicine: Diagnosis and Treatment,* 8th ed. Lynch MA (editor). Lippincott, 1983.

## PHARYNGITIS & TONSILLITIS

Streptococcal tonsillitis is common and is distinguished from streptococcal pharyngitis by the presence of erythematous and enlarged tonsils, often covered with a white exudate. Although an elevated white blood cell count with a leftward shift and the presence of cervical adenopathy suggest that pharyngitis is bacterial and not viral, the diagnosis is best made by throat culture. An exudative pharyngitis accompanied by marked cervical lymphadenitis in a young adult suggests infectious mononucleosis. A Monospot or heterophil agglutination test or anti-Epstein-Barr virus titer measurement will assist in making this diagnosis. About one-third of patients with mononucleosis have secondary streptococcal tonsillitis as well. This may be very severe but responds dramatically to oral steroids. Diphtheria, which is rare today, presents with high fever and a gray tonsillar pseudomembrane. Vincent's angina and herpangina have been previously discussed and complete the differential diagnosis in most cases.

Treatment is with oral penicillin for a full 10-day course. In patients allergic to penicillin, erythromycin is recommended. Adequate antibiotic treatment usually avoids the streptococcal complications of scarlet fever, glomerulonephritis, and myocarditis. When odynophagia is severe, hospitalization may be needed for intravenous hydration and antibiotics. Topical anesthetic gargles and lozenges (eg, benzocaine) may provide symptomatic relief.

## PERITONSILLAR ABSCESS & CELLULITIS

When infection penetrates the tonsillar capsule and involves the surrounding tissues, peritonsillar cellulitis results. Peritonsillar abscess and cellulitis present with severe sore throat, odynophagia, trismus, medial deviation of the soft palate and peritonsillar fold, and a ''hot potato'' voice. Following therapy, peritonsillar cellulitis usually either resolves over several days or evolves into peritonsillar abscess. The existence of an abscess may be confirmed by aspirating pus from the peritonsillar fold just superior and medial to the upper pole of the tonsil. A No. 19 or No. 21 needle should be passed no deeper than 1 cm, because the internal carotid artery passes posterior and deep to the tonsillar fossa. There is controversy about the best way to treat peritonsillar abscesses. Some incise and drain the area and continue with parenteral antibiotics, whereas others aspirate only and follow as an outpatient. At times it is appropriate to consider immediate tonsillectomy (quinsy tonsillectomy) both to drain the abscess and to avoid recurrence. Both approaches are rational and have support in the literature. Whichever approach is taken, one must be sure the abscess is adequately drained, since complications such as extension to the retropharyngeal, deep neck, and posterior mediastinal spaces is possible. Pus may also be aspirated into the lungs, resulting in pneumonia. While there is controversy about whether a single abscess is sufficient indication for tonsillectomy, most would agree that patients with recurrent abscesses should have their tonsils removed.

## TONSILLECTOMY

Despite the frequency with which tonsillectomy is performed, the indications for the procedure remain controversial. Most would agree that airway obstruction causing sleep apnea or cor pulmonale is an absolute indication for tonsillectomy. Similarly, persistent marked tonsillar asymmetry should prompt an excisional biopsy to rule out lymphoma. Relative indications include recurrent streptococcal tonsillitis, causing considerable loss of time from school or work, recurrent peritonsillar abscess, and chronic tonsillitis.

Tonsillectomy is not an entirely benign procedure. Postoperative bleeding occurs in 2–8% of cases and on rare occasions can lead to laryngospasm and airway obstruction. Pain may be considerable, especially in the adult. The pros and cons of the procedure need to be discussed with each prospective patient. Although reports in the 1970s suggested an association of tonsillectomy with Hodgkin's disease, careful review of this literature reveals no causative association whatever.

Blum DJ: Current thinking on tonsillectomy and adenoidectomy. *Compr Ther* 1983;**9**:48.

Kornblut AD (editor): The tonsils and adenoids. *Otolaryngol Clin North Am* 1987:**20**:207. [Entire issue.]

Mandel JH: Pharyngeal infections: Causes, findings, and management. *Postgrad Med* (Feb) 1985;**77**:187.

## DEEP NECK SPACE INFECTIONS

Deep neck abscesses are emergencies because they may rapidly compromise the airway. They may also spread to the mediastinum or cause septicemia. Most commonly, they originate from odontogenic infections. Other causes include suppurative lymphadenitis, direct spread of pharyngeal infection, penetrating trauma, pharyngoesophageal foreign bodies, and intravenous injection of the internal jugular vein, especially in drug abusers. Fundamentals of treatment include securing the airway, intravenous antibiotics, and incision and drainage. The airway may be secured either by intubation or tracheostomy. Tracheostomy is preferable in the patient with substantial pharyngeal edema, since attempts at intubation may precipitate acute airway obstruction. CT scan may be helpful in defining the extent of the abscess. Bleeding in association with a deep neck abscess suggests the possibility of carotid artery or internal jugular vein involvement and requires prompt neck exploration both for drainage of pus and for vascular ligation.

Ludwig's angina is the most commonly encountered neck space infection. It is a cellulitis of the sublingual and submaxillary spaces, often arising from infection of the tooth roots that extend below the mylohyoid line of the mandible. Clinically, there is edema and erythema of the upper neck under the chin and often of the floor of the mouth. The tongue may be displaced upward and backward by the posterior spread of cellulitis. This may lead to occlusion of the airway and necessitate tracheostomy. Hospitalization and intravenous antibiotics effective against streptococci and staphylococci are necessary. Dental consultation is advisable. External drainage via bilateral submental incisions is required immediately if the airway is threatened and when medical therapy has not reversed the process.

Stiernberg CM: Deep-neck space infections. *Arch Otolaryngol Head Neck Surg* 1986;**112**:1274.

White B: Deep neck infections and respiratory distress in children. *Ear Nose Throat J* 1985;**64**:30.

# DISEASES OF THE SALIVARY GLANDS

The salivary glands are divided into the 2 large parotid glands, 2 submandibular glands, several sublingual glands, and 600–1000 minor salivery glands located throughout the upper aerodigestive tract.

## ACUTE INFLAMMATORY SALIVARY GLAND DISORDERS

### 1. SIALADENITIS

Acute bacterial sialadenitis in the adult most commonly affects either the parotid or submandibular gland. It typically presents with acute swelling of the gland, increased pain and swelling with meals, and tenderness and erythema of the duct opening. Pus often can be massaged from the duct. Sialadenitis often occurs in the setting of dehydration, either postsurgical or associated with chronic illness. The pathogenesis is ductal obstruction, often by an inspissated mucous plug, followed by salivary stasis and secondary infection. The most common organism recovered from purulent draining saliva is *S aureus*. Treatment consists of intravenous antibiotics such as nafcillin and measures to increase salivary flow, including hydration, warm compresses, sialagogues (eg, lemon drops), and massage of the gland. Failure of the process to resolve on this regimen suggests abscess formation, ductal stricture, stone, or tumor causing obstruction. Ultrasound or CT scan may be helpful in establishing the diagnosis. Sialography is best avoided in acute cases.

Children are also subject to acute bacterial sialadenitis, and at times this is a recurrent problem. There need to be no underlying pathologic process. Treatment is similar to that outlined for adults, though outpatient management is worth a try. Usually even recurrent sialadenitis of childhood resolves. Epidemic viral parotitis, better known as mumps, is uncommon today because of immunizations.

Rice DH: Advances in diagnosis and management of salivary gland diseases. *West J Med* 1984;**140**:238.

Travis LW, Hecht DW: Acute and chronic inflammatory diseases of the salivary glands: Diagnosis and management. *Otolaryngol Clin North Am* 1977;**10**:329.

### 2. SIALOLITHIASIS

Calculus formation is more common in Wharton's duct (draining the submandibular glands) than in Stensen's duct (draining the parotid glands). Clinically, a patient may note postprandial pain and local swelling, often with a history of recurrent acute sialadenitis.

Stones in Wharton's duct are usually large and radiopaque, whereas those in Stensen's duct are usually radiolucent and smaller. Those very close to the orifice of Wharton's duct may be removed intraorally by dilating or incising the distal duct. Those more than 1.5–2 cm from the duct are too close to the lingual nerve to be removed safely in this manner. Similarly, dilation of Stensen's duct, located on the buccal surface opposite the second maxillary molar, may relieve distal stricture or allow a small stone to pass. The location of the facial nerve makes intraoral retrieval of more proximal parotid stones unsafe.

Repeated episodes of sialadenitis invariably lead to stricture and chronic infection. If the obstruction cannot be safely removed or dilated, excision of the gland parenchyma is necessary.

## CHRONIC INFLAMMATORY & INFILTRATIVE DISORDERS OF THE SALIVARY GLANDS

Numerous infiltrative disorders may cause unilateral or bilateral parotid gland enlargement. Sjögren's disease and sarcoidosis are examples of lymphoepithelial and granulomatous diseases that may affect the salivary glands. Metabolic disorders including alcoholism, diabetes mellitus, vitamin deficiencies, and certain thyroid disorders may also cause diffuse enlargement. Several drugs have been associated with parotid enlargement, including thioureas, iodine, and drugs with cholinergic effects (eg, phenothiazines), which stimulate flow and cause more viscous saliva.

Moutsopoulos HM et al: Sjögren's syndrome (Sicca syndrome): Current issues. *Ann Intern Med* 1980;**92**:212.

## SALIVARY GLAND TUMORS

Approximately 80% of salivary gland tumors occur in the parotid gland. In adults, about 80% of these are benign. In the submandibular triangle, it is sometimes difficult to distinguish a primary submandibular gland tumor from a metastatic submandibular space node. Only about 50–60% of primary submandibular tumors are benign. Tumors of the minor salivary glands are most likely to be malignant, with adenoid cystic carcinoma predominating.

In children, the likelihood of salivary gland cancer is considerably greater than in the adult. Watchful waiting is not recommended management of a parotid mass in a child. Mucoepidermoid carcinoma is the most common salivary gland cancer in children.

Most parotid tumors present as an asymptomatic mass in the superficial part of the gland. Their presence may have been noted by the patient for months or years. Facial nerve involvement correlates strongly with malignancy. Tumors may extend deep to the plane of the facial nerve or may originate in the parapharyngeal space. In such cases, medial deviation of the soft palate is visible on intraoral examination. MRI and CT scans have largely replaced sialography in defining the extent of tumor.

Although the accuracy of fine-needle aspiration is improving, superficial parotidectomy with facial nerve dissection is required for both diagnosis and treatment of most primary tumors. Similarly, submandibular gland masses generally require excision of the gland. In benign and small low-grade malignant tumors, no additional treatment is needed. Postoperative irradiation is required for larger and high-grade cancers.

Johns ME, Kaplan MJ: Malignant neoplasms (of the salivary glands). Page 1035 in: *Otolaryngology: Head and Neck Surgery*. Cummings CW, Frederickson J (editors). Mosby, 1986.

# DISEASES OF THE LARYNX

The primary symptoms of laryngeal disease are hoarseness and stridor. Hoarseness is caused by an abnormal flow of air past the vocal cords. The voice is "breathy" when too much air passes incompletely apposed vocal cords, as in unilateral vocal cord paralysis. The voice is harsh when turbulence is created by irregularity of the vocal cords, as in laryngitis or a mass lesion. Stridor, a high-pitched sound, is produced by lesions that narrow the airway. Airway impairment above the vocal cords produces predominantly inspiratory stridor. Lesions below the vocal cord level produce either expiratory or mixed stridor.

Fried MP (editor): The larynx. *Otolaryngol Clin North Am* 1984;**17**:1. [Entire issue.]

## CONGENITAL LESIONS OF THE LARYNX

Although many congenital laryngeal lesions are strongly suggested by their clinical presentations, laryngoscopy and bronchoscopy are recommended investigative procedures for all pediatric patients with stridor. This is important both to ensure the diagnosis and because multiple abnormalities may be present.

By far the most common cause of congenital stridor is laryngomalacia, which is caused by an immature omega-shaped epiglottis that prolapses into the airway during inspiration. Stridor is often louder when supine. It resolves with time, usually within the first 18 months of life, and requires no additional treatment.

Stridor in an infant with a cutaneous hemangioma suggests the presence of a subglottic hemangioma. These tumors often involute in time without treatment but may require laser excision or tracheostomy if critical airway obstruction occurs. Other causes of congenital stridor include laryngeal webs, subglottic stenosis, and vocal cord paralysis.

## INFECTIONS OF THE LARYNX

### 1. CROUP
#### (Laryngotracheobronchitis)

Croup is a viral infection of the subglottic region and tracheobronchial tree. It presents with inspiratory and expiratory stridor accompanied by a barking cough. The child with croup often has had a preceding upper respiratory infection. An anteroposterior soft tissue radiograph of the neck may show a narrowed subglottic airway (pencil sign), but this is not needed to make the diagnosis. Treatment is with cool humidity in a mist tent and hydration. In most severe cases, racemic epinephrine and intubation may be necessary.

It should be kept in mind that an aspirated foreign body may mimic the symptoms of croup.

Differentiation of croup and epiglottitis is shown in Table 6–2.

Baugh R, Gilmore BB Jr: Infectious croup: A critical review. *Otolaryngol Head Neck Surg* 1986;**95**:40.
Goldhagen JL: Croup: Pathogenesis and management. *J Emerg Med* 1983;**1**:3.
Levy ML, Ericsson CD, Pickering LK: Infections of the upper respiratory tract. *Med Clin North Am* 1983;**67**:153.

### 2. EPIGLOTTITIS
#### (Supraglottitis)

Epiglottitis is an infection involving the supraglottic region of the larynx. In children, it is usually caused by *H influenzae* type B. Fever, odynophagia, dysphagia, and inspiratory stridor are prominent. In severe cases, the child may be leaning forward and drooling and have little stridor owing to severe airway compromise. In a patient suspected of having epiglottitis, no attempt should be made to view the epiglottis, as doing so may precipitate acute obstruction. The child should be kept with its parents, giving humidified oxygen, and transported to the operating room for direct laryngoscopy and intubation once an appropriate team has been assembled. After control of the airway, blood cultures (which are usually positive) may be obtained. Treatment includes hydration and intravenous antibiotics effective against *H influenzae*. Racemic epinephrine and steroids may hasten extubation, usually in 48 hours.

Differentiation of epiglottitis and croup is shown in Table 6–2.

Epiglottitis in adults should be suspected when odynophagia seems out of proportion to pharyngeal findings. It may be viral or bacterial in origin. In contrast to children, indirect laryngoscopy is generally safe and may demonstrate the swollen, erythematous epiglottis. Initial treatment is hospitalization for intravenous antibiotics, steroids, and observation of the airway. When epiglottitis is recognized early, it is usually possible to avoid intubation.

Selbst SM: Epiglottitis: A review of 13 cases and a suggested protocol for management. *J Fam Pract* 1984;**19**:333.
Warner JA, Finlay WE: Fulminating epiglottitis in adults: Report of three cases and review of the literature. *Anaesthesia* 1985;**40**:348.

### 3. LARYNGEAL PAPILLOMAS

Papillomas, thought to be caused by human papovavirus, are common lesions of the larynx in both children and adults. Patients present with hoarseness that progresses to stridor over weeks to months. Repeated laser excisions are often needed to control the disease. Tracheostomy should be avoided, as this may lead to seeding of papillomas in the tracheobronchial tree, a potentially lethal complication.

Dedo HH, Jackler RK: Laryngeal papilloma: Results of treatment with the $CO_2$ laser and podophyllum. *Ann Otol Rhinol Laryngol* 1982;**91**:425.

### 4. VIRAL LARYNGITIS

Viral laryngitis is probably the most common cause of hoarseness, which may persist for a week or so after other symptoms of upper respiratory infection have cleared. The patient should be warned to avoid vigorous use of the voice (singing, shouting) while

**Table 6–2.** Differential diagnosis of croup (laryngotracheobronchitis) and epiglottitis.

|  | Croup | Epiglottitis |
|---|---|---|
| Age | 6 months to 3 years | 3–6 years |
| Stridor | Inspiratory and expiratory | Inspiratory only |
| Pace | Days, then bark | Hours |
| Agent | Viral (often) | *H influenzae* type B (parainfluenzae) |
| Site | Subglottis | Supraglottis |

laryngitis is present, since this may foster the formation of vocal nodules.

## TUMORS OF THE LARYNX

### 1. BENIGN TUMORS OF THE LARYNX

Vocal cord nodules are smooth, paired lesions that form at the junction of the anterior one-third and posterior two-thirds of the vocal cords. They are a common cause of hoarseness resulting from vocal abuse. In adults, they are referred to as "singer's nodules"; in children, "screamer's nodules." Treatment requires modification of voice habits, and referral to a speech therapist is indicated. Recalcitrant nodules may require surgical excision.

Polypoid changes of the vocal cords may result from vocal abuse, smoking, or chemical industrial irritants or may be seen in hypothyroidism. Attention to the underlying problem may resolve the polypoid changes. Inhaled steroid spray (eg, beclomethasone) may hasten resolution. At times, removal of the hyperplastic vocal cord mucosa may be indicated.

A common but often unrecognized cause of hoarseness is contact ulcers on the vocal processes of the arytenoid cartilages secondary to esophageal reflux. Treatment of the underlying reflux with antacids or histamine $H_2$-receptor antagonists and elevation of the head of the bed is often curative. Intubation granulomas may also be seen posteriorly between the vocal processes.

### 2. LARYNGEAL LEUKOPLAKIA

Leukoplakia is a frequent cause of hoarseness, most commonly arising in smokers. Direct laryngoscopy with biopsy is advised. Histologic examination usually demonstrates mild, moderate, or severe dysplasia. Cessation of smoking may reverse dysplastic changes. A certain percentage of patients—estimated to be less than 5% of those with mild dysplasia and about 35–60% of those with severe dysplasia—will subsequently develop squamous cell carcinoma. In some cases, invasive squamous cell carcinoma is present on initial biopsy.

### 3. SQUAMOUS CELL CARCINOMA OF THE LARYNX

Squamous cell carcinoma is the most common cancer seen in the larynx. It occurs predominantly in heavy smokers, with alcohol an apparent cocarcinogen. It is most common between ages 50 and 70. Hoarseness is the usual presenting symptom. Any patient with hoarseness that has persisted beyond 2 weeks must be evaluated by indirect laryngoscopy. Odynophagia, hemoptysis, weight loss, referred otal-

gia, vocal cord immobility, and cervical adenopathy suggest more advanced disease.

Early squamous cell carcinoma is best treated with radiation, with cure rates in excess of 85–95%. Conservation surgery or total laryngectomy is necessary for radiation failures and for more advanced disease. Today, the use of tracheoesophageal valves following total laryngectomy restores useful speech for most laryngectomy patients.

Bryce DP: Cancer of the larynx. Page 194 in: *Head and Neck Cancer*. Chretien PB et al (editors). Mosby, 1985.

## VOCAL CORD PARALYSIS

Most cases of vocal cord paralysis result from lesions of the recurrent laryngeal nerve. In the adult, unilateral vocal cord paralysis generally presents as hoarseness with a breathy character. The most common cause is thyroid surgery. In left vocal cord paralysis, it is important to eliminate a mediastinal or pulmonary apical lesion (Pancoast's tumor) as the causative factor. Involvement of the vagus nerve by tumors involving the jugular foramen may cause vocal cord paralysis that is usually accompanied by additional cranial neuropathies (IX, XI). When no cause can be found, function may return spontaneously within a year. Hoarseness secondary to unilateral vocal cord paralysis may be improved by injecting Teflon into the paralyzed cord.

Bilateral vocal cord paralysis usually causes stridor. The voice may be quite good, as the cords are apposed in the midline. Thyroid surgery, neck trauma, and tumor invasion from anaplastic thyroid or esophageal carcinoma are among the more common causes. Immobility of the vocal cords may also result from cricoarytenoid arthritis, as seen in advanced rheumatoid arthritis. When airway obstruction is severe, tracheostomy is indicated. Various procedures, which open the glottis by lateralizing a vocal cord, have been used in order to remove the tracheostomy. A less powerful, breathy voice often accompanies these procedures.

Snow JB Jr: Surgical therapy for vocal dysfunction. *Otolaryngol Clin North Am* 1984;**17**:91.

Tyler HR: Neurology of the larynx. *Otolaryngol Clin North Am* 1984;**17**:75.

## TRACHEOSTOMY & CRICOTHYROTOMY

There are 2 primary indications for tracheostomy: airway obstruction at or above the level of the larynx and respiratory failure requiring ventilation. In an acute emergency, cricothyrotomy secures an airway more rapidly than tracheostomy, with fewer potential immediate complications such as pneumothorax and hemorrhage. In order to reduce the chance of subglottic stenosis, cricothyrotomy should be converted to tracheostomy as soon as the patient is stable.

The most common indication for elective tracheostomy is the need for mechanical ventilation. There is no firm rule about how many days a patient must be intubated before conversion to tracheostomy should be advised. The incidence of serious complications such as subglottic stenosis increases with extended endotracheal intubation. As soon as it is apparent that the patient will require protracted ventilatory support, tracheostomy should replace the endotracheal tube. Less frequent indications for tracheostomy are life-threatening aspiration pneumonia, the need to improve pulmonary toilet to correct problems related to insufficient clearing of tracheobronchial secretions, and sleep apnea.

Posttracheostomy care requires humidified air to prevent secretions from crusting and occluding the inner cannula of the tracheostomy tube. The tracheostomy tube should be cleaned several times daily. The most frequent early complication of tracheostomy is dislodgment of the tracheostomy tube. Surgical creation of an inferiorly based tracheal flap sutured to the inferior neck skin may make reinsertion of a dislodged tube easier. It should be recalled that the act of swallowing requires elevation of the larynx, which is prevented by tracheostomy. Therefore, frequent tracheal and bronchial suctioning is often required to clear the aspirated saliva as well as the increased tracheobronchial secretions. Care of the skin around the stoma is important to prevent maceration and secondary infection.

Berlauk JF: Prolonged endotracheal intubation vs tracheostomy. *Crit Care Med* 1986;**14**:742.

Thawley SE (editor). Sleep apnea disorders. *Med Clin North Am* 1985;**69**:1121. [Entire issue.]

# FOREIGN BODIES IN THE UPPER AERODIGESTIVE TRACT

## FOREIGN BODIES OF THE TRACHEA & BRONCHI

Aspiration of foreign bodies is not rare in young children. Tracheal foreign bodies produce immediate symptoms of obstruction and choking, while bronchial foreign bodies often have an initial asymptomatic period generally lasting a few hours. Following this, symptoms of obstruction and inflammation appear, ie, wheezing and coughing that may mimic asthma.

Plain chest radiographs may reveal a radiopaque foreign body, such as a coin. Detection of radiolucent foreign bodies may be aided by inspiration-expiration films that demonstrate air trapping distal to the obstructed segment. Atelectasis and pneumonia may occur later.

Tracheal and bronchial foreign bodies should be removed under general anesthesia by a skilled endoscopist working with an experienced anesthesiologist.

Brown TC, Clark CM: Inhaled foreign bodies in children. *Med J Aust* 1983;**2**:322.

Hoffman JR: Treatment of foreign body obstruction of the upper airway. *West J Med* 1982;**136**:11.

## ESOPHAGEAL FOREIGN BODIES

Foreign bodies in the esophagus generally produce immediate symptoms of gagging and coughing. Dysphagia is often nearly complete. Patients can often point to the exact level of the obstruction. Indirect laryngoscopy often shows pooling of saliva at the esophageal inlet. Plain films may detect radiopaque foreign bodies such as chicken bones. Coins tend to align in the coronal plane in the esophagus and sagitally in the trachea. If a foreign body is suspected but not certainly known to be present, barium swallow may help make the diagnosis.

Although some have suggested that a Foley catheter may be used to remove an esophageal foreign body, this method risks displacing it into the larynx with resultant airway obstruction. Endoscopic removal under general anesthesia is safer.

Nardi P, Ong GB: Foreign bodies in the oesophagus: Review of 2394 cases. *Br J Surg* 1978;**65**:5.

O'Neill JA Jr, Holcomb GW Jr, Neblett WW: Management of tracheobronchial and esophageal foreign bodies in childhood. *J Pediatr Surg* 1983;**18**:475.

# DISEASES PRESENTING AS NECK MASSES

The differential diagnosis of neck masses is heavily dependent on the location in the neck, the age of the patient, and the presence of associated disease processes. Rapid growth and tenderness suggest an inflammatory process, while firm, painless, and slowly enlarging masses are often neoplastic. In children, most neck masses are benign, arising due to congenital problems (eg, branchial cleft cysts, lymphangioma, hemangioma) or infection. The most common pediatric tumors involving the neck are neuroblastoma and rhabdomyosarcoma. In adults, the incidence of cancer is much greater. Among neoplasms, squamous cell carcinomas arising in the upper aerodigestive tract predominate. Persistent neck masses, especially when enlarging, deserve attention. Most important are a comprehensive otolaryngologic examination and histologic evaluation of the lesion, often via fine-needle biopsy.

Miller DM et al: The differential diagnosis of the mass in the neck: A fresh look. *Laryngoscope* 1981;**91**:140.

## CONGENITAL LESIONS PRESENTING AS NECK MASSES

### 1. HEAD & NECK HEMANGIOMA

Hemangiomas are common on the face and neck, with most appearing at birth or by age 1. Intervention should be delayed, as most hemangiomas will involute over the first few years of life. In those persisting beyond the age of 5 years, conventional surgical excision or photocoagulation with an argon laser should be considered. Intervention is mandatory in the rare cases where hemangioma interferes with swallowing or breathing.

### 2. HEAD & NECK LYMPHANGIOMA

Lymphangiomas, also known as cystic hygromas, present at birth in two-thirds of cases and by age 2 in 90%. They are palpable as a lobulated soft and transilluminable mass involving the subcutaneous and deep tissues of the neck. When large, they may compress the esophagus or trachea, causing dysphagia or stridor. Fine-needle aspiration yields a mucoid yellow fluid. Unlike hemangiomas, lymphangiomas do not regress. Meticulous dissection is required for complete excision with preservation of cranial nerves and important vascular structures.

### 3. BRANCHIAL CLEFT CYSTS

Branchial cleft cysts usually present as a soft cystic mass along the anterior border of the sternocleidomastoid muscle. These lesions are usually recognized in the second or third decades of life, often when they suddenly swell or become infected. To prevent recurrent infection and possible carcinoma, they should be completely excised, along with their fistulous tracts.

First branchial cleft cysts present high in the neck, sometimes just below the ear. A fistulous connection with the floor of the external auditory canal may be present. Second cleft cysts, which are far more common, may communicate with the tonsillar fossa. Third cleft cysts, which may communicate with the piriform sinus, are rare.

### 4. THYROGLOSSAL DUCT CYST

Thyroglossal duct cysts are remnants occurring along the embryologic course of the thyroid's descent from the tuberculum impar of the tongue base to its usual position in the low neck. Although they may occur at any age, they are commonest before age 20. They present as a midline neck mass, often just below the hyoid bone, that moves with swallowing. Surgical excision is recommended to prevent recurrent infection. This requires removal of the entire fistulous tract along with the middle portion of the hyoid bone.

## INFECTIOUS & INFLAMMATORY NECK MASSES

### 1. REACTIVE CERVICAL LYMPHADENOPATHY

The normal cervical lymphatic chain is not palpable. Infections involving the pharynx, salivary glands, and scalp usually cause tender enlargement of neck nodes. In children with frequent upper respiratory tract infections, it is common to palpate small, soft, and mobile nodes in the neck. Reactive nodes are especially prominent in infectious mononucleosis. Except for the occasional node that suppurates and requires incision and drainage, treatment is directed against the underlying infection. Enlarged lymph nodes that persist beyond several months, are firm in consistency, or show steady growth should be examined histologically.

### 2. NECK INFECTIONS WITH ATYPICAL MYCOBACTERIA (Scrofula)

Scrofula is most common in children, in whom it presents as persistent adenopathy that may become fixed to the skin and drain externally. Treatment requires excision and antituberculous antibiotics. Cat-scratch disease and sarcoidosis are also in the differential diagnosis of granulomatous neck masses.

## TUMOR METASTASES

In older adults, 80% of firm, persistent, and enlarging neck masses are metastatic in origin. The great majority of these arise from squamous cell carcinoma of the upper aerodigestive tract. A complete head and neck examination may reveal the tumor of origin, but examination under anesthesia with direct laryngoscopy, esophagoscopy, and bronchoscopy is usually required to fully evaluate the tumor and exclude second primaries.

The initial evaluation of most persistent neck masses is fine-needle aspiration. It is important not to perform open biopsy on a neck mass when squamous cell carcinoma is in the differential diagnosis unless the surgeon is prepared to proceed immediately with a definitive procedure. There is an increased risk of recurrence and decreased survival when premature biopsy is performed.

Other than thyroid carcinoma, non-squamous cell metastases to the neck are infrequent. While tumors not involving the head and neck seldom metastasize to the middle or upper neck, the supraclavicular region is quite often involved by lung and breast tumors. Infradiaphragmatic tumors, with the exception of renal carcinoma, rarely metastasize to the neck.

## LYMPHOMA

About 10% of lymphomas present in the head and neck. Multiple rubbery nodes, especially in the young adult, are suggestive of this disease. A thorough physical examination may demonstrate other sites of nodal involvement. Needle aspiration may be diagnostic, but open biopsy is often required.

# OTOLARYNGOLOGIC MANIFESTATIONS OF AIDS

## MANIFESTATIONS OF AIDS IN THE ORAL CAVITY & PHARYNX

Severe gingivitis and stomatitis are frequent presenting symptoms in AIDS patients. Candidiasis is common and may require prolonged ketoconazole and topical nystatin for control. Giant intraoral ulcers have been seen in some patients. Hairy leukoplakia occurring on the lateral border of the tongue is often an early finding. Kaposi's sarcoma is commonest on the hard palate but may not be seen anywhere in the oral cavity and pharynx. It usually appears as a raised violaceous lesion beneath an intact mucosa, although it may be ulcerated, erythematous, and bleeding. Radiation therapy may control the tumor. A brisk mucositis can be expected.

In addition to Kaposi's sarcoma, an increased incidence of non-Hodgkin's lymphoma is seen in AIDS. An increase in squamous cell carcinoma is also seen

in the homosexual population, possibly related to AIDS.

## MANIFESTATIONS OF AIDS IN THE NECK

Persistent generalized lymphadenopathy is extremely common in HIV infection. In this setting, a tender or growing node may represent secondary infection, lymphoma, or other tumor. Fine-needle aspiration for culture and biopsy is the best initial diagnostic step. Open biopsy will be needed if granulomatous disease or lymphoma is suspected.

## MANIFESTATIONS OF AIDS IN THE PARANASAL SINUSES

Sinusitis is common in AIDS, and the causative organisms are diverse. Early sinus irrigation, with aspirates sent for cytologic examination as well as fungal, viral, *Legionella,* and aerobic and anaerobic cultures, is warranted. Initial antibiotic coverage should be based on the aspirate smear.

## OTOLOGIC MANIFESTATIONS OF AIDS

Given the common neurological manifestations in AIDS, it is not surprising that there is a higher incidence of sensorineural hearing loss and auditory brain stem response abnormalities in AIDS patients than in the general population. Kaposi's sarcoma of the auricle is not uncommon. Seborrheic dermatitis, more common in AIDS, may be more difficult to treat in the external auditory canal.

Cooke D, Jahn A, Oleske J: Ear, nose, and throat manifestations in acquired immunodeficiency syndrome in children. *Otolaryngol Head Neck Surg* 1985;**94:**68.

Greenspan D, Silverman S Jr: Oral lesions: Dentists play key role in early AIDS detection. *Calif Dent Assn J* 1987;**15:**28.

Greenspan D et al: Relation of oral hairy leukoplakia to infection with the human immunodeficiency virus and the risk of developing AIDS. *J Infect Dis* 1987;**155:**475.

Marcusen DC, Sooy CD: Otolaryngologic and head and neck manifestations of acquired immunodeficiency syndrome (AIDS). *Laryngoscope* 1985;**95:**401.

Rosenberg RA, Schneider KL, Cohen NL: Head and neck presentations of acquired immunodeficiency syndrome. *Laryngoscope* 1984:**94:**642.

## REFERENCES

Cummings CW, Frederickson J: *Otolaryngology: Head and Neck Surgery.* Mosby, 1986.

Gates GA: *Current Therapy in Otolaryngology Head and Neck Surgery.* Mosby, 1986.

Hughes GB: *Textbook of Clinical Otology.* Thieme-Stratton, 1985.

Wilson WR, Nadol JB: *Quick Reference to Ear, Nose, and Throat Disorders.* Lippincott, 1982.

# Pulmonary Diseases

*John L. Stauffer, MD*

## DIAGNOSTIC METHODS

### SYMPTOMS OF PULMONARY DISEASES

The history is the foundation of a precise diagnosis of pulmonary disease. Attention is paid not only to the respiratory system but also to other organ systems. Pulmonary diseases often have extrapulmonary manifestations, and diseases in other organ systems may affect the lungs. Previous treatment for respiratory complaints, previous chest x-rays and other diagnostic studies, travel, and exposure to occupational and environmental insults are all important.

**Dyspnea** is the subjective sensation of breathlessness or air hunger that is excessive for any given level of physical activity. The severity of dyspnea can be graded by the patient but can only be inferred by the physician on the basis of signs of respiratory distress. Nevertheless, the physician should record the level of activity that induces dyspnea, to serve as a basis for assessing the results of therapy. Dyspnea of pulmonary origin may be due to disorders of the airway, lung parenchyma, pleura, respiratory muscles, or chest wall. Extrapulmonary disorders causing dyspnea include heart disease, shock, anemia, hypermetabolic states, and anxiety. **Paroxysmal nocturnal dyspnea** and **orthopnea** usually are caused by left ventricular failure but may also be observed in asthma, aspiration, and chronic obstructive pulmonary disease.

**Persistent cough** should always be considered abnormal. The cough reflex may be triggered by stimulation of receptors located in the tracheobronchial tree, the upper airway (larynx, pharynx, nose, mouth), and in other sites such as the sinuses, auditory canal, pleura, pericardium, stomach, and diaphragm. Thus, the differential diagnosis of cough is considerable. Complications of severe cough include worsening of bronchospasm, vomiting, rib fractures, urinary incontinence, and, occasionally, syncope.

**Stridor** is a crowing sound during breathing caused by turbulent airflow through a narrowed upper airway. Inspiratory stridor suggests extrathoracic variable airway obstruction, while expiratory stridor indicates intrathoracic variable airway obstruction. Inspiratory

and expiratory stridor occurring together suggest fixed obstruction anywhere in the upper airway. **Snoring** is an inspiratory sound due to vibration in the pharynx.

**Wheezes** are continuous musical or whistling noises caused by turbulent airflow through narrowed intrathoracic airways. Most, but not all, complaints of wheezing are due to asthma. Wheezing may be accompanied by a sensation of **chest tightness,** a nonspecific feeling of labored breathing that implies airway obstruction.

**Hemoptysis**—the expectoration of blood or blood-tinged sputum—is often the first indication of serious bronchopulmonary disease; the history distinguishes it from hematemesis and from nasopharyngeal bleeding. The duration of symptoms, the appearance of the expectorated blood, and accompanying symptoms help narrow the differential diagnosis. Bright red, frothy blood implies a bronchopulmonary origin of bleeding. Massive hemoptysis is defined arbitrarily as the coughing up of more than 600 mL of blood in 24 hours; carcinoma is its most likely cause. Patients are rarely able to accurately localize the site of bronchopulmonary bleeding. Though bronchitis and bronchiectasis overall may be more common causes of hemoptysis, carcinoma must be excluded in all types.

Adelman M et al: Cryptogenic hemoptysis: Clinical features, bronchoscopic findings, and natural history in 67 patients. *Ann Intern Med* 1985;**102:**829.

Altose MD: Assessment and management of breathlessness. *Chest* 1985;**88(Suppl):**77.

Stulbarg M: Evaluating and treating intractable cough. (Medical Staff Conference, University of California, San Francisco.) *West J Med* 1985;**143:**223.

### SIGNS OF PULMONARY DISEASES

**Tachypnea** may be defined arbitrarily as a respiratory rate greater than 25/min; a sudden onset or persistence of tachypnea is particularly alarming.

The thorax is normally symmetric and both sides expand equally on inspiration. **Asymmetry** at rest is observed in scoliosis, chest wall deformity, severe fibrothorax, and conditions with unilateral loss of lung volume. Symmetrically reduced chest expansion is seen in such conditions as neuromuscular disease, emphysema, and ankylosis of the spine. Asymmetric chest expansion during inspiration suggests unilateral airway obstruction, pleural or pulmonary fibrosis, or splinting due to chest pain. Expansion of the chest but collapse of the abdomen on inspiration indicates weakness or paralysis of the diaphragm. If the chest collapses and the abdomen rises on inspiration, airway obstruction or a flail deformity of the chest wall may be present.

The arterial blood pressure normally falls about 5 mm Hg on inspiration. **Paradoxic pulse,** an exaggeration of the normal response, is defined as a fall in systolic arterial blood pressure of more than 10 mm Hg on inspiration. This occurs in severe asthma or emphysema, upper airway obstruction, pulmonary embolism, pericardial constriction or tamponade, and restrictive cardiomyopathy.

**Cyanosis** is a bluish discoloration of skin or mucous membranes caused by increased amounts of unsaturated hemoglobin in the blood.

**Central cyanosis,** which is usually caused by hypoxemia from respiratory failure or a right-to-left intracardiac or intrapulmonary shunt, is apparent on inspection of the oral mucous membranes; **peripheral cyanosis** is more likely due to nonrespiratory causes such as reduced cardiac output and vasoconstriction.

**Digital clubbing** is present when the anteroposterior thickness of the index finger at the base of the fingernail exceeds the thickness at the distal interphalangeal joint. Nail bed sponginess, rounding of the nail plate, and flattening of the angle between the nail plate and proximal nail skin fold are helpful clues to clubbing. Symmetric clubbing occurs in lung cancer, bronchiectasis, lung abscess, pulmonary arteriovenous malformation, idiopathic pulmonary fibrosis, and cystic fibrosis. It is rarely seen in chronic obstructive pulmonary disease and asthma. Nonpulmonary causes of symmetric clubbing include cyanotic congenital heart disease, infective endocarditis, cirrhosis, and inflammatory bowel disease. Clubbing may be familial.

**Hyperresonance to percussion** occurs in diseases accompanied by hyperinflation (asthma, emphysema) and in pneumothorax. **Dullness to percussion** is observed in thickening of the chest wall or pleura, pleural effusion, atelectasis, parenchymal infiltration or consolidation, elevation of the diaphragm, or displacement of abdominal contents into the thorax.

**Vesicular breath sounds** are normal and heard at the periphery of the lung. The finding of **bronchial (tracheal) breath sounds** in areas where vesicular sounds are normally heard implies consolidation, compression, or infiltration of the lung with a patent bronchus. **Bronchovesicular breath sounds** are intermediate in quality between vesicular and bronchial sounds. Diminished breath sounds imply obstruction to airflow, pleural disease (especially effusion), or pneumothorax.

**Adventitious sounds** may be classified as continuous **(wheezes, rhonchi)** or discontinuous **(crackles or rales).** Wheezes result from bronchospasm, bronchial mucosal edema, or airway obstruction by mucus, tumors, or foreign bodies. Rhonchi are often caused by sputum in large airways and frequently clear after cough. Crackles are probably generated by the snapping open of small airways during inspiration. Fine crackles are heard in interstitial diseases and in early pneumonia or congestive heart failure. Coarse crackles are heard late in the course of pulmonary edema or pneumonia.

**Tactile (vocal) fremitus** consists of palpable voice vibrations on the chest wall. Localized reduction in fremitus occurs in pleural effusion, pneumothorax, or thickening of the chest wall. Increased fremitus suggests lung consolidation.

**Rhonchal fremitus** consists of palpable coarse vibrations on the chest wall in patients with loud rhonchi.

**Bronchophony** refers to increased intensity and clarity of the spoken word during auscultation; it is heard over areas of consolidation or lung compression. **Whispered pectoriloquy** is an extreme form of bronchophony in which softly spoken words are readily heard by auscultation. **Egophony** refers to auscultation of an ''a'' sound when the patient speaks an ''e'' sound. It is demonstrated over compressed lung above a pleural effusion, and in consolidation.

Kraman SS (editor): Lung sounds. *Sem Respir Med* 1985;**6**:157. [Entire issue.]

## PULMONARY FUNCTION TESTS & BRONCHOSCOPY

Pulmonary function tests objectively measure the ability of the respiratory system to perform gas exchange by assessing its ventilation, diffusion, and mechanical properties.

Indications for pulmonary function testing include the following:

(1) Evaluation of the type and degree of pulmonary dysfunction.

(2) Evaluation of dyspnea, cough, and other symptoms.

(3) Early detection of lung dysfunction.

(4) Surveillance in occupational settings.

(5) Follow-up of response to therapy.

(6) Preoperative evaluation.

(7) Disability assessment.

Relative contraindications to pulmonary function testing include severe acute asthma or respiratory distress, chest pain aggravated by testing, pneumothorax, brisk hemoptysis, and active tuberculosis. Most of the tests depend on the efforts of the patient; some patients may be too ill to make an optimal effort.

Spirometry and measurement of lung volumes allow determination of the presence and severity of *obstructive* and *restrictive* pulmonary dysfunction. The hallmark of obstructive pulmonary dysfunction is reduction in airflow rates. Causes include asthma, chronic bronchitis, emphysema, small airway dysfunction, bronchiolitis, bronchiectasis, cystic fibrosis, and upper airway obstruction. Restrictive pulmonary dysfunction is characterized by reduction in lung volumes. Pulmonary infiltrates, lung resection, pleural diseases, chest wall disorders, reduced diaphragm movement, and neuromuscular disease may be responsible.

Obstructive dysfunction is graded according to the reduction in the ratio of forced expiratory volume in 1 second ($FEV_1$) to forced vital capacity (FVC). Restrictive dysfunction is graded by reduction in the FVC or total lung capacity. Grading the severity of dysfunction according to decrements of 95% confidence intervals has been proposed (see Wilson reference).

Wilson A (editor): *Pulmonary Function Testing: Indications and Interpretations.* Grune & Stratton, 1985.

## Pulmonary Exercise Stress Testing

Pulmonary exercise testing is usually performed to evaluate patients with unexplained exertional dyspnea. A bicycle ergometer or treadmill is used. Minute ventilation, expired oxygen and carbon dioxide tension, heart rate, blood pressure, and respiratory rate are monitored. The exercise protocol is determined by the indications for the test and the ability of the patient to exercise. Complications are rare.

Exercise testing in the dyspneic patient. (Symposium.) *Am Rev Respir Dis* 1984;**129(Suppl):**1. [Entire issue.]

## Bronchoscopy

Flexible fiberoptic bronchoscopy is an essential step in the diagnosis and management of many pulmonary diseases. Bronchoscopy is of value for diagnosis and staging of bronchogenic carcinoma, evaluation of hemoptysis, biopsy of diffuse lung infiltrates, diagnosis of opportunistic pulmonary infections, facilitation of bronchoalveolar lavage, and removal of retained secretions and foreign bodies from the airway. The procedure is contraindicated in patients with severe bronchospasm. A bleeding diathesis is a contraindication to biopsy and brushing. Complications include hemoptysis, fever, and a transient reduction in $P_{O2}$ ($< 10$ mm Hg). The rate of major complications is less than 2%, and deaths are rare. Hospitalization for fiberoptic bronchoscopy is not necessary in all cases.

# DEVELOPMENTAL DISORDERS

## PULMONARY AGENESIS, APLASIA, & HYPOPLASIA

The development of the lungs is complex, so that the potential for developmental anomalies is consider-

able. Bilateral arrested lung development is usually incompatible with extrauterine life. An entire lung is more commonly affected by agenesis, aplasia, or hypoplasia than is a single lobe, and the condition is usually asymptomatic. Most patients with arrested development of a lung have associated anomalies in other organs. Isolated agenesis, aplasia, or hypoplasia is usually detected on routine chest x-ray, which shows volume loss and absence of aerated lung in the affected hemithorax.

# BRONCHOPULMONARY SEQUESTRATION

The term bronchopulmonary sequestration denotes an area of nonfunctioning lung tissue that is discontinuous with the remainder of the lung and derives its blood supply from the systemic circulation, usually a branch of the descending aorta. Bronchopulmonary sequestration is located in the posterior basal segment of the lower lobes, more often on the left side than on the right. If no communication exists between the bronchial tree and the sequestration, the latter appears on x-ray as a soft tissue mass or infiltrate. If such communication exists, x-ray demonstrates a cystic, air-containing structure with or without air-fluid levels.

Bronchopulmonary sequestration is usually asymptomatic until pneumonia occurs and leads to infection of the sequestration; chronic infection follows.

Once sequestration becomes symptomatic, it should be resected. The aberrant systemic vessel supplying the sequestration is identified by preoperative aortography, so that the possibility of bleeding from an unrecognized anomalous artery is reduced. MRI has been proposed as a noninvasive method to diagnose intralobar pulmonary sequestration. Asymptomatic sequestration requires no treatment.

Oliphant L et al: Magnetic resonance imaging to diagnose intralobar pulmonary sequestration. *Chest* 1987;**91:**500.

# BRONCHOGENIC CYSTS

Bronchogenic cysts are thin-walled cystic structures lined with bronchial epithelium and filled with mucus. They arise when a portion of the bronchial tree becomes detached during organogenesis. Bronchogenic cysts are recognized on chest x-ray as round, sharply circumscribed structures containing fluid, air, or both. They usually are located near the trachea or main bronchi.

Patients with bronchogenic cysts are usually asymptomatic. However, hemoptysis, infection, or rupture into the trachea, lung, esophagus, or pleural space may occur; large proximal cysts occasionally compress major airways or blood vessels. The major clinical significance of bronchogenic cysts lies in their presentation as pulmonary nodules in patients at risk for more serious disorders. Surgical excision is often necessary.

## PULMONARY ARTERIOVENOUS MALFORMATIONS

Pulmonary arteriovenous malformation is a direct communication between a pulmonary artery and a pulmonary vein, producing a right-to-left shunt. They are multiple in as many as a third of cases and may be associated with hereditary hemorrhagic telangiectasias (Osler-Weber-Rendu disease). Pulmonary arteriovenous malformations are often asymptomatic, but they may cause hemoptysis or dyspnea. Potential physical findings include cyanosis, clubbing, and a continous murmur heard over the malformation. Laboratory studies reveal hypoxemia and often erythrocytosis. The severity of the shunt may vary as blood flow through the malformation is altered by changes in body position or lung volume. Complications include paradoxic systemic emboli, brain abscess, and hemothorax.

Arteriovenous malformations appear radiographically as sharply circumscribed round or lobulated densities within the lung parenchyma. Dilated vessels (''feeder'' vessels) connecting the arteriovenous malformation to the hilum may be visible. Changes in size of the lesion induced by alterations in intrathoracic pressure (Valsalva and Müller maneuvers) during fluoroscopy suggest the diagnosis. CT scan may reveal the feeder vessels if they are not visible on the conventional chest x-ray. Pulmonary angiography is necessary to confirm the diagnosis and to rule out the presence of additional malformations. Arteriovenous malformation must be considered in the differential diagnosis of pulmonary nodules, because failure to do so may lead to excessive bleeding after transthoracic needle aspiration or transbronchial biopsy. Single symptomatic arteriovenous malformations should be resected; multiple arteriovenous malformations that are unresectable may be treated with therapeutic embolization.

Burke CM et al: Pulmonary arteriovenous malformations: A critical update. *Am Rev Respir Dis* 1986;**134**:334.

Moser RJ, Tenholder MF: Diagnostic imaging of pulmonary arteriovenous malformations. *Chest* 1986;**89**:587.

## DISORDERS OF THE AIRWAYS

Diseases of the airways have diverse causes but share certain pathophysiologic and clinical features. Limitation of airflow is characteristic and results from intraluminal airway obstruction, thickening of airway walls, or the loss of distending support by interstitial tissues necessary to maintain patency of the airways. Hypersecretion of mucus, airway irritability, and gas exchange abnormalities are common and result in cough, sputum production, wheezing, and dyspnea.

## ASTHMA

### Essentials of Diagnosis

- Episodic or chronic wheezing, dyspnea, cough, and feeling of tightness in the chest.
- Prolonged expiration and diffuse wheezing on physical examination.
- Limitation of airflow on pulmonary function testing, or positive bronchoprovocation challenge test.
- Complete or partial reversibility of obstructive dysfunction after bronchodilator therapy.

### General Considerations

Asthma is defined as a ''disease characterized by an increased responsiveness of the trachea and bronchi to various stimuli, and manifested by widespread narrowing of the airways that changes in severity either spontaneously or as a result of treatment'' (American Thoracic Society). Asthma is characterized by such pathologic changes as hypertrophy of bronchial smooth muscle, mucosal edema and hyperemia, thickening of epithelial basement membrane, hypertrophy of mucous glands, acute inflammation, and plugging of airways by thick, viscid mucus. These changes result in obstruction of airways of all calibers.

The pathogenesis of asthma is poorly understood. Mast cells, neutrophils, eosinophils, and platelets are important in various phases of bronchoconstriction. Putative chemical mediators of asthma include histamine, leukotrienes, prostaglandins and thromboxanes, bradykinin, neutrophil and eosinophil chemotactic factors, and platelet-activating factor. Neural factors also influence bronchoconstriction and mucus secretion.

Asthma is common in adults and even more common in children. Men and women are equally affected. About 3% of the population has asthma. Death rates are increasing. It is useful to distinguish **extrinsic** from **intrinsic** asthma (Table 7–1).

Several other asthma syndromes have been identified. **Exercise-induced asthma** occurs mainly in patients with a known diagnosis of asthma. Attacks occur 5–10 minutes after the patient starts to exercise and may be related to heat loss or water loss from the bronchial surface. **Triad asthma,** a combination of intrinsic asthma, aspirin sensitivity, and nasal polyposis, occurs in fewer than 10% of asthma patients. Bronchoconstriction in this condition is due to the effects on arachidonic acid metabolism of aspirin and other compounds, including indomethacin, ibuprofen, and tartrazine dyes. **Occupational asthma** may be triggered by various agents found in the workplace (see p 175) and occurs a few weeks to many years after initial exposure to an offending agent. Nocturnal

**Table 7–1.** Features distinguishing extrinsic from intrinsic asthma.

| | Extrinsic | Intrinsic |
|---|---|---|
| Etiology | Mainly atopy | Complex |
| Antigen-related | Yes | No |
| IgE-mediated | Yes | No |
| Eczema, hay fever | Common | Uncommon |
| Family history | Usually positive | Often negative |
| Hypersensitivity skin tests | Often positive | Usually negative |
| Typical attack | Acute, mild | Often severe |
| Results of treatment | Effective | Variable |
| Environmental control | Useful | Not useful |
| Desensitization | Occasionally helpful | Not helpful |
| Relief between attacks | Complete | Often incomplete |
| Prognosis | Usually good | Less favorable |

cough may be the only symptom. **Cardiac asthma** represents bronchospasm precipitated by congestive heart failure. **Asthmatic bronchitis** denotes chronic bronchitis with features of bronchospasm that quickly responds to bronchodilator therapy. **Drug-induced asthma** is caused by many commonly used agents (Table 7–15).

## Clinical Findings

**A. Symptoms and Signs:** Asthma is characterized by episodic wheezing, feelings of tightness in the chest, dyspnea, and cough. Attacks occur spontaneously or result from various "trigger factors," including nonspecific irritants (dusts, odors, sulfur dioxide fumes), emotional stress, infection, exertion, exposure to aeroallergens, sulfites, aspiration, and abrupt changes in weather.

Physical findings vary with the severity of the attack. A mild attack may produce only slight tachycardia and tachypnea, with prolonged expiration and mild diffuse wheezing. More severe attacks are associated with use of accessory muscles of respiration, distant breath sounds, loud wheezing, hyperresonance, and intercostal retraction. Ominous signs in severe asthma include fatigue, pulsus paradoxus (> 20 mm Hg), diaphoresis, inaudible breath sounds with diminished wheezing, inability to maintain recumbency, and cyanosis.

**B. Laboratory Findings:** The total white blood cell count may be slightly increased during an acute attack, and eosinophilia is common though not invariably frequent. Expectorated sputum is viscid on gross examination; uncommon but characteristic microscopic findings include mucus casts of small airways (Curschmann's spirals), eosinophils, and elongated

rhomboid crystals derived from eosinophil cytoplasm (Charcot-Leyden crystals). Pulmonary function tests reveal abnormalities typical of obstructive dysfunction. Arterial blood gas measurements in asthma (Table 7–2) may be normal during a mild attack, but respiratory alkalosis and mild hypoxemia are usually observed. In more severe cases, respiratory alkalosis disappear when respiratory muscle fatigue prevents hyperventilation. This is a poor prognostic sign that usually indicates the need for mechanical ventilation.

**C. Imaging:** Routine chest radiographs in adults and children with uncomplicated attacks reveal only hyperinflation; they are unnecessary unless pneumothorax or pneumonia is suspected.

**D. Special Examinations:** Skin testing for allergens that trigger attacks is most useful in young patients with extrinsic asthma. Bronchial provocation testing with methacholine or histamine is helpful in confirming asthma when the diagnosis is uncertain.

## Differential Diagnosis

Wheezing occurs not only in bronchial asthma but also in chronic obstructive pulmonary disease (COPD), left ventricular failure, pulmonary embolism, and bronchogenic carcinoma. Stridor in upper airway obstruction or in vocal cord dysfunction may simulate wheezing. Reversible bronchial obstruction with eosinophilia occurs in infestations with parasitic infection (particularly *Strongyloides*), bronchopulmonary aspergillosis, and Churg-Strauss syndrome.

## Complications

Complications of asthma include exhaustion, dehydration, airway infection, cor pulmonale, and tussive syncope. Acute respiratory failure with hypoxemia and hypercapnia occurs in severe disease. Asthma has an overall mortality rate of about 0.1%.

## Prevention

Asthma is often preventable if environmental and occupational agents and other "trigger factors" known to provoke asthma attacks can be identified and eliminated. Early treatment of chest infections, recognition and effective management of nasal and paranasal disorders, discontinuation of cigarette smoking, and a sympathetic attitude on the part of the physician are essential aspects of preventive care.

**Table 7–2.** Arterial blood gas measurements in asthma.

| Severity of Attack | pH | $P_{CO_2}$ | $P_{O_2}$ |
|---|---|---|---|
| Mild | N | N | N |
| Moderate | ↑ | ↓ | ↓ |
| Severe | N | N | ↓↓ |
| Very severe | ↓ | ↑ | ↓↓↓ |

N = normal; ↑ = increased; ↓ = reduced.

## Treatment

**A. Ambulatory Patients With Asthma:** Most patients eventually require bronchodilator therapy to control symptoms. Patients with infrequent attacks may use, on an "as needed" basis, inhaled sympathomimetic bronchodilator drugs. These include albuterol, metaproterenol, bitolterol, terbutaline, isoetharine, and isoproterenol. Metered-dose inhaler (MDI) devices are the most convenient and practical way of administering these drugs; since many patients cannot use them properly, "spacer" devices are quite valuable (see below). Oral sympathomimetics should, in general, be avoided because of cardiac and neuromuscular side effects, but they may be useful in patients unable to use inhalers. Continuous treatment with theophylline derivatives is not recommended for infrequent, mild attacks of asthma; however, a long-acting theophylline compound taken at bedtime may be helpful for patients with nocturnal asthma. Exercise-induced asthma may be avoided by treatment with inhaled bronchodilators or cromolyn sodium before exercise.

Patients with more frequent or more severe attacks of asthma require maintenance bronchodilator therapy with inhaled sympathomimetics, oral theophylline drugs, or both; most clinicians favor regular use of inhaled sympathomimetics both to prevent and to treat asthma. Table 7–3 summarizes drugs used in the treatment of asthma and COPD.

**1. Inhaled sympathomimetics**–Albuterol, bitolterol, and terbutaline are relatively long-acting and may be administered every 4–6 hours. Metaproterenol may be administered as often as every 3–4 hours. One or 2 inhalations suffice to prevent most attacks, but as many as 4 inhalations every 4 hours may be required to treat acute illness or status asthmaticus (see below).

The metered-dose inhaler is the preferred means of delivery of sympathomimetic and corticosteroid aerosol drugs. Various extension devices ("spacers") may be attached to the inhaler to facilitate use and enhance aerosol deposition in the lung. Hand-bulb nebulizers have no practical advantage. Compressed air or oxygen may be used to nebulize certain sympathomimetic drug solutions and cromolyn solution. Several liquid solutions may be mixed together in the nebulizer unit. IPPB is rarely indicated to deliver inhaled drugs.

**2. Oral theophylline**–Long-acting oral theophylline preparations allow infrequent dosing. The usual starting dose for adults is 400–1000 mg/d in 2 divided doses. Serum theophylline levels should be measured 3–5 days after therapy is started. Therapeutic levels of theophylline are 10–20 $\mu$g/mL; higher concentrations are associated with gastrointestinal, cardiac, and central nervous system side effects. Mild hypercalcemia may also occur. Short-acting theophylline derivatives such as aminophylline and oxtriphylline require dosing every 6 hours and are rarely (if ever) indicated.

**3. Cromolyn sodium**–Inhaled cromolyn sodium is particularly useful in preventing exercise-induced asthma and seasonal extrinsic asthma but is ineffective in acute exacerbations of asthma. Cromolyn is sometimes effective in reducing the amount of corticosteroids needed by patients with severe asthma. Unlike sympathomimetics, cromolyn inhibits late phase allergen-induced bronchospasm. Aerosol (2 puffs, 1 mg each), powder (20 mg per capsule), and nebulizer solution (20 mg/2 mL) formulations are available and should be used 4 times daily or 10–15 minutes before exposure to the precipitating factor. Toxicity is minimal.

**4. Anticholinergics**–Ipratropium bromide, an atropine derivative, is a second-line drug for asthma. It may benefit selected ambulatory patients with asthma, such as those whose symptoms are poorly controlled by sympathomimetics alone. This drug is less effective than sympathomimetics in counteracting bronchospasm from specific stimuli, and experience with it in asthma is limited. The dose is 2–4 inhalations by metered-dose inhaler every 6 hours. Systemic toxicity is minimal. The availability of ipratropium bromide has rendered inhaled atropine for outpatient treatment of asthma practically obsolete.

**5. Corticosteroids**–Corticosteroid therapy is used only when other measures fail to relieve symptoms. Prednisone or prednisolone is preferred; the dosage is 40–60 mg/d orally to start, tapered in increments of 5–10 mg every 2–3 days over 1–3 weeks. Early treatment of severe asthma attacks with adequate doses of corticosteroids usually relieves symptoms and prevents hospitalization. Chronic maintenance therapy with corticosteroids is rarely necessary and is associated with many adverse effects. Inhaled corticosteroids may eliminate the need for oral corticosteroids or permit a substantial reduction in their dosage. Choices include beclomethasone, beginning with 2 inhalations (84 $\mu$g) 4 times daily progressing, if necessary, to 6 inhalations 4 times daily; flunisolide, beginning with 2 inhalations (500 $\mu$g) every 12 hours and progressing to 4 inhalations every 12 hours; or triamcinolone, beginning with 2 inhalations (200 $\mu$g) 4 times daily and progressing to 4 inhalations 4 times daily. Use of spacer devices for inhalation and mouth rinsing after dosing help prevent oral candidiasis. If inhalation provokes cough and wheezing, prescribe these drugs 20 minutes after inhalation of a sympathomimetic agent. Too rapid transfer from systemic to inhaled corticosteroids may precipitate adrenal insufficiency.

**6. Hyposensitization**–Desensitization therapy is indicated for patients with extrinsic asthma who fail to respond to conventional therapy and who have specific skin reactivity to allergens that have consistently induced asthma attacks. Overall, only a few patients with bronchial asthma are likely to benefit from hyposensitization.

**B. Patients With Acute, Severe Asthma:** Patients with acute, severe asthma are often exhausted, irritable, and apprehensive. Dehydration and toxic effects resulting from overuse of medications are com-

**Table 7–3.** Selected drugs for obstructive airway diseases.

| Drug | Formulation | Usual Adult Dosage | Comments |
|---|---|---|---|
| **Bronchodilators**<br>**Sympathomimetics**<br>Albuterol (Proventil, Ventolin) | Metered-dose inhaler (90 μg/puff; 200 puffs/inhaler) | 1–4 puffs every 4–6 hours | Preferred formulation in most cases. |
| | Nebulized solution (0.5%) | 0.5 mL plus 2.5 mL normal saline every 6–8 hours | Administer with powered nebulizer or, rarely, by IPPB. |
| | Syrup (2 mg/5 mL) | 1–2 tsp orally every 6–8 hours | |
| | Tablets (2 mg, 4 mg) | 2–4 mg orally every 6–8 hours | |
| Metaproterenol (Alupent, Metaprel) | Metered-dose inhaler (0.65 mg/puff; 300 puffs/inhaler) | 1–4 puffs every 3–4 hours | Preferred formulation in most cases. |
| | Nebulized solution (5%) | 0.3 mL plus 2.5 mL normal saline every 3–4 hours | Administer with powered nebuilized or, rarely, by IPPB. Also available as unit dose vial. |
| | Syrup (10 mg/5 mL) | 2 tsp orally every 6–8 hours | |
| | Tablets (10 mg, 20 mg) | 20 mg orally every 6–8 hours | |
| Bitolterol (Tornalate) | Metered-dose inhaler (0.37 mg/puff; 300 puffs/inhaler) | 2–3 puffs every 4–6 hours | |
| Terbutaline (Brethaire) | Metered-dose inhaler (0.2 mg/puff; 300 puffs/inhaler) | 2–3 puffs every 4–6 hours | |
| (Brethine, Bricanyl) | Tablets (2.5 mg, 5 mg) | 2.5–5 mg orally 3 times daily | Tremor, nervousness, palpitations common. Oral formulation therefore not recommended. |
| | Subcutaneous injection (1 mg/mL) | 0.25 mg subcutaneously; may be repeated once in 30 minutes | Slow onset of action (30 minutes). Not limited to $\beta_2$-adrenergic stimulation. |
| Isoetharine (Bronkometer) | Metered-dose inhaler (340 μg/puff; 200 puffs/10-mL inhaler) | 1–4 puffs every 3–4 hours | |
| (Bronkosol) | Nebulized solution (1%) | 0.5 mL plus 1.5 mL normal saline every 3–4 hours | Administer with powered nebulizer or, rarely, by IPPB. |
| Isoproterenol (Isuprel and others) | Metered-dose inhaler (131 μg/puff; 200 puffs/10 mL) | 1–3 puffs every 2–4 hours | |
| | Nebulized solution (0.5%; 1% also available) | 0.5 mL of 0.5% solution plus 1.5 mL normal saline every 2–4 hours | Administer with powered nebulizer or, rarely, by IPPB. |
| Epinephrine (many brands) | Metered dose inhaler (0.2 mg/puff ) | 1–2 puffs every 2–4 hours | Available without prescription. $\beta_1$ and $\alpha$ stimulation limit usefulness. |
| | Subcutaneous injection (0.1%, 1:1000) | 0.3–0.5 mL subcutaneously; may be repeated once in 30 minutes | Use with caution in older patients or those with tachycardia, hypertension, or arrhythmia. No more effective than inhaled $\beta_2$ agonist. |
| **Anticholinergics**<br>Ipratropium bromide (Atrovent) | Metered dose inhaler (18 μg/puff; 200 puffs/inhaler) | 2–4 puffs every 6 hours | More potent than sympathomimetics in COPD. Minimal side effects. |
| Atropine sulfate | Nebulized solution (1 mg/mL) | 0.025 mg/kg by inhalation every 6 hours; volume diluted to 2.5 mL with normal saline | Administer with powered nebulizer. Side effects common. Contraindicated in narrow-angle glaucoma or prostatic hypertrophy. |

**Table 7–3 (cont'd).** Selected drugs for obstructive airway diseases.

| Drug | Formulation | Usual Adult Dosage | Comments |
|---|---|---|---|
| **Theophyllines**<br>Theophylline, oral (many brands) | Sustained-release tablets and bead-filled capsules | 200 mg orally every 12 hours initially; thereafter, 200–600 mg orally every 8–12 hours | Maintenance dose is guided by serum theophylline level. Therapeutic level 10–20 μg/ml. Absorption varies with brand. Formulations are also available for administration every 24 hours. |
| Aminophylline | Intravenous | Loading dose is 5.6 mg/kg over 30 minutes for a person not using oral theophylline; maintenance dose is 0.7 mg/ kg/h by constant infusion pump, lower if patient has liver disease, heart failure, or erythromycin or cimetidine therapy | Calculate dose on lean body mass. Monitor serum theophylline level. |
| **Antimediators**<br>Cromolyn sodium (Intal) | Metered-dose inhaler (800 μg/puff; 200 puffs/14.2-g cannister) | 2 puffs 4 times daily | Clinical response may require 2–4 weeks of treatment. Useful only for prophylaxis. To prevent bronchospasm, cromolyn may be used 15–30 minutes before exercise or exposure to cold air or allergens. |
| | Nebulized solution (20 mg/ 2-mL ampule) | 20 mg 4 times daily by powered nebulizer | |
| | Powder for inhalation (20 mg/ capsule) | 20 mg 4 times daily by turboinhaler (Spinhaler) | Cough and airway irritation common with powder. |
| **Corticosteroids**<br>Prednisone (many names) | Tablets (2.5, 5, 10, 20, 50 mg) | Acute bronchospasm: 10–40 mg every 8 hours to 60 mg every 24 hours<br>Chronic bronchospasm: 5–40 mg daily to every other day | |
| Methylprednisolone sodium succinate (several brands) | Intravenous injection (40, 125, 500 mg, and larger vials) | 0.5–1 mg/kg every 6 hours | Clinical response may be delayed for several hours. |
| Hydrocortisone sodium succinate (several brands) | Intravenous injection (vials of 100, 250, 500, and 1000 mg) | 4 mg/kg every 6 hours | Clinical response may be delayed for several hours. |
| Beclomethasone dipropionate (Beclovent, Vanceril) | Metered-dose inhaler (42 μg/puff; 200 puffs/inhaler) | 2–4 puffs every 6–8 hours | Rinse mouth with water after use to prevent oral candidiasis; use 30 seconds after inhaled sympathomimetic to control cough and airway irritation. Spacer devices also helpful to prevent oral candidiasis. |
| Triamcinolone acetonide (Azmacort) | Metered-dose inhaler with spacer (100 μg/puff; 240 puffs/inhaler) | 2–4 puffs every 6–8 hours | |
| Flunisolide (AeroBid) | Metered-dose inhaler (250 μg/puff; 100 puffs/inhaler) | 2–4 puffs every 12 hours | |

mon. Objective measurement of airflow is important in patients with acute asthma because the intensity of wheezing on auscultation is an unreliable indicator of the extent of airflow limitation; however, in severe cases, patients may be unable to cooperate. The peak expiratory flow rate (PEFR), the preferred index of airflow in an emergency setting, is measured initially to provide a baseline and then obtained at successive intervals during treatment. A PEFR under 100 L/min indicates severe airway obstruction.

All patients with acute, severe asthma should receive supplemental oxygen, 1–3 L/min by nasal cannula. An inhaled sympathomimetic drug such as metaproterenol (0.3 mL of 5% solution) or albuterol (0.5

mL of 0.5% solution) may be tried, diluted in 2.5 mL sterile normal saline, using a powered nebulizer. A metered-dose inhaler is satisfactory if the patient is able to inspire deeply. If the patient fails to respond within 30 minutes, the dose may be repeated. Inhaled sympathomimetic therapy is superior to intravenous aminophylline in improving airflow. Subcutaneous epinephrine (0.3 mL of 1:1000 dilution) or terbutaline (0.25 mg) is an alternative form of sympathomimetic therapy, indicated only in patients unable to use aerosolized drugs.

Patients with severe, acute asthma who fail to respond to oxygen and sympathomimetic therapy are often given intravenous aminophylline, although data supporting the efficacy of this approach are lacking. Simultaneous administration of intravenous aminophylline and sympathomimetic may increase toxicity. If aminophylline is used at all, treatment is guided by serum theophylline levels. If the patient has not been receiving oral theophylline compounds, a loading dose of 5.6 mg/kg is administered intravenously over 30 minutes; the loading dose is eliminated or reduced if these agents are already part of the patient's ongoing regimen. Maintenance doses of aminophylline, 0.7 mg/kg/h intravenously, are given if the patient is a nonsmoking, otherwise healthy adult. The dose is reduced substantially in patients with congestive heart failure, liver disease, or concurrent use of erythromycin or cimetidine.

Corticosteroids are administered intravenously if the patient fails to respond to sympathomimetic therapy. Hydrocortisone (4 mg/kg) or methylprednisolone (0.5–1 mg/kg) is given initially and every 6 hours thereafter. A lag period of 4–6 hours before improvement occurs is common. Larger doses have no proved benefit. Inhaled corticosteroids have no role in acute, severe asthma.

Failure to respond to the above regimen, a persistently low PEFR, respiratory acidosis, electrocardiographic abnormalities, and pneumothorax or pneumomediastinum are indications for hospitalization. Respiratory fatigue, suspected airway infection, and a history of status asthmaticus are also reasons for hospitalization.

**Status asthmaticus** is severe, prolonged asthma refractory to conventional modes of therapy. Management is similar to that for acute, severe asthma; it consists of controlled-flow oxygen therapy, rehydration, corticosteroids, inhaled sympathomimetics, and antibiotics for presumed or proved airway infection; intravenous aminophylline may add marginally to the regimen. Treatment in an intensive care unit is necessary. The role of ipratropium bromide has not been established, but this agent may hold promise.

Most patients with status asthmaticus improve with this regimen; however, some develop progressive respiratory acidemia and require tracheal intubation and mechanical ventilation. The decision to intubate is a complex one and is better based on the general appearance of the patient (fatigue, apprehension) than on any single laboratory datum. Status asthmaticus not controlled after intubation and mechanical ventilation requires highly aggressive therapy, eg, sedation with morphine or diazepam, paralysis with pancuronium, general anesthesia with a bronchodilating anesthetic agent, such as halothane, or segmental bronchial lavage to remove plugs of mucus.

**Prognosis**

The outlook for patients with bronchial asthma is excellent. Attention to general health measures and use of pharmacologic agents permit control of symptoms in nearly all cases. The outlook is better for patients with extrinsic asthma and for those who develop asthma early in life. Pneumococcal and yearly influenzal immunization should be part of every patient's regimen.

Drugs for asthma. *Med Lett Drugs Ther* (Jan 30) 1987;**29:**11.
Goldstein RA (editor): Advances in the diagnosis and treatment of asthma. (Symposium.) *Chest* 1985;**87(Suppl):**1. [Entire issue.]
Gross NJ, Skorodin MS: Anticholinergic, antimuscarinic bronchodilators. *Am Rev Respir Dis* 1984;**129:**856.
Hodgkin JE (editor): International scope of asthma. (Symposium.) *Chest* 1986;**90(Suppl):**39S. [Entire issue.]
Littenberg B, Gluck EH: A controlled trial of methylprednisolone in the emergency treatment of acute asthma. *N Engl J Med* 1986;**314:**150.
Newhouse MT, Dolovich MB: Control of asthma by aerosols. *N Engl J Med* 1986;**315:**870.

# CHRONIC OBSTRUCTIVE PULMONARY DISEASE (COPD)

## Essentials of Diagnosis

- History of cigarette smoking (most cases).
- Chronic cough and sputum production (in chronic bronchitis) and dyspnea (in emphysema).
- Rhonchi, decreased intensity of breath sounds, and prolonged expiration on physical examination.
- Airflow limitation on pulmonary function testing.

## General Considerations

The term chronic obstructive pulmonary disease (COPD) identifies patients with emphysema (type A COPD) or chronic bronchitis (type B COPD). Although emphysema and chronic bronchitis must be diagnosed and treated as specific diseases, most patients with COPD have features of both conditions. About 10 million Americans are affected.

**Chronic bronchitis** is characterized by excessive secretion of bronchial mucus and is manifested by productive cough for 3 months or more in at least 2 consecutive years in the absence of any other disease that might account for this symptom. **Emphysema** denotes permanent and abnormal enlargement of the acinus (primary lobule of the lung), with destruction of alveolar walls. The cause of both chronic bronchitis and emphysema is obscure. Cigarette smoking is clearly the most important cause of COPD. Air pollution, airway infection, familial factors, and allergy have also been implicated in chronic bronchitis, and hereditary factors (deficiency of alpha$_1$-antitrypsin) have been implicated in emphysema.

## Clinical Findings

**A. Symptoms and Signs:** The clinical, roentgenographic, and laboratory findings in chronic bronchitis and emphysema are summarized in Table 7–4.

Patients with the 2 combined forms of COPD characteristically present in the fifth or sixth decade of life complaining of excessive cough, sputum production, and shortness of breath that have often been present for 10 years or more. Productive cough usually occurs in the morning. Dyspnea is noted initially only on extreme exertion, but as the condition progresses, it becomes more severe and occurs with mild activity. In severe disease, dyspnea occurs at rest. Frequent exacerbations of illness are common and result in absence from work and eventual disability. Pneumonia, pulmonary hypertension, cor pulmonale, and chronic respiratory failure characterize the late stage of COPD. Death usually occurs during an exacerbation of illness in association with acute respiratory failure.

Clinical findings may be completely absent early in the course of COPD. Diminished breath sounds and prolonged expiration may be detectable during exacerbations of the disease. The physical findings presented in Table 7–4 become apparent as the disease progresses.

**B. Laboratory Findings.** Secondary polycythemia may be found in advanced COPD as a result of hypoxemia. During exacerbations of illness, examination of the sputum may reveal *Streptococcus pneumoniae* or *Haemophilus influenzae,* though these may be present in the carrier state between episodes of deterioration. The ECG may show sinus tachycardia, and in advanced disease, chronic pulmonary hypertension may produce electrocardiographic abnormalities typical of cor pulmonale. Supraventricular arrhythmias (multifocal atrial tachycardia, atrial flutter, and atrial fibrillation) and ventricular irritability also occur.

Arterial blood gas measurements characteristically show no abnormalities early in COPD; indeed, they are unnecessary unless hypoxia or hypercapnia is suspected. Hypoxemia occurs in advanced disease, particularly when chronic bronchitis predominates. Compensated respiratory acidosis occurs in patients with chronic respiratory failure, particularly in chronic bronchitis, with worsening of acidemia during acute exacerbations.

Spirometry provides objective information about pulmonary function and assesses the results of therapy. Pulmonary function tests early in the course of COPD reveal only evidence of dysfunctional small airways (abnormal closing volume, reduced midexpiratory flow rate). Reduction in forced expiratory volume in 1 second (FEV$_1$) and in the ratio of forced

**Table 7–4.** Clinical, roentgenographic, and laboratory findings distinguishing emphysema and chronic bronchitis.

| | Emphysema (Type A COPD) | Chronic Bronchitis (Type B COPD) |
|---|---|---|
| **History** | | |
| Onset of symptoms | After age 50. | After age 35. |
| Dyspnea | Progressive, constant, severe. | Intermittent, mild to moderate. |
| Cough | Absent or mild. | Persistent, severe. |
| Sputum production | Absent or mild. | Copious. |
| Sputum appearance | Clear, mucoid. | Mucopurulent or purulent. |
| Other features | Weight loss.* | Airway infections, right heart failure, obesity. |
| **Physical examination** | | |
| Body habitus | Thin, wasted.* | Stocky, obese. |
| Central cyanosis | Absent. | Present.* |
| Plethora | Absent. | Present. |
| Accessory respiratory muscles | Hypertrophied. | Unremarkable. |
| Anteroposterior chest diameter | Increased. | Normal. |
| Percussion note | Hyperresonant. | Normal. |
| Auscultation | Diminished breath sounds. | Wheezes, rhonchi. |
| **Chest x-ray** | | |
| Bullae, blebs | Present. | Absent. |
| Overall appearance | Decreased markings in periphery. | Increased markings ("dirty lungs"). |
| Hyperinflation | Present. | Absent. |
| Heart size | Normal or small, vertical | Large, horizontal. |
| Hemidiaphragms | Low, flat. | Normal, rounded. |
| **Laboratory studies** | | |
| Hematocrit | Normal. | Increased. |
| ECG | Normal. | Right axis deviation, right ventricular hypertrophy, "p" pulmonale.* |
| Hypoxemia | Absent, mild. | Moderate, severe. |
| Hypercapnia | Absent. | Moderate, severe. |
| Respiratory acidosis | Absent. | Present. |
| Total lung capacity | Increased. | Normal. |
| Static lung compliance | Increased. | Normal. |
| Diffusing capacity | Decreased. | Normal. |

* In advanced disease.

expiratory volume to forced vital capacity ($FEV_1$:FVC) occurs later. In severe disease, the forced vital capacity is markedly reduced. Lung volume measurements reveal increase in the total lung capacity (TLC), marked increase in the residual volume (RV), and elevation of the RV/TLC ratio, indicative of air trapping, particularly in emphysema.

**C. Imaging:** When emphysema is the main clinical feature, hyperinflation is apparent. Parenchymal bullae or subpleural blebs are pathognomonic of emphysema. Radiographs of patients with chronic bronchitis may show only nonspecific peribronchial and perivascular markings. Pulmonary hypertension becomes evident in advanced disease.

## Differential Diagnosis

Clinical, roentgenographic, and laboratory findings usually enable the clinician to distinguish COPD from other obstructive pulmonary disorders such as bronchial asthma, bronchiectasis, cystic fibrosis, bronchopulmonary aspergillosis, and central airway obstruction. Bronchiectasis is distinguished from COPD by features such as recurrent pneumonia and hemoptysis, 3-layered sputum, digital clubbing, and radiographic abnormalities. Cystic fibrosis occurs in children and younger adults. Rarely, mechanical obstruction of the central airways simulates COPD. Flow-volume curves may help separate patients with central airway obstruction from those with diffuse intrathoracic airway obstruction characteristic of COPD.

## Complications

Acute bronchitis, pneumonia, pulmonary embolization, and concomitant left ventricular failure may worsen otherwise stable COPD. Pulmonary hypertension, cor pulmonale, and chronic respiratory failure are common in advanced COPD. Spontaneous pneumothorax occurs in a small fraction of patients with emphysema. Hemoptysis may result from chronic bronchitis or may signal potential bronchogenic carcinoma.

## Prevention

COPD is largely preventable. Many believe that early recognition of small airway dysfunction in patients who smoke, combined with appropriate treatment and cessation of smoking, may prevent relentless progression of the disease. Early treatment of airway infections and vaccination against influenza and pneumococcal disease may also be of benefit but have no effect on the progression of the disease.

## Treatment

Successful therapy of COPD depends on skillful use of community resources and a comprehensive respiratory care program with realistic goals of treatment. Basic principles of management include discontinuation of cigarette smoking, education about the disease, relief of bronchospasm, aerosol therapy, chest physiotherapy, treatment of complications such as airway infections and heart failure, use of supplemental oxygen, and other measures designed to promote rehabilitation.

**A. Ambulatory Patients:** The general health maintenance measures for patients with bronchial asthma (see p 137) are also important for patients with COPD. Goals in the treatment of COPD include control of symptoms, improvement in ability to carry out daily activities, reduction in the need for hospitalization, and rehabilitation.

A trial of bronchodilator drugs is warranted in all patients with symptomatic COPD. Inhaled sympathomimetic drugs are the mainstay of this therapy; long-acting theophylline compounds may be of some added value. Although theophylline has value as a bronchodilator in COPD patients with partial reversibility of airflow limitation, its principal value in COPD may relate to improving contractility of the diaphragm and decreasing diaphragmatic fatigue. The response to therapy is assessed with spirometry. Patients with asthmatic bronchitis and those with partially reversible airflow obstruction, frequent acute exacerbations of disease, or wheezing may benefit the most from bronchodilator therapy. The routine use of maintenance bronchodilator drugs in all patients with COPD is controversial. These drugs probably have little value in patients with pure emphysema. If a clinical trial of bronchodilators over several months demonstrates no objective (spirometric) or symptomatic improvement, they may be discontinued; however, this is not often the case.

A newly available anticholinergic aerosol, **ipratropium bromide,** appears superior to sympathomimetic aerosols in effecting bronchodilation in COPD and may become the inhaled bronchodilator of choice. In combination with other bronchodilators, it enhances and prolongs bronchodilation. Side effects are minimal, and effects on sputum production and viscosity are negligible. Two to 4 inhalations every 6 hours is recommended.

Corticosteroids are prescribed in the same fashion as in asthma (see p 137). Candidates for a trial of corticosteroid therapy include patients with asthmatic bronchitis and those with frequent exacerbations or disabling symptoms who fail to respond to conventional therapy with sympathomimetics and theophylline; eosinophils in peripheral blood or sputum may also predict a response. Corticosteroids should be discontinued after 2–4 weeks if there is no objective improvement. Inhaled corticosteroids (see p 137) may be of value for patients who require some maintenance dose ($<$ 15 mg of prednisone) and allow the systemic administration to be discontinued. Cromolyn has no role in treatment of chronic bronchitis or emphysema.

Bronchial hygiene decreases production of bronchopulmonary secretions and enhances their mobilization and clearance. Smoking cessation, avoiding airway irritants and allergens, controlling airway infection with broad-spectrum oral antimicrobials (ampicillin, tetracycline, trimethoprim-sulfamethoxazole), and preventing pulmonary aspiration are ways of decreasing production of mucus. Ampicillin and tetracycline are given in dosages of 250–500 mg 4 times daily and trimethoprim-sulfamethoxazole in dosages of 160/800 mg every 12 hours. Seven to 10 days of treatment is usually adequate.

Increased mobilization of secretions may be accomplished through the use of adequate systemic hydration, effective ("staircase") coughing methods, and postural drainage, sometimes with chest percussion or vibration. Inhalation of bland water aerosols is sometimes helpful. Postural drainage and chest percussion should be used only in selected patients with excessive amounts of retained secretions that cannot be cleared by coughing and other methods; these measures are of no benefit in pure emphysema. Expectorants and mucolytic drugs are rarely useful. Cough suppressants and sedatives should be avoided as routine measures.

Graded aerobic physical exercise programs (eg, walking 20 minutes 3 times weekly, or bicycling) are helpful to prevent deterioration of physical condition and to improve the patient's ability to carry out daily activities. Pursed-lip breathing to slow the rate of breathing and abdominal breathing exercises to relieve fatigue of accessory muscles of respiration are helpful in reducing dyspnea in some patients. Training of inspiratory muscles by having patients inspire against resistive loads improves exercise tolerance in some but not all patients.

Severe dyspnea in spite of optimal medical management may respond to a trial of an opiate drug (eg, hydrocodone, 5 mg orally 4 times daily). Constipation is a common side effect. Sedative-hypnotic drugs (eg, diazepam, 5 mg 3 times daily) are controversial in intractable dyspnea but may benefit very anxious patients. Bilateral carotid body resection is unacceptable because of the severe hypoxemia that ensues. Intermittent negative-pressure (cuirass) ventilation is a promising new approach to improve respiratory muscle function and reduce dyspnea in patients with severe COPD.

Home oxygen therapy is prescribed for selected patients with COPD or other severe lung diseases who have significant hypoxemia. Requirements for Medicare coverage for a patient's home use of oxygen and oxygen equipment are listed in Table 7–5. Arterial blood gas measurements, not ear or pulse oximetry, should be used to guide initial oxygen therapy. Oxygen may be prescribed for continuous use, only at night, or with exercise. Cardiovascular disorders without hypoxemia are not indications for this expensive therapy. Hypoxemic patients with pulmonary hypertension, chronic cor pulmonale, erythrocytosis, impaired cognitive function, exercise intolerance, nocturnal restlessness, or morning headache are particularly good candidates for home oxygen therapy. Benefits from home oxygen delivery have been shown in each of these conditions.

Home oxygen may be supplied by liquid oxygen cylinders, gas tanks, or oxygen concentrators. Most patients benefit from having both stationary and portable systems. Oxygen by nasal prongs must be given at least 15 hours a day unless therapy is intended only for exercise or sleep. For most patients, a flow rate of 1–3 L/min achieves a $PaO_2 > 55$ mm Hg. Transtracheal oxygen is a new and promising alternative method of delivery. Reservoir nasal cannulas or "pendants" and demand oxygen delivery systems are also available to conserve oxygen.

**B. Hospitalized Patients:** Hospitalization is indicated for acute worsening of COPD that fails to respond to measures for ambulatory patients. Patients with acute respiratory failure or complications such as cor pulmonale and pneumothorax should also be hospitalized.

Management of the hospitalized patient with an exacerbation of COPD uses a comprehensive approach similar to that for patients hospitalized with asthma. Therapeutics modalities include supplemental oxygen, inhaled sympathomimetics, ipratropium bromide, and intravenous aminophylline, as well as broad-spectrum antibiotics, corticosteroids, and, in selected cases, chest physiotherapy. Oxygen therapy should not be withheld for fear of suppressing ventilatory drive; hypoxemia is more detrimental than hypercapnia. Cor pulmonale is treated with salt restriction and diuretics. Cardiac arrhythmias are managed with antiarrhythmic drugs as indicated but usually respond

**Table 7–5.** Requirements for Medicare coverage of home oxygen therapy.

I. Significant hypoxemia in spite of optimal medical management

Awake (breathing room air)

At rest: $PaO_2 \leq 55$ mm Hg or $SaO_2 \leq 85\%$
or
$PaO_2$ 56–59 mm Hg or $SaO_2$ 85–89% with
(1) Dependent edema suggesting congestive heart failure, or
(2) "P" pulmonale on ECG (P wave > 3 mm in standard leads II, III, or aVF), or
(3) Hematocrit > 56%

With exercise: $PaO_2 \leq 55$ mm Hg or $SaO_2 \leq 85\%$ with proof that oxygen improves hypoxemia induced by exercise

Asleep (breathing room air): Signs and symptoms of hypoxemia with a decrease in $PaO_2$ of > 10 mm Hg or in $SaO_2$ of > 5%

II. Severe chronic lung disease

COPD
Diffuse interstitial lung disease
Cystic fibrosis
Bronchiectasis
Widespread pulmonary neoplasm

III. Features of hypoxemia that might be expected to improve with oxygen therapy

Dyspnea, exercise intolerance
Impaired cognitive processes
Nocturnal restlessness
Morning headache
Pulmonary hypertension
Congestive heart failure (cor pulmonale)
Erythrocytosis

to aggressive treatment of COPD itself. Recent experience indicates that verapamil (240–480 mg/d in divided doses every 8 hours, or 0.075 mg/kg given intravenously at a rate of 1–2 mg/min) is especially effective in multifocal atrial tachycardia. If progressive respiratory failure ensues, tracheal intubation and mechanical ventilation are necessary (see p 180).

## Prognosis

The outlook for patients with clinically significant COPD is poor. The median survival time of patients with severe COPD ($FEV_1 \leq 1$ L) is about 4 years. The degree of pulmonary dysfunction (as measured by $FEV_1$) at the time the patient is first seen is probably the most important predictor of survival. Comprehensive care programs and cessation of smoking apparently reduce the rate of decline of pulmonary function, but therapy with bronchodilators and other approaches probably has little, if any, impact on the natural course of COPD. Survival time varies widely and cannot be easily predicted.

Christopher KL et al: Transtracheal oxygen therapy for refractory hypoxemia. *JAMA* 1986;**256**:494

Cropp A, Dimarco AF: Effects of intermittent negative pressure ventilation on respiratory muscle function in patients with severe chronic obstructive pulmonary disease. *Am Rev Respir Dis* 1987;**135**:1056.

Eliasson O et al: Corticosteroids in COPD: A clinical trial and reassessment of the literature. *Chest* 1986;**89**:484.

Hodgkin JE, Petty TL (editors): *Chronic Obstructive Pulmonary Disease: Current Concepts.* Saunders, 1987.

O'Donohue WJ Jr: Oxygen conserving devices. *Respir Care* 1987;**32**:37.

Tashkin DP et al: Comparison of the anticholinergic bronchodilator ipratropium bromide with metaproterenol in chronic obstructive pulmonary disease: A 90-day multi-center study. *Am J Med* 1986;**81(Suppl 5A)**:81.

Snider GL: Chronic obstructive pulmonary disease: A continuing challenge. *Am Rev Respir Dis* 1986;**133**:942.

## CYSTIC FIBROSIS
## (See also Chapter 31.)

### Essentials of Diagnosis

- Chronic pulmonary disease in childhood and early adulthood.
- Pancreatic insufficiency.
- Positive family history.
- Increased $Na^+$ and $Cl^-$ in sweat.

### General Considerations

Cystic fibrosis is a generalized autosomal recessive disorder of the exocrine glands. The basic genetic defect is obscure, and it is possible that more than one genetic error is involved. Almost all exocrine glands are affected by secretion of an abnormal mucus that obstructs glands and ducts in various organs. Obstruction results in dilation of the secretory glands and eventual damage to exocrine tissue. Pulmonary manifestations, which occur in all patients who survive infancy, include acute and chronic bronchitis, bronchiectasis, pneumonia, atelectasis, and peribronchial and parenchymal scarring. Pneumothorax and mild hemoptysis are common.

Cystic fibrosis is the most common fatal hereditary disorder of Caucasians in the USA and is the most common cause of chronic lung disease in children and young adults. About half of children with cystic fibrosis live beyond age 20, and although it is unusual, survival to age 30 and beyond now occurs. About one-third of the 25,000 cystic fibrosis patients in the United States are adults.

### Clinical Findings

**A. Symptoms and Signs:** The diagnosis should be suspected in a young adult presenting with a history of chronic lung disease. Cough, exercise intolerance, and recurrent pneumonia are typical. Steatorrhea is common. Digital clubbing, increased anteroposterior chest diameter, hyperresonance to percussion, and basilar crackles are noted on physical examination. Nasal polyps occur in as many as 15% of patients with cystic fibrosis. Biliary cirrhosis and gallstones are common.

**B. Laboratory Findings:** Arterial blood gas studies reveal hypoxemia. Pulmonary function studies show reduction in forced vital capacity, airflow rates, and total lung capacity.

**C. Imaging:** Common radiographic abnormalities include peribronchial thickening, obstructive emphysema, bronchiectasis, atelectasis, and cysts.

**D. Special Examinations:** The pilocarpine iontophoresis "sweat test" reveals elevated sodium and chloride levels ($> 60$ meq/L) in the sweat of patients with cystic fibrosis. Values higher than 80 meq/L are diagnostic. Two separate tests on consecutive days are required for accurate diagnosis.

### Treatment

Early recognition and comprehensive, multidisciplinary therapy lengthen survival time and ameliorate symptoms. Treatment of the psychosocial aspects is of paramount importance in young people; genetic and occupational counseling is also critical. Antibiotics are used to treat active airway infections based on results of culture and susceptibility testing of sputum. *Staphylococcus aureus* and a mucoid variant of *Pseudomonas aeruginosa* are commonly present. *Haemophilus influenzae* and *Pseudomonas cepacia*—the latter a highly drug-resistant organism—are occasionally isolated. Inhaled aerosols, chest physiotherapy, and inhaled bronchodilators are used to promote clearance of inspissated airway secretions. Daily postural drainage and chest percussion are very helpful for patients with copious sputum production.

### Prognosis

Survival beyond age 30 is unusual. Death occurs from pulmonary complications, eg, pneumonia, pneumothorax, or hemoptysis, or as a result of terminal chronic respiratory failure and cor pulmonale.

Davis PB (editor): Cystic fibrosis. *Semin Respir Med* 1985; **6**:243.

## UPPER AIRWAY OBSTRUCTION

Acute upper airway obstruction may cause life-threatening asphyxia and must be relieved promptly. Acute upper airway obstruction due to foreign body aspiration is discussed below. Emergency treatment of food choking and other causes of acute airway obstruction are discussed in the Appendix. Other causes of acute upper airway obstruction include laryngospasm, trauma to the larynx and pharynx, laryngeal edema from airway burns, and various inflammatory conditions (Ludwig's angina, peritonsillar and retropharyngeal abscess, acute epiglottitis, and acute allergic larnygitis).

Chronic obstruction of the upper airway may be caused by carcinoma of the pharynx or larynx, laryngeal or subglottic stenosis, laryngeal granulomas or webs, or vocal cord paralysis. Inspiratory stridor, intercostal retractions on inspiration, and a palpable inspiratory thrill over the throat are characteristic findings. Flow-volume curves may reveal evidence of fixed airway obstruction or variable extrathoracic obstruction. Helpful diagnostic studies include endoscopy and conventional tomography of the upper airway.

Occasionally, a functional disorder of the larynx may mimic bronchial asthma. This condition, variously called "episodic laryngeal dyskinesis," "factitious asthma," and "emotional laryngeal wheezing," may be distinguished from true asthma by the finding of variable extrathoracic airway obstruction on the flow-volume loop, a normal alveolar-arterial oxygen tension gradient, laryngoscopic evidence of adduction of the vocal cords on both inspiration and expiration, and lack of response to bronchodilator therapy. Pulmonary function testing is normal immediately after the attack resolves. Treatment consists of speech therapy and psychotherapy. Bronchodilator drugs are of no benefit.

Haponik EF et al: Acute upper airway injury in burn patients: Serial changes of flow-volume curves and nasopharyngoscopy. *Am Rev Respir Dis* 1987;**135**:360.

Ramírez J, Leon I, Rivera LM: Episodic laryngeal dyskinesia: Clinical and psychiatric characterization. *Chest* 1986; **90**:716.

## LOWER AIRWAY OBSTRUCTION

**Tracheal obstruction** may be intrathoracic (below the suprasternal notch) or extrathoracic. Fixed tracheal obstruction may be caused by acquired or congenital tracheal stenosis, primary and secondary tracheal neoplasms, compression by extrinsic diseases (tumors of the lung, thymus, or thyroid; lymphadenopathy; congenital vascular rings; aneurysms; etc), foreign body aspiration, tracheal granulomas and papillomas, and tracheal trauma.

Acquired **tracheal stenosis** is usually secondary to tracheostomy or endotracheal intubation. Dyspnea, cough, and inability to clear pulmonary secretions occur weeks to months after tracheal decannulation or extubation. Stridor implies severe stenosis. Physical findings may be absent until tracheal diameter is reduced 50% or more, when wheezing, a palpable tracheal thrill, and harsh breath sounds may be detected. The diagnosis is usually confirmed by conventional tomography of the trachea, CT scan, and characteristic findings of the flow-volume curve. Complications include recurring pulmonary infection and life-threatening respiratory failure. Management is directed toward ensuring adequate ventilation and oxygenation and avoiding manipulative procedures that may increase edema of the tracheal mucosa. Surgical reconstruction or laser photoresection is required in severe cases.

**Bronchial obstruction** is caused by retained pulmonary secretions, aspiration, primary lung cancer, compression by extrinsic masses, and (rarely) tumors metastatic to the airway. Clinical and radiographic findings vary depending on the location of the obstruction and the degree of airway narrowing. Symptoms include dyspnea, cough, wheezing, and if infection is present, fever and chills. A history of recurrent pneumonia in the same lobe or segment or slow resolution ($> 3$ months) of pneumonia on successive x-rays suggests the possibility of bronchial obstruction. Complete obstruction of a main stem bronchus may be obvious on physical examination (asymmetric chest expansion, mediastinal shift, absence of breath sounds on the affected side, and dullness to percussion), but partial obstruction is often difficult to detect. Prolonged expiration and localized wheezing may be the only clues. Segmental or subsegmental bronchial obstruction may produce no abnormalities on physical examination.

Roentgenographic findings range from **atelectasis** (lung collapse) to air trapping. The latter may be caused by unidirectional expiratory obstruction. Expiratory films are particularly useful to show air trapping. Hilar tomograms may delineate the nature and location of obstruction of the central bronchi. Bronchoscopy is helpful, particularly if tumor or foreign body aspiration is suspected. An air bronchogram on chest radiography in an area of atelectasis rules out complete airway obstruction. Bronchoscopy is unlikely to be of benefit in this situation.

**Right middle lobe syndrome** is recurrent or persistent atelectasis of the right middle lobe, probably related to inadequate collateral ventilation. Fiberoptic bronchoscopy is necessary to rule out obstructing tumor or foreign body.

## ALLERGIC BRONCHOPULMONARY ASPERGILLOSIS

Allergic bronchopulmonary aspergillosis is a pulmonary hypersensitivity disorder that is being recognized with increasing frequency in the USA. It is caused by allergy to antigens of *Aspergillus* species and usually occurs in atopic asthmatic individuals who are 20–40 years of age. Primary criteria for the diagnosis of allergic bronchopulmonary aspergillosis include a clinical history of asthma, peripheral eosinophilia, immediate skin reactivity to *Aspergillus* antigen, precipitating antibodies to *Aspergillus* antigen, elevated serum IgE levels, pulmonary infiltrates, and central bronchiectasis. If the first 6 of these 7 primary criteria are present, the diagnosis is almost certain. Secondary diagnostic criteria include identification of *Aspergillus* in sputum, a history of brown-flecked sputum, and late skin reactivity to *Aspergillus* antigen. Corticosteroids are the treatment of choice, and the response is usually excellent. Prednisone (0.5 mg/kg/d) is given as a single morning dose for several weeks before the change is made to alternate-day dosing. Several months of prednisone therapy may be required. Bronchodilators (see Table 7–31) are also helpful. Complications include hemoptysis, severe bronchiectasis, and pulmonary fibrosis.

Ricketti AJ et al: Allergic bronchopulmonary aspergillosis. *Chest* 1984;**86**:773.

## BRONCHIECTASIS

Bronchiectasis is a congenital or acquired disorder of the large bronchi characterized by permanent, abnormal dilatation and destruction of bronchial walls. It is caused by recurrent inflammation or infection of the airways and is primarily a disorder of childhood and young adulthood, with most cases being recognized during the first 2 decades of life. Cystic fibrosis causes about half of all cases of bronchiectasis. Acquired primary bronchiectasis is now uncommon in the USA because of improved control of bronchopulmonary infections.

Symptoms of bronchiectasis include chronic cough, production of copious amounts of purulent sputum, hemoptysis, and recurrent pneumonia. Weight loss, anemia, and other systemic manifestations are common. Physical findings are nonspecific, but persistent crackles at the lung bases are common. Clubbing is infrequent. Foul-smelling, purulent sputum that separates into 3 layers in a sputum cup is characteristic. Obstructive pulmonary dysfunction with hypoxemia is seen in moderate or severe disease. Roentgenographic abnormalities include crowded bronchial markings related to peribronchial fibrosis and small cystic spaces at the base of the lungs. Thin-section (1.5-mm) CT scanning may detect moderate to severe cases. Bronchography is usually not performed unless surgery is planned.

Treatment consists of antibiotics (selected on the basis of sputum smears and cultures), chest physiotherapy with postural drainage and chest percussion, and inhaled bronchodilators. Bronchoscopy is sometimes necessary to remove retained secretions and rule out obstructing airway lesions. Surgical resection is reserved for a few patients with localized bronchiectasis who fail to respond to conservative management. Surgery is also indicated for massive hemoptysis. Complications of bronchiectasis include cor pulmonale, amyloidosis, and secondary visceral abscesses at distant sites, eg, brain.

Davis AL (chairman): Bronchiectasis. (Symposium.) *Am Rev Respir Dis* 1986;**134**:824.
Mootoosamy IM et al: Assessment of bronchiectasis by computed tomography. *Thorax* 1985;**40**:290.

## IMMOTILE CILIA SYNDROME (Primary Ciliary Dyskinesia)

Immotile cilia syndrome is an autosomal recessive disorder characterized by ultrastructural defects in the microtubular apparatus of both ciliated epithelial cells and spermatozoa, resulting in abnormal mucociliary clearance, reduced fertility in women, and male infertility. Cough productive of copious mucopurulent sputum, sinusitis, and otitis occur in almost all patients. Situs inversus is present in half of cases (Kartagener's syndrome). Nasal stuffiness, rhinorrhea, and childhood nasal polyposis are common. Bronchiectasis and signs of COPD occur in severe disease. Clubbing occurs occasionally. Chest radiography reveals features of chronic bronchitis and bronchiectasis. Paranasal sinus films reveal sinusitis. Definitive diagnosis requires biopsy of nasal or tracheal mucosa with electron microscopic examination of the ultrastructure of the cilia.

Treatment consists of maintenance of bronchial hygiene through coughing and chest physiotherapy and antibiotics (selected on the basis of sputum smears and cultures) for acute airway infections. Bronchodilator drugs and mucolytic agents are not effective. Surgical resection may be considered if severe saccular bronchiectasis is present.

Newhouse MT, Rossman C: Primary ciliary dyskinesia. *Semin Respir Med* 1984;**5**:341.

## BRONCHOCENTRIC GRANULOMATOSIS & MUCOID IMPACTION SYNDROME

**Bronchocentric granulomatosis** is a rare chronic idiopathic disorder in which bronchi and bronchioles are destroyed and replaced by granulomas. Symptoms include fever, cough, chest pain, anorexia, malaise, and hemoptysis of short duration. In patients with bronchocentric granulomatosis and chronic asthma, the condition resembles allergic bronchopulmonary aspergillosis; eosinophilia is common. Chest radiography reveals mass lesions or alveolar or reticular nodular infiltrates that are more common in the upper lung. The diagnosis of bronchocentric granulomatosis is confirmed by lung resection, which is also therapeutic.

**Mucoid impaction syndrome** is characterized by obstruction of large, proximal bronchi by plugs of inspissated mucus. This syndrome has clinical features similar to those of bronchocentric granulomatosis, eosinophilic pneumonia, and allergic bronchopulmonary aspergillosis, but the cause of this condition and its relationship to hypersensitivity to fungal antigens are not clear. Most patients with mucoid impaction syndrome have symptoms of chronic bronchitis or asthma. Expectoration of large, rubbery plugs of mucus suggests the diagnosis. Radiographs show densities shaped like branching central airways in the upper lung; atelectasis or consolidation is a common associated feature. Mucolytic therapy (inhaled acetylcysteine, 10% solution, 5 mL 4 times daily by nebulizer) may be tried if bland aerosols fail to relieve mucus plugging. Pretreatment with bronchodilators is recommended, since acetylcysteine may provoke bronchospasm. Corticosteroids are not helpful.

## BRONCHIOLITIS

Bronchiolitis is a common, often severe respiratory illness of infants and young children caused by respiratory syncytial virus, other viruses (occasionally), and *Mycoplasma pneumoniae*. The child presents with combined bronchospasm and pneumonia.

Bronchiolitis in adults may occur as a result of viral infections or inhalation of toxic fumes, or it may occur in association with connective tissue disease. However, most cases are idiopathic. Acute episodes are characterized by wheezing, cough, and sputum production. Chest x-ray reveals severe hyperinflation. Poorly defined small opacities, focal atelectasis, and pneumonia have been described in adults with bronchiolitis associated with asthma. Pulmonary function studies reveal a severe obstructive—and, less commonly, restrictive—ventilatory defect.

The severity and clinical course of the disease are unpredictable. Most patients recover after an acute episode. Bronchodilators (see Table 7–3) are indicated in symptomatic patients. Corticosteroids are effective in some patients. **Bronchiolitis obliterans with organizing pneumonia** is an idiopathic form of bronchiolitis with diffuse, patchy "ground-glass" or alveolar infiltrates and lung restriction. Response to corticosteroids is favorable. **Respiratory bronchiolitis** is an inflammatory disorder of respiratory bronchioles in cigarette smokers characterized by accumulation of pigmented macrophages and thickening of the peribronchiolar interstitium. Cough, dyspnea, restrictive pulmonary dysfunction, and peribronchiolar interstitial infiltrates on chest radiographs suggest the diagnosis and may avoid the need for open lung biopsy. Corticosteroids are not helpful. The prognosis is good after smoking cessation.

**Unilateral hyperlucent lung** (Swyer-James or MacLeod's syndrome) is a rare disorder attributed to an episode of acute infectious bronchiolitis in infancy or childhood. Unilateral hyperlucency is related to oligemia and obliteration of bronchioles and small bronchi on the affected side, a small hilum, and redistribution of blood flow to the opposite lung. Expiratory films reveal air trapping on the affected side and subsequent mediastinal shift. No specific treatment is recommended.

McLoud TC, Epler GR, Colby TV: Bronchiolitis obliterans. *Radiology* 1986;**159**:1

Myers JL et al: Respiratory bronchiolitis causing interstitial lung disease: A clinicopathologic study of six cases. *Am Rev Respir Dis* 1987;**135**:880.

## BRONCHOLITHIASIS

In broncholithiasis, a calcified mass (broncholith) lies in the lumen of a bronchus or a cavity derived from a bronchus. Broncholiths are usually calcified hilar lymph nodes that have migrated through the wall of a bronchus into the lumen of the airway. Tuberculosis and histoplasmosis are the most common causes. Broncholiths may be expectorated or retained in the airway, in which case they cause hemoptysis, atelectasis, and postobstructive pneumonia.

Broncholithiasis should be suspected in any patient with hilar calcification who complains of worsening cough or hemoptysis. Late complications include bronchoesophageal or aortotracheal fistula, erosion into the pleura, and bronchiectasis. The diagnosis is confirmed by examination of expectorated material or by disappearance of a calcified hilar or intracavitary density on serial chest x-rays. Management includes observation, appropriate treatment of central airway obstruction or hemoptysis, bronchoscopic removal of the broncholith, and surgery (lung resection, debridement, or fistula repair) as required. Successful laser treatment has been reported.

Miks VM et al: Broncholith removal using the YAG laser. *Chest* 1986;**90**:295.

# PLEUROPULMONARY INFECTIONS

## ACUTE TRACHEOBRONCHITIS

Acute tracheobronchitis is a common condition caused by acute inflammation of the trachea and bronchi due to viruses or *Mycoplasma;* secondary bacterial infection may occur. Symptoms of upper respiratory infection often precede the manifestations of tracheobronchitis by several days. *S pneumoniae* or *H influenzae* is commonly recovered from sputum cultures. Clinical manifestations include cough (initially nonproductive but later productive of mucopurulent sputum) and substernal discomfort worsened by coughing. Fever may occur. Signs of pulmonary consolidation are absent. Chest x-ray is normal. Treatment is symptomatic; broad-spectrum antibiotics may be used if sputum is purulent.

## PNEUMONIA

Pneumonia continues to be a major health problem despite the availability of potent antimicrobial drugs. Microorganisms gain access to the lower respiratory tract in 1 of 3 ways, of which **aspiration of oropharyngeal secretions** and associated bacterial flora occurs most commonly. Viruses, *Mycoplasma,* and other infectious organisms that cause pneumonia also reach the lungs through **inhalation of infected aerosols.** Pneumonia also occurs when lung parenchyma is infected as a result of **hematogenous dissemination** (eg, spread of septic emboli from rightsided bacterial endocarditis). Characteristics of pneumonia caused by specific agents and appropriate antimicrobial therapy are presented in Table 7–6.

### Approach to the Patient With Possible Pneumonia

A chest radiograph is included in the initial evaluation of a patient with symptoms and signs suggestive of pneumonia. The pattern of the infiltrate is not pathognomonic of a specific cause of pneumonia.

The attempt to establish a specific causative diagnosis should begin with a Gram-stained smear of expectorated sputum, which often reveals the predominant organism. Cultures of sputum representative of lower respiratory tract secretions (ie, devoid of epithelial cells) should be obtained. Results of sputum cultures may be misleading because of contamination with flora of the upper respiratory tract; cultures are most helpful when correlated with Gram-stained smears. In patients appearing especially ill, blood cultures should also be obtained before antimicrobial therapy is started; if cultures are positive, the causative organism has been definitively identified.

Thoracentesis should be performed if an associated pleural effusion is present. Gram-stained smears and cultures of pleural fluid may reveal the causative organism. Pleural fluid with characteristics diagnostic of empyema (see p 151) represents an indication for tube thoracostomy in most cases.

Therapy should be started after initial diagnostic procedures (including smears and cultures) have been performed. If data are inconclusive, the physician must decide whether to start empiric antimicrobial therapy or use more invasive diagnostic techniques such as transtracheal or transthoracic aspiration, or bronchoscopy. Invasive procedures are not necessary

in most patients with uncomplicated community-acquired pneumonia, but are justified in immunodeficient patients or patients who fail to respond to conventional therapy. Knowledge of indigenous hospital flora and their antimicrobial sensitivities is vital in selecting empiric therapy for nosocomial pneumonia; therapy is modified when antimicrobial sensitivities become known or if the patient fails to respond.

Perrino TA, Stollerman GH: The management of pneumonia. *Adv Intern Med* 1984;**30:**113.

### Prevention

Polyvalent pneumococcal vaccine (containing capsular polysaccharide antigens of 23 strains of *S pneumoniae*) has the potential to prevent or lessen the severity of 85–90% of pneumococcal infections in immunocompetent patients. Although routine vaccination remains controversial, the vaccine's potential value and proved safety have led the Centers for Disease Control to recommend vaccination of the following adults:

(1) Those with chronic illnesses (eg, chronic cardiovascular and pulmonary diseases) that lead to increased morbidity from respiratory infections.

(2) Those with underlying illnesses associated with an increased risk of pneumococcal disease (eg, asplenia or splenic dysfunction, Hodgkin's disease, multiple myeloma, cirrhosis, alcoholism, renal failure, cerebrospinal fluid leaks, sickle cell anemia, and conditions associated with immunosuppression).

(3) Those aged 65 years and older in general good health.

Local discomfort at the injection site occurs in about 50% of those immunized. Systemic reactions (fever, malaise) are rare in those vaccinated for the first time but are common in those who are revaccinated. Pneumococcal vaccine should therefore be administered only once to each individual.

Annual vaccination against influenza is recommended for those at risk. Guidelines are updated yearly by the Centers for Disease Control.

Health and Public Policy Committee, American College of Physicians: Pneumococcal vaccine. *Ann Intern Med* 1986; **104:**118.

## 1. ACUTE BACTERIAL PNEUMONIA

### Essentials of Diagnosis

- Fever, chills, pleuritic chest pain, cough, purulent sputum.
- Evidence of consolidation on examination of the chest.
- Leukocytosis with leftward shift; leukopenia in some.
- Patchy or lobar infiltrates on chest x-ray.

### General Considerations

Information about the cause of acute bacterial pneumonia is incomplete because of the difficulty

Table 7–6. Characteristics of selected pneumonias.

| Organism | Clinical Setting | Gram-stained Smears of Sputum | Chest Radiograph[1] | Laboratory Studies | Complications | Antimicrobial Therapy[2] |
|---|---|---|---|---|---|---|
| *Streptococcus pneumoniae* (pneumococcus) | Age 60–70 years; chronic cardiopulmonary disease; follows upper respiratory tract infection. | Gram-positive diplococci. | Lobar consolidation. | Gram-stained smear of sputum; culture of blood, pleural fluid. | Bacteremia, meningitis, endocarditis, pericarditis, empyema. | Preferred: Penicillin G (or V, oral). Alternative: Erythromycin, cephalosporin. |
| *Haemophilus influenzae* | Age 60–70 years; chronic cardiopulmonary disease; follows upper respiratory tract infection. | Pleomorphic gram-negative coccobacilli. | Lobar consolidation. | Culture of sputum, blood, pleural fluid. | Empyema, endocarditis. | Preferred: Ampicillin (or amoxicillin). Alternative: Chloramphenicol; second-generation cephalosporin (eg, cefamandol, cefuroxime); trimethoprimsulfamethoxazole. |
| *Staphylococcus aureus* | Influenza epidemics; nosocomial. | Plump gram-positive cocci in clumps. | Patchy infiltrates. | Culture of sputum, blood, pleural fluid. | Empyema, cavitation. | Preferred: Nafcillin. Alternative: Vancomycin. |
| *Klebsiella pneumoniae* | Alcohol abuse, diabetes mellitus; nosocomial. | Plump gram-negative encapsulated rods. | Lobar consolidation. | Culture of sputum, blood, pleural fluid. | Cavitation, empyema. | Preferred: Aminoglycoside plus cephalosporin. Alternative: Chloramphenicol. |
| *Escherichia coli* | Nosocomial; rarely community-acquired. | Gram-negative rods. | Patchy infiltrates, pleural effusion. | Culture of sputum, blood, pleural fluid. | Empyema. | Preferred: Aminoglycoside. Alternative: Ampicillin, cephalosporin, chloramphenicol. |
| *Pseudomonas aeruginosa* | Nosocomial. | Gram-negative rods. | Patchy infiltrates, cavitation. | Culture of sputum, blood. | Cavitation. | Preferred: Aminoglycoside plus anti-*Pseudomonas* penicillin. Alternative: Aminoglycoside plus anti-*Pseudomonas* cephalosporin. |
| Anaerobes | Aspiration, periodontitis. | Mixed flora. | Patchy infiltrates in dependent lung zones. | Culture of pleural fluid or material obtained by transtracheal or transthoracic aspiration. | Necrotizing pneumonia, abscess, empyema. | Preferred: Penicillin G. Alternative: Clindamycin, chloramphenicol. |
| *Mycoplasma pneumoniae* | Young adults; summer and fall. | PMNs and monocytes; no bacterial pathogens. | Extensive patchy infiltrates. | Complement fixation titer.[3] | Skin rashes, bullous myringitis; hemolytic anemia. | Preferred: Erythromycin. Alternative: Tetracycline. |
| *Legionella* species | Summer and fall; exposure to contaminated construction site, water source, air conditioner; community-acquired or nosocomial. | Few PMNs; no bacteria. | Patchy or lobar consolidation. | Direct immunofluorescent examination of sputum or tissue; immunofluorescent antibody titer;[3] culture of sputum or tissue.[4] | Empyema, cavitation, endocarditis, pericarditis. | Preferred: Erythromycin, with or without rifampin. Alternative: Trimethoprimsulfamethoxazole. |

[1] See p 146 regarding the lack of specificity of x-ray findings.
[2] Antimicrobial sensitivities should guide therapy when available.
[3] Four-fold rise in titer is diagnostic.
[4] Selective media are required.

encountered in isolating the responsible organisms. Sputum cultures may fail to reveal the bacterial pathogen while demonstrating other organisms that have merely colonized the upper respiratory tract. Blood cultures and cultures of pleural fluid are positive in a minority of patients. Most studies of community-acquired acute bacterial pneumonia identify *S pneumoniae* (pneumococcus) as the causative organism in about two-thirds of cases; *H influenzae, S aureus,* enteric gramnegative rods, and anaerobes account for most of the remainder.

The bacterial pathogens of nosocomial acute bacterial pneumonia differ from those of the community-acquired variety. Hospitalized patients commonly develop oropharyngeal colonization with enteric gram-negative rods, particularly *pseudomonas aeruginosa,* and *S aureus,* which are usually responsible for lower respiratory tract infections in these patients. *S pneumoniae* is an infrequent cause of nosocomial pneumonia.

### Clinical Findings

**A. Symptoms and Signs:** Acute bacterial pneumonia is manifested by the abrupt onset of fever, chills, cough productive of purulent sputum, and pleuritic chest pain. Physical examination reveals a toxic-appearing, febrile patient with tachypnea and tachycardia. Evidence of consolidation may be present. In elderly patients, acute pneumonia may be heralded only by an alteration in mental status or an apparent worsening of underlying disease such as chronic obstructive pulmonary disease or congestive heart failure. Unless the patient is otherwise healthy and has disease limited to one lobe, hospitalization is advised.

**B. Laboratory Findings:** An initial pair of blood cultures is necessary in these patients. Hematologic evaluation reveals leukocytosis with a shift to the left or sometimes leukopenia. Sputum is purulent or mucopurulent. Gram-stained smears of sputum reveal neutrophils and (usually) a single predominant organism. They should not be interpreted unless epithelial cells are absent from the specimen. Quantitative bacteriologic methods may increase the reliability of cultures of sputum and tracheal aspirates in the diagnosis of pneumonia.

**C. Imaging:** Chest radiography shows lobar or segmental ("patchy") infiltrates. Ipsilateral pleural effusion may be present.

### Treatment

See Table 7–6.

Austrian R: Pneumococcal pneumonia: Diagnostic, epidemiologic, therapeutic, and prophylactic considerations. *Chest* 1986;**90**:738.
Salata RA et al: Diagnosis of nosocomial pneumonia in intubated, intensive care unit patients. *Am Rev Respir Dis* 1987;**135**:426.

## 2. ATYPICAL PNEUMONIA

The clinical picture in atypical pneumonia is dominated by constitutional symptoms such as fever, malaise, and headache rather than by respiratory symptoms, though a nonproductive cough is usually present. Unfortunately, overlap of these symptoms with similar ones in bacterial processes precludes their use in establishing a diagnosis. Physical findings of consolidation are absent. Leukocytosis, if present, is mild. Gram-stained smears of sputum (if obtainable) reveal neutrophils or mononuclear cells but no predominant bacterial pathogens. Chest radiograph reveals patchy nonlobar infiltrates that are more extensive than might be predicted from the clinical presentation.

The most common cause of atypical pneumonia is *M pneumoniae.* Other less common causative agents include *Legionella* species, *Chlamydia psittaci* (psittacosis), *Coxiella burnetii* (Q fever), adenovirus, and, in endemic areas, *Coccidioides immitis* and *Histoplasma capsulatum.* A newly recognized "TWAR" strain of *Chlamydia* is the most common cause of human *Chlamydia* infection. Viral pneumonia produces a similar clinical picture; adenoviruses are the most common cause.

Amantidine is 65–80% effective in prevention of symptomatic influenza A infection during outbreaks. If given during the first 1–2 days of illness, it also shortens the duration of symptoms of influenza A infection. Treatment guidelines are available from the Centers for Disease Control.

Barnes DW, Whitley RJ: Antiviral therapy and pulmonary disease. *Chest* 1987;**91**:246.
Edelstein PH, Meyer RD: Legionnaires' disease: A review. *Chest* 1984;**85**:114.
Grayston JT et al: A new *Chlamydia psittaci* strain, TWAR, isolated in acute respiratory tract infections. *N Engl J Med* 1986;**315**:161.

## 3. ANAEROBIC PNEUMONIA & LUNG ABSCESS

### Essentials of Diagnosis
- Predisposition to aspiration.
- Poor dental hygiene.
- Fever, weight loss, malaise.
- Foul-smelling sputum (fewer than half of patients).
- Infiltrate in dependent lung zone, with single or multiple areas of cavitation or pleural effusion.

### General Considerations
Aspiration of small amounts of oropharyngeal secretions occurs during sleep in normal individuals and rarely causes disease. Sequelae of aspiration of larger amounts of material include nocturnal asthma, bronchiectasis, chemical pneumonitis, mechanical obstruction of airways by particulate matter, and pleuropulmonary infection. Individuals predisposed to disease induced by aspiration include those with depressed levels of consciousness due to drug or alco-

hol use, seizures, general anesthesia, or central nervous system disease; those with impaired deglutition due to esophageal disease or neurologic disorders; and those with endotracheal or nasogastric tubes, that disrupt the mechanical defenses of the airways.

Periodontal disease, which increases the number of anaerobic bacteria in aspirated material, is associated with a greater likelihood of anaerobic pleuropulmonary infection. Aspiration of infected oropharyngeal contents initially leads to pneumonia in dependent lung zones, such as the posterior segments of the upper lobes and superior and basilar segments of the lower lobes. Body position at the time of aspiration determines which lung zones are dependent. The onset of symptoms is insidious. By the time the patient seeks medical attention, necrotizing pneumonia, lung abscess, or empyema may be apparent.

About two-thirds of patients with necrotizing pneumonia, lung abscess, and empyema are found to be infected with multiple species of anaerobic bacteria only. Most of the remainder are infected with both anaerobic and aerobic bacteria. *Bacteroides melaninogenicus,* anaerobic streptococci, and *Fusobacterium nucleatum* are commonly isolated anaerobic bacteria.

### Clinical Findings

**A. Symptoms and Signs:** Patients with anaerobic pleuropulmonary infection usually present with constitutional symptoms such as fever, weight loss, and malaise. Cough with expectoration of foul-smelling purulent sputum suggests anaerobic infection, though the absence of productive cough does not rule out such an infection. Dental hygiene is poor, but patients are rarely edentulous; if the patient is edentulous, an obstructing bronchial lesion is commonly present.

**B. Laboratory Findings:** Expectorated sputum is inappropriate for culture of anaerobic organisms because of mouth contaminants. Culture material can be obtained only by transtracheal or transthoracic aspiration, thoracentesis, or bronchoscopy with a protected brush. Transthoracic or transtracheal aspiration is rarely indicated, because anaerobic pleuropulmonary infections respond well to penicillin or clindamycin.

**C. Imaging:** The different types of anaerobic pleuropulmonary infection are distinguished on the basis of their radiographic appearance. **Lung abscess** appears as a thick-walled solitary cavity surrounded by consolidation. An air-fluid level is usually present. Other causes of cavitary lung disease should be excluded. **Necrotizing pneumonia** is distinguished by multiple areas of cavitation within an area of consolidation. **Empyema** is characterized by the presence of pleural fluid and may accompany either of the other 2 radiographic findings. Ultrasonography is of value in locating fluid and may also reveal pleural loculations.

### Treatment

Penicillin G (1–2 million units intravenously every 4 hours) is the usual treatment for anaerobic pleuropulmonary infections; clindamycin may be equally or more effective. Penicillin V (0.5–1 g orally every 6 hours) may be used after improvement with intravenous penicillin G has occurred. Antimicrobials should be given until the chest x-ray stabilizes. The treatment of anaerobic pleuropulmonary disease requires adequate drainage. Tube thoracostomy is required for the treatment of empyema, but open pleural drainage is often necessary because of the propensity of these infections to produce loculations in the pleural space.

Levison ME et al: Clindamycin compared with penicillin for the treatment of anaerobic lung abscess. *Ann Intern Med* 1983;**98**:466.

Sosenko A, Glassroth J: Fiberoptic bronchoscopy in the evaluation of lung abscesses. *Chest* 1985;**87**:489.

## PULMONARY TUBERCULOSIS

### Essentials of Diagnosis

- Fatigue, weight loss, fever, night sweats.
- Productive cough.
- Pulmonary infiltrates on chest radiograph.
- Positive tuberculin skin test reaction (most cases).
- Acid-fast bacilli on smear of sputum.
- Sputum culture positive for *Mycobacterium tuberculosis.*

### General Considerations

Infection with *Mycobacterium tuberculosis* begins when aerosolized droplets containing viable organisms are inhaled by a person susceptible to the disease. When they reach the lungs, the organisms are ingested by macrophages and either die or persist and multiply. Widespread lymphatic and hematogenous dissemination of organisms occurs before development of an effective immune response when mycobacteria throughout the body are walled off by granulomatous inflammation. Dormant but viable organisms persist for years, and reactivation of disease in any of these sites may occur if the host's defense mechanisms become impaired. Most cases of tuberculosis in adults are due to reactivation of disease and not to recent infection. As the number of reported cases decreases, however, the percentage of patients with atypical presentations—particularly elderly patients and those in nursing homes—has increased.

Persons infected with the human immunodeficiency virus (HIV) appear to be at increased risk of developing tuberculosis. Tuberculosis is also common in the homeless and in refugees from Asia and Central America.

### Clinical Findings

**A. Symptoms and Signs:** The patient typically presents with constitutional symptoms of fatigue, weight loss, anorexia, low-grade fever, and night sweats. Pulmonary symptoms include cough, which is initially dry but later productive of purulent sputum and (sometimes) blood. Occasionally, there may be no symptoms. On physical examination, patients often appear chronically ill and exhibit evidence of weight loss. Examination of the chest may reveal findings such as posttussive apical rales or may be normal.

**B. Laboratory Findings:** A high index of suspicion is critical to the diagnosis of tuberculosis. Definitive diagnosis depends on recovery of *M tuberculosis* from cultures. Diagnosis therefore starts with collection of a series of early morning sputum specimens for stain and culture. Induction of sputum may be helpful in patients who cannot voluntarily produce good specimens. Multiple sputum specimens are often required to identify acid-fast bacilli. Demonstration of acid-fast bacilli on sputum smear does not confirm a diagnosis of tuberculosis, since saprophytic nontuberculous mycobacteria may colonize the airways or cause pulmonary disease. False-positive sputum cultures of *Mycobacterium tuberculosis* are, however, very rare.

If attempts to obtain sputum are unsuccessful, gastric washings may be useful, although they are suitable only for culture and not for stained smear, because nontuberculous mycobacteria may be present in the stomach in the absence of tuberculous infection. Fiberoptic bronchoscopy with bronchial washings may also lead to diagnosis in patients who are unable to produce adequate amounts of sputum or in those who are still thought to have tuberculosis despite negative results on sputum smears.

Cultures require 6–8 weeks for final interpretation. A radiometric culture system (Bactec) may allow detection of mycobacterial growth in as little as several days.

In primary tuberculosis, needle biopsy of the pleura reveals granulomas in a high percentage of patients, though pleural fluid culture is usually not revealing.

**C. Imaging:** Pulmonary tuberculosis is associated with various radiographic manifestations, including fibrocavitary apical disease, nodules, and pneumonic infiltrates. The usual location is in the apical or posterior segments of the upper lobes or in the superior segments of the lower lobes; as many as 30% of patients may present with radiographic evidence of disease in other locations, however. This is especially true in elderly patients, in whom lower lobe infiltrates with or without pleural effusion are encountered with increasing frequency. Lower lung zone tuberculosis, which may occur with endobronchial tuberculosis, may masquerade as pneumonia or lung cancer. Finally, unexplained pleural effusion may be the sole radiographic abnormality; this occurs with primary infection.

**D. Special Examinations:** The tuberculin skin test (5 tuberculin units of purified protein derivative [PPD] intradermally) identifies individuals who have been infected at some time with *M tuberculosis,* but does not distinguish between current disease and past infection. Patients with a high likelihood of infection with *M tuberculosis,* eg, those who are known contacts of an individual with active disease or those

with findings consistent with tuberculosis on chest x-ray, should be considered to have ''significant'' tuberculin skin test results if induration is 5 mm or more. Patients with a lower likelihood of tuberculous infection and a high likelihood of infection with atypical mycobacteria should be considered to have significant results on tuberculin skin testing if induration is 10 mm or more.

Both false-positive and false-negative tuberculin reactions occur. False-positive reactions are due to infection with nontuberculous mycobacteria. False-negative reactions occur in patients with malnutrition, immunologic defects, renal failure, overwhelming tuberculosis, or old age.

''Boosting'' of the skin test reaction by serial testing may cause a false impression of conversion, as dormant mycobacterial sensitivity is restored by the antigenic challenge of the initial skin test.

## Treatment

**A. Hospitalization:** Hospitalization for initial therapy of tuberculosis is not necessary in most patients, though it should be considered if a patient is incapable of self-care or is likely to expose susceptible individuals to the risk of tuberculosis. A private room with appropriate ventilation and instruction in the importance of covering the mouth while coughing are sufficient infection control measures for hospitalized patients receiving effective chemotherapy. If patient noncompliance is demonstrated or anticipated, direct supervision of drug treatment is required.

**B. Drug Therapy:** (Table 7–7.) The standard therapy of pulmonary tuberculosis currently consists of isoniazid (INH) and rifampin for 9 months. Drugs may be given daily for the entire 9 months or daily for 4 weeks, followed by supervised biweekly administration for the remaining months. The initial use of a third drug such as ethambutol or streptomycin is probably not necessary in the absence of microbial drug resistance. A 6-month regimen of isoniazid and rifampin, with the addition of pyrazinamide for the first 2 months, is equally effective if the organism is not resistant and the patient is compliant. If isoniazid resistance is suspected, ethambutol is added during the first 2 months of therapy.

Resistance to isoniazid should be suspected if tuberculosis was acquired in an area with a high prevalence of *isoniazid-resistant organisms* (Asia, Latin America); if the patient has been previously treated with isoniazid; or if the patient has been exposed to tuberculosis known to be drug-resistant. In these situations, initial therapy should consist of at least 2 bactericidal drugs in addition to isoniazid. If resistance to isoniazid is documented, give rifampin and ethambutol for at least 12 months, perhaps supplemented by pyrazinamide in the initial phase of treatment. Re-treatment of tuberculosis requires at least 2 drugs (bactericidal if possible) to which the patient has not been exposed and against which microbial resistance has not been demonstrated (see pp 980–982).

**C. Chemoprophylaxis:** Patients infected with

**Table 7–7.** First-line antituberculous drugs.[*]

| | Dosage | | Most Common Side Effects | Tests for Side Effects | Drug Interactions | Remarks |
|---|---|---|---|---|---|---|
| | **Daily** | **Twice Weekly** | | | | |
| Isoniazid (INH) | 5–10 mg/kg, up to 300 mg orally or intramuscularly. | 15 mg/kg orally or intramuscularly. | Peripheral neuritis, hepatitis, hypersensitivity. | SGOT (AST)/SGPT (ALT) | Phenytoin (synergistic); disulfiram. | Bactericidal to both extracellular and intracellular organisms. Pyridoxine, 10 mg orally as prophylaxis for neuritis; 50–100 mg as treatment. |
| Rifampin | 10 mg/kg, up to 600 mg orally. | 10 mg/kg, up to 600 mg orally. | Hepatitis, febrile reaction, purpura (rare). | SGOT (AST)/SGPT (ALT) | Rifampin inhibits the effect of oral contraceptives, quinidine, corticosteroids, coumarin anticoagulants, methadone, digoxin, oral hypoglycemics; PAS may interfere with absorption of rifampin. | Bactericidal to all populations of organisms. Colors urine and other body secretions orange. Discoloring of contact lenses. |
| Streptomycin | 15–20 mg/kg, up to 1 g intramuscularly. | 25–30 mg/kg. | Eighth nerve damage, nephrotoxicity. | Vestibular function (audiograms); blood urea nitrogen and creatinine. | Neuromuscular blocking agents may be potentiated and cause prolonged paralysis. | Bactericidal to extracellular organisms. Use with caution in older patients or those with renal disease. |
| Pyrazinamide | 15–30 mg/kg, up to 2 g orally. | 50–70 mg/kg. | Hyperuricemia, hepatotoxicity. | Uric acid, SGOT (AST)/SGPT (ALT). | · · · | Bactericidal to intracellular organisms. Combination with an aminoglycoside is bactericidal. |
| Ethambutol | 15–25 mg/kg orally. | 50 mg/kg orally. | Optic neuritis (reversible with discontinuation of drug; rare at 15 mg/kg), rash. | Red-green color discrimination and visual acuity (difficult to test in children under 3 years of age). | | Bacteriostatic to both intracellular and extracellular organisms. Mainly used to inhibit development of resistant mutants. Use with caution in renal disease or when ophthalmologic testing is not feasible. |

[*]Modified and reproduced, with permission, from Bailey WC et al: Treatment of tuberculosis and other mycobacterial diseases. *Am Rev Respir Dis* 1983:**127**:790.

*M tuberculosis* but without active disease harbor small numbers of organisms. Recent data confirm that isoniazid prophylaxis for 12 months in such patients may reduce the expected incidence of reactivated tuberculosis by 93%.

The following groups of individuals should be offered isoniazid prophylaxis if they have significant results on tuberculin skin tests:

(1) Household members and other close contacts of individuals with potentially infectious tuberculosis. Children should be treated even if their skin test results are nonsignificant, and such tests should be repeated after 3 months of isoniazid therapy. Isoniazid should be continued for a total of 12 months if the skin test reaction becomes significant.

(2) Newly infected persons (conversion of skin test reaction from nonsignificant to significant within 2 years).

(3) Individuals with positive skin test reactions and chest x-ray abnormalities consistent with tuberculosis but without bacteriologic evidence of active disease.

(4) Individuals with previous or current positive skin test reactions and underlying conditions that increase the risk of reactivated tuberculosis, including silicosis, diabetes mellitus, prolonged corticosteroid therapy, immunosuppressive therapy, end-stage renal disease, chronic undernutrition (including that following gastrectomy), hematologic and reticuloendothelial cancers, and AIDS or positive tests for antibodies to AIDS virus.

(5) Individuals with positive skin test reactions who are under 35 years of age and who have none of the risk factors discussed above.

The major risk of isoniazid prophylaxis is drug-induced hepatitis, the incidence of which increases with age. Isoniazid should be discontinued if a patient develops clinical evidence of hepatitis during therapy. Failure to discontinue the drug may result in progressive and possibly fatal hepatic necrosis. The routine monitoring of biochemical tests of liver function periodically during isoniazid prophylaxis is recommended for persons 35 and older. Elevations of transaminase up to twice normal without symptoms do not constitute an indication to stop therapy. Rifampin rather than isoniazid should be given for chemoprophylaxis if the patient has had contact with someone known to have isoniazid-resistant organisms.

**D. Vaccine:** A number of live tuberculosis vaccines are available and are known collectively as BCG after the original strain of bacterium used in the vaccine (bacillus Calmette-Guérin). Current recommendations are that BCG vaccination be considered for tuberculin-negative persons, especially children, who are repeatedly exposed to individuals with untreated or ineffectively treated tuberculosis. Vaccination should be considered for communities or groups in which a high rate of new infections occurs despite aggressive treatment and surveillance programs.

## Prognosis

Almost all properly treated patients with tuberculosis are cured. Relapse rates are less than 5% with current regimens. The only important cause of treatment failure is noncompliance.

American Thoracic Society: Treatment of tuberculosis and tuberculosis infection in adults and children. *Am Rev Respir Dis* 1986;**134:**355.

Centers for Disease Control: Diagnosis and management of mycobacterial infection and disease in persons with human immunodeficiency virus infection. *Ann Intern Med* 1987; **106:**254.

Slutkin G, Perez-Stable EJ, Hopewell PC: Time course and boosting of tuberculin reactions in nursing home residents. *Am Rev Respir Dis* 1986;**134:**1048.

## DISEASE CAUSED BY NONTUBERCULOUS MYCOBACTERIA

Mycobacteria other than *M tuberculosis* ("atypical" mycobacteria) are ubiquitous in nature. Only *M kansasii* and *M avium-intracellulare* complex are important causes of pulmonary disease in humans, which is clinically indistinguishable from tuberculosis. The diagnosis rests on recovery of the pathogen from cultures. Infections with *M avium-intracellulare* are being seen with increasing frequency in patients with AIDS, in whom the disease is likely to be disseminated.

Sputum cultures positive for atypical mycobacteria do not in themselves prove the presence of atypical tuberculosis, because atypical bacteria may exist as saprophytes in the airways or as environmental contaminants. Sputum cultures are meaningful if the following criteria are met: (1) The patient has clinical and radiographic evidence of disease compatible with a diagnosis of pulmonary tuberculosis; and (2) multiple colonies are present on more than one culture. A positive result on culture of material obtained from tissue biopsies or pleural fluid is also diagnostic.

Disease caused by *M kansasii* responds well to drug therapy. Recent data suggest that a regimen of rifampin, isoniazid, and ethambutol for 12 months, with streptomycin added for the first 3 months, is sufficient.

In contrast, *M avium-intracellulare* is resistant in vitro to most antituberculosis drugs. Traditional chemotherapeutic regimens have taken an aggressive approach using 5 or 6 drugs, but these have been associated with drug-induced side effects and patient noncompliance. An alternative regimen uses isoniazid, ethambutol, and rifampin for 18–24 months, plus streptomycin during the first 2–3 months. This regimen may yield successful results in 40–60% of cases. Most of the remaining patients will have active but stable disease despite the discontinuation of drugs. Surgical resection is an alternative for the patient with progressive disease that responds poorly to chemotherapy. In patients with AIDS, *M avium-intracel-*

*lulare* infections are systemic and tend to occur late in the course. The prognosis is dismal in such cases.

Ahn CH et al: Short course chemotherapy for pulmonary disease caused by *Mycobacterium kansasii. Am Rev Respir Dis* 1983;**128**:1048.

Ahn CH et al: A four-drug regimen for initial treatment of cavitary disease caused by *Mycobacterium avium* complex. *Am Rev Respir Dis* 1986;**134**:438.

## PULMONARY INFILTRATES IN THE COMPROMISED HOST

Pneumonia in immunocompromised patients may be caused by bacterial, mycobacterial, fungal, protozoal, helminthic, or viral pathogens, but not all pulmonary infiltrates in compromised hosts are due to infection. Noninfectious processes such as pulmonary edema, drug reaction, pulmonary infarction, underlying malignant disease, and radiation pneumonitis may mimic infection. Although almost any pathogen can cause pneumonia in a compromised host, 2 clinical tools help the clinician narrow the differential diagnosis. The first of these is knowledge of the underlying immunologic defect: specific types of immunologic defects predispose to particular infections; eg, defects in humoral immunity predispose mainly to bacterial infections against which antibodies play an important role, whereas defects in cellular immunity predispose to infections with viruses, fungi, mycobacteria, and protozoa. Chest radiography is also helpful in clarifying the differential diagnosis. Diffuse infiltrates are usually seen with *Pneumocystis carinii* or viral pneumonias. Bacterial and fungal infections are typically associated with more localized infiltrates.

Diagnostic procedures should include blood cultures and examination and culture of sputum and pleural fluid, if present. Routine evaluation often fails to identify the causative organism. The clinician must then either begin empiric antimicrobial therapy or proceed to invasive procedures such as bronchoscopy, transthoracic aspiration, or open lung biopsy. Selection must be based on the severity of the pulmonary infection, the underlying disease, the risks of empiric therapy, and local expertise and experience with the diagnostic procedures. Open lung biopsy is considered the "gold standard" for diagnosis of pulmonary infiltrates in the compromised host, but choice of this procedure should be tempered by the realization that the information obtained rarely affects the ultimate outcome. Moreover, a specific diagnosis is obtained in only about two-thirds of cases in which this test is performed. Therefore, empiric treatment is generally preferred, especially when the risk-benefit ratio of lung biopsy is high.

Masur H, Shelhamer J, Parillo JE: The management of pneumonias in immunocompromised patients. *JAMA* 1985; **253**:1769.

Robin ED, Burke CM: Lung biopsy in immunosuppressed patients. *Chest* 1986;**89**:276.

# NEOPLASTIC & RELATED DISEASES

## BRONCHOGENIC CARCINOMA

### Essentials of Diagnosis
- Cough, dyspnea, hemoptysis, anorexia, or weight loss in most patients.
- Variable findings on physical examination depending on stage of disease.
- Enlarging mass, infiltrate, atelectasis, cavitation, or pleural effusion on chest x-ray in most patients.
- Cytologic or histologic findings diagnostic of primary lung cancer in sputum, pleural fluid, or tissue.

### General Considerations
About 150,000 new cases of lung cancer are expected in the USA in 1988. Lung cancer accounts for 35% of cancer deaths in men and 20% of cancer deaths in women, and its incidence in women is rising rapidly. Most cases present between the ages of 50 and 70. Fewer than 5% of lung cancer patients are under 40 years of age; cigarette smoke is the most common cause of lung cancer. Lung scars, air pollution, and genetic factors are also implicated, but the data supporting these associations are not conclusive. Chronic obstructive pulmonary disease may represent a risk factor for lung cancer even after controlling for cigarette smoking. Primary lung cancer in nonsmokers is uncommon.

More than 20 benign and malignant primary neoplasms of the lung have been identified and classified histologically. Ninety percent of malignant cancers belong to one of the 4 major cell types of bronchogenic carcinoma, a term denoting primary malignant tumors of the airway epithelium. **Squamous cell carcinoma** and **adenocarcinoma** are the most common types of bronchogenic carcinoma and account for about 35% of primary tumors each. **Small cell carcinoma** and **large cell carcinoma** account for about 20% and 10%, respectively.

Squamous cell carcinoma of the lung tends to originate in the central bronchi as an intraluminal growth and is thus more amenable to early detection through cytologic examination of sputum than are the other types of carcinoma. Doubling time (time required for a spherical tumor to double its volume) is about 100 days. Squamous cell carcinoma tends to metastasize in regional lymph nodes, and about 10% of such tumors cavitate. Small-cell carcinoma also occurs centrally, has a doubling time of about 33 days, and tends to narrow bronchi by extrinsic compression; wide-spread metastases are common. Adenocarcinoma and large-cell carcinoma resemble each other in their clinical behavior. These tumors usually appear in the periphery of the lung and therefore are not amenable to early detection through examination of sputum. They typically metastasize to distant organs. Doubling times are about 180 days for adenocarcinoma and 100 days for large-cell carcinoma. **Bronchioloalveolar cell carcinoma,** a subtype of adenocarcinoma, is a low-grade carcinoma that represents about 2% of cases of bronchogenic carcinoma and presents as single or multiple pulmonary nodules or an alveolar infiltrate.

## Clinical Findings

The clinical features of lung cancer depend on the primary cancer itself, its metastases, systemic effects of the cancer, and any coexisting paraneoplastic syndromes.

**A. Symptoms and Signs:** Only 10–25% of patients are asymptomatic at the time of diagnosis of lung cancer. Symptomatic lung cancer is generally advanced and often not resectable. Initial symptoms include nonspecific complaints such as cough, weight loss, dyspnea, chest pain, and hemoptysis that are associated with other disorders. Any change in the pattern of cough, blood-streaked sputum, anorexia with weight loss, and hoarseness are symptoms that point to a diagnosis of bronchogenic carcinoma in the appropriate clinical setting.

Physical findings vary and may be totally absent. Central tumors that obstruct segmental, lobar, or main stem bronchi may cause atelectasis and postobstructive pneumonitis with typical physical findings. Peripheral tumors may cause no abnormalities on physical examination. Extension of the tumor to the pleural surface may cause pleural effusion. In one large series, lymphadenopathy, hepatomegaly, and clubbing were noted in about 20% of patients with lung cancer. Superior vena cava syndrome, Horner's syndrome (miosis, ptosis, enophthalmos, and loss of sweating on the affected side), Pancoast's syndrome (neurovascular complications of superior pulmonary sulcus tumor), recurrent laryngeal nerve palsy with hoarseness, phrenic nerve palsy with hemidiaphragm paralysis, and skin metastases are each seen in fewer than 5% of cases.

**Paraneoplastic syndromes** (extrapulmonary organ dysfunction not related to space-occupying metastases) occur in 15–20% of lung cancer patients. A number of tumor secretory products have been associated with lung cancer. The manifestations of paraneoplastic syndromes may precede, coincide with, or follow the diagnosis of lung cancer. Recognition of paraneoplastic syndromes in lung cancer is important, because treatment of the associated symptoms may improve the patient's well-being even though the primary tumor itself is not curable; occasionally, resection of the tumor is followed by immediate resolution of the paraneoplastic syndrome. Table 7–8 lists important paraneoplastic syndromes associated with lung cancer.

**B. Laboratory Findings:** All patients with suspected lung cancer should receive a complete blood count, liver function tests, and measurement of serum electrolytes and calcium in addition to a chest radio-

**Table 7–8.** Paraneoplastic syndromes in lung cancer.

| Classification | Syndrome | Common Histologic Type of Cancer |
|---|---|---|
| Endocrine and metabolic | Cushing's syndrome | Small-cell |
| | Inappropriate secretion of antidiuretic hormone (SIADH) | Small-cell |
| | Hypercalcemia | Squamous cell |
| | Gynecomastia | Large-cell |
| Connective tissue and osseous | Clubbing and hypertrophic pulmonary osteoarthropathy | Squamous cell, adenocarcinoma, large-cell |
| Neuromuscular | Peripheral neuropathy (sensory, sensorimotor) | Small-cell |
| | Subacute cerebellar degeneration | Small-cell |
| | Myasthenia (Eaton-Lambert syndrome) | Small-cell |
| | Dermatomyositis | All |
| Cardiovascular | Thrombophlebitis | |
| | Nonbacterial verrucous (marantic) endocarditis | Adenocarcinoma |
| Hematologic | Anemia | |
| | Disseminated intravascular coagulation | |
| | Eosinophilia | |
| | Thrombocytosis | |
| Cutaneous | Acanthosis nigricans | |
| | Erythema gyratum repens | |

graph. Definitive diagnosis requires cytologic or histologic evidence of cancer.

Cytologic examination of sputum permits definitive diagnosis of lung cancer in many cases, especially in centrally located tumors. Examination of pleural fluid reveals cytologic findings positive for cancer in 40–50% of patients with malignant pleural effusion from lung cancer. Closed pleural biopsy (Cope or Abrams needle) yields a histologic diagnosis of cancer in about 55% of patients. Biopsy and cytologic study of pleural fluid combined establish a diagnosis of cancer in about 80% of patients with malignant pleural effusion.

Tissue for histologic confirmation of lung cancer may be obtained by various techniques, including bronchoscopy, percutaneous needle aspirate, mediastinoscopy, scalene lymph node biopsy, or biopsy of other metastatic sites (eg, skin), and thoracotomy. Biopsy of mediastinal lymph nodes reveals cancer in about a third of lung cancer patients. Fine-needle aspiration of supraclavicular or cervical lymph nodes is useful if these nodes are enlarged on palpation. Thoracotomy is occasionally necessary to diagnose lung cancer when simpler cytologic and histologic evaluations are negative.

**C. Imaging:** Chest radiography demonstrates abnormal findings in nearly all patients with lung cancer. Comparison of old and current chest radiographs enables calculation of the doubling time. A doubling time of less than 30 days or more than 500 days makes the diagnosis of primary lung cancer unlikely.

Radiographic abnormalities in primary lung cancer are not specific. Common abnormalities are hilar masses or enlargement, peripheral masses, atelectasis, infiltrates, cavitation, and pleural effusions. Multiple masses, consolidation, and chest wall involvement are unusual. Squamous cell and small cell carcinoma commonly produces a hilar mass and mediastinal widening. Cavitation suggests squamous cell carcinoma and is exceedingly rare in small-cell carcinoma. Small peripheral masses usually are adenocarcinomas.

**D. Special Examinations:** Early detection of lung cancer in an asymptomatic stage is feasible with cytologic examination of sputum and chest radiography. Small-cell carcinoma, however, is nearly always metastatic when first detected. Routine screening for lung cancer with chest radiography or cytologic studies of sputum is not recommended because the mortality rate from lung cancer is not appreciably reduced by early detection.

**Staging of lung cancer** utilizes the TNM staging system for non-small-cell carcinoma, in which T describes the primary tumor, N the nodal involvement, and M any distant metastases. Small-cell carcinoma is staged as "limited" (tumor confined to one hemithorax and ipsilateral hilar, mediastinal, and supraclavicular nodes) or "extensive" (spread to more distant sites). CT scan of the lungs, mediastinum, and upper abdomen (liver, adrenal glands, and periaortic lymph nodes) is usually helpful in staging lung cancer. In a patient with known lung cancer, the finding of mediastinal lymph nodes larger than 2 cm in diameter on CT scan is strong evidence of mediastinal spread of the tumor; however, occasional false-positive results occur with this technique. Nodes smaller than 1 cm have a low probability of tumor involvement. At least 85% of lung cancer patients with negative results on mediastinal CT scans have no evidence of mediastinal lymphadenopathy at the time of surgery.

History, physical examination, and simple laboratory studies are usually sufficient to detect metastases to distant sites such as liver, brain, bone, heart, abdomen, and skin. Radionuclide scans to detect occult distant metastases are not recommended.

**Complications**

**A. Superior Vena Cava Syndrome:** This syndrome is partial or complete obstruction of the thin-walled superior vena cava with associated symptoms and signs. Cancer (mainly bronchogenic carcinoma) accounts for 85–95% of cases of superior vena cava syndrome. Symptoms include swelling of the neck and face, headache, dizziness, visual disturbances, stupor, and syncope. Abnormalities on physical examination include facial plethora and edema and dilatation of venous channels over the upper chest, shoulders, and neck. Superior vena cava syndrome is usually managed initially with radiation therapy for immediate control, followed by chemotherapy if the disease is due to small-cell carcinoma. Patients with superior vena cava syndrome are not candidates for surgical resection of the underlying tumor, and the overall prognosis is poor.

**B. Phrenic Nerve Palsy:** Tumor destruction of the phrenic nerve, which courses through the mediastinum to innervate the hemidiaphragm, occurs in about 1% of patients with lung cancer and results in hemidiaphragmatic paralysis.

**C. Recurrent Laryngeal Nerve Palsy:** Recurrent laryngeal nerve palsy due to destruction of the recurrent laryngeal nerve by tumor causes paralysis of the muscles of the larynx, resulting in hoarseness. This palsy almost always occurs on the left side and is seen in fewer than 3% of patients with lung cancer.

**Treatment**

The main treatment options in lung cancer include surgery, chemotherapy, and radiation therapy. Laser photocoagulation has been performed on obstructing central tumors to relieve dyspnea and control hemoptysis.

Surgery remains the treatment of choice for patients with non-small-cell carcinoma. Unfortunately, only about 25% of patients with lung cancer are appropriate candidates for surgery, and many of these are found to have unresectable disease at the time of thoracotomy. Contraindications to surgery include extrathoracic metastases; tumor involving the trachea, carina, or proximal main stem bronchi ($<$ 2 cm from the carina); malignant pleural effusion; recurrent laryngeal nerve or phrenic nerve palsy; superior vena cava syndrome; tumor involving the esophagus or pericardium; spread to contralateral mediastinal lymph nodes; poor general health; and extensive involvement of the chest wall.

Combination chemotherapy (see Chapter 32) is the treatment of choice for small-cell carcinoma and results in considerable improvement in median survival times. Occasionally, posttreatment surgical debulking of primary lesions is carried out. Prophylactic cranial radiation is performed in patients with small-cell carcinoma who have responded to chemotherapy. Single-agent chemotherapy has no proved value. Although tumor regression in non-small-cell carcinoma is possible with combination chemotherapy, median survival time is not prolonged.

External beam radiation therapy is often used to palliate symptoms of lung cancer such as cough, hemoptysis, pain due to bone metastases, and dyspnea from bronchial or tracheal obstruction. Superior vena cava syndrome and central nervous system involvement by metastatic tumor are also treated with radiation. Symptomatic brain metastases are treated with radiation therapy and corticosteroids. Selected patients with unresectable lung cancer also receive external beam radiation to the primary tumor site. In patients with limited-stage small cell carcinoma, this improves complete response rates and survival when compared to chemotherapy alone. However, in non-small cell lung cancer, survival is not improved. Intraluminal radiation ("brachytherapy") is a new approach to relief of symptoms of recurrent endobronchial lung cancer.

## Prognosis

The overall 5-year survival rate for lung cancer is 10–15%. Determinants of survival include the stage of disease at the time of presentation, the patient's general health, age, histologic type of tumor, tumor growth rate, and type of therapy. Overall, the 5-year survival rate after "curative" resection of squamous cell carcinoma is 35–40%, compared with 25% for adenocarcinoma and large-cell carcinoma. Patients with small-cell carcinoma rarely live for 5 years after the diagnosis is made.

Bunn PA et al: Chemotherapy alone or chemotherapy with chest radiation therapy in limited stage small cell lung cancer: A prospective, randomized trial. *Ann Intern Med* 1987; **106:**655.

Iannuzzi MC, Scoggin CH: Small cell lung cancer. *Am Rev Respir Dis* 1986;**134:**593.

Perry MC et al: Chemotherapy with or without radiation therapy in limited small-cell carcinoma of the lung. *N Engl J Med* 1987;**316:**912.

McKenna RJ Jr et al: Roentgenographic evaluation of mediastinal lymph nodes for preoperative assessment in lung cancer. *Chest* 1985;**88:**206.

Seagren SL, Harrell JH, Horn RA: High dose rate intraluminal irradiation in recurrent endobronchial carcinoma. *Chest* 1985;**88:**810.

## SOLITARY PULMONARY NODULE

A solitary pulmonary nodule is a round or oval sharply circumscribed pulmonary lesion (up to 5 cm in diameter; larger lesions are termed "masses") surrounded by normal lung tissue. Central cavitation, calcification, or surrounding ("satellite") lesions may occur. Finding a solitary pulmonary nodule on chest x-ray is important, because about 25% of cases of bronchogenic carcinoma present as solitary pulmonary nodule, and the 5-year survival rate for bronchogenic carcinoma that is detected in this form approaches 50%, which is considerably higher than the 10–15% 5-year survival rate of lung cancer overall.

In large surgical series, about 60% of solitary pulmonary nodules are benign lesions and 40% are malignant. Infectious granulomas account for most benign lesions, whereas primary lung cancer accounts for more than three-quarters of all malignant solitary pulmonary nodules. Solitary pulmonary nodules occasionally represent metastases from another primary tumor. Determining whether the lesion is likely to be benign or malignant preoperatively is more important than establishing its precise cause.

A lesion is almost certainly benign if the doubling time is less than 30 days or more than 500 days or if the lesion is calcified (central, "clustered," or laminated calcium pattern). Factors favoring a benign diagnosis are young age, absence of symptoms, small size (< 2 cm in diameter), smooth margins on tomography, and presence of satellite lesions, but none of these criteria are foolproof. Malignant solitary pulmonary nodules are occasionally symptomatic, tend to occur in patients over 45 years of age, are usually larger than 2 cm, often have indistinct margins, and are rarely calcified. Typical features of solitary pulmonary metastases include smooth or lobulated margins, peripheral location, location in the lower lobe, and absence of satellite lesions.

Cytologic examination of sputum, skin tests, and serologic studies for fungal infection are generally not helpful. Radiographic studies and *comparisons with old chest radiographs* are the most important aspects of the evaluation. Conventional tomograms and CT scan are particularly useful approaches. Investigations for primary cancer elsewhere in the body are not indicated unless abnormal symptoms, signs, and results of simple laboratory studies suggest an extrapulmonary cancer. Routine percutaneous needle aspiration of all solitary pulmonary nodules is not advised; it seldom changes subsequent therapy, and false negatives are common.

## Treatment

As a general rule, all solitary pulmonary nodules should be considered potentially malignant and should be resected unless calcification typical of benign lesions or stability on radiography for 2 years is documented. Prospective evaluation ("watchful waiting") is generally not appropriate if calcification is not present or if stability cannot be documented. However, strong indications of a benign diagnosis or contraindications to surgery may justify a conservative approach. Otherwise, exploratory thoracotomy is advised as soon as possible after a solitary pulmonary nodule is detected.

Khouri NF et al: The solitary pulmonary nodule: Assessment, diagnosis, and management. *Chest* 1987;**91:**128.

Stauffer JL: What to do when you detect a solitary pulmonary nodule. *J Respir Dis* (Feb) 1986;**7:**17.

## SECONDARY LUNG CANCER

Secondary lung cancers represent metastases from extrapulmonary malignant neoplasms that spread to the lungs through vascular or lymphatic channels or by direct extension. Metastases to the lung usually occur via the pulmonary artery and typically present as multiple masses on chest radiograph. **Lymphangitic carcinoma** denotes diffuse involvement of the pulmonary lymphatic network by secondary lung cancer, probably a result of extension of tumor from lung capillaries to the lymphatics. **Tumor embolism** from extrapulmonary cancer (renal cell carcinoma, hepatoma, choriocarcinoma) is an uncommon way that tumor is spread to the lungs. Secondary lung cancer also presents as malignant pleural effusion.

## Clinical Findings

**A. Symptoms and Signs:** Almost any cancer may metastasize to the lung. Symptoms are uncommon but include cough, hemoptysis, and in advanced cases, dyspnea. Symptoms are usually referable to the site of the primary tumor. Endobronchial metastases occur in fewer than 5% of patients dying of nonpulmonary cancer; most metastases are intraparenchymal. Carcinoma of the kidney, breast, colon, and cervix and malignant melanoma are the tumors most likely to cause endobronchial metastases.

There are no physical findings specific to secondary lung cancer. Hypertrophic pulmonary osteoarthropathy is rare.

**B. Laboratory Findings:** The diagnosis of secondary lung cancer is usually established by identifying the primary tumor. Cytologic examination of sputum is not often helpful. If history and physical examination fail to reveal the site of the primary tumor, an expensive radiographic and endoscopic search for the primary lesion is ill advised. Attention is better focused on the lung, where tissue samples obtained at aspiration bronchoscopy, needle or thoracotomy establish the histologic diagnosis and suggest the most likely primary. Occasionally, cytologic studies of pleural fluid or pleural biopsy reveal the diagnosis. If a solitary lung lesion is detected in a patient with known extrapulmonary cancer, primary lung cancer is the most likely diagnosis. Patients with sarcoma or melanoma are exceptions to this rule. Only about 3% of all solitary pulmonary nodules represent solitary metastases, and about a third of these are metastases from rectosigmoid tumors.

**C. Imaging:** Chest radiographs usually show multiple spherical densities with sharp margins. Solitary metastases occur in fewer than 25% of cases of secondary lung cancer. The size of metastatic lesions varies from a few millimeters (miliary densities) to large masses. The lesions are usually bilateral, peripheral, and more common in lower lung zones. Cavitation suggests primary squamous cell tumor; calcification suggests osteosarcoma. Conventional chest radiography is less sensitive than whole-lung tomography and CT scan in detecting pulmonary metastases. The radiographic differential diagnosis of multiple pulmonary nodules includes pulmonary arteriovenous malformation, pulmonary abscesses, granulomatous infection, sarcoidosis, rheumatoid nodules, and Wegener's granulomatosis.

## Treatment

Surgical resection is often prudent in the patient with known current or previous extrapulmonary cancer. A solitary pulmonary nodule in such patients is more often primary lung cancer than a single metastasis.

Once the diagnosis of secondary lung cancer has been proved, management consists of treatment of the primary neoplasm and any pulmonary complications. Local resection of one or more pulmonary metastases via thoracotomy or median sternotomy is feasible in a few carefully selected patients with various sarcomas and carcinomas (breast, testis, colon, kidney, and head and neck). Surgical resection should be considered only if the primary tumor is under control, if the patient is a good surgical risk, if all of the metastatic tumor can be resected, if nonsurgical approaches are not available, and if there are no metastases elsewhere in the body. The overall 5-year survival rate in secondary lung cancer treated surgically is 20–35%. Surgery is not advised if the primary lesion is a melanoma, if metastases are synchronous, if pneumonectomy is required, or if there is pleural involvement.

Lefor AT et al: Multiple malignancies of the lung and head and neck: Second primary tumor or metastasis? *Arch Surg* 1986;**121:**265.

Mountain CF, McMurtrey MJ, Hermes KE: Surgery for pulmonary metastasis: A 20-year experience. *Ann Thorac Surg* 1984;**38:**323.

## MESOTHELIOMA

Mesotheliomas are primary tumors arising from the surface lining of the pleura (80% of cases) or peritoneum (20% of cases). About three-fourths of pleural mesotheliomas are diffuse (usually malignant) tumors, and the remaining one-fourth are localized (usually benign). Men outnumber women by a 3:1 ratio. Numerous studies have confirmed the association of malignant pleural mesothelioma with exposure to asbestos (particularly the crocidolite form). About 7% of asbestos workers are affected.

The mean age of onset of symptoms of malignant pleural mesothelioma is about 60 years. The latent period between exposure and onset of symptoms ranges from 20 to 40 years. Symptoms include the insidious onset of shortness of breath, nonpleuritic chest pain, and weight loss. Physical findings include dullness to percussion, diminished breath sounds, and finger clubbing. Radiographic abnormalities consist of nodular, irregular, unilateral pleural thickening and varying degrees of pleural effusion. CT scan helps demonstrate the extent of pleural involvement and the magnitude of pleural effusion.

Pleural fluid is exudative and often hemorrhagic. Open pleural biopsy is usually necessary to obtain an adequate specimen for histologic diagnosis; even then, it is difficult to distinguish benign from malignant disease, making it essential to observe for progression.

Malignant pleural mesothelioma progresses rapidly as the tumor spreads quickly along the pleural surface to involve the pericardium, mediastinum, and contralateral pleura. The tumor may eventually extend beyond the thorax to involve abdominal lymph nodes and organs. Progressive pain and dyspnea are characteristic. Median survival time from onset of symptoms is 8–14 months, and about 75% of patients are dead within 1 year of diagnosis. Treatment with surgery, radiotherapy, chemotherapy, and a combination of methods has been attempted but is generally unsuccessful.

Antman KH, Corson JM: Benign and malignant pleural mesothelioma. *Clin Chest Med* 1985;**6**:127.

## BENIGN TUMORS OF THE LUNG

Benign neoplasms of the lung typically present as asymptomatic solitary pulmonary nodules detected on routine chest radiography. They account for about 2% of all solitary pulmonary nodules.

Hamartoma is the most common benign lung tumor. Fibromas, lipomas, leiomyomas, hemangiomas, and papillomas account for most of the remainder. The clustered ("popcorn") pattern of calcification on chest x-ray or tomograms is a helpful diagnostic clue to hamartoma.

The medical history, physical examination, and radiographic studies do not permit reliable differentiation of malignant and benign lung tumors. Most patients with benign lung tumors require thoracotomy for definitive diagnosis. Patients who are poor operative risks may be followed with serial chest films for progression. Even if cancer is present, short periods of observation do not appreciably affect the prognosis.

## BRONCHIAL CARCINOID TUMORS

Carcinoid and bronchial gland tumors are sometimes termed "bronchial adenomas," but this classification is a misnomer, because it implies that the lesions are benign, when in fact carcinoid tumors and bronchial gland carcinomas are low-grade malignant neoplasms.

Carcinoid tumors are about 6 times more common than bronchial gland carcinomas, and most of them occur as pedunculated or sessile growths in central bronchi. Men and women are equally affected. Most patients are between 50 and 60 years of age. Common symptoms of bronchial carcinoid tumors are hemoptysis, cough, wheezing, and recurrent pneumonia. Carcinoid syndrome (flushing, diarrhea, wheezing, hypotension, etc) is rare. Most carcinoid tumors are diagnosed at the time of fiberoptic bronchoscopy, the characteristic finding being a pink or purplish tumor

protruding into the lumen of main stem, lobar, or segmental bronchi. Bronchoscopic biopsy is occasionally complicated by significant bleeding, because these lesions have a well-vascularized stroma.

Bronchial carcinoid tumors grow slowly and rarely metastasize. Complications involve bleeding and airway obstruction rather than invasion by tumor and metastases. Surgical excision is necessary in some cases, and the prognosis is generally favorable. Most bronchial carcinoid tumors are resistant to radiation and chemotherapy.

Hurt R, Bates M: Carcinoid tumours of the bronchus: A 33 year experience. *Thorax* 1984;**39**:617.

## MEDIASTINAL MASSES

Various developmental, neoplastic, infectious, traumatic, and cardiovascular disorders may cause masses that appear in the mediastinum on chest x-ray (Table 7–9). A useful convention arbitrarily divides the mediastinum into 3 compartments—anterior, middle, and posterior—in order to classify mediastinal masses and assist in differential diagnosis. Specific mediastinal masses have a predilection for one or more of these compartments; most mediastinal masses are located in the anterior or middle compartment.

Symptoms and signs of mediastinal masses are nonspecific and are usually caused by the effects of the mass on surrounding structures. Insidious onset of retrosternal chest pain, dysphagia, or dyspnea is often an important clue to the presence of a mediastinal mass. In about half of cases, symptoms are absent, and the mass is detected on routine chest x-ray. Physical findings vary depending upon the nature and location of the mass.

CT scan is helpful in management; additional radiographic studies of benefit include barium swallow if esophageal disease is suspected, Doppler sonography or venography of brachiocephalic veins and the superior vena cava, and arteriography. Tissue diagnosis is necessary if a neoplastic disorder is suspected. Treatment and prognosis depend on the underlying cause of the mediastinal mass.

Inouye SK, Sox HC Jr: Standard and computed tomography in the evaluation of neoplasms of the chest: A comparative efficacy assessment. *Ann Intern Med* 1986;**105**:906.
LeRoux BT, Kallichurum S, Shama DM: Mediastinal cysts and tumors. *Curr Probl Surg* 1984;**21**:1. [Entire issue.]

## INTERSTITIAL LUNG DISEASES

Interstitial lung diseases comprise a heterogeneous group of disorders that have in common the features of inflammation and fibrosis of the interalveolar sep-

**Table 7–9.** Radiographic and clinical features of selected mediastinal masses.

| Mass | Radiographic Features | Clinical Features |
|---|---|---|
| **Anterior compartment**<br>Thymoma | Smooth or lobulated, round or oval homogeneous density; calcified rim in some cases. | A fourth to a half of patients have myasthenia gravis; otherwise, usually asymptomatic. Local symptoms suggest cancer (50% of thymomas). |
| Teratomas and dermoid cysts | Same as thymoma; teeth, bone may be present. | Asymptomatic young adults; expectoration of cyst contents may occur. Surgical excision advised because of potential for malignancy. |
| **Middle compartment**<br>Lymph node enlargement | Common cause of mediastinal masses; single or multiple lobulated masses; variable size; unilateral or bilateral. | Symptoms are those of underlying diseases, including bronchogenic carcinoma, lymphoma and leukemia, sarcoidosis, granulomatous infections. |
| Bronchogenic cysts | Oval or round, sharp margins; near carina or main bronchi. | Asymptomatic young adults; expectoration of contents, secondary infection may occur; surgery often warranted. |
| Pleuropericardial cysts | Round or oval, smooth margins; most at cardiophrenic angle; more common on right side; fluid contents move with change in position. | Asymptomatic. |
| Foramen of Morgagni hernia | Abdominal contents in thorax; round or oval mass; usually on right side of pericardium. | Usually asymptomatic. |
| Enlarged pulmonary arteries | Smooth structures; usually bilateral and contiguous with hili; CT scan or angiography may be necessary for clarification. | Clinical evidence of pulmonary hypertension; rarely, pulmonic stenosis or aneurysm. |
| Dilatation of superior vena cava | Right-sided smooth-walled density; azygos vein usually dilated as well; size changes with change in intrapleural pressure. | Findings of right-sided heart disease or constrictive pericardial disease. |
| Aneurysm of aorta or innominate artery | Variable saccular or fusiform masses adjacent to aorta or innominate artery; calcification common; angiography or CT scan required for clarification. | Symptoms vary depending on cause, location, and size. |
| **Posterior compartment**<br>Neurogenic tumors | Round or oval homogeneous densities with sharp margins; paravertebral location; usually unilateral. | Usually asymptomatic; occasional pain and dyspnea; surgical excision usually required. |
| Esophageal tumors | Usually not visible on plain chest x-ray; barium swallow required. | Dysphagia; pain under sternum; bleeding. |
| Esophageal hiatus hernia | Retrocardiac location slightly to the right of midline; air and fluid contents; confirmation by barium swallow. | Dysphagia; postprandial pain on bending over or lying down. |
| Thoracic spine diseases | Bone tumors produce round, paravertebral soft tissue masses; occasional destruction of vertebra; tomograms and CT scan helpful. | Variable; back pain common. |

tum, which represent a nonspecific reaction of the lung to injury of diverse cause. Some 130 disease entities share the manifestations of interstitial lung disease (Table 7–10); most are of unknown cause.

Interstitial lung diseases share common clinical, physiologic, and radiographic features. Dyspnea and cough of insidious onset are the usual presenting symptoms. Chest examination is notable for fine inspiratory crackles at the bases of the lung. Digital clubbing is common. Pulmonary function testing reveals a restrictive ventilatory defect and a decreased diffusing capacity for carbon monoxide. Hypoxemia, especially with exercise, is common. Diffuse reticular, reticulonodular, or ground-glass infiltrates that may progress to "honeycomb lung" are noted on chest x-ray.

History, physical examination, chest x-ray, and laboratory studies may provide evidence of a specific cause of interstitial lung disease. The role of lung biopsy (open or transbronchial), bronchoalveolar lavage, and Ga 67 lung scanning in the diagnostic evaluation of patients with interstitial lung disease is controversial; histopathologic examination of lung tissue is generally required for the definitive diagnosis of any interstitial lung disease.

Transbronchial biopsy using a fiberoptic bronchoscope is easily performed and is associated with a low morbidity rate, but the tissue specimens obtained are small, and sampling errors may result. Open lung biopsy produces large specimens but has a higher rate of complications. Transbronchial biopsies and washings may be adequate to permit the diagnosis of diseases such as sarcoidosis, histiocytosis X, *Pneumocystis carinii* pneumonia, miliary tuberculosis, pulmonary alveolar proteinosis, and lymphangitic carcinomatosis. On the other hand, patients who are rapidly deteriorating may be best served by definitive open lung biopsy rather than potentially nondiagnostic transbronchial biopsy. The choice between transbronchial biopsy and open lung biopsy depends on the following factors: (1) the probable diagnosis, (2) the patient's condition, (3) the operator's expertise in these biopsy procedures, (4) the risks of empiric therapy, and (5) the risk of biopsy procedures. It is probably reasonable to begin with transbronchial biopsy in most patients because of the low rate of complications associated with this procedure. If no specific diagnosis can be reached and the patient is a good candidate for surgery, open lung biopsy may then be performed.

The pathogenesis of interstitial lung disease of unknown etiology is believed to be lung injury that leads to inflammation of the interalveolar septum (alveolitis). Persistent alveolitis is thought to lead to eventual irreversible interstitial fibrosis. Techniques to evaluate the progression of alveolitis have been devised in an attempt to identify patients suitable for anti-inflammatory therapy. These techniques include bronchoalveolar lavage, lung biopsy, and Ga 67 lung scanning.

Bronchoalveolar lavage is useful in the diagnosis of *Pneumocystis carinii* pneumonia and in selected patients with lung infection from other organisms (mycobacteria, fungi, cytomegalovirus, and *Legionella* species). It is occasionally employed for specific diagnosis of lung cancer, pulmonary alveolar proteinosis, or pulmonary hemorrhage in thrombocytopenic patients. In ongoing studies, a very high percentage of T lymphocytes in bronchoalveolar lavage fluid suggests sarcoidosis or hypersensitivity pneumonitis; a predominance of neutrophils, eosinophils, and macrophages suggests idiopathic pulmonary fibrosis. Lung scanning with Ga 67 is nonspecific and has no proved value in diagnosis or management of patients with interstitial lung disease.

**Table 7–10.** Interstitial lung diseases.[*]

| Known Cause | Unknown Cause |
|---|---|
| Inorganic dusts | Cryptogenic fibrosing |
|   Silica |   alveolitis |
|   Silicates (including | Sarcoidosis |
|     asbestos) | Histiocytosis X |
|   Aluminum | Rheumatic disease- |
|   Antimony |   associated |
|   Carbon | Goodpasture's syndrome |
|   Beryllium | Idiopathic pulmonary |
|   Hard metal dusts |   hemosiderosis |
| Organic dusts | Wegener's granulomatosis |
|   (hypersensitivity | Lymphomatoid |
|   pneumonitis) |   granulomatosis |
| Gases, fumes, vapors | Churg-Strauss syndrome |
|   Chlorine | Angioimmunoblastic |
|   Sulfur dioxide |   lymphadenopathy |
|   Mercury | Inherited diseases |
| Drugs |   Tuberous sclerosis |
|   Antineoplastic agents |   Neurofibromatosis |
|   Antibiotics | Pulmonary veno-occlusive |
|     Sulfonamides |   disease |
|     Penicillins | Ankylosing spondylitis |
|     Nitrofurantoin | Amyloidosis |
|   Drugs inducing lupus | Chronic eosinophilic |
|     erythematosus |   pneumonia |
|   Sulfonylureas | Pulmonary |
|   Gold |   lymphangiomyomatosis |
|   Phenytoin | Whipple's disease |
|   Penicillamine | Alveolar proteinosis |
|   Amiodarone | Inflammatory bowel disease- |
| Poisons |   associated |
|   Paraquat | |
| Radiation | |
| Infections | |
|   Disseminated | |
|     mycobacterial or fungal | |
|     infections | |
|   Viral pneumonia | |
|   *Pneumocystis carinii* | |
|     pneumonia | |
|   Residue of active infection | |
|     of any type | |
| Pulmonary edema | |
| Lymphangitic carcinoma | |

[*] Modified and reproduced, with permission, from Crystal RG et al: Interstitial lung disease: Current concepts of pathogenesis, staging, and therapy. *Am J Med* 1981;**70**:542.

Crystal RG et al: Interstitial lung diseases of unknown cause: Disorders characterized by chronic inflammation of the lower respiratory tract. (2 parts.) *N Engl J Med* 1984;**310**:154,235.

Reynolds HY: Bronchoalveolar lavage. *Am Rev Respir Dis* 1987;**135**:250.

Schwarz MI (editor): Twenty-Eighth Annual ASPEN Lung Conference: Interstitial lung diseases. *Chest* 1986;**89**:1075

## CRYPTOGENIC FIBROSING ALVEOLITIS
## (Idiopathic Pulmonary Fibrosis)

Cryptogenic fibrosing alveolitis is the most common diagnosis among patients presenting with interstitial lung disease. Patients usually present in the sixth or seventh decade. The disease is more common in men than in women. A familial form of the disease (autosomal dominant trait with variable penetrance) has been described. Serologic tests for antinuclear antibody and rheumatoid factor are frequently positive. Symptoms, physical findings, and results on pulmonary function tests are typical of those of interstitial lung disease and are described above. The diagnosis is based on the clinical presentation and exclusion of other specific diagnoses, usually by means of lung biopsy. Histologic examination of lung tissue reveals a combination of cellular infiltration and fibrosis of the alveolar septum. Desquamated mononuclear cells, mainly macrophages, may be observed within alveoli; it is likely that fibrosis is preceded by other histologic stages (desquamative interstitial pneumonitis, then usually interstitial pneumonitis) in many of these patients.

High doses of oral corticosteroids (eg, prednisone, 40–80 mg daily) are the usual treatment. Cytotoxic drugs such as cyclophosphamide and azathioprine have also been used. Controlled clinical trials have not demonstrated any beneficial effect of therapy, but clinical experience with these drugs suggests that about 20% of patients will improve. The response to corticosteroids is better in patients with more inflammation and less fibrosis noted on lung biopsy. Relentless progression of the disease with eventual respiratory insufficiency is the rule, and the average survival time is about 4 years. Lung transplantation for highly selected patients with end-stage pulmonary fibrosis has been reported.

Bitterman PB et al: Familial idiopathic pulmonary fibrosis: Evidence of lung inflammation in unaffected family members. *N Engl J Med* 1986;**314**:1343.

## SARCOIDOSIS

Sarcoidosis is a systemic disease of unknown cause characterized by granulomatous inflammation that affects the lung in about 90% of patients. The incidence is highest in North American blacks and northern European whites; among blacks, women are more frequently affected than men. Onset of disease is usually in the third or fourth decade.

Patients may present with malaise, fever, and dyspnea of insidious onset. Alternatively, sarcoidosis may present with symptoms referable to the skin, eyes, peripheral nerves, liver, or heart. Some patients are asymptomatic and come to medical attention after abnormal findings on routine chest radiographs. Physical findings in the chest are typical of those associated with interstitial lung involvement, if the parenchyma is involved. Other findings may include skin rashes, erythema nodosum, parotid gland enlargement, hepatosplenomegaly, and lymphadenopathy.

Laboratory tests may show leukopenia, eosinophilia, an elevated erythrocyte sedimentation rate, and hypercalcemia (about 10% of patients) or hypercalciuria. Angiotensin-converting enzyme levels may be elevated with active sarcoidosis, but this finding is neither sensitive nor specific enough to have diagnostic significance. Physiologic testing may reveal evidence of airflow obstruction, but decreased lung volumes and diffusing capacity are more common signs. Skin test anergy is present in 70%.

Radiographic findings are variable and include bilateral hilar adenopathy alone (stage I), hilar adenopathy and parenchymal involvement (stage II), or parenchymal involvement alone (stage III). Parenchymal involvement is usually manifested radiographically by diffuse reticular infiltrates, but focal infiltrates, nodules, and, rarely, cavitation may be seen. Pleural effusion is noted in fewer than 10% of patients.

The diagnosis of sarcoidosis generally requires histologic demonstration of noncaseating granulomas in biopsies from a patient with other typical associated manifestations. Other granulomatous diseases must be ruled out. Biopsy of easily accessible sites, eg, palpable lymph nodes, skin lesions, or salivary glands, is likely to provide positive findings. Transbronchial lung biopsy has a high yield of positive findings, especially in patients with radiographic evidence of parenchymal involvement.

Indications for treatment with corticosteroids include constitutional symptoms, hypercalcemia, iritis, arthritis, central nervous system involvement, granulomatous hepatitis, cutaneous lesions, and symptomatic pulmonary lesions. About 20% of patients with lung involvement suffer irreversible lung impairment. The outlook is best for patients with hilar adenopathy alone; radiographic involvement of the lung parenchyma is associated with a worse prognosis. Death due to pulmonary insufficiency occurs in about 5% of patients.

Bascom R, Johns CJ: The natural history and management of sarcoidosis. *Adv Intern Med* 1986;**31**:213.

Thomas PD, Hunninghake GW: Current concepts of the pathogenesis of sarcoidosis. *Am Rev Respir Dis* 1987;**135**:747.

## HISTIOCYTOSIS X
## (Eosinophilic Granuloma)

Histiocytosis X is a generic term embracing 3 clinical syndromes that share a common histologic characteristic and are defined by age of onset, clinical course, and organ involvement. Letterer-Siwe disease is a rapidly fatal disseminated disorder occurring in children. Hand-Schüller-Christian disease is a slowly progressive disorder occurring in children and adolescents that involves bone and the posterior pituitary and may be disseminated. Pulmonary histiocytosis X (eosinophilic granuloma) is characterized by bronchiolitis and small-vessel vasculitis that progresses to fibrosis and destruction of alveolar walls; bone and posterior pituitary are uncommonly involved. Most patients present in the third and fourth decade. Symptoms may be absent or include cough, dyspnea, chest pain, fever, and weight loss. Spontaneous pneumothorax occurs in about 10% of patients and may be bilateral. Chest x-ray is characterized by finely nodular interstitial infiltrates mostly in the upper lung zones. A honeycomb pattern may evolve. Physiologic testing may reveal a restrictive defect, obstructive defect with hyperinflation, or a combination of these patterns.

The diagnosis is confirmed by the demonstration of characteristic pentalaminar structures (''X bodies'') within histiocytosis X cells (mononuclear phagocytes similar to Langerhans cells in normal skin). The disease spontaneously stabilizes or improves in about half of patients and progresses to permanent loss of lung function in the other half. Corticosteroids are the usual form of therapy, although their efficacy has not been established.

## INTERSTITIAL LUNG INVOLVEMENT IN OTHER DISEASES

Interstitial lung disease that clinically resembles cryptogenic fibrosing alveolitis has been described in a variety of rheumatic diseases. It also occurs with chronic active hepatitis, inflammatory bowel disease, biliary cirrhosis, autoimmune thrombocytopenia, and hemolytic anemia. Although other manifestations of these diseases usually dominate the clinical picture, interstitial lung disease may be symptomatic and progress to respiratory insufficiency, in which case treatment with anti-inflammatory drugs similar to those used in cryptogenic fibrosing alveolitis should be started.

## MISCELLANEOUS INFILTRATIVE LUNG DISEASES

### PULMONARY ANGIITIS & GRANULOMATOSIS

**Wegener's granulomatosis** is an idiopathic disease manifested by a combination of glomerulonephri-

tis, necrotizing granulomatous vasculitis of the upper and lower respiratory tracts, and varying degrees of small vessel vasculitis. Complaints of chronic sinusitis are a common presentation; pulmonary symptoms occur less often. Multiple nodular infiltrates, often with cavitation, are present on chest radiography. Diagnosis depends on histologic identification of the characteristic necrotizing granulomatous vasculitis in biopsies of lung or sinus tissue; lung biopsy is more specific but is associated with greater morbidity.

**Lymphomatoid granulomatosis** is a systemic disease manifested by granulomatous angiitis and a polymorphic cellular infiltrate consisting of atypical lymphocytoid and plasmacytoid cells. Any organs may be involved, but lung, brain, and skin are the most frequently affected. In contrast to Wegener's granulomatosis, the upper airway and kidneys are rarely involved clinically, though histologic evidence of cellular infiltration of the kidneys is frequently seen. The glomeruli are spared. Radiographic manifestations may include multiple nodular infiltrates or diffuse reticular infiltrates. The diagnosis is suggested by the characteristic pattern of organ system involvement and is confirmed by histologic findings. Treatment and prognosis are controversial. Lymphomatoid granulomatosis has a poor prognosis, since it evolves into malignant lymphoma in nearly half of patients.

**Allergic angiitis and granulomatosis (Churg-Strauss syndrome)** is an idiopathic multisystem vasculitis of small and medium-sized arteries that occurs in patients with asthma. Histologic features include fibrinoid necrotizing epithelioid and eosinophilic granulomas. The skin and lungs are most often involved, but other organs, including the heart, gastrointestinal tract, liver, and peripheral nerves, may also be affected. Marked peripheral eosinophilia is the rule. Abnormalities on chest radiographs range from transient infiltrates to multiple nodules. This illness may be part of a spectrum that includes polyarteritis nodosa.

Treatment of these disorders consists of combination therapy with corticosteroids and cyclophosphamide. Oral prednisone (1 mg/kg/d initially, tapering slowly to alternate-day therapy over 3–6 months) is the corticosteroid of choice; in Wegener's granulomatosis, some clinicians may omit the use of steroids. For fulminant vasculitis, therapy may be initiated with intravenous methylprednisolone for several days. Cyclophosphamide (2 mg/kg/d initially, with dosage adjustments to avoid neutropenia) is given daily by mouth for at least 1 year after complete remission is obtained. Five-year survival rates have been improved to about 90% by this combination therapy.

Leavitt RY, Fauci AS: Pulmonary vasculitis. *Am Rev Respir Dis* 1986;**134**:149.

### GOODPASTURE'S SYNDROME

Goodpasture's syndrome is idiopathic recurrent pulmonary hemorrhage and rapidly progressive glomerulonephritis. The disease is mediated by anti-glomerular basement membrane antibodies detected as a linear fluorescent pattern on immunofluorescence studies of the lung and kidneys. Goodpasture's syndrome occurs mainly in men who are in their 30s and 40s. Hemoptysis is the usual presenting symptom, but pulmonary hemorrhage may be occult. Iron deficiency anemia is often present. The diagnosis is based on characteristic histologic patterns in the kidneys or lungs and on the presence of immunofluorescent anti-glomerular basement membrane antibody eluted from tissue or circulating in serum. Combinations of immunosuppressive drugs and plasmapheresis have yielded excellent results in recent years.

Albelda SM et al: Diffuse pulmonary hemorrhage: A review and classification. *Radiology* 1985;**154:**289.

## IDIOPATHIC PULMONARY HEMOSIDEROSIS

Idiopathic pulmonary hemosiderosis is a disease of children or young adults characterized by recurrent pulmonary hemorrhage; unlike Goodpasture's syndrome, renal involvement and anti-glomerular basement membrane antibodies are absent. Treatment of acute episodes of hemorrhage with corticosteroids may be useful. Recurrent episodes of pulmonary hemorrhage may result in interstitial fibrosis.

## PULMONARY ALVEOLAR PROTEINOSIS

Pulmonary alveolar proteinosis is a disease in which a phospholipid material similar to surfactant accumulates within alveolar spaces. Progressive dyspnea is the usual presenting symptom, and chest x-ray shows bilateral alveolar infiltrates suggestive of pulmonary edema. The diagnosis is based on demonstration of characteristic intra-alveolar phospholipid on open lung biopsy. Analysis of bronchoalveolar lavage fluid holds promise as a less invasive diagnostic method.

The course of the disease varies; some patients experience spontaneous remission, whereas in others, progressive respiratory insufficiency develops. Pulmonary infection with *Nocardia* or fungi may occur. Therapy for alveolar proteinosis consists of periodic whole lung lavage, which is effective in reducing exertional dyspnea.

Claypool WD, Rogers RM, Matuschak GM: Update on the clinical diagnosis, management, and pathogenesis of pulmonary alveolar proteinosis (phospholipidosis). *Chest* 1984; **85:**550.

## EOSINOPHILIC PNEUMONIA

The term "eosinophilic pneumonia" denotes a syndrome characterized by eosinophilia and peripheral lung infiltrates. Symptoms may be mild and transient and can include fever, cough, and wheezing (Löffler's syndrome); or severe and progressive (chronic eosinophilic pneumonia). Fever, weight loss, and dyspnea may occur in chronic eosinophilic pneumonia.

Eosinophilic pneumonia may be associated with exposure to various drugs or infestation with roundworm parasites such as filariae, *Ascaris,* or *Strongyloides.* No precipating cause may be apparent in as many as one-third of cases. If an extrinsic cause is identified, therapy consists of removal of the offending drug or treatment of the underlying parasitic infestation. Corticosteroid treatment should be instituted if no treatable extrinsic cause is discovered. The response to corticosteroids is usually dramatic.

Lynch JP, Flint A: Sorting out the pulmonary eosinophilic syndromes. *J Respir Dis* (July) 1984;**5:**61.

## AMYLOIDOSIS

Amyloid may accumulate in the lungs of patients with primary amyloidosis. Tracheobronchial, parenchymal nodular, and diffuse interstitial patterns of pulmonary involvement are seen. The tracheobronchial form may present with airflow obstruction mimicking asthma or with focal obstruction leading to atelectasis. The nodular form is usually asymptomatic. The diffuse interstitial form usually presents with dyspnea. The diagnosis requires the demonstration of amyloid deposits in tissue. Treatment is unsatisfactory; the prognosis of the diffuse interstitial form is poor.

# DISORDERS OF THE PULMONARY CIRCULATION

## PULMONARY THROMBOEMBOLISM

### Essentials of Diagnosis

- Predisposition to venous thrombosis, usually of the lower extremities.
- Abrupt onset of dyspnea, chest pain, apprehension, hemoptysis, or syncope.
- Acute respiratory alkalosis and hypoxemia in most patients.
- Characteristic defects on ventilation-perfusion lung scan.
- Diagnostic findings on pulmonary angiogram.

## General Considerations

Pulmonary emboli arise from thrombi in the venous circulation or right side of the heart (thromboembolism), from tumors that have invaded the venous circulation (tumor emboli), or from other sources (amniotic fluid, air, fat, bone marrow, and foreign intravenous material).

Pulmonary embolism is associated with as many as 200,000 deaths per year; about 10% of victims die within the first hour. Fewer than 10% of patients who die of pulmonary embolism have received treatment for the condition, a fact underscoring the difficulty encountered in diagnosis.

More than 90% of pulmonary emboli originate as clots in the deep veins of the lower extremities. Most deep venous thrombi originate in the calves, and some 80% of these spontaneously resolve without embolizing. The remainder may propagate into the iliofemoral veins. Fracture of the propagating thrombus in these proximal veins allows a clot to migrate into the inferior vena cava and ultimately to the lungs. One-third to one-half of patients with deep venous thrombosis of the iliofemoral system have clinically significant pulmonary embolism.

Physiologic risk factors for venous thrombosis include venous stasis, venous endothelial injury, and hypercoagulability (eg, oral contraceptives, cancer, antithrombin III deficiency). Clinical risk factors include prolonged bed rest or inactivity, surgery, stroke, myocardial infarction, congestive heart failure, abdominal or pelvic surgery, obesity, and fractures of the hip or femur. Occasionally, in situ thrombosis in the pulmonary arteries occurs without embolization; predisposing factors include sickle cell anemia, chest trauma, and certain congenital cardiac anomalies.

Discharge of thrombus into the pulmonary artery has both hemodynamic and pulmonary consequences. The hemodynamic consequences of pulmonary thromboembolism are related to mechanical obstruction of the pulmonary vascular bed and obscure neurohumoral reflexes causing vasoconstriction. Both factors result in increased pulmonary vascular resistance and, in severe cases, pulmonary hypertension and right ventricular failure. The pulmonary consequences of thromboembolism result from reflex bronchoconstriction in the embolized lung zone, wasted ventilation (increased physiologic dead space), and loss of alveolar surfactant. Frank pulmonary infarction is uncommon.

## Clinical Findings

**A. Symptoms and Signs:** The clinical findings in pulmonary thromboembolism depend on the size of the embolus and the patient's preexisting cardiopulmonary status. In pulmonary embolism that is less than massive, clot obstructs less than two-thirds of the pulmonary arterial tree. In massive pulmonary embolism, acute right ventricular failure and systemic hypotension result. Recognizing pulmonary thromboembolism is more difficult in patients with underlying cardiopulmonary disease, and the cardiovascular effects of pulmonary emboli are usually more profound in these patients.

Symptoms of pulmonary thromboembolism include chest pain, which is often pleuritic, dyspnea, apprehension, cough, hemoptysis, and diaphoresis. In massive embolization, pulmonary embolism occasionally presents as syncope.

The signs of pulmonary thromboembolism include tachycardia, tachypnea, crackles, and accentuation of the pulmonic component of the second heart sound. Low-grade fever occurs in about 40% of cases. Evidence of thrombophlebitis, diaphoresis, and cardiac gallop is noted in about a third of cases. The clinician should be alert to other conditions that mimic thrombophlebitis of the calf, including cellulitis, muscle strain or rupture, lymphangitis, and rupture of a Baker's cyst. Cyanosis, wheezing, and cardiac arrhythmias are noted in fewer than a fourth of the cases. Shock is unusual. Signs and symptoms do not generally differ between massive and less severe thromboembolism. It can be seen that this constellation is far from specific; pulmonary embolism may mimic pneumonia, myocardial infarction, pneumothorax, and even rib fractures, among others.

**B. Laboratory Findings:** The results of routine laboratory tests are not helpful in diagnosing pulmonary thromboembolism. Arterial blood gas measurements usually reveal acute respiratory alkalosis due to hyperventilation. About 90% of patients with proved pulmonary embolism have an arterial $Po_2$ under 80 mm Hg. Electrocardiographic findings are likewise not diagnostic. Nearly all patients with pulmonary thromboembolism have an abnormal ECG; tachycardia and nonspecific ST-T wave changes are the most common abnormalities. A pattern of acute right heart strain ($S_1Q_3$, $S_{1-3}$, T wave inversion in leads $V_{1-3}$) is more characteristic but uncommon. Pulmonary function tests are not specific.

**C. Imaging and Special Examinations:**

**1. Chest radiography**–The chest radiograph is usually abnormal in patients with pulmonary embolism, but the abnormalities are often related to chronic pulmonary or cardiac disease. There are no findings pathognomonic of pulmonary embolism on conventional chest radiography. Elevation of a hemidiaphragm and pulmonary infiltration are the most common abnormalities. Platelike atelectasis, oligemia in the embolized lung zone (Westermark sign), and prominence of the pulmonary artery are sometimes seen. A small unilateral pleural effusion is occasionally present. A homogeneous, wedge-shaped density based in the pleura and pointing toward the hilum (Hampton's hump) is highly suggestive of pulmonary infarction but is uncommon.

**2. Lung scanning**–Most if not all patients with suspected pulmonary embolism should undergo a perfusion scan. Though perfusion lung scans may be abnormal in other diseases, including COPD, asthma, pneumonia, and heart failure, their results may be used to direct subsequent pulmonary arteriography and reduce the load of contrast media in these patients.

A ventilation scan may be performed prior to the perfusion scan if concurrent disease of the airways or lung parenchyma is present. It is important to recognize that a "low-probability" ventilation/perfusion scan does *not* rule out pulmonary thromboembolism. However, a high probability (85–90%) of pulmonary embolism exists when there is a lobar perfusion defect with ventilation mismatch.

The following are additional important considerations in the interpretation of lung scans:

(1) A normal perfusion scan rules out pulmonary embolism, and no further diagnostic studies are necessary.

(2) A *single* segmental or subsegmental defect on the perfusion scan is unlikely to represent pulmonary embolism.

(3) *Multiple* segmental or larger perfusion defects are more likely to represent pulmonary emboli.

(4) Mismatched ventilation-perfusion defects (hypoperfusion with normal ventilation) involving segments or larger amounts of lung are likely to represent pulmonary embolism; this is least likely to be the case in subsegmental defects, more likely in segmental defects, and most likely in lobar defects.

(5) Perfusion defects in locations matching abnormalities on chest x-ray do not reliably predict either the presence or the absence of pulmonary embolism. If the infiltrate on chest x-ray is substantially larger than the perfusion defect, however, the likelihood of pulmonary embolism is low. If the defect on chest x-ray is substantially smaller than the perfusion defect, however, the likelihood of pulmonary embolism is high.

(6) Perfusion defects persist 7–14 days after pulmonary embolism, so a follow-up perfusion-ventilation scan is sometimes helpful in diagnosis. Resolution of a perfusion defect in less than 5 days suggests an alternative diagnosis.

**3. Venous thrombosis studies**–Because the history and physical examination are neither sensitive nor specific in detecting thrombi in the deep veins of the lower extremities, specific tests such as contrast venography, radionuclide venography, impedance plethysmography, and Doppler ultrasonography are necessary. None of these tests is ideal, and there is no consensus about which should be used. However, documentation of deep venous thrombosis in a patient with suspected pulmonary thromboembolism may preclude the need for pulmonary angiography.

Because of its high sensitivity and specificity, contrast venography remains the "gold standard" in testing for venous thrombosis. An intraluminal filling defect is pathognomonic of venous thrombosis. Disadvantages of contrast venography include discomfort, difficulty in interpretation expense, difficult technical requirements, and complications such as phlebitis; it is less accurate below the knee. Bilateral radionuclide venography has a sensitivity similar to that of contrast venography but lacks its specificity. This procedure may be combined with perfusion lung scanning and does not cause phlebitis. Impedance plethys-

mography has both a sensitivity and a specificity of about 95% in the detection of thrombi in the popliteal, femoral, and iliac veins. Serial impedance plethysmography is a safe, effective, noninvasive, and inexpensive approach to detection of proximal thrombi in outpatients with suspected acute deep venous thrombosis. Doppler ultrasound is an alternative approach with similar sensitivity and specificity. [125]I fibrinogen scanning is not useful in the diagnosis of acute deep venous thrombosis.

**4. Pulmonary angiography**–Pulmonary angiography—which can detect emboli as small as 3 mm in diameter—remains the definitive test for diagnosis of pulmonary embolism, because of its high sensitivity and specificity. Emboli smaller than 3 mm in diameter are unlikely to be of clinical significance. The finding of an intraluminal defect or an arterial cutoff on the pulmonary angiogram is diagnostic. Oligemia and asymmetry of blood flow are suggestive but not specific. After 5 days, negative results on angiography do not rule out the possibility that an embolism has occurred.

Pulmonary angiography is expensive and invasive, occasionally difficult to interpret, and may be associated with complications; in experienced hands, however, the procedure is associated with a morbidity and mortality rate of less than 1%. The procedure is advised when the diagnosis of pulmonary embolism must be established with certainty. Pulmonary angiography is required if any type of surgical procedure is planned, eg, interruption of the inferior vena cava. It is indicated in patients with suspected embolism if the diagnosis remains in doubt after preliminary studies (clinical evaluation, lung scans, tests for deep venous thrombosis) have been performed. Allergy to the contrast medium is an absolute contraindication to pulmonary angiography. Relative contraindications include severe pulmonary hypertension, ventricular arrhythmias, left bundle branch block, and renal failure.

## Prevention

Prevention of deep venous thrombosis and pulmonary thromboembolism may be accomplished by using physical measures, low-dose heparin, and antiplatelet drugs in patients at risk.

Custom-fitted leg stockings are probably effective in preventing deep venous thrombosis in immobilized patients. Postoperative intermittent external pneumatic compression of the legs is recommended for patients undergoing neurosurgery, prostate surgery, or major knee surgery. Early ambulation after surgery, elevation of the legs for immobilized patients, and active and passive leg exercises are reasonable approaches to preventing deep venous thrombosis.

Low-dose heparin is of proved benefit in reducing the risk of deep vein thrombosis and fatal pulmonary embolism in patients undergoing thoracoabdominal surgery and in patients who have suffered myocardial infarction, respiratory failure and acute spinal cord injury. Low-dose heparin is *not* effective in preventing pulmonary embolism in patients with major long bone fractures or those undergoing hip surgery or above-the-knee amputation. Intravenous dextran, adjusted-dose heparin, and moderate-dose warfarin are effective approaches to prophylaxis against postoperative venous thrombosis in these high-risk patients. If low-dose heparin is indicated, 5000 units subcutaneously is given every 8–12 hours, beginning 2 hours before surgery or upon admission to the hospital and continuing until the risk for deep vein thrombosis has lessened. Continuous monitoring of clotting studies is not necessary, though the partial thromboplastin time should be checked occasionally, since some patients show increased sensitivity to heparin.

The role of antiplatelet drugs in the prevention of deep vein thrombosis is unsettled. Aspirin prophylaxis may have a role in male patients scheduled for treatment of high-risk orthopedic problems, eg, total hip replacement, knee replacement, and, possibly, hip fracture.

## Treatment

**A. Anticoagulation:** Anticoagulation for established pulmonary embolism is preventive rather than definitive therapy. For acute pulmonary thromboembolism, heparin is the anticoagulant of choice. Heparin inhibits thrombin and other clotting factors by potentiating antithrombin III; it does not dissolve established thrombi but does prevent their distal propagation. Heparin reduces the rate of recurrence of pulmonary embolism; it may reduce the incidence of death due to recurrence.

Heparin is given intravenously by continuous infusion. Intermittent subcutaneous heparin is clearly less effective in patients with acute proximal deep vein thrombosis. After a loading dose of 5000–10,000 units by bolus intravenous injection, the drug is given at a rate of 1000–1500 units/h. The activated partial thromboplastin time is determined 4–6 hours after therapy has been started and is maintained at 1.5–2 times the pretreatment control value until it has stabilized; the requirements for heparin are greater early in the clinical course. The platelet count is monitored every 2–3 days, because heparin may induce thrombocytopenia.

Oral anticoagulant therapy with warfarin is started either concurrently with heparin or 1–3 days after heparin has been started. A 4- to 5-day overlap is preferred to allow time for warfarin to exert its full anticoagulant effects. Heparin is usually discontinued after 7–10 days. Warfarin alters the synthesis of vitamin K-dependent procoagulants (factors II, VII, IX, and X) and requires 6–7 days to achieve full effectiveness; it is given in a daily dose of 10–15 mg orally until the prothrombin time is 1.2–1.5 times the baseline value (rabbit brain thromboplastin test). This is equivalent to 2 or 3 times the baseline value using human brain thromboplastin. If warfarin is contraindicated or inconvenient, subcutaneous heparin may be substituted for warfarin, the dose being adjusted to maintain an activated partial thromboplastin time of half-again the control value at the mid dosing interval. Warfarin is contraindicated in pregnancy. The prothrombin time may be lengthened by several seconds by concurrent administration of intravenous heparin.

The duration of warfarin therapy after thromboembolic disease has been diagnosed depends on the clinical situation, but a minimum of 4–6 weeks is advised. Warfarin may be discontinued if a risk factor for pulmonary embolism has been eliminated (eg, immobilization, oral contraceptives). If the patient has slowly resolving risk factors (eg, heart failure, prolonged immobility), 3–6 months of warfarin therapy are advised. If the patient has continuing, unresolvable risk factors or a second pulmonary embolism after discontinuation of warfarin, permanent anticoagulant therapy is recommended.

The major risk of anticoagulant therapy is bleeding. Major hemorrhage occurs in about 5% of patients receiving intravenous heparin, and the death rate is 0.6%. The risk of hemorrhage is increased in women over 60 years of age and in patients taking aspirin. The rate of major hemorrhage is similar for warfarin (2–10%), but serious hemorrhage is unusual in patients with adequately controlled prothrombin times. Subcutaneous heparin, administered in adjusted doses, may be as effective as warfarin in long-term treatment of deep venous thrombosis and is less likely to cause bleeding.

**B. Thrombolytic Therapy:** Lysis of pulmonary thromboemboli in situ represents the only available definitive medical treatment and is achieved by use of streptokinase and urokinase, which enhance endogenous fibrinolysis by activating plasmin. Plasmin directly lyses thrombi both in the pulmonary artery and in the venous circulation and also has a secondary anticoagulant effect. Thrombolytic therapy, when compared to heparin alone, accelerates the resolution of pulmonary emboli, reduces pulmonary artery and right heart pressures, and improves right and left ventricular function in patients with established pulmonary embolism. Thrombolytic therapy may also protect the pulmonary microcirculation, and preserves the anatomy and function of the valves in deep veins of the lower extremities. It has not been shown to affect the mortality rate from pulmonary thrombembolism, however.

The use of thrombolytic therapy in clinical practice is controversial. Most physicians reserve its use for patients with acute massive pulmonary embolism confirmed by pulmonary angiography and for selected patients with established deep venous thrombosis. Suitable candidates for thrombolytic therapy include patients with hemodynamic compromise due to pulmonary embolism, those with underlying severe cardiopulmonary disease, and those who fail to show hemodynamic improvement after heparin therapy.

Care and expertise in monitoring therapy, managing bleeding, and controlling subsequent anticoagulation are essential. The duration of symptoms prior to starting thrombolytic therapy should be less than

7 days. Puncture of noncompressible arteries or veins, or intramuscular injections are not permitted during thrombolytic therapy. Anticoagulants and antiplatelet drugs should not be given concurrently.

Urokinase or streptokinase is given as a continuous intravenous infusion by an infusion pump. Streptokinase is usually preferred because it is less expensive, but development of antibodies may prevent future use of the drug. Streptokinase, 250,000 units intravenously over 30 minutes as a loading dose, is followed by a maintenance dose of 100,000 units/h for 24–72 hours. The effectiveness of therapy is monitored by measuring the thrombin time every 4 hours to assure the presence of a fibrinolytic state. Too high a dose may produce a paradoxic normalization of the thrombin time, so that use of this test must be correlated with clinical assessment of bleeding. Administration of intravenous heparin is resumed upon completion of thrombolytic therapy.

Absolute contraindications to thrombolytic therapy include active internal bleeding and recent (within 2 months) cerebrovascular accident. Other major contraindications include severe hypertension, recent trauma, gastrointestinal bleeding, and major surgical or obstetric procedures. Hemorrhage is the major complication of thrombolytic therapy and can usually be avoided by strict adherence to treatment guidelines.

**C. Additional Measures:** Rarely, surgical interruption of the inferior vena cava is indicated when recurrent pulmonary embolism would be life-threatening in a patient with major contraindications to anticoagulation or failure or complications of anticoagulant or thrombolytic therapy. Life-threatening paradoxic thromboembolism or septic thromboembolism may also justify surgical interruption, which may be achieved by ligation, plication, clipping, and insertion of intraluminal umbrellas or filters. The Greenfield filter is now widely used. It is inserted percutaneously through the internal jugular vein and advanced below the renal veins, where it is lodged in place. Its use is quite effective, but the device requires considerable experience in placement.

Surgical removal of acute pulmonary embolism (pulmonary embolectomy) is now rarely performed.

**Prognosis**

Pulmonary embolism may cause sudden death, though the prognosis for survivors is generally favorable. The prognosis depends on the underlying disease and on proper diagnosis and treatment. The mortality rate in patients with undiagnosed pulmonary thromboembolism is about 30%, compared to 10% when appropriate therapy for definitively diagnosed pulmonary embolism is initiated—though these figures do not reflect controlled studies. Perfusion defects resolve in most survivors. Pulmonary hypertension may be a complication of chronic recurrent pulmonary thromboembolism.

Dalen JE, Hirsh J (editors): American College of Chest Physicians–National Heart, Lung and Blood Institute: National conference on antithrombotic therapy. *Chest* 1986;**89** (**Suppl**):1. [Entire issue.]

Hirsh J (editor): Venous thromboembolism: Prevention, diagnosis and treatment. *Chest* 1986;**89(Suppl):**369. [Entire issue.]

Hull RD et al: Diagnostic value of ventilation-perfusion lung scanning in patients with suspected pulmonary embolism. *Chest* 1985;**88:**819.

Hull RD et al: Continuous intravenous heparin compared with intermittent subcutaneous heparin in the initial treatment of proximal-vein thrombosis. *N Engl J Med* 1986;**315:**1109.

Salzman EW: Venous thrombosis made easy. (Editorial.) *N Engl J Med* 1986;**314:**847.

## PULMONARY HYPERTENSION

### Essentials of Diagnosis

- Dyspnea, fatigue, chest pain, and occasionally syncope on exertion.
- Narrow splitting of second heart sound with loud pulmonic component; findings of right ventricular hypertrophy and cardiac failure in advanced disease.
- Hypoxemia; wasted ventilation on pulmonary function tests in most cases.
- Electrocardiographic evidence of right ventricular strain or hypertrophy and right atrial enlargement.
- Enlarged central pulmonary arteries on chest x-ray.

### General Considerations

The pulmonary circulation is unique because of its high blood flow, low pressure (normally 25/8 mm Hg, mean 12), and low resistance (normally 200–250 dynes/sec/cm$^{-5}$). It can accommodate large increases in blood flow during exercise with only modest increases in pressure because of its ability to recruit and distend blood vessels. The normal pulmonary circulation is also largely passive, since its pressures are determined mainly by the function of the right and left ventricles. Contraction of smooth muscle in the walls of pulmonary arteriolar resistance vessels becomes an important factor in numerous pathologic states.

Pulmonary hypertension is present when pulmonary artery pressure rises to a high level inappropriate for a given level of cardiac output. Primary (idiopathic) pulmonary hypertension (see Chapter 8) is a rare disorder of the pulmonary circulation occurring in young and middle-aged women; it is characterized by progressive dyspnea, a rapid downhill course, and invariably fatal outcome. Secondary pulmonary hypertension is more common and clinically more important, because it is found in a wide variety of medical conditions and often responds to therapy.

Selected mechanisms responsible for pulmonary hypertension and examples of corresponding clinical conditions are set forth in Table 7–11. Pulmonary hypertension is usually caused by reduction of the cross-sectional area of the pulmonary vasculature at the arterial, capillary, or venous level. Hypoxia of any cause is the most important and potent stimulus

**Table 7–11.** Mechanisms of pulmonary hypertension and examples of corresponding clinical conditions.

**Reduction in cross-sectional area of pulmonary arterial bed**
Vasoconstriction
  Hypoxia of any cause
  Acidosis
Loss of vessels
  Lung resection
  Emphysema
  Vasculitis
  Pulmonary fibrosis
  Connective tissue disease
Obstruction of vessels
  Pulmonary embolism (thromboemboli, tumor emboli, foreign body emboli, etc)
  In situ thrombosis
  Schistosomiasis
Narrowing of vessels
  Secondary structural changes due to pulmonary hypertension
**Increased pulmonary venous pressure**
Constrictive pericarditis
Left ventricular failure or reduced compliance
Mitral stenosis
Left atrial myxoma
Pulmonary veno-occlusive disease
Mediastinal diseases compressing pulmonary veins
**Increased pulmonary blood flow**
Congenital left-to-right intracardiac shunts
**Increased blood viscosity**
Polycythemia
**Miscellaneous**
Pulmonary hypertension occurring in association with hepatic cirrhosis and portal hypertension

of pulmonary arterial vasoconstriction. The mechanisms by which hypoxia causes pulmonary hypertension are poorly understood. Factors operating at the alveolar level and direct stimulation of arteriolar smooth muscle have been implicated. Hypoxia is partially or fully responsible for the pulmonary hypertension observed in chronic bronchitis, infiltrative lung disease due to various causes, kyphoscoliosis, obesity-hypoventilation syndrome, chronic mountain sickness, obstructive sleep apnea, and neuromuscular disease. Acidosis is also a potent stimulus of pulmonary hypertension and exerts a synergistic vasoconstrictive effect with hypoxia.

Obliteration and obstruction of the pulmonary arterial tree may cause pulmonary hypertension. At least two-thirds of the pulmonary arterial bed must be obstructed or destroyed before pulmonary hypertension occurs. Once present, pulmonary hypertension is self-perpetuating. It introduces secondary structural abnormalities in pulmonary vessels, including smooth muscle hypertrophy and intimal proliferation, and these may eventually stimulate atheromatous changes and in situ thrombosis, leading to further narrowing of the arterial bed.

Increased pulmonary venous pressure, when sustained, may cause "postcapillary" pulmonary hypertension; left ventricular failure is the most common cause.

Pulmonary hypertension is readily recognized when an obvious cause, such as severe COPD, is present. In adults, pulmonary hypertension in the absence of COPD is often caused by chronic pulmonary thromboembolism, interstitial fibrosis, sleep apnea, or obesity-hypoventilation syndrome. Other disorders listed in Table 7–11 should be excluded before the diagnosis of primary pulmonary hypertension is entertained.

**Pulmonary veno-occlusive disease** is a rare cause of postcapillary pulmonary hypertension occurring in children and young adults. The cause is unknown. The disease is characterized by progressive fibrotic occlusion of pulmonary veins and venules. Nodular areas of pulmonary congestion, edema, hemorrhage, and hemosiderosis are found. Chest radiography reveals prominent, symmetric interstitial markings, Kerley B lines, pulmonary artery dilatation, and normally sized left atrium and left ventricle. Premortem diagnosis is often difficult but is occasionally established by open lung biopsy. There is no effective therapy, and most patients die within 2 years as a result of progressive pulmonary hypertension.

## Clinical Findings:

**A. Symptoms and Signs:** Secondary pulmonary hypertension is difficult to recognize clinically in the early stages, when symptoms and signs are primarily those of the underlying disease. Pulmonary hypertension may cause or contribute to dyspnea, which is present initially on exertion and later at rest. Dull, retrosternal chest pain resembling angina pectoris may be present. Fatigue and syncope on exertion also occur.

The signs of pulmonary hypertension include narrow splitting of the second heart sound, accentuation of the pulmonic component of the second heart sound, and a systolic ejection click. In advanced cases, tricuspid and pulmonic valve insufficiency and signs of right ventricular failure and cor pulmonale are found.

**B. Laboratory Findings:** Polycythemia is found in many cases of pulmonary hypertension that are associated with chronic hypoxemia. Electrocardiographic changes are those of right ventricular hypertrophy, right ventricular strain, or right atrial enlargement.

**C. Imaging and Special Examinations:** Radiographic findings depend on the cause of pulmonary hypertension. In chronic disease, dilatation of the right and left main and lobar pulmonary arteries and enlargement of the pulmonary outflow tract are seen; in advanced disease, right ventricular and right atrial enlargement are seen. Peripheral "pruning" of large pulmonary arteries is characteristic of pulmonary hypertension in severe emphysema.

Selected special studies may help in the management of patients with pulmonary hypertension.

Echocardiography is helpful in evaluating patients thought to have mitral stenosis, left atrial myxoma, and pulmonary valvular disease. Echocardiography may also reveal right ventricular enlargement and paradoxic motion of the interventricular septum. Doppler echocardiography is a reliable noninvasive means of estimating right ventricular and pulmonary artery pressures. However, precise hemodynamic measurements can only be obtained with right heart catheterization, which is often helpful when postcapillary pulmonary hypertension, intracardiac shunting, or thromboembolic disease is considered as part of the differential diagnosis.

Routine pulmonary function tests reveal no findings diagnostic of pulmonary hypertension. Diminution of the pulmonary capillary bed may cause reduction in the single breath diffusing capacity.

Depending upon the suspected cause of pulmonary hypertension, perfusion lung scanning, pulmonary angiography, and open lung biopsy are occasionally helpful. Transbronchial biopsy carries an increased risk of bleeding.

Early recognition of pulmonary hypertension is crucial to interrupt the self-perpetuating cycle responsible for the rapid progression of this disorder. By the time most patients present with signs and symptoms of pulmonary hypertension, however, the condition is far advanced. Treatable causes and underlying diseases should be aggressively sought; these include hypoxemia, pulmonary thromboembolism, intracardiac right-to-left shunts, and mitral stenosis (Table 7–11).

### Treatment

Treatment of primary pulmonary hypertension is discussed in Chapter 8. Treatment of secondary pulmonary hypertension consists mainly of treating the underlying disorder, such as COPD, sleep apnea, obesity-hypoventilation syndrome, and mitral stenosis. If hypoxemia or acidosis is detected, corrective measures should be started immediately. Supplemental oxygen administered for at least 15 hours per day has been demonstrated to be of benefit in patients with hypoxemic COPD (see p 142).

Other disorders responsible for pulmonary hypertension should be treated appropriately. Patients with documented recurrent pulmonary thromboembolism should receive permanent anticoagulation therapy; some clinicians employ this therapy in pulmonary hypertension of unknown cause, since multiple, very small pulmonary emboli may produce this picture. Postcapillary pulmonary hypertension usually responds to treatment of the underlying cardiac disease.

Vasodilator therapy using various pharmacologic agents (eg, calcium antagonists, hydralazine, isoproterenol, diazoxide, nitroglycerin) has been tried in primary pulmonary hypertension and a few patients with secondary pulmonary hypertension with inconsistent results. Short-term benefits have been demonstrated with some of these agents, but long-term benefits are unclear. Complications of pulmonary vasodilator therapy have occurred, including systemic hypotension, hypoxemia, and even death. Routine clinical use of these agents is not currently recommended.

However, it is important to distinguish primary pulmonary hypertension with pulmonary vasoconstriction, a potentially reversible condition, from fixed obstruction of the pulmonary vascular bed. Patients most likely to benefit from long-term pulmonary vasodilator therapy are those who respond favorably to a vasodilator challenge at right heart catheterization.

Patients with marked polycythemia (hematocrit > 60%) should undergo repeated phlebotomy in an attempt to reduce blood viscosity. Cor pulmonale complicating pulmonary hypertension is treated by managing the underlying pulmonary disease and by using diuretics, salt restriction, and, in appropriate patients, supplemental oxygen. The use of digitalis in cor pulmonale remains controversial. Pulmonary thromboendarterectomy may benefit selected patients with pulmonary hypertension secondary to chronic thrombotic obstructions of major pulmonary arteries.

### Prognosis

The prognosis in secondary pulmonary hypertension depends on the course of the underlying disease. Patients with pulmonary hypertension due to fixed obliteration of the pulmonary vascular bed generally respond poorly to therapy; development of cor pulmonale in these cases implies a poor prognosis. The prognosis is favorable when pulmonary hypertension is detected early and the conditions leading to it are readily reversed.

D'Alonzo GE, Bower JS, Dantzker DR: Differentiation of patients with primary and thromboembolic pulmonary hypertension. *Chest* 1984;**85**:457.

Hecht SR et al: Use of continuous-wave Doppler ultrasound to evaluate and manage primary pulmonary hypertension. *Chest* 1986;**90**:781.

Packer M: Vasodilator therapy for primary pulmonary hypertension: Limitations and hazards. *Ann Intern Med* 1985;**103**:258.

Reeves JT, Groves BM, Turkevich D: The case for treatment of selected patients with primary pulmonary hypertension. *Am Rev Respir Dis* 1986;**134**:342.

Reid LM: Structure and function in pulmonary hypertension: New perceptions. *Chest* 1986;**89**:279.

Voelkel NF: Mechanisms of hypoxic pulmonary vasocontriction. *Am Rev Respir Dis* 1986;**133**:1186.

# DISORDERS DUE TO CHEMICAL & PHYSICAL AGENTS

## INHALATION OF AIR POLLUTANTS & TOXIC SUBSTANCES

The respiratory tract is exposed to numerous potentially harmful substances in the environment, including air pollutants and toxic gases and fumes. Whereas air pollutants are ubiquitous, particularly in urban areas, toxic gases and fumes are usually encountered in the workplace or as the result of an environmental accident. Respiratory tract defense mechanisms protect the lung from noxious substances, but when these defenses are breached, serious respiratory tract injury may result. Selected air pollutants and toxic substances and their adverse effects are set forth in Table 7–12.

## Clinical Findings

Exposure to low levels of air pollutants is usually inconsequential; exposure to higher levels produces symptoms of upper and lower respiratory tract irritation, particularly in patients with asthma and COPD. Exposure to the toxic substances listed in Table 7–12 results in profound illness characterized by upper respiratory complaints (sneezing, irritation of the eyes and nose, stridor) and features of tracheobronchitis (cough, wheezing, dyspnea). Systemic symptoms such as nausea and vomiting, headache, and fever are common; in severe disease, pulmonary edema may develop. Chest radiographs may be normal; however, bilateral diffuse infiltrates progressing to consolidation, atelectasis, and pulmonary edema are common.

## Treatment

Healthy persons exposed to the usual ambient levels of air pollutants need not observe special precautions. Patients with severe COPD or asthma should be advised to stay indoors and not engage in strenuous activity when high concentrations of air pollutants are present. If exposure to toxic chemicals is documented or suspected, patients should be observed carefully for as long as 24 hours after exposure. Respiratory distress may be absent initially, only to appear after a 12- to 24-hour delay.

If admitted to the hospital, the patient should be followed closely with arterial blood gas measurements. Hypoxemia may occur before clinical and radiographic evidence of pulmonary edema develops and should be managed appropriately with supplemental oxygen. Because laryngeal edema and severe, exudative tracheobronchitis are common following inhalation of toxic substances, maintaining the patency of the airway is of paramount importance. Respiratory therapy may be required to clear the airway of tenacious secretions and sloughed fragments of mucosa. Acute respiratory failure is common and should be managed appropriately (see p 179). Intubated patients require frequent suctioning to remove airway se-

**Table 7–12.** Major air pollutants and toxic gases and fumes, their sources, and adverse effects.

| Noxious Agent | Sources | Adverse Effects |
|---|---|---|
| **Air pollutants**<br>Oxides of nitrogen | Automobile exhaust; gas stoves and heaters, wood-burning stoves, kerosene space heaters. | Respiratory tract irritation, bronchial hyperreactivity, impaired lung defenses, bronchiolitis fibrosa obliterans. |
| Hydrocarbons | Automobile exhaust, cigarette smoke. | Lung cancer. |
| Ozone | Automobile exhaust, high-altitude aircraft cabins. | Cough, substernal discomfort, bronchoconstriction, decreased exercise performance, respiratory tract irritation. |
| Sulfur dioxide | Power plants, smelters, oil refineries, kerosene space heaters. | Exacerbation of asthma and COPD, respiratory tract irritation. Hospitalization may be necessary and death may occur in severe exposure. |
| **Toxic gases and fumes**<br>Carbon monoxide | Cigarette smoke, incomplete combustion of organic fuels. | Headache, nausea and vomiting, dyspnea, dizziness, ataxia, convulsions, coma, death. |
| Sulfur dioxide | Leakage from storage tanks. | Airway irritation, exacerbation of COPD and asthma. |
| Ozone | Arc welding. | Cough, chest pain, eye and nose irritation. |
| Oxides of nitrogen ($NO_2$, $N_2O_4$) | Silage; arc welding, chemical industry. | Silo-filler's disease, pulmonary edema, hypotension, bronchiolitis fibrosa obliterans. |
| Cyanide | Production of synthetic rubber; extraction of gold and silver; electroplating. | Severe, rapidly progressive systemic toxicity with coma, convulsions, death within 4 hours. |
| Phosgene | Plastics and chemical industry. | Pulmonary edema after asymptomatic period. |
| Ammonia | Leakage from storage containers and railroad cars. | Severe inflammation of respiratory tract, laryngeal edema. |
| Cadmium | Welding, smelting of ores. | Pulmonary edema, tracheobronchitis, metal fume fever. |
| Chlorine | Spillage from storage containers; chemical and plastics industry. | Bronchitis, pulmonary edema. |

cretions. Intravenous fluids and vasopressor agents are necessary in some patients, but excessive amounts of fluids should be avoided because of the tendency to worsen pulmonary edema. Antibiotics are administered only if lower respiratory tract infection develops; bronchodilators are administered if bronchospasm is apparent. The use of corticosteroids in the management of acute lung injury due to inhalation of toxic substances is controversial; most authorities feel they are contraindicated in burn patients with smoke inhalation because of the risk of secondary infection.

## Prognosis

The prognosis following acute lung injury from inhalation of toxic substances depends on the severity of exposure and the nature of the toxic substance. Death may occur as a result of acute respiratory failure. Survivors have an excellent prognosis, with full recovery of lung function expected in most cases. Bronchiolitis fibrosa obliterans may occur 1–6 weeks after apparent recovery from inhalation of nitrogen dioxide and should be managed with oral corticosteroids.

Beeley JM et al: Mortality and lung histopathology after inhalation lung injury: The effect of corticosteroids. *Am Rev Respir Dis* 1986;**133:**191.

Cohen MA, Guzzardi LJ: Inhalation of products of combustion. *Ann Emerg Med* 1983;**12:**628.

## PULMONARY ASPIRATION SYNDROMES

Aspiration of foreign material into the tracheobronchial tree results from various disorders that impair normal deglutition, especially disturbances of consciousness and esophageal dysfunction.

### Aspiration of Inert Material

Aspiration of inert material may cause asphyxia if the amount aspirated is massive and if cough is impaired, in which case immediate tracheobronchial suctioning is necessary. Most patients suffer no serious sequelae from aspiration of inert material.

### Aspiration of Toxic Material

Aspiration of toxic material into the lung usually results in clinically evident pneumonia. **Hydrocarbon pneumonitis** is caused by ingestion of petroleum distillates, eg, gasoline, kerosene, furniture polish, and other household petroleum products. Lung injury results mainly from vomiting and secondary aspiration. Therapy is supportive. The lung should be protected from repeated aspiration with a cuffed endotracheal tube if necessary. **Lipid pneumonia** is a chronic syndrome related to the repeated aspiration of oily materials, eg, mineral oil, cod liver oil, and oily nose drops; it often occurs in elderly patients with impaired swallowing. Patchy infiltrates in dependent lung zones and lipid-laden macrophages in expectorated sputum are characteristic findings.

### "Café Coronary"

Acute obstruction of the upper airway by food usually occurs in intoxicated individuals. Other predisposing factors include difficulty in swallowing, old age, poor dentition, dental problems that impair chewing, and use of sedative drugs. The Heimlich procedure may be lifesaving (see Appendix).

### Retention of an Aspirated Foreign Body

Retention of an aspirated foreign body in the tracheobronchial tree may produce various acute and chronic conditions, including recurrent pneumonia, bronchiectasis, lung abscess, atelectasis, and postobstructive hyperinflation. Occasionally, a misdiagnosis of asthma, COPD, or lung cancer is made in patients who have aspirated a foreign body. Bronchoscopy is usually necessary to establish the diagnosis and attempt removal of the foreign body.

### Chronic Aspiration of Gastric Contents

Chronic aspiration of gastric contents may result from primary disorders of the esophagus, eg, achalasia, esophageal stricture, scleroderma, esophageal carcinoma, esophagitis, and gastroesophageal reflux. In the last condition, relaxation of the tone of the lower esophageal sphincter allows reflux of gastric contents into the esophagus and predisposes to chronic pulmonary aspiration, especially at night. Cigarette smoking, consumption of alcohol, and use of theophylline are known to relax the lower esophageal sphincter. Pulmonary disorders linked to gastroesophageal reflux and chronic aspiration include bronchial asthma, idiopathic pulmonary fibrosis, bronchiectasis, and, in young children, apnea. Even in the absence of aspiration, acid in the esophagus may trigger bronchospasm through reflex mechanisms.

The diagnosis of chronic aspiration is difficult, and barium swallow is usually necessary to rule out esophageal disease. Management consists of elevation of the head of the bed, cessation of smoking, weight reduction, and antacids or $H_2$ receptor antagonists (eg, cimetidine, 300–400 mg) at night. Metoclopramide (10–20 mg at bedtime) or bethanechol (10–25 mg at bedtime) is helpful in some patients with gastroesophageal reflux, as they elevate pressure in the lower esophageal sphincter.

### Acute Aspiration of Gastric Contents (Mendelson's Syndrome)

Acute aspiration of gastric contents is often catastrophic. The pulmonary response depends on the characteristics and amount of the gastric contents aspirated. The more acidic the material, the greater the degree of chemical pneumonitis. Aspiration of pure gastric acid (pH < 2.5) causes extensive desquamation of the bronchial epithelium, bronchiolitis, hemorrhage, and pulmonary edema. Acute gastric aspiration is one of the commonest causes of adult respiratory distress syndrome (see p 182). The clinical picture is one of abrupt onset of respiratory distress, with cough, wheezing, fever, and tachypnea. Crackles are audible at the bases of the lungs. Hypoxemia may be noted immediately after aspiration occurs. Radiographic abnormalities, consisting of patchy alveolar infiltrates in dependent lung zones, appear within a few hours. If particulate food matter has been aspirated along with gastric acid, radiographic features of bronchial obstruction may be observed. Even without superinfection, fever and leukocytosis occur.

Treatment of acute aspiration of gastric contents consists of supplemental oxygen, measures to maintain the airway, and the usual measures for treatment of acute respiratory failure (see p 179). There is no evidence to support the routine use of corticosteroids or prophylactic antibiotics after gastric aspiration has occurred. Secondary pulmonary infection, which occurs in about a fourth of patients, typically appears 2–3 days after aspiration. Management of this complication depends upon the observed flora of the tracheobronchial tree (Table 7–6). Hypotension secondary to alveolocapillary membrane injury and intravascular volume depletion is common and is managed with the judicious administration of intravenous fluids.

Allen CJ, Newhouse MT: Gastroesophageal reflux and chronic respiratory disease. *Am Rev Respir Dis* 1984;**129**:645.

Ducolone A et al: Gastroesophageal reflux in patients with asthma and chronic bronchitis. *Am Rev Respir Dis* 1987;**135**:327.

Weissberg D, Schwartz I: Foreign bodies in the tracheobronchial tree. *Chest* 1987;**91**:730.

**Table 7–13.** Selected pneumoconioses.

| Disease | Agent | Occupational Source |
|---|---|---|
| **Metal dusts** | | |
| Siderosis | Metallic iron or iron oxide | Mining, welding, foundry work. |
| Stannosis | Tin, tin oxide | Mining, tinwork, smelting. |
| Baritosis | Barium salts | Glass and insecticide manufacturing. |
| **Coal dust** | | |
| Coal worker's pneumoconiosis | Coal dust | Coal mining. |
| **Inorganic dusts** | | |
| Silicosis | Free silica (silicon dioxide) | Rock mining, quarrying, stone cutting, tunneling, sandblasting, pottery, diatomaceous earth. |
| **Silicate dusts** | | |
| Asbestosis | Asbestos | Mining, insulation, construction, shipbuilding. |
| Talcosis | Magnesium silicate | Mining, milling, rubber industry. |
| Kaolin pneumoconiosis | Sand, mica, aluminum silicate | Mining of china clay; pottery and cement work. |
| Shaver's disease | Aluminum powder | Manufacture of corundum. |

# OCCUPATIONAL PULMONARY DISEASES

Many acute and chronic pulmonary diseases are directly related to inhalation of noxious substances encountered in the workplace; those disorders that are due to chemical agents may be classified as follows: (1) pneumoconioses, (2) hypersensitivity pneumonitis, (3) obstructive airway disorders, (4) toxic lung injury, (5) lung cancer, (6) pleural diseases, and (7) miscellaneous disorders.

## Pneumoconioses

Pneumoconioses are chronic fibrotic lung diseases caused by the inhalation of coal dust and various inert, inorganic, or silicate dusts (Table 7–13). Pneumoconioses due to inhalation of inert dusts are usually asymptomatic disorders with diffuse nodular infiltrates on chest x-ray. Clinically important pneumoconioses include coal worker's pneumoconiosis, silicosis, and asbestosis. Treatment for each is supportive.

**A. Coal Worker's Pneumoconiosis:** In coal worker's pneumoconiosis, ingestion of inhaled coal dust by alveolar macrophages leads to the formation of coal macules, usually 2–5 mm in diameter, which appear on chest x-ray as small opacities throughout the lungs but are especially prominent in the upper lung. In complicated coal worker's pneumoconiosis ("progressive massive fibrosis"), conglomeration and contraction in the upper lung zones occur, with radiographic and clinical features resembling complicated silicosis. **Caplan's syndrome** is a rare condition characterized by the presence of necrobiotic rheumatoid nodules (1–5 cm in diameter) in the periphery of the lung in coal workers with rheumatoid arthritis.

**B. Silicosis:** In silicosis, extensive or prolonged inhalation of free silica (silicon dioxide) particles in the respirable range (0.3–5 μm) causes the formation of small rounded opacities (silicotic nodules) throughout the lung. Calcification of the periphery of hilar lymph nodes ("eggshell" calcification) is an unusual finding that strongly suggests silicosis. Simple silicosis is usually asymptomatic and has no effect on routine pulmonary function tests; in complicated silicosis, large conglomerate densities appear in the upper lung and are accompanied by dyspnea and obstructive and restrictive pulmonary dysfunction. The incidence of tuberculosis is increased in patients with chronic silicosis.

**C. Asbestosis:** Asbestosis, a nodular interstitial fibrosis occurring in asbestos workers and miners, is characterized by dyspnea, inspiratory crackles, and in some cases, clubbing and cyanosis. The radiographic features include interstitial fibrosis, thickened pleura, and calcified plaques (pleural) on the diaphragms or lateral chest wall. The lower lungs are more often involved than the upper. Pulmonary function studies show restrictive dysfunction and reduced diffusing capacity.

## Hypersensitivity Pneumonitis

The term hypersensitivity pneumonitis (''extrinsic allergic alveolitis'') denotes nonatopic, nonasthmatic, allergic pulmonary disease. Hypersensitivity pneumonitis is manifested mainly as occupational disease (Table 7–14), in which exposure to inhaled organic agents leads to acute and eventually chronic pulmonary disease; lung injury is produced by antibodies directed against the inhaled agent. Acute illness is characterized by sudden onset of malaise, chills, fever, cough, dyspnea, and nausea 4–8 hours after exposure to the offending agent. This may occur after the patient has left work or even at night, and thus may mimic paroxysmal nocturnal dyspnea. Bibasilar crackles, tachypnea, tachycardia, and (occasionally) cyanosis are noted. Small nodular densities sparing the apexes and bases of the lungs are noted on chest x-ray. Pulmonary function studies reveal restrictive dysfunction and reduced diffusing capacity. Laboratory studies reveal an increase in the white blood cell count with a shift to the left, hypoxemia, and

the presence of precipitating antibodies to the offending agent in serum. A subacute syndrome has been described that is characterized by the insidious onset of chronic cough and slowly progressive dyspnea, anorexia, and weight loss. Chronic respiratory insufficiency and the appearance of pulmonary fibrosis on radiographs may or may not occur after repeated exposure to the offending agent. Acute hypersensitivity pneumonitis is characterized by interstitial infiltrates of lymphocytes and plasma cells, with noncaseating granulomas in the interstitium and air spaces. Diffuse fibrosis is the hallmark of the subacute and chronic phases.

Treatment of hypersensitivity pneumonitis consists of identification of the offending agent, avoidance of further exposure, and, in severe acute or protracted cases, oral corticosteroids (prednisone, 0.5 mg/kg daily as a single morning dose, tapered to nil over 4–6 weeks). Change in occupation is advisable in some cases.

## Obstructive Airway Disorders

Occupational pulmonary diseases manifested as obstructive airway disorders include occupational asthma, industrial bronchitis, and byssinnosis.

**A. Occupational Asthma:** It has been estimated that about 2% of all cases of asthma are related to occupation. Offending agents include grain dust, tobacco, pollens, enzymes, gum arabic, synthetic dyes, isocyanates (particularly toluene diisocyanate), wood dust, rosin (soldering flux), inorganic chemicals (salts of nickel, platinum, and chromium), trimellitic anhydride, phthallic anhydride, formaldehyde, and various pharmaceutical agents, including penicillin, cimetidine, and sulfonamides. Diagnosis of occupational asthma depends on a high index of suspicion, an appropriate history, spirometric studies before and after exposure to the offending substance, and peak flow rate measurements in the workplace. Bronchial provocation testing (a pulmonary function laboratory test demonstrating bronchial hyperreactivity to pharmacologic or antigenic agents) is helpful in some cases. Treatment consists of avoidance of further exposure to the offending agent and bronchodilators (see p 137), but symptoms may persist for years after workplace exposure has been terminated.

**B. Industrial Bronchitis:** Industrial bronchitis is chronic bronchitis found in coal miners and others exposed to cotton, flax, or hemp dust. Chronic disability does not occur from industrial bronchitis.

**C. Byssinnosis:** Byssinnosis is an asthmalike disorder in textile workers caused by inhalation of cotton dust. The pathogenesis is obscure. Chest tightness, cough, and dyspnea are characteristically worse on Mondays or the first day back at work, with symptoms subsiding later in the week. Repeated exposure leads to chronic bronchitis.

## Toxic Lung Injury

Toxic lung injury from inhalation of irritant gases

**Table 7–14.** Selected causes of hypersensitivity pneumonitis.

| Disease | Antigen | Source |
|---------|---------|--------|
| Farmer's lung | *Micropolyspora faeni, Thermoactinomyces vulgaris.* | Moldy hay. |
| "Humidifier lung" | Thermophilic actinomycetes. | Contaminated humidifiers, heating systems, or air conditioners. |
| Bird-fancier's lung ("pigeon-breeder's disease") | Avian proteins. | Bird serum and excreta. |
| Bagassosis | *Thermoactinomyces sacchari* and *T vulgaris.* | Moldy sugarcane fiber (bagasse). |
| Sequoiosis | *Graphium, Aureobasidium,* and other fungi. | Moldy redwood sawdust. |
| Maple bark stripper's disease | *Cryptostroma (Coniosporium) corticale.* | Rotting maple tree logs or bark. |
| Mushroom picker's disease | Same as farmer's lung. | Moldy compost. |
| Suberosis | *Penicillium frequentans.* | Moldy cork dust. |
| Detergent worker's lung | *Bacillus subtilis* enzyme. | Enzyme additives. |

is discussed on p 171. **Silo-filler's disease** is acute toxic noncardiogenic pulmonary edema caused by inhalation of nitrogen dioxide encountered in recently filled silos. Bronchiolitis fibrosa obliterans is a common late complication, which perhaps can be prevented by early treatment of the acute reaction with corticosteroids. Extensive exposure to silage gas may cause sudden death.

## Lung Cancer

Many industrial pulmonary carcinogens have been identified, including asbestos, radon gas, arsenic, iron, chromium, nickel, coal tar fumes, petroleum oil mists, isopropyl oil, mustard gas, and printing ink. Cigarette smoking acts as a cocarcinogen with asbestos and radon gas to cause bronchogenic carcinoma. Asbestos alone causes malignant mesothelioma. Almost all histologic types of lung cancer have been associated with these carcinogens. Chloromethylmethyl ether specifically causes small-cell carcinoma of the lung.

## Pleural Diseases

Occupational diseases of the pleura may result from exposure to asbestos (see above) or talc. Inhalation of talc causes pleural plaques that are similar to those caused by asbestos.

## Other Occupational Pulmonary Diseases

Occupational agents are also responsible for other pulmonary disorders. These include **berylliosis,** an acute or chronic pulmonary disorder related to exposure to beryllium, which is absorbed through the lungs or skin and widely disseminated throughout the body. Acute berylliosis is a toxic, ulcerative tracheobronchitis and chemical pneumonitis following intense and severe exposure to beryllium. Chronic berylliosis, a systemic disease closely resembling sarcoidosis, is more common.

Chan-Yeung M, Lam S: Occupational asthma. *Am Rev Respir Dis* 1986;**133**:686.

Cormier Y, Bélanger J: Long-term physiologic outcome after acute farmer's lung. *Chest* 1987;**87**:796.

Dodge R: Sensitivity of methacholine testing in occupational asthma. *Chest* 1986;**89**:324.

Moller D et al: Persistent airways disease caused by toluene diisocyanate. *Am Rev Respir Dis* 1986;**134**:175.

Mundie TG, Ainsworth SK: Etiopathogenic mechanisms of bronchoconstriction in byssinosis: A review. *Am Rev Respir Dis* 1986;**133**:1181.

Schuyler M, Salvaggio JE: Hypersensitivity pneumonitis. *Sem Respir Med* 1984;**5**:246.

## DRUG-INDUCED LUNG DISEASE

Typical patterns of pulmonary response to various drugs implicated in drug-induced respiratory disease are summarized in Table 7–15. Pulmonary injury due to drugs occurs as a result of allergic reactions, idio-

**Table 7–15.** Pattern of response to selected drugs causing lung disease.

| Asthma | Pulmonary edema |
|---|---|
| Propranolol and other beta blockers | Noncardiogenic* |
| | Aspirin |
| Aspirin | Chlordiazepoxide |
| Nonsteroidal anti-inflammatory drugs | Ethchlorvynol |
| | Cardiogenic |
| Histamine | Propranolol |
| Methacholine | **Pleural effusion** |
| Acetylcysteine | Nitrofurantoin |
| Any nebulized medication | Any drug inducing |
| **Pulmonary infiltration** | systemic lupus |
| Without eosinophilia | erythematosus |
| Amitriptyline | Methysergide |
| Azathioprine | Chemotherapeutic agents |
| Amiodarone | **Mediastinal widening** |
| With eosinophilia | Phenytoin |
| Sulfonamides | Corticosteroids |
| Nitrofurantoin | Methotrexate |
| Penicillin | **Respiratory failure** |
| Methotrexate | Neuromuscular blockade |
| **Drug-induced systemic lupus erythematosus** | Aminoglycosides |
| | Succinylcholine |
| Hydralazine | Gallamine |
| Procainamide | Dimethyltubocurarine |
| Isoniazid | (metocurine) |
| Chlorpromazine | Central nervous system |
| Phenytoin | depression |
| **Interstitial fibrosis** | Sedatives |
| Nitrofurantoin | Hypnotics |
| Bleomycin | Narcotics |
| Busulfan | Alcohol |
| Cyclophosphamide | Tricyclic antidepressants |
| Methysergide | Oxygen |

* Heroin overdose also causes noncardiogenic pulmonary edema.

syncratic reactions, overdose, or undesirable side effects. In most patients, the mechanism of pulmonary injury is unknown.

Precise diagnosis of drug-induced pulmonary disease is often difficult, because results of routine laboratory studies are not helpful and radiographic findings are not specific. A high index of suspicion and a thorough medical history of drug usage are critical to establishing the diagnosis of drug-induced lung disease. The clinical response to cessation of the suspected offending agent is also helpful. Acute episodes of drug-induced pulmonary disease usually disappear 24–48 hours after the drug has been discontinued, but chronic syndromes may take longer to resolve. Challenge tests to confirm the diagnosis are risky and rarely performed.

Treatment of drug-induced lung disease consists of discontinuing the offending agent immediately and managing the pulmonary symptoms appropriately.

Cooper JAD Jr, White DA, Matthay RA: Drug-induced pulmonary disease. (2 parts.) *Am Rev Respir Dis* 1986;**133**:321, 488.

## RADIATION LUNG INJURY

The lung is a radiosensitive organ that can be affected by external beam radiation therapy. The pulmonary response is determined by the volume of lung radiated, the dose and rate of therapy, and potentiating factors, eg, concurrent chemotherapy, previous radiation therapy in the same area, and simultaneous withdrawal of corticosteroid therapy. Symptomatic radiation lung injury occurs in about 10% of patients treated with megavoltage therapy for carcinoma of the breast, 5–15% of patients treated for carcinoma of the lung, and 5–35% of patients treated for lymphoma. Two phases of the pulmonary response to radiation are apparent: an acute phase (radiation pneumonitis) and a chronic phase (radiation fibrosis).

### Radiation Pneumonitis

Radiation pneumonitis usually occurs 2–3 months (range 1–6 months) after completion of radiotherapy and is characterized by insidious onset of dyspnea, intractable dry cough, chest fullness or pain, weakness, and fever. Physical findings are usually absent, but inspiratory crackles may be heard in the involved area. In severe disease, respiratory distress and cyanosis occur that are characteristic of adult respiratory distress syndrome (ARDS). An increased white blood cell count and elevated sedimentation rate are common. Pulmonary function studies reveal reduced lung volumes, reduced lung compliance, hypoxemia, reduced diffusing capacity, and reduced maximum voluntary ventilation. Chest x-ray, which correlates poorly with the presence of symptoms, usually demonstrates an alveolar or nodular infiltrate with a ground-glass opacification limited to the irradiated area. Air bronchograms are often observed. The sharp borders of the infiltrate help distinguish radiation pneumonitis from other conditions, eg, infectious pneumonia, lymphangitic spread of carcinoma, and recurrent tumor.

Treatment of radiation pneumonitis consists of aspirin, cough suppressants, and bed rest. Acute respiratory failure, if present, is treated appropriately. Although there is no proof that corticosteroids are effective in radiation pneumonitis, prednisone (1 mg/kg/d orally) is usually given immediately and tapered slowly over several weeks. Radiation pneumonitis usually resolves in 2–3 weeks. Death from ARDS is unusual.

### Pulmonary Radiation Fibrosis

Pulmonary radiation fibrosis occurs in nearly all patients who receive a full course of radiation therapy for cancer of the lung and breast. Patients who experience radiation pneumonitis develop pulmonary fibrosis after an intervening period (6–12 months) of wellbeing. Most patients are asymptomatic, though slowly progressive dyspnea occurs in some. Cor pulmonale and chronic respiratory failure are rare. Radiographic findings include obliteration of normal lung markings, dense interstitial and pleural fibrosis, reduced lung volumes, tenting of the diaphragm, and sharp delineation of the irradiated area. No specific therapy is necessary, and corticosteroids have no value.

### Other Complications of Radiation Therapy

Other complications of radiation therapy directed to the thorax include pericardial effusion, constrictive pericarditis, tracheoesophageal fistula, esophageal candidiasis, radiation dermatitis, and rib fractures. Small pleural effusions, radiation pneumonitis outside the irradiated area, spontaneous pneumothorax, and complete obstruction of central airways are unusual occurrences.

# DISORDERS OF VENTILATION

The principal influences on ventilatory demand are arterial $P_{CO_2}$, pH and $P_{O_2}$. These variables are monitored by **peripheral** and **central chemoreceptors.** Under normal conditions, the ventilatory control system maintains arterial pH and $P_{CO_2}$ within narrow limits; arterial $P_{O_2}$ is more loosely controlled.

The function of the ventilatory control system may be assessed by observing ventilatory responses to hypoxemia and hypercapnia. The marked variability of these responses in the normal population reduces their diagnostic value in individual patients, but characterization of ventilatory drives has been a valuable tool in the investigation of groups of patients with disorders of ventilatory control. Deviations from normal ventilation are considered primary if they are not explained by disorders of ventilatory effectors or by diseases of the central nervous system, or if they do not represent compensatory responses to other physiologic derangements.

## PRIMARY ALVEOLAR HYPOVENTILATION

Primary alveolar hypoventilation is an uncommon syndrome of unknown cause characterized by inadequate alveolar ventilation despite normal airways, lungs, chest wall, and ventilatory muscles. Hypoventilation is even more marked during sleep. Individuals with this disorder are usually nonobese males in their third or fourth decades who present with lethargy, headache, and somnolence. Dyspnea is absent. Physical examination may reveal cyanosis and evidence of pulmonary hypertension and cor pulmonale. Hypoxemia and hypercapnia are present and improve with voluntary hyperventilation. Erythrocytosis is common. Results of pulmonary function tests are normal, but responses to induced hypercapnia and hypoxemia are reduced or absent. Central sleep apnea (see below) may occur and lead to severe nocturnal hypoxemia. Treatment with ventilatory stimulants such as medroxyprogesterone acetate, theophylline, acetazolamide, or methylphenidate may be of benefit. Augmentation of spontaneous ventilation has been beneficial in selected patients. Adequate oxygenation should be maintained with supplemental oxygen, but nocturnal oxygen therapy should be prescribed only if diagnostic nocturnal polysomnography has demonstrated its efficacy. Some patients show longer apneic intervals and increased $CO_2$ retention during sleep when given supplemental oxygen.

## OBESITY-HYPOVENTILATION SYNDROME

A few obese individuals demonstrate waking hypoventilation, which is distinguished from primary alveolar hypoventilation by the presence of extreme obesity. Symptoms, physical findings, and laboratory data are otherwise similar in the 2 syndromes. In obesity-hypoventilation syndrome, hypoventilation appears to result from a synergistic combination of blunted ventilatory drives and the mechanical load imposed upon the ventilatory apparatus by obesity. Most, if not all, patients with obesity-hypoventilation syndrome also suffer from obstructive sleep apnea (see below). Therapy of obesity-hypoventilation syndrome consists mainly of weight loss, which improves hypercapnia and hypoxemia as well as the ventilatory responses to hypoxia and hypercapnia; and medroxyprogesterone acetate, 10–20 mg every 8 hours orally. Marked improvement in hypoxemia, hypercapnia, erythrocytosis, and cor pulmonale may result.

## SLEEP-RELATED BREATHING DISORDERS

Abnormal ventilation during sleep is manifested by apnea (breath cessation for at least 10 seconds) or hypopnea (decrement in airflow with drop in oxyhemoglobin saturation of at least 4%). Episodes of apnea are **central** if ventilatory effort is absent for the duration of the apneic episode, **obstructive** if ventilatory effort persists throughout the apneic episode but no airflow occurs because of transient obstruction of the upper airway, and **mixed** if absent ventilatory effort precedes upper airway obstruction during the apneic episode. Central sleep apnea is rare; it may occur in patients with primary alveolar hypoventilation or in patients with lesions of the brain stem. Obstructive and mixed sleep apneas are more common and may be associated with life-threatening cardiac arrhythmias, severe hypoxemia, and consequences of hypoxemia, including cor pulmonale and secondary erythrocytosis.

**Polysomnography,** the monitoring of multiple physiologic factors during sleep, is used to evaluate sleep-related breathing disorders. Electroencephalography, electro-oculography, electromyography, electrocardiography, oximetry, and measurement of respiratory effort and airflow are performed in a complete evaluation, but screening may be performed using oximetry and electrocardiography only. Indications for study include a suggestive history of nocturnal breath cessation and loud snoring from a bed partner, daytime hypersomnolence, unexplained erythrocytosis or cor pulmonale, and nocturnal cardiac arrhythmias noted on Holter monitoring.

### Obstructive Sleep Apnea

Upper airway obstruction during sleep occurs when loss of normal pharyngeal muscle tone allows the pharynx to collapse passively during inspiration. Patients with anatomically narrowed upper airways (eg, micrognathia, macroglossia, obesity, tonsillar hypertrophy) are predisposed to the development of obstructive sleep apnea. Alcohol or sedatives before sleeping may precipitate or worsen the condition.

Most patients with obstructive or mixed sleep apnea are obese middle-aged men. Patients complain of excessive daytime somnolence, morning headaches, impotence, and enuresis. Bed partners usually report loud snoring as well as thrashing of the extremities during sleep. Personality changes and intellectual deterioration may also be observed. Physical examination may be normal or may reveal systemic and pulmonary hypertension with cor pulmonale. The pharynx may be narrowed by facial deformities, macroglossia, or abnormalities of pharyngeal soft tissue. Erythrocytosis is common. Observation of the sleeping patient reveals loud snoring interrupted by episodes of increasingly vigorous ventilatory effort that fail to produce airflow. A loud snort accompanies the first breath following an apneic episode. Polysomnography reveals apneic episodes associated with continued ventilatory effort of increasing vigor lasting as long as 1–2 minutes. Oxygen saturation falls, often to very low levels. Bradyarrhythmias such as sinus bradycardia, sinus arrest, or atrioventricular block may occur. Tachyarrhythmias, including paroxysmal supraventricular tachycardia, atrial fibrillation, and ventricular tachycardia, are common once airflow is reestablished.

**Tracheostomy** relieves upper airway obstruction and its physiologic consequences and represents the definitive treatment for obstructive sleep apnea. **Uvulopalatopharyngoplasty,** a procedure consisting of resection of pharyngeal soft tissue and amputation of the soft palate and uvula, may be helpful in selected patients with retropalatal airway occlusion during sleep. Indentifying such patients is difficult. Only about half of these operations are successful. **Nasal septoplasty** is performed if gross anatomic nasal septal deformity is present. These surgical approaches are reserved for those patients with life-threatening arrhythmias or severe disability who have failed to respond to conservative therapy. Alcohol and sedatives should be avoided before sleeping. Sleeping with the head of the bed elevated to 45 degrees or on one's side is often helpful. Weight loss is an important first step in obese patients with obstructive sleep apnea. Pharmacologic therapy with medroxyprogesterone acetate, protriptyline, or acetazolamide may be attempted but is usually not effective. Supplemental oxygen may lessen severe desaturation but may also lengthen apneic episodes. The effects of supplemental oxygen should be assessed during polysomnography before it is prescribed. Prevention of upper airway obstruction by using mechanical devices (nasopharyngeal airways, tongue retainers) or continuous positive airway pressure through the nose ("nasal CPAP") has been successful in selected patients but compliance is usually poor.

Kales A, Vela-Bueno A, Kales JD: Sleep disorders: sleep apnea and narcolepsy. *Ann Intern Med* 1987;**106**:434.
Kryger MH (editor): Sleep disorders. (Symposium.) *Clin Chest Med* 1985;**6**:553. (Entire issue.)

| **Acronyms in This Section** | |
| --- | --- |
| **A/C** | Assist/control |
| **AMV** | Assisted mechanical ventilation |
| **ARDS** | Adult respiratory distress syndrome |
| **CMV** | Continuous mechanical ventilation |
| **COPD** | Chronic obstructive pulmonary disease |
| **CPAP** | Continuous positive airway pressure |
| **DLV** | Differential lung ventilation |
| **EMMV** | Extended mandatory minute ventilation |
| **HFV** | High-frequency ventilation |
| **IMV** | Intermittent mandatory ventilation |
| **IRV** | Inverse ratio ventilation |
| **PEEP** | Positive end expiratory pressure |
| **PSV** | Pressure support ventilation |
| **SIMV** | Synchronized intermittent mandatory ventilation |

## HYPERVENTILATION SYNDROME

Hyperventilation may be caused by a variety of organic disorders. Functional hyperventilation may be acute or chronic. Acute hyperventilation presents with hyperpnea, paresthesias, carpopedal spasm, tetany, and anxiety. Chronic hyperventilation may present with various nonspecific symptoms, including fatigue, dyspnea, anxiety, palpitations, and dizziness. The diagnosis of chronic hyperventilation syndrome is established if symptoms are reproduced during voluntary hyperventilation. Once organic causes of hyperventilation have been excluded, treatment of acute hyperventilation consists of rebreathing expired gas in order to decrease respiratory alkalemia and its associated symptoms.

## ACUTE RESPIRATORY FAILURE

Respiratory failure is defined as respiratory dysfunction resulting in abnormalities of oxygenation or $CO_2$ elimination severe enough to impair or threaten function of vital organs. Arterial blood gas criteria for respiratory failure are not absolute but may be arbitrarily established as a $P_{O_2}$ under 50 mm Hg and a $P_{CO_2}$ over 50 mm Hg. Acute respiratory failure may occur in both pulmonary and nonpulmonary disorders (Table 7–16). Respiratory failure may be considered a failure of oxygenation, failure of ventilation, or both. Appropriate treatment is guided by assessment of the relative contributions of each of these components to the overall clinical picture.

### Clinical Findings

Symptoms and signs of acute respiratory failure are those of the underlying disease combined with those of hypoxemia and hypercapnia. The chief symptom of hypoxemia is dyspnea, though profound hypoxemia may exist in the absence of complaints. Signs of hypoxemia include cyanosis, restlessness, confusion, anxiety, delirium, tachypnea, tachycardia, hypertension, cardiac arrhythmias, and tremor. Dyspnea and headache are the cardinal symptoms of hypercapnia. Signs of hypercapnia include peripheral and conjunctival hyperemia, hypertension, tachycardia, tachypnea, impaired consciousness, papilledema, and asterixis. The symptoms and signs of acute respiratory failure are both insensitive and nonspecific; therefore, the physician must maintain a high index of suspicion and request an arterial blood gas analysis if respiratory failure is suspected.

### Treatment

Treatment of the patient with acute respiratory failure consists of (1) specific therapy directed toward

**Table 7–16.** Selected causes of acute respiratory failure in adults

**Airway disorders**
  Asthma
  Chronic bronchitis or emphysema in acute exacerbation
  Bronchiolitis
**Parenchymal lung disorders**
  Adult respiratory distress syndrome
  Congestive heart failure
  Pneumonia
  Hypersensitivity pneumonitis
**Pulmonary vascular disorders**
  Pulmonary thromboembolism
**Chest wall and pleural disorders**
  Flail chest
  Pneumothorax
**Neuromuscular disorders**
  Narcotic or sedative-hypnotic overdose
  Guillain-Barré syndrome
  Botulism
  Spinal cord injury
  Myasthenia gravis
  Poliomyelitis

the underlying disease; (2) respiratory supportive care directed toward the maintenance of adequate gas exchange; and (3) general supportive care. Only the last 2 aspects are discussed below.

**A. Respiratory Support:** Respiratory support has both nonventilatory and ventilatory aspects.

**1. Nonventilatory aspects**–*The main therapeutic goal in acute hypoxemic respiratory failure is to ensure adequate oxygenation of vital organs.* Inspired oxygen concentration should be the lowest value that results in an oxygen saturation of $\geq 90\%$ ($P_{a_{O_2}}$ about 60 mm Hg). Higher arterial oxygen tensions are of no benefit and may cause hypoventilation in patients with chronic hypercapnia; however, *oxygen therapy should not be withheld for fear of suppressing ventilatory drive.* Hypoxemia in patients with obstructive airway disease is usually easily corrected by administering low-flow oxygen by nasal cannulas (1–3 L/min) or Venturi mask (24–28%). Higher concentrations of oxygen are usually necessary to correct hypoxemia in patients with adult respiratory distress syndrome (ARDS), pneumonia, and other parenchymal lung diseases and may be administered without fear of causing hypoventilation in these disorders. Higher concentrations of oxygen may be delivered by Venturi mask or a mask with a reservoir bag.

**2. Ventilatory aspects**–Ventilatory support consists of maintaining patency of the airway and ensuring adequate alveolar ventilation. Tracheal intubation and mechanical ventilation are often required.

Indications for tracheal intubation are (1) hypoxemia which is not quickly reversed by supplemental oxygen, (2) upper airway obstruction, (3) impaired airway protection, (4) poor handling of secretions, and (5) need for positive pressure mechanical ventilation. Indications for mechanical ventilation include (1) apnea, (2) acute hypercapnia that is not quickly reversed by appropriate specific therapy, and (3) progressive patient fatigue despite appropriate conservative treatment.

The trachea may be intubated by means of the oral or the nasal route. In general, orotracheal intubation is preferred in urgent or emergency situations because it is easier, faster, and less traumatic. Nasotracheal tubes are more comfortable and may be preferable if prolonged intubation is anticipated. The largest tube that can be easily passed through the glottis should be used. Successful intubation may be enhanced by preoxygenation and preventilation with a bag and mask before intubation and use of adequate topical anesthesia. The position of the tip of the endotracheal tube at the level of the aortic arch should be verified by chest x-ray immediately following intubation, and auscultation should be performed to verify that both lungs are being ventilated.

In general, positive-pressure, volume-cycled ventilators should be used to provide mechanical ventilatory support. Critical ventilator settings include mode of ventilation, tidal volume, frequency, inspiratory flow rate, sensitivity, and inspired oxygen concentration. Although all ventilator settings must be modified to fit the clinical situation, general guidelines for initial ventilator settings are listed in Table 7–17. Patients with hyperinflation caused by airflow obstruction should be ventilated at the lower end of the indicated range for tidal volume, whereas patients with disease characterized by alveolar filling and collapse should be ventilated toward the higher end of this range. After about 20 minutes of mechanical ventilation, arterial blood gas analysis should be performed to provide guideline measurements for possible changes in ventilator settings. The inspired oxygen concentration should be quickly reduced to the lowest value compatible with an acceptable arterial oxygen tension or saturation. Arterial pH reflects the appropriateness of minute ventilation. Ventilation should be directed toward a pH within the normal range rather than toward normal arterial $P_{CO_2}$. Changes in minute ventilation are accomplished mainly by manipulating ventilatory frequency rather than tidal volume.

Several modes of ventilation are available. Assisted mechanical ventilation (AMV), or assist/control (A/C), is a ventilatory mode in which the ventilatory frequency set on the ventilator serves as a backup rate, but the patient may trigger the ventilator to deliver additional positive-pressure breaths. Continuous mechanical ventilation (CMV) provides ventilation at a specified rate for patients who are apneic. Intermittent mandatory ventilation (IMV) is a ventilatory technique in which the rate set on the ventilator serves as a backup rate, but the patient is able to augment the minute ventilation by taking spontaneous breaths through a one-way valve from a reservoir. Ventilator breaths are customarily delivered between spontaneous breaths (synchronized IMV, or SIMV). Intermittent mandatory ventilation may be of value for patients whose breathing cannot be synchronized with the ventilator; for tachypneic or agitated patients who develop respiratory alkalemia on assist/control ventilation; and for patients in whom strictly positive-pressure ventilation results in a reduction of cardiac output and in whom the occasional negative-pressure breaths of intermittent mandatory ventilation produce an improvement in cardiac output. New modes of mechanical ventilation are being developed, but clinical experience with them is limited. These include pressure support ventilation (PSV), high-frequency ventilation (HFV), inverse ratio ventilation (IRV), differential lung ventilation (DLV), and extended mandatory min-

**Table 7–17.** Initial ventilator settings in acute respiratory failure.

| Mode of ventilation | Assist/control |
|---|---|
| Tidal volume | 10–15 mL/kg ideal weight |
| Frequency | 12–14/min |
| Inspiratory flow rate | 50 L/min |
| Sensitivity | −3 cm water |
| Inspired $O_2$ concentration | 100% |

ute ventilation (EMMV). All require the use of new, expensive, microprocessor-based mechanical ventilators.

Positive end-expiratory pressure (**PEEP**) is useful in improving oxygenation in patients with diffuse parenchymal lung disease such as ARDS (see p 182). It should be avoided in patients with localized parenchymal disease, hyperinflation, or very high airway pressure requirements during mechanical ventilation.

Predictors of successful termination of mechanical ventilation include clinical stability or improvement and the patient's ability to meet certain "weaning criteria" that test the reserve of the ventilatory system (Table 7–18). These criteria are not applicable in patients with acute respiratory failure complicating COPD. In such patients, judgment about overall respiratory status becomes more important with respect to attempts to extubate.

Patients capable of adequate spontaneous ventilation can be identified through the use of the "T-piece trial," in which the patient first undergoes thorough suctioning and then breathes humidified and oxygen-enriched gas spontaneously through the tracheal tube while in the sitting position. After 30 minutes, arterial blood gas measurements are obtained. If ventilation and oxygenation are adequate, the trial is prolonged and a second analysis is performed. If oxygenation and ventilation remain adequate, mechanical ventilation may be discontinued. If the patient has no other indications for intubation, the tracheal tube may be removed. Microatelectasis leading to hypoxemia without hypercapnia may occur when mechanical ventilation using large tidal volume is replaced by spontaneous breathing. Continuous positive airway pressure (**CPAP**) applied through the tracheal tube during spontaneous ventilation may prevent this.

Those patients who fail one or more T-piece trials may require a more prolonged weaning process. Repeated episodes of spontaneous T-piece breathing of increasing duration are instituted and continued until the patient can maintain spontaneous ventilation. An alternative method is to ventilate the patient using intermittent mandatory ventilation and gradually re-duce the frequency of mechanical breaths. Although convenient, IMV weaning may actually slow the weaning process and increase the patient's work of breathing against the ventilator's valve systems. Weaning with PSV, which reduces the patient's work of breathing, is a promising new approach to weaning.

Potential complications of mechanical ventilation are numerous. Migration of the tip of the endotracheal tube into the right main bronchus can cause atelectasis of the left lung and overdistention of the right lung. Barotrauma manifested by subcutaneous emphysema, pneumomediastinum, subpleural air cysts, or pneumothorax is common in patients whose lungs are overdistended by excessive tidal volumes, especially those with hyperinflation caused by airflow obstruction or PEEP. Subtle parenchymal lung injury due to overdistention of alveoli is another potential hazard. Acute respiratory alkalosis caused by overventilation is common. Hypotension induced by elevated intrathoracic pressure that results in decreased return of systemic venous blood to the heart may occur in patients treated with PEEP, those with severe airflow obstruction, and those with intravascular volume depletion.

Negative pressure ventilation with chest cuirass and similar devices and continuous positive-pressure ventilation via tracheostomy tubes are acceptable approaches to treatment of chronic ventilatory failure when repeated attempts at weaning have failed. Mechanical ventilation in the home is feasible, but logistical problems are enormous. Nocturnal positive-pressure ventilation via nasal mask is a new experimental approach to management of patients with nocturnal hypoventilation from neuromuscular disease.

**B. General Supportive Care:** Patients with acute respiratory failure are seriously ill, and careful attention must be paid to general supportive measures. Maintenance of adequate nutrition is vital; parenteral nutrition should be used only when conventional feeding methods are not possible. Overfeeding, especially with carbohydrate, should be avoided, because it increases $CO_2$ production and may potentially worsen or induce hypercapnia in patients with limited ventilatory reserve; however, failure to provide adequate nutrition is more common. Hypokalemia and hypophosphatemia may worsen hypoventilation due to muscle weakness. The hematocrit should be determined regularly and transfusions given if necessary. Sedative-hypnotics and narcotic analgesics are avoided if possible. If sedation is necessary, short-acting drugs such as triazolam are preferred.

Attention must also be paid to preventing complications associated with serious illness. Stress gastritis and ulcers may be avoided by administering histamine $H_2$ receptor antagonists. The risk of deep venous thrombosis and pulmonary embolism may be reduced by the administration of subcutaneous heparin (5000 units every 12 hours).

## Course & Prognosis

The course and prognosis of acute respiratory fail-

**Table 7–18.** Predictors of successful termination of mechanical ventilation.

| | |
|---|---|
| Forced vital capacity | ≥ 10 mL/kg |
| Tidal volume | ≥ 5 mL/kg |
| Minute ventilation | ≤ 10 L |
| Maximum voluntary ventilation | ≥ Twice minute ventilation |
| Peak inspiratory pressure | More negative than −20 cm water |
| "T"-piece trial | No evidence of rapid, shallow breathing; adequate ventilation and oxygenation |

ure vary and depend on the underlying disease. The prognosis of acute respiratory failure caused by uncomplicated sedative or narcotic drug overdose is excellent. Acute respiratory failure in patients with COPD who do not require intubation and mechanical ventilation has a good immediate prognosis. On the other hand, ARDS associated with sepsis has an extremely poor prognosis, with mortality rates of about 90%.

Cane RD, Shapiro BA: Mechanical ventilatory support. *JAMA* 1985;**254:**87.

Kerby GR, Mayer LS, Pingleton SK: Nocturnal positive pressure ventilation via nasal mask. *Am Rev Respir Dis* 1987;**135:**738.

Tobin MJ et al: The pattern of breathing during successful and unsuccessful trials of weaning from mechanical ventilation. *Am Rev Respir Dis* 1986;**134:**1111.

Weisman IM et al: Intermittent mandatory ventilation. *Am Rev Respir Dis* 1983;**127:**641.

Wissing DR, Romero MD, George RB: Comparing the newer modes of mechanical ventilation. *J Crit Illness* 1987;**2:**41.

**Table 7–19.** Disorders associated with ARDS.

| Systemic Insults | Pulmonary Insults |
|---|---|
| Trauma | Embolism of thrombus, fat, or |
| Sepsis | amniotic fluid |
| Pancreatitis | Miliary tuberculosis |
| Shock | Aspiration of gastric contents |
| Multiple transfusions | Diffuse pneumonia |
| Disseminated intravascular | Viral |
|   coagulation | *Mycoplasma* |
| Burns | Legionnaire's |
| Drugs |   (*Pneumophila*) |
|   Narcotics | *Pneumocystis* |
|   Aspirin | Near-drowning |
|   Chlordiazepoxide | Toxic gas inhalation |
|   Phenylbutazone |   Nitrogen dioxide |
|   Colchicine |   Chlorine |
|   Ethchlorvynol |   Sulfur dioxide |
|   Hydrochlorothiazide |   Ammonia |
|   Paraldehyde | Smoke inhalation |
|   Lidocaine | Oxygen toxicity |
| Thrombotic thrombocytopenic | Lung contusions |
|   purpura | Radiation |
| Cardiopulmonary bypass | High altitude |
| Venous air embolism | Hanging |
| Head injury | Reexpansion |
| Paraquat | |

# ADULT RESPIRATORY DISTRESS SYNDROME (ARDS)

## Essentials of Diagnosis

- History of systemic or pulmonary insult.
- Respiratory distress.
- Diffuse pulmonary infiltrates.
- Severe hypoxemia refractory to treatment with supplemental oxygen.
- Normal pulmonary capillary wedge pressure.

## General Considerations

Adult respiratory distress syndrome denotes acute respiratory failure following a systemic or pulmonary insult; it is characterized by respiratory distress, diffuse infiltrates, hypoxemia, noncompliant lungs, and normal pulmonary capillary wedge pressure. ARDS may follow a wide variety of catastrophic clinical events (Table 7–19). Common risk factors for ARDS include sepsis, aspiration of gastric contents, shock, trauma, severe pneumonia, and multiple blood transfusions. Although the mechanism of lung injury varies with the cause, damage to capillary endothelial cells and alveolar epithelial cells (type I pneumonocytes) is common to ARDS regardless of cause. Damage to these cells causes increased vascular permeability and inactivation of surfactant; both of these lead to interstitial and alveolar pulmonary edema and alveolar collapse.

## Clinical Findings

ARDS is marked by the rapid onset of profound dyspnea that usually occurs 12–48 hours after the initiating event. Labored breathing, tachypnea, intercostal retractions, and crackles are noted on physical examination. Chest radiograph shows diffuse or patchy bilateral infiltrates that are initially interstitial but rapidly become alveolar; these characteristically spare the costophrenic angles. Air bronchograms occur in about 80% of cases. Upper lung zone venous engorgement (flow inversion) is distinctly uncommon. Heart size is normal, and pleural effusions are uncommon. Marked hypoxemia occurs that is refractory to treatment with supplemental oxygen, indicating shunting.

## Differential Diagnosis

Since ARDS is a physiologic and radiographic syndrome rather than a specific disease, the concept of differential diagnosis does not strictly apply. Normal-permeability ("cardiogenic") pulmonary edema must be ruled out, however, because specific therapy is available for that disorder. Measurement of pulmonary capillary wedge pressure by means of a flow-directed pulmonary artery catheter may be required, though routine use of the Swan-Ganz catheter in ARDS is discouraged.

## Prevention

No measures that effectively prevent ARDS have been identified; specifically, prophylactic use of PEEP in patients at risk for ARDS has not been shown to be effective.

## Treatment

Treatment of ARDS must include identification and specific treatment of the underlying condition (eg, sepsis). Aggressive supportive care must then be provided to compensate for the severe dysfunction of the respiratory system associated with ARDS. Supportive therapy almost always includes tracheal intubation and mechanical ventilation. The use of **positive end expiratory pressure (PEEP)** usually improves oxygenation in patients with ARDS but does not affect the natural history of this condition. PEEP should be used if the $F_{IO_2}$ required to produce an acceptable level of oxygenation exceeds 0.6. The lowest level of PEEP that produces adequate oxygenation combined with an acceptable $F_{IO_2}$ should be used. High levels of PEEP may improve arterial $Po_2$ but may depress cardiac output and reduce oxygen delivery. Cardiac output must therefore be monitored with a thermodilution pulmonary artery catheter if PEEP in excess of 10 cm water is required. Cardiac output that falls when PEEP is used may be improved by reducing the level of PEEP or by administering inotropic drugs (eg, dopamine); administering fluids to increase intravascular volume should be a treatment of last resort.

Elevated pulmonary capillary pressure worsens pulmonary edema in the presence of increased capillary permeability; therefore, the goal of fluid management is to maintain pulmonary capillary wedge pressure at the lowest possible level compatible with adequate cardiac output. Crystalloid solutions should be used when intravascular volume expansion is necessary. Diuretics should be used to reduce intravascular volume if pulmonary capillary wedge pressure is elevated.

Oxygenation in patients with ARDS may be improved by turning them from the supine to the prone position.

Corticosteroids have no proved efficacy in ARDS, with the possible exception of fat embolism syndrome. Broad-spectrum antimicrobial treatment should be started promptly when infection is known or suspected.

### Course & Prognosis

The mortality rate associated with ARDS exceeds 50%. If ARDS is accompanied by sepsis, the mortality rate may reach 90%. The major cause of death in ARDS is nonpulmonary multiple organ system failure, often with sepsis. Median survival is about 2 weeks. Most survivors are asymptomatic within a few months, though abnormalities of oxygenation, diffusing capacity, and lung mechanics are present in many survivors.

Elliott CG et al: Prediction of pulmonary function abnormalities after adult respiratory distress syndrome (ARDS). *Am Rev Respir Dis* 1987;**135:**634.

Rinaldo JE, Rogers RM: Adult respiratory distress syndrome. *N Engl J Med* 1986;**315:**578.

Robin ED: The cult of the Swan-Ganz catheter: Overuse and abuse of pulmonary flow catheters. *Ann Intern Med* 1985;**103:**445.

# PLEURAL DISEASES

## PLEURITIS

Pain due to acute pleural inflammation is caused by irritation of the parietal pleura. Such pain is localized, sharp, and fleeting and is made worse by cough, sneezing, deep breathing, or movement. When the central portion of the diaphragmatic parietal pleura is irritated, pain may be referred to the shoulder. There are numerous causes of pleuritis. The setting in which pleuritic pain develops helps to narrow the differential diagnosis; eg, in young, otherwise healthy individuals, pleuritis is usually caused by viral respiratory infections or pneumonia. The presence of pleural effusion, pleural thickening, or air in the pleural space requires further diagnostic and therapeutic measures. It should also be recalled that simple rib fracture may cause severe pleurisy.

Treatment of pleuritis consists of treating the underlying disease. Simple analgesics and anti-inflammatory drugs are often helpful for pain relief. Codeine (30–60 mg orally every 8 hours) may be used to control cough associated with pleuritic chest pain if retention of airway secretions is not a likely complication. Intercostal nerve blocks are sometimes helpful when simple measures fail; postinjection chest radiography is necessary to exclude pneumothorax.

Branch WT Jr, McNeil BJ: Analysis of the differential diagnosis and assessment of pleuritic chest pain in young adults. *Am J Med* 1983;**75:**671.

## PLEURAL EFFUSION

### Essentials of Diagnosis

- Asymptomatic in many cases; pleuritic chest pain if pleuritis is present; dyspnea if effusion is large.
- Decreased tactile fremitus; dullness to percussion; distant breath sounds; egophony if effusion is large.
- Radiographic evidence of pleural effusion.
- Diagnostic findings on thoracentesis.

### General Considerations

Pleural fluid is formed in the normal individual mostly on the parietal pleural surface at the rate of about 0.1 ml/kg/h. Absorption of this fluid on the visceral pleural surface is thought to occur, keeping the pleural space nearly dry. However, the parietal pleura may also contribute to absorption. A few milliliters of pleural fluid ($< 25$ mL) is normally present in the pleural space and is not detectable on conventional chest radiographs. Movement of fluid into and out of the pleural space is dependent mostly on hydrostatic and osmotic forces in parietal and visceral pleural capillaries. **Pleural effusion** is an abnormal accumulation of fluid in the pleural space. The 5 major types of pleural effusion are transudates, exudates, empyema, hemorrhagic pleural effusion or hemothorax, and chylous or chyliform effusion.

Pleural effusions are classified as **transudates** or **exudates** to help in differential diagnosis. An exudate is a pleural fluid having *one or more* of the following features:

(1) Pleural fluid protein to serum protein ratio greater than 0.5.

(2) Pleural fluid LDH to serum LDH ratio greater than 0.6.

(3) Pleural fluid LDH greater than two-thirds the upper limit of normal of serum LDH.

Transudates have none of these features.

Causes of transudates and exudates are listed in Table 7–20. Congestive heart failure accounts for most transudates and is the most common cause of pleural effusion. Bacterial pneumonia and cancer are the commonest causes of exudative effusion. Mechanisms (and examples) leading to formation of transudates include increase in hydrostatic pressure (congestive heart failure), decreased oncotic pressure (hypoalbuminemia), and greater negative intrapleural pressure (acute atelectasis). Exudates form as a result of disease of the pleura itself in association with increased capillary permeability (pneumonia) or reduced lymphatic drainage (carcinoma obstructing lymphatic drainage).

The gross appearance of pleural fluid helps to identify the other major types of pleural effusion. **Empyema** is an exudative pleural effusion caused by direct infection of the pleural space. **Hemothorax** is the presence of gross blood in the pleural space, usually a result of chest trauma. **Hemorrhagic pleural effusion** is a mixture of blood and pleural fluid. About 10,000 red blood cells per microliter are necessary to create blood-tinged pleural fluid;

100,000 red blood cells per microliter make pleural fluid appear grossly bloody. If the hematocrit of pleural fluid is more than 50% of the hematocrit of peripheral blood, hemothorax is present. In the absence of trauma, grossly bloody pleural fluid suggests cancer or, less commonly, pulmonary embolism.

Pleural fluid that is milky in appearance should be centrifuged. Clearing of the milky appearance from the supernatant suggests empyema, whereas persistent cloudy or turbid supernatant signifies **chylous** or **chyliform pleural effusion.** Chylous pleural effusion occurs acutely in chylothorax as a result of disruption of the thoracic duct. Chyliform pleural effusion occurs in pseudochylothorax as a result of accumulation of cholesterol complexes in a chronically thickened pleural space, a phenomenon sometimes seen in cases of trapped lung (entrapment of lung by a fibrous "peel" on the visceral pleura), tuberculous pleuritis (especially with previous therapeutic pneumothorax), or rheumatoid pleural effusion. Chylous pleural effusion may be distinguished from chyliform pleural effusion on the basis of lipid analysis of the fluid. A chylous pleural effusion has chylomicrons and a high triglyceride level, usually above 100 mg/dL.

### Clinical Findings

**A. Symptoms and Signs:** Small pleural effusions are usually asymptomatic, whereas large pleural effusions may cause dyspnea, particularly in the presence of underlying cardiopulmonary disease. Pleuritic chest pain and dry cough may occur; any pleural fluid found in association with pleuritic chest pain is invariably an exudate. Physical findings are absent if less than 200–300 mL of pleural fluid is present. Findings consistent with the presence of a larger pleural effusion include decrease in tactile fremitus, dullness to percussion, and diminution of breath sounds over the effusion. In large effusions that compress the lung, accentuation of breath sounds and egophony may be noted just above the effusion. A pleural friction rub indicates pleuritis. A massive pleural effusion with high intrapleural pressure may cause contralateral shift of the trachea and bulging of the intercostal spaces.

**B. Laboratory Findings:** Transudates lack the distinguishing protein and LDH findings described above and are usually identified on the basis of other characteristics (white blood cell count $< 1000/\mu L$, predominance of mononuclear cells in the differential, glucose level in pleural fluid equal to that of serum, and normal pH). Laboratory findings in exudative pleural effusions are more variable and are summarized in Table 7–21. If an exudate is suspected, thoracentesis should be performed. One should have a low threshold for performing pleural biopsy at this time. This procedure is particularly useful in the diagnosis of tuberculosis and cancer and reduces the duration of hospitalization. The presence of malignant cells or positive results on smear or culture are pathognomonic findings in pleural fluid; determination of other causes depends on a constellation of findings

**Table 7–20.** Causes of pleural fluid transudates and exudates.

| Transudates | Exudates |
|---|---|
| Congestive heart failure | Parapneumonic effusion |
| Cirrhosis with ascites | Cancer |
| Nephrotic syndrome | Pulmonary embolism |
| Peritoneal dialysis | Empyema |
| Myxedema | Tuberculosis |
| Acute atelectasis | Connective tissue disease |
| Constrictive pericarditis | Viral infection |
| Superior vena cava obstruction | Fungal infection |
| Pulmonary embolism | Rickettsial infection |
| | Parasitic infection |
| | Asbestos pleural effusion |
| | Meigs' syndrome |
| | Pancreatic disease |
| | Uremia |
| | Chronic atelectasis |
| | Trapped lung |
| | Chylothorax |
| | Sarcoidosis |
| | Drug reaction |
| | Postmyocardial infarction syndrome |

Table 7–21. Characteristics of important exudative pleural effusions.

| Etiology or Type of Effusion | Gross Appearance | White Blood Cell Count (cells/µL) | Differential* | Red Blood Cell Count (cells/µL) | Glucose | Comments |
|---|---|---|---|---|---|---|
| Malignant effusion | Turbid to bloody; occasionally serous. | 1000– <100,000 | M | 100 to several hundred thousand. | Equal to serum levels; <60 mg/dL in 15% of cases. | Eosinophilia uncommon; positive results on cytologic examination. |
| Uncomplicated parapneumonic effusion | Clear to turbid. | 5000–25,000 | P | <5000 | Equal to serum levels. | Tube thoracostomy unnecessary. |
| Empyema | Turbid to purulent. | 25,000–100,000 | P | <5000 | Less than serum levels; often very low. | Drainage necessary; putrid odor suggests anaerobic infection. |
| Tuberculosis | Serous to serosanguineous. | 5000–10,000 | M | <10,000 | Equal to serum levels; occasionally <60 mg/dl. | Protein may exceed 5 g/dL; eosinophils (>10%) or mesothelial cells (>5%) make diagnosis unlikely. |
| Rheumatoid effusion | Turbid; greenish-yellow. | 1000–20,000 | M or P | <1000 | <40 mg/dL. | Secondary empyema common; high LDH, low complement, high rheumatoid factor, high cholesterol levels or cholesterol crystals are characteristic. |
| Pulmonary infarction | Serous to grossly bloody. | 1000–50,000 | M or P | 100–>100,000 | Equal to serum levels. | Variable findings; no pathognomonic features. |
| Esophageal rupture | Turbid to purulent; red-brown. | <5000– >50,000 | P | ... | Usually low. | High amylase level (salivary origin); pneumothorax in 25% of cases; effusion usually on left side; pH <6.0 strongly suggests diagnosis. |
| Pancreatitis | Turbid to serosanguineous. | 1000–50,000 | P | 1000–10,000 | Equal to serum levels. | Usually left-sided; high amylase level. |

* M = mononuclear cell predominance; P = polymorphonuclear leukocyte predominance.

on gross examination and laboratory studies or on biopsy results. Routine laboratory tests of pleural fluid should include total and differential white blood cell count, protein, glucose, and LDH. Additional tests may be ordered as required after thoracentesis. Pleural fluid pH is helpful in narrowing the differential diagnosis of exudative effusions. A pH less than 7.30 indicates cancer, complicated parapneumonic effusion, lupus or rheumatoid effusion, tuberculosis, or esophageal rupture. A high percentage of lymphocytes in pleural fluid suggests tuberculosis or cancer. Low levels of glucose in pleural fluid point toward cancer, empyema, tuberculosis, esophageal rupture, or connective tissue disease (rheumatoid pleuritis or systemic lupus erythematosus). Elevated levels of amylase in pleural fluid suggest one of 4 diagnoses: pancreatitis, pancreatic pseudocyst, cancer, or esophageal rupture.

**C. Imaging:** About 250 mL of pleural fluid must be present before effusion can be detected on conventional erect posteroanterior chest x-ray. Lateral decubitus views can detect much smaller amounts of pleural fluid. Free pleural fluid collects in the subpulmonic area. Larger amounts of fluid spill over into the costophrenic sulcus to form a meniscus. Thickening of major and minor fissures is common. Atypical collections of pleural fluid are frequently seen. Lateral displacement of the apex of the diaphragm and abrupt obliteration of lung markings at the level of the diaphragm are features of subpulmonic effusion. Round or oval-shaped collections of fluid in fissures resemble pseudotumor. Ultrasound guidance of thoracentesis is the most reliable method of tapping small amounts of fluid or identifying loculations. Massive pleural effusion (opacification of an entire hemithorax) is usually caused by cancer but has been observed in tuberculosis and other diseases.

## Treatment

Treatment addresses the disease causing the pleural effusion as well as the effusion itself. Because a specific diagnosis can be established in most cases of pleural effusion, a diagnosis of "idiopathic" effusion may delay or even prevent successful therapy.

**A. Malignant or Paramalignant Pleural Effusion:** Pleural effusion in a patient with known cancer may be either malignant or paramalignant. In malignant pleural effusion, the tumor causing the effusion is unresectable, and treatment with chemotherapy or radiotherapy is directed at the underlying cancer. In paramalignant pleural effusion, the pleural space is not directly invaded by tumor, and repeated thoracentesis and needle biopsy of the pleura give negative results. In this situation, the underlying tumor may or may not be resectable. Chemical pleurodesis is advised for selected patients with symptomatic malignant pleural effusion who fail to respond to chemotherapy or mediastinal radiation or who are not candidates for these forms of therapy. Intrapleural tetracycline is now the method of choice for chemical pleurodesis. Repeated therapeutic thoracentesis and surgical pleurectomy are alternative approaches for certain patients with rapidly recurring malignant pleural effusion.

**B. Transudative Pleural Effusion:** Transudative pleural effusions generally respond to treatment of the underlying condition; therapeutic thoracentesis is indicated only if massive effusion causes dyspnea. Pleurodesis and tube thoracostomy are rarely if ever indicated.

**C. Parapneumonic Pleural Effusion:** Pleural effusion in the setting of pneumonia ("parapneumonic effusion") usually responds to systemic antibiotic therapy. Management steps include sputum Gram stain and culture, blood cultures, diagnostic thoracentesis, antibiotic therapy, and a decision regarding closed chest drainage (tube thoracostomy). *Effective therapy requires early intervention* to avoid progression of the effusion from the exudative to subsequent (fibrinopurulent and organized) stages. Laboratory findings—especially the pH, glucose concentration, and the white cell count of pleural fluid—are important in guiding additional therapy. In "uncomplicated" parapneumonic effusion, no pleural infection is present, and the pleural fluid glucose and pH are normal. Such effusion is likely to resolve spontaneously, and chest tube drainage is not required. In "complicated" parapneumonic effusion, pleural fluid is either frank empyema or has the potential to organize into a fibrous "peel." A low pH ($< 7.2$), low glucose ($< 50$ mg/dL), and high LDH ($> 1000$ IU/L)—but not pleural fluid white blood cell count or protein concentration—help to separate complicated from uncomplicated parapneumonic effusions.

Tube thoracostomy is required for parapneumonic effusion if any of the following are present: (1) the fluid resembles frank pus, (2) an organism is evident on Gram stain, or (3) glucose $< 40$ mg/dL or (4) pH $< 7.0$. If the pleural fluid pH is between 7.0 and 7.2 or the LDH is $> 1000$ IU/L, the physician should strongly consider chest tube placement or should monitor the effusion carefully with serial thoracentesis. A thick pleural "peel" developing after treatment of complicated parapneumonic effusion may resolve slowly over several months. Surgical decortication should be reserved for selected patients with established fibrothorax.

**D. Hemothorax:** Hemothorax is managed by the immediate insertion of one or more large chest tubes in order to control bleeding by causing apposition of pleural surfaces; chest tubes help the physician determine the amount of bleeding and decrease the risk of complications such as empyema and eventual fibrothorax. As much blood as possible should be drained before the chest tube is removed. Thoracotomy is occasionally required to control bleeding, remove large volumes of blood clots, and treat coexisting complications of trauma such as bronchopleural fistula.

**E. Other Types of Pleural Effusion:** Management of patients with exudative pleural effusion due to other causes consists mainly of treating the underlying disease. Pleural fluid acidosis outside the setting of pneumonia is not an automatic indication for chest tube drainage. Patients with rheumatoid pleural effusions should be watched closely for the development of secondary empyema.

## Prognosis

The prognosis of patients with pleural effusion depends on the prognosis of the underlying disease. The prognosis of patients with documented malignant pleural effusion is poor, particularly if pleural fluid pH or glucose levels are low.

American College of Physicians: Diagnostic thoracentesis and pleural biopsy in pleural effusions. *Ann Intern Med* 1985;**103**:799.

Epstein DM et al: Tuberculous pleural effusions. *Chest* 1987;**91**:106.

Light RW (editor): Symposium on Pleural Diseases. *Clin Chest Med* 1985;**6**:1. [Entire issue.]

Miller KS, Sahn SA: Chest tubes: Indications, technique, management, and complications. *Chest* 1987;**91**:258.

## SPONTANEOUS PNEUMOTHORAX

### Essentials of Diagnosis

- Acute onset of ipsilateral chest pain and dyspnea, often of several days' duration.
- Minimal physical findings in mild cases; unilateral chest expansion, decreased tactile fremitus, hyperresonance, diminished breath sounds, mediastinal shift, cyanosis in tension pneumothorax.
- Presence of pleural air on chest x-ray.

### General Considerations

Pneumothorax, or accumulation of air in the pleural space, is classified as spontaneous (primary or secondary) or traumatic. Primary pneumothorax occurs in the absence of an underlying cause, whereas secondary pneumothorax is a complication of preexisting pulmonary disease. Traumatic pneumothorax results from penetrating or nonpenetrating trauma and is often iatrogenic.

Secondary pneumothorax occurs as a complication of COPD, asthma, cystic fibrosis, tuberculosis, and certain infiltrative lung diseases. Pneumothorax in association with menstruation (catamenial pneumothorax) is another well-established form of secondary pneumothorax. Because of underlying disease, secondary pneumothorax is usually a more serious condition than primary spontaneous pneumothorax.

The incidence of primary pneumothorax is about 9 per 100,000 per year; the disease affects mainly tall, thin men between the ages of 20 and 40 years. Primary pneumothorax is thought to occur from rupture of subpleural apical blebs in response to high negative intrapleural pressures. Familial factors and cigarette smoking may also be important.

### Clinical Findings

**A. Symptoms and Signs:** Chest pain on the affected side and dyspnea occur in nearly all patients. Symptoms usually begin during rest or sleep. Many patients wait for several days before seeking medical attention. Alternatively, this may be present with life-threatening respiratory failure if underlying COPD or asthma is present; this is true irrespective of the size of the pneumothorax.

If pneumothorax is small, physical findings, other than mild tachycardia, are unimpressive. If pneumothorax is large, diminished breath sounds, decreased tactile fremitus, and hyperresonance are noted. Tension pneumothorax should be suspected in the presence of severe tachycardia, hypotension, and mediastinal or tracheal shift.

**B. Laboratory Findings:** Arterial blood gas analysis reveals hypoxemia in most patients but is often unnecessary. Left-sided primary pneumothorax may produce QRS axis and precordial T wave changes on the ECG.

**C. Imaging:** Demonstration of a visceral pleural line is diagnostic and is best revealed on an expiratory film. A few patients have secondary pleural effusion that demonstrates a characteristic air-fluid level on chest radiography. In tension pneumothorax, chest radiographs show a large amount of air in the affected hemithorax and contralateral shift of mediastinal structures.

### Differential Diagnosis

If the patient is a young, tall, thin cigarette-smoking man, the diagnosis of primary spontaneous pneumothorax is usually obvious and can be confirmed by chest x-ray. In secondary pneumothorax, it is sometimes difficult to distinguish loculated pneumothorax from an emphysematous bleb. Occasionally, pneumothorax may mimic myocardial infarction, pulmonary embolization, or pneumonia.

### Complications

Tension pneumothorax may result in acute respiratory failure. Cardiopulmonary arrest and death are extremely rare. Pneumomediastinum may occur as a complication of spontaneous pneumothorax. If this is detected, rupture of the esophagus or a bronchus should be considered.

### Treatment

Treatment depends upon the severity of pneumothorax. The patient with a small ($< 15\%$) pneumothorax should be hospitalized and placed at bed rest, treated symptomatically for cough and chest pain, and followed with serial chest x-rays every 12–24 hours. Many small pneumothoraces resolve spontaneously as air is absorbed from the pleural space; however, pneumothorax may unpredictably progress to tension pneumothorax. In this situation, or in patients who are severely symptomatic or who have a larger pneumothorax ($> 15\%$), tube thoracostomy is performed. The chest tube is placed under water-seal drainage, and suction is applied until the lung expands. Intravenous catheters and emergency pneumothorax treatment tubes should not be used in the hospital setting because of a high rate of technical failures. Air leaks persisting after 3 days are unusual. Tube thoracostomy alone does not cause enough pleural scarification to prevent recurrence of spontaneous pneumothorax. Pulmonary edema on the affected side may follow abrupt evacuation of pneumothorax. If tension pneumothorax is suspected, a large-bore needle should be inserted immediately in the affected side; tube thoracostomy may be performed thereafter.

Chemical pleurodesis with instillation of tetracycline into the pleural space by chest tube has been recommended by some authorities for management of a first episode of spontaneous pneumothorax, but this procedure causes considerable pain, and no long-term studies have evaluated its effectiveness.

All patients should be advised to discontinue smoking and warned that the risk of recurrence is 50%. Exposure to high altitudes, flying in unpressurized aircraft, and scuba diving should be avoided. If spontaneous pneumothorax recurs, the second episode should be managed in a manner similar to that of the first episode. Some experts advocate thoracotomy for any recurrence.

Indications for open thoracotomy include a third episode of spontaneous pneumothorax, any occurrence of bilateral pneumothorax, and failure of tube thoracostomy for the first episode (failure of lung to reexpand or persistent air leak). Open thoracotomy permits oversewing of the ruptured blebs responsible for the pneumothorax and greatly reduces the risk of recurrence. Pleural symphysis may be obtained by scarification from abrasion of the pleural surface. Pleurectomy is of no particular value.

## Prognosis

About half of patients with spontaneous pneumothorax experience recurrence of the disorder after either observation or tube thoracostomy for the first episode. Recurrence after open thoracotomy is rare. Following successful therapy, there are no long-term complications.

Nakamura H et al: Epidemiology of spontaneous pneumothorax in women. *Chest* 1986;**89:**378.

Stephenson LW: Treatment of pneumothorax with intrapleural tetracycline. *Chest* 1985;**88:**803.

## REFERENCES

Brenner BE (editor): *Comprehensive Management of Respiratory Emergencies.* Aspen Systems Corporation, 1985.

Burton GG, Hodgkin JE (editors): *Respiratory Care: A Guide to Clinical Practice,* 2nd ed. Lippincott, 1984.

Cherniak RM (editor): *Current Therapy of Respiratory Disease-2.* Marcel Decker, 1986.

Clausen JL (editor): *Pulmonary Function Testing Guidelines and Controversies: Equipment, Methods, and Normal Values.* Grune & Stratton, 1984.

Fraser RG, Pare' JAP: *Diagnosis of Diseases of the Chest,* 2nd ed. Vols I–IV. Saunders, 1978.

Goldhaber SZ (editor): *Pulmonary Embolism and Deep Venous Thrombosis.* Saunders, 1985.

Hodgkin JE, Zorn EG, Connors GL (editors): *Pulmonary Rehabilitation: Guidelines to Success.* Butterworth, 1984.

Light RW: *Pleural Diseases.* Lea & Febiger, 1983.

Luce JM, Tyler ML, Pierson DJ: *Intensive Respiratory Care.* Saunders, 1984.

Morgan WKC, Seaton A (editors): *Occupational Lung Diseases,* 2nd ed. Saunders, 1984.

Murray JF: *The Normal Lung,* 2nd ed. Saunders, 1986.

Rippe JM et al (editors): *Intensive Care Medicine.* Little, Brown, 1985.

Shoemaker WC, Thompson WL, Holbrook PR: *Textbook of Critical Care.* Saunders, 1984.

Simmons DH (editor): *Current Pulmonology.* Vol 6. Year Book, 1985.

Weir EK, Reeves JT (editors): *Pulmonary Hypertension.* Futura, 1984.

Weiss EB, Segal MS, Stein M (editors): *Bronchial Asthma: Mechanisms and Therapeutics,* 2nd ed. Little, Brown, 1985.

West JB: *Respiratory Physiology: The Essentials,* 3rd ed. Williams & Wilkins, 1985.

Wilson AF (editor): *Pulmonary Function Testing Indications and Interpretations.* Grune and Stratton, 1985.

# 8

# Heart & Great Vessels

*Maurice Sokolow, MD, & Barry Massie, MD*

Evaluation of the patient with cardiovascular disease requires (1) identification of the physiologic abnormality, (2) delineation of the underlying structural abnormality and its cause, (3) assessment of the severity of functional impairment and its potential for progression or reversal, and (4) determination of the need for treatment and the type of treatment. Such an evaluation implies a medical history, physical examination, laboratory testing, and, in most cases, noninvasive diagnostic procedures.

## COMMON SYMPTOMS

The most common symptoms of heart disease are dyspnea, chest pain, palpitations, presyncope or syncope, and fatigue. None of these are specific, and their interpretation depends on systematic inquiry and diagnostic studies.

### Dyspnea

Dyspnea (shortness of breath) due to heart disease is precipitated or worsened by exertion and results from elevated left atrial and pulmonary venous pressures or hypoxia. The former are most commonly caused by left ventricular systolic dysfunction (due to congestive heart failure or transient myocardial ischemia), left ventricular diastolic dysfunction (elevated diastolic pressures due to hypertrophy, fibrosis, or pericardial disease), or valvular obstruction. The acute onset or worsening of left atrial hypertension may result in **pulmonary edema,** or leaking of fluid into the interstitial or alveolar spaces. Hypoxia may be due to pulmonary edema or intracardiac shunting. Dyspnea should be quantified by the kind of activity that precipitates it. Dyspnea is also a common symptom of pulmonary disease, and the etiologic distinction may be very difficult. Shortness of breath is also found in deconditioned or obese individuals, anxiety states, and many illnesses.

**Orthopnea** is dyspnea that occurs or increases in recumbency and results from an increase in central blood volume. However, orthopnea may also result from pulmonary disease. **Paroxysmal nocturnal dyspnea** interrupting sleep is relieved by sitting up or standing. It too results from increase of central intravascular volume in patients with already elevated left atrial pressures. This symptom is usually diagnostic of cardiac disease.

### Chest Pain

Chest pain is a common nonspecific symptom that can occur as a result of pulmonary or musculoskeletal disease, esophageal or other gastrointestinal disorders, cervicothoracic nerve root irritation, or anxiety states, as well as many cardiovascular diseases. The commonest cause of cardiac chest pain is myocardial ischemia due to obstructive coronary artery disease. This is characteristically described as dull, aching, or as a sensation of "pressure," "tightness," "squeezing," or "gas," rather than as sharp or spasmodic; and it is often perceived as an uncomfortable sensation rather than "pain." Ischemic pain may last up to an hour; it is neither fleeting (lasting only a few seconds) nor persistent (lasting hours to days). It is commonly accompanied by a sense, often profound, of anxiety or uneasiness. The location is usually retrosternal or left precordial. Though the pain may radiate to or be localized in the throat, lower jaw, shoulders, inner arms, upper abdomen, or back, it nearly always also involves the sternal region. It is often precipitated by exertion, cold temperature, large meals, emotional stress, or combinations of these factors and is usually relieved by rest. Ischemic pain is not related to position or respiration.

Hypertrophy of either ventricle and aortic valvular disease may also give rise to ischemic pain or pain with less typical features. Mitral valve prolapse is associated with chest pain of a more fleeting yet sharp nature. Pericarditis may produce pain that changes with position or respiration. Aortic dissection produces an instantaneous tearing pain of great intensity that usually is felt in or radiates to the back (see below).

### Palpitations, Dizziness, Syncope

Awareness of the heartbeat may be a normal phenomenon or may reflect increased cardiac or stroke output in patients with many noncardiac conditions (eg, exercise, thyrotoxicosis, anemia, anxiety). It may also be due to cardiac abnormalities that increase stroke volume (regurgitant valvular disease, bradycardia) or may be a manifestation of cardiac arrhythmias. Ventricular premature beats may be sensed as extra or "missed" beats. Supraventricular or ventricular tachycardia may be felt as rapid, regular or irregular palpitations or fluttering; many patients with these rhythms do not sense them, however.

If dysrhythmia is associated with a sufficient decline in arterial pressure or cardiac output, it may—especially in the upright position—impair cerebral blood flow, causing dizziness, blurring of vision or narrowing of the visual fields, and loss of consciousness (syncope).

Cardiogenic syncope most commonly results from loss of sinus node impulse, atrioventricular conduction block, or ventricular tachycardia or fibrillation. It is usually associated with few prodromal symptoms and may thus be an occasion for head injuries or other injuries. The absence of premonitory symptoms helps distinguish cardiogenic syncope from vasovagal faint, postural hypotension, or seizure disorder. Aortic valve disease and hypertrophic obstructive cardiomyopathy may also cause syncope, usually exertional or postexertional.

## Edema

Subcutaneous fluid collections appear first in the ankles and lower extremities in ambulatory patients or in the sacral region of bedridden individuals. In heart disease, edema results from elevated right atrial pressures that may indicate valvular disease or myocardial dysfunction of the right heart or pulmonary hypertension (cor pulmonale). Right heart failure most commonly results from left heart failure, although the right-sided signs may predominate. Edema may also be due to peripheral venous insufficiency, nephrotic syndrome, cirrhosis, or premenstrual fluid retention, or it may be idiopathic. Advanced right heart failure can rarely produce ascites.

## Fatigue

Fatigue is the least specific of cardiac symptoms, but it may result from low-output states. The underlying cardiac disorder is easily demonstrated on examination or by diagnostic testing.

## FUNCTIONAL CLASSIFICATION OF HEART DISEASE

As a means of quantifying the limitation on activity of cardiac patients imposed by their symptoms, the classification system of the New York Heart Association is commonly employed.

Class I: No limitation of physical activity. Ordinary physical activity does not cause undue fatigue, palpitation, dyspnea, or anginal pain.

Class II: Slight limitation of physical activity. Comfortable at rest, but ordinary physical activity results in symptoms.

Class III: Marked limitation of physical activity. Comfortable at rest, but less than ordinary activity causes symptoms.

Class IV: Unable to engage in any physical activity without discomfort. Symptoms may be present even at rest. If any physical activity is undertaken, discomfort is increased.

## SIGNS OF HEART DISEASE

Valuable information pertaining to the cause, nature, and extent of heart disease—as well as the presence of other conditions that may mimic it—is gathered during physical examination. Although the cardiovascular examination centers on the heart, peripheral signs are often invaluable.

### Cyanosis, Pallor

Cyanosis may be central, due to arterial desaturation, or peripheral, reflecting impaired tissue delivery of adequately saturated blood either in low-output states, polycythemia, or peripheral vasoconstriction. Central cyanosis may be caused by pulmonary disease, left heart failure, or right-to-left shunting; the latter will not be improved by increasing the inspired oxygen concentration. Pallor usually indicates anemia but may be a sign of low cardiac output.

### Peripheral Pulses & Venous Pulsations

Diminished peripheral pulsations most commonly result from arteriosclerotic peripheral vascular disease and may be accompanied by localized bruits. Asymmetry of pulses should arouse suspicion of coarctation of the aorta or aortic dissection. Generalized weak pulses may reflect reduced stroke volume, while exaggerated pulses may indicate aortic regurgitation, coarctation, or patent ductus arteriosus. The carotid pulse is a valuable aid to assessment of left ventricular ejection. It has a delayed upstroke in aortic stenosis and a bisferiens quality in mixed aortic valvular disease or hypertrophic obstructive cardiomyopathy. Pulsus paradoxus (greater than the normal 10 mm Hg decline in systolic blood pressure with inspiration) can be recognized by palpation or measurement and is a valuable sign of pericardial tamponade, though it also occurs in asthma or chronic obstructive pulmonary disease.

Jugular venous pulsations provide insight into right atrial pressure. They indicate (1) elevated central venous pressure if they are more than 3 vertical centimeters above the angle of Louis, (2) increased central blood volume if they rise more than 1 cm with sustained upper abdominal pressure (**hepatojugular reflux**), (3) tricuspid obstruction or pulmonary hypertension if the *a* wave is exaggerated, and (4) tricuspid regurgitation if large *cv* waves are seen. The latter may be associated with hepatic pulsations. Atrioventricular dissociation due to conduction block or ventricular dysrhythmia can be recognized by intermittent cannon *a* waves.

### Pulmonary Examination

Crackles heard at the lung bases and extending upward are a classic sign of congestive heart failure but may be caused by similarly localized pulmonary disease. Expiratory wheezing and rhonchi suggest obstructive pulmonary disease but may occur in left heart failure. Pleural effusions with bibasilar percussion dullness and reduced breath sounds are common in congestive heart failure.

## Precordial Pulsations

A parasternal lift or heave usually indicates right ventricular hypertrophy or pulmonary hypertension (systolic pressure > 50 mm Hg) or left atrial enlargement; pulmonary artery pulsations may also be visible. The left ventricular apical impulse provides an indication of heart position and, if sustained and enlarged, of myocardial hypertrophy or dysfunction. The atrial filling *a* wave may be palpated or seen in the presence of impaired left ventricular compliance. If forceful but not sustained, the apical impulse may indicate volume overload or high-output states. Additional precordial pulsations reflect regional abnormalities of left ventricular contraction (aneurysms or akinetic segments).

## Heart Sounds & Murmurs

Auscultation is of primary diagnostic value in many congenital and valvular heart diseases and in cardiac failure. Specific findings are discussed under diagnostic headings.

The first heart sound ($S_1$) may be diminished with severe left ventricular dysfunction or accentuated in mitral stenosis or short PR intervals. $S_2$ is usually split, at least in younger individuals, with the 2 components (aortic preceding pulmonary) being separated more during inspiration; splitting is fixed in atrial septal defect, wide with right bundle branch block, and absent or reversed with aortic stenosis, left ventricular failure, or left bundle branch block. With normal splitting, an accentuated $P_2$ is an important sign of pulmonary hypertension. Third and fourth heart sounds (ventricular and atrial gallops, respectively) indicate ventricular volume overload or impaired compliance and may be heard over either ventricle. The $S_3$ is a normal finding in younger individuals and in pregnancy. Additional auscultatory findings include sharp, high-pitched sounds classified as "clicks." These may be early systolic and represent ejection sounds (as with a bicuspid aortic valve or pulmonary stenosis) or may occur in mid or late systole, indicating myxomatous changes in the mitral valve.

While many heart murmurs indicate valvular disease, a soft, short systolic murmur, usually localized along the left sternal border or toward the apex, may be innocent, reflecting pulmonary flow. Systolic murmurs are classified as pansystolic (holosystolic) when they merge with the first sound and persist through all of systole or as "ejection" murmurs when they begin after the first sound, end before the second sound, and peak in early or mid systole (diamond-shaped). The former usually represent mitral regurgitation if maximal at the apex or in the axilla, or tricuspid regurgitation if best heard at the sternal border. Ejection murmurs which are maximal at the aortic area of the apex usually are caused by aortic flow, while those localized over the pulmonary area are caused by flow through that valve. Louder systolic murmurs and association of murmurs with palpable vibrations ("thrills") are clinically significant as are all diastolic murmurs.

## LABORATORY TESTING

The chest radiograph will provide information about heart size, the pulmonary circulation (with characteristic signs suggesting both pulmonary artery or pulmonary venous hypertension), primary pulmonary disease, and aortic abnormalities. The echocardiogram has replaced the radiograph in Western countries in the assessment of individual chamber size and valvular disease. The electrocardiogram (ECG) remains a standard part of cardiac evaluation, indicating cardiac rhythm and revealing conduction abnormalities and evidence of ventricular hypertrophy, myocardial infarction, or ischemia. Nonspecific ST segment and T wave changes may reflect these processes but are also noted with electrolyte imbalance, drug effects, and many other conditions.

## SPECIAL DIAGNOSTIC TESTS

### Echocardiography

Despite its cost, echocardiography has become the most readily available and clincially useful diagnostic aid for most cardiovascular diseases. **M-mode echocardiography** yields quantitative measurements of left ventricular size, function, and thickness and qualitative information about aortic and mitral stenosis. It may be diagnostic for hypertrophic cardiomyopathy, pericardial effusion, mitral valve prolapse, valvular vegetations, and cardiac tumors. **Two dimensional echocardiograms** visualize more of the heart. Left ventricular segmental wall motion can be assessed, and the size of both atria and the right ventricle can be determined. Absolute valve areas can be measured. **Doppler ultrasound** now permits the qualitative assessment of valvular regurgitation, an assessment of pulmonary artery pressure, and measurement of transvalvular gradients.

Belkin RN, Kisslo J: Clinical applications of echocardiography in myocardial and valvular heart disease. *Prog Cardiovasc Dis* 1986;**29**:81.

### Exercise Electrocardiography

The resting ECG is often insensitive for ischemic heart disease, but exercise-induced ST segment depression, particularly when it exceeds 0.1 mV and is of horizontal or downsloping configuration, is strongly suggestive of ischemia. Exercise-induced chest pain and hypotension also suggest coronary disease, and changes occurring at low levels of exercise suggest more severe disease. Overall, exercise testing has a sensitivity of 60–80% and a specificity of 80–

90%. This procedure helps to diagnose or exclude disease, to estimate its severity, and to provide guidelines for activity in patients with known ischemic heart disease. Exercise testing may also be useful to assess arrhythmia and to quantify exercise capacity in heart disease not involving the coronary arteries.

## Ambulatory Electrocardiographic (Holter) Monitoring

Holter monitoring is most useful for determining the need for therapy in patients with symptoms consistent with dysrhythmia. Since these symptoms are often nonspecific, their temporal association with a conduction abnormality or rhythm disturbance provides a definitive indication for treatment. Documentation of asymptomatic "premonitory" abnormalities such as second-degree atrioventricular block, transient sinus node arrest, or nonsustained ventricular tachycardia is also possible. Ambulatory monitoring may assess the benefit of treatment, but its use in the evaluation of asymptomatic individuals should be limited. There is growing interest in the use of this technique for diagnosing harmless ischemia by ST segment shifts, but this also is best limited to patients with known coronary disease.

## Radionuclide Techniques

Several nuclear medicine studies are useful in the assessment of heart disease.

**Thallium-201 scintigraphy** demonstrates relative myocardial perfusion. It is most commonly employed in conjunction with exercise testing to detect ischemia, which appears as a perfusion defect. After 3–24 hours, the defect will fill in or "redistribute" if it reflects reversible ischemia but will remain fixed in regions of infarction. Thallium scintigraphy following dipyridamole-induced vasodilatation provides similar information in patients unable to exercise. The sensitivity and specificity of this technique are superior to those of exercise electrocardiography, but its expense limits its use to situations in which ordinary exercise testing needs corroboration or is not accurate (eg, bundle branch block, digitalis effect, baseline repolarization changes). Tomographic techniques have slightly improved the accuracy of thallium scintigraphy.

**Radionuclide angiography** provides accurate measurements of left and, in some laboratories, right ventricular ejection fractions. Segmental wall motion may be examined, and semiquantitative estimates of valvular regurgitation are possible. Radionuclide angiography may be performed during exercise, so that changes in global or segmental left ventricular function can be employed to diagnose ischemia or impaired functional reserve. Thallium scintigraphy is a more accurate test for evaluating ischemic heart disease. Radionuclide angiography can also be used to quantify the pulmonary-to-systemic flow ratio in left-to-right shunts. Ratios have 1.3–1.5 can be accurately detected.

**Technetium-99m pyrophosphate scintigraphy** produces radiotracer uptake in areas of recent infarction. Its usefulness is limited by an 18- to 24-hour lag time after acute infarction before the test becomes positive and a limited sensitivity for small, especially nontransmural infarctions. This technique is most useful when the ECG and cardiac enzymes are nondiagnostic, such as after cardiac surgery or when chest pain has occurred more than 48 hours prior to assessment.

## Newer Imaging Modalities

Many new imaging techniques have been developed, but their application in cardiovascular disease remains to be determined. **Computed tomography (CT scan)** can image the heart and, with contrast medium, the vascular system, but the relatively slow speed of most instruments limits its utility. The main applications of CT scan appear to be evaluation of aortic dissection, pericardial disease, and bypass graft patency, though the images are often suboptimal in the latter condition. **Ultrafast** or **cine CT** involves a specially designed instrument with high temporal resolution. Its availability is limited, but early reports indicate that it will provide accurate assessment of cardiac size and function and bypass graft patency and perhaps useful data on myocardial perfusion. **Digital subtraction angiography,** a once promising technique, has proved to be chiefly an adjunct to cardiac catheterization.

**Magnetic resonance imaging (MRI)** is an expensive evolving modality that provides high-resolution images of the heart and vascular bed without radiation exposure or use of contrast media. It provides excellent anatomic definition, permitting assessment of pericardial disease, myocardial thickness, and chamber size and of many congenital heart defects. The impact of MRI will increase if assessment of tissue metabolism becomes feasible.

**Positron emission tomography (PET)** can provide both qualitative and quantitative information concerning myocardial metabolism and blood flow, but its availability is limited, and a nearby cyclotron is required for most applications. Recent data indicate that PET can accurately distinguish between myocardium which is transiently dysfunctional ("stunned") due to ischemia and infarcted myocardium—a distinction that is important in considering revascularization.

## Cardiac Catheterization

**Right heart catheterization** is convenient to perform and allows measurement of right atrial, right ventricular, pulmonary artery, and pulmonary capillary wedge pressures (the latter an indicator of left atrial pressure), oxygen saturation, and cardiac output. These data are vital in the management of critically ill patients and may diagnose intracardiac shunts, physiologically signficant pericardial disease, and right-sided valve lesions and can distinguish between cardiac and pulmonary disease.

**Left heart catheterization** permits quantitative assessment of mitral and aortic stenosis. With contrast angiography, valvular regurgitation and global and regional left ventricular function can be examined. Its main application is to produce selective coronary arteriograms.

Despite the increasing capability of noninvasive investigations, cardiac catheterization remains the standard against which most of them are evaluated. With the advent of coronary angioplasty and balloon valvuloplasty, the catheterization laboratory has become a major source of therapeutic intervention as well.

### Electrophysiologic Testing

Intracardiac electrocardiographic recording and stimulation studies have revolutionized the diagnosis and treatment of severe arrhythmias. Electrophysiologic testing is important for evaluating unexplained syncope or presyncope. The location and severity of atrioventricular conduction disturbances and sinus node dysfunction can be assessed in symptomatic patients in whom diagnostic information cannot be obtained by ambulatory monitoring. The mechnism and optimal therapy of complex supraventricular arrhythmias—particularly those associated with accessory conduction pathways—can be elucidated. The commonest procedure has become ventricular stimulation to induce ventricular tachycardia, which in some settings may provide specific diagnostic information and guide subsequent treatment. The value of this procedure in asymptomatic patients has not been confirmed.

---

# CONGENITAL HEART DISEASES

---

Congenital lesions account for only about 2% of heart disease in adults. Following corrective surgery, many patients are symptom-free, but few are completely normal. They may develop cardiac arrhythmias or conduction defects, cardiac failure, and infective endocarditis and often show residual defects.

The reader is referred to the references below for full discussions.

Graham TP Jr (chairman): Fourteenth Bethesda Conference Report: Noninvasive diagnostic instrumentation in the assessment of cardiovascular disease in the young. *J Am Coll Cardiol* 1985;**5(Suppl):**1. [Entire issue].

Reeder GS et al: Use of Doppler techniques (continuous-wave, pulsed-wave, and color flow imaging) in the noninvasive hemodynamic assessment of congenital heart disease. *Mayo Clin Proc* 1986;**61:**725.

## PULMONARY STENOSIS

Stenosis of the pulmonary valve or infundibulum increases the resistance to outflow, raises the right ventricular pressure, and limits pulmonary blood flow. In the absence of associated shunts, arterial saturation is normal, but severe stenosis causes peripheral cyanosis by reducing cardiac output. Clubbing and polycythemia do not develop unless a patent foramen ovale or atrial septal defect is present, permitting right-to-left shunting.

### Clinical Findings

**A. Symptoms and Signs:** Mild cases (right ventricular-pulmonary artery gradient < 50 mm Hg) are asymptomatic. Moderate to severe stenosis (gradients > 80 mm Hg) may cause dyspnea on exertion, syncope, chest pain, and eventually right ventricular failure.

There is a palpable right ventricular heave. A loud, harsh systolic murmur and a prominent thrill are present in the left second and third interspaces parasternally; the murmur is in the third and fourth interspaces in infundibular stenosis. The second sound is obscured by the murmur in severe cases; the pulmonary component is diminished, delayed, or absent. Both components are audible in mild cases. A right-sided $S_4$ and a prominent *a* wave in the venous pulse are present in severe cases.

**B. Imaging:** Heart size may be normal on radiographs, or there may be a prominent right ventricle and atrium or gross cardiac enlargement, depending upon the severity. There is often poststenotic dilatation of the pulmonary artery. Pulmonary vascularity is normal or diminished. Echocardiography usually demonstrates the anatomic abnormality and assesses right ventricular size and function. Doppler ultrasound can measure the gradient accurately, which is usually confirmed by cardiac catheterization.

**C. Electrocardiographic Findings:** Right axis deviation or right ventricular hypertrophy is noted; peaked P waves provide evidence of right atrial overload.

### Treatment

Pure pulmonary stenosis with evidence of progressive hypertrophy and resting gradients of over 75–80 mm Hg may be treated surgically, with an operative mortality rate of 3–4% and excellent long-term results in most cases. Percutaneous balloon valvuloplasty has proved successful and may become the treatment of choice.

### Prognosis

Patients with mild stenosis may have normal life expectancy. Severe stenosis is associated with sudden death and can cause refractory heart failure in the 20s and 30s. Moderate stenosis may be asymptomatic in childhood and adolescence, but symptoms increase as patients become older.

## COARCTATION OF THE AORTA

Coarctation of the aorta consists of localized narrowing of the aortic arch just distal to the origin of the left subclavian artery. A bicuspid aortic valve is present in 25% of cases. Blood pressure is elevated in the aorta and its branches proximal to the coarctation and decreased distally. Collateral circulation develops through the intercostal arteries and branches of the subclavian arteries.

### Clinial Findings

**A. Symptoms and Signs:** There are no symptoms until the hypertension produces left ventricular failure or cerebral hemorrhage; the latter may also occur from associated cerebral aneurysms. Strong arterial pulsations are seen in the neck and suprasternal notch. Hyptertension is present in the arms, but the pressure is normal or low in the legs. This difference is exaggerated by exercise. Femoral pulsations are weak and are delayed in comparison with the brachial pulse. Patients with large collaterals may have relatively small gradients but still have severe coarctation. Late systolic ejection murmurs at the base are often heard better posteriorly, especially over the spinous processes. There may be an associated aortic insufficiency murmur due to a bicuspid aortic valve.

**B. Imaging:** Radiography shows scalloping of the ribs due to enlarged collateral intercostal arteries, dilatation of the left subclavian artery and poststenotic aortic dilatation, and left ventricular enlargement. Measurement of the gradient across the lesion by catheterization and aortography remain the primary methods of diagnosis. Doppler ultrasound can also estimate the severity of obstruction.

**C. Electrocardiographic Findings:** The ECG usually shows left ventricular hypertrophy; it may be normal in mild cases.

### Treatment

Resection of the coarcted site has a surgical mortality rate near 1–4%. The risks of the disease are such, however, that all coarctations in patients up to age 20 years should be resected. In patients under 40 years of age, surgery is advisable if the patient has refractory hypertension or significant left ventricular hypertrophy. The surgical mortality rate rises considerably in patients over age 50 and is of doubtful value. Balloon angioplasty of the stenosis has been accomplished successfully and may become the procedure of choice, but aortic tears have been described; these have lessened with the use of 2 small balloons rather than one large balloon.

### Prognosis

Cardiac failure is common in infancy and in older untreated patients; it is uncommon in late childhood and young adulthood. Most untreated patients with the adult form of coarctation die before age 40 from the complications of hypertension, rupture of the aorta, infective endarteritis, or cerebral hemorrhage (congenital aneurysms). About one-fourth of patients continue to be hypertensive years after surgery, and they have all the complications associated with hypertension. However, 25% have a normal cardiovascular prognosis and die of causes unrelated to the coarctation. Aortic dissection also occurs with increased frequency in coarctation.

Cooper RS et al: Angioplasty for coarctation of the aorta: Long-term results. *Circulation* 1987;**75**:600.

## ATRIAL SEPTAL DEFECT

The most common form of atrial septal defect (80% of cases) is persistence of the ostium secundum in the mid septum; less commonly, the ostium primum (which is low in the septum) persists, in which case mitral or tricuspid abnormalities may also be present. A third form is the sinus venosus defect of the upper part of the septum. This is often associated with partial anomalous drainage of the pulmonary veins into the superior vena cava. In all cases, normally oxygenated blood from the left atrium passes into the right atrium, increasing right ventricular output and pulmonary blood flow.

### Clinical Findings

**A. Symptoms and Signs:** Most patients with moderate secundum defects are asymptomatic. With large shunts, exertional dyspnea or cardiac failure may develop. Prominent right ventricular pulsations are readily visible and palpable. A moderately loud systolic ejection murmur can be heard in the second and third interspaces parasternally as a result of increased pulmonary artery flow. $S_2$ is widely split and does not vary with breathing.

**B. Imaging:** The chest radiograph shows large pulmonary arteries (with vigorous pulsations fluoroscopically), increased pulmonary vascularity, an enlarged right atrium and ventricle, and a small aortic knob. Echocardiography can demonstrate right ventricular volume overload with a large right ventricle and atrium, and sometimes the defect itself. Echocardiography with contrast and Doppler flow studies can demonstrate shunting and increased pulmonary flow. Radionuclide flow studies quantify left-to-right shunting, and MRI can also elucidate the anatomy. Cardiac catheterization remains the definitive diagnostic procedure, since it can demonstrate an oxygen saturation "step-up," quantify the shunt, and measure pulmonary vascular resistance.

**C. Electrocardiographic Findings:** Right axis or right ventricular hypertrophy may be present in ostium secundum defects. Incomplete or complete right bundle branch block is present in nearly all cases of atrial septal defect, and superior axis deviation is noted in ostium primum defect. With sinus venosus defects, the P axis is leftward of +15 degrees.

### Treatment

Small atrial septal defects do not require surgery.

The risks are now sufficiently low so that patients with pulmonary to systemic flow ratios between 1.5 and 2.0 may be operated on if the total clinical picture warrants. Ratios exceeding 2.0 are an indication for surgical closure of the defect.

Surgery should be withheld from patients with pulmonary hypertension with reversed shunt because of the risk of acute right heart failure. Relocation of pulmonary veins is required in patients with partial anomalous venous drainage. In ostium primum defects, in addition to closure of the defect, suture of the valve clefts—especially those of the mitral valve— is advisable if mitral regurgitation of any significant degree is present.

## Prognosis

Patients with small shunts may live a normal life span. Large shunts cause disability by age 40. Raised pulmonary vascular resistance secondary to pulmonary hypertension rarely occurs in childhood or young adult life in secundum defects but is more common in primum defects; after age 40, pulmonary hypertension, cardiac arrhythmias, and left ventricular failure may occur in secundum defects. Infective endocarditis does not occur with increased frequency.

The surgical mortality rate is low (< 1%) in patients under age 45, those who are not in cardiac failure, those who have pulmonary artery pressures less than 60 mm Hg. It increases to 5–10% in patients over age 40, with cardiac failure, or with pulmonary artery pressures greater than 60 mm Hg. Most survivors show considerable improvement.

Shub C et al: Sensitivity of two-dimensional echocardiography in the direct visualization of atrial septal defect utilizing the subcostal approach: Experience with 154 patients. *J Am Coll Cardiol* 1983;**2:**127.

## PATENT DUCTUS ARTERIOSUS

The embryonic ductus arteriosus fails to close normally and persists as a shunt connecting the left pulmonary artery and aorta, usually near the origin of the left subclavian artery. Blood flows continuously from the aorta through the ductus into the pulmonary artery in both systole and diastole; the defect is a form of arteriovenous fistula, increasing the work of the left ventricle. In some patients, obliterative changes in the pulmonary arterioles cause pulmonary hypertension. Then the shunt is bidirectional or right-to-left (Eisenmenger's syndrome). This complication does not correlate with shunt size.

### Clinical Findings

**A. Symptoms and Signs:** There are no symptoms unless left ventricular failure develops. The heart is of normal size or slightly enlarged, with a hyperdynamic apical impulse. The pulse pressure is wide, and diastolic pressure is low. A continuous rough "machinery" murmur, accentuated in late systole

at the time of $S_2$, is heard best in the left first and second interspaces at the left sternal border. Thrills are common.

**B. Imaging:** On chest radiographs, the heart is normal in size and contour, or there may be left ventricular and left atrial enlargement. The pulmonary artery, aorta, and left atrium are prominent. Cardiac catheterization establishes the presence and severity of a left-to-right shunt; angiography can define its anatomy. The magnitude of the shunt can also be determined by radionuclide flow studies, and the pulmonary artery pressure can be estimated by Doppler ultrasound, while left ventricular and atrial size is assessed by echocardiography.

**C. Electrocardiographic Findings:** A normal pattern or left ventricular hypertrophy is found, depending upon the magnitude of shunting.

### Treatment

Surgical correction rather than medical treatment is recommended for children or adults with symptoms or large shunts. Asymptomatic adults with no left ventricular hypertrophy and small left-to-right shunts are at low risk of developing complications such as pulmonary hypertension or congestive heart failure, and surgery may not be indicated. The indications for ligation or division of a patent ductus arteriosus in the presence of pulmonary hypertension are controversial. Opinion favors ligation whenever the pulmonary vascular resistance is low and the flow through the ductus is from left to right.

Large shunts cause a high mortality rate from cardiac failure early in life. Smaller shunts are compatible with long survival, congestive heart failure being the most common complication. Infective endocarditis or endarteritis may also occur. A small percentage of patients develop pulmonary hypertension and reversal of shunt, such that the lower legs, especially the toes, appear cyanotic and clubbed in contrast to normally pink fingers. At this stage, the patient is inoperable.

## VENTRICULAR SEPTAL DEFECT

In this lesion, a persistent opening in the upper interventricular septum resulting from failure of fusion with the aortic septum permits blood to pass from the high-pressure left ventricle into the low-pressure right ventricle. The subsequent natural history and pathophysiology depend on the size of the defect and the magnitude of left-to-right shunting. Large defects are associated with early left ventricular failure. Chronic but more moderate left-to-right shunts may led to pulmonary vascular disease and right-sided failure. Many ventricular defects close spontaneously in early childhood.

### Clinical Findings

**A. Symptoms and Signs:** The clinical features are dependent upon the size of the defect and the presence or absence of a raised pulmonary vascular resistance. Large shunts are associated with loud, harsh holosystolic murmurs in the left third and fourth interspaces along the sternum and in some cases mid-diastolic flow murmurs and an $S_3$ at the apex. Smaller shunts may produce only an early systolic murmur or a diamond-shaped murmur. A systolic thrill is common. Clinical evidence of pulmonary hypertension is often more informative than the murmur itself. High defects may be associated with aortic regurgitation owing to prolapse of a valve leaflet.

**B. Imaging:** With large shunts, the right or left ventricle (or both), the left atrium, and the pulmonary arteries are enlarged, and pulmonary vascularity is increased on chest radiographs. If pulmonary vascular disease evolves, an enlarged pulmonary artery with diminished distal vascularity is seen. Echocardiography can demonstrate chamber size and may demonstrate the defect. Doppler ultrasound can qualitatively assess the magnitude of shunting and the pulmonary artery pressure. Magnetic resonance imaging can often visualize the defect, while radionuclide flow studies quantify pulmonary-to-systemic flow ratios. Cardiac catheterization permits definitive diagnosis in all but the most trivial defects; it is the only technique that can measure pulmonary vascular resistance.

**C. Electrocardiographic Findings:** The ECG may be normal or may show right, left, or biventricular hypertrophy, depending on the size of the defect and the pulmonary vascular resistance.

Ventricular septal defects vary in severity from trivial asymptomatic lesions with normal cardiac hemodynamics to extensive lesions causing death from cardiac failure in infancy. The former do not require surgery. Defects causing large shunts should be repaired to prevent irreversible pulmonary vascular disease or late heart failure. When severe pulmonary hypertension is present (pulmonary arterial pressures > 85 mm Hg) and the left-to-right shunt is small, the surgical mortality risk is at least 50%. If the shunt is reversed, surgery is contraindicated. If surgery is required because of unrelenting cardiac failure in infancy due to a large left-to-right shunt, early closure of the defect is now the preferred procedure. The surgical mortality rate is 2–3% for primary repair. Some defects (perhaps as many as 30%) close spontaneously. Therefore, surgery should be deferred until late childhood unless the disability is severe or unless pulmonary hypertension is observed to progress or to develop.

**Prognosis**

Patients with the typical murmur as the only abnormality have a normal life expectancy except for the threat of infective endocarditis. The latter is more typical of smaller shunts. With large shunts, congestive heart failure may develop early in life, and survival beyond age 40 is unusual. Shunt reversal occurs in an estimated 25%, producing Eisenmenger's syndrome.

Blake RS et al: Conduction defects, ventricular arrhythmias, and late death after surgical closure of ventricular septal defect. *Br Heart J* 1982;**47**:305.

# ACUTE RHEUMATIC FEVER & RHEUMATIC HEART DISEASE

Rheumatic fever is a systemic immune process which is a sequela to hemolytic streptococcal infection. It may be self-limiting or may lead to slowly progressive valvular deformity. Rheumatic fever is the most common precursor of heart disease in people under age 50 years in less developed countries, but it has become uncommon in the USA. The peak incidence is between ages 5 and 15; rheumatic fever is rare before age 4 and after age 40. The characteristic lesion is a perivascular granulomatous reaction with vasculitis. The mitral valve is attacked in 75–80% of cases, the aortic valve in 30%, and the tricuspid and pulmonary valves in under 5%. Healing may be complete, or progressive scarring may develop.

**Clinical Findings**

**A. Major Criteria:**

**1. Carditis**—Carditis is most likely to be evident in children and adolescents. Any of the following signs establishes the presence of carditis. (1) Pericarditis, uncommon in adults and diagnosed by detection of a friction rub or evidence of effusion by echocardiogram. (2) Cardiomegaly, detected by physical signs, radiography, or echocardiography. (3) Congestive failure, right- or left-sided—the former perhaps more prominent in children, with painful liver engorgement due to tricuspid regurgitation. (4) Mitral or aortic regurgitation murmurs, indicative of dilatation of a valve ring with or without associated valvulitis. The Carey-Coombs short middiastolic mitral murmur should be sought.

In the absence of any of the above definitive signs, the diagnosis of carditis depends upon the following less specific abnormalities. (1) Electrocardiographic changes: The most significant abnormality in PR prolongation greater than 0.04 s above the patient's normal. Changing contour of P waves or inversion of T waves is less specific. (2) Changing quality of heart sounds. (3) Sinus tachycardia persisting during sleep and markedly increased by slight activity. (4) Arrhythmias, shifting pacemaker, ectopic beats.

**2. Erythema marginatum and subcutaneous nodules**—The former begin as rapidly enlarging macules that assume the shape of rings or crescents with clear centers. They may be raised, confluent, and either transient or persistent.

Subcutaneous nodules are uncommon except in children. The nodules are usually small (2 cm or less in diameter), firm, and nontender and are attached to fascia or tendon sheaths over bony prominences. They persist for days or weeks, are usually recurrent, and are clinically indistinguishable from the nodules of rheumatoid arthritis.

**3. Sydenham's chorea**–Sydenham's chorea may occur suddenly and may be the only clinically apparent manifestation; half of cases have other overt signs of rheumatic fever. Girls are more frequently affected, and occurrence in adults is rare. This is the least common (3% of cases) but most diagnostic of the manifestations of rheumatic fever.

**4. Arthritis** This is a migratory polyarthritis that involves the large joints sequentially. In adults, only a single joint may be affected. The acute arthritis lasts 1–5 weeks and usually subsides without residual deformity. Prompt response of arthritis to therapeutic doses of salicylates is characteristic.

**B. Minor Criteria:** These include fever, polyarthralgias, reversible prolongation of the PR interval, rapid erthyrocyte sedimentation rate, evidence of an antecedent β-hemolytic streptococcal infection, or a history of rheumatic fever.

**C. Laboratory Findings:** There is nonspecific evidence of inflammatory disease, as shown by a rapid sedimentation rate. High or increasing titers of antistreptococcal antibodies, especially antistreptolysin O (ASO), are used to confirm recent infection; 10% of cases lack this serologic evidence.

## Differential Diagnosis

Rheumatic fever may be confused with the following: rheumatoid arthritis, osteomyelitis, infective endocarditis, chronic meningococcemia, disseminated lupus erythematosus, Lyme disease, sickle cell anemia, inactive rheumatic heart disease, congenital heart disease, "surgical abdomen," and many other diseases.

## Complications

Congestive heart failure, often due to acute mitral regurgitation, occurs in severe cases. In the longer term, the development of rheumatic heart disease is the major problem. Other complications include cardiac arrhythmias, pericarditis with effusion, and rheumatic pneumonitis.

## Treatment
### A. Medical Measures:

**1. Salicylates**–The salicylates markedly reduce fever and relieve joint pain and swelling. They have no effect on the natural course of the disease. Adults may require 0.6–0.9 g every 4 hours; children are treated with lower doses. Toxicity includes tinnitus, vomiting, and gastrointestinal bleeding.

**2. Penicillin**–Penicillin should be employed to eradicate streptococcal infection if present.

**3. Corticosteroids**–There is no proof that cardiac damage is prevented or minimized by corticosteroids. Corticosteroids are effective anti-inflammatory agents for reversing the acute exudative phase of rheumatic fever and are probably more potent for this

purpose than salicylates. A short course of corticosteroids usually causes rapid improvement and may be indicated in severe cases.

**B. General Measures:** Bed rest should be enforced until all signs of active rheumatic fever have disappeared. The criteria for this are as follows: return of temperature to normal with the patient at bed rest and without medications; normal sedimentation rate; normal resting pulse rate (< 100/min in adults); and return of ECG to normal or reversed abnormalities.

## Prevention of Recurrent Rheumatic Fever

The goals of prevention are to avoid β-hemolytic streptococcal infections if possible and to treat streptococcal infections promptly and intensively.

**A. Penicillin:** The preferred method of prophylaxis is with benzathine penicillin G, 1.2 million units intramuscularly every 4 weeks. Oral penicillin (200,000–250,000 units daily before breakfast) is less reliable. Prophylaxis is advocated especially for children who have had one or more acute attacks and should be given through the school years and continued until about age 25. Adults should receive preventive therapy for about 5 years after an attack or until about age 30.

**B. Sulfonamides or Erythromycin:** If the patient is allergic to penicillin, sulfadiazine, 1 g daily throughout the year, may be substituted, as may erythromycin, 250 mg orally twice daily.

## Prognosis

Initial episodes of rheumatic fever last months in children and weeks in adults. Twenty percent of children have recurrences within 5 years. Recurrences are uncommon after 5 years of well-being and infrequent after age 21. The immediate mortality rate is 1–2%. Persistent rheumatic activity with cardiomegaly, heart failure, and pericarditis imply a poor prognosis; 30% of children thus affected die within 10 years after the initial attack. Otherwise, the prognosis for life is good. Eighty percent of all patients attain adult life, and half of these have little if any limitation of activity. After 10 years, two-thirds of surviving patients will have detectable valvular disease. In adults, residual heart damage occurs in less than 20%, with mitral insufficiency the commonest; aortic insufficiency is more common than in children. In underdeveloped countries, acute rheumatic fever appears earlier in life, and the evolution to chronic valvular disease is accelerated, because of the frequency of recurrent streptococcal infections and the consequent recrudescences of rheumatic fever.

Gotsman MS: Rheumatic fever in the 80's. (Two parts.) *Cardiovasc Rev Rep* 1985;**6**:861, 935.

## RHEUMATIC HEART DISEASE

Chronic rheumatic heart disease results from single or repeated attacks of rheumatic fever that produce rigidity and deformity of the cusps, fusion of the commissures, or shortening and fusion of the chordae tendineae. Stenosis or insufficiency results, and the two often coexist, although one or the other predominates. The mitral valve alone is affected in 50–60% of cases; combined lesions of the aortic and mitral valves occur in 20%; pure aortic lesions are seen in only 10%. Tricuspid involvement occurs only in association with mitral or aortic disease in about 10% of cases. The pulmonary valve is rarely affected. A history of rheumatic fever is obtainable in only 60% of patients with rheumatic heart disease.

The first clue to organic valvular disease is a murmur. Physical examination permits accurate diagnosis of most valve lesions. Echocardiography will reveal thickened valves of decreased area in stenosis, estimate the magnitude of regurgitation, and demonstrate the earliest stages of specific chamber enlargement.

Recurrences of acute rheumatic fever can be prevented (see above). The patient should also be advised about prophylactic antibiotics preceding dental extraction, urologic and surgical procedures, etc, to prevent bacteremia and possible infective endocarditis. Once a valvular abnormality is identified, regular follow-up at yearly or more frequent intervals is necessary. Follow-up observations should emphasize maintenance of general health, avoidance of smoking and obesity, and excessive physical exertion. It is important to identify the onset of atrial fibrillation in order to institute anticoagulation and to assess the need for valve surgery at the appropriate time (see next section for discussion of specific lesions).

The important findings in each of the major valve lesions are summarized in Table 8–1. The hemodynamic changes, symptoms, associated findings, and course are discussed below.

## VALVULAR HEART DISEASE

While most cases of valvular disease were at one time due to rheumatic heart disease (still true in underdeveloped countries), other causes are now more common. The typical findings of each lesion are described in Fig 8–1 and Table 8–1.

### MITRAL STENOSIS

Nearly all patients with mitral stenosis have underlying rheumatic heart disease, though a history of rheumatic fever is often absent.

#### Clinical Findings

**A. Symptoms and Signs:** A characteristic finding of mitral stenosis is a localized middiastolic murmur low in pitch whose duration varies with the severity of the stenosis and the heart rate (Table 8–1). Because it is thickened, the valve opens in early diastole with an opening snap. The sound is sharp, is widely distributed over the chest, and occurs early after $A_2$ in severe and later in milder varieties of mitral stenosis. In severe mitral stenosis with low flow across the mitral valve, the murmur may be soft and difficult to find, but the opening snap can usually be heard. If the patient has both mitral stenosis and mitral insufficiency, the dominant features may be the systolic murmur of mitral regurgitation with or without a short diastolic murmur and a delayed opening snap.

When the valve has narrowed to less than 1.5 $cm^2$ (normal, 4 $cm^2$), the left atrial pressure must rise to maintain normal flow across the valve and a normal cardiac output. This results in a pressure difference between the left atrium and left ventricle during diastole. The pressure gradient and the length of the diastolic murmur reflect the severity of mitral stenosis; they persist throughout diastole when the lesion is severe or when the ventricular rate is rapid.

In mild cases, left atrial pressure and cardiac output may be essentially normal and the patient asymptomatic, but in moderate stenosis (valve area < 1.5 $cm^2$)—especially with tachycardia, which increases mitral flow—dyspnea and fatigue appear as the left atrial pressure rises. With severe stenosis, the left atrial pressure is high enough to produce pulmonary venous congestion at rest and reduce cardiac output, with resulting fatigue and right heart failure. Recumbency at night further increases the pulmonary blood volume, causing orthopnea, paroxysmal nocturnal dyspnea, or actual transudation of fluid into the alveoli, leading to acute pulmonary edema. Severe pulmonary congestion may also be initiated by any acute respiratory infection, excessive salt and fluid intake, infective endocarditis, or recurrence of rheumatic carditis. As a result of long-standing pulmonary venous hypertension, anastomoses develop between the pulmonary and bronchial veins in the form of bronchial submucosal varices. These often rupture, producing mild or severe hemoptysis.

Fifty to 80% of patients develop paroxysmal or chronic atrial fibrillation that, until the venticular rate is controlled, may precipitate dyspnea or pulmonary edema. Twenty to 30% of these patients will later have major emboli in the cerebral, visceral, or peripheral arteries as a consequence of thrombus formation in the left atrium.

In a few patients, the pulmonary arterioles become narrowed; this greatly increases the pulmonary artery pressure and accelerates the development of right ventricular hypertrophy and failure. These patients have relatively little dyspnea but experience fatigue on exertion.

**B. Imaging:** Echocardiography is the most valuable technique for assessing mitral stenosis. The valve is thickened, opens poorly, and closes slowly. The anterior and posterior leaflets are fixed and move together, rather than in opposite directions. Left atrial

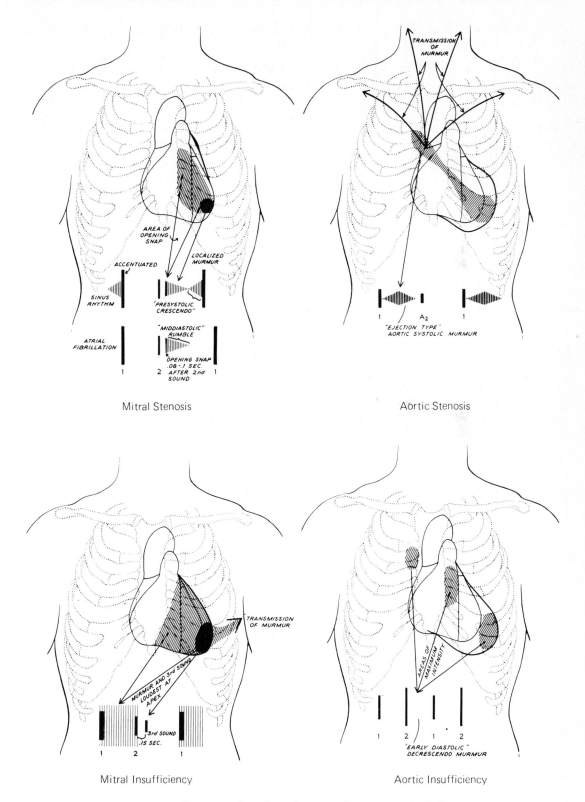

**Figure 8–1.** Murmurs and cardiac enlargement in common valve lesions.

**Table 8–1.** Differential diagnosis of rheumatic heart disease.

| | Mitral Stenosis | Mitral Insufficiency | Aortic Stenosis | Aortic Insufficiency | Tricuspid Stenosis | Tricuspid Insufficiency |
|---|---|---|---|---|---|---|
| Inspection | Malar flush, precordial bulge and diffuse pulsation in young patients. | Usually forceful apical impulse to left of MCL. | Localized heaving PMI. Carotid pulsations weak, exhibiting slow rise. | Generalized pallor. Strong, abrupt carotid pulsations. Forceful PMI to left of MCL and down. Capillary pulsations. | Giant a wave in jugular pulse with sinus rhythm. Often olive-colored skin (mixed jaundice and local cyanosis). | Large v wave in jugular pulse. |
| Palpation | "Tapping" sensation over area of expected PMI. Middiastolic and/or presystolic thrill at apex. Small pulse. Right ventricular pulsation left third to fifth ICS parasternally when pulmonary hypertension is present. | Forceful, brisk PMI; systolic thrill over PMI. Pulse normal, small, or slightly collapsing. | Powerful, heaving localized PMI to left of MCL and slightly down. Systolic thrill over aortic area (best felt with patient leaning forward, breath held in maximum expiration). Plateau pulse, small and slowly rising; best appreciated in the carotid pulse. | Apical impulse forceful and displaced significantly to left and down. Water-hammer pulses. | Middiastolic thrill between lower left sternal border and PMI. Presystolic pulsation of liver (sinus rhythm only). | Right ventricular pulsation. Occasionally systolic thrill at lower left sternal edge. Systolic pulsation of liver. |
| Percussion | Dullness in left third ICS parasternally. ACD normal or slightly enlarged to left only. | ACD increased to left of MCL and slightly down. | ACD slightly enlarged to left and down. | Definite cardiac enlargement to left and down. | | Usually cardiac enlargement to left and right. |
| Heart sounds, rhythm, and blood pressure | Loud snapping $M_1$. Opening snap along left sternal border or at apex. Atrial fibrillation common. Blood pressure normal. | $M_1$ normal or buried in murmur. Third heart sound. Delayed opening snap occasionally present. Atrial fibrillation common. Blood pressure normal. | $A_2$ normal, or delayed and weak; may be absent. Blood pressure normal or systolic pressure normal with high diastolic level. Ejection click occasionally present just preceding murmur. | Sounds normal or $A_2$ loud. Wide pulse pressure with diastolic pressure < 60 mm Hg. | $M_1$ often loud. | Atrial fibrillation usually present. |
| Murmurs: Location and transmission | Sharply localized at or near apex. Graham Steell murmur along lower left sternal border in severe pulmonary hypertension. | Loudest over PMI; transmitted to left axilla, left infrascapular area. | Right second ICS parasternally and/or at apex; heard in carotids and occasionally in upper interscapular area. | Loudest along left sternal border in third to fourth interspace. Heard over aortic area and apex. | Third to fifth ICS along left sternal border out to apex. | As for tricuspid stenosis. |
| Timing | Onset at opening snap ("middiastolic") with presystolic accentuation if in sinus rhythm. Graham Steell begins with $P_2$ (immediate diastolic). | Pansystolic: begins with $M_1$ and ends at or after $A_2$. | Midsystolic: begins after $M_1$, ends before $A_2$, reaches maximum intensity in mid systole. | Begins immediately after aortic second sound and ends before first sound. | As for mitral stenosis. | As for mitral insufficiency. |
| Character | Low-pitched, rumbling; presystolic murmur merges with loud $M_1$ in a "crescendo." Graham Steell high-pitched, blowing. | Blowing, high-pitched; occasionally harsh or musical. | Harsh, rough. | Blowing, often faint. | As for mitral stenosis. | Blowing, coarse, or musical. |

| | | | | | | |
|---|---|---|---|---|---|---|
| **Optimum auscultatory conditions** | After exercise, left lateral recumbency. Bell chest piece lightly applied. | | Patient resting, leaning forward, breath held in full expiration. Bell chest piece, lightly applied. | Slow heart rate; patient leaning forward, breath held in full expiration. Diaphragm chest piece. | Murmur usually louder during and at peak of inspiration. Patient recumbent. Bell chest piece. | Murmur usually becomes louder during inspiration. |
| **X-ray and fluoroscopy*** | Straight left heart border. Large left atrium sharply indenting esophagus. Large right ventricle and pulmonary artery if pulmonary hypertension present. Elevation of left branches. Occasional calcification seen in mitral valve. | Enlarged left ventricle and left atrium; systolic expansion of left atrium if enlargement not extreme. | Concentric left ventricular hypertrophy. Prominent ascending aorta, small knob. Calcified valve common. | Moderate to great left ventricular hypertrophy. Prominent ascending aorta, small knob. Strong aortic pulsation on fluoroscopy. | Enlarged right atrium only. | Enlarged right atrium and ventricle. |
| **ECG** | Broad P waves in standard leads; broad negative phase of diphasic P in $V_1$. Normal axis. If pulmonary hypertension is present, tall peaked P waves, right axis deviation or right ventricular hypertrophy appear. | Left axis deviation or frank left ventricular hypertrophy. P waves broad, tall, or notched in standard leads; broad negative phase of diphasic P in $V_1$. | Left ventricular hypertrophy. | Left ventricular hypertrophy. | Wide, tall peaked P waves. Normal axis. | Right axis usual. |
| **Echocardiography†** **M mode** | Slow early diastolic filling slope, left atrial enlargement, normal to small left ventricle. | Loss of the A wave with only minimal reduction of the early diastolic filling slope, hyperdynamic enlarged left ventricle. | Dense persistent echoes from the aortic valve with poor leaflet excursion, left ventricular hypertrophy (LVH) with preserved contractile functions. | Low-frequency diastolic vibrations of the anterior leaflet of the mitral valve and septum, early closure of the mitral valve when condition is severe, dilated left ventricle with normal contractility. | Tricuspid valve thickening, decreased early diastolic filling slope of the tricuspid valve. | Systolic reflux of intravenous contrast agent (saline) from the superior vena cava to the inferior vena cava. |
| **Two-dimensional** | Maximum diastolic orifice size reduced, subvalvular apparatus foreshortened, variable thickening of other valves. | Portions of the mitral valve fail to collapse in systole. | Above plus poststenotic dilatation of the aorta, restricted opening of the aortic leaflets, bicuspid aortic valve in about 30%. | Above plus may show vegetations in endocarditis. | Above plus enlargement of the right atrium. | Same as above. |

\* Technetium 99m pertechnetate radioisotope scans and echocardiography are being increasingly used to augment x-ray studies.

† With the assistance of Dr Nelson B Schiller.

| | | |
|---|---|---|
| $A_2$ = Aortic second sound | | MCL = Midclavicular line |
| ACD = Area of cardiac disease | | $P_2$ = Pulmonary second sound |
| ICS = Intercostal space | | PMI = Point of maximal impulse |
| $M_1$ = Mitral first sound | | |

size can be determined by echocardiography: increased size denotes an increased likelihood of atrial fibrillation or systemic emboli. The mitral valve area can be measured, and the gradient and pulmonary artery pressure can be estimated by Doppler techniques. Echocardiography also detects atrial myxoma, which is clinically similar to mitral stenosis.

Because echocardiography provides most of the needed information, cardiac catheterization is employed primarily to detect associated valve, coronary, or myocardial disease—usually preoperatively.

## Treatment & Prognosis

Mitral stenosis may be present for a lifetime with few or no symptoms, or it may become severe in a few years. In most cases, there is a long asymptomatic phase, followed by subtle limitation of activity. The onset of atrial fibrillation often precipitates more severe symptoms, although with return to sinus rhythm (using digoxin and, often, type I antiarrhythmic agents) or ventricular rate control the patient may be stabilized. Once atrial fibrillation has occurred, the patient should receive anticoagulation therapy to prevent systemic embolization. Systemic embolization in the presence of only mild to moderate disease is not an indication for surgery but should be treated with anticoagulants.

Patients whose activity remains limited despite ventricular rate control and diuretics need valve surgery. Open mitral commissurotomy may be effective in patients without substantial mitral regurgitation. Closed commissurotomy is less commonly performed, although it is still used in underdeveloped countries. Replacement of the valve is indicated when combined stenosis and insufficiency are present or when the mitral valve is so distorted and calcified that a satisfactory valvulotomy is not possible. Operative mortality rates are low: 1–5% in most institutions.

Balloon valvuloplasty has been performed successfully but remains investigational. It should be reserved for patients with contraindications for surgery.

Indications for surgery include the following: (1) uncontrollable pulmonary edema, (2) disabling dyspnea and occasionally pulmonary edema, and (3) evidence of pulmonary hypertension with right ventricular hypertrophy and early congestive failure.

Problems associated with prosthetic valves are thrombosis (especially at the mitral position), paravalvular leak, endocarditis, and degenerative changes in porcine valves. Anticoagulant therapy is preferable for all patients following valve replacement and mandatory with mechanical prostheses.

MacMahon SW, Devereux RB, Schron E (guest editors): Proceedings of a National Heart, Lung, and Blood Institute Symposium: Clinical and epidemiological issues in mitral valve prolapse. *Am Heart J* 1987;**113**:1265. [Entire issue.]

Rahimtoola SH: Catheter balloon valvuloplasty of aortic and mitral stenosis in adults. *Circulation* 1987;**75**:895.

Scott WE et al: Operative risk of mitral valve replacement: Discrimination analysis of 1329 procedures. *Circulation* 1985;**72(Suppl II)**:108.

## MITRAL REGURGITATION
### (Mitral Insufficiency)

Mitral regurgitation may result from many processes. Rheumatic disease is associated with a thickened valve with reduced mobility and often a mixed picture of stenosis and regurgitation. Other common causes are myxomatous degeneration (eg, **mitral valve prolapse** with or without connective tissue diseases such as Marfan's syndrome), infective endocarditis, and subvalvular dysfunction (due to papillary muscle infarction or dysfunction or ruptured chordae tendineae). Cardiac tumors, chiefly left atrial myxoma, are a rare cause of mitral regurgitation.

### Clinical Findings
**A. Symptoms and Signs:** During left ventricular systole, the mitral leaflets do not close normally, and blood is ejected into the left atrium as well as through the aortic valve. The net effect is an increased volume load on the left ventricle. The left atrium enlarges progressively, but the pressure in pulmonary veins and capillaries rises only transiently during exertion. Unless the regurgitant volume increases acutely, exertional dyspnea and fatigue progress gradually over many years.

Mitral regurgitation, like mitral stenosis, predisposes to atrial fibrillation; but this arrhythmia is less likely to provoke acute pulmonary congestion, and fewer than 5% of patients have peripheral arterial emboli. Mitral regurgitation more often predisposes to infective endocarditis.

Clinically, mitral regurgitation is characterized by a pansystolic murmur maximal at the apex, radiating to the axilla and occasionally to the base; a hyperdynamic left ventricular impulse and a brisk carotid upstroke; and a prominent third heart sound. The magnitude of the left ventricular hypertrophy is usually moderate, and much of the enlargement of the cardiac shadow on radiographs may be due to left atrial dilatation. Calcification of the mitral valve is less common than in pure mitral stenosis. The same is true of enlargement of the main pulmonary artery on radiographs. Hemodynamically, overwork of the left ventricle ultimately leads to left ventricular failure and reduced cardiac output, but for many years the left ventricular end-diastolic pressure and the cardiac output may be normal at rest, even with considerable increase in left ventricular volume.

In contrast to rheumatic mitral regurgitation, nonrheumatic disease may develop abruptly. In acute mitral insufficiency, patients are in sinus rhythm rather than atrial fibrillation, have little or no enlargement of the left atrium, no calcification of the mitral valve, no associated mitral stenosis, and in many cases little left ventricular dilatation.

Myxomatous mitral valve ("floppy" or "billowing" mitral valve, or **mitral valve prolapse**) is usually asymptomatic but may be associated with nonspecific chest pain, dyspnea, fatigue, or palpitations. Most patients are female, many are thin, and many have minor chest wall deformities. There are characteristic midsystolic clicks, which may be multiple, often but not always followed by a late systolic murmur. These findings are accentuated in the standing position. The diagnosis is primarily clinical but can be confirmed echocardiographically. Its significance is in dispute because of the frequency (up to 10%) with which it is diagnosed in healthy young men and women, but in occasional patients this lesion is not benign. Patients who have only a midsystolic click usually have no sequelae, but patients with a late or pansystolic murmur may develop significant mitral insufficiency, often due to rupture of chordae tendineae. Infective endocarditis may occur in 5–10% of cases, chiefly in those with murmurs. Sudden death is rare and is perhaps related to supraventricular and ventricular tachycardias shown by ambulatory echocardiographic monitoring; β-adrenergic blocking agents are often effective for supraventricular arrhythmias. If ventricular tachycardia or fibrillation is present, amiodarone may be the most effective treatment. An association between mitral prolapse and embolic cerebrovascular events has also been reported.

**Papillary muscle dysfunction** or infarction following acute myocardial infarction is less common. When mitral regurgitation is due to papillary dysfunction, it may subside as the infarction heals or left ventricular dilatation diminishes.

**B. Imaging:** Echocardiography is useful in demonstrating the underlying pathologic process (rheumatic, prolapse, flail leaflet) but provides only estimates of its severity, even by Doppler techniques. The accompanying information concerning left ventricular size and function, left atrial size, pulmonary artery pressure, and right ventricular function can be invaluable in planning treatment as well as in recognizing associated lesions. Nuclear medicine techniques permit measurement of left ventricular function and estimation of the severity of regurgitation.

Cardiac catheterization provides the best assessment of regurgitation and, additionally, of left ventricular function and pulmonary artery pressure. Coronary arteriography is often indicated to determine the cause of the lesion and for preoperative evaluation.

### Treatment & Prognosis

Acute mitral regurgitation due to endocarditis, myocardial infarction, and ruptured chordae tendineae often requires surgery to reverse heart failure. Some patients can be stabilized with vasodilators or intraortic balloon counterpulsation. Patients with chronic lesions may remain symptomatic for many years. Operation is necessary when activity becomes limited or if left ventricular function deteriorates progressively. When left ventricular function is poor (ejection fraction < 40%), due either to chronic volume overload or to another process, the surgical risk is high and the subsequent outcome poor. There has been growing interest in valve repair in nonrheumatic lesions. This is preferable to valve replacement because of the complications of prosthetic valves described earlier.

Blumlein S et al: Quantitation of mitral regurgitation by Doppler echocardiography. *Circulation* 1986;**74**:306.

Hochreiter C et al: Mitral regurgitation: Relationship of noninvasive descriptors of right and left ventricular performance to clinical and hemodynamic findings and to prognosis in medically and surgically treated patients. *Circulation* 1986;**73**:900.

## AORTIC STENOSIS

Aortic valvular stenosis may follow rheumatic fever but is more commonly caused by progressive valvular calcification superimposed upon a congenitally bicuspid valve or, in the elderly, a previously normal valve. Aortic stenosis has become the commonest valvular lesion in developed countries with aging populations. Over 80% of patients are men. Valvular stenosis must be distinguished from supravalvular obstruction and from outflow obstruction of the left ventricular infundibulum.

### Clinical Findings

**A. Symptoms and Signs:** Slight narrowing, roughened valves, or aortic dilatation may produce the typical murmur and thrill without causing significant hemodynamic effects. In mild or moderate cases, the characteristic signs are a systolic ejection murmur at the aortic area transmitted to the neck and apex; in severe cases, a palpable left ventricular heave, a weak to absent aortic second sound, or reversed splitting of the second sound are present (see Table 8–1). When the valve area is less than one-fifth of normal (3–4 cm$^2$), ventricular systole becomes prolonged and the typical carotid pulse pattern of delayed upstroke and low amplitude are present. Left ventricular hypertrophy increases progressively, with resulting elevations in diastolic pressure. Cardiac output is maintained until the stenosis is severe. Patients may present with left ventricular failure, angina pectoris, or syncope.

Angina pectoris frequently occurs in aortic stenosis. One-third to one-half of patients with calcific aortic stenosis and angina have significant coronary artery disease, whereas coronary disease is noted at only half this rate in the absence of angina. The prognosis is worse with coexisting coronary disease. Syncope is typically postexertional and may be due to arrhythmias (usually ventricular tachycardia), hypotension, or decreased cerebral perfusion resulting from increased blood flow to exercising muscle without compensatory increase in cardiac output. Sudden death may occur even in previously asymptomatic individuals.

**B. Imaging:** The clinical assessment of aortic stenosis may be difficult. The chest radiograph may show a normal or enlarged cardiac silhouette as well as dilatation and calcification of the ascending aorta. Echocardiography can visualize the aortic valve; in older patients, it usually is thickened and immobile. The Doppler technique measures the aortic valve gradient. However, in patients with low cardiac output or concomitant regurgitation, these evaluations may be inaccurate.

Cardiac catheterization is the ultimate diagnostic procedure. The valve gradient is measured, and the valve area is calculated from the relation between gradient and flow. The critical valve area is 0.6–0.7 cm$^2$. Aortic regurgitation can be quantified by aortic root angiography. Coronary arteriography should be performed in most older patients with aortic stenosis, especially if angina is present.

**C. Electrocardiographic Findings:** The ECG reveals some evidence of left ventricular hypertrophy in most patients but is normal in almost 10%.

## Treatment & Prognosis

Following the onset of heart failure, angina, or syncope, the prognosis without surgery is poor (50% 3-year mortality rate). Even asymptomatic patients with severe stenosis are at risk for sudden death, so that consideration for surgery is appropriate; however, the surgical mortality rate usually exceeds this risk.

The surgical mortality rate for valve replacement is 3–5%. Once left ventricular failure has occurred in aortic stenosis, surgery should not be postponed in favor of continued conservative treatment. Even severe left ventricular dysfunction may be reversed postoperatively and is not a contraindication to surgery. The late mortality rate reflects both associated illnesses in older people and the complications of prosthetic valves. Anticoagulation is required for mechanical prostheses but is not essential with bioprostheses. The latter undergo degenerative changes and usually require reoperation in 5–10 years. Many patients continue to exhibit conduction system disease or ventricular arrhythmias postoperatively.

Recently, many centers have performed balloon valvuloplasty with some success, though restenosis is common. This should be considered an alternative approach limited to individuals who are poor candidates for surgery.

Cribier A et al: Percutaneous transluminal balloon valvuloplasty of adult aortic stenosis: Report of 92 cases. *J Am Coll Cardiol* 1987;**9**:381.

Lund O: Determinants of long-term survival after isolated aortic valve replacement: A 10- to 17-year follow-up. *Tex Heart Inst J* 1987;**14**:144.

Magovern JA et al: Aortic valve replacement and combined aortic valve replacement and coronary artery bypass grafting: Predicting high risk groups. *J Am Coll Cardiol* 1987;**9**:38.

## AORTIC REGURGITATION
(Aortic Insufficiency)

Rheumatic aortic regurgitation has become less common than in the preantibiotic era, but nonrheumatic causes are frequent. These include congenitally bicuspid valves, infective endocarditis, and hypertension. Some patients have aortic regurgitation secondary to aortitis or aortic root disease, such as syphilis, Marfan's syndrome, aortic dissection, ankylosing spondylitis, and Reiter's syndrome.

## Clinical Findings

**A. Symptoms and Signs:** For many years, the only sign may be a soft aortic diastolic murmur. As the valve deformity increases, larger amounts regurgitate, diastolic blood pressure falls, and the left ventricle progressively enlarges. Most patients remain asymptomatic even at this point, and an often prolonged plateau phase, characterized by stable left ventricular dilatation, occurs. Left ventricular failure is a late event. Fatigue, weakness, and exertional dyspnea are the most frequent symptoms, but paroxysmal nocturnal dyspnea and pulmonary edema may also be present. Angina pectoris or atypical chest pain may be present. Syncope is less common than in aortic stenosis.

Hemodynamically, because of marked left ventricular dilatation, patients eject a large stroke volume which is adequate to maintain cardiac output until late in the course of the disease. Left ventricular diastolic pressure remains normal also but may abruptly rise when heart failure occurs. Abnormal left ventricular systolic function, as manifested by reduced ejection fraction and increasing end-systolic left ventricular volume, is a late sign of aortic regurgitation.

The major physical findings relate to the wide arterial pulse pressure. The pulse characteristically has a rapid rise and fall (Corrigan's pulse), with an elevated systolic and low diastolic pressure. The apical impulse is prominent, laterally displaced, and usually hyperdynamic, though it may be sustained. The murmur itself may be quite soft and localized; it is high-pitched and decrescendo. A mid or late diastolic low-pitched mitral murmur (Austin Flint murmur) may be heard in advanced aortic insufficiency of nonrheumatic origin. A fourth heart sound is unusual in chronic aortic insufficiency.

When aortic insufficiency develops acutely (as in dissecting aortic dissection or infective endocarditis), left ventricular failure may develop rapidly, and surgery may be urgently required. Patients with acute aortic insufficiency do not have the large dilated left ventricle characteristic of chronic aortic insufficiency. In the same way, the diastolic murmur is shorter and may be minimal in intensity, making clinical diagnosis difficult.

**B. Imaging:** Radiographs show cardiomegaly with left ventricular prominence.

Echocardiography can demonstrate diastolic fluttering of the anterior mitral leaflet or septum produced by the regurgitant jet. Serial assessments of left ventricular size and function are critical. Doppler techniques can qualitatively estimate the severity of regurgitation. Scintigraphic studies can quantify left ventricular function and functional reserve during exercise—a useful predictor of prognosis.

Cardiac catheterization can help quantify the severity of regurgitation and is used to evaluate the coronary anatomy.

**C. Electrocardiographic Findings:** The ECG usually shows moderate to severe left ventricular hypertrophy.

## Treatment & Prognosis

Aortic regurgitation that appears or worsens during or after an episode of infective endocarditis may lead to acute severe left ventricular failure or subacute progression over weeks or months. The former usually presents as pulmonary edema; surgical removal of the valve is indicated even during active infection. Chronic regurgitation has a long natural history, but the prognosis is poor when significant symptoms occur. Medical therapy may stabilize or improve symptoms but should be employed only as a preliminary to surgical correction. Surgery is also indicated for those who exhibit progressive deterioration of left ventricular function, irrespective of symptoms.

The operative mortality rate is usually in the 3–10% range. Following surgery, left ventricular size usually decreases and left ventricular function improves, except where dysfunction has been present chronically.

Perry GJ et al: Evaluation of aortic insufficiency by Doppler color flow mapping. *J Am Coll Cardiol* 1987;**9**:952.

Stone PH et al: Determinants of prognosis of patients with aortic regurgitation who undergo aortic valve replacement. *J Am Coll Cardiol* 1984;**3**:1118.

## TRICUSPID STENOSIS

Tricuspid stenosis is usually rheumatic in origin. It should be suspected when "right heart failure" appears early in the course of mitral valve disease, marked by hepatomegaly, ascites, and dependent edema. The typical diastolic rumble along the lower left sternal border must be differentiated from the murmur of mitral stenosis. In the presence of sinus rhythm, a presystolic liver pulsation can be found in half of patients.

Hemodynamically, a diastolic pressure gradient of 5–15 mm Hg is found across the tricuspid valve in conjunction with raised pressure in the right atrium and jugular veins, with prominent *a* waves and a slow *y* descent because of slow right ventricular filling.

Echocardiography usually demonstrates the lesion, and Doppler flow studies can measure the gradient; accompanying valve lesions can also be detected. Right heart catheterization is diagnostic.

Acquired tricuspid stenosis may be amenable to valvotomy under direct vision, but it usually requires a prosthetic valve replacement. There may be a role for balloon valvuloplasty.

## TRICUSPID REGURGITATION

Tricuspid regurgitation may occur in a variety of situations other than disease of the tricuspid valve itself. The most common is right ventricular overload resulting from left ventricular failure due to any cause. Tricuspid insufficiency occurs in association with right ventricular and inferior myocardial infarction. Tricuspid valve endocarditis and resulting regurgitation are common in intravenous drug abusers. The symptoms and signs of organic tricuspid valve disease are identical to those resulting from right ventricular failure due to any cause. In the presence of mitral valve disease, the tricuspid valvular lesion can be suspected on the basis of early onset of right heart failure and a harsh systolic murmur along the lower left sternal border which is separate from the mitral murmur and which often increases in intensity during and just after inspiration.

Hemodynamically, tricuspid insufficiency is characterized by a prominent regurgitant systolic (*v*) wave in the right atrium and jugular venous pulse, with a rapid *y* descent and a small or absent *x* descent. The regurgitant wave, like the systolic murmur, is increased with inspiration, and its size depends upon the size of the right atrium. In tricuspid regurgitation, especially with right ventricular failure, a right ventricular $S_3$ may be present.

Replacement of the tricuspid valve is infrequently done now. Tricuspid insufficiency secondary to severe mitral valve disease or other left-sided lesions may regress when the underlying disease is corrected. When surgery is required, valve repair or valvuloplasty of the tricuspid ring are often preferable to valve replacement.

Yock PG, Popp RL: Noninvasive estimation of right ventricular systolic pressure by Doppler ultrasound in patients with tricuspid regurgitation. *Circulation* 1984;**70**:657.

## INFECTIVE ENDOCARDITIS
*Ernest Jawetz, MD, PhD*

Traditionally, endocarditis was called "acute" or "subacute," but it is more desirable to group endocarditis according to the causative microorganism. The traditional "subacute" infective endocarditis has an insidious onset, with low-grade fever, anemia, weight loss, and valve damage. It requires preexisting congenital, rheumatic, or calcific abnormalities of the heart valves. Bacteremia occurring frequently with dental procedures and endoscopic or other manipulations of the respiratory, urinary, or gastrointestinal tract results in organisms adhering to the valve. Viridans (50%) and fecal (10%) streptococci are common causative agents, but virtually any microorganism can cause endocarditis.

The initial event is an abnormality in blood flow resulting in endothelial damage. A thrombotic lesion develops, consisting of fibrin, platelets, and leukocytes. Pieces of vegetation may break off, sending emboli to various organs and sites. Immune complex nephritis often develops and may lead to renal failure.

The traditional "acute" infective endocarditis is a rapidly progressive, destructive infection of normal, abnormal, or prosthetic valves, often developing in the course of intense bacteremia secondary to intravenous narcotic abuse. Staphylococci and gram-negative enteric bacteria are common pathogens. Among intravenous drug users, staphylococci, *Candida,* enterococci, and gram-negative bacteria are prominent causes of endocarditis. Right-sided valvular lesions are common in these patients; pulmonary infiltrates with pneumonia are an important predominant manifestation.

Acute endocarditis produces large, friable vegetations, with severe embolic episodes with metastatic abscess formation early in the course. Local invasion leads to rapid perforation, affected valve rupture of chordae tendineae, or valve ring abscess.

### Clinical Findings

**A. Symptoms and Signs:** Fever is present in most cases, but afebrile periods may occur, especially in the aged. Any or all of the following may occur also: night sweats, chills, malaise, anorexia, weight loss; myalgias, arthralgia, or redness and swelling of joints; stroke due to cerebral emboli; pain in the abdomen, chest, or flanks due to mesenteric, splenic, pulmonary, or renal emboli; and symptoms of heart failure. In acute infective endocarditis, the course is more fulminating, and the patient more acutely ill.

In subacute infective endocarditis, evidence of rheumatic or congenital heart disease is often present. Occasionally, mitral valve prolapse is the underlying lesion. Findings include splenomegaly; petechiae of the skin, mucous membranes, and ocular fundi; clubbing of the fingers and toes; pallor; manifestations of cerebral emboli; and tender red nodules of the finger or toe pads. Heart murmurs may be absent in infection of the tricuspid and pulmonary valves, where recurrent pulmonary infarction suggesting pneumonia may be prominent. The clinical picture is often atypical in older persons; fever, chills, and heart murmurs may be unimpressive, but stroke or renal failure may be prominent.

Acute infective endocarditis presents as a severe infection associated with chills, high fever, prostration, and multiple serious embolic phenomena. These may be superimposed on the antecedent causative infection (eg, pneumonia) or may appear abruptly following instrumentation, surgery, or self-injection of narcotics. Heart murmurs may change rapidly, and heart failure occurs early.

Infective endocarditis may develop during "prophylactic" or inadequate therapeutic antibiotic administration. In these circumstances, the onset is cryptic, and a sudden embolic episode, the appearance of petechiae, unexplained heart failure, changing murmurs, or fever may be the first clue.

**B. Laboratory Findings:** In suspected infective endocarditis, 4–6 blood cultures are obtained at different times, although bacteremia is constant. Within 2–7 days of incubation, over 90% of these cultures will grow organisms and permit specific drug selection. In acute infective endocarditis, cultures are obtained during the emergency workup, and antibiotic treatment is then instituted. The administration of an antimicrobial drug may interfere with positive blood cultures for 7–10 days.

Normochromic anemia, a markedly elevated sedimentation rate, variable leukocytosis, microscopic hematuria, proteinuria, and casts are commonly present in infective endocarditis. Nitrogen retention may be present, especially in older patients. Echocardiography shows vegetation in most cases, but false-positives and false-negatives occur.

### Differential Diagnosis

Infective endocarditis must be differentiated from various seemingly primary disease states. Stroke, intractable heart failure, anemia, or uremia may be caused by infective endocarditis. If a patient presenting with any of these illnesses has fever or a heart murmur, blood cultures should be taken.

Specific diseases that require differentiation are lymphomas, leukemias, acute rheumatic fever, disseminated lupus erythematosus, polyarteritis nodosa, chronic meningococcemia, brucellosis, septic thrombophlebitis, disseminated tuberculosis, mycoses, and nonbacterial thrombotic endocarditis.

**In summary:** Endocarditis must be considered in the differential diagnosis of any patient with an unexplained multisystem illness.

### Prevention

**A. Medical Measures:** Some cases of endocarditis arise after dental procedures or surgery of the upper respiratory, genitourinary, or intestinal tract. Patients with known cardiac anomalies who are to have any of these procedures should be prepared in one of the following ways, although failures sometimes occur.

**1. For dental and upper respiratory tract procedures–**

**a. Oral–**Penicillin V, 2 g 1 hour before the procedure and 1 g 6 hours later. In patients with penicillin allergy, give erythromycin, 1 g 1 hour before the procedure and 0.5 g 6 hours later.

**b. Parenteral–**Ampicillin, 1 g, or penicillin G, 2 million units, intramuscularly or intravenously, plus gentamicin, 1.5 mg/kg intramuscularly or intravenously, each given 1 hour before the procedure and again 8 hours later. In patients with penicillin allergy, give vancomycin, 1 g intravenously as a 1-hour infusion beginning 1 hour before the procedure, and repeat once 8 hours later.

**2. For gastrointestinal or genitourinary tract procedures–**

**a. Parenteral–**Ampicillin, 2 g intravenously or intramuscularly, plus gentamicin, 1.5 mg/kg intravenously or intramuscularly, each given 1 hour before the procedure and once 8 hours later. In patients with penicillin allergy, give vancomycin alone or with gentamicin as above.

**b. Oral**–Oral prophylaxis (amoxicillin, 3 g 1 hour before the procedure and 1.5 g 6 hours later) is probably less desirable than parenteral prophylaxis.

Many alternative regimens have been proposed. For none of them is there absolute proof of efficacy. Any form of antimicrobial prophylaxis may favor the selection of resistant organisms in the normal flora, with subsequent involvement of such organisms in infective endocarditis.

**B. Surgical Measures:** Surgery is warranted for prevention of infective endocarditis in selected patients with surgically correctable congenital lesions (patent ductus arteriosus). It should also be offered to patients with acute infective endocarditis who develop congestive heart failure. It is not necessary to complete a course of antibiotics preoperatively; indeed, delay of surgery is unwise in such patients. Mycotic aneurysms may also be treated surgically.

## Treatment

**A. Specific Measures:** The most important consideration in the treatment of infective endocarditis is a bactericidal concentration of antibiotics in contact with the infecting organism, which is often localized in avascular tissues or in vegetations. Penicillins, because of their high degree of bactericidal activity against many bacteria that produce endocarditis and because of their low toxicity, are by far the most useful drugs. Synergistic combinations of antibiotics have proved valuable.

Positive blood cultures are invaluable to confirm the diagnosis and to guide treatment with tests of susceptibility of the infecting organism to various antibiotics or combinations of antibiotics. See ¶ B, p 206, for blood culture directions.

*Note:* **Control of antimicrobial treatment.** Negative blood cultures are a minimal goal of effective therapy. Assay of serum bactericidal activity is the best guide to support the selection of drugs and the daily dose after treatment has been started. During therapy, the patient's serum diluted 1:10 or 1:5 should (at least during part of the interval between drug doses) be rapidly bactericidal in vitro under standardized laboratory conditions for the organisms originally grown from the patient's bloodstream. Drugs are initially administered by the intravenous route. If clinical and laboratory response is good, drugs may later be given orally, under control of serum bactericidal tests.

Specific antimicrobial regimens are as follows:

**1. Endocarditis Due to S viridans (Streptococcus Salivarius, Streptococcus Mutans, Streptococcus Sanguis, Streptococcus Bovis)**–Viridans streptococci (usually originating in the oropharynx) are the infecting organisms in over 60% of spontaneously arising cases of typical slow-onset endocarditis. Most such organisms are susceptible to 0.1–1 unit/mL penicillin G in vitro. Penicillin G, 5–10 million units daily (in divided doses given as a bolus every 4 hours into an intravenous infusion) continued for 3–4 weeks, is generally curative. Enhanced bactericidal action is obtained if an aminoglycoside (eg, gentamicin, 3–5 mg/kg/d intramuscularly) is added during the first 10–14 days of treatment. More resistant organisms may require daily doses of 20–40 million units of penicillin G. Probenecid, 0.5 g orally 3 times daily, enhances blood levels of penicillin by interfering with its tubular excretion.

**2. Endocarditis due to *Streptococcus faecalis* (enterococcus)**–This organism causes 5–10% of cases of spontaneously arising endocarditis and rarely also follows abuse of intravenous drugs. Treatment requires the simultaneous use of penicillin and an aminoglycoside. Penicillin G, 20 million units daily, or ampicillin, 6–12 g daily, is given in divided doses as bolus injections every 2–4 hours into an intravenous infusion. An aminoglycoside (eg, gentamicin, 5 mg/kg/d) selected by laboratory test is injected intramuscularly 2–3 times daily in divided doses. The cell wall-inhibitory drug (eg, penicillin, vancomycin) enhances the entry of the aminoglycoside and permits killing of the enterococci. Treatment must be continued for 4–5 weeks; cephalosporins cannot be substituted for penicillins, and tobramycin and amikacin appear less effective than gentamicin. Vancomycin may be substituted for penicillin if allergy is present.

**3. Endocarditis due to staphylococci (*Staphylococcus aureus, Staphylococcus epidermidis*)**–If the infecting staphylococci are *not* penicillinase producers, penicillin G, 10–20 million units in divided doses, is the treatment of choice; these organisms are unusual causes of endocarditis, however. If the staphylococci produce penicillinase, as is usually the case, nafcillin, 8–12 g daily, given as a bolus every 2 hours into an intravenous infusion, is the drug of choice. In probable or established hypersensitivity to penicillin, the alternative drug is vancomycin, 2–3 g intravenously daily in divided doses every 4 hours. This treatment must be continued for 6 weeks, and a frequent careful check for metastatic lesions or abscesses must be conducted (and lesions drained) to avoid reseeding of cardiac sites from such reservoirs of infectious organisms.

**4. Endocarditis due to gram-negative bacteria**–The susceptibility of these organisms to antimicrobial drugs varies so greatly that effective treatment must be based on laboratory tests. An aminoglycoside (gentamicin, 5–7 mg/kg/d; amikacin, 15 mg/kg/d; or tobramycin, 5–7 mg/kg/d) is often combined with a cell wall-inhibitory drug (ticarcillin, 18 g/d; cefotaxime or cefoperazone, 12 g/d) to enhance penetration of the aminoglycoside. Laboratory guidance is essential not only for susceptibility tests but also to establish the presence of sufficient bactericidal activity in serum obtained during treatment. The dosage of aminoglycosides must be adjusted if renal function is impaired (Chapter 28). Each of these drugs can also cause eighth nerve damage, and the patient should be monitored often for hearing loss and vestibular function.

Whenever large doses of penicillins or cephalosporins are given, the following must be considered: (1) Each million units of potassium penicillin G contains about 1.7 meq of potassium, which might give rise to toxicity, especially in the presence of renal failure. (2) At very high concentrations of penicillin, there is enough diffusion into the central nervous system to cause neurotoxicity. (3) With *any* intravenous infusions of long duration, there is a significant risk of superinfection; to minimize this possibility, injection sites must be changed every 48–72 hours and must be kept scrupulously clean. Prolonged high concentrations of antimicrobials are irritating and favor the development of thrombophlebitis. Therefore, bolus injection of a portion of the total daily dose over a 20- to 30-minute period (through a Volutron or similar device) every 2–6 hours into a continuous infusion (drip) of 5% glucose in water is preferable to a steady flow of antibiotic.

**5. Endocarditis due to yeasts and fungi–** This type is seen with increasing frequency in abusers of intravenous drugs and after cardiac surgery. *Candida parapsilosis* is encountered commonly, but virtually any fungus, including *Aspergillus* and even *Histoplasma,* can be seen. Fungal endocarditis is often associated with bulky, friable vegetations that tend to produce massive emboli in large arteries. *Candida* endocarditis has occurred early after the insertion of prosthetic valves, and the diagnosis may be based on the finding of pseudohyphae in emboli surgically removed from large vessels. Blood cultures may require 1–3 weeks to grow these organisms.

The drugs most active against yeasts and fungi are amphotericin B (0.4–0.8 mg/kg/d) and flucytosine (150 mg/kg/d orally). However, these drugs rarely eradicate fungal endocarditis. Early surgical excision of the involved valve tissue during antifungal therapy and continuation of the latter for several weeks offer the best opportunity for cure.

**6. Prosthetic valve endocarditis–** This may occur early, within days after insertion of a valve, and then is usually caused by staphylococci, gram-negative enteric bacteria, or *Candida.* The most common organism may be *S epidermidis* resistant to lactamase-resistant penicillins (eg, nafcillin); it requires treatment with vancomycin plus rifampin. Fungal infections on prosthetic valves are incurable medically and require replacement of the prosthesis.

Late prosthetic valve endocarditis is similar microbiologically to infection on native valves and occurs as a consequence of bacteremia. Antimicrobial treatment may or may not eradicate the infection. Drugs aimed at the infecting organisms are given before, during, and after removal of the infected prosthesis and its replacement. There is a substantial mortality rate (> 10%) with such a replacement.

**7. Culture-negative endocarditis–** With a clinical picture suggestive of infective endocarditis but with persistently negative blood cultures, empiric treatment with penicillin G, 20 million units/d intravenously, plus an aminoglycoside (eg, gentamicin, 5 mg/kg/d intramuscularly), can be given for 4 weeks. There should be significant clinical improvement within 7–10 days. If not, other causes such as Q fever must be considered. The diagnosis of Q fever endocarditis rests on a serum complement fixation titer of more than 1:200 or an immunofluorescent titer of 1:400 with phase I *Coxiella burnetii* antigen. That diagnosis requires continuous treatment with tetracyclines for an indefinite period and sometimes valve replacement.

**8. Follow-up and recurrences–** At the end of the established treatment period of 3–6 weeks, all antimicrobial therapy should be stopped. Blood cultures are then taken once weekly for 4 weeks while the patient is observed carefully. Most bacteriologic relapses occur during this time. Embolic phenomena and fever may occur both during and after successful treatment and—by themselves—are not adequate grounds for re-treatment. An initial adequate course of therapy in culture-positive infective endocarditis can result in microbiologic cure in up to 90% of cases. If relapse occurs, the organism must be isolated and tested again, and a second—and often longer—course of treatment administered with properly selected drugs.

In spite of microbiologic cure, 50% of patients treated for infective endocarditis progress to cardiac failure in 5–10 years. This mechanical failure can be attributed in part to valvular deformities (eg, perforation of cusp, tearing of chordae) caused by the infection and in part to the healing and scarring process. Therefore, surgical correction of abnormalities in cardiovascular dynamics and possible valvular prostheses must be considered as part of the follow-up.

**B. General Measures:** Anticoagulants (eg, heparin, warfarin) are contraindicated in uncomplicated infective endocarditis and contribute to hemorrhagic complications. In prosthetic endocarditis, despite the risk, these drugs should be continued unless serious bleeding occurs, because of the greater risk of thrombosis on the mechanical infected valves.

**C. Treatment of Complications:**

**1. Acute valvular regurgitation–** The acute onset of aortic regurgitation due to perforation of the valve or adjacent sinus of Valsalva may be catastrophic. Early valve replacement is indicated. Mitral regurgitation may be tolerated better, but this valve may need to be replaced also. Tricuspid regurgitation is usually tolerated adequately.

**2. Cardiac failure–** Myocarditis, which frequently accompanies infective endocarditis of long duration, and increasing deformity of heart valves may precipitate cardiac failure and require diuretics, vasodilators, or digoxin. Valvular regurgitation as the primary problem should be excluded by echo-Doppler studies. The conduction system may also be involved with resultant atrioventricular block; this is more common in staphylococcal endocarditis or in infections on prosthetic valves.

**3. Infarctions–** Infarctions of organs in the systemic circulation usually result from emboli originating in vegetations in the left heart. In acute infective endocarditis, these may be indication for valve replacement; blood emboli may occur after bacteriologic cure in subacute disease but require no additional antibiotics. Emboli derived from right heart lesions may produce pulmonary infarction. Treatment is symptomatic.

**4. Renal failure**—Infective endocarditis often leads to renal failure resulting from immune complex glomerulonephritis. Rising serum creatinine requires adjustment of drug dosage and—rarely—temporary dialytic treatment of uremia until renal function improves during antimicrobial therapy.

## Prognosis

Infective endocarditis is uniformly fatal unless the infection can be eradicated, but in some cases surgical removal of an infected arteriovenous fistula, patent ductus arteriosus, or infected prosthesis has been curative. Patients with the poorest prognosis for microbiologic cure are those with consistently negative blood cultures and long delay in therapy, those with highly resistant organisms, and those with infected prostheses. If microbiologic cure is accomplished, the prognosis depends on the adequacy of cardiovascular function, since mechanical distortions and impairment of dynamics develop during infection and healing. Only about 60% of patients with microbiologically cured infective endocarditis are well 5 years after treatment. Among valve lesions, aortic insufficiency carries the worst outlook and merits early evaluation for surgery. Among embolic events, those to the brain have the poorest prognosis. Cerebral emboli and rupture of mycotic aneurysms may occur even after microbiologic cure. Renal functional impairment is generally reversible.

Baddour LM, Bisno AL: Infective endocarditis complicating mitral valve prolapse. *Rev Infect Dis* 1986;**8**:117.

Brandenburg RO et al: Infective endocarditis: A 25-year overview of diagnosis and therapy. *J Am Coll Cardiol* 1983;**1**:280.

Kaye D: Prophylaxis for infective endocarditis: An update. *Ann Intern Med* 1986;**104**:419.

Wilson WR: Symposium on infective endocarditis. (2 parts.) *Mayo Clin Proc* 1982;**57**:3, 81.

# SYSTEMIC HYPERTENSION

Most authorities define hypertension as diastolic pressure consistently greater than 100 mm Hg in a person more than 60 years of age or 90 mm Hg in a person under 50 years of age. WHO criteria require pressures exceeding 160/95 mm Hg. Between 140/90 and 160/95 mm Hg is considered to be borderline hypertension. The vascular complication of hyperten-

sion are thought to result from the raised arterial pressure and associated atherosclerosis of major arterial circuits.

Hypertension is uncommon before age 20. In young people it is commonly caused by renal insufficiency, renal artery stenosis, or coarctation of the aorta.

Transient elevation of blood pressure caused by excitement or apprehension does not constitute hypertensive disease. However, sustained systolic elevation suggests atherosclerosis of the aorta, and the prognosis is therefore less good. Treatment with antihypertensive agents has not been established as effective in decreasing the mortality rate in this group, and the drugs must be used cautiously and in small doses to prevent hypotension and decreased cardiac output.

Hypertension is an important preventable cause of cardiovascular disease; prospective studies have shown that without treatment, hypertension greatly increases the incidence of cardiac failure, coronary heart disease with angina pectoris and myocardial infarction, hemorrhagic and thrombotic stroke, and renal failure. Epidemiologic studies have shown that only a portion of the hypertensive population is receiving effective therapy. It is essential to identify patients with hypertension and to ensure compliance with the treatment program. The prevention of hypertensive complications by antihypertensive therapy is a major public health concern.

## Etiology & Classification

**A. Primary (Essential) Hypertension:** In about 95% of cases of hypertensive cardiovascular disease, no cause can be established. The condition occurs in 10–15% of white adults and 20–30% of black adults in the USA. The onset of essential hypertension is usually between ages 25 and 55. The family history is often suggestive of hypertension (stroke, "sudden death," heart failure). Women are affected more often than men.

Elevations in pressure are transient early in the course of the disease but eventually become permanent. Even in established cases, the blood pressure fluctuates widely in response to emotional stress and physical activity. The resting blood pressure is lower than single casual office readings. Blood pressures taken by the patient at home or during daily activities using a portable apparatus are lower than those recorded in the office, clinic, or hospital and are more reliable in estimating prognosis.

The pathogenesis of essential hypertension is multifactorial. Genetic factors play an important role. Children with one—and even more so with two—hypertensive parents tend to have higher blood pressures from a very early age. Abnormal $Na^+-K^+$ exchange in red blood cells has been suggested to be a potential marker of a genetic defect.

Environmental factors also appear to play an important role. Increased dietary salt intake has long been incriminated as a possible pathogenic factor in some patients ("salt-prone") with essential hypertension. Increased salt intake alone is probably not sufficient to elevate blood pressure to abnormal levels: a combination of too much salt plus a genetic predisposition is probably required. $Cl^-$ may be as important as $Na^+$ in the pathogenesis of hypertension.

**1. Sympathetic nervous system hyperactivity–**Sympathetic nervous system hyperactivity is most apparent in younger hypertensives, who may exhibit tachycardia and an elevated cardiac output. However, this is usually a transient phase, and correlations between plasma catecholamines and blood pressure have generally been poor. Sympathetic activation may also play a role in "labile" hypertension, characterized by marked blood pressure fluctuations under differing, or even similar, circumstances.

**2. Renin-angiotensin system–**Renin, a proteolytic enzyme, is secreted by the juxtaglomerular cells surrounding afferent arterioles in response to a number of stimuli, including reduced renal perfusion pressure, diminished intravascular volume, circulating catecholamines, increased sympathetic nervous system activity, increased arteriolar stretch, and hypokalemia. Renin acts on angiotensinogen or renin substrate to cleave off the 10-amino-acid peptide angiotensin I. This peptide is then acted upon by angiotensin-converting enzyme to create the 8-amino-acid peptide angiotensin II, a potent vasoconstrictor and a major stimulant of aldosterone release from the adrenal glands. Despite the important role of this system in the regulation of blood pressure, it does not play a primary role in the pathogenesis of essential hypertension in most individuals. Plasma renin activity levels can be best classified in relation to dietary sodium intake or urinary sodium excretion. Approximately 10% of essential hypertension patients have relatively high levels, 60% have essentially normal levels, and 30% have relatively low levels. Black hypertensives and older patients tend to have lower plasma renin activity. Nonetheless, it could be postulated that even normal levels are inappropriately high for the level of blood pressure. Patients with low plasma renin activity may have higher intravascular volumes.

**3. Defect in natriuresis–**Normal individuals increase their renal sodium excretion in response to elevations in arterial pressure and to a sodium or volume load. Hypertensive patients, particularly when their blood pressure is normal, exhibit a diminished ability to excrete a sodium load. This defect may result in increased plasma volume and hypertension. However, during chronic hypertension, a sodium load is usually handled normally. This may reflect increased levels of natriuretic hormones.

**4. Intracellular sodium and calcium–**There is growing evidence that intracellular $Na^+$ is elevated in blood cells and other tissues in essential hypertension. This may result from abnormalities in $Na^+$-$K^+$ exchange and other $Na^+$ transport mechanisms. Some data indicate that circulating "digitalislike" substances may be responsible. An increase in intracellular $Na^+$ may lead to increased intracellular $Ca^{2+}$ concentrations as a result of facilitated exchange. This could explain the increase in vascular smooth muscle tone that is characteristic of established hypertension.

**5. Exacerbating conditions–**A number of conditions exacerbate or precipitate hypertension in predisposed individuals. The best-documented of these is **obesity,** which is associated with an increase in intravascular volume and an appropriately high output. Weight reduction in the obese lowers blood pressure slightly. Excessive use of **alcohol** also raises blood pressure by increasing plasma catecholamines. Hypertension can be difficult to control in people with high alcohol intake. **Cigarette smoking** acutely raises blood pressure, again by increasing plasma norepinephrine, but the long-term effect of smoking in essential hypertension is less clear. The relationship of **exercise** to hypertension is also uncertain, although exercise training can lower blood pressure modestly. **Polycythemia** increases the viscosity, whether it be primary or due to diminished plasma volume. This may raise blood pressure.

**B. Secondary Hypertension:** With complete evaluation, approximately 5% of patients with hypertension can be found to have specific causes. These are labeled secondary hypertension.

**1. Estrogen use–**The most common definable cause is the chronic use of oral contraceptive pills. A small increase in blood pressure occurs in most women taking oral contraceptives. This is caused by volume expansion due to increased activity of the renin-angiotensin-aldosterone system. The primary abnormality is an increase in the hepatic synthesis of renin substrate. Approximately 5% of women taking oral contraceptives chronically will exhibit a rise in blood pressure above 140/90 mm Hg; this represents twice the expected prevalence. Contraceptive-related hypertension is more common in women over 35 years of age and in the obese. It is less common in those taking low-dose estrogen tablets. In most cases, hypertension is reversible by discontinuing the contraceptive, but it may take several weeks. Nonetheless, hypertension is associated with a number of vascular complications of oral contraceptive use. There is no evidence that hypertension is related to postmenopausal estrogen use.

**2. Renal disease–**Virtually any disease of the renal parenchyma can produce secondary hypertension. These processes include glomerulonephritis, chronic interstitial pyelonephritis, autoimmune disease, polycystic kidney disease, hydronephrosis, and diabetic nephropathy as well as most other renal disorders. The mechanism of renal hypertension is multifaceted, but most instances are related to increased intravascular volume or increased activity of the renin-angiotensin-aldosterone system. Hypertension exaggerates progression of renal insufficiency, so its early recognition and vigorous treatment is important. Hypertension may be reversed if plasma volume is controlled by drugs or dialysis or after bilateral nephrectomy (rarely necessary) and is often improved by renal transplantation. However, posttransplantation hypertension is also a problem; this is now recognized to be in part precipitated by immunosuppressive therapy with cyclosporin.

**3. Renal vascular hypertension**–Renal artery stenosis is a common cause of secondary hypertension and is present in 1–2% of hypertensive patients. The cause in younger individuals is most commonly fibromuscular hyperplasia. This accounts for approximately 30% of renal vascular disease, though it is more common in women under 50. The remainder of renal vascular disease is due to atherosclerotic stenoses of the proximal renal arteries. The mechanism of renal vascular hypertension is excessive renin release due to reduction in renal blood flow and perfusion pressure. Renal vascular hypertension may occur when a single branch of the renal artery is obstructed, but in as many as 25% of patients both arteries are obstructed.

Renal vascular hypertension may present in the same manner as essential hypertension but may be suspected in the following circumstances: (1) if the onset is after age 50, (2) if there are epigastric or renal artery bruits, (3) if there is atherosclerosis elsewhere, or (4) if there is abrupt deterioration in renal function after administration of captopril or enalapril. Renal angiograms should be performed if anatomic stenosis is strongly suggested by the history and signs and if the hypertensive disease is difficult to control medically. Reconstructive surgery or transluminal angioplasty may offer a good prognosis.

There is no ideal "screening" test for renal vascular hypertension. All tests are sufficiently nonspecific so that in populations with a low incidence of the disease, false-positive results will exceed true-positives. In addition, none of these tests have more than 80% sensitivity. Additional diagnostic testing is appropriate only in the high-risk population described in the previous paragraph. If the suspicion of renal vascular hypertension is sufficiently high, renal arteriography, the definitive diagnostic test, is the best approach. In patients in whom suspicion is moderate, the rapid-sequence intravenous urogram, which demonstrates smaller renal size, delayed appearance of contrast, and late hyperconcentration of contrast in the affected kidney, is appropriate. Radioisotope renography, particularly following a test dose of captopril, has shown decreased renal blood flow on the side of the lesion. Measurement of plasma renin activity in the renal veins is used by some workers to identify and lateralize physiologically significant renal artery stenosis.

The treatment of patients with recognized renal vascular hypertension is controversial. Young individuals and good-risk patients of any age who have not responded to medical therapy should have the lesion corrected. Older individuals, particularly if they have bilateral disease or other risk factors, may be managed medically if renal function does not deteriorate. The use of converting enzyme inhibitors has improved the success rate of medical therapy, but these have been associated with marked hypotension and deterioration of renal function in individuals with bilateral renal artery stenosis. Although the surgical results from renal vascular hypertension are generally good, the use of percutaneous transluminal angioplasty is growing.

**4. Primary hyperaldosteronism**–Most patients with adrenal hypertension have excess aldosterone secretion as the underlying pathophysiologic process. This makes up less than 0.5% of all cases of hypertension. The usual lesion is an adrenal adenoma, although a minority of patients have bilateral adrenal hyperplasia. The diagnosis should be suspected when patients present with hypokalemia prior to diuretic therapy and when this is associated with excessive urinary potassium excretion and suppressed levels of plasma renin activity. Aldosterone concentrations in urine and blood are elevated. The lesion can be demonstrated by CT scanning as well as by MRI and abdominal ultrasound. Even less commonly, patients with **Cushing's syndrome** (glucocorticoid excess) manifest hypertension as a first sign (see Chapter 18).

**5. Pheochromocytoma**–Pheochromocytoma is an often sought but uncommon cause of hypertension. Blood pressure elevations result from excessive catecholamine secretion by the adrenal medulla or from extra-adrenal chromaffin tissue. The lesion is usually an adrenal tumor, which may be bilateral; approximately 10% are malignant. The clinical presentation characteristically includes fluctuating blood pressure associated with headache, palpitations, pallor, sweating, orthostatic hypotension, and hyperglycemia. Severe hypertensive episodes may accompany anesthesia induction, surgery, ingestion of phenothiazines or tricyclic antidepressants, or beta-blocker therapy (which leaves alpha-adrenergic stimulation unopposed). However, many patients exhibit sustained hypertension, often associated with one or more of these features. Screening for pheochromocytoma is by measurement of metabolities of norepinephrine such as urinary metanephrine excretion, although urinary vanillylmandelic acid (VMA) assays are still performed. Plasma catecholamine levels provide valuable confirmatory information, especially during hypertensive episodes, but they may be elevated in some individuals without pheochromocytoma. Nonspecifically elevated plasma norepinephrine levels are usually suppressed after an oral dose of clonidine. The tumors can usually be demonstrated by CT scanning or by uptake of adrenal specific radionuclides. Surgical excision is usually successful in nonmalignant cases.

**6. Coarctation of the aorta**–This uncommon cause of hypertension has been discussed previously.

**7. Hypertension associated with pregnancy**–Hypertension occurring de novo or worsening during pregnancy is one of the commonest causes of maternal and fetal morbidity and mortality. This problem is discussed in Chapter 13.

**8. Other causes of secondary hypertension**–Hypertension has also been associated with hyperparathyroidism, acromegaly, hypercalcemia due to any cause, and a variety of neurologic disorders causing increased intracranial pressure.

## Natural History of Untreated Hypertension

A number of complications are associated with hypertension. These are related either to sustained elevations of blood pressure, with consequent changes in the vasculature and heart, or to the accelerated atherosclerosis that accompanies long-standing hypertension. The excess morbidity and mortality related to hypertension is progressive over the whole range of systolic and diastolic blood pressures. However, end-damage varies markedly between individuals with similar levels of office hypertension. In general, blacks of both sexes and white males have a higher incidence of complications from hypertension. In addition, the presence of other risk factors such as hyperlipidemia, smoking, diabetes, and obesity modulates individual risks. Specific complications include the following.

**A. Hypertensive Cardiovascular Disease:** Left ventricular hypertrophy is found in 10–30% of chronic hypertensives, depending on the level of blood pressure, the duration of hypertension, the technique of diagnosis (echocardiography is more sensitive than electrocardiography), and additioanl factors that remain poorly understood. Once established, left ventricular hypertrophy is an indication of increased risk for morbidity and mortality; for any level of blood pressure, its presence is associated with a severalfold increase in risk. In the past, hypertension was the major cause of congestive heart failure, but this complication is rare in patients receiving adequate treatment and is decreasing in prevalence. Hypertension remains an important exacerbating factor in patients with congestive heart failure due to other causes.

**B. Hypertensive Cerebrovascular Disease:** Hypertension is the major predisposing cause of cerebrovascular accidents, including intracerebral hemorrhage and cerebral infarction. Cerebrovascular complications are more closely correlated with the systolic than the diastolic blood pressure. The incidence of these complications is markedly reduced by antihypertensive therapy.

**C. Hypertensive Renal Disease:** Chronic hypertension leads to nephrosclerosis, a common cause of renal insufficiency. Hypertensive renal damage is limited or prevented by successful therapy.

**D. Aortic Dissection:** Hypertension is a major cause and exacerbating factor in dissection of the aorta. This complication is largely prevented by successful therapy, except in patients with underlying disease of the aortic media or pregnancy. The diagnosis and treatment of aortic dissection is discussed in Chapter 9.

**E. Atherosclerotic Complications:** The linkage between hypertension and atherosclerotic cardiovascular disease is much less close than that with the previously discussed complications. This reflects the multifactorial origin of atherosclerosis. Therefore, it is not surprising that effective antihypertensive therapy is less successful in preventing coronary heart disease. Furthermore, because the duration of most antihypertensive therapeutic trials has been relatively short, it is likely that most coronary events occurred in patients with preexisting coronary artery disease. Most patients with hypertension in the USA die of atherosclerotic complications.

**F. Malignant Hypertension:** Any form of sustained hypertension, primary or secondary, may abruptly become accelerated, with diastolic pressure rising rapidly above 130 mm Hg and causing widespread arteriolar necroses and hyperplasia of the intima of the interlobular arteries of the kidney, in turn causing ischemia of the nephron. Without treatment, there is rapidly progressive renal failure, left ventricular failure, and stroke. The raised arterial pressure results in papilledema and hemorrhages and exudates in the retinas; these signs may precede clinical evidence of renal impairment and are the most reliable definitive clincial signs of malignant hypertension. Examination of the retina for evidence of accelerated hypertension is necessary in all hypertensive patients because the early stages of the malignant phase may be essentially asymptomatic.

## Clinical Findings

The clinical and laboratory findings are mainly referable to the degree of vascular deterioration and involvement of the "target organs": heart, brain, kidneys, eyes, and peripheral arteries.

**A. Symptoms:** Mild to moderate essential hypertension is compatible with normal health and wellbeing for many years. Vague symptoms usually appear after patients learn they have "high blood pressure." Suboccipital pulsating headaches, characteristically occurring early in the morning and subsiding during the day, are common, but any type of headache may occur. Severe hypertension may be associated with somnolence, headache, confusion, visual disturbances, and nausea and vomiting (hypertensive encephalopathy).

Patients with pheochromocytomas that secrete predominantly norepinephrine usually have sustained hypertension but may have intermittent hypertension. Intermittent release of catecholamines causes attacks (lasting minutes to hours) of anxiety, palpitation, profuse perspiration, pallor, tremor, and nausea and vomiting; blood pressure is markedly elevated during the attack, and angina or acute pulmonary edema may occur. In primary aldosteronism, patients may have recurrent episodes of generalized muscular weakness or paralysis as well as paresthesias, polyuria, and nocturia due to associated hypokalemia; malignant hypertension, however, is rare.

Cardiac involvement secondary to increased work of the left ventricle in overcoming the raised systemic vascular resistance often leads to paroxysmal nocturnal dyspnea. Angina pectoris or myocardial infarction may develop.

Progressive renal involvement may not produce striking symptoms, but nocturia or intermittent hematuria may ultimately occur (especially during the malignant phase).

Cerebral involvement causes (1) stroke due to thrombosis or (2) sudden hemorrhage from microaneurysms of small penetrating intracranial arteries, leading to death in hours or days. In malignant hypertension, hypertensive encephalopathy is probably caused by acute capillary congestion and exudation with cerebral edema. The findings are usually reversible if adequate treatment is given promptly. There is no strict correlation of diastolic blood pressure with hypertensive encephalopathy.

**B. Signs:** Physical findings depend upon the cause of hypertension, its duration and severity, and the degree of effect on target organs.

**1. Blood pressure–**A diagnosis of hypertension is not warranted in patients under age 50 unless the blood pressure exceeds 140/90 mm Hg on at least 3 separate occasions after the patient has rested 10–20 or more minutes in familiar, quiet, warm surroundings. Readings taken in the usual fashion may be much higher than this in the absence of hypertensive disease, since with rest the pressures return to normal; though not true hypertension, these transient rises may often represent a precursor to sustained hypertension. On the initial observation, pressure should be examined in both arms and, if lower extremity pulses are diminished, in the legs. Supine and standing measurements should be made to detect postural changes.

**2. Retinas–**The Keith-Wagener (KW) classification of retinal changes in hypertension, in spite of deficiencies, has prognostic significance.

KW1 = Focal arteriolar narrowing
KW2 = More marked narrowing and arteriovenous nicking (atherosclerotic as well as hypertensive changes)
KW3 = Flame-shaped or circular hemorrhages and fluffy "cotton wool" exudates
KW4 = Any of the above plus papilledema, ie, elevation of the optic disk, obliteration of the physiologic cup, or blurring of the lateral disk margins. By definition, malignant hypertension is always associated with papilledema.

**3. Heart and arteries–**A loud aortic second sound and an early systolic ejection click may occur. Left ventricular enlargement with a left ventricular heave indicates well-established disease. A presystolic gallop alone does not imply failure but is due to decreased compliance of the left ventricle; it is quite common.

**4. Pulses–**Direct bilateral comparison should be made of both carotid, radial, femoral, popliteal, and pedal pulses; and the presence or absence of bruits over major vessels, including the abdominal aorta and iliacs, should be determined.

**C. Laboratory Findings:** Though normal early in essential hypertension, the urine may show a low, fixed specific gravity compatible with advanced renal parenchymal disease or hypokalemic nephropathy of primary aldosteronism. In renal disease, blood urea nitrogen and serum creatinine are elevated, and anemia due to advanced azotemia may be present. In aldosteronism, however, the serum potassium is low and the serum sodium and $HCO_3^-$ elevated; the reverse is true in uremia associated with primary renal disease.

Proteinuria, granular casts, and microhematuria may occur in either nephrosclerosis or chronic renal failure of other origin. (See Chapter 18 and the Appendix for laboratory findings associated with endocrine abnormalities.)

Appropriate laboratory tests should seek other risk factors for the development of atherosclerosis, particularly serum cholesterol and blood glucose determinations.

**D. Imaging:** Chest radiographs may disclose rib notching and the small aortic knob of coarctation. Intravenous urograms yield valuable information on renal size, rate of appearance and disappearance of the contrast material, and obstruction and are diagnostic of polycystic disease. However, they should not be performed unless preliminary evaluation suggests a secondary cause.

Though unnecessary in uncomplicated essential hypertension, echocardiography can assess the degree of left ventricular hypertrophy because it demonstrates increased ventricular septal and posterior free wall thickness and increased left ventricular mass. These abnormalities may be found even in patients without symptoms; they appear earlier and are a more sensitive index of left ventricular hypertrophy than electrocardiographic signs. Decreased diastolic function may also be noted.

**E. Electrocardiographic Findings:** Electrocardiography can predict left ventricular hypertrophy and may show signs of associated coronary artery disease. In aldosteronism and Cushing's disease, the QT interval is prolonged and the ST segment may be depressed (hypokalemia).

**F. Summary:** Since most hypertension is "primary," an extensive diagnostic evaluation is not indicated before starting therapy. Most clinicians obtain only a blood count, renal function study, electrolyte panel and urinalysis, chest film, and ECG after establishing the diagnosis. If conventional therapy is unsuccessful or if symptoms suggest a secondary cause, further studies are indicated.

## Who Should Be Treated?

Recommendations concerning which patients should be treated remain controversial. Factors that unfavorably influence the prognosis in chronic arterial hypertension and so determine the nature of drug therapy include the following: (1) the level of diastolic and systolic blood pressure, (2) male gender, (3) early age at onset, (4) black race, (5) retinal abnormalities, (6) cardiac abnormalities (eg, electrocardiographic changes, cardiomegaly, angina), (7) stroke, (8) renal dysfunction, and (9) family history of hypertension.

Appropriate drug treatment of asymptomatic chronic hypertension of moderate degree (> 105 mm Hg diastolic) results in significantly lower morbidity and mortality rates from cardiovascular disease (heart failure, hemorrhagic stroke, renal failure) than occur in untreated control patients. In patients with diastolic pressures under 105 mm Hg, the 5-year mortality rate from all causes was 20% lower in a stepped-care experimental group than in similar patients treated in the community. The conclusion that treatment of hypertension decreases the incidence of clinical coronary disease has been suggested but not established by some studies; another concluded that treatment of mild hypertension decreased the incidence of stroke but not that of coronary disease. Current insurance data have shown that even slight increases in blood pressure reduce longevity, especially by causing premature atherosclerosis.

Most recommendations are based upon the diastolic blood pressure, although as noted previously the systolic pressure is at least as good an indicator of risk. Virtually all patients should have 3 or more blood pressure measurements on different occasions prior to a final decision on therapy, since many patients will exhibit lower pressures. There is agreement that individuals with diastolic blood pressures greater than 100 mm Hg warrant treatment. At present, most authorities recommend treatment for patients who consistently exhibit diastolic pressures above 95 mm Hg despite nonpharmacologic measures. In these— and in individuals with blood pressures between 90 and 95 mm Hg—the presence of the additional risk factors noted above lowers the threshold for instituting therapy. White women tend to develop fewer complications, and a threshold of 100 mm Hg may be appropriate in otherwise low-risk members of this group.

## Nonpharmacologic Therapy

Because of growing appreciation of the toxicity of antihypertensive drugs, more serious attempts at nonpharmacologic therapy of mild hypertension are being made. Approaches of proved but modest value include weight reduction, reduced alcohol consumption, and in some patients reduced salt intake. Exercise conditioning programs also appear to be somewhat effective. Calcium and potassium supplements have been advocated, but their ability to lower blood pressure is limited and probably not applicable to most patients.

## Antihypertensive Drug Therapy

An ideal antihypertensive drug would be effective as a single agent or in combination with other agents in all classes of patients; would lower blood pressure by a physiologic mechanism; would reduce morbidity and mortality rates; would have no long-term toxicity; could be taken once a day; and would not require multiple-dose titration steps. In addition, the cost would be moderate. No such agent currently exists, but the growing number of available drugs has increasingly allowed the physician to tailor treatment to the needs of individual patients. These agents are listed in Table 8–2.

**A. The Stepped Care Approach:** Over the past 2 decades, the "stepped care" approach to treatment of hypertension has been advocated. Patients were initially started on a diuretic agent, and sympatholytic and vasodilator drugs were added later in that order if required. More recently, beta-blockers have been suggested as alternative starting agents. This approach has been highly effective, with approximately 80% of compliant patients exhibiting adequate blood pressure control. It has also been relatively inexpensive and straightforward.

However, a number of considerations have led experts to question this as a universal treatment plan. These include recognition of the frequency of adverse effects with diuretics and beta-blockers, concern over the long-term implications of the metabolic changes induced by these agents, realization that patients not controlled by one agent may be controlled by another without moving directly to combined therapy, and the more recent availability of other agents suitable for initial therapy.

**B. Potential Initial Medications:** Four classes of agents have been demonstrated to be effective and suitable for initial antihypertensive therapy: diuretics, beta-blockers, angiotensin-converting enzyme (ACE) inhibitors, and calcium channel blockers. The 4 classes of drugs produce comparable lowering of blood pressure, so that selection is based upon other factors such as the presence of accompanying illnesses and cost. In addition, the alpha-adrenergic blockers and central sympatholytic agents are sometimes employed as single therapy.

**C. Current Antihypertensive Agents:**

**1. Diuretics–**The diuretics are the most widely used hypertensive medications. They are effective in patients with all levels of blood pressure and in all demographic groups. Relative to the beta-blockers and the ACE inhibitors, they are more potent in blacks, older individuals, the obese, and other subgroups with increased plasma volume or low plasma renin activity. Overall, when administered alone, they control blood pressure in 50–60% of patients, and they can be used effectively with all other agents.

Diuretics lower blood pressure initially by decreasing plasma volume (by suppressing tubular reabsorption of sodium, thus increasing the excretion of sodium and water) and cardiac output, but during chronic therapy their major hemodynamic effect is reduction of peripheral vascular resistance by an as yet unknown mechanism. It is now generally appreciated that most of the effect of these agents is achieved at lower dosages than used previously but that their

**Table 8–2.** Antihypertensive medications.

| Class (Drug) | Initial Dosage | Usual Range | Common Adverse Effects | Comments |
|---|---|---|---|---|
| **Diuretics** Hydrochlorothiazide | 12.5–25 mg daily | 12.5–100 mg daily | $\downarrow$ $K^+$, $Mg^{2+}$, $\uparrow$ glucose, $Ca^{2+}$ cholesterol, uric acid | Concern over long-term consequences of metabolic changes |
| Other thiazides | Various | Various | | |
| Chlorthalidone | 12.5–25 mg | 12.5–50 mg daily | Rash, impotence, metabolic changes | $K^+$ replacement often necessary |
| Metolazone | 2.5 mg daily | 2.5–5 mg daily | | |
| Indapamide | 2.5 mg | 2.5–5 mg daily | | |
| **Combination agents** Dyazide | 1–2 capsules daily | 1–4 capsules in 1 or 2 doses | Same as diuretics plus gastrointestinal disturbances | |
| Maxide | ½ tablet daily | ½–2 tablets | | |
| Moduretic | ½ tablet daily | ½–2 tablets daily | | |
| **Beta-blockers** Propranolol | 20 mg twice daily | 20–160 mg twice daily | Bradycardia, fatigue, bronchospasm, sleep disturbances, cold extremities, impotence, triglycerides, $\uparrow$ HDL cholesterol | See Table 8–3. |
| Metoprolol | 50 mg twice daily | 50–200 mg twice daily | | |
| Nadolol | 20 mg daily | 20–160 mg daily | | |
| Atenolol | 50 mg twice daily | 50–200 mg daily | | |
| Timolol | 5 mg twice daily | 5–10 mg twice daily | | |
| Pindolol | 5 mg twice daily | 5–20 mg twice daily | | |
| Labetalol | 100 mg twice daily | 100–600 mg twice daily | | Combined beta- and alpha-blocker |
| Acebutolol | 400 mg daily | 400–1200 mg in 1 or 2 doses | | |
| **ACE inhibitors** Captopril | 12.5–25 mg twice daily | 50–300 mg in 2 or 3 doses | Skin rash, taste disturbances, cough, angioneurotic edema, hypotension, renal insufficiency | |
| Enalapril | 5 mg daily | 5–40 mg in 1 or 2 doses | | |
| **Calcium blockers** Verapamil | 240 mg daily | 240–480 mg in 1 or 2 doses | Constipation, headache, edema, bradycardia | Slow-release form |
| Diltiazem | 120 mg twice daily | 120–240 mg twice daily | Headache, eczema, bradycardia | Approval pending |
| Nifedipine | 10 mg 3 times daily | 10–30 mg twice daily | Headache, palpitations, edema | Approval pending |
| Nitrendipine | 10 mg daily | 10–40 mg in 1 or 2 doses | Same as nifedipine | Approval pending |
| **Central sympatholytics** Methyldopa | 250 mg twice daily | 250 mg–1 gm twice daily | Sedation, dry mouth, hemolytic anemia, hepatitis | |
| Clonidine | 0.1 mg twice daily | 0.1–0.3 twice daily | Sedation, dry mouth | Rebound hypertension |
| Guanabenz | 4 mg twice daily | 4–16 mg twice daily | Same as clonidine | Rebound hypertension |
| **Peripheral sympatholytics** Prazosin | 1 mg twice daily | 1–10 mg twice daily | First dose syncope, palpitations, headaches | |
| Guanethidine | 10 mg daily | 10–100 mg daily | Orthostatic hypotension, diarrhea | |
| Guanadrel | 5 mg twice daily | 5–20 mg twice daily | Same as guanethedine | |
| Reserpine | 0.1 mg daily | 0.1–0.25 mg daily | Depression, peptic disease | |
| **Arteriolar dilators** Hydralazine | 25 mg twice daily | 25–200 mg twice daily | Gastrointestinal intolerance, headache, tachycardia | |
| Minoxidil | 5 mg daily | 5–20 mg twice daily | Headache, fluid retention, hirsutism | |

biochemical effects are dose-related. The thiazide diuretics are the most widely used. The loop diuretics (such as furosemide) may lead to electrolyte and volume depletion more readily than the thiazides and have short durations of action; therefore, they are not ordinarily used in hypertension except in the presence of renal failure (serum creatinine above 2.5 mg/dL).

Combinations of thiazide diuretics and potassium-sparing agents (spironolactone, triamterine, amiloride) are often employed, but these medications are considerably more expensive, have additional side effects, impose a risk of hyperkalemia if potassium supplements are given, are often unnecessary in patients receiving low diuretic dosages, and are dangerous in the presence of oliguria. Their use should be restricted to individuals demonstrating hypokalemia (serum $K^+$ < 3.5 mmol/L or a reduction greater than 0.6 mmol/L from baseline).

The adverse effects of diuretics relate chiefly to the metabolic changes listed in Table 8–2. Impotence, skin rashes, and photosensitivity are also frequent. Hypokalemia leads to decreased renal blood flow with a potential rise in serum creatinine, especially in older patients. The rise in serum creatinine is usually reversible, but the evidence is unclear about its long-term significance and reversibility. Hypokalemia can be avoided by a high-potassium diet with fresh fruit and green vegetables. Diuretics also increase serum uric acid and may facilitate acute gout. An increase in blood glucose is common as well.

**2. Beta-adrenergic blocking agents–**(Table 8–3.) These drugs are effective in hypertension because they decrease the heart rate and cardiac output. Even after continued use of beta-blockers for a number of years, cardiac output remains decreased and systemic vascular resistance increased. The beta-blockers also decrease renin release, and they are in general more efficacious in populations likely to have elevated plasma renin activity, such as younger white patients. They neutralize the reflex tachycardia caused by vasodilators such as hydralazine and prazosin in the treatment of hypertension.

Although all beta-blockers appear to be approximately equivalent in antihypertensive potency, they differ in a number of pharmacologic properties (these differences are summarized in Table 8–3). They differ with respect to whether their effect is relatively specific to the cardiac $\beta_1$ receptors (cardioselectivity) or whether they also block the $\beta_2$ receptors in the bronchi and vasculature; at higher dosages, however, all agents are nonselective. The beta-blockers also differ in their pharmacokinetics, lipid solubility—which determines whether they enter the brain and cause cerebral symptoms—and mechanism of elimination. The effect on the pulse rate varies; pindolol or acebutolol, with intrinsic sympathetic activity, may be preferable in patients who develop more pronounced bradycardia (< 45/min) when given other beta-blockers. Labetalol is a combined alpha- and beta-blocker and decreases peripheral resistance more than the other agents. Experience leads physicians to prefer one over another.

The side effects of all beta-blockers include development of bronchial asthma in predisposed patients; severe bradycardia; atrioventricular conduction defects; left ventricular conduction defects; left ventricular failure, because of the negative inotropic action of the sympatholytic action of the drug; nasal congestion; cold hands and feet or Raynaud's phenomenon, especially in women in cold weather; and, rarely, central nervous system symptoms with nightmares, excitement, and confusion. Fatigue and lethargy may occur.

The beta-blockers are most useful in patients with associated conditions that benefit from this mode of therapy. These include patients with angina pectoris, patients with previous myocardial infarction, individuals with migraine headaches, and somatic manifestations of anxiety. These agents are contraindicated in patients with congestive heart failure, symptomatic bronchospasm, and peripheral vascular disease.

**3. Angiotensin converting enzyme (ACE) inhibitors–**These drugs are being increasingly used in mild to moderate hypertension, often as the initial medication. Their mode of action relates to inhibition of the renin-angiotensin-aldosterone system and decreased inhibition of bradykinin. They exhibit some effect even in patients with low plasma renin activity and may increase the synthesis of vasodilating prostaglandins responsible for the side effect of cough (see below). The ACE inhibitors appear to be most effective in younger individuals, whites, and those with increased plasma renin activity. They are relatively less effective in blacks and in the elderly. While as single therapy they achieve adequate antihypertensive control in only about 40–50% of patients, the combination of an ACE inhibitor and a diuretic is potent.

The major advantage of the ACE inhibitors is their relative freedom from troublesome side effects. Hypotension is most severe in patients with bilateral renal artery stenosis; acute renal failure may ensue. A chronic dry cough due to bronchial or laryngeal irritation is seen in 5–10% of patients and may require stopping the drug. Skin rashes and taste alterations are seen more often with captopril than enalapril but

**Table 8–3.** Pharmacologic properties of beta-blockers.

| | Cardio-selectivity | Intrinsic Sympathomimetic Activity | Lipid Solubility |
|---|---|---|---|
| Propranolol | 0 | 0 | ++ |
| Metoprolol | + | 0 | ++ |
| Nadolol | 0 | 0 | 0 |
| Atenolol | + | 0 | 0 |
| Timolol | 0 | 0 | + |
| Pindolol | 0 | ++ | + |
| Acebutolol | + | + | + |
| Labetalol* | 0 | 0 | ++ |

0 = absent; + = moderate; ++ = marked
* Labetalol has additional alpha-adrenergic blocking properties.

often disappear with continued therapy. Angioneurotic edema is an uncommon but potentially dangerous side effect of all agents of this class. Proteinuria and neutropenia are very uncommon at the lower dosages now employed except in individuals with preexisting renal insufficiency or autoimmune disease. ACE inhibitors do not produce impotence or fatigue and therefore, unlike many other medications, do not impair quality of life.

**4. Calcium channel blockers–**All the agents of this class reduce blood pressure, although at this time only verapamil has been approved for this indication in the United States. They do so by peripheral vasodilation, which is associated with less reflex tachycardia, increase in myocardial contractility, or fluid retention than with other vasodilators. These agents are effective as single-drug therapy in approximately 50% of patients and appear to be beneficial in all demographic groups and all grades of hypertension. As a result, they may be preferable to beta-blockers and ACE inhibitors in blacks and older subjects. Calcium channel blockers and diuretics are less additive when given together than when either is combined with beta-blockers or ACE inhibitors. However, calcium channel blockers should be combined cautiously with beta-blockers because of their potential for depressing atrioventricular conduction and sinus node automaticity.

The most common side effects of calcium channel blockers are headache, peripheral edema, bradycardia, and constipation (especially with verapamil in the elderly). The dihydropyridine agents, such as nifedipine and nitrendipine, are more likely to produce symptoms of vasodilation, such as headache, flushing, and palpitations. All calcium channel blockers have negative inotropic effects and may cause heart failure in patients with cardiac dysfunction. All of these agents are being developed in preparations that can be administered once or twice daily, but their high cost will limit their use in hypertension.

**5. Drugs with central sympatholytic action–** Methyldopa, clonidine, and guanabenz lower blood pressure by stimulating alpha-adrenergic receptors in the central nervous system, thus reducing efferent peripheral sympathetic outflow. These agents may be effective as single therapy in a minority of patients, but they are often associated with fluid retention and subsequent "pseudotolerance." They are thus most useful in combination with diuretics or ACE inhibitors. In addition, these agents produce frequent side effects, including sedation, fatigue, dry mouth, postural hypotension, and impotence. An important concern is rebound hypertension following abrupt withdrawal. The first dose of clonidine may cause marked drowsiness; therefore, it should be given at bedtime at a dose no greater than 0.1 mg. Methyldopa also causes hepatitis and hemolytic anemia and should be avoided except in individuals who have already tolerated chronic therapy.

**6. Alpha-receptor antagonists–**Prazosin blocks postsynaptic alpha receptors, relaxes smooth muscle,

and reduces blood pressure by lowering peripheral vascular resistance. This agent is effective as single-drug therapy in some individuals, but tachyphylaxis may appear during long-term therapy. The major side effects are marked hypotension and syncope after the first dose, which, therefore, should be given at bedtime; palpitations and headache also occur. Unlike the beta-blockers and diuretics, prazosin has no adverse effect on serum lipid levels—in fact, it appears to lower total cholesterol—and does not impair exercise tolerance. Prazosin is most useful in combination with diuretics or in multidrug combinations in refractory patients.

**7. Arteriolar dilators–**Hydralazine and minoxidil relax vascular smooth muscle and produce peripheral vasodilatation. When given alone, they stimulate reflex tachycardia, increase myocardial contractility, and cause headache, palpitations, and fluid retention. They are usually given in combination with diuretics and beta-blockers in resistant patients. Hydralazine produces frequent gastrointestinal disturbances and may induce a lupuslike syndrome. Minoxidil causes hirsutism and marked fluid retention; this agent is reserved for the most refractory of patients.

**8. Peripheral sympathetic inhibitors–**These agents are now used infrequently. Reserpine remains an effective antihypertensive agent and a cost-effective one. Its reputation for inducing mental depression and its other side effects—sedation, nasal stuffiness, sleep disturbances, and gastroduodenal ulcers—have made it unpopular, though these problems are uncommon at low dosages. Guanethidine and guanadrel inhibit catecholamine release from peripheral neurons but frequently cause orthostatic hypotension (especially in the morning or after exercise), diarrhea, and fluid retention. These agents are used chiefly in refractory hypertension.

**9. Combination therapy–**The vast majority of patients with hypertension can be controlled with one agent or combinations such as diuretics plus beta-blockers, diuretics plus ACE inhibitors, diuretics plus calcium channel blockers, calcium blockers plus ACE inhibitors, or diuretics plus central sympatholytic agents. A minority of patients may require triple-drug therapy. Patients who are compliant with their medications and who do not respond to these combinations should usually be evaluated for secondary hypertension before proceeding to more complex regimens.

### Goal of Treatment

The goal of treatment should be to reduce blood pressure to normal levels (ie, less than 140/90 mm Hg). Since there may be additional benefits from further lowering of blood pressure, most authorities also seek to achieve a minimum of 10 mm Hg reduction in diastolic pressure in patients with mild hypertension (90–99 mm Hg). In older patients with predominantly systolic hypertension, a systolic pressure of 150–160 mm Hg is a satisfactory end point. However, a significant decrease in hypertension-related morbidity from blood pressure reduction is possible even if these therapeutic goals are not achieved. Thus, a compromise between goal blood pressure and an adequately tolerated therapeutic regimen may be necessary in some individuals.

The effectiveness of therapy often cannot be determined by casual blood pressure readings in the physician's office. Ideally, home blood pressure readings should be recorded and shown to the physician at regular visits. Ambulatory blood pressure recordings taken throughout the day give a more representative record of the patient's usual pressures and may predict clinical outcome more reliably than office pressures. The apparatus is commercially available.

### Acute Hypertensive Crises

**A. Parenteral Agents:** Several parenteral antihypertensive drugs are available for management of acute hypertensive crisis (see Table 8–4), but none can be called the drug of choice. The treatment goal should be relatively gradual reduction in blood pressure to levels near normal. Rapid reduction of pressure is best avoided.

**1. Sodium nitroprusside**–0.5–10 µg/kg/min

is given by controlled intravenous infusion gradually titrated to the desired effect. It lowers the blood pressure within seconds by direct arteriolar and venous dilatation, thus decreasing preload as well as afterload. Monitoring with an intra-arterial line is essential to avoid hypotension. The drug—in combination with a beta-blocker—is especially useful in patients with aortic dissection.

**2. Trimethaphan (Arfonad)**–The ganglionic blocking agent trimethaphan (1–5 mg/min intravenously) is titrated with the patient sitting; its activity depends upon this. The patient can be placed supine if the hypotensive effect is excessive. The effect occurs within a few minutes and persists for the duration of the infusion.

**3. Diazoxide (Hyperstat)**–Diazoxide, 75–300 mg intravenously in a single dose or in multiple smaller doses, acts promptly as a vasodilator without decreasing renal blood flow. It has been used often in preeclampsia-eclampsia. Side effects include hypotension, which may be severe; this necessitates starting with a smaller dose in elderly patients or administering by slow infusion over 30 minutes, which is

**Table 8–4.** Drugs for hypertensive crises.

| Agent | Action | Dosage | Onset | Duration | Adverse Effects | Comments |
|---|---|---|---|---|---|---|
| **Parenteral agents (intravenously unless noted)** | | | | | | |
| Nitroprusside | Vasodilator | 0.5–10 µg/kg/min | Seconds | 3–5 minutes | Gastrointestinal, central nervous system | Most effective treatment. Use with beta-blocker in aortic dissection. |
| Diazoxide | Vasodilator | 15–30 mg/min to 300 mg | 1–5 minutes | 4–12 hours | Nausea, excessive hypotension, tachycardia | Avoid in coronary artery disease and dissection. Use with beta-blocker and diuretic. |
| Trimethaphan | Ganglionic blocker | 1–5 mg/min | 1–3 minutes | 10 minutes | Hypotension, ileus | Useful in aortic dissection. |
| Labetalol | Beta- and alpha-blocker | 20 mg every 10 minutes to 300 mg | 5 minutes | 3–6 hours | Gastrointestinal, hypotension | Avoid in congestive heart failure, asthma. |
| Hydralazine | Vasodilator | 5–20 mg intravenously or intramuscularly | 10–30 minutes | 2–6 hours | Tachycardia, headache, gastrointestinal | Avoid in coronary artery disease, dissection. |
| Propranolol | Beta-blocker | 1 mg/min to 10 mg | 1 minute | 2–3 hours | Bradycardia | Avoid in congestive heart failure, asthma. Useful in combination with vasodilator. |
| Furosemide | Diuretic | 10–80 mg | 15 minutes | 4 hours | | Adjunct to vasodilator. |
| **Oral agents** | | | | | | |
| Nifedipine | $Ca^{2+}$ blocker | 10 mg initially | 15 minutes | 2–6 hours | Excessive hypotension, tachycardia, headache | Response variable. |
| Clonidine | Central sympatholytic | 0.2 mg initially; 0.1 mg every hour to 0.8 mg | 30–60 minutes | 6–8 hours | Sedation | Rebound may occur. |
| Captopril | ACE inhibitor | 6–50 mg | 15–30 minutes | 4–6 hours | Excessive hypotension | |

usually just as effective and better tolerated. Hyperglycemia and sodium and water retention may occur. The drug should be used only for short periods and is best combined with a powerful diuretic such as furosemide.

**4. Labetalol**–This combined beta- and alpha-adrenergic blocking agent is the only beta-blocker that can lower blood pressure rapidly enough for emergency treatment. The usual intravenous dose is 20 mg over 5–10 minutes, followed by additional 20-mg increments each 10–20 minutes to a maximum of 300 mg.

**5. Hydralazine**–Hydralazine can be given intravenously or intramuscularly, but its effect is less predictable than that of other drugs in this group. It produces reflex tachycardia and should not be given without beta-blockers in patients with possible coronary disease or aortic dissection. Hydralazine is also valuable in children and pregnant women.

**6. Diuretics**–Diuretics can be very helpful when the patient has signs of heart failure or fluid retention. They facilitate the response to vasodilators, which often stimulate fluid retention.

**B. Oral Agents:** Patients with less severe acute hypertensive syndromes can often be treated with oral therapy. They should be closely monitored until a therapeutic end point is achieved.

**1. Clonidine**–Clonidine, 0.2 mg orally initially, followed by 0.1 mg every hour to a total of 0.8 mg will usually lower blood pressure over a period of several hours. Sedation is frequent, and rebound hypertension may occur unless the agent is continued.

**2. Nifedipine**–Nifedipine, 5–10 mg orally or sublingually, will reduce blood pressure within 5–20 minutes in most patients. An additional 10-mg dose may be needed. Excessive hypotensive responses may occur, and reflex tachycardia may induce angina.

**3. Captopril**–Captopril, 12.5–25 mg orally, will also lower blood pressure in 15–30 minutes. The response is variable and may be excessive.

**C. Subsequent Therapy:** When the blood pressure has been brought under control, combinations of oral antihypertensive agents can be added as parenteral drugs are tapered off over a period of 2–3 days.

## Hypertension in the Presence of Renal Failure

In the presence of renal failure, hypertension is highly dependent on blood volume. If the blood pressure is not reduced by vigorous use of antihypertensive drugs—including furosemide, beta-blocking drugs, minoxidil, or diazoxide—dialysis should be employed; in most instances, the blood pressure will be reduced as the patient achieves a dry weight state. The presence of renal failure is an adverse prognostic sign, but vigorous therapy often can prolong life.

## Prognosis

Although many patients with slight elevation of blood pressure live a normal life span, most patients with untreated hypertension die of complications within 20 years. Before effective antihypertensive drugs were available, 70% of patients died of heart failure or coronary artery disease, 15% of cerebral hemorrhage, and 10% of uremia.

Buck C et al: The prognosis of hypertension according to age at onset. *Hypertension* 1987;**9**:204.

Contemporary considerations in the treatment of hypertension: Cost, efficacy, and preference. (Symposium.) Stason WB, Pauly MV (guest editors). *Am J Med* 1986;**81(Suppl 6C):**1.[Entire issue.]

Cressman MD, Gifford RW: Hypertension and stroke. *J Am Coll Cardiol* 1983;**1(2-Part 1):**521.

Frishman WH et al: Comparison of hydrochlorothiazide and sustained-release diltiazem for mild-to-moderate systemic hypertension. *Am J Cardiol* 1987;**59**:615.

Houston MC: Treatment of hypertensive urgencies and emergencies with nifedipine. *Am Heart J* 1986;**11**:963.

Lang RE, Unger T, Ganten D: Atrial natriuretic peptide: A new factor in blood pressure control (editorial review). *J Hypertens* 1987;**5**:255.

Liebson PR, Devereux RB, Horan MJ (guest editors): Hypertension research: Echocardiography in the measurement of left ventricular wall mass. *Hypertension* 1987;**9(Suppl II).** [Entire issue.]

Medical Research Council Working Party: MRC trial of treatment of mild hypertension: Principal results. *Br Med J* 1985;**291**:97.

Parati GF et al: Relationship of 24-hour blood pressure mean and variability to severity of target-organ damage in hypertension. *J Hypertens* 1987;**5**:93.

Perloff D: Hypertensive emergencies. Chap 9, pp 181–201, in: *Cardiac Emergencies*. Scheinman MM (editor). Saunders, 1984.

Perloff D, Sokolow M, Cowan R: The prognostic value of ambulatory blood pressures. *JAMA* 1983;**249**:2792.

Reams GP, Bauer JH, Gaddy P: Use of the converting enzyme inhibitor enalapril in renovascular hypertension: Effect on blood pressure, renal function, and the renin-angiotensin-aldosterone system. *Hypertension* 1986;**8**:290.

Sos TA et al: Percutaneous transluminal renal angioplasty in renovascular hypertension due to atheroma or fibromuscular dysplasia. *N Engl J Med* 1983;**309**:274.

Szlachcic J: Diltiazem versus propranolol in essential hypertension: Responses of rest and exercise blood pressure and effects on exercise capacity. *Am J Cardiol* 1987;**59**:393.

# CORONARY HEART DISEASE (Arteriosclerotic Coronary Artery Disease; Ischemic Heart Disease)

Coronary atherosclerotic heart disease is the commonest cause of cardiovascular disability and death in the United States. Altered lipid metabolism or excessive intake of cholesterol and saturated fats, together with changes in the vascular endothelium and smooth muscle proliferation, lead to localized subintimal accumulations of fatty and fibrous tissue that progressively obstruct the coronary arteries and their main branches. Elevated total serum cholesterol and low-density lipoproteins are involved in the development of atherosclerosis and are markers of high risk. High-density lipoproteins may play an equally important protective role, and the concentrations of the apoproteins A-I and B (the protein moieties of the lipoproteins) are also important markers of risk.

While atherosclerosis is a chronic process occurring over decades, it is becoming increasingly clear that plaque ulceration, intimal hemorrhage and dissection, and vascular thrombosis accelerate the process and are responsible for most acute ischemic syndromes, such as infarction and unstable angina.

Additional risk factors for the development of ischemic heart disease include age, genetic predisposition, arterial hypertension, cigarette smoking, and diabetes mellitus. Other factors of less certain importance include obesity, poor physical fitness, and personality type.

## Prevention of Ischemic Heart Disease in Patient With High-Risk Factors

Risk factors are less significant in patients over 50. It is not clear to what extent treating risk factors will prevent further progression of disease once it has started, but favorable trends are becoming clear; for example, the treatment of type II hypercholesterolemia has decreased the incidence of coronary events in affected patients. Cessation of smoking, treatment of hyperlipidemia, and amelioration of hypertension have reduced coronary risk in some studies. Control of blood pressure has less impact on coronary morbidity but remains an important goal. The decrease in number of coronary deaths over the last 2 decades may be due to a decrease in the prevalence of risk factors but also probably reflects the role of coronary care units, better treatment of arrhythmias and heart failure, and improved survival after coronary revascularization in some patient subsets.

## Pathophysiology

Men are more often affected than women by an overall ratio of 4:1, but before age 40, the ratio is 8:1, and beyond age 70 it is 1:1. In men, the peak incidence of clinical manifestations is at age 50–60; in women, at age 60–70. Advanced stages of atherosclerotic coronary artery disease—even complete occlusion—may remain clinically silent, being discovered incidentally after death due to other causes. At present, the only means of determining the location and extent of narrowing is coronary arteriography, although ischemia can be recognized by other studies. There is only a modest correlation between the clinical symptoms and the extent of disease. Functional myocardial ischemia may be documented even in asymptomatic individuals by electrocardiographic stress tests, by reversible thallium-201 perfusion defects, or by reversible segmental wall motion abnormalities at echocardiography. Some episodes of myocardial ischemia are painful, causing angina pectoris; others are completely silent. In preliminary studies, the prognosis is similar whether or not pain occurs.

Anderson KM, Castelli WP, Levy D: Cholesterol and mortality: 30 years follow-up from the Framingham Study. *JAMA* 1987;**257**:2176.

Beller GA, Gibson RS: Sensitivity, specificity, and prognostic significance of noninvasive testing for occult or known coronary disease. *Prog Cardiovasc Dis* 1987;**26**:241.

Berkoff HA, Levine RL: Management of the vascular patient with multisystem atherosclerosis. *Prog Cardiovasc Dis* 1987;**29**:347.

Bigger JT et al: Prevalence, characteristics and significance of ventricular tachycardia detected by 24-hour continuous electrocardiographic recordings in the late hospital phase of acute myocardial infarction. *Am J Cardiol* 1986;**58**:1151.

Fuster V et al: Platelet-inhibitor drugs' role in coronary artery disease. *Prog Cardiovasc Dis* 1987;**29**:325.

Gottlieb SO et al: Silent ischemia as a marker for early unfavorable outcomes in patients with unstable angina. *N Engl J Med* 1986;**314**:1214.

Hoeg JM et al: Comparison of six pharmacologic regimens for hypercholesterolemia. *Am J Cardiol* 1987;**59**:812.

Kane JP, Havel RJ: Treatment of hypercholesterolemia. *Ann Rev Med* 1986;**37**:427.

Kottke BA et al: Apolipoproteins and coronary artery disease. *Mayo Clin Proc* 1986;**61**:313.

Kromhout D, Bosschieter EB, de Lezenne Coulander C: The inverse relation between fish consumption and 20-year mortality from coronary heart disease. *N Engl J Med* 1985;**312**:1205.

Lipid Research Clinics Program: The lipid research clinics coronary primary prevention trial results. 1. Reduction in incidence of coronary heart disease. 2. The relationship of reduction in incidence of coronary heart disease to cholesterol lowering. *JAMA* 1984;**251**:351, 365.

Silverman KJ, Grossman W: Angina pectoris: Natural history and strategies for evaluation and management. *N Engl J Med* 1984;**310**:1712.

## SUDDEN DEATH

Sudden death may be the first clinical manifestation of coronary disease in as many as one-fourth of patients but is more likely to occur in patients with prior infarction and moderate to severe left ventricular dysfunction. In addition, 25% of patients with acute myocardial infarction will die before reaching a hospital. Most of these deaths are caused by ventricular fibrillation. See p 213 for management of patients at risk for sudden death and the management of survivors.

Kannel WB, Cupples LA, D'Agostino RB: Sudden death risk in overt coronary heart disease: The Framingham Study. *Am Heart J* 1987;**113**:799.

## ANGINA PECTORIS

Angina pectoris is usually due to atherosclerotic heart disease, but in rare instances it may occur in the absence of coronary artery obstruction as a result of coronary spasm, severe aortic stenosis or insufficiency, syphilitic aortitis, or vasculitis, or in response to increased metabolic demands, as in hyperthyroidism, marked anemia, or paroxysmal tachycardias with rapid ventricular rates. The underlying mechanism is a discrepancy between the myocardial requirements for oxygen and the amount delivered through the coronary arteries: either increased demand (as in exercise) or diminished coronary flow (increased vascular tone or platelet deposition) or both.

## Clinical Findings

**A. History:** The diagnosis of angina pectoris depends principally upon the history; the patient should describe the symptoms without prompting by the examiner, using gestures to characterize the location and quality of the symptom. The history should specifically include the following information.

**1. Circumstances that precipitate and relieve angina**–Angina occurs most commonly during activity and is relieved by resting. Exertion that involves straining the thoracic or upper extremity muscles (eg, lifting) or walking rapidly uphill precipitates an attack most rapidly. Patients prefer to remain upright rather than lie down. The amount of activity required to produce angina may be relatively consistent under comparable physical and emotional circumstances but may vary from day to day. It is usually less after meals, during excitement, or on exposure to cold. The threshold for angina is often lower in the morning or after strong emotion; the latter can provoke attacks in the absence of exertion. In addition, discomfort may occur at rest or at night as a result of coronary spasm.

**2. Characteristics of the discomfort**–Patients often do not refer to angina as ''pain'' but as a sensation of tightness, squeezing, burning, pressing, choking, aching, bursting, ''gas,'' indigestion, or an ill-characterized discomfort. It is often characterized by clenching a fist over the mid chest. The distress of angina is never sharply localized and is not spasmodic.

**3. Location and radiation**–The distribution of the distress may vary widely in different patients but is usually the same for each patient unless unstable angina or myocardial infarction supervenes. In 80–90% of cases, the discomfort is felt behind or slightly to the left of the mid sternum. When it begins farther to the left or, uncommonly, on the right, it characteristically moves centrally to include the sternum. Although angina may radiate to any dermatome from C8 to T4, it radiates most often to the left shoulder and upper arm, frequently moving down the inner volar aspect of the arm to the elbow, forearm, wrist, or fourth and fifth fingers. Radiation to the right shoulder and distally is less common, but the characteristics are the same. Occasionally, angina may be felt initially in the lower jaw, the back of the neck, the interscapular area, high in the left back, or in the volar aspect of the wrist. If the patient identifies the site of pain by pointing to the area of the apical impulse with one finger, angina is an unlikely diagnosis.

**4. Duration of attacks**–Angina is of short duration and subsides completely without residual discomfort. If the attack is precipitated by exertion and the patient promptly stops to rest, the distress usually lasts less than 3 minutes (although most patients think it is longer). Attacks following a heavy meal or brought on by anger often last 15–20 minutes. Attacks lasting more than 30 minutes are unusual and suggest the development of unstable angina or myocardial infarction.

**5. Effect of nitroglycerin**–The diagnosis of angina pectoris is strongly supported if sublingual nitroglycerin invariably shortens an attack and if prophylactic nitrates permit greater exertion or prevent angina entirely.

**B. Signs:** Examination during a spontaneous or induced attack frequently reveals a significant elevation in systolic and diastolic blood pressure, although hypotension may also occur; occasionally, gallop rhythm and an apical systolic murmur are present during pain only. Supraventricular or ventricular arrhythmias may be present, either as the precipitating factor or as a result of ischemia.

It is important to detect signs of diseases that may contribute to or accompany atherosclerotic heart disease, eg, diabetes mellitus (retinopathy or neuropathy), xanthelasma, tendinous xanthomas, hypertension, thyrotoxicosis, or peripheral vascular disease. Aortic stenosis or regurgitation, hypertrophic cardiomyopathy, and mitral valve prolapse should be sought, since they may produce angina or other forms of chest pain.

**C. Laboratory Findings:** It is wise to evaluate risk factors associated with the development of atherosclerosis, particularly serum cholesterol. Contributing factors such as anemia, renal disease, thyrotoxicosis, or myxedema may be sought if history and physical examination warrant.

**D. Electrocardiography:** The resting ECG is normal in about a quarter of patients with angina. In the remainder, abnormalities include old myocardial infarction, nonspecific ST-T changes, atrioventricular or intraventricular conduction defects, and patterns of left ventricular hypertrophy.

**E. Exercise Electrocardiography:** Exercise testing is the most useful readily available procedure to assess the patient with angina. Ischemia is detected by precipitation of typical chest pain or ST segment depression (or, rarely, elevation). Exercise testing is often combined with scintigraphic studies (see below), but in patients without baseline ST segment abnormalities or in whom anatomic localization is not necessary, the exercise ECG should be the initial procedure because of considerations of cost and convenience.

Exercise testing can be done on a motorized treadmill (Bruce protocol) or with a bicycle ergometer. At least 2 electrocardiographic leads should be monitored continuously.

**1. Precautions and risks**–Patients should not undergo exercise testing if they are clinically unstable. The usually quoted risk is one infarction or death per 1000 tests, but individuals with pain at rest or minimal activity are at higher risk and should not be tested. Many of the tradtional exclusions, such as recent myocardial infarction or congestive heart failure, are no longer employed *if the patient is stable and ambulatory,* but aortic stenosis remains a contraindication. A physician should monitor the test, and full resuscitation equipment should be available. While most tests are carried to a symptom-limited endpoint (except submaximal testing early postinfarction), the test should be terminated when hypotension, significant ventricular or supraventricular arrhythmias, more than mild to moderate angina, or more than 3- to 4-mm ST segment depression occurs.

**2. Indications**–Exercise testing is employed (1) to diagnose angina; (2) to determine the severity of limitation due to angina; (3) to assess prognosis in patients with known coronary disease, by detecting groups at high or low risk; and (4) less successfully, to screen asymptomatic populations, in whom false-positive results are common. Nevertheless, silent ischemia may be demonstrated.

**3. Interpretation**–The usual electrocardiographic criterion for a positive test is 1 mm (0.1 mV) horizontal or downsloping ST segment depression (beyond baseline) measured 80 ms after the J point. By this criterion, 60–80% of patients with anatomically significant coronary disease will have a positive test, but 10–20% of those without significant disease will also be positive. False-positives are uncommon when a 2-mm depression is required. Additional information is inferred from the time of onset and duration of the electrocardiographic changes, their magnitude and configuration, blood pressure and heart rate changes, the duration of exercise, and the presence of associated symptoms. In general, patients exhibiting more severe ST segment depression (> 2 mm) at low workloads (< 6 min on the Bruce protocol) or heart rates (< 85% of age-predicted maximum)—especially when the duration of exercise and rise in blood pressure are limited—have more severe disease and a poorer prognosis. Depending on symptom status, age, and other factors, such patients are often referred for coronary arteriography and possible revascularization. On the other hand, less impressive positive tests in asymptomatic patients are often "false positives." Therefore, exercise testing results that do not conform to the clinical picture should be confirmed by scintigraphic study (see below).

**F. Scintigraphic Assessment of Ischemia:** Two nuclear medicine studies provide additional information about the presence, location, and extent of coronary disease.

**1. Thallium-201 scintigraphy**–This test provides images in which radionuclide uptake is proportionate to blood flow at the time of injection. Areas of diminished uptake reflect relative hypoperfusion (compared to other myocardial regions). If the radiotracer is injected during exercise or dipyridamole (Persantine)-induced coronary vasodilation, thallium-201 defects indicate a zone of ischemia or hypoperfusion. Over time, as relative blood flow equalizes, these defects "fill in" if the abnormality is transient, indicating reversible ischemia. Defects observed when the radiotracer is injected at rest or still present 3–4 hours after an injection during exercise or dipyridamole vasodilatation usually indicate myocardial infarction (old or recent) but may be present with severe ischemia. Occasionally, other conditions, including infiltrative diseases (sarcoidosis, amyloidosis) and dilated cardiomyopathy, may produce resting or persistent perfusion defects.

In experienced laboratories, thallium-201 scintigraphy is positive in 75–85% of patients with anatomically significant coronary disease and in only about 10% of those without it. False-positive tests in women may be due to attenuation through breast tissue. Although semiquantitative methods of analysis are available, the value of this test is dependent on the expertise of the laboratory involved.

Thallium-201 scintigraphy is indicated (1) when the resting ECG makes an exercise ECG difficult to interpret (LBBB, baseline ST-T changes, low voltage, etc); (2) for confirmation of the results of the exercise ECG when they are contrary to the clinical impression (eg, a positive test in an asymptomatic patient); (3) to anatomically localize the region of ischemia; (4) to distinguish ischemic from infarcted myocardium; or (5) as a prognostic indicator in patients with known coronary disease.

**2. Radionuclide Angiography**–This procedure images the left ventricle and measures its ejection fraction and wall motion. In coronary disease, resting abnormalities usually represent infarction, and those that occur with exercise usually indicate stress-induced ischemia. Normal subjects usually exhibit an increase in ejection fraction with exercise or no change; patients with coronary disease may exhibit a decrease. Exercise radionuclide angiography has approximately the same sensitivity as thallium-201 scintigraphy, but it is less specific in that older individuals and those with other forms of heart disease may have abnormal responses. The indications are similar to those for thallium-201 scintigraphy, and the choice of study usually depends on the expertise of the laboratory.

**G. Coronary Angiography:** Selective coronary arteriography is the definitive diagnostic procedure for coronary artery disease. It can be performed with low mortality (about 0.2%) and morbidity (1–7%), but the cost is high, and with currently available noninvasive techniques it is rarely indicated solely for diagnosis.

Coronary arteriography should be performed in the following patients:

(1) Those being considered for coronary artery revascularization because of disabling stable angina who have failed to improve on an adequate medical regimen.

(2) Those in whom coronary revascularization is being considered because the clinical presentation (unstable angina, postinfarction angina, etc) or noninvasive testing suggests high-risk disease (see Indications for Revascularization).

(3) Those with aortic valve disease who also have angina pectoris, in order to determine whether the angina is due to accompanying coronary disease. Coronary angiography is usually performed in older patients undergoing valve surgery, even if these patients have no chest pain, so that concomitant bypass may be done if the anatomy is propitious.

(4) Those who have had coronary revascularization with initial improvement and subsequent relapse of symptoms, to determine whether bypass grafts or native vessels are occluded.

(5) Those with ischemic cardiomyopathy and cardiac failure in whom a surgically correctable lesion, such as left ventricular aneurysm, mitral insufficiency, or reversible dysfunction, is suspected.

(6) Those with chest pain of uncertain cause or cardiomyopathy of unknown cause.

Coronary arteriography visualizes the location and severity of stenoses. Narrowing greater than 50% of the luminal diameter is considered clinically significant, although most lesions producing ischemia cause narrowing in excess of 70%. This information has important prognostic value, since mortality rates are progressively higher in patients with one-, 2-, and 3-vessel disease and those with left main coronary artery obstruction (ranging from 1% per year to 25% per year). Among stable patients, 20%, 30%, and 50% have one-, 2-, and 3-vessel involvement, respectively, while left main disease is present in 10%. In those with strongly positive exercise ECGs or scintigraphic studies, 3-vessel or left main disease may be present in 75–95% depending upon the criteria employed. Coronary arteriography also shows whether the obstructions are amenable to bypass surgery or percutaneous transluminal coronary angioplasty (PTCA).

**H. Left Ventricular Angiography:** Left ventricular angiography is usually performed at the same time as coronary arteriography. Global and regional left ventricular function are visualized, as well as mitral regurgitation if present. Left ventricular function is the major determinant of prognosis in stable coronary disease and of the risk of bypass surgery.

**I. Coronary Spasm:** Although most symptoms of myocardial ischemia result from fixed stenosis of the coronary arteries or thrombosis or hemorrhage at the site of lesions, some ischemic events may be precipitated by increases in coronary vasoconstrictive tone.

Spasm of the large coronary arteries with resulting decreased coronary blood flow may occur spontaneously or may be induced by mechanical irritation from a coronary catheter, by exposure to cold, or by ergot derivative drugs. Spasm may occur both in normal and in stenosed coronary arteries and may be silent or result in angina pectoris. Even myocardial infarction may occur as a result of spasm in the absence of visible obstructive coronary heart disease, although most instances of coronary spasm occur in the presence of coronary stenosis.

**Prinzmetal's (variant) angina** is a clinical syndrome in which chest pain occurs without the usual precipitating of factors such as exertion and is associated with ST segment elevation rather than depression. It affects a proportionately large number of women under age 50. It characteristically occurs in the early morning, awakening patients from sleep, and is apt to be associated with arrhythmias or conduction defects. There may be no fixed stenoses.

Patients with this pattern of pain or any chest pain syndrome associated with ST segment elevation should usually undergo coronary arteriography to determine whether fixed stenotic lesions are present. If they are, aggressive medical therapy or revascularization is indicated, since this may represent an unstable phase of the disease. If significant lesions are not seen and spasm is suspected, ergonovine may be administered intravenously to precipitate vasospasm. This must be done cautiously and with nitroglycerin prepared for intracoronary administration, since irreversible spasm may lead to infarction. Episodes respond well to nitrates or calcium channel blockers, and both drugs are effective prophylactically. Beta-blockers have exacerbated coronary vasospasm, but they have also been effective when it is associated with fixed stenoses.

### Differential Diagnosis

With an appropriate history, the diagnosis of angina pectoris is more than 90% certain. When atypical features are present—such as duration for hours or days; often aggravated by exertion but not promptly relieved by rest; or darting, knifelike pains at the apex or over the precordium—the pain is often due to functional disorders. Dyspnea or hyperventilation, palpitation, fatigue, headache, and exhaustion may be associated.

"Anterior chest wall syndrome" is characterized by sharply localized tenderness of intercostal muscles. Sprain or inflammation of the chondrocostal junctions, which may be warm, swollen, and red, may result in diffuse chest pain that is also reproduced by local pressure (Tietze's syndrome). Intercostal neuritis (herpes zoster, diabetes mellitus, etc) also mimics angina.

Cervical or thoracic spine disease involving the dorsal roots produces sudden sharp, severe chest pain suggesting angina in location and "radiation" but related to specific movements of the neck or spine, recumbency, and straining or lifting. Pain due to cervical or thoracic disk disease involves the outer or dorsal aspect of the arm and the thumb and index fingers rather than the ring and little fingers.

Peptic ulcer, chronic cholecystitis, esophageal spasm, and functional gastrointestinal disease may produce pain suggestive of angina pectoris. Reflux esophagitis is characterized by lower chest and upper abdominal pain after heavy meals, occurring in recumbency or upon bending over. The pain is relieved by antacids, Fowler's position, $H_2$ receptor antagonists. The picture may be especially confusing because ischemic pain may also be associated with upper gastrointestinal symptoms, and esophageal motility disorders may be improved by nitrates and calcium channel blockers. Detailed assessment of esophageal motility may be necessary.

Degenerative and inflammatory lesions of the left shoulder, cervical rib, and the scalenus anticus syndrome differ from angina in that the pain is precipitated by movement of the arm and shoulder; paresthesias are present in the left arm, and postural exercises and pillow support to the shoulders in bed give relief.

Spontaneous pneumothorax may cause chest pain as well as dyspnea and may create confusion with angina as well as myocardial infarction. The same is true of pneumococcal pneumonia and pulmonary embolization. Dissection of the thoracic aorta can cause severe chest pain, but the discomfort is more commonly felt in the back, is described as "tearing," is sudden in onset, and may be associated with changes in pulses. Other cardiac disorders such as mitral valve prolapse, hypertrophic cardiomyopathy, myocarditis, pericarditis, aortic valve disease, or right ventricular hypertrophy may cause atypical chest pain or even myocardial ischemia. Noninvasive testing and, in many cases, cardiac catheterization may be required to establish the diagnosis and appropriate treatment.

## Treatment

**A. Treatment of Acute Attack:** Sublingual nitroglycerin is the drug of choice; it acts in about 1–2 minutes. Nitrates decrease arteriolar and venous tone, reduce preload and afterload, and lower the oxygen demand of the heart. Nitrates may also improve myocardial blood flow by dilating collateral channels and, in the presence of increased vasomotor tone, coronary stenoses. As soon as the attack begins, one fresh tablet is placed under the tongue and allowed to dissolve. This may be repeated at 3- to 5-minute intervals. The dosage (0.3, 0.4, or 0.6 mg) and the number of tablets to be used before seeking further medical attention must be individualized. Nitroglycerin should also be used prophylactically before activities likely to precipitate angina. Pain not responding

to 3–4 tablets or lasting more than 20 minutes may represent evolving infarction.

**B. Prevention of Further Attacks:**

**1. Aggravating factors–**Angina may be aggravated by hypertension, left ventricular failure, arrhythmia (usually tachycardias), and emotional states.

**2. Nitroglycerin–**Nitroglycerin, 0.3–0.6 mg sublingually, should be taken just before activity. Sublingual isosorbide dinitrate (2.5–10 mg) is only slightly longer-acting than sublingual nitroglycerin.

**3. Long-acting nitrates–**Many longer-acting nitrate preparations are available. These include isosorbide dinitrate (Isordil, Sorbitrate), 10–40 mg orally 4 times daily; oral sustained-release nitroglycerin preparations, 6.25–12.5 mg 2–4 times daily; and nitroglycerin ointment, 6.25–25 mg applied 4 times daily. Transdermal nitroglycerin patches deliver nitroglycerin through the skin at a predetermined rate (usually 5–20 mg/24 h). Growing evidence indicates that continuous nitrate levels are associated with pharmacologic tolerance, so it is probably preferable to avoid nitrates overnight except in patients with nocturnal pain.

Nitrate therapy is often limited by headache, gastrointestinal side effects, or, if the dosage is too large and the patient remains erect, hypotension.

**4. Beta-blockers–**The beta-blockers prevent angina by reducing myocardial oxygen requirements during exertion and stress. This is accomplished by reducing the heart rate, cardiac muscle contractility, and, to a lesser extent, blood pressure. All available beta-blockers appear to be effective for angina. The pharmacology of the beta-blockers is discussed under Hypertension (Table 8–3).

Because the beta-blockers improve survival after myocardial infarction and, to a small degree, after acute infarction, they are a reasonable initial choice for chronic antianginal therapy. The side effects of the beta-blockers are discussed above.

**5. Calcium entry blocking agents–**(See Table 8–5.) Nifedipine, verapamil, and diltiazem are chemically and pharmacologically heterogeneous agents that prevent angina by reducing myocardial oxygen requirements and by inducing coronary artery vasodilatation. The former is accomplished by reducing blood pressure, left ventricular wall stress, and, in the case of verapamil and diltiazem, increment

**Table 8–5.** Oral calcium entry-blocking drugs.

| Agent | Inhibition of Atrioventricular Conduction | Coronary Vasodilatation | Negative Inotropic Action | Hypotension, Edema | Dosage Initial (Range) |
|---|---|---|---|---|---|
| Verapamil (Calan, Isoptin) | +++ | ++ | +++ | ++ | 80 mg 3 times daily (240–480 mg daily) |
| Diltiazem (Cardizem) | + to ++ | ++ | + | + | 60 mg 3 times daily (180–480 mg daily) |
| Nifedipine (Procardia) | 0 to + | +++ | + | +++ | 10 mg 3 times daily (30–120 mg daily) |

in heart rate caused by vasodilatation. Though these agents are all potent coronary vasodilators, it is unclear whether they improve myocardial blood flow in most patients with stable exertional angina. In those with coronary vasospasm, the calcium entry blockers may be the agent of choice.

The currently available calcium channel blockers all have negative inotropic, chronotropic, and dromotropic properties in vitro, but the reflex sympathetic response obscures these effects in vivo, especially in the case of nifedipine except in the presence of beta blockade or severely depressed left ventricular function. Diltiazem appears to have fewer side effects, whereas—because of its reflex activation—nifedipine is better tolerated when combined with beta-blockers. Each of these agents must be titrated upward at intervals of at least several days, since the range of dosages employed is wide.

**6. Combination therapy–**Patients remaining symptomatic when given one class of preventive agent should be treated with combinations. A beta-blocker and a long-acting nitrate or a beta-blocker and either nifedipine or diltiazem (rather than verapamil, where the risk of atrioventricular block or heart failure is higher) are the commonest combinations. A few patients will have a further response to a regimen including all 3 agents.

**7. Platelet-inhibiting agents–**It has become clear that coronary thrombosis is responsible for most episodes of myocardial infarction and many unstable ischemic syndromes. It seems reasonable to extrapolate the findings of several studies that have demonstrated the benefit of antiplatelet drugs following unstable angina and infarction to those patients with stable angina. Ingestion of one aspirin tablet daily is an innocuous and possibly helpful measure. The ingestion of fish oil supplements or fish itself several times weekly has also become popular, since highly unsaturated omega-3 fats may reduce platelet aggregation.

**8. Revascularization–**The indications for coronary artery revascularization and the choice of procedure are discussed below.

## Prognosis

The prognosis of angina pectoris has improved with advances in the understanding of its pathophysiology and improvements in pharmacologic therapy. Mortality rates range from 1% to 25% per year depending on the number of vessels diseased, the severity of obstruction, the status of left ventricular function, and the presence of complex arrhythmias. In patients with stable symptoms and normal ejection fractions (> 55%, depending on the laboratory), the mortality rate is less than 4% per year. However, the outlook in individual patients is unpredictable, and nearly half of the deaths are sudden. Therefore, risk stratification is often attempted. Patients with accelerating symptoms have a poorer outlook. Among stable patients, those whose exercise tolerance is severely limited by ischemia (less than 6 minutes on

the Bruce treadmill protocol) and those with extensive ischemia by exercise electrocardiography or scintigraphy have more severe anatomic disease and a poorer prognosis. In younger and otherwise healthy patients with these findings, revascularization is often indicated.

Braunwald E (guest editor): Surgery in the treatment of coronary artery disease. *Circulation* 1985;**72 (6-Part 2.)** [Entire issue.]

Kemp HG et al: Seven year survival of patients with normal or near normal coronary angiograms: A CASS registry study. *J Am Coll Cardiol* 1986;**7**:479.

Pigott JD et al: Late results of surgical and medical therapy for patients with coronary artery disease and depressed left ventricular function. J Am Coll Cardiol 1985;**5**:1036.

Reeder GS et al: Angioplasty for aortocoronary bypass graft stenosis. *Mayo Clin Proc* 1986;**61**:14.

Scanlon PJ et al: Urgent surgery for ventricular septal rupture complicating acute myocardial infarction. *Circulation* 1985;**72(Suppl II)**:185.

Tracy CM et al: Determinants of ventricular arrhythmias in mildly symptomatic patients with coronary artery disease and influence of inducible left ventricular dysfunction on arrhythmia frequency. *J Am Coll Cardiol* 1987;**9**:483.

## REVASCULARIZATION PROCEDURES FOR PATIENTS WITH ANGINA PECTORIS

### Indications

The indications for coronary artery revascularization in patients with stable angina pectoris are often debated. There is general agreement that otherwise healthy patients with one of the first 3 presentations that follow should undergo revascularization. The last group is controversial. (1) Patients with unacceptable symptoms despite maximally tolerated medical therapy. (2) Patients with left main coronary artery stenosis greater than 50% with or without symptoms. (3) Patients with 3-vessel disease with left ventricular dysfunction (ejection fraction < 50%, old myocardial infarction). (4) Patients with multivessel disease with objective evidence of severe exercise-induced ischemia.

### Type of Procedure
**A. Coronary Artery Bypass Grafting (CABG):** The number of CABG procedures has grown enormously since the late 1960s, and the results have improved greatly as surgical and anesthesiologic techniques have been improved. Grafts employing one or both internal mammary arteries (usually to the left anterior descending artery or its branches) provide the best long-term results in terms of patency and flow. Alternatively (and usually), grafts employ segments of the saphenous vein placed between the aorta and the coronary arteries distal to the obstructions. One to 5 distal anastomoses are commonly performed.

In uncomplicated cases, the operative mortality rate is 1–3%, but it may be much higher in patients with poor left ventricular function, those over 70 years of age, those needing other surgical procedures (valve replacement, aneurysmectomy), or those with severe noncardiac disease. Operative mortality and morbidity rates are higher in these patients, and full recovery is slow. Thus, CABG should be reserved for severely symptomatic patients in this group. Early (1–6 months) graft patency rates average 85–90% (higher for internal mammary grafts), and subsequent graft closure rates are about 4% annually. Early graft failure is common in vessels with poor distal flow, while late closure is more frequent in patients who continue smoking and those with hyperlipidemia. Antiplatelet therapy with aspirin alone or combined with dipyridamole improves graft patency rates. Repeat CABG or angioplasty (see below) is often necessitated by progressive native vessel disease and graft occlusions. Reoperation is technically demanding and less often fully successful than the initial operation.

**B. Percutaneous Transluminal Coronary Angioplasty (PTCA):** Coronary artery stenoses can be effectively dilated by inflation of a balloon under high pressure. This procedure is performed in the cardiac catheterization laboratory under local anesthesia either at the same time as coronary arteriography or at a later time. The mechanism of dilation is rupture of the atheromatous plaque, with subsequent resorption of intraluminal debris.

This procedure was at one time reserved for proximal single-vessel disease, but now it is widely employed in multivessel disease with multiple lesions, though not in left main disease. PTCA is also effective in CABG stenoses. In the USA, the number of PTCA procedures is approaching that of CABG surgeries. With improved catheter systems, experienced operators are able to cross approximately 90% of lesions and successfully dilate 90% of those. The major early complication is plaque dissection with vessel occlusion. This can sometimes be treated by repeat PTCA, but urgent CABG is required in 3–5% of cases. Therefore, these procedures must be done in a laboratory where surgery is available on short notice.

The major limitation with PTCA has been restenosis, which occurs in the first 6 months in 20–30% of vessels dilated. The mechanism of restenosis is unclear, and it can often be treated successfully by repeat PTCA.

**C. Investigational Revascularization Procedures:** There is considerable interest in the use of laser energy to "vaporize" atherosclerotic plaques. This approach is technically feasible and has been employed in peripheral arteries and in coronary arteries (in the operating room). It remains investigational. Catheters designed to physically remove obstructing plaques are also under investigation.

## Results

The mortality rates of PTCA and CABG are comparable in stable angina. Recovery after PTCA is obviously faster, but the early success rate of CABG is probably higher. The increasing popularity of PTCA primarily reflects its lower cost, shorter hospitalization, the perception that CABG is best done only once and can be reserved for later, and the preference of patients for less invasive treatment.

Becker LC, Ambrosio G: Myocardial consequences of reperfusion. *Prog Cardiovasc Dis* 1987;**30**:23.

Mabin TA et al: Follow-up clinical results in patients undergoing percutaneous transluminal coronary angioplasty. *Circulation* 1985;**71**:754.

## UNSTABLE ANGINA

Most clinicians use the term "unstable angina" to denote an accelerating or "crescendo" pattern of pain in cases where previously stable angina occurs with less exertion or at rest, lasts longer, and is less responsive to medication. Coronary angioscopy has shown that a high proportion of patients with this pattern of symptoms have "complex" coronary stenosis characterized by plaque ulceration, hemorrhage, or thrombosis. This inherently unstable situation may progress to complete occlusion and infarction or may heal, with reendotheliazation and a return to a stable though possibly more severe pattern of ischemia.

### Diagnosis

Most patients with unstable angina will exhibit electrocardiographic changes during pain—commonly ST segment depression or T wave flattening or inversion but sometimes, and more ominously, ST segment elevation. They may exhibit signs of left ventricular dysfunction during pain and for a time thereafter.

### Treatment

**A. General Measures:** Treatment of unstable angina should be multifaceted and vigorous. Patients should be hospitalized, maintained at bed rest or at very limited activity, monitored, and given supplemental oxygen. Light sedation with a benzodiazepine agent is usually indicated. The systolic blood pressure is usually maintained at 100–120 mm Hg, except in previously severe hypertensives; this can be achieved with the specific agents described below, and previous antihypertensive therapy is generally continued. Patients with heart rates above 70–80/min should be given beta-blockers unless heart failure is present.

**B. Nitroglycerin:** The nitrates are first-line therapy for unstable angina. Nonparenteral therapy with sublingual or oral agents or nitroglycerin ointment is usually sufficient. If pain persists despite the addition of other agents, intravenous nitroglycerin should be started. The usual initial dosage is 0.25–0.5 μg/kg/min. The dosage should be titrated to 1–2 μg/kg/min over 5–30 minutes and further increased as tolerated if pain recurs. Dosages up to 10 μg/kg/min or higher may be used. Tolerance to continuous nitrate infusion has been noted. Careful—usually continuous—blood pressure monitoring is required when intravenous nitroglycerin is used.

**C. Calcium Entry Blockers:** Since alterations in coronary vasomotor tone more frequently play a role in unstable ischemic syndromes, these agents are often the second line of therapy. In the presence of nitrates and without accompanying beta-blockers, diltiazem or verapamil is preferred, since nifedipine is more likely to cause reflex tachycardia or hypotension. The initial dosage should be low, but up-titration should proceed rapidly. (See Table 8–5.)

**D. Beta-Blockers:** These agents are effective in unstable angina, particularly when tachycardia is present or precipitated by other medications. The goal of acute treatment is to reduce the heart rate below 60–70/min. Again, the dosage can be titrated upward at intervals of several hours with careful monitoring.

**E. Anticoagulation and Antiplatelet Therapy:** As noted above, intravascular thrombosis plays a prominent role in the pathophysiology of unstable angina and its progression to myocardial infarction. Therefore, most authorities recommend intravenous heparin treatment and low-dose aspirin (325 mg daily).

**F. Intra-aortic Balloon Counterpulsation (IABC):** If pain persists with accompanying electrocardiographic changes despite the above measures, IABC should be considered both to reduce myocardial energy requirements (systolic unloading) and to improve diastolic blood flow. While this approach is often effective, other experts will proceed directly to coronary arteriography and revascularization. It is best applied only if proceeding to a more definitive therapy is complicated. Aortic insufficiency is a contraindication, and IABC must be used cautiously in patients with peripheral vascular disease.

**G. Chronic Treatment:** If pain is eliminated, ambulation should be gradual. Long-term therapy should follow the guidelines for stable angina but should generally include aspirin as well.

## Prognosis

Over 90% of patients can be rendered pain-free with these measures. Controlled trials have not shown any advantage in increased survival or lower infarction rates with CABG compared to medical therapy, although many patients treated medically will need surgery later for recurrent symptoms. However, these studies are from the early era of surgery and precede the availability of PTCA; furthermore, more sophisticated medical regimens are available. Depending on the stringency of the definition of unstable angina, 10–30% of patients will have an early infarction, and the 1-year mortality rate of these patients exceeds 10% (and may be as high as 20% in some severe subsets). Recent data from ambulatory monitoring indicates that many patients without pain continue to have "silent" episodes of ST segment depression or, less commonly, elevation. These individuals have a poorer prognosis.

Because the outlook is poor following relief of unstable angina, most cardiologists recommend either (1) coronary arteriography before discharge or when the patient is stabilized or (2) early submaximal exercise testing to identify high-risk subsets for further invasive evaluation. The artery responsible for the ischemia can usually be determined from electrocardiographic changes during pain, and the lesion is often amenable to PTCA.

Braunwald E: The thrombolysis in myocardial infarction (TIMI) trial: Phase I findings. (Special report.) *N Engl J Med* 1985;**312**:932.

Cairns JA et al: Aspirin, sulfinpyrazone, or both in unstable angina: Results of a Canadian Multicenter Trial. *N Engl J Med* 1985;**313**:1369.

deFeyter PJ et al: Emergency coronary angioplasty in refractory unstable angina. *N Engl J Med* 1985;**313**:342.

Haines DE et al: A prospective clinical, scintigraphic, angiographic and functional evaluation of patients after inferior myocardial infarction with and without right ventricular dysfunction. *J Am Coll Cardiol* 1985;**6**:995.

Health and Public Policy Committee, American College of Physicians: Thrombolysis for evolving myocardial infarction. *Ann Intern Med* 1985;**103**:463.

Nishimura RA et al: Early repair of mechanical complications after acute myocardial infarction. *JAMA* 1986;**256**:47.

Pell S, Fayerweather WE: Trends in the incidence of myocardial infarction and in associated mortality and morbidity in a large employed population, 1957–1983. *N Engl J Med* 1985;**312**:1005.

Pigott JD et al: Late results of surgical and medical therapy for patients with coronary artery disease and depressed left ventricular function. *J Am Coll Cardiol* 1985;**5**:1036.

Simoons ML et al: Early thrombolysis in acute myocardial infarction: Limitation of infarct size and improved survival. *J Am Coll Cardiol* 1986;**7**:717.

Vigilante GJ et al: Improved survival with coronary bypass surgery in patients with three-vessel coronary disease and abnormal left ventricular function: Matched case-control study in patients with potentially operable disease. *Am J Med* 1987;**82**:697.

Visser CA et al: Incidence, timing and prognostic value of left ventricular aneurysm formation after myocardial infarction: A prospective, serial echocardiographic study of 158 patients. *Am J Cardiol* 1986;**57**:729.

## ACUTE MYOCARDIAL INFARCTION

### Pathophysiology

Myocardial infarction results from prolonged myocardial ischemia, precipitated in most cases by an occlusive coronary thrombus at the site of a preexisting atherosclerotic stenosis. More rarely, infarction may result from prolonged vasospasm, inadequate myocardial blood flow (eg, hypotension), or excessive metabolic demand. These processes also occur most commonly in patients with atherosclerotic disease. Very rarely, myocardial infarction may be caused by embolic occlusion, vasculitis, aortic root dissection, and aortitis.

The location and extent of infarction depend upon the anatomic distribution of the occluded vessel, the presence of additional occlusions, and the adequacy of collateral circulation. Thrombosis in the anterior descending branch of the left coronary artery results in infarction of the anterior left ventricle and interventricular septum. Occlusion of the left circumflex artery produces anterolateral or posterolateral infarction. Right coronary thrombosis leads to infarction of the posteroinferior portion of the left ventricle and may involve the right ventricular myocardium and interventricular septum. However, because there are great individual variations in coronary anatomy and because associated lesions and collaterals may confuse the picture, prediction of coronary anatomy from the infarct location may be inaccurate.

The size and anatomic location of the infarction determines the acute clinical picture, the early complications, and the long-term prognosis. The hemodynamic findings are related directly to the extent of necrosis (together with the amount of damage from previous infarctions). In small infarctions, cardiac function is normal, whereas with more extensive damage, early heart failure and hypotension (cardiogenic shock) may appear. Additional myocardium beyond that initially infarcted is often in jeopardy, being maintained by collateral circulation or by blood flow through a partially recanalized vessel. Thus, preventing extension of the infarct is one of the major goals of early management. The complications of acute infarction are discussed below.

## Clinical Findings

### A. Symptoms:

**1. Premonitory pain**–One-third of patients give a history of alteration in the pattern of angina, recent onset of typical or atypical angina, or unusual "indigestion" felt in the chest.

**2. Pain of infarction**–Most infarctions occur at rest—unlike anginal episodes, most commonly in the early morning. The pain is similar to angina in location and radiation but is more severe, and it builds up rapidly or in waves to maximum intensity over a few minutes or longer. Nitroglycerin has little effect. The pain may last for hours if unrelieved by narcotics and is often unbearable. Patients break out in a cold sweat, feel weak and apprehensive, and move about, seeking a position of comfort. They prefer not to lie quietly. Lightheadedness, syncope, dyspnea, orthopnea, cough, wheezing, nausea and vomiting, or abdominal bloating may be present singly or in any combination.

**3. Painless infarction**–In a minority of cases, pain is absent or minor and is overshadowed by the immediate complications. As many as 25% of infarctions are detected on routine ECG without there having been any recallable acute episode.

**4. Sudden death and early arrhythmias**–Approximately 25% of patients with acute infarction will die before reaching the hospital; these deaths are usually in the first hour and are chiefly due to ventricular fibrillation.

### B. Signs:

**1. General**–Patients usually appear anxious and are often sweating profusely. The heart rate may range from marked bradycardia (most commonly in inferior infarction) to tachycardia due to low cardiac output or anxiety. The blood pressure may be high, especially in former hypertensives, or low in patients with shock. Respiratory distress usually indicates heart failure. Fever, usually low-grade, may appear after 12 hours and persist for several days.

**2. Chest**–Clear lung fields are a good prognostic sign, but basilar rales are common and do not necessarily indicate heart failure. More extensive rales or diffuse wheezing may indicate pulmonary edema.

**3. Heart**–The cardiac examination may be unimpressive or very abnormal. An abnormally located ventricular impulse often represents the dyskinetic infarcted region. Soft heart sounds may indicate left ventricular dysfunction. Atrial gallops ($S_4$) are the rule, whereas ventricular gallops ($S_3$) are less common and indicate significant left ventricular dysfunction. Mitral regurgitation murmurs are not uncommon and usually indicate papillary muscle dysfunction or, rarely, rupture. Pericardial friction rubs are uncommon in the first 24 hours but may appear later.

**4. Extremities**–Edema is usually not present. Cyanosis and cold temperature indicate low output. The peripheral pulses should be noted, since later shock or emboli may alter the examination.

**C. Laboratory Findings:** Leukocytosis of 10,000–20,000/$\mu$L often develops on the second day and disappears in 1 week. The most valuable diagnostic test is serial measurement of cardiac enzymes, of which creatine kinase (CK) or creatine phosphokinase (CPK) rises the earliest and is the most specific for infarction. The MB isoenzyme is very specific for the heart. The peak CK value correlates with the size of the infarction. Serum lactic acid dehydrogenase may remain elevated for 5–7 days, and fraction 1 is relatively specific for myocardial damage. Serial determinations may be helpful in equivocal instances.

**D. Electrocardiography:** Most patients with acute infarction have electrocardiographic changes, and a normal ECG is rare. The extent of the electrocardiographic abnormalities provides only a crude estimate of the magnitude of infarction. The classic evolution of changes is from peaked ("hyperacute") T waves, to ST segment elevation, to Q wave development, to T wave inversion. This may occur over a few hours to several days. The evolution of new Q waves (> 30 ms in duration and 25% of the R wave amplitude) is diagnostic. Patients with appropriate clinical presentation and characteristic cardiac enzymes who exhibit ST segment changes (usually depression) or T wave inversion lasting at least 48 hours are classified as having non-Q wave infarctions.

**E. Scintigraphic Studies: Technetium-99m pyrophosphate scintigraphy** can be used to diagnose acute myocardial infarction. When injected at least 18 hours postinfarction, the radiotracer complexes with calcium in necrotic myocardium to provide a "hot spot" image of the infarction. This test is insensitive to small infarctions, and false-positive studies occur, so its use is limited to patients in whom the diagnosis by electrocardiography and enzymes is not possible—principally those who present several days after the event or have intraoperative infarctions.

**Thallium-201 scintigraphy** will demonstrate "cold spots" in regions of diminished perfusion, which usually represent infarction when the radio-tracer is administered at rest, but abnormalities do not distinguish recent from old damage.

Radionuclide angiography demonstrates akinesis or dyskinesis in areas of infarction and also measures ejection fraction, which can be valuable. Right ventricular dysfunction may indicate infarction of this chamber.

**F. Echocardiography:** Echocardiography provides convenient bedside assessment of left ventricular global and regional function. This can help with the diagnosis and management of infarction. Doppler echocardiography is probably the easiest method for diagnosing postinfarction mitral regurgitation or ventricular septal defect.

**G. Hemodynamic Measurements:** These can be invaluable in managing the complicated patient. Their use is described below.

## Treatment

**A. Thrombolytic Therapy:** Thrombolytic therapy appears to reduce the mortality rate and limit infarct size when started within 3 hours following the onset of infarction, and it may have an effect in some patients (probably in those with extensive collateral circulation) up to 6 hours. The benefit is greatest in patients with potentially large infarcts, ie, those with anterior or multifocal electrocardiographic changes. Benefit is difficult to demonstrate in patients with inferior infarctions, who have a relatively good prognosis in any case. Patients with non-Q wave infarctions generally have incomplete or partially recanalized occlusions and have not benefited from thrombolysis. Complications are more frequent in patients with a history of hemorrhagic disorders and in older patients. Therefore, the current recommendation is to administer thrombolytic therapy to patients under 70 years of age with anterior or multifocal ST elevation or Q waves who present within 6 hours of the onset of pain, unless otherwise contraindicated. This can be initiated in the emergency room or ambulance if personnel are appropriately trained and equipped.

Intracoronary administration was the initial approach, but the difficulty in maintaining laboratories at readiness and the critical delay have led most centers to abandon this procedure. Intravenous streptokinase is the most widely used thrombolytic (until tissue plasminogen activation is approved and available). To avoid bleeding, any intravenous or intra-arterial catheters or access ports should be inserted prior to administration. The dosage is 750,000 units of streptokinase infused over 20–30 minutes. Hypotension is common and is minimized by slow administration. A second dose is usually given unless signs of reperfusion are obvious.

Although investigational at this time, intravenous recombinant tissue plasminogen activation (TPA) is more successful in lysing coronary thrombi. Where available, it is the preferred thrombolytic agent. Newer agents such as antibody-targeted TPA are being investigated.

Reperfusion rates of 40–80% can be expected, determined primarily by the interval between onset of the infarction and treatment. Reperfusion is recognized clinically by the abrupt cessation of pain, ventricular arrhythmias (most characteristically accelerated idioventricular rhythm), rapid evolution of the ECG to Q waves, and an early peak of CK (by 12 hours); however, all of these signs may be misleading. Following thrombolytic therapy, intravenous heparin should be started. Even with anticoagulation, 10–20% of reperfused vessels will reocclude during hospitalization. This has led many authorities to advocate early coronary arteriography and PTCA of the vessel responsible for the infarction. Ongoing trials should establish whether and when such measures should be routinely employed.

**B. Acute PTCA:** A number of centers are now performing immediate coronary arteriography in patients presenting within 3 hours after infarction. Either without or with the aid of thrombolytic agents, the occlusion can often be opened and the residual stenosis, if significant, dilated. This approach, though highly effective, is not widely available.

**C. General Measures:** Patients are best treated in a coronary care unit equipped with continuous monitoring, readily available resuscitation equipment, and properly trained nurses and physicians. The risk of ventricular fibrillation and sudden death is greatest in the first few hours after onset of myocardial infarction. Uncomplicated patients can be transferred to less intensively monitored settings after 24–48 hours. Activity should initially be limited to bed rest, with the availability of a nearby toilet or commode in more stable patients. Progressive ambulation should be started after 48–72 hours if tolerated. Low-flow oxygen therapy (2–4 L/min) is usually given. A liquid diet is recommended during the initial 24 hours.

**D. Analgesia:** An initial attempt should be made to relieve pain with sublingual nitroglycerin. However, if no response occurs after 2 or 3 tablets, this approach should be abandoned. The opiates provide the most rapid and effective analgesia. Intravenous treatment is optimal, so that the onset and duration of effect are known. Morphine sulfate, 4–8 mg, or meperidine, 50–75 mg, should be given slowly intravenously. Subsequent small doses can be given every 15 minutes. Respiration and blood pressure should be monitored.

**E. Antiarrhythmic Prophylaxis:** The incidence of ventricular fibrillation in hospitalized patients is approximately 5%, with 80% of episodes occurring in the first 12–24 hours. Prophylactic lidocaine infusions (1–2 mg/min) prevent most episodes, though they do not improve overall survival since most episodes are effectively treated by DC cardioversion.

Nonetheless, in younger patients at relatively low risk for lidocaine toxicity, such treatment is worthwhile.

**F. Beta-Adrenergic Blocking Agents:** Several studies have shown modestly improved short-term survival when beta-blockers are given immediately after acute myocardial infarction. Long-term beta-blocker therapy is discussed below.

**G. Anticoagulation:** With the exception of patients undergoing thrombolysis and subsequent heparin therapy, the use of anticoagulation remains controversial. Patients who will be at bed rest or on limited activity status for some time should be given 5000 units of heparin subcutaneously every 8–12 hours unless contraindicated.

## Complications

Most patients have one or more complications of myocardial infarction, although the response to treatment is usually prompt.

**A. Postinfarction Angina:** Pain from the initial infarction usually subsides within 4–8 hours following treatment, although a dull ache may persist. Further ischemic pain may reflect extension of the infarct. The general approach is that described for unstable angina. The nitrates are usually used first. Beta-blockers or calcium channel blockers (or both) are added as needed, with the former being favored if tachycardia without pulmonary edema is present. Particular care should be taken in patients with left ventricular dysfunction or atrioventricular block. Full anticoagulation may be helpful, and intra-aortic balloon counterpulsation is of value if early revascularization is being considered. Pericarditis should be excluded when pain recurs postinfarction.

**B. Arrhythmias:** Abnormalities of rhythm and conduction are common.

**1. Sinus bradycardia–**This is most common in inferior infarctions or may be precipitated by medications. Observation or withdrawal of the offending agent is usually sufficient. If accompanied by signs of low cardiac output, atropine, 0.5–1 mg intravenously, is usually effective. A pacemaker is rarely required.

**2. Supraventricular tachyarrhythmias–**Sinus tachycardia is common and may reflect hemodynamic compromise due to hypovolemia or pump failure. If the latter, beta blockade is contraindicated. Supraventricular premature beats are common and may be premonitory for atrial fibrillation. Electrolyte and oxygenation abnormalities should be corrected and causative agents (especially aminophylline) stopped. Atrial fibrillation should be rapidly controlled or converted to sinus rhythm. Intravenous verapamil (given cautiously in 2- to 5-mg increments up to 20 mg) or the newly released short-acting beta-blocker esmolol (Brevibloc) (500 μg/kg, followed by 50–200 μg/kg/min) is the agent of choice if cardiac function is adequate. Digoxin (0.5 mg initial dosage; 0.25 mg every 90–120 minutes up to 1–1.25 mg) is preferable if heart failure is present. Cardio-

version may be necessary, but the arrhythmia often recurs. A type I agent may be required in addition to verapamil, a beta-blocker, or digoxin to maintain sinus rhythm.

**4. Intraventricular block–**Intraventricular conduction abnormalities occur principally in anterior infarctions and reflect the extent of myocardial damage, thus carrying a poor prognosis. New conduction abnormalities such as right or left bundle branch block or posterior or anterior fascicular blocks may presage progression, often sudden, to second- or third-degree atrioventricular block. Prophylactic temporary ventricular pacing is recommended for new-onset alternating bilateral bundle branch block, bifascicular block, or bundle branch block with worsening first-degree atrioventricular block. Patients with anterior infarction who progress to second- or third-degree block even transiently should be considered for insertion of a prophylactic permanent ventricular pacemaker before discharge.

**5. Ventricular arrhythmias–**Ventricular arrhythmias are most common in the first few hours after infarction.

Ventricular premature beats (VPB) may be premonitory for ventricular tachycardia or fibrillation. If prophylactic lidocaine has not been employed, it should be started (1 mg/kg bolus followed by an infusion of 2 mg/min) if more than 6 VPB/min, early (R or T wave) VPB, or couplets are observed. Additional boluses of 0.5 mg/kg followed by an increased infusion rate (up to 4 mg/min) may be necessary, but toxicity (tremor, anxiety, confusion, seizures) is common, especially in older patients and those with hypotension, heart failure, or liver disease. The infusion rate should be reduced after 3–4 hours, since blood levels tend to rise, but generally, once initiated, lidocaine should be continued for at least 24 hours.

Ventricular tachycardia should be treated with a 1 mg/kg bolus of lidocaine if the patient is stable or by electrical cardioversion (100–200 J) if not. If the arrhythmia cannot be suppressed with lidocaine, procainamide should be initiated (100-mg boluses over 1–2 minutes every 5 minutes to a cumulative dose of 750–1000 mg, followed by an infusion of 20–80 μg/kg/min). Hypotension may occur acutely, and depression of myocardial function or conduction may complicate maintenance therapy. Refractory ventricular arrhythmias may rarely respond to beta blockade (esmolol is recommended because of its rapid onset and short duration of action), phenytoin (loading dose: boluses of 100 mg over 5 minutes every 5–10 minutes to a total of 1000 mg; maintenance 300–500 mg/d in divided doses), or bretylium tosylate (5 mg/kg intravenously over 3–5 minutes, repeated after 20 minutes if necessary, followed by an infusion of 1–2 mg/min). Ventricular fibrillation is treated electrically (300–400 J). Unresponsive ventricular fibrillation should be treated by bretylium and repeat cardioversion while CPR is administered. Accelerated idioventricular rhythm is a regular, wide complex rhythm at a rate of 70–100/min. It often follows reperfusion after thrombolytic therapy. The need for treating it in the absence of other ventricular arrhythmias is controversial.

**C. Myocardial Dysfunction:** The severity of cardiac dysfunction is proportionate to the extent of myocardial necrosis but is exacerbated by preexisting dysfunction and ongoing ischemia. Patients who have no signs of heart failure, normal blood pressure, and normal urine output have a good prognosis. Patients with hypotension or evidence of more than mild heart failure should have bedside right heart catheterization and continuous measurements of arterial pressure. These measurements permit the accurate assessment of cardiac function, facilitate the correct choice of therapy, and provide important prognostic information. Table 8–6 categorizes patients based upon these hemodynamic findings.

**1. Left ventricular failure**–Basilar rales are common in acute myocardial infarction, but dyspnea, more diffuse rales, and arterial hypoxemia usually indicate left ventricular failure. Since both the physical examination and chest radiograph correlate poorly with hemodynamic measurements and since the central venous pressure does not correlate with the pulmonary capillary wedge pressure (PCWP), right heart catheterization may be essential in monitoring therapy. General measures include supplemental oxygen to increase arterial saturation to above 95% and elevation of the trunk. Diuretics are usually the initial therapy unless right ventricular infarction is present. Intravenous furosemide (10–40 mg) or bumetanide (0.5–1 mg) is preferred because of the reliably rapid

onset and short duration of action of these drugs. Higher dosages can be given if an inadequate response occurs. Morphine sulfate (4 mg intravenously followed by increments of 2 mg) is valuable in acute pulmonary edema.

Diuretics are usually effective; however, since most patients with acute infarction are not volume overloaded, the hemodynamic response may be limited and may be associated with hypotension. Vasodilators will reduce PCWP and improve cardiac output by a combination of venodilation (increasing venous capacitance) and arteriolar dilation (reducing afterload and left ventricular wall stress). In mild heart failure, sublingual isosorbide dinitrate (2.5–10 mg every 2 hours) or topical nitroglycerin ointment (6.25–25 mg every 4 hours) may be adequate to lower PCWP. In more severe failure, especially if cardiac output is reduced, sodium nitroprusside is the preferred agent. It should be initiated only with hemodynamic monitoring; the initial dosage should be low (0.25 μg/kg/min) to avoid excessive hypotension, but dosage can be increased by increments of 0.5 μg/kg/min every 5–10 minutes up to 5–10 μg/kg/min until the desired hemodynamic response (PCWP < 18 mm Hg, CI > 2.5) is obtained. Excessive hypotension (mean blood pressure < 65–75 mm Hg) or tachycardia (> 10/min increase) should be avoided. Combination with inotropic agents may be necessary to preserve blood pressure or maximize benefit.

Intravenous nitroglycerin (starting at 0.25 μg/kg/min and titrating up to 10 μg/kg/min) is usually less effective but may lower PCWP with less hypoten-

**Table 8–6.** Hemodynamic subsets in acute myocardial infarction.

| Category | CI or SWI | PCWP | Treatment | Comment |
|----------|-----------|------|-----------|---------|
| Normal | > 2.2, > 30 | < 15 | None | Mortality rate < 5%. |
| Hyperdynamic | > 3.0, > 40 | < 15 | Beta-blockers | Characterized by tachycardia; mortality rate < 5%. |
| Hypovolemic | < 2.5, < 30 | < 10 | Volume expansion | Hypotension, tachycardia, but preserved left ventricular function by echocardiography; mortality rate 4–8%. |
| Left ventricular failure | < 2.2, < 30 | > 15 | Diuretics | Mild dyspnea, rales, normal blood pressure; mortality rate 10–20%. |
| Severe | < 2.0, < 20 | > 20 | Diuretics, vasodilators | Pulmonary edema, mild hypotension; inotropic agents, IABC may be required; mortality rate 20–40%. |
| Shock | < 1.8, < 20 | > 18 | Inotropic agents, IABC | IABC early unless rapid reversal; mortality rate > 60%. |

CI = cardiac index (L/min/min$^2$); SWI = stroke work index (g-m/m$^2$, calculated as [mean arterial pressure—PCWP] × stroke volume index × 0.0136); PCWP = pulmonary capillary wedge pressure (in mm Hg; pulmonary artery diastolic pressure may be used instead); IABC = intra-aortic balloon counterpulsation.

sion. Oral or nonparenteral vasodilator therapy with nitrates or angiotensin converting enzyme inhibitors is often necessary after the initial 24–48 hours (see below).

Inotropic agents should be avoided if possible, because they often increase heart rate and myocardial oxygen requirements. Dobutamine has the best hemodynamic profile, increasing cardiac output and modestly lowering PCWP, usually without excessive tachycardia, hypotension, or arrhythmias. The initial dosage is 2.5 μg/kg/min, and it may be increased by similar increments up to 15–20 μg/kg/min at intervals of 5–10 minutes. Dopamine is more useful in the presence of hypotension (see below), since it produces peripheral vasoconstriction, but it has a less beneficial effect on PCWP. Amrinone is a positive inotrope and vasodilator that produces hemodynamic effects similar to those of dobutamine but with a greater decrease in PCWP. However, its longer duration of action makes it less useful in unstable situations, and it may cause thrombocytopenia. Milrinone is a more potent and newer congener of amrinone with fewer side effects but remains investigational. Digoxin has not been helpful in acute infarction except to control the ventricular response in atrial fibrillation, but it may be beneficial if chronic failure persists.

**2. Hypotension and shock**–Patients with hypotension (systolic blood pressure < 100 mm Hg, individualized depending on prior blood pressure) and signs of diminished perfusion (low urine output, confusion, cold extremities) should be hemodynamically monitored. Up to 20% will have findings indicative of intravascular hypovolemia (due to diaphoresis, vomiting, decreased venous tone, medications such as nitrates or morphine, and lack of oral intake). These should be treated with successive boluses of 100 mL of normal saline until PCWP exceeds 15–18 mm Hg to determine whether cardiac output and blood pressure respond. Right ventricular infarction, characterized by a normal PCWP but elevated right atrial pressure, can produce hypotension. This is discussed below.

Most hypotensive patients will have moderate to severe left ventricular dysfunction; pathologic studies indicate that more than 20% of the left ventricle is infarcted (> 40% in cardiogenic shock). If hypotension is only modest (systolic pressure > 90 mm Hg) and the PCWP is elevated, diuretics and an initial trial of nitroprusside (see above) are indicated. If the blood pressure falls, inotropic support will need to be added or substituted. Such patients may also be treated with intra-aortic balloon counterpulsation. This device unloads the left ventricle during systole and increases diastolic coronary artery filling pressure. It often facilitates the use of vasodilators in patients who previously did not tolerate them.

Dopamine is an effective pressor for cardiogenic hypotension. It should be initiated at a rate of 2 μg/kg/min and increased at 5-minute intervals to the appropriate hemodynamic end point. At low dosages (< 5 μg/kg/min), it improves renal blood flow;

at medium dosages (2.5–10 μg/kg/min), it stimulates myocardial contractility; at higher dosages (> 8 μg/kg/min), it is a potent α₁-adrenergic agonist. In general, blood pressure and cardiac index rise, but PCWP does not fall. Dopamine may be combined with nitroprusside or dobutamine (see above), or the latter may be used in its place if hypotension is not severe. Amrinone has effects similar to those of dobutamine, but its longer duration of action precludes rapid dosage adjustment.

Patients with cardiogenic shock have a poor prognosis. Operation to repair mechanical defects (see below), revascularize ischemic myocardium, and resect aneurysms should be considered. Cardiac transplantation is indicated in appropriate individuals.

**D. Right Ventricular Infarction:** Right ventricular infarction is present in one-third of patients with inferior wall infarction but is clinically significant in less than 50% of these. It presents as hypotension with relatively preserved left ventricular function and should be considered whenever patients with inferior infarction exhibit signs of low cardiac output and raised venous pressure. Hypotension is often exacerbated by medications that decrease intravascular volume or produce venodilation, such as diuretics, nitrates, and narcotics. Right atrial pressure and JVP are high, while PCWP is normal or low and the lungs are clear. The diagnosis is suggested by right precordial ST segment elevation and confirmed by echocardiography or hemodynamic measurements. When hypotension is present, hemodynamic measurements are necessary to monitor therapy. Treatment consists of fluid loading to improve left ventricular filling; inotropic agents may also be useful.

**E. Mechanical Defects:** Partial or complete rupture of a papillary muscle or of the interventricular septum occurs in less than 1% of acute myocardial infarctions and carries a poor prognosis. These complications occur in both anterior and inferior infarctions, usually a 3–7 days after the acute event. They are detected by the appearance of a new systolic murmur and clinical deterioration, often with pulmonary edema. The 2 lesions are distinguished by the location of the murmur (apical versus parasternal) and by Doppler echocardiography. Hemodynamic monitoring is essential for appropriate management and demonstrates an increase in oxygen saturation between the right atrium and pulmonary artery in ventricular septal defect and, often, a large *v* wave with mitral regurgitation. Treatment by nitroprusside and, preferably, intra-aortic balloon counterpulsation reduces the regurgitation or shunt, but surgical correction is mandatory. There is controversy over whether this should be done acutely or after a period of stabilization; the better surgical results with the latter approach primarily reflect preoperative mortality in the highest-risk patients.

**F. Myocardial Rupture:** Complete rupture of the left ventricular free wall occurs in less than 1% of patients and usually results in immediate death. It occurs 2–7 days postinfarction, most often of the anterior wall, and is more frequent in older women. Incomplete or gradual rupture may be sealed off by the pericardium, creating a pseudoaneurysm. These may be recognized by echocardiography, radionuclide angiography, or left ventricular angiography, often as an incidental finding. They demonstrate a narrow-neck connection to the left ventricle. Early surgical repair is indicated, since delayed rupture is common.

**G. Left Ventricular Aneurysm:** Ten to 20% of patients surviving an acute infarction develop a left ventricular aneurysm, a sharply delineated area of scar that bulges paradoxically during systole. This usually follows anterior Q wave infarctions. Aneurysms are recognized by persistent ST segment elevation (beyond 4–8 weeks), and a wide neck from the left ventricle can be demonstrated by echocardiography, scintigraphy, or contrast angiography. They rarely rupture but may be associated with arterial emboli, ventricular arrhythmias, and congestive heart failure. Surgical resection may be performed for these indications if other measures fail. The best results are obtained when the residual myocardium contracts well and when significant coronary lesions supplying adjacent regions are bypassed.

**H. Pericarditis:** The pericardium is involved in approximately 50% of infarctions, but pericarditis is often not clinically significant. Twenty percent of patients with Q wave infarctions will have an audible friction rub if examined repetitively. Pericardial pain occurs in approximately the same proportion after 2–7 days and is recognized by its variation with respiration and position (improved by sitting). Often, no treatment is required, but aspirin (650 mg every 4–6 hours) or indomethacin (25 mg 3–4 times daily) will usually relieve the pain. Anticoagulation should be avoided, since hemorrhagic pericarditis may result.

From 1 to 12 weeks after infarction, Dressler's syndrome (post-myocardial infarction syndrome) occurs in less than 5% of patients. This is an autoimmune phenomenon and presents as pericarditis with associated fever, leukocytosis, and, occasionally, pericardial or pleural effusion.

**I. Mural Thrombus:** Mural thrombi are common in large anterior infarctions but not in infarctions at other locations. They can be detected by echocardiography but with only moderate reliability. Arterial emboli occur in approximately 5% of patients with known infarction, usually within 6 weeks. Anticoagulation appears to limit the incidence of arterial emboli, but since these occur nearly as frequently in patients with negative as with positive echocardiograms, they are best prevented by short-term (3-month) anticoagulation with heparin followed by warfarin in patients with large anterior infarctions.

## Postinfarction Prognosis

Twenty-five percent of patients with acute myocardial infarction die before they reach the hospital. Mortality rates in hospitalized patients range from 8% to 15% and are determined chiefly by the size of the infarction. Patients developing heart failure or hypotension have high early mortality rates. Several classification criteria have been developed to estimate early prognosis for survival. The most accurate is hemodynamic subsetting (see Table 8–6). The prognosis after discharge is determined by 3 major factors: the degree of left ventricular dysfunction, the extent of residual ischemic myocardium, and the presence of ventricular arrhythmias. The mortality rate in the first year after discharge is approximately 8%, with over half of deaths occurring in the first 3 months, chiefly in patients with postinfarction heart failure. Subsequently, the mortality rate averages 4% per year.

**A. Risk Stratification:** A number of findings indicate increased risk after infarction. These include: (1) postinfarction angina; (2) non-Q wave infarction; (3) heart failure; (4) left ventricular ejection fraction less than 40%; (5) exercise-induced ischemia, diagnosed by electrocardiography or scintigraphy; and (6) ventricular ectopy.

Authorities differ about which tests should be performed routinely. Significant left ventricular dysfunction is most likely with anterior infarction or multiple infarctions. In these, noninvasive assessment of left ventricular function will help assess prognosis and facilitate medical management. Submaximal exercise testing before discharge or a maximal test after 3–6 weeks may help patients and physicians plan the return to normal activity. Ambulatory monitoring is of less clear value; though it has some prognostic value beyond measurements of left ventricular function, no benefit from antiarrhythmic therapy has been demonstrated.

**B. Prophylactic Therapy:** Many drugs have been studied, and some have been shown to be beneficial in preventing death or reinfarction. However, their usefulness in the era of thrombolysis and revascularization is unclear. Beta-blockers improve survival rates, primarily by reducing the incidence of sudden death in high-risk subsets of patients. Beta-blockers should be given to such individuals, except those with heart failure but are of limited value in uncomplicated patients with small infarctions and normal exercise tests. No advantage of any one agent over another has been demonstrated. Calcium channel blockers have not been shown to improve prognosis, but diltiazem prevents reinfarction after non-Q wave infarction. Antiplatelet agents probably are beneficial; low-dose aspirin (325 mg daily) is recommended. Anticoagulants have not been shown to improve prognosis, though they do reduce peripheral emboli in the early postdischarge phase (see above). Treatment of hyperlipidemia improves the prognosis of affected patients. Antiarrhythmic therapy other than with beta-blockers has not been shown to be effective except in patients with symptomatic arrhythmias. Cardiac rehabilitation programs and exercise training can be of considerable psychologic benefit but have not been shown to alter prognosis.

**C. Revascularization:** Because of the increasing use of thrombolytic therapy and accumulating experience with PTCA, the indications for revascularization are rapidly evolving. Postinfarction patients who appear likely to benefit from early revascularization if the anatomy is appropriate are (1) those who have undergone thrombolytic therapy and have residual symptoms or laboratory evidence of ischemia; (2) patients with left ventricular dysfunction and evidence of ischemia; (3) patients with non-Q wave infarction and evidence of more than mild ischemia; and (4) patients with markedly positive exercise tests and multivessel disease. The value of revascularization in the following groups is less clear: (1) patients treated with thrombolytic agents, with little evidence of reperfusion or residual ischemia; (2) patients with left ventricular dysfunction but no detectable ischemia; and (3) patients with preserved left ventricular function who have mild ischemia and are not symptom-limited. Patients who survive infarctions without complications, have preserved left ventricular function (ejection fraction > 50%), and have no exercise-induced ischemia have an excellent prognosis and do not require invasive evaluation.

Blankenhorn DH et al: Beneficial effects of combined colestipol-niacin therapy on coronary atherosclerosis and coronary venous bypass grafts. *JAMA* 1987;**257**:3233.

Bosch X et al: Early postinfarction ischemia: Clinical, angiographic, and prognostic significance. *Circulation* 1987;**75**:988.

Genton R, Jaffe AS: Management of congestive heart failure in patients with acute myocardial infarction. *JAMA* 1986;**256**:2556.

Gibson RS et al: The prevalence and clinical significance of residual myocardial ischemia 2 weeks after uncomplicated non-Q wave infarction: A prospective natural history study. *Circulation* 1986;**73**:1186.

Glasser SP: Predischarge post-myocardial infarction testing: Exercise electrocardiography. *Cardiovasc Rev Rep* 1985;**6**:128.

Gold HK et al: A randomized, blinded, placebo-controlled trial of recombinant human tissue-type plasminogen activator in patients with unstable angina pectoris. *Circulation* 1987;**75**:1192.

Gruentzig AR et al: Long-term follow-up after percutaneous transluminal coronary angioplasty: The early Zurich experience. *N Engl J Med* 1987;**316**:1127.

Holmes DR et al: The effect of medical and surgical treatment on subsequent sudden cardiac death in patients with coronary artery disease: A report from the Coronary Artery Surgery Study. *Circulation* 1986;**73**:1254.

Hugenholtz PG: Acute coronary artery obstruction in myocardial infarction: Overview of thrombolytic therapy. *J Am Coll Cardiol* 1987;**9**:1375.

Moss AJ, Bigger JT Jr, Odoroff CL: Postinfarct risk stratification. *Prog Cardiovasc Dis* 1987;**29**:389.

Patel B, Kloner RA: Analysis of reported randomized trials of streptokinase therapy for acute myocardial infarction in the 1980s. *Am J Cardiol* 1987;**59**:501.

Sheehan FH et al: The effect of intravenous thrombolytic therapy on left ventricular function: A report on tissue-type plasminogen activator and streptokinase from the Thrombolysis in Myocardial Infarction (TIMI phase I) trial. *Circulation* 1987;**75**:817.

Stone PH et al: Prognostic significance of treadmill exercise test performance 6 months after myocardial infarction. *J Am Coll Cardiol* 1986;**8**:1007.

Visser CA et al: Incidence, timing and prognostic value of left ventricular aneurysm formation after myocardial infarction: A prospective, serial echocardiographic study of 158 patients. *Am J Cardiol* 1986;**57**:729.

Zipes DP: A consideration of antiarrhythmic therapy. (Editorial.) *Circulation* 1985;**72**:949.

Zipes DP et al: Task Force VI: Arrhythmias. *J Am Coll Cardiol* 1985;**6**:1225.

# DISTURBANCES OF RATE & RHYTHM

Arrhythmias are harmful to the extent that they reduce cardiac output, lower blood pressure, and interfere with perfusion of the vital territories of the brain, heart, and kidney. Patients with otherwise normal hearts may tolerate rapid rates with no symptoms other than palpitations or fluttering, but prolonged attacks usually cause weakness, exertional dyspnea, and precordial aching. Whether slow heart rates produce symptoms at rest or on exertion depends upon the underlying state of the cardiac muscle and its ability to increase its stroke output. If the heart rate abruptly slows, as with the onset of complete heart block or transient standstill, syncope or convulsions may result.

The final diagnosis of an arrhythmia depends upon the surface ECG or, in complex arrhythmias, electrophysiologic studies involving intracardiac electrocardiographic recordings and atrial and ventricular stimulation. Intracardiac recordings aid in the interpretation of complex arrhythmias, especially when there is a question about whether the rhythm is atrial or ventricular, by demonstrating the supraventricular or ventricular origin of wide QRS complexes. If the QRS complex follows the His bundle spike, ventricular aberrancy is present, and treatment is influenced accordingly. His bundle recordings and intracardiac electrograms from both chambers also aid in the recognition of abnormal conduction pathways (as in Wolff-Parkinson-White syndrome). Electrical stimulation is used to induce arrhythmias and assess therapy.

## Mechanisms of Arrhythmias

Electrophysiologic studies have greatly increased our understanding of the mechanisms underlying most arrhythmias. These include disorders of impulse formation or automaticity, which is the mechanism for sinus node arrest, premature beats, and automatic rhythms as well as the initiating factor in many reentry arrhythmias. Abnormalities of impulse conduction can occur at the sinus or atrioventricular node, in the intraventricular conduction system, and within the atria or ventricle. These are responsible for sinoatrial exit block, for atrioventricular block at the node or below, and for establishing reentry circuits.

Reentry is the underlying mechanism for many

arrhythmias, including premature beats, most paroxysmal supraventricular tachycardias, and atrial flutter and fibrillation. For reentry to occur, there must be an area of unidirectional block with an appropriate delay to allow repeat depolarization at the site of origin. Reentry is confirmed if the arrhythmia can be terminated by interruption of the circuit by a spontaneous or induced premature beat.

Less common mechanisms included triggered activity, where the abnormal impulse is related to the preceding depolarization; and parasystole, where a focus is protected from conducted depolarization by entry block—ie, its spontaneous depolarizations are intermittently conducted outward.

## Antiarrhythmic Drugs
## (Table 8–7)

Antiarrhythmic drugs have limited efficacy and produce frequent side effects. Although the in vitro electrophysiologic effects of most of these agents have been defined, their use remains largely empirical. All can exacerbate arrhythmias (proarrhythmic effect), and most (except Ib agents and bretylium) depress left ventricular function. Their use is discussed below.

Horowitz LN, Morganroth J: Second generation antiarrhythmic agents: Have we reached antiarrhythmic nirvana? *J Am Coll Cardiol* 1987;**9**:459.

Wellens HJJ, Brugada P, Stevenson WG: Programmed electrical stimulation: Its role in the management of ventricular arrhythmias in coronary heart disease. *Prog Cardiovasc Dis* 1986;**29**:165.

## SUPRAVENTRICULAR ARRHYTHMIAS

### 1. SINUS ARRHYTHMIAS

Sinus arrhythmia is a cyclic increase in normal heart rate with inspiration and decrease with expiration. It results from reflex changes in vagal influence on the normal pacemaker and disappears with breath-holding or increase of heart rate due to any cause. It has no clinical significance. It is common in both the young and the elderly.

### 2. SINUS BRADYCARDIA

Sinus bradycardia is a heart rate slower than 50/min due to increased vagal influence on the normal pacemaker or organic disease of the sinus node. The rate usually increases during exercise or administration of atropine. Slight degrees have no significance, especially in youth or in athletes; it is of more concern if there is underlying heart disease, especially coronary heart disease or acute myocardial infarction. Elderly patients may develop weakness, confusion, or even syncope with slow heart rates due to degenera-

tive disease of the sinus node. Atrial and ventricular ectopic rhythms are more apt to occur with slow ventricular rates. Rarely, pacing is required if symptoms correlate with the bradycardia.

### 3. SINUS TACHYCARDIA

Sinus tachycardia is defined as a heart rate faster than 100 beats/min that is caused by rapid impulse formation by the normal pacemaker; it occurs with fever, exercise, emotion, anemia, shock, thyrotoxicosis, or drug effect. The onset and termination are usually gradual, in contrast to paroxysmal supraventricular tachycardia due to reentry. The rate may reach 180/min in young persons but infrequently exceeds 160/min. The rhythm is basically regular, but serial 1-minute counts of the heart rate indicate that it varies 5 or more beats per minute with changes in position, with breath-holding or sedation, or with correction of the underlying disorder.

### 4. ATRIAL PREMATURE BEATS
### (Atrial Extrasystoles)

Atrial premature beats occur when an ectopic focus in the atria fires before the next sinus node impulse or a reentry circuit is established. The contour of the P wave usually differs from the patient's normal complex. Ventricular systole occurs prematurely, and the compensatory pause following this is only slightly longer than the normal interval between beats. Such premature beats occur with equal frequency in normal and diseased hearts and are never a sufficient basis for a diagnosis of heart disease. Speeding of the heart rate by any means usually abolishes most premature beats. Early atrial premature beats may cause aberrant QRS complexes (wide and bizarre) or may be nonconducted to the ventricle because the latter is still refractory.

### 5. PAROXYSMAL SUPRAVENTRICULAR
### TACHYCARDIA
### (Atrial or Junctional Tachycardia)

This is the commonest paroxysmal tachycardia. It occurs more often in young patients with normal hearts. Attacks begin and end abruptly and usually last up to several hours. The heart rate may be 140–240/min (usually 170–220/min) and is perfectly regular (despite exercise or change in position). The P wave usually differs in contour from sinus beats. Patients may be asymptomatic except for awareness of rapid heart action, but some experience mild chest pain or shortness of breath, especially when episodes are prolonged, even in the absence of associated cardiac abnormalities. Paroxysmal supraventricular tachycardia may result from digitalis toxicity and then is commonly associated with atrioventricular block.

Table 8-7. Antiarrhythmic drugs.

| | Intravenous Dosage | Oral Dosage | Therapeutic Plasma Level | Route of Elimination | Mechanism | Indications | Side Effects |
|---|---|---|---|---|---|---|---|
| Quinidine | 6–10 mg/kg over 20 min | 325–650 mg every 6–8 h | 2–6 µg/mL | Hepatic | Class Ia: sodium channel blockers: Depress phase 0 depolarization; slow conduction; prolong repolarization. | APB, VPB, SVT, VT, prevent VF | Gastrointestinal, ↓ LVF, ↑ Dig |
| Procainamide | 100 mg/1–3 min to 500–1000 mg; maintain at 2–6 mg/min | 500–1500 mg every 3–6 h | 4–10 µg/mL | Renal | | | Systemic lupus erythematosus, hypersensitivity, ↓ LVF |
| Disopyramide | — | 100–200 mg every 6–8 hr | 2–6 µg/mL | Renal | | | Urinary retention, dry mouth, ↓ LVF |
| Lidocaine | 1–2 mg/kg at 50 mg/min; maintain at 1–4 mg/min | — | 1–5 µg/mL | Hepatic | Class Ib: Shorten repolarization. | VPB, VT, prevent VF | Central nervous system, gastrointestinal |
| Tocainide | — | 200–300 mg every 6–8 hr | 0.5–2 µg/mL | Hepatic | | | Central nervous system, gastrointestinal, leukopenia |
| Mexiletine | — | 400–600 mg every 6–8 hr | 6–12 µg/mL | Hepatic | | | Central nervous system, gastrointestinal, leukopenia |
| Phenytoin | 100 mg/5 min to 1000 mg; maintain at 100–500 mg/d | 200–400 mg every 12–24 hr | 10–20 µg/mL | Hepatic | | | Central nervous system, gastrointestinal |
| Flecainide | — | 50–200 mg twice daily | 0.2–0.8 µg/mL | Hepatic | Class Ic: Depress phase 0 repolarization; slow conduction. | VPB, VT, SVT | Central nervous system, ↓ LVF |
| Encainide | — | 25–75 mg every 6–8 h | 0.5–1 µg/mL | Hepatic | | | Central nervous system, ↓ LVF |
| Esmolol | 500 µg/kg over 1–2 min; maintain at 50–200 µg/kg/min | — | — | Hepatic | Class II: Beta-blockers slow AV conduction. | SVT; may prevent VF | ↓ LVF, bronchospasm |
| Amiodarone | Same as oral | 1200 mg/d for 7–14 days; maintain at 200–800 mg/d | 1–5 µg/mL | Hepatic | Class III: Prolong action potential. | Refractory VT, SVT, prevent VT, VF | Pulmonary fibrosis, thyroid abnormalities, corneal and skin deposits, hepatitis, ↑ Dig |
| Bretylium | 5–10 mg/kg over 5–10 min; maintain at 0.5–2 mg/min | — | 0.5–1.5 µg/mL | Renal | | VF, VT | Hypotension, nausea |
| Verapamil | 10–20 mg over 2–20 min; maintain at 5 µg/kg/min | 80–120 mg every 6–8 hr | 0.1–0.15 µg/mL | Hepatic | Class IV: Slow calcium channel blocker | SVT | ↓ LVF, constipation, ↑ Dig |

APB = atrial premature beats; ↑ Dig = elevation of serum digoxin level; ↓ LVF = reduced left ventricular function; SVT = supraventricular tachycardia; VF = ventricular fibrillation; VPB = ventricular premature beats; VT = ventricular tachycardia.

The most common mechanism for paroxysmal supraventricular tachycardia is reentry from an atrial premature beat through an atrioventricular node whose conduction has been slowed, combined with unidirectional block in a neighboring fiber. In addition to the atrioventricular node, the reentry circuit may include the sinoatrial node, the atrium, or an accessory bypass tract (see below). Recent evidence indicates that about one-third of patients have aberrant pathways to the ventricles. A single fortuitously timed atrial or ventricular premature beat may set up the reentry cycle or may terminate it.

## Treatment of the Acute Attack

In the absence of heart disease, serious effects are rare. Most attacks subside spontaneously, and the physician should not use remedies that are more dangerous than the disease. Particular effort should be made to terminate the attack quickly if cardiac failure, syncope, or anginal pain develops or if there is underlying cardiac or (particularly) coronary disease. Because reentry is the most common mechanism for paroxysmal atrial tachycardia, effective therapy requires that conduction be interrupted at some point in the reentry circuit.

**A. Mechanical Measures:** A variety of methods have been used to interrupt attacks, and patients may learn to perform these themselves. These include Valsalva's maneuver, stretching the arms and body, lowering the head between the knees, coughing, and breath-holding. These maneuvers, as is true also of carotid sinus pressure (see below), stimulate the vagus, delay atrioventricular conduction, and block the reentry mechanism, terminating the arrhythmias.

**B. Vagal Stimulation With Carotid Sinus Pressure: Caution:** *This procedure should not be performed if the patient has carotid bruits or a history of transient cerebral ischemic attacks.* With the patient relaxed in the semirecumbent position, firm but gentle pressure and massage are applied first over one carotid sinus for 10–20 seconds and then over the other. Pressure should not be exerted on both carotid sinuses at the same time. Continuous electrocardiographic or auscultatory monitoring of the heart rate is required so that carotid sinus pressure can be relieved as soon as the attack ceases or if excessive slowing occurs. Carotid sinus pressure will interrupt about half of the attacks, especially if the patient has been digitalized or sedated. *Do not apply eyeball pressure.*

**C. Drug Therapy:** Verapamil intravenously is the drug of choice if mechanical measures fail; it terminates 90% of episodes. An initial 2.5 mg bolus is employed to ensure that no untoward responses in blood pressure or rhythm occur. An additional 2.5 mg every 1–3 minutes up to 10 mg is then infused. If the blood pressure is stable, another 10 mg may be given. If the rhythm recurs, further doses can be given. Minimally symptomatic outpatients can be treated with 80–120 mg orally every 4–6 hours. Para-

sympathetic stimulating drugs such as edrophonium (Tensilon), 5–10 mg intravenously, which delay atrioventricular conduction, may break the reentry mechanism. Esmolol (Brevibloc), a short-acting beta-blocker, is also highly effective; the initial dose is 500 μg/kg intravenously over 1 minute followed by an infusion of 50–200 μg/min. Metaraminol or phenylephrine, alpha-adrenergic stimulants that activate the baroreceptors by raising the blood pressure and causing vagal stimulation, can break attacks but should be used cautiously. Digoxin is effective, but it often requires several hours to safely administer an adequate dose. An initial dose of 0.5–0.75 mg intravenously, followed by 0.25 or 0.125 increments every 3–4 hours up to a total of 1–1.25 mg, is used. Minimally symptomatic outpatients can be treated by oral digitalis. Intravenous procainamide may terminate supraventricular tachycardia; however, since it facilitates atrioventricular conduction and an initial increase in rate may occur, it is usually not given until after digoxin, verapamil, or a beta-blocker has been administered. Procainamide is the drug of choice for acute episodes of supraventricular tachycardia with antegrade conduction down an accessory pathway in Wolff-Parkinson-White syndrome.

**D. Cardioversion:** If the clinical situation is severe enough to warrant immediate termination and verapamil is contraindicated or ineffective, synchronized electrical cardioversion (beginning at 50–100 J) is almost universally successful. If digitalis toxicity is present or strongly suspected, as in the case of paroxysmal tachycardia with block, atrial pacing is preferable therapy. If digitalis has been given but toxicity is doubtful, electric shock can be used in progressively increasing amounts beginning with 10 J. If ventricular premature beats develop, lidocaine (1 mg/kg intravenously) is given. If the premature beats disappear, one can repeat the shock.

## Prevention of Attacks

**A. Drugs:** Digoxin orally is the usual drug of first choice because of its convenience and efficacy. Verapamil, alone or in combination with digitalis, is a second choice, though oral therapy is not as effective as intravenous therapy. *(Note:* Verapamil increases digoxin serum levels.) Beta-blockers are also effective. Patients who do not respond to these agents should be treated with a type Ia agent such as quinidine, perhaps in combination with digoxin or another agent that inhibits atrioventricular conduction. In patients taking quinidine, digoxin levels also increase by about 30%.

Procainamide and disopyramide are also effective, but the latter may cause or worsen cardiac failure. The newer type Ic agents, flecainide and encainide, are especially successful in patients with bypass tracts.

Amiodarone is highly effective, but because of its toxicity it should be employed only in refractory and symptomatic patients.

**B. His Bundle Ablation:** In patients with repeated or near-incessant symptomatic attacks that are difficult to control, ablation of the His bundle or accessory pathways has been accomplished by surgical interruption and catheter electrical ablation in order to prevent reentry. A ventricular pacemaker is necessary, because complete atrioventricular block is often produced.

**C. Antitachycardia Pacemakers:** Programmable permanent pacemakers have been employed to sense the appearance of supraventricular tachycardia and pace to interrupt the reentry circuit and stop the arrhythmia.

Luceri RM et al: The arrhythmias of dual-chamber cardiac pacemakers and their management. *Ann Intern Med* 1983;**99:**354.

Parsonnet V, Bernstein A: Pacing in perspective concepts and controversies. *Circulation* 1986;**73:**1087.

## 6. ATRIAL FIBRILLATION

Atrial fibrillation is the commonest chronic arrhythmia. It occurs in rheumatic heart disease, dilated cardiomyopathy, atrial septal defect, hypertension, mitral valve prolapse, and hypertrophic cardiomyopathy. Atrial fibrillation may be the initial presenting sign in thyrotoxicosis. Atrial fibrillation often appears paroxysmally before becoming the established rhythm. Pericarditis, chest trauma or surgery, or excessive alcohol intake may cause attacks in patients with normal hearts.

Atrial fibrillation is the only common arrhythmia in which the ventricular rate is rapid and the rhythm very irregular. The atrial rate is 400–600/min, but most impulses are blocked at the atrioventricular node. The ventricular response is completely irregular, ranging from 80 to 160/min in the untreated state. Because of the varying stroke volumes resulting from varying periods of diastolic filling, not all ventricular beats produce a palpable peripheral pulse. The difference between the apical rate and the pulse rate is the "pulse deficit"; this deficit is greater when the ventricular rate is high.

The major morbidity from atrial fibrillation (other than precipitation of cardiac failure) is arterial emboli from the poorly contracting and often enlarged left atrium. Anticoagulation should be initiated in patients with atrial fibrillation and mitral valve disease; its use is debated if the atrium is of normal size.

**A. Acute Ventricular Rate Control:** The initial goal of therapy is to control the ventricular response. Intravenous verapamil is the agent of choice and will control the ventricular response in 90% of patients. It selectively increases atrioventricular block and slows the ventricular rate. Because of its negative inotropic action, it may cause cardiac failure or hypotension, especially if it is used in combination with beta-blockers of disopyramide. The short-acting beta-blocker esmolol is an alternative approach. Digoxin remains highly effective, albeit control takes longer to accomplish. Digoxin is particularly appropriate if chronic therapy is planned. None of these agents should be given to patients with Wolff-Parkinson-White syndrome conducting antegrade through the accessory pathway (wide ventricular complexes), since conduction may accelerate. Procainamide is preferable.

**B. Cardioversion:** Immediate cardioversion required for patients with hemodynamic instability, most commonly when hypotension or heart failure prevents the use of verapamil. However, once the ventricular rate is controlled, a decision must be made about whether to attempt conversion to sinus rhythm. In general, if atrial fibrillation is of recent onset and the left atrium is not markedly enlarged, conversion is recommended. In patients with mitral valve disease or with a markedly dilated left ventricle and atrium, the risk of embolization is high, so most authorities initiate anticoagulation for 2–4 weeks prior to electric cardioversion. Quinidine, 300 mg every 6 hours, is often given for 24 hours before the procedure to prevent recurrence. Synchronized DC shock should be employed, with the initial dosage being 100 J, though more current may be needed. Quinidine can be used for conversion to sinus rhythm if electrical cardioversion is not available. Although digoxin alone often maintains sinus rhythm, the addition of a type Ia agent such as quinidine may be required. Procainamide and disopyromide are also effective. Amiodarone is perhaps the most effective agent, but its use is limited by its toxicity.

**C. Treatment of Chronic Atrial Fibrillation:** Digoxin is the preferred drug for chronic ventricular rate control in the absence of preexcitation. Higher than normal dosages and serum levels are often required to maintain the resulting ventricular response in the 60- to 80/min range and to prevent excessive rise with modest exertion. Often a second agent, such as verapamil or a beta-blocker, facilitates ventricular rate control, especially with activity.

Flegel KM, Shipley MJ, Rose G: Risk of stroke in non-rheumatic atrial fibrillation. *Lancet* 1987;**1:**526.

Mancini JGB, Goldberger AL: Cardioversion of atrial fibrillation: Consideration of embolization, anticoagulation, prophylactic pacemaker, and long-term success. *Am Heart J* 1982;**104:**617.

Morady F et al: Electrophysiologic testing in the management of patients with Wolff-Parkinson-White syndrome and atrial fibrillation. *Am J Cardiol* 1983;**51:**1623.

Scheinman MM: Atrioventricular nodal or atrio-junctional reentrant tachycardia. *J Am Coll Cardiol* 1985;**6:**1393.

## 7. ATRIAL FLUTTER

Atrial flutter is less common than fibrillation and usually occurs in patients with COPD, rheumatic or coronary heart disease, congestive heart failure, or atrial septal defect; it may also occur as result of quinidine effect on atrial fibrillation. Ectopic impulse formation occurs at atrial rates of 250–350/min, with transmission of every second, third, or fourth impulse through the atrioventricular node to the ventricles. When the ventricular rate is 75 (4:1 block), standing or exercise may cause sudden doubling of the rate to 150 (2:1 block).

Atrial flutter is unpredictably responsive to pharmacologic therapy, though verapamil may transiently increase atrioventricular block, and a combination of digoxin and quinidine may cause the rhythm to revert to sinus rhythm. In contrast, the rhythm is exquisitely sensitive to electrical cardioversion, which can usually be accomplished with less than 50 J, and is therefore the treatment of choice for acute episodes. Type Ia or Ic agents should be avoided unless an agent that delays atrioventricular conduction has been administered, because they can lead to 1:1 conduction. The same approaches discussed under atrial fibrillation are used to prevent further episodes.

## 8. ATRIOVENTRICULAR JUNCTIONAL RHYTHM

The atrial-nodal junction or the nodal-His bundle junctions may assume pacemaker activity for the heart, usually at a rate of 40–60/min. This may occur in normal hearts in patients with myocarditis, coronary artery disease, or as a result of digitalis toxicity. The rate responds normally to exercise, and the diagnosis is often an incidental finding on electrocardiographic monitoring, but it can be suspected if the jugular venous pulse shows cannon waves. Junctional rhythm is often an escape rhythm because of depressed sinus node function with sinoatrial block or delayed conduction in the atrioventricular node. **Nonparoxysmal junctional tachycardia** results from increased automaticity of the junctional tissues in digitalis toxicity or ischemia and is associated with a narrow QRS complex and a rate usually less than 120–130/min. It is usually considered benign when it occurs in acute myocardial infarction, but the ischemia that induces it may also induce ventricular tachycardia and ventricular fibrillation.

## 9. MULTIFOCAL (CHAOTIC) ATRIAL TACHYCARDIA

This is a rhythm characterized by varying P-wave morphology and markedly irregular PP intervals. The rate is usually between 100 and 140/min, and atrioventricular block is unusual. Most patients have severe associated illnesses, especially COPD. Treatment of the underlying condition is the most effective approach; verapamil may also be of value.

## 10. DIFFERENTIATION OF ABERRANTLY CONDUCTED SUPRAVENTRICULAR BEATS FROM VENTRICULAR BEATS

This distinction can be very difficult in patients with a wide QRS complex; it is important because of the differing prognostic and therapeutic implications of each type. Changes favoring a ventricular origin include (1) a QRS duration exceeding 0.14 s; (2) left axis deviation; (3) atrioventricular dissociation; (4) capture or fusion beats (infrequent); (5) monophasic (R) or biphasic (qR, QR, or RS) complexes in $V_1$; and (6) a qR or QS complex in $V_6$. Supraventricular origin is favored by (1) a triphasic QRS complex, especially if there was initial negativity in leads I and $V_6$; (2) ventricular rates exceeding 170/min; (3) QRS duration longer than 0.12 s but not longer than 0.14 s; and (4) the presence of preexcitation syndrome (Wellens, 1978).

The relationship of the P waves to the tachycardia complex is helpful. A 1:1 relationship usually means a supraventricular origin except in the case of ventricular tachycardia with retrograde P waves. If the P waves are not clearly seen, Lewis leads—in which the right arm electrode is placed in the $V_1$ position 2 interspaces higher than usual and the left arm electrode is placed in the usual $V_1$ position—may be employed. This accentuates the size of the P waves. Esophageal leads, in which the electrode is placed directly posterior to the left atrium, achieve the same effect even more clearly. Right atrial electrograms may also help to clarify the diagnosis by accentuating the P waves.

## 11. PREEXCITATION SYNDROME

### Pathophysiology & Clinical Findings

Preexcitation occurs as a result of abnormal or accessory pathways between the atria and the ventricle which avoid the conduction delay of the atrioventricular node. These may be wholly or partly within the node (Mahaim fibers), yielding a short PR internal and normal QRS morphology (**Lown-Ganong-Levine syndrome**). More commonly, they make direct connections between the atria and ventricle, through Kent bundles (**Wolff-Parkinson-White syndrome**). This produces a short PR interval but an early delta wave at the onset of the wide, slurred QRS complex owing to early ventricular depolarization of the region adjacent to the pathway. While the morphology and polarity of the delta wave can suggest the location of the bypass tract, mapping by intracardiac recordings is required for precise anatomic localization.

Accessory pathways occur in 0.1–0.3% of the population and predispose to reentry arrhythmias owing to the disparity in refractory periods of the atrioventricular node and accessory pathway. Whether the tachycardia is associated with a narrow or wide QRS complex is determined by whether antegrade conduction is through the node (narrow) or the bypass tract (wide). Many patients with Wolff-Parkinson-White syndrome never conduct antegrade through the bypass tract which is therefore "concealed." Although reentry supraventricular tachycardias involving the AV node are commonest, 20–30% of patients with tachyarrhythmias have atrial fibrillation or flutter. Many have no arrhythmia. A minority of patients conduct antegrade through the accessory pathway, but these individuals may develop very fast rates, especially during atrial fibrillation, and the rhythm may deteriorate into ventricular fibrillation. Patients with RR intervals less than 220 ms are at highest risk. Digoxin and, to a lesser extent, verapamil and beta-blockers may decrease accessory pathway refractoriness and increase ventricular response and should be avoided in atrial fibrillation with accessory pathways to prevent ventricular tachycardia or ventricular fibrillation.

## Pharmacologic Therapy

Narrow complex reentry rhythms can be managed as discussed for paroxysmal supraventricular tachycardias other than atrial fibrillation or flutter, though digoxin is best avoided in patients with known Wolff-Parkinson-White syndrome. The type 1a antiarrhythmics, as well as the newer class Ic and class III agents, will increase the refractoriness of the bypass tract and are the drugs of choice for wide-complex tachycardias. If hemodynamic compromise is present, cardioversion is warranted.

Long-term therapy often involves a combination of agents that increase refractoriness in the bypass tract (type Ia or Ic agents) and in the atrioventricular node (verapamil, digoxin, and beta-blockers). Amiodarone is effective in refractory cases. Patients who are difficult to manage should undergo electrophysiologic evaluation.

## Electrophysiologic Evaluation & Specialized Treatment

Patients who do not have arrhythmias or who have only rare episodes characterized by narrow complex paroxysmal supraventricular tachycardia do not require further evaluation.

Patients who have episodes of atrial fibrillation or flutter should be tested by induction of atrial fibrillation in the electrophysiologic laboratory, noting duration of the RR cycle; if it is less than 220 ms, a short refractory period is present, and these individuals are at highest risk for sudden death. Patients with frequent tachycardia, especially if refractory to therapy, and those who conduct antegrade through the accessory pathway should be evaluated by electrophysiologic studies. These can assess the risk of excessively rapid conduction and facilitate appropriate drug selection. The accessory pathway can be localized and its refractory period determined. In difficult patients, if the bypass tract is accessible, endocardial electroablation or surgical interruption may be the treatment of choice. Some patients can be managed with antitachycardia pacemakers that deliver properly timed impulses to interrupt the reentry cycle.

Alpert MA, Flaker GC: Arrhythmias associated with sinus node dysfunction: Pathogenesis, recognition, and management. JAMA 1983;250:2160.

Horowitz LN et al: Risks and complications of clinical cardiac electrophysiologic studies: A prospective analysis of 1,000 consecutive patients. J Am Coll Cardiol 1987;9:1261.

Kennedy HL et al: Long-term follow-up of asymptomatic healthy subjects with frequent and complex ventricular ectopy. N Engl J Med 1985;312:193.

McGovern B, Garan H, Ruskin JN: Precipitation of cardiac arrest by verapamil in patients with Wolff-Parkinson-White syndrome. Ann Intern Med 1986;104:791.

Wellens HJJ, Bär FWHM, Lie KI: The value of the electrocardiogram in the differential diagnosis of a tachycardia with a widened QRS complex. Am J Med 1978;64:27.

Wellens HJJ, Brugada P, Penn OC: The management of preexcitation syndromes. JAMA 1987;257:2325.

# VENTRICULAR ARRHYTHMIAS

## 1. VENTRICULAR PREMATURE BEATS (Ventricular Extrasystoles)

Ventricular premature beats are similar to atrial premature beats in mechanism and manifestations but are more common. They are characterized by wide QRS complexes that differ in morphology from the patient's normal beats. They are usually not preceded by a P wave, although retrograde ventriculoatrial conduction may occur. Unless the latter is present, there is a fully compensatory pause. Bigeminy and trigeminy are arrhythmias in which every second or third beat is premature. The extra beat can be noted at the apex but may not be felt at the wrist, in contrast to dropped beats (see below). Exercise generally abolishes premature beats in normal hearts, and the rhythm becomes regular. The patient may or may not sense the irregular beat.

Premature beats have questionable significance in the absence of coronary disease, hypertrophic cardiomyopathy, or prolapse of the mitral valve. Sudden death occurs more frequently (presumably as a result of ventricular fibrillation) when ventricular premature beats occur in the presence of known disease but not in individuals with no known cardiac disease in the middle-aged normal population.

Ambulatory electrocardiographic monitoring or continuous electrocardiography during graded exercise reveals more frequent and complex ventricular premature beats than occur in a single routine ECG. Exercise-induced premature beats may have a worse prognosis than those which occur spontaneously.

If no associated cardiac disease is present and if the ectopic beats are asymptomatic, no specific therapy is indicated. If they are frequent, electrolyte abnormalities and occult heart disease should be considered. Treatment is indicated for patients who are symptomatic. Though most clinicians treat ectopic beats in patients with known heart disease, the value of treatment is controversial. In general, if the beats are single, even though frequent, observation without therapy is usually indicated. If there are couplets or runs or if beats are multiform, treatment may be worthwhile. If the underlying condition is mitral prolapse, hypertrophic cardiomyopathy, left ventricular hypertrophy, or coronary disease—or if the QT interval is prolonged—a trial of a beta-blocker may be worthwhile even though these agents are often unsuccessful. The type Ia, Ib, and Ic agents are all effective in reducing ventricular premature beats but often cause side effects and may exacerbate arrhythmias in 5–20% of patients. Amiodarone should not be given to patients unless more severe arrhythmias are present.

## 2. VENTRICULAR TACHYCARDIA

Ventricular tachycardia is defined as 3 or more consecutive ventricular premature beats. The usual rate is 160–240/min and is moderately regular, but less so than atrial tachycardia. Carotid sinus pressure has no effect. The distinction from aberrant conduction of supraventricular tachycardia may be difficult and is discussed above. The usual mechanism is reentry, but abnormally triggered rhythms occur. Ventricular tachycardia is either nonsustained (lasting less than 30 seconds) or sustained. It may be asymptomatic or associated with chest pain, syncope, or milder symptoms of impaired cerebral perfusion.

Ventricular tachycardia is a frequent complication of acute myocardial infarction and dilated cardiomyopathy but may occur in hypertrophic cardiomyopathy or mitral valve prolapse. Torsade de pointes, a form of ventricular tachycardia in which QRS morphology varies, may occur after quinidine or any drug that prolongs the QT interval. In nonacute settings, most patients with ventricular tachycardia have known or easily detectable cardiac disease, and the finding of ventricular tachycardia is an unfavorable prognostic sign.

### Treatment

**A. Acute Ventricular Tachycardia:** The treatment of acute ventricular tachycardia is determined by the degree of hemodynamic compromise and the duration of the arrhythmia. The management of ventricular tachycardia in acute infarction has been discussed. In other patients, if severe hypotension is present, synchronized DC cardioversion with 100–400 J should be performed immediately. If the patient is tolerating the rhythm, lidocaine can be infused first and may terminate it. If the patient is stable and lidocaine is not effective, a trial of intravenous procainamide or bretylium may be successful; the latter is most effective in digitalis toxicity. Ventricular tachycardia can be terminated by ventricular overdrive pacing, and this approach is useful when the rhythm is recurrent.

Amiodarone takes time to achieve a therapeutic level, but intravenous or oral loading with 1000–2000 mg/d may deliver a therapeutic response in 24–72 hours in refractory patients.

**B. Chronic Recurrent Ventricular Tachycardia:** The treatment of recurrent, nonsustained ventricular tachycardia (runs of 3 or more beats lasting less than 30 seconds) not associated with symptoms is controversial. In subjects without heart disease, this rhythm is not clearly associated with a poor prognosis, whereas in patients with cardiac problems, it

is a marker for increased mortality rate from the underlying disease and, in some studies, for arrhythmic death. Whether antiarrhythmic therapy is beneficial in these patients in **nonsustained ventricular tachycardia** is unclear, but it is recommended. Type Ia agents are usually employed, but type Ib and Ic drugs are alternatives (see Table 8–7). Beta-blockers are occasionally beneficial. The efficacy of treatment is assessed by ambulatory monitoring. Some authorities recommend ventricular stimulation; if sustained tachycardia of similar morphology is induced, they undertake more aggressive management with the goal of complete suppression of the arrhythmia. Amiodarone should probably not be used for asymptomatic, nonsustained tachycardia unless sustained ventricular tachycardia is inducible.

Patients with symptomatic or asymptomatic **sustained ventricular tachycardia** require effective suppressive therapy. To develop an effective therapeutic regimen, it is essential that the rhythm either be present spontaneously or be induced by programmed stimulation in the electrophysiology laboratory. Various antiarrhythmic drugs can then be given in sequence to determine which agents prevent ventricular tachycardia. Drugs that prevent the electrical induction of ventricular tachycardia in the laboratory or suppress its occurrence during monitoring are more likely to be effective in vivo for long-term therapy; long-term use of a particular drug may still be effective even if the arrhythmia is not fully prevented in the laboratory. This is the case especially with amiodarone, which has emerged as a very effective though toxic agent for this select group of patients. The potential of all antiarrhythmia drugs to exacerbate ventricular arrhythmias in some patients should be kept in mind in initiating and monitoring therapy.

Patients with refractory ventricular tachycardia should be evaluated and treated in specialized centers. Endocardial mapping using intracardiac catheters is employed in patients who have frequent recurrences with life-threatening symptoms that fail to respond to drugs. The origin and sequence of activation can be determined; this is essential if surgical treatment or transcatheter electrical ablation is being considered. The indications for surgical treatment and the various approaches are still being developed, but the results have occasionally been dramatic when all else has failed.

In selected patients in whom ventricular tachycardia can be reproducibly terminated by overdrive pacing, a specially programmed pacemaker can be inserted that will automatically sense the arrhythmia and interrupt it. There has also been a growing experience with automatic implantable defibrillators, which deliver an electric shock when ventricular tachycardia is sensed. These devices require sophisticated electrophysiologic studies prior to their insertion.

Gabry MD et al: Automatic implantable cardioverter-defibrillator: Patient survival, battery longevity and shock delivery analysis. *J Am Coll Cardiol* 1987;**9**:1349.

Hammill SC et al: Clinical intracardiac electrophysiologic testing: Technique, diagnostic indications, and therapeutic uses. *Mayo Clin Proc* 1986;**61**:478.

Kupersmith J, Reder RF, Slater W: New antiarrhythmic drugs. *Cardiovasc Rev Rep* 1985;**6**:35.

Likoff ML, Chandler SL, Kay HR: Clinical determinants of mortality in chronic congestive heart failure secondary to idiopathic dilated or to ischemic cardiomyopathy. *Am J Cardiol* 1987;**59**:634.

McGovern BA, Ruskin JN: Ventricular tachycardia: Initial assessment and approach to treatment. *Mod Concepts Cardiovasc Dis* 1987;**56**:13.

Mirowski M: The automatic implantable cardioverter-defibrillator: An overview. *J Am Coll Cardiol* 1985;**6**:461.

National Conference on Cardiopulmonary Resuscitation (CPR) and Emergency Cardiac Care (ECC): Standards and guidelines for cardiopulmonary resuscitation (CPR) and emergency cardiac care (ECC). *JAMA* 1986;**255**:2905.

Stewart RB, Bardy GH, Greene HL: Wide complex tachycardia: Misdiagnosis and outcome after emergent therapy. *Ann Intern Med* 1986;**104**:766.

## 3. VENTRICULAR FIBRILLATION

The management of ventricular fibrillation is discussed under complications of myocardial infarction and is similar in all clinical settings.

## 4. ACCELERATED IDIOVENTRICULAR RHYTHM

Accelerated idioventricular rhythm is a relatively regular wide complex rhythm with a rate of 60–120/min, usually with a gradual onset. Because the rate is often similar to the sinus rate, fusion beats and alternating rhythms are common. Two mechanisms have been invoked: (1) an escape rhythm due to suppression of higher pacemakers resulting from sinoatrial and atrioventricular block or from depressed sinus node function; and (2) slow ventricular tachycardia due to increased automaticity or, less frequently, reentry. It occurs commonly in acute infarction and following reperfusion after thrombolytic drugs. The incidence of associated ventricular fibrillation is much less than that of ventricular tachycardia with a rapid rate, and treatment is not indicated unless there is hemodynamic compromise or more serious arrhythmias. This rhythm also is common in digitalis toxicity.

Accelerated idioventricular rhythm must be distinguished from the idioventricular or junctional rhythm with rates less than 40–45/min that occurs in the presence of complete atrioventricular block. Atrioventricular dissociation—where ventricular rate exceeds sinus—but not atrioventricular block occurs in most cases of accelerated idioventricular rhythm.

## 5. LONG QT SYNDROME

Idiopathic long QT syndrome is an uncommon disease that was first described in deaf siblings. It is characterized by recurrent syncope, a long QT interval (usually 0.5–0.7 s), documented ventricular arrhythmias, and sudden death. Recent research emphasizes the role of the sympathetic nervous system (especially the left stellate ganglion) in pathogenesis.

Beta-blockers are the most effective therapy for "congenital" long QT syndrome, though phenytoin and the type Ib agents have also been beneficial. Agents that prolong the QT (types Ia, Ic, and III) are contraindicated. Refractory acute arrhythmic episodes may be treated by local anesthetic block of the left stellate ganglion, and recurrent episodes can be treated by resection of this ganglion as well as of the first 3–5 thoracic ganglia.

**Acquired long QT.** Acquired prolongation of the QT interval secondary to use of antiarrhythmic agents or antidepressant drugs, electrolyte abnormalities, myocardial ischemia, or significant bradycardia may result in ventricular tachycardia (torsade de pointes, ie, twisting about the baseline into varying QRS morphology). The role of a prolonged QT interval is difficult to evaluate because types Ia, Ic, and III antiarrhythmic agents increase the QT interval and yet are effective in treating the ventricular tachyarrhythmias; it may be the reason that these drugs parodoxically cause ventricular tachycardia in some patients. Acquired QT interval prolongation requires further study, but prudence speaks against continuing therapy that prolongs the QT interval beyond 500 ms.

Jackman WM et al: Ventricular tachyarrhythmias in the long QT syndromes. *Med Clin North Am* 1984;**68**:1079.

# CONDUCTION DISTURBANCES

Abnormalities of conduction can occur between the sinus node and atrium, within the atrioventricular node, and in the intraventricular conduction pathways.

## SINOATRIAL EXIT BLOCK

Sinoatrial exit block produces a pause of a duration equal to a multiple of the underlying PP interval. Often there is progressive shortening of the PP interval prior to the pause (sinoatrial Wenckebach). This disturbance may be due to excessive vagal tone, ischemia, fibrosis or calcification of the conduction fibers, or drug effect (especially digitalis or calcium blockers). Sinoatrial exit block is usually asymptomatic, though prolonged pauses equivalent to sinus arrest rarely occur as part of the sick sinus syndrome and are treated as outlined below.

## SICK SINUS SYNDROME

This imprecise diagnosis is applied to patients with sinus arrest, sinoatrial exit block, or persistent sinus bradycardia. These rhythms are often caused or exacerbated by drug therapy (digitalis, calcium channel blockers, beta-blockers, sympatholytic agents, antiarrhythmics), and agents that may be responsible should be withdrawn prior to making the diagnosis.

Pathologic causes of the syndrome include degenerative fibrotic lesions of the cardiac conduction system and other conditions in which sclerotic or granulomatous lesions may occur, including scleroderma, Chagas' disease, and various cardiomyopathies. Coronary disease is an uncommon cause. In conjunction with a slow atrial rate resulting from these abnormalities, paroxysmal atrial or junctional arrhythmias and perfusion abnormalities may occur. There may be alteration of a slow rate (which may not be adequate to perfuse the vital organs) with rapid atrial or junctional tachycardia or atrial fibrillation. Treatment of atrial arrhythmias with drugs such as quinidine or digitalis may enhance the automaticity or conduction abnormalities of the sinus node.

Most patients with electrocardiographic evidence of sick sinus syndrome are asymptomatic, but rare individuals may experience syncope, dizziness, confusion, palpitations, heart failure, or angina. Because these symptoms are either nonspecific or have other causes, it is essential that they be demonstrated to coincide with arrhythmias. This may require prolonged ambulatory monitoring or the use of an event recorder. In such cases, permanent pacing is indicated; since atrioventricular node disease is often also present, ventricular or dual chamber pacing is preferred unless electrophysiologic studies indicate normal atrioventricular conduction. Unfortunately, symptomatic relief has not been consistent, largely because of inadequate documentation of the etiologic role of bradyarrhythmias in producing the symptom. Furthermore, many of these patients may have associated ventricular arrhythmias that may require treatment; however, carefully selected patients may become asymptomatic with permanent pacing alone.

Tresch DD, Fleg JL: Unexplained sinus bradycardia: Clinical significance and long-term prognosis in apparently healthy persons older than 40 years. *Am J Cardiol* 1986;**58**:1009.

## ATRIOVENTRICULAR BLOCK

Atrioventricular block is categorized as first degree (PR interval $\geq$ 0.21 s with all atrial impulses conducted), second degree (intermittent blocked beats), or third degree (complete heart block), in which no supraventricular impulses are conducted to the ventricles.

Second-degree block is subclassified. In **Mobitz type I (Wenckebach)** atrioventricular block, the atrioventricular conduction time (PR interval) progressively lengthens, with the RR interval shortening, before the blocked beat; this phenomenon is almost always due to abnormal conduction within the node. **Mobitz type II** atrioventricular block is abrupt and is not preceded by a lengthening atrioventricular conduction time; it is usually due to block within the

His bundle system. The classification as Mobitz type I or Mobitz type II is only partially reliable, because patients may have both types in the same lead, and one cannot predict the site or origin of the 2:1 atrioventricular block from the ECG. The width of the QRS complexes assists in determining whether the block is nodal or infranodal. When they are narrow, the block is usually nodal; when they are wide, the block is usually infranodal. His bundle readings may be necessary for accurate localization. Management of atrioventricular block in acute myocardial infarction has already been discussed. This section deals with patients in the nonacute setting.

**First-degree** and **Mobitz type I block** may occur in normal individuals with heightened vagal tone. They may also occur as a drug effect (especially digitalis, calcium channel blockers, beta-blockers, or other sympatholytic agents), often superimposed on organic disease. These disturbances also occur transiently or chronically due to ischemia, infarction, inflammatory processes, fibrosis, calcification, or infiltration. The prognosis is usually good, since lower reliable pacemakers are available if higher degrees of block occur.

**Mobitz type II block** is almost always due to organic disease involving the infranodal conduction system. In the event of progression to complete heart block, lower pacemakers are not reliable. Thus, prophylactic ventricular pacing is required.

**Complete (third-degree) heart block** is a more advanced form of block often due to a lesion distal to the His bundle and associated with bilateral bundle branch block. The QRS is wide and the ventricular rate is slower, usually less than 50/min. Transmission of atrial impulses through the atrioventricular node is completely blocked, and a ventricular pacemaker maintains a slow, regular ventricular rate, usually less than 45/min. Exercise does not increase the rate. The first heart sound varies in intensity; wide pulse pressure, a changing systolic blood pressure level, and cannon venous pulsations (abrupt, large, rapid upstroke and downstroke) in the neck are also present. Patients may be asymptomatic or may complain of weakness or dyspnea if the rate is less than 35/min; symptoms may occur at higher rates if the left ventricle cannot increase its stroke output. During periods of transition from partial to complete heart block, some patients have ventricular asystole that lasts several seconds to minutes. Syncope occurs abruptly, and if asystole is prolonged beyond a few seconds, convulsive movements appear **(Stoke-Adams syndrome).** Asystole of 2–3 minutes is usually fatal.

Patients with episodic or chronic infranodal complete heart block require permanent pacing, and temporary pacing is indicated if implantation is delayed.

## ATRIOVENTRICULAR DISSOCIATION

When a ventricular pacemaker is firing at a rate faster than or close to the sinus rate (accelerated idioventricular rhythm, ventricular premature beats, or ventricular tachycardia), atrial impulses arriving at the atrioventricular node when it is refractory may not be conducted. This phenomenon is atrioventricular dissociation but does not necessarily indicate atrioventricular block. No treatment is required aside from management of the causative arrhythmia.

## INTRAVENTRICULAR BLOCK

Intraventricular conduction defects, including bundle branch block, are common in individuals with otherwise normal hearts and in many disease processes, including ischemic heart disease, inflammatory disease, infiltrative disease, cardiomyopathy, and postcardiotomy. Below the atrioventricular node and bundle of His, the conduction system trifurcates into a right bundle and anterior and posterior fascicles of the left bundle. Conduction block in each of these fascicles can be recognized on the surface ECG. Although such conduction abnormalities are often seen in normal hearts, they are more commonly due to organic heart disease—either an isolated process of fibrosis and calcification (Lev's or Lenegre's disease) or more generalized myocardial disease. Bifascicular block is present when 2 of these—right bundle, left anterior and posterior hemibundle—are involved. Trifascicular block is defined as right bundle branch block with alternating left hemiblock, alternating right and left bundle branch block, or bifascicular block with documented prolonged infranodal conduction (long HV interval).

The prognosis of intraventricular block is generally that of the underlying myocardial process. Even in bifascicular block, the incidence of occult complete heart block or progression to it is low, and pacing is not usually warranted. In patients with symptoms (eg, syncope) consistent with heart block and intraventricular block, pacing should be reserved for those with documented concomitant complete heart block on monitoring or those with a very prolonged HV interval ($\geq$ 90 ms) with no other cause for symptoms. Even in the latter group, prophylactic pacing has not improved the prognosis significantly, probably because of the high incidence of ventricular arrhythmias in the same population.

## PERMANENT PACING

The indications for permanent pacing have been discussed: symptomatic bradyarrhythmias, asymptomatic Mobitz II AV block, or complete heart block. The versatility of pacemaker generator units has increased markedly, and dual-chamber multiple programmable units are readily available. Conceptually, a pacemaker that senses and paces in both chambers is the most physiologic approach to pacing patients who remain in sinus rhythm. However, because of the added cost and complexity of dual-chamber pacing

and the shorter projected battery life, their use should be limited to patients who are most likely to benefit, ie, those in whom atrial contraction produces a substantial increment in stroke volume. In general, the device is most useful for individuals with left ventricular systolic or—perhaps more importantly—diastolic dysfunction. The latter may lead to the so-called pacemaker syndrome, in which the patient experiences signs of low cardiac output while upright from loss of an atrial "kick." Patients with intermittent or potential bradyarrhythmias or conduction disturbances in whom pacing is primarily prophylactic should undergo ventricular pacing. The newer dual-chamber pacemakers are complicated, and it is wise to refer patients to cardiologists experienced in their use. Regular follow-up after pacemaker implantation, usually by telephonic monitoring, is essential. All pulse generators and lead systems have an early failure rate as well as a finite life expectancy.

Dewey RC, Capeless MA, Levy AM: Use of ambulatory electrocardiographic monitoring to identify high-risk patients with congenital complete heart block. *N Engl J Med* 1987;**316:**835.

Flowers NC: Left bundle branch block: A continuously evolving concept. *J Am Coll Cardiol* 1987;**9:**684.

Parsonnet V, Bernstein A: Pacing in perspective: Concepts and controversies. *Circulation* 1986;**73:**1087.

---

# EVALUATION OF SYNCOPE & SURVIVORS OF SUDDEN DEATH

---

## EVALUATION OF SYNCOPE

Syncope is especially common in the elderly. Virtually any bradyarrhythmia, tachyarrhythmia, or conduction disturbance sufficient to impair cardiac output may produce it. Atrioventricular block and sick sinus syndrome are the commonest causes. Cardiac syncope also occurs in aortic stenosis, pulmonary stenosis, hypertrophic cardiomyopathy, and left atrial myxoma. Hypersensitive carotid sinus syndrome may cause syncope by either bradyarrhythmia or hypotension. Despite these observations, most syncopal episodes are not cardiogenic. Other causes include vasovagal fainting, postural hypotension, autonomic neuropathy, epilepsy, posterior circulation ischemia, and hyperventilation. Cardiac syncope is characterized by its abrupt onset, lack of premonitory symptoms, and rapid recovery.

In general, the cause of syncope is suggested by the history and initial clinical evaluation. Most patients with cardiogenic syncope have known or easily diagnosable heart disease. The physical examination should seek valvular disease. The ECG is valuable for showing baseline rhythm, rate, and conduction patterns. Complete heart block usually is accompanied by evidence of intraventricular conduction abnormality. Recent or old infarction enhances the likelihood of ventricular tachycardia. If the cause is not clear, 24 hours of monitoring in the hospital is sometimes diagnostic. Echocardiography and exercise testing are helpful when other findings raise the possibility of undiagnosed or possibly related cardiac disease. Ambulatory monitoring is the key to diagnosis and management of patients with recurrent syncope. Ideally, an event is recorded. If not, evidence of an arrhythmia that might cause syncope if it were more severe or sustained is helpful.

Patients with recurrent syncope may be referred for electrophysiologic studies when noncardiac causes have been excluded, no episode has been monitored, nonarrhythmic cardiac causes have been ruled out, and a related rhythm disorder has not been detected. The yield is highest in patients with organic heart disease and low when no heart disease is present. Such an evaluation should include assessment of sinus node and atrioventricular conduction and atrial and ventricular stimulation studies.

Treatment of the potentially causative arrhythmias has been discussed previously. Even after complete cardiac and noncardiac evaluation, the cause remains undiagnosed in 10–25% of patients with recurrent syncope—though this proportion falls when syncope is more frequent.

Hammill SC et al: Clinical intracardiac electrophysiologic testing: Technique, diagnostic indications, and therapeutic uses. *Mayo Clin Proc* 1986;**61**:478.

## SURVIVORS OF SUDDEN DEATH

Sudden cardiac death is defined as unexpected nontraumatic death in clinically well or stable patients who die with 1 hour after onset of symptoms. Primary prevention is the obvious goal, best accomplished by eliminating the risk factors for coronary disease, the most common underlying cause.

Over 75% of victims of sudden cardiac death have had severe coronary artery disease ($\geq$ 60% have 3-vessel disease). Many have old infarctions. Sudden death may be the initial manifestation of coronary disease in up to 25% of patients and occurs in 30–40% of patients with acute myocardial infarction. Survivors of sudden death require careful evaluation and management. When ventricular fibrillation occurs in the initial 24 hours after infarction, long-term management is no different from that of other patients with acute infarction. Other patients, whether they have coronary disease, other forms of heart disease, or apparently normal hearts, are at high risk of recurrence.

Underlying diagnoses should be made and treatment optimized, but unless an unusual correctable process was present (such as an electrolyte abnormality, drug toxicity, or aortic stenosis), these patients should undergo intensive investigation. Conduction

disturbances should be managed as described above. If serious prodromal ventricular arrhythmias such as sustained or nonsustained ventricular tachycardia or frequent ventricular premature beats are found by monitoring, their elimination by therapy *may* prevent further episodes—the evidence is conflicting. Most experts believe that ventricular stimulation studies are also indicated, especially if monitoring does not reveal significant arrhythmias. If sustained ventricular tachycardia or fibrillation is induced, therapy should be undertaken to prevent it. Pharmacologic therapy should follow the guidelines described under ventricular tachycardia. If inducibility cannot be prevented by the usual agents or if monitored arrhythmias are not obliterated, amiodarone may still be effective. Alternatively, either surgical or catheter ablation or implantation of an automatic implantable defibrillator may be attempted. Patients in whom ventricular tachycardia cannot be detected or induced are usually treated empirically with beta-blockers and antiarrhythmic therapy.

Patients being managed in a carefully designed therapeutic program who have recurrent sudden death, syncope, or documented sustained ventricular tachycardia should be referred for ablation of foci or implantation of an automatic defibrillator.

Holmes DR et al: The effect of medical and surgical treatment on subsequent sudden cardiac death in patients with coronary artery disease: A report from the Coronary Artery Surgery Study. *Circulation* 1986;**73**:1254.

Platia EV et al: Treatment of malignant ventricular arrhythmias with endocardial resection and implantation of the automatic cardioverter-defibrillator. *N Engl J Med* 1986;**314**:213.

## CARDIAC FAILURE

The function of the heart is governed by 4 major determinants: the contractile state of the myocardium, the preload of the ventricle (the end-diastolic volume and the resultant fiber length of the ventricles prior to onset of the contraction), the afterload applied to the ventricles (the impedance to left ventricular ejection), and the heart rate.

Cardiac function may be inadequate as a result of alterations of these determinants. In most instances, the primary derangement is depression of myocardial contractility caused either by loss of functional muscle (due to myocardial infarction, etc) or by processes diffusely affecting the myocardium. However, the heart may fail as a pump because preload is excessively elevated, such as in valvular regurgitation or when left ventricular filling is restricted for any reason, or when afterload is excessive, such as in aortic stenosis or in severe hypertension. Pump function may also be inadequate when the heart rate is too slow or too rapid. While the normal heart can tolerate wide variations in preload, afterload, and heart rate, the diseased heart often has limited reserve for such alterations. Finally, cardiac pump function may be supranormal but nonetheless inadequate when metabolic demands or requirements for blood flow are excessive. This situation is termed high-output heart failure and, though uncommon, should be identified and treated specifically. Causes of high output include thyrotoxicosis, beriberi, severe anemia, arteriovenous shunting, and Paget's disease of bone.

## Pathophysiology

When the heart fails, a number of adaptations occur both in the heart and systemically. If the stroke volume of either ventricle is reduced by depressed contractility or excessive afterload, end-diastolic volume and pressure in that chamber will rise. This increases end-diastolic myocardial fiber length, resulting in a greater systolic shortening (Starling's law of the heart). If the condition is chronic, ventricular dilatation will occur. While this may restore resting cardiac output, the resulting chronic elevation of diastolic pressures will be transmitted to the atria and to the pulmonary and systemic venous circulation. Ultimately, increased capillary pressure may lead to transudation of fluid with resulting pulmonary or systemic edema. Reduced cardiac output, particularly if associated with reduced arterial pressure or perfusion of the kidneys, will also activate several neural and humoral systems. Increased activity of the sympathetic nervous system will stimulate myocardial contractility, heart rate, and venous tone; the latter change results in a rise in the effective central blood volume, which serves to further elevate preload. Though these adaptations are designed to increase cardiac output, they may themselves be deleterious. Thus, tachycardia and increased contractility may precipitate ischemia in patients with underlying coronary artery disease, and the rise in preload may worsen pulmonary congestion. Sympathetic nervous system activation also increases peripheral vascular resistance; this adaptation is designed to maintain perfusion to vital organs, but when it is excessive it may itself reduce renal and other tissue blood flow. Peripheral vascular resistance is also a major determinant of left ventricular afterload, so that excessive sympathetic activity may further depress cardiac function.

One of the more important effects of lower cardiac output is reduction of renal blood flow and glomerular filtration rate, which leads to sodium and fluid retention. In moderate to severe heart failure, the renin-angiotensin-aldosterone system is also activated, leading to further increases in peripheral vascular resistance and left ventricular afterload as well as sodium and fluid retention. Heart failure is associated with increased circulating levels of arginine vasopressin, which also serves as a vasoconstrictor and inhibitor of water excretion. While release of atrial natriuretic peptide is increased in heart failure owing to the elevated atrial pressures, there is evidence of resistance to its natriuretic and vasodilating effects.

## Hemodynamic Alterations

Myocardial failure is characterized by 2 hemodynamic derangements, and the clinical presentation is determined by their severity. Resting cardiac output or—in cases where compensatory mechanisms are relatively effective—the ability to increase cardiac output in response to increased demands imposed by exercise or even ordinary activity (cardiac reserve) is usually reduced. The second abnormality, elevation of ventricular diastolic pressures, is primarily a result of the compensatory processes.

Heart failure is sometimes classified as being forward or backward. **Forward heart failure** is a manifestation of low cardiac output and includes symptoms and signs of reduced perfusion of vital organs, including the kidneys (renal dysfunction, sodium and water retention), the brain (fatigue, depressed mental status), and skeletal muscle (weakness and exercise intolerance). The term **"backward heart failure"** denotes manifestations of elevated intracardiac diastolic pressures and the resulting transudation of fluid. These include dyspnea and pulmonary edema, peripheral edema, hepatic congestion and ascites, and edema of the gastrointestinal tract, with resulting impaired absorption and digestion. Manifestations of forward and backward failure are closely linked.

Heart failure may be right-sided or left-sided. Patients with the picture of **left heart failure** have symptoms of low cardiac output and elevated pulmonary venous pressure; dyspnea is the predominant symptom. Signs of fluid retention predominate in **right heart failure,** with the patient exhibiting edema, hepatic congestion, and, on occasion, ascites. Most patients exhibit signs of both right- and left-sided failure, and left ventricular dysfunction is the primary cause of right ventricular failure. Surprisingly, some individuals with severe left ventricular dysfunction and secondary right ventricular failure will display few signs of left heart failure and appear to have isolated right heart failure. Indeed, they may be clinically indistinguishable from patients with cor pulmonale, who have right heart failure secondary to pulmonary disease.

Although this section concerns cardiac failure due to systolic left ventricular dysfunction, patients with diastolic dysfunction experience many of the same symptoms and may be difficult to distinguish clinically. These patients have normal contractility but "stiff" or noncompliant hearts. Therefore, diastolic pressures are elevated even though diastolic volumes are normal or small. These pressures are transmitted to the pulmonary and systemic venous systems, resulting in dyspnea and edema. The commonest cause of diastolic cardiac dysfunction is left ventricular hypertrophy, but conditions such as hypertrophic or restrictive cardiomyopathy, diabetes, and pericardial disease can produce the same clinical picture. While diuretics are often useful in these patients, the other therapies discussed in this section (digitalis, vasodilators, inotropic agents) may be inappropriate.

## Causes of Cardiac Failure

The syndrome of cardiac failure can be produced by many diseases. In developed countries, coronary artery disease with resulting myocardial infarction and loss of functioning myocardium (ischemic cardiomyopathy) is the commonest cause. A number of processes may present with dilated or congestive cardiomyopathy, which is characterized by left ventricular or biventricular dilatation and generalized systolic dysfunction. These are discussed in subsequent sections, but the most common are alcoholic cardiomyopathy, viral myocarditis, and dilated cardiomyopathies with no obvious underlying cause (idiopathic cardiomyopathy). Rare causes of dilated cardiomyopathy include infiltrative diseases (hemochromatosis, sarcoidosis, amyloidosis, etc), other infectious agents, cardiotoxins, and drug toxicity. Systemic hypertension remains an important cause of congestive heart failure and, even more commonly in the USA, an exacerbating factor in patients with cardiac dysfunction due to other causes.

Patients with chronic volume overload of the left ventricle, such as mitral or aortic regurgitation, may develop progressive myocardial dysfunction and have a picture of cardiomyopathy even after the underlying condition is corrected. This form of congestive heart failure is preventable by early diagnosis and treatment of the valvular lesion.

## Clinical Findings

**A. Symptoms:** The symptoms of cardiac failure have been discussed in part in earlier sections. The most common complaint is shortness of breath often chiefly exertional dyspnea at first and progressing to orthopnea, paroxysmal nocturnal dyspnea, and rest dyspnea. A more subtle and often overlooked symptom of heart failure is a chronic nonproductive cough often worse in the recumbent position. Nocturia due to excretion of fluid retained during the day and increased renal perfusion in the recumbent position is a common nonspecific symptom of heart failure. Patients with heart failure also complain of fatigue and weakness, which result from reduced blood flow to skeletal muscle and the central nervous system. These symptoms may be exacerbated by electrolyte changes induced either by the heart failure or by diuretic treatment. Patients with right heart failure may experience right upper quadrant pain due to passive congestion of the liver, loss of appetite and nausea due to edema or impaired gastrointestinal perfusion, and peripheral edema.

Cardiac failure may present acutely in a previously asymptomatic patient. The most common cause of acute heart failure is myocardial infarction or rapidly progressive myocarditis or cardiomyopathy. Acute valvular regurgitation due to endocarditis or other conditions may also present as acute heart failure. These patients usually present with pulmonary edema. The management of acute heart failure has been discussed under myocardial infarction and centers around initial stabilization with diuretics and parenteral vaso-dilators or inotropic agents. After stabilization, the underlying disease should be determined and corrected, or the patient should be managed as outlined below for chronic heart failure.

Patients may also present with acute exacerbations of chronic, stable heart failure. Exacerbations are usually caused by alterations in therapy (or patient noncompliance), excessive salt and fluid intake, arrhythmias, excessive activity, pulmonary emboli, intercurrent infection, or progression of the underlying disease.

**B. Signs:** Many patients with heart failure, including some with severe symptoms, appear comfortable at rest. Others will be dyspneic during conversation or minor activity, and those with long-standing severe heart failure may appear cachetic or cyanotic. The vital signs may be normal, but tachycardia, hypotension, and reduced pulse pressure may be present. Patients often show signs of increased sympathetic nervous system activity, including cold extremities and diaphoresis. Important peripheral signs of heart failure can be detected by examination of the neck, the lungs, the abdomen, and the extremities. Right atrial pressure may be estimated through the height of the pulsations in the jugular venous system. In addition to the height of the venous pressure, abnormal pulsations such as regurgitant $v$ waves should be sought. Examination of the carotid pulse allows estimation of pulse pressure as well as detection of aortic stenosis. The thyroid examination is important, since occult hyperthyroidism is a readily treatable cause of heart failure. In the lungs, crackles at the bases reflect transudation of fluid into the alveoli. Pleural effusions may cause bibasilar dullness to percussion. Expiratory wheezing and rhonchi may be signs of heart failure. Patients with severe right heart failure may have hepatic enlargement—tender or nontender—due to passive congestion. Systolic pulsations may be felt in tricuspid regurgitation. Sustained moderate pressure on the liver may increase jugular venous pressure (a positive hepatojugular reflux is an increase of $> 1$ cm). Ascites may also be present. Peripheral pitting edema is a common sign in patients with right heart failure and may extend into the thighs and abdominal wall.

The cardiac examination has been discussed. Cardinal signs in heart failure are a parasternal lift, indicating pulmonary hypertension; an enlarged and sustained left ventricular impulse, indicating left ventricular dilatation and hypertrophy; a diminished first heart sound, suggesting impaired contractility; and $S_3$ gallops originating in the left and sometimes the right ventricle. Murmurs should be sought to exclude primary valvular disease; secondary mitral regurgitation and tricuspid regurgitation murmurs are common in patients with dilated ventricles.

**C. Laboratory Findings:** A blood count may reveal anemia, a cause of high-output failure and an exacerbating factor in other forms of cardiac dysfunction, or polycythemia. Biochemical studies may show renal insufficiency as a possible exacerbating factor. Renal function tests also determine whether cardiac failure has been associated with reduced renal blood flow (recognized by azotemia). Electrolytes may disclose heightened neuroendocrine activity with resultant hyponatremia. Particularly in older patients and in those with atrial fibrillation, thyroid function should be assessed to detect occult thyrotoxicosis. The additional diagnostic assessment of patients with dilated cardiomyopathy may include iron studies to exclude hemochromatosis.

**D. Electrocardiographic Findings:** Electrocardiography may indicate an underlying or secondary arrhythmia, myocardial infarction, or nonspecific changes that often include low voltage, intraventricular conduction defects, left ventricular hypertrophy, and nonspecific repolarization changes.

**E. Imaging:** Chest radiographs provide information about the size and shape of the cardiac silhouette. Cardiomegaly is an important finding. Evidence of pulmonary venous hypertension includes relative dilatation of the upper lobe veins, perivascular edema (haziness of vessel outlines), interstitial edema, and alveolar fluid. In acute heart failure, these findings correlate moderately well with pulmonary venous pressure, and when present in chronic failure they indicate elevated pressures. However, patients with chronic heart failure may show relatively normal pulmonary vasculature and have markedly elevated pressures. Pleural effusions are common and tend to be bilateral or right-sided.

Most patients with heart failure should undergo noninvasive cardiac testing because many of the symptoms are nonspecific and many studies have indicated that the clinical diagnosis of systolic myocardial dysfunction is often inaccurate. The primary confounding conditions are diastolic dysfunction of the heart with decreased relaxation and filling of the left ventricle (particularly in hypertension and in hypertrophic states) and pulmonary disease.

The most useful test is the echocardiogram. This will reveal the size and function of both ventricles and of the atria. It will also allow detection of pericardial effusion, valvular abnormalities, intracardiac shunts, and segmental wall motion abnormalities suggestive of old myocardial infarction as opposed to more generalized forms of dilated cardiomyopathy.

Radionuclide angiography measures left ventricular ejection fraction and permits analysis of regional wall motion. This test is especially useful when echocardiography is technically suboptimal, such as in patients with severe pulmonary disease.

**F. Cardiac Catheterization:** Cardiac catheterization is not necessary in most patients with heart failure. Clinical examination and noninvasive tests can determine left ventricular size and function well enough to confirm the diagnosis. Left heart catheterization is necessary when valvular disease must be excluded and when the presence and extent of coronary artery disease must be determined. The latter is particularly important when surgery to excise a left ventricular aneurysm is contemplated or when it is believed that left ventricular dysfunction may be partially reversible by revascularization. Right heart catheterization may be useful to select and monitor therapy in patients refractory to standard therapy.

## Treatment

**A. Correction of Reversible Causes:** While most cases of congestive heart failure are due to irreversible damage to the left ventricle, it is important to detect the minority of cases with reversible lesions and those who do not have impaired systolic performance as the underlying pathophysiologic mechanism. The major reversible causes have been discussed earlier and include thyrotoxicosis, valvular lesions, intracardiac shunts, high-output states, arrhythmias, and drug-induced myocardial depression. Reversible causes of diastolic dysfunction include pericardial disease and left ventricular hypertrophy due to hypertension. In addition, factors that may produce acute deterioration—alterations in medications, intercurrent illnesses, changes in activity and diet, and arrhythmias—should be managed appropriately. Once it is established that there is no reversible component to the heart failure and that the underlying pathophysiologic process is impaired contractility of the left ventricle, the measures outlined below are appropriate.

**B. Diet and Activity:** Sodium and fluid retention are an important part of the pathophysiology of heart failure. Patients should routinely be under moderate sodium restriction (1.5–2 g sodium). Patients with more severe heart failure, particularly those with hyponatremia, may benefit from fluid restriction, since they are unable to excrete a water load normally. More severe sodium restriction is usually difficult to achieve and unnecessary because of the availability of potent diuretic agents. Some patients with mild or moderate heart failure are symptomatic only with exertion. Alterations in life-style that moderate symptoms and reduce the need for additional medications are appropriate. In severe heart failure, restriction of activity, including bed rest if necessary, often facilitates temporary recompensation. With such limitations, these patients may exhibit profound diuresis even though fluid retention was previously refractory. There is no convincing evidence that prolonged bed rest alters the natural history of congestive heart failure. However, restricted activity decreases the work of the heart and provides symptomatic relief.

**C. Diuretic Therapy:** Diuretics are the most effective means of providing symptomatic relief to patients with moderate to severe congestive heart failure. When fluid retention is mild, thiazide diuretics or a similar type of agent (hydrochlorothiazide, 25–100 mg; metolazone, 2.5–10 mg; chlorothalidone, 25–100 mg; etc) may be sufficient. These agents block sodium reabsorption in the cortical diluting segment at the terminal portion of the loop of Henle and in the proximal portion of the distal convoluted tubule. The result is natriuresis and kaliuresis. These agents also have weak carbonic anhydrase inhibitor activity, which results in proximal tubule inhibition of sodium reabsorption.

The thiazides are generally ineffective when the glomerular filtration rate falls below 30 mL/min, a not infrequent occurrence in patients with severe heart failure. Metolazone maintains its efficacy down to a glomerular filtration rate of approximately 10 mL/min. Adverse reactions to the thiazide diuretics include hypokalemia and intravascular volume depletion with resulting prerenal azotemia, skin rashes, neutropenia and thrombocytopenia, hyperglycemia, hyperuricemia, and hepatic dysfunction.

Patients with more severe heart failure should be treated with one of the "loop diuretics." These include furosemide (40–320 mg daily in single or divided doses), bumetanide (1–8 mg daily in single or divided doses), and ethacrynic acid (25–200 mg daily in single or divided doses). These agents have a rapid onset and short duration of action. In acute situations or when gastrointestinal absorption is in doubt, they should be given intravenously. The loop diuretics inhibit chloride reabsorption in the ascending limb of the loop of Henle, which results in natriuresis, kaliuresis, and metabolic alkalosis.

They are active even in severe renal insufficiency. The major adverse reaction to the loop diuretics relates to their potency; patients often develop excessive diuresis with resultant intravascular volume depletion, prerenal azotemia, and hypotension. Hypokalemia, particularly with accompanying digitalis therapy, is a major problem. Thus, common side effects include skin rashes, gastrointestinal distress, and ototoxicity (the latter more common with ethacrynic acid).

The potassium-sparing agents spironolactone, triamterene, and amiloride are often useful in combination with the loop diuretics and thiazides. Triamterene and amiloride act on the distal tubule to reduce potassium secretion. Their diuretic potency is only mild and not adequate for most patients with heart failure, but they may minimize the hypokalemia induced by more potent agents. Side effects include hyperkalemia, gastrointestinal symptoms, and renal dysfunction. Spironolactone is a specific inhibitor of aldosterone, which is often increased in congestive heart failure. Its onset of action is slower than the other potassium-sparing agents, and its side effects include gynecomastia. Potassium supplements should be avoided when potassium-sparing drugs are used in order to prevent hyperkalemia.

Patients with refractory edema often respond to combinations of a loop diuretics and thiazidelike agents. Metolazone, because of its continued activity with renal insufficiency, is the most useful agent for such a combination. Extreme caution must be observed with this approach, since massive diuresis and electrolyte imbalances often occur; 2.5 mg of metolazone should be added to the previous dosage of loop diuretic. In many cases this is necessary only once or twice a week, but dosages up to 10 mg daily have been used in some patients.

**D. Digitalis Glycosides:** Although digitalis was once the mainstay of treatment in congestive heart failure, it is now used somewhat more judiciously. This change in attitude toward digitalis reflects a number of factors. Its efficacy in patients with normal sinus rhythm has been repeatedly questioned. Several retrospective analyses have indicated that patients with underlying coronary artery disease are at greater risk of death when treated with digitalis, but this remains to be confirmed. Finally, the availability of potent diuretics that more consistently relieve symptoms has made digitalis the second line of therapy in patients with normal sinus rhythm.

**1. Mechanism of action–**Digitalis has a number of effects on the heart. The positive inotropic effect is accomplished by increasing intracellular calcium and enhancing actin-myosin cross-bridge formation. Intracellular potassium rises as a result of inhibition of the sodium pump, with the resulting increase in intracellular sodium facilitating sodium-calcium exchange. Digitalis also inhibits sodium-potassium ATPase, but this may play a lesser role in its inotropic action.

The digitalis glycosides have a number of electrophysiologic effects that may be beneficial or deleterious in individual patients. These effects are primarily the result of its inhibition of sodium-potassium exchange and enhancement of the cardiac effects of the parasympathetic nervous system. Its primary therapeutic effect is inhibition of atrioventricular conduction. This will decrease the ventricular response to supraventricular arrhythmias, such as atrial fibrillation or flutter. In addition, digitalis decreases sinus node automaticity and may increase the automaticity of pacemakers in the His-Purkinje system and ventricles. The increased automaticity of latent pacemakers and increased excitability of ventricular myocardium underlie many of the arrhythmias associated with digitalis toxicity. Digitalis effect and toxicity are increased by reduced intracellular potassium concentrations and increased extracellular calcium concentrations.

**2. Pharmacokinetics–**Digitalis glycosides are available in a variety of preparations, but of these only digoxin (intravenously and orally) and digitoxin (primarily orally) are usually employed. The intravenous route is preferable if a rapid effect is desired; this is necessary chiefly in the setting of rapid supraventricular arrhythmias when early control of the ventricular rate is desirable. Intravenous digoxin begins to have an effect after 15–30 minutes, and the peak effect is seen after 1½–3 hours. The usual initial dose is 0.5 mg given slowly over 10–20 minutes to avoid an immediate hypertensive response. Additional 0.25-mg or 0.125-mg doses may be administered after 3 hours. A total dosage of 1–1.25 mg is usually required to achieve full digitalis effect, but smaller dosages are sometimes adequate in older patients and in individuals with small lean body masses.

Therapeutic concentrations may also be achieved by the oral route. If a full effect is desired fairly rapidly, 1–1.25 mg are administered in divided dosages over the initial 24 hours. An additional 0.5 mg is added during the second 24 hours. In most instances, maximum effect is accomplished more gradually by administering 0.5 mg daily for 3 days, followed by the usual maintenance dosage. Digoxin is excreted principally by the kidneys and has a half-life ranging from 36 to 48 hours. The oral maintenance dose may range from 0.125 to 0.5 mg daily, depending on renal function, body size, age, thyroid function, and gastrointestinal absorption (ordinarily, approximately 60–70% of the oral dose is absorbed). Unless the end point of therapy is control of the ventricular response in atrial fibrillation, it is worthwhile to measure serum digoxin levels after approximately 1 week of maintenance therapy; individual absorption rates and excretion rates may vary considerably. Digitoxin is less frequently used because of its long half-life (4–6 days), which will prolong the duration of toxicity if it occurs. Digitoxin is excreted by the liver, so blood levels may fluctuate less in patients with varying degrees of renal insufficiency.

A number of drugs have been found to affect digoxin absorption and blood levels. Cholestyramine, some broad spectrum oral antibiotics, antacids, and kaolin-pectin mixtures (eg, Kaopectate) may decrease plasma absorption of digoxin. Quinidine, verapamil, and amiodarone increase plasma levels of digoxin by reducing both the volume of distribution and the renal excretion of the agent. As noted previously, hypokalemia, hypercalcemia, and hypomagnesemia enhance the digitalis effect and potentiate its toxicity.

**3. Digitalis toxicity–**The therapeutic-to-toxic ratio of digitalis is quite narrow, and digitalis toxicity remains a common problem. Its frequency has diminished as a result of improved understanding of its pharmacology, a trend toward employing lower dosages, and the availability of measurements of digoxin levels. Digoxin toxicity is uncommon with serum levels below 1.4 ng/mL and is present in approximately 50% of patients with levels above 3 ng/mL. Symptoms of digitalis toxicity include anorexia, nausea and vomiting, headache, visual symptoms (changes in color perception, halos, and scotomas), and disorientation. These symptoms may precede cardiotoxic effects, and if any are present the agent should be stopped until a serum sample is drawn to determine whether they reflect glycoside toxicity.

Cardiac toxicity may take many forms, the most common being atrioventricular conduction disturbances, arrhythmias reflecting increased automaticity, and reentry arrhythmias. Arrhythmias due to digitalis toxicity include sinus node arrest, Mobitz type I second-degree atrioventricular block, ventricular premature beats or bigeminy, atrioventricular junctional tachycardia, paroxysmal supraventricular tachycardia with associated atrioventricular block, and ventricular tachycardia or fibrillation. When these arrhythmias are seen, digitalis toxicity should be suspected and the medication withheld. This, together with electrocardiographic monitoring, is adequate for many arrhythmias. Hypokalemia, if present, should be corrected, and tachyarrhythmias if present may respond after blood potassium levels increase to the high-normal range. Potassium administration may exacerbate atrioventricular blook, however. Ventricular tachycardia and very frequent ventricular premature beats should be treated with lidocaine or phenytoin. Type Ia and Ib agents are often less effective, and quinidine may exacerbate toxicity. Second-degree atrioventricular block usually does not require treatment, but complete heart block should be managed with atropine followed by temporary transvenous pacing. Electrical cardioversion should be avoided if possible, since digitalis toxicity may predispose to intractable ventricular fibrillation or cardiac standstill. If it cannot be avoided, patients should be pretreated with lidocaine and low energy levels should be employed initially.

Life-threatening episodes of digitalis toxicity or massive overdosages are characterized by severe hyperkalemia. They can be treated with digoxin-specific Fab antibody fragments. These are now commercially available (though expensive) and will rapidly reverse all manifestations of digitalis toxicity.

**E. Vasodilators:** Agents that dilate arteriolar smooth muscle and lower peripheral vascular resistance reduce left ventricular afterload. Medications that diminish venous tone and increase venous capacitance reduce the preload of both ventricles as their principal effect. Since, as noted earlier, most patients with moderate to severe heart failure have both elevated preload and reduced cardiac output, the maximum benefit of vasodilator therapy can be achieved by an agent or combination of agents with both actions. Many patients with heart failure have mitral or tricuspid regurgitation; agents that reduce resistance to left or right ventricular outflow tend to redirect regurgitant flow in a forward direction.

The intravenous vasodilating drugs and their dosages have been discussed in the section on complications in acute myocardial infarction.

**1. Nitrates–**Sodium nitroprusside is a potent dilator of both the arteriolar resistance and venous capacitance vessels, and it consistently increases cardiac output and reduces ventricular filling pressures. It is only occasionally employed in the management of chronic heart failure, usually during episodes of acute decompensation. In such cases it may produce excessive hypotension, and it has been combined with dopamine or dobutamine to produce optimal hemodynamic improvement. Intravenous nitroglycerin is less useful in chronic heart failure, since it produces only a limited increase in cardiac output.

Long-term, nonparenteral vasodilator therapy has become a standard approach in patients with congestive heart failure. A number of medications with vasodilating activity have been studied in this setting. The longest experience has been with the various nitrate preparations. Isosorbide dinitrate, 2.5–10 mg sublingually every 2–3 hours or 20–80 mg orally every 4–6 hours, has proved effective in several small studies. Nitroglycerin ointment, 12.5–50 mg (1–4 in) every 4–6 hours, appears to be equally effective although somewhat inconvenient for long-term therapy. The optimal nitrate regimen probably consists of oral isosorbide dinitrate during the daytime and nitroglycerin applied overnight, since the latter has a longer duration of action. The nitrates are moderately effective in relieving shortness of breath, especially in patients with mild to moderate symptoms, but less successful—probably because they have little effect on cardiac output—in advanced heart failure. Nitrate therapy is generally well tolerated, but headaches and hypotension may limit the dose of all agents. The development of tolerance to chronic nitrate therapy is now generally accepted. This is minimized by intermittent therapy but probably develops to some extent in most patients receiving these agents. Transdermal nitroglycerin patches have no sustained effect in patients with heart failure and should not be employed for this indication.

**2. Hydralazine**–Oral hydralazine is a potent arteriolar dilator and markedly increases cardiac output in patients with congestive heart failure. However, as a single agent, it has not been shown to improve symptoms or exercise tolerance during chronic treatment. The combination of nitrates and oral hydralazine does appear to be effective, and this combination may improve survival in patients with mild to moderate symptoms.

Hydralazine therapy is frequently limited by side effects. Approximately 30% of patients are unable to tolerate the relatively high doses required to produce hemodynamic improvement in heart failure (100–400 mg daily in divided doses). The major side effect is gastrointestinal distress, but headaches, tachycardia, hypotension, and the drug-induced lupus syndrome are also relatively common.

**3. Prazosin**–Oral prazosin, a postsynaptic alpha-adrenergic blocking agent, was previously thought to be beneficial in patients with heart failure, but long-term benefits have not been demonstrated.

**4. Angiotensin converting enzyme (ACE) inhibitors**–Captopril and enalapril are the most effective vasodilators for congestive heart failure. These agents block the renin-angiotensin-aldosterone system. They produce vasodilation by blocking angiotensin II-induced vasoconstriction, but they also inhibit the degradation of bradykinin, increase the production of vasodilating prostaglandins, and indirectly inhibit the adrenergic nervous system. They also increase sodium excretion by inhibiting aldosterone production and improve the ability of the kidneys to excrete free water by unknown mechanisms. Although the other vasodilators tend to stimulate the renin-angiotensin system and often lose part of their effect due to the resulting fluid retention, tolerance to the ACE inhibitors is uncommon.

Acute hemodynamic studies show that both captopril and enalapril reduce left ventricular filling pressure and right atrial pressure and moderately increase cardiac output. During long-term follow-up, these hemodynamic benefits are maintained or increased. ACE inhibitors lessen symptoms and increase exercise

tolerance. They also correct the electrolyte abnormalities that characterize severe heart failure, such as hyponatremia and diuretic-induced hypokalemia, which may reduce the propensity to arrhythmias. Survival may be improved by ACE inhibitor therapy in patients with severe heart failure.

Because the ACE inhibitors may produce significant hypotension in some patients with congestive heart failure, particularly after the initial doses, they must be started with caution. Hypotension is most prominent in patients with hyponatremia (an indicator of activation of the renin-angiotensin system) and prerenal azotemia. Before therapy with the ACE inhibitors is started, other vasodilators should be discontinued and the dosages of diuretics should be reduced or the drugs withheld for 24 hours. Captopril is the preferred agent for beginning ACE inhibitor therapy because of its predictable onset and short duration of action (peak effect in 30–90 minutes). Treatment should be started with a low dose: either 12.5 mg or, in patients with hyponatremia or preexisting low blood pressure, 6.25 mg. The blood pressure should be monitored for the first 2–3 hours after dosing; if symptomatic or clinically significant hypotension does not occur, the patient may be sent home on a dosage of 12.5 mg 3 times daily. In patients with borderline blood pressure, renal function should be checked during the first week. The chronically effective dose of captopril appears to be 25 to 50 mg 3 times daily, although some patients will not tolerate this high a dose.

Enalapril is less convenient for initiating ACE inhibitor therapy in heart failure because its onset of action may be delayed beyond the time of convenient observation, and hypotension, if it occurs, may be prolonged. Because enalapril must be deesterified in the liver, which may be affected by passive congestion, its pharmacokinetics are less predictable in heart failure. However, maintenance therapy with enalapril in patients who do not develop hypotension has been effective. The chronic dosage of enalapril ranges from 2.5 to 20 mg twice daily.

The major limitation to ACE inhibitor therapy in heart failure is hypotension and renal insufficiency due to inadequate renal perfusion pressures. Other side effects such as skin rashes, taste alterations, cough, neutropenia, and proteinuria are less troublesome or very uncommon. The ACE inhibitors tend to increase serum potassium concentrations, and hyperkalemia may occur, particularly since many patients are also receiving potassium supplements. Potassium-sparing agents should be withdrawn before ACE inhibitor therapy is started; and although potassium supplements may be required in individuals receiving diuretics and digitalis, their dosage should be decreased and subsequently adjusted as needed.

Vasodilator therapy was at one time reserved for patients not helped by digitalis and diuretics, but many experts now consider them a second line of therapy after diuretics. Studies are under way to determine whether vasodilator therapy, particularly with the

ACE inhibitors, is indicated with patients with mild symptoms or those with asymptomatic left ventricular dysfunction.

**F. Newer Positive Inotropic Agents:** Digoxin is the only available oral inotropic agent at this time in the United States. However, a number of agents that increase myocardial contracility in experimental preparations are under investigation. These include beta-adrenergic agonists, dopaminergic agents, and a group of nondigitalis, noncatecholamine agents that increase myocardial contractility by inhibiting myocardial phosphodiesterase. One of the latter class, amrinone, has been approved for intravenous use; another, milrinone, shows promise. These drugs have been discussed previously.

The value of positive inotropic agents for chronic treatment is in doubt.

**G. Beta-Blocker Therapy:** A number of investigators have suggested that beta-blockers in very low dosages may produce symptomatic improvement in patients with chronic congestive heart failure. Metoprolol may be started at extremely low doses (often as low as 2.5 or 5 mg twice daily). Obviously, this approach carries the risk of worsening heart failure; however, in patients with dilated cardiomyopathy of nonischemic origin with persistent tachycardia (> 100 beats/min), some data suggest a beneficial effect. The efficiency and safety of beta-blockers is now under investigation in multicenter trials.

**H. Anticoagulation:** Patients with severe left ventricular failure are prone to development of systemic arterial emboli, particularly when they are in atrial fibrillation. While these may be catastrophic, the routine use of anticoagulants is controversial, since these patients are taking multiple medications that may interfere with optimal regulation of anticoagulation and have short life expectancies. Most experts prescribe anticoagulants to patients who have had embolic episodes, those with large atria, and those with atrial fibrillation. Some also anticoagulate patients with dilated cardiomyopathy in normal sinus rhythm.

## Prognosis

Despite advances in treatment of patients with congestive heart failure, their prognosis remains poor (upward of 60% 1-year mortality rate). Poorer prognosis is associated with severe left ventricular dysfunction (ejection fractions < 20%), severe symptoms and limitation of exercise capacity (maximal oxygen consumption < 10 mL/kg/min), and secondary renal insufficiency, hyponatremia, and elevated plasma catecholamine levels. About 40–50% of patients with heart failure die suddenly, presumably due to ventricular arrhythmias. Ambulatory electrocardiographic monitoring shows that patients with moderate to severe heart failure have frequent ventricular premature beats and high-grade ventricular ectopy. However, the prevalence of these arrhythmias is so high that, again, they cannot be used to predict which individuals are at risk of sudden death. The question when to institute antiarrhythmic therapy is discussed in a separate section below.

Bigger, JT Jr: Why patients with congestive heart failure die: Arrhythmias and sudden cardiac death. *Circulation* 1987;**75** (**Suppl 5**):IV-28.

Cohn JN et al: Effect of vasodilator therapy on mortality in chronic congestive heart failure. Results of a Veterans Administration Cooperative Study. *N Engl J Med* 1986;**314:** 1547.

Colucci WS, Wright RF, Braunwald E: New positive inotropic agents in the treatment of congestive heart failure: Mechanisms of action and recent clinical developments. (2 Parts.) *N Engl J Med* 1986;**314:**290, 349.

Consensus Trial Study Group: Effects of enalapril on mortality in severe congestive heart failure: Results of the Cooperative North Scandinavian Enalapril Survival Study (CONSENSUS). *N Engl J Med* 1987;**316:**1429.

Gheorghiade M et al: Hemodynamic effects of intravenous digoxin in patients with severe heart failure initially treated with diuretics and vasodilators. *J Am Coll Cardiol* 1987; **9:**849.

Massie BM, Conway M: Survival of patients with congestive heart failure: Past, present, and future prospects. *Circulation* 1987;**75** (**Suppl 5**):IV-11.

Packer M (editor): Physiologic determinants of survival in congestive heart failure. *Circulation* 1987;**75** (**Suppl 5**):IV-1. [Entire issue.]

Parmley WW: Medical treatment of congestive heart failure: Where are we now? *Circulation* 1987;**75** (**Suppl 5**):IV-4.

## Cardiac Transplantation

Because of the poor prognosis in patients with advanced heart failure, cardiac transplantation has become increasingly popular. Since the advent of cyclosporine immunosuppressive therapy, the survival of patients after cardiac transplantation has increased considerably. Many centers now have 1-year survival rates exceeding 80–90%, and 5-year survival rates are likely to be in the 50–70% range. Clearly, cardiac transplantation is effective in selected individuals, but the high cost and limited number of donor organs require careful patient selection.

Goodwin JF: Cardiac transplantation. *Circulation* 1986;**74:**913.

## SPECIAL PROBLEMS IN THE MANAGEMENT OF CONGESTIVE HEART FAILURE

## 1. ACUTE PULMONARY EDEMA

Cardiogenic pulmonary edema occurs when pulmonary venous pressure rises to a point where the resulting transudation of fluid cannot be compensated for by reabsorption of fluid or lymphatic drainage. The most common causes of cardiogenic pulmonary edema are acute myocardial infarction, acute volume overload of the left ventricle (valvular regurgitation or ventricular septal defect), and mitral stenosis.

## Clinical Findings

Acute pulmonary edema presents with a characteristic clinical picture of severe dyspnea (associated with profound air hunger or a feeling of drowning and attendant anxiety), the production of pink, frothy sputum, and diaphoresis and cyanosis. Examination of the lungs reveals rales in all lung fields or generalized wheezing and rhonchi. Pulmonary edema may appear suddenly in the setting of chronic heart failure or may be the first manifestation of cardiac disease, usually acute myocardial infarction, which may be painful or silent.

The chest radiograph reveals signs of pulmonary vascular redistribution, blurriness of vascular outlines, increased interstitial markings, and, characteristically, the butterfly pattern of alveolar edema. The heart may be enlarged or normal in size depending on whether heart failure was previously present. An acute assessment of cardiac function by echocardiography or right heart catheterization is helpful in determining the cause. In cardiogenic pulmonary edema, PCWP is universally elevated, usually over 25 mm Hg. Cardiac output may be normal or depressed. In noncardiogenic pulmonary edema, the acute respiratory distress syndrome, or severe pulmonary disease masquerading as pulmonary edema, PCWP may be normal or even low.

## Treatment

Oxygen should be delivered by mask to obtain an arterial $PO_2$ greater than 60 mm Hg. If respiratory distress is severe, endotracheal intubation and mechanical ventilation may be necessary.

Morphine sulfate is highly effective in pulmonary edema. The initial dosage should be 4–8 mg intravenously (subcutaneous administration is effective in milder cases), and this may be repeated after 2–4 hours. Morphine increases venous capitance, lowering left atrial pressure, and relieves anxiety, which can reduce the efficiency of ventilation. However, morphine may lead to $CO_2$ retention and reduce the ventilatory drive, thus necessitating artificial ventilation. Morphine should be avoided in patients with narcotic-induced pulmonary edema, who may improve with narcotic antagonists, and in those with neurogenic pulmonary edema.

Intravenous diuretic therapy (furosemide, 40 mg, or bumetanide, 1 mg—or higher doses if the patient has been receiving chronic diuretic therapy) is usually indicated even if the patient has not exhibited prior fluid retention. These agents produce immediate venodilation even prior to the onset of diuresis. Other approaches to therapy include further measures to reduce left ventricular preload. This may be accomplished by the administration of sublingual or intravenous nitrates, the use of rotating tourniquets to decrease venous return from the extremities, and, in otherwise refractory cases, phlebotomy of approximately 500 mL of blood. Intravenous aminophylline may relieve the associated bronchospasm. The usual dose is 5 mg/kg intravenously over approximately

10 minutes, followed by a constant infusion of approximately 1 mg/kg/h. Aminophylline may exacerbate tachycardia or tachyarrhythmias, however. Particularly in patients with elevated arterial pressures, vasodilators such as intravenous nitroprusside may be worthwhile. In patients with low-output states, particularly when hypotension is present, positive inotropic agents are indicated. These approaches to treatment have been discussed previously.

## 2. ARRHYTHMIAS IN PATIENTS WITH HEART FAILURE

Patients with moderate to severe heart failure have a high incidence of both symptomatic and asymptomatic arrhythmias. Although fewer than 10% of patients have syncope or presyncope resulting from ventricular tachycardia and a smaller number have survived cardiac arrest, ambulatory monitoring reveals that upward of 70% of patients have asymptomatic episodes of nonsustained ventricular tachycardia. As noted previously, these arrhythmias indicate a poor prognosis, but it is not clear that they are an important independent predictor of mortality rates over and above the severity of left ventricular dysfunction or that antiarrhythmic therapy improves prognosis.

Patients with symptomatic ventricular arrhythmias should be treated vigorously as outlined previously. Whether patients with asymptomatic nonsustained ventricular tachycardia warrant therapy remains controversial, largely because such treatment is not without risk. Most effective antiarrhythmic agents may depress left ventricular function or may themselves worsen the arrhythmia. While most experts will not initiate treatment for frequent ventricular premature beats, they will attempt to suppress frequent episodes of nonsustained ventricular tachycardia. Usually the first approach is with a type Ia agent (procainamide or quinidine; disopyramide should be avoided because of its negative inotropic effect). The type Ib agents have proved less effective; the type of Ic agents may be effective but are more likely to depress left ventricular function. Amiodarone is perhaps the most effective agent, but because of its toxicity it should probably be reserved for individuals with symptomatic arrhythmias. A definitive trial to determine the value of antiarrhythmec therapy in patients with heart failure and asymptomatic venticular arrhythmias is sorely needed.

## DISEASES OF THE PERICARDIUM

### ACUTE PERICARDITIS
### (For Pericardial Effusion, see p 255)

### Essentials of Diagnosis

- Pleuritic, substernal, or precordial pain referred to the left neck, shoulder, or back.

- Pericardial friction rub.
- Electrocardiography: Early, concordant ST elevation; late, general symmetric T wave inversion without Q waves or reciprocal changes except in aVR.

## General Considerations

Infectious pericarditis may be caused by viruses, pyogenic bacteria (pneumococcus, hemolytic *Streptococcus, Staphylococcus aureus,* meningococcus, gonococcus), *Mycobacterium tuberculosis,* and *Brucella.* Immune pericarditis is seen with systemic lupus erythematosus, acute rheumatic fever, rheumatoid arthritis, and serum sickness. A miscellaneous group includes pericarditis that occurs after pericardiotomy, myocardial infarction, or trauma; pericarditis associated with uremia, metastatic tumors, and the lymphomas (or to radiation therapy); and hemorrhagic pericarditis due to aortic dissection. Varying degrees of myocarditis accompany pericarditis and are responsible for the electrocardiographic changes in ST-T contours.

## Clinical Findings

**A. Symptoms and Signs:** Acute viral pericarditis is more common in men age 20–50 years and often follows an upper respiratory infection. The onset of pain is usually sudden; it is precordial or substernal, pleuritic or steady (or both), and radiates to the left neck, shoulder, back, or epigastrium. It is worse in the supine position and may be accentuated by swallowing. Fever of 37.8–39.4 °C (100–103 °F) is always present in infectious pericarditis. Tachycardia and a pericardial or pleuropericardial friction rub are present.

Pericardial biopsy through a subxiphoid incision may be particularly useful in toxic patients in whom mycobacterial or other bacterial pericarditis is suspected.

**B. Laboratory Findings:** Leukocytosis of 10,000–20,000/ μL is usually present in acute viral pericarditis; leukopenia may be noted in pericarditis associated with disseminated lupus erthematosus.

**C. Imaging:** An enlarged cardiac silhouette, pneumonitis, and pleural effusion may be seen on chest radiographs. Echocardiography is most valuable in the diagnosis of pericardial effusion. The fluid occupies an echo-free space separating the anterior wall of the right ventricle from the chest and the posterior wall of the left ventricle from the lung. The procedure may differentiate between cardiac dilatation and pericardial effusion, especially in the presence of suspected cardiac tamponade.

**D. Electrocardiography:** Initial changes consist only of ST-T segment elevation in all leads, with preservation of normal upward concavity. Return to the baseline in a few days is followed by T wave inversion. Reciprocal changes are absent except in aVR, and Q waves do not appear.

## Differential Diagnosis

**A. Acute Myocardial Infarction:** Acute viral pericarditis usually follows a respiratory infection, occurs in the age group from 20 to 50 years, and characteristically presents with pleuritic pain. Fever, friction rub, leukocytosis, and an elevated sedimentation rate are found at the onset rather than 24–72 hours later. Electrocardiographic changes are usually distinctive. SGOT (AST), CK and CPK, and LDH are rarely elevated even in severe pericarditis.

**B. Pleurisy Due to Other Causes:** Pericardial friction rub is differentiated from pleural friction rub by its persistence upon breath-holding. Electrocardiographic changes may be diagnostic of pericarditis in the absence of a rub.

**C. Confusion of Rub With Murmurs:** Pericardial friction rubs are differentiated by their presence with the breath held, changing character, lack of association with the usual areas of murmurs, high-pitched or "scratchy" quality, asynchrony with heart sounds, and often triple character.

## Complications

Pericardial effusion is the most noteworthy complication, but if myocarditis is present there may be cardiac dilatation as well. Arrhythmias, especially atrial fibrillation, are frequent. The pericarditis may be recurrent for weeks or months. Pericardial constriction may complicate pericarditis due to any cause.

## Treatment

Analgesics as necessary are given for relief of pain. Salicylates and the corticosteroids are useful in rheumatic pericarditis. In severe acute myocarditis or if cardiac failure develops rapidly, corticosteroids combined with immunosuppressive drugs may be tried, but results have been inconclusive. If the pericarditis is of bacterial cause, specific antimicrobials are administered.

## Prognosis

The prognosis of viral pericarditis is usually excellent. Recovery occurs in 2 weeks or 3 months; recurrences, however, are relatively common. Residual pericardial thickening or persistent electrocardiographic abnormalities are rare. Constrictive pericarditis has been reported following viral pericarditis, but this is rare. Similarly, dilated cardiomyopathy has been described, but it is also rare following acute infection. The promptness and adequacy of antibiotic and surgical treatment determine the outcome in tuberculous and purulent pericarditis. Other manifestations of disseminated lupus erythematosus may become apparent after an attack of presumed "viral" pericarditis. In the miscellaneous group, the basic disorder determines the prognosis.

Lee DC et al: Heart failure in outpatients: A randomized trial of digoxin versus placebo. *N Engl J Med* 1983;**306:**699.

Permanyer-Miralda G, Sagrista-Sauleda J, Soler-Soler J: Primary acute pericardial disease: A prospective series of 231 consecutive patients. *Am J Cardiol* 1985;**56**:623.

# PERICARDIAL EFFUSION

The speed of accumulation of a pericardial effusion determines the physiologic importance of the effusion. Massive pericardial effusions (> 1000 mL) that accumulate slowly may produce no symptoms. However, hemorrhage into the pericardium or sudden accumulation of relatively small effusions (about 200 mL) may raise the intrapericardial pressure to the point of cardiac tamponade, in which the fluid limits venous inflow and diastolic filling of the heart. In tamponade, the cardiac output falls, the pulse pressure narrows, and tachycardia and elevation of the central venous pressure appear as the compensatory mechanisms. Shock and death may result.

## Clinical Findings

**A. Symptoms and Signs:** Pain is often absent but may be present, as in acute pericarditis, or may be described as a dull, diffuse, oppressive precordial or substernal distress. Dyspnea and cough cause the patient to sit up and lean forward for relief. Dysphagia is prominent. Fever and other symptoms depend upon the primary disease (eg, septicemia, empyema, cancer).

The area of "cardiac" dullness is enlarged, and the apex beat is often not palpable or is well within the lateral border of dullness. Friction rub may persist despite a large effusion. In tamponade, the clinical findings include dyspnea, sinus tachycardia, falling blood pressure, narrow pulse pressure, distended neck veins (increased with inspiration), decrease in blood pressure ($\geq$ 10 mm Hg) with inspiration (paradoxic pulse) owing to decreased dimensions of the left ventricular cavity, and decreased stroke output. This is an exaggerated form of the normal respiratory response and can be demonstrated by echocardiography. Paradoxic pulse is absent when pericardial effusion complicates atrial septal defect. Liver enlargement, ascites, and leg edema depend upon the degree and duration of tamponade. Acute cardiac tamponade produces shock.

**B. Laboratory Findings:** The cause of acute effusion is determined by bacteriologic and cytologic study of aspirated fluid and by the presence of primary disease elsewhere. The cause of chronic effusion is determined by pericardial biopsy. Leukocytosis and a rapid sedimentation rate are present when the effusion is infectious or inflammatory. In myxedema, pericardial effusion and prolongation of the circulation time are present without tamponade.

**C. Imaging:** On radiographs, a rapidly enlarging "cardiac" silhouette with sharply defined margins, an acute right cardiophrenic angle, clear lung fields, and pleural effusion are common.

Echocardiography is the best and simplest method of diagnosis. It also demonstrates diastolic compression of the right ventricle, a sensitive and specific sign.

**D. Electrocardiographic Findings:** The T waves are low, flat, diphasic, or inverted in all leads; the QRS voltage is uniformly low. Electrical alternans may be present.

## Differential Diagnosis

Cardiac dilatation with congestive heart failure may be difficult to differentiate from pericardial effusion if pleural effusion is also present. Pulmonary crackles, gallop rhythm, and raised jugular venous pressure may help in assessing cardiac failure. Echocardiography is definitive in the diagnosis of pericardial effusion. In a patient with "heart failure," the absence of significant murmurs, arrhythmias, gallop sounds, and hypertension should suggest pericardial effusion.

## Treatment

**A. Emergency Treatment (Paracentesis):** The indications for pericardial paracentesis are the symptoms and signs of cardiac tamponade. If pericardial fluid increases rapidly, the hemodynamic compromise is typical. Under these circumstances, removal of pericardial fluid may be lifesaving; fluid should be removed slowly to avoid cardiac dilatation or sudden reflex changes in rate and rhythm. Fluid should be removed in the catheterization laboratory, with resuscitation equipment available. It is best to totally remove the pericardial fluid with catheter drainage. If the patient has carcinomatous effusion, consideration should be given to inserting sclerosing agents such as tetracycline or perhaps antineoplastic agents such as thiotepa or fluorouracil after the fluid has been removed to prevent recurrence of the effusion. If fluid reaccumulates, partial pericardiectomy may be necessary.

**B. Specific Measures:**

**1. Tuberculous pericarditis**–Antituberculosis chemotherapy is instituted. If signs of pericardial effusion do not rapidly subside and are still obvious in 1 month, surgical decortication of the pericardium should be considered in order to prevent chronic constrictive pericarditis.

**2. Hydropericardium due to heart failure**–Treatment of congestive failure is usually sufficient.

**3. Hemopericardium due to rupture of adjacent structures**–This is invariably an indication for pericardiocentesis and for surgical treatment of the cause (eg, aortic dissection).

**4. Infection**–Infection is treated with appropriate chemotherapeutic agents and paracentesis is performed as needed. Chemotherapeutic agents are administered systemically, aimed at anticipated organisms or dictated by antimicrobial sensitivities once isolated. If the patient is not responding to therapy, the fluid may be encapsulated, and surgical drainage via pericardiotomy may be necessary.

**5. Uremic pericarditis**–Pericardial Effusion is Associated With Uremia With Aggressive Dialysis Therapy. Severe Tamponade May Require Pericardiotomy.

**6. Myxedema**–Replacement of thyroid hormone is invariably successful, and pericardiocentesis is seldom necessary.

**7. Autoimmune disorders**–Therapy for the specific disorders is adequate; generally, pericardial effusions are small and hemodynamically insignificant.

**8. Others**–Sarcoidosis is treated with corticosteroids. Lymphoma and tumors may be treated with radiotherapy or chemotherapy; it should be remembered that irradiation itself may cause pericarditis, usually several months after therapy.

### Prognosis

Tuberculous pericarditis causes chronic constrictive pericarditis in many patients. The mortality rate is low with early and adequate treatment; the effect of early treatment on the incidence of constrictive pericarditis is not known. Acute benign pericarditis is only rarely fatal. Purulent pericarditis is usually associated with a systemic infection; though patients are seriously ill, they may respond satisfactorily to antibiotics and pericardial drainage when necessary.

Cogswell TL et al: Effects of intravascular volume state on the value of pulsus paradoxus and right ventricular diastolic collapse in predicting cardiac tamponade. *Circulation* 1986;**72:**1076.

Kralstein J, Frishman W: Malignant pericardial diseases: Diagnosis and treatment. *Am Heart J* 1987;**113:**785.

Singh S et al: Usefulness of right ventricular diastolic collapse in diagnosing cardiac tamponade and comparison to pulsus paradoxus. *Am J Cardiol* 1986;**57:**652.

## CHRONIC CONSTRICTIVE PERICARDITIS

### Essentials of Diagnosis

- Markedly elevated venous pressure.
- Slight to moderate cardiac enlargement and quiet heart action.
- Paradoxic pulse.
- Ascites out of proportion to degree of ankle edema.

### General Considerations

In the past, tuberculosis was the most common cause of constriction of the pericardium, and this is still true in areas of the world where tuberculosis remains a public health problem. Now, constriction can occur following viral pericarditis but is uncommon. Radiation therapy of the mediastinum (eg, Hodgkin's disease), trauma, and other malignant involvement of the pericardium may lead to subacute constriction, which with time will become fibrous and perhaps calcified. In many cases the cause is not determined, perhaps because the inciting incident occurred years previously.

Encasement of the myocardium by an adherent, dense fibrous pericardium may be asymptomatic or may prevent ventricular expansion during diastole. If this happens, the stroke volume is low and fixed, and cardiac output can be increased only by tachycardia. Venous pressure rises as in congestive heart failure; together with renal retention of sodium and water, this suggests right heart failure.

### Clinical Findings

**A. Symptoms and Signs:** The principal symptoms are slowly progressive dyspnea, fatigue, and weakness on exertion; abdominal distention; and leg edema. Examination shows markedly distended neck veins, with a characteristic rapid y descent. The precordium is quiet in the presence of tachycardia; the heart sounds are faint and there may be a palpable and audible pericardial knock in early diastole. The pulse pressure is low, and paradoxic pulse is often present. Hepatosplenomegaly, ascites, and edema of both legs are common. Atrial fibrillation is frequently present.

**B. Laboratory Findings:** None are diagnostic.

**C. Imaging:** The heart is either normal in size or moderately enlarged as shown on radiographs. Its shape is not consistent with valvular or hypertensive heart disease. Lung fields are clear. Pericardial calcification is common but is not diagnostic of constrictive pericarditis.

The abrupt cessation of ventricular filling and decreased excursion of the left ventricular endocardium occurring in chronic constrictive pericarditis can be seen on 2-dimensional echocardiography and contrasts with the ventricular dilatation and decreased ejection rate associated with restrictive cardiomyopathy, which is the major disease to be considered in the differential diagnosis. Thickening of the pericardium may be seen.

CT scans of the chest may show pericardial thickening or fluid and appear to be more sensitive for this purpose than echocardiography. Demonstration of a thickened pericardium in patients with constriction can thus differentiate patients with restrictive cardiomyopathy and a normal pericardium.

**D. Electrocardiographic Findings:** T waves are flat or inverted; low voltage of QRS complexes is variable. Atrial fibrillation is common.

### Differential Diagnosis

Marked venous engorgement in the neck without systolic pulsation, slight to moderate cardiac enlargement, absence of significant murmurs or hypertension, paradoxic pulse, and electrocardiographic changes distinguish chronic constrictive pericarditis from congestive heart failure. Restrictive cardiomyopathy, as seen in diabetes or cardiac amyloidosis, may be identical clinically. In these instances, CT scans of the chest may be diagnostic by demonstrating a thickened pericardium. Cirrhosis of the liver, mediastinal tumor, nephrosis, and obstruction of the vena cava must also be considered. Diagnosis may be difficult and may require cardiac catheterization.

## Complications

Thrombophlebitis of the leg veins may occur secondary to elevated venous pressure, venous stasis, and inactivity.

## Treatment

Diuresis may be due to further reduction of an already precarious preload. Digitalis is of no value unless the patient has atrial fibrillation.

Surgical removal of the constricting pericardium can frequently restore a patient to normal health. It is the only method offering possible cure. The surgical mortality rate is 3–5%.

## Prognosis

Most patients with constrictive pericarditis due to any cause have increasing disability because of ascites and edema and die of mechanical "heart failure." A few patients show no progression of symptoms or signs for years.

Cameron J et al: The etiologic spectrum of constrictive pericarditis. *Am Heart J* 1987;**113**:354.

Seifert FC et al: Surgical treatment of constrictive pericarditis: Analysis of outcome and diagnostic error. *Circulation* 1986;**72(Suppl II)**:264.

# DISEASES OF THE MYOCARDIUM

## PRIMARY PULMONARY HYPERTENSION

Primary pulmonary hypertension is defined as pulmonary hypertension and raised pulmonary vascular resistance in the absence of any other disease of the lungs or heart. Pathologically, it is characterized by diffuse narrowing of the pulmonary arterioles without obvious reason. Late in the course of the disease, thrombi may develop in the pulmonary arterioles, and there may be evidence of superimposed pulmonary embolism as a result of chronic low-output failure. Primary pulmonary hypertension must be distinguished from chronic pulmonary heart disease, recurrent pulmonary emboli, mitral stenosis, and other conditions.

The clinical picture is similar to that of pulmonary hypertension from any other cause. Patients—often young women—present with evidence of right heart failure that is usually progressive, leading to death in 2–8 years. Patients have the manifestations of low cardiac output, with weakness and fatigue, as well as edema and ascites as right heart failure advances. Peripheral cyanosis is present, and syncope on effort may occur.

Exclusion of secondary causes by echocardiography and lung scanning—and if necessary, pulmonary angiography—is essential. Vasodilator drugs are the mainstay of medical treatment and are most effective when secondary vasoconstriction and not structural obstruction is the cause of pulmonary hypertension. Virtually all vasodilators have been tried with temporary but rarely durable benefit.

The prognosis in primary pulmonary hypertension is poor. Although most patients have a downhill course within a few years, some patients survive for 5 to 6 years. Heart-lung transplantation is being employed more frequently now with encouraging successes, resulting primarily from the availability of cyclosporine to decrease rejection.

Packer M: Vasodilator therapy for primary pulmonary hypertension. *Ann Intern Med* 1985;**103**:258.

## PULMONARY HEART DISEASE (Cor Pulmonale)

### Essentials of Diagnosis

- Symptoms and signs of chronic bronchitis and pulmonary emphysema.
- No significant murmurs or hypertension; neck vein distention, right ventricular lift, edema prominent.
- Electrocardiography: Tall, peaked P waves; right axis deviation; and right ventricular hypertrophy.
- Chest radiograph: Enlarged right ventricle and pulmonary artery.

### General Considerations

The term "cor pulmonale" denotes right ventricular hypertrophy and eventual failure resulting from pulmonary disease. Its clinical features depend upon both the primary disease and its effects on the heart.

Cor pulmonale is most commonly caused by chronic obstructive pulmonary emphysema. Rare causes include pneumoconiosis, pulmonary fibrosis or schistosomiasis, kyphoscoliosis, primary pulmonary hypertension, repeated episodes of subclinical or clinical pulmonary embolization, Pickwickian syndrome, and obliterative pulmonary capillary or lymphangitic infiltration from metastatic carcinoma. Hypoxia is the common denominator of these conditions which ultimately lead to cor pulmonale.

### Clinical Findings

**A. Symptoms and Signs:** The predominant symptoms of compensated cor pulmonale are chronic productive cough, exertional dyspnea, wheezing respirations, easy fatigability, and weakness. When the pulmonary disease causes right ventricular failure, these symptoms may be intensified. Dependent edema and right upper quadrant pain may also appear. The signs of cor pulmonale include cyanosis, clubbing, distended neck veins, right ventricular heave or gallop (or both), prominent lower sternal or epigastric pulsations, an enlarged and tender liver, and dependent edema.

**B. Laboratory Findings:** Polycythemia is often present in cor pulmonale secondary to emphysema. The arterial oxygen saturation is below 85%; $P_{CO_2}$

is often elevated. Venous pressure is significantly elevated in right ventricular failure. Pulmonary function studies define the nature of the pulmonary disease.

**C. Imaging:** The chest radiograph discloses the presence or absence of parenchymal disease and a prominent or enlarged right ventricle, pulmonary conus, and artery.

CT and MRI scans may demonstrate central pulmonary artery thrombi noninvasively in the uncommon instances where this process causes cor pulmonale. In chronic pulmonary hypertension, echocardiography may show right ventricular enlargement and hypertrophy.

**D. Electrocardiographic Findings:** The ECG may show right axis deviation and peaked P waves. Deep S waves are present in lead $V_6$. Left axis deviation and low voltage may be noted in patients with pulmonary emphysema. Frank right ventricular hypertrophy is uncommon except in "primary pulmonary hypertension." The ECG often mimics myocardial infarction; Q waves may be present in leads II, III, and aVF because of the vertically placed heart, but they are rarely deep or wide, as in inferior myocardial infarction. Arrhythmias are frequent and nonspecific.

**E. Other Studies:** Pulmonary function studies may demonstrate increased airway resistance in chronic bronchitis and emphysema (see section on pulmonary disease). Perfusion pulmonary scans are rarely of value, but, if negative, they exclude pulmonary emboli, an occasional cause of cor pulmonale. Pulmonary angiography is the most specific method of diagnosis of pulmonary emboli, but it carries increased risk when performed in patients with pulmonary hypertension.

## Differential Diagnosis

In its early stages, cor pulmonale can be diagnosed on the basis of radiologic, echocardiographic, or electrocardiographic evidence. Catheterization of the right heart will establish a definitive diagnosis but is usually performed to exclude left-sided heart failure. Differential diagnostic considerations relate chiefly to the specific pulmonary disease that has produced right ventricular failure (see above).

## Treatment

The details of the treatment of chronic pulmonary disease (chronic respiratory failure) are discussed in Chapter 7. Otherwise, therapy is directed at the pulmonary process responsible for right heart failure. Oxygen, salt and fluid restriction, and diuretics are mainstays; digitalis has no place in right heart failure unless atrial fibrillation is present.

## Prognosis

Compensated cor pulmonale has the same outlook as the underlying pulmonary disease. Once congestive signs appear, the average life expectancy is 2–5 years, but survival is significantly longer when uncomplicated emphysema is the cause. Left ventricular failure secondary to coronary artery disease or hypertension

may develop and shorten life expectancy accordingly; it has also been established that right heart failure may lead to left-sided dysfunction absent these conditions, but the mechanisms are uncertain.

## SYPHILITIC CARDIOVASCULAR DISEASE (See also Chapter 24)

### Essentials of Diagnosis

- Linear calcification or localized dilatation of the ascending aorta on radiographs.
- Aortic valvular insufficiency without stenosis or mitral valve disease.
- Aneurysm of the aorta.
- Coronary ostial stenosis.
- Diagnosis of syphilis.

### General Considerations

Syphilitic "heart disease" may consist of aortic valvular insufficiency (most common), aortic dilatation or aneurysm, or narrowing of the coronary ostia. It comprises less than 5% of all heart disease in population groups that have ready access to effective treatment of syphilis; it has become rare in the USA. It is more common in men (3:1) and is usually diagnosed between ages 35 and 55 (10–20 years after the primary infection). Serologic tests for syphilis are positive in nearly 100% of cases with the fluorescent treponemal antibody absorption test (FTA-ABS). The ascending aorta, arch, and descending aorta are most commonly affected; the abdominal aorta is rarely involved. Aortic valve insufficiency occurs in about 10% of cases of untreated syphilitic aortitis.

### Clinical Findings

**A. Aortitis:** There are no symptoms or physical signs unless dilatation has occurred. In a patient under age 40 without hypertension or demonstrable arteriosclerosis, a ringing or accentuated second aortic sound with or without a soft aortic systolic murmur is "suggestive" of syphilitic aortitis. Linear calcification that is limited to the root of the aorta and arch is a diagnostic sign. There is echocardiographic evidence of aortic root dilatation.

**B. Aortic Insufficiency:** Clinical, radiographic, and electrocardiographic manifestations are as described for rheumatic aortic insufficiency. Ten percent of cases are associated with saccular aneurysm of the aorta.

**C. Aortic Aneurysm:** Symptoms and signs are dependent upon the site and size of the aneurysm. Aneurysm of the ascending aorta is characterized by visible pulsation of dullness on palpation at the manubrium and in the first to third interspaces parasternally, lowered blood pressure in the right arm, and an aortic systolic murmur and thrill without peripheral signs of aortic stenosis. Aneurysm of the aortic arch produces cough, dyspnea, and recurrent pulmonary infections (compression of trachea or right main stem bronchus); hoarseness (compression of recurrent laryngeal nerve); tracheal tug, edema of the face and neck, distended neck veins, and prominent veins over the upper chest (compression of superior vena cava); and dysphagia (compression of the esophagus). Aneurysm of the descending aorta is usually asymptomatic; when it is large it may erode the ribs or spine, producing pain that is worse in recumbency and visible or palpable pulsations medial to the left scapula.

Radiographic and echocardiographic findings consist of saccular or sharply defined fusiform bulging of the thoracic aorta with increased pulsation. Clot formation or periaortic fibrosis may dampen the pulsation and simulate a solid tumor. Aortography demonstrates continuity of the aorta with the lumen of the aneurysm.

**D. Narrowing of the Coronary Artery Ostia:** Angina pectoris is identical to that seen in coronary heart disease. Its syphilitic origin can only be inferred in the presence of one of the other manifestations of syphilitic aortitis.

### Differential Diagnosis

The clinical picture can mimic rheumatic heart disease, ankylosing spondylitis, Reiter's disease, and rheumatoid arthritis. Syphilitic aneurysms are indistinguishable clinically from those caused by atherosclerosis.

### Treatment

Syphilis is treated as outlined in Chapter 24 if the patient has not had a full course of treatment.

Bed rest may be desirable at the beginning of treatment with penicillin because of the possibility of Herxheimer's reaction.

Surgical repair of the aneurysm has been attempted but is hazardous. Successful surgical aortocoronary bypass for coronary ostia stenosis has been accomplished. An aortic valve prosthesis may be necessary for aortic insufficiency.

### Prognosis

**A. Aortitis:** Ten to 20% of patients develop aortic insufficiency and other manifestations of syphilitic cardiovascular disease; in the remainder, life expectancy is not affected.

**B. Aortic Insufficiency:** If penicillin is given when the signs of aortic insufficiency are purely auscultatory, the progress of the lesion may be slowed or even arrested; this significantly improves the prognosis for survival.

**C. Aortic Aneurysm:** Once aneurysms have reached sufficient size to produce symptoms by compression of adjacent structures, life expectancy is measured in months. Longer survival is possible when the aneurysm is small and effective therapy for syphilis has been given. Death is usually due to rupture of the aneurysm.

**D. Narrowing of the Coronary Artery Ostia:** This condition tends to aggravate the heart failure due to syphilitic aortic insufficiency and predisposes to sudden death. Surgical aortocoronary bypass has been successfully accomplished.

## ACUTE MYOCARDITIS

Acute myocarditis is a focal or diffuse inflammation of the myocardium occurring during or after many viral, bacterial, rickettsial, spirochetal, fungal, and parasitic diseases or after administration of various drugs. Mild forms are common and recognizable only by serial electrocardiographic changes. Severe symptomatic myocarditis occurs most commonly in acute rheumatic fever, diphtheria, scrub typhus, and Chagas' disease (*Trypanosoma cruzi* infection). Bacteremia, viral pneumonia and encephalitis, and trichinosis may be associated with it.

The most common cause of acute viral myocarditis is coxsackie B virus, usually type B3 or B5. The disease is diagnosed by isolating the virus from throat washings, feces, or blood; by detecting a 4-fold increase in serum antibody titers from paired sera; or, in fatal cases, by isolating the virus from the myocardium.

### Clinical Findings

**A. Symptoms and Signs:** In acute myocarditis, the patient usually presents with an acute febrile illness associated with fever, malaise, arthralgias, chest pain, dyspnea, and palpitations. The patient may have associated pericarditis, with characteristic chest pain. The chest pain is frequently vague. An acute febrile illness with symptoms suggesting cardiac involvement should provoke a meticulous search for signs of heart disease. The patient may experience syncope (Stokes-Adams attacks) if conduction defects are present.

Tachycardia out of proportion to the fever suggests the diagnosis of acute myocarditis. There may be no abnormalities on examination except for displacement of the cardiac impulse to the left. The blood pressure is usually normal. Auscultation may reveal a tictac rhythm, a "functional" systolic murmur, and a gallop rhythm, with $S_3$. In the presence of cardiac failure, the patient may have a raised pulmonary venous or jugular venous pressure. Various types of ventricular arrhythmias or atrioventricular conduction defects may be found.

Acute circulatory collapse, with hypotension, cold and clammy extremities, oliguria, and obtundation, may occur when myocardial damage is severe. Systemic emboli and sudden death are possible.

**B. Imaging:** The chest film may show an enlarged and globular heart and pericardial or pleural effusion or pulmonary venous congestion.

Echocardiography may reveal enlargement of the left ventricle, E point separation in severe cardiac failure, and pericardial effusion. It is a means of ruling out other diseases (eg, hypertrophic cardiomyopathy and mitral stenosis).

**C. Electrocardiographic Findings:** ST-T changes, often in the inferior leads, are the most common abnormalities. If the inflammatory or infiltrative process affects the conduction system, the patient may have conduction defects.

**D. Endomyocardial Biopsy:** Right ventricular

endomyocardial biopsy may establish the specific cause of the myocarditis but more commonly shows a nonspecific inflammatory infiltrate. Biopsy is not recommended in the usual case, but if the clinical course is severe with cardiac failure, and aggressive therapy is considered (see below), serial biopsies may assist in determining the benefit of such therapy.

## Differential Diagnosis

Acute myocarditis resulting from infection with viruses (eg, coxsackieviruses), protozoa (eg, trypanosomes), or bacteria (eg, pneumococci) must be distinguished from acute toxic myocarditis due to alcohol, drugs (eg, doxorubicin), or diphtheria and from myocarditis associated with acute rheumatic fever and other autoimmune disorders.

Nonviral myocarditis is recognized on the basis of the manifestations of the underlying disease. The use of drugs for treatment of an underlying disease, their dosage, and the nature of the disease being treated help differentiate myocardial drug toxicity from acute myocarditis. In patients with acute lupus erythematosus with fever and pericarditis, evidence for renal and central nervous system involvement help distinguish the disorder from primary myocarditis.

## Treatment

In the absence of effective specific antiviral therapy, treatment consists of general supportive care, avoidance of vigorous exercise, and management of cardiac failure, arrhythmias, or conduction defects if they occur. Immunosuppressive drugs combined with corticosteroids may be used in severe cases in patients with rapidly developing cardiac failure.

In nonviral acute myocarditis, treatment is directed toward the underlying cause if known.

## Prognosis

Depending upon the cause, the cardiac failure of myocardial disease may differ from that due to ischemic cardiomyopathy or severe valvular disease. In acute viral myocarditis, for example, cardiac failure may be completely reversible over a period of 1–2 months; alternatively, it may be progressive and disabling.

Dec GW Jr et al: Active myocarditis in the spectrum of acute dilated cardiomyopathies: Clinical features, histologic correlates, and clinical outcome. *N Engl J Med* 1985;**312**:885.

Fowles RE, Mason JW: Role of cardiac biopsy in the diagnosis and management of cardiac disease. *Prog Cardiovasc Dis* 1984;**27**:153.

## ACUTE MYOCARDIAL DAMAGE DUE TO DRUG TOXICITY

Acute myocardial damage has been noted in the past after use of a variety of drugs, notably chemotherapeutic agents, emetine, digitalis, sympathomimetic drugs, corticosteroids, arsenic, antimony, amphetamines, and tricyclic antidepressants (amitriptyline and imipramine, among others). The negative inotropic action of beta-adrenergic blocking drugs (including timolol eye drops), verapamil, and disopyramide (Norpace) has also caused cardiac failure, especially when there is underlying heart disease.

Myocardial toxicity is occurring with greater frequency as a result of the use of high doses of multiple cytotoxic drugs in the treatment of serious diseases. About one-fourth of patients receiving high-dose multiple chemotherapy may die of acute myocardial failure during treatment as a result of endothelial injury, pericardial effusion, cardiac failure, and cardiac arrhythmias. The toxic effects of cytotoxic agents are dose-related and more apt to occur when such drugs are used in combination. The total dose of doxorubicin in adults should not exceed 500 mg/m$^2$ body surface—less in patients receiving other potentially cardiotoxic agents. Radionuclide angiography may demonstrate impaired left ventricular diastolic filling, which may be an early sign of toxicity.

As in any other variety of acute myocardial disease or toxicity, the patient may present with cardiac failure, arrhythmias, conduction defects, postural hypotension, or electrocardiographic T wave abnormalities. Patients receiving emetine (for amebiasis) or antimony (for schistosomiasis) may demonstrate electrocardiographic abnormalities without clinical symptoms or signs; it is then desirable to use alternative drugs or proceed with smaller dosages and close observation. Onset of failure may be rapid or delayed.

Serial ECGs, chest radiographs, and echocardiograms, cautious restriction of total dosage, and close clinical observation for early evidence of cardiac involvement are advised. Endomyocardial biopsy may demonstrate inflammatory changes reflecting early injury. In addition, decrease in the height of the R wave is an early sign of cardiac toxicity, and the risk/benefit ratio of continued therapy must be assessed.

## Treatment

Cardiotoxic drugs are withdrawn, and the heart failure is otherwise treated conventionally.

## Prognosis

The prognosis is good if appropriate measures are taken before severe cardiac failure occurs; it is poor if the offending drug is continued after early cardiac toxicity is manifest. Mild to moderate cardiac failure subsides gradually after the cardiotoxic drug is stopped.

Kantrowitz NE, Bristow MR: Cardiotoxicity of antitumor agents. *Prog Cardiovasc Dis* 1984;**27**:195.

## CHRONIC CARDIOMYOPATHIES

This is a miscellaneous group of heart muscle diseases of unknown cause, divided on the basis of the clinical and hemodynamic features into 3 types:

(1) congestive dilated cardiomyopathy (see below); (2) hypertrophic cardiomyopathy (see p 262); and (3) restrictive cardiomyopathy, with infiltrative myocardial disease associated with endomyocardial fibrosis, amyloid disease, scleroderma, hemochromatosis, and other disorders that interfere with left ventricular filling and emptying (decreased distensibility). Restrictive cardiomyopathy is uncommon, and no further discussion will be offered here; it may also be caused by the small-vessel disease of diabetes.

Schoenfeld MH et al: Restrictive cardiomyopathy versus constrictive pericarditis: Role of endomyocardial biopsy in avoiding unnecessary thoracotomy. *Circulation* 1987;**75**: 1012.

## 1. CONGESTIVE (IDIOPATHIC) DILATED OR PRIMARY CARDIOMYOPATHY

Idiopathic dilated congestive cardiomyopathy is a nonspecific diagnosis, and there are no characteristics that distinguish it from congestive cardiomyopathy caused by a variety of myocardial diseases that have a similar end point: congestive failure. Excessive alcohol intake over a period of many years is a possible cause in many cases, as is ischemic coronary disease.

### Clinical Findings

**A. Symptoms:** The disease is suspected early in patients who have paroxysmal nocturnal dyspnea, orthopnea, or palpitations. Symptoms of right heart failure, eg, edema, occur early.

Associated chest pain is nondescript and not typical of angina pectoris. It may be related to pulmonary congestion or, if pleuritic, to complicating pulmonary embolism. Pericardial pain is rare.

Patients who complain of palpitations may have chronic atrial fibrillation or paroxysmal atrial or ventricular arrhythmia. The arrhythmias may be incidental or may dominate the clinical picture. Ventricular premature beats occur in about half of cases; ventricular tachycardia or fibrillation usually occurs late.

Dizziness or syncope may occur from bradyarrhythmia or ventricular conduction defects secondary to fibrosis.

Symptoms of pulmonary or systemic emboli may occur, sometimes dominating the clinical features.

**B. Signs:** The signs are those of cardiac failure and do not differ from those seen in congestive heart failure from other causes. The blood pressure is usually normal. A history of hypertension is present in 30–40% of patients with cardiomyopathy, but hypertension is not usually present in patients presenting with cardiac failure.

Signs of pulmonary emboli or systemic emboli may be found when these complications occur.

**C. Laboratory Findings:** There are no specific laboratory findings unless the congestive cardiomyopathy is due to a specific disease.

**D. Imaging:** Radiography shows diffuse cardiac enlargement, chiefly left ventricular, with pulmonary congestion but without disproportionate left atrial enlargement, calcified valves, or abnormalities of the aorta.

Echocardiography can rule out pericardial effusion, aortic stenosis, and mitral valve disease, as well as estimate left ventricular volume and ejection fraction. Marked increases in diastolic volume or decreases in ejection fraction ($< 20\%$) are poor prognostic signs.

**E. Electrocardiographic Findings:** These include left ventricular hypertrophy, conduction defects, and nonspecific ST-T abnormalities.

**F. Hemodynamic Findings and Angiography:** In advanced cases the heart has a large volume, poor contractions and generalized hypokinesis, decreased ejection fraction (usually 30–40% or less), and increased left ventricular filling pressure. The latter may be raised out of proportion to right ventricular filling pressure, which helps to differentiate congestive or hypertrophic cardiomyopathy from constrictive pericarditis. However, the filling pressure may be approximately equal in the 2 ventricles.

### Differential Diagnosis

**A. Ischemic Cardiomyopathy:** Increased left ventricular volume with decreased ejection fraction and hypokinesis are seen on left ventricular angiography in both idiopathic cardiomyopathy and ischemic cardiomyopathy. The latter, however, may have segmental defects in contraction rather than symmetric hypokinesis. A history of myocardial infarction may be elicited, and myocardial ischemia may be induced by exercise.

**B. Other Disorders:** Other forms of cardiac disease (eg, valvular heart disease), hypertension, and secondary cardiomyopathies are discussed elsewhere.

### Treatment

There are no specific measures for idiopathic dilated cardiomyopathy or endomyocardial fibrosis other than the treatment of cardiac failure. Anticoagulants, if the patient is reliable, and antiarrhythmic treatment may be valuable in some cases.

Cardiac failure may be severe and unrelenting in idiopathic congestive cardiomyopathy, and the use of intravenous and oral vasodilators should be considered if the usual therapeutic agents fail.

### Prognosis

The prognosis of advanced idiopathic cardiomyopathy is poor. Even with the best of care, survival for only 2–3 years is the rule. Prolonged bed rest and intensive treatment of cardiac failure has not been shown to improve the prognosis.

Eisenberg JD, Sobel BE, Geltman EM: Differentiation of ischemic from nonischemic cardiomyopathy with positron emission tomography. *Am J Cardiol* 1987;**59**:1410.

Guerra HAC et al: Clinical, histochemical, and ultrastructural correlation in septal endomyocardial biopsies from chronic chagasic patients: Detection of early myocardial damage. *Am Heart J* 1987;**113**:716.

Johnson RA, Palacios I: Dilated cardiomyopathies of the adult. (2 parts.) *N Engl J Med* 1982;**307**:1051, 1119.

Kyle RA, Greipp PR: Amyloidosis (AL): Clinical and laboratory features in 229 cases. *Mayo Clin Proc* 1983;**58**:665.

## 2. HYPERTROPHIC (OBSTRUCTIVE) CARDIOMYOPATHY
### (Idiopathic Hypertrophic Subaortic Stenosis [IHSS]; Asymmetric Septal Hypertrophy)

Hypertrophic cardiomyopathy, may be associated with asymmetric hypertrophy of the septum and free wall of the left ventricle. There may be decreased diastolic function and variable obstruction of the left ventricular outflow tract associated with apposition of the anterior mitral valve leaflet to the ventricular septum. In some cases, left ventricular hypertrophy may be slight; the major defect resulting in cardiac failure may be impaired left ventricular diastolic filling and relaxation rather than severe systolic abnormality, although the latter may be present concurrently. Hypertrophy of the right ventricle with obstruction of the right ventricular outflow tract may coexist. The degree of obstruction is highly variable and is related to the contractile force of the left ventricle, the systemic vascular resistance, and the left ventricular diastolic volume. Factors that increase the force of left ventricular contraction, such as inotropic agents (digitalis, isoproterenol) or the first beat following a postextrasystolic pause, potentially increase obstruction. Similarly, decrease in the systemic vascular resistance (such as occurs with amyl nitrite) decreases the impedance to left ventricular outflow, and a pressure gradient, if present, becomes increased as obstruction develops.

### Clinical Findings

**A. Symptoms:** Dyspnea on exertion and chest pain are the commonest presenting symptoms. The pain is similar but not identical to that of angina pectoris but is not relieved by nitroglycerin. Fatigue and dizziness not related to exertion are often present. Hypertrophic cardiomyopathy may be the most common cause of sudden death in young athletes. The symptoms may be related to the degree of obstruction in the infundibulum of the left ventricle or to the presence of complex ventricular arrhythmias or ventricular tachycardia, which may be demonstrated on ambulatory ECG monitoring. Anything that reduces systemic vascular resistance, such as a hot environment, pregnancy, exercise, or suddenly assuming the erect position, may induce symptoms. Left ventricular failure is a late manifestation, sometimes following atrial fibrillation.

**B. Signs:** The abnormal position of the anterior leaflet also results in mitral insufficiency with its characteristic pansystolic murmur; patients have as well a late crescendo systolic ejection murmur resulting from the left ventricular outflow tract obstruction. The carotid pulse and the left ventricular pressure pulse have a rapid upstroke time, since forceful contraction of the hypertrophied left ventricle ejects most of the blood during the first part of systole. When the increased force of contraction results in obstruction of the outflow tract, ejection of blood is abruptly slowed, and a slower (bisferiens) wave then appears. The palpable fourth heart sound due to decreased compliance of the left ventricle causes a "triple-humped" pressure pulse that can be demonstrated by palpation and by the apexcardiogram.

**C. Laboratory Findings and Special Studies:** Patients with hypertrophic cardiomyopathy demonstrate left ventricular hypertrophy, electrocardiographically and radiologically. Left ventricular catheterization and angiography demonstrate the variable pressure gradient (which can be induced during the study; see above) across the ventricular outflow tract; the narrow systolic left ventricular outflow tract with marked, irregular septal hypertrophy; delayed left ventricular diastolic filling and relaxation; and abnormalities of systolic contraction that differ from those seen in valvular aortic stenosis. Amyl nitrite inhalation and isoproterenol induce or exaggerate the outflow obstruction murmur by reducing systemic vascular resistance and exaggerating the outflow obstruction. Phenylephrine increases the systemic vascular resistance, decreases the outflow obstruction, and reduces the pressure gradient across the outflow tract. The left ventricular end-diastolic pressure is almost always raised, especially after exercise, owing to the considerably decreased diastolic compliance of the hypertrophied left ventricle. A characteristic feature is impaired diastolic function with general and regional abnormalities of relaxation. Inflow obstruction from decreased distensibility causes slow filling of the left ventricle, a large *a* wave, a slow *y* descent, and a small *v* wave in the left atrium. Decreased left ventricular filling due to decreased diastolic compliance is in contrast to the "pump failure" of dilated idiopathic cardiomyopathy. Coronary arteriograms are usually normal.

Echocardiographic findings are the most practical means of making the diagnosis, obviating the need for cardiac catheterization in asymptomatic or mild cases. The 4 diagnostic features are hypertrophy of the posterior wall of the left ventricle, asymmetric hypertrophy of the ventricular septum (the width of the septum is at least 1.3 times as great as the width of the posterior myocardium), systolic anterior motion of the anterior cusp of the mitral valve, which approaches or impinges on the ventricular septum, and decreased filling and delayed relaxation of the left ventricle. The aortic valve is normal on echocardiography. The echocardiographic signs may be too sensitive and may occur in other conditions, but when combined with Doppler flow studies they are reliable for estimating gradients, the degree of mitral regurgitation, and the morphology of the left ventricle.

## Course of the Disease

The course of the disease is variable. It may be first recognized by symptoms of dyspnea, angina, or dizziness, which indicate a more advanced stage of the disease; by the pansystolic murmur of mitral insufficiency; by the presence of left ventricular hypertrophy; or by the demonstration of echocardiographic abnormalities. About half of patients have multiform or complex ventricular premature beats, including ventricular tachycardia, which may explain the frequency of syncope and sudden death in this syndrome. Sudden death cannot be clearly related to the severity of symptoms or obstruction or to the degree of left ventricular hypertrophy. Sudden death can sometimes be associated with a family history of the disease, with rapidly worsening symptoms and signs, or with complex arrhythmias and ventricular tachycardia; but it may also occur in apparently healthy individuals, especially during vigorous exercise. Ambulatory electrocardiographic monitoring and appropriate antiarrhythmic drugs may prove helpful.

Atrial fibrillation may, by further interfering with left ventricular filling, precipitate congestive failure; it is an uncommon arrhythmia in hypertrophic cardiomyopathy. The disease may also end in systemic embolism, angina pectoris, syncope, and sudden death. Infective endocarditis may involve the mitral valve.

## Treatment

Treatment is often not satisfactory, because it may not prevent progression of the disease or increase survival rates. Treatment begins with beta-adrenergic blocking agents. Verapamil may be beneficial by improving left ventricular diastolic function. The effects have not been dramatic, and in some patients, sinus bradycardia and sinus arrest may occur. Vasodilatation induced by the drug may increase left ventricular obstruction and induce symptoms. Antiarrhythmic therapy should be considered in order to prevent sudden death. Amiodarone has been used with some success in these patients. If the patient remains symptomatic and receives no benefit from propranolol, surgery may be advised. Myotomy and limited resection of the hypertrophied muscle have occasionally produced gratifying results.

Betocchi S et al: Isovolumic relaxation period in hypertrophic cardiomyopathy: Assessment by radionuclide angiography. *J Am Coll Cardiol* 1986;**7**:74.

Maron BJ et al: Hypertrophic cardiomyopathy: Interrelations of clinical manifestations, pathophysiology, and therapy. (2 parts.) *N Engl J Med* 1987;**316**:780, 844.

Wigle ED: Hypertrophic cardiomyopathy: A 1987 viewpoint. (Editorial.) *Circulation* 1987;**75**:311.

## PRIMARY CARDIAC TUMORS

Primary cardiac tumors are rare and constitute only a small fraction of all tumors that involve the heart or pericardium. Metastases from malignant tumors elsewhere are more frequent and may appear in the myocardium or pericardium. When pericardial effusion occurs, the patient may show manifestations of pericardial tamponade. The most common primary cancers of the heart are sarcomas of various types.

A cardiac tumor may obstruct the venous or arterial vessels in the region of the heart, may obstruct the superior or inferior vena cava, or may interfere with left ventricular filling or left ventricular output.

The diagnosis is suggested by bizarre outlines of the cardiac shadow on plain films; by a malignant tumor elsewhere; by the relationship of posture to symptoms of syncope or vertigo as well as to murmurs; and, in pericardial effusion, by finding malignant cells in the fluid. Definitive diagnosis is by cineangiocardiography, which may demonstrate obstruction of any chamber.

The most common benign tumor of the heart is myxoma, usually left atrial myxoma. The patient usually presents in one of 3 ways: (1) With intermittent symptoms of syncope, vertigo, and dyspnea as well as signs suggesting mitral valve disease. There may be changing murmurs. The tumor is usually on a stalk and is mobile, and the degree of mitral valve obstruction varies depending upon its position, the position of the patient, and varying hemodynamic events. (2) With systemic emboli in about one-third of cases. The diagnosis can be made by histologic recognition of myxoma in the embolic tissue removed at surgery. (3) With systemic symptoms and signs of fever, tachycardia, raised sedimentation rate, anemia, clubbed fingers, protein abnormalities, raised serum globulin, etc.

The diagnosis of left atrial myxoma is made by echocardiography, which shows multiple dense echoes representing a mass with its stalk posterior to the anterior mitral valve leaflet in diastole, and by cineangiocardiography, in which a filling defect is demonstrated.

Treatment of myxoma consists of surgical excision, including removal of the base of the stalk to prevent recurrences.

Sutton MGSJ et al: Atrial myxomas: A review of clinical experience in 40 patients. *Mayo Clin Proc* 1980;**55**:371.

## THE CARDIAC PATIENT & SURGERY

Major surgery in the cardiac patient is inevitably more hazardous than in patients with normal hearts. When shock, hemorrhage, hypoxia, induction of anesthesia, thromboembolism, and hypoventilation occur in a patient with heart disease, the danger of myocardial infarction, cardiac failure, and arrhythmias is increased.

The major cardiac lesions that increase the risks of surgery are rheumatic heart disease (especially aortic stenosis); coronary heart disease (about 5% additional hazard); and syphilitic cardiovascular disease, especially if there is involvement of the coronary ostia. Hypertension without cardiac or renal involvement does not usually add to the surgical risk. Surgery for atherosclerotic vascular disease is a major risk factor for postoperative myocardial infarction. Previous infarction, abnormal exercise stress tests, and dipyridamole-thallium perfusion redistribution after exercise may predict the likelihood of cardiac events following peripheral vascular surgery. Myocardial ischemia demonstrated by these noninvasive tests indicates a high-risk group in whom cardiac revascularization should be considered prior to vascular surgery.

If possible, elective surgery of significant magnitude and duration in patients with recent congestive failure should be delayed until 3 weeks after recovery; in patients with recent myocardial infarction, a delay of 3–6 months is advisable.

In inducing and maintaining anesthesia in a cardiac patient, adequate ventilation, oxygenation, and smooth induction are important.

During surgery, hypotension should be treated promptly and fluid therapy given to maintain optimal cardiac reserve. In high-risk patients, intraoperative monitoring of PCWP and esophageal echocardiography should be considered to detect cardiac complications early.

Improvements in anesthesia and surgical skill have reduced the risk of major surgery. The presence of cardiac disease increases the risk but should not per se deny patients the benefits of elective surgery.

Boucher CA et al: Determination of cardiac risk by dipyridamolethallium imaging before peripheral vascular surgery. *N Engl J Med* 1985;**312:**389.

Goldman L: Cardiac risks and complications of non-cardiac surgery. *Ann Intern Med* 1983;**98:**504.

Leppo J et al: Noninvasive evaluation of cardiac risk before elective vascular surgery. *J Am Coll Cardiol* 1987;**9:**269.

# THE CARDIAC PATIENT & PREGNANCY*

The following information will assist in estimating the likelihood of cardiac failure in a pregnant woman: (1) the functional class before pregnancy, (2) the age of the patient, (3) the size of the heart, (4) the structural lesion of the heart, (5) the presence of arrhythmias, (6) the patient's socioeconomic status (eg, if children are at home or if the patient must work),

_____

* See also Chapter 13 for discussion of hypertension of pregnancy and other obstetric subjects.

(7) the cooperation of the patient, and (8) the presence of associated disease.

## Assessment of Risk of Heart Disease in Pregnancy

**A. Little or No Functional Incapacity:** Most patients who are asymptomatic or who have only mild symptoms with ordinary activities can continue to term under close medical supervision. If the patient develops more severe symptoms with activity, she should be hospitalized, treated for cardiac failure, and kept in bed until term.

**B. Moderate or Marked Functional Incapacity:** If the patient has pure mitral stenosis and develops acute pulmonary edema or has moderate to marked symptoms with activity, mitral valvulotomy should be considered. This has been successfully accomplished up to the eighth month. If the patient does not have an operable lesion, she should be hospitalized, treated for cardiac failure, and kept in bed until term.

**C. Severe Functional Incapacity:** Patients seen during the first trimester who have symptoms upon little or no activity and who do not have an operable cardiac lesion should be counseled about the desirability of termination of pregnancy because of the high incidence of recurrent failure and death in this group of patients. Tubal ligation should be considered.

## Physiologic Load Pregnancy Imposes on the Heart

The work of the heart increases by about 50% at the beginning of the third month, when the blood volume and cardiac output increase. In a normal pregnant woman, these physiologic factors can produce systolic "flow" murmurs. These murmurs, together with a normal physiologic $S_3$, can lead to a false diagnosis of heart disease. The placenta acts as an arteriovenous fistula. Cardiac failure may occur at any time from the end of the first trimester up to 2–3 weeks before term, at which time the load for some reason decreases. Cardiac arrhythmias are apt to occur, especially in patients with mitral valve or congenital heart disease.

Sodium should be restricted after the second month. Anticoagulants should be avoided. Care should be taken with the use of any drugs during pregnancy.

## Management of Labor

Vaginal delivery is to be preferred except when there is an obstetric indication for cesarean section. Coarctation of the aorta may be the only cardiac disease that contraindicates vaginal delivery, because of the danger of aortic rupture.

The second stage should be made as short as possible, with forceps if feasible. Ergonovine maleate should probably not be used because it increases the work of the heart.

## Postpartum Cardiac Failure

Cardiac failure days or weeks after delivery in an apparently normal woman has been observed particularly in the tropics, where it is thought to be a distinct entity. However, it also occurs in temperate climates. The cause is unknown, but the condition is thought by some to be a form of myocarditis. Hemodynamic and echocardiographic studies indicate that left ventricular function is relatively normal despite edema and dyspnea. The clinical findings are not characteristic of congestive cardiomyopathy. The combination of fluid retention from high salt intake and increased cardiac output resulting from lying in heated beds (a tribal custom) may be the cause in tropical countries; many patients promptly improve when they are hospitalized under normal environmental circumstances. Late follow-up indicates a good prognosis in many cases.

Ben-Ismail M et al: Cardiac valve prostheses, anticoagulation, and pregnancy. *Br Heart J* 1986;**55**:101.

Julian DH, Szekely P: Peripartum cardiomyopathy. *Prog Cardiovasc Dis* 1985;**27**:223.

Rotmensch HH, Elkayam U, Frishman W: Antiarrhythmic drug therapy during pregnancy. *Ann Intern Med* 1983;**98**:487.

Shapiro EP et al: Safety of labor and delivery in women with mitral valve prolapse. *Am Heart J* 1985;**56**:806.

Sullivan JM, Ramanathan KB: Management of medical problems in pregnancy: Severe cardiac disease. *N Engl J Med* 1985;**313**:304.

Svensson A: Hypertension in pregnancy: State of the art lecture. *J Hypertension* 1985;**3(Suppl 3)**:395.

## REFERENCES

Applefeld MM (guest editor): Contemporary issues in the management of chronic congestive heart failure. *Am J Med* 1986;**80**:1. [Entire issue.]

Blaufox MD (guest editor): Results and implications of the hypertension detection and follow-up program. *Prog Cardiovasc Dis* 1986;**29 (Suppl 1)**. [Entire issue.]

Braunwald E (editor): Calcium antagonists: Emerging clinical opportunities. (Symposium.) *Am J Cardiol* 1987;**59**:1. [Entire issue.]

Braunwald E (editor): *Heart Disease: A Textbook of Cardiovascular Medicine,* 2nd ed. Saunders, 1984.

Cohn JN (editor): A symposium: Role of nitrates in congestive heart failure. *Am J Cardiol* 1985;**56**:1A. [Entire issue.]

Colucci WS et al: Calcium channel blockers in congestive heart failure: Theoretic considerations and clinical experience. *Am J Med* 1985;**78 (Suppl 2B)**:9.

Dzau VJ: Significance of vascular renin-angiotension pathway. (Editorial.) *Hypertension* 1986;**8**:553.

Epstein SE et al: Task Force V: Ischemic heart disease. *J Am Coll Cardiol* 1985;**6**:1222.

Frohlich ED: A symposium: Role of calcium entry-blocking drugs in hypertension. *Am J Cardiol* 1985;**56**:1H.

Goldman MJ: *Principles of Clinical Electrocardiography,* 12th ed. Lange, 1985.

Hall JE, Mizelle HL, Woods LL: The renin-angiotension system and long-term regulation of arterial pressure. (Editorial Review). *J Hypertension* 1986;**4**:387.

Hatle L, Angelsen B: *Doppler Ultrasound in Cardiology,* 2nd ed. Lea & Febiger, 1985.

Health and Public Policy Committee: Automated ambulatory blood pressure monitoring. *Ann Intern Med* 1986;**104**:275.

Hurst JW, Logue RB: *The Heart, Arteries and Veins,* 6th ed. McGraw-Hill, 1986.

MacMahon SW, Devereux RB, Schron E (guest editors): Proceedings of a National Heart, Lung, and Blood Institute Symposium: Clinical and epidemiological issues in mitral valve prolapse. *Am Heart J* 1987;**113**:1265. [Entire issue.]

Marcus ML: *The Coronary Circulation in Health and Disease.* McGraw-Hill, 1983.

Maron BJ et al: Task Force III: Hypertrophic cardiomyopathy, other myopericardial diseases and mitral valve prolapse. *J Am Coll Cardiol* 1985;**6**:1215.

Mitchell JH, Maron BJ, Epstein SE (co-chairman): 16th Bethesda Conference: Cardiovascular abnormalities in the athlete: Recommendations regarding eligibility for competition. *J Am Coll Cardiol* 1985;**6**:1189.

Morganroth J, Parisi AF, Pohost GM: *Noninvasive Cardiac Imaging.* Year Book, 1983.

Nikkila EA, Tikkanen MJ (guest editors): Lipoprotein metabolism in relation to coronary heart disease. (Symposium.) *Am Heart J* 1987;**113**:1.

O'Connell JB et al: Peripartum cardiomyopathy: Clinical hemodynamic, histologic and prognostic characteristics. *J Am Coll Cardiol* 1986;**8**:52.

O'Rourke RA (guest editor): Calcium-entry blockade: Basic concepts and clinical implications. *Circulation* 1987;**75(Suppl)**:V-1.

A report of the American College of Cardiology/American Heart Association Task Force on Assessment of Cardiovascular Procedures (Subcommittee on Exercise Testing): Guidelines for exercise testing. *J Am Coll Cardiol* 1986;**8**:725.

Selzer A: *Principles and Practice of Clinical Cardiology: An Analytical Approach,* 2nd ed. Saunders, 1983.

Smith TW (editor): *Digitalis Glycosides.* Grune & Stratton, 1986.

Sokolow M, McIlroy MB: *Clinical Cardiology,* 4th ed. Appleton & Lange, 1986.

Whelton A (editor): A symposium: Current trends in diuretic therapy. *Am J Cardiol* 1986;**57**:1A. [Entire issue.]

# Blood Vessels & Lymphatics

*Lawrence M. Tierney, Jr., MD, & John M. Erskine, MD*

---

## ARTERIAL DISEASES

Atherosclerosis causes most degenerative arterial disease. Its incidence increases with age; although manifestations of the disease may appear in the fourth decade, people over 40 (particularly men) are most commonly affected. Risk factors include hypercholesterolemia, diabetes mellitus, smoking, and hypertension. Atherosclerosis tends to be a generalized disease, with some degree of involvement of all major arteries, but it produces its clinical manifestations by critical involvement of a limited number of arteries. Narrowing and occlusion of the artery are the most common manifestations of the disease, but weakening of the arterial wall, with aneurysmal dilatation of the arterial segment, also occurs, and both may be present in the same individual. Less common arterial diseases that must be considered are arteritis (of both large and small arteries), thromboangiitis obliterans (Buerger's disease), fibrodysplasia of visceral arteries, syphilitic aortitis, and radiation arteritis.

## DISEASES OF THE AORTA

### ANEURYSMS OF THE ABDOMINAL AORTA

#### Essentials of Diagnosis

- Most are asymptomatic, detected at incidental physical examination or sonography.
- Back or abdominal pain often precedes rupture.
- Peripheral atherosclerotic disease (aortoiliac) uncommonly associated.

#### General Considerations

The vast majority of aneurysms of the abdominal aorta are below the origin of the renal arteries and generally involve the bifurcation of the aorta and thus the proximal end of the common iliac arteries. Aneurysms of the upper abdominal aorta are rare. Most aneurysms of the distal aorta are atherosclerotic in origin and fusiform in shape. Eighty percent of aortic aneurysms are in the distal aorta.

#### Clinical Findings

**A. Symptoms and Signs:** Three phases can be recognized:

**1. Asymptomatic**–A pulsating mid and upper abdominal mass may be discovered on a routine physical examination, most frequently in men over 50. Also, sonography done for other purposes often detects asymptomatic aneurysms. It is also the most cost-effective test for confirming a suspicion of aneurysm aroused during physical examination.

**2. Symptomatic**–Pain is present in some form in one-fourth to one-third of cases and varies from mild midabdominal or lumbar discomfort to more severe constant or intermittent abdominal and back pain requiring narcotics for relief. Intermittent pain may be associated with enlargement or intramural dissection. Peripheral emboli may occur, even from small and unsuspected aneurysms, and symptomatic arterial insufficiency in the legs may result.

**3. Rupture**–Pain is usually severe and sudden in onset. Because the hemorrhage is most often into the retroperitoneal tissues, which offer some resistance, shock and other manifestations of blood loss may at first be mild or absent; but free uncontrolled bleeding inevitably follows, resulting in death. There is an expanding, pulsating abdominal and flank mass, and subcutaneous ecchymosis is occasionally present in the flank or groin. Many such patients can be saved by emergency surgery.

**B. Laboratory Findings:** Cardiac and renal function should be evaluated by means of electrocardiography, urinalysis, and blood urea nitrogen determination. Ultrasonic studies are of value and can be used to follow extension of aneurysms that are not removed following diagnosis.

**C. Imaging:** Curvilinear calcifications outlining portions of the aneurysm wall may be visible on plain films of the aortic area in approximately three-fourths of those with an aneurysm. If distal occlusive disease or renal artery involvement by the aneurysm is suspected, an aortogram may be indicated. CT scanning coupled with contrast-enhanced scanning may also define the mass and its vascularity and may make arteriography unnecessary. Occasionally, CT is valuable in the detection of subacute rupture; in most instances, its use is confined to preoperative assessment.

#### Treatment

Surgical excision and grafting of the defect is indicated for most aneurysms of the distal abdominal aorta in good-risk patients. Most aneurysms continue to enlarge and will rupture if left untreated. The size of the aneurysm correlates best with the risk of rupture; in asymptomatic patients, surgery is advised when the aneurysm is 6 cm in size. It is also advisable in all symptomatic aneurysms. Opinions differ as to whether asymptomatic small aneurysms in poor-risk patients with significant cardiovascular, pulmonary, or renal disease should be removed or should be followed closely by means of ultrasound measurements to detect any signs of growth. Patients with significant symptomatic coronary or carotid artery disease are at risk during and following aneurysm resection, and surgery to lessen the chance of myocardial infarction or stroke prior to elective aneurysm surgery is sometimes advisable. If surgery is not performed, hypertension, if present, should be controlled. Individuals over age 80 with good preoperative risk factors can undergo elective surgery with an acceptable mortality rate; those with significant associated disease generally should not undergo operation without compelling indications.

## Complications

Irreversible renal injury can occur if hemodynamic instability is allowed to develop through inadequate monitoring during surgery. The rather high incidence of early and late myocardial infarction in this group of patients may be diminished by preoperative coronary angiography in those with evidence of coronary disease and preoperative bypass grafting or angioplasty if indicated. Ischemia of the distal colon and of one or both legs occasionally occurs following this surgery; in most cases, it can be prevented by meticulous attention to detail before and during surgery.

## Prognosis

The mortality rate following elective surgical resection is 3–8%, though in certain clinics it has recently approached 1%. Of those who survive surgery, approximately 60% are alive 5 years later, and of those who died, myocardial infarction was the leading cause of death. Among unoperated patients, less than 20% survive 5 years, and aneurysm rupture is the cause of 60% of the deaths. In general, a patient with an aortic aneurysm has a 3-fold greater chance of dying as a consequence of rupture of the aneurysm than of dying from surgical resection.

Bernstein EF et al: Growth rates of small abdominal aortic aneurysms. *Surgery* 1986;**80**:765.

Crawford ES et al: Infrarenal abdominal aortic aneurysm:Factors influencing survival after operation performed over a 25-year period. *Ann Surg* 1983;**193**:699.

Donaldson MC, Rosenberg JM, Bucknam CA: Factors affecting survival after ruptured abdominal aortic aneurysm. *J Vasc Surg* 1986;**3**:564.

Fortner G, Johansen K: Abdominal aortic aneurysms. *West J Med* 1984;**140**:50.

## ANEURYSMS OF THE THORACIC AORTA

Thoracic aortic aneurysms are most commonly due to atherosclerosis; syphilis is now a rare cause. Vasculitis and annuloaortic ectasia (with or without Marfan's syndrome) may also result in thoracic aneurysm. Traumatic aneurysms may occur just beyond the origin of the left subclavian artery when the wall of the aorta is incompletely torn as a result of a rapid deceleration accident. Only one-sixth of aortic aneurysms are thoracic.

### Clinical Findings

Manifestations depend largely on the size and position of the aneurysm and its rate of growth.

**A. Symptoms and Signs:** There may be no symptoms. Substernal, back, or neck pain may occur, as well as symptoms and signs due to pressure on (1) the trachea (dyspnea, stridor, a brassy cough), (2) the esophagus (dysphagia), (3) the left recurrent laryngeal nerve (hoarseness), or (4) the superior vena cava (edema in the neck and arms, distended neck veins). The findings of regurgitation at the aortic valve may be present, together with manifestations of coronary or myocardial insufficiency.

**B. Imaging:** In addition to routine chest x-rays, aortography may be necessary to substantiate the diagnosis and to delineate the precise location and extent of the aneurysm and its relation to the vessels arising from the arch. CT scan is of more use than ultrasound in scanning thoracic aneurysms and may be as sensitive and specific as aortography. Digital subtraction angiography or magnetic resonance imaging, if available, may be of value. The coronary vessels and the aortic valve should also be studied if the ascending aorta is involved.

### Differential Diagnosis

It may be difficult to determine whether a mass in the mediastinum is an aneurysm, a neoplasm, or a cyst. The x-ray studies mentioned above (B) will distinguish an aneurysm. Radioactive isotope studies may be helpful in diagnosing a substernal goiter ($^{125}$I) or certain malignant tumors that also simulate aneurysm.

### Treatment

Aneurysms of the thoracic aorta often progress, with increasing symptoms, and finally rupture. Resection of aneurysms is now considered the treatment of choice if a skilled surgical team is available and if the patient's general condition is such that the major surgical procedure usually required can be done with an acceptable risk. This is especially true if an aneurysm is large, associated with symptoms and signs, and limited to the ascending or descending aorta. Small asymptomatic aneurysms, especially in poor-risk patients, are perhaps better treated only if progressive enlargement occurs. Hypertension—if present—should be controlled. The overall mortality rate of thoracic aneurysmectomy, however, is considerably higher than the 3–5% rate for abdominal aneurysms.

Saccular aneurysms with narrow necks can often be excised without occluding the aorta. Fusiform aortic aneurysms require resection and grafting of the aortic defect, often with the patient on partial or complete cardiac bypass. If the aortic valve is involved, an aortic valve replacement may be necessary, and reattachment of the coronary arteries or aortocoronary bypass grafts may also be indicated. Paraplegia is a dreaded complication of excision and graft replacement of aneurysms involving the descending thoracic aorta (3% of cases) and is due to compromise of the anterior spinal artery.

### Prognosis

Small aneurysms may change very little over a period of years, and death may result from causes other than rupture. If the aneurysm is large, symptomatic, and associated with hypertension or arteriosclerotic cardiovascular disease, the prognosis is poor. Saccular aneurysms, those distal to the left subclavian artery, and those limited to the ascending aorta can now be removed with an acceptable mortality rate. Resection of aneurysms of the transverse aortic arch involves major technical problems that can be dealt with only by skilled surgical teams using hypothermia to protect the nervous system.

Crawford ES et al: Thoracoabdominal aortic aneurysms: Preoperative and intraoperative factors determining immediate and long term results of operations in 605 patients. *J Vasc Surg* 1986;**3**:389.

## PERIPHERAL ARTERY ANEURYSMS (Popliteal & Femoral)

Popliteal artery aneurysms rank third in frequency among aneurysmal lesions; most of the other peripheral aneurysms are femoral. Almost all are atherosclerotic and occur in men. They are often multiple and bilateral, and aneurysmal disease of the aortoiliac vessels is commonly associated with the more peripheral aneurysms.

### Popliteal Aneurysms

Almost half are asymptomatic when diagnosed, and they are generally discovered in the popliteal fossa as a pulsating mass 2 cm or more in diameter. When a popliteal aneurysm is diagnosed, abdominal aneurysm is also likely and should be excluded by ultrasonography. Most aneurysms present with symptoms generally related to varying degrees of arterial insufficiency to the lower leg and foot, ie, intermittent claudication if insufficiency develops slowly, or severe ischemic manifestations with rest pain, pregangrene, or gangrene if sudden thrombosis of the aneurysm has developed or, less commonly, if distal embolization has occurred. (See below.) When complete thrombosis has occurred, a nonpulsatile popliteal mass

is noted. The large aneurysms may be associated with a degree of venous obstructive manifestations or pain from pressure on the nerves; thrombophlebitis is infrequent, and rupture is rare.

Angiography is of value in defining the distal arterial tree and the collateral vessels. The actual size of the aneurysm is more clearly determined by ultrasound examination.

Popliteal aneurysms rank second to abdominal aortic aneurysms in the incidence of potentially serious complications. Even small aneurysms (2 cm in size) can become thrombosed or give rise to emboli, particularly if laminated clot is demonstrated within the lumen of the aneurysm. When thrombosis occurs, over 40% will require amputation; its incidence is difficult to assess, since the prevalence of this problem is unknown. No amputation should be necessary when the aneurysm is treated surgically in the asymptomatic stage. Thus, surgery is advisable, and a reversed saphenous vein bypass graft with proximal and distal ligation of the aneurysm is generally employed. In large aneurysms with manifestations of vein or nerve compression, resection of the aneurysm with grafting of the arterial defect may be necessary.

### Femoral Aneurysms

Femoral aneurysms, as manifested by a pulsatile mass in the femoral area on one or both sides, have the potential for the same complications as popliteal aneurysms, although rupture is a more frequent complication and limb-threatening episodes are less frequent in femoral aneurysms. Because the incidence of serious complications in the asymptomatic group seems to be considerably less than for popliteal aneurysms, there is more reason to follow rather than operate on smaller, asymptomatic femoral aneurysms and to deal first with aortoiliac and then popliteal aneurysms in preference to femoral aneurysms when aneurysmal disease exists in all of these areas.

Anton GE et al: Surgical management of popliteal aneurysms: Trends in presentation, treatment and results from 1952 to 1984. *J Vasc Surg* 1986;**3**:1986.
Melliere D et al: Should all spontaneous popliteal aneurysms be operated on? *J Cardiovasc Surg* 1986;**27**:273.

## ACUTE AORTIC DISSECTION

### Essentials of Diagnosis

- Sudden severe chest pain with radiation to the back, abdomen, and hips.
- Patient appears to be in shock, but blood pressure is normal or elevated.
- A history of hypertension is usually present.
- Aortic insufficiency may be present.
- A history of hypertension is usually present.
- Dissection occurs most frequently in males.

### General Considerations

Extravasation of blood into and along the wall of the aorta may occur, resulting in aortic dissection.

Dissection generally begins either in the proximal aorta just above the aortic valve (type A, or proximal dissection) or at a site just beyond the origin of the left subclavian artery (type B, or distal dissection). The initial intimal tear probably results from the constant movement of the ascending and proximal descending aorta that occurs at these 2 points as a result of the pulsatile blood flow from the heart. Dissection occurs on rare occasions in an aorta even without an intimal tear; these aortas invariably show histologic abnormalities of the media. Proximal dissections are more often in aortas involved with abnormalities of the smooth muscle, elastic tissue, or collagen; distal dissections often occur in older patients with long-standing hypertension. Pregnancy (types A and B), bicuspid aortic valves and coarctation (types A and B), and Marfan's syndrome (type A) are associated with dissection in younger individuals. Both hypertension and a forceful pulse are important in the progression, which may extend from the ascending aorta distally to the abdominal aorta or beyond. It may remain limited to the ascending aorta and the aortic valve area, especially if hypertension is not present or is controlled early, and the distal dissections may progress not only distally but also proximally. Death may occur after hours, days, or weeks and is usually due to rupture of the aorta into the pericardial sac (and cardiac tamponade), into the left pleural cavity, or into the retroperitoneal area. The dissections may rupture back into the true lumen of the aorta (recanalization) with blood flow through both the true and false lumens; long-term survival can thus occur.

## Clinical Findings

**A. Symptoms and Signs:** Severe, persistent pain of sudden onset is almost always present, most often in the anterior and posterior chest, although it may be limited to one or the other, and may later progress to the abdominal and hip areas. Radiation down the arms may or may not occur. Usually there is only a mild decrease in the prerupture hypertensive level. Partial or complete occlusion of the arteries arising from the aortic arch or of the intercostal and lumbar arteries may lead to such central nervous system findings as syncope, hemiplegia, or paralysis of the lower extremities. Peripheral pulses and blood pressures may be diminished or unequal. Murmurs may appear over arteries along with signs of acute arterial insufficiency. An aortic diastolic murmur may develop as a result of dissection close to the aortic valve, resulting in secondary valvular insufficiency, heart failure, and cardiac tamponade.

**B. Laboratory Findings:** Electrocardiographic changes indicating left ventricular hypertrophy are often present; acute changes may not develop unless the dissection involves the coronary ostium. Indeed, the ECG may be perfectly normal.

**C. Imaging:** Chest radiographs often reveal an abnormal aortic contour or a wide superior mediastinum, with changes in the configuration and thickness of the aortic wall in successive films. There may be findings of pleural or pericardial effusion. CT scan with contrast enhancement and magnetic resonance imaging (MRI) are sensitive studies but are too time-consuming if dissection is clinically likely. These patients should have immediate angiography, because emergency surgery may be lifesaving in type A dissection; most surgeons require angiographic confirmation preoperatively. CT and MRI effectively exclude the diagnosis and are excellent first tests if dissection is believed to be possible but unlikely.

## Differential Diagnosis

Aortic dissection is most commonly confused with myocardial infarction (see Chapter 8). However, it may simulate numerous neurologic lesions, pulmonary emboli, and even various abdominal conditions.

## Treatment

**A. Medical Measures:** A combined and detailed program of intensive medical and surgical monitoring should be established promptly in an individual with severe spontaneous truncal pain; and, if hypertension is present, aggressive measures to lower the pressure should probably be initiated even before diagnostic studies have been completed. Treatment generally includes the simultaneous reduction of the systolic blood pressure to 100 mm Hg and reduction of the pulsatile aortic flow by means of the following:

(1) A rapid-acting antihypertensive agent as an intravenous infusion at a flow rate regulated by very frequent blood pressure determinations. Nitroprusside and trimethaphan (Arfonad) are the most commonly used drugs and may be given as follows: (a) Nitroprusside (50 mg in 1000 mL of 5% dextrose in water and shielded from light by foil) is started at a rate of 0.5 mL/min, and the infusion rate may be increased by 0.5 mL every 5 minutes until adequate control of the pressure has been achieved. Thiocyanate levels should be obtained, and the infusion should be stopped if the drug level reaches 10 mg/dL. (b) Trimethaphan (1 or 2 mg/mL) may be infused at a flow rate determined by the blood pressure response and the possible side effects of the drug; the patient must be in the semi-Fowler's position for the drug to work, as it is a ganglionic blocker.

(2) Intravenous propranolol, 0.15 mg/kg given over a 5-minute period and repeated as necessary to maintain the pulse rate at 60/min. Intravenous reserpine may be used if beta blockers are contraindicated.

Failure of this pharmacologic approach is suggested if chest pain is not relieved or if it reappears; if saccular aneurysm appears; if significant compromise or occlusion of a major branch of the aorta develops; or if progressive enlargement with impending rupture or leakage from the aneurysm occurs.

**B. Surgical Measures:** The emphasis in treatment has shifted toward surgery, as a result of increased proficiency in handling these very difficult technical problems. If a skilled cardiovascular team is available, all acute dissections involving the ascending aorta (type A) should be treated promptly with surgery to relieve or to prevent aortic valve insufficiency and to prevent rupture. Other indications for surgery are noted above. Using total body hypothermia and circulatory arrest, the ascending aorta and, if necessary, the aortic valve and arch may be replaced with reattachment of the coronaries and brachiocephalic vessels.

Surgical treatment is increasingly popular for the dissections arising in the descending thoracic aorta (type B); surgery may be delayed until the hypertension and dissection have been stabilized by medical means. The origin of the dissection is then removed; the false lumen is closed; and a graft is inserted to deliver all blood flow through the normal lumen, thus relieving the occlusive pressure on the aortic branches.

Since patients with type B dissections tend to be poor surgical risks, permanent medical therapy may be offered. Regimens should include beta blockers and antihypertensive drugs; vasodilators are contraindicated unless beta blockade has been effected.

### Prognosis

Without treatment, the mortality rate at 3 months is over 90%, but only 3% die immediately; 21% are dead in 24 hours, and 60% in 2 weeks. Survival without treatment, usually due to recanalization, does occasionally occur, and intensive pharmacologic methods to lower the pulse wave and blood pressure have led to healing of the dissected aorta in 50–80% of patients with an acute dissection and will convert others to a subacute or chronic form, which may then be treated by surgery. After 3 years, only 30% of the medically treated patients are alive as compared to 60% of those treated surgically. With the significant improvement in operative mortality rate, surgery by a skilled team now appears to be the treatment of choice.

Roberts WC: Aortic dissection: Anatomy, consequences, and cause. *Am Heart J* 1981;**101**:195.

Weingarten J, Tierney LM Jr: Aortic dissection. *West J Med* 1986;**144**:728.

# ATHEROSCLEROTIC OCCLUSIVE DISEASE

Occlusive disease of the aorta and its branches is an exceptionally common cause of disability. It is essential for the primary physician to emphasize its prevention, particularly in light of what is known about etiologic factors. Smoking must be interdicted in all individuals, and serum cholesterol should be determined in all adults under the care of physicians. Discontinuation of smoking and dietary or pharmacologic management when the serum cholesterol exceeds 200 mg/dL are prudent and inexpensive measures likely to reduce morbidity from atherosclerosis if more widely used.

## OCCLUSIVE DISEASE OF THE AORTA & ILIAC ARTERIES (Leriche Syndrome)

Occlusive disease of the aorta and the iliac arteries begins most frequently just proximal to the bifurcation of the common iliac arteries and at or just distal to the bifurcation of the aorta. Atherosclerotic changes occur in the intima and media, often with associated perivascular inflammation and calcified plaques in the media. Progression involves the complete occlusion of one or both common iliac arteries and then the abdominal aorta up to the segment just below the renal vessels. Although atherosclerosis is a generalized disease, occlusion tends to be segmental in distribution, and when the involvement is in the aortoiliac vessels there may be minimal atherosclerosis in the more distal external iliac and femoral arteries. The best candidates for arterial reconstructive surgery are those with localized occlusions at or just beyond the aortic bifurcation with relatively normal vessels proximally and distally. Conversely, patients with multisegmented arterial disease usually have more symptoms and are at greater risk of losing a limb. In planning therapy for these patients, it is important to carefully evaluate the relative significance of each segmental stenosis.

### Clinical Findings

Intermittent claudication is almost always present in the calf muscles and is usually present in the thighs and buttocks. It is most often bilateral and progressive. Some complain only of weakness in the legs when walking or a feeling of "tiredness" in the buttocks. Impotence is a common complaint in men. Rest pain is infrequent.

Femoral pulses are absent or very weak, and distal pulses are absent. A bruit may be heard over the aorta or over the iliac or femoral arteries. Atrophic changes of the skin, subcutaneous tissues, and muscles of the distal leg are usually minimal, as are dependent rubor and coolness of the skin, unless distal arterial disease is also present. Aortography including oblique views of the thigh and leg arteries demonstrates the level and extent of the occlusion and the condition of the vessels distal to the block.

### Treatment

Surgical treatment is indicated if claudication interferes appreciably with the patient's essential activities or work. If significant distal occlusive disease exists as well, more extensive surgery may be required.

Because many of these patients have coexisting ischemic heart disease, their medical management should be maximized preoperatively. The roles of exercise testing and coronary angiography have not been established. Some surgeons perform these studies with an eye toward prophylactic bypass grafting, but grafting has not been conclusively shown to be of benefit in this situation if patients are minimally symptomatic.

Patients with this disorder should quit smoking and undertake a graded exercise program to achieve and maintain ideal body weight.

**A. Arterial Graft (Prosthesis):** An arterial prosthesis bypassing the occluded segment is the treatment of choice in the more extensive aortoiliac occlusions. In general, the bifurcation graft extends from the infrarenal abdominal aorta, usually by means of an end-to-end anastomosis, to the distal external iliac or common femoral arteries as end-to-side anastomoses. A patient with leg ischemia who is considered to be too poor a risk for the major surgical procedure in the aortoiliac area can be treated with little risk but less favorable results by means of a graft from the axillary artery to one or both femoral arteries or, in the case of iliac unilateral disease, from the femoral artery with normal blood flow to the femoral artery distal to the stenotic iliac vessel.

**B. Thromboendarterectomy:** This procedure, which avoids the use of a prosthesis, is generally used when the occlusion is limited to the common iliac arteries and when the external iliac and common femoral arteries are free of significant occlusive disease.

**C. Percutaneous Transluminal Angioplasty:** This is a means of dealing with symptomatic iliac artery stenoses by the transfemoral artery approach. It should not be used in complete common iliac artery occlusion because of the danger of embolization. Postsurgical sexual problems in men are avoided by this technique, and in those already affected with impotence, relief of the problem may occur.

**Prognosis**

The operative mortality rate is 2–6%, and the immediate and long-term benefits are often impressive, particularly if there is no significant distal occlusive disease. In those with no distal occlusive disease, improvement is both subjective and objective, with relief of all or most of the claudication and, usually, return of all of the pulses in the extremities. Late occlusions in this group of patients are infrequent, and if proper judgment is used in patient selection, results are comparable for angioplasty, endarterectomy, and arterial grafting techniques.

Szilagyi DE et al: A thirty year survey of the reconstructive surgical treatment of aortoiliac occlusive disease. *J Vasc Surg* 1986;3:421.

**OCCLUSIVE DISEASE OF THE FEMORAL & POPLITEAL ARTERIES**

In the region of the thigh and knee, the vessels most frequently blocked by occlusive disease are the superficial femoral artery and the popliteal artery.

Atherosclerotic changes usually appear first at the most distal point of the superficial femoral artery, where it passes through the adductor magnus tendon into the popliteal space. In time, the whole superficial femoral artery may become occluded; the disease progresses into the popliteal artery less frequently. The common femoral and deep femoral arteries are usually patent and relatively free of disease, although the origin of the profunda femoris is sometimes narrowed. The distal popliteal and its 3 terminal branches may also be relatively free of occlusive disease.

**Clinical Findings**

**A. Symptoms and Signs:** Intermittent claudication is confined to the calf and foot. Atrophic changes in the lower leg and foot are distinct, with loss of hair, thinning of the skin and subcutaneous tissues, and diminution in the size of the muscles. Dependent rubor and blanching on elevation of the foot are usually present. When the leg is lowered after elevation, venous filling on the dorsal aspect of the foot may be slowed to 15–20 seconds or more. The foot is usually cool. The common femoral pulsations are usually of fair or good quality, although a bruit may be heard. No popliteal or pedal pulses can be felt. Pressure measurements in the distal leg, using ultrasound, will supply an objective functional assessment of the circulation and will aid in the decision whether to follow the patient or to go on to x-ray studies and possibly surgery.

**B. Imaging:** Radiographs of the thigh and leg may show calcification of superficial femoral and popliteal vessels. A femoral arteriogram will show the location and extent of the block as well as the status of the distal vessels, and lateral or oblique views will reveal whether the origin of the profunda femoris is narrow. It is important to know the condition of the aortoiliac vessels also, since a relatively normal inflow as well as an adequate distal "run-off" is important in determining the likelihood of success of an arterial procedure. Added oblique and leg and foot views at aortography will supply important information.

**Treatment**

The patient should be instructed to walk slowly, take short steps, avoid stairs and hills, and stop for brief rests to avoid pain. Walking, however, is the most effective way to develop collateral circulation, and walking up to the point of claudication, followed by a 3-minute rest, should be done at least 8 times a day. Smoking must be discontinued.

Surgery is indicated (1) if intermittent claudication is progressive or incapacitating and thus interferes significantly with the patient's essential physical activities such as ability to work or (2) if there is rest pain or if there are pregangrenous or gangrenous lesions on the foot.

**A. Arterial Graft:** An autogenous vein graft using a reversed segment of the great saphenous vein can be placed, bypassing the occluded segment. The distal anastomosis is usually to the popliteal artery, below the site of major occlusive disease. When the entire popliteal artery is occluded and gangrene or advanced ischemic changes are present in the foot, it is generally better to perform an amputation below the knee rather than an anastomosis to one of the leg arteries, though in rare patients anastomosis to a tibial or peroneal artery may save the extremity. Synthetic arterial prostheses, with the possible exception of the PTFE (polytetrafluoroethylene) grafts, have not proved to be very successful in this area because of the relatively high incidence of early or late thrombosis.

**B. Thromboendarterectomy:** Thromboendarterectomy with removal of the central occluding core may be successful if the occluded and stenotic segment is very short.

When significant aortoiliac or common femoral occlusive disease exists as well as superficial femoral and popliteal occlusions, it is usually better to relieve the obstructions in the larger, proximal arteries and deliver more blood flow to the profunda femoris than to operate on the smaller distal vessels, where the chances of success are less. If the origin of the profunda femoris is narrowed, a limited procedure at that site—a profundoplasty—may be successful in improving blood flow to the leg and foot and may be used, especially in poor-risk patients with rest pain.

**C. Percutaneous Transluminal Angioplasty:** Under radiographic control, the Grüntzig balloon catheter can be placed across a stenosis, which can then be disrupted by dilating the balloon. In the process, the intima is split, the media overstretched, and the stenosis generally eliminated. Fibrous healing results in a normal-sized lumen that persists for months or years. Although stenosis may recur, it may again be dilated, and failure of the procedure does not generally result in significant complications, nor does it interfere with surgical bypass procedures to deal with the arterial insufficiency should bypass become necessary. This technique can also be used in conjunction with direct arterial surgery and may be preferable in poor-risk patients.

1. Most favorable lesions—Single, short, discrete stenosis in medium-sized arteries such as the iliac-femoral-popliteal vessels.

2. Less favorable lesions—Multiple stenosis in series, those longer than 5 cm, complete occlusions less than 5 cm long, small arteries, recent acute occlusions (in conjunction with local intra-arterial streptokinase infusion).

3. Stenotic arterial anastomoses or grafts may sometimes be dilated.

Complications, though infrequent, include embolism, thrombosis of the dilated stenosis, and arterial perforation or rupture; a surgical team should be available to deal with such problems on an emergency basis. In the femoral-popliteal area, where arterial spasm following the dilatation may be a problem, heparin is often used. Antiplatelet therapy is usually employed for several months following the procedure.

Immediate and long-term success rates in properly selected cases are comparable to those achieved by surgical means, and the expense of this form of therapy is considerably less. Results in diabetics and in those who continue to smoke are less favorable.

## Prognosis

Thrombosis of the "bypass" graft or of the endarterectomized vessel either in the immediate postoperative period or months or years later is relatively frequent in the superficial femoral-popliteal area. This is particularly true if iliac arterial stenosis exists or if one or more of the 3 terminal branches of the distal popliteal artery are badly diseased. It is also observed after endarterectomy or when a synthetic prosthesis is used. For this reason, operation is usually not recommended for mild or moderate claudication, and approximately 80% of these patients will have relatively stable symptoms and will go for years without much progression of their symptoms or the development of ischemia or gangrene. Some may improve as collateral circulation develops. The chances of improvement after surgery are less in patients with ischemia or early gangrene, but surgery is often justified because some limbs can be saved from amputation. Failure of the graft or the endarterectomy may make the condition of the limb worse than it was before the procedure and may complicate a subsequent amputation, particularly if the distal anastomosis is to a lower leg artery. The 5-year overall patency rate for the saphenous vein bypass grafts is in the range of 60–80%, or less if the bypass is to a tibial artery. The 2-year patency rate after transluminal angioplasty is over 80% and thus compares favorably with the venous bypass results over that period, although the long-term results may not be as good. Only about 50% of these patients survive 5 years; most deaths are due to complications of atherosclerosis, especially myocardial infarction. After 5 years, the yearly mortality rate exceeds the rate of loss of patency of the graft.

Barry R et al: Prognostic indicators in femoropopliteal and distal bypass grafts. *Surg Gynecol Obstet* 1985;**161:**129.
Morin JF et al: Factors that determine the long term results of percutaneous transluminal dilatation for peripheral arterial occlusive disease. *J Vasc Surg* 1986;**4:**68.

## OCCLUSIVE DISEASE OF THE ARTERIES IN THE LOWER LEG & FOOT

Occlusive processes in the lower leg and foot may involve, in order of incidence, the tibial and common peroneal arteries, the pedal vessels, and occasionally the small digital vessels. Symptoms depend upon the vessels that are narrowed or thrombosed, the suddenness and extent of the occlusion, and the status of the proximal and collateral vessels. The clinical picture may be a rather stable or a slowly progressive form of vascular insufficiency that over months or

## INFECTIONS, ULCERS, & GANGRENE
## OF THE TOES OR FEET

### Early Treatment of Acute Infections

The patient is placed at bed rest with the leg in a horizontal or slightly depressed position. An open or discharging lesion should be covered with a light gauze dressing, but tape should not be used on the skin. If advancing infection is present, an appropriate antibiotic should be started immediately. Dicloxacillin and clindamycin are good choices.

Ulcerations covered with necrotic tissue can often be prepared for spontaneous healing or grafting with wet dressings of sterile saline changed 3–4 times a day. Petrolatum or Xeroform gauze and a bacitracinneomycin ointment may also help soften crusted infected areas and aid drainage.

### Early Management of Established Gangrene

In most instances an area of gangrene will progress to a point where the circulation provided by the inflammatory reaction is sufficient to prevent progressive tissue death. The process will at least temporarily demarcate at that level. This can be encouraged by measures similar to those outlined in the preceding section on the treatment of acute infection. If the skin is intact and the gangrene is dry and due only to arterial occlusion, antibiotics should be withheld. If infection is present or if the gangrene is moist, antibiotics should be used in an effort to limit the process and prevent septicemia.

If the gangrene involves only a segment of skin and the underlying superficial tissue, sympathectomy and, if possible, and artery graft may reverse the process. The necrotic tissue can then be removed and the ulcer grafted or allowed to heal. If amputation is required, it can sometimes be carried out at a more distal level because of those procedures.

### Amputations for Gangrene

(1) A toe that is gangrenous to its base can sometimes be amputated through the necrotic tissue and left open; this procedure may be employed to establish adequate drainage when there is active infection with undrained pus in addition to the gangrene.

(2) When the distal part of the toe is gangrenous and there is sufficient circulation in the proximal toe, closed amputation can be carried out after the area has become well demarcated and inflammation has subsided.

(3) Transmetatarsal amputation can be considered if the gangrene involves one or more toes down to but not into the foot and if the circulation in the distal foot seems adequate to support healing.

(4) Below the knee is the amputation level of choice when gangrene or ischemia in the foot is so distributed that local amputation is not possible. The preservation of the knee and proximal part of the lower leg is most important in that a more useful prosthesis can be applied and the patient can walk. Even when the circulation below the knee is quite poor, successful healing of the stump is often achieved by the use of a meticulous and gentle technique and often a rigid cast to support a well-padded stump dressing. Amputation below the knee should be attempted if there is a chance of success. Amputation through the knee joint will sometimes succeed when a below-knee amputation would fail and provides a much more useful stump than the above-knee amputation.

(5) Amputation above the knee (through the distal thigh in the supracondylar area) is indicated in patients with very advanced peripheral vascular disease requiring amputation because of gangrene, particularly if the leg as well as the foot is extensively involved with infection. It is also employed if an attempted below-knee amputation has failed to heal. Even if the femoral artery is obliterated, there will be sufficient collateral circulation to allow healing provided gentle technique with good hemostasis is used. Few of these patients have the strength and coordination to walk with a prosthesis; most are limited to wheelchair and bed.

(6) Guillotine amputation—Infection with bacteremia or septicemia occasionally develops secondary to gangrene of the lower extremity. This usually requires emergency amputation, and the mortality rate is 30%. In such a situation, it is often wise to leave the stump open so that it can heal by second intention or be revised or reamputated with the infection has been controlled. The mortality rate of a major amputation in this group of poor-risk patients is approximately 10%.

years may ultimately result in atrophy, ischemic pain, and, occasionally, gangrene.

### Clinical Findings

Although all of the possible manifestations of vascular disease in the lower leg and foot cannot be described here, there are certain significant clinical aspects that enter into the evaluation of these patients.

**A. Symptoms and Signs:** Intermittent claudication is the commonest presenting symptom. Aching fatigue during exertion usually appears first in the calf muscles; in more severe cases, a constant or cramping pain may be brought on by walking only a short distance. Less commonly, the feet are the site of most of the pain. The distance the patient can walk before onset of pain is indicative of the degree of circulatory inadequacy: 2 blocks (360–460 m) or more is mild, one block is moderate, and one-half block or less is severe. Rest pain may occur at night and is a dull, persistent ache. As in the case of femoral and popliteal disease, rest pain implies severe involvement. A degree of relief can often be obtained by uncovering the foot and letting it hang over the side of the bed.

Although the popliteal pulse may be present, both pedal pulses are usually absent. Exercise may make pedal pulses disappear in some patients.

Dependent rubor and elevation are prominent. The skin is cool, atrophic, and hairless. Again, these findings may be indistinguishable from those of occlusive disease higher in the leg. The presence of a popliteal pulse points to more distal occlusion when these symptoms and signs are present.

**B. Imaging:** Films of the lower leg and foot may show calcification of the vessels. If there is a draining sinus or an ulcer close to a bone or joint, osteomyelitis may be apparent on the film. If fairly strong popliteal pulses can be felt, arteriography is of little value.

### Treatment

**A. Medical Measures:** Low-dose aspirin has theoretical value and is innocuous as an antiplatelet agent. Pentoxifylline (Trental) is a new drug that affects vessel rheology. It may allow more exercise before claudication develops but does not affect the natural history of the disease.

**B. Circulatory Insufficiency in the Foot and Toes:** Lumbar sympathectomy may be indicated when ischemic or pregangrenous changes are present in the distal foot or when small ulcers are present in a foot with diminished circulation. There is no change in the circulation to the muscles and thus no relief from claudication. Patients who cannot tolerate the surgical procedure may be considered for chemical sympathectomy with 6% phenol. Vasodilator drugs are of little or no value. The general care of the feet is most important (see Chapter 19).

### ARTERIAL DISEASE IN DIABETIC PATIENTS

Atherosclerosis develops more often and earlier in patients with diabetes mellitus, especially if the patient smokes. Either the large or small vessels may be involved, but occlusion of the smaller vessels is more frequent than in the nondiabetic, and diabetics thus more often have the form of the disease that may not be suitable for arterial surgery. Cigarette smoking is particularly harmful and must be strongly interdicted. Ulcers, when present, are more likely to be moist and infected, and healing, if it occurs at all, may be very slow, and healed areas may break down easily.

Diabetic neuropathy with diminished or absent sensation of the toes or feet may occur, predisposing to injury or pressure ulcerations that may be neglected because of the absence of pain. These patients may not necessarily have diminished circulation to the feet.

Poor vision due to diabetic retinopathy makes the care of the feet more difficult and injury more likely. See Chapter 19 for instructions on care of the feet.

Delbridge L: Factors associated with development of foot lesions in the diabetic. *Surgery* 1983;**93**:78.

Samson RH et al: Combined segment arterial disease. *Surgery* 1985;**97**:385.

### OCCLUSIVE CEREBROVASCULAR DISEASE

Although episodes of weakness or dizziness, blurred vision, or sudden complete hemiplegia may be due to a variety of causes, atherosclerotic occlusive or ulcerative disease accounts for many of these problems (see Chapter 16). Single or multiple segmental lesions are often located in the extracranial arteries and account for many ischemic stroke syndromes. The extracranial areas most often involved are (1) the common carotid bifurcation, including the origins of the internal and external carotid arteries (approximately 90%); (2) the origin of the vertebral artery; and (3) the intrathoracic segments of the aortic arch branches.

### Clinical Findings

**A. Symptoms:** Transient ischemic attacks (TIAs) may be the earliest manifestation of carotid arterial stenosis or ulceration, and the episode may last minutes or up to 24 hours. Significant carotid artery stenosis with temporary diminished blood flow to the brain or ulcerations with microemboli from the ulcer to the brain or the ipsilateral retinal artery are responsible for approximately half of TIAs and may precede a complete stroke in many of these patients. The classic manifestations include contralateral weakness or sensory changes, speech alterations, and visual disturbance (usual temporary partial or complete loss of vision in the ipsilateral eye, known as amaurosis fugax. Vertebrobasilar TIAs are characterized by brain stem and cerebellar symptoms, including dysarthria, diplopia, vertigo, ataxia, and alternating hemiparesis or quadriparesis.

Dizziness and unsteadiness, particularly when associated with a quick change in position, are nonspecific and more often the result of postural hypotension than of vertebrobasilar problems. Atypical neurologic symptoms or personality changes are seldom symptoms of cerebral ischemia.

**B. Signs:** Bruits, diminished or absent pulsations, and a blood pressure difference in the 2 arms of more than 10 mm Hg may be indications of occlusive disease in the brachiocephalic arteries. The most significant bruit is one that is sharply localized high in the lateral neck close to the angle of the jaw (overlying the common carotid bifurcation), but a major stenosis sufficient to reduce the blood flow through the vessel is present in only a fourth of these arteries. The murmur of aortic stenosis may be heard as a bruit over the subclavian and carotid arteries; when there is no such heart murmur, the bruit generally denotes disease in these arteries. Bruits are often present without central nervous system symptoms, and the absence of a bruit does not exclude the possibility of carotid artery stenosis. Microemboli can arise from ulcerations of arteries without stenosis or bruit, particularly if the ulcer is large. Only the common carotid and superficial temporal pulses can be felt with accuracy; the internal carotid pulses cannot usually be palpated.

A reduction in the retinal artery pressure as determined by oculoplethysmography may be present on the side of the significant carotid stenosis. The Doppler ultrasound devices are useful in determining information about the collateral flow to the brain by recording the direction of flow in the supraorbital artery with and without compression of the superficial temporal artery. Ultrasonic arteriography, sometimes used with Doppler spectral analysis, may yield a good image of the stenosis provided it is significant in degree. The noninvasive tests presently available are accurate in about 90% of cases and can be helpful in determining which patients need the more definitive x-ray studies. However, even large plaques capable of embolization produce normal results with these studies, which detect only stenosis.

**C. Imaging:** Arteriographic visualization of the brachiocephalic arteries defines the location and degree of stenoses and plaques, the presence of arterial occlusions, and the nature of the collateral flow to the brain in the presence of significant stenoses or thromboses. The study includes the carotid vessels with their intracranial branches and the vertebral-basilar system, usually by means of transfemoral percutaneous catheterization of the aortic arch and its branches (Seldinger technique). Selective arterial injections are safer than aortic arch studies, and digital subtraction angiography, if available, allows for a lower dose of contrast; it is not as sensitive as conventional angiography if used by intravenous injection. It may be a valuable screening test in the latter instance.

## Treatment

**A. Medical Measures:** Acute strokes, most progressive or evolving strokes, and those with major neurologic deficits are treated by medical means as discussed in the section on cerebrovascular accidents in Chapter 16. Patients with transient ischemic attacks may be treated with antiplatelet drugs (dipyridamole [Persantine], 50–75 mg/d, and aspirin, 100–325 mg/d) or with oral anticoagulants (see p 168), though there is now some evidence that the former are both safer and more effective than the latter, particularly in men.

**B. Surgical Measures:** Carotid endarterectomy, when expertly performed, may be offered for properly evaluated transient ischemic attacks of the anterior circulation if the onset of symptoms has been within the previous 2 months. It is crucial that symptoms be specific for cerebral ischemia, that the surgeon be experienced, and that the patient not have any complicating medical illness. There are those who recommend the same treatment for individuals with asymptomatic bruits in the neck who, on further investigation, prove to have carotid stenosis greater than 60–75% of the diameter of the internal carotid; this area remains controversial. Others recommend antiplatelet medication and periodic neurologic evaluation for these patients, supplemented by high-resolution ultrasound or digital subtraction angiography to determine if the carotid stenosis is static or progressing.

Carotid endarterectomy may be employed both for stenosing lesions and for nonstenosing plaques that are embolizing. In the case of the latter, antiplatelet therapy may be more effective.

Endarterectomy may be indicated as an emergency procedure in patients with very early and fluctuating neurologic deficits with significant carotid stenosis. It is not indicated in acute stroke or progressing stroke or when there is also severe intracranial disease. The surgical technique is of great importance in achieving good results, and many advocate the use of a temporary inlying bypass shunt to support cerebral circulation during the endarterectomy. Great care should be taken to avoid hypotension in these patients; general anesthesia is used by many, but others prefer local anesthesia. As in the case of aortic and femoral popliteal disease needing operation, the approach to coexistent coronary artery disease is controversial.

Occlusions at or close to the aortic arch can generally be treated using extrathoracic bypass grafts in the neck connecting a subclavian artery to the ipsilateral carotid artery. If both carotid and vertebral artery stenoses exist, the carotid lesion should be selected for treatment. When the internal carotid artery is completely occluded, microsurgical technique has been used to anastomose the superficial temporal artery to the middle cerebral artery on the surface of the brain; the efficacy of this operation is unproved.

## Prognosis

The prognosis and results of therapy are related to the number of vessels involved, the degree of stenosis in each, the collateral flow in the circle of Willis, and the specific effects of the occlusive disease on the function of the brain. Expertly performed surgery can be done in carefully selected patients with an acceptable mortality rate of 1–2% or less and with 1–4% permanent major or minor neurologic complications. Transient ischemic attacks known to be secondary to significant carotid artery stenosis or ulceration can usually be eliminated by surgery, and although future strokes can occur in such patients, other arterial lesions, such as a contralateral carotid stenosis or intracranial arterial lesions, are usually responsible.

The coronary vessels are generally responsible for a mortality rate that is rather similar in operated and unoperated groups. The operative procedure in patients with transient ischemic attacks is thought to reduce the chance of developing a permanent neurologic deficit within 5 years from 15–35% to 3–5%. The incidence of a later stroke after an uncomplicated endarterectomy is around 5–10%. Significant carotid artery stenosis without symptoms entails no more than a 6–18% stroke risk over 3–5 years.

Hertzer NR et al: Surgical versus non-operative treatment of symptomatic carotid stenosis. *Am Surg* 1986;**204**:154.

Stewart G, Ross-Russell RW, Browse NL: The long-term results of carotid endarterectomy for transient ischemic attacks. *J Vasc Surg* 1986;**4**:600.

Whisnant JP et al: Carotid endarterectomy for unilateral carotid system transient cerebral ischemia. *Mayo Clin Proc* 1983;**58**:171.

## VISCERAL ARTERY INSUFFICIENCY

**Chronic intestinal ischemia** generally results from atherosclerotic occlusive lesions at or close to the origins of the superior mesenteric, celiac, and inferior mesenteric arteries, leading to a significant reduction of blood flow to the intestines. Symptoms may be mild initially, more severe later, and typically consist of epigastric or periumbilical postprandial pains that last for 1–3 hours. To avoid pain, the patient limits oral intake, and weight loss results; at this stage of the illness, pain may be absent. Diarrhea may be present. Such a history in a person over 45 years of age who appears chronically ill and who may have epigastric bruit or findings of peripheral arterial disease is probably an indication for arteriography or digital subtraction angiography, including lateral views of the aorta if the patient is felt to be a candidate for surgery.

**Acute intestinal ischemia** results from (1) embolic occlusions of the visceral branches of the abdominal aorta, generally in patients with heart disease; (2) thrombosis of one or more of the visceral vessels involved with arteriosclerotic occlusive changes, sometimes in patients with a history of abdominal angina as described in Chapter 11; or (3) nonocclusive mesenteric vascular insufficiency, generally in patients with congestive heart failure receiving digitalis therapy or in patients in shock. The acute onset of crampy or steady epigastric and periumbilical abdominal pain combined with minimal or no findings on examination and often a high leukocyte count should suggest one of these 3 events in the superior mesenteric system. Emergency angiography of the superior mesenteric artery is essential for the early diagnosis and treatment of both occlusive and nonocclusive intestinal ischemia and should be performed, if possible, before physical findings develop. Intra-arterial vasodilators may be valuable in rare instances of spasm. If occlusion is present, antibiotics specific for intestinal flora should be instituted (eg, aminoglycoside plus clindamycin or metronidazole) and laparotomy performed to reestablish blood flow and remove necrotic bowel.

Through early diagnosis and aggressive treatment, the very poor prognosis of the past should yield somewhat lower morbidity and mortality rates. If systemic lactic acidosis, hypotension, and abdominal distention develop, frank infarction of bowel has probably occurred. In this instance, salvage of the patient is possible only if the necrotic bowel can be thoroughly resected.

**Ischemic colitis** develops when the diminished circulation is most prominent in the distribution of the inferior mesenteric artery. Because of the nature of the collaterals, infarction is uncommon in this instance. However, the patient may have episodic bouts of crampy lower abdominal pain associated with mild diarrhea, often bloody. This picture may be indistinguishable from inflammatory bowel disease. Colonoscopy shows inflamed areas most commonly in the rectosigmoid and at the splenic flexure (''watersheds'' of collateral circulation). Treatment consists of maintenance of hydration but otherwise does not differ from that of other occlusive diseases. Any surgery is dictated by events elsewhere in the circulation.

Jaxheimer EC et al: Chronic intestinal ischemia. *Surg Clin North Am* 1985;**65**:123.

Rapp JH et al: Durability of endarterectomy and antegrade grafts in the treatment of chronic visceral ischemia. *J Vasc Surg* 1986;**3**:799.

## ACUTE ARTERIAL OCCLUSION

### Essentials of Diagnosis

- Symptoms and signs depend on the artery occluded, the organ or region supplied by the artery, and the adequacy of the collateral circulation to the area primarily involved.
- Occlusion in an extremity usually results in pain, numbness, tingling, weakness, and coldness. There is pallor or mottling; motor, reflex, and sensory alteration; and collapsed superficial veins. Pulsations are absent in arteries distal to the occlusion.
- Occlusions in other areas result in such conditions as cerebrovascular accidents, intestinal ischemia and gangrene, and renal or splenic infarcts.

### Differential Diagnosis

The primary differentiation is between arterial embolism and thrombosis. In an older individual with both arteriosclerotic vascular disease and cardiac disease, the differentiation may be very difficult, and in 10–20% a definite diagnosis either cannot be made or turns out to be incorrect. Arterial trauma may result in either occlusion or spasm.

# 1. ARTERIAL EMBOLISM

Arterial embolism is generally a complication of heart disease; a minority of those with embolism have rheumatic heart disease, but most have ischemic heart disease, with or without myocardial infarction. Atrial fibrillation is often present. Other forms of heart disease and miscellaneous causes account for the rest. In 10%, there is more than one embolism, and recurrent emboli after initial successful treatment may occur.

Emboli tend to lodge at the bifurcation of major arteries, with over half going to the aortic bifurcation or the vessels in the lower extremities; the carotid system is involved in 20%, and the upper extremity and the mesenteric arteries in the remainder. Emboli from arterial ulcerations are usually small, giving rise to transient symptoms in the toes or brain.

## Clinical Findings

In an extremity, the initial symptoms are usually pain (sudden or gradual in onset), numbness, coldness, and tingling. Signs include absence of pulsations in the arteries distal to the block, coldness, pallor or mottling, hypesthesia or anesthesia, and weakness, rigidity, or muscle paralysis. The superficial veins are collapsed. Later, blebs and skin necrosis may appear, and gangrene may occur.

Emboli to the carotid system resulting in stroke cannot be treated surgically.

## Treatment

Immediate embolectomy is the treatment of choice in almost all early cases of emboli in extremities. It should be done within 4–6 hours of the embolic episode if possible. If a longer delay has occurred or if there is clinical evidence of tissue necrosis (particularly in muscle, noted as an area of rigidity), embolectomy may be associated with an unacceptably high mortality rate related to the release of substances from the revascularized but previously ischemic limb; in such circumstances, nonoperative measures (as outlined below) should be employed, and the possibility of amputation at a later date must be accepted in some of these cases. Embolectomy many days after the initial episode may occasionally be successful.

**A. Emergency Preoperative Care:**

**1. Heparin**–Heparin sodium, 5000 units intravenously, should be given as soon as the diagnosis is made or suspected in an effort to prevent distal thrombosis and continued until the time of surgery, maintaining the partial thromboplastin time (PTT) at twice the normal level.

**2. Protect the part**–The extremity is kept at or below the horizontal plane, and neither heat nor cold is applied. The limb must be protected from hard surfaces and overlying bedclothes.

**3. Arteriography**–Arteriography is often of value either before or during surgery. There may be more than one embolus in an extremity; x-ray studies may help locate a distal embolus or determine the extent of the thrombosis.

**B. Surgical Measures:** Local anesthesia is generally used if the occlusion is in an artery to an extremity. After removing the embolus through the arteriotomy, the proximal and distal artery should be explored for additional emboli or secondary thrombi by means of a specially designed catheter with a small inflatable balloon at the tip (Fogarty catheter). An embolus at the aortic bifurcation or in the iliac artery can often be removed under local anesthesia through common femoral arteriotomies with the use of these same catheters. Laparotomy is necessary for emboli to the mesenteric circulation. Heparinization for a week or more postoperatively is indicated, and prolonged anticoagulation with warfarin is usually desirable after that to prevent recurrence.

Delayed embolectomy carried out more than 12 hours following the embolism and when there is also evidence of a considerable degree of ischemia, as shown by mottled cyanosis, muscle paralysis and rigidity, anesthesia, or early evidence of tissue necrosis, involves a high risk of acute respiratory distress syndrome or acute renal shutdown; rapid deterioration and death may result. Anticoagulation in liberal doses rather than surgery is the proper approach under such circumstances even though amputation may become necessary later.

## Prognosis

Arterial embolism is a threat not only to the limb (5–25% amputation rate) but also to the life of the patient (25–30% hospital mortality rate, with the underlying heart disease responsible for over half of these deaths). Emergency surgery, even under local anesthesia, is poorly tolerated by patients with advanced cardiopulmonary disease.

Emboli in the aortoiliac area are more dangerous than more peripheral emboli, and the mortality rate rises if there are multiple peripheral emboli or carotid or visceral emboli; the mortality rate is essentially 100% if all 3 areas are involved. Emboli associated with hypertensive or arteriosclerotic heart disease have a poorer prognosis than those arising from rheumatic valvular disease, and congestive heart failure significantly increases the mortality rate.

In patients with atrial fibrillation, an attempt may be made to restore normal rhythm with quinidine or cardioversion, although restoration of normal rhythm tends to be permanent only in patients with recent or transitory fibrillation. Long-term anticoagulant therapy definitely diminishes the danger of further emboli and in the majority of patients is the only long-term prophylactic measure that can be instituted.

If no heart disease exists, arteriography may reveal an arteriosclerotic ulcer or small aneurysm to be the origin of the embolus; such a defect should be removed.

## 2. ACUTE ARTERIAL THROMBOSIS

Acute arterial thrombosis generally occurs in an artery extensively involved with arteriosclerosis, resulting in almost complete obliteration of the channel. Blood flowing through such a narrow, irregular, or ulcerated lumen may clot, leading to a sudden, complete occlusion of the narrow segment. The thrombosis may then propagate either up or down the artery to a point where the blood is flowing rapidly through a somewhat less diseased artery (usually to a significant arterial branch proximally or one or more functioning collateral vessels distally). Occasionally, the thrombosis is precipitated when the bloodstream dissects and displaces an arteriosclerotic plaque, blocking the lumen; trauma to the artery may precipitate a similar event. Inflammatory involvement of the arterial wall will also lead to acute thrombosis. Chronic mechanical irritation of the subclavian artery compressed by a cervical rib may also lead to a complete occlusion. Thrombosis in a diseased artery may be secondary to an episode of hypotension or cardiac failure. Polycythemia and dehydration also increase the chance of thrombosis.

Chronic, incomplete arterial obstruction usually results in the establishment of some collateral flow, and further flow will develop relatively rapidly through the collaterals once complete occlusion has developed. The extremity may go through an extremely critical period of hours or days, however, while the additional collateral circulation develops around the block. The survival of the tissue distal to the block depends on the development of adequate collateral circulation, which in turn depends on the location and length of the arterial thrombosis and whether conditions such as shock, heart failure, anemia, or hemoconcentration can be corrected promptly.

### Clinical Findings

The local findings in the extremity are usually very similar to those described in the section on arterial embolism. The following differential points should be checked: (1) Are there manifestations of advanced occlusive arterial disease in other areas, especially the opposite extremity (bruit, absent pulses, secondary change as described on p 276)? Is there a history of intermittent claudication? These clinical manifestations are suggestive but not diagnostic of thrombosis. (2) Is there a history or are there findings of rheumatic heart disease or of a recent episode of atrial fibrillation or myocardial infarction? If so, an embolism is more likely than a thrombosis. (3) Electrocardiography and serum enzyme studies may give added information regarding the presence of a silent myocardial infarction and its likelihood as a source of an embolus. Ultimately, arteriography is necessary for accurate differential diagnosis and for planning therapy.

### Treatment

Whereas emergency embolectomy is the usual approach in the case of an early occlusion from an embolus, a nonoperative approach is generally used in the case of thrombosis for 2 reasons: (1) The segment of thrombosed artery may be quite long, requiring rather extensive and difficult surgery (thromboendarterectomy or artery graft). The removal of a single embolus in a normal or nearly normal artery is, by comparison, relatively easy and quick. (2) The extremity is more likely to survive without development of gangrene because some collateral circulation has usually formed during the stenotic phase before acute thrombosis. With an embolism, this is not usually the case; the block is most often at a major arterial bifurcation, occluding both branches, and the associated arterial spasm is usually more acute. There has been recent interest in the direct infusion of streptokinase into thrombotic arterial occlusion of the lower extremities. Much lower doses of the thrombolytic agent can be used. Further study is required to document the efficacy of this procedure.

Treatment is therefore as outlined under emergency preoperative care for arterial embolism. Gradual improvement in the circulation of the distal areas of the extremity is usually noted. If this does not occur or if muscle tenderness and swelling are prominent, early angiography and surgery may be considered, but attempts at revascularization of an ischemic extremity often result in death of the patient. In most cases it is best not to risk the patient's life for the sake of an extremity and to accept the loss of the limb if tissue necrosis is present.

### Prognosis

Limb survival usually occurs with acute thrombosis of the iliac or superficial femoral arteries; gangrene is more likely if the popliteal is suddenly occluded, especially if the period between occlusion and treatment is long or if there is considerable arterial spasm or proximal arterial occlusive disease. If the limb does survive the acute occlusion, a period of observation and evaluation is usually advisable, for significant functional recovery may occur gradually over a number of weeks. The later treatment and prognosis are outlined above in the section on occlusive disease of the iliac, femoral, and popliteal arteries.

Gregg RO et al: Embolectomy or heparin therapy for arterial emboli? *Surgery* 1983;**93**:377.

McPhair NV et al: Management of acute thromboembolic limb ischemia. *Surgery* 1983;**93**:381.

## THROMBOANGIITIS OBLITERANS (TAO) (Buerger's Disease)

### Essentials of Diagnosis

- Almost always in young men who smoke.
- Extremities involved with inflammatory occlusions of the more distal arteries, resulting in circulatory insufficiency of the toes or fingers.
- Thromboses of superficial veins may also occur.
- Course is intermittent and amputation may be necessary, especially if smoking is not stopped.

## General Considerations

Buerger's disease is an episodic and segmental inflammatory and thrombotic process of the arteries and veins, principally in the limbs. The cause is not known. It is seen most commonly in men between ages 25 and 40 who smoke. The effects of the disease are almost solely due to occlusion of the arteries. The symptoms are primarily due to ischemia, complicated in the later stages by infection and tissue necrosis. The inflammatory process is intermittent, with quiescent periods lasting weeks, months, or years.

The arteries most commonly affected are the plantar and digital vessels in the foot and those in the lower leg. The arteries in the hands and wrists may also become involved. Different arterial segments may become occluded in successive episodes; a certain amount of recanalization occurs during quiescent periods. Superficial migratory thrombophlebitis is a common early indication of the disease.

## Clinical Findings

The signs and symptoms are primarily those of arterial insufficiency, and the differentiation from arteriosclerotic peripheral vascular disease may be difficult; however, the following findings suggest Buerger's disease:

(1) The patient is a man between ages 20 and 40 who smokes.

(2) There is a history or finding of small, red, tender cords resulting from migratory superficial segmental thrombophlebitis, usually in the saphenous tributaries rather than the main vessel. A biopsy of such a vein often gives microscopic proof of Buerger's disease.

(3) Intermittent claudication is common and is frequently noted in the palm of the hand or arch of the foot. Rest pain is frequent and persistent. It tends to be more pronounced than in the patient with atherosclerosis. Numbness, diminished sensation, and pricking and burning pains may be present as a result of ischemic neuropathy.

(4) The digit or the entire distal portion of the foot may be pale and cold, or there may be rubor that may remain relatively unchanged by posture; the skin may not blanch on elevation, and on dependency the intensity of the rubor is often more pronounced than that seen in the atherosclerotic group. The distal vascular changes are often asymmetric, so that not all of the toes are affected to the same degree. Absence or impairment of pulsations in the dorsalis pedis, posterior tibial, ulnar, or radial artery is frequent.

(5) Trophic changes may be present, often with painful indolent ulcerations along the nail margins.

(6) There is usually evidence of disease in both legs and possibly also in the hands and lower arms. There may be a history or findings of Raynaud's phenomenon in the finger or distal foot.

(7) The course is usually intermittent, with acute and often dramatic episodes followed by rather definite remissions. When the collateral vessels as well as the main channels have become occluded, an exacerbation is more likely to lead to gangrene and amputation. The course in the patient with atherosclerosis tends to be less dramatic and more persistent.

## Differential Diagnosis

Differences between thromboangiitis obliterans and arteriosclerosis obliterans are discussed above.

Scleroderma causes characteristic skin changes prior to definite vascular findings.

Raynaud's disease causes symmetric bilateral color changes, primarily in young women. There is no impairment of arterial pulsations.

Livedo reticularis and acrocyanosis are vasospastic diseases that do not affect peripheral pulsations.

## Treatment

The principles of therapy are the same as those outlined for atherosclerotic peripheral vascular disease, but the long-range outlook is better in patients with Buerger's disease, so that when possible the approach should be more conservative and tissue loss kept to a minimum.

**A. General Measures:** Smoking must be stopped; the physician must insist on it. The disease is almost sure to progress if this advice is not followed.

See the discussion of instructions in the care of the feet in Chapter 19.

**B. Surgical Measures:**

**1. Sympathectomy–**Sympathectomy may be useful in eliminating the vasospastic manifestations of the disease and aiding in the establishment of collateral circulation to the skin. It may also relieve the mild or moderate forms of rest pain. If amputation of a digit is necessary, sympathectomy may aid in healing of the surgical wound.

**2. Arterial grafts–**Arterial grafting procedures are seldom indicated in patients with Buerger's disease because they do not usually have significant occlusive disease in the iliofemoral region.

**3. Amputation–**The indications for amputation are similar in many respects to those outlined for the atherosclerotic group, although the approach should be more conservative from the point of view of preservation of tissue. Most patients with Buerger's disease who are managed carefully and who stop smoking do not require amputation of the fingers or toes. It is almost never necessary to amputate the entire hand, but amputation below the knee is occasionally necessary because of gangrene or severe pain in the foot.

## Prognosis

Except in the case of the rapidly progressive form of the disease—and provided the patient stops smoking and takes good care of his or her feet—the prognosis for survival of the extremities is good. Buerger's disease rarely results in death.

## IDIOPATHIC ARTERITIS OF TAKAYASU ("Pulseless Disease")

Pulseless disease, most frequent in young women, is an occlusive polyarteritis of unknown cause with a special predilection for the branches of the aortic arch. It occurs most commonly in Asians. Manifestations, depending upon the vessel or vessels involved, may include evidence of cerebrovascular insufficiency, with transient ischemic attacks and visual disturbances; and absent pulses in the arms, with a rich collateral flow in the shoulder, chest, and neck areas.

Pulseless disease must be differentiated from vascular lesions of the aortic arch due to atherosclerosis. Histologically, the arterial lesions are indistinguishable from those of giant cell arteritis. Unless this disease is treated by bypass grafts ensuring adequate blood flow beyond the arterial occlusions, blindness and hemiplegia can result.

## GIANT CELL ARTERITIS

This disorder is discussed in Chapter 16.

## CHOLESTEROL ATHEROEMBOLIC DISEASE

In some patients with severe atherosclerosis involving the aorta and its branches, a distinct syndrome resulting from repeated microembolization has been observed. Patients complain of pain in the abdomen and legs and of mottled lower extremities. Physical examination reveals cholesterol plaques in the optic fundi, livedo reticularis, and reduced arterial pulses (with or without bruits). Laboratory investigations disclose microhematuria, renal insufficiency, eosinophilia, and an accelerated sedimentation rate. Biopsies of the kidney show cholesterol clefts in the small vessels.

Although no specific therapy exists, it is important to recognize this disease, since its similarity to systemic vasculitis may result in inappropriate use of immunomodulating drugs.

---

# VASOMOTOR DISORDERS

---

## RAYNAUD'S DISEASE & RAYNAUD'S PHENOMENON

### Essentials of Diagnosis

- Paroxysmal bilateral symmetric pallor and cyanosis followed by rubor of the skin of the digits.
- Precipitated by cold or emotional upset; relieved by warmth.
- Primarily a disorder of young women.

### General Considerations

Raynaud's disease is the primary, or idiopathic, form of paroxysmal digital cyanosis. Raynaud's phenomenon, which is more common than Raynaud's disease, may be due to a number of regional or systemic disorders. In Raynaud's disease the digital arteries respond excessively to vasospastic stimuli. The cause is not known, but some abnormality of the sympathetic nervous system seems to be active in this entity.

### Clinical Findings

Raynaud's disease and Raynaud's phenomenon are characterized by intermittent attacks of pallor or cyanosis—or pallor followed by cyanosis—in the fingers (and rarely the toes), precipitated by cold or occasionally by emotional upsets. In early attacks of Raynaud's phenomenon, only 1–2 fingertips may be affected; as it progresses, all the fingers down to the distal palm may be involved. The thumbs are rarely affected. General as well as local body cooling may be necessary to cause such attacks. Recovery usually begins near the base of the fingers as a bright red return of color to the cyanotic or pale digit. During recovery there may be intense rubor, throbbing, paresthesia, and slight swelling. Attacks usually terminate spontaneously or upon returning to a warm room or putting the extremity in warm water. Between attacks there may be no abnormal findings. Sensory changes that often accompany vasomotor manifestations include numbness, stiffness, diminished sensation, and aching pain. The condition may progress to atrophy of the terminal fat pads and the digital skin, and gangrenous ulcers may appear near the fingertips; they may heal during warm weather. Although the radial and ulnar pulses are present, these arteries as well as the palmar and particularly the digital vessels may be involved with significant organic obstructive disease. Other patients may have only increased vasomotor tone without organic arterial disease.

Raynaud's disease appears first between ages 15 and 45, almost always in women. It tends to be progressive, and, unlike Raynaud's phenomenon (which may be unilateral and may involve only 1–2 fingers), symmetric involvement of the fingers of both hands is ultimately the rule. Spasm gradually becomes more frequent and prolonged, but the severe changes that may develop in those with Raynaud's phenomenon generally do not occur.

### Differential Diagnosis

Raynaud's disease must be differentiated from the numerous disorders that may be associated with Raynaud's phenomenon. The history and examination lead to the diagnosis of rheumatoid arthritis, systemic sclerosis, systemic lupus erythematosus, and mixed connective tissue disease, with which Raynaud's phenomenon is commonly associated. Raynaud's phenomenon is occasionally the first manifestation of these disorders.

The differentiation from thromboangiitis obliterans

is usually not difficult, since thromboangiitis obliterans is generally a disease of men; peripheral pulses are often diminished or absent; and, when Raynaud's phenomenon occurs in association with thromboangiitis obliterans, it is usually in only one or two digits.

Raynaud's phenomenon may occur in patients with the thoracic outlet syndromes. In these disorders, involvement is generally unilateral, and symptoms referable to brachial plexus compression tend to dominate the clinical picture. Carpal tunnel syndrome should also be considered, and nerve conduction tests are appropriate.

In acrocyanosis, cyanosis of the hands is permanent and diffuse. Frostbite may lead to chronic Raynaud's phenomenon. Ergot poisoning, particularly the prolonged or excessive use of ergotamine, must also be considered.

Finally, Raynaud's phenomenon may be mimicked by cryoglobulinemia, in which serum proteins aggregate in the cooler distal circulation. Cryoglobulinemia may be idiopathic or associated with multiple myeloma and other hyperglobulinemic states.

### Treatment

**A. General Measures:** The body should be kept warm, and the hands especially should be protected from exposure to cold; gloves should be worn when out in the cold. The hands should be protected from injury at all times; wounds heal slowly, and infections are consequently hard to control. Softening and lubricating lotion to control the fissured dry skin should be applied to the hands frequently. Smoking should be stopped.

**B. Vasodilators:** Vasodilators drugs are of limited value but may be of some benefit in those patients who are not adequately controlled by general measures and when there is peripheral vasoconstriction without significant organic vascular disease. With the relatively large doses used, side effects are troublesome. Shortening of temperature recovery time may occur with the use of reserpine, methyldopa, topical nitroglycerin (Transderm-Nitro 5) or a longer-acting oral nitrate, or phenoxybenzamine. Recently, nifedipine has been employed with good effect in the treatment of Raynaud's phenomenon and disease. It may be preferable to other medical measures. Regional medical sympathectomy can be achieved by intravenous injection of reserpine (0.5 mg in 50 mL of saline) into a hand vein after the venous blood has been drained from the extremity and a tourniquet has been inflated to hold the drug in the distal extremity for 20 minutes. If vasospasm is present, a good response may be achieved for about 2 weeks and will often get the patient through an acute exacerbation. The procedure can be easily repeated at intervals as necessary for symptomatic relief.

**C. Surgical Measures:** Sympathectomy may be indicated when attacks have become frequent and severe, interfering with work and well-being—and particularly if trophic changes have developed and

medical measures have failed. In the lower extremities, complete and permanent relief usually results, whereas dorsal sympathectomies generally result in only temporary improvement in approximately 80% of patients treated with operation. Although vascular tone of the vessels in the hands usually ultimately reappears, the symptoms in the fingers that may thus recur in 1–5 years are usually milder and less frequent. When the symptoms do recur, carefully selected drugs may be of help. If the process is due to collagen vascular disease, sympathectomy may be used as an adjuvant to systemic therapy. Sympathectomies are of very limited value in far-advanced cases, particularly if significant digital artery obstructive disease or scleroderma is present.

### Prognosis

Raynaud's disease is usually benign, causing mild discomfort on exposure to cold and progressing very slightly over the years. In a few cases rapid progression does occur, so that the slightest change in temperature may precipitate color changes. It is in this situation that sclerodactyly and small areas of gangrene may be noted, and such patients may become quite disabled by severe pain, limitation of motion, and secondary fixation of distal joints.

## LIVEDO RETICULARIS

Livedo reticularis is a vasospastic disorder of unknown cause that results in constant mottled discoloration on large areas of the extremities, generally in a fishnet pattern with reticulated cyanotic areas surrounding a paler central core. It occurs primarily in young women. It may be associated with an occult malignant neoplasm, polyarteritis nodosa, or atherosclerotic microemboli to the skin.

Livedo reticularis is most apparent on the thighs and forearms and occasionally on the lower abdomen and is most pronounced in cold weather. The color may change to a reddish hue in warm weather but never entirely disappears spontaneously. A few patients complain of paresthesias, coldness, or numbness in the involved areas. In severe cases there may be recurrent ulcerations in the lower extremities.

Bluish mottling of the extremities is diagnostic. The peripheral pulses are normal. The extremity may be cold, with increased perspiration.

Treatment consists of protection from exposure to cold; use of vasodilators is seldom indicated. In most instances, livedo reticularis is entirely benign. The rare patient who develops ulcerations or gangrene should be studied for underlying systemic disease.

## ACROCYANOSIS

Acrocyanosis is an uncommon symmetric condition that involves the skin of the hands and feet and, to a lesser degree, the forearms and legs. It is associated with arteriolar vasoconstriction combined with dilatation of the subpapillary venous plexus of the skin, through which deoxygenated blood slowly circulates. It is worse in cold weather but does not completely disappear during the warm season. It occurs in either sex, is most common in the teens and 20s, and usually improves with advancing age or during pregnancy. It is characterized by coldness, sweating, slight edema, and cyanotic discoloration of the involved areas. Pain, trophic lesions, and disability do not occur, and the peripheral pulses are present. The individual may thus be reassured and encouraged to dress warmly in cold weather.

## ERYTHROMELALGIA
## (Erythermalgia)

Erythromelalgia is a paroxysmal bilateral vasodilative disorder of unknown cause. Idiopathic (primary) erythromelalgia occurs in otherwise healthy persons, rarely in children, and affects men and women equally. A secondary type is occasionally seen in patients with polycythemia vera, hypertension, gout, and organic neurologic diseases.

The chief symptom is bilateral burning distress that lasts minutes to hours, involving circumscribed areas on the soles or palms first and, as the disease progresses, the entire extremity. The attack occurs in response to stimuli producing vasodilatation (eg, exercise, warm environment), especially at night when the extremities are warmed under bedclothes. Reddening or cyanosis as well as heat may be noted. Relief may be obtained by cooling the affected part and by elevation.

No findings are generally present between attacks. With onset of an attack, heat and redness are noted in association with the typical pain. Skin temperature and arterial pulsations are increased, and the involved areas may sweat profusely.

In primary erythromelalgia, aspirin may give excellent relief. The patient should avoid warm environments. In severe cases, if medical measures fail, section or crushing of peripheral nerves may be necessary to relieve pain.

Primary idiopathic erythromelalgia is uniformly benign.

Rodeheffer RJ et al: Controlled double blind trial of nifedipine in the treatment of Raynaud's phenomenon. *N Engl J Med* 1983**308**:880.

## POSTTRAUMATIC SYMPATHETIC DYSTROPHY (Causalgia)

## Essentials of Diagnosis

- Burning or aching pain following trauma to an extremity of a severity greater than that expected from the initiating injury.
- Manifestations of vasomotor instability are gener-

ally present and include temperature, color, and texture alterations of the skin of the involved extremity.

## General Considerations

Pain—usually burning or aching—in an injured extremity is the single most common finding, and the disparity between the severity of the inciting injury and the degree of pain experienced is the most characteristic feature. Crushing injuries with lacerations and soft tissue destruction are the most common causes, but closed fractures, simple lacerations, burns (especially electric), and elective operative procedures are also responsible for this syndrome. It is rare in children. The manifestations of pain and the associated objective changes may be relatively mild or quite severe, and the initial manifestations often change if the condition proceeds to a chronic stage.

## Clinical Findings

In the early stages, the pain, tenderness, and hyperesthesia may be strictly localized to the injured area, and the extremity may be warm, dry, swollen, and red or slightly cyanotic. The involved extremity is held in a splinted position by the muscles, and the nails may become ridged and the hair long. In advanced stages, the pain is more diffuse and worse at night; the extremity becomes cool and clammy and intolerant of temperature changes (particularly cold); and the skin becomes glossy and atrophic. The joints become stiff, generally in a position that makes the extremity useless. The bones become osteoporotic. The dominant concern of the patient may be to avoid the slightest stimuli to the extremity and especially to the trigger points that may develop.

## Prevention

During operations on an extremity, peripheral nerves should be handled only when absolutely necessary and then with utmost gentleness. Splinting of an injured extremity for an adequate period during the early, painful phase of recovery, together with adequate analgesics, may help prevent this condition.

## Treatment & Prognosis

**A. Conservative Measures:** It is most important that the condition be recognized and treated in the early stages, when the manifestations are most easily reversed and major secondary changes have not yet developed. In mild, early cases with minimal skin and joint changes, physical therapy involving active and passive exercises combined with diazepam, 2 mg twice daily, may relieve symptoms. Protecting the extremity from irritating stimuli is important, and the use of nonaddicting analgesics may be necessary.

**B. Surgical Measures:** If the condition fails to respond to conservative treatment or if there are more severe or advanced objective findings, sympathetic blocks (stellate ganglion or lumbar) may be helpful. Intensive physical therapy may be used during the pain-free periods following effective blocks. Patients who achieve significant temporary relief of symptoms after sympathetic blocks but fail to obtain permanent relief by the blocks may be cured by sympathectomy. In the advanced forms—particularly in association with major local changes and emotional reactions—the prognosis for a useful life is poor. The newer neurosurgical approaches using implantable electronic biostimulator devices to block pain impulses in the cervical spinal cord have met with some success.

Garrett WV et al: Posttraumatic pain syndromes: Causalgia and mimocausalgia. In: *Vascular Surgery: Principles and Practice.* Wilson SE et al (editors). McGraw-Hill, 1987.

# VENOUS DISEASES

## VARICOSE VEINS

### Essentials of Diagnosis

- Dilated, tortuous superficial veins in the lower extremities.
- May be asymptomatic or may be associated with fatigue, aching discomfort, or pain.
- Edema, pigmentation, and ulceration of the skin of the distal leg may develop.

### General Considerations

Varicose veins develop predominantly in the lower extremities. They consist of abnormally dilated, elongated, and tortuous alterations in the saphenous veins and their tributaries. These vessels lie immediately beneath the skin and superficial to the deep fascia; they therefore do not have as adequate support as the veins deep in the leg, which are surrounded by muscles. An inherited defect seems to play a major role in the development of varicosities in many instances, but it is not known whether the basic valvular incompetence that exists is secondary to defective valves in the saphenofemoral veins or to a fundamental weakness of the walls of the vein, resulting in dilatation of the vessel. Periods of high venous pressure related to prolonged standing or heavy lifting are contributing factors, and the highest incidence is in women who have been pregnant. Fifteen percent of adults develop varicosities.

Secondary varicosities can develop as a result of obstructive changes and valve damage in the deep venous system following thrombophlebitis, or occasionally as a result of proximal venous occlusion due to neoplasm. Congenital or acquired arteriovenous fistulas are also associated with varicosities.

The long saphenous vein and its tributaries are most commonly involved, but the short saphenous vein may also be affected. There may be one or many incompetent perforating veins in the thigh and lower leg, so that blood can reflux into the varicosities not only from above, by way of the saphenofemoral junction, but also from the deep system of veins through the incompetent perforators in the mid thigh or lower leg. Largely because of these valvular defects in the most proximal valve of the long saphenous vein or in the distal communicating veins, venous pressure in the superficial veins does not fall appreciably on walking; over the years, the veins progressively enlarge, and the surrounding tissue and skin develop secondary changes such as fibrosis, chronic edema, and skin pigmentation and atrophy.

### Clinical Findings

**A. Symptoms:** The severity of the symptoms caused by varicose veins is not necessarily correlated with the number and size of the varicosities; extensive varicose veins may produce no subjective symptoms, whereas minimal varicosities may produce many symptoms, especially in women. Dull, aching heaviness or a feeling of fatigue brought on by periods of standing is the most common complaint. Cramps may occur, often at night, and elevation of the legs typically relieves symptoms. One must be careful to distinguish between the symptoms of arteriosclerotic peripheral vascular disease, such as intermittent claudication and coldness of the feet, and symptoms of venous disease, since occlusive arterial disease usually contraindicates the operative treatment of varicosities distal to the knee. Itching from an associated eczematoid dermatitis may occur above the ankle.

**B. Signs:** Dilated, tortuous, elongated veins beneath the skin in the thigh and leg are generally readily visible in the standing individual, although in very obese patients palpation may be necessary to detect their presence and location. Secondary tissue changes may be absent even in extensive varicosities; but if the varicosities are of long duration, brownish pigmentation and thinning of the skin above the ankle are often present. Swelling may occur, but signs of severe chronic venous stasis such as extensive swelling, fibrosis, pigmentation, and ulceration of the distal lower leg usually denote the postphlebitic state.

**C. Trendelenburg's Test:** This test is of use in determining competence at the proximal end of the long saphenous vein close to the saphenofemoral junction, in the long saphenous vein in the thigh and leg, and in the communicating veins between superficial and deep vessels.

1. With the patient supine, elevate the leg. If there is no organic venous obstruction, varicosities will empty immediately.

2. Place a rubber tourniquet around the upper thigh and ask the patient to stand.

a. If the long saphenous vein remains empty for 30 seconds or more and then fills very slowly from below over a period of 1–2 minutes, the valves close to the saphenofemoral junction are incompetent, the valves in the communicating veins are competent, and the blood is flowing through them in the normal direction (superficial to deep). On release of the tourniquet, if the veins fill rapidly from above, the incompetence of the proximal valves is confirmed.

b. If the varicosities fill rapidly, the communicating veins between the deep and the superficial vessels are incompetent and blood is refluxing into the varicosed vessels. If, on release of the tourniquet, no additional filling of the varicosities occurs, the valves in the saphenous vein close to the saphenofemoral junction are competent; if, on the other hand, further distention of the varicosities occurs when the tourniquet is released, the valves at the upper end of the long saphenous vein are also incompetent. The precise site of these defective perforating veins can often be determined by repetition of this maneuver while placing the tourniquet at successively lower levels or using 2 or 3 tourniquets at different levels. If varices in the posterior leg fill within less than 30 seconds with the tourniquet at the level of the mid thigh but remain relatively empty with the tourniquet at the level of the knee, an incompetent short saphenous vein should be suspected.

## Differential Diagnosis

Primary varicose veins should be differentiated from those secondary to (1) chronic venous insufficiency of the deep system of veins (the postphlebitic syndrome); (2) retroperitoneal vein obstruction from extrinsic pressure or fibrosis; (3) arteriovenous fistula (congenital or acquired)—a bruit is present and a thrill is often palpable; and (4) congenital venous malformation. Venography may be of value in the investigation of some of these problems. Pain or discomfort secondary to arthritis, radiculopathy, or arterial insufficiency should be distinguished from symptoms associated with coexistent varicose veins.

## Complications

If thin, atrophic, pigmented skin has developed at or above the ankle, secondary ulcerations may occur—often as a result of little or no trauma. An ulcer will occasionally extend into the varix, and the resulting fistula will be associated with profuse hemorrhage unless the leg is elevated and local pressure is applied to the bleeding point.

Chronic stasis dermatitis with fungal and bacterial infection may be a problem.

Thrombophlebitis may develop in the varicosities, particularly in postoperative patients, pregnant or postpartum women, or those taking oral contraceptives. Local trauma or prolonged periods of sitting may also lead to superficial venous thrombosis. Extension of the thrombosis into the deep venous system by way of the perforating veins or through the saphenofemoral junction may occur.

## Prevention

Individuals with early or minimal varicosities, particularly if there is a family history of varicosities and their activities involve a great deal of standing, should use elastic stockings to protect their veins from the chronic venous hypertension that is not reduced by walking. Elastic stockings are particularly important in these individuals if pregnancy occurs. They are best put on before getting out of bed.

## Treatment

**A. Nonsurgical Measures:** The use of elastic stockings (medium or heavy weight) to give external support to the veins of the proximal foot and leg up to but not including the knee is the best nonoperative approach to the management of varicose veins. When elastic stockings are worn during the hours that involve much standing and when this is combined with the habit of elevation of the legs when possible, reasonably good control can be maintained and progression of the condition and the development of complications can often be avoided. This approach may be used in elderly patients, in those who refuse or wish to defer surgery, sometimes in women with mild or moderate varicosities who plan to have more children, and in those with mild asymptomatic varicosities.

**B. Surgical Measures:** The surgical treatment of varicose veins consists of interruption or removal of the varicosities and the incompetent perforating veins. Accurate delineation and division of the latter are required to prevent recurrence in the varicosities that are not to be removed. The most important phase of the procedure is transection and ligation of the incompetent long saphenous vein precisely at its junction with the common femoral vein, combined with ligation and division of the 5 or 6 tributaries joining the terminal 3–10 cm of this vein. The previously marked incompetent perforating veins and the large varicosed tributaries of the saphenous system can then be ligated and the long saphenous vein removed by the stripping method. The same technique may be applied to the short saphenous vein if varicosed, as it occasionally is. If the stripping procedure is not considered necessary or desirable, as in older individuals or those with minimal varicosities, the entire operation can be done under local anesthesia. Venous segments that are not demonstrated to be incompetent and varicosed should not be ligated or removed; they may be needed as artery grafts later in the patient's life.

Varicose ulcers that are small generally heal with local care, frequent periods of elevation of the extremity, and compression bandages or some form of compression boot dressing for the ambulatory patient. It is best to defer a stripping procedure until healing has been achieved and stasis dermatitis has been controlled. Some ulcers require skin grafting.

**C. Compression Sclerotherapy:** Sclerotherapy to obliterate and produce permanent fibrosis of the collapsed veins is generally reserved for the treatment of residual small varicosities following definitive varicose vein surgery, although it is used by some who have become very competent in this technique as a primary form of treatment. With the patient reclining and following the aspiration of all blood from an isolated segment of vein, an injection of 0.5 mL sclerosing solution into the vein is made (3% sodium tetradecyl sulfate [Sotradecol] is often used), and this is followed by ambulation with continuous pressure to that segment of vein for 1–4 weeks. Complications such as phlebitis, tissue necrosis, or infection may occur.

## Prognosis

Patients should be informed that even extensive and carefully performed surgery may not prevent the development of additional varicosities and that further (though usually more limited) surgery or scleropathy may be necessary in later years. Good results with relief of symptoms are usually obtained in most patients. If extensive varicosities reappear after surgery, the completeness of the high ligation should be questioned, and reexploration of the saphenofemoral area may be necessary. Even after adequate treatment, secondary tissue changes may not regress.

## THROMBOPHLEBITIS

Thrombophlebitis is partial or complete occlusion of a vein by a thrombus with secondary inflammatory reaction in the wall of the vein. The thrombotic process, once established, is generally quite similar in all cases no matter what the cause, although the initiating factors may be quite variable. Trauma to the endothelium of the vein wall resulting in exposure of subendothelial tissues to platelets in the venous blood may initiate thrombosis, especially if a degree of venous stasis also exists. Platelet aggregates form on the vein wall followed by the deposition of fibrin, leukocytes, and finally erythrocytes; a thrombus results that can then propagate along the veins as a free-floating clot. Within 7–10 days, this thrombus becomes adherent to the vein wall, and secondary inflammatory changes develop, although a free-floating tail may persist. The thrombus is ultimately invaded by fibroblasts, resulting in scarring of the vein wall and destruction of the valves. Central recanalization may occur later, with restoration of flow through the vein; however, because the valves do not recover function, directional flow is not reestablished, leading in turn to secondary functional and anatomic problems.

## 1. THROMBOPHLEBITIS OF THE DEEP VEINS

### Essentials of Diagnosis

- Pain in the calf or thigh, occasionally associated with swelling; or may be clinically silent.
- History of congestive heart failure, recent surgery, neoplasia, oral contraceptive use, or varicose veins.
- Physical signs unreliable.
- Ultrasound and plethysmography are abnormal; venography is diagnostic.

### General Considerations

The deep veins of the lower extremities and pelvis are most frequently involved. The process begins approximately 80% of the time in the deep veins of the calf, although it can arise in the femoral or iliac veins. Radioisotope fibrinogen uptake studies on postoperative or posttrauma patients reveal the development of small thrombi in the deep calf veins within 24 hours in 27% of patients studied, and propagation of the thrombosis into the popliteal and femoral veins takes place in approximately 10% of these cases. The process may become clinically detectable 4–14 days following major surgery or trauma or the end of pregnancy. Approximately 3% of patients undergoing major general surgical procedures will develop clinical manifestations of thrombophlebitis; many others with the process will have no detectable findings. Many patients undergoing total hip replacement develop evidence of thromboembolic complications. Illnesses that involve periods of bed rest, such as cardiac failure, stroke, sepsis, or cancer, are associated with a high incidence of thrombophlebitis, especially if shock, obesity, or dehydration is also present. Use of oral contraceptive drugs, especially by women over 30 and by those who smoke, may be associated with hypercoagulability, resulting in thrombophlebitis in some women. These drugs should not be prescribed for women with a history of phlebitis.

### Clinical Findings

Approximately half of patients with thrombophlebitis have no symptoms or signs in the extremity in the early stages. The patient often suffers a pulmonary embolism, presumably from the leg veins, without symptoms or demonstrable abnormalities in the extremities.

**A. Symptoms:** The patient may complain of a dull ache, a tight feeling, or frank pain in the calf or, in more extensive cases, the whole leg, especially when walking.

**B. Signs:** Typical findings, though variable and unreliable and in about half of cases absent, are as follows: slight swelling in the involved calf, distention of the superficial venous collaterals; and slight fever and tachycardia. Any of these signs may occur without deep vein thrombosis. When the femoral and iliac veins are also involved, there may be tenderness over these veins, and the swelling in the extremity may be marked. The skin may be cyanotic if venous obstruction is severe, or pale and cool if a reflex arterial spasm is superimposed.

**C. Diagnostic Techniques:** Because of the difficulty in making a precise diagnosis by history and examination and because of the morbidity associated with treatment, diagnostic studies are essential.

1. Ascending contrast venography, the most accurate and complete method of diagnosis thus far available, will define by x-ray means the location, extent, and degree of attachment of the thrombosis (thrombi in the profunda femoris and internal iliac veins will not be demonstrated). Bilateral studies are

of importance in planning therapy. Because of the time, expense, and discomfort involved, this test is not used as a screening study and is unsuitable for repeated monitoring. It is particularly useful when the clinical picture strongly suggests calf vein thromboses but noninvasive tests are equivocal. It may on occasion produce or exacerbate a thrombotic process, but this occurs in less than 5% of patients.

2. The Doppler ultrasound blood flow detector allows the major veins in an extremity to be examined for thrombosis. This test is of value as a rapid screening procedure for the detection of thrombosis in large veins in high-risk patients, and it may be particularly helpful in detecting an extension of small thrombi in the calf veins (see ¶ 2 above) into the popliteal and femoral veins. This test is inexpensive but operator-dependent; it relies on sonic differences in flow rates that occur with inspiration in normal veins. Incompetent venous valves in the legs may also be inferred from this investigation. Venous plethysmography may similarly be used to detect the alteration of venous flow by obstruction of thrombi. Small thrombi in calf veins when collateral channels are patent or even large thrombi in the main channel if not fully obstructing may be missed. The combination of a Doppler examination and plethysmography is more sensitive and specific than either test alone. Because the accuracy of these methods in detecting main channel deep venous obstruction is approaching 85–95%, the decision to start anticoagulation therapy can be based in most cases on one or more of these tests. If available, these tests should be employed rather than starting anticoagulant therapy on the basis of clinical impression only.

3. Radionuclide venography may be performed at the time of lung scanning. The isotope may be injected into a foot vein and immediate views obtained as the radionuclide moves up the circulation. In venous thrombosis, isotope accumulates at the clot and is not cleared. This test may also detect intra-abdominal venous thrombi—an advantage over Doppler ultrasound and plethysmography.

## Differential Diagnosis

Calf muscle strain or contusion may be difficult to differentiate from thrombophlebitis; phlebography may be required to determine the correct diagnosis.

Cellulitis may be confused with thrombophlebitis; with infection, there is usually an associated wound, and inflammation of the skin is more marked.

Obstruction of the lymphatics or the iliac vein in the retroperitoneal area from tumor or irradiation may lead to unilateral swelling, but it is usually more chronic and painless. An acute arterial occlusion is more painful, the distal pulses are absent, there is usually no swelling, and the superficial veins in the foot fill slowly when emptied.

Bilateral leg edema is more likely to be due to heart or kidney disease.

Occasionally, a ruptured or dissected Baker cyst may produce unilateral pain and swelling in the calf.

A history of arthritis in the knee of the same leg is a clue to diagnosis, and the patient may report disappearance of the popliteal cyst at the time symptoms develop.

## Complications

**A. Pulmonary Thromboembolism:** See p 165.

**B. Chronic Venous Insufficiency:** Chronic venous insufficiency with or without secondary varicosities is a late complication of deep thrombophlebitis. (See Chronic Venous Insufficiency, below.)

## Prevention

Prophylactic measures may diminish the incidence of venous thrombosis in hospitalized patients.

**A. Nonpharmacologic Means:** Venous stasis may be avoided by the following measures–

1. Elevation of the foot of the bed 15–20 degrees will encourage venous flow from the legs, particularly if the head of the bed is kept low or horizontal. Slight flexion of the knees is desirable. This position is also maintained on the operating table and in the recovery room.

2. Leg exercises, carried out by the surgical team immediately following major surgery and during the early postoperative period and practiced by the patient when in bed, are important. A few minutes every hour of leg exercises against a footboard are helpful. The importance of frequent leg movements and exercises as well as ambulation and very limited chair sitting should be explained to patients so as to secure their cooperation.

3. Elastic antiphlebitic stockings may be employed, particularly in patients with varicose veins or a history of phlebitis who will require bed rest for a number of days.

4. Walking for brief but regular periods postoperatively and during long airplane and automobile trips should be encouraged, because active, healthy travelers may sometimes develop thrombotic problems.

**B. Anticoagulation:** Anticoagulants may be used in patients considered at high risk for venous thrombosis.

1. Low-dose heparin, 5000 units every 12 hours subcutaneously 2 hours preoperatively and during the postoperative period of bed rest and limited ambulation, appears to be effective in reducing the incidence of thromboembolic complications in high-risk patients, although its effectiveness in major pelvic and hip procedures has been disappointing. Significant postoperative or posttrauma bleeding is not generally a problem. The partial thromboplastin time (PTT) should be used to monitor therapy; a minimum of 1½ times control elevation may be adequate. Heparin should not be given whenever limited bleeding would be dangerous, such as in brain and eye surgery.

2. Aspirin, 150 mg daily, may have a prophylactic value when used both pre- and postoperatively.

## Treatment

**A. Local Measures:** The legs should be elevated

15–20 degrees, the trunk should be kept horizontal, and the head and shoulders may be supported with pillows. The legs should be slightly flexed at the knees. Bed rest should be maintained until local tenderness and swelling have disappeared, by which time the thrombus has generally become adherent to the vein wall; a week may be adequate for calf thrombosis and 10–14 days for thigh or pelvic thrombosis. Walking but not standing or sitting is then permitted; the time out of bed and walking is increased each day.

Below-the-knee elastic support may be started soon after diagnosis and should be used when ambulation is started and continued for a number of months, or years if the process has been extensive. Intermittent elevation of the legs is also important.

**B. Medical Measures (Anticoagulants):** Therapy with anticoagulants is considered to be the preferred treatment in most cases of deep thrombophlebitis with or without pulmonary embolism. There is evidence that the incidence of fatal pulmonary embolism secondary to venous thrombosis is reduced by adequate anticoagulant therapy, and the incidence of death from additional emboli following an initial embolism is apparently reduced from approximately 20% to 1–2%. Progressive thrombosis with its associated morbidity is also reduced considerably, and the chronic secondary changes in the involved leg are probably also less severe. When embolic fatalities do occur during well-established and adequate heparin therapy, it is likely that the thrombus responsible has already developed to the point of insensitivity to heparin. Heparin acts rapidly and must be considered the anticoagulant of choice for short-term therapy; it can only be given parenterally, so hospitalization is necessary. After the initial phase of therapy with heparin, and if a prolonged period of anticoagulation is advisable, an oral drug can be used.

Treatment with heparin does not affect thrombi that have already developed but stops propagation and allows fibrinolysis to occur. The duration of therapy is purely an empirical decision—most clinicians administer heparin for 7–10 days and oral anticoagulants for at least 6 weeks, but data to support these regimens are sparse. Permanent anticoagulation is probably justified if the stimulus to thrombosis is chronic—eg, congestive heart failure, postphlebitic syndrome—or if previous episodes have occurred. As experience with thrombolysis develops (see below), it may replace heparin as the treatment of first choice.

**1. Heparin**–Before starting heparin therapy, baseline coagulation studies should be obtained that should include a prothrombin time, a partial thromboplastin time, a bleeding time, a blood urea nitrogen measurement, and a platelet count. The therapeutic range of the commonly used partial thromboplastin time (PTT) is considered to be $1\frac{1}{2}$–$2\frac{1}{2}$ times the baseline pretreatment value. Because the test can be done easily, any necessary adjustment in the heparin dose can be made immediately. Serious bleeding com-

plications, such as bleeding into the brain or retroperitoneum, are more likely to occur in patients with other serious concomitant illnesses; in patients over age 60 (especially women); in patients with hypertension, uremia, hemostatic defects, or duodenal ulcer; or in patients who have had recent trauma or surgery.

The dose of heparin required to maintain the PTT at a therapeutic level may vary considerably with individuals or even in the same patient at different times during the course of treatment. The required dose is typically highest within the first days of therapy. Platelet counts should be performed every 2–3 days, and if thrombocytopenia develops, heparin should be discontinued. A hematocrit and a test on urine and stool for occult blood every 2–3 days may help detect bleeding. Aspirin and similar anti-inflammatory drugs and intramuscular medication should be avoided during heparin therapy.

Continuous intravenous infusion of heparin by means of a reliable infusion pump is favored over intermittent intravenous or subcutaneous therapy. Before starting the constant infusion, an initial loading dose of heparin should be given intravenously as a bolus (100 units/kg is often used). The constant infusion may then be started so that the average-sized adult receives 1500 units of heparin per hour (250–500 mL of 5% dextrose solution containing 100 units/mL is a convenient concentration), and the hourly dose is subsequently adjusted depending on laboratory determinations performed every 2–3 hours on blood drawn from the arm not being infused. A heparin algorithm combined with an easily interpreted flowchart giving specific instructions with respect to the volume per hour required to deliver the desired dose of heparin is a great help to personnel who administer this potentially dangerous drug. After a stable infusion rate has been achieved, as determined by at least 2 successive PTTs in the therapeutic range, subsequent laboratory control may be repeated every 8–12 hours or possibly less often if a stable state develops. The therapeutic dose of heparin usually becomes less within 2–4 days.

**2. Oral anticoagulants**–The shift to the prothrombin depressant drugs usually occurs after the symptoms and signs of thrombosis have largely or completely subsided and after the patient becomes ambulatory. Heparin may thus be used for the first 7–14 days and withdrawn only when the prothrombin time is therapeutic for 3–4 days, by which time the full anticoagulant effects of the drug will have taken place.

Prothrombin depressant drugs include coumarin and indandione derivatives; of these, warfarin sodium (Coumadin) is most commonly used now. The dose during the first 48 hours of therapy is usually 10–15 mg/d. The usual maintenance dose is 2.5–7.5 mg daily and must be determined for each individual patient. The approximate duration of effect of the drug is 2–3 days. A pretreatment prothrombin time should be determined, and if it is prolonged as compared with the control value, less drug should be used. Smaller doses should be used in the elderly, in patients with kidney or liver disease, and in those with congestive heart failure or chronic illness. These drugs are contraindicated during pregnancy. Interaction with many other drugs does occur, and the anticoagulant effect may be either potentiated or reduced; this possibility must be considered if the individual is already receiving other drugs at the time the anticoagulant is started. Attention to the maintenance dose is also required when a new drug which enhances or inhibits the anticoagulant effect is added or one which was in use is withdrawn. Interacting drugs should be avoided if possible. Many of the drugs that increase and decrease the sensitivity to coumarins are listed in Table 2 of the Appendix.

A good therapeutic effect can usually be achieved in 3–5 days and exists when the prothrombin time is around one and one-half to two and one-half times the control value. Further prolongation of the prothrombin time may result in bleeding complications (ie, hematuria, ecchymosis, epistaxis, gastrointestinal bleeding); even within the therapeutic range, complications are less common when prothrombin time is near 1½ times control, without loss of benefit. At the beginning of treatment, daily prothrombin times should be determined and the subsequent dose withheld until the report is received. In well-stabilized patients, weekly to monthly determination may be adequate.

**3. Treatment of bleeding and overdosage–** Any new development that occurs in a patient receiving anticoagulant therapy should be considered to be a complication of the anticoagulant until proved otherwise. Whereas bleeding complications will occur in at least 3% and death will result in 0.3% of patients receiving anticoagulants, the incidence of complications is considerably higher with heparin therapy and may be as high as 25–35% in some groups. Complications appear most frequently after the first 3 days of heparin; they are infrequent when heparin is being given while diagnostic studies are in progress to determine whether thrombophlebitis is present. Phytonadione (Mephyton [oral] or AquaMephyton [intravenous]) will counteract the effect of prothrombin depressant drugs, and if transfusion is necessary, fresh frozen plasma should be used. When the vitamin K analogs are given subcutaneously, their duration of action may be very long. Thus, if reanticoagulation is contemplated, intravenous phytonadione in low dosage (1 mg) should be used. When gastrointestinal or urologic bleeding occurs in a patient receiving anticoagulant therapy, investigation for an anatomic lesion is mandated.

**4. Thrombolytic therapy–**The ideal treatment for thrombophlebitis involving the iliac, femoral, or popliteal veins or for a major pulmonary embolism would involve removal of the thrombus and restoration of blood flow through vessels that have been cleaned of the thrombus with little or no damage to their walls or valves. Heparin will not remove a thrombus and only serves to halt an ongoing thrombotic process. Streptokinase and urokinase, potent and expensive thrombolytic agents, will clear the vessels of fresh clots and may restore them to normal function. As experience with these drugs increases, it appears that their safety approaches that of heparin. Since streptokinase is much less expensive than urokinase, it is preferable; however, since it is antigenic, subsequent use may not be possible. Treatment of deep venous thrombophlebitis with thrombolytic agents preserves valvular function in a fashion superior to heparin, and it may be less likely that patients so treated will develop postphlebitic syndrome. Concomitant arterial thrombi in the cerebral circulation contraindicate the use of the thrombolytics. After the initial treatment, anticoagulation is maintained with warfarin (see above). A loading dose of 250,000 units of streptokinase is administered over a 30-minute period, and 100,000 units per hour is given for 72 hours. The thrombin time (TT) is monitored for efficacy and kept at 2–5 times control. After discontinuation—and until TT is less than twice normal—heparin is begun until therapeutic levels of concomitantly given warfarin are achieved as outlined.

**C. Surgical Measures:** An inferior vena caval filter device may be inserted under local anesthesia through the right internal jugular vein to the third lumbar level, using radiologic control. This approach is considerably safer than surgical ligation, is quite effective in trapping further emboli, generally does not result in later caval occlusion, and is now the preferred means of preventing embolism in those who require mechanical protection.

**1. Vein interruption–**Ligation or plication of the inferior vena cava with a partially occluding plastic clip may be recommended when anticoagulant therapy is contraindicated or if a filter cannot be placed. Examples are patients with bleeding peptic ulcer, those with malignant hypertension with retinopathy; those with a history of cerebrovascular hemorrhage or recent head trauma; or those who are 1–3 days postoperative, especially if the operation has involved extensive dissection or surgery on the brain or spinal cord. Caval interruption is also indicated if emboli continue to occur during adequate anticoagulant therapy (3–16% of patients) or if septic phlebitis is present. After ligation, emboli may still occur, and the surgical mortality rate is about 7–20%. Although some degree of chronic edema of the legs may develop as a result of ligation (15–30%), it can usually be minimized if anticoagulant therapy can be resumed 1–2 days following surgery and if follow-up care, consisting of elastic supports to the lower legs and elevation of the legs at intervals, is continued for at least 1 year (see next section).

**2. Femoral vein thrombectomy–**In the rare case of massive venous occlusion that has not responded to elevation of the leg, heparin, and fluid and electrolyte replacement, thrombectomy to remove the iliofemoral thrombosis with the use of balloon-tipped catheters may be considered if the condition is of recent onset (1–2 days) and venous gangrene is considered a possibility.

## Prognosis

With adequate treatment the patient usually returns to normal health and activity within 3–6 weeks. The prognosis in most cases is good once the period of danger of pulmonary embolism has passed. Occasionally, recurrent episodes of phlebitis will occur in spite of good local and anticoagulant management. Such cases may even have recurrent pulmonary emboli as well. Chronic venous insufficiency may result, with its associated complications.

Conti S et al: A comparison of high-dose versus conventional-dose heparin therapy for deep vein thrombosis. *Surgery* 1982;**92:**972.

Greenfield LJ et al: Greenfield vena caval filter experience: Late results in 156 patients. *Arch Surg* 1981;**116:**1451.

Hirsch J: Therapeutic range for the control of oral anticoagulant therapy. (Editorial.) *Arch Intern Med* 1985;**145:**1187.

O'Donnell TF et al: Diagnosis of deep venous thrombosis in the outpatient by venography. *Surg Gynecol Obstet* 1980;**150:**69.

Salzman EW, Davies GC: Prophylaxis of venous thromboembolism, *Ann Surg* 1980;**191:**207.

Wessler S, Gitel SN: Warfarin: From bedside to bench. *N Engl J Med* 1984;**311:**645.

## 2. THROMBOPHLEBITIS OF THE SUPERFICIAL VEINS

### Essentials of Diagnosis

- Induration, redness, and tenderness along a superficial vein.
- Often a history of recent intravenous line or trauma.
- No significant swelling of the extremity.

### General Considerations

Superficial thrombophlebitis may occur spontaneously, as in pregnant or postpartum women or in individuals with varicose veins or thromboangiitis obliterans; or it may be associated with trauma, as in the case of a blow to the leg or following intravenous therapy with irritating solutions. It may also be a manifestation of abdominal cancer such as carcinoma or the pancreas and may be the earliest sign. The long saphenous vein is most often involved. Superficial thrombophlebitis may be associated with occult deep vein thrombosis in about 20% of cases. Pulmonary emboli are rare.

Short-term plastic venous catheterization of superficial arm veins is now in routine use. The catheter should be observed daily for signs of local inflammation. It should be removed if a local reaction develops in the veins. Serious thrombotic or septic complications can occur if this policy is not followed. The steel intravenous needle with the anchoring flange (butterfly needle) is less likely to be associated with phlebitis and infection than the plastic catheter, but this may be due to its remaining in place for shorter periods.

### Clinical Findings

The patient usually experiences a dull pain in the region of the involved vein. Local findings consist of induration, redness, and tenderness along the course of a vein. The process may be localized, or it may involve most of the long saphenous vein and its tributaries. The inflammatory reaction generally subsides in 1–2 weeks; a firm cord may remain for a much longer period. Edema of the extremity and deep calf tenderness are absent unless deep thrombophlebitis has also developed. If chills and high fever develop, septic thrombophlebitis exists.

### Differential Diagnosis

The linear rather than circular nature of the lesion and the distribution along the course of a superficial vein serve to differentiate superficial phlebitis from cellulitis, erythema nodosum, erythema induratum, panniculitis, and fibrositis. Lymphangitis and deep thrombophlebitis must also be considered.

### Treatment

If the process is well localized and not near the saphenofemoral junction, local heat and bed rest with the leg elevated are usually effective in limiting the thrombosis. The resolution of the inflammatory process may be aided by use of one of the nonsteroidal anti-inflammatory drugs.

If the process is very extensive or is progressing upward toward the saphenofemoral junction, or if it is in the proximity of the saphenofemoral junction initially, ligation and division of the saphenous vein at the saphenofemoral junction are indicated. The inflammatory process usually regresses following this procedure, though removal of the involved segment of vein (stripping) may result in a more rapid recovery.

Anticoagulation therapy is usually not indicated unless the disease is rapidly progressing. It is indicated if there is extension into the deep system.

Septic thrombophlebitis requires excision of the involved vein up to its junction with an uninvolved vein in order to control bacteremia.

### Prognosis

The course is generally benign and brief, and the prognosis depends on the underlying pathologic process. Phlebitis of a saphenous vein occasionally extends to the deep veins, in which case pulmonary embolism may occur.

## CHRONIC VENOUS INSUFFICIENCY

### Essentials of Diagnosis

- A history is often obtained of phlebitis or leg injury.
- Ankle edema is the earliest sign.

- Stasis pigmentation, dermatitis, subcutaneous induration, and often varicosities occur later.
- Ulceration at or above the ankle is common (stasis ulcer).

## General Considerations

Chronic venous insufficiency generally results from changes secondary to deep thrombophlebitis, although a definite history of phlebitis is not obtainable in about 25% of these patients. There is often a history of leg trauma. It can also occur in association with varicose veins and as a result of neoplastic obstruction of the pelvic veins or congenital or acquired arteriovenous fistula.

When insufficiency is secondary to deep thrombophlebitis (the postphlebitic syndrome), the valves in the deep venous channels of the lower leg have been damaged or destroyed by the thrombotic process. The recanalized, nonelastic deep veins are functionally inadequate because of the damaged valves in the deep and perforating veins. The antegrade venous flow ensured by the valves and the calf muscle pump is lost, resulting in bidirectional flow and abnormally high ambulatory venous pressures in the calf veins in particular. The high ambulatory venous pressure transmitted through the communicating veins to the subcutaneous veins and tissues of the calf and ankle areas results in a series of deleterious secondary changes, including edema, fibrosis of subcutaneous tissue and skin, pigmentation of skin, and, later, dermatitis, cellulitis, and ulceration. Dilatation of the superficial veins may occur, leading to varicosities. Whereas primary varicose veins with no abnormality of the deep venous system may be associated with some similar changes, the edema is more pronounced in the postphlebitic extremities, and the secondary changes are more extensive and encircling.

## Clinical Findings

Chronic venous insufficiency is characterized first by progressive edema of the leg (particularly the lower leg) and later also by secondary changes in the skin and subcutaneous tissues. The usual symptoms are itching, a dull discomfort made worse by periods of standing, and pain if an ulceration is present. The skin is usually thin, shiny, atrophic, and cyanotic; and a brownish pigmentation often develops. Eczema may be present, with superficial weeping dermatitis. The subcutaneous tissues become thick and fibrous. Recurrent ulcerations may occur, usually just above the ankle, on the medial or anterior aspect of the leg; healing results in a thin scar on a fibrotic base that often breaks down with minor trauma. Varicosities frequently appear that are associated with incompetent perforating veins.

## Differential Diagnosis

Congestive heart failure and chronic renal disease may result in bilateral edema of the lower extremities, but generally there are other clinical or laboratory findings of heart or kidney disease.

Lymphedema is associated with a brawny thickening in the subcutaneous tissue that does not respond readily to elevation; varicosities are absent, and there is often a history of recurrent episodes of cellulitis.

Primary varicose veins may be difficult to differentiate from the secondary varicosities that often develop in this condition, as discussed above. It may be impossible to exclude superimposed acute phlebitis from chronic venous insufficiency without diagnostic tests.

Other conditions associated with chronic ulcers of the leg include autoimmune diseases (eg, Felty's syndrome), arterial insufficiency (often very painful), sickle cell anemia, erythema induratum (bilateral and usually on the posterior aspect of the lower part of the leg), and fungal infections (cultures specific; no chronic swelling or varicosities).

## Prevention

Irreversible tissue changes and associated complications in the lower legs can be minimized through early and energetic treatment of acute thrombophlebitis with anticoagulants that may minimize the occlusive and valve damage, particularly in the calf, and specific measures to avoid chronic edema in subsequent years, as described in A, below. Thrombolytic therapies of acute phlebitis may be of greater value than other anticoagulants in prevention.

## Treatment

**A. General Measures:** Bed rest, with the legs elevated to diminish chronic edema, is fundamental in the treatment of the acute complications of chronic venous insufficiency. Measures to control the tendency toward edema include (1) intermittent elevation of the legs during the day and elevation of the legs at night (kept above the level of the heart with pillows under the mattress); (2) avoidance of long periods of sitting or standing; and (3) the use of well-fitting, heavy-duty elastic supports worn from the mid foot to just below the knee during the day and evening if there is any tendency for swelling to develop.

**B. Stasis Dermatitis:** Eczematous eruption may be acute or chronic; treatment varies accordingly. (See also Chapter 4.)

**1. Acute weeping dermatitis–**

a. Wet compresses for 1 hour 4 times daily of solutions containing boric acid, potassium permanganate, buffered aluminum acetate (Burow's solution), or isotonic saline.

b. Compresses are followed with a local corticosteroid such as 0.5% hydrocortisone cream in a water-soluble base. (Neomycin and nystatin may be incorporated into this cream.)

c. Systemic antibiotics are indicated only if active infection is present.

**2. Subsiding or chronic dermatitis–**

a. Continue the hydrocortisone cream for 1–2 weeks or until no further improvement is noted. Cordran tape, a plastic tape impregnated with flurandrenolide, is a convenient way to apply both medication and dressing.

b. Zinc oxide ointment with ichthammol (Ichthyol), 3%, 1–2 times a day, cleaned off as desired with mineral oil.

c. Carbolfuchsin (Castellani's) paint to the toes and nails 1–2 times a week may help control dermatophytosis and onychomycosis. Miconazole cream (2%) may also be used.

3. Energetic treatment of chronic edema, as outlined in sections A and C, with almost complete bed rest is important during the acute phase of stasis dermatitis.

**C. Ulceration:** Ulcerations are preferably treated with compresses of isotonic saline solution, which aid the healing of the ulcer or may help prepare the base for a skin graft. A lesion can often be treated on an ambulatory basis by means of a semirigid boot applied to the leg after much of the swelling has been reduced by a period of elevation. The pumping action of the calf muscles on the blood flow out of the lower extremity is enhanced by a circumferential nonelastic bandage on the ankle and lower leg. The boot must be changed every 1–2 weeks, depending to some extent on the amount of drainage from the ulcer. The ulcer, tendons, and bony prominences must be adequately padded. Special ointments on the ulcer are not necessary. The semirigid boot may be made with Unna's paste (Gelocast, Medicopaste) or Gauztex bandage (impregnated with a nonallergenic self-adhering compound). After the ulcer has healed, heavy below-the-knee elastic stockings are used in an effort to prevent recurrent edema and ulceration. Occasionally, the ulcer is so large and chronic that total excision of the ulcer, with skin graft of the defect, is the best approach. This is often combined with ligation of all incompetent perforating veins.

**D. Secondary Varicosities:** Varicosities secondary to damage to the deep system of veins may in turn contribute to undesirable changes in the tissues of the lower leg. Varicosities should occasionally be removed and the incompetent veins connecting the superficial and deep system ligated, but the tendency toward edema will persist, because the chronic high venous pressure is usually not effectively lowered during walking by the procedure, and thus the measures outlined above (¶ A) will be required for life. Varicosities can often be treated along with edema by elastic stockings and other nonoperative measures, and only about 15–20% require surgery. If the obstructive element in the deep system appears to be severe, phlebography may be of value in mapping out the areas of venous obstruction or incompetence in the deep system as well as the number and location of the damaged perforating veins. A decision about whether to treat with surgery may be influenced by such a study; if the varicosities furnish the chief route of venous return, they should not be removed. Venous valvular reconstructive surgery is now in an investigative stage.

**Prognosis**

Individuals with chronic venous insufficiency often

have recurrent problems, particularly if measures to counteract persistent venous hypertension, edema, and secondary tissue changes are not conscientiously adhered to throughout life. Additional episodes of acute thrombophlebitis may occur, and in reliable patients permanent anticoagulation is a reasonable therapeutic objective.

Huse JF et al: Direct venous surgery for venous valvular insufficiency of the lower extremity. *Arch Surg* 1983;**118**:719.

## SUPERIOR VENA CAVAL OBSTRUCTION

Obstruction of the superior vena cava is a relatively rare condition that is usually secondary to the neoplastic or inflammatory process in the superior mediastinum. The most frequent causes are (1) neoplasms, such as lymphomas, primary malignant mediastinal tumors, or carcinoma of the lung with direct extension (over 80%); (2) chronic fibrotic mediastinitis, either of unknown origin or secondary to tuberculosis, histoplasmosis, or pyogenic infections; (3) thrombophlebitis, often by extension of the process from the axillary or subclavian vein into the innominate vein and vena cava and often associated with catheterization of these veins for central venous pressure measurements or for hyperalimentation; (4) aneurysm of the aortic arch; and (5) constrictive pericarditis.

**Clinical Findings**

**A. Symptoms and Signs:** There usually is an insidious onset as progressive obstruction of the venous drainage of the head, neck, and upper extremities develops. The cutaneous veins of the upper chest and lower neck become dilated, and edema develops around the eyes. Later, edema of the face, neck, and arms develops, and cyanosis of these areas then appears. Cerebral and laryngeal edema ultimately results in impaired function of the brain as well as respiratory insufficiency. Bending over or lying down accentuates the symptoms; sitting quietly is generally preferred. The manifestations are more severe if the obstruction develops rapidly and if the azygos junction or the vena cava between that vein and the heart is obstructed.

**B. Laboratory Findings:** The venous pressure is elevated (often > 20 cm of water) in the arm and is normal in the leg.

**C. Imaging:** Chest radiographs and a CT scan will define the location and often the nature of the obstructive process, and phlebography will map out the extent and degree of the venous obstruction and the collateral circulation. Estimation of blood flow around the occlusion, as well as serial evaluation of the response to therapy, may be obtained by means of radionuclear scans using intravenous injection of technetium Tc 99m pertechnetate.

**Treatment**

If the primary problem is due to a malignant neoplasm, radiation therapy or chemotherapy may relieve the pressure on the superior vena cava. Surgical procedures to bypass the obstruction are complicated by bleeding relating to high venous pressure. In cases secondary to mediastinal fibrosis or pericardial constriction, excision of the fibrous tissue around the great vessels may reestablish flow.

## Prognosis

The prognosis depends upon the nature and degree of obstruction and its speed of onset. Slowly developing forms secondary to fibrosis may be tolerated for years. A high degree of obstruction of rapid onset secondary to cancer is often fatal in a few days or weeks, but treatment of the tumor with radiation and drugs may result in significant palliation.

Parish JM et al: Etiologic considerations in superior vena cava syndrome. *Mayo Clin Proc* 1981;**56**:407.

# DISEASES OF THE LYMPHATIC CHANNELS

## LYMPHANGITIS & LYMPHADENITIS

### Essentials of Diagnosis

- Red streak from wound or area of cellulitis toward regional lymph nodes, which are usually enlarged and tender.
- Chills, fever, and malaise may be present.

### General Considerations

Lymphangitis and lymphadenitis are common manifestations of a bacterial infection that is usually caused by hemolytic streptococci and usually arises from an area of cellulitis, generally at the site of an infected wound. The wound may be very small or superficial, or an established abscess may be present, feeding bacteria into the lymphatics. The involvement of the lymphatics is often manifested by a red streak in the skin extending in the direction of the regional lymph nodes, which are, in turn, generally tender and enlarged. Systemic manifestations include fever, chills, and malaise. The infection may progress rapidly, often in a matter of hours, and may lead to septicemia and even death.

### Clinical Findings

**A. Symptoms and Signs:** Throbbing pain is usually present in the area of cellulitis at the site of bacterial invasion. Malaise, anorexia, sweating, chills, and fever of 37.8–40 °C (100–104 °F) develop rapidly. The red streak, when present, may be definite or may be very faint and easily missed. It is not usually tender or indurated, as is the area of cellulitis.

The involved regional lymph nodes may be significantly enlarged and are usually quite tender. The pulse is often rapid.

**B. Laboratory Findings:** Leukocytosis with a leftward shift is usually present. Later, a blood culture may be positive. Culture and sensitivity studies on the wound exudate or pus may be helpful in treatment of the more severe or refractory infections.

### Differential Diagnosis

Lymphangitis may be confused with superficial thrombophlebitis, but the erythematous reaction associated with thrombosis overlies the induration of the inflammatory reaction in and around the thrombosed vein. Venous thrombosis is not associated with lymphadenitis, and a wound of entrance with the secondary cellulitis is generally absent. Superficial thrombophlebitis frequently arises as a result of intravenous therapy, particularly when the needle or catheter is left in place for more than 2 days; if bacteria have also been introduced, suppurative thrombophlebitis may develop.

Cat-scratch fever should be considered when lymphadenitis is present in which the nodes, though often very large, are relatively nontender. Exposure to cats is common, but the scratch may be forgotten by the patient.

It is extremely important to differentiate cellulitis from soft tissue infections that require early and aggressive incision and often resection of necrotic infected tissue, eg, acute streptococcal hemolytic gangrene, necrotizing fasciitis, gram-negative anaerobic cutaneous gangrene, and progressive bacterial synergistic gangrene. These are deeper infections that are more anatomically extensive.

### Treatment

**A. General Measures:** Prompt treatment should include heat (hot, moist compresses or heating pad), elevation when feasible, and immobilization of the infected area. Analgesics may be prescribed for pain.

**B. Specific Measures:** Antibiotic therapy should always be instituted when local infection becomes invasive, as manifested by cellulitis and lymphangitis. A culture of any purulent discharge available should be obtained (often there is nothing to culture), and antibiotic therapy should be started in full doses at once. The initial drug may have to be replaced by a second antibiotic if a clinical response is not apparent in 36–48 hours or if the culture and sensitivity studies indicate that it is not effective. Because the causative organism is so frequently the streptococcus, penicillin is usually the drug of choice. If the patient is allergic to penicillin, erythromycin may be substituted. (See Chapter 28.)

**C. Wound Care:** Drainage of pus from an infected wound should be carried out, generally after the above measures have been instituted and only when it is clear that there is an abscess associated with the site of initial infection. An area of cellulitis should not be incised, because the infection may be spread by attempted drainage when pus is not present.

## Prognosis

With proper therapy and particularly with the use of an antibiotic effective against the invading bacteria, control of the infection can usually be achieved in a few days. Delayed or inadequate therapy can still lead to overwhelming infection with septicemia.

## LYMPHEDEMA

### Essentials of Diagnosis

- Painless edema of one or both lower extremities, primarily in young women.
- Initially, pitting edema, which becomes brawny and often nonpitting with time.
- Ulceration, varicosities, and stasis pigmentation do not occur.
- There may be episodes of lymphangitis and cellulitis.

### General Considerations

The underlying mechanism in lymphedema is impairment of the flow of lymph from an extremity. When due to congenital developmental abnormalities consisting of hypo- or hyperplastic involvement of the proximal or distal lymphatics, it is referred to as the primary form. The obstruction may be in the pelvic or lumbar lymph channels and nodes when the disease is extensive and progressive. The secondary form results when an inflammatory or mechanical obstruction of the lymphatics occurs from trauma, regional lymph node resection or irradiation, or extensive involvement of regional nodes by malignant disease or filariasis. Secondary dilatation of the lymphatics that occurs in both forms leads to incompetence of the valve system, disrupting the orderly flow along the lymph vessels, and results in progressive stasis of a protein-rich fluid, with secondary fibrosis. Episodes of acute and chronic inflammation may be superimposed, with further stasis and fibrosis. Hypertrophy of the limb results, with markedly thickened and fibrotic skin and subcutaneous tissue and diminution in the fatty tissue.

Lymphangiography and radioactive isotope studies are often useful in defining the specific lymphatic defect.

### Treatment

The treatment of lymphedema is often not very satisfactory. The majority of patients can be treated conservatively with some of the following measures: (1) The flow of lymph out of the extremity, with a consequent decrease in the degree of stasis, can be aided through intermittent elevation of the extremity, especially during the sleeping hours (foot of bed elevated 15–20 degrees, achieved by placing pillows beneath the mattress); the constant use of elastic bandages or carefully fitted heavy-duty elastic stockings; and massage toward the trunk—either by hand or by means of pneumatic pressure devices designed to milk edema out of an extremity. (The Wright linear pump delivers sequential pressure cycles that effectively milk fluid out of the foot and leg and then out of the thigh.) (2) Secondary cellulitis in the extremity should be avoided by means of good hygiene and treatment of any trichophytosis of the toes. Once an infection starts, it should be treated by very adequate periods of rest, elevation, and antibiotics. Infection can be a serious and recurring problem and is often difficult to control. Intermittent prophylactic antibiotics may occasionally be necessary. (3) Intermittent courses of diuretic therapy, especially in those with premenstrual or seasonal exacerbations. (4) In carefully selected cases, there are operative procedures that may give satisfactory functional results. Lymphaticovenous anastomosis using microsurgery has yielded some satisfactory cosmetic and functional results, particularly in those with primary lymphedema. This technique may replace the more deforming procedures and those aimed at introducing lymphatic bridges or lymphatic venous connections. Amputation is used as a last resort in very severe forms or when lymphangiosarcoma develops in the extremity.

Savage RC: The surgical management of lymphedema. *Surg Gynecol Obstet* 1985;**160**:283.

## REFERENCES

Bergan JJ, Yao JST (editors): *1986 Year Book of Vascular Surgery.* Year Book, 1986.

Moore WS (editor): *Vascular Surgery: A Comprehensive Review,* 2nd ed. Grune & Stratton, 1986.

Kempczinski RF (editor): *The Ischemic Leg.* Year Book, 1985.

Wilson SE et al (editors): *Vascular Surgery: Principles and Practice.* McGraw-Hill, 1987.

# 10

# Blood

*Charles Linker, MD*

## ANEMIAS

### General Approach to Anemias

Anemia is a common problem in clinical medicine. Anemias should be characterized initially as to type and evaluated subsequently to determine the underlying cause. Anemia is said to be present in adults if the hematocrit is less than 41% in males or 37% in females. In taking the history, one should consider the possibility of congenital anemia based on the patient's personal and family history. One should consider whether the patient has been anemic in the past or has received treatment for anemia. The dietary history may help explain iron deficiency or folic acid deficiency. The possibility of prior or ongoing bleeding should always be considered. Physical examination should include careful attention to signs of primary hematologic diseases (lymphadenopathy, hepatosplenomegaly, or bone tenderness). Mucosal changes such as a smooth tongue raise the possibility of megaloblastic anemia.

Initial laboratory evaluation consists of obtaining a complete blood count, including measurement of red cell indices—chiefly the mean corpuscular volume (MCV). The reticulocyte count on the peripheral blood smear is an index of red blood cell production. Further laboratory tests may be ordered depending on the diagnostic possibilities in individual cases.

Anemias are classified according to their pathophysiologic basis, ie, whether related to diminished production or accelerated loss of red blood cells (Table 10–1); or according to cell size (Table 10–2). The diagnostic possibilities in microcytic anemia are iron deficiency, thalassemia, and anemia of chronic disease. A severely microcytic anemia (MCV < 70 fL) is always due either to iron deficiency or to thalassemia. Macrocytic anemia may be due to megaloblastic (folate or vitamin $B_{12}$ deficiency) or nonmegaloblastic causes. A severely macrocytic anemia (MCV > 125 fL) is almost always due to megaloblastic causes; rare exceptions are the myelodysplastic syndromes, either before or after chemotherapy.

Rapaport SI: *Introduction to Hematology.* Lippincott, 1987.

Wallerstein RO Jr.: Laboratory evaluation of anemia. *West J Med* 1987;**146**:443.

Williams WJ et al: *Hematology,* 3rd ed. McGraw-Hill, 1983.

**Table 10–1.** Classification of anemias by pathophysiology.

**Decreased production**
  Hemoglobin synthesis: Iron deficiency, thalassemia, anemia of chronic disease
  DNA synthesis: Megaloblastic anemia
  Stem cell: Aplastic anemia, myeloproliferative leukemia
  Bone marrow infiltration: Carcinoma, lymphoma
  Pure red cell aplasia
**Increased destruction**
  Blood loss
  Hemolysis (intrinsic)
    Membrane: Hereditary spherocytosis, elliptocytosis
    Hemoglobin: Sickle cell, unstable hemoglobin
    Glycolysis: Pyruvate kinase, etc
    Oxidation: G6PD deficiency
  Hemolysis (extrinsic)
    Immune: Warm antibody, cold antibody
    Microangiopathic: Thrombotic thrombocytopenic purpura, hemolytic-uremic syndrome, valve
    Infection: Clostridial
    Hypersplenism

## IRON DEFICIENCY ANEMIA

### Essentials of Diagnosis

- Absent bone marrow iron stores or serum ferritin less than 12 pg/L.
- Microcytic anemia.
- Response to iron therapy.

### General Considerations

Iron deficiency is the most common cause of anemia worldwide. The anemia is usually mild, but it may become moderate or even severe. It is important

**Table 10–2.** Classification of anemias by MCV.

**Microcytic**
  Iron deficiency
  Thalassemia
  Anemia of chronic disease
**Macrocytic**
  Megaloblastic
    Vitamin $B_{12}$ deficiency
    Folate deficiency
  Nonmegaloblastic
    Myelodysplasia, chemotherapy
    Liver disease
    Increased reticulocytosis
    Myxedema
**Normocytic**
  Many causes

to make the diagnosis so that the underlying cause (usually gastrointestinal blood loss) can be identified and treated (Table 10–3).

Iron is necessary for the formation of heme and other enzymes. Total body iron stores range between 2 and 4 g: approximately 50 mg/kg in men and 35 mg/kg in women. The vast majority (70–95%) of total body iron is present in hemoglobin in circulating red blood cells. One milliliter of packed red blood cells (not whole blood) contains approximately 1 mg of iron. In men, red blood cell volume is approximately 30 mL/kg. A 70-kg man will therefore have approximately 2100 mL of packed red blood cells and consequently 2100 mg of iron in his circulating blood. In women, the red cell volume is about 27 mL/kg; a 50-kg woman will thus have 1350 mg of iron circulating in her red blood cells. Only 200–400 mg of iron is present in myoglobin and nonheme enzymes. The amount of iron present in plasma is negligible. Aside from circulating red blood cells, the major location of iron in the body is the storage pool. Iron is deposited either as ferritin or as hemosiderin and is located largely in macrophages. Iron stores are normally 0.5–2 g, larger in men than in women. However, the range for storage iron is wide; approximately 25% of women in the USA have no storage iron.

The average American diet contains 10–15 mg of iron per day. About 10% of this amount is absorbed, which means that the net daily intake is 1–2 mg. Absorption occurs in the stomach, duodenum, and upper jejunum. Dietary iron present as heme is efficiently absorbed (10–20%) but nonheme iron less so (1–5%), largely because of interference by phosphates, tannins, and other food constituents. Small amounts of iron—approximately 1 mg/d—are normally lost through exfoliation of skin and mucosal cells. There is no mechanism for increasing normal body iron losses.

Menstrual blood loss in women plays a major role in iron metabolism. The average monthly menstrual blood loss is approximately 50 mL, or about 0.7 mg/d. However, menstrual blood loss may be 5 times the average. In order to maintain adequate iron stores, women with heavy menstrual losses must absorb 3–4 mg of iron from the diet each day. This strains the upper limit of what may reasonably be absorbed,

and women with menorrhagia of this degree will almost always become iron-deficient.

In general, iron metabolism is balanced between absorption of 1 mg/d and loss of 1 mg/d. Pregnancy may also upset iron balance, since requirements increase to 2–5 mg of iron per day during pregnancy and lactation. Normal dietary iron cannot supply these requirements, and medicinal iron is needed during pregnancy.

It is possible to become iron-deficient because of dietary deficiency, though this is uncommon in adults. Decreased iron absorption can cause iron deficiency and is usually due to gastric surgery. Repeated pregnancy (especially with breast feeding) is a common cause of iron deficiency if increased requirements are not met with supplemental medicinal iron.

By far the most important cause of iron deficiency anemia is blood loss, especially gastrointestinal blood loss. Chronic aspirin use may cause chronic iron loss even without a documented structural lesion. It cannot be overemphasized that iron deficiency should prompt a search for a potential source of gastrointestinal bleeding unless another cause is identified. Other sources of blood loss include menorrhagia or other uterine bleeding and repeated blood donation.

Chronic hemoglobinuria may lead to iron deficiency, since more than 1 mg/d of iron can be lost by this route. The most common cause is traumatic hemolysis due to an abnormally functioning cardiac valve. Other causes of intravascular hemolysis (eg, paroxysmal nocturnal hemoglobinuria) should also be considered if hemoglobinuria is documented.

Rare causes of iron deficiency include sequestration of iron in pulmonary macrophages in the syndrome of idiopathic pulmonary hemosiderosis.

## Clinical Findings

**A. Symptoms and Signs:** As a rule, the only symptoms of iron deficiency anemia are those of the anemia itself (easy fatigability, tachycardia, palpitations and tachypnea on exertion). Severe iron deficiency (uncommon in the USA) causes progressive skin and mucosal changes. These include a smooth tongue, brittle nails, and cheilosis. Advanced iron deficiency may cause dysphagia because of the formation of esophageal webs (Plummer-Vinson syndrome). Many iron-deficient patients develop pica, an unusual craving for specific foods (ice cubes, etc).

**B. Laboratory Findings:** Laboratory data are important in diagnosis and often reflect the severity of the anemia.

Iron deficiency develops slowly and in stages. The first stage is depletion of iron stores. At this point, there is anemia and no changes in red blood cell size. Iron stores in the marrow will become depleted and eventually disappear. The serum ferritin will become abnormally low. Ferritin values less than 30 μg/L usually indicate absent iron stores. The serum total iron-binding capacity (TIBC) will gradually rise.

After iron stores have been depleted, red blood cell formation will continue with deficient supplies

**Table 10–3.** Causes of iron deficiency.

| |
|---|
| Deficient diet |
| Decreased absorption |
| Increased requirements |
|     Pregnancy |
|     Lactation |
| Blood loss |
|     Gastrointestinal |
|     Menstrual |
|     Blood donation |
| Hemoglobinuria |
| Iron sequestration |
|     Pulmonary hemosiderosis |

of iron. Serum iron values will begin to fall to less than 30 μg/dL, and transferrin saturation will fall to less than 15%.

Eventually, anemia will develop. In the mildest state of anemia, the MCV remains normal. With progressive development of anemia, MCV will fall and the blood smear will show hypochromic microcytic cells. With further progression, anisocytosis (variations in red blood cell size) followed by poikilocytosis (variation in shape of red cells) will develop. Severe iron deficiency will produce a bizarre peripheral blood smear, with severely hypochromic cells, target cells, hypochromic pencil-shaped cells, and occasionally small numbers of nucleated red blood cells. The platelet count may rise above normal.

### Differential Diagnosis

Other causes of microcytic anemic that need to be excluded include anemia of chronic disease, thalassemia, and (less commonly) sideroblastic anemia. Anemia of chronic disease is characterized by normal or increased iron stores in the bone marrow and a normal ferritin level. The TIBC is either normal or low. Thalassemia characteristically produces a greater degree of microcytosis (lower MCV) for any given level of anemia than does iron deficiency. Red blood cell morphology on the peripheral smear becomes abnormal earlier in the evolution of anemia, and iron parameters should be normal.

### Treatment

To make the diagnosis of iron deficiency anemia, one can either demonstrate an iron-deficient state or evaluate the response to a therapeutic trial of iron replacement.

Since the anemia itself is rarely life-threatening, the most important part of treatment is identification of the cause—especially a source of occult blood loss. Iron deficiency cannot be overcome by increasing dietary iron; medicinal iron is always required.

**A. Oral Iron:** There is no better treatment than ferrous sulfate, 325 mg 3 times daily, which provides 180 mg of iron daily of which 20–40 mg may be absorbed. Although ferrous sulfate is optimally taken 3 times a day on empty stomach, compliance is often improved by introducing the medicine more slowly in a gradually escalating dose. Patients who cannot tolerate iron on an empty stomach should take it with food. An appropriate response is a return of the hematocrit level halfway toward normal within 3 weeks. It is advisable to see the patient after 3 weeks both to monitor the hematologic response and to answer questions about the medication that may improve compliance. In general, hematologic values return to normal after 2 months of treatment. Iron therapy should continue for 3–6 months after restoration of normal hematologic values in order to replenish iron stores. Failure of response to iron therapy is usually due to noncompliance, although occasional patients may absorb iron poorly. Other reasons for failure to respond include incorrect diagnosis (anemia of chronic dis-

ease, thalassemia) and ongoing gastrointestinal blood loss that exceeds the rate of new erythropoiesis.

**B. Parenteral Iron:** The indications are intolerance to oral iron, refractoriness to oral iron (poor absorption), gastrointestinal disease precluding the use of oral iron, continued blood loss, and replacement of depleted iron stores when oral iron fails. Parenteral iron should be given only in the amounts necessary to correct the deficiency. Calculate the total dosage as follows: 250 mg for each g of hemoglobin below normal. (Normal: men, 14; women, 12 g.)

Iron dextran injection (Imferon) for intramuscular use contains 5% metallic iron (50 mg/mL). Give 50 mg (1 mL) at first and then 100–250 mg intramuscularly daily or every other day until the total dose has been given. Inject deeply with a 5-cm needle into the upper outer quadrant of the buttock, using the Z technique (pulling the skin to one side before inserting the needle) to prevent leakage of the solution and discoloration of the skin. This preparation may also be given intravenously; it is best administered in doses of 250–500 mg. A test dose of 0.5 mL should be given first; if the patient experiences no unusual reaction, the entire amount may be given over 3–5 minutes. The intravenous route is preferred if repeated injections must be given, eg, in hereditary telangiectasia.

Cook JD: Clinical evaluation of iron deficiency. *Semin Hematol* 1982;**19**:6.

Finch CA, Huebers H: Perspectives in iron metabolism. *N Engl J Med* 1982;**306**:1520.

## ANEMIA OF CHRONIC DISEASE

Many chronic systemic diseases are associated with mild or moderate anemia. Common causes include chronic infection or inflammation, cancer, and liver disease. The anemia of chronic renal failure is somewhat different in pathophysiology and is usually more severe.

Red blood cell survival is modestly reduced, and the bone marrow fails to compensate adequately by increasing red blood cell production. Failure to increase red cell production is largely due to sequestration of iron within the reticuloendothelial system. Decrease in erythropoietin is rarely an important cause of underproduction of red cells except in renal failure, when decreased erythropoietin is the rule.

### Clinical Findings

**A. Symptoms and Signs:** The clinical features are those of the anemia, which is usually modest. The diagnosis should be suspected in cases of modest anemia in patients with known chronic diseases; it is confirmed by the findings of low serum iron, low TIBC, and normal or increased serum ferritin (or normal or increased bone marrow iron stores). In cases of significant anemia, coexistent iron deficiency or folic acid deficiency should be suspected. Decreased dietary intake of folate or iron is common in these ill patients, and many will also have ongoing gastrointestinal blood losses. Patients undergoing hemodialysis regularly lose both iron and folate during dialysis.

**B. Laboratory Findings:** The hematocrit rarely falls below 25% (except in renal failure). The MCV is usually normal but may be slightly reduced, though rarely to less than 70 fL. Red blood cell morphology is nondiagnostic, and the reticulocyte count is neither strikingly reduced or increased. Characteristically, both the serum iron values and the TIBC are reduced. Serum iron values may be unmeasurable, and transferrin saturation may be extremely low. A mistaken diagnosis of iron deficiency anemia may be made if overemphasis is placed on the reduced serum iron and reduced transferrin saturation. A low serum iron and percentage saturation are diagnostic of iron deficiency only when the TIBC is also increased. In contrast to iron deficiency, serum ferritin values should be normal or increased. A serum ferritin value of less than 25 μg/L should suggest coexistent iron deficiency. A Prussian blue stain of the bone marrow should show normal or increased amounts of iron in macrophages.

## Treatment

No specific treatment is available, and none is usually needed. The exception is the anemia of renal insufficiency. Purified recombinant erythropoietin appears to be safe and effective in eliminating the need for red blood cell transfusions in these patients.

Eschbach JW et al: Correction of the anemia of end-stage renal disease with recombinant human erythropoietin: Results of a combined phase I and II clinical trial. *N Engl J Med* 1987;**316**:73.
Lee GR: The anemia of chronic disease. *Semin Hematol* 1983;**20**:61.

## THE THALASSEMIAS

### Essentials of Diagnosis

- Microcytosis out of proportion to the degree of anemia.
- Positive family history or lifelong personal history of microcytic anemia.
- Abnormal red blood cell morphology with microcytes, acanthocytes, and target cells.
- In beta thalassemia, elevated levels of hemoglobin $A_2$ or F.

### General Considerations

The thalassemias are hereditary disorders characterized by reduction in the synthesis of globin chains (alpha or beta). Reduced globin chain synthesis causes reduced hemoglobin synthesis and eventually produces a hypochromic microcytic anemia because of defective hemoglobinization of red blood cells. Thalassemias can be considered among the hypoproliferative anemias, the hemolytic anemias, and the anemias related to abnormal hemoglobin, since all of these factors may play a role.

Normal adult hemoglobin is primarily hemoglobin A, which represents approximately 98% of circulating hemoglobin. Hemoglobin A is formed from a tetramer—2 alpha chains and 2 beta chains—and can be designated $\alpha_2\beta_2$. Two copies of the alpha globin gene are located on chromosome 16, and there is no substitute for alpha globin in the formation of hemoglobin. The beta globin gene residues on chromosome 11 adjacent to genes encoding the betalike globin chains, delta and gamma. The tetramer of $\alpha_2\delta_2$ forms a hemoglobin $A_2$, which normally comprises 1–2% of adult hemoglobin. The tetramer $\alpha_2\gamma_2$ forms hemoglobin F, which is the major hemoglobin of fetal life but which comprises less than 1% of normal adult hemoglobin.

Alpha thalassemia is due primarily to gene deletion directly causing reduced alpha globin chain synthesis (Table 10–4). Since all adult hemoglobins are alpha-containing, alpha thalassemia produces no change in the percentage distribution of hemoglobins A, A2, and F. In severe forms of alpha thalassemia, excess beta chains may form a $\beta_4$ tetramer called hemoglobin H. Hemoglobin H has high oxygen affinity and delivers oxygen to tissues poorly. It is also unstable and subject to oxidative denaturation under conditions of infection or exposure to oxidative drugs (sulfonamides, etc).

Beta thalassemias are usually caused by point mutations rather than large deletions (Table 10–5). These mutations result in premature chain termination or in problems with transcription of RNA and ultimately result in reduced or absent beta globin chain synthesis. The molecular defects leading to beta thalassemia are numerous and heterogeneous. Defects that result in absent globin chain expression are termed $B^0$, whereas defects causing reduced synthesis are termed $B^+$. The reduced beta globin chain synthesis in beta thalassemia results in a relative increase in the percentages of hemoglobins $A_2$ and F compared to hemoglobin A, as the betalike globins (gamma and delta) substitute for the missing beta chains. In the presence of reduced beta chains, the excess alpha chains are unstable and precipitate, leading to damage to red blood cell membranes. This damage causes marked intramedullary hemolysis (destruction of developing erythroid cells within the bone marrow) as well as

**Table 10–4.** Alpha thalassemia syndromes.

| Alpha Globin Genes | Syndrome | Hematocrit | MCV |
|---|---|---|---|
| 4 | Normal | Normal | |
| 3 | Silent carrier | Normal | |
| 2 | Thalassemia minor | 32–40% | 60–75 fL |
| 1 | Hemoglobin H disease | 22–32% | 60–70 fL |
| 0 | Hydrops fetalis | | |

**Table 10–5.** Beta thalassemia syndromes.

| | Beta Globin Genes | Hgb A | Hgb A$_2$ | Hgb F |
|---|---|---|---|---|
| Normal | Homozygous β | 97–99% | 1–3% | <1% |
| Thalassemia major | Homozygous β$^0$ | 0 | 4–10% | 90–96% |
| | Homozygous β$^+$ | | 4–10% | |
| Thalassemia intermedia | Homozygous β$^+$ (mild) | 0–30% | 0–10% | 6–100% |
| Thalassemia minor | Heterozygous β$^0$ | 80–95% | 4–8% | 1–5% |
| | Heterozygous β$^+$ | 80–95% | 4–8% | 1–5% |

hemolysis in the peripheral blood. The bone marrow becomes markedly hyperplastic under the drive of severe anemia and the ineffective erythropoiesis that results from destruction of the developing erythroid cells. This marked expansion of the erythroid element in the bone marrow causes severe bony deformities, osteopenia, and pathologic fractures.

## Clinical Findings

**A. Symptoms and Signs:** The alpha thalassemia syndromes are seen primarily in persons from southeast Asia and China, and, less commonly, in blacks. Normally, adults have 4 copies of the alpha globin chain. When 3 alpha globin genes are present, the patient is hematologically normal and is called a silent carrier. When 2 alpha globin genes are present, the patient is said to have alpha thalassemia trait, one form of thalassemia minor. These patients are clinically normal and have normal life expectancy and performance status. They have a very mild microcytic anemia with no harmful consequences. When only one alpha globin chain is present, the patient has hemoglobin H disease. This is a chronic hemolytic anemia of variable severity (thalassemia minor or intermedia). Physical examination will reveal pallor and splenomegaly. Although affected individuals do not usually require transfusions, they may need transfusions during periods of hemolytic exacerbation caused by infection or other stresses. When all 4 alpha globin genes are deleted, the affected fetus is stillborn as a result of hydrops fetalis.

Beta thalassemia affects persons of Mediterranean origin (Italian, Greek) and to a lesser extent Chinese, other Asians, and blacks. Patients homozygous for beta thalassemia have the syndrome of thalassemia major, formerly called Cooley's anemia. Affected children are normal at birth but during the first year of life develop severe anemia requiring transfusion. Numerous clinical problems ensue, including growth failure, bony deformities (abnormal facial structure, pathologic fractures), hepatosplenomegaly, and jaundice. The clinical course has been modified significantly by transfusion therapy. Children with severe thalassemia may grow normally until puberty, when they experience hypogonadism, growth failure, and clinical consequences of iron overload from years of transfusion. The transfusional iron overload (hemosiderosis) results in cardiomyopathy, progressive hepatomegaly, and numerous endocrine dysfunctions.

Death from cardiac failure usually occurs between ages 20 and 30.

Patients homozygous for a milder form of beta thalassemia (allowing a higher rate of globin gene synthesis) may have the syndrome of thalassemia intermedia. These patients have chronic hemolytic anemia but usually do not require transfusions except under periods of stress. These patients develop iron overload because of increased gut absorption of iron and periodic transfusion. They survive into adult life but with hepatosplenomegaly and bony deformities.

Patients heterozygous for beta thalassemia had thalassemia minor. These patients have a mild microcytic anemia that is not clinically significant.

Prenatal diagnosis is available for couples at risk of producing a child with one of the severe thalassemia syndromes. Asian couples whose parents on both sides have alpha thalassemia trait are at risk of producing an infant with hydrops fetalis. Mediterranean people (and, less commonly, Chinese or blacks) with 2 parents heterozygous for beta thalassemia are at risk of producing a child with Cooley's anemia. Genetic counseling should be offered, and the opportunity for prenatal diagnosis should be discussed.

**B. Laboratory Findings:**

**1. Alpha thalassemia trait**–Patients with 2 alpha globin genes have mild anemia, with hematocrits between 28% and 40%. The MCV is strikingly low (60–75 fL) despite the modest degree of anemia, and the red blood count is usually normal. The peripheral blood smear shows mild abnormalities, including microcytes, hypochromia, occasional target cells, and acanthocytes (cells with irregularly spaced bulbous projections). The reticulocyte count is normal, and iron parameters are normal. Hemoglobin electrophoresis will show no increase in the percentage of hemoglobins A$_2$ or F and no hemoglobin H. Alpha thalassemia trait is usually diagnosed by exclusion in a patient with modest anemia, significant microcytosis, and no elevation of hemoglobins A$_2$ or F. Definitive diagnosis depends upon hemoglobin gene mapping demonstrating a reduced number of alpha globin genes.

**2. Hemoglobin H disease**–These patients have a variably severe hemolytic anemia, with hematocrits between 22% and 32%. The MCV is strikingly low (60–70 fL). the peripheral blood smear is markedly abnormal, with hypochromia, microcytosis, target cells, and poikilocytosis. The reticulocyte count is elevated. Hemoglobin electrophoresis will show the presence of a fast migrating hemoglobin (hemoglobin H), which comprises 10–40% of the hemoglobin. A peripheral blood smear can be stained with supravital dyes to demonstrate the presence of hemoglobin H.

**3. Beta thalassemia minor**–Like patients with alpha thalassemia trait, these patients have a modest anemia with hematocrit between 28% and 40%. The MCV ranges from 55 to 75 fL, and the red blood cell count is usually normal. The peripheral blood smear is mildly abnormal, with hypochromia, microcytosis, and occasional target cells. In contrast to alpha thalassemia, basophilic stippling may be present. The reticulocyte count may be normal or slightly elevated. Hemoglobin electrophoresis (using quantitative techniques) may show an elevation of hemoglobin $A_2$ to 4–8% and occasional elevations of hemoglobin F to 1–5%.

**4. Beta thalassemia major**–Beta thalassemia major produces a severe life-threatening anemia, and without transfusion the hematocrit may fall to less than 10%. The peripheral blood smear is bizarre, showing severe poikilocytosis, hypochromia, microcytosis, target cells, basophilic stippling, and nucleated red blood cells. Little or no hemoglobin A is present. Variable amounts of hemoglobin $A_2$ are seen, and the major hemoglobin present is hemoglobin F.

## Differential Diagnosis

Mild forms of thalassemia must be differentiated from iron deficiency. Compared to iron deficiency anemia, patients with thalassemia have a lower MCV, a more normal red blood count, and a more abnormal peripheral blood smear at modest levels of anemia. Iron parameters are normal. The diagnosis of beta thalassemia can be shown by demonstrating increased levels of hemoglobin $A_2$ (or, less commonly, hemoglobin F), while the diagnosis of alpha thalassemia is made by exclusion. Severe forms of thalassemia may be confused with other hemoglobinopathies. The diagnosis will be made by hemoglobin electrophoresis.

## Treatment

Patients with mild thalassemia (alpha thalassemia trait or beta thalassemia minor) are clinically normal and require no treatment. Most importantly, patients with microcytosis should be identified so that they will not be subjected to repeated evaluations for iron deficiency and inappropriately given supplemental iron. Patients with hemoglobin H disease should take folate supplementation and avoid medicinal iron and oxidative drugs such as sulfonamide drugs. They may occasionally need transfusion during pregnancy or under periods of stress. Patients with severe thalassemia should be maintained on a regular transfusion schedule and should receive folate supplementation. Splenectomy is occasionally performed when hypersplenism causes a marked increase in the transfusion requirement. Deferoxamine is routinely given as an iron-chelating agent to avoid or postpone hemosiderosis.

Forget BG: Molecular genetics of human hemoglobin synthesis. *Ann Intern Med* 1979;**91**:605.

Nienhuis AW, Anagnou NP, Ley TJ: Advances in thalassemia research. *Blood* 1984;**63**:738.

## SIDEROBLASTIC ANEMIA

The sideroblastic anemias are a heterogeneous group of disorders in which hemoglobin synthesis is reduced because of failure to incorporate heme into protoporphyrin to form hemoglobin. Iron accumulates, particularly in the mitochondria. A Prussian blue stain of the bone marrow will reveal ringed sideroblasts, cells with iron deposits (in the mitochondrium) encircling the red cell nucleus. Rare cases are congenital, but the disorder is usually acquired. Sometimes it represents a stage in evolution of a generalized bone marrow disorder that may ultimately terminate in acute leukemia. Other important causes include chronic alcoholism, drug toxicity (antituberculous agents, chloramphenicol), and lead poisoning.

Patients have no specific clinical features other than those related to anemia. The anemia is usually moderate, with hematocrits of 20–30%, but transfusions may occasionally be required. Although the MCV is usually normal or slightly increased, it may occasionally be low, leading to confusion with iron deficiency. The peripheral blood smear characteristically shows a dimorphic population of red blood cells, one normal and one hypochromic. It is the presence of hypochromic cells on peripheral smear combined with a low MCV that may raise the consideration of iron deficiency. In cases of lead poisoning, coarse basophilic stippling of the red cells is seen.

The diagnosis is made by examination of the bone marrow. Characteristically, there is marked erythroid hyperplasia, a sign of ineffective erythropoiesis (expansion of the erythroid compartment of the bone marrow that does not result in the production of reticulocytes in the peripheral blood). The iron stain of the bone marrow shows a generalized increase in iron stores and the presence of ring sideroblasts. Other characteristic laboratory features include a high serum iron and a high transferrin saturation. In the presence of lead poisoning, serum lead levels will be elevated.

The offending drug or toxin (lead) should be eliminated. Occasional patients will respond to pharmacologic doses of folate or pyridoxine, but most patients do not respond to therapy. Occasionally, the anemia is so severe that support with red cell transfusion is required.

Cheng DS, Kushner JP, Wintrobe MM: Idiopathic refractory sideroblastic anemia: Incidence and risk factors for leukemic transformation. *Cancer* 1979;**44**:724.

Kushner JP et al: Idiopathic refractory sideroblastic anemia: Clinical and laboratory investigation of 17 patients and review of the literature. *Medicine* 1971;**50**:139.

## VITAMIN B$_{12}$ DEFICIENCY

### Essentials of diagnosis

- Macrocytic anemia.
- Macro-ovalocytes and hypersegmented neutrophils on peripheral blood smear.
- Serum vitamin B$_{12}$ level less than 100 pg/mL.

### General Considerations

Vitamin B$_{12}$ belongs to the family of cobalamins and serves as a cofactor for 2 important reactions in humans. As methylcobalamin, it serves as a cofactor for methionine synthetase in the conversion of homocysteine to methionine. As adenosylcobalamin, it serves as a cofactor for the conversion of methylmalonyl CoA to succinyl CoA. All vitamin B$_{12}$ comes from the diet, and vitamin B$_{12}$ is present in all foods of animal origin. We absorb approximately 5 μg/d of vitamin B$_{12}$ from the diet.

After being ingested, vitamin B$_{12}$ becomes bound to intrinsic factor, a protein secreted by gastric parietal cells. Other cobalamin-binding proteins (called R factors) compete with intrinsic factor for vitamin B$_{12}$. Vitamin B$_{12}$ bound to R factors cannot be absorbed. The vitamin B$_{12}$-intrinsic factor complex travels through the intestine and is absorbed in the terminal ileum by specific receptors for the complex. It is then transported through plasma and stored in the liver. Three plasma transport proteins have been identified. Transcobalamins I and III (differing only in carbohydrate structure) are secreted by white blood cells. Although approximately 90% of plasma vitamin B$_{12}$ circulates bound to these proteins, only transcobalamin II is capable of transporting vitamin B$_{12}$ into cells. The liver contains 2000–5000 μg of stored vitamin B$_{12}$. Since daily losses are 3–5 μg/d, the body usually has sufficient stores of vitamin B$_{12}$ so that vitamin B$_{12}$ deficiency develops more than 3 years after vitamin B$_{12}$ absorption ceases.

Since vitamin B$_{12}$ is present in all foods of animal origin, dietary vitamin B$_{12}$ deficiency is extremely rare and seen only in vegans—strict vegetarians who avoid all dairy products as well as meat and fish (Table 10–6). Abdominal surgery may lead to vitamin B$_{12}$ deficiency in several ways. Gastrectomy will eliminate that site of intrinsic factor production; blind loop syndrome will cause competition for vitamin B$_{12}$ by bacterial overgrowth in the lumen of the intestine; and surgical resection of the ileum will eliminate the site of vitamin B$_{12}$ absorption. Rare causes of vitamin B$_{12}$ deficiency include Scandinavian fish tapeworm disease (rarely seen in the United States) and severe Crohn's disease causing sufficient destruction of the ileum to retard vitamin B$_{12}$ absorption.

By far the most common cause of vitamin B$_{12}$ deficiency is that associated with **pernicious anemia.** This is a hereditary autoimmune disorder historically seen chiefly in patients of Scandinavian or Northern European ancestry but now seen with increased frequency in young black and Hispanic women. Although the disease is hereditary, it is rarely manifested before age 35. Pernicious anemia produces a number of clinical findings in addition to vitamin B$_{12}$ deficiency. Atrophic gastritis is invariably present and results in histamine-fast achlorhydria. These patients may also have a number of other autoimmune diseases, including IgA deficiency, rheumatoid arthritis, and Graves' disease. Over time, the atrophic gastritis is associated with an increased risk of gastric carcinoma.

### Clinical Findings

**A. Symptoms and Signs:** The hallmark of vitamin B$_{12}$ deficiency is megaloblastic anemia. The anemia may be severe, with hematocrits as low as 10–15%. The megaloblastic state also produces changes in mucosal cells, leading to glossitis, as well as other vague gastrointestinal disturbances such as anorexia and diarrhea. Vitamin B$_{12}$ deficiency also leads to a complex neurologic syndrome. Peripheral nerves are usually affected first, and patients complain initially of paresthesias. The posterior columns next become impaired, and patients complain of difficulty with balance. In more advanced cases, cerebral function may be altered as well.

On examination, patients are usually pale and may be mildly icteric. Neurologic examination will reveal decreased vibration and position sense.

**B. Laboratory Findings:** The megaloblastic state produces an anemia of variable severity that on occasion may be very severe. The MCV is usually strikingly elevated, between 110 and 140 fL. However, it is possible to have vitamin B$_{12}$ deficiency with a normal MCV. Occasionally, the normal MCV may be explained by coexistent thalassemia or iron deficiency, but in other cases the reason for the normal MCV is obscure. Patients with neurologic signs or symptoms that suggest possible vitamin B$_{12}$ deficiency should be thoroughly evaluated for the possibility of that deficiency despite a normal MCV and the absence of anemia. The peripheral blood smear is usually strikingly abnormal, with anisocytosis and poikilocytosis. A characteristic finding is the macro-ovalocyte, but numerous other abnormal shapes are usually seen. Because of the strikingly abnormal red blood cell morphology, it is often mistakenly assumed that the anemia is hemolytic. The neutrophils are hy-

**Table 10–6.** Causes of vitamin B$_{12}$ deficiency.

Dietary deficiency (rare)
Decreased production of intrinsic factor
   Pernicious anemia
   Gastrectomy
Competition for vitamin B$_{12}$ in gut
   Blind loop syndrome
   Fish tapeworm (rare)
Decreased ileal absorption of vitamin B$_{12}$
   Surgical resections
   Crohn's disease
Transcobalamin II deficiency (rare)

persegmented. The reticulocyte count is reduced. Because vitamin $B_{12}$ deficiency affects all hematopoietic cell lines, in severe cases the white blood cell count and platelet count are reduced, and pancytopenia is present.

Bone marrow morphology is characteristically abnormal. Marked erythroid hyperplasia is present as a response to defective red blood cell production (ineffective erythropoiesis). Characteristic megaloblastic changes in the erythroid series include abnormally large cell size and asynchronous maturation of the nucleus and cytoplasm—ie, cytoplasmic maturation continues while impaired DNA synthesis causes retarded nuclear development. In the myeloid series, giant metamyelocytes are characteristically seen.

Other laboratory abnormalities include markedly elevated LDH and a modest increase in indirect bilirubin. These 2 findings are a reflection of intramedullary destruction of developing erythroid cells (ineffective erythropoiesis).

The diagnosis of vitamin $B_{12}$ deficiency is made by finding an abnormally low vitamin $B_{12}$ serum level. Whereas the normal vitamin $B_{12}$ level is 150–350 pg/mL, most patients with overt vitamin $B_{12}$ deficiency will have serum levels less than 100 pg/mL. The Schilling test is used to document the decreased absorption of oral vitamin $B_{12}$ characteristic of pernicious anemia. Initially, a large intramuscular dose of vitamin $B_{12}$ is given to saturate plasma transport proteins. Radiolabeled vitamin $B_{12}$ is given orally, and a 24-hour urine collection is performed to determine how much vitamin $B_{12}$ is absorbed and subsequently excreted. Normally, more than 7% of an administered dose is present in the urine; most patients with imparied absorption will have less than 3% of the dose present in the urine. The second stage of the Schilling test is to administer radiolabeled vitamin $B_{12}$ together with intrinsic factor. If pernicious anemia (a lack of intrinsic factor) is the cause of vitamin $B_{12}$ deficiency, the combined use of vitamin $B_{12}$ and intrinsic factor should correct the abnormally low absorption. However, the full-blown megaloblastic state causes abnormalities in intestinal epithelium that may lead to generalized malabsorption. In these cases, the second stage of the Schilling test will remain abnormal until the intestinal mucosal defect is first corrected by vitamin $B_{12}$ replacement (in approximately 2 months).

## Differential Diagnosis

Vitamin $B_{12}$ deficiency should be differentiated from folic acid deficiency, the other common cause of megaloblastic anemia. The differentiation is based on a low serum vitamin $B_{12}$ level and a normal serum folate level. Differentiation of vitamin $B_{12}$ deficiency from myelodysplasia (the other common cause of macrocytic anemia with abnormal morphology) is based on the characteristic morphology and the low vitamin $B_{12}$ level.

It should be emphasized that any neurologic signs or symptoms suggestive of vitamin $B_{12}$ deficiency

should be evaluated for that disorder even in the absence of anemia or macrocytosis.

## Treatment

Patients with pernicious anemic cannot absorb oral vitamin $B_{12}$ and require parenteral therapy. Intramuscular injections of 200 μg are adequate for each dose. Replacement is usually given daily for the first week, weekly for the first month, and then monthly for life. It should be stressed that pernicious anemia is a lifelong disorder and that if patients discontinue their monthly therapy, the vitamin deficiency will recur.

Patients respond to therapy with an immediate improvement in their sense of well-being. Hypokalemia may complicate the first several days of therapy, particularly if the anemia is severe. A brisk reticulocytosis occurs in 5–7 days, and the hematologic picture normalizes in 2 months. Central nervous system symptoms and signs are reversible if they are of relatively short duration (less than 6 months), but they may be permanent if treatment is not initiated promptly.

Carmel R, Johnson CS: Racial patterns in pernicious anemia: Early age at onset and increased frequency of intrinsic-factor antibody in black women. *N Engl J Med* 1978;**298**:647.

Green R et al: Masking of macrocytosis by alpha-thalassemia in blacks with pernicious anemia. *N Engl J Med* 1982;**307**:1322.

Kapadia CP, Donaldson RM Jr: Disorders of cobalamin (vitamin $B_{12}$) absorption and transport. *Annu Rev Med* 1985;**36**:93.

Lindenbaum J: Status of laboratory testing in the diagnosis of megaloblastic anemia. *Blood* 1983;**61**:624.

## FOLIC ACID DEFICIENCY

### Essentials of Diagnosis

- Macrocytic anemia.
- Macro-ovalocytes and hypersegmented neutrophils on peripheral blood smear.
- Normal serum vitamin $B_{12}$ levels.
- Reduced folate levels in red blood cells or serum.

### General Considerations

Folic acid is the term commonly used for pterylmonoglutamic acid. In its reduced form of tetrahydrofolate, it serves as an important mediator of many reactions involving one-carbon transfers. Important reactions include the conversion of homocysteine to methionine and of deoxyuridylate to thymidylate, an important step in DNA synthesis.

Folic acid is present in most fruits and vegetables (especially citrus fruits and green leafy vegetables) and daily requirements of 50–100 μg/d are usually met in the diet. Total body stores of folate are approximately 5000 μg, enough to supply requirements for 2–3 months.

By far the most common cause of folate deficiency is inadequate dietary intake (Table 10–7). Alcoholics, anorectic cancer patients, elderly persons who do not

**Table 10–7.** Causes of folate deficiency.

| |
|---|
| Dietary deficiency |
| Decreased absorption |
|    Tropical sprue |
|    Drugs: Phenytoin, sulfasalazine |
| Increased requirement |
|    Chronic hemolytic anemia |
|    Pregnancy |
|    Exfoliative skin disease |
| Loss: Dialysis |
| Inhibition of reduction to active form |
|    Methotrexate |

buy fresh fruits and vegetables, and persons who overcook their food are candidates for folate deficiency. Reduced folate absorption is rarely seen except in the case of tropical sprue. However, drugs such as phenytoin or sulfasalazine may interfere with folate absorption. Folic acid requirements are increased in pregnancy, chronic hemolytic anemia, and exfoliative skin disease, and in these cases the increased requirements (5–10 times normal) may not be met by a normal diet. Patients with increased folate requirements should receive oral medicinal supplementation with 1 mg/d of folic acid.

### Clinical Findings

**A. Symptoms and Signs:** The clinical features are similar to those of vitamin $B_{12}$ deficiency, with megaloblastic anemia and megaloblastic changes in mucosa. However, there are none of the neurologic abnormalities associated with vitamin $B_{12}$ deficiency.

**B. Laboratory Findings:** The megaloblastic anemia is identical to that resulting from vitamin $B_{12}$ deficiency (see above). However, the serum vitamin $B_{12}$ level is normal. In contrast, the serum folic acid level is low, usually less than 3 ng/mL (normal: > 6 ng/mL). However, serum folate levels are often misleading, since one meal containing folate will cause a transient correction of the low serum level. For these reasons, the red blood cell folate level, which reflects folic acid intake over the previous months, is often more reliable. A red blood cell folate level of less than 150 ng/mL is diagnostic of folate deficiency.

### Differential Diagnosis

The megaloblastic anemia of folic deficiency should be differentiated from vitamin $B_{12}$ deficiency by the finding of a normal vitamin $B_{12}$ level and a reduced serum folate or red blood cell folate level. Alcoholics, who often have folate deficiency, may also have anemia of liver disease. This latter macrocytic anemia does not cause megaloblastic morphologic changes but rather produces target cells in the peripheral blood.

### Treatment

Folic acid deficiency is treated with folic acid, 1 mg/d orally. The response is similar to that seen in the treatment of vitamin $B_{12}$ deficiency, with rapid improvement and a sense of well-being, reticulocytosis in 5–7 days, and total correction of hematologic abnormalities within 2 months.

Lindenbaum J: Status of laboratory testing in the diagnosis of megaloblastic anemia. *Blood* 1983;**61**:624.

## PURE RED CELL APLASIA

Adult acquired pure red cell aplasia is extremely rare. It appears to be an autoimmune disease in which an IgG antibody specifically attacks erythroid precursors. A congenital form (Diamond-Blackfan syndrome) has been identified. In adults, the disease is usually idiopathic. However, cases have been seen in association with systemic lupus erythematosus, chronic lymphocytic leukemia, lymphomas, or thymoma. Some drugs (phenytoin, chloramphenicol) may cause red cell aplasia. Transient episodes of red cell aplasia are probably common in response to viral infections, especially parvovirus infections. However, these acute episodes will go unrecognized unless the patient has a chronic hemolytic disorder, in which case the hematocrit may fall precipitously.

Clinically, the only signs are those of anemia, unless the patient has an associated autoimmune or lymphoproliferative disorder. The anemia is often severe and is normochromic. Reticulocytes are very low or absent. Red blood cell morphology is normal, and the myeloid and platelet lines are unaffected. The bone marrow is normocellular. All elements present are normal, but erythroid percursors are markedly reduced or absent.

Occasionally, other signs of autoimmune disorder such as hypogammaglobulinemia or a positive antinuclear antibody test are seen. In some cases, the chest radiograph will reveal a thymoma.

The disorder should be distinguished from aplastic anemia (in which the marrow was generally hypocellular and other cell lines are affected) and from myelodysplasia. This latter disorder is recognized by the presence of morphologic abnormalities that should not be present in pure red cell aplasia.

If the thymoma is present, it should be resected, and in some cases the anemia will remit. In other cases, suppression of the autoimmune phenomenon with prednisone, cyclophosphamide, and plasmapheresis should be considered.

Clark DA, Dessypris EN, Krantz SB: Studies on pure red cell aplasia. 11. Results of immunosuppressive treatment of 37 patients. *Blood* 1984;**63**:277.

## HEMOLYTIC ANEMIAS

The hemolytic anemias are a group of disorders in which red blood cell survival is reduced, either episodically or continuously. The bone marrow has the ability to increase erythroid production up to 8-

fold in response to reduced red cell survival, so anemia will be present only when the ability of the bone marrow to compensate is outstripped. This will occur when red cell survival is extremely short or when the ability of the bone marrow to compensate is impaired for some second reason.

Hemolysis is an uncommon cause of anemia. In assessing whether hemolytic anemia is present, one must determine whether the rate of fall of the hematocrit is faster than can be accounted for by lack of production alone. Since red blood cell survival is normally 120 days, in the absence of red cell production the hematocrit will fall at the rate of approximately 1/100 of the hematocrit per day, which translates to a decrease in the hematocrit reading of approximately 3% per week. For example, a fall of hematocrit from 45% to 36% over 3 weeks' time need not indicate hemolysis, since this rate of fall would result simply from cessation of red blood cell production. If the hematocrit is falling at a faster rate than that due to decreased production, blood loss or hemolysis is the cause. Consequently, hemolysis can be defined as a hematocrit falling at a rate faster than can be accounted for by lack of production alone in the absence of bleeding.

Reticulocytosis is an important clue to the presence of hemolysis, since in most hemolytic disorders the bone marrow will respond with increased red blood cell production. However, hemolysis can be present without reticulocytosis when a second disorder (infection, folate deficiency) is superimposed on hemolysis; in these circumstances, the hematocrit will fall rapidly. However, reticulocytosis also occurs during recovery from hypoproliferative anemia or bleeding. Hemolysis is correctly diagnosed (when bleeding is excluded) when the hematocrit is either falling or stable despite reticulocytosis.

Hemolytic disorders are generally classified according to whether the defect is intrinsic to the red cell or due to some external factor (Table 10–8). Intrinsic defects have been described in all compo-

nents of the red blood cell, including the membrane, glycolytic and other enzymes, and hemoglobin. Most of these disorders are hereditary. The vast majority of hemolytic anemias due to external factors are the immune hemolytic anemias.

Certain laboratory features are common to all the hemolytic anemias. Haptoglobin, a normal plasma protein that binds and clears hemoglobin released into plasma, may be depressed in hemolytic disorders. When intravascular hemolysis occurs, transient hemoglobinemia occurs. Hemoglobin is filtered through the glomerulus and usually reabsorbed by tubular cells. Hemoglobinuria will be present only when the capacity for reabsorption of hemoglobin by these cells is exceeded. In the absence of hemoglobinuria, evidence for prior intravascular hemolysis is the presence of hemosiderin in shed renal tubular cells (positive urine hemosiderin). With severe intravascular hemolysis, hemoglobinemia and methemalbuminemia may be present. Hemolysis increases the indirect bilirubin, and the total bilirubin may rise to as high as 4 mg/dL. Bilirubin levels higher than this indicate some degree of hepatic dysfunction.

Dacie JV: *The Hemolytic Anemias: Congenital and Acquired,* 2nd ed. Grune & Stratton, 1960.

## HEREDITARY SPHEROCYTOSIS

### Essentials of Diagnosis

- Spherocytes and increased reticulocytes on peripheral blood smear.
- Negative Coombs test.
- Positive family history.

### General Considerations

Hereditary spherocytosis is a disorder of the red blood cell membrane, leading to chronic hemolytic anemia. Normally, the red blood cell is a biconcave disk with a diameter of 7–8 μm. The red blood cells must be both strong and deformable—strong to withstand the stress of circulating for 120 days and deformable so as to pass through capillaries 3 μm in diameter and splenic fenestrations in the cords of the red pulp of approximately 2 μm. The red blood cell skeleton, made up primarily of the proteins spectrin and actin, gives the red cells these characteristics of strength and deformability.

The membrane defect in hereditary spherocytosis has not been defined but is most likely an abnormality in spectrin. The result is a decrease in surface-to-volume ratio that results in a spherical shape of the cell. These spherical cells are less deformable and unable to pass through 2-μm fenestrations in the splenic red pulp. Hemolysis takes place because of trapping of red blood cells within the spleen.

Family members should be screened to detect those with spherocytosis (see laboratory findings).

### Clinical Findings

**A. Symptoms and Signs:** Hereditary spherocy-

---

**Table 10–8.** Classification of hemolytic anemias.

**Intrinsic**
  Membrane defects: Hereditary spherocytosis, hereditary elliptocytosis, paroxysmal nocturnal hemoglobinuria
  Glycolytic defects: Pyruvate kinase deficiency, severe hypophosphatemia
  Oxidation vulnerability: G6PD deficiency, methemoglobinemia
  Hemoglobinopathies: Sickle syndromes, unstable hemoglobins, methemoglobinemia
**Extrinsic**
  Immune: Autoimmune, lymphoproliferative disease, drug toxicity
  Microangiopathic: Thrombotic thrombocytopenic purpura, hemolytic-uremic syndrome, disseminated intravascular coagulation, valve hemolysis, metastatic adenocarcinoma, vasculitis
  Infection: Malaria, *Clostridia, Borrelia*
  Hypersplenism
  Burns

tosis is an autosomal dominant disease of variable severity. It is often diagnosed during childhood, but milder cases may be discovered incidentally late in adult life. Anemia may or may not be present, since the bone marrow may be able to compensate for shortened red cell survival. Severe anemia (aplastic crisis) may occur when bone marrow compensation is impaired by infection or folate deficiency. Chronic hemolysis may cause jaundice and pigment gallstones, leading to attacks of cholecystitis. Examination may reveal icterus and a palpable spleen.

**B. Laboratory Findings:** The anemia is of variable severity, and the hematocrit may be normal. Reticulocytosis is always present. The peripheral blood smear shows the presence of spherocytes, small cells that have lost their central pallor. Spherocytes usually make up only a small percentage of red blood cells on the peripheral smear. One clue to hereditary spherocytosis is that the mean corpuscular hemoglobin concentration (MCHC) may be abnormally high, often greater than 36 g/dL. Hereditary spherocytosis is one of the few disorders associated with increased MCHC. As with other hemolytic disorders, there may be an increase in direct bilirubin. The Coombs test is negative.

The presence of spherocytes may be confirmed by the osmotic fragility test. Spherocytes are red cells that have lost some membrane surface and are abnormally vulnerable to swelling induced by hypotonic media. Increased osmotic fragility merely reflects the presence of spherocytes and does not distinguish hereditary spherocytosis from other spherocytic hemolytic disorders such as autoimmune hemolytic anemia.

## Treatment

These patients should receive uninterrupted supplementation with folic acid, 1 mg/d. The treatment of choice is splenectomy. Splenectomy will not correct the membrane defect or remove the spherocytes but will eliminate the site of hemolysis. In very mild cases discovered late in adult life, splenectomy may not be necessary.

Palek J, Lux SE: Red cell membrane skeletal defects in hereditary and acquired hemolytic anemias. *Semin Hematol* 1983;**20**:189.

## HEREDITARY ELLIPTOCYTOSIS

Hereditary elliptocytosis is a congenital disorder of the red blood cell membrane and probably is due to abnormalities in spectrin tetramer formation. The disorder is autosomal dominant and of variable severity. In the most common form of hereditary elliptocytosis, the mild hemolytic disorder is well compensated, and there is little or no anemia. However, more severe varieties do produce anemia, splenomegaly, and pigment gallstones.

In the common mild variety, the hallmark of the disorder is the elliptical shape of the majority of red blood cells on peripheral blood smear. Reticulocytosis may be present. In the rare severe varieties of the disorder (hereditary pyropoikilocytosis), the peripheral blood smear is extremely bizarre; and in addition to elliptocytes, microspherocytes and a variety of unusually shaped red cells are present.

No treatment is usually indicated. Severe variants are treated with splenectomy and folate supplementation.

## PAROXYSMAL NOCTURNAL HEMOGLOBINURIA

Paroxysmal nocturnal hemoglobinuria is an acquired clonal stem cell disorder that results in abnormal sensitivity of the red blood cell membrane to lysis by complement. The exact nature of the defect is unknown but involves both increased binding of C3b and increased vulnerability to lysis by complement.

The best screening test for paroxysmal nocturnal hemoglobinuria is the sucrose hemolysis test. The diagnosis can be confirmed by Ham's (acidified serum) test. Paroxysmal nocturnal hemoglobinuria is a very rare disorder and should be suspected in confusing cases of hemolytic anemia.

### Clinical Findings

**A. Symptoms and Signs:** The anemia is of variable severity and may be severe. Classically, patients report episodic hemoglobinuria resulting in reddish brown urine. Hemoglobinuria may be present in the first morning urine, since the mild respiratory acidosis of sleep leads to enhanced complement activity. In addition to anemia, these patients may be affected by thrombosis, especially mesenteric and hepatic vein thromboses. The reason for thombus formation is unclear but may be related to platelet activation by complement. As this is a stem cell disorder, paroxysmal nocturnal hemoglobinuria may progress either to aplastic anemia or to acute myeloid leukemia.

**B. Laboratory Findings:** Anemia is of variable severity, and reticulocytosis may or may not be present. Abnormalities on the blood smear are nondiagnostic and may include macro-ovalocytes. As with other hemolytic disorders, haptoglobin may be decreased or absent. Since the episodic hemolysis in paroxysmal nocturnal hemoglobinuria is intravascular, the finding of urine hemosiderin is a useful test. Serum LDH is characteristically elevated. Iron deficiency is commonly present and is related to chronic iron loss from hemoglobinuria.

The white blood cell count and platelet count may be decreased. A decreased leukocyte alkaline phosphatase—evidence for qualitative abnormality in the myeloid series—is good evidence for paroxysmal nocturnal hemoglobinuria. Bone marrow morphology is variable and may show either hypoplasia or erythroid hyperplasia.

## Treatment

Iron replacement is often indicated for treatment of iron deficiency. This may improve the anemia but may also cause a transient increase in hemolysis. For unclear reasons, prednisone is effective in decreasing hemolysis, and some patients can be managed effectively with alternate-day steroids. In severe cases, bone marrow transplantation has been used to correct the disorder.

Rosse WF: Paroxysmal nocturnal hemoglobinuria: Present status and future prospects. *West J Med* 1980;**132:**219.

Rosse WF: Treatment of paroxysmal nocturnal hemoglobinuria. *Blood* 1982;**60:**20.

## PYRUVATE KINASE DEFICIENCY

The red blood cell obtains 90% of its energy from anaerobic glycolysis. Defects in glycolytic enzymes produce a chronic hemolytic anemia because of depletion of ATP. Severe hypophosphatemia may result in hemolysis for the same reason.

Pyruvate kinase deficiency is a very rare autosomal recessive disorder that causes chronic hemolytic anemia, usually with onset in childhood. In addition to the anemia, splenomegaly and pigment gallstones may be present. The red blood cell smear is normal, and the diagnosis is made by specific enzyme assays available only in specialized laboratories. Splenectomy is the treatment of choice.

Valentine WN, Tanaka KR, Paglia DE: Hemolytic anemias and erythrocyte enzymopathies. *Ann Intern Med* 1985; **103:**245.

## GLUCOSE-6-PHOSPHATE DEHYDROGENASE DEFICIENCY

### Essentials of Diagnosis

- X-linked recessive disorder seen commonly in American black males.
- Episodic hemolysis in response to oxidant drugs or infection.
- Minimally abnormal peripheral blood smear.
- Reduced levels of G6PD.

### General Considerations

Glucose-6-phosphate dehydrogenase (G6PD) deficiency is a hereditary enzyme defect that causes episodic hemolytic anemia because of decreased ability of red blood cells to deal with oxidative stresses. The hexose monophosphate shunt is not an important source of energy generation in red cells but is important in generating reduced glutathione, which protects hemoglobin from oxidative denaturation. The first step in this pathway is the generation of NADPH by the action of G6PD on glucose 6-phosphate.

NADPH serves as a cofactor for glutathione reductase in generating reduced glutathione, which detoxifies hydrogen peroxide. In the absence of reduced glutathione, hemoglobin may become oxidized. Oxidized hemoglobin denatures and forms precipitants called Heinz bodies. These Heinz bodies cause membrane damage, which leads to removal of these cells by the spleen.

Numerous types of G6PD enzymes have been described. The normal type found in Caucasians is designated G6PD-B. Most American blacks have G6PD-A, which is normal in function. Ten to 15% of American blacks have the variant G6PD designated A$^-$, in which there is only 15% of normal enzyme activity, and enzyme activity declines rapidly as the red blood cell ages past 40 days. Many other G6PD variants have been described, including some Mediterranean variants with extremely low enzyme activity.

### Clinical Findings

G6PD deficiency is an X-linked recessive disorder affecting 10–15% of American black males. Female carriers are rarely affected—only when an unusually high percentage of cells producing the normal enzyme are inactivated.

**A. Symptoms and Signs:** Patients are usually healthy, without chronic hemolytic anemia or splenomegaly. Hemolysis occurs as a result of oxidative stress on the red blood cells, generated either by infection or exposure to certain drugs. Common drugs initiating hemolysis include primaquine, quinidine, quinine, sulfonamides, and nitrofurantoin. When hemolysis occurs, the patient may become jaundiced and have dark urine. Even with continuous use of the offending drug, the hemolytic episode is usually self-limited because older red blood cells (with low enzyme activity) are removed and replaced with a population of young red blood cells with adequate functional levels of G6PD.

Severe G6PD deficiency (as in Mediterranean variants) may produce a chronic hemolytic anemia, and hemolytic crises may be severe or even fatal.

**B. Laboratory Findings:** Between hemolytic episodes, the blood is normal. During episodes of hemolysis, there is reticulocytosis and increased serum indirect bilirubin. The red blood cell smear is not diagnostic but may reveal a small number of "bite" cells—cells that appear to have had a bite taken out of their periphery. This in fact indicates pitting of hemoglobin aggregates by the spleen. Heinz bodies may be demonstrated by staining a peripheral blood smear with crystal violet. Specific enzyme assays for G6PD may reveal a low level. Results for G6PD assays may be misleading if they are performed during a hemolytic episode when the enzyme-deficient cohort of cells has been removed and replaced with a young cohort with nearly normal enzyme activity. In these cases, the enzyme assays should be repeated after hemolysis has resolved. In severe cases of G6PD deficiency, enzyme levels are always low.

## Treatment

No treatment is necessary except to avoid known oxidant drugs.

Luzzatto L: Inherited hemolytic states: Glucose-6-phosphate dehydrogenase deficiency. *Clin Haematol* 1975;**4**:83.

Valentine WM, Tanaka KR, Paglia DE: Hemolytic anemias and erythrocyte enzymopathies. *Ann Intern Med* 1985;**103**:245.

# SICKLE CELL ANEMIA & RELATED SYNDROMES

## Essentials of Diagnosis

- Irreversibly sickled cells on peripheral blood smear.
- Positive family history and lifelong history of hemolytic anemia.
- Recurrent painful episodes.
- Hemoglobin S is the major hemoglobin seen on electrophoresis.

## General Considerations

Sickle cell anemia is an autosomal dominant disorder in which an abnormal hemoglobin (hemoglobinopathy) leads to chronic hemolytic anemia with a variety of severe clinical consequences. The disorder is a classic example of disease caused by a point mutation in DNA. A single DNA base change leads to an amino acid substitution of valine for glutamine in the sixth position on the beta globin chain. The abnormal beta chain is designated $\beta^s$ and the tetramer of $\alpha_2\beta^s_2$ is designated hemoglobin S.

When in the deoxy form, hemoglobin S forms polymers that damage the red blood cell membrane. Both polymer formation and membrane damage are reversible. However, red blood cells that have undergone repeated sickling are damaged beyond repair and become irreversibly sickled cells.

The rate of sickling is influenced by a number of factors, most importantly by the concentration of hemoglobin S in the individual red blood cell. Red cell dehydration makes the cell quite vulnerable to sickling. Sickling is also strongly influenced by the presence of other hemoglobins within the cell. Hemoglobin F cannot participate in polymer formation, and its presence markedly retards sickling. Other factors that increase sickling are those which lead to formation of deoxyhemoglobin S, eg, acidosis and hypoxemia.

Prenatal diagnosis is now available for couples at risk of producing a child with sickle cell anemia. DNA from fetal cells can be directly examined, and the presence of the sickle cell mutation can be accurately and definitively diagnosed. Genetic counseling should be made available to such couples.

## Clinical Findings

**A. Symptoms and Signs:** The hemoglobin S gene is carried in 8% of American blacks, and one birth out of 400 in American blacks will produce a child with sickle cell anemia. The disorder has its onset during the first year of life, when hemoglobin F levels fall.

Chronic hemolytic anemia produces jaundice, pigment gallstones, splenomegaly, and poorly healing ulcers over the lower tibia. The chronic anemia may become life-threatening when severe anemia is produced by hemolytic or aplastic crises. Aplastic crises occur when the ability of the bone marrow to compensate is reduced by viral or other infection or by folate deficiency. Hemolytic crises may be related to splenic sequestration of sickled cells (primarily in childhood, before the spleen has been infarcted) or with coexistent disorders such as G6PD deficiency.

Acute painful episodes due to acute vaso-occlusion may occur spontaneously or be provoked by infection, dehydration, or hypoxia. Clusters of sickled red cells occlude the microvasculature of the organs involved. These episodes last hours to days and produce acute pain and low-grade fever. Common sites of acute painful episodes include the bones (especially the back and long bones) and the chest. Acute vaso-occlusion may also cause strokes and priapism. Vaso-occlusive episodes are not associated with increased hemolysis.

Repeated episodes of vascular occlusion cause chronic organ damage affecting a large number of organs, especially the heart and liver. Ischemic necrosis of bone occurs, rendering the bond susceptible to osteomyelitis due to staphylococci or (less commonly) salmonellae. In adult life, the spleen is infarcted. Infarction of the papillae of the renal medulla causes renal tubular defects and gross hematuria. Retinopathy is often present and may lead to blindness.

These patients are prone to delayed puberty and may rarely have an increased incidence of infection. Infections are related to hyposplenism as well as to defects in the alternative pathway of complement.

On examination, patients are often chronically ill and jaundiced. There is hepatomegaly, but the spleen is not palpable in adult life. The heart is enlarged, with a hyperdynamic precordium and systolic murmurs. Nonhealing ulcers of the lower leg and retinopathy may be present.

Sickle cell anemia becomes a chronic multisystem disease, with death from organ failure commonly occurring between ages 20 and 40.

**B. Laboratory Findings:** Chronic hemolytic anemia is present. The hematocrit is usually 20–30%. The peripheral blood smear is characteristically abnormal, with irreversibly sickled cells comprising 5–50% of red cells. Other findings include reticulocytosis (10–25%), nucleated red blood cells, and hallmarks of hyposplenism such as Howell-Jolly bodies and target cells. The white blood cell count is characteristically elevated to 12,000–15,000/$\mu$L, and thrombocytosis may occur. Indirect bilirubin levels are high, and haptoglobin is absent.

The presence of hemoglobin S can be demonstrated by a screening test. The sodium metabisulfite test has now largely been replaced by a solubility test in high-ionic-strength media. Normal hemoglobin will produce a clear solution, whereas hemoglobin S will produce a turbid solution. The diagnosis of sickle cell anemia may be confirmed by hemoglobin electrophoresis (Table 10–9). Hemoglobin S has an abnormal migration pattern on electrophoresis and will usually comprise 85–98% of hemoglobin. In homozygous S disease, no hemoglobin A will be present. Hemoglobin F levels are variably increased.

## Treatment

No specific treatment is available for the primary disease. However, both longevity and quality of life may be improved by comprehensive medical management by a concerned physician. Patients are maintained chronically on folic acid supplementation and should not routinely be given transfusions. Transfusions are indicated for aplastic or hemolytic crises and during the third trimester of pregnancy.

When acute painful episodes occur, precipitating factors should be identified and infections treated if present. The patient should be kept well hydrated, and oxygen should be given if the patient is hypoxic. Otherwise, treatment is supportive (hydration and analgesics).

Acute vaso-occlusive crises can be treated with exchange transfusion, in which the patient's blood containing a sickled hemoglobin is removed and replaced with normal blood. However, this should not be performed as a routine procedure, because of risks of transfusion including iron overload and stimulation of alloantibody production. Exchange transfusions are indicated for the treatment of intractable crises, priapism, and stroke and as a preventive measure for patients undergoing general anesthesia.

Chang JC, Kan YW: A sensitive new prenatal test for sickle-cell anemia. *N Engl J Med* 1982;**307**:30.

Embury SH et al: Concurrent sickle-cell anemia and alpha-thalassemia: Affect on severity of anemia. *N Engl J Med* 1982;**306**:270.

Steinberg MH, Hebbel RP: Clinical diversity of sickle cell anemia: Genetic and cellular modulation of disease severity. *Am J Hematol* 1983;**14**:405.

## SICKLE CELL TRAIT

Patients with the heterozygous genotype (AS) have sickle cell trait. These persons are clinically normal and have acute painful episodes only under extreme conditions such as vigorous exertions at high altitudes (or in unpressurized aircraft). The patients are hematologically normal, with no anemia and normal red blood cells on peripheral blood smear. They may, however, have a defect in renal tubular function, causing an inability to concentrate the urine. A screening test for sickle hemoglobin (sodium metabisulfite or solubility test) will be positive, and hemoglobin electrophoresis will reveal that approximately 40% of hemoglobin is hemoglobin S (Table 10–9).

No treatment is necessary. These patients should be considered normal in all respects.

## SICKLE THALASSEMIA

Patients with homozygous sickle cell anemia and alpha thalassemia have a somewhat milder form of hemolysis because of a slower rate of sickling related to reduced hemoglobin concentration (MCHC) within the red blood cell.

Patients who are double heterozygotes for sickle cell anemia and beta thalassemia are clinically affected with sickle cell syndromes. Sickle $\beta^0$ thalassemia is clinically very similar to homozygous SS disease. Vaso-occlusive crises may be somewhat less severe, and the spleen is usually not infarcted. Hematologically, the MCV is usually low—in contrast to the normal MCV of sickle cell anemia—and the smear usually reveals fewer irreversibly sickled cells. Hemoglobin electrophoresis (Table 10–9) reveals no hemoglobin A but will show an increase in hemoglobin $A_2$ which is not present in sickle cell anemia.

Sickle $\beta^+$ thalassemia is a milder disorder than homozygous SS disease, with fewer crises. The spleen is usually palpable. The hemolytic anemia is less severe, and the hematocrit is usually 30–38%, with reticulocytes of 5–10%. Hemoglobin electrophoresis shows the presence of some hemoglobin A.

## HEMOGLOBIN C DISORDERS

Hemoglobin C is formed by a single amino acid substitution at the same site of substitution as in sickled hemoglobin but with lysine instead of valine substituted for glutamine at the $\beta6$ position. Hemoglobin C is nonsickling but may participate in polymer formation in association with hemoglobin S. Homozygous

**Table 10–9.** Hemoglobin distribution in sickle cell syndromes.

| Genotype | Diagnosis | Hgb A | Hgb S$_3$ | Hgb A$_2$ | Hgb F |
|----------|-----------|-------|-----------|-----------|-------|
| AA | Normal | 97–99% | 0 | 1–2% | < 1% |
| AS | Sickle trait | 60% | 40% | 1–2% | < 1% |
| SS | Sickle cell anemia | 0 | 85–98% | 1–3% | 5–15% |
| SB$^0$ thal | Sickle B thalassemia | 0 | 70–80% | 3–5% | 10–20% |
| SB$^+$ thal | Sickle B thalassemia | 10–20% | 60–75% | 3–5% | 10–20% |
| AS, $\alpha$ thalassemia | Sickle trait | 70–75% | 25–30% | 1–2% | < 1% |

hemoglobin C disease produces a mild hemolytic anemia with splenomegaly, mild jaundice, and pigment gallstones. The peripheral blood smear shows numerous target cells as well as occasional cells with rectangular crystals of hemoglobin C. Persons heterozygous for hemoglobin C are clinically normal.

Patients with hemoglobin SC disease are double heterozygotes for beta S and beta C. These patients, like those with sickle $\beta^+$ thalassemia, have a milder hemolytic anemia and milder clinical course than those with homozygous SS disease. There are fewer vaso-occlusive events, and the spleen remains palpable in adult life. However, persons with hemoglobin SC disease have more retinopathy and more ischemic necrosis of bone than those with SS disease. The hematocrit is usually 30–38%, with 5–10% reticulocytes and few irreversibly sickled cells on the blood smear. Target cells are more numerous than in SS disease. Hemoglobin electrophoresis will show approximately 50% hemoglobin C, 50% hemoglobin S, and no increase in hemoglobin F levels.

## UNSTABLE HEMOGLOBINS

Unstable hemoglobins are prone to oxidative denaturation even in the presence of a normal G6PD system. The disorder is autosomal dominant and of variable severity. Most patients have a mild chronic hemolytic anemia with splenomegaly, mild jaundice, and pigment gallstones. Less severely affected patients are not anemic except under conditions of oxidative stress.

The diagnosis is made by the finding of Heinz bodies and a normal G6PD level. Hemoglobin electrophoresis is usually normal, since these hemoglobins characteristically do not have a change in their migration pattern. These hemoglobins can be shown to precipitate in isopropanol. Usually no treatment is necessary. Patients with chronic hemolytic anemia should receive folate supplementation and avoid known oxidative drugs. In rare severe cases, splenectomy may be required.

## AUTOIMMUNE HEMOLYTIC ANEMIA

### Essentials of Diagnosis
- Spherocytes and reticulocytosis on peripheral blood smear.
- Positive Coombs test.

### General Considerations
Autoimmune hemolytic anemia is an acquired disorder in which an IgG autoantibody is formed that binds to the red blood cell membrane. The antibody is most commonly directed against a basic component of the Rh system and is present on virtually all human red blood cells. When IgG antibodies coat the red blood cell, the Fc portion of the antibody is recognized by macrophages (with Fc reception) present in the spleen and other portions of the reticuloendothelial system. The interaction between splenic macrophage and the antibody-coated red blood cell results in removal of red blood cell membrane and the formation of a spherocyte because of the decrease in surface-to-volume ratio of the red blood cell. These spherocytic cells have decreased deformability and become trapped in the red pulp of the spleen because of their inability to squeeze through the 2- to 3-$\mu$m fenestrations. When large amounts of IgG are present on red blood cells, complement may be fixed. Direct lysis of cells is rare, but the presence of C3b on the surface of red blood cells allows Kupffer cells in the liver to participate in the hemolytic process because of the presence of C3b receptors on Kupffer cells.

Approximately half of all cases of autoimmune hemolytic anemia are idiopathic. The disorder may also be seen in association with systemic lupus erythematosus, chronic lymphocytic leukemia, or diffuse lymphomas. It must be distinguished from drug-induced hemolytic anemia. Methyldopa commonly stimulates the production of an autoantibody with the same specificity as that in idiopathic autoimmune hemolytic anemia. Other drugs (penicillin, quinidine) become associated with the red blood cell membrane, and the antibody is directed against the membrane-drug complex.

The Coombs antiglobulin test forms the basis for diagnosis of these immune hemolytic disorders. The Coombs reagent is a rabbit IgM antibody raised against human IgG or human complement. The direct Coombs test is performed by mixing the patient's red blood cells with the Coombs reagent and looking for agglutination. Agglutination (a positive test) indicates the presence of antibody on the red blood cell surface. Initially, a polyspecific antibody is used that detects the presence of either IgG or complement. Subsequently, specific reagents against either IgG or complement can be used to determine which component is present. The indirect Coombs test is performed by mixing the patient's serum with a panel of type O red blood cells. After incubation of the test serum and panel red blood cells, the Coombs reagent is added and one looks for agglutination. Agglutination in this system indicates the presence of free antibody in the patient's serum. The indirect Coombs test can be modified to make the diagnosis of drug-induced hemolytic anemia. An indirect Coombs test which is initially negative but becomes positive when the offending drug is added to the initial incubation makes the diagnosis of penicillin type drug-induced immune hemolytic anemia. Because the traditional Coombs test relies on visible agglutination as an end point, the test is not very sensitive and will not detect immune hemolytic anemias, in which only a small amount of IgG is present on red blood cells. More sensitive tests (micro-Coombs) are now available.

### Clinical Findings
**A. Symptoms and Signs:** Autoimmune hemo-

lytic anemia typically produces an anemia of rapid onset that may be life-threatening in severity. Patients complain of fatigue and may present with angina or congestive heart failure. On examination, jaundice and splenomegaly are usually present. If the patient has an underlying disorder such as systemic lupus erythematosus or chronic lymphocytic leukemia, features of these diseases may be present.

**B. Laboratory Findings:** The anemia is of variable severity but may be severe, with hematocrit of less than 10%. Reticulocytosis is usually present, and spherocytes are seen on the peripheral blood smear. As with other hemolytic disorders, indirect bilirubin is increased. Approximately 10% of patients with autoimmune hemolytic anemia have co-incident immune thrombocytopenia (Evans's syndrome).

The direct Coombs test is positive for IgG and possibly for complement as well. The indirect Coombs test may or may not be positive. A positive indirect Coombs test indicates the presence of a large amount of autoantibody that has saturated binding sites in the red blood cell and consequently appears in the serum. A patient with acquired spherocytic hemolytic anemia that may be of the autoimmune variety who has a negative Coombs test should be tested with a micro-Coombs test (which is necessary to make the diagnosis in approximately 10% of cases). Because the patient's serum usually contains the autoantibody, it may be difficult to obtain a compatible cross-match with donor's cells. Suitable donors may be selected by special laboratory methods.

## Treatment

Initial treatment is with prednisone, 1–2 mg/kg/d in divided doses. If anemia is life-threatening, transfusions should be given cautiously. Most transfused blood will survive no more poorly than the patient's own red blood cells. However, because of difficulty in performing the cross-match, it is possible that incompatible blood will be given, and patients must be monitored carefully during transfusion. If prednisone is ineffective or if the disease recurs on tapering the dose of prednisone to an acceptable chronic dose, splenectomy should be performed. Patients with autoimmune hemolytic anemia refractory to prednisone and splenectomy may be treated with a variety of immunosuppressive agents.

The long-term prognosis for patients with this disorder is good. Splenectomy is often successful in controlling or at least ameliorating the disorder.

Frank MM et al: Pathophysiology of immune hemolytic anemia. *Ann Intern Med* 1977;**87**:210.

Petz LD, Garratty G: *Acquired Immune Hemolytic Anemia.* Churchill Livingstone, 1980.

Sokol RJ, Hewitt S, Stamps BK: Autoimmune haemolysis: An 18-year study of 865 cases referred to a regional transfusion centre. *Br Med J* 1981;**282**:2023.

# COLD AGGLUTININ DISEASE

## Essentials of Diagnosis

- Increased reticulocytes and spherocytes on peripheral blood smear.
- Coombs test positive only for complement.
- Positive cold agglutinin test.

## General Considerations

Cold agglutinin disease is an acquired hemolytic anemia due to an IgM autoantibody usually directed against the I antigen on red blood cells. These IgM autoantibodies characteristically will not react with cells at 37 °C but only at lower temperatures. Since the blood temperature (even in the most peripheral parts of the body) rarely goes lower than 20 °C, only antibodies active at higher temperatures than this will produce clinical effects. In the cooler parts of the body (fingers, nose, ears), agglutination of red blood cells by the IgM antibodies will transiently occur. Hemolysis results indirectly from attachment of IgM, which in the cooler parts of the circulation binds and fixes complement. When the red blood cell returns to a cooler temperature, the IgM antibody dissociates, leaving complement on the cell. Lysis of cells rarely occurs. Rather, C3b present on the red cells is recognized by Kupffer cells (which have receptors for C3b), and red blood cell sequestration ensues.

Most cases of chronic cold agglutinin disease are idiopathic. Others occur in association with Waldenström's macroglobulinemia, an indolent lymphoproliferative disease in which a monoclonal IgM paraprotein is produced. Acute postinfectious cold agglutinin disease occurs following mycoplasmal pneumonia or infectious mononucleosis.

## Clinical Findings

**A. Symptoms and Signs:** In chronic cold agglutinin disease, symptoms related to red blood cell agglutination occur on exposure to cold, and patients may complain of mottled or numb fingers or toes. Hemolytic anemia is rarely severe, but episodic hemoglobinuria may occur on exposure to cold. The hemolytic anemia in acute postinfectious syndromes is rarely severe.

**B. Laboratory Findings:** Mild anemia is present with reticulocytosis and spherocytes. The direct Coombs test will be positive for complement only. Occasionally, a micro-Coombs test is necessary to reveal bound complement (low-titer cold agglutinin disease).

## Treatment

Treatment is largely symptomatic, based on avoiding exposure to cold. Patients with severe involvement may be treated with alkylating agents such as chlorambucil. Splenectomy is ineffective, since hemolysis takes place in the liver. Prednisone is ineffective in reducing Kupffer cell function.

Schreiber AD, Herskovitz BS, Goldwein M. Low-titer cold-hemagglutinin disease: Mechanism of hemolysis and response to corticosteroids. *N Engl J Med* 1977;**296**:1490.

## MICROANGIOPATHIC HEMOLYTIC ANEMIAS

The microangiopathic hemolytic anemias are a group of disorders in which red blood cell fragmentation takes place. The anemia is intravascular, producing hemoglobinemia, hemoglobinuria, and, in severe cases, methemalbuminemia. The hallmark of the disorder is the finding of fragmented red blood cells (schistocytes, helmet cells) on the peripheral blood smear.

These fragmentation syndromes can be caused by a variety of disorders (Table 10–8). Thrombotic thrombocytopenic purpura is the most important of these and is discussed below. Clinical features of the fragmentation syndromes are variable and depend on the underlying disorder. Coagulopathy and thrombocytopenia are variably present.

Chronic microangiopathic hemolytic anemia (such as is present with a malfunctioning cardiac valve prosthesis) may cause iron deficiency anemia because of continuous low-grade hemoglobinuria. This can be diagnosed by measuring 24-hour excretion of iron in the urine.

Antman KH et al: Microangiopathic hemolytic anemia and cancer: A review. *Medicine.* 1979;**58**:377.

## HEMOLYSIS RELATED TO INFECTION

Clostridial infections may cause severe intravascular hemolysis, presumably because of the action of a clostridial toxin on the red blood cell membrane. Malaria may cause intravascular hemolysis because of parasitism of red blood cells; falciparum malaria causes the severest form (blackwater fever).

Other infections associated with hemolysis are bartonellosis and babesiosis.

## APLASTIC ANEMIA

### Essentials of Diagnosis
- Pancytopenia.
- No abnormal cells seen.
- Hypocellular bone marrow.

### General Considerations
All hematopoietic cells are derived from a pluripotent stem cell that gives rise to precursors of erythroid, myeloid, and platelet forms. Injury to or suppression of this hematopoietic stem cell will result in pancytopenia—reduction in all 3 hematopoietic cell lines (red blood cells, neutrophils, and platelets). Aplastic anemia is a condition of bone marrow failure that arises from injury to or abnormal expression of the stem cell. The bone marrow becomes hypoplastic, and pancytopenia develops.

There are a number of causes of aplastic anemia (Table 10–10). Direct stem cell injury may be caused by radiation, chemotherapy, toxins, or pharmacologic agents. Systemic lupus erythematosus may rarely cause suppression of the hematopoietic stem cell by an IgG autoantibody directed against the stem cell. However, the most common pathogenesis of aplastic anemia appears to be autoimmune suppression of hematopoiesis by a T cell-mediated cellular mechanism.

### Clinical Findings
**A. Symptoms and Signs:** Patients come to medical attention because of the consequences of bone marrow failure. Anemia leads to symptoms of weakness and fatigue; neutropenia causes vulnerability to bacterial infections; and thrombocytopenia results in mucosal and skin bleeding. Physical examination may reveal signs of pallor, purpura, and petechiae. Other abnormalities such as hepatosplenomegaly, lymphadenopathy, or bone tenderness should *not* be present, and their presence should lead one to question the diagnosis of aplastic anemia.

**B. Laboratory Findings:** The hallmark of aplastic anemia is pancytopenia. However, early in the evolution of aplastic anemia, only one or 2 cell lines may be reduced.

Anemia may be severe and is always associated with decreased reticulocytes. Red blood cell morphology is remarkable. The MCV is usually normal but occasionally may be increased. Neutrophils and platelets are reduced in number, and no immature or abnormal forms are seen. The bone marrow aspirate and the bone marrow biopsy appear hypocellular, with only scant amounts of normal hepatopoietic progenitors. No abnormal cells are seen.

### Differential Diagnosis
The diagnosis of aplastic anemia is made in cases of pancytopenia with a hypocellular marrow biopsy containing no abnormal cells. Aplastic anemia must be differentiated from other causes of pancytopenia (Table 10–11). Myelodysplastic disorders or acute leukemia may occasionally be confused with aplastic anemia. These are differentiated by the presence of morphologic abnormalities or increased blasts. Hairy cell leukemia has been misdiagnosed as aplastic ane-

**Table 10–10.** Causes of aplastic anemia.

| |
| --- |
| Congenital (rare) |
| "Idiopathic" (probably autoimmune) |
| Systemic lupus erythematosus |
| Chemotherapy, radiotherapy |
| Toxins: Benzene, toluene, insecticides |
| Drugs: Chloramphenicol, phenylbutazone, gold salts, sulfonamides, phenytoin, carbamazepine, quinacrine, tolbutamide |
| Posthepatitis |
| Pregnancy |
| Paroxysmal nocturnal hemoglobinuria |

**Table 10–11.** Causes of pancytopenia.

**Bone marrow disorders**
  Aplastic anemia
  Myelodysplasia
  Acute leukemia
  Myelofibrosis
  Infiltrative disease: Lymphoma, myeloma, carcinoma, hairy
    cell leukemia
  Megaloblastic anemia
**Nonmarrow disorders**
  Hypersplenism
  Systemic lupus erythematosus
  Infection: Tuberculosis, AIDS, leishmaniasis, brucellosis

mia and should be recognized by a high incidence of splenomegaly and by the presence of abnormal lymphoid cells on the bone marrow biopsy. Pancytopenia in the presence of a normal bone marrow is usually due to systemic lupus erythematosus, disseminated infection, or hypersplenism. Isolated thrombocytopenia may occur early as aplastic anemia develops and be confused with immune thrombocytopenia.

## Treatment

Mild cases of aplastic anemia may be treated with supportive care. Red blood cell transfusions and platelet transfusions are given as necessary, and antibiotics are used to treat infections.

Severe aplastic anemia is defined by the presence of neutrophils less than 500/µL, platelets less than 20,000/µL, reticulocytes less than 1%, and bone marrow cellularity less than 20%. When this constellation (or 3 of the 4) of features is present, the median survival is approximately 3 months, and only 20% of patients will survive 1 year. Severe aplastic anemia is a life-threatening condition that requires urgent treatment. The treatment of choice for adults under age 40 who have HLA-matched siblings is allogeneic bone marrow transplantation. The best results occur in younger patients who have not been previously transfused. Prior transfusion increases the risk of graft rejection, apparently because of prior sensitization to antigens present on hematopoietic progenitors. Young patients may tolerate severe anemia and thrombocytopenia and should not be transfused unless there is imminent bleeding or cardiorespiratory distress. These patients and their siblings should be HLA-typed promptly and referred for further evaluation by a hematologist.

For adults over age 40 or those without HLA-matched siblings, the treatment of choice for severe aplastic anemia is antithymocyte globulin (ATG). ATG is a horse serum containing polyclonal antibodies against human T cells. The success of this form of treatment has helped confirm the notion that most cases of aplastic anemia are immunologically mediated rather than caused by irreversible stem cell injury. ATG is given in the hospital over 7–10 days in conjunction with transfusion and antibiotic support. Responses usually occur in 4–12 weeks. Responses to ATG are usually only partial, but the blood counts

rise high enough to give patients a safe and transfusion-free life.

Androgens have been widely used in the past, with a low response rate. However, a few patients can be maintained successfully with this form of treatment. One regimen is oxymethalone, 2–3 mg/kg orally daily. In the rare syndrome of systemic lupus erythematosus causing humorally mediated aplastic anemia, the combination of plasmapheresis and high-dose prednisone may be successful.

## Course & Prognosis

Patients with severe aplastic anemia have a rapidly fatal illness if left untreated. Allogeneic bone marrow transplantation is highly successful in young adults with HLA-matched siblings. For this group of patients, the durable complete response rate is 80%. For older adults or those who have previously been exposed to blood products, long-term survival rates are between 40% and 70%. ATG treatment leads to partial response in approximately 60% of adults, and the long-term prognosis of responders appears to be very good.

Camitta BM, Storb R, Thomas ED: Aplastic anemia: Pathogenesis, diagnosis, treatment, and prognosis. (2 parts.) *N Engl J Med* 1982;**306**:645, 712.

Champlin R, Ho W, Gale RP: antithymocyte globulin treatment in patients with aplastic anemia: A prospective randomized trial. *N Engl J Med* 1983;**308**:113.

Storb R et al: Marrow transplantation in 30 ''untransfused'' patients with severe aplastic anemia. *Ann Intern Med* 1980;**92**:30.

Storb R et al: Marrow transplantation with or without donor buffy coat cells for 65 transfused aplastic anemia patients. *Blood* 1982;**59**:236.

# NEUTROPENIA

Neutropenia exists when the neutrophil count falls below 1500/µL. However, blacks and other specific population groups may normally have neutrophil counts as low as 1200/µL. The neutropenic patient is increasingly vulnerable to infection by gram-positive and gram-negative bacteria and by the fungi *Candida* and *Aspergillus*. The risk of infection is related to the severity of neutropenia. Patients with ''chronic benign neutropenia'' are free of infection for years despite very low neutrophil levels.

A variety of bone marrow disorders and nonmarrow conditions may cause neutropenia (Table 10–12). All the causes of aplastic anemia (Table 10–10) and pancytopenia (Table 10–11) may cause neutropenia as part of their overall picture. Isolated neutropenia is often due to an idiosyncratic reaction to a drug, and agranulocytosis (complete absence of neutrophils in the peripheral blood) is almost always

**Table 10–12.** Causes of neutropenia.

**Bone marrow disorders**
  Aplastic anemia
  Pure white cell aplasia
  Congenital (rare)
  Cyclic neutropenia
  Drugs: Sulfonamides, chlorpromazine, procainamide, peni-
    cillin, cephalosporins, cimetidine, methimazole, phenytoin,
    chlorpropamide
  Benign chronic
**Peripheral disorders**
  Hypersplenism
  Sepsis
  Immune
  Felty's syndrome

due to a drug reaction or to exposure to a variety of chemicals (eg, pesticides). In these cases, examination of the bone marrow shows virtual absence of myeloid precursors, with other cell lines undisturbed. Pure white cell aplasia is a rare condition in which an autoantibody is formed against myeloid progenitors. Neutropenia in the presence of a normal bone marrow may be due to immunologic peripheral destruction, sepsis, or hypersplenism.

## Clinical Findings

Neutropenia results in stomatitis and in infections. Infections are usually due to gram-positive or gram-negative aerobic bacteria or to fungi such as *Candida* or *Aspergillus*. The most common infections are septicemia, cellulitis, and pneumonia. It should be emphasized that in the presence of severe neutropenia the usual signs of inflammatory response to infection may be absent. Infection (especially septicemia) in the presence of severe neutropenia is a medical emergency, and death may occur within hours without appropriate antibiotic therapy.

Felty's syndrome is a combination of neutropenia with seropositive rheumatoid arthritis. The bone marrow is usually normal, and the neutropenia appears to be related to antineutrophil antibodies causing peripheral destruction of these cells. The disorder is clinically manifested as repeated infections and nonhealing ulcers on the lower legs.

## Treatment

Infections in a neutropenic patient should be treated on an emergent basis. Many combinations of broad-spectrum antibiotics can be used, but particular attention should be paid to enteric gram-negative bacteria. Combined treatment with aminoglycosides and a semisynthetic penicillin is commonly used. Offending drugs should be immediately discontinued.

When Felty's syndrome leads to repeated bacterial infections, splenectomy is the treatment of choice. Splenectomy usually leads to healing of leg ulcers and to reduction in the rate of infection whether or not the neutrophil count rises.

The prognosis of patients with neutropenia depends on the underlying cause. Most patients with drug-

induced agranulocytosis can be supported with broad-spectrum antibiotics and will recover completely.

Blumfelder TM, Logue GL, Shimm DS: Felty's syndrome: Effects of splenectomy upon granulocyte count and granulocyte-associated IgG. *Ann Intern Med* 1981;**94**:623.
Dale DC et al: Chronic neutropenia. *Medicine* 1979;**58**:128.

# LEUKEMIAS & OTHER MYELOPROLIFERATIVE DISORDERS

Myeloproliferative disorders are due to acquired clonal abnormalities of the hematopoietic stem. Since the stem cell gives rise to myeloid, erythroid, and platelet cells, one sees qualitative and quantitative changes in all these cell lines. In some disorders (chronic myeloid leukemia), specific characteristic chromosomal changes are seen. In others, although the disorder is presumed to be related to a defect in DNA, no characteristic cytogenetic abnormalities are seen.

Classically, the myeloproliferative disorders produce characteristic syndromes with well-defined clinical and laboratory features (Tables 10–13 and 10–14). However, these disorders are grouped together because the disease may evolve from one form into another and because hybrid disorders are commonly seen. All of the myeloproliferative disorders may progress to acute myeloid leukemia.

## POLYCYTHEMIA VERA

### Essentials of Diagnosis

- Increased red blood cell mass.
- Splenomegaly.
- Normal arterial oxygen saturation.
- Usually elevated white blood count and platelet count.

### General Considerations

Polycythemia vera is an acquired myeloproliferative disorder that causes overproduction of all 3 hematopoietic cell lines, most prominently the red blood cells. The hematocrit is elevated (at sea level) when

**Table 10–13.** Classification of myeloproliferative disorders.

  Myeloproliferative syndromes
    Polycythemia vera
    Myelofibrosis
    Essential thrombocytosis
    Chronic myeloid leukemia
  Myelodysplastic syndromes
  Acute myeloid leukemia

**Table 10–14.** Laboratory features of myeloproliferative disorders.

| | White Count | Hematocrit | Platelet Count | Red Cell Morphology |
|---|---|---|---|---|
| Chronic myeloid leukemia | ↑ ↑ | Normal | Normal or ↑ | Normal |
| Myelofibrosis | Normal or ↓ or ↑ | Normal or ↓ | ↓ or normal or ↑ | Abnormal |
| Polycythemia vera | Normal or ↑ | ↑ | Normal or ↑ | Normal |
| Essential thrombocytosis | Normal or ↑ | Normal | ↑ ↑ | Normal |

values exceed 54% in males or 51% in females (Table 10–15).

When the hematocrit is elevated, the red blood cell mass should be measured to determine whether true polycythemia or relative polycythemia exists. Normal values for red blood cell mass are 26–34 mL/kg in men and 21–29 mL/kg in women. Relative ("spurious") polycythemia characteristically presents in middle-aged men who are overweight and hypertensive; the hematocrit is almost always less than 60%.

If the red blood cell mass is increased, one must determine whether the increase is primary or secondary. Primary polycythemia (polycythemia vera) is a bone marrow disorder characterized by autonomous overproduction or erythroid cells. Erythroid production is independent of erythropoietin, and the serum erythropoietin level is low. In vitro, erythroid progenitor cells grow without added erythropoietin, a finding not seen in normal individuals.

Polycythemia vera is a relatively common disorder. Sixty percent of patients are male, and the median age at presentation is 60. Polycythemia vera rarely occurs in adults under age 40.

## Clinical Findings

**A. Symptoms and Signs:** Most patients present with symptoms related to expanded blood volume and increased blood viscosity. Common complaints include headache, dizziness, tinnitus, blurred vision, and fatigue. Generalized pruritus, especially that occurring following a warm shower or bath, may be a striking symptom and is related to histamine release from the increased number of basophils present. Patients may also initially complain of epistaxis. This is probably related to engorgement of mucosal blood vessels in combination with abnormal hemostasis due to qualitative abnormalities in platelet function.

**Table 10–15.** Causes of polycythemia.

Spurious polycythemia
Secondary polycythemia
  Hypoxia: Cardiac disease, pulmonary disease, high altitude
  Carboxyhemoglobin: Smoking
  Renal lesions
  Erythropoietin-secreting tumors (rare)
  Abnormal hemoglobins (rare)
Polycythemia vera

Physical examination reveals plethora and engorged retinal veins. The spleen is palpably enlarged in 75% of cases, but splenomegaly is nearly always present if assayed by an isotope scan. Less commonly, the liver is mildly enlarged.

Thrombosis is the most common complication of polycythemia vera and the major cause of morbidity and death in this disorder. Thrombosis appears to be related to increased blood viscosity and abnormal platelet function. Uncontrolled polycythemia leads to a very high incidence of thrombotic complications of surgery, and elective surgery should be deferred until the condition has been treated. Paradoxically, in addition to thrombosis, increased bleeding also occurs. There is a high incidence of peptic ulcer disease as well as gastrointestinal bleeding. Overproduction of uric acid may lead to gout.

**B. Laboratory Findings:** The hallmark of polycythemia vera is a hematocrit above normal, at times greater than 60%. Red blood cell morphology is normal. The white blood count is characteristically elevated to 10,000–20,000/μL and the platelet count is variably elevated, sometimes with counts exceeding 1,000,000/μL. Platelet morphology is usually normal, but large hypogranular forms may be seen. White blood cells are usually normal, but basophilia is frequently present. By definition, the red blood cell mass is elevated.

The bone marrow is hypercellular, with panhyperplasia of all hematopoietic elements. A characteristic finding is increased numbers of megakaryocytes. Iron stores are usually absent from the bone marrow, having been exhausted by exuberant red cell production. Iron deficiency may result from chronic gastrointestinal blood loss.

Vitamin $B_{12}$ levels are strikingly elevated because of increased levels of transcobalamin III (secreted by white blood cells). The leukocyte alkaline phosphatase is characteristically elevated as a marker of qualitative abnormalities in the myeloid line. Uric acid levels may be increased. There is no characteristic chromosomal abnormality in this disorder.

Although red blood cell morphology is usually normal at presentation, microcytosis, hypochromia, and poikilocytosis may result from iron deficiency following treatment by phlebotomy (see below). Progressive hypersplenism may also lead to elliptocytosis.

## Differential Diagnosis

A secondary cause of polycythemia should be suspected if splenomegaly is absent and the high hematocrit is not accompanied by increases in other cell lines. Arterial oxygen saturation should be measured to determine if hypoxia is the cause. A smoking history should be taken and carboxyhemoglobin levels measured when indicated. An intravenous urogram or renal sonogram may be indicated to evaluate the kidneys for abnormalities. A positive family history should lead to investigation for congenital high-affinity hemoglobin.

Polycythemia vera should be differentiated from other myeloproliferative disorders (Table 10–14). Marked elevation of the white blood count above 30,000/μL) should lead to consideration of chronic myeloid leukemia. This disorder is confirmed by the finding of a low leukocyte alkaline phosphatase and by the presence of the Philadelphia chromosome. Abnormal red blood cell morphology and nucleated red blood cells in the peripheral blood should lead to the consideration of myelofibrosis. This condition is diagnosed by bone marrow biopsy showing fibrosis of the marrow. Essential thrombocytosis is diagnosed when the platelet count is strikingly elevated and the red blood cell count is normal.

## Treatment

The treatment of choice is phlebotomy. One unit of blood (approximately 500 mL) is removed weekly until the hematocrit is less than 45%; the hematocrit is maintained at less than 45% by repeated phlebotomy as necessary. Because repeated phlebotomy produces iron deficiency, the requirement for phlebotomy should gradually decrease. It is important to avoid medicinal iron supplementation, as this can thwart the goals of a phlebotomy program. It is not necessary to manipulate the diet to decrease iron intake. Patients will usually feel much better as soon as the hematocrit is lowered. Maintaining the hematocrit at normal levels has been shown to decrease the incidence of thrombotic complications.

Occasionally, myelosuppressive therapy is indicated. Indications include a high phlebotomy requirement, marked thrombocytosis, and intractable pruritus. Alkylating agents and radiophosphorus ($^{32}$P) have been shown to increase the risk of conversion of this disease to acute leukemia. Hydroxyurea is now being widely used when myelosuppressive therapy is indicated because of the presumption that antimetabolites will not be leukemogenic. Busulfan may also be used.

The role of antiplatelet agents such as aspirin in preventing thrombotic complications is controversial, but this treatment may be warranted in selected patients who have recurrent thromboses despite control of their platelet count with myelosuppressive therapy.

Allopurinol may be indicated for hyperuricemia. Antihistamine therapy with diphenhydramine and cimetidine may be helpful for control of pruritus.

## Prognosis

Polycythemia is an indolent disease with median survival of 10–15 years. The major cause of morbidity and mortality is arterial thrombosis. Over time, polycythemia vera may convert to myelofibrosis or to chronic myeloid leukemia. In approximately 10% of cases, the disorder progresses to acute myeloid leukemia, which is usually refractory to therapy.

Berk PD et al: Therapeutic recommendations in polycythemia vera based on Polycythemia Vera Study Group protocols. *Semin Hematol* 1986;**23**:132.

Golde DW et al: Polycythemia: Mechanisms and management. *Ann Intern Med* 1981;**95**:71.

## MYELOFIBROSIS

### Essentials of Diagnosis

- Teardrop poikilocytosis on peripheral smear.
- Leukoerythroblastic blood picture; giant abnormal platelets.
- Hypercellular bone marrow with reticulin or collagen fibrosis.

### General Considerations

Myelofibrosis (myelofibrosis with myeloid metaplasia, agnogenic myeloid metaplasia) is a myeloproliferative disorder characterized by fibrosis of the bone marrow, splenomegaly, and a leukoerythroblastic peripheral blood picture with teardrop poikilocytosis. In response to bone marrow fibrosis, extramedullary hematopoiesis (hematopoietic cell development outside the bone marrow) takes place in the liver, spleen, and lymph nodes. In these sites, mesenchymal cells responsible for fetal hematopoiesis can be reactivated.

### Clinical Findings

**A. Symptoms and Signs:** Myelofibrosis develops in adults over age 50 and is usually insidious in onset. Patients most commonly present with fatigue related to their anemia or abdominal fullness related to splenomegaly. Uncommon presentations include bleeding and bone pain. On examination, splenomegaly is almost invariably present and is sometimes massive. The liver is enlarged in more than half of cases.

Later in the course of the disease, progressive bone marrow failure takes place as the marrow becomes progressively more fibrotic. Anemia becomes severe, and red cell transfusion becomes necessary. Progressive thrombocytopenia leads to bleeding. The spleen continues to enlarge, which leads to early satiety. Painful episodes of splenic infarction may occur. Late in the course of the disease, the patient becomes cachectic and may experience severe bone pain, especially in the lower legs. Hematopoiesis in the liver leads to portal hypertension with ascites, esophageal varices, and eventually liver failure.

**B. Laboratory Findings:** Patients are almost invariably anemic at presentation. The white blood count is variable—either low, normal, or elevated—and may be increased to 50,000/µL. The platelet count is variable. The peripheral blood smear is characteristic, consisting of significant poikilocytosis with numerous teardrop forms. Immature myeloid and erythroid forms are present (leukoerythroblastic blood picture). Nucleated red blood cells are present and the myeloid series is less strikingly shifted, with immature forms including a small percentage of promyelocytes or myeloblasts. Platelet morphology may be bizarre, and giant degranulated platelet forms (megakaryocyte fragments) may be seen. The triad of teardrop poikilocytosis, leukoerythroblastic blood, and giant abnormal platelets is almost diagnostic of myelofibrosis.

The bone marrow is usually inaspirable (dry tap). Early in the course of the disease, the bone marrow is hypercellular, with a marked increase in megakaryocytes. Fibrosis at this stage is detected only by a silver stain demonstrating increased reticulin fibers. Later in the course of the disease, bone marrow biopsy reveals that fibrosis becomes more severe, with eventual replacement of hematopoietic precursors by collagen fibrosis. There is no characteristic chromosomal abnormality.

### Differential Diagnosis

A leukoerythroblastic blood picture may be seen in response to severe infection or inflammation. However, teardrop poikilocytosis and giant abnormal platelet forms will not be present. Bone marrow fibrosis may be seen in metastatic carcinoma, Hodgkin's disease, and hairy cell leukemia. These disorders are diagnosed by characteristic tissue morphology.

Myelofibrosis is distinguished from other myeloproliferative disorders by the characteristic constellation of findings (Table 10–14). Chronic myeloid leukemia is diagnosed when there is marked elevation of the white blood count, a low leukocyte alkaline phosphatase, normal red blood cell morphology, and the presence of the Philadelphia chromosome. Polycythemia vera is characterized by an elevated hematocrit, and patients with essential thrombocytosis should have normal red blood cell morphology. Ultimately, the diagnosis is made by examination of the bone marrow biopsy.

### Treatment

There is no specific treatment for this disorder. Anemic patients are supported with red blood cells in transfusion. Androgens such as oxymetholone may help reduce the transfusion requirement. Splenectomy is not routinely performed but is indicated for splenic enlargement that causes recurrent painful episodes, severe thrombocytopenia, or an unacceptably high red blood cell transfusion requirement.

### Course & Prognosis

It is often hard to date the onset of myelofibrosis, but the median survival from time of diagnosis is approximately 5 years. End-stage myelofibrosis is a wasting illness characterized by generalized debility, liver failure, and bleeding from thrombocytopenia. Some cases may terminate in acute myeloid leukemia.

Silverstein MN, ReMine WH: Splenectomy in myeloid metaplasia. *Blood* 1979;**53:**515.

Varki A et al: The syndrome of idiopathic myelofibrosis: A clinicopathologic review with emphasis on the prognostic variables predicting survival. *Medicine* 1983;**62:**353.

## CHRONIC MYELOID LEUKEMIA

### Essentials of Diagnosis

- Markedly elevated white blood count.
- Markedly left-shifted myeloid series with a low percentage of promyelocytes and blasts.
- Presence of Philadelphia chromosome.

### General Considerations

Chronic myeloid leukemia is a myeloproliferative disorder characterized by overproduction of myeloid cells. These myeloid cells retain the capacity for differentiation, and normal bone marrow function is retained during the early phases. The disease usually remains stable for years and then transforms to a more overtly malignant disease.

Chronic myeloid leukemia is associated with a characteristic chromosomal abnormality, the Philadelphia chromosome, and was the first disease associated with a specific karyotypic abnormality. The Philadelphia chromosome is now recognized to be a reciprocal translocation between the long arms of chromosomes 9 and 22. A large portion of 22q is translocated to 9q, and a smaller piece of 9q is moved to 22q. This translocation is thought to be pathogenically significant, based on recent evidence that oncogene activation occurs. The portion of 9q that is translocated contains *abl*, a proto-oncogene that is the cellular homolog of the Ableson murine leukemia virus. The *abl* gene is received at a specific site on 22q, the break point cluster (BCR). The fusion gene *abl*-BCR produces a novel protein that differs from the normal transcript of the *abl* gene in that it possesses tyrosine kinase activity (a characteristic activity of transforming genes).

Usually at the time of diagnosis, the Philadelphia chromosome-positive clone dominates and may be the only one detected. However, a normal clone is present and may express itself either in vivo, after certain forms of therapy, or in vitro, in long-term bone marrow cultures. Approximately 5% of cases of chronic myeloid leukemia are Philadelphia chromosome-negative. In some cases, although the characteristic karyotype is not seen at the light mcrioscopic level, gene mapping demonstrates translocation of *abl* to 22q. In other cases of Philadelphia-negative chronic myeloid leukemia, the disease is atypical and is better described as chronic myelomonocytic leukemia. Philadelphia chromosome-negative disease has a poor prognosis.

Early chronic myeloid leukemia ("chronic phase") does not behave like a malignant disease. Normal bone marrow function is retained, white blood cells differentiate, and, despite some qualitative abnormalities (low leukocyte alkaline phosphatase), the neutrophils combat infection normally. However, chronic myeloid leukemia is inherently unstable, and the disease progresses to accelerated phase and finally to blast crisis. This progression of the disease is often associated with added chromosomal defects superimposed on the Philadelphia chromosome. Blast crisis chronic myeloid leukemia is an overtly malignant process that becomes indistinguishable from acute leukemia.

## Clinical Findings

**A. Symptoms and Signs:** Chronic myeloid leukemia is a disorder of middle age (median age at presentation is 42 years). Patients usually present with fatigue, night sweats, and low-grade fever related to the hypermetabolic state caused by overproduction of white blood cells. At other times, the patient complains of abdominal fullness related to splenomegaly, or an elevated white blood count is discovered incidentally. Rarely, the patient will present with a clinical syndrome related to leukostasis with blurred vision, respiratory distress, or priapism. The white blood count in these cases is usually greater than 500,000/μL.

On examination, the spleen is enlarged (often markedly so), and sternal tenderness may be present as a sign of marrow overexpansion.

Acceleration of the disease is often associated with fever in the absence of infection, bone pain, and splenomegaly. In blast crisis, patients may experience bleeding and infection related to bone marrow failure.

**B. Laboratory Findings:** The hallmark of chronic myeloid leukemia is an elevated white blood count; the median white blood count at diagnosis is 150,000/μL. The peripheral blood is characteristic. The myeloid series is left-shifted, with mature forms dominating and with cells usually present in proportion to their degree of maturation. Blasts are usually less than 5%. Basophilia of granulocytes may be present. The peripheral blood smear gives the impression that the bone marrow has spilled over into the blood. At presentation, the patient is usually not anemic. Red blood cell morphology is normal, and nucleated red blood cells are rarely seen. The platelet count may be normal or elevated (sometimes to strikingly high levels). Platelet morphology is usually normal, but abnormally large forms may be seen.

The bone marrow is hypercellular, with markedly left-shifted myelopoiesis. Myeloblasts comprise less than 5% of marrow cells.

The leukocyte alkaline phosphatase score is invariably low and is a sign of qualitative abnormalities in neutrophils. The vitamin $B_{12}$ level is usually markedly elevated because of increased secretion of transcobalamin III. Uric acid levels may be high.

The Philadelphia chromosome is almost invariably present and may be detected in the peripheral blood or bone marrow.

With progression to the accelerated and blast phases, progressive anemia and thrombocytopenia occur, and the percentage of blasts in the blood and bone marrow increases. Blast phase chronic myeloid leukemia is diagnosed when blasts comprise more than 30% of bone marrow cells.

## Differential Diagnosis

Early chronic myeloid leukemia must be differentiated from the reactive leukocytosis associated with infection, inflammation, or cancer. In these reactive disorders, the white blood count is usually less than 50,000/μL, splenomegaly is absent, the leukocyte alkaline phosphatase is normal or increased, and the Philadelphia chromosome is not present. If one is in doubt whether leukocytosis is due to chronic myeloid leukemia or a reactive condition, the patient should be observed, since there is no advantage to early therapy for asymptomatic patients.

Chronic myeloid leukemia must be distinguished from other myeloproliferative disease (Table 10–14). The hematocrit should not be elevated, the red blood cell morphology should be normal, and nucleated red blood cells should be rare or absent. Definitive diagnosis is made by finding the Philadelphia chromosome.

## Treatment

Treatment is usually not an emergent necessity even with white blood counts over 200,000/μL. In the rare instances in which extreme hyperleukocytosis is associated with the clinical syndrome of leukostasis (priapism, respiratory distress, visual blurring, altered mental status), leukapheresis should be performed on an emergency basis in conjunction with myelosuppressive therapy.

The usual treatment is palliative and improves the patient's sense of well-being without altering the natural history of the disease. Myelosuppressive therapy consists of giving either busulfan or hydroxyurea in combination with allopurinol. When busulfan is used, the usual dose is 4–8 mg daily for 4–8 weeks. One aims to lower the white count to 10,000–20,000/μL. Busulfan has a notoriously prolonged duration of action, and it is important not to lower the white blood count too much because this will expose the patient to an unnecessary risk of infection. Patients are managed either intermittently or continuously. When hydroxyurea is used, the initial dose is usually 2–4 g/d orally, and the maintenance dose varies between 0.5 and 2 g/d as necessary to maintain the white blood count at 10,000–20,000/μL. Hydroxyurea must be given without interruption, since the white blood count will rise within days after discontinuing this medication. The response to hydroxyurea or busulfan is usually gratifying. The white blood count decreases, the spleen decreases in size, and the patient becomes asymptomatic. Most patients in the chronic phase of chronic myeloid leukemia will have no symptoms either from the disease or their chemotherapy. Recently, recombinant alpha interferon has been used in the treatment of the chronic phase with good results. Interestingly, in some patients the Philadelphia chromosome-positive clone has decreased or disappeared—changes not seen in response to treatment with busulfan or hydroxyurea. The ultimate significance of this finding is unclear.

Although the response to myelosuppressive therapy of the chronic phase is gratifying, the treatment is only palliative, and the disease is invariably fatal. Curative therapy is available with high-dose chemotherapy in association with allogeneic bone marrow transplantation. This treatment is available for adults under age 50 who have HLA-matched siblings. Approximately 60% of adults have long-term disease-free survival following bone marrow transplantation and appear to be cured of their disease. All young patients should be given the opportunity for allogeneic bone marrow transplantation in chronic phase if they have suitable bone marrow donors.

Blast crisis of chronic myeloid leukemia is a notoriously difficult form of acute leukemia to treat. Lymphoid blast crisis (present in one-third of cases) should be identified because chemotherapy for this disorder is less toxic and more effective.

## Course & Prognosis

Median survival is 3–4 years. Once the disease has progressed to the accelerated or blast phase, survival is measured in months. Approximately 60% of young adults who have successful allogeneic bone marrow transplantation appear to be cured.

Champlin RE, Golde DW: Chronic myelogenous leukemia: Recent advances. *Blood* 1985;**65**:1039.

Sokal JE et al: Prognostic discrimination in "good risk" chronic granulocytic leukemia. *Blood* 1984;**63**:789.

Thomas ED et al: Marrow transplantation for the treatment of chronic myelogenous leukemia. *Ann Intern Med* 1986; **104**:155.

## MYELODYSPLASTIC SYNDROMES

### Essentials of Diagnosis

- Cytopenias with a hypercellular bone marrow.
- Morphologic abnormalities in 2 or more hematopoietic cell lines.

### General Considerations

The myelodysplastic syndromes are a group of acquired clonal disorders of the hematopoietic stem cell. They are characterized by the constellation of cytopenias, a hypercellular marrow, and a number of morphologic abnormalities. The disorders are usually idiopathic but may be seen after cytotoxic chemotherapy—especially procarbazine for Hodgkin's disease and melphalan for multiple myeloma or ovarian carcinoma.

Despite the presence of adequate numbers of hematopoietic progenitor cells, "ineffective hematopoi-

esis" occurs, resulting in various cytopenias. Ultimately, the disorder may evolve into frank acute myeloid leukemia, and the term "preleukemia" has been used to describe these disorders. Although no specific chromosomal abnormality is seen in myelodysplasia, there are frequently abnormalities involving the long arm of chromosome 5, which contains a number of genes encoding both growth factors and receptors involved in myelopoiesis.

### Clinical Findings

**A. Symptoms and Signs:** Elderly patients are usually affected except in cases of postchemotherapy myelodysplasia. Patients usually present with fatigue, infection, or bleeding related to bone marrow failure. The course may be indolent, and the disease may present as a wasting illness with fever, weight loss, and general debility. On examination, splenomegaly may be present in combination with pallor, bleeding, and various signs of infection.

**B. Laboratory Findings:** Anemia may be severe and may require transfusion support. The MCV is normal or increased, and macro-ovalocytes may be seen on the peripheral blood smear. The reticulocyte count is usually reduced. The white blood cell count is usually normal or reduced, and neutropenia is common. The neutrophils may exhibit morphologic abnormalities, including deficient numbers of granules or a bilobed nucleus (Pelger-Huet). The myeloid series may be left-shifted, and small numbers of promyelocytes or blasts may be seen. The platelet count is normal or reduced, and hypogranular platelets may be present.

The bone marrow is characteristically hypercellular. Erythroid hyperplasia is common, and signs of abnormal erythropoiesis include melagoblastic features, nuclear budding, or multinucleated erythroid precursors. The Prussian blue stain may demonstrate ringed sideroblasts. The myeloid series is often left-shifted, with variable increases in blasts. Deficient or abnormal granules may be seen. A characteristic abnormality is the presence of dwarf megakaryocytes with a unilobed nucleus.

### Differential Diagnosis

As the number of blasts increase in the bone marrow, myelodysplasia is arbitrarily separated from acute myeloid leukemia by the presence of less than 30% blasts.

### Treatment

Patients affected primarily by anemia are best supported with red blood cell transfusions. Patients with severe neutropenia or thrombocytopenia or those with marked constitutional symptoms may be treated with low-dose chemotherapy, although results of such treatment are poor.

### Course & Prognosis

Myelodysplasia is an ultimately fatal disease. Patients most commonly succumb to infections or bleeding. The risk of transformation to acute myeloid leukemia depends on the percentage of blasts in the bone marrow. Patients with more than 5% blasts in the bone marrow will almost invariably develop leukemia if they do not die of their cytopenias first.

Bennett JM et al: Proposals for the classification of the myelodysplastic syndromes. *Br J Haematol* 1982;**51**:189.

## ACUTE LEUKEMIA

### Essentials of Diagnosis

- Cytopenias or pancytopenia.
- Bone marrow failure causing infection, bleeding, or fatigue.
- More than 30% blasts in the bone marrow.

### General Considerations

Acute leukemia is a malignancy of the hematopoietic progenitor cell. The malignant cell loses its ability to mature and differentiate. These cells proliferate in an uncontrolled fashion and ultimately replace normal bone marrow elements. Most cases arise with no clear cause. However, radiation and some toxins (benzene) are clearly leukemogenic. In addition, a number of chemotherapeutic agents (especially procarbazine, melphalan, and other alkylating agents) may cause leukemia. The leukemias seen after toxin or chemotherapy exposure often develop from a myelodysplastic prodrome and are associated with abnormalities in chromosomes 5 and 7. Although a number of other cytogenetic abnormalities are seen in certain types of acute leukemia, their exact role in pathogenesis remains unclear.

Most of the clinical findings in acute leukemia are due to bone marrow failure, which results from replacement of normal bone marrow elements by the malignant cell. Less common manifestations include direct organ infiltration (skin, gastrointestinal tract, meninges).

Acute leukemia is one of the outstanding examples of a once invariably fatal disease that is now treatable and potentially curable with combination chemotherapy.

Acute lymphoblastic leukemia (ALL) comprises 80% of the acute leukemias of childhood. The peak incidence is between 3 and 7 years of age. However, ALL is also seen in adults and comprises approximately 20% of adult acute leukemias. Acute myeloid leukemia (AML; acute nonlymphocytic leukemia [ANLL]) is chiefly an adult disease with a median age at presentation of 50 years and an increasing incidence with advanced age. However, it is also seen in young adults and children.

### Clinical Findings

**A. Symptoms and Signs:** Most patients with acute leukemia present with an acute illness and have been ill only for days or weeks. The most common presenting complaints are those due to bone marrow

failure: fatigue, bleeding, and infection. Bleeding (usually due to thrombocytopenia) is usually in the skin and mucosal surfaces, manifested as gingival bleeding, epistaxis, or menorrhagia. Less commonly, widespread severe bleeding is seen in patients with disseminated intravascular coagulation (seen in acute promyelocytic leukemia and monocytic leukemia). Infection is due to neutropenia, with the risk of infection becoming high as the neutrophil count falls below 500/µL. Patients with neutrophil counts less than 100/ µL almost invariably become infected within several days. The most common pathogens are gram-negative bacteria (*E coli, Klebsiella, Pseudomonas*) or fungi (*Candida, Aspergillus*). Common presentations include cellulitis, pneumonia, and perirectal infections. Septicemia in severely neutropenic patients is a medical emergency and can cause death within a few hours if treatment with appropriate antibiotics is delayed.

Patients may also seek medical attention because of gum hypertrophy and bone and joint pain. The most dramatic presentation is hyperleukocytosis, in which a markedly elevated circulating blast count (usually greater than 200,000/uL) leads to imparied circulation, presenting as headache, confusion, and dyspnea. Leukostasis is a medical emergency, and patients require emergent leukapheresis and chemotherapy.

On examination, patients are usually pale and have purpura, petechiae, and various signs of infection. Stomatitis and gum hypertrophy may be seen in patients with monocytic leukemia. There is variable enlargement of the liver, spleen, and lymph nodes. Bone tenderness, particularly in the sternum and tibia, may be present.

**B. Laboratory Findings:** The hallmark of acute leukemia is the combination of pancytopenia with circulating blasts. However, blasts may be absent from the peripheral smear in as many as 10% of cases (''aleukemic leukemia'').

The bone marrow is usually hypercellular and dominated by blasts. More than 30% blasts are required to make a diagnosis of acute leukemia.

A number of other laboratory abnormalities may be present. Hyperuricemia and hypokalemia may be seen. If disseminated intravascular coagulation is present, the fibrinogen level will be reduced, the prothrombin time prolonged, and fibrin degradation products present. Patients with acute lymphoblastic leukemia (especially T cell) may have a mediastinal mass visible on chest radiograph. Patients with meningeal leukemia will have blasts present in the spinal fluid.

The diagnosis of acute leukemia is made by finding more than 30% blasts in the bone marrow. Acute leukemia should then be classified as either acute lymphoblastic or acute myeloid leukemia, also called acute nonlymphocytic leukemia. Patients with acute myeloid leukemia may have granules visible in the blast cells. The Auer rod, an eosinophilic needlelike inclusion in the cytoplasm, is pathognomonic of acute myeloid leukemia. To confirm the myeloid nature of the cells, histochemical stains demonstrating myeloid enzymes such as peroxidase or chloroacetate esterase may be useful. Monocytic lineage can be demonstrated by the finding of butyrate esterase. Acute lymphoblastic leukemia should be considered when there is no morphologic or histochemical evidence of myeloid or monocytic lineage. The diagnosis is confirmed by demonstrating surface markers characteristic of primitive lymphoid cells. Terminal deoxynucleotidal transferase (TdT) is present in 95% of cases of acute lymphoblastic leukemia. A variety of monoclonal antibodies have been used to define other phenotypes of acute lymphoblastic leukemia. Primitive B lymphocyte antigens include CALLA, B1, and BA1. T cell acute lymphoblastic leukemia is diagnosed by the finding of rosette formation with sheep erythrocytes or identification of cell markers by monoclonal antibodies such as Leu-1 or Leu-9.

Acute myeloid leukemia is usually so categorized on the basis of morphology and histochemistry as follows: Acute myeloblastic leukemia (M1), acute myeloblastic leukemia with differentiation (M2), acute promyelocytic leukemia (M3), acute myelomonocytic leukemia (M4), acute monoblastic leukemia (M5), and erythroleukemia (M6).

Acute lymphoblastic leukemia is most usefully classified by immunologic phenotype as follows: common, early B lineage, and T cell.

## Differential Diagnosis

Acute myeloid leukemia must be distinguished from other myeloproliferative disorders, chronic myeloid leukemia, and myelodysplastic syndromes. The diagnosis is made by finding more than 30% blasts in the bone marrow. It is important to distinguish acute leukemia from a left-shifted bone marrow that is recovering from a previous toxic insult. If the question is in doubt, a bone marrow study should be repeated in several days to see if maturation has taken place. Acute lymphoblastic leukemia must be distinguished from other lymphoproliferative disease such as chronic lymphocytic leukemia, lymphomas, and hairy cell leukemia. It may also be confused with the atypical lymphocytosis of mononucleosis. An experienced observer can distinguish these entities based on morphology.

## Treatment

Acute leukemia may present as a medical emergency. Sepsis in a neutropenic patient must be treated immediately with broad-spectrum antibiotics. Leukostasis must be treated immediately with leukapheresis and chemotherapy. Disseminated intravascular coagulation must be treated with replacement of platelets, coagulation factors, and fibrinogen in combination with heparin (discussed below).

Most young patients with acute leukemia are treated with the objective of effecting a cure. The first step in treatment is to obtain complete remission, defined as normal peripheral blood with resolution of cytopenias, normal bone marrow with no excess in blasts, and normal clinical status. However, complete remission is not synonymous with cure, and leukemia will invariably recur if no further treatment is given.

Acute myeloid leukemia is treated with intensive combination chemotherapy, including daunorubicin and cytarabine, and sometimes thioguanine. Effective treatment produces aplasia of the bone marrow, which takes 2–3 weeks to recover. During this period, intensive supportive care, including transfusion and antibiotic therapy, is required. Once complete remission has been achieved, several different types of postremission therapy are potentially curative. Options include repeated intensive chemotherapy, high-dose chemoradiotherapy with allogeneic bone marrow transplantation, and high-dose chemotherapy with autologous bone marrow transplantation.

Acute lymphoblastic leukemia is treated initially with combination chemotherapy, including daunorubicin, vincristine, prednisone, and sometimes asparaginase. Remission induction therapy for acute lymphoblastic leukemia is less myelosuppressive than treatment for acute myeloid leukemia and does not necessarily produce marrow aplasia. After achieving complete remission, patients receive central nervous system prophylaxis with cranial irradiation and intrathecal methotrexate so that meningeal sequestration of leukemic cells does not develop. As with acute myeloid leukemia, patients may be treated with either chemotherapy or high-dose chemotherapy plus bone marrow transplantation.

## Prognosis

Approximately 70% of adults with acute myeloid leukemia under age 50 achieve complete remission. Chemotherapy leads to long-term disease-free survival in 20–30% of cases. Allogeneic bone marrow transplantation (for younger adults with HLA-matched siblings) is curative in approximately 50% of cases. The role of autologous bone marrow transplantation remains to be defined. Older adults with acute myeloid leukemia achieve complete remission approximately 50% of the time. A selected older patient may be treated with intensive chemotherapy with curative intent.

Eighty percent of adults with acute lymphoblastic leukemia achieve complete remission. Subsequent postremission chemotherapy is curative in 30–50% of adults. Acute lymphoblastic leukemia in children is much more responsive to therapy, with 95% achieving complete remission and 50–60% of these being cured with postremission treatment that is far less toxic than that necessary for adults.

Champlin RE et al: Treatment of acute myelogenous leukemia: A prospective controlled trial of bone marrow transplantation vs consolidation chemotherapy. *Ann Intern Med* 1985; **102**:285.

Foon KA, Todd RF: Immunologic classification of leukemia and lymphoma. *Blood* 1986;**68**:1.

Jacobs AD, Gale RP: Recent advances in the biology and treatment of acute lymphoblastic leukemia in adults. *N Engl J Med* 1984;**311**:1219.

Linker CA et al: Improved results of treatment of adult acute lymphoblastic leukemia. *Blood* 1987;**69**:1242.

Schauer P et al: Treatment of acute lymphoblastic leukemia in adults: Results of the L-10 and L-10M protocols. *J Clin Oncol* 1983;**1**:462.

# CHRONIC LYMPHOCYTIC LEUKEMIA

## Essentials of Diagnosis

- Lymphocytosis greater than 15,000/μL.
- "Mature" appearance of lymphocytes.

## General Considerations

Chronic lymphocytic leukemia is a clonal malignancy of B lymphocytes (rarely T lymphocytes). The disease is usually indolent, with slowly progressive accumulation of long-lived small lymphocytes. These cells are immunoincompetent and respond poorly to antigenic stimulation.

Chronic lymphocytic leukemia is manifested clinically by immunosuppression, bone marrow failure, and organ infiltration with lymphocytes. Immunosuppression, bone marrow failure, and infiltration of organs account for most clinical manifestations. Immunodeficiency is also related to inadequate antibody production by the abnormal B cells. With advanced disease, chronic lymphocytic leukemia may cause damage by direct tissue infiltration.

## Clinical Findings

**A. Symptoms and Signs:** Chronic lymphocytic leukemia is a disease of the elderly, with 90% of cases occurring after age 50 and a median age at presentation of 65. Many patients will be incidentally discovered to have lymphocytosis. Others present with fatigue or lymphadenopathy. On examination, 80% of patients will have lymphadenopathy and half will have enlargement of the liver or spleen.

A prognostically useful staging system has been developed as follows: stage 0, lymphocytosis only; stage I, lymphocytosis plus lymphadenopathy; stage II, organomegaly; stage III, anemia; stage IV, thrombocytopenia.

Chronic lymphocytic leukemia usually pursues an indolent course but occasionally will present as a rapidly progressive disease. These patients usually have larger, less mature-appearing lymphocytes and are said to have "prolymphocytic" leukemia. In 5–10% of cases, chronic lymphocytic leukemia may be complicated by autoimmune hemolytic anemia or autoimmune thrombocytopenia. In approximately 5% of cases, while the systemic disease remains stable, an isolated lymph node will be transformed into an aggressive large cell lymphoma (Richter's syndrome).

**B. Laboratory Findings:** The hallmark of chronic lymphocytic leukemia is isolated lymphocyto-sis. The white blood count is usually greater than 20,000/μL and may be markedly elevated. Usually 75–98% of the circulating cells are lymphocytes. Lymphocytes appear small and "mature," with condensed nuclear chromatin, and are morphologically indistinguishable from normal small lymphocytes. The hematocrit and platelet count are usually normal at presentation. The bone marrow is variably infiltrated with small lymphocytes. The malignant cells weakly express surface immunoglobulin, and the monoclonal nature of the cells can be demonstrated by the finding of a single light chain type on the surface.

Hypogammaglobulinemia is present in half of cases and becomes more common with advanced disease. In some instances, a small amount of IgM paraprotein is present in the serum. Pathologic changes in lymph nodes are the same as in diffuse small cell lymphocytic lymphoma.

## Differential Diagnosis

Few syndromes can be confused with chronic lymphocytic leukemia. Viral infections producing lymphocytosis should be obvious from the presence of fever and other clinical findings. Other lymphoproliferative diseases such as Waldenström's macroglobulinemia, hairy cell leukemia, or lymphoma in the leukemic phase are distinguished on the basis of the morphology of circulating lymphocytes and bone marrow.

## Treatment

Most cases of early indolent chronic lymphocytic leukemia require no specific therapy. Indications for treatment include progressive fatigue, troublesome lymphadenopathy, or the development of anemia or thrombocytopenia. Initial therapy includes chlorambucil and prednisone. A common regimen is chlorambucil, 0.6–1 mL/kg, in combination with 4 days of prednisone every 3 weeks. Complications such as autoimmune hemolytic anemia or immune thrombocytopenia may be treated with high-dose prednisone but often require splenectomy for control.

## Prognosis

Median survival is approximately 6 years, and 25% of patients live more than 10 years. Patients with stage 0 or I disease have a median survival of 10 years. It is important to reassure these patients that despite the frightening diagnosis of "leukemia," they can live a normal life for many years. Patients with stage III or IV disease have a median survival of less than 2 years. Chronic lymphocytic leukemia is managed in palliative fashion. Patients with advanced disease benefit only briefly from intensive therapy.

Gale RP, Foon KA: Chronic lymphocytic leukemia: Recent advances in biology and treatment. *Ann Intern Med* 1985;**103**:101.

## HAIRY CELL LEUKEMIA

### Essentials of Diagnosis
- Pancytopenia.
- Splenomegaly, often massive.
- Hairy cells present on blood smear and bone marrow biopsy.

### General Considerations
Hairy cell leukemia, an uncommon form of leukemia, is an indolent cancer of B lymphocytes.

### Clinical Findings
**A. Symptoms and Signs:** The disease characteristically presents in middle-aged men. The median age at presentation is 55 years, and there is a striking 5:1 male predominance. Most patients present with gradual onset of fatigue, but others complain of symptoms related to markedly enlarged spleen and still others come to attention because of infection.

On physical examination, splenomegaly is almost invariably present and may be massive. The liver is enlarged in half of cases, but lymphadenopathy is uncommon.

**B. Laboratory Findings:** The hallmark of hairy cell leukemia is pancytopenia. Anemia is nearly universal, and 75% of patients have thrombocytopenia and neutropenia as well. The "hairy cells" are usually present in small numbers on the peripheral blood smear and have a characteristic appearance with numerous cytoplasmic projections. Less commonly, a "leukemic form" of the disorder exists in which large numbers of hairy cells dominate the peripheral blood smear. The bone marrow is usually inaspirable (dry tap), and the diagnosis is made by characteristic morphology on bone marrow biopsy. The hairy cells have a characteristic histochemical staining pattern, with tartrate-resistant acid phosphatase (TRAP). Pathologic examination of the spleen shows marked infiltration of the red pulp with hairy cells. This is in marked contrast to the usual predilection of lymphomas to involve the white pulp of the spleen.

Hairy cell leukemia is usually an indolent disorder whose course is dominated by pancytopenia and recurrent infections. For unclear reasons, these patients have a particular predilection for mycobacterial infections.

### Differential Diagnosis
Hairy cell leukemia should be distinguished from other lymphoproliferative diseases such as chronic lymphocytic leukemia, Waldenström's macroglobulinemia, and non-Hodgkin's lymphomas.

### Treatment
Many patients with indolent disease require no specific therapy. In the past, the treatment of choice has been splenectomy, indicated for severe cytopenias or recurrent infections. More recently, interferon has produced responses in a high proportion of patients and has led to disappearance of the disease for some time. Most recently, the experimental drug deoxycoformycin has produced encouraging results with a high percentage of complete remissions, some of which appear to be durable. The ultimate role of deoxycoformycin remains to be defined.

### Course & Prognosis
The median survival of patients with hairy cell leukemia is approximately 6 years, and one-third of patients survive more than 10 years. It remains to be seen whether recently developed treatments such as interferon and deoxycoformycin will improve the survival rates of these patients.

Quesada JR et al: Alpha interferon for induction of remission in hairy-cell leukemia. *N Engl J Med* 1984;**310**:15.

Spiers ASD et al: Remissions in hairy-cell leukemia with pentostatin (2'-deoxycoformycin). *N Engl J Med* 1987;**316**:825.

# LYMPHOMAS

## NON-HODGKIN'S LYMPHOMAS

### Essentials of Diagnosis
- Tumors in lymph nodes or extranodal sites.
- Pathologic diagnosis by lymph node biopsy.

### General Considerations
The non-Hodgkin's lymphomas are a heterogeneous group of cancers of the white cells. The disorders are variable in clinical presentation and course, varying from indolent disease to rapidly progressive devasting illnesses.

Results of studies using techniques of molecular biology have provided clues to the pathogenesis of these disorders. The best-studied example is Burkitt's lymphoma, in which a characteristic cytogenetic abnormality of translocation between the long arms of chromosomes 8 and 14 has been identified.

Classification of the lymphomas is a controversial area still undergoing evolution. Recently, the National Cancer Institute has sponsored a "working formulation" that characterizes these lymphomas according to their biologic behavior, whether indolent or aggressive (Table 10–16).

### Clinical Findings
**A. Symptoms and Signs:** Patients with indolent lymphomas usually present with painless lymphadenopathy, which may be isolated or widespread. However, the indolent lymphomas are almost always disseminated at the time of diagnosis, and bone marrow involvement is frequent.

Patients with high-grade lymphomas may present with adenopathy or with constitutional symptoms such as fever, drenching night sweats, or weight loss. On

**Table 10–16.** Classification of lymphomas; "working formulation."

Low-grade
   Small lymphocytic
   Small lymphocytic, plasmacytoid
   Follicular, small cleaved cell
   Follicular mixed cell
Intermediate-grade
   Follicular large cell
   Diffuse small cleaved cell
   Diffuse mixed cell
   Diffuse large cell
High-grade
   Immunoblastic
   Small noncleaved (Burkitt's)
   Small noncleaved (non-Burkitt's)
   Lymphoblastic
   True histiocytic
Other
   Cutaneous T cell
   Adult T cell leukemia/lymphoma
   T γ lymphocytosis

examination, lymphadenopathy may be isolated, or extranodal sites of disease (skin, gastrointestinal tract) may be found. Patients with Burkitt's lymphoma frequently deteriorate, with abdominal pain or abdominal fullness because of the predilection of the disease for the abdomen.

**B. Laboratory Findings:** The peripheral blood is usually normal, but a number of lymphomas may present in a "leukemic" phase. In these situations, the distinction between leukemia and lymphoma is arbitrary, as the malignant cell is the same. Examples of the diseases that may present as lymphoma or leukemia are small cell lymphoma versus chronic lymphocytic leukemia, small cell plasmacytic lymphoma versus Waldenström's macroglobulinemia, follicular small cleaved cell lymphoma versus lymphosarcoma cell leukemia, cutaneous T cell lymphoma versus Sezary syndrome, lymphoblastic lymphoma versus T cell acute lymphoblastic leukemia, and Burkitt's lymphoma versus B cell acute lymphoblastic leukemia.

Bone marrow involvement is usually manifested as paratrabecular lymphoid aggregates. In some high-grade lymphomas, the meninges may be involved and the spinal fluid may contain malignant cells. The chest radiograph may show a mediastinal mass in lymphoblastic lymphoma.

## Treatment

Once a pathologic diagnosis is established, the patient should be evaluated ("staged") to determine the extent of disease. The primary purpose of staging is to determine whether regional therapy such as surgery or radiation therapy is appropriate or whether the disease must be approached in a systemic fashion with chemotherapy.

The indolent lymphomas are not curable and are approached with palliative therapy. If patients are asymptomatic, no initial treatment may be necessary.

However, in 1–3 years, the disease will usually progress and require treatment. Initial therapy is based on the alkylating agents, and a regimen such as chlorambucil, 0.6–1 mg/kg every 3 weeks, may be used.

The high-grade lymphomas should be managed with curative intent. Although radiation therapy is occasionally indicated for localized disease, intensive multiagent chemotherapy is most commonly used.

## Prognosis

The median survival of patients with indolent lymphomas is 6–8 years. These diseases ultimately become refractory to chemotherapy. This often occurs at the time of histologic progression of the disease to a more aggressive form of lymphoma. The prognosis of patients with high-grade lymphomas depends on their response to chemotherapy. Depending on the initial pathologic subtype and initial bulk of disease, these patients are variably curable. Patients who do not respond well to chemotherapy have a very short survival.

Coleman M: Chemotherapy for large-cell lymphoma: Optimism and caution. *Ann Intern Med* 1985;**103:**140.
Horning SJ, Rosenberg SA: The natural history of initially untreated low-grade non-Hodgkin's lymphomas. *N Engl J Med* 1984;**311:**1471.

## HODGKIN'S DISEASE

### Essentials of Diagnosis

- Painless lymphadenopathy.
- Constitutional symptoms may be present.
- Pathologic diagnosis by lymph node biopsy.

### General Considerations

Hodgkin's disease is a group of cancers characterized by Reed-Sternberg cells in an appropriate reactive cellular background. The nature of the malignant cell is a subject of controversy, but recent evidence suggests that it is of macrophage origin.

### Clinical Findings

There is a bimodal age distribution, with one peak in the 20s and a second peak over age 50. Most patients present because of a painless mass, commonly in the neck. Others may seek medical attention because of constitutional symptoms such as fever, weight loss, or drenching night sweats, or because of generalized pruritus. An unusual symptom of Hodgkin's disease is pain in an involved lymph node following alcohol ingestion.

An important clinical feature of Hodgkin's disease is its tendency to arise within lymph node areas and to spread in an orderly fashion to contiguous areas of lymph nodes. Only late in the course of the disease will vascular invasion lead to widespread hematogenous dissemination.

The diagnosis is made by examination of lymph node tissue by an experienced hematopathologist.

Hodgkin's disease is divided into several subtypes: lymphocyte predominance, nodular sclerosis, mixed cellularity, and lymphocyte depletion. Hodgkin's disease should be distinguished pathologically from other malignant lymphomas. It may also occasionally be confused with reactive lymph nodes seen in infectious mononucleosis, cat-scratch disease, or drug reactions (phenytoin).

Patients should initially undergo a "staging" evaluation to determine the extent of disease. The purpose of this evaluation is to determine whether localized treatment (radiotherapy) is indicated or if systemic chemotherapy must be given. The staging nomenclature is as follows: stage I, one lymph node involved; stage II, involvement of 2 lymph node areas on one side of the diaphragm; stage III, lymph nodes involved on both sides of the diaphragm; Stage IV, disseminated disease with bone marrow or liver involvement. In addition, patients are designated stage A if they lack constitutional symptoms and stage B if significant weight loss, fever, or night sweats are present.

## Treatment

Patients with localized disease (stages IA, IIA) are treated with radiation therapy. Patients with disseminated disease (IIIB, IV) are treated with aggressive combination chemotherapy. The optimal management of patients with stages IIB or IIIA is controversial. Both radiotherapy and systemic chemotherapy have their proponents.

## Prognosis

Hodgkin's disease is no longer invariably fatal, and patients with both localized and disseminated disease should be treated with curative intent. The prognosis of patients with stage IA or IIA disease treated by radiotherapy is excellent, with 10-year survival rates in excess of 80%. Patients with disseminated disease (IIIB, IV) have 5-year survival rates of 20–50%. The poorer results are seen in patients who are elderly, those who have bulky disease, and those with lymphocyte depletion or mixed cellularity on histologic examination. The prognosis of patients with stage IIB or stage IIIA disease is intermediate, with 5-year survival rates between 30% and 60%.

Bonadonna G, Valagussa P, Santoro A: Alternating non-cross-resistant combination chemotherapy or MOPP in stage IV Hodgkin's disease: A report of 8-year results. *Ann Intern Med* 1986;**104**:739.

DeVita VT Jr et al: Curability of advanced Hodgkin's disease with chemotherapy: Long-term follow-up of MOPP-treated patients at the National Cancer Institute. *Ann Intern Med* 1980;**92**:587.

Kaplan HS: Hodgkin's disease: Biology, treatment, prognosis. *Blood* 1981;**57**:813.

## MULTIPLE MYELOMA

### Essentials of Diagnosis

- Monoclonal paraprotein by serum or urine protein electrophoresis or immunoelectrophoresis.
- Bone Pain and destruction.
- Replacement of bone marrow by malignant plasma cells.

## General Considerations

Multiple myeloma is a malignancy of plasma cells characterized by replacement of the bone marrow, bone destruction, and paraprotein formation. Myeloma is a complex disease that causes clinical signs and symptoms through a variety of mechanisms.

Replacement of the bone marrow (and perhaps humoral suppression of myelopoiesis) leads initially to anemia and later to general bone marrow failure. Bone destruction causes bone pain, osteoporosis, and pathologic fractures. Erosion of bone causes hypercalcemia. Some bone destruction is mediated by osteoclast activating factor (OAF). The malignant plasma cells can form tumors (plasmacytomas) that have a predilection for causing spinal cord compression.

The paraproteins secreted by the malignant plasma cells may cause problems in their own right. Very high paraprotein levels (either IgG or IgA) may cause the hyperviscosity syndrome. The light chain component of the immunoglobulin may cause renal failure (often aggravated by hypercalcemia). Paraproteins may become catabolized into amyloid, causing heart failure or neuropathy.

Myeloma patients are prone to recurrent infections for a number of reasons, including neutropenia and the immunosuppressive effects of chemotherapy. Additionally, there is a failure of antibody production in response to antigen challenge, and myeloma patients are especially prone to infections with encapsulated organisms such as *Streptococcus pneumoniae* and *Haemophilus influenzae*.

## Clinical Findings

**A. Symptoms and Signs:** Myeloma is a disease of older adults (median age at presentation, 60 years). The classic picture of myeloma is anemia, back pain, and an elevated sedimentation rate in an older man, and the most common presenting complaints are those related to anemia, bone pain, and infection. Bone pain is most common in the back or ribs or may present as a pathologic fracture, especially of the femoral neck. Patients may also come to medical attention because of renal failure; spinal cord compression, or the hyperviscosity syndrome (mucosal bleeding, vertigo, nausea, visual disturbances, alterations in mental status). Occasionally, patients are diagnosed as having myeloma because of initial laboratory findings of hypercalcemia, proteinuria, elevated sedimentation rate, or abnormalities on serum protein electrophoresis.

Examination may reveal pallor, bone tenderness, and soft tissue masses. Patients may have neurologic signs related to neuropathy or spinal cord compression. Patients with amyloidosis may have an enlarged tongue, neuropathy, or congestive heart failure.

**B. Laboratory Findings:** Anemia is nearly universal. Red blood cell morphology is normal, but rouleau formation is common and may be marked. The neutrophil and platelet counts are usually normal at presentation. Only rarely will plasma cells be visible on peripheral smear (plasma cell leukemia).

The hallmark of myeloma is the finding of a paraprotein on serum protein electrophoresis (SPEP). The majority of patients will have a monoclonal spike visible in the beta or gamma globulin region. Immunoelectrophoresis (IEP) will reveal this to be a monoclonal protein. Approximately 20% of patients will have no demonstrable paraprotein in the serum. SPEP or IEP of the urine will reveal either complete immunoglobulin or light chains. Overall, approximately 60% of myeloma patients will have an IgG paraprotein, 25% on IgA, and 15% light chains only.

The bone marrow will be infiltrated by variable numbers of plasma cells ranging from 5% to 100%. Occasionally, the plasma cells may be morphologically indistinguishable from normal cells but more commonly will appear abnormal. Bone radiographs are important in establishing the diagnosis of myeloma. Lytic lesions are most commonly seen in the axial skeleton: skull, spine, proximal long bones, and ribs. At other times, only generalized osteoporosis is seen. The radionuclide bone scan is not useful in detecting bone lesions in myeloma, as there is usually no osteoblastic component.

Other laboratory features include hypercalcemia, renal failure, and an elevated erythrocyte sedimentation rate. The urinalysis may reveal proteinuria, but the dipstick test (which detects primarily albumin) is notoriously unreliable.

## Differential Diagnosis

When a patient is discovered to have a monoclonal paraprotein, the distinction between myeloma and benign monoclonal gammopathy must be made. Benign monoclonal gammopathy can be considered an adenoma of plasma cells and is present in 1% of all adults and 3% of adults over age 70. Thus, if one considers all patients with paraproteins, benign monoclonal gammopathy is far more common than myeloma. Most commonly, patients with benign monoclonal gammopathy will have a monoclonal IgG spike less than 2.5 g/dL, and the height of the spike remains stable. In approximately 25% of cases, benign monoclonal gammopathy progresses to overt malignant disease, but this may take years or even decades.

Myeloma is distinguished from benign monoclonal gammopathy by findings of replacement of the bone marrow, bone destruction, and progression over time. Although the height of the paraprotein spike should not be used by itself to distinguish benign from malignant disease, in practice all patients with IgG spikes greater than 3.5 g/dL prove to have myeloma. If there is doubt about whether paraproteinemia is benign

or malignant, the patient should be observed without therapy, since there is no advantage to early treatment of asymptomatic multiple myeloma.

Myeloma should be distinguished from polyclonal hypergammaglobulinemia seen in reactive conditions. The distinction is made by finding the polyclonal as opposed to the monoclonal spike. Myeloma may also need to be distinguished from other malignant lymphoproliferative diseases such as Waldenström's macroglobulinemia, lymphomas, and primary amyloidosis.

## Treatment

The goal of treatment of myeloma is palliation. Patients with minimal disease or in whom the diagnosis of malignancy is in doubt should be observed without treatment. Most commonly, patients require treatment at diagnosis because of bone pain or other symptoms related to the disease. In the past, standard therapy has been melphalan plus prednisone; more recently, combination chemotherapy with alkylating agents has been used. The optimal chemotherapy regimen has not been determined. The height of the paraprotein spike on SPEP is a useful marker for monitoring response to therapy.

A number of other ancillary measures are important in the treatment of myeloma. Localized radiotherapy may be very useful for palliation of bone pain or for eradicating tumor at the site of pathologic fracture. Hypercalcemia should be treated aggressively and prolonged immobilization and dehydration avoided. Recently, allogeneic bone marrow transplantation has been tried for the few young patients with multiple myeloma. Initial results appear promising, but this is currently experimental treatment.

## Prognosis

The median survival of patients with myelomas is 3 years. The prognosis is markedly affected by a number of prognostic features, with shorter survivals in those with high paraprotein spikes, renal failure, hypercalcemia, or extensive bony disease. Patients are said to have a "low tumor burden" if the IgG spike is less than 5 g/dL and there is no more than one lytic bone lesion and no evidence of severe anemia, hypercalcemia, or renal failure. These patients have a median survival of 5–6 years. Conversely, patients with a "high tumor burden" have an IgG spike greater than 7 g/dL, hematocrit less than 25%, calcium greater than 12 mg/dL, or more than 3 lytic bone lesions. Median survival for this group is approximately 1 year.

Bergsagel DE et al: The chemotherapy of plasma cell myeloma and the incidence of acute leukemia. *N Engl J Med* 1979;**301**:743.

Kyle RA: Monoclonal gammopathy of undetermined significance: Natural history in 241 cases. *Am J Med* 1978;**64**:814.

Kyle RA, Greipp PR: "Idiopathic" Bence Jones proteinuria; Long-term follow-up in 7 patients. *N Engl J Med* 1982;**306**:564.

# WALDENSTRÖM'S MACROGLOBULINEMIA

## Essentials of Diagnosis
- Monoclonal IgM paraprotein.
- Infiltration of bone marrow by plasmacytic lymphocyte.

## General Considerations
Waldenström's macroglobulinemia is a malignant disease of B cells that appear to be a hybrid of lymphocytes and plasma cells. These cells characteristically secrete an IgM paraprotein, and many clincial manifestations of the disease are related to this macroglobulin.

## Clinical Findings
**A. Symptoms and Signs:** This disease characteristically presents insidiously in patients in their 60s or 70s. Patients usually present with fatigue related to anemia. Hyperviscosity of serum may be manifested in a number of ways. Mucosal and gastrointestinal bleeding is related to engorged blood vessels and platelet dysfunction. Other complaints include nausea, vertigo, and visual disturbances. Alterations in consciousness vary from mild lethargy to stupor and coma. The IgM paraprotein may also cause symptoms of cold agglutinin disease or peripheral neuropathy.

On examination, there may be hepatosplenomegaly or lymphadenopathy. The retinal veins are characteristically engorged. Purpura may be present. There should be no bone tenderness.

**B. Laboratory Findings:** Anemia is nearly universal, and rouleau formation is common. The anemia is related in part to expansion of the plasma volume by 50–100% due to the presence of the paraprotein. Other blood counts are usually normal. The abnormal plasmacytic lymphocyte usually appears in small numbers on the peripheral blood smear. The bone marrow is characteristically infiltrated by the plasmacytic lymphocytes.

The hallmark of macroglobulinemia is the presence of a monoclonal IgM spike seen on serum protein electrophoresis (SPEP) in the beta or gamma globulin region. The serum viscosity is usually increased above the normal of 1.4–1.8 times that of water. Symptoms of hyperviscosity usually develop when the serum viscosity is over 4 times that of water, and marked symptoms usually arise when the viscosity is over 6 times that of water. Because paraproteins vary in their physicochemical properties, there is no strict correlation between the concentration of paraprotein and serum viscosity. However, after a certain threshold, viscosity rises exponentially with small increments in paraprotein amounts.

The IgM paraprotein may cause a positive Coombs test or have cold agglutinin or cryoglobulin properties. If one suspects macroglobulinemia but the SPEP shows only hypogammaglobulinemia, one should repeat the test while taking special measures to maintain the blood at 37 °C, since the paraprotein may precipitate out at room temperature.

Bone radiographs should be normal, and there should be no evidence of renal failure.

## Differential Diagnosis
Waldenström's macroglobulinemia is differentiated from benign monoclonal gammopathy by the finding of bone marrow infiltration. It is differentiated from chronic lymphocytic leukemia and multiple myeloma by bone marrow morphology and the finding of the characteristic IgM spike.

## Treatment
Patients who present with marked hyperviscosity syndrome (stupor or coma) should be treated on an emergency basis with plasmapheresis. Pheresis will usually rapidly reduce the paraprotein level below the threshold required to produce symptoms. On a chronic basis, some patients can be managed with periodic plasmapheresis alone. Others are treated with intermittent chemotherapy with chlorambucil or cyclophosphamide.

## Prognosis
Waldenström's macroglobulinemia is an indolent disease with a median survival rate of 3–5 years. However, patients may survive 10 years or longer.

Dellagi K et al: Waldenström's macroglobulinemia and peripheral neuropathy: A clinical and immunologic study of 25 patients. *Blood* 1983;**62**:280.

McKenzie MR, Fudenberg HH: Macroglobulinemia: An analysis for 40 patients. *Blood* 1972;**39**:874.

# COAGULATION DISORDERS

# IDIOPATHIC (AUTOIMMUNE) THROMBOCYTOPENIC PURPURA

## Essentials of Diagnosis
- Isolated thrombocytopenia. Other hematopoietic cell lines normal.
- No systemic illness.
- Normal bone marrow with normal or increased megakaryocytes.

## General Considerations
Idiopathic thrombocytopenic purpura is an autoimmune disorder in which an IgG autoantibody is formed that binds to platelets. It is not clear which antigen on the platelet surface is involved. Although the antiplatelet antibody may bind complement, platelets are not destroyed by direct lysis. Rather, destruction takes place in the spleen, where splenic macrophages with Fc receptors bind to antibody-coated platelets. Since

the pathogenesis of this disorder is now well understood, the term idiopathic is no longer appropriate, but the term idiopathic thrombocytopenic purpura is deeply entrenched in the literature.

The spleen plays a major role in the pathogenesis of idiopathic thrombocytopenic purpura. The spleen is the major site both of antibody production and platelet sequestration. This explains the high degree of effectiveness of splenectomy in treating this disorder.

## Clinical Findings

**A. Symptoms and Signs:** Idiopathic thrombocytopenic purpura occurs commonly in childhood, frequently precipitated by viral infection and usually self-limited. In contrast, the adult form is usually a chronic disease and only infrequently follows a viral infection. It is a disease of young persons, with peak incidence between ages 20 and 50, and there is a 2:1 female predominance.

Patients are systemically well and not febrile. The presenting complaint is mucosal or skin bleeding. Common types of bleeding are epistaxis, oral bleeding, menorrhagia, purpura, and petechiae.

On examination, the patient appears well, and there are no abnormal findings other than those related to bleeding. An enlarged spleen should lead one to doubt the diagnosis. Common signs of bleeding are purpura, petechiae, and hemorrhagic bullae in the mouth.

**B. Laboratory Findings:** The hallmark of the disease is thrombocytopenia, which may be severe. This is one of the few disorders that will produce a platelet count less than $10,000/\mu L$. The other blood counts are usually normal except for mild anemia, which can be explained by bleeding. Peripheral blood cell morphology is normal except that platelets are slightly enlarged (megathrombocytes). These larger platelets are young platelets produced in response to enhanced platelet destruction. Approximately 10% of patients will have coexistent autoimmune hemolytic anemia, and in these cases one will see anemia, reticulocytosis, and spherocytes on peripheral smear. Red blood cell fragmentation should not be seen.

The bone marrow will appear normal, with a normal or increased number of megakaryocytes. Coagulation studies will be entirely normal. Tests now available to quantitate platelet-associated IgG may help in the diagnosis. At present, although these tests are highly sensitive (95%), they are very nonspecific, and 50% of all patients with thrombocytopenia from any cause may have increased levels of IgG on the platelet.

## Differential Diagnosis

Thrombocytopenia may be produced either by abnormal bone marrow function or by peripheral destruction (Table 10–17). Although most bone marrow disorders produce abnormalities in addition to isolated thrombocytopenia, diagnoses such as myelodysplasia can only be excluded by examining the bone marrow.

**Table 10–17.** Causes of thrombocytopenia.

| |
|---|
| **Bone marrow disorders** |
|   Aplastic anemia |
|   Hematologic malignancies |
|   Myelodysplasia |
|   Megaloblastic anemia |
|   Chronic alcoholism |
| **Nonmarrow disorders** |
|   Immune disorders |
|     Idiopathic thrombocytopenic purpura |
|     Drug-induced |
|     Secondary |
|     Posttransfusion purpura |
|   Hypersplenism |
|   Disseminated intravascular coagulation |
|   Thrombotic thrombocytopenic purpura |
|   Hemolytic-uremic syndrome |
|   Sepsis |
|   Hemangiomas |
|   Viral infection, AIDS |

Most causes of thrombocytopenia resulting from peripheral destruction can be ruled out by initial evaluation. Disorders such as disseminated intravascular coagulation, thrombotic thrombocytopenic purpura, hemolytic-uremic syndrome, hypersplenism, and sepsis are easily excluded by the absence of systemic illness. Thus, patients with isolated thrombocytopenia with no other abnormal findings almost certainly have immune thrombocytopenia. Patients should be questioned regarding drug use, especially sulfonamides, quinidine, quinine, thiazides, cimetidine, gold, and heparin. Heparin is now the most common cause of drug-induced thrombocytopenia in hospitalized patients. Systemic lupus erythematosus and a lymphoproliferative disorder are common causes of secondary idiopathic thrombocytopenic purpura.

## Treatment

Few adults with idiopathic thrombocytopenic purpura will have spontaneous remissions, and most will require treatment. Initial treatment is with prednisone, 1–2 mg/kg/d. Prednisone works primarily by decreasing the affinity of splenic macrophages for antibody-coated platelets. High-dose prednisone therapy also reduces the binding of antibody to the platelet surface, and long-term therapy may decrease antibody production. Bleeding will often diminish within 1 day after beginning prednisone—even before the platelet count begins to rise. This effect has been attributed to "enhanced vascular stability" produced by prednisone. The platelet count will usually begin to rise within a week, and responses are almost always seen within 3 weeks. About 80% of patients will respond to prednisone therapy, and the platelet count will usually return to normal. High-dose prednisone therapy should be continued until the platelet count is normal, and the dose should then be gradually tapered. In most patients, thrombocytopenia will recur if prednisone is completely withdrawn, and one aims to find a low prednisone dose that will maintain an adequate platelet count. It is not necessary for the platelet count to be entirely normal; the risk of bleeding is small with platelet counts above 50,000/μL.

Splenectomy is the most definitive treatment for idiopathic thrombocytopenic purpura, and most adult patients will ultimately undergo splenectomy. High-dose prednisone therapy should not be prolonged unduly in an attempt to avoid surgery. Splenectomy is indicated if patients do not respond to prednisone initially or require unacceptably high doses to maintain an adequate platelet count. Other patients may be intolerant of prednisone or may simply prefer the surgical alternative. Splenectomy can be performed safely even with platelet counts less than 10,000/μL. Approximately 80% of patients benefit from splenectomy with either complete or partial remission.

High-dose intravenous immunoglobulin, 400 mg/kg/d for 3–5 days, is highly effective in rapidly raising the platelet count. The response rate is approximately 90%, and the platelet count rises within 1–5 days. However, this treatment is very expensive (approximately $5000), and the beneficial effect lasts only 1–2 weeks. Immunoglobulin treatment should be reserved for emergency situations such as preparing a severely thrombocytopenic patient for surgery.

For patients who fail to respond to prednisone and splenectomy, danazol, 600 mg/d, has been used, with responses obtained in about half of cases. Immunosuppressive agents employed in refractory cases include vincristine, vinblastine infusions, azathioprine, and cyclophosphamide. In using any of these more toxic treatments, one must carefully balance the risks against the anticipated benefits.

Platelet transfusions are rarely used in the treatment of idiopathic thrombocytopenic purpura, since exogenous platelets will survive no better than the patient's own platelets and in many cases will survive less than a few hours. Platelet transfusion should be reserved for cases of life-threatening bleeding in which enhanced hemostasis for even an hour may be of benefit.

## Prognosis

The prognosis for remission is good. In most cases, the disease is initially controlled with prednisone, and splenectomy offers definitive therapy for most patients. The major concern during the initial phases is cerebral hemorrhage, which becomes a risk when the platelet count is less than 5000/μL. However, at these very low platelet counts, fatal bleeding is rare. Chronic disease that has failed to respond to prednisone and splenectomy has a waxing and waning course over years and usually requires continued management. However, bleeding is rarely life-threatening.

Bussel JB et al: Intravenous gammaglobulin treatment of chronic idiopathic thrombocytopenic purpura. *Blood* 1983; **62**:480.

DiFino SM et al: Adult idiopathic thrombocytopenic purpura: Clinical findings and response to therapy. *Am J Med* 1980;**69**:430.

McMillan R: Chronic idiopathic thrombocytopenic purpura. *N Engl J Med* 1981;**304**:1135.

## THROMBOTIC THROMBOCYTOPENIC PURPURA

### Essentials of Diagnosis

- Microangiopathic hemolytic anemia and thrombocytopenia.
- Neurologic abnormalities.
- Fever in the absence of infection.
- Normal coagulation test.

### General Considerations

Thrombotic thrombocytopenic purpura is an uncommon syndrome characterized by the triad of microangiopathic hemolytic anemia, thrombocytopenia, and neurologic abnormalities, as well as fever and renal abnormalities. The cause is unknown. A platelet-agglutinating factor has recently been identified in the plasma of these patients. Its role in pathogenesis remains controversial.

Thrombotic thrombocytopenic purpura is seen primarily in young adults between ages 20 and 50, and there is a slight female predominance. The syndrome is occasionally precipitated by estrogen use or pregnancy.

### Clinical Findings

**A. Symptoms and Signs:** Patients come to medical attention because of anemia, bleeding, or neurologic abnormalities. The neurologic signs and symptoms are unusual in that they may wax and wane over minutes. Neurologic symptoms include headache, confusion, aphasia, and alterations in consciousness from lethargy to coma. With more advanced disease, one may see hemiparesis and seizures.

On examination, the patient appears acutely ill and is usually febrile. One may detect pallor, purpura, petechiae, and signs of neurologic dysfunction. Patients may have abdominal pain and tenderness due to pancreatitis.

**B. Laboratory Findings:** Anemia is universal and may be extremely severe. There is usually marked reticulocytosis and occasionally nucleated red blood cells. The hallmark of thrombotic thrombocytopenic purpura is a microangiopathic blood picture with fragmented red blood cells (schistocytes, helmet cells, triangle forms) on the smear. One cannot make the diagnosis without significant red blood cell fragmentation. Thrombocytopenia is invariably present and may be severe. White blood cells may show increased band neutrophils.

Hemolysis may be manifested by increasing indirect bilirubin, absent haptoglobin, and occasionally hemoglobinemia and hemoglobinuria. In severe cases, methemalbuminemia may impart a brown color to the plasma. The LDH is usually markedly elevated in proportion to the severity of hemolysis. The Coombs test should be negative.

Coagulation tests (prothrombin time, partial thromboplastin time, fibrinogen) are normal. Elevated fibrin degradation products may be seen, as in other acutely ill patients. Renal insufficiency may be present, and the urinalysis may be abnormal.

Pathologically, one may see the characteristic hyaline thrombus in capillaries and small arteries.

## Differential Diagnosis

The normal values of coagulation tests differentiate thrombotic thrombocytopenic purpura from disseminated intravascular coagulation (DIC). Other conditions causing microangiopathic hemolysis (Table 10–18) should be excluded. Evans' syndrome is characterized by the combination of autoimmune thrombocytopenia and autoimmune hemolytic anemia, but the peripheral smear will show spherocytes and not red blood cell fragments. Skin or muscle biopsy is usually not necessary for diagnosis but may be helpful when vasculitis is a consideration.

## Treatment

Thrombotic thrombocytopenic purpura should be treated on an emergency basis with large-volume plasmapheresis. Sixty to 80 mL/kg of plasma should be removed and replaced with fresh frozen plasma. Treatment should be continued daily until the patient is in complete remission. Prednisone and antiplatelet agents (aspirin and dipyridamole) have been used in addition to plasmapheresis, but their role is unclear.

Patients who do not respond to plasmapheresis or who have rapid recurrences require splenectomy. The combination of splenectomy, steroids, and dextran has been used with success.

## Prognosis

With the advent of plasmapheresis, the formerly dismal prognosis of thrombotic thrombocytopenic purpura has been dramatically changed. Eighty to 90% of patients now recover completely. Most complete responses are durable, but in 10–20% of cases, the disease will be chronic and relapsing.

Bukowski RM et al: Therapy of thrombotic thrombocytopenic purpura: An overview. *Semin Thromb Hemost* 1981;**7**:1.

Byrnes JJ: Thrombotic thrombocytopenic purpura. *Adv Intern Med* 1980;**26**:131.

Kacich R, Linker C: Thrombotic thrombocytopenic purpura. *West J Med* 1982;**136**:513.

Liu ET, Linker CA, Shuman MA: Management of treatment failures in thrombotic thrombocytopenic purpura. *Am J Hematol* 1986;**23**:347.

**Table 10–18.** Causes of microangiopathic hemolytic anemia.

| |
|---|
| Thrombotic thrombocytopenic purpura |
| Hemolytic-uremic syndrome |
| Disseminated intravascular coagulation |
| Prosthetic valve hemolysis |
| Metastatic adenocarcinoma |
| Malignant hypertension |
| Vasculitis |

## HEMOLYTIC-UREMIC SYNDROME

### Essentials of Diagnosis

- Microangiopathic hemolytic anemia, thrombocytopenia, and renal failure.
- Normal coagulation test.
- Absence of neurologic abnormalities.

### General Considerations

Hemolytic-uremic syndrome is an uncommon disorder consisting of microangiopathic hemolytic anemia, thrombocytopenia, and renal failure. The cause is unclear. The disease is similar to thrombotic thrombocytopenic purpura except that different vascular beds are involved. The pathogenesis of the 2 disorders is probably similar, and a platelet-agglutinating factor found in plasma may be involved. In children, hemolytic-uremic syndrome frequently occurs after a diarrheal illness. In adults, this syndrome is frequently precipitated by estrogen use or pregnancy (especially postpartum).

### Clinical Findings

**A. Symptoms and Signs:** Patients present with anemia, bleeding, or renal failure. The renal failure may or may not be oliguric. In contrast to thrombotic thrombocytopenic purpura, there are no neurologic manifestations other than those due to the uremic state.

**B. Laboratory Findings:** As in thrombotic thrombocytopenic purpura, there is microangiopathic hemolytic anemia and thrombocytopenia, but the thrombocytopenia is often less severe. The peripheral blood smear should show striking red blood cell fragmentation, and the diagnosis of hemolytic-uremic syndrome is untenable without this finding. The LDH is usually strikingly elevated in proportion to the severity of hemolysis, and the Coombs test is negative. Coagulation tests are normal with the exception of elevated fibrin degradation products.

Renal insufficiency is invariably present, and anuric renal failure requiring dialysis may be seen. Kidney biopsy will show hyaline thrombi in the afferent arterioles and glomeruli.

### Differential Diagnosis

Disseminated intravascular coagulation is excluded by normal coagulation results. Other causes of microangiopathic hemolytic anemia (Table 10–19) should be considered. Occasionally, vasculitis or acute glomerulonephritis is considered, and in these cases renal biopsy may be necessary to establish the diagnosis.

Hemolytic-uremic syndrome is arbitrarily distinguished from thrombotic thrombocytopenic purpura by the presence of renal failure and the lack of neurologic findings.

### Treatment

In children, hemolytic-uremic syndrome is almost always self-limited and requires only supportive treat-

**Table 10–19.** Qualitative platelet disorders.

Congenital
    Glanzmann's thrombasthenia
    Bernard-Soulier syndrome
    Storage pool disease
Acquired
    Myeloproliferative disorders
    Uremia
    Drugs: Aspirin, anti-inflammatory agents
    Autoantibody
    Paraproteins
    Acquired storage pool
    Fibrin degradation products
Von Willebrand's disease

ment. In adults, however, without treatment, there is a high rate of permanent renal insufficiency and death. The treatment of choice (as in thrombotic thrombocytopenic purpura) is large-volume plasmapheresis performed daily with fresh frozen plasma replacement.

**Prognosis**

The prognosis of hemolytic-uremic syndrome in adults remains unclear. Early institution of aggressive therapy with plasmapheresis promises to be beneficial.

Misiani R et al: Haemolytic uraemic syndrome: Therapeutic effect of plasma infusion. *Br Med J* 1982;**285:**1304.

## CONGENITAL QUALITATIVE PLATELET DISORDERS

Bleeding disorders characterized by prolonged bleeding times despite a normal platelet count are called qualitative platelet disorders. Patients have a positive family history or lifelong personal history of the defect. The disorders may be classified as (1) acquired and congenital disorders intrinsic to the platelet and (2) von Willebrand's disease (see next section), a disorder of a plasma protein necessary for platelet adhesion (Table 10–19).

### Glanzmann's Thrombasthenia

This is a rare autosomal recessive intrinsic platelet disorder causing bleeding. Platelets are unable to aggregate because of lack of receptors (containing glycoproteins IIb and IIIa) for fibrinogen, which forms the bridges between platelets during aggregation. Clinically, it is manifested chiefly as mucosal bleeding (epistaxis, gingival bleeding, menorrhagia) and postoperative bleeding. The bleeding defect is of variable severity but may be severe.

Platelet numbers and morphology are normal, but the bleeding time is markedly prolonged. Platelets fail to aggregate in response to typical agonists (ADP, collagen, thrombin) but aggregate normally in response to ristocetin, which causes platelet clumping by a separate mechanism.

Patients are treated with platelet transfusions when necessary. Platelet transfusion therapy is limited by the tendency of these patients to develop multiple alloantibodies.

### Bernard-Soulier Syndrome

This is a rare autosomal recessive intrinsic platelet disorder causing bleeding. Platelets cannot adhere to subendothelium because they lack receptors (composed of glycoprotein Ib) for von Willebrand factor, which mediates platelet adhesion. This is often a severe bleeding disorder with mucosal and postoperative bleeding.

Thrombocytopenia may be present, and platelets on smear are abnormally large. The bleeding time is markedly prolonged. Platelet aggregation is normal in response to standard agonists (collagen, ADP, thrombin), but platelets fail to aggregate in response to ristocetin. Measurements of von Willebrand factor in the plasma are normal. Patients are treated with platelet transfusion when necessary.

### Storage Pool Disease

This is a group of mild bleeding disorders characterized by defective secretion of platelet granule contents (especially ADP) that stimulate platelet aggregation. Most patients are mildly affected and have increased bruising and postoperative bleeding.

Platelets are normal in number and morphology, but the bleeding time is slightly prolonged. In some cases, the baseline bleeding time is normal, but it becomes markedly prolonged after aspirin. There are variable abnormalities in platelet aggregation studies.

Most patients do not require treatment but should avoid aspirin. Platelet transfusions transiently correct the bleeding tendency. Some patients respond to infusions of cryoprecipitate, and some respond transiently to desmopressin acetate (DDAVP), 0.3 μg/kg.

George JN, Nurden AT, Phillips DR: Molecular defects in interactions of platelets with the vessel wall. *N Engl J Med* 1984;**311:**1084.
Shattil SJ, Bennett JS: Platelets and their membranes in hemostasis: Physiology and pathophysiology. *Ann Intern Med* 1980;**94:**108.

## VON WILLEBRAND'S DISEASE

### Essentials of Diagnosis

- Family history with autosomal dominant pattern of inheritance.
- Prolonged bleeding time, either at baseline or after challenge with aspirin.
- Reduced levels of factor VIII antigen or ristocetin cofactor.
- May have reduced levels of factor VIII coagulant activity.

### General Considerations

Von Willebrand's disease is a group of disorders characterized by deficient or defective von Willebrand factor (vWF), a protein that mediates platelet adhesion. Adhesion is a process separate from platelet aggregation. Platelets adhere to the subendothelium via vWF, which is bound to a specific receptor composed of glycoprotein Ib (and missing in Bernard-Soulier syndrome). Platelets aggregate via fibrinogen, which binds to a different receptor composed of glycoproteins IIb and IIIa (deficient in Glanzmann's thrombasthenia). The platelet aggregation system is entirely normal in von Willebrand's disease.

Von Willebrand factor is synthesized in megakaryocytes and endothelial cells and circulates in plasma as multimers of varying size. Only the large multimeric forms are functional in mediating platelet adhesion. Von Willebrand factor has a separate function of binding the factor VIII coagulant protein and protecting it from degradation. The factor VIII coagulant protein (factor VIII:C), a protein encoded by a gene on the X chromosome, is the protein deficient in classic hemophilia. Any of the multimeric forms of vWF can bind and protect factor VIII:C. Von Willebrand's disease, which is primarily a disorder of platelet function, may secondarily cause a coagulation disturbance because of deficient levels of factor VIII:C. However, this coagulopathy is rarely severe.

There are several subtypes of von Willebrand's disease. The most common type (type I) is caused by a quantitative decrease in vWF. Type IIa is caused by a qualitative abnormality in protein that prevents multimer formation. Only small multimers are present, and both intermediate and large forms that mediate platelet adhesion are missing. Type IIb von Willebrand's disease is caused by a qualitative abnormality in the protein that causes rapid clearance of the large multimeric forms. Type III von Willebrand's disease is a rare autosomal recessive disorder in which vWF is nearly absent. Pseudo-von Willebrand disease is a rare disorder in which an abnormal platelet membrane has excessive avidity for the large multimeric forms of vWF, causing their clearance from plasma.

## Clinical Findings

**A. Symptoms and Signs:** Von Wildebrand's disease is the most common congenital coagulation abnormality. Most cases are mild. It is autosomal dominant and, unlike hemophilia, occurs in women as well as men. Most bleeding is mucosal (epistaxis, gingival bleeding, menorrhagia), but gastrointestinal bleeding may occur. In most cases, incisional bleeding occurs after surgery or dental extractions. Von Willebrand's disease is rarely as severe as hemophilia, and spontaneous hemarthroses do not occur.

The bleeding tendency is exacerbated by aspirin. Characteristically, bleeding decreases during pregnancy or estrogen use.

**B. Laboratory Findings:** Platelet number and morphology are normal, and the bleeding time is usually (not always) prolonged. When the bleeding time is normal, it is prolonged markedly by aspirin. In the most common form of von Willebrand's disease

(type I), vWF levels in plasma are reduced. This may be measured by factor VIII antigen, which measures the immunologic presence of vWF, or by ristocetin cofactor activity, which measures functional properties of vWF in mediating platelet adhesion.

When factor VIII antigen is reduced, one may also see a decrease in factor VIII coagulant (factor VIII:C) levels. When factor VIII:C levels are less than 25%, the partial thromboplastin time (PTT) will be prolonged. Platelet aggregation studies with standard agonists (ADP, collagen, thrombin) are normal, but platelet aggregation in response to ristocetin is usually subnormal.

In difficult cases, it may be helpful to assay directly the multimeric composition of vWF.

## Differential Diagnosis

When patients present with a prolonged bleeding time, one must distinguish von Willebrand's disease from other qualitative platelet disorders (Table 10–19). Acquired qualitative platelet disorders can usually be diagnosed by recent onset of the bleeding tendency and other characteristic clinical features. Congenital intrinsic platelet disorders may present with a positive family history and lifelong history of bleeding episodes. Von Willebrand's disease is diagnosed by the finding of abnormal measurements of vWF and by normal results of platelet aggregation.

When patients present with a prolonged PTT, measurements of factor VIII:C will distinguish von Willebrand's disease from all disorders except hemophilia (Table 10–20). Hemophilia is diagnosed when factor VIII:C is reduced but all measurements of vWF (factor VIII antigen, ristocetin cofactor activity) are normal.

Patients with a suspicious bleeding history but with normal bleeding time and PTT pose a diagnostic problem. On occasion, the postaspirin bleeding time can be used to unmask a bleeding disorder. At other times, one must perform further plasma assays of vWF to make the diagnosis. Von Willebrand's disease waxes and wanes in severity and may be difficult to diagnose, especially in a woman taking estrogens (which raises plasma vWF levels).

It is often useful to distinguish between subtypes of von Willebrand's disease (Table 10–21).

**Table 10–20.** Causes of prolonged partial thromboplastin time.

| |
|---|
| **Congenital factor deficiencies** |
| Contact factors |
| Factor XII |
| Factor XI |
| Factor IX |
| Factor VIII |
| Hemophilia |
| Von Willebrand's disease |
| **Anticoagulants** |
| Anti-VIII |
| Lupus |
| Heparin |

**Table 10–21.** Types of Von Willebrand's disease.

| | Bleeding Time | Factor VIII Antigen | Ristocetin Cofactor Activity | Factor VIII Coagulant Activity | Multimer |
|---|---|---|---|---|---|
| Type I | ↑ or N | ↓ or N | ↓ or N | ↓ or N | N |
| Type IIa | ↑ | ↓ or N | 0 | ↓ or N | Abn |
| Type IIb | ↑ | ↓ or N | ↓ or N | ↓ or N | Abn |
| Type III | ↑ | 0 | 0 | 0 | — |
| Pseudo-vW disease | ↑ | ↓ or N | ↓ or N | ↓ or N | Abn |
| Hemophilia A | N | N | N | ↓ | N |

N = normal; Abn = abnormal.

## Treatment

The bleeding disorder is characteristically mild, and no treatment is routinely given other than avoidance of aspirin. However, patients often need to be prepared for surgical or dental procedures. The bleeding time is probably the best indicator of the likelihood of bleeding, and prophylactic therapy may be reasonably withheld if the procedure is minor and the bleeding time is normal.

Standard therapy for von Willebrand's disease is transfusion of plasma cryoprecipitate. It should be noted that factor VIII concentrates (using the treatment of hemophilia A) cannot be used, as they do not contain functional vWF. Each unit of cryoprecipitate will raise vWF levels approximately 3%, and thus 10–15 units of cryoprecipitate are commonly used to raise vWF levels by 30–50%. Factor VIII antigen levels decline, with a half-life of 12–18 hours, but the duration of corrected bleeding time is usually shorter than this. In some instances the prolonged bleeding time may be completely corrected.

Desmopressin acetate (DDAVP, Stimate) is a useful treatment for mild type I von Willebrand's disease. The dose is 0.3 μg/kg, after which vWF levels usually rise 2- to 3-fold in 30–90 minutes. Desmopressin acetate appears to cause release of stored vWF from endothelial cells. The treatment can be given only every 24 hours as stores of vWF become depleted. The drug is not effective in type IIa von Willebrand's disease, in which no endothelial stores are present, and may be harmful in type IIb or may lead to thrombocytopenia and increased bleeding.

The antifibrinolytic agent aminocaproic acid (EACA; Amicar) is useful as adjunctive therapy during dental procedures. After either cryoprecipitate of desmopressin acetate, the patient is given 4 g orally every 4 hours for several days to reduce the likelihood of bleeding.

## Prognosis

The prognosis is excellent. In most cases, the bleeding disorder is mild, and in the more serious cases replacement therapy is effective.

De la Fuente B et al: Response of patients with mild and moderate hemophilia A and von Willebrand's disease to treatment with desmopressin. *Ann Intern Med* 1985;**103**:6.

Zimmerman TS, Ruggeri ZM: Von Willebrand's disease. *Prog Hemost Thromb* 1982;**6**:203.

## ACQUIRED QUALITATIVE PLATELET DISORDERS

A number of acquired disorders lead to abnormal platelet function (Table 10–19).

### Uremia

Uremia causes abnormal platelet function by unknown mechanisms. The severity of the bleeding tendency is roughly proportionate to the degree of renal insufficiency. Bleeding is most commonly mucosal and gastrointestinal and may occasionally be severe. Dialysis is effective in reducing the bleeding tendency but may not completely eliminate it. Patients appear to respond to transfusion with cryoprecipitate, 10 units every 12 hours. Desmopressin acetate, 0.3 μg/kg every 24 hours, appears to be just as effective as cryoprecipitate.

### Myeloproliferative Disorders

All the myeloproliferative disorders can produce abnormalities in platelet function. A number of biochemical abnormalities are present in these platelets, but the cause of the bleeding tendency is unclear. The severity of the bleeding tendency correlates roughly with the height of the platelet count. Bleeding decreases when the platelet count is controlled with myelosuppressive therapy. In cases of life-threatening bleeding with high platelet counts, plateletpheresis may be necessary to control bleeding. Platelet transfusion will also be helpful temporarily.

### Other Disorders

Aspirin causes a mild bleeding tendency by irreversibly acetylating cyclooxygenase, an enzyme that participates in platelet aggregation. Aspirin by itself does not cause significant bleeding, but it may unmask bleeding disorders such as mild von Willebrand's disease or mild thrombocytopenia. Certain antibiotics (ticarcillin, some cephalosporins) cause a mild bleeding tendency, presumably by coating the surface of platelets. Nonsteroidal anti-inflammatory drugs cause a transient aspirinlike effect.

Patients with autoantibodies against platelets may have prolonged bleeding times even in the absence of thrombocytopenia. Platelet-associated IgG levels should be high, and the bleeding tendency responds quickly to modest doses of prednisone such as 20 mg/d. Acquired storage pool disease refers to the circulation of "exhausted platelets" that have been stimulated to release their granule contents and hence are no longer functional. Such granule release occurs in response to cardiopulmonary bypass and severe vasculitis.

Janson PA et al: Treatment of the bleeding tendency in uremia with cryoprecipitate. *N Engl J Med* 1980;**303**:1318.

Livio M et al: Conjugated estrogens for the management of bleeding associated with renal failure. *N Engl J Med* 1986;**315**:731.

Mannucci PM et al: Deamino-8-D-arginine vasopressin shortens the bleeding time in uremia. *N Engl J Med* 1983;**308**:8.

Weiss HJ et al: Acquired storage pool deficiency with increased platelet-associated IgG: Report of 5 Cases. *Am J Med* 1980;**69**:711.

## HEMOPHILIA A

### Essentials of Diagnosis

- X-linked recessive pattern of inheritance with only males affected.
- Low factor VIII coagulant activity.
- Normal factor VIII antigen.
- Spontaneous hemarthroses.

### General Considerations

Hemophilia A (classic hemophilia, factor VIII deficiency hemophilia) is a hereditary disorder in which bleeding is due to deficiency of the coagulation factor VIII (VIII:C). In most cases, the factor VIII coagulant protein is quantitatively reduced, but in a small number of cases the coagulant protein is present by immunoassay but defective.

Hemophilia is a classic example of an X-linked recessive disease, and as a rule only males are affected. In rare instances, female carriers are clinically affected if their normal X chromosomes are disproportionately inactivated. Females may also become affected if they are the offspring of a hemophilic father and carrier mother.

Hemophilia is classified as severe if factor VIII:C levels are less than 1%, moderate if levels are 1–5%, and mild if levels are greater than 5%. Families tend to breed true in the severity of hemophilia produced.

### Clinical Findings

**A. Symptoms and Signs:** Hemophilia A is the most common severe bleeding disorder and after von Willebrand's disease is the most common congenital bleeding disorder overall. Approximately one in 10,000 males is affected. The bleeding tendency is related to factor VIII:C levels. Bleeding may occur anywhere. The most common sites of bleeding are into joints (knees, ankles, elbows), into muscles, and from the gastrointestinal tract. Spontaneous hemarthroses are so characteristic of severe hemophilia that they are almost diagnostic of the disorder. Patients with mild hemophilia bleed only in response to major trauma or surgery. Patients with moderately severe hemophilia bleed in response to mild trauma or surgery, and those with severe hemophilia bleed spontaneously.

**B. Laboratory Findings:** The partial thromboplastin time (PTT) is prolonged, and other measures of coagulation, including prothrombin time, bleeding time, and fibrinogen level, are normal. Levels of factor VIII:C are reduced, but measurements of von Willebrand factor are normal (Table 10–21).

If one mixes plasma from a hemophilic patient with normal plasma, the PTT will become normal. Failure of the PTT to normalize in such a mixing test is diagnostic of the presence of a factor VIII inhibitor.

### Differential Diagnosis

The finding of a reduced factor VIII:C level will distinguish this disorder from other causes of prolonged PTT (Table 10–20). Clinically, factor VIII hemophilia is indistinguishable from factor IX hemophilia, and only specific factor assays can distinguish these disorders. In cases of mild hemophilia, the disorder needs to be distinguished from von Willebrand's disease by VIII:A assay, which shows normal levels of factor VIII antigen in the latter.

An important issue for the families of hemophilic patients is identifying which females are carriers. Female carriers can usually be identified by the presence of low or normal levels of factor VIII:C with normal levels of factor VIII antigen.

### Treatment

Patients with hemophilia should try to live as nearly normal lives as possible. Activities associated with a risk of trauma should be avoided, however, and aspirin should never be used.

Standard treatment is based on infusion of factor VIII concentrates, now heat-treated to reduce the likelihood of transmission of AIDS. The level of factor VIII one aims to achieve in plasma depends on the severity of the bleeding problem. In response to minor bleeding, it may be necessary only to raise factor VIII:C levels to 25% with one infusion. For moderate bleeding (such as deep muscle hematomas), it is adequate to raise the level initially to 50% and maintain the level at greater than 25% with repeated infusion for 2–3 days. When major surgery is to be performed, one raises the factor VIII:C level to 100% and then maintains the factor level at greater than 50% continuously for 10–14 days. Head injuries (with or without neurologic signs) should be emergently treated as though major bleeding were present.

The dose of factor VIII concentrate is calculated on the basis that one unit of factor VIII is the amount present in 1 mL of plasma. Plasma volume is 40 mL/kg, and the volume of distribution of factor VIII:C is 1.5 times the plasma volume. Thus, to raise the level 100%, the dose should be $40 \times 1.5 = 60$ units/kg, or approximately 4000 units. To raise the levels to 25% would require 1000 units. The half-life of factor VIII:C is approximately 12 hours. Thus, during major surgery, to achieve an initial level of 100% and maintain it continuously at greater than 50%, a dose of 60 units/kg (approximately 4000 units) initially followed by 30 units/kg (approximately 2000 units) every 12 hours should be adequate. During surgery, one should initially verify that these doses give the anticipated levels. If factor VIII levels fail to rise as expected, one should suspect an inhibitor. Patients with inhibitors require specialized therapy under direction of an experienced hematologist.

Mild hemophilia may be treated with cryoprecipitate in place of factor VIII concentrates. One unit of cryoprecipitate contains about 100 units of factor VIII:C. For mild hemophiliacs, desmopressin acetate, 0.3 μg/kg every 24 hours, may be useful in preparing for minor surgical procedures. Desmopressin acetate causes release of factor VIII:C and will raise the factor VIII:C levels 2- to 3-fold for several hours. In the management of persistent bleeding following use of either desmopressin acetate or factor VIII concentrate, patients may be treated with aminocaproic acid (EACA; Amicar), 4 g orally every 4 hours for several days.

The ongoing care of patient with hemophilia should be coordinated with an orthopedic surgeon who can help manage the chronic joint deformities of these patients.

### Prognosis

The prognosis of patients with hemophilia has been transformed by the availability of factor VIII replacement. The major limiting factors are disability from recurrent joint bleeding and viral infections (hepatitis B, AIDS) from recurrent transfusion. Approximately 15% of patients develop inhibitors to factor VIII, and these patients may die of bleeding because they cannot be adequately supported with factor VIII.

Kasper CK, Dietrich SL: Comprehensive management of haemophilia. *Clin Haematol* 1985;**14**:489.

Kasper CK et al: Hematologic management of hemophilia A for surgery. *JAMA* 1985;**253**:1279.

Klein HG et al: A cooperative study for the detection of the carrier state of classic hemophilia. *N Engl J Med* 1977;**296**:959.

## HEMOPHILIA B

### Essentials of Diagnosis

- X-linked recessive inheritance, with only males affected.
- Low levels of factor IX coagulant activity.
- Spontaneous hemarthroses.

### General Considerations

Hemophilia B (Christmas disease, factor IX hemophilia) is a hereditary bleeding disorder due to deficiency of coagulation factor IX. Most commonly, factor IX is quantitatively reduced, but in one-third of cases an abnormally functioning molecule is immunologically present. Factor IX deficiency is one-seventh as common as factor VIII deficiency hemophilia but is otherwise clinically and genetically identical.

The PTT is prolonged, and factor IX levels are reduced when measured by specific factor assays. Other laboratory features are the same as for factor VIII hemophilia.

### Treatment

Factor IX hemophilia is managed with factor IX concentrates. Factor VIII concentrates are ineffectual in this type of hemophilia; therefore it is imperative to distinguish between the two. The same dosing considerations apply as in factor VIII hemophilia, with the exception that the volume of distribution of factor IX is twice the plasma volume, so that 80 units/kg are necessary to achieve a 100% level. In addition, the half-life of factor IX is 18 hours. Thus, to maintain a patient through major surgery, the dosage should be 80 units/kg (approximately 6000 units) initially followed by 40 units/kg (3000 units) every 18 hours. Factor levels should be measured to ensure that expected levels are achieved and that an inhibitor is not present.

Unlike factor VIII concentrates, factor IX concentrates contain a number of other proteins, including activated coagulating factors that appear to contribute to a risk of thrombosis with recurrent usage of factor IX concentrates. Because of the risk of thrombosis, more care is needed in deciding to use these concentrates. Desmopressin acetate is not useful in this disorder.

### Prognosis

The prognosis for these patients is the same as for those with factor VIII hemophilia.

## OTHER CONGENITAL COAGULATION DISORDERS

### Factor XI Deficiency

This disorder is seen primarily among Ashkenazi Jews and is autosomal recessive. The PTT may be markedly prolonged, and specific assays of factor XI will show reduced levels. This is usually a mild bleeding disorder manifested primarily by postoperative bleeding. Factor replacement is given with fresh-frozen plasma when necessary.

## Afibrinogenemia

In this rare disorder, fibrinogen is absent and both prothrombin time and partial thromboplastin time are markedly prolonged. These patients may have a severe bleeding disorder similar to hemophilia. Fibrinogen is replaced with cryoprecipitate.

## Other Coagulation Disorders

Bleeding disorders due to isolated deficiency of factors II, V, X, or VII are extremely rare. Deficiencies of factor XII and the contact pathway factors cause a markedly prolonged PTT but are not associated with any increased bleeding.

Factor XIII deficiency results in delayed bleeding after trauma or surgery. All coagulation tests are normal. The disorder is diagnosed by showing instability of the fibrin clot in 8-molar urea. Factor XIII is replaced with cryoprecipitate or plasma.

## COAGULOPATHY OF LIVER DISEASE

### Essentials of Diagnosis

- Prothrombin time more prolonged than PTT.
- No response to Vitamin K.

### General Considerations

The liver is the site of synthesis of all the coagulation factors except factor VIII. As hepatic insufficiency develops, the vitamin K-dependent factors (factors II, VII, IX, X) and factor V are the first to be affected. Because of its rapid turnover (half-life 6 hours), factor VII levels are the first to decline. Conversely, fibrinogen levels are remarkably well conserved, and decreased fibrinogen synthesis does not occur unless liver disease is very severe.

Liver disease has a number of other effects on the hemostatic system. Increased fibrinolysis occurs because the liver synthesizes $\alpha_2$ antiplasmin (the main inhibitor of fibrinolysis), which is responsible for the clearance of plasminogen activator. Biliary tract disease may lead to malabsorption of vitamin K, and congestive splenomegaly may produce mild thrombocytopenia. A variety of chronic liver diseases cause abnormal posttranslation modification of fibrinogen with resultant dysfibrinogenemia.

### Clinical Findings

**A. Symptoms and Signs:** The coagulopathy of liver disease may lead to bleeding at any site. Excessive fibrinolysis may lead to oozing at venipuncture sites.

**B. Laboratory Findings:** Hepatic coagulopathy produces a more marked abnormality in the prothrombin time (PT) than the partial thromboplastin time

**Table 10–22.** Causes of isolated prolonged prothrombin time.

| |
|---|
| Liver disease |
| Vitamin K deficiency |
| Warfarin therapy |
| Factor VII deficiency |

(PTT). Early in the course of liver disease, only the PT will become affected. Fibrinogen levels should be normal, and the thrombin time should be normal unless dysfibrinogenemia is present. The platelet count should be normal unless production is suppressed by acute alcohol ingestion or unless hypersplenism is present. The peripheral blood smear may show target cells.

### Differential Diagnosis

Hepatic coagulopathy can be distinguished from vitamin K deficiency only by demonstrating the failure of vitamin K to correct the abnormal values. Liver disease is distinguished from disseminated intravascular coagulation by the normal fibrinogen level and lack of thrombocytopenia. End-stage liver disease almost invariably leads to some element of disseminated intravascular coagulation, and the disorders overlap (see Tables 10–22 and 10–23).

### Treatment

Long-term treatment of hepatic coagulopathy with factor replacement is usually ineffective. Fresh-frozen plasma is the treatment of choice, and volume overload will limit one's ability to maintain hemostatic factor levels. For example, to maintain factor levels greater than 25%, one must initially raise the level to 50% with 50% of the plasma volume (20 mL/kg) and then replace 10 mL/kg every 6 hours to maintain adequate factor VII levels. In average-sized persons, this will require transfusion of 1400 mL of plasma initially followed by 700 mL every 6 hours. Factor IX concentrates are contraindicated in liver disease because of their tendency to cause disseminated intravascular coagulation. If thrombocytopenia is present, platelet transfusion may be of some help, but platelet recovery is usually disappointing because of hypersplenism.

### Prognosis

The prognosis is that of the underlying liver disease.

**Table 10–23.** Causes of prolonged prothrombin time and partial thromboplastin time.

| |
|---|
| Liver disease |
| Vitamin K deficiency |
| Disseminated intravascular coagulation |
| Heparin |
| Warfarin |
| Isolated factor deficiencies (rare): II, V, X, I |

## VITAMIN K DEFICIENCY

### Essentials of Diagnosis
- Prothrombin time more prolonged than PTT.
- Rapid correction with vitamin K replacement.
- Underlying dietary deficiency or antibiotic use.

### General Considerations
Vitamin K plays a role in coagulation by acting as a cofactor for the posttranslational γ-carboxylation of zymogens II, VII, IX, and X. The modified zymogens (with γ-carboxyglutamic acid residues) are able to bind to platelets in a calcium-dependent reaction and consequently better participate in the complex reactions that activate factors X and II (Fig 10–1). Without γ-carboxylation, these reactions on the platelet surface occur slowly and hemostasis is impaired.

Vitamin K is supplied in the diet primarily in leafy vegetables and endogenously from synthesis from intestinal bacteria. Factors that contribute to vitamin K deficiency include poor diet, malabsorption, and broad-spectrum antibiotics suppressing colonic flora. A characteristic setting for vitamin K deficiency is a postoperative patient who is not eating and who is receiving antibiotics. Body stores of vitamin K are small, and deficiency may develop in as little as 1 week.

### Clinical Findings
**A. Symptoms and Signs:** There are no specific clinical features, and bleeding may occur at any site.

**B. Laboratory Findings:** The prothrombin time is prolonged to a greater extent than the PTT, and with mild vitamin K deficiency only the PT is defective (Tables 10–22 and 10–23). Fibrinogen level, thrombin time, and platelet count are not affected.

### Differential Diagnosis
Vitamin K deficiency can be distinguished from hepatic coagulopathy only by assessing the response to vitamin K therapy. Surreptitious warfarin use will produce laboratory features indistinguishable from those of vitamin K deficiency.

Vitamin K deficiency is distinguished from disseminated intravascular coagulation by the normal platelet count and normal fibrinogen level in the former.

### Treatment
Vitamin K deficiency responds rapidly to subcutaneous vitamin K, and a single dose of 15 mg will completely correct laboratory abnormalities in 12–24 hours.

### Prognosis
The prognosis is excellent, as vitamin K deficiency can be completely corrected with replacement.

## DISSEMINATED INTRAVASCULAR COAGULATION (DIC)

### Essentials of Diagnosis
- Hypofibrinogenemia, thrombocytopenia, fibrin degradation products, and prolonged prothrombin time.
- Underlying serious illness.
- Microangiopathic hemolytic anemia may be present.
- Fibrin monomer may be present.

### General Considerations
Coagulation is usually confined to a localized area by the combination of blood flow and circulating inhibitors of coagulation, especially antithrombin III. If the stimulus to coagulation is too great, these control mechanisms can be overwhelmed, leading to the syndrome of disseminated intravascular coagulation. In pathophysiologic terms, disseminated intravascular coagulation can be thought of as the consequence of the presence of circulating thrombin (normally confined to a localized area). The effects of thrombin are to cleave fibrinogen to fibrin monomer, stimulate

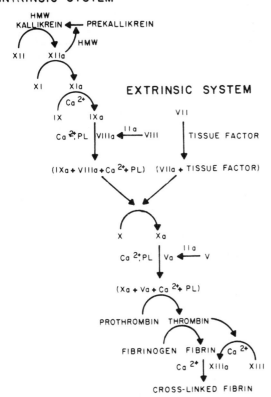

**Figure 10–1.** Cascade mechanism of blood coagulation. PL, phospholipid; Ca²⁺, calcium ion; HMW, high-molecular-weight kininogen. (Adapted from Davie and Ratnoff. Reproduced, with permission from Baugh RF, Hougie C: The chemistry of blood coagulation. *Clin Haematol* 1979;**8**:3.)

platelet aggregation, activate factors V and VIII, and release plasminogen activator, which generates plasmin. Plasmin in turn cleaves fibrin, generating fibrin degradation products, and further inactivates factors V and VIII. Thus, the excess thrombin activity produces hypofibrinogenemia, thrombocytopenia, depletion of coagulation factors, and fibrinolysis.

Disseminated intravascular coagulation can be caused by a number of serious illnesses, including sepsis (especially with gram-negative bacteria but possible with any widespread bacterial or fungal infection), severe tissue injury (especially burns and head injury), obstetric complications (amniotic fluid embolus, septic abortion, retained dead fetus), cancer (acute promyelocytic leukemia, mucinous adenocarcinomas), and major hemolytic transfusion reactions.

## Clinical Findings

**A. Symptoms and Signs:** Disseminated intravascular coagulation leads to both bleeding and thrombosis. Bleeding is far more common than thrombosis, but the latter may dominate if coagulation is activated to a far greater extent than fibrinolysis. Bleeding may occur at any site, but spontaneous bleeding and oozing at venipuncture sites or wounds are important clues to the diagnosis. Thrombosis is most commonly manifested by digital ischemia and gangrene, but catastrophic events such as renal cortical necrosis and hemorrhagic adrenal infarction may occur. Disseminated intravascular coagulation may also secondarily produce microangiopathic hemolytic anemia.

Subacute disseminated intravascular coagulation is seen primarily in cancer patients and is manifested primarily as recurrent superficial and deep venous thromboses (Trousseau's syndrome).

**B. Laboratory Findings:** Disseminated intravascular coagulation produces a complex coagulopathy with the characteristic constellation of hypofibrinogenemia, elevated fibrin degradation products, thrombocytopenia, and a prolonged prothrombin time. Hypofibrinogenemia is the most important diagnostic laboratory feature, because few disorders (congenital hypofibrinogenemia, severe liver disease) will lower the fibrinogen level. In some cases of disseminated intravascular coagulation, when the patient's baseline fibrinogen level is markedly elevated, the initial fibrinogen level may be normal. However, since the half-life of fibrinogen is approximately 4 days, a noticeably falling fibrinogen level will confirm the diagnosis of disseminated intravascular coagulation.

Other laboratory abnormalities are variably present. The partial thromboplastin time may or may not be prolonged. Fibrin monomer is present in approximately one-third of cases. Although not very sensitive, its presence is highly specific for disseminated intravascular coagulation. In approximately one-fourth of cases, a microangiopathic hemolytic anemia is present, and fragmented red blood cells are seen on the peripheral smear. Antithrombin III levels may be markedly depleted. When fibrinolysis is activated,

levels of plasminogen and $\alpha_2$-antiplasmin may be low.

Subacute disseminated intravascular coagulation produces a very different laboratory picture. Thrombocytopenia and elevated fibrin degradation products are usually the only abnormalities. Fibrinogen levels are normal, and the PTT may be short.

## Differential Diagnosis

Liver disease may prolong both the PT and PTT, but fibrinogen levels are usually normal, and the platelet count is usually normal or only slightly reduced. However, severe liver disease may be difficult to distinguish from disseminated intravascular coagulation. Vitamin K deficiency will not affect the fibrinogen level or platelet count and will be completely corrected by vitamin K replacement.

Sepsis may produce thrombocytopenia and digital ischemia, and coagulopathy may be present because of vitamin K deficiency. However, in these cases, the fibrinogen level should be normal.

Thrombotic thrombocytopenic purpura may produce fever and microangiopathic hemolytic anemia. However, fibrinogen levels and other coagulation tests should be normal.

## Treatment

The primary focus should be the diagnosis and treatment of the underlying disorder that has given rise to disseminated intravascular coagulation. In many cases, disseminated intravascular coagulation will produce laboratory abnormalities with only mild clinical manifestations, and in these cases no specific therapy is required.

When the underlying cause of disseminated intravascular coagulation is rapidly reversible (such as in obstetric cases), replacement therapy alone may be indicated. The role of heparin in the treatment of disseminated intravascular coagulation is controversial. In some cases, when any increase in bleeding is unacceptable (neurosurgical procedures), heparin therapy is contraindicated. However, when disseminated intravascular coagulation is producing serious clinical consequences and the underlying cause is not rapidly reversible, heparin therapy may be necessary to control the syndrome. In cases where disseminated intravascular coagulation causes thrombosis, heparin therapy is mandatory.

In replacement therapy, platelet transfusion should be used to maintain a platelet count greater than $50,000/\mu L$. Fibrinogen is replaced with cryoprecipitate, and one should aim for a level of 150 mg/dL. One unit of cyroprecipitate usually raises the fibrinogen level by 6–8 mg/dL, so that 15 units of cryoprecipitate will raise the level from 50 to 150 mg/dL. Coagulation factor deficiency may require replacement with fresh-frozen plasma.

Heparin therapy must be used in combination with replacement therapy, since administering heparin on its own will lead to an unacceptable increase in bleeding. Heparin therapy usually requires a dose of 500–

750 units per hour. Heparin cannot be effective if antithrombin III levels are markedly depleted. Antithrombin III levels should be measured, and fresh-frozen plasma should be used to raise levels to greater than 50%. In using heparin, it is not necessary to prolong the PTT. Successful therapy is indicated by a rising fibrinogen level. Fibrin degradation products will decline over 1–2 days. Improvement in the platelet count may lag as much as 1 week behind control of the coagulopathy.

In some cases, when disseminated intravascular coagulation is complicated by excessive fibrinolysis, even the combination of heparin and replacement therapy may not be adequate to control bleeding. In these cases, aminocaproic acid, 1 g intravenously per hour, should be added to decrease the rate of fibrinolysis, raise the fibrinogen level, and control bleeding. *Caution:* It must be emphasized that aminocaproic acid can *never* be used without heparin in disseminated intravascular coagulation, since fatal thrombosis will occur.

## Prognosis

The prognosis is that of the underlying disease. Severe disseminated intravascular coagulation can be lethal.

Coleman R, Robboy SJ, Minna JD: Disseminated intravascular coagulation (DIC): An approach. *AM J Med* 1972;**52**:679.
Feinstein DI: Diagnosis and management of disseminated intravascular coagulation: The role of heparin therapy. *Blood* 1982;**60**:284.

## LUPUS ANTICOAGULANT

The lupus anticoagulant is an IgM or IgG immunoglobulin that produces a prolonged PTT by binding to the phospholipid used in the in vitro PTT assay. As such, it is a laboratory artifact and does not cause a clinical bleeding disorder. The "lupus anticoagulant" is seen in 5–10% of patients with systemic lupus erythematosus. More commonly, it is seen without an underlying disorder or in patients taking phenothiazines.

There is no bleeding defect unless a second disorder such as thrombocytopenia, hypoprothrombinemia, or a prolonged bleeding time is present. Paradoxically, the lupus anticoagulant has been associated with an increased risk of thrombosis and of recurrent spontaneous abortions.

The PTT is prolonged and fails to correct when the patient's plasma is mixed in a 1:1 dilution with normal plasma. The PT is either normal or slightly prolonged. The fibrinogen level and thrombin time are normal. The Russel viper venom (RVV) time is a more sensitive assay and is specifically designed to demonstrate the presence of a lupus anticoagulant. An antiphospholipid, the lupus anticoagulant, will cause a false-positive VDRL test for syphilis.

Lupus anticoagulant should be suspected in cases of a markedly prolonged PTT without clinical bleeding (other causes are factor XII or contact factor deficiency). The plasma mixing test will demonstrate the presence of an inhibitor by the failure of normal plasma to correct the PTT. When acquired factor VIII inhibitors are being considered, a factor VIII:C level may be measured; this will be normal in patients with lupus anticoagulant.

No specific treatment is necessary. Prednisone will usually rapidly eliminate the lupus anticoagulant, and it has been suggested that prednisone therapy reduces spontaneous abortions in this syndrome. It is not clear whether prednisone has any effect on the thrombotic tendency associated with lupus anticoagulant. Patients with thromboses should be treated with anticoagulation in a standard manner.

Branch DW et al: Obstetric complications associated with the lupus anticoagulant. *N Engl J Med* 1985;**313**:1322.
Mueh JR, Herbst KD, Rapaport SI: Thrombosis in patients with the lupus anticoagulant. *Ann Intern Med* 1980;**92**:156.

## ACQUIRED FACTOR VIII ANTIBODIES

Antibodies to factor VIII may develop either postpartum or with no underlying illness. Factor VIII antibodies also develop in 15% of patients with factor VIII hemophilia who have received infusions of plasma concentrates.

Acquired factor VIII antibodies usually produce a severe bleeding disorder. The PTT is prolonged, and the fibrinogen level, prothrombin time, and platelet count are not affected. A plasma mixing test will usually reveal the presence of an inhibitor by the failure of normal plasma to correct the prolonged PTT. However, the mixing test may require incubation for 2–4 hours to reveal the inhibitor. Factor VIII coagulant levels are low.

Factor VIII antibodies should be suspected in any acquired severe bleeding disorder associated with a prolonged PTT. Factor VIII antibodies are distinguished from lupus anticoagulants both by the presence of clinical bleeding and more importantly by the reduced factor VIII:C level. The diagnosis is confirmed by mixing tests and in vivo by the failure of factor VIII concentrates to raise factor VIII:C levels by the expected amount.

The treatment of choice is cyclophosphamide, usually combined with prednisone. In the interim, aggressive factor VIII replacement may be necessary. Plasmapheresis to reduce inhibitor levels may be useful. Treatment of factor VIII antibodies is complex and should be done in consultation with a hematologist.

The prognosis of these patients is poor, and many die of overwhelming bleeding.

Feinstein DI, Rapaport SI: Acquired inhibitors of blood coagulation. *Prog Hemost Thromb* 1972;**1**:75.

## THROMBOTIC DISEASES

Thrombosis is a common event in clinical medicine. Most thromboses are due to local factors and not to hematologic disorders. Factors predisposing to venous thrombosis include stasis due to structural lesions, general immobility, and damage to vessel walls. Arterial thromboses are most commonly superimposed on underlying atherosclerosis.

Less commonly, thromboses are manifestations of hematologic disorders causing an increased risk of clotting. A variety of acquired and congenital disorders lead to a "hypercoagulable state" (Table 10–24).

## THE HYPERCOAGULABLE STATES

*Ralph O. Wallerstein, MD*

Some patients who appear unusually prone to develop thromboembolism have specific laboratory abnormalities. Others have clinical conditions associated with an increased risk of thromboembolic complications. Among the primary coagulable states are deficiency of antithrombin III, protein C, or protein S; disorders of the fibrinolytic system; dysfibrinogenemia; and the presence of lupus anticoagulant. All of these conditions are rare, but in a relatively young person with recurrent thrombosis, an attempt may have to be made to detect an abnormality of one of these clotting factors.

The estimated incidence of antithrombin III deficiency may be as high as 1 in 2000. Heterozygotes have levels of antithrombin III between 25 and 60% of normal; the homozygous state is incompatible with life. Lifelong prophylaxis with an oral anticoagulant is indicated. Low levels of antithrombin III may be seen in association with advanced liver disease and with a nephrotic syndrome.

Very much rarer are deficiencies of either protein C or protein S. Moderate reductions can cause severe thrombotic complications. Protein C is a vitamin K-dependent, naturally occurring anticoagulant. Protein C, when activated by thrombin, inactivates the acti-

vated coagulation cofactors Va and VIIIa. It may also stimulate fibrinolysis. Protein S appears to act as a cofactor to protein C. Patients with a heterozygous deficiency of protein S have a clinical appearance similar to that of patients with deficiencies of antithrombin III or protein C. Plasminogen deficiency may also be associated with recurrent thrombosis. While most patients with dysfibrinogenemia have abnormal bleeding, a few have recurrent thromboses, which may be caused by the formation of fibrin pathologically resistant to the lytic effect of plasmin. Finally, the lupus anticoagulant has on rare occasions been associated with increased thrombosis.

The secondary hypercoagulable states are clinical disorders historically associated with a high risk of thromboembolic complications. This includes patients with cancer, especially of the pancreas and lung. Pregnancy and the use of oral contraceptives are associated with an increased incidence of thrombosis. Patients with a nephrotic syndrome have an increased risk of venous thrombosis, thought to be due to renal loss of antithrombin III along with other proteins. The incidence of thrombosis is also increased in the myeloproliferative diseases, especially when the platelet count is elevated.

Clouse LH, Comp PC: The regulation of hemostasis: The protein C system. *N Engl J Med* 1986;**314**:1298.

Schafer AI: The hypercoagulable states. *Ann Intern Med* 1985;**102**:814.

---

# BLOOD TRANSFUSIONS

*Ralph O. Wallerstein, MD*

Blood transfusions are used to restore blood volume after hemorrhage; to improve the oxygen-carrying capacity of the blood in severe anemia; and to combat shock in acute hemolytic anemia. Blood volume or red cell mass should be restored to approximately 70% of normal after hemorrhage. Adequate oxygen-carrying capacity can usually be maintained in chronic anemia by raising the hemoglobin value to 50–70% of normal. Shock in acute hemolytic or acute aplastic anemia can be prevented by maintaining hemoglobin values at 50–70% of normal.

### Rate of Transfusion

Except in the case of emergencies, blood should be given at a rate of 80–100 drops/min, or 500 mL in 1½–2 hours. For rapid transfusions, it is best to use a 15-gauge needle and allow the blood to run freely. The use of pressure is dangerous unless it can be applied by gentle compression of collapsible plastic blood containers.

### Serologic Considerations

The antigens for which routine testing is always

**Table 10–24.** Causes of hypercoagulability.

| |
|---|
| **Acquired** |
| Cancer |
| Inflammatory disorders: Ulcerative colitis |
| Myeloproliferative disorders |
| Postoperative |
| Estrogens, pregnancy |
| Lupus anticoagulant |
| Heparin-induced thrombocytopenia |
| **Congenital** |
| Antithrombin III deficiency |
| Protein C deficiency |
| Protein S deficiency |
| Dysfibrinogenemia |
| Abnormal plasminogen |

performed in donors and recipients are A, B, and D ($Rh_0$). Pretransfusion compatibility tests use the serum of the recipient and the cells of the donor (major cross-match). To ensure a maximal margin of safety, each transfusion should be preceded by a 3-part compatibility procedure: (1) at room temperature in saline; (2) at 37 °C fortified by the addition of albumin; and (3) at 37 °C followed by an antiglobulin test.

## Miscellaneous Considerations

The age of the blood (within the expiration period) is relatively unimportant in restoring volume deficits or repairing oxygen-carrying capacity defects. Fresh blood is required only if functioning platelets are needed. Red cell mass (hematocrit about 70%), infused through 17- to 18-gauge needles, is the treatment of choice in chronic anemias. Precipitates of platelets, leukocytes, and fibrinogen or fibrin in some bank bloods may clog the filters in administration sets and cause the infusion rate to slow down; when this happens, the filters should be replaced.

Barton JC: Nonhemolytic, noninfectious transfusion reactions. *Semin Hematol* 1981;**18**:95.

Boral LI et al: The type and antibody screen, revisited. *Am J Clin Pathol* 1979;**71**:578.

Collins JA: Pertinent recent developments in blood banking. *Surg Clin North Am* 1983;**63**:483.

Mollison PL: *Blood Transfusion in Clinical Medicine,* 6th ed. Davis, 1979.

Tibor JG: Pathogenesis and management of hemolytic transfusion reaction. *Semin Hematol* 1981;**18**:84.

## FRESH BLOOD TRANSFUSIONS

Concern about the freshness of blood has to do with 4 considerations: **(1) Platelets:** Platelets are in adequate supply in whole blood up to about 24 hours after collection. **(2) Factors V and VIII:** All coagulation factors except V and VIII are stable in banked blood for at least 21 days; factors V and VIII decline fairly rapidly within a few days after collection. **(3) Levels of 2,3-diphosphoglycerate (2,3-DPG):** As red cells age—usually after a week or so—levels of 2,3-diphosphoglycerate decline; this causes increased affinity of hemoglobin for oxygen and results in less supply to the tissues. Although normal affinity is restored in a few hours after transfusion, massive infusions of older blood may make a critically ill patient worse. The problem of declining 2,3-diphosphoglycerate levels may be largely solved when citrate-phosphate-dextrose (CPD) replaces acid-citrate-dextrose (ACD) as the standard anticoagulant in blood banking. **(4) Levels of plasma potassium, lactic acid, and ammonia:** Plasma levels rise very little above the baseline for the first 4–5 days of storage and become potentially important only after 2 weeks. Most transfusions are given for acute blood loss—either posttraumatic, during surgery where blood loss

is inevitable, or in patients with acute hemorrhage from the gastrointestinal tract. In none of these 3 categories is the age of blood particularly important, and fresh blood should not be ordered.

The recognized occasions when the age of the blood may be specified are the following:

(1) Open heart surgery, where heparinized blood is needed. Heparinized blood cannot be used later than 24 hours after procurement.

(2) Massive transfusions, ie, more than 10 units in a few hours. Platelets may become a problem (see next section).

(3) In renal dialysis and in patients with liver failure, blood can be given within a week after procurement.

## PLATELET TRANSFUSIONS

Platelet transfusions may be indicated in patients with aplastic anemia or whose platelet counts have fallen below 10,000/$\mu$L after chemotherapy for acute leukemia. Platelets do not have to be ABO type-specific; concentrates do not contain enough red cells to cause a reaction. These transfusions raise the platelet count by 10,000 platelets per microliter per platelet unit given; survival is usually about 2 days. After repeated transfusions of platelets, recipients may become immunized to random platelets; HLA-matched platelets should then be given. Platelet transfusions are of little value in conditions associated with rapid destruction of platelets such as idiopathic thrombocytopenic purpura.

## WHITE CELL TRANSFUSIONS

Granulocyte concentrates can now be transfused. They are obtained by leukapheresis from a single donor who must be ABO-compatible but need not be matched for HLA or granulocyte-specific antigens. If the patient has been alloimmunized, granulocyte transfusions may induce severe chill and fever reactions and will fail to have a clinical effect. In such cases, HLA typing of family members may yield a compatible match. Indications for granulocyte transfusions are a granulocyte count of less than 500/$\mu$L, with fever and infection that have failed to respond to antibiotics administered for 48 hours, and a marrow that shows no sign of imminent recovery.

## TRANSFUSIONS IN BLEEDING PROBLEMS

Fresh-frozen plasma, which contains all the clotting factors except platelets, may be used in a patient who continues to ooze postoperatively for several days if the suspicion of some type of hemophilia is strong and diagnostic results are not immediately available. Plasma is not a clinically useful source of fibrinogen because its fibrinogen concentration is too low.

When over 10 units of bank blood have to be given in a few hours, the levels of factors V and VIII may decrease sufficiently to cause prolongation of the PTT, but they usually do not fall below hemostatically adequate levels. Thrombocytopenic bleeding may become a problem. Platelet concentrates may have to be given. Central venous pressure should be monitored to protect against overtransfusion.

Higby DJ, Burnett D: Granulocyte transfusions: Current status. *Blood* 1980;**55**:2.

## HEMOLYTIC TRANSFUSION REACTIONS

### Essentials of Diagnosis
- Chills and fever during blood transfusion.
- Pain in the back, chest, or abdomen.
- Hemoglobinemia and hemoglobinuria.

### General Considerations
In all significant hemolytic transfusion reactions there is immediate, easily visible hemoglobinemia with pinkish or red plasma. A normal serum color during or immediately after a transfusion rules out hemolysis as the cause of even severe symptoms.

In transfusion reaction due to ABO incompatibility the donor cells are hemolyzed instantaneously in the general circulation. Reactions caused by some of the other blood groups (such as Rh) have more gradual hemolysis and may last hours, most of the destruction occurring in the reticuloendothelial tissues.

Serious transfusion reactions are often caused by clerical errors such as improper labeling of specimens or improper identification of patients.

### Clinical Findings
**A. Symptoms and Signs:** There may be chills and fever, and pain in the vein at the local injection site or in the back, chest, or abdomen. Anxiety, apprehension, and headache are common. In the anesthetized patient, spontaneous bleeding from different areas may be the only sign of a transfusion reaction.

**B. Laboratory Findings:** Posttransfusion blood counts fail to show the anticipated rise in hemoglobin; spherocytes may be present on the blood smear; and initial leukopenia at 1–2 hours is followed by a slight leukocytosis. Free hemoglobin can be detected within a few minutes. Methemalbumin, an acid hematin-albumin complex giving a brown color to the serum, may appear after a few hours and persist for several days. Elevated bilirubin levels, when present, are usually greatest 3–6 hours after the transfusion. Haptoglobin disappears from the serum. Hemoglobinuria and oliguria may occur.

After the reaction occurs it is essential to draw a fresh specimen from the patient, perform a direct Coombs test, and check it against the blood in the transfusion bottle (not the pilot tube) by the indirect Coombs test. If the indirect Coombs test is positive, exact identification of the offending antibody may be made by matching the patient's serum against a panel of known test cells. Usual antibodies found in transfusion reactions are anti-c, anti-K (Kell), anti-E, anti-Fy$^a$ (Duffy), anti-Le$^a$ (Lewis), anti-Jk$^a$ (Kidd), anti-C, and anti-P.

### Differential Diagnosis
Transfusion in the presence of leukoagglutinins, which usually develop after 5 or more transfusions or after previous pregnancy, may cause severe chills and high fever and pulmonary infiltrates. There is no fall in hematocrit, a cross-match is compatible, and there are no pigmentary changes in the serum; leukoagglutinins can be demonstrated by cytotoxicity studies. All subsequent transfusions must be in the form of packed red cells, "white cell-poor," ie, with the buffy coat removed.

In allergic transfusion reactions, the above tests also are negative, and no leukoagglutinins are present; recipients who lack IgA develop hives on the basis of anti-IgA.

### Complications
Acute tubular necrosis and azotemia may follow a hemolytic transfusion reaction.

### Treatment
Hives, chills, and fever following the transfusion of blood are not necessarily due to hemolysis; if the patient's serum remains clear, the transfusion may be continued. However, once the diagnosis of hemolysis is established by appropriate tests, the main problems are to combat shock and treat possible renal damage.

**A. Treatment of Shock:** After antibody screening of the patient's serum, transfusions with properly matched blood may be advisable. If no satisfactory answer can be found to account for the transfusion reaction, plasma expanders, such as dextran, and plasma may have to be used instead of whole blood. Pressor agents may be necessary.

**B. Treatment of Renal Failure:** Some studies suggest that osmotic diuretics such as mannitol can prevent renal failure following a hemolytic transfusion reaction. After an apparent reaction and in oliguric patients, a test dose of 12.5 g of mannitol (supplied as 25% solution in 50-mL ampules) is administered intravenously over a period of 3–5 minutes; this dose may be repeated if no signs of circulatory overload develop. A satisfactory urinary output following the use of mannitol is 60 mL/h or more. Mannitol can be safely administered as a continuous intravenous infusion; each liter of 5–10% mannitol should be alternated with 1 L of normal saline to which 40 meq of KCl has been added to prevent serious potassium depletion. If oliguria develops, treat as for acute renal failure.

## Prognosis

The hemolysis is self-limited. Renal involvement is comparatively infrequent. The death rate from hemolytic transfusion reactions is about 10%.

## POSTTRANSFUSION HEPATITIS

The risk of clinical hepatitis following transfusion is approximately 1%; subclinical hepatitis occurs in about 10% of patients transfused. Current donor testing includes check for hepatitis B surface antigen (HBsAG), for antibody to core antigen (anti-HBc), and for serum levels of alanine aminotransferase (ALT). Most cases of posttransfusion hepatitis are now of the non-A, non-B (NANB) type; screening donors for anti-HBc has resulted in reduction of NANB in recipients by 40%.

Koziol DE et al: Antibody to hepatitis B core antigen as a paradoxical marker for non-A, non-B hepatitis in donated blood. *Ann Intern Med* 1986;**104**:488.

Miller DJ: Seroepidemiology of viral hepatitis: Correlation with clinical findings. *Postgrad Med* (Sept) 1980;**68**:137.

Ratey GG: Transfusions and hepatitis, update 1978. (Editorial.) *N Engl J Med* 1978;**298**:1413. [This editorial reviews the status of hepatitis and transfusions and points out the role of non-A, non-B transfusional hepatitis.]

## ACQUIRED IMMUNODEFICIENCY SYNDROME (AIDS) ASSOCIATED WITH BLOOD TRANSFUSION

The risk of contracting acquired immunodeficiency syndrome (AIDS) from a blood transfusion is estimated at 4 per million patients transfused, compared to a 1 per million risk in the general population. For comparison, in the male homosexual population, the risk of contracting AIDS is 1 per 100. The incidence of transfusion-associated AIDS is expected to decrease substantially now that blood banks are routinely using the HTLV-III antibody test to screen all donations for evidence of past exposure to the AIDS virus. The test is not infallible but reduces the risk of transfusing AIDS-contaminated blood to almost nil.

Weiss SH et al: Screening test for HTLV-III (AIDS agent) antibodies: Specificity, sensitivity, and applications. *JAMA* 1985;**253**:221.

## REFERENCES

Carter SK, Bakowski MT, Hellman K: *Chemotherapy of Cancer,* 2nd ed. Wiley, 1981.

Chanarin I: *The Megaloblastic Anemias,* 2nd ed. Blackwell, 1979.

Colman RW et al: *Hemostasis and Thrombosis: Basic Principles and Clinical Practice.* Lippincott, 1982.

Mollison PL: *Blood Transfusion in Clinical Medicine.* 7th ed. Mosby, 1983.

Ratnoff OD, Forbes CD (editors): *Disorders of Hemostasis.* Grune & Stratton, 1984.

Stites DP, Stobo JD, Wells JV (editors): *Basic & Clinical Immunology,* 6th ed. Appleton & Lange, 1987.

Williams WJ et al: *Hematology,* 3rd ed. McGraw-Hill, 1983.

Wintrobe MM et al: *Clinical Hematology,* 8th ed. Lea & Febiger, 1981.

# 11

# Alimentary Tract & Liver

*C. Michael Knauer, MD, & Sol Silverman, Jr., DDS*

## NAUSEA & VOMITING

These intensely disagreeable symptoms may occur singly or concurrently and may be due to a wide variety of factors (see below). The pathophysiology of vomiting is not completely understood. Vomiting appears to involve 2 functionally distinct medullary centers: the vomiting center, which initiates and controls the act of emesis; and the chemoreceptor trigger zone, which is activated by many drugs and endogenous and exogenous toxins. The vomiting center may receive stimuli from the alimentary tract and other organs, from the cerebral cortex, from the vestibular apparatus, and from the chemoreceptor trigger zone. Two or more stimuli may coexist.

An oversimplified classification of causes of vomiting is as follows:

(1) Alimentary disorders: Irritation, inflammation, or mechanical disturbance at any level of the gastrointestinal tract.

(2) Hepatobiliary and pancreatic disorders.

(3) Acute systemic infection.

(4) Central nervous system disorders: Increased intracranial pressure, stroke, migraine, infection, toxins, radiation sickness.

(5) Labyrinthine disorders: Motion sickness, infection, Meniere's syndrome.

(6) Endocrine disorders: Diabetic acidosis, adrenocortical crisis, pregnancy, starvation, lactic acidosis.

(7) Genitourinary disorders: Uremia, infection, obstruction.

(8) Cardiovascular disorders: Acute myocardial infarction, congestive heart failure.

(9) Drugs: Morphine, meperidine, codeine, excess alcohol, anesthetics, anticancer drugs, many others.

(10) Psychologic disorders: Reaction to pain, fear, or displeasure, chronic anxiety reaction, anorexia nervosa, bulimia, psychosis.

Complications of vomiting include fluid and electrolyte disturbances, pulmonary aspiration of vomitus, gastroesophageal mucosal tear (Mallory-Weiss syndrome), malnutrition, and postemetic rupture of the esophagus (Boerhaave's syndrome).

## Treatment

Simple acute vomiting such as occurs following dietary or alcoholic indiscretion or during morning sickness of early pregnancy (see p 479) may require little or no treatment. Avoiding known aggravating factors and taking simple corrective dietary measures usually suffice.

Severe or prolonged nausea and vomiting usually require careful medical management in the hospital. Attempt to determine and correct the causes of the vomiting as soon as possible. The vomiting patient should be checked to see if aspiration has occurred. The following general measures may be used as adjuncts to specific medical or surgical treatment:

**A. Fluids and Nutrition:** Maintain adequate hydration and nutrition, and correct any electrolyte imbalance that may occur. Hypokalemia and metabolic alkalosis are common in patients with severe vomiting. Withhold food temporarily and give intravenously 5% dextrose in saline with appropriate KCl supplementation (see pp 36 and 37). If vomiting continues, employ a nasogastric tube to intermittent suction for gastric decompression. When oral feedings are resumed, begin with dry foods in small quantities, eg, salted crackers, graham crackers. With "morning sickness," these foods may best be taken before arising. Later, change to frequent small feedings of simple palatable foods. Hot beverages (tea and clear broths) and cold beverages (iced tea and carbonated liquids, especially ginger ale) are tolerated quite early. Avoid lukewarm beverages. Always consider the patient's food preferences.

**B. Medical Measures:** *Note:* All unnecessary medication should be withheld from pregnant women during the critical early phase of fetal development. Unless nausea and vomiting of pregnancy are severe or progressive, avoid using medication for this purpose. The possible teratogenic effects of many classes of drugs are now being investigated.

Antiemetic drugs are usually better for preventing vomiting, but they may be employed selectively if the cause of vomiting cannot be treated effectively. The drugs should be used cautiously to avoid masking the development of serious illness. The choice of drug treatment depends on the reasons for the vomiting, the needs of the patient, and the known pharmacology of the available drugs:

(1) Sedatives, alone or with anticholinergics, may be helpful in patients with psychogenic vomiting.

(2) Antihistamines, eg, dimenhydrinate, 50 mg orally or intramuscularly every 4 hours or 100 mg by suppository twice daily, may be useful for patients with vestibular disorders (eg, Meniere's syndrome, motion sickness).

(3) Phenothiazines, eg, prochlorperazine, 5–10 mg orally or intramuscularly 3 times daily or 25 mg by suppository twice daily, may be preferred for vomiting caused by drugs, radiation sickness, or surgery.

(4) Metoclopramide, 10 mg orally or intravenously, is particularly helpful for the nausea and vomiting of diabetic gastroparesis and for the prevention of the nausea and vomiting of cancer chemotherapy.

(5) Tetrahydrocannabinol (from marihuana) is currently under investigation as treatment for refractory vomiting induced by cancer chemotherapy.

**C. Psychotherapy:** Attempt to determine the possible psychic basis of prolonged nausea and vomiting, but avoid aggressive psychotherapy during the acute phase of the illness. Hospitalization and restricted visiting may be necessary. Avoid unpleasant psychic stimuli such as strange odors, foul-smelling or foul-tasting medication, unattractive objects, and foods that are improperly prepared or served.

Clarke RSJ: Nausea and vomiting. *Br J Anaesth* 1984;**56**:19.

Hanson JS et al: The diagnosis and management of nausea and vomiting: A review. *Am J Gastroenterol* 1985;**80**:210.

Malagelada J-R, Camilleri M: Unexplained vomiting: A diagnostic challenge. *Ann Intern Med* 1984;**101**:211.

Uribe M et al: Successful administration of metoclopramide for the treatment of nausea in patients with advanced liver disease: A double-blind controlled trial. *Gastroenterology* 1985;**88**:757.

# HICCUP
## (Singultus)

Hiccup, although usually transient and benign, may be caused by or associated with a wide range of disorders. Of importance are disease processes just above and below the diaphragm, such as (1) inflammation (pneumonia, esophagitis, subphrenic abscess, pancreatitis); (2) gastric distention; (3) neoplasms; (4) myocardial infarction or pericardial disease; (5) metabolic derangements (azotemia); (6) central nervous system disorders (infection, tumors); and (7) idiopathic disorders. Correction of potentially remediable causes will be most effective in the management of hiccup.

## Treatment

Countless measures have been suggested for interrupting the rhythmic reflex that produces hiccup. At times, however, none of these may be successful, and the symptom may be so prolonged and severe as to jeopardize the patient's life.

**A. Simple Home Remedies:** These measures probably act by diverting the patient's attention; they consist of distracting conversation, fright, painful or unpleasant stimuli, or of having the patient perform such apparently purposeless procedures as breath-holding, sipping ice water, or inhaling strong fumes.

**B. Medical Measures:**

**1. Sedation**–Any of the common sedative drugs may be effective, eg, pentobarbital sodium, 100 mg orally or 120 mg by rectal suppository.

**2. Stimulation of nasopharynx**–A soft catheter introduced nasally to stimulate the nasopharynx and pharynx is often successful.

**3. Local anesthetics**–Viscous 2% lidocaine, 15 mL orally, may be of some use. General anesthesia may be tried in intractable cases.

**4. Antispasmodics**–Atropine sulfate, 0.3–0.6 mg, may be given subcutaneously.

**5. Amyl nitrate** inhalations may be effective.

**6. $CO_2$ inhalations**–Have the patient rebreathe into a paper bag for 3–5 minutes, or give 10–15% $CO_2$ mixture by face mask for 3–5 minutes.

**7. Tranquilizers**–Phenothiazine drugs have been used successfully for prolonged hiccup.

**8. Antacids.**

**C. Surgical Measures:** Various phrenic nerve operations, including bilateral phrenicotomy, may be indicated in extreme cases that fail to respond to all other measures and are considered to be a threat to life.

Shay SS et al: Hiccups associated with reflux esophagitis. *Gastroenterology* 1984;**87**:204.

# CONSTIPATION

The frequency of defecation and the consistency and volume of stools vary so greatly from individual to individual that it is often difficult to determine what is "normal." Familial, social, and dietary customs may help determine individual differences in bowel habits. Normal bowel movements may range in frequency from 3 to 12 stools per week, and the weights may range from 35 to 235 g of stool per day. The complaint of constipation often reflects the attitude of the patient with respect to the expected pattern of bowel movements. The patient should be considered to be constipated only if defecation is unexplainably delayed for days or if the stools are unusually hard, dry, and difficult to express. Constipation may result from repeatedly ignoring the urge to defecate because of unwillingness to interrupt social, recreational, or occupational activities.

Because there are many specific organic causes of constipation (see below), it is essential to explore such possibilities in patients with unexplained constipation. Be especially suspicious of organic causes when there have been sudden and unaccountable changes in bowel habits, or blood in the stools.

## Causes of Constipation

(1) Dietary factors: Highly refined and low-fiber foods, inadequate fluids.

(2) Physical inactivity: Inadequate exercise, prolonged bed rest.

(3) Pregnancy.

(4) Advanced age (often multifactorial).

(5) Drugs: Analgesics (codeine, oxycodone [Per-

codan]), anesthetics, antacids (aluminum and calcium salts), anticholinergics, anticonvulsants, antidepressants (tricyclics, monoamine oxidase inhibitors), antihypertensives (ganglionic blocking agents), antiparkinsonism drugs, antipsychotic drugs (phenothiazines), beta-adrenergic blocking agents, bismuth salts, calcium channel blockers, diuretics, iron salts, laxatives and cathartics (chronic use), metallic intoxications (arsenic, lead, mercury), muscle relaxants, opiates.

(6) Metabolic abnormalities: Hypokalemia, hyperglycemia, uremia, porphyria, amyloidosis.

(7) Endocrine abnormalities: Hypothyroidism, hypercalcemia, panhypopituitarism, pheochromocytoma, glucagonoma.

(8) Lower bowel abnormality: (a) Colon: prediverticular disease, diverticulosis, diverticulitis of sigmoid colon, neoplasm, extrinsic obstruction, inflammatory disease, especially with stricture. (b) Rectum: Disturbances in the defecatory mechanism, aganglionosis, pelvic floor spasm, neoplasm, inflammation. (c) Anus: Stricture, fissure, neoplasm.

(9) Neurogenic abnormalities: Innervation disorders of the bowel wall (aganglionosis, autonomic neuropathy), spinal cord disorders (trauma, multiple sclerosis, tabes dorsalis), disorders of the splanchnic nerves (tumors, trauma), cerebral disorders (strokes, parkinsonism, neoplasm).

(10) Psychogenic disorders.

(11) Enemas (Chronic use).

## Diagnosis

The history is all-important in the evaluation of this problem. If the cause is not obvious (no tumors, no stricture, etc) and the patient does not respond to simple measures (see below), further workup may be indicated to determine whether the problem is decreased motility or "outlet obstruction."

**A. Motility Disorders:** Assess transit through the colon with radiopaque markers (see Metcalf reference).

**B. Obstruction:** Barium enema to assess for possible distal aganglionic segment, rectal biopsy to assess the presence of ganglion cells, defecography to assess for rectal intussusception (usual mechanism for solitary rectal ulcer), anorectal manometry.

## Treatment

The patient should be told that a daily bowel movement is not essential to health or well-being and that many symptoms (eg, lack of "pep") attributed to constipation have no such relationship.

**A. Reestablishment of Regular Evacuation:** A regular period should be set aside after a meal for a bowel movement, even when the urge to defecate is not present. Cathartics and enemas should not be used for simple constipation, since they interfere with the normal bowel reflexes. If it seems inadvisable to withdraw such measures suddenly from a patient who has employed them for a long time, the milder laxatives and enemas (see below) can be used tempo-

rarily. Cathartic and enema "addicts" often defy all medical measures, and treatment is especially difficult when there is a serious underlying psychiatric disturbance.

**B. Diet:** The diet may be modified to satisfy the following requirements:

**1. Adequate volume**–Often "constipation" is merely due to inadequate food intake.

**2. Adequate bulk or residue**–Foods with high fiber content such as bran and raw fruits and vegetables may be helpful.

**3. Vegetable irritants**–Unless there is a specific contraindication (eg, intolerance), stewed or raw fruits (particularly prunes and figs) or vegetables may be of value, especially in the "atonic" type of constipation.

**4. Adequate fluids**–The patient should be encouraged to drink adequate quantities of fluids to permit passage of intestinal contents. Six to 8 glasses of fluid per day, in addition to the fluid content of foods, are ordinarily sufficient. A glass of hot water taken one-half hour before breakfast seems to exert a mild laxative effect.

**C. Exercise:** Moderate physical exercise is essential. Bed patients may require active and passive exercises. Good tone of the external abdominal muscles is important. Corrective physical therapy may be employed in patients with protuberant abdomens.

**D. Laxatives:** Laxatives may be classified as (1) stimulants (irritants), (2) bulk-forming agents, (3) osmotic laxatives, (4) wetting agents, and (5) lubricants. They are intended for temporary use on a selective basis by patients with simple constipation. Laxatives should *never* be given to patients with undiagnosed abdominal pain or when there is a possibility of intestinal obstruction or fecal impaction. Prolonged use of laxatives is seldom justified unless definitive therapy for specific disease is not possible. Chronic laxative use interferes with normal bowel motility and reflexes, thereby setting up a pattern for persistent constipation. Habitual use may also result in damage to the myenteric plexus of the colon and rectum. Melanosis coli may occur with certain laxatives but is probably not functionally important. There are no advantages— and there may be serious disadvantages—to mixing various laxatives.

**1. Stimulant (irritant) laxatives**–

a. Docusate sodium (eg, Colace, Doxinate), 50– 350 mg/d. This agent interferes with sodium resorption in the colon, leading to increased water content in stool. Docusate sodium is also an "irritant" that produces mucosal changes in the small bowel, but the effect of this action on stool character or frequency is unclear.

b. Cascara sagrada aromatic fluid extract, a mild agent; 4–8 mL acts within 6–12 hours.

c. Bisacodyl (Dulcolax, etc), a mild to moderate laxative that stimulates sensory nerve endings of the colon to produce parasympathetic reflexes; 10–15 mg acts within 6 hours. Efficacious in suppository form as well; particularly useful in patients with spinal cord injury.

d. Phenolphthalein, a potent over-the-counter laxative; 30–240 mg acts within 4–6 hours.

e. Glycerin suppository, an agent for lubricating hard fecal material and stimulating the rectocolic reflex; 3 g acts within 30 minutes.

**2. Bulk-forming agents–**

a. Psyllium hydrophilic mucilloid (Hydrocil, Konsyl, Metamucil), more than 14 g (1–2 rounded teaspoonfuls), 2–3 times daily after meals in a full glass of water, is probably one of the least harmful mild laxatives when administered with an adequate or high fluid intake. It is particularly useful in elderly patients and in those with irritable colon syndrome.

b. Unprocessed bran, one-fourth cup daily with cereal or in unsweetened applesauce.

**3. Osmotic laxatives–**

a. Milk of magnesia (magnesium hydroxide), 15–30 mL at bedtime, is a common mild-to-moderate generically available laxative. It should not be used by patients with impaired renal function.

b. Citrate of magnesia, 120–240 mL. Avoid use for patients with renal impairment.

c. Sodium phosphate, 4–8 g in hot water before breakfast.

d. Lactulose syrup, 15–60 mL daily.

**4. Wetting agents–**Docusate sodium is a detergent; see ¶ 1(a) above.

**5. Lubricants–**Liquid petrolatum (mineral oil), 15–30 mL per rectum, may help soften stool. Administration orally should be avoided because of risk of aspiration with resulting lipid pneumonia, and because petrolatum may interfere with intestinal absorption of fat-soluble vitamins.

**E. Enemas:** Because they interfere with restoration of a normal bowel reflex, enemas should ordinarily be used only as a temporary expedient in chronic constipation or fecal impaction. Infrequently, it may be necessary to administer enemas for prolonged periods.

**1. Saline enema (nonirritating)–**Warm physiologic saline solution, 500–2000 mL.

**2. Warm tap water (irritating)–**500–1000 mL.

**3. Soapsuds (SS) enema (irritating)–**75 mL of soap solution per liter of water.

**4. Oil retention enema–**180 mL of mineral oil or vegetable oil instilled in the rectum in the evening, retained overnight, and evacuated the next morning.

Akdamar K, Maumus LT: Management of constipation in the elderly. *Geriatrics* (Dec) 1984;**39**:81.

Cummings JH: Constipation, dietary fibre and the control of large bowel function. *Postgrad Med J* 1984;**60**:811.

Levine DA: "Solitary" rectal ulcer syndrome. *Gastroenterology* 1987;**92**:243.

Metcalf AM et al: Simplified assessment of segmental colonic transit. *Gastroenterology* 1987;**92**:40.

Shouler P, Keighly MRB: Changes in colorectal function in severe chronic constipation. *Gastroenterology* 1986;**90**:414.

# FECAL IMPACTION

Hardened or puttylike stools in the rectum or colon may interfere with the normal passage of feces; if the impaction is not removed manually, by enemas, or by surgery, it can cause partial or complete intestinal obstruction. The impaction may be due to organic causes (painful anorectal disease, tumor, or neurogenic disease of the colon) or to functional causes (bulk laxatives, antacids, residual barium from x-ray study, low-residue diet, starvation, drug-induced colonic stasis, or prolonged bed rest and debility). The patient may give a history of obstipation, but more frequently there is a history of watery diarrhea. There may be blood or mucus in the stool. Physical examination may reveal a distended abdomen, palpable "tumors" in the abdomen, and a firm stool in the rectum. The impaction may be broken up digitally or dislodged with a sigmoidoscope. Cleansing enemas (preferably in the knee-chest position) or, in the case of impaction higher in the colon, colonic irrigations may be of value. Daily oil retention enemas followed by digital fragmentation of the impaction and saline enemas may be necessary.

Bustin MP, Iber F: Management of common nonmalignant GI problems in the elderly. *Geriatrics* (March) 1983;**38**:69.

# GASTROINTESTINAL GAS (Flatulence)

The amount of gastrointestinal gas varies considerably from individual to individual. Subjective estimates by patients may be at considerable variance from observed findings, which indicate the average to be 17 passages of flatus per 24 hours. Five gases—nitrogen and oxygen from swallowed air, and carbon dioxide, hydrogen, and methane produced in the gut—constitute more than 99% of gastrointestinal gas. Excessive belching or eructation is usually due to air swallowed during eating or drinking, or it may be due to a nervous habit of sucking in air; the latter may be severe.

Excessive passage of flatus per rectum is due largely to gases formed by bacterial fermentation of maldigested carbohydrates and cellulose in the intestine. Rectal gas consists predominantly of $H_2$, $CO_2$, $CH_4$—all odorless; there is little objective information on the malodorous gases. Many problems of abdominal bloating or distention with pain appear to be caused by disordered bowel motility rather than by excessive gas. Since excessive gastrointestinal gas may be due to both functional and organic disease, complaints of unusual belching, bloating, and flatulence may require search for specific causes.

## Treatment

**A. Specific Treatment:** Eliminate specific causes, if known.

**B. Correction of Aerophagia:** Anxiety states are often associated with deep breathing and sighing and consequent swallowing of considerable quantities of air. When possible, treat underlying anxiety.

**C. Correction of Physical Defects:** These sometimes interfere with normal swallowing or breathing: (1) Structural deformities of the nose and nasopharynx, eg, nasal obstruction and adenoids. (2) Spatial defects of the teeth or ill-fitting dentures.

**D. Good Hygiene and Eating Habits:** Instruct the patient to avoid dietary indiscretions, eating too rapidly and too much, eating while under emotional strain, drinking large quantities of liquids with meals, taking laxatives, and chewing gum.

**E. Diet:** The diet should be nutritious as tolerated and enjoyed by the patient, but eliminate foods that may lead to excessive flatulence in susceptible individuals. An initial trial of a lactose-free diet is often rewarding.

**F. Medications:** Drugs (including charcoal, simethicone, and antiflatulence tablets) are generally unsatisfactory and at times are only of placebo value. Anticholinergic-sedative drugs serve to diminish the flow of saliva (which is often excessive in some patients), thereby reducing the aerophagia that accompanies swallowing; bowel motility is reduced.

Levitt MD: Gastrointestinal gas and abdominal symptoms. (Part 2.) *Pract Gastroenterol* (Jan/Feb) 1984;**8**:6.
Van Ness MM, Cattau EL Jr: Flatulence: Pathophysiology and treatment. *Am Fam Physician* (April) 1985;**31**:198.

## DIARRHEA

Diarrhea is defined as an increase in the frequency, fluidity, and volume of bowel movements. Normal bowel function varies from individual to individual, and the definition of diarrhea must take this variation into account. Factors influencing stool consistency are poorly understood; water content is not the sole determinant. Thus, the definition of diarrhea in a clinical sense is an increase in frequency or increased fluidity of bowel movements in a given individual. In pathophysiologic terms, diarrhea results from the passage of stools containing excess water, ie, from malabsorption or secretion of water. Although daily stool weight or water is probably the best single index to diarrhea, "small-volume diarrhea" with frequent evacuations of blood, mucus, or exudate is a syndrome often signifying disease of the distal colon.

### Pathophysiology
**A. Types of Diarrhea:**
**1. With excess fecal water–**
**a. Osmotic diarrhea–**Excess water-soluble molecules in the bowel lumen cause osmotic retention of intraluminal water.

**b. Secretory diarrhea–**Excessive active ion secretion by the mucosal cells of the intestine.

**c. Deletion or interference with normal ion absorption–**This is usually a congenital problem.

**d. Exudative disease–**Abnormal mucosal permeability, with intestinal loss of serum proteins, blood, mucus, or pus.

**e. Impaired contact between intestinal chyme and absorbing surface–**Rapid transit, short bowel syndromes.

**2. Without excess fecal water–**Frequent small, painful evacuations are usually a result of disease of the left colon or rectum.

**B. Causes of Diarrhea:** Most diarrheal states are self-limited and pose no special diagnostic problem. They are often due to dietary indiscretions or mild gastrointestinal infections. The following list of the causes of diarrhea is indicative of the extensive diagnostic evaluation that may be required in patients with unexplained, profound, or chronic diarrhea.

**1. Psychogenic disorders–**"Nervous" diarrhea.

**2. Drugs–**Antacids, antibiotics, laxatives, sorbitol (excess diet drinks, sugarless gum, etc), metoclopramide.

**3. Intestinal Infections:**
**a. Viral infections–**Enterovirus, Norwalk virus.
**b. Bacterial infections–**Most common are *Campylobacter jejuni, Shigella, Salmonella,* and *Yersinia enterocolitica.*
**c. Bacterial toxins–***Clostridium difficile,* enterotoxigenic *Escherichia coli, Staphylococcus, V parahaemolyticus,* and *V cholerae* (see Table 23–1).

**4. Parasitic infections–***Giardia lamblia, Entamoeba histolytica, Cryptosporidium,* and *Isospora* are the most common.

**5. Other intestinal factors–**Fecal impaction, lactase deficiency (milk intolerance), antibiotic therapy, inflammatory bowel disease, catharsis habituation, vagotomy, carcinoma, heavy metal poisoning, and gastrocolic fistula.

**6. Cholestatic syndromes–**Hepatitis and bile duct obstruction may result in steatorrhea and mild diarrhea.

**7. Malabsorption states–**Primary small bowel mucosal diseases (eg, celiac sprue), short small bowel states, and intestinal blind loop syndrome (eg, diverticula, afferent loop).

**8. Pancreatic disease–**Pancreatic insufficiency, diabetes mellitus, pancreatic endocrine tumors.

**9. Reflex from other viscera–**Pelvic disease (extrinsic to gastrointestinal tract).

**10. Neurologic disease–**Tabes dorsalis, diabetic neuropathy.

**11. Metabolic disease–**Hyperthyroidism.

**12. Immunodeficiency disease–**IgA deficiency.

**13. Malnutrition–**Marasmus, kwashiorkor.

**14. Food allergy.**

**15. Dietary factors–**Excessive fresh fruit intake.

**16. Factitious–**Surreptitious laxative ingestion.

**17. Unknown.**

## Diagnosis

Specific diagnosis is based on careful examination of diarrheal material for polymorphonuclear cells, parasites, culture for bacterial pathogens, and assay for toxin of *Clostridium difficile*. This is best accomplished at sigmoidoscopy prior to preparation with a cleansing enema. Cotton swabs should not be used in making slides, as both polymorphonuclear cells and parasites cling to cotton. The presence of polymorphonuclear cells indicates an inflammatory process. Rectal biopsy may prove helpful, particularly when *Entamoeba histolytica* is being considered and there is colitis. These studies should be performed prior to barium studies and treatment.

## Treatment

Culture for bacterial pathogens and examination of several stools for polymorphonuclear cells and parasites must be done before barium studies or treatment is begun.

**A. Treat Specific Disease if Possible.**

**B. Correct Physiologic Changes Induced by Diarrhea:**

1. Acid-base disturbance, fluid loss.

2. Electrolyte depletion (hyponatremia, hypokalemia, hypocalcemia, hypomagnesemia).

3. Malnutrition, vitamin deficiencies.

4. Psychogenic disturbances (eg, fixation on gastrointestinal tract or anxiety regarding incontinence in cases of long-standing diarrhea).

**C. Diet:**

**1. Acute severe**–Food should be withheld for the first 24 hours or restricted to lukewarm clear liquids—a physiologic glucose and salt solution, sipped slowly as needed to replace large fluid and electrolyte losses, may be especially useful in patients with severe watery diarrhea. Frequent small soft feedings are added as tolerated. Milk and milk products are the last foods to be added, since lactase deficiency frequently is present after an ''insult'' to the small intestine.

**2. Convalescent**–Food should be incorporated into the diets of patients convalescing from acute diarrhea as tolerated. Nutritious food, preferably all cooked, in small frequent meals, is usually well tolerated. *Avoid* raw vegetables and fruits, fried foods, bran, whole grain cereals, preserves, syrups, candies, pickles, relishes, spices, coffee, and alcoholic beverages.

A diet free of milk and milk products and with no uncooked foods is a restricted diet. These patients may require vitamin supplements if the diet is prolonged.

**3. Chronic diarrhea**–Chronic diarrhea is due to many causes. Nutritional disturbances range from none to marked depletion of electrolytes, water, protein, fat, and vitamins. Treat specific disease when known (eg, gluten-free diet in celiac sprue and enzyme replacement in pancreatic insufficiency). Give fat-soluble vitamins (vitamins A, D, E, K) when steator-

rhea is present. Some patients are so ill that they require parenteral alimentation, sometimes at home.

**D. Antidiarrheal Agents:**

**1. Pepto-Bismol**–Give 30 mL 3–6 times per day for symptomatic treatment of diarrhea. Remind the patient that this agent causes black stools.

**2. Narcotic analogs**–Avoid with possible acute infectious diarrhea, as they may worsen and prolong the course.

**a. Lomotil (diphenoxylate with atropine),** 2.5 mg 3–4 times daily as needed. It must be used cautiously in patients with advanced liver disease and in those who are addiction-prone or who are taking sedatives.

**b. Loperamide (Imodium),** 2 mg 2–4 times daily, is effective in acute and chronic diarrhea.

**3. Narcotics**–Narcotics must be avoided in chronic diarrheas and are preferably avoided in acute diarrheas unless there is intractable diarrhea, vomiting, and colic. Always exclude the possibility of acute surgical abdominal disease before administering opiates. Give any of the following:

**a. Paregoric,** 4–8 mL after liquid movements as needed or with bismuth.

**b. Codeine phosphate,** 15–60 mg subcutaneously, if the patient is vomiting, after liquid bowel movements as needed.

**c. Strong opiates**–Morphine should be reserved for selected patients with severe acute diarrhea who fail to respond to more conservative measures.

**4. Anticholinergic drugs,** particularly when used in combination with sedatives, exert a mild antiperistaltic action in acute and chronic diarrheas associated with anxiety tension states. It may be necessary to administer the various drugs to a point near toxicity in order to achieve the desired effect.

Antidiarrheal drugs must be used with great caution in inflammatory bowel disease and amebiasis because of the risk of ''toxic'' dilatation of the colon. They should usually be avoided in bacillary dysentery, since they may prolong or worsen the course of the acute illness.

**E. Psychotherapy:** Many cases of chronic diarrhea are of psychogenic origin. A survey of anxiety-producing mechanisms should be made in all patients with this complaint. Antidepressant drug therapy may be useful, particularly since many of these agents have an anticholinergic effect.

**F. Prophylaxis:** Traveler's diarrhea, most commonly due to enterotoxigenic *E coli* and *Shigella*, can frequently be prevented with the prophylactic use of doxycycline or trimethoprim-sulfamethoxazole. However, the low incidence and moderate morbidity among travelers to developing countries probably do not warrant the risks of prophylactic treatment of all travelers.

DuPont HL, Ericsson CD, Johnson PC: Chemotherapy and chemoprophylaxis of traveler's diarrhea. (Editorial.) *Ann Intern Med* 1985;**102**:260.

Fedorak RN, Field M, Chang EB: Treatment of diabetic diarrhea with clonidine. *Ann Intern Med* 1985;**102**:197.

Tolle SW: The evaluation and management of acute diarrhea. *West J Med* 1984;**140**:293.

Wolfson JS et al: Cryptosporidiosis in immunocompetent patients. *N Engl J Med* 1985;**312**:1278.

# MASSIVE UPPER GASTROINTESTINAL HEMORRHAGE

Massive upper gastrointestinal hemorrhage is a common emergency. It may be defined as rapid loss of sufficient blood to cause hypovolemic shock. The actual volume of blood loss required to produce shock varies with the size, age, and general condition of the patient and with the rapidity of bleeding. Sudden loss of 20% or more of blood volume (blood volume is approximately 75 mL/kg of body weight) produces hypotension, tachycardia, and other signs of shock. For example, a previously well 70-kg man who develops shock as a result of gastrointestinal hemorrhage will have lost at least 1000–1500 mL of blood. The immediate objectives of management are (1) to restore an effective blood volume and (2) to establish a diagnosis on which definitive treatment can be based.

The major causes of upper gastrointestinal bleeding are peptic ulceration of the duodenum, stomach, or esophagus, esophageal varices, and gastritis. In addition, bleeding may be due to Mallory-Weiss syndrome and hemorrhagic gastritis due to ulcerogenic drugs such as aspirin, nonsteroidal anti-inflammatory drugs, or alcohol. Vascular lesions are a rare cause of massive upper gastrointestinal hemorrhage.

## Clinical Findings

**A. Symptoms and Signs:** There is usually a history of sudden weakness or fainting associated with or followed by tarry stools or vomiting of blood. Melena occurs in most patients and hematemesis in over half. Hematemesis is especially common in esophageal varices (90%), gastritis, and gastric ulcer. The patient may or may not be in shock when first seen but will at least be pale and weak if major blood loss has occurred. If the patient is not vomiting, a nasogastric tube will often help determine if the bleeding is in the upper gastrointestinal tract. There may be a history of peptic ulcer, chronic liver disease, other predisposing disease, alcoholic excess, or severe vomiting.

There is usually no pain, and the pain of peptic ulcer disease often stops with the onset of bleeding. Abdominal findings are not remarkable except when hepatomegaly, splenomegaly, or a mass (neoplasm) is present. Bowel sounds may be increased due to blood in the gut.

The cause of bleeding should be established as promptly as possible, since management will in part be dependent on the findings. This is particularly true if emergency surgery is anticipated, so that surgical approach and type of procedure can be determined.

A history of peptic ulcer or of antacid ingestion suggests duodenal ulcer. Ingestion of aspirin or other nonsteroidal anti-inflammatory agents on a regular or intermittent basis suggests gastric ulcer or hemorrhagic erosive gastritis. A history of alcoholism or evidence of chronic liver disease, such as jaundice, hepatosplenomegaly, spider angioma, liver palms, ascites, or encephalopathy, indicates probable portal hypertension and possible variceal bleeding. Aspiration of gastric contents by nasogastric tube is diagnostically useful and permits estimation of the continued rate of bleeding.

The principal diagnostic procedures that should be carried out after necessary emergency treatment has been given are outlined below.

**B. Laboratory Findings:** In addition to the baseline studies of a complete blood count, urinalysis, and serum electrolyte and creatinine measurements, the following may prove helpful in selected patients.

**1. Liver tests**–Serum bilirubin, transaminase, albumin/globulin, alkaline phosphatase, and prothrombin time may help support a diagnosis of chronic liver disease (portal hypertension).

**2. Coagulation studies**–In addition to the prothrombin time, other tests may sometimes be indicated. Determine bleeding time in cases of suspected ingestion of aspirin or nonsteroidal anti-inflammatory agents or of azotemia; a platelet count when platelets are low on the complete blood count; and a partial thromboplastin time when there is a history of excessive dental, gynecologic, or other bleeding.

**C. Endoscopy:** Fiberoptic oral panendoscopy should be the first definitive examination performed if an experienced endoscopist is available. This procedure permits visualization of the upper gastrointestinal tract from the cricopharyngeus to the second or third portion of the duodenum and can identify mucosal lesions not readily seen by other techniques. Sometimes, sclerosis of bleeding esophageal varices or other treatment can be accomplished during panendoscopy. When it is unclear that bleeding is from the upper gastrointestinal tract, sigmoidoscopy should be the first diagnostic procedure.

**D. Imaging:** If upper gastrointestinal endoscopy does not reveal the bleeding site, selective angiography should be considered if the bleeding persists. Arteriography may not be successful if the bleeding is less than 1 mL/min.

If angiography fails to demonstrate the site of bleeding, then an upper gastrointestinal series is done. The patient's vital signs should be monitored during the procedure.

## Treatment

**A. General Measures:** The patient should be under the observation of both the primary care physician and a surgeon from the outset. Bed rest and charting of fluid intake, urine output, and temperature are ordered. Insert a large-bore nasogastric tube to verify the source of hemorrhage and to remove gastric contents (see below). If bleeding continues or if tachycardia or hypotension is present, monitor and treat the patient for shock (see Chapter 1). Insert a Foley catheter and a central venous pressure or pulmonary artery wedge pressure line. Blood is obtained immediately for complete blood count, hematocrit, and crossmatching of at least 3 or 4 units of packed red blood cells. In interpreting the hematocrit, it should be kept in mind that after acute blood loss, a period of 24–36 hours may be required for reequilibration of body fluids. Meanwhile, the hematocrit poorly reflects extent of blood loss. Frequent determination of vital signs, especially those associated with postural changes, is helpful in estimating acute blood loss. Replacement therapy through a large-bore intravenous needle (18-gauge minimum) or catheter is started immediately with normal saline. If shock is severe or if the patient has portal hypertension, fresh frozen plasma is given while a blood transfusion is being prepared.

Aqueous vasopressin (Pitressin), 20 units in 200–250 mL of 5% glucose in water intravenously over a 30- to 40-minute period, may cause temporary arteriolar vasoconstriction and lowering of the portal venous pressure for variceal bleeding. Infusion of vasopressin through the angiographic catheter may be effective in controlling hemorrhage, if the bleeding is from small vessels. The entire matter of using vasopressin therapy to control hemorrhage is unclear at present.

Water-soluble vitamin K (menadiol sodium diphosphate [Synkayvite]), 5–10 mg intramuscularly, is given empirically if hepatobiliary disease is suspected. Restlessness may be due to continued hemorrhage, shock, or hypoxia.

**B. Blood Replacement:** Treatment of shock by transfusion with blood cells or fresh frozen plasma (or both) is begun without delay. Hematocrit determinations are done every few hours until they are stabilized. The objective of blood replacement is to relieve shock and restore blood volume. The amount of blood required is estimated on the basis of vital signs, measured loss, central venous pressure, and renal perfusion as measured by urine output, usually with the aim of a minimum hematocrit of 30%. While a patient is actively bleeding, at least 6 units of packed red blood cells should be available for emergency transfusion; rapid administration will control shock. When blood pressure and pulse have been restored to relatively normal levels and clinical signs of hypovolemia are no longer present, the rate of transfusion can be slowed. The total volume of blood given is determined by the course of the disease. A poor response usually means continued bleeding (see below) or inadequate replacement. Venous pressure or pulmonary artery wedge pressure is useful in gauging adequacy of blood replacement and detecting overtransfusion and congestive heart failure in the clinically fragile patient.

**C. Medical Measures:** Acid peptic digestion is a causative or aggravating factor in many cases of massive upper gastrointestinal hemorrhage, perhaps including varices. Feedings and oral medications for ulcer are begun as soon as shock and nausea have subsided. Continued slight bleeding is not a contraindication for the following regimen:

**1. Diet–**Liquid diet for the first 24 hours, followed by a soft or regular diet, depending on the clinical situation.

**2. Acid reduction–**While a nasogastric tube is still in place, antacids such as aluminum hydroxide-magnesium hydroxide mixtures can be administered hourly by mouth in a dose of 30 mL to protect the distal esophagus from reflux and to help neutralize gastric contents not suctioned by the tube. In the fasting patient, an $H_2$ antagonist by constant infusion (cimetidine, 37.5 mg/h, or ranitidine, 8.3 mg/h) reduces acid output, although it does not appear to affect the incidence of acute rebleeding. For the nonfasting patient with ulcer disease, the $H_2$ receptor antagonists (cimetidine, ranitidine), antacids, and sucralfate are equally efficacious in inducing healing. Therapeutic doses of antacids, 1 and 3 hours after meals and at bedtime, may cause diarrhea.

**3. Mild sedation.**

**4. A nasogastric tube** may be useful to permit continued decompression of the stomach and evacuation of blood by lavage with saline. The tube is also useful to monitor the rate of continued bleeding. Whenever the tube is placed, the patient should be in a moderate reversed Trendelenburg position, if possible, to minimize reflux around the tube. See above concerning antacid use.

**D. Management of Bleeding Esophageal Varices:** When varices are the cause of bleeding, special measures are indicated (see p 410).

**E. Indications for Emergency Operation:** Emergency surgery to stop active bleeding should be considered under any of the following circumstances: (1) When the patient has received 6 units of packed cells or more of blood but shock is not controlled or recurs promptly. (2) When acceptable blood pressure and hematocrit cannot be maintained with a maximum of 2 units of packed red blood cells every 8 hours. (3) When bleeding is slow but persists more than 2–3 days. (4) When bleeding stops initially but recurs while the patient is receiving adequate medical treatment. (5) When the patient is over age 50. The death rate from exsanguination in spite of conservative measures is greater in the older age group.

Some patients have visible vessels on endoscopy. About half of these patients will have uncontrolled or recurrent bleeding and are therefore candidates for urgent surgery.

**Prognosis**

The overall mortality rate of about 14% indicates the seriousness of massive upper gastrointestinal hemorrhage. Fatality rates vary greatly, depending upon the cause of bleeding and the presence of other serious systemic disease. The overall operative mortality rate for emergency surgery to stop bleeding is high, and best results are obtained when bleeding can be controlled medically and surgery deferred until the patient has recovered from the effects of bleeding. Hemorrhage from duodenal ulcer causes death in about 3% of treated cases, whereas in bleeding varices the mortality rate may be as high as 50%.

Bernuau J, Rueff B: Treatment of acute variceal bleeding. *Clin Gastroenterol* 1985;**14**:185.

Fleischer D: Endoscopic therapy of upper gastrointestinal bleeding in humans. *Gastroenterology* 1986;**90**:217.

Hussey KP: Vasopressin therapy for upper gastrointestinal hemorrhage. *Arch Intern Med* 1985;**145**:1263.

Ostro MJ et al: Control of gastric pH with cimetidine: Boluses versus primed infusion. *Gastroenterology* 1985;**89**:532.

Zucherman G et al: Controlled trial of medical therapy for active upper gastrointestinal bleeding and prevention of rebleeding. *Am J Med* 1984;**76**:361.

## MASSIVE LOWER GASTROINTESTINAL HEMORRHAGE

Massive lower gastrointestinal bleeding occurs most frequently in older, poor-risk patients and is always a *medical emergency*. Colonic diverticulosis and angiodysplasia (acquired arteriovenous malformation) are the most common causes of hemodynamically significant lower gastrointestinal bleeding, but other possibilities—including massive upper gastrointestinal hemorrhage—must be considered (see above).

### Causes of Massive Lower Abdominal Hemorrhage

**A. Colonic Disorders:**

**1. Inflammatory**–Ulcerative colitis, regional enteritis, infectious diarrhea (eg, shigellosis), radiation colitis.

**2. Diverticular**–Diverticulosis.

**3. Vascular**–Hemorrhoids, angiodysplasia (vascular ectasia), bowel ischemia, colonic varices, aortic aneurysm.

**4. Neoplastic**–Benign and malignant disorders.

**5. Hereditary**–Telangiectasias, arteriovenous malformations.

**6. Coagulopathies**–Anticoagulant drugs, blood dyscrasias.

**B. Upper Gastrointestinal Disorders:**

**1. Vascular**–Esophageal varices, telangiectasias, aortoduodenal fistula.

**2. Ulcerative**–Peptic ulceration.

**3. Neoplastic**–Benign and malignant disorders.

### Management of Hemorrhage

The patient usually has a sudden onset of weakness and fainting, combined with or followed by passage of grossly bloody stools (which may be either bright red or dark red according to the time elapsed since the beginning of the hemorrhage). There may be a history and physical findings of one or more of the disorders listed above. The patient may appear pale and weak and may rapidly develop signs of shock.

If rectal bleeding is copious or if there is evidence of shock, the patient should be resuscitated with intravenous fluids and blood products before and during the diagnostic evaluation. Colonic bleeding stops spontaneously in about 75% of patients treated with bed rest and simple resuscitative measures.

A nasogastric tube should be inserted to rule out upper gastrointestinal bleeding (see above). However, unless bile is aspirated via this tube, one cannot be certain that bleeding is not duodenal in origin. Rectal examination and proctosigmoidoscopy may identify bleeding lesions of the anorectal region as well as of the sigmoid mucosa. Lesions may require biopsy so that appropriate therapy can be instituted.

If several blood transfusions are necessary, further definitive diagnostic study is warranted. Radionuclide localization of shed technetium Tc 99m-labeled red cells is proving to be helpful in localizing lower gastrointestinal bleeding. Pertechnetate Tc 99m scintigraphy can be used to localize ectopic gastric mucosa, such as in Meckel's diverticulum, with an accuracy of about 90%. Meckel's diverticulum is an occasional cause of lower gastrointestinal bleeding in young patients. Colonoscopy may sometimes be useful for identifying and fulgurating bleeding sites. Selective mesenteric angiography can often demonstrate and localize the site of hemorrhage in patients who are actively bleeding. Once the bleeding site is identified, selective intra-arterial infusion of vasopressin into the affected portion may control the bleeding, at least temporarily, in 75–80% of cases. If no bleeding site can be determined, laparotomy and appropriate surgical treatment may be required.

Cello JP et al: Diagnosis and management of lower gastrointestinal tract hemorrhage: Medical Staff Conference UCSF. *West J Med* 1985;**143**:80.

Koval G et al: Aggressive angiographic diagnosis in acute lower gastrointestinal hemorrhage. *Dig Dis Sci* 1987;**32**:248.

Richter JM et al: Angiodysplasia: Clinical presentation and colonoscopic diagnosis. *Dig Dis Sci* 1984;**29**:481.

Sfakianakis GN, Conway JJ: Detection of ectopic gastric mucosa in Meckel's diverticulum and in other aberrations by scintigraphy. 1. Pathophysiology and 10-year chemical experience. *J Nucl Med* 1981;**22**:647.

# DISEASES OF THE MOUTH

## DISCOLORED TEETH

The most common causes of discolored teeth are food stains, bacteria, tobacco use, and drugs. These can be managed by altering habits and by practicing dental prophylaxis. There may be pulpal hemorrhage induced by trauma, resulting in a deposition of hemosiderin on the internal crown surface. This causes a darkening of the tooth, which usually remains sterile and asymptomatic but nonvital. These teeth can be effectively bleached for aesthetic reasons. Occasionally, however, discoloration is due to changes in tooth structure caused by tetracyclines, congenital defects of enamel or dentin, fluorosis, and erythroblastosis fetalis.

Tetracycline discoloration occurs in some patients when these antibiotics are given during the period of tooth development, particularly in the fetus and during the first 8 years of life. Since an entire layer of dentin may be calcified in a few days, a small dosage over a short period may be incorporated into and appear to involve an entire tooth. The discoloration is gray-brown or yellow-brown and is permanent. A typical yellow fluorescence is seen under ultraviolet light.

Dental fluorosis occurs most frequently when the fluoride in the water supply exceeds 2 ppm (1 ppm is the recommended concentration). Fluorosis can also be caused when the daily ingestion of fluoride-vitamin combinations exceeds the recommended levels (maximum of 1 mg of fluoride). The frequency and intensity of the discoloration are proportionate to the concentration in the water and the amount consumed during tooth development. The discoloration can vary from chalky-white to yellow-brown stains, often irregular in appearance. These teeth can be effectively bleached as required with 30% hydrogen peroxide.

Rare hereditary congenital defects may cause brownish discoloration of the teeth. Treatment is primarily for aesthetic reasons.

Black JB: Esthetic restoration of tetracycline-stained teeth. *J Am Dent Assoc* 1982;**104**:846.

Driscoll WS et al: Prevalence of dental caries and dental fluorosis in areas with optimal and above-optimal water fluoride concentrations. *J Am Dent Assoc* 1983;**107**:42.

## ABSCESSES OF THE TEETH
### (Periapical Abscess)

Dental decay is not self-limiting; unless it is removed, it will lead to infection of the pulp and subsequent periapical abscess. Pulp infection may also result from physical and chemical trauma. The only treatment is root canal therapy (cleansing and filling of the canal) or extraction.

In the early stage of pulp infection, the symptoms may not be localized to the infected tooth. Intermittent throbbing pain is usually present and is intensified by local temperature change. In the later putrescent stage, the pain is extreme and continuous and may be accentuated by heat but is often relieved by cold. After the infection reaches the bone, the typical syndrome is localization, pain upon pressure, and looseness of the tooth. Symptoms may then disappear completely, and, if drainage occurs, a parulis (gumboil) may be the only finding. When drainage is inadequate, swelling, pain, lymphadenopathy, and fever are often present. At this stage, antibiotics are advisable before local therapy is undertaken. Diagnosis depends upon symptoms, pulp testing (hot, cold, electricity), percussion, x-rays (may not show the diagnostic periapical radiolucency), looseness, deep decay or fillings, parulis, and swelling. Rule out sinusitis, neuralgia, and diseases affecting the cervical lymph nodes.

Incision and drainage are indicated whenever possible. Antibiotics and analgesics may be given as necessary. Unless contraindicated from a history of hypersensitivity, penicillin is the antibiotic of choice. Do not use antibiotic troches.

If not eventually treated by root canal therapy or extraction, the abscess may develop into a more extensive osteomyelitis or cellulitis (or both) or may eventually become cystic, expand, and slowly destroy bone without causing pain.

## VINCENT'S INFECTION
### (Necrotizing Ulcerating Gingivitis, Trench Mouth)

Vincent's infection is an acute inflammatory disease of the gums that may be accompanied by pain, bleeding, fever, and lymphadenopathy. The cause is not known, and it is doubtful if the disease is communicable. It may occur as a response to many factors, such as poor mouth hygiene, inadequate diet and sleep, alcoholism, and various other diseases such as infectious mononucleosis, nonspecific viral infections, bacterial infections, thrush, blood dyscrasias, and diabetes mellitus.

Management depends upon ruling out underlying systemic factors and treating the signs and symptoms as indicated with systemic antibiotics, oxygenating mouth rinses (3% hydrogen peroxide in an equal volume of warm water), analgesics, rest, and appropriate dietary measures. Refer the patient to a dentist for further treatment (eg, curettage).

## PERIODONTAL DISEASE

Periodontal disease is related to accumulations of microorganisms and substrate (plaque) on tooth surfaces. These may calcify and be recognized as calculus. Food, bacteria, and calculi that are present between the gums and teeth in areas called "dental pockets" may cause an inflammatory process and the formation of pus (pyorrhea) with or without discomfort or other symptoms. If this continues unchecked, the involved teeth will become loose and eventually will be lost as a result of resorption of supporting alveolar bone. If there is no drainage, accumulation of pus will lead to acute swelling and pain (lateral abscess).

The diagnosis depends upon a combination of findings, including localized pain, loose teeth, dental pockets, erythema, and swelling or suppuration. Radiography may reveal destruction of alveolar bone.

As in periapical abscess, the severity of signs and symptoms will determine the advisability of antibiotics. Local drainage and oxygenating mouth rinses (3% hydrogen peroxide in an equal volume of warm water) will usually reverse the acute symptoms and allow for routine follow-up procedures. Curettage or gingivectomy (or both) to reduce excess gum tissue helps prevent formation of the "dental pockets" that predispose to acute periodontal infections. In some cases, because of the advanced nature of the lesion (bone loss) or the position of the tooth (third molars in particular), extraction is indicated.

In some cases, periodontal disease occurs even in the presence of good hygiene and without obvious cause. Programs of regular dental care (periodic curettage and gingival or bone procedures) and home care (brushing, flossing, and rinsing) to remove dental plaque will at least slow alveolar bone destruction.

Joseph CE, Farnoush A: Current concepts of periodontitis. *J Calif Dent Assoc* 1984;**12**:43.

## APHTHOUS ULCER
### (Canker Sore, Ulcerative Stomatitis)

An aphthous ulcer is a shallow mucosal ulcer with flat, fairly even borders surrounded by erythema. The ulcer is often covered with a pseudomembrane. It has never been adequately demonstrated that this lesion is due to a virus or any other specific chemical, physical, or microbial agent. One or more ulcers may be present, and they tend to be recurrent. They are often painful. Nuts, chocolates, and irritants such as citrus fruits often cause flare-ups of aphthous ulceration, but abstinence will not prevent recurrence. Aphthous ulcers may be associated with inflammatory bowel disease, Behçet's syndrome, infectious mononucleosis, and prolonged fever. The diagnosis depends mainly upon ruling out similar but more readily identifiable disease, a history of recurrence, and inspection of the ulcer.

Bland mouth rinses and hydrocortisone-antibiotic ointments reduce pain and encourage healing. Fluocinonide ointment (Lidex 0.05%) mixed in equal parts in an adhesive base (Orabase) has been particularly useful. Sedatives and analgesics may be of help. Vaccines and gamma globulins have not proved significantly beneficial. Although caustics relieve pain by cauterizing the fine nerve endings, they also cause necrosis and scar tissue. Systemic antibiotics are contraindicated. Systemic prednisone (20–40 mg/d) for a short period of time may be very helpful for severe debilitating recurrent attacks.

Healing, which usually occurs in 1–3 weeks, may be only slightly accelerated by treatment. Occasionally, aphthous ulcers take the form of periadenitis,

in which they are larger, persist sometimes for months, and may leave a scar. This form can be confused with carcinoma.

Ulcerative stomatitis is a general term for multiple ulcerations on an inflamed oral mucosa. It may be secondary to blood dyscrasias, erythema multiforme (allergies), bullous lichen planus, acute herpes simplex infection, pemphigoid, pemphigus, and drug reactions. If the lesions cannot be classified, they are referred to as aphthae.

Brown RB, Clinton D: Vesicular and ulcerative infections of the mouth and oropharynx. *Postgrad Med* (Feb) 1980; **67**:107.

Olson JA, Greenspan JS, Silverman S Jr: Recurrent aphthous ulcerations. *J Calif Dent Assoc* 1982;**10**:53.

Silverman S Jr, Lozada-Nur F, Migliorati C: Clinical efficacy of prednisone in the treatment of patients with oral inflammatory ulcerative diseases: A study of fifty-five patients. *Oral Surg* 1985;**59**:360.

## HERPETIC STOMATITIS

Herpetic infections of the mouth can be primary (one episode) or secondary (recurrent attacks).

Primary gingivostomatitis due to herpesvirus hominis type 1 occurs in about 90% of the population before age 10. The disease has diverse manifestations, ranging from mild, almost unrecognizable signs and symptoms to multiple intraoral and lip ulcerations, erythema, edema, fever, cervical lymphadenopathy, and malaise. The course of the illness usually entails an increase in signs and symptoms for 1 week and then 1 week of progressive improvement as antibodies are produced (serum antibody titers will increase at least 4-fold). Adults who have never been infected or who have not developed adequate immunity may develop similar disease. Increasing susceptibility is seen in patients on immunosuppressive drugs. Infection with herpesvirus confers permanent immunity.

Herpetic gingivostomatitis must be differentiated from aphthous stomatitis, which is not due to a virus. The diagnosis is established by the history (no prior attack and short duration), characteristic signs and symptoms, and a confirmatory cytologic smear (pathognomonic pseudogiant cells). Direct cultures for herpes simplex virus are positive but impractical.

There is no evidence that the disease is contagious; however, this might be explained by existing immunologic resistance among the contacts.

Treatment is palliative (analgesics, bland mouth rinses, fluids, soft diet, and rest). In the differential diagnosis, erythema multiforme, infectious mononucleosis, and pemphigus must be considered.

Recurrent intraoral herpetic infections are extremely rare and only occur on the mucosa covering bone (gingiva and palate). The ulcers are small, shallow, and irregular in size and shape. They can be mistaken for traumatic abrasions. There is no effective therapy; the infection is self-limiting within 2 weeks.

Herpes labialis (cold sore) is due to recurrent herpesvirus infections. These lesions usually have a burning premonitory stage and are first manifested by small vesicles that soon rupture and scab. Factors that trigger herpesvirus migration by nerve pathways to the lip range from unidentifiable stimuli to temperature changes, chemical and physical irritants, or "stress."

The diagnosis is based on the history and appearance of the lesions. The differential diagnosis includes carcinoma, syphilitic chancre, and erythema multiforme. No method of treatment has been uniformly successful. Improvement has been claimed with the use of idoxuridine and acyclovir ointments, chloroform, ether applications, lysine, and vitamin C.

When any of the above herpetic infections are severe, acyclovir (200 mg orally 5–6 times daily) may be helpful.

There is no firm evidence that type 1 herpesvirus is associated with oral carcinoma.

Hirsch MS, Schooley RT: Treatment of herpesvirus infections. (2 parts.) *N Engl J Med* 1983;**309**:963, 1034.

Park NH: Current aspects of anti-herpes research. *J Calif Dent Assoc* 1984;**12**:167.

## CANDIDIASIS
## (Moniliasis, Thrush)

Thrush is due to overgrowth of *Candida albicans*. It is characterized by creamy-white curdlike patches anywhere in the mouth. The adjacent mucosa is usually erythematous, and scraping the lesions often uncovers a raw, bleeding surface. Quite commonly, a candidal lesion may appear as a slightly granular or irregularly eroded erythematous patch. Pain is commonly present; fever and lymphadenopathy are uncommon. This fungus appears in most normal-appearing mouths, but overgrowth does not occur unless the "balance" of the oral microbial flora is disturbed.

Candidiasis is most commonly seen in denture wearers, with the appliances serving as a nutrient reservoir to foster fungal growth. It is also frequently seen in patients with debilitating or acute illness or in those being treated with antibiotics and corticosteroids. Candidal growth also is favored by xerostomia (eg, after head and neck irradiation), diabetes mellitus, anemia, and immunosuppressed status. Unexplained thrush in a high-risk group for AIDS is a portent of AIDS (see p 818). Concomitant candidiasis of the gastrointestinal tract (including the pharynx and the esophagus) may occur.

The diagnosis is based upon the varied clinical picture of surface white patches or erythematous changes and may be confirmed by culture. A smear frequently will reveal characteristic spores and sometimes the more suggestive hyphae. Biopsy from active lesions will often reveal pseudomycelia of *Candida* invading surface epithelium.

## Treatment

Treatment is usually successful; however, the infection will often return in spite of treatment as long as causative factors are present. Antibiotics should be discontinued if possible. Diabetes, if present, must be carefully controlled. Local treatment often should be prolonged well beyond the period of signs or symptoms. Mouth rinses made up of equal parts of hydrogen peroxide and saline solution every 2 hours provide local relief and promote healing. Specific antifungal therapy consists of any of the following: nystatin mouth rinses, 500,000 units 3 times daily (100,000 units/mL in a flavored vehicle), held in the mouth and then swallowed; nystatin vaginal troches (100,000 units) to be dissolved orally 4 times daily; clotrimazole troches (Mycelex) (10 mg) to be dissolved orally 5 times a day; and ketoconazole tablets (Nizoral), 200–400 mg with breakfast for 7–14 days. In denture wearers, nystatin powder (100,000 units/g) applied to the dentures 3–4 times daily for several weeks, can be helpful in reversing signs and symptoms.

Chronic angular cheilitis is often a manifestation of candidiasis. It is best treated with nystatin powder or Mycolog (nystatin-triamcinolone acetonide) cream. Mucocutaneous candidiasis is rare and frequently does not respond well to any form of treatment, including immunostimulation.

Budtz-Jorgensen E: Clinical aspects of *Candida* infection in denture wearers. *J Am Dent Assoc* 1978;**96**:474.

Kirkpatrick CH, Alling DW: Treatment of chronic oral candidiasis with clotrimazole troches. *N Engl J Med* 1978;**299**:1201.

Klein RS et al: Oral candidiasis in high-risk patients as the initial manifestation of the acquired immunodeficiency syndrome. *N Engl J Med* 1984;**311**:354.

## LEUKOPLAKIA

Leukoplakia (a white patch) of the oral mucous membranes is occasionally a sign of carcinoma; it is important to rule out cancer. The most common cause of leukoplakia is epithelial hyperplasia and hyperkeratosis, usually in response to an irritant. In many cases the etiology cannot be determined.

Leukoplakia is usually asymptomatic. It is often discovered upon routine examination or by patients feeling roughness in their mouths. Because there is no reliable correlation between clinical features and microscopic findings, a definitive diagnosis may be established only by histopathologic examination. However, because of the extensiveness of some intraoral leukoplakias, cytologic smears from the surface are helpful in supplementing both clinical and biopsy information.

Remove all irritants (eg, tobacco, ill-fitting dentures). If the leukoplakia is not reversible, perform excision when feasible. Since some leukoplakias occur so diffusely that complete excision is impractical, careful examination and follow-up are essential. The diagnosis must be reaffirmed periodically, since a leukoplakia may unpredictably be transformed into a malignant tumor. Electrodesiccation, cryosurgery, vitamin A, and proteolytic enzymes have not been predictably effective.

Silverman S Jr et al: Oral leukoplakia and malignant transformation: A follow-up study of 257 patients. *Cancer* 1984;**53**:563.

## SIALADENITIS

Acute inflammation of a parotid or submandibular salivary gland is usually due to viral or bacterial infection or, less commonly, blockage of the duct. The gland is swollen and tender. Observation of Wharton's and Stensen's ducts may show absent or scanty secretion, with fluctuation of swelling, especially during meals, which indicates blockage; or a turbid secretion, which suggests infection. Clinical examination and x-ray may disclose ductal or glandular calcific deposits. Sialograms are of help in differentiating normal and diseased glands. Probing the ducts may reveal an inorganic plug or organic stenosis.

Dryness of the mouth (xerostomia) may be due to inflammation of the salivary glands, mouth breathing, dehydration, anticholinergic and psychotropic drugs, Sjögren's syndrome, and radiation injury. Mouth dryness is a common complaint in the elderly. Correct specific causes when possible. Frequent mouth rinsing and local troches may help.

Tumors may be confused with nonneoplastic inflammation. In these situations, biopsy (usually excisional) should be performed, but only after other diagnostic and therapeutic procedures have failed to yield a diagnosis. Neoplasms are usually not associated with an acute onset and, at least in the early phases, are not painful. The lymph nodes are intimately associated with the salivary glands, and consideration must be given to diseases in which lymphadenopathy is a prominent finding, eg, lymphomas and metastatic cancer.

In the acute stage, antibiotics, heat, and analgesics are indicated. Ductal stones that are too large for removal by massage and manipulation must be removed surgically (when the acute phase has subsided). If calcification or infection of the gland recurs often, extirpation of the gland must be considered. Radiation therapy may be effective in curing acute or recurrent sialadenitis that does not respond to other types of therapy.

McKenna RJ: Tumors of the major and minor salivary glands. *CA* 1984;**34**:24.
Rice DH: Advances in the management of salivary gland disease. *West J Med* 1984;**140**:238.

## GLOSSITIS

Inflammation of the tongue (usually associated with partial or complete loss of the filiform papillae, which creates a red, smooth appearance) may be secondary to a variety of diseases such as anemia, nutritional deficiency, drug reactions, systemic infection, and physical or chemical irritations. Treatment is based on identifying and correcting the primary cause if possible and palliating the tongue symptoms as required. Many obscure cases are due to such conditions as geographic tongue and median rhomboid glossitis.

The diagnosis is usually based on the history and laboratory studies, including cultures as indicated. Empiric therapy may be of diagnostic value in obscure cases.

When the cause cannot be determined and there are no symptoms, therapy is not indicated.

Dreizen S: The telltale tongue. *Postgrad Med* (March) 1984;**75**:150.

## GLOSSODYNIA, GLOSSOPYROSIS
### (Chronic Lingual Papillitis)

Burning and pain, which may involve the entire tongue or isolated areas and may occur with or without glossitis, may be associated findings in hypochromic or pernicious anemia, nutritional disturbances, or diabetes mellitus and may be the presenting symptoms. Xerostomia, drugs (frequently diuretics), and candidiasis may be responsible. Smoking can be a causative irritant. Allergens (eg, in dentifrices) are rare causes of tongue pain. Certain foods may cause flare-ups but are not the primary causes. Dental prostheses, caries, and periodontal disease are usually of no causative significance.

Although most cases occur in postmenopausal women, these disorders are neither restricted to this group nor indicative of hypoestrogenemia.

In most cases a primary cause cannot be identified. Cultures are of no value, since the offending organisms are usually present also in normal mouths. Many clinicians believe that these symptoms occur on a primarily functional basis.

Treatment is mainly empiric, since causative factors usually are not identified. Important approaches include ruling out systemic conditions sometimes associated with these symptoms, changing the drugs being given for other disorders, and reassuring patients that there is no evidence of infection or neoplasia. Antidepressants and tranquilizers are occasionally of value. Ointments and mouth rinses are of no value.

Partial xerostomia may be remedied by sucking on nonmedicated troches or by the administration of pilocarpine, 10–20 mg daily in divided doses, or bethanechol, 100–200 mg daily in divided doses.

Gorsky M, Silverman S Jr, Chinn H: Burning mouth syndrome: A review of 98 cases. *J Oral Med* 1987;**42**:7.

## PIGMENTATION OF GINGIVAE

Abnormal pigmentation of the gingiva is most commonly a racially controlled melanin deposition in the epithelial cytoplasm. It is most prevalent in non-white peoples. The color varies from brown to black, and the involvement may be in isolated patches or a diffuse speckling. Nongenetic causes include epithelial or dermal nevi (rare), drugs (eg, bismuth, arsenic, mercury, or lead), and amalgam fragments that become embedded in the gums during dental work. (Mercury from this source has not been determined to be a health hazard.) Similar lesions may also appear during the menopause or in Addison's disease, intestinal polyposis, neurofibromatosis, and several other disorders associated with generalized pigmentations.

The most important consideration is to rule out malignant melanoma (extremely rare in the mouth), which is suggested by rapid growth and slight elevation.

Buchner A, Hansen LS: Pigmented nevi of the oral mucosa: A clinicopathologic study of 32 new cases and review of 75 cases from the literature. *Oral Surg* 1980;**49**:55.

## ORAL CANCER

Cancers of the lips, tongue, floor of the mouth, buccal mucosa, palate, gingivae, and oropharynx account for about 4% of all cancers. Estimates from various surveys indicate that the average 5-year survival rate for all patients with oral cancer is less than 30%. However, with early detection, the 5-year survival rates are almost doubled. (By definition, detection is "early" when lesions are less than 3 cm in size, without evidence of metastases.) Therefore, early diagnosis followed by adequate treatment appears to be the most effective means of controlling oral cancer.

The lips and tongue are the most frequent sites of involvement. Squamous cell carcinoma is the most common type, accounting for over 90% of all oral cancers. Oral cancer is a disease of older people; over 90% of all cases occur after age 45, and the average age is about 60. The male/female ratio is about 2:1.

The cause of oral cancer is not known. A genetic factor is not apparent. There is a definite increased risk with the use of tobacco and alcohol. Oral leukoplakia is an important precancerous lesion.

Red to purple submucosal lesions on the gingiva, palate, and tongue may be due to disseminated Kaposi's sarcoma associated with AIDS.

### Clinical Findings

There are no reliable signs or symptoms in early oral carcinoma, although pain is the most frequent first complaint. An early cancer may appear as a small white patch (leukoplakia), an aphthouslike or traumatic ulcer, an erythematous plaque, or a small swelling. Biopsy is the only method of definitely diagnosing a carcinoma. However, immediate biopsy of every ill-defined or innocuous-appearing lesion is impractical and not indicated. Exfoliative cytology is a simple, reliable, and acceptable means of differentiating benign and early malignant neoplasms. In the case of small lesions whose gross appearance would be altered by biopsy, the clinician who will give the treatment should see the lesion before the biopsy is taken in order to determine the extent of resection or radiation required. Lymph nodes should not be incised for biopsy for fear of causing dissemination of tumor cells.

### Treatment

Curative treatment consists of surgery and radiation, alone or in combination. An attempt should be made to save the teeth necessary to support prostheses. The periodontium is maintained in optimal condition by periodic routine dental procedures. When areas that have been directly in the beam of irradiation are treated, extreme care is exercised and antibiotics may be selectively administered. Frequent fluoride applications appear to aid in minimizing tooth decalcification and caries. Alterations of taste and saliva formation are usually not permanent. Pilocarpine solution, 5 mg 2–4 times daily, or bethanechol, 25 mg tablets, 100–200 mg daily in divided doses, will often selectively increase salivation.

Decker J, Goldstein JC: Current concepts in otolaryngology: Risk factors in head and neck cancer. *N Engl J Med* 1982;**306**:1151.

Silverman S Jr et al: Oral findings in people with or at high risk for AIDS: A study of 375 homosexual males. *J Am Dent Assoc* 1986;**112**:187.

Silverman S, Greenspan D: Early detection and diagnosis of oral cancer. *J Calif Dent Assoc* 1985;**13**:29.

# DISEASES OF THE ESOPHAGUS

## REFLUX ESOPHAGITIS (Peptic Esophagitis)

### Essentials of Diagnosis

- Substernal burning, cramping, severe pain, or pressure (any or all).
- Symptoms aggravated by recumbency or increase of abdominal pressure; relieved by upright position.
- Nocturnal regurgitation, cough, dyspnea, aspiration may be present.

### General Considerations

Reflux esophagitis results from regurgitation of gastric contents into the esophagus. Acid, pepsins, or bile reflux is essential in pathogenesis. Hyperemia or exudates with erosions may be seen at endoscopy. The pathophysiology includes a permanently or intermittently incompetent lower esophageal sphincter, frequency and duration of reflux, and the inability of the esophagus to generate secondary peristaltic waves that normally prevent prolonged contact of the mucosa with acid and pepsin. A hiatal hernia may or may not be present. The presence of a hiatal hernia is of no consequence unless it is associated with reflux.

## Clinical Findings

**A. Symptoms and Signs:** Pyrosis (''heartburn'') is the most common symptom and is inconstantly indicative of the degree of esophagitis that is secondary to reflux. It is frequently severe, occurring 30–60 minutes after eating, and is initiated or accentuated by recumbency and relieved by sitting upright. Pain at the lower sternal level or xiphoid frequently radiates into the interscapular area, neck, jaw, or down the arms and may closely mimic angina pectoris.

The symptoms are the result of reflux of acid or alkaline gastric contents into the esophagus because of an incompetent lower esophageal sphincter. The conditions associated with an incompetent esophageal sphincter are hiatal hernia, pregnancy, obesity, recurring or persistent vomiting, and nasogastric tubes. Other symptoms include water brash (combination of regurgitation and increased salivation), dysphagia, and odynophagia due to diffuse spasm, stricture, or ulceration; hematemesis; and melena. Iron deficiency anemia may occur with chronic occult bleeding. Aspiration may cause cough, dyspnea, or pneumonitis.

**B. Imaging:** Esophageal reflux may be seen on radiographs. Unless stricture, ulcer, or motor abnormalities are present, esophagitis usually cannot be diagnosed by x-ray. In some patients, reflux may be impossible to document by radiographic techniques.

**C. Special Examinations:** Most patients with reflux can be managed effectively with the usual measures set forth below. Patients who do not respond fully or have atypical or complicated presentations should be investigated further.

**1. Acid perfusion test (Bernstein)**–During perfusion of the distal esophagus with 0.1-N HCl, the patient's symptoms will be reproduced if due to esophagitis.

**2. Peroral endoscopy**–Thirty percent of patients with symptoms of esophagitis will have normal-appearing mucosa upon endoscopic inspection of the esophagus. Biopsy of the mucosa (at least 3 cm proximal to the esophagogastric junction) will establish the diagnosis of esophagitis in most of these patients. Biopsy can identify those with Barrett's esophagus (see below). All patients with complaints of dysphagia should undergo esophagoscopy.

**3. Esophageal manometry**–This test is useful for assessing lower esophageal sphincter function, the ability of the esophagus to clear refluxed acid, and the presence of esophageal dysmotility. Symptomatic patients with no functioning lower esophageal sphincter are usually surgical candidates.

**4. Esophageal pH monitoring**–This is the most objective means of demonstrating esophageal reflux and the clearing time of refluxed acid—a determinant of esophagitis. pH is usually monitored at night with the patient asleep.

## Differential Diagnosis

The differentiation of the retrosternal chest pain of esophagitis from that of angina pectoris or myocardial infarction may require sequential ECGs, enzyme determinations, and close clinical observation. Gastroduodenal ulcer disease, presenting with similar symptoms, can usually be distinguished by radiographic or endoscopic study.

## Complications

Esophagitis, stricture, and esophageal ulcer are the most common complications. However, significant gastritis in the herniated portion of the stomach is sometimes a cause of occult bleeding and anemia.

## Treatment

**A. General Measures:** Since obesity is often an associated or precipitating factor in esophagitis, weight reduction is essential. Other conditions that predispose to increased intra-abdominal pressure, eg, tight belts or corsets, should be avoided. The patient should also be advised to avoid lying down immediately after meals and to sleep with the head of the bed elevated 20–25 cm with wooden blocks. Medication should be taken with an ample amount of water, preferably when the patient is in an upright position. Foods that decrease lower esophageal sphincter pressure should be avoided as much as possible, eg, dietary fat, chocolate, peppermint, and possibly caffeine. Tobacco and alcohol also decrease lower esophageal sphincter pressure and are best avoided. Many patients become symptomatic when they ingest citrus or tomato products and should avoid these foods.

**B. Medical Measures:**

**1. Antacids**–Thirty milliliters taken 1 and 3 hours after meals and at bedtime is effective in neutralizing residual acidic peptic gastric contents. Combination antacids containing aluminum hydroxide, magnesium salts (hydroxide, carbonate, or trisilicate), or alginic acid, 1 or 2 tablets chewed thoroughly after meals and at bedtime, may be effective in relieving the effects of reflux.

**2. Histamine $H_2$ receptor blockers**–Cimetidine (Tagamet), 400 mg, ranitidine (Zantac), 150 mg, or famotidine (Pepcid), 20 mg, at dinnertime, will suppress gastric secretions and thereby minimize nocturnal reflux.

**3. Cholinergic agents**–Bethanechol chloride, 10–20 mg at mealtime, may increase esophageal and gastric motility and speed gastric emptying, thereby decreasing reflux.

**4. Gastrointestinal stimulants**–Metoclopramide (Reglan), 10–20 mg/d, will increase the rate of gastric and esophageal emptying by stimulating the smooth muscle of the intestine. Its exact role in treatment has not been defined.

**C. Surgical Measures:** Antireflux operations may be indicated in a small number of patients who have persistent or recurrent symptoms despite adequate medical therapy. The most commonly performed antireflux procedure is Nissen fundoplication, which produces good results though with some recurrences reported after 5 years. Placement of an Angelchik ring around the distal esophagus in the infradiaphragmatic region is occasionally done. The long-term results of this procedure are unknown.

### Prognosis

Most patients (85–90%) with esophagitis respond to management of weight reduction, antacids, elevation of the head of the bed, and other nonsurgical measures. Even those with strictures (see below) can usually be managed successfully with these measures plus bougienage. For those who cannot be managed medically, fundoplication produces good results in most instances.

Kahrilas PJ et al: Esophageal peristaltic dysfunction in peptic esophagitis. *Gastroenterology* 1986;**91**:897.

Nath BJ, Warshaw AL: Alkaline reflux gastritis and esophagitis. *Annu Rev Med* 1984;**35**:383.

Navab F, Texter EC Jr: Gastroesophageal reflux: Pathophysiologic concepts. *Arch Intern Med* 1985;**145**:329.

Richter JE, Castell DO: Gastroesophageal reflux: Pathogenesis, diagnosis and therapy. *Ann Intern Med* 1982;**97**:93.

## BARRETT'S ESOPHAGUS

Barrett's esophagus is a disorder in which the esophagus is lined with columnar epithelium for varying lengths. It probably represents healing of esophagitis by replacement of the normal squamous epithelium with columnar cells. The symptoms are pyrosis or dysphagia. The incidence of this condition is 3 times greater in males than in females. The entity should be thought of when there is radiographic evidence of a high, benign stricture or a discrete "peptic ulcer" of the lower gullet. Esophagoscopy and biopsy are required to establish the histologic characteristics.

Treatment is the same as for esophagitis. These patients have about a 10% risk of developing adenocarcinoma in this abnormal epithelium. Criteria for follow-up are unclear, but upper endoscopy with biopsies—looking for neoplasm or dysplasia—at 1- to 2-year intervals appears reasonable at this time. The columnar epithelium may regress after successful antireflux surgery, possibly decreasing the chance of malignant degeneration.

Spechler SJ, Goyal RK: Barrett's esophagus. *New England J Med* 1986;**315**:362.

Winters C Jr et al: Barrett's esophagus: A prevalent, occult complication of gastroesophageal reflux disease. *Gastroenterology* 1987;**92**:118.

## CORROSIVE ESOPHAGITIS

### Essentials of Diagnosis

● History of ingestion of corrosive substance.
● Oral, pharyngeal, or substernal pain.
● Odynophagia.
● Evidence of mucosal injury.

### General Considerations

This disorder results from inadvertent or deliberate (suicidal) ingestion of a liquid or crystalline alkali (Plumber's Helper, Drano, etc) or acid (toilet bowl cleaners, hydrochloric acid, etc) substance.

### Clinical Findings

There is usually an almost immediate sensation of severe burning pain of the oropharynx. Gagging secondary to spasm of the cricopharyngeus is common, and some of the material may be regurgitated. Much of the ingested material will traverse the esophagus, causing burning substernal pain that may last for days. The stomach is often affected as well.

Physical findings may include obvious mucosal burns of the lips, mouth, or hypopharynx as well as acute distress due to the pain. Drooling is common. In severe cases, marked hypotension and a shocklike state may be present. With ammonia or formaldehyde ingestion, the odor will be apparent.

### Treatment

Treatment is supportive, with fluids plus narcotics for pain relief. Avoid maneuvers that may induce vomiting, so that there will be no secondary mucosal exposure to the noxious material. Administration of water by mouth may help dilute the corrosive substance. No antidotes are available, and nasogastric tubes are to be avoided because of the risks of inducing retching and perforation.

Indications for peroral endoscopy are controversial. Perhaps endoscopy is most helpful in patients with a history of ingestion and a normal-appearing oropharynx, in whom endoscopy can help determine the extent of injury, if any. In patients with obvious oropharyngeal burns and substernal chest pain, little appears to be gained by endoscopy.

Although corticosteroids and antibiotics have been used in cases of acute corrosive esophagitis, there is only slight justification for these agents in the published reports. Severe injuries may require esophagogastrectomy with colon interposition.

### Prognosis & Course

Mild to moderate burns of the esophagus usually heal without sequelae. Patients with more severe injuries have a small risk of perforation in the short term and a greater risk of stricture formation in the long term. If the stricture is localized, it can often be managed with bougienage. If it is long and tight, surgical replacement of the esophagus with colon interposition may be necessary.

Friedman EM et al: The emergency management of caustic ingestions. *Emerg Med Clin North Am* 1984;**2**:77.

Goldman LP et al: Corrosive substance ingestion: A review. *Am J Gastroenterol* 1984;**79**:85.

## BENIGN STRICTURE OF THE ESOPHAGUS

Healing of any inflammatory lesion of the esophagus may result in stricture formation. Common causes are peptic esophagitis secondary to gastroesophageal reflux, indwelling nasogastric tube, Barrett's epithelium and ulcer formation, ingestion of corrosive substances, acute viral or bacterial infectious diseases, sclerotherapy of varices, and, rarely, injuries caused by endoscopes.

The principal symptom is dysphagia, which may not appear for years after the initial insult. Ability to swallow liquids is maintained the longest.

Odynophagia (painful swallowing) occurs not infrequently in association with dysphagia (difficult swallowing). The patient's description of the point at which the ''hang-up'' of food is perceived conforms with amazing accuracy to the level of the obstruction.

Radiographic demonstration of smooth narrowing with no evidence of mucosal irregularity is usually diagnostic. However, esophagoscopy, biopsy, and cytologic examination are mandatory in all cases to rule out the possibility of cancer.

Dilatation is the definitive form of treatment, using Puestow dilators or mercury-filled (Maloney or Hurst) bougies to attain a lumen size of 44–60F. However, both patient and physician must be prepared for continuing bougienage, since recurrence of stenosis may occur if dilatation is terminated once swallowing again becomes normal. Monthly passage of the largest bougie the patient can tolerate usually prevents regression. If dilatation is unsuccessful, surgical replacement of the esophagus with a segment of stomach, jejunum, or colon will be indicated.

Patterson DJ et al: Natural history of benign esophageal stricture treated by dilatation. *Gastroenterology* 1983;**85**:346.

## LOWER ESOPHAGEAL RING
### (Schatzki's Ring)

The finding of a static but distensible lower esophageal ring signifies the presence of a sliding hiatal hernia that may or may not be symptomatic. Most rings histologically represent the esophagogastric junction. Manometric studies have also confirmed that the lower esophageal ring physiologically repre-

sents the point at which the esophagus and stomach meet. Some rings can be purely esophageal in origin.

The classic ring is 4 mm or less in thickness, is composed of a connective tissue core with muscularis mucosae, and is covered on the upper side by squamous epithelium and on the lower side by columnar epithelium. Submucosal fibrosis is present, but esophagitis is usually absent. Significant gastroesophageal reflux is not present.

Not all lower esophageal rings are mucosal in nature. Some are due to muscular contractions of the esophagus. Distention of the lower esophagus with barium does not obliterate a mucosal ring but accentuates it. Dysphagia is usually present when the ring reduces the internal esophageal lumen to a diameter of 13 mm or less and is often present with a diameter of 18 mm or less.

Most rings can be seen at endoscopy with fiberoptic instruments and can frequently be successfully treated simply by passing an esophagoscope through the ring, thereby dilating it. With a tight ring, one or 2 biopsies can be taken around its circumference, followed either by endoscopic bougienage or bougienage with mercury-filled dilators.

Hill M et al: The management of symptomatic Schatzki ring: A report of 7 cases. *Gastrointest Endosc* 1975;**21**:116.

Ott DJ et al: Review: Esophagogastric region and its rings. *AJR* 1984;**142**:281.

## MOTILITY DISORDERS OF THE ESOPHAGUS

Motility disorders of the esophagus range from absent peristalsis (aperistalsis) to hyperperistalsis and spasm. Combinations of all of these with abnormal lower or upper esophageal sphincter function complete the clinical picture. The abnormalities as determined by radiography or esophageal manometry may be either symptomatic or asymptomatic.

### Aperistalsis of the Esophagus

This is absence of motor activity of the esophagus as determined fluoroscopically and, more exactly, by esophageal motility/manometry studies. The clinical corollary may be a sensation of esophageal fullness, dysphagia, or symptoms of reflux with heartburn. Aperistalsis is commonly associated with Raynaud's phenomenon (80%) and thus is common in patients with scleroderma (about 80%), systemic lupus erythematosus (20–25%), and polymyositis (10–15%). Aperistalsis may also occur in the elderly.

The clinical consequences of aperistalsis are failure to clear refluxed gastric contents, leading to esophagitis, decreased lower esophageal sphincter function, and, in some cases, esophageal ulceration and stricture. The scleroderma patient, in addition to having aperistalsis, usually has dysfunction of the lower esophageal sphincter secondary to muscle displacement by the fibrosing process, leading to an incompetent sphincter and increased reflux.

Management is basically that of reflex esophagitis and should be anticipatory, ie, before symptoms appear, in patients likely to have aperistalsis and an incompetent lower esophageal sphincter (eg, patients with Raynaud's phenomenon or scleroderma).

## Presbyesophagus

This refers to the radiographic demonstration of esophageal dysmotility as characterized by nonpropulsive contractions (tertiary contractions), usually as an incidental finding during an upper gastrointestinal study. Presbyesophagus is usually asymptomatic and requires no therapy.

## Diffuse Esophageal Spasm (Nutcracker Esophagus)

Symptomatic diffuse esophageal spasm is characterized by substernal pain or dysphagia. The pain may be indistinguishable from angina and may include radiation of pain into the neck, jaws, right arm, left arm, or to the back. There may be hypersalivation and reflux of recently swallowed food. A specific cause is seldom found, but there may be associated reflux esophagitis. Very cold or very hot foods may trigger an episode. Diffuse esophageal spasm may be part of the spectrum of achalasia (see below).

Radiographically and endoscopically, vigorous nonpropulsive esophageal contractions are noted. Manometrically, they may be high-pressure sustained contractions. Diagnosis is essentially based on the clinical picture, since all of the objective findings can be seen in asymptomatic patients. A high resting lower esophageal sphincter pressure is common, but, as is not the case in achalasia, the sphincter will relax normally.

Sublingual nitroglycerin is usually effective for the acute episode, and long-acting nitroglycerin (isosorbide) or calcium channel blockers (nifedepine, diltiazem)—or both—are often effective. In severely symptomatic patients unresponsive to medical management, a long esophageal myotomy may prove helpful.

## Achalasia of the Esophagus

Achalasia is a motor disorder of the esophagus characterized by loss of primary peristalsis, presence of a hypertonic lower esophageal sphincter that does not relax in response to a swallow, and evidence of denervation of the esophagus as shown by an exaggerated esophageal response to cholinergic agents. It is, in part, the result of impaired integration of parasympathetic stimulation. There is difficulty in swallowing both liquids and solids, at first of variable frequency and degree but later usually persistent and severe and characterized by dysphagia, occasional odynophagia, frequent regurgitation of food, and dilatation of the esophagus, as shown by radiography. Although achalasia may appear in infancy or old age, it most commonly afflicts patients in the third to fifth decades. It may predispose to esophageal carcinoma.

Two types of achalasia of the esophagus can be defined by differences in pathologic anatomy, symptoms, and radiographic findings. The first type (about 75% of cases) is characterized by a beaklike narrowing of the distal 2–4 cm of the esophagus. The more proximal portion is markedly dilated and tortuous, with the ultimate appearance of an elongated sigmoid configuration. Stasis of intraluminal contents is responsible for varying degrees of esophagitis. Patients with this form of achalasia characteristically experience dysphagia without chest pain. However, regurgitation may cause aspiration, with resultant pneumonitis, bronchiectasis, lung abscess, or pulmonary fibrosis.

The second form of achalasia, vigorous achalasia, is characterized by recurring esophageal spasm, which may result in retrosternal and subxiphoid pain with frequent associated dysphagia or hypersalivation. The circular muscle of the esophagus appears hypertrophied, and the dilatation proximal to the lower esophageal sphincter is not as marked as with the first type of achalasia.

Dysphagia may initially be intermittent, with food apparently sticking at the level of the xiphoid cartilage, and is associated with variable discomfort in the retrosternal or subxiphoid areas. Precipitation or accentuation of difficult swallowing may inconstantly follow the ingestion of solids or cold beverages and may be related to emotionally stressful situations. Continued esophageal dilatation with retention of food and liquids results in a sensation of fullness behind the sternum. Pain (when present) may also radiate to the back, neck, and arms and may occur independently of swallowing. Increased hydrostatic pressure within the esophagus will overcome the high resting pressure of the lower esophageal sphincter, and patients should therefore drink extra water and perform the Valsalva maneuver so that the esophageal contents will more readily enter the stomach. However, prolonged impairment of alimentation may cause varying degrees of malnutrition.

Radiographic diagnosis is based on the characteristic tapering of the distal esophagus in a conical fashion to a markedly narrowed distal segment, 1–3 cm long, which usually lies above the diaphragm. Fluoroscopy, cinefluorography, and films of the proximal esophagus reveal purposeless and ineffectual contractions as well as varying degrees of dilatation. Esophageal motility and manometric studies provide characteristic findings and may be required to establish a diagnosis of achalasia.

After the patient has consumed a clear liquid diet for 24–36 hours and undergone preendoscopic aspiration and lavage, esophagoscopy should be performed at least once in every case of achalasia to ascertain the severity of esophagitis and to eliminate the possibility of occult carcinoma.

Passage of a pneumatic dilator under fluoroscopic

guidance—designed to split muscle fibers of the lower esophageal sphincter—has been recommended as appropriate nonsurgical treatment. Passage of mercury-filled bougies is only a palliative measure at best but may be employed in a preparatory way to enable easier emptying of esophageal contents before pneumatic dilation is performed. Treatment of achalasia with long-acting nitrates (eg, isosorbide dinitrate) or calcium channel blockers (eg, nifedipine), which lower the resting pressure of the lower esophageal sphincter, has met with modest success. Esophagocardiomyotomy is ultimately required in approximately 20–25% of patients.

## Upper Esophageal Sphincter Dysfunction

Dysfunction of the upper esophageal sphincter may give rise to symptoms of a "lump in the throat" as well as reflux of dysphagia. A hypotensive sphincter has on occasion been associated with the "lump in the throat" sensation as well as reflux of stomach contents into the mouth. In the elderly patient with cervical dysphagia, the upper esophageal sphincter usually functions normally, but there is ineffective swallowing, most likely due to a lacunar or larger cerebrovascular accident. The gag reflex in this latter setting is often decreased or absent.

The hypertensive upper esophageal sphincter, often with poor relaxation on deglutition, is associated with dysphagia and may well be the underlying abnormality that gives rise to Zenker's diverticulum—a posterior out-pouching of the cervical esophagus just cephalad to the upper esophageal sphincter. These diverticula may harbor inspissated food, giving rise to halitosis, regurgitation of food eaten 1 or 2 days before, and increasing dysphagia secondary to pressure on the esophagus.

Management of these disorders is difficult. For the hypotensive upper esophageal sphincter, little but antireflux measures can be offered. For the stroke patient with dysphagia, a feeding tube (nasogastric or gastric) can be offered to provide nutrition until there is return of function. For the hypertensive upper esophageal sphincter that is symptomatic or with an associated Zenker's diverticulum, surgical myotomy is the treatment of choice.

Chuong JJH et al: Achalasia as a risk factor for esophageal carcinoma: A reappraisal. *Dig Dis Sci* 1985;**29**:1105.

Richter JE, Barish CF, Castell DO: Abnormal sensory perception in patients with esophageal chest pain. *Gastroenterology* 1986;**91**:845.

Richter JE, Castell DO: Diffuse esophageal spasm: A reappraisal. *Ann Intern Med* 1984;**100**:242.

Traube M et al: Effects of nifedipine in achalasia and in patients with high-amplitude peristaltic esophageal contractions. *JAMA* 1984;**152**:1733.

Vantrappen G, Hellmans J: Treatment of achalasia and related motor disorders. *Gastroenterology* 1980;**79**:144.

## ESOPHAGEAL DIVERTICULA

### Essentials of Diagnosis

- Dysphagia progressing as more is eaten; bad breath, foul taste in mouth.
- Regurgitation of undigested or partially digested food representing first portion of a meal.
- Radiography (barium) confirms diagnosis.

### General Considerations

The clinical picture and pathologic effects of an esophageal diverticulum are to a large extent dictated by the location of the lesion. It is therefore convenient to distinguish pharyngoesophageal (pulsion or Zenker's), midesophageal (traction), and epiphrenic (traction-pulsion) diverticula by their locations. The first (pharyngoesophageal) develops through the space at the junction of the hypopharynx and esophagus just proximal to the cricopharyngeal sphincter, occurs chiefly in middle-aged men, and may attain large size. The second (midesophageal) type rarely is larger than 2 cm, may be multiple, frequently arises opposite the pulmonary hilar region, occurs with equal frequency in men and women, and usually causes no symptoms. The third and least common (epiphrenic) type occurs primarily in men in the esophageal segment immediately proximal to the hiatus, may be congenital in origin, and progressively enlarges, so that symptoms develop in middle age. Pharyngoesophageal and epiphrenic diverticula frequently produce nocturnal regurgitation and aspiration, with resultant bronchitis, bronchiectasis, and lung abscess.

### Clinical Findings

**A. Symptoms and Signs:** The main symptoms of pharyngoesophageal (Zenker's) diverticula are dysphagia, regurgitation, gurgling sounds in the neck, nocturnal coughing, halitosis, and weight loss. Enlargement of the pouch results in its downward dissection between the postesophageal septum of the deep cervical fascia and the prevertebral fascia. When filled with food, the pouch may appear as a swelling at the side of the neck and internally may cause compression and obstruction of the proximal esophagus. There is occasionally so much compression of the esophagus that its entrance becomes slitlike, making it difficult to find endoscopically, and this readily explains the difficulty in swallowing and impaired nutrition.

Epiphrenic diverticula, which are occasionally associated with peptic strictures, usually cause no symptoms at first but ultimately may produce dysphagia, pain, and pulmonary complications.

Although midesophageal diverticula may rarely be responsible for mediastinal abscess or esophagobronchial fistulas and inconstantly may cause dysphagia, these lesions generally produce no symptoms.

**B. Imaging:** Barium swallow will usually demonstrate the 3 types of diverticula.

### Differential Diagnosis

Regurgitation and difficult swallowing associated

with diverticula must be distinguished from that caused by neoplasm, vascular anomalies, strictures, or motility dysfunction of the esophagus. Epiphrenic diverticula must also be differentiated from esophageal ulcer. Physical examination, radiography, and endoscopy will clarify the diagnosis.

## Treatment & Prognosis

Large and symptom-producing pharyngoesophageal and epiphrenic diverticula should be treated surgically by amputation. Although recurrence or postoperative dysphagia is occasionally seen following operation for the former, long-term results are usually excellent. Cricopharyngeal sphincter myotomy has been advocated for pharyngoesophageal diverticula secondary to an abnormal sphincter. Since midesophageal pouches rarely produce complications or significant symptoms, therapy is usually not required.

Knuff TE, Benjamin SB, Castell DO: Pharyngoesophageal (Zenker's) diverticulum: A reappraisal. *Gastroenterology* 1982;**82:**734.

## CARCINOMA OF THE ESOPHAGUS

In the USA, carcinoma of the esophagus is predominantly a disease of men in the fifth to eighth decades. It usually arises from squamous epithelium. There is increased incidence of squamous cell carcinoma of the esophagus among smokers and in association with other otolaryngologic neoplasms. Stasis-induced inflammation such as is seen in achalasia or esophageal stricture and chronic irritation induced by excessive use of alcohol seemingly are etiologically important in the development of this neoplasm. Malignant tumors of the distal esophagus are frequently adenocarcinomas that originate in the stomach and spread cephalad to the gullet. Conversely, squamous cell carcinoma of the esophagus rarely invades the stomach. Primary adenocarcinoma of the esophagus is rare and probably arises in Barrett's epithelium. Regardless of cell type, the prognosis for cancer of the esophagus is usually poor.

### Clinical Findings

**A. Symptoms and Signs:** Dysphagia, which is progressive and ultimately prevents swallowing of even liquids, is the principal symptom. Anterior or posterior chest pain that is unrelated to eating implies local extension of the tumor, whereas significant weight loss over a short period is an ominous sign.

**B. Imaging:** Barium swallow is positive for an irregular, frequently annular space-occupying lesion. CT scan of the esophagus can delineate extraesophageal involvement (eg, mediastinum, lymph nodes).

**C. Special Examinations:** Esophagoscopy, biopsy, and cytologic examination are confirmatory.

## Differential Diagnosis

Achalasia can be differentiated by endoscopy, esophageal manometry, and cinefluorography. Since there is a significant association of stricture with malignant neoplasms, any narrowing of the lumen should be evaluated by esophagoscopy and biopsy.

## Treatment & Prognosis

Although it was once considered a hopeless disease, improvements during the last 2–3 decades in anesthesia, surgical techniques, and radiation therapy have improved survival of patients with esophageal carcinoma. Irradiation generally is the best form of therapy, particularly for lesions in the proximal half of the esophagus. When there is no evidence of metastases, tumors of the lower half of the esophagus may be treated by resection and esophagogastrostomy or jejunal or colonic interpositions. After dilatation of tumor-bearing portions of the esophagus, effective palliation and improved survival can often be accomplished by the use of prosthetic tubes that are inserted through the mouth to facilitate swallowing. Cure rates are still dismal, however, and do not exceed 5–10%.

Gastrostomy may improve nutrition but does not prolong survival, and the inability of completely obstructed patients to swallow even saliva makes the operation of questionable value for palliation. Anticancer drugs have not proved to be of value.

Mellow MH, Pinkas H: Endoscopic laser therapy for malignancies affecting the esophagus and gastroesophageal junction. *Arch Intern Med* 1985;**145:**1443.
Picus D et al: Computed tomography in the staging of esophageal carcinoma. *Radiology* 1983;**146:**433.

## BENIGN NEOPLASMS OF THE ESOPHAGUS

Benign tumors of the esophagus are quite rare and are generally found accidentally by either the radiologist or prosector in the lower half of the esophagus. The most common of the benign neoplasms is the leiomyoma, which arises from one of the smooth muscle coats of the esophagus. This lesion may be circumferential or multiple, gradually increases in size (up to 2–2.5 cm), and may ultimately compromise the esophageal lumen or normal peristalsis, producing dysphagia. Other uncommon benign tumors are fibromas, lipomas, lymphangiomas, hemangiomas, and schwannomas. The diagnosis is made by barium swallow and esophagoscopy. Cytologic examination is not definitive, and biopsy may be inadequate or technically not feasible. Surgical removal is curative.

## ESOPHAGEAL WEBS

Esophageal webs are thin membranous structures that include in their substance only mucosal and submucosal coats. They are occasionally congenital but more commonly appear to be the sequelae of ulceration, local infection, hemorrhage, or mechanical trauma. Cervical vertebral exostoses are sometimes mentioned as a common cause. Most webs are found in the proximal portion of the esophagus and produce significant dysphagia with occasional laryngospasm secondary to aspiration. Difficult swallowing secondary to a web—when combined with iron deficiency anemia, splenomegaly, glossitis, and spooning of the nails and occurring almost invariably in premenopausal women—is called Plummer-Vinson syndrome. In this condition, a diaphanous web is usually located immediately below the cricopharyngeus and is associated with an atrophic pharyngoesophagitis. Esophagoscopy (essential to rule out carcinoma) ameliorates dysphagia by disrupting the web. Bougienage with Maloney or Hurst dilators may occasionally be necessary.

## ESOPHAGEAL CYSTS

Esophageal cysts probably result from buds of the primitive foregut or tracheobronchial branches. They may be asymptomatic but can cause dysphagia, dyspnea, cough, cyanosis, or chest pain, either because of their location or because they tend to contain acid-secreting epithelium that may produce peptic ulceration. The cysts are in the lower half of the esophagus between the muscle layers of the esophageal wall. Diagnosis is made by demonstration of a mediastinal mass on x-ray or at surgery. Surgical excision may be necessary.

Heithoff K et al: Bronchopulmonary foregut malformations: A unifying etiological concept. *Am J Roentgenol* 1976; **126**:46.

## MALLORY-WEISS SYNDROME
## (Mucosal Lacerations of the Esophagus or Cardioesophageal Junction)

Forceful or prolonged vomiting followed by the vomiting of bright-red blood suggests Mallory-Weiss syndrome. The bleeding is due to a vertical tear involving the mucosa of the cardioesophageal junction or, more commonly, the most proximal portion of the stomach. A hiatal hernia is frequently present. The diagnosis is based on the history of vomiting followed by hematemesis. The diagnosis is confirmed by endoscopic demonstration of the mucosal tear. Usually no active intervention is required, as most lesions stop bleeding spontaneously. Rarely, endoscopic injection with epinephrine, balloon tamponade, or surgery is required to control bleeding.

Sugawa C et al: Mallory-Weiss syndrome: A study of 224 patients. *Am J Surg* 1983;**145**:30.

# DISEASES OF THE STOMACH

## GASTRITIS

Gastritis is a descriptive term often used by clinicians for vague, self-limited illnesses characterized by nausea, anorexia, epigastric distress with or without vomiting, and some systemic symptoms. The cause is usually obscure and, because of the self-limited nature of the disorder, usually not important. For the gastroenterologist, gastritis is an endoscopic finding of varying specificity seen both with and without associated clinical symptoms. For the pathologist, gastritis means the presence of inflammatory cells, acute or chronic (or both), in the gastric mucosa with or without additional mucosal abnormalities.

There are many causes of gastritis; some are listed in Table 11–1.

### Clinical Findings
**A. Symptoms and Signs:** The manifestations of gastritis are variable depending on the cause, but persistent anorexia is often a major feature. Epigastric fullness or easy satiety as well as nausea and vomiting may be present. Upper gastrointestinal bleeding, occasionally major, may occur, particularly with drug-, stress-, or corrosive-induced erosive hemorrhagic gastritis. In patients with gastritis secondary to acute infections or bacterial toxins (staphylococcal toxin),

**Table 11–1.** Causes of gastritis.

**Common causes**
  Drugs (eg, nonsteroidal anti-inflammatory agents [including aspirin], alcohol)
  Gastric ulcer (peptic ulcer)
  Stress (especially in patients in intensive care or coronary care units)
  Aging
  Idiopathic disorders
**Uncommon causes**
  Postgastrectomy
  Bile reflux
  Infection (? *Campylobacter*)
**Very uncommon causes**
  Allergy (usually specific, eg, nuts, chocolate)
  Bacterial infections (tuberculosis, syphilis)
  Corrosive substances (Clinitest tablet, ingestion of lye or acid)
  Crohn's disease
  Eosinophilia
  Epidermic gastritis of unknown cause (one series reported)
  Granulomatosis
  Parasitic diseases (eg, strongyloidiasis, anisakiasis, schistosomiasis)
  Pseudolymphoma
  Radiation therapy or exposure to radiation
  Sarcoidosis
  Viral diseases (eg, herpesvirus, cytomegalovirus, varicella virus)

malaise, diarrhea, colic, fever, chills, and headache may be associated, with resultant dehydration. Examination may show epigastric tenderness.

**B. Laboratory Findings:** The laboratory findings may be normal or may reflect the underlying process—infectious, hemorrhagic, etc.

**C. Special Examinations:** For those who present with acute upper gastrointestinal hemorrhage, early endoscopy (within 24 hours) permits accurate identification of the source: hemorrhagic erosive gastritis, drug-induced ulcerations, etc. The clinical preendoscopic diagnosis of the source of bleeding is correct no more than half the time. In patients with corrosive gastritis, endoscopy permits determination of the extent of injury. In the dyspeptic patient with normal radiographic studies who is unresponsive to the usual treatment, peroral endoscopy may demonstrate the presence or absence of motility disorders or mucosal abnormalities.

## Differential Diagnosis

In addition to the conditions listed in Table 11–1, peptic ulcer, neoplasms, cholecystitis, esophageal spasm, angina pectoris, abdominal angina, pancreatic disease, and psychologic gastrointestinal disorders must be considered.

## Treatment & Prognosis

**A. Drug-Induced Gastritis:** Remove the offending agent. If bleeding is a major part of the clinical picture—ie, requiring transfusion—serious consideration must be given to administration of platelets, since the endogenous platelets are ineffective for up to 5 days after stopping aspirin. Sucralfate, 1 g before meals 3 times a day and at bedtime, or a liquid antacid, 30 mL, is often effective. In the absence of ulcer disease, a week's course should be sufficient.

**B. Gastric Ulcer-Associated Gastritis:** Gastritis is almost always present in patients with peptic gastric ulcer. The treatment is that of the ulcer.

**C. Stress Gastritis:** This is best managed by prevention. In the stressed noneating patient (burn center, intensive care unit, coronary care unit), gastric ulcer should be prevented by hourly titrations of the intragastric pH to at least 4.0–5.0. This is achieved by instillation of antacids or by continuous intravenous infusions of an $H_2$ antagonist (the usual bolus dose given by infusion) or, in the enterally fed patient, by continuous nasogastric infusion of the liquid diet (Ensure, Osmolyte, etc).

Once the patient has developed erosive bleeding gastritis, support with transfusions and intragastric neutralization with antacids or $H_2$ antagonists seems reasonable. Sucralfate may be of benefit as well. Various prostaglandin agents are currently undergoing clinical trials to test the efficacy of their cytoprotective and antisecretory properties.

**D. Gastritis Associated With Aging:** Endoscopically, many individuals past age 65 have what is termed "chronic gastritis" or "atrophic gastritis," often verified by biopsy as a thinning of the mucosa

and decrease in the glandular elements. These conditions are rarely symptomatic and require no treatment unless there is associated malabsorption of vitamin $B_{12}$. They are incidental findings in patients undergoing endoscopy for other reasons. If vitamin $B_{12}$ deficiency is present, supplementation is required.

**E. Idiopathic Gastritis:** Endoscopic evaluation of epigastric distress commonly discloses varying degrees of erythema and mucosal irregularities without erosions or bleeding. Biopsies often will show an increase in chronic inflammatory cells and occasionally polymorphonuclears as well. The cause is obscure, and management is difficult. Avoidance of gastric irritants is usually advised, along with antacids or sucralfate, but only modest benefits have been reported.

**F. Postgastrectomy Gastritis:** Symptomatic postgastrectomy gastritis is uncommon, though acute gastritis (redness) is frequently seen by endoscopy at the anastomosis. When more extensive gastritis is seen, it is often associated with bile reflux (see below) or uncommonly with a bezoar. Owing to poor gastric motility there is a tendency after resection for vegetable bezoars to form, and this not only helps produce a mechanically induced gastritis but causes sensations of fullness, obstruction, and easy satiety. The bezoar can usually be broken with the endoscope. Kanulase tablets, which contain the enzyme cellulase (9 mg per tablet), are often helpful in breaking down the cellulose of a vegetable/fruit bezoar. Two tablets every 2–3 hours during the day for a week may be necessary. Avoidance of large quantities of cellulose-containing foods is important.

**G. Bile Reflux:** This is an occasional cause of severe gastritis after pyloroplasty or gastric resection, particularly following Billroth II anastomosis. It is characterized by almost constant epigastric pain, and endoscopy shows a fiery red mucosa. Although bile sequestrants have been tried, they have been at best only marginally successful. If symptoms persist, operation is necessary and consists of implanting the afferent loop 20–25 cm below the gastrojejunostomy so that bile does not bathe the gastric pouch. The success rate with this procedure is high but less than 100%.

**H. Acute Corrosive Esophagitis and Gastritis:** Ingestion of corrosive substances is most common in children but may occur in cases of attempted suicide. The substances most commonly swallowed are strong acids (sulfuric, nitric), alkalies (lye, potash), oxalic acid, iodine, bichloride of mercury, arsenic, silver nitrate, and carbolic acid. The esophagus is most severely injured. Gastric changes vary from superficial edema and hyperemia to deep necrosis and sloughing or even perforation.

Corrosion of the lips, tongue, mouth, and pharynx, along with pain and dysphagia due to esophageal lesions, is usually present. Nitric acid causes brown discoloration; oxalic acid causes white discoloration of mucous membranes. There is severe epigastric burning and cramping pain, nausea and vomiting, and diarrhea. The vomitus is often blood-tinged. Severe prostration with a shocklike picture and thirst may occur. Palpation of the abdomen may show epigastric tenderness or extreme rigidity. Leukocytosis and proteinuria are present.

Immediate treatment is supportive, including analgesics, intravenous fluids and electrolytes, sedatives, and antacids. Although the specific antidote (see Chapter 30) should be administered immediately, supportive measures must not be neglected. The benefit to be expected from the antidote appears minuscule if a large amount of corrosive has been ingested, and the benefit is doubtful considering that tissue damage occurs almost immediately. Avoid emetics and lavage if corrosion is severe, because of the danger of perforation.

The outcome depends upon the extent of tissue damage. Careful fiberoptic endoscopy may serve to determine the extent of injury. Emergency laparotomy may be indicated to resect the area of gangrene and potential perforation. If alkali has been ingested, prednisone, 20 mg every 8 hours started immediately, may prevent esophageal stricture. This dose should be tapered slowly over several weeks.

After the acute phase has passed, place the patient on a peptic ulcer regimen. If perforation has not occurred, recovery is the rule. However, pyloric stenosis may occur early or late, requiring gastric aspiration, parenteral fluid therapy, and surgical repair.

The amount of the corrosive substance, its local and general effects, and the speed with which it is removed or neutralized determine the outcome. If the patient survives the acute phase, gastric effects are usually overshadowed by esophageal strictures, although chronic gastritis or stricture formation at the pylorus may follow.

**I. Uncommon Conditions:** Treatment of some cases of gastritis depends in part on making the diagnosis. Endoscopy and biopsy must be performed to confirm a suspected diagnosis.

Dilawari JB et al: Corrosive acid ingestion in man: Clinical and endoscopic study. *Gut* 1984;**25**:183.

Maull KI: Surgical implications of acid ingestion. *Surg Gynecol Obstet* 1979;**148**:893.

Ritchie WP: Alakaline reflux gastritis: A critical reappraisal. *Gut* 1984;**25**:975.

Rumack BH, Burrington JD: Caustic ingestions: A rational look at diluents. *Clin Toxicol* 1977;**11**:27.

Strickland RG: Acute and chronic gastritis. *Hosp Med* (June) 1983;**19**:148.

Weinstein WM: Gastritis. Page 559 in: *Gastrointestinal Disease: Pathophysiology, Diagnosis, Management*, 3rd ed. Sleisenger MH, Fordtran JS (editors). Saunders, 1983.

# PEPTIC ULCER

A peptic ulcer is an acute or chronic benign ulceration occurring in a portion of the digestive tract that is accessible to gastric secretions. An active peptic ulcer does not occur in the absence of acid-peptic gastric secretions. Other than the requirement for acid and pepsin, the cause of peptic ulcer at any level of the gut remains obscure.

Other factors in peptic ulceration (besides the presence of gastric acid) include hypersecretion of hydrochloric acid and decreased tissue resistance.

Peptic ulcer may occur during the course of drug therapy (salicylates and other nonsteroidal anti-inflammatory drugs, reserpine). It may occur as a result of critical illness or severe tissue injury such as extensive burns or intracranial surgery (stress ulcer), and may be associated with endocrine tumors producing gastrin, which stimulates hypersecretion of hydrochloric acid and results in a very refractory peptic ulcer diathesis (Zollinger-Ellison syndrome, gastrinoma).

## 1. DUODENAL ULCER

### Essentials of Diagnosis

- Epigastric distress 45–60 minutes after meals, or nocturnal pain, both relieved by food, antacids, or vomiting.
- Epigastric tenderness and guarding.
- Chronic and periodic symptoms.
- Gastric analysis shows acid in all cases and hypersecretion in some.
- Ulcer crater or deformity of duodenal bulb on x-ray or with oral endoscopy.

### General Considerations

The incidence of duodenal ulcer has been declining at a rate of about 8% per year for the past decade. It still remains a major health problem. Although the average age at onset is 33 years, duodenal ulcer may occur at any time from infancy to the later years. It is twice as common in males as in females. Occurrence during pregnancy is unusual.

Duodenal ulcer is 4 or 5 times as common as benign gastric ulcer.

About 95% of duodenal ulcers occur in the duodenal bulb or cap. The remainder are between this area and the ampulla. Ulcers below the ampulla are rare. The ulceration varies from a few mm to 1–2 cm in diameter and extends at least through the muscularis mucosae, often through to the serosa and into the pancreas. The margins are sharp, but the surrounding mucosa is often inflamed and edematous. The base consists of granulation tissue and fibrous tissue, representing healing and continuing digestion.

### Clinical Findings

**A. Symptoms and Signs:** Symptoms may be absent, or vague and atypical. In the typical case, pain is described as gnawing, burning, cramplike, or aching, or as "heartburn"; it is usually mild to moderate, located over a small area near the midline in the epigastrium near the xiphoid. The pain may radiate below the costal margins, into the back, or, rarely, to the right shoulder. Nausea may be present, and vomiting of small quantities of highly acid gastric juice with little or no retained food may occur. The distress usually occurs 45–60 minutes after a meal; is usually absent before breakfast; worsens as the day progresses; and may be most severe between 12 midnight and 2:00 AM. It is relieved by food, milk, alkalies, and vomiting, generally within 5–30 minutes.

Spontaneous remissions and exacerbations are common. Precipitating factors are often unknown but may include trauma, infections, or physical or emotional distress.

Signs include superficial and deep epigastric tenderness, voluntary muscle guarding, and unilateral (rectus) spasm over the duodenal bulb.

**B. Laboratory Findings:** Bleeding, hypochromic anemia, and occult blood in the stools may occur in chronic ulcers. Gastric analysis shows acid in all cases and a basal and maximal gastric hypersecretion of hydrochloric acid in some.

**C. Imaging:** An ulcer crater is demonstrable by Radiography in 50–70% of cases but may be obscured by deformity of the duodenal bulb. When no ulcer is demonstrated, the following are suggestive of ulceration: (1) irritability of the bulb, with difficulty in retaining barium there, (2) point tenderness over the bulb, (3) pylorospasm, (4) gastric hyperperistalsis, and (5) hypersecretion or retained secretions.

**D. Special Examinations:** Duodenoscopy has proved to be a valuable adjunct in the diagnosis of duodenal ulcer not demonstrated radiographically. Duodenoscopy may also demonstrate duodenitis, a disorder that may have a pathogenetic mechanism in common with duodenal ulcer.

### Differential Diagnosis

When symptoms are typical, the diagnosis of peptic ulceration can be made with assurance; when symptoms are atypical, duodenal ulcer may be confused clinically with functional gastrointestinal disease, gastritis, gastric carcinoma, and irritable colon syndrome. The final diagnosis often depends upon x-ray or endoscopic observation.

### Complications

**A. Intractability to Treatment:** Most cases of apparently intractable ulcer are probably due to an inadequate medical regimen or failure of cooperation on the part of the patient. The designation "intractable" should be reserved for patients who have received an adequate supervised trial of therapy. The possibility of gastrinoma as well as complications of the ulcer must always be considered.

**B. Hemorrhage Due to Peptic Ulcer:** Hemorrhage is caused either by erosion of an ulcer into an artery or vein or, more commonly, by bleeding from granulation tissue. Most bleeding ulcers are on the posterior wall. The sudden onset of weakness, faintness, dizziness, chills, thirst, cold moist skin, desire to defecate, and the passage of loose tarry or even red stools with or without coffee-ground vomitus is characteristic of acute duodenal ulcer hemorrhage.

The blood findings (hemoglobin, red cell count, and hematocrit) lag behind the blood loss by several hours and may give a false impression of the quantity of blood lost. Postural hypotension and tachycardia and central venous pressure are more reliable indicators of hypovolemia than the hematocrit (see p 348).

**C. Perforation:** Perforation occurs almost exclusively in men 25–40 years of age. The symptoms and signs are those of peritoneal irritation and peritonitis; ulcers that perforate into the lesser peritoneal cavity cause less dramatic symptoms and signs. A typical description of perforated peptic ulcer is an acute onset of epigastric pain, often radiating to the shoulder or right lower quadrant and sometimes associated with nausea and vomiting, followed by a lessening of pain for a few hours and then by boardlike rigidity of the abdomen, fever, rebound tenderness, absent bowel sounds, leukocytosis, tachycardia, and even signs of marked prostration. Radiographic demonstration of free air in the peritoneal cavity confirms the diagnosis.

**D. Penetration:** Extension of the crater beyond the duodenal wall into contiguous structures but not into the free peritoneal space occurs fairly frequently with duodenal ulcer and is one of the important causes of failure of medical treatment. Penetration usually occurs in ulcers on the posterior wall, and extension is usually into the pancreas; but the liver, biliary tract, or gastrohepatic omentum may be involved.

Radiation of pain into the back, night distress, inadequate or no relief from eating food or taking alkalies, and, in occasional cases, relief upon spinal flexion and aggravation upon hyperextension—any or all of these findings in a patient with a long history of duodenal ulcer usually signify penetration.

**E. Obstruction:** Minor degrees of pyloric obstruction are present in about 20–25% of patients with duodenal ulcer, but clinically significant obstruction is much less common. The obstruction is generally caused by edema and spasm associated with an active ulcer, but it may occur as a result of scar tissue contraction even in the presence of a healed ulcer.

The occurrence of epigastric fullness or heaviness and, finally, copious vomiting after meals—with the vomitus containing undigested food from a previous meal—suggests obstruction. The diagnosis is confirmed by the presence of an overnight gastric residual exceeding 50 mL containing undigested food, and x-ray evidence of obstruction, gastric dilatation, and hyperperistalsis. A succussion splash on pressure in the left upper quadrant may be present, and gastric peristalsis may be visible.

### Treatment

Currently, antacids, histamine $H_2$ receptor antagonists, and sucralfate have all been shown to be equally effective in the treatment of duodenal ulcers when compared with placebos. These regimens provide symptomatic relief in the vast majority of patients. Less clear has been the therapeutic efficacy of various dietary measures. The limiting factor with existing therapies is that although the ulcers heal, the ulcer diathesis remains and recurrence rates are high.

**A. Acute Phase:**

**1. General measures**–The patient should be encouraged to have adequate rest and sleep, and it may sometimes be necessary to recommend 2 or 3 weeks' rest from work if that can be managed. In some instances, if the home situation is unsuitable or if the patient is unable to cooperate, hospitalization is recommended. The patient who must continue to work should be given careful instructions about the medical program. Arrangements should be made for rest periods and sufficient sleep. Anxiety should be relieved whenever possible.

Alcohol, a gastric secretagogue and irritant, should be strictly forbidden. The patient should also quit smoking, since smoking has been shown to markedly decrease the healing rate of duodenal ulcer even when optimal treatment is being given.

The following drugs may aggravate peptic ulcer or may even cause perforation and hemorrhage: rauwolfia, salicylates, phenylbutazone, indomethacin, and other nonsteroidal anti-inflammatory analgesics. They should be discontinued if possible.

**2. Diet**–All controlled clinical studies have documented that neither the type nor the consistency of diet will affect the healing of ulcers. The important principles of dietary management of peptic ulcer are as follows: (1) nutritious diet; (2) regular meals; (3) restriction of coffee, tea, cola beverages, decaffeinated beverages, and alcohol; and (4) avoidance of foods that are clearly known to produce unpleasant symptoms in a given individual.

In the acute phase, when there is partial gastric outlet obstruction, it is often useful to begin with a full liquid diet, provided that 1-hour postprandial gastric residuals are less than 100 mL. Milk, because of its secretagogue effect, should be avoided. Large amounts of milk and cream in the diet are associated with a striking increase in deaths from myocardial infarction in ulcer patients. Interval feedings should be avoided. Food of any type or consistency has been shown to markedly stimulate gastric acid secretion and to be ineffective as a buffer against acid in the stomach.

It is doubtful that any dietary measures other than elimination of known aggravating factors play a significant role in preventing ulcer recurrence.

**3. Antacids**–Antacids usually relieve ulcer pain promptly. Antacid dosage should be selected on the basis of neutralizing capacity. The response to antacids varies widely according to the preparation, the dosage, and the individual patient. Tablet preparations must be thoroughly chewed and dissolved to have effectiveness.

In order to be effective, antacids must be taken frequently. During the acute phase, a full dose 1 and 3 hours after meals and at bedtime should be sufficient. If pain relief is not achieved on this regimen, the stomach is emptying too rapidly or the patient

is secreting more acid than the antacid can neutralize. (Suspect Zollinger-Ellison syndrome.)

Magnesium hydroxide-aluminum hydroxide mixtures (many preparations available) are effective and widely used antacids. The usual dose is 30 mL. When full therapeutic doses are given, the magnesium in the mixtures may produce diarrhea; it may be necessary to alternate with a straight aluminum hydroxide gel preparation (eg, Alternagel), which tends to be constipating. Prolonged ingestion of aluminum hydroxide gels may lead to phosphate depletion and osteoporosis. Magnesium salts should be used cautiously in patients with renal insufficiency.

Calcium carbonate has an excellent neutralizing action and may be used at times when the magnesium-aluminum gel antacids are inadequate. Antacid mixtures containing aluminum hydroxide, calcium carbonate, and magnesium hydroxide are available (Camalox), and the usual dose is 15–30 mL. A paradoxic calcium-induced gastric hypersecretion has been reported but probably has no clinical significance with this combination agent. However, when calcium carbonate (Tums) alone is used, there may be hypercalcemia and its attendant complications.

**4. Sucralfate (Carafate)**–This nonabsorbable aluminum salt of sucrose octasulfate is a mucosal protective agent that has antipepsin activity and tends to adhere to areas of gastric and duodenal mucosal injuries, eg, ulcers. It is as effective with duodenal ulcer as antacids or $H_2$ receptor blockers and has the advantage of being nonsystemic. The only side effect reported to date is mild constipation in about 5% of patients. Dosage is 1 g 30–60 minutes before meals and at bedtime. Antacids may be used when necessary but not within 1 hour of sucralfate.

**5. Histamine $H_2$ receptor antagonists**–

**a. Cimetidine (Tagamet)**–This drug markedly inhibits gastric secretion stimulated by food, gastrin, histamine, and caffeine. Cimetidine is approved in the USA for short-term treatment of duodenal ulcer and gastric ulcer, for use in preventing recurrence of duodenal ulcer (up to 1 year), for management of Zollinger-Ellison syndrome, and for treatment of other hypersecretory states such as systemic mastocytosis. The dosage is 300 mg 4 times daily before meals and at bedtime. An alternative dosage is 400 mg twice daily. The dose must be reduced by half in patients with renal insufficiency. An intravenous form is available. The dosage, depending on the indication, is usually 300 mg every 6 hours, or, preferably, the same dosage by drip, ie, at a rate of 50 mg/h.

Rare side effects have included gynecomastia, galactorrhea, impotence, skin rashes, leukopenia, agranulocytosis, hepatitis, elevated serum creatinine, decreased IgA and IgM, and confusion in the elderly. Of more concern are interactions between cimetidine and warfarin, theophylline, lidocaine, phenytoin, and other drugs, which occur via the P-450 cytochrome system of the liver.

**b. Ranitidine (Zantac)**–This $H_2$ receptor antagonist is more potent than cimetidine and does not interfere with the metabolism of drugs that use the P-450 cytochrome system of the liver. Ranitidine is of value in treatment of duodenal ulcer, benign gastric ulcer, and Zollinger-Ellison syndrome. It is approved in the USA for treatment of active duodenal ulcer disease and Zollinger-Ellison syndrome. The dosage is 150 mg every 12 hours or 300 mg at dinnertime. An intravenous form of ranitidine is available; the dosage is 50 mg every 6 hours or (and preferably) 8.3 mg/h by continuous infusion.

Rare side effects have included mild serum transaminase elevation (more common with intravenous administration), decreases in white blood cell and platelet counts, false-positive tests for proteinuria with Multistix, and some increase in headaches. Gynecomastia and impotence secondary to cimetidine have reversed when ranitidine is substituted. There have been no reports of galactorrhea or definite drug interactions.

**c. Famotidine (Pepcid)**–This newly released $H_2$ receptor antagonist is more potent than either ranitidine or cimetidine. The full therapeutic dose is 40 mg at dinnertime. Clinical experience with this drug is still limited.

**6. Sedatives**–Tense and apprehensive patients will usually benefit greatly from sedation. Hypnotic doses of the drugs may be necessary to ensure sleep.

**7. Parasympatholytic (anticholinergic) drugs**–Although the parasympatholytic drugs have been widely used over a long period of time for treatment of peptic ulcer, their effectiveness is questionable. Their usefulness is limited largely to the relief of refractory pain. The dosage necessary to produce significant gastric antisecretory effect may cause blurring of vision, constipation, urinary retention, and tachycardia. If patients have gastric retention, these drugs are contraindicated.

*Note:* Belladonna and other anticholinergic drugs should be avoided in patients with glaucoma, esophageal reflux, gastric ulcer, pyloric obstruction, cardiospasm, gastrointestinal hemorrhage, bladder neck obstruction, or serious myocardial disease.

a. Belladonna extract (tincture, 0.25 mg/mL), 10–15 drops, or atropine, 0.25–0.5 mg, 20–30 minutes before meals and at bedtime with or without sedatives.

b. Synthetic parasympatholytics—Numerous proprietary tertiary and quaternary amines are available as belladonna or atropine substitutes. Although they do not have central nervous system side effects, it is difficult to substantiate other therapeutic advantages. They are also more expensive.

**B. Convalescent Phase:**

**1. Reexamination**–Once the diagnosis is established, it is unnecessary to repeat the gastrointestinal series unless complications develop. Anticholinergic therapy, if used, should be discontinued 72 hours prior to x-ray examination for duodenal ulcer.

**2. Education of patient regarding recurrences**–The patient should be informed about the chronic and recurrent nature of the illness and warned about the complications of careless or improper treatment. Although the cause of ulcer recurrence is not known, it may be associated with irregular eating habits, irregular living habits (long or irregular hours), use of alcohol or tobacco, emotional stress, and infections, particularly of the upper respiratory tract. The patient should be instructed to return to the ulcer regimen if symptoms recur or if conditions known to aggravate the ulcer cannot be avoided. Antacids or other medications should be readily available.

**3. Rest and recreation**–Provisions should be made for rest and recreation to promote physical and mental relaxation.

**C. Treatment of Complications:**

**1. Hemorrhage**–Institute immediate emergency measures for treatment of hemorrhage and shock (see p 348).

**2. Perforation**–Acute perforation constitutes a surgical emergency. Immediate surgical repair, preferably by simple surgical closure, is indicated. More extensive operations may be unwise at the time of the acute episode because of the increased operative hazard due to the patient's poor physical condition. If the patient has had no previous therapy or if previous therapy has been inadequate, conservative medical treatment should be instituted.

The morbidity and mortality rates depend upon the amount of spillage and especially the time lapse between perforation and surgery. Surgical closure of the perforation is indicated as soon as possible. If surgery is delayed beyond 24 hours, gastric suction, antibiotics, and intravenous fluids are the treatment of choice.

**3. Obstruction**–Obstruction due to spasm and edema can usually be treated adequately by gastric decompression and ulcer therapy; obstruction due to scar formation requires surgery. It must be remembered that the obstruction may not represent a complication of an ulcer but may be due to a primary neoplastic disease, especially in those patients with no history or only a short history of peptic ulcer.

**a. Medical measures** (for obstruction due to spasm or edema) consist of bed rest, preferably in a hospital; continuous gastric suction for 72 hours; and parenteral administration of electrolytes and fluids. After 72 hours, test the degree of residual obstruction with the saline load test. Instill 700 mL of normal saline into the stomach with the patient at least sitting, and aspirate the contents after 30 minutes. If less than 200 mL is recovered, begin liquid feeding. If the residual volume is greater than 200 mL, obstruction is still present and the patient is usually a surgical candidate. Do not use anticholinergic drugs, since they delay gastric emptying. Give sedative-tranquilizer drugs and a progressive diet as tolerated. Use antacids as with uncomplicated ulcer.

**b. Surgical measures** (for obstruction due to scarring) are indicated only after a thorough trial of conservative measures.

## Prognosis

Duodenal ulcer tends to have a chronic course with remissions and exacerbations. Many patients can be adequately controlled by medical management. About 25% develop complications, and 5–10% ultimately require surgery for obstruction, uncontrollable pain, or recurrent bleeding. The recurrence rate is substantially reduced if the patient stops smoking and is given an $H_2$ receptor blocking agent at dinnertime or sulcralfate twice a day for at least 1 year.

Blum AL: Therapeutic approach to ulcer healing. *Am J Med* 1985;**79 (Suppl 2C):**8.

Collen MJ et al: Comparison of ranitidine and cimetidine in the treatment of gastric hypersecretion. *Ann Intern Med* 1984;**100:**52.

Collier DSJ, Pain JA: Non-steroidal anti-inflammatory drugs and peptic ulcer perforation. *Gut* 1985;**26:**359.

Dooley CP et al: Double contrast barium meal and upper gastrointestinal endoscopy: A comparative study. *Ann Intern Med* 1984;**101:**538.

Forsell H et al (editors): Symposium on antacids. *Scand J Gastroenterol* 1982;**17 (Suppl 75):**1.

Isenberg JI, Johanssen C: Peptic ulcer disease. *Clin Gastroenterol* 1984;**13:**287.

Johansson C et al (editors): Symposium: Frontiers in gastroduodenal disease. *Scand J Gastroenterol* 1985;**20 (Suppl 110):**1.

Kurata JH, Haile BM, Elashoff JD: Sex differences in peptic ulcer disease. *Gastroenterology* 1985;**88:**96.

Legerton CW (editor): Symposium on management of the ulcer patient: Therapeutic advances. *Am J Med* 1984;**17 (Nov Suppl):**1.

Peura DA, Johnson LF: Cimetidine for prevention and treatment of gastroduodenal mucosal lesions in patients in an intensive care unit. *Ann Intern Med* 1985;**103:**173.

Sedman AJ: Cimetidine-drug interactions. (Review.) *Am J Med* 1984;**76:**109.

Wormsley KG: Assessing the safety of drugs for the long-term treatment of peptic ulcers. *Gut* 1984;**25:**1416.

## 2. ZOLLINGER-ELLISON SYNDROME (Gastrinoma)

### Essentials of Diagnosis

- Severe peptic ulcer disease.
- Gastric hypersecretion.
- Elevated serum gastrin.
- Gastrinoma of pancreas, duodenum, or other ectopic site.

### General Considerations

Zollinger-Ellison peptic ulceration syndrome, although uncommon, is not rare. Sixty percent of patients are males. Onset may be at any age from early childhood on but is most common in persons 20–50 years old. Most patients have the gastrin-secreting tumor in the pancreas; a few have tumors in the submucosa of the duodenum and stomach, the hilum of the spleen, and the regional lymph nodes. They may be either single or multiple. Approximately two-thirds of Zollinger-Ellison tumors are malignant with respect either to their biologic behavior or to their histologic appearance.

## Clinical Findings

**A. Symptoms and Signs:** Pain is of the typical peptic ulcer variety but is more difficult to control by medical means. Diarrhea may occur secondary to the hypersecretion or as a result of inactivation of lipase when the intraluminal pH of the small bowel falls below 6.5, thus interfering with fat digestion. Hemorrhage, perforation, and obstruction occur commonly.

**B. Laboratory Findings:** The most reliable means of establishing the diagnosis of Zollinger-Ellison syndrome is measurement of serum gastrin by radioimmunoassay. Patients with Zollinger-Ellison syndrome usually have serum gastrin levels higher than 300 pg/mL. Serum calcium levels are useful in revealing hypercalcemia to evaluate the possibility of hyperparathyroidism and multiple endocrine adenomatosis. Gastric analysis reveals basal gastric hypersecretion ($>$ 15 meq/h). Maximal acid output following stimulation with pentagastrin does not show the increased rate of gastric acid secretion as much as in normal people or in patients with peptic ulcer disease not of the Zollinger-Ellison type. In the Zollinger-Ellison patient, the basal acid output is greater than 60% of the maximal output, while in ordinary peptic ulcer disease the basal output is usually substantially less than 60% of the maximal. Intravenous secretin causes a marked elevation of serum gastrin in patients with gastrinomas and is of use in diagnosis.

**C. Imaging:** Gastrointestinal series reveal that 75% of the ulcers are in the first part of the duodenum and that the ulcers are usually not multiple. Ulcers occurring in the second, third, or fourth portion of the duodenum or in the jejunum are strongly suggestive of Zollinger-Ellison syndrome. Coarseness of the proximal jejunal folds and radiographic evidence of gastric hypersecretion also suggest Zollinger-Ellison syndrome.

## Treatment

$H_2$ receptor blockers have been shown to markedly inhibit gastric acid secretion in patients with gastrinoma and have brought about healing of ulcers, but doses 4–10 times higher than conventional ones may be required. In patients poorly controlled with $H_2$ receptor blockers alone, vagotomy and pyloroplasty may also be necessary.

Jin GL, Braasch JW, Rossi RL: Surgical management of gastrinoma. *Surg Clin North Am* 1985;**65:**285.

Townsend CM Jr, Thompson JC: Surgical management of tumors that produce gastrointestinal hormones. *Annu Rev Med* 1985;**36:**111.

## 3. GASTRIC ULCER

### Essentials of Diagnosis

- Epigastric distress on an empty stomach, relieved by food, antacids, or vomiting.
- Epigastric tenderness and voluntary muscle guarding.

- Anemia, occult blood in stool, gastric acid.
- Ulcer demonstrated by x-ray or gastroscopy.
- Acid present on gastric analysis.

## General Considerations

Benign gastric ulcer is in many respects similar to duodenal ulcer. Acid gastric juice is necessary for its production, but decreased tissue resistance appears to play a more important role than hypersecretion. Most patients have a history of aspirin or other nonsteroidal anti-inflammatory drug use.

About 60% of benign gastric ulcers are found within 6 cm of the pylorus. The ulcers are generally located at or near the lesser curvature and most frequently on the posterior wall. Another 25% of the ulcers are located higher on the lesser curvature.

If the radiographic appearance of the ulcer is benign, the occurrence of carcinoma is about 3.3%. If it is indeterminate (features of both benignancy and malignancy), it is approximately 9.5%. With evidence of associated duodenal ulcer, it is about 1%.

## Clinical Findings

**A. Symptoms and Signs:** There may be no symptoms, or only vague and atypical symptoms. The epigastric distress is typically described as gnawing, burning, aching, or "hunger pangs," referred at times to the left subcostal area. Episodes occur usually 45–60 minutes after a meal and are relieved by food, alkalies, or vomiting. Nausea and vomiting are frequent complaints. There may be a history of remissions and exacerbations, especially if patients are taking aspirin or other nonsteroidal analgesics. Weight loss and fatigue are common.

Epigastric tenderness or voluntary muscle guarding is usually the only finding.

**B. Laboratory Findings:** If bleeding has occurred, there may be hypochromic anemia or occult blood in the stool. The gastric analysis always shows an acid pH after pentagastrin and usually the presence of low normal to normal secretion.

**C. Other Examinations:** An upper gastrointestinal series is the usual initial diagnostic procedure for the non-actively bleeding patient suspected of having a gastric ulcer. When the radiographic appearance of the ulcer is not clearly benign or when an ulcer is not 75% healed by 8 weeks or completely healed by 12 weeks, peroral endoscopy with multiple biopsies (6–10) of the ulcer margin and base is indicated to rule out cancer.

## Differential Diagnosis

The symptoms of gastric ulcer, especially if atypical, must be differentiated from those of gastritis and functional gastrointestinal distress.

Most important is the differentiation of benign from malignant gastric ulcer. A favorable response to adequate medical management is presumptive evidence that the lesion is not malignant. Malignant ulcers may respond initially, but residual changes at the site usually demonstrate the nature of the process.

## Complications

Hemorrhage, perforation, and obstruction may occur. (See Complications of Duodenal Ulcer, p 365.)

## Treatment

Ulcer treatment (as for duodenal ulcer) should be intensive. Aspirin and other nonsteroidal anti-inflammatory agents must be avoided. Repeat x-rays should be obtained to document the rate of healing at 4- to 8-week intervals. Failure to respond in 8–12 weeks with significant healing may be an indication for surgical resection in the patient who has no contraindication to surgery. Gastroscopy and biopsy should be repeated. Histamine $H_2$ receptor antagonists or sucralfate are as effective as antacids in healing gastric ulcer. However, even a carcinoma may show improvement on an ulcer regimen, and clinical relief does not necessarily mean that the ulcer is benign. Follow-up at 3 and 6 months after apparently complete healing is therefore indicated. In the event of recurrence under intensive medical management, perforation, obstruction, or massive uncontrollable hemorrhage, surgery is mandatory.

## Prognosis

Gastric ulcers tend to be recurrent. There is no evidence that malignant degeneration of gastric peptic ulceration ever occurs. Recurrent uncomplicated ulcer is not a serious event, and, in fact, it may heal more readily than the previous ulcer.

Adkins RB et al: The management of gastric ulcers: A current review. *Ann Surg* 1985;**201**:741.
Gastric ulcer or cancer? (Editorial.) *Lancet* 1985;**1**:202.
Kelly KA, Malagelada JR: Medical and surgical treatment of chronic gastric ulcer. *Clin Gastroenterol* 1984;**13**:621.

## 4. STOMAL (MARGINAL) ULCER (Jejunal Ulcer)

Marginal ulcer should be suspected when there is a history of operation for an ulcer followed by recurrence of abdominal symptoms after a symptom-free interval of months to years. The marginal ulcer incidence after simple gastroenterostomy is 15–20%; after subtotal gastrectomy or vagotomy and antrectomy, about 2%. Nearly all of the ulcers are jejunal, and the others are located on the gastric side of the anastomosis.

## Clinical Findings

The abdominal pain is burning or gnawing, often more severe than the preoperative ulcer pain, and is located lower in the epigastrium, even below the umbilicus and often to the left. The pain often covers a wider area and may radiate to the back.

The "food-pain rhythm" of peptic ulcer distress frequently occurs earlier (within an hour) in marginal ulcer as a result of more rapid emptying time; and relief with antacids, food, and milk may be incomplete and of short duration. Nausea, vomiting, and weight loss are common. Hematemesis occurs frequently. Low epigastric tenderness with voluntary muscle guarding is usually present. An inflammatory mass may be palpated. Anemia and occult blood in the stool are common. On radiography, the ulcer niche at the stoma is often difficult to demonstrate or differentiate from postsurgical defects, despite use of compression films. Gastroscopy is the most effective means of diagnosing stomal ulcer.

## Differential Diagnosis

Stomal ulcer must be differentiated from functional gastrointestinal distress, especially in a patient concerned about the possibility of recurrence of an ulcer after surgery. Atypical symptoms must be differentiated from "bile" gastritis and from biliary tract or pancreatic disease. Consider the possibility of Zollinger-Ellison syndrome.

## Complications

Complications include gross hemorrhage, perforation, stenosis of the stoma, and gastrojejunocolic fistula.

## Treatment

Stomal ulcers are often resistant to medical therapy; vagotomy or a more extensive gastrectomy is usually necessary to decrease the acid secretion of the stomach.

Histamine $H_2$ receptor antagonists as used in treatment of duodenal and gastric ulcer often lead to healing.

X-ray therapy to the stomach will substantially reduce the gastric secretion of hydrochloric acid and in some instances may induce achlorhydria for varying periods of time. Since the advent of $H_2$ antagonists, the use of x-ray therapy has been restricted to a few instances of complicating disease leading to increased surgical risk and to elderly patients.

Kennedy T, Green WER: Stomal and recurrent ulceration: Medical or surgical management? *Am J Surg* 1980;**139:**18.

## POSTGASTRECTOMY SYNDROMES

### Dumping Syndrome

Postgastrectomy dumping syndrome probably occurs in about 10% of patients after partial gastrectomy. The pathogenesis is complex and incompletely understood. The disorder is provoked mainly by soluble hypertonic carbohydrates, which, when present in the small intestine, have an osmotic effect resulting in rapid flow of fluid into the small intestine; increase in free plasma kinins; increase in peripheral blood flow; and a modest drop in plasma volume with a corresponding increase in hematocrit and a mild decrease in serum potassium. Whether sympathetic vasomotor responses contribute to the syndrome is uncertain.

One or more of the following symptoms occur within 20 minutes after meals: sweating, tachycardia, pallor, epigastric fullness and grumbling, warmth, nausea, abdominal cramps, weakness, and, in severe cases, syncope, vomiting, or diarrhea. Nonspecific electrocardiographic changes may be noted. Plasma glucose is not low during an attack.

It is important to distinguish this syndrome from the reactive hypoglycemia that occurs in some postgastrectomy patients. This latter syndrome occurs much later after the meal (1–3 hours) and is relieved by the ingestion of food.

Changing the diet to frequent (6) small, equal feedings high in protein, moderately high in fat, and low in simple carbohydrates usually lessens the severity of symptoms. Fluids should not be taken with meals. Sedative and anticholinergic drugs may be of value.

### Afferent (Blind) Loop Syndrome

The afferent loop syndrome occurs after Billroth II gastrectomy or gastrojejunostomy. The syndrome may occur acutely early in the postoperative period or months to years following operation. An acute abdominal catastrophe (rare) may require emergency operation to release the obstruction and follow-up measures to prevent recurrence. More commonly, afferent loop syndrome is caused by chronic or recurring partial obstruction, although the exact etiologic mechanisms are not clear. The symptoms are caused by distention of and stasis within the afferent loop of the gastrojejunostomy. Typically, abdominal pain occurs 15–30 minutes after eating and is relieved by vomiting of bile fluid that does not contain food.

Poor emptying of the afferent loop may result in stasis of contents, leading to bacterial overgrowth. This in turn may lead to deficiency of vitamin $B_{12}$ because of bacterial uptake of vitamin $B_{12}$. Deconjugation of bile salts may also occur, with subsequent impairment of micelle formation, leading to steatorrhea and its attendant complications. This complication is not usually associated with obstructive symptoms.

Avoidance of the Billroth II procedure will prevent the afferent loop from occurring. Surgical reconstruction of the afferent loop to produce better emptying is the treatment of choice. Bacterial overgrowth can be temporarily controlled with repeated 7- to 10-day courses of a broad-spectrum antibiotic, such as tetracycline, 250 mg 4 times daily. With vitamin $B_{12}$ deficiency, vitamin $B_{12}$ should be administered.

### Bile Reflux

Bile reflux is one of the most debilitating complications following gastric surgery. Bile reflux may occur after cholecystectomy and occasionally with no prior surgery. Typically, the patient experiences nausea, substernal distress, and anorexia. Vomiting or reflux of clear bile-stained fluid may occur.

Medical management is unsatisfactory. The surgical approach is a diversion of bile from the stomach. The Roux-en-Y gastrojejunostomy procedure serves this end.

## Other Postgastrectomy Syndromes

Other complications that may follow gastric surgery include reflux esophagitis, gastric retention, postvagotomy diarrhea, and the development of carcinoma in the gastric stump many years after surgery. Iron deficiency anemia occurs in 50% of patients 5 years or longer after a Billroth II gastrectomy, because of the bypassing of the duodenum, the major locus for iron absorption. The incidence of pulmonary tuberculosis is thought to be increased after gastrectomy.

Buxbaum KL: Bile gastritis occurring after cholecystectomy. *Am J Gastroenterol* 1982;**77:**305.
Horowitz M, Collins PJ, Shearman DJC: Disorders of gastric emptying in humans and the use of radionuclide techniques. *Arch Intern Med* 1985;**145:**1467.
Meyer JH: Chronic morbidity after ulcer surgery. Pages 757–779 in: *Gastrointestinal Disease: Pathophysiology, Diagnosis, Management,* 3rd ed. Sleisenger MH, Fordtran JS (editors). Saunders, 1983.
Thompson SC, Wiener I: Evaluation of surgical treatment of duodenal ulcer: Short-term and long-term effects. *Clin Gastroenterol* 1984;**13:**564.

## CARCINOMA OF THE STOMACH

### Essentials of Diagnosis

- Upper gastrointestinal symptoms with weight loss in patients over age 40.
- Palpable abdominal mass (very late).
- Anemia, occult blood in stools, positive cytologic examination.
- Gastroscopic and x-ray abnormality.

### General Considerations

Carcinoma of the stomach is a common cancer of the digestive tract. It occurs predominantly in males over 40 years of age. Delay of diagnosis is caused by absence of definite early symptoms and by the fact that patients treat themselves instead of seeking early medical advice. Further delays are due to the equivocal nature of early findings and to temporary improvement with symptomatic therapy.

A history of the following possibly precancerous conditions should alert the physician to the danger of stomach cancer:

**(1) Atrophic gastritis of pernicious anemia:** The incidence of adenomas and carcinomas is *significantly increased.*

**(2) Chronic gastritis, particularly atrophic gastritis:** There is a wide variation in the reported incidence of gastritis with cancer, and a definite relationship has not been proved.

**(3) Gastric ulcer:** The major problem is in the differentiation between benign and malignant ulcer.

**(4) Achlorhydria:** The incidence of lowered secretory potential in early life is higher in those patients who later develop carcinoma.

**(5)** Patients who have had a partial gastrectomy for peptic ulcer 10–15 years previously may have an increased risk of gastric cancer.

Carcinoma may originate anywhere in the stomach. Grossly, lesions tend to be of 4 types (Borrman):

**Type I:** Polypoid, intraluminal mass.

**Type II:** Noninfiltrating ulcer.

**Type III:** Infiltrating ulcer.

**Type IV:** Diffuse infiltrating process (to linitis plastica).

Gross typing generally correlates better with prognosis than the histologic grading of malignancy, ie, type I has a better prognosis than type II, etc.

### Clinical Findings

**A. Symptoms and Signs:** Early gastric carcinoma, such as is detected in the mass surveys in Japan, causes no symptoms. The appearance of symptoms implies relatively advanced disease. The patient may complain of vague fullness, nausea, a sensation of pressure, belching, and heartburn after meals, with or without anorexia (especially for meat). These symptoms in association with weight loss and a decline in general health and strength in a man over age 40 years should suggest the possibility of stomach cancer. Diarrhea, hematemesis, and melena may be present.

Specific symptoms may be determined in part by the location of the tumor. A peptic ulcer-like syndrome generally occurs with ulcerated lesions (types II and III) and in the presence of acid secretion but may occur with complete achlorhydria. Unfortunately, symptomatic relief from antacids tends to delay diagnosis. Symptoms of pyloric obstruction are progressive postprandial fullness to vomiting of almost all ingested foods. Lower esophageal obstruction causes progressive dysphagia and regurgitation. Early satiety usually occurs with linitis plastica but may be seen with other cancers.

Physical findings are usually limited to weight loss and, if anemia is present, pallor. In about 20% of cases, a palpable abdominal mass is present; this does not necessarily mean that the lesion is inoperable. Liver or peripheral metastases may also be present.

**B. Laboratory Findings:** Achlorhydria (gastric pH > 6.0) after stimulation with pentagastrin, 6 $\mu$g/kg intramuscularly or subcutaneously, in the presence of a gastric ulcer is virtually pathognomonic of cancer; but this finding is present in only about 20% of patients with gastric cancer. The presence of acid does not exclude cancer. If bleeding occurs, there will be occult blood in the stool and mild to severe anemia. With bone marrow invasion, the anemia rarely may be normochromic and normocytic.

**C. Other Examinations:** Endoscopic biopsy and directed cytology and expert lavage cytology with chymotrypsin will provide the correct diagnosis in almost every case. These methods will also establish the important differential diagnosis between adenocarcinoma and the malignant lymphomas.

### Differential Diagnosis

The symptoms of carcinoma of the stomach are often mistaken for those of benign gastric ulcer, chronic gastritis, irritable colon syndrome, or functional gastrointestinal disturbance; x-ray and gastroscopic findings must be differentiated from those of benign gastric ulcer or tumor. Nonhealing ulcers or ulcers that are enlarging with a strict ulcer regimen require surgery. Most of these will still be benign.

The clinical history of gastric leiomyosarcoma may be indistinguishable from that of carcinoma. Bleeding, particularly massive, is more common. These tumors account for approximately 1.5% of gastric cancers. A palpable mass is more frequent than in gastric carcinoma, and the x-ray picture is characteristically that of a well-circumscribed intramural mass with, frequently, a central crater.

With the decreasing incidence of carcinoma of the stomach in the USA, gastric lymphoma now accounts for about 10% of gastric malignant disease. It is an important consideration in patients presenting with enlarged gastric folds, masses, or ulcerations. Biopsy and cytologic examination are essential in establishing the diagnosis. The prognosis is much more favorable than in patients with carcinoma; cure may be anticipated in over half of patients if the tumor is confined to the stomach.

### Treatment

Surgical resection is the only curative treatment. Signs of metastatic disease include a hard, nodular liver, enlarged left supraclavicular (Virchow's) nodes, skin nodules, ascites, rectal shelf, and x-ray evidence of osseous or pulmonary metastasis. If none of these are present and there is no other contraindication to operation, exploration is indicated. The presence of an abdominal mass is not a contraindication to laparotomy, since bulky lesions can often be totally excised. Palliative resection or gastroenterostomy is occasionally helpful. High-voltage x-ray therapy may be of some value. Multiple-drug regimens are under study. Mitomycin C, 5-fluorouracil, adriamycin, and cytarabine (cytosine arabinoside) in various combinations have been reported to be beneficial.

For gastric lymphoma, the treatment is surgical excision, radiation, or a combination of the two.

### Prognosis

There is wide variation in the biologic malignancy of gastric carcinomas. In many, the disease is widespread before symptoms are apparent; in a fortunate few, slow growth may progress over years and be resectable even at a late date. Approximately 10% of all patients with gastric carcinoma will be cured by surgical resection.

Scott HW Jr, Adkins RB Jr, Sawyers JL: Results of an aggressive surgical approach to gastric carcinoma during a twenty-three-year period. *Surgery* 1985;**97**:55.

Yan C, Brooks JR: Surgical management of gastric adenocarcinoma. *Am J Surg* 1985;**149**:771.

## BENIGN TUMORS OF THE STOMACH

Most benign tumors do not cause symptoms and often are so small that they are overlooked on x-ray examination. Their importance lies in the problem of differentiation from malignant lesions, their precancerous possibilities, and the fact that they occasionally cause symptoms.

These tumors may be of epithelial origin (eg, adenomas, papillomas) or mesenchymal origin (eg, leiomyomas, fibromas, hemofibromas, lipomas, hemangiomas). The mesenchymal tumors, which are intramural, rarely undergo malignant change. Most polyps of the stomach are hyperplastic ones with no malignant potential. Adenomas have a small but unknown potential for malignant change.

### Clinical Findings

**A. Symptoms and Signs:** Large tumors may cause a vague feeling of epigastric fullness or heaviness; tumors located near the cardia or pylorus may produce symptoms of obstruction. If bleeding occurs, it will cause symptoms and signs of acute gastrointestinal hemorrhage (eg, tarry stools, syncope, sweating, vomiting of blood). Chronic blood loss will cause symptoms of anemia (fatigue, dyspnea). If the tumor is large, a movable epigastric mass may be palpable.

**B. Laboratory Findings:** The usual laboratory findings may be present.

**C. Imaging:** The radiograph is characterized by a smooth filling defect, clearly circumscribed, which does not interfere with normal pliability or peristalsis. Larger tumors may show a small central crater, especially leiomyomas.

### Treatment & Prognosis

If symptoms occur (particularly hemorrhage), surgical resection is necessary. If there are no symptoms, the patient does not require surgery. These tumors may even regress spontaneously. Polyps may be excised by endoscopic electroresection.

Feczko PJ et al: Gastric polyps: Radiological evaluation and clinical significance. *Radiology* 1985;**155**:581.

# DISEASES OF THE INTESTINES

## REGIONAL ENTERITIS
### (Regional Ileitis, Granulomatous Ileocolitis, Crohn's Disease)
### (See also Granulomatous Colitis, Below.)

### Essentials of Diagnosis
- Insidious onset.
- Intermittent bouts of diarrhea, low-grade fever, and right lower quadrant pain.
- Fistula formation or right lower quadrant mass and tenderness (late finding).
- Radiographic evidence of abnormality of the terminal ileum.

### General Considerations
Regional enteritis is a chronic inflammatory disease that may involve the alimentary tract anywhere from the mouth to the anus. The ileum is the principal site of the disease, either alone or in conjunction with the colon and jejunum. It generally occurs in young adults and runs an intermittent clinical course with mild to severe disability and frequent complications.

There is marked thickening of the submucosa with lymphedema, lymphoid hyperplasia, nonspecific granulomas, and often ulceration of the overlying mucosa. A marked lymphadenitis occurs in the mesenteric nodes.

The cause is unknown. Genetic factors appear to play a role. There is a higher than normal incidence in monozygotic twins and a greater than random familial incidence. The most common familial pattern involves 2 or more affected siblings. Regional enteritis and chronic ulcerative colitis occur in the same families. The possibility of an infectious origin for regional enteritis has been raised by studies demonstrating transmission of an agent from tissues with regional enteritis into immunologically deficient mice and rabbits, but no agent to date has been substantiated.

### Clinical Findings
**A. Symptoms and Signs:** The disease is characterized by exacerbations and remissions. Colicky or steady abdominal pain is present in the right lower quadrant or periumbilical area at some time during the course of the disease and varies from mild to severe. Diarrhea may occur, usually with intervening periods of normal bowel function or constipation. Patients with these symptoms are often diagnosed as having irritable or functional bowel disease. Fever may be low-grade or, rarely, spiking with chills. Anorexia, flatulence, malaise, and weight loss are present. Milk products and chemically or mechanically irritating foods may aggravate symptoms.

Abdominal tenderness is usually present, especially in the right lower quadrant, with signs of peritoneal irritation and an abdominal or pelvic mass in the same area. The mass is tender and varies from a sausagelike thickened intestine to matted loops of intestine.

Regional enteritis may pursue various clinical patterns. In certain instances, the course is indolent and the symptomatology mild. In other instances, the course is toxic, with fever, toxic erythema, arthralgia, anemia, etc. Still other patients pursue courses complicated by stricture or perforations of the bowel and suppurative complications of intra-abdominal perforation.

**B. Laboratory Findings:** There is usually a hypochromic (occasionally macrocytic due to vitamin $B_{12}$ malabsorption) anemia and occult blood in the stool. The small bowel x-ray may show mucosal irregularity, ulceration, stiffening of the bowel wall, and luminal narrowing. Barium enema may show fissures or deep ulcers. Eccentric involvement, skipped areas of involvement, and strictures suggest Crohn's disease of the colon. Sigmoidoscopic examination may show an edematous hyperemic mucosa or a discrete ulcer when the colon is involved.

### Differential Diagnosis
Acute regional enteritis may simulate acute appendicitis. Location in the terminal ileum requires differentiation from intestinal tuberculosis, *Yersinia enterocolitica* infection, and lymphomas. Regional enteritis involving the colon must be distinguished from idiopathic ulcerative colitis, amebic colitis, ischemic colitis, and infectious disease of the colon. The sigmoidoscopic and x-ray criteria distinguishing these various entities may not be absolute, and definitive diagnosis may require cultures, examinations of the stool for parasites, and biopsy in selected instances.

### Complications
Ischiorectal and perianal fistulas occur frequently. Fistulas may occur to the bladder or vagina and even to the skin in the area of a previous scar. Mechanical intestinal obstruction may occur. Nutritional deficiency caused by malabsorption and maldigestion (the latter caused by a decreased bile salt pool) may produce a spruelike syndrome. Generalized peritonitis is rare because perforation occurs slowly, is locally contained, or results in internal fistulization. The incidence of colon or rectal cancer in regional enteritis patients is greater than in a control population, but less than for ulcerative colitis. Migratory peripheral synovitis and axial arthropathy indistinguishable from sporadic ankylosing spondylitis may occur.

### Treatment & Prognosis
**A. General Measures:** The diet should be high in calories and vitamins and adequate in protein. Raw fruits and vegetables should be avoided in patients who have obstructive symptoms. These patients may benefit from a nonresidue, well-balanced diet to main-

tain nutrition until obstructive symptoms subside. Anemia, dehydration, diarrhea, and avitaminosis should be treated as indicated.

**B. Antimicrobial Agents:** In our present state of knowledge about this disease, antimicrobials are indicated only for specific infectious problems, ie, abscess, fistulas.

**1. Sulfasalazine**–Sulfasalazine (Azulfidine), 2–8 g/d orally, has been shown to be effective. The salicylate moiety of sulfasalazine, 5-aminosalicylic acid, appears to be of equal efficacy without the side effects attributable to the sulfapyridine portion of sulfasalazine. 5-Aminosalicylic acid will soon be available for use.

**2. Antibiotics**–In cases of acute suppuration (manifested by tender mass, fever, leukocytosis), ampicillin, 4–8 g/d intravenously or 2–4 g/d orally, may be useful. Clindamycin and aminoglycosides are also effective. In cases where internal fistulization has led to a defunctionalized loop with bacterial overgrowth or where stricture formation has led to small bowel stasis with malabsorption, tetracycline, 1–2 g/d orally, may be valuable in combating bacterial overgrowth in the bowel and correcting absorptive malfunction.

**3. Metronidazole**–Metronidazole, 20 mg/kg/d, has been advocated for enterocutaneous fistulas.

**C. Adrenocortical Hormones:** These agents are often of use in the diffuse form of the disease and are particularly helpful in the toxic forms (arthritis, anemia, toxic erythemas). The complications of long-term therapy can be minimized by administering the drug on an alternate-day schedule (eg, prednisone, 15–40 mg every other day) once the patient's clinical symptoms have been brought under control. The National Cooperative Crohn's Disease Study conducted a randomized double-blind study comparing prednisone, sulfasalazine, and azathioprine in the treatment of regional enteritis. These data indicated that sulfasalazine and prednisone are effective in the acute phase of the disease but do not exert a prophylactic effect. In the national cooperative study, azathioprine proved to be of no value, though perhaps the observation period may have been too short. More recent studies indicate that mercaptopurine, the active metabolite of azathioprine, has a beneficial effect on the fistulas of Crohn's disease as well as on other features of the disease.

**D. Other Medical Measures:** When terminal ileal disease is present, vitamin B$_{12}$ supplementation is often necessary. Calcium supplementation in the form of calcium gluconate or Os-Cal will alleviate the frequent calcium deficiency seen in these patients and is also helpful in decreasing excessive oxalate absorption, resulting in lowered incidence of oxalate urinary tract stones.

**E. Surgical Measures:** Surgical treatment of this disease is best limited to the management of its complications. Resection of the small bowel, particularly the extensive resection often necessary in regional enteritis, leads to a "short bowel" syndrome

(diminished absorptive surface), ie, malabsorption of vitamin B$_{12}$ to varying degrees (loss of terminal ileum), hyperoxaluria, steatorrhea, osteomalacia, and macrocytic anemia (due to folic acid and vitamin B$_{12}$ deficiency). Short-circuiting operations may lead to blind loops (intestinal defunctionalization with bacterial overgrowth) with similar difficulties in absorption. When surgery is necessary in this disease, study of postsurgical bowel function is indicated to detect the possibility of impaired bowel function. If defects in absorption are present, appropriate therapy may prevent serious complications.

Dworken HJ: Crohn disease. (Editorial.) *Ann Intern Med* 1984;**101**:258.

Farmer RG, Whelan G, Fazio VW: Longterm follow-up of patient with Crohn's disease: Relationship between the clinical pattern and prognosis. *Gastroenterology* 1985;**88**:1818.

Glotzer DJ: The risk of cancer in Crohn's disease. *Gastroenterology* 1985;**89**:438.

Korelitz BI, Present DH: Favorable effect of 6-mercaptopurine on fistulae of Crohn's disease. *Dig Dis Sci* 1985;**30**:58.

Lee ECG: Aim of surgical treatment of Crohn's disease. *Gut* 1984;**25**:217.

Puntis J, McNeish AS, Allan RN: Long-term prognosis of Crohn's disease with onset in childhood and adolescence. *Gut* 1984;**25**:329.

Singleton JW (editor): The National Cooperative Crohn's Disease Study. *Gastroenterology* 1979;**74**:825.

Ursing B et al: A comparative study of metronidazole and sulfasalazine for active Crohn's disease: The cooperative Crohn's disease study in Sweden. 2. Result. *Gastroenterology* 1982;**83**:550.

Whelan G et al: Recurrence after surgery in Crohn's disease: Relationship to location of disease (clinical pattern) and surgical indications. *Gastroenterology* 1985;**88**:1826.

## TUMORS OF THE SMALL INTESTINE

Benign and malignant tumors of the small intestine are rare. There may be no symptoms or signs, but bleeding or obstruction (or both) may occur. The obstruction consists of either an intussusception with the tumor in the lead or a partial or complete occlusion in the lumen by growth of the tumor. Bleeding may cause weakness, fatigability, lightheadedness, syncope, pallor, sweating, tachycardia, and tarry stools. Obstruction causes nausea, vomiting, and abdominal pains. The abdomen is tender and distended, and bowel sounds are high-pitched and active. Malignant lesions produce weight loss and extraintestinal manifestations (eg, pain due to stretching of the liver capsule, flushing due to carcinoid). In the case of a duodenal carcinoma, a peptic ulcer syndrome may be present. A palpable mass is rarely found.

If there is bleeding, melena and hypochromic anemia occur. X-ray (small bowel series) may show the tumor mass or dilatation of the small bowel if obstruction is present; in the absence of obstruction, it is extremely difficult to demonstrate the mass.

## Benign Tumors

Benign tumors may be symptomatic or may be incidental findings at operation or autopsy. Treatment consists of surgical removal.

Benign **adenomas** constitute 25% of all benign bowel tumors. **Lipomas** occur most frequently in the ileum; the presenting symptom is usually obstruction due to intussusception. **Leiomyomas** are usually associated with bleeding and may also cause intussusception. **Angiomas** behave like other small bowel tumors but have a greater tendency to bleed.

Multiple intestinal polyposis of the gastrointestinal tract (any level) associated with mucocutaneous pigmentation (Peutz-Jeghers syndrome) is a benign condition. Malignant change has been reported but is rare, and the entity becomes a problem only with complications such as obstruction or bleeding. The polyps are hamartomas, and the pigment is melanin. The pigment is most prominent over the lips and buccal mucosa (see p 391).

## Malignant Tumors

The treatment of malignant tumors and their complications is usually surgical.

**Adenocarcinoma** is the most common cancer of the small bowel, occurring most frequently in the duodenum and jejunum. Symptoms are due to obstructions or hemorrhage. The prognosis is very poor. **Lymphomas** are also first manifested by obstruction or bleeding. Perforation or malabsorption may also occur. Postoperative radiation therapy may occasionally be of value. **Sarcomas** occur most commonly in the mid small bowel and may first be manifested by mass, obstruction, or bleeding. The prognosis is guarded.

**Carcinoid tumors** arise from the argentaffin cells of the gastrointestinal tract. Ninety percent of these tumors occur in the appendix, and 75% of the remainder occur in the small intestine (usually the distal ileum). Carcinoids may arise in other sites, including the stomach, colon, bronchus, pancreas, and ovary. Most small bowel carcinoids do not produce carcinoid syndrome. The main problem is metastases. In general, carcinoid syndrome occurs only with malignant tumors that have metastasized. The tumor may secrete serotonin and bradykinin. The systemic manifestations may consist of (1) paroxysmal flushing and other vasomotor symptoms, (2) dyspnea and wheezing, (3) recurrent episodes of abdominal pain and diarrhea, and (4) symptoms and signs of right-sided valvular disease of the heart. The diagnosis is confirmed by finding elevated levels of 5-hydroxyindoleacetic acid in the urine. The primary tumor is usually small, and obstruction is unusual. The metastases are usually voluminous and surprisingly benign. Treatment is symptomatic and supportive; surgical excision may be indicated if the condition is recognized before widespread metastases have occurred. Response to treatment with serotonin antagonists has been irregular. Repeated administration of corticotropin or the corticosteroids may occasionally be of value. The prognosis for cure is poor, but long-term survival is not unusual.

Johnson AM, Harman PK, Hanks JB: Primary small bowel malignancies. *Am Surg* 1985;**51**:31.

## MECKEL'S DIVERTICULITIS

Meckel's diverticulum, a remnant of the omphalomesenteric duct, is found in about 2% of persons, more frequently in males. It arises from the ileum 60–90 cm from the ileocecal valve and may or may not have an umbilical attachment. Most are silent, but various abdominal symptoms may occur. The blind pouch may be involved by an inflammatory process similar to appendicitis; its congenital bands or inflammatory adhesions may cause acute intestinal obstruction; it may induce intussusception; or, in the 16% that contain heterotopic islands of gastric mucosa, it may form a peptic ulcer.

The symptoms and signs of the acute appendicitis-like disease and the acute intestinal obstruction caused by Meckel's diverticulitis cannot be differentiated from other primary processes except by exploration. Ulcer type distress, if present, is localized near the umbilicus or lower and, more importantly, is not relieved by alkalies or food. If ulceration has occurred, blood will be present in the stool. Massive gastrointestinal bleeding and perforation may occur (see p 350). The presence of Meckel's diverticulum can frequently be determined in patients with gastric mucosa by a technetium radioisotope scan.

Meckel's diverticulitis should be resected, either for relief or for differentiation from acute appendicitis. Surgery is curative.

Mackey WC, Dineen P: A fifty year experience with Meckel's diverticulum. *Surg Gynecol Obstet* 1983;**156**:56.

## MESENTERIC VASCULAR INSUFFICIENCY

### 1. CHRONIC MESENTERIC VASCULAR INSUFFICIENCY (Abdominal Angina)

The syndrome of intestinal angina has received increasing attention of late. Progress in angiographic techniques and vascular surgery has led to effective diagnostic and therapeutic approaches. The entity may be secondary to atherosclerosis and may precede vascular occlusion (see below). In some instances it is secondary to compression of the vessels either by the crura of the diaphragm or by anomalous bands.

Localized or generalized postprandial pain is the classic picture. The intensity of pain may be related to the size of the meal; the relationship to eating leads to a diminution in food intake and, eventually, weight loss. An epigastric bruit may be heard. Laboratory evidence of malabsorption may be present. The small bowel series may reveal a motility disorder. Visceral angiograms are necessary to confirm narrowing of the celiac and mesenteric arteries. It is generally believed that 2 of the 3 main vessels must be involved in order for symptoms to occur.

Surgical revascularization of the bowel is the treatment of choice if the patient's condition permits. Small, frequent feedings may prove helpful.

Jaxheimer EC, Jewell ER, Persson AV: Chronic intestinal ischemia: The Lahey Clinic approach to management. *Surg Clin North Am* 1985;**64**:123.

## 2. ACUTE MESENTERIC VASCULAR INSUFFICIENCY

### Essentials of Diagnosis

- Severe abdominal pain with nausea and bloody diarrhea.
- Severe prostration and shock.
- Abdominal distention, tenderness, rigidity.
- Leukocytosis, hemoconcentration.

### General Considerations

Mesenteric arterial or venous occlusion is a catastrophic abdominal disorder. Arterial occlusion is occasionally embolic but is more frequently thrombotic. Both occur more frequently in men and in the older age groups. Acute mesenteric vascular occlusion may also be a small vessel phenomenon, particularly in patients with vasculitis in association with a variety of collagen diseases. In patients with sudden onset of pain in the setting of recent myocardial infarction or in the presence of an arrhythmia, serious consideration must be given to the possibility of an embolic event.

Involvement of the superior mesenteric artery or its branches is common. The affected bowel becomes congested, hemorrhagic, and edematous, and may cease to function, producing intestinal obstruction. True ischemic necrosis then develops.

Intestinal infarction may occur in the absence of mesenteric vascular thrombosis; nonocclusive disease may in fact be a more common cause of infarction than is occlusion. Most patients have been in severe congestive heart failure or shock or in a state of hypoxia. Although many patients with this syndrome have been receiving digitalis glycosides, the relationship of this agent to the bowel problem is unclear. Occlusive vascular disease may also play a role in reducing perfusion of the bowel in these patients.

### Clinical Findings

**A. Symptoms and Signs:** Generalized abdominal pain often comes on abruptly and is usually steady and severe, but it may begin gradually and may be intermittent, with colicky exacerbations. Nausea and vomiting occur; the vomitus is rarely bloody. Bloody diarrhea and marked prostration, sweating, and anxiety may occur. For a period following the occlusion, symptoms are severe but the physical findings meager.

Shock may be evident. Abdominal distention occurs early, and audible peristalsis (evident early) may later disappear. As peritoneal irritation develops, diffuse tenderness, rigidity, and rebound tenderness appear.

**B. Laboratory Findings:** Hemoconcentration, leukocytosis ($> 15,000/\mu$L with a shift to the left), and blood in the stool may be present.

**C. Imaging:** A plain film of the abdomen shows moderate gaseous distention of the small and large intestines and evidence of peritoneal fluid.

### Differential Diagnosis

Differentiate from acute pancreatitis and a perforated viscus. The elevated amylase in pancreatitis and free peritoneal air in perforation may help to differentiate these conditions. Amylase may be elevated in intestinal infarction. When an embolic event is a possibility, visceral angiography must be done to locate the obstruction and assess for operation.

### Treatment & Prognosis

The treatment of acute mesenteric arterial thrombosis consists of the measures necessary to (1) restore fluid, colloid, and electrolyte balance; (2) decompress the bowel; and (3) prevent sepsis by administration of antimicrobial drugs. Angiography must be done if embolus is suspected. Unless there are absolute contraindications to surgery, laparotomy should be done as soon as possible and gangrenous bowel resected. If the infarction is due to an isolated thrombus or embolus of the superior mesenteric artery, embolectomy or thrombectomy may be possible. Anticoagulants are not indicated. The mortality rate is extremely high in the acute disease. The treatment of nonthrombotic intestinal infarction poses a therapeutic dilemma. Basically, the principles are the same, ie, maintenance of fluid, electrolyte, and colloid balance. However, in the face of congestive failure, this can be most difficult. Careful hemodynamic monitoring provides useful information but is not the solution to this problem. Surgical resection of gangrenous bowel in a patient with congestive failure is a formidable undertaking but should be tried if at all possible. The prognosis in either event is grave; survival is unusual.

Camilleri M et al: Gastrointestinal manifestation of systemic vasculitis. *Q J Med* 1983;**52**:141.
Gillespie IE: Intestinal ischemia. *Gut* 1985;**26**:653.
Khan AH, Rubinstein PC: Ischemic bowel disease: Diagnosis and prognosis. *Geriatrics* 1984;**39(11)**:63.

## ACUTE ORGANIC SMALL INTESTINAL OBSTRUCTION

### Essentials of Diagnosis

- Colicky abdominal pain, vomiting, constipation, borborygmus.

- Tender distended abdomen without peritoneal irritation.
- Audible high-pitched tinkling peristalsis or peristaltic rushes.
- Radiographic evidence of dilated loops of small intestine with or without fluid levels.
- Little or no leukocytosis.

## General Considerations

Acute organic intestinal obstruction usually involves the small intestine, particularly the ileum. Major inciting causes are external hernia and postoperative adhesions. Less common causes are gallstones, neoplasms, granulomatous processes, intussusception, volvulus, internal hernia, and foreign bodies.

## Clinical Findings

**A. Symptoms and Signs:** Colicky abdominal pain in the periumbilical area becomes more constant and diffuse as distention develops. Vomiting, at first of a reflex nature associated with the waves of pain, later becomes fecal in obstruction of the distal bowel. Borborygmus and consciousness of intestinal movement, obstipation, weakness, perspiration, and anxiety are often present. The patient is restless, changing position frequently with pain, and is often in a shock-like state, with sweating, tachycardia, and dehydration. Abdominal distention may be localized, with an isolated loop, but usually is generalized. The higher the obstruction, the less the distention; the longer the time of obstruction, the greater the distention. Audible peristalsis, peristaltic rushes with pain paroxysms, high-pitched tinkles, and visible peristalsis may be present. Moderate generalized abdominal tenderness may be present, and there are no signs of peritoneal irritation. Fever is absent or low-grade. A tender hernia may be present.

**B. Laboratory Findings:** Hemoconcentration may occur with true dehydration or may reflect sequestration of fluid in the obstructed loop or third space. Leukocytosis is absent or mild. Vomiting may cause electrolyte disturbances.

**C. Imaging:** Abdominal radiography reveals gas- and fluid-filled loops of bowel, and the gas does not progress downward on serial radiographs. Fluid levels may be visible.

## Differential Diagnosis

Differentiate from other acute abdominal conditions such as inflammation and perforation of a viscus or renal or gallbladder colic. The absence of peritoneal signs, ie, rigidity and rebound tenderness, should aid in differentiating small bowel obstruction from ileus secondary to peritonitis. The absence of leukocytosis and the presence of high-pitched bowel sounds or intestinal rushes are also helpful. Differentiate also from mesenteric vascular disease and torsion of an organ (eg, ovarian cyst). In the late stages of obstruction it may be impossible to distinguish acute organic intestinal obstruction from the late stage of peritonitis with ileus.

## Complications

Strangulation (necrosis of the bowel wall) occurs with impairment of the blood supply to the gut. Strangulation is difficult to determine clinically, but fever, marked leukocytosis, and signs of peritoneal irritation should alert the clinician to this possibility. Strangulation may lead to perforation, peritonitis, and sepsis. Strangulation increases the mortality rate of intestinal obstruction to about 25%.

## Treatment

**A. Supportive Measures:**

1. Decompression of the intestinal tract by nasogastric suction should relieve vomiting, reduce intestinal distention, and prevent aspiration. Endoscopic decompression alone may relieve obstruction in many patients.

2. Correct fluid, electrolyte, and colloid deficits.

3. Give broad-spectrum antibiotics (gentamicin, ampicillin, or clindamycin) if strangulation is suspected.

4. The level of obstruction must be delineated; this is often best achieved initially by a barium enema.

**B. Surgical Measures:** Complete obstruction of the intestine is treated surgically after appropriate supportive therapy. Strangulation is always a danger as long as obstruction persists, and fever, leukocytosis, peritoneal signs, or blood in the feces means that strangulation may have occurred and that immediate surgery is required.

If the bowel is successfully decompressed during the preoperative preparation period, with cessation of pain and passage of flatus and feces, surgery may be delayed. Otherwise, surgical relief of the obstruction is indicated. Surgery consists of relieving the obstruction and removing gangrenous bowel with reanastomosis.

## Prognosis

Prognosis varies with the causative factor and the presence of strangulation.

## FUNCTIONAL OBSTRUCTION
## (Adynamic Ileus, Paralytic Ileus)

## Essentials of Diagnosis

- Continuous abdominal pain, distention, vomiting, and obstipation.
- History of a precipitating factor (surgery, peritonitis, pain, anticholinergic drugs, pneumonia, inferior myocardial infarction).
- Minimal abdominal tenderness; decreased to absent bowel sounds.
- X-ray evidence of gas and fluid in bowel.

## General Considerations

Adynamic ileus is a neurogenic impairment of peristalsis that may lead to intestinal obstruction. It is a common disorder that may be due to a variety of intra-abdominal causes, eg, gastrointestinal surgery, peritoneal irritation (hemorrhage, ruptured viscus, pancreatitis, peritonitis), or anoxic organic obstruction. Drugs with anticholinergic properties, renal colic, vertebral fractures, spinal cord injuries, severe infections, uremia, diabetic coma, and electrolyte abnormalities also may cause adynamic ileus.

## Clinical Findings

**A. Symptoms and Signs:** There is mild to moderate abdominal pain, continuous rather than colicky, associated with vomiting (which may later become fecal) and obstipation. Borborygmus is absent. Symptoms of the initiating condition may also be present (eg, fever; prostration due to ruptured viscus).

Abdominal distention is generalized and may be massive, with nonlocalized minimal abdominal tenderness and no signs of peritoneal irritation unless due to the primary disease. Bowel sounds are decreased to absent. Dehydration may occur after prolonged vomiting or from sequestration of fluid in bowel loops. Other signs of the initiating disorder may be present.

**B. Laboratory Findings:** With prolonged vomiting, hemoconcentration and electrolyte imbalance may occur. Leukocytosis, anemia, and elevated serum amylase may be present, depending upon the initiating condition.

**C. Imaging:** Radiography of the abdomen shows distended gas-filled loops of bowel in the small and large intestines and even in the rectum. There may be evidence of air-fluid levels in the distended bowel. When the underlying clinical problem is unclear, a barium enema and subsequent small bowel x-ray will rule out organic obstruction.

## Differential Diagnosis

The symptoms and signs of obstruction with absent bowel sounds and a history of a precipitating condition leave little doubt about the diagnosis. It is important to make certain that the adynamic ileus is not secondary to an organic obstruction, especially anoxic, where conservative management is harmful and immediate surgery may be lifesaving.

## Treatment

Most cases of adynamic ileus are postoperative and respond to restriction of oral intake with gradual liberalization of the diet as the bowel function returns. Severe and prolonged ileus may require gastrointestinal suction and complete restriction of oral intake. Parenteral restoration of fluids and electrolytes is essential in such instances. When conservative therapy fails, it may be necessary to operate for the purpose of decompressing the bowel by enterostomy or cecostomy and to rule out mechanical obstruction.

Those cases of adynamic ileus secondary to other disorders (eg, electrolyte imbalance, severe infection, intra-abdominal or back injury, pneumonitis) are managed as above plus treatment of the primary disease.

## Prognosis

The prognosis varies with that of the initiating disorder. Adynamic ileus may resolve without specific therapy when the cause is removed. Intubation with decompression is usually successful in causing return of function.

## INTESTINAL PSEUDO-OBSTRUCTION

This idiopathic disorder, usually seen in teenagers or young adults, is characterized by recurring symptoms of small bowel obstruction but no evidence of organic obstruction on x-ray or with surgical exploration. All previously mentioned causes of functional obstruction are absent. The clinical course is progressively downhill unless the patient is treated with nasogastric suction, intravenous fluids, and parenteral nutrition as required.

Esquivel CO et al: Postoperative small bowel intussusception. *West J Med* 1985;**143**:108.

Gowen GF: Endoscopic decompression in partial small-bowel obstruction. *Am J Surg* 1985;**149**:252.

Rohrmann CA et al: Radiologic and histologic differentiations of neuromuscular disorders of the gastrointestinal tract: Visceral myopathies, visceral neuropathies, and progressive systemic sclerosis. *Am J Roentgenol* 1984;**143**:933.

Sarr MG, Bulkley GB, Zuidema GD: Preoperative recognition of intestinal strangulation obstruction: Prospective evaluation of diagnostic capability. *Am J Surg* 1983;**145**:176.

Schuffler MD et al: Chronic intestinal pseudo-obstruction: A report of 27 cases and review of the literature. *Medicine* 1981;**60**:173.

## MALABSORPTION SYNDROMES (Primary Mucosal Disease)

Malabsorption syndromes may be associated with a wide variety of small intestine mucosal disease processes that have in common the malabsorption of nutrients by the gastrointestinal tract. These syndromes should be contrasted to states of maldigestion where intraluminal abnormalities result in failure to absorb nutrients, such as pancreatic insufficiency, bile salt deficiency, and a variety of postsurgical abnormalities. The clinical and laboratory manifestations are summarized in Table 11–2.

Sleisenger MH et al: Malabsorption and nutritional support. *Clin Gastroenterol* 1983;**12**:323.

## 1. CELIAC SPRUE & TROPICAL SPRUE

### Essentials of Diagnosis

- Bulky, pale, frothy, foul-smelling, greasy stools with increased fecal fat on chemical analysis of the stool.
- Weight loss and signs of multiple vitamin deficiencies.

**Table 11–2.** Clinical and laboratory manifestations of malabsorption.[*]

| Manifestation | Laboratory Findings | Malabsorbed Nutrient |
|---|---|---|
| Steatorrhea (bulky, light-colored) | Increased fecal fat; decreased serum cholesterol | Fat |
| Diarrhea (increased fecal water) | Increased fecal fat and/or positive bile salt breath test | Fatty acids and/or bile salts |
| Weight loss; malnutrition (muscle wasting); weakness, fatigue | Increased fecal fat and nitrogen; decreased glucose and xylose absorption | Calories (fat, protein, carbohydrates) |
| Abdominal distention | | |
| Iron deficiency anemia | Hypochromic anemia; low serum iron | Iron |
| Megaloblastic anemia | Macrocytosis; decreased vitamin $B_{12}$ absorption ($^{67}$Co-labeled $B_{12}$); decreased serum vitamin $B_{12}$ and folic acid activity (microbiologic assay) | Vitamin $B_{12}$ and/or folic acid |
| Paresthesia; tetany; positive Trousseau and Chvostek signs | Decreased serum calcium, magnesium, and potassium | Calcium, vitamin D, magnesium, potassium |
| Bone pain; pathologic fractures; skeletal deformities | Osteoporosis; osteomalacia on x-ray | Calcium, protein |
| Bleeding tendency (ecchymoses, melena, hematuria) | Prolonged prothrombin time | Vitamin K |
| Edema | Decreased serum albumin; increased fecal loss of $^{51}$Cr-labeled albumin | Protein (and/or protein-losing enteropathy) |
| Nocturia; abdominal distention | Increased small bowel fluid on x-ray | Water |
| Milk intolerance (cramps, bloating, diarrhea) | Flat lactose tolerance test; decreased mucosal lactase levels | Lactose |

[*] Modified from Bayless TM: Malabsorption in the elderly. *Hosp Pract* (Aug) 1979;**14**:57.

- Impaired intestinal absorption of vitamins, fat; large amounts of fat in the stool.
- Hypochromic or megaloblastic anemia; small bowel x-ray pattern that of small bowel dilatation and dilution of barium.

## General Considerations

Sprue syndromes are diseases of disturbed small intestine function characterized by impaired absorption, particularly of fats, and motor abnormalities. Celiac sprue responds to a gluten-free diet, whereas tropical sprue does not. The polypeptide gliadin is the offending substance in gluten. Although an infectious cause has not been conclusively demonstrated, tropical sprue behaves clinically like an infectious disease. It responds to folic acid and broad-spectrum antibiotics.

The clinical severity of sprue syndrome varies depending upon the extent of the lesion in the small intestine and the duration of the disease. Severe wasting, gastrointestinal protein loss, multiple vitamin deficiencies, and adrenal and pituitary deficiency may be associated with the severe forms of the disease. A flat intestinal mucosa without villi in the small intestine is noted, and some observers have described degenerative changes in the myenteric nerve plexuses. With the loss of villi, the microvilli are also lost, leading to disaccharidase deficiency, particularly lactase deficiency.

Rare secondary varieties of sprue syndrome in which the cause of the small intestine dysfunction is known include gastrocolic fistulas, obstruction of intestinal lacteals by lymphoma, Whipple's disease, extensive regional enteritis, and parasitic infections such as giardiasis, cryptosporidiasis, strongyloidiasis, and coccidiosis.

## Clinical Findings

**A. Tropical Sprue:** Patients with tropical sprue are either residents of, or have had prolonged visits in, tropical regions. The main symptom is diarrhea; at first it is explosive and watery; later, stools are fewer and more solid and characteristically pale, frothy, foul-smelling, and greasy, with exacerbations on high-fat diet. Indigestion, flatulence, abdominal cramps, weight loss (often marked), pallor, asthenia, irritability, paresthesias, and muscle cramps may occur. Quiescent periods with or without mild symptoms may occur especially on leaving the tropics. Symptoms may appear years after the patient has left endemic areas.

Vitamin deficiencies cause glossitis, cheilosis, angular stomatitis, cutaneous hyperpigmentation, and dry, rough skin. Abdominal distention and mild tenderness are present. Edema occurs late.

Anemia is usually macrocytic, and, with blood loss or malabsorption of iron, may be hypochromic, microcytic, or mixed. The fecal fat is increased. Serum proteins, calcium, phosphorus, cholesterol, and prothrombin are low. Gastric hypochlorhydria is frequent. The pancreatic enzymes are normal.

Radiographs using nonflocculating barium show dilatation of the intestine and occasionally excess fluid and gas.

**B. Celiac Sprue:** This disorder is characterized by defective absorption of fat, protein, carbohydrates, iron, and water. Absorption of fat-soluble vitamins A, D, and K is impaired. Osteomalacia may ensue. Protein loss from the intestine may occur. Elimination of gluten from the diet causes dramatic improvement. Gluten is found in wheat, barley, oats, and rye and is used as a filler in many prepared foods. Diligent elimination of this substance from the diet is important in achieving remission.

In one-third of patients with celiac sprue, symptoms begin in early childhood. Symptoms may persist into adult life, but there is usually a latent phase of apparent good health. The anemia is usually hypochromic and microcytic. The complications of impaired absorption are more severe: infantilism, dwarfism, tetany, vitamin deficiency signs, and even rickets may be seen. The definitive diagnosis of steatorrhea requires quantitative measurement of fecal fat, preferably on a known fat intake, and a characteristic small bowel biopsy.

Patients presenting with dermatitis herpetiformis frequently have associated celiac sprue, usually symptomatic. Both the sprue and the dermatitis herpetiformis are responsive to a gluten-free diet—the latter only after many months, and rechallenge with gluten results in recurrence of the rash within weeks.

A small group of patients with apparent celiac sprue are nonresponsive to a gluten-free diet. On closer inspection of the small bowel mucosal biopsy, a collagenous layer is found between the surface absorptive cells and the lamina propria. No consistently helpful medical therapy has yet been found.

## Differential Diagnosis

It is necessary to differentiate between the various causes of malabsorption to permit selection of specific therapy, if any. Anatomic abnormalities such as fistulas, blind loops, and jejunal diverticulosis may be found on radiography. Regional enteritis usually has a characteristic radiographic appearance but must be distinguished from intestinal tuberculosis and lymphoma. The small bowel x-ray appearance in Whipple's disease, nodular lymphoid hyperplasia, intestinal lymphoma, and amyloidosis is abnormal but not specific or diagnostic. In primary diseases of the small intestine, mucosal suction biopsy is the most effective way of making the diagnosis. The pathologic response in some diseases is patchy, and multiple specimens may be required. Pancreatic insufficiency due to obstruction may be diagnosed by a low water and bicarbonate secretion in response to intravenous administration of secretin.

## Treatment

**A. Tropical Sprue:** Folic acid, 10–20 mg daily orally or intramuscularly for a few weeks, corrects diarrhea, anorexia, weight loss, glossitis, and anemia. Tetracycline, 250 mg orally 4 times daily, is given at the outset of treatment. When complete remission occurs, the patient may be maintained on 5 mg of folic acid daily. If the patient has achlorhydria, giving vitamin $B_{12}$ intramuscularly should also be considered. Hypochromic anemia can be treated with oral iron. A high-calorie, high-protein, low-fat diet can be given.

**B. Celiac Sprue:** Strict elimination of gluten from the diet will lead to clinical recovery. If there is no response, another diagnosis must be sought. The diet should be high in calories and protein, low in fat, and gluten-free. Prothrombin deficiency is treated by means of water-soluble vitamin K orally or, if urgent, parenterally. Treat hypocalcemia or tetany with calcium phosphate or gluconate, 2 g orally or intravenously 3 times daily, and vitamin D, 5–20 thousand units. Multiple vitamin supplements may also be advisable. Macrocytic anemia usually responds to vitamin $B_{12}$, 100 $\mu$g intramuscularly every month until the disease is in clinical remission.

The corticosteroids may be advantageous in certain patients with sprue, particularly the severely ill, since they increase the absorption of nitrogen, fats, and other nutrients from the gastrointestinal tract. They have a nonspecific effect in increasing appetite and inducing mild euphoria. Cortisol is best given in dosages of 100–300 mg/24 h intravenously and tapered off according to the patient's response.

## Prognosis

With proper treatment, the response is good. Patients with celiac sprue have a late increased incidence of abdominal lymphoma and carcinomas. Patients who develop gastrointestinal symptoms while in remission on a gluten-free diet should be carefully evaluated for cancer.

Gawkrodger DJ et al: Dermatitis herpetiformis: Diagnosis, diet and dermography. *Gut* 1984;**25**:151.

Klipstein FA: Tropical sprue in travelers and expatriates living abroad. *Gastroenterology* 1981;**80**:590.

Kumar PJ: The enigma of celiac disease. *Gastroenterology* 1985;**89**:214.

Trier JS: Celiac sprue. Pages 1050–1067 in: *Gastrointestinal Disease: Pathophysiology, Diagnosis, Management*, 3rd ed. Sleisenger MH, Fordtran JS (editors). Saunders, 1983.

## 2. DISACCHARIDASE DEFICIENCY

Lactase deficiency may occur in a congenital or adult-onset form. With the congenital form, the absence of lactase leads to acidic diarrhea (fecal pH 4.5–6). There are large amounts of lactic acid in the stool secondary to bacterial breakdown of lactose. The infant fails to thrive until lactose-containing foods are eliminated from the diet.

Lactase deficiency in the adult is common worldwide. It has been estimated from many studies that the incidence of lactase deficiency is 70–90% in Orientals, blacks, American Indians, and Mediterranean populations. The incidence of lactase deficiency in northern and western Europeans is 10–15%. Symptoms may vary from minor abdominal bloating, distention, flatulence, and discomfort to markedly severe diarrhea in response to even small amounts of lactose. The diagnosis is confirmed by a lactose tolerance test; marked diarrhea usually occurs with this test. Onset in the adult may follow gastroduodenal surgery and may be associated with regional enteritis. The primary mucosal diseases of the small intestine usually have associated lactase deficiency.

Intercurrent acute illnesses, such as viral and bacterial enteritis, particularly in children, will frequently injure the microvilli of the mucosal cells of the small intestine, resulting in temporary lactase deficiency.

Other congenital defects described thus far are sucrose-isomaltose and glucose-galactose intolerance. Secondary disaccharidase deficiencies have been described in patients with giardiasis, celiac disease, ulcerative colitis, short bowel syndrome, and cystic fibrosis and postgastrectomy. Removal of the offending sugar from the patient's diet will often result in remission.

Levitt MD, Savaiano DA: Lactose intolerance and yogurt: Diagnosis and treatment. *Pract Gastroenterol* (March-April) 1985;**9**:41.

## 3. WHIPPLE'S DISEASE

Whipple's disease is an uncommon malabsorption disorder due to an infection of the gut with widespread systemic manifestations. Histologic examination of a small bowel mucosal biopsy specimen reveals characteristic large, foamy mononuclear cells filled with cytoplasmic material that gives a positive periodic acid-Schiff staining reaction. Electron microscopy reveals Whipple's bacilli in the intestines and in the eyes, heart, lungs, synovia, kidneys, and central nervous system. The disease occurs primarily in middle-aged men and is of insidious onset; without treatment, it is usually fatal. The manifestations include abdominal pain, diarrhea, steatorrhea, gastrointestinal bleeding, fever, lymphadenopathy, polyarthritis, edema, gray to brown skin pigmentation, and severe central nervous system manifestations. Anemia and hypoproteinemia are common.

Treatment programs are somewhat controversial but should be continued for at least 1 year and should include administration of agents that cross the blood-brain barrier. Current options are trimethoprim-sulfamethoxazole (TMP-SMX) alone or parenteral penicillin and streptomycin followed by TMP-SMX. Reappearance of symptoms after or during therapy suggests emergence of resistant organisms, and the antibiotic should be changed.

Keinath RD et al: Antibiotic treatment and relapse in Whipple's disease: Long-term follow-up of 88 patients. *Gastroenterology* 1985;**88**:1867.

## PROTEIN-LOSING ENTEROPATHY

Leakage of plasma proteins into the intestinal lumen is an integral phase of the metabolism of plasma proteins. In certain intestinal disease states, excessive protein loss into the intestinal lumen may be responsible for the hypoproteinemia that occurs. Excessive loss of plasma protein may be due to increased mucosal permeability to protein, inflammatory exudation, excessive cell desquamation, or direct leakage of lymph from obstructed lacteals. Gastrointestinal diseases associated with protein-losing enteropathy include all of the primary mucosal diseases of the small bowel, as well as gastric carcinoma, lymphoma, gastric rugal hypertrophy, sprue, and others.

Treatment consists of management of the primary disorder.

Sleisinger MH, Kim YS: Protein digestion and absorption. *N Engl J Med* 1979;**300**:659.

## APPENDICITIS

### Essentials of Diagnosis
- Right lower quadrant abdominal pain and tenderness with signs of peritoneal irritation.
- Anorexia, nausea and vomiting, and constipation.
- Low-grade fever and mild polymorphonuclear leukocytosis.

### General Considerations
Appendicitis is initiated by obstruction of the appendiceal lumen by a fecalith, inflammation, foreign body, or neoplasm. Obstruction is followed by infection, edema, and, frequently, infarction of the appendiceal wall. Intraluminal tension develops rapidly and tends to cause early mural necrosis and perforation. All ages and both sexes are affected, but appendicitis is more common in males between 10 and 30 years of age.

Appendicitis is one of the most frequent causes of acute surgical abdomen. The symptoms and signs usually follow a fairly stereotyped pattern, but appendicitis is capable of such protean manifestations that it should be considered in the differential diagnosis of every obscure case of intra-abdominal sepsis and pain.

### Clinical Findings
**A. Symptoms and Signs:** An attack of appendicitis usually begins with epigastric or periumbilical pain associated with 1–2 episodes of vomiting. Within 2–12 hours, the pain shifts to the right lower quadrant, where it persists as a steady soreness that is aggravated by walking or coughing. There is anorexia, moderate malaise, and slight fever. Constipation is usual, but diarrhea occurs occasionally, as does nausea and vomiting.

At onset there are no localized abdominal findings.

Within a few hours, however, progressive right lower quadrant tenderness can be demonstrated; careful examination will usually identify a single point of maximal tenderness. The patient can often place a finger precisely on this area, especially if asked to accentuate the soreness by coughing. Light percussion over the right lower quadrant is helpful in localizing tenderness. Rebound tenderness and spasm of the overlying abdominal muscles are usually present. Psoas and obturator signs, when positive, are strongly suggestive of appendicitis. Rectal tenderness is common and, in pelvic appendicitis, may be more definite than abdominal tenderness. Peristalsis is diminished or absent. Slight to moderate fever is present.

**B. Laboratory Findings:** Moderate leukocytosis (10,000–20,000/$\mu$L) with an increase in neutrophils is usually present. It is not uncommon to find microscopic hematuria and pyuria.

**C. Imaging:** There are no characteristic changes on plain films of the abdomen. However, visualization in the right lower quadrant of a radiopaque shadow consistent with fecalith in the appendix may heighten the suspicion of appendicitis. In uncertain cases, barium enemas are being used, as visualization of the entire appendix rules out acute appendicitis.

## Factors That Cause Variations From the "Classic" Clinical Picture

**A. Anatomic Location of Appendix:** Abdominal findings are most definite when the appendix is in the iliac fossa or superficially located. When the appendix extends over the pelvic brim, abdominal signs may be minimal, greatest tenderness being elicited on rectal examination. Right lower quadrant tenderness may be poorly localized and slow to develop in retrocecal or retroileal appendicitis. Inflammation of a high-lying lateral appendix may produce maximal tenderness in the flank, and in the left lower quadrant in situs inversus. Bizarre locations of the appendix may rarely occur in association with a mobile or undescended cecum; in such cases, symptoms and signs may localize in the right upper or left lower quadrant.

**B. Age:**

**1. Infancy and childhood**–In infancy, appendicitis is relatively rare. When it does occur, history and physical findings are difficult to interpret. The disease tends to progress rapidly, and rupture results in generalized peritonitis.

**2. Old age**–Elderly patients frequently have few or no prodromal symptoms. Abdominal findings may be unimpressive, with slight tenderness and negligible muscle guarding, until perforation occurs. Fever and leukocytosis may also be minimal or absent. When the white count is not elevated, a shift to the left is significant evidence of inflammation.

**C. Obesity:** Obesity frequently increases the difficulty of evaluation by delaying the appearance of abdominal signs and by preventing sharp localization.

**D. Pregnancy:** See discussion in Chapter 13.

## Differential Diagnosis

Acute gastroenteritis is the disorder most commonly confused with appendicitis. In rare cases it either precedes or is coincident with appendicitis. Vomiting and diarrhea are more common. Fever and the white blood count may rise sharply and may be out of proportion to abdominal findings. Localization of pain and tenderness is usually indefinite and shifting. Hyperactive peristalsis is characteristic. Gastroenteritis frequently runs an acute course. A period of observation usually serves to clarify the diagnosis.

Mesenteric adenitis may cause signs and symptoms identical with appendicitis. Usually, however, there are some clues to the true diagnosis. Mesenteric adenitis is more likely to occur in children or adolescents; respiratory infection is a common antecedent; localization of right lower quadrant tenderness is less precise and constant; and true muscle guarding is infrequent. In spite of a strong suspicion of mesenteric adenitis, it is often safer to advise appendectomy than to risk a complication of appendicitis by delay.

Meckel's diverticulitis may mimic appendicitis. The localization of tenderness may be more medial, but this is not a reliable diagnostic criterion. Because operation is required in both diseases, the differentiation is not critical. When a preoperative diagnosis of appendicitis proves on exploration to be erroneous, it is essential to examine the terminal 150 cm of ileum for Meckel's diverticulitis and mesenteric adenitis.

Regional enteritis, amebiasis, acute ileitis due to *Yersinia pseudotuberculosis*, perforated duodenal ulcer, ureteral colic, acute salpingitis, mittelschmerz, ruptured ectopic pregnancy, and twisted ovarian cyst may also be confused with appendicitis.

## Complications

**A. Perforation:** Appendicitis may rarely subside spontaneously, but it is an unpredictable disease with a marked tendency (about 95%) to progression and perforation. Because perforation rarely occurs within the first 8 hours, diagnostic observation during this period is relatively safe. Signs of perforation include increasing severity of pain, tenderness, and spasm in the right lower quadrant followed by evidence of generalized peritonitis or of a localized abscess. Ileus, fever, malaise, and leukocytosis become more marked. If perforation with abscess formation or generalized peritonitis has already occurred when the patient is first seen, the diagnosis may be quite obscure.

The treatment of perforated appendicitis is appendectomy unless a well-localized right lower quadrant or pelvic abscess has already walled off the appendix. Supportive measures are as for acute peritonitis.

**1. Generalized peritonitis**–This is a common sequela to perforation. Clinical findings and treatment are discussed elsewhere in this chapter.

**2. Appendiceal abscess**–This is one of the possible complications of untreated appendicitis. Malaise, toxicity, fever, and leukocytosis vary from minimal to marked. Examination discloses a tender mass in the right lower quadrant or pelvis. Pelvic abscesses tend to bulge into the rectum or vagina.

Abscesses usually become noticeable 2–6 days after onset, but antibiotic therapy may delay their appearance. Appendiceal abscess is occasionally the first and only sign of appendicitis and may be confused with neoplasm of the cecum, particularly in older persons, who may have little or no systemic reaction to the infection.

Treatment of early abscess is by intensive combined antibiotic therapy (eg, penicillin and gentamicin or clindamycin). On this regimen, the abscess will frequently resolve. Appendectomy should be performed 6–12 weeks later. A well-established progressive abscess in the right lower quadrant should be drained without delay. Pelvic abscess requires drainage when it bulges into the rectum or vagina and has become fluctuant.

**B. Pylephlebitis:** Suppurative thrombophlebitis of the portal system with liver abscess is a rare but highly lethal complication. It should be suspected when septic fever, chills, hepatomegaly, and jaundice develop after appendiceal perforation. Intensive combined antibiotic therapy with surgical drainage of the abscesses is indicated.

**C. Other Complications:** These include subphrenic abscess and other foci of intra-abdominal sepsis. Intestinal obstruction may be caused by adhesions.

### Treatment

**A. Preoperative Care:**

**1. Observation for diagnosis**–Within the first 8–12 hours after onset, the symptoms and signs of appendicitis are frequently indefinite. Under these circumstances a period of close observation is essential. The patient is placed at bed rest and given nothing by mouth. *Note:* Laxatives should not be prescribed when appendicitis or any form of peritonitis is suspected. Parenteral fluid therapy is begun as indicated. Narcotic medications are avoided if possible, but sedation with tranquilizing agents is not contraindicated. Abdominal and rectal examinations, white blood count, and differential count are repeated periodically. Abdominal films and an upright chest film must be obtained as part of the investigation of all difficult diagnostic problems. In most cases of appendicitis, the diagnosis is clarified by localization of signs to the right lower quadrant within 12 hours after onset of symptoms.

**2. Intubation**–Preoperatively, a nasogastric tube is inserted if there is sufficient peritonitis or toxicity to indicate that postoperative ileus may be troublesome. In such patients the stomach is aspirated and lavaged if necessary, and the patient is sent to the operating room with the tube in place.

**3. Antibiotics**–In the presence of a marked systemic reaction with severe toxicity and high fever, preoperative administration of antibiotics (eg, penicillin and cephalothin or gentamicin) is advisable.

**B. Surgical Treatment:** In uncomplicated appendicitis, appendectomy is performed as soon as fluid imbalance and other significant systemic disturbances are controlled. Little preparation is usually required. Early surgery has a mortality rate of a fraction of 1%. The morbidity and mortality rates associated with this disease reflect the occurrence of gangrene and perforation that occur when operation is delayed.

**C. Postoperative Care:** In uncomplicated appendicitis, postoperative gastric suction is usually not necessary. Ambulation is begun on the first postoperative day. The diet is advanced from clear liquids to soft solids during the second to fifth postoperative days depending upon the rapidity with which peristalsis and gastrointestinal function return. Parenteral fluid supplements are administered as required. Enemas are contraindicated. Milk of magnesia or a similar mild laxative may be given orally at bedtime daily from about the third day onward if necessary. Antibiotic therapy (eg, penicillin and gentamicin or clindamycin) is advisable for 5–7 days, or longer if abdominal fluid at operation was purulent or malodorous, if culture was positive, or if the appendix was gangrenous. Primary wound healing is the rule, and the period of hospitalization is usually 1 week or less. Normal activity can usually be resumed in 2–3 weeks after surgery in uncomplicated cases.

**D. Emergency Nonsurgical Treatment:** When surgical facilities are not available, treat as for acute peritonitis. On such a regimen, acute appendicitis may subside, and complications will be minimized.

### Prognosis

With accurate diagnosis and early surgical removal, mortality and morbidity rates are minimal. Delay of diagnosis produces significant mortality and morbidity rates if complications occur.

Recurrent acute attacks may occur if the appendix is not removed. "Chronic appendicitis" does not exist.

Bongard F, Landers DV, Lewis F: Differential diagnosis of appendicitis and pelvic inflammatory disease: A prospective analysis. *Am J Surg* 1985;**150**:90.

Burns RP et al: Appendicitis in mature patients. *Ann Surg* 1985;**201**:695.

Lee BW et al: Recurrent appendiceal colic. *Surg Gynecol Obstet* 1985;**161**:21.

### INTESTINAL TUBERCULOSIS (Tuberculous Enterocolitis)

Gastrointestinal tuberculosis may occur anywhere along the gastrointestinal tract. Involvement of the intestine frequently complicates pulmonary tuberculosis. Ingestion of milk containing tubercle bacilli is another means of infection.

The mode of infection is by ingestion of tubercle bacilli, with the formation of ulcerating lesions in the intestine, particularly the ileocecal region, and involvement of the mesenteric lymph nodes.

## Clinical Findings

Symptoms may be absent or minimal even with extensive disease. When present, they usually consist of fever, anorexia, nausea, flatulence, distention after eating, and food intolerance. There may be abdominal pain and mild to severe cramps, usually in the right lower quadrant and often after meals. Constipation may be present, but mild to severe diarrhea is more characteristic. Tuberculosis may involve the peritoneum. It may appear as a primary infection, and the disease course is chronic.

Findings on abdominal examination are not characteristic, although there may be mild right lower quadrant tenderness. Fistula in ano may be evident. Weight loss occurs.

There are no characteristic laboratory findings. The presence of tubercle bacilli in the feces does not correlate with intestinal involvement.

Radiographic examination of the involved bowel reveals irritability and spasm, particularly in the cecal region; irregular hypermotility of the intestinal tract; ulcerated lesions and irregular filling defects, particularly in the right colon and ileocecal region; and usually pulmonary tuberculosis.

## Treatment & Prognosis

The prognosis varies with that of the pulmonary disease. The intestinal lesions usually respond to chemotherapy and rest when reexposure to infecting material is prevented. Operation may be required for intestinal obstruction or for diagnosis.

Kasulke RJ et al: Primary tuberculous enterocolitis: Report of 3 cases and review of literature. *Arch Surg* 1981;**116**:110.

---

# DISEASES OF THE COLON & RECTUM

---

## IRRITABLE BOWEL SYNDROME

Irritable bowel syndrome is a term denoting a clinical entity characterized by some combination of (1) abdominal pain; (2) altered bowel function, constipation, or diarrhea; (3) hypersecretion of colonic mucus; (4) dyspeptic symptoms (flatulence, nausea, anorexia); and (5) varying degrees of anxiety or depression. This common group of disorders has many names, eg, nervous indigestion, functional dyspepsia, pylorospasm, irritable colon, spastic "colitis," functional "colitis," mucous "colitis," intestinal neurosis, and laxative or cathartic "colitis."

## Pathogenesis

Three main factors appear significant in the pathogenesis of irritable bowel syndrome.

(1) Colonic motor activity: There is no abnormality of either motility or electrical activity of the colon specific to the irritable bowel syndrome. However, prediverticular disease can be frequently demonstrated and is characterized by increased width of the sigmoid circular muscles, increased segmentation, and increased nonpropulsive intraluminal pressures. Colonic motor activity is abnormally increased in patients with colonic pain, eg, after meals, after administration of cholecystokinin or cholinergic drugs, or after emotional stress.

(2) Psychologic stress: Many patients with irritable bowel syndrome exhibit colonic symptoms at times of stress. The changes in colonic function are common manifestations of emotional tension. The reaction, however, may be more severe in patients with irritable bowel.

(3) Diet: A low-residue diet in some patients may be a prominent predisposing factor. Intolerance of lactose and other sugars may account for irritable bowel syndrome in certain patients.

It is essential to eliminate the possibility of organic gastrointestinal disease. A history of "nervousness," neuropathic traits, and emotional disturbances can usually be obtained. Bowel consciousness and cathartic and enema habits are prominent features. There is a highly variable complex of gastrointestinal symptoms: nausea and vomiting, anorexia, foul breath, sour stomach, flatulence, cramps, and constipation or diarrhea; hysteria and depression are the most prevalent syndromes.

Nocturnal diarrhea, awakening the patient from a sound sleep, is frequently a result of organic disease of the bowel.

## Clinical Findings

Examination discloses variable abdominal tenderness, particularly along the course of the colon. Sigmoidoscopy often reveals marked spasm and mucus in the colonic lumen and will frequently provoke the patient's spontaneously occurring symptoms. Laboratory studies should include a complete blood count and stool examination to rule out the presence of occult blood, ova, parasites, and pathogenic bacteria. Gastrointestinal x-rays may show altered gastrointestinal motility without other evidence of abnormalities.

## Treatment

**A. Diet:** No single diet is applicable to all patients with irritable bowel syndrome. Some patients may respond to an increase in dietary fiber. Exclusion of milk and milk products may prove helpful. Irrational fear of foods must be dispelled.

**B. Personal Habits:** Regular hours and meals and adequate sleep, exercise, and recreation are important. Restriction of alcohol and tobacco may be indicated.

**C. Psychotherapy:** Reassurance is important. Once the diagnosis has been established, the patient should be reassured that the symptoms are not due to an organic disease. Anxiety states or depression should be treated appropriately.

**D. Symptomatic Treatment:** Sedative-antispasmodic medication may be of value.

**E. Vegetable Mucilages:** Psyllium hydrophilic mucilloid (Metamucil) may be useful.

Goldsmith G, Patterson M: Irritable bowel syndrome: Treatment update. *Am Fam Physician* (Jan) 1985;**31**:191.

Schuster MM: Irritable bowel syndrome. Pages 880–895 in: *Gastrointestinal Disease: Pathophysiology, Diagnosis, Management*, 3rd ed. Sleisenger MH, Fordtran JS (editors). Saunders, 1983.

Thompson WG: Progress report: The irritable bowel. *Gut* 1984;**25**:305.

## INFECTIOUS COLITIS

Bacterial infections are common causes of acute colitis and are usually associated with fever, cramps, and diarrhea with tenesmus and often with blood in the stool. The most common causes are *Campylobacter jejuni, Shigella, Salmonella,* and *Yersinia enterocolitica.* (See Chapter 23.) Diarrhea due to the toxins of *E coli* (a common cause of "turista") should be considered, but this is a secretory diarrhea without evidence of colitis. Anal intercourse may be responsible for additional infectious diseases of the rectum, including gonorrhea, syphilis, lymphogranuloma venereum, condyloma latum, herpes simplex, and acquired immunodeficiency syndrome (AIDS).

AIDS (see Chapter 22) is a multisystem disorder, and the impaired immune function of the intestinal tract makes it particularly vulnerable to damage because of the large number of potential pathogens usually found in the intestinal lumen. Diarrhea and weight loss may precede the other manifestations of AIDS. Rectal and jejunal biopsies may show histologic abnormalities in AIDS patients with diarrhea.

Sigmoidoscopy will usually reveal acute colitis with small ulcerations; a mucus smear will reveal a preponderance of polymorphonuclear neutrophils; and cultures may reveal the organism. Tuberculosis is an uncommon cause.

Acute and chronic colitis caused by parasites such as the protozoan *Entamoeba histolytica* is common worldwide and not uncommon in the USA. It may be clinically indistinguishable from other types of acute and chronic colitis; differentiation can often be made by smears of aspirates at sigmoidoscopy, multiple stool examinations, and, in patients with sigmoidoscopic abnormalities, mucosal biopsy. In chronic forms, the areas of involvement are most commonly the cecum, sigmoid colon, or rectum. The chronic form may mimic granulomatous colitis or neoplasm. Complications include local abscess, liver abscess, and fistula formation. For treatment, see p 898.

Kotler DP et al: Enteropathy associated with the acquired immunodeficiency syndrome. *Ann Intern Med* 1984;**101**:421.

Pai CH et al: Sporadic cases of hemorrhagic colitis associated with *Escherichia coli* 0157:H7: Clinical, epidemiologic and bacteriologic features. *Ann Intern Med* 1984;**101**:738.

Quinn TC et al: Infections with *Campylobacter jejuni* and *Campylobacter*-like organisms in homosexual men. *Ann Intern Med* 1984;**101**:187.

## ANTIBIOTIC-ASSOCIATED COLITIS

Antibiotic-associated colitis may occur during antibiotic usage or up to 2 weeks subsequent to usage. The disease usually subsides when the offending antibiotic is withdrawn, but it is potentially lethal and diagnosis should be pursued.

**Pseudomembranous colitis** is characterized by profuse watery diarrhea with cramps, tenesmus, low-grade fever, and, rarely, blood per rectum. Current or recent antibiotic therapy is a usual part of the history. Almost all antibiotics have been implicated; clindamycin, ampicillin, and the cephalosporins are most common. Metronidazole has been reported to be effective in treatment of pseudomembranous enterocolitis, but it has also been reported to be a cause of this disease. Uncommonly, the disease occurs without antibiotic usage.

Diarrhea occurs secondary to selective overgrowth of the bacterium *Clostridium difficile,* which produces a toxin that causes the lesion of pseudomembranous colitis. Laboratory assays for detecting this toxin in stool are now available and are important in establishing the diagnosis.

Physical findings may be minimal but can include a distended, tender abdomen with a dilated bowel. Sigmoidoscopy may reveal a pseudomembrane characterized by adherent plaques (mushroom caps) of exudate with intervening normal mucosa. Occasionally the exudate is confluent. When the pseudomembrane is stripped away, capillary type bleeding will occur from the denuded mucosa. In a few patients, routine sigmoidoscopy is normal but colonoscopy shows involvement of the sigmoid colon or more proximal areas. Sometimes only the right colon is involved.

Vancomycin, 500–1000 mg/d orally for 7–10 days, is the drug of choice; it is very expensive but about 90% effective. Metronidazole, 0.5 g orally 3 times a day for 7–14 days, has been shown to be effective and is less expensive.

Complications include dehydration with electrolyte imbalance, perforation, toxic megacolon, and death.

A similar colitis without pseudomembrane is clinically indistinguishable from pseudomembranous colitis and may be more common. It is usually (not always) *Clostridium difficile* toxin-related. Sigmoidoscopy and occasionally colonoscopy will show evidence of acute colitis, usually right-sided. Ampicillin is often associated. All antibiotics should be withdrawn, and treatment should proceed as with pseudomembranous colitis if the toxin is demonstrated. Otherwise, treat expectantly.

Bartlett JG: Treatment of antibiotic-associated pseudomembranous colitis. *Rev Infect Dis* 1984;(**Suppl 6**):S235.

Daly JJ, Chowdary KVS: Pseudomembranous colitis secondary to metronidazole. *Dig Dis Sci* 1983;**28**:573.

George WL: Antimicrobial agent-associated colitis and diarrhea: Historical background and clinical aspects. *Rev Infect Dis* 1984;(**Suppl 6**):S208.

# NONSPECIFIC ULCERATIVE COLITIS

## Essentials of Diagnosis

- Bloody diarrhea with lower abdominal cramps.
- Mild abdominal tenderness, weight loss, fever.
- Anemia; no stool pathogens.
- Specific x-ray and sigmoidoscopic abnormalities.

## General Considerations

Ulcerative colitis is a chronic inflammatory disease of the colon of unknown cause characterized by bloody diarrhea, a tendency to remissions and exacerbations, and involvement mainly of the left colon. It is primarily a disease of adolescents and young adults but may have its onset in any age group.

The pathologic process is that of acute nonspecific inflammation in the colon, particularly the rectosigmoid area, with multiple irregular superficial ulcerations. Repeated episodes lead to thickening of the wall with scar tissue, and the proliferative changes in the epithelium may lead to polypoid structures. Pseudopolyps are usually indicative of severe ulceration. The cause is not known; it may be multiple.

## Clinical Findings

**A. Symptoms and Signs:** This disease may vary from mild cases with relatively minimal symptoms to acute and fulminating, with severe diarrhea and prostration. Diarrhea is characteristic; there may be up to 30 or 40 discharges daily, with blood and mucus in the stools, or blood and mucus may occur without feces. Blood in the stool is the cardinal manifestation of ulcerative colitis. Constipation may occur instead of diarrhea.

Nocturnal diarrhea is usually present when daytime diarrhea is severe. Rectal tenesmus may be severe, and anal incontinence may be present. Cramping lower abdominal pain often occurs but is generally mild. Anorexia, malaise, weakness, and fatigability may also be present. A history of intolerance to dairy products can often be obtained, and there is a tendency toward remissions and exacerbations.

Fever, weight loss, and evidence of toxemia vary with the severity of the disease. Abdominal tenderness is generally mild and occurs without signs of peritoneal irritation. Abdominal distention may be present in the fulminating form and is a poor prognostic sign. Rectal examination may show perianal irritation, fissure, hemorrhoids, and, uncommonly, fistulas and abscesses.

**B. Laboratory Findings:** Hypochromic microcytic anemia due to blood loss is usually present. In acute disease, a polymorphonuclear leukocytosis may also be present. The sedimentation rate is usually elevated. Stools contain blood, pus, and mucus but no pathogenic organisms. Hypoproteinemia may occur. In the fulminating disease, electrolyte disturbances may be evident.

**C. Imaging:** As shown by air contrast barium enema, the involvement may be regional to generalized and may vary from irritability and fuzzy margins to pseudopolyps, decreased size of colon, shortening and narrowing of the lumen, and loss of haustral markings. When the disease is limited to the rectosigmoid area, the barium enema may even be normal.

**D. Special Examinations:** Sigmoidoscopic changes are present in over 95% of cases and vary from mucosal hyperemia, petechiae, and minimal granularity in mild cases to ulceration and polypoid changes in severe cases. The mucosa, even when it appears grossly normal, is almost invariably friable when wiped with a cotton sponge. Colonoscopic examination may prove useful in defining the extent of ulcerative colitis. Colonoscopy with multiple biopsies looking for dysplasia and cancer should be considered on an annual basis after the tenth year of disease.

## Differential Diagnosis

Differentiate from bacillary dysentery and amebic dysentery on the basis of specific stool pathogens and (for amebiasis) the indirect hemagglutination test. When rectal strictures have developed, differentiate from lymphogranuloma venereum by history and complement fixation test. Other entities that must be distinguished are functional diarrhea, granulomatous colitis, intestinal neoplasm, and diverticulitis. It is imperative that any cultures and parasitology specimens be obtained before barium examinations are performed or before therapy is begun. Rectal abscesses and fistulas are considerably less frequent than in granulomatous colitis.

## Complications

**A. Local Complications:** Local complications in and around the large bowel include ischiorectal abscess, fistula in ano, rectovaginal fistula, rectal prolapse, fibrous stricture of the rectum or colon, colonic perforation, toxic dilatation of the colon, carcinoma, and massive colonic hemorrhage.

The incidence of carcinoma is significantly greater in patients with ulcerative colitis. It appears to be related to 2 factors. The first is the extent of involvement. Involvement of the entire colon carries a greater risk than minimal disease. The second factor is duration of the disease. The risk rises from approximately 2% at 10 years to 10–15% at 20 years, although a more recent study suggests a considerably lower risk.

**B. Systemic Complications:** Systemic complications include pyoderma gangrenosum, erythema nodosum, polyarthritis, ankylosing spondylitis, ocular lesions (episcleritis, iritis, uveitis), liver disease (fatty liver, pericholangitis, sclerosing cholangitis), anemia, pleuropericarditis, thrombophlebitis, and impaired growth and sexual development in children.

## Treatment

Ulcerative colitis is characterized by recurrent exacerbations, varying degrees of damage to the colonic mucosa, and complications both intestinal and extraintestinal. The treatment programs should attempt to (1) terminate the acute attack, (2) prevent recurrent attacks, and (3) promote healing of the damaged mucosa. Long-term therapy may be modified by considerations relating to complications, eg, carcinoma and ocular disease. Symptomatic remission should not be the only index of therapeutic response.

The choice and intensity of therapy should be determined by the clinical severity of the disease.

**A. Severe (Fulminant) Disease:**

**1. Hospitalization–**Hospitalization is indicated. Patients with severe disease may deteriorate rapidly, with hemorrhage, perforation, toxic megacolon, and sepsis developing over a short period of time.

**2. General measures–**

a. Restore circulating blood volume with fluids, plasma, and blood as indicated.

b. Discontinue opiates and anticholinergics.

c. Correct electrolyte abnormalities.

d. Discontinue all oral intake. Institute nasogastric suction if the colon has become dilated.

**3. Antimicrobial therapy–**The clinical course of fulminant ulcerative colitis is associated with extensive necrosis of colonic mucosa, and perforation with sepsis is not uncommon in this form of the disease. Intravenous antibiotics are given these patients for presumed or potential sepsis. Ampicillin, a cephalosporin, clindamycin, metronidazole, and gentamicin have been used singly or in appropriate combinations.

**4. Adrenocorticosteroids–**Give intravenous hydrocortisone, 300 mg daily, or prednisone, 60 mg daily, in divided doses at 6- to 8-hour intervals.

**5. Surgery–**If the patient with toxic colonic dilatation does not improve within 24 hours, colonic resection is usually indicated. In those patients who have fulminant disease but are not toxic, intravenous therapy is continued for 5–7 days. If improvement occurs, oral therapy can be substituted. If the patient fails to respond or deteriorates, colectomy should be considered. Malnourished patients may be benefited by total parenteral nutrition during this phase.

**B. Moderate Disease:** This group of patients has substantial evidence of activity, ie, diarrhea, abdominal cramping, weight loss, and anemia, and hospitalization should be advised. However, they are not in a toxic condition, ie, they do not have severe hypoproteinemia, fever, or leukocytosis.

**1. Diet–**Food served should be appealing and nutritious and contain adequate protein. Avoid foods known to exacerbate the individual patient's diarrhea or cramping. Some patients appear to be lactase-deficient and should avoid milk and milk products.

**2. Adrenocorticosteroids–**Give prednisone, 20–60 mg orally daily, and reduce by 5 mg per day per week when there is clinical and sigmoidoscopic evidence of improvement. Hydrocortisone enemas, 100 mg each night, may provide additional benefit.

**3. Sulfasalazine–**Sulfasalazine, 2–4 g daily in divided doses, has been shown to be beneficial in reducing inflammation and in decreasing the frequency of recurrent attacks in this form of the disease. It has been suggested that 5-aminosalicylic acid is the active moiety of sulfasalazine and that it does not have the side effects attributed to the sulfonamide moiety. 5-Aminosalicylic acid preparations will soon be available for use in enemas as well as orally. Sulfasalazine has been shown to produce oligospermia and infertility in men during the treatment period.

**C. Mild Disease:** These patients have minimal evidence of inflammatory bowel disease, ie, asymptomatic rectal bleeding, minimal involvement by sigmoidoscopic examination, and no systemic signs.

**1. Diet–**See ¶ 1 above.

**2. Sulfasalazine–**Sulfasalazine, 2–4 g daily in divided doses, as prolonged maintenance therapy.

**3. Adrenocorticosteroids–**Hydrocortisone enemas or suppositories, 100 mg each night until lesion heals or treatment proves ineffective.

**D. Surgical Measures:** Surgical excision of the colon is required for patients with refractory disease, severe extracolonic complications (growth suppression), prolonged widespread colon disease, massive hemorrhage, or extensive perirectal disease. The usual procedure is total colectomy with a permanent ileostomy. In some instances, the rectum may be preserved (stripped of its mucosa) and an ileoproctostomy performed with ileal mucosa replacing the stripped rectal mucosa. This allows intestinal continuity and avoids an ileostomy, but most of these patients will have 4–7 liquid stools per day.

## Prognosis

The course may be characterized by remissions and exacerbations over a period of many years, or it may be fulminant. Permanent and complete cure on medical therapy is unusual, and life expectancy is shortened. The incidence of bowel cancer in patients with active disease rises with each decade after the diagnosis. Medical measures control the majority of cases, but colectomy is often necessary for fulminant, refractory disease and for complications. Because of potential complications with chronic ulcerative colitis, close follow-up is indicated, particularly after the disease has been present for 8–10 years. It is recommended that after 10 years of disease, colonoscopy be performed annually, and that on these occasions multiple biopsies should be examined for dysplasia. Dysplasia is considered a precancerous lesion and if severe is thought to be an indication for colectomy.

Bailar JC III: Cigarettes, ulcerative colitis, and inferences from uncontrolled data. (Editorial.) *N Engl J Med* 1983;**308:**275.

Dobbins WO III: Dysplasia and malignancy in inflammatory bowel disease. *Annu Rev Med* 1984;**35:**33.

Hendriksen C, Kreiner S, Binder V: Long-term prognosis in ulcerative colitis: Based on results from a regional patient group from the County of Copenhagen. *Gut* 1985;**26:**158.

Lennard-Jones JE et al: Cancer surveillance in ulcerative colitis. *Gastroenterology* 1984;**86:**770.

Peppercorn MA: Sulfasalazine: Pharmacology, clinical use, toxicity and related new drug development. *Ann Intern Med* 1984;**101**:377.

Sales DJ, Kirsner JB: The prognosis of inflammatory bowel disease. (Review.) *Arch Intern Med* 1983;**143**:294.

Sandberg-Gertzen H et al: Azodisal sodium in the treatment of ulcerative colitis: A study of tolerance and relapse-prevention properties. *Gastroenterology* 1986;**90**:1024.

Taylor BM, Beart RW Jr: Alternatives to ileostomy after colectomy for inflammatory bowel disease. *Annu Rev Med* 1985;**36**:315.

Waterhouse JAH et al: Survival of patients with colorectal cancer complicating ulcerative colitis. *Gut* 1984;**25**:228.

## TOXIC DILATATION OF THE COLON
### (Toxic Megacolon)

Toxic megacolon is a life-threatening complication of idiopathic ulcerative colitis or Crohn's disease of the colon. The disease has also been observed in amebiasis, pseudomembranous colitis, typhoid fever, cholera, and bacillary dysentery. It results from extensive damage to the mucosa, with areas of mucosal denudation and inflammation of the submucosal layers. Contributing factors include cathartics, opiates, anticholinergics, and hypokalemia. It is manifested clinically by evidence of systemic toxicity, fever, leukocytosis, tachycardia, and abdominal distention. Radiographically, the colon is seen to be dilated. Colonic dilatation per se without signs of systemic toxicity may be the result of potassium deficiency or anticholinergic or opiate therapy. The mortality rate of this fulminant complication is high, and treatment, both medical and surgical, should be instituted as soon as possible.

Treatment consists of the following urgent measures: (1) Decompress the bowel and pass an intestinal tube to prevent swallowed air from further distending the colon. (2) Replace lost fluids and electrolytes and restore colloid and blood volume. Remember that diarrhea and adrenal steroid therapy significantly reduce total body potassium and that this has an adverse effect on colonic function. (3) Suppress the inflammatory reaction with hydrocortisone, 100 mg intravenously every 8 hours. (4) Prevent sepsis with broad-spectrum antibiotics (gentamicin, clindamycin).

Careful observation with frequent abdominal films during the period of 8–12 hours while the above therapy is being given determines whether or not the patient will require surgical treatment. If the colon decompresses, medical therapy is continued; if not, colectomy should be considered. These patients are desperately ill, and if surgery is necessary the procedure of choice is subtotal colectomy. This reduces operating time and the extent of operative trauma. Most of the patients who develop toxic dilatation of the colon but do not require emergency colectomy will require colectomy at a later time because of continuing disease.

Grant CS et al: Toxic megacolon: Ultimate fate of patients after successful medical management. *Am J Surg* 1984;**147**:106.

Greenstein AJ et al: Outcome of toxic dilatation in ulcerative and Crohn's colitis. *J Clin Gastroenterol* 1985;**7**:137.

## GRANULOMATOUS COLITIS*
### (Crohn's Disease of the Colon)

Granulomatous colitis (transmural colitis; Crohn's disease of the colon) may be difficult or impossible to distinguish from the mucosal form of colitis (idiopathic ulcerative colitis) by clinical criteria alone. The most distinguishing feature is transmural involvement in Crohn's colitis. Table 11–3 briefly summarizes the features of these 2 entities. However, the differential diagnostic criteria, when tested against the pathologic findings following colectomy, show a substantial overlap in clinical, radiographic, and histologic criteria.

The most common clinical manifestations are abdominal cramping, diarrhea, and weight loss. Extracolonic manifestations such as erythema nodosum, spondylitis, polyarthritis, and perirectal disease may antedate the colonic manifestations of the disease.

The treatment of granulomatous colitis is essentially the same as for idiopathic ulcerative colitis.

Binder V, Hendriksen C, Kreiner S: Prognosis in Crohn's disease: Based on results from the County of Copenhagen. *Gut* 1985;**26**:146.

Farmer RG, Whelan G, Fazio VW: Long-term follow-up of patients with Crohn's disease: Relationship between the clinical pattern and prognosis. *Gastroenterology* 1985;**88**:1818.

Korelitz BI: Carcinoma of the intestinal tract in Crohn's disease: Results of a survey conducted by the National Foundation for Ileitis and Colitis. *Am J Gastroenterol* 1983;**78**:44.

## ISCHEMIC COLITIS

Interference with blood flow to the colon causes ischemic colitis. The rectum is usually spared because of its dual blood supply from the inferior mesenteric artery and, via the rectal (hemorrhoidal) vessels, from the internal iliac artery. Most patients are 50–70 years old. Younger women taking oral contraceptives are also at risk.

Presenting symptoms are lower abdominal pain of sudden onset, fever, vomiting, and the passage of bright red blood and clots per rectum. A neutrophil leukocytosis is usual. The sigmoidoscopic examination is often normal, since involvement is usually of the more proximal portions of the colon, particularly the cecum, splenic flexure, and sigmoid colon. When the sigmoid colon is involved, a demarcation in mucosal color can often be seen at the rectosigmoid junction. Involvement of the sigmoid colon or the rectum (rare) may have the appearance on sigmoidos-

---

* See also p 373.

**Table 11–3.** Differential features of ulcerative colitis and granulomatous colitis.[*]

|  | Ulcerative Colitis | Granulomatous Colitis |
|---|---|---|
| **Clinical** | | |
| Toxicity | Common | Rare |
| Bleeding | Common | Rare |
| Perianal disease | Rare | Common |
| Fistula | Rare | Common |
| Perforation | Rare | Common |
| Sigmoidoscopy | Diffuse, friable superficial ulceration | Discrete, occasionally diffuse |
| **X-ray** | | |
| Distribution | Continuous | Segmental |
| Mucosa | Serrated | Fissures to deep ulcers |
| Stricture | Rare | Common |
| **Pathology** | Mucosal microabscesses | Transmural involvement, granulomas |

[*] Reference: Margulis AR et al: The overlapping spectrum of ulcerative and granulomatous colitis: A roentgenographic-pathologic study. *Am J Roentgenol* 1971;**113**:325.

copy of nonspecific proctocolitis or multiple ulcers, polypoid or nodular lesions, or, in some instances, hemorrhagic or necrotic membrane formation.

Plain films of the abdomen may show generalized dilatation of the colon. Barium enema normally shows a segmental area of involvement occurring, in descending order of frequency, in the splenic flexure, sigmoid colon, and ascending colon. The involved area is characterized by a variable combination of thumbprinting (edematous mucosal folds), sawtoothed mucosal irregularity, tubular narrowing, and sacculation. Angiograms may be helpful in showing vascular occlusions, particularly in patients who may have embolic potential. Most ischemic disease is nonocclusive, and angiograms will not be helpful. Inflammatory bowel involvement by Crohn's disease, idiopathic ulcerative colitis, and infection and stricture due to carcinoma must be ruled out.

Severe ischemia leading to gangrene is treated by replacement of blood volume, antibiotics (eg, ampicillin, clindamycin, metronidazole, or gentamicin), and excision of necrotic bowel. Less severe ischemia leading to stricture formation is treated by resection of the stricture. Transient ischemia requires no specific treatment.

The prognosis is good in transient proctocolitis. The mortality rate is high when gangrene occurs.

Anderson R et al: Acute intestinal ischemia. A 14 year retrospective investigation. *Acta Chir Scand* 1984;**150**:217.

Brandt LJ et al: Simulations of colonic carcinoma by ischemia. *Gastroenterology* 1985;**88**:1137.

Ottinger LW: Mesenteric ischemia. *N Engl J Med* 1982; **307**:535.

# DIVERTICULAR DISEASE OF THE COLON

## Essentials of Diagnosis

- Intermittent, cramping left lower abdominal pain.
- Constipation or alternating constipation and diarrhea.
- Tenderness in the left lower quadrant.
- X-ray evidence of diverticula, thickened interhaustral folds, narrowed lumen.

## General Considerations

Diverticula of the colon occur with increasing frequency after age 40—5% in the tenth decade and 50% in the ninth decade. Although diverticula may occur throughout the gut, excluding the rectum, they are most common in the high-pressure areas of the colon (eg, sigmoid). They tend to dissect along the course of the nutrient vessels, and they consist of a mucosal coat and a serosa. The inflammatory complication, diverticulitis, probably affects 10–20% of patients at some time.

Inflammatory changes in diverticulitis vary from mild polymorphonuclear infiltration in the wall of the sac to extensive inflammatory change in the surrounding area (peridiverticulitis), with perforation or abscess formation. The changes are comparable to those that occur in appendicitis.

## Clinical Findings

**A. Symptoms and Signs:** Left lower quadrant pain may be steady and severe and last for days or may be cramping and intermittent and relieved by a bowel movement. Constipation is usual, but diarrhea may occur. Occult blood is found in the stool in about 20% of cases. Diverticulosis coli is the most common cause of colonic hemorrhage; lower gastrointestinal hemorrhage is uncommon in diverticulitis.

**B. Laboratory Findings:** Noncontributory in uncomplicated diverticular disease.

**C. Imaging:** Radiographic examination reveals diverticula and in some cases spasm, interhaustral thickening, or narrowing of the colonic lumen.

## Complications

Diverticulitis is a complication of diverticular disease in which gross or microscopic perforation of the diverticulum has occurred. The clinical manifestations vary with the extent of the inflammatory process and may include pain, signs of peritoneal irritation, chills, fever, sepsis, ileus, and partial or complete colonic obstruction. Peritonitis and abscess formation may also occur. Urinary frequency and dysuria are associated with bladder involvement in the inflammatory process. Fistula formation usually involves the bladder (usually vesicosigmoid) but may also be to the skin, perianal area, or small bowel. The white blood count shows polymorphonuclear leukocytosis. Red and white blood cells may be seen in the urine. Blood cultures may be positive.

## Differential Diagnosis

The constrictive lesion of the colon seen on x-ray or at sigmoidoscopy must be differentiated from carcinoma of the colon. The appearance of a short lesion with abrupt transition to normal bowel suggests carcinoma. Colonoscopy with biopsy can be very useful in these instances.

## Treatment

The treatment of uncomplicated diverticular disease consists primarily of increasing bulk in the diet by means of the following: (1) high-residue diet; (2) unprocessed bran, ¼ cup daily in fruit juice or muffins; or (3) bulk additives such as psyllium hydrophilic mucilloid (Hydrocil, Konsyl, Metamucil, and others). Other measures that may be helpful are (1) stool softeners such as docusate sodium (Colace and others), 240 mg per day; and (2) anticholinergic drugs to decrease "spasm" in the sigmoid colon.

The treatment of acute diverticulitis requires antibiotic therapy. The antibiotic of choice is ampicillin or cefoxitin. Other useful antibiotic drugs include metronidazole and combined treatment with penicillin and gentamicin.

Recurrent attacks of diverticulitis or the presence of perforation, fistula formation, or abscess formation requires surgical resection of the involved portion of the colon.

Massive diverticular hemorrhage usually stops spontaneously. Adequate blood replacement and careful endoscopic and barium studies are indicated to rule out other causes of bleeding. In certain instances, selective arteriography may localize the site of the bleeding and make it possible to control the bleeding with vasopressin. Operation may be required for uncontrolled bleeding.

## Prognosis

The usual case is mild and responds well to dietary measures and antibiotics.

Almy TP, Naitove A: Diverticular disease of the colon. Pages 896–911 in: *Gastrointestinal Disease: Pathophysiology, Diagnosis, Management*, 3rd ed. Sleisenger MH, Fordtran JS (editors). Saunders, 1983.

Hackford AW, Veidenheimer MC: Diverticular disease of the colon: Current concepts and management. *Surg Clin North Am* 1985;**65**:347.

## ANGIODYSPLASIA OF THE COLON

Angiodysplasia of the colon as a cause of acute and chronic lower gastrointestinal bleeding is being increasingly recognized. It is seen chiefly in patients over age 50 (most of them over 70) with a prevalence of approximately 2% and is characterized by painless, usually self-limited intermittent rectal bleeding. The bleeding is usually of dark red blood but may be occult. There may be tarry stools. Up to 30% of patients have a history of surgery for gastrointestinal

bleeding—eg, vagotomy and pyloroplasty, gastrectomy. Patients with angiodysplasia have an incidence of aortic stenosis of up to 25%. Most lesions of angiodysplasia are in the cecum and right colon.

## Treatment

**A. Medical Treatment:** The patient must be stabilized with fluids and packed red cells as clinically dictated and then evaluated for bleeding diatheses: ask about aspirin and warfarin ingestion, perform liver function tests, and check prothrombin time. To rule out an upper gastrointestinal site, upper endoscopy should be seriously considered even when the gastric aspirate is negative for blood and positive for bile. The sequence of additional evaluation is controversial, partly depending upon the resources available, but would include the following:

1. Technetium-labeled red cell scan to attempt to localize the site of bleeding. This is more sensitive than angiography; it has been shown to identify bleeding at a rate of 0.05 mL/min in experimental settings and at a rate of 0.5 mL/min clinically.

2. Colonoscopy after appropriate cleansing of the colon. In some studies, over 80% of patients with angiographically proved angiodysplasia are identified in this way.

3. Angiography provides definitive diagnosis at centers where experts with the procedure are available.

**B. Surgical Treatment:** The major options are cautery or sclerosis of the vascular lesion via colonoscopy, or surgical resection.

Boley SJ, Brandt LJ, Mitsudo SM: Vascular lesions of the colon. *Adv Intern Med* 1984;**29**:301.

Richter JM et al: Angiodysplasia: Clinical presentation and colonoscopic diagnosis. *Dig Dis Sci* 1984;**29**:481.

## POLYPS OF THE COLON & RECTUM
## (Intestinal Polyps)

Adenomatous polyps of the colon and rectum are common benign neoplasms that are usually asymptomatic but may cause painless rectal bleeding. They may be single or multiple, occur most frequently in the sigmoid and rectum, and are found incidentally in about 9% of autopsies. The incidence of polyps increases with age. The diagnosis is established by sigmoidoscopy, double contrast barium enema, and colonoscopy. When a polyp is found in the rectum, the colon should be studied by x-ray or colonoscopy.

Whether polyps are precancerous is an important question. Pedunculated adenomatous polyps less than 1 cm in diameter have very slight malignant potential and can usually be managed by simple polypectomy through the colonoscope. Larger adenomatous polyps impose a greater risk and must be removed. Villous adenomas are usually sessile and become malignant in 10% of cases if they are 2 cm in diameter or less and in up to 50% of cases if they are larger. These too require removal, which can often be accomplished with the colonoscope; if not, surgical resection is required. Because colonic polyps tend to recur and because of their malignant potential, colonscopic surveillance should be scheduled at 1 year postpolypectomy. If no polyps are found at that time, a repeat examination is indicated 2 years later unless clinically indicated sooner. Most cancers of the colon and rectum arise de novo. For polyps removed by colonoscopic polypectomy that are determined to be malignant, the sufficiency of polypectomy as the sole treatment is determined by the histologic characteristics of the cancer and the extent of invasion of the stalk and the mucosa.

There are several familial polyp syndromes, some of which have a strong predilection for carcinoma (Table 11–4). These need to be identified and treated and genetic counseling provided. For polyps with high malignant potential, colectomy with ileostomy or ileoproctostomy—after stripping of the rectal mucosa—is indicated.

Boland CR: Familial colonic cancer syndromes. (Medical Staff Conference.) *West J Med* 1983;**139**:351.

Bülow S: Colorectal polyposis syndromes. *Scand J Gastroenterol* 1984;**19**:289.

Cranley JP et al: When is endoscopic polypectomy adequate therapy for colonic polyps containing invasive carcinoma? *Gastroenterology* 1986;**91**:419.

Sherlock P, Winawer SJ: Are there markers for the risk of colorectal cancer? *N Engl J Med* 1984;**311**:118.

## COLONIC OBSTRUCTION

Colonic obstruction may be acute or chronic. It may be simple, strangulating, paralytic, or closed loop. The most common cause of subacute and chronic obstruction of the colon is carcinoma. Other causes include drugs (phenothiazine, tricyclic antidepressants, morphine derivatives), fecal impaction, scleroderma, strictures caused by granulomatous colitis, and diverticular disease of the colon. Acute obstruction is usually due to volvulus, intussusception, or

**Table 11–4.** Gastrointestinal polyposis syndromes.[*]

| Syndrome | Histology | Distribution | Malignant Potential | Other Manifestations | Genetic Mechanism |
|---|---|---|---|---|---|
| Familial polyposis | 150–5000 adenomas | Colorectum | High | None, but included in many syndromes | Autosomal dominant |
| Gardner syndrome | 25–200 scattered adenomas | Colorectum, occasionally esophagus, stomach, small bowel | High | Osteomas, epidermoid cysts, fibromas, desmoid tumors, mesenteric fibromatosis, dental abnormalities | Autosomal dominant |
| Turcot syndrome | Scattered adenomas | Colorectum | High | Central nervous system tumors | Autosomal recessive |
| Familial discrete polyps | 1–6 scattered adenomas | Colorectum | High | None | Autosomal dominant |
| Peutz-Jeghers syndrome | Hamartomas | Entire gastrointestinal tract, mainly stomach, small bowel, colorectum | Low or absent | Pigmentation of lips and skin | Autosomal dominant |
| Juvenile polyposis | Most hamartomas, few adenomas | Entire gastrointestinal tract, most common in colorectum | Low | Anemia, protein-losing enteropathy | Some familial |
| Multiple hamartoma syndrome (Cowden disease) | Multiple hamartomas | Gastrointestinal tract | None | Warty papules on mucosa and skin, multiple malformations | Autosomal dominant |
| Basal cell nevus syndrome | Multiple hamartomas | Stomach | None from gastrointestinal polyps (skin cancer) | Benign mesenteric cysts | Autosomal dominant |
| Cronkhite-Canada syndrome | Thickened mucosa, likened to juvenile polyps | Stomach, small bowel, colon | None | Skin pigmentation, nail atrophy, alopecia, protein-losing enteropathy | All cases sporadic, probably nongenetic |

[*] Reproduced, with permission, from: Gardner EJ et al: Gastrointestinal polyposis: Syndromes and genetic mechanisms. *West J Med* 1980;**132**:488.

inguinal herniation of the colon. Idiopathic pseudo-obstruction may also occur (Ogilvie's syndrome).

## Clinical Findings

**A. Symptoms and Signs:** Simple obstruction with constipation or obstipation may lead to the insidious development of pain. Severe continuous pain suggests strangulation. Borborygmus may be prominent. Nausea and vomiting are late signs. Physical examination discloses abdominal distention and tympany. High-pitched tinkles may be heard on auscultation. A localized mass suggests carcinoma, intussusception, or strangulated closed loop. Peritoneal signs suggest perforation. Blood in the rectum suggests intussusception or carcinoma.

**B. Laboratory Findings:** Noncontributory unless strangulation has occurred.

**C. Imaging:** Colonic distention can be demonstrated by plain abdominal films. The barium enema will demonstrate the site of obstruction, but this procedure is contraindicated if there is ischemia with necrosis of the bowel wall. Barium by upper gastrointestinal series should never be given if there is any possibility of colonic obstruction.

## Differential Diagnosis

In paralytic ileus the abdomen is silent, and cramping does not occur. Signs of peritonitis are present, or there is a history of drug ingestion or trauma to the back or pelvis.

In small bowel obstruction, vomiting is more common and occurs earlier. The abdominal pain is usually more severe, and x-ray may reveal the ladder configuration of distended small bowel with little or no colonic distention.

## Complications

Delay in treatment may lead to strangulation with perforation, peritonitis, and sepsis.

## Treatment

The treatment of colonic obstruction is usually surgical. However, sigmoid volvulus or pseudo-obstruction often can be decompressed with sigmoidoscopy or colonoscopy and intussusception by barium enema. The baseline medical treatment is to decompress the patient from above with nasogastric suction and to stabilize fluid, electrolyte, cardiac, and pulmonary status. Even patients acutely decompressed by nonsurgical means usually require surgery for definitive care.

Ballantyne GH: Review of sigmoid volvulus: History and results of treatment. *Dis Colon Rectum* 1982;**25**:494.

Fausel CS, Goff JS: Nonoperative management of acute idiopathic colonic pseudo-obstruction (Ogilvie's syndrome). *West J Med* 1985;**143**:50.

# CANCER OF THE COLON & RECTUM

## Essentials of Diagnosis

- Altered bowel function (constipation or diarrhea).
- Blood in the feces, unexplained anemia, weight loss.
- Palpable mass involving colon or rectum.
- Sigmoidoscopic or radiographic evidence of neoplasm.

## General Considerations

Carcinoma is the only common cancer of the colon and rectum. Lymphoma, carcinoid, melanoma, fibrosarcoma, and other types of sarcoma occur rarely. The treatment of all is essentially the same.

Carcinoma of the colon and rectum accounts for about 15% of cancer deaths, second only to cancer of the lung. Predisposing causes are listed in Table 11–5. Males are affected slightly more commonly than females. The highest incidence is in patients about 50 years of age, but occasional cases have been reported in younger persons and even in children. The anatomic distribution of cancer of the large bowel is approximately 16% in the cecum and ascending colon, 5% in the transverse colon, 9% in the descending colon, 20% in the sigmoid, and 50% in the rectum.

Many lesions of the rectum and colon lie within reach of the examining finger or sigmoidoscope and therefore can be biopsied on the first visit.

## Clinical Findings

Symptoms vary depending upon whether the lesion is in the right or the left side of the colon. In either case, a persistent change in the customary bowel habits almost always occurs and should invariably alert the physician to investigate the colon. Bleeding is a cardinal diagnostic point. An acute abdominal emergency may be precipitated by perforation or colonic obstruction (due to circumferential narrowing, not intussusception). The diagnosis of colonic and rectal cancer is established by sigmoidoscopy and colonoscopy with biopsy and barium enema. Polyps and carcinoma not detected by barium enema may be detected by colonoscopy.

**Table 11–5.** Factors associated with increased risk of colonic cancer.

| Standard Risk | High Risk[*] |
|---|---|
| After age 40 (both men and women) | Rectocolonic polyps (familial polyposis, villous polyps, adenomatous polyps, history of juvenile polyps)<br>Cancer elsewhere in the body<br>Familial history of colon cancer<br>Ulcerative colitis<br>Granulomatous colitis<br>Immunodeficiency disease |

[*] Listed in approximate decreasing frequency of importance.

**A. Carcinoma of the Right Colon:** Because the fecal stream is fluid and the bowel lumen large in the right half of the colon, symptoms of obstruction occur less frequently than in left-sided tumors. Vague abdominal discomfort is often the only initial complaint. This may progress to cramplike pain, occasionally simulating cholecystitis or appendicitis. Secondary anemia with associated weakness and weight loss is found in half of patients with right colon lesions. The stools are usually positive for occult blood but rarely show gross blood. The patient is likely to have diarrhea. The first indication of cancer may be the discovery of a palpable mass in the right lower quadrant.

**B. Carcinoma of the Left Colon:** Obstructive symptoms predominate, particularly increasing constipation. There may be short bouts of diarrhea. Occasionally the first sign is acute colonic obstruction. A small amount of bright red blood with bowel movements is common, and anemia is found in about 20% of cases. At times a mass is palpable. About half of patients give a history of weight loss.

### Differential Diagnosis

Diverticulitis is usually associated with fever and has a different x-ray appearance. Functional bowel distress may also simulate cancer of the colon symptomatically.

### Treatment

The only curative treatment in cancer of the large bowel is wide surgical resection of the lesion and its regional lymphatics after adequate bowel preparation and appropriate supportive measures. When a significant degree of mechanical obstruction is present, a preliminary transverse colostomy or cecostomy is necessary. Even in the presence of metastatic disease, palliative resection may be of value to relieve obstruction, bleeding, or the symptoms of local invasion. Preoperative irradiation, 2000–2500 R in 10 fractions given over 12 days, has been shown to increase resectability and improve survival in patients undergoing abdominoperineal resection.

### Prognosis

Over 90% of patients with carcinoma of the colon and rectum are suitable for either curative or palliative resection, with an operative mortality rate of 3–6%. The overall 5-year survival rate after resection is about 50%. If the lesion is confined to the bowel and there is no evidence of lymphatic or blood vessel invasion, the 5-year survival rate is 60–70%. Local recurrence of carcinoma in the anastomotic suture line or wound area occurs in 10–15% of cases. The incidence of local recurrence can be decreased if special precautions are taken at operation to avoid implantation of malignant cells. About 5% of patients develop multiple primary colon cancers. Early identification of resectable local recurrence or a new neoplasm depends upon careful follow-up with sigmoidoscopy and barium enema every 6 months for 2 years and yearly

thereafter. Carcinoembryonic antigen (CEA) is also a marker for detection of recurrent tumor (levels increase) in patients with normal levels after resection and may prove useful if monitored at 6-month intervals.

Gastrointestinal Tumor Study Group: Prolongation of the disease-free interval in surgically treated rectal carcinoma. *N Engl J Med* 1985;**312:**1465.

Love RR, Morrissey JF: Colonoscopy in asymptomatic individuals with a family history of colorectal cancer. *Arch Intern Med* 1984;**144:**2209.

Markovitz JF, Aiges HW, Cunningham-Rundles S: Cancer family syndrome: Marker studies. *Gastroenterology* 1986; **91:**581.

Moore JRL, LaMont JT: Colorectal cancer: Risk factors and screening strategies. *Arch Intern Med* 1984;**144:**1819.

Third International Symposium on Colorectal Cancer. *CA* 1984;**34:**130.

Winawer SJ, Miller DG, Sherlock P: Risk and screening for colorectal cancer. *Adv Intern Med* 1985;**30:**471.

# ANORECTAL DISEASES

## HEMORRHOIDS

### Essentials of Diagnosis

- Rectal bleeding, protrusion, and vague discomfort.
- Mucoid discharge from rectum.
- Characteristic findings on external anal inspection or anoscopic examination.

### General Considerations

Internal hemorrhoids are varices of the portion of the venous hemorrhoidal plexus that lies submucosally just proximal to the dentate margin. External hemorrhoids arise from the same plexus but are located subcutaneously immediately distal to the dentate margin. There are 3 primary internal hemorrhoidal masses: right anterior, right posterior, and left lateral. Three to 5 secondary hemorrhoids may be present between the 3 primaries. Straining at stool, constipation, prolonged sitting, and anal infection are contributing factors and may precipitate complications such as thrombosis. The diagnosis is suspected on the history of protrusion, anal pain, or bleeding and is confirmed by proctologic examination.

Carcinoma of the colon or rectum not infrequently aggravates hemorrhoids or produces similar complaints. Polyps may be present as a cause of bleeding that is wrongly attributed to hemorrhoids. For these reasons, the treatment of hemorrhoids is always preceded by sigmoidoscopy and barium enema. When portal hypertension is suspected as a causative factor, investigations for liver disease should be carried out. Hemorrhoids that develop during pregnancy or parturition tend to subside thereafter and should be treated conservatively unless persistent.

## Clinical Findings

The symptoms of hemorrhoids are usually mild and remittent, but a number of disturbing complications may develop and call for active medical or surgical treatment. These complications include pruritus; incontinence; recurrent protrusion requiring manual replacement by the patient; fissure, infection, or ulceration; prolapse and strangulation; and secondary anemia due to chronic blood loss. Carcinoma has been reported to develop very rarely in hemorrhoids.

## Treatment

Conservative treatment suffices in most instances of mild hemorrhoids, which may improve spontaneously or in response to a high-roughage diet, psyllium seed preparation, or nonirritating laxatives to produce soft stools. Local pain and infection are managed with warm sitz baths and insertion of a soothing anal suppository 2 or 3 times daily. Benzocaine and similar types of anal ointments should be avoided so as not to sensitize the patient to these agents. Prolapsed or strangulated hemorrhoids may be treated conservatively by gentle reduction with a lubricated gloved finger; by rubber band ligation or cryosurgery, or both; or by immediate surgical resection.

For severe symptoms or complications, complete internal and external hemorrhoidectomy is advisable and is a highly satisfactory procedure when properly done. Excision of a single external hemorrhoid, evacuation of a thrombosed pile, and the injection treatment of internal hemorrhoids fall within the scope of office practice. Injection therapy is effective, but there is a recurrence rate of more than 50%.

## Evacuation of Thrombosed External Hemorrhoid

This condition is caused by the rupture of a vein at the anal margin, forming a clot in the subcutaneous tissue. The patient complains of a painful lump, and examination shows a tense, tender, bluish mass covered with skin. If the patient is seen after 24–48 hours when the pain is subsiding—or if symptoms are minimal—hot sitz baths are prescribed. If discomfort is marked, removal of the clot is indicated. With the patient in the lateral position, the area is prepared with antiseptic, and 1% lidocaine is injected intracutaneously around and over the lump. An ellipse of skin is then excised and the clot evacuated. A dry gauze dressing is held in place for 12–24 hours by taping the buttocks together, and daily sitz baths are then begun.

## CRYPTITIS & PAPILLITIS

Anal pain and burning of brief duration with defecation is suggestive of cryptitis and papillitis. Digital and anoscopic examination reveals hypertrophied papillae and indurated or inflamed crypts. Treatment consists of adding bulk agents, such as psyllium seed preparations, to the diet; sitz baths; and anal suppositories containing hydrocortisone after each bowel movement. Some recommend local application of 5% phenol in oil or carbolfuchsin compound to the crypts. If these measures fail, surgical excision of involved crypts and papillae should be considered.

## Anorectal Infections

Anorectal infections are seen chiefly in homosexual men and can be divided into 2 clinical syndromes: proctitis and proctocolitis.

**Proctitis** is characterized by anorectal pain, mucopurulent or bloody discharge, tenesmus, constipation, and an inflamed, often mucopurulent rectal mucosa. The most common pathogens are *Neisseria gonorrhoeae,* chlamydiae and herpesvirus. The diagnosis can be made on sigmoidoscopy, with specimens obtained for Gram's stain and culture as well as by biopsy. Syphilis may cause proctitis, with a chancre appearing 2–6 weeks after anal intercourse. Secondary syphilis may be characterized by condyloma latum, which must be differentiated from anal warts.

The differential diagnosis should include traumatic proctitis.

Treatment depends upon the cause.

**Proctocolitis** implies involvement beyond the rectum to include at least the sigmoid colon. The causes may include those of proctitis, but more commonly are due to *Shigella, Campylobacter,* or amebiasis. Symptoms usually include diarrhea, abdominal cramping, and fever—in addition to the symptoms of proctitis.

Ulcerative colitis and granulomatous colitis must be considered in the differential diagnosis.

Treatment depends upon the specific bacteriologic diagnosis.

## Rectal Prolapse & Solitary Ulcer

Rectal prolapse is a not uncommon problem, particularly among the elderly, and is associated with a long history of constipation and straining. The support structures of the anorectal area have usually become weakened, leading to rectal intussusception with straining. An early manifestation may be solitary rectal ulcer—a painful condition with ulcerogenesis apparently secondary to the intussusception.

Management consists of surgical correction of the lax support system.

## FISSURA IN ANO (Anal Fissure)

Acute fissures represent linear disruption of the anal epithelium due to various causes. They usually clear if bowel movements are kept regular and soft (eg, with a bulk agent, bran, or psyllium seed preparation). The local application of a mild styptic such as 1–2% silver nitrate or 1% gentian violet solution may be of value.

Chronic fissure is characterized by (1) acute pain during and after defecation; (2) spotting of bright red blood at stool, with occasional more abundant bleeding; (3) tendency to constipation through fear of pain; and (4) the late occurrence of a sentinel pile, a hypertrophied papilla, and spasm of the anal canal (usually very painful on digital examination). Regulation of bowel habits with use of bran or psyllium seed preparation in the diet or use of stool softeners, sitz baths, or anal suppositories (eg, Anusol) twice daily should be tried. If these measures fail, the fissure, sentinel pile, or papilla and the adjacent crypt must be excised surgically. Postoperative care is along the lines of the preoperative treatment.

## ANAL ABSCESS

Perianal abscess should be considered the acute stage of an anal fistula until proved otherwise. The abscess should be adequately drained as soon as localized. Hot sitz baths may hasten the process of localization. The patient should be warned that the fistula may persist after drainage of the abscess. It is painful and fruitless to search for the internal opening of a fistula in the presence of acute infection. The presence of an anal abscess should alert the clinician to the possibility of inflammatory bowel disease, especially Crohn's disease.

## FISTULA IN ANO

About 95% of all anal fistulas arise in an anal crypt, and they are often preceded by an anal abscess. If an anal fistula enters the rectum above the pectinate line and there is no associated disease in the crypts, granulomatous colitis, regional ileitis, rectal tuberculosis, lymphogranuloma venereum, cancer, or foreign body should be considered in the differential diagnosis.

Acute fistula is associated with a purulent discharge from the fistulous opening. There is usually local itching, tenderness, or pain aggravated by bowel movements. Recurrent anal abscess may develop. The involved crypt can occasionally be located anoscopically with a crypt hook. Probing the fistula should be gentle because false passages can be made with ease, and in any case demonstration of the internal opening by probing is not essential to the diagnosis.

Treatment is by surgical incision or excision of the fistula under general anesthesia. If a fistula passes deep to the entire anorectal ring, so that all the muscles must be divided in order to extirpate the tract, a 2-stage operation must be done to prevent incontinence.

## ANAL CONDYLOMAS
## (Genital Warts)

These wartlike papillomas of the perianal skin and anal canal flourish on moist, macerated surfaces, particularly in the presence of purulent discharge. They are not true tumors but are infectious and autoinoculable, probably owing to a sexually transmitted papovavirus. They must be distinguished from condylomata lata caused by syphilis. The diagnosis of the latter rests on a positive serologic test for syphilis or discovery of *Treponema pallidum* on darkfield examination.

Treatment consists of *cautious* accurate application of liquid nitrogen or 25% podophyllum resin in tincture of benzoin to the lesion (with bare wooden or cotton-tipped applicator sticks to avoid contact with uninvolved skin). The compound should be washed off after 2–4 hours. Condylomas in the anal canal are treated through the anoscope and the painted site dusted with powder to localize the application and minimize discomfort. Electrofulguration under local anesthesia is useful if there are numerous lesions. Local cleanliness and the frequent use of a talc dusting powder are essential.

Condylomas tend to recur. The patient should be observed for several months and advised to report promptly if new lesions appear.

## BENIGN ANORECTAL
## STRICTURES

### Traumatic

Acquired stenosis is usually the result of surgery or trauma that denudes the epithelium of the anal canal. Hemorrhoid operations in which too much skin is removed or which are followed by infection are the commonest cause. Constipation, ribbon stools, and pain on defecation are the most frequent complaints. Stenosis predisposes to fissure, low-grade infection, and, occasionally, fistula.

Prevention of stenosis after radical anal surgery is best accomplished by local cleanliness, hot sitz baths, and gentle insertion of the well-lubricated finger twice weekly for 2–3 weeks beginning 2 weeks after surgery. When stenosis is chronic but mild, graduated anal dilators of increasing size may be inserted daily by the patient. For marked stenosis, a plastic operation on the anal canal is advisable.

### Inflammatory

**A. Lymphogranuloma Venereum:** This disease is caused by certain immunotypes of *Chlamydia* and is the commonest cause of an infectious inflammatory stricture of the anorectal region. It is most common in women and in male homosexuals and occurs in about 3% of patients in sexually transmitted disease clinics. Acute proctitis due to lymphatic spread of the organism occurs early and may be followed by perirectal infections, sinuses, and formation of scar tissue (resulting in stricture). Swollen, often painful, purple discolored inguinal lymph nodes appear early in the course. Frei and complement fixation tests are positive.

The tetracycline drugs are curative in the initial phase of the disease. When extensive chronic secondary infection is present or when a stricture has formed, repeated biopsies are essential because epidermoid carcinoma develops in about 4% of strictures. Local operation on a stricture may be feasible, but a colostomy or an abdominoperineal resection is often required.

**B. Granuloma Inguinale:** This disease may cause anorectal fistulas, infections, and strictures. The Donovan body is best identified in tissue biopsy when there is rectal involvement. Epidermoid carcinoma develops in about 4% of cases with chronic anorectal granuloma.

The early lesions respond to tetracyclines. Destructive or constricting processes may require colostomy or resection.

## ANAL INCONTINENCE

Obstetric tears, anorectal operations (particularly fistulotomy), and neurologic disturbances are the most frequent causes of anal incontinence. Diarrhea due to any cause or fecal impaction may contribute to incontinence. When incontinence is due to surgery or trauma, surgical repair of the divided or torn sphincter is indicated. Repair of anterior childbirth lacerations should be delayed for 6 months or more. In those with manometrically demonstrated decreased anal sphincter tone, biofeedback therapy has been moderately successful in achieving continence.

## SQUAMOUS CELL CARCINOMA OF THE ANUS

These tumors are relatively rare, comprising only 1–2% of all cancers of the anus and large intestine. Bleeding, pain, and local tumor are the commonest symptoms. Because the lesion is often confused with hemorrhoids or other common anal disorders, immediate biopsy of any suspicious lesion or mass in the anal area is essential. These tumors tend to become annular, invade the sphincter, and spread upward into the rectum.

Except for very small lesions (which can be adequately excised locally), treatment is by combined abdominoperineal resection. Radiation therapy is reserved for palliation and for patients who refuse or cannot withstand operation. Metastases to the inguinal nodes are treated by radical groin dissection when clinically evident. The 5-year survival rate after resection is about 50%.

Adams D, Kovalcik PJ: Fistula in ano. *Surg Gynecol Obstet* 1981;**153**:731.

Crooms JW, Kovalcik PJ: Anal lesions: When to suspect carcinoma. *Postgrad Med* (April) 1985;**77**:85.

Hoffman MS, Kodner IJ, Fry RD: Internal intussusception of the rectum: Diagnosis and surgical management. *Dis Colon Rectum* 1984;**27**:435.

Lieberman DA: Common anorectal disorders. *Ann Intern Med* 1984;**101**:837.

MacLeod JH: Rational approach to treatment of hemorrhoids based on a theory of etiology. *Arch Surg* 1983;**118**:29.

Marzuk PM: Biofeedback for gastrointestinal disorders: A review of the literature. *Ann Intern Med* 1985;**103**:240.

Rompalo AM, Stamm WE: Anorectal and enteric infections in homosexual men. *West J Med* 1985;**142**:647.

Salmon RJ et al: Treatment of epidermoid anal canal cancer. *Am J Surg* 1984;**147**:43.

Schoetz DJ: Operative therapy for anal incontinence. *Surg Clin North Am* 1985;**65**:35.

# DISEASES OF THE LIVER & BILIARY TRACT

## JAUNDICE (Icterus)

Since antiquity, a yellowish appearance of the skin and scleras has been recognized as a manifestation of liver disease. Jaundice is evidence of accumulation of bilirubin—a red pigment product of heme metabolism—in the body tissues; it has extrahepatic as well as hepatic causes. Hyperbilirubinemia may be due to abnormalities in the formation, transport, metabolism, and excretion of bilirubin. Total serum bilirubin is normally 0.2–1.2 mg/dL, and jaundice may not be clinically recognizable until levels are about 3 mg/dL.

From an anatomic standpoint, elevation of serum bilirubin levels is prehepatic, hepatic, or posthepatic. Prehepatic jaundice is due to excess production of bilirubin (eg, hemolysis). In hepatic jaundice, elevated serum bilirubin may be caused by qualitative or quantitative dysfunction of liver cells (eg, faulty uptake, metabolism, or excretion of bilirubin). Posthepatic jaundice results from interference with the physiologic removal of bilirubin from the hepatobiliary system (eg, obstruction of the common bile duct).

Because of the great diversity of causes of jaundice, no classification is entirely satisfactory; one that includes anatomy, biochemistry, and etiology is presented in Table 11–6.

### Manifestations of Diseases Associated With Jaundice

**A. Prehepatic:** Weakness or abdominal or back pain may occur with acute hemolytic crises. There is normal stool and urine color, jaundice, indirect (unconjugated) hyperbilirubinemia, and splenomegaly, except in sickle cell anemia. Hepatomegaly is variable. Hemolysis is present.

**Table 11–6.** Classification of jaundice.

| Type of Hyperbilirubinemia | Location and Cause |
|---|---|
| Unconjugated hyperbilirubinemia (predominant indirect-acting bilirubin) | **PREHEPATIC**<br><br>Increased bilirubin production (eg, hemolytic anemias, hemolytic reactions, hematoma, infarction).<br><br>**HEPATIC**<br><br>Impaired bilirubin uptake and storage (eg, posthepatitis hyperbilirubinemia, Gilbert's syndrome, drug reactions).<br><br>Impaired glucuronyl transferase activity (eg, Crigler-Najjar syndrome, Gilbert's syndrome). |
| Conjugated hyperbilirubinemia (predominant direct-acting bilirubin) | Faulty excretion of bilirubin conjugates (eg, Dubin-Johnson syndrome, Rotor's syndrome).<br><br>Biliary epithelial damage (eg, hepatitis, hepatic cirrhosis).<br><br>Intrahepatic cholestasis (eg, viral hepatitis, alcoholic hepatitis, certain drugs, biliary cirrhosis).<br><br>Hepatocellular damage or intrahepatic cholestasis resulting from miscellaneous causes (eg, viral hepatitis, spirochetal infections, infectious mononucleosis, cholangitis, sarcoidosis, lymphomas, industrial toxins).<br><br>**POSTHEPATIC**<br><br>Gallstones, biliary atresia, carcinoma of biliary duct, sclerosing cholangitis, choledochal cyst, external pressure on common duct, pancreatitis, pancreatic neoplasms. |

**B. Hepatic:**

**1. Acquired**–Malaise, anorexia, low-grade fever, and right upper quadrant discomfort are manifestations. Dark urine, jaundice, and amenorrhea occur. An enlarged, tender liver; vascular spiders; palmar erythema; ascites; gynecomastia; sparse body hair; fetor hepaticus; and asterixis may be present.

**2. Congenital**–This form may be asymptomatic; the intermittent cholestasis is often accompanied by pruritus, light-colored stools, and, occasionally, malaise.

**C. Posthepatic:** There is colicky right upper quadrant pain, weight loss (carcinoma), jaundice, dark urine, and light-colored stools. Fluctuating jaundice and intermittently colored stools indicate intermittent obstruction owing to stone or to carcinoma of the ampulla or junction of the intrahepatic ducts. Blood in the stools suggests cancer. Hepatomegaly, visible and palpable gallbladder (Courvoisier's sign), ascites, rectal (Blumer's) shelf, and weight loss also indicate cancer. Chills and fever suggest stone with cholangitis.

## Diagnostic Methods for Evaluation of Jaundice (Table 11-7)

**A. Laboratory Studies:** SGOT (AST) is valuable in the assessment of liver disease. Diagnostic usefulness is enhanced when the test is combined with complementary studies such as alkaline phosphatase and serum bilirubin. SGPT (ALT) may be useful in differentiating alcoholic from viral hepatitis, because SGPT levels are disproportionately low in alcoholic hepatitis.

**B. Liver Biopsy:** Percutaneous liver biopsy is a safe and accurate way of diagnosing diffuse hepatic

**Table 11–7.** Liver function tests: Normal values and changes in 2 types of jaundice.

| Tests | Normal Values | Hepatocellular Jaundice | Uncomplicated Obstructive Jaundice |
|---|---|---|---|
| Bilirubin<br>  Direct | 0.1–0.3 mg/dL | Increased | Increased |
|   Indirect | 0.2–0.7 mg/dL | Increased | Increased |
| Urine bilirubin | None | Increased | Increased |
| Serum albumin/<br> total protein | Albumin, 3.5–5.5<br>Total protein, 6.5–8.4 | Albumin decreased | Unchanged |
| Alkaline phosphatase | 30–115 IU | Increased (++) | Increased (++++) |
| Cholesterol<br>  Total | 100–250 mg/dL | Decreased if damage severe | Increased |
|   Esters | 60–70% of total | Decreased if damage severe | Normal |
| Prothrombin time | 60–100%. After vitamin K, 15% increase in 24 hours. | Prolonged if damage severe and does not respond to parenteral vitamin K | Prolonged if obstruction marked but responds to parenteral vitamin K |
| SGPT (ALT)<br>SGOT (AST) | SGPT, 5–35 IU<br>SGOT, 5–40 IU | Increased in hepatocellular damage, viral hepatitis | Minimally increased |

disease. It is of less value in differentiating intrahepatic from extrahepatic cholestasis and is moderately successful in defining liver metastases.

**C. Imaging:** When the cause of jaundice cannot be determined on the basis of the patient's history and clinical and laboratory findings, it may be possible to differentiate hepatocellular and obstructive jaundice in 80–90% of cases by ultrasonography, CT scan, or radionuclide imaging, all of which are noninvasive (but the latter 2 are expensive). Dilated bile ducts demonstrated by these techniques indicate biliary obstruction, which helps distinguish between obstructive and hepatocellular disease. These methods do not depend on the presence of normal hepatic function— an important point, since conventional oral cholecystography is unsatisfactory when total bilirubin levels are greater than 3 mg/dL. Ultrasonography and CT scan can be used to demonstrate hepatomegaly, intrahepatic tumors, and dilated hepatic ducts. Ultrasonography can also identify gallbladders and detect even 2-mm gallstones.

If surgical (obstructive) jaundice is initially suspected, some clinicians proceed directly from clinical and laboratory findings to percutaneous transhepatic cholangiography; this fine-needle technique often pinpoints the cause, location, and extent of the biliary obstruction. Unusual complications may include fever, bacteremia, bile peritonitis, and intraperitoneal hemorrhage. Endoscopic retrograde cholangiopancreatography, which requires a skilled endoscopist, is a fiberoptic technique comparable in accuracy to percutaneous cholangiography. It may also be utilized to demonstrate pancreatic causes of jaundice or, if choledocholithiasis is present, to carry out papillotomy and stone extraction. Complications of the endoscopic procedure include pancreatitis and cholangitis, which occur in less than 3% of cases.

Corless JK, Middleton HM III: Normal liver function: A basis for understanding hepatic disease. *Arch Intern Med* 1983;**143**:2291.

Ferrucci JT et al: Advances in the radiology of jaundice. *Am J Radiol* 1983;**141**:1.

Scharschmidt BF, Goldberg HI, Schmid R: Current concepts in diagnosis: Approach to the patient with cholestatic jaundice. *N Engl J Med* 1983;**308**:1515.

Venu RP et al: Endoscopic retrograde cholangiopancreatography: Diagnosis of cholelithiasis in patients with normal gallbladder x-ray and ultrasound studies. *JAMA* 1983;**249**:758.

Wolkoff AW et al: Bilirubin metabolism and hyperbilirubinemia. *Semin Liver Dis* 1983;**3**:1.

## VIRAL HEPATITIS

### Essentials of Diagnosis

- Anorexia, nausea, vomiting, malaise, symptoms of upper respiratory throat infection or "flu"-like syndrome, aversion to smoking.
- Fever; enlarged, tender liver; jaundice.
- Normal to low white cell count; abnormal liver tests and liver function.

- Liver biopsy shows characteristic hepatocellular necrosis and mononuclear infiltrate but is rarely indicated.

### General Considerations

Hepatitis can be caused by many drugs and toxic agents as well as by numerous viruses, the clinical manifestations of which may be quite similar. The development of serologic tests has made possible the identification of a growing number of specific viruses causing viral hepatitis. The more common of these are (1) hepatitis A virus (HAV: "infectious," or short-incubation period disease); (2) hepatitis B virus (HBV; "serum," or long-incubation period disease); and (3) non-A, non-B hepatitis virus (NANBH; "post-transfusion" disease, probably due to 2 or more viruses).

**A. Hepatitis A:** (Fig 11–1) Hepatitis A is a viral infection of the liver that may occur sporadically or in epidemics. The liver involvement is part of a generalized infection but dominates the clinical picture. Although transmission of the virus may occur by contaminated needles, it is usually by the fecal-oral route. The excretion of hepatitis A virus (HAV) as determined by immune electron microscopy of stool occurs up to 2 weeks prior to illness. HAV is rarely demonstrated in feces after the third week of illness. There is no known carrier state with HAV. Blood and stools are infectious during the incubation period (2–6 weeks) and early illness until peak transaminase levels are achieved. Although theoretically possible, the short duration of viremia makes posttransfusion hepatitis unlikely. In fact, posttransfusion hepatitis due to HAV has not been documented. Although the mortality rate with hepatitis A is low, it may cause fulminant disease. The mortality rate (as with hepatitis B) appears to be age-related.

**1. Hepatitis A viral agent–**The viral agent of hepatitis A is a small, 27-nm RNA virus that belongs

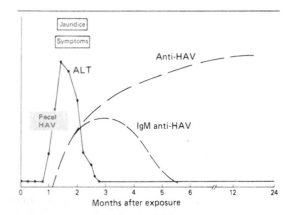

**Figure 11–1.** The typical course of acute type A hepatitis. HAV = hepatitis A antigen; anti-HAV = antibody to hepatitis A virus; ALT = alanine aminotransferase. (Reproduced, with permission, from Schafer DF, Hoofnagel JH: *Viewpoints on Digestive Diseases* 1982;**14**:5.)

to the picornavirus group, which also includes poliomyelitis virus and coxsackievirus. The agent is inactivated by ultraviolet light, by heating to 100 °C for 5 minutes, and by exposure to 1:4000 formalin solution.

**2. HAAg**–The presence of HAV is unequivocally established by demonstration of the hepatitis A virus antigen (HAAg) in the stool. The absence of HAAg in the stool does not rule out HAV infection, and the test is not commonly done.

**3. Hepatitis A antibodies**–Antibodies to type A hepatitis appear early in the course of the illness and tend to persist in the serum. Immune electron microscopy and radioimmunoassay detect both IgM and IgG antibodies and are positive soon after the onset of the illness. Immune adherence hemagglutination reflects an IgG response and is positive later in the course of the disease. Peak titers of IgG antibodies occur after 1 month of disease and may persist for years. Peak titers of IgM antibodies occur during the first week of clinical disease and usually disappear within an 8-week period; therefore, measurement of these antibodies is an excellent test for demonstrating acute hepatitis A infection. The presence of anti-HAV activity indicates (1) previous exposure to HAV, (2) noninfectivity, and (3) immunity to recurring HAV infection. It does not imply previous clinically apparent hepatitis, nor does it establish a relationship to ongoing liver disease unless seroconversion has been demonstrated.

**B. Hepatitis B:** (Fig 11–2) Hepatitis B is a viral infection of the liver usually transmitted by inoculation of infected blood or blood products. However, the antigen has been found in most body secretions,

and it is known that the disease can be spread by oral or sexual contact. Hepatitis B virus (HBV) is highly prevalent in homosexuals and intravenous drug abusers. Other groups at high risk include patients and staff at hemodialysis centers, physicians, dentists, nurses, and personnel working in clinical and pathology laboratories and blood banks. Approximately 5–10% of infected individuals become carriers, providing a substantial reservoir of infection. Forty to 70% of infants born to HBsAg-positive mothers will develop antigens to hepatitis B in the bloodstream. Fecal-oral transmission of virus B has also been documented. The incubation period of hepatitis B is 6 weeks to 6 months but may be prolonged by the administration of hyperimmune globulin. Clinical features of hepatitis A and B are similar; however, the onset in hepatitis B tends to be more insidious.

Hepatitis B virus is pleomorphic and occurs in spherical and tubular forms of different sizes. The largest of these, the Dane particle, is thought to be the complete infectious virus. The 42-nm Dane particle is composed of a core (27-nm particle) found in the nucleus of infected liver cells, and a double-shelled surface particle found in the cytoplasm. The other particles form an excess coating of the virus and contain no nucleic acid.

There are 3 distinct antigen-antibody systems that relate to HBV infection. In addition, DNA polymerase activity can be measured as a sensitive index of viral replication and infectivity.

**1. HBsAg**–The surface antigen (HBsAg) is the antigen routinely measured in blood. HBsAg is unaffected by repeated freezing and thawing or by heating at 56 °C overnight or at 60 °C for 1 hour. It is inactivated by heating between 85 and 100 °C for 15–30 minutes. HBsAg can exist in serum as 3 antigenically identical forms: (1) the outer coat of the intact Dane particle, (2) a spherical 22-nm particle, and (3) elongated tubular particles. The spherical and tubular particles do not contain nucleic acid and are not infectious. Four major antigenic subtypes of HBsAg have been recognized. Subtyping of HBsAg is primarily of epidemiologic importance. The presence of HBsAg is the first manifestation of HBV infection occurring before biochemical evidence of liver disease. HBsAg persists throughout the clinical illness. Persistence of HBsAg is usually associated with clinical and laboratory evidence of chronic hepatitis. The presence of HBsAg establishes infection with HBV and implies infectivity. Specific antibody to HBsAg (anti-HBs) occurs in most individuals after clearance of HBsAg. Anti-HBs is usually delayed after clearance of HBsAg. During this serologic gap, infectivity has been demonstrated. Development of anti-HBs signals recovery from HBV, noninfectivity, and protection from HBV infection.

**2. HBcAg**–Disruption of the Dane particle releases an antigenically distinct inner core structure (HBcAg). Antibodies against core antigen (anti-HBc) localize the core antigen primarily to the nucleus of infected human and primate liver cells. The core parti

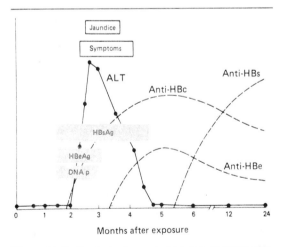

**Figure 11–2.** The typical course of acute type B hepatitis. HBsAg = hepatitis B surface antigen; anti-HBs = antibody to HBsAg; HBeAg = hepatitis Be antigen; anti-HBe = antibody to HBeAg; anti-HBc = antibody to hepatitis B core antigen; DNA p = DNA polymerase; ALT = alanine aminotransferase. (Reproduced, with permission, from Schafer DF, Hoofnagel JH: *Viewpoints on Digestive Diseases* 1982;**14:**5.)

cles are not found in the serum. Core particles may be present in liver tissue in the absence of HBsAg, and recovery from HBV is complete only when core particles are no longer detected in the liver. Anti-HBc appears shortly after HBsAg is detected and persists throughout the period of HBs antigenemia. It fills the serologic gap in patients who have cleared the HBsAg but have not demonstrated detectable amounts of anti-HBs. Anti-HBc can be found alone or in any combination with HBsAg or anti-HBs. Anti-HBc has been shown in all instances of acute HBV infection and appears simultaneously with the onset of clinical illness. Infectivity has been demonstrated in instances where donors are HBsAg-negative and positive for anti-HBc.

**3. HBeAg**–HBeAg is distinct from HBsAg. It is a soluble protein found only in HBsAg-positive sera. All patients with HBV infection demonstrate HBe antigenemia. HBeAg appears during the incubation period shortly after the detection of HBsAg and only during HBsAg reactivity. HBeAg may be a sensitive index of viral replication and infectivity. Anti-HBe is detected as early as the fourth week of illness. The clinical usefulness of this antigen-antibody system lies in its predictive value of infectivity.

**4. DNA polymerase**–DNA polymerase activity is first detectable at the time of peak HBsAg titer, suggesting that this enzyme is a manifestation of viremia and viral replication. DNA polymerase activity is usually transient but may persist for years in chronic carriers and is an indication of continued infectivity.

**C. Delta Agent:** The delta agent has an RNA genome, smaller than all known RNA animal viruses. The delta agent appears to be defective and depends upon external help to initiate and maintain replication. To date, it has been identified only in association with hepatitis B infection and specifically only in the presence of HBsAg; it is cleared when the latter is cleared. The distribution of the delta agent is global.

Clinically, the delta agent appears to be invariably pathogenic and may increase the severity of an acute HBV infection, aggravate previously existing HBV liver disease, or cause new disease in asymptomatic HBsAg carriers. When the delta agent is coincident with an acute HBV infection, the infection appears to be more severe, and the delta agent has recently been found in up to 50% of fulminant HBV infections. In chronic active hepatitis B, presence of the delta agent appears to carry a more severe prognosis. Vertical transmission of this agent appears to be much less frequent than that of HBV.

At present, there are no unique preventive or therapeutic measures for delta agent infections.

**D. Hepatitis Non-A, Non-B:** Although it has been generally accepted that virus A and virus B accounted for most instances of viral hepatitis, recent evidence provided by specific immunologic tests for virus types A and B, epidemiologic analysis of posttransfusion hepatitis, and response to prophylactic gamma globulin offers substantial evidence for the existence of one or more additional types of viral hepatitis (non-A, non-B hepatitis). These observations are of major importance in the problem of posttransfusion hepatitis. Although routine screening of HBsAg has appreciably reduced the incidence of posttransfusion type B hepatitis, its overall incidence has not changed. The incidence of posttransfusion hepatitis is approximately 7–10%. About 90% of the posttransfusion cases are caused by non-A, non-B hepatitis. The chronic carrier state of non-A, non-B hepatitis has been identified. The usual incubation period is 7–8 weeks, but it may vary from 2 to 20 weeks. Epidemiologic studies suggest that there are at least 2 non-A, non-B viruses. Aside from the exclusive use of volunteer blood donors, further reduction in the incidence of posttransfusion hepatitis will require development of serologic techniques to detect the agent or agents of non-A, non-B viral hepatitis.

The histologic findings in hepatitis A, B, and non-A, non-B are those of varying degrees of necrosis of the liver parenchymal cells and variable numbers of lymphocytes and monocytes in the portal areas and in areas of hepatocellular necrosis. The reticulum framework is well preserved, although there may be varying degrees of collapse if the insult is severe. In severe hepatitis, strands of collapsed reticulum may bridge from portal to portal, portal to central vein, or central vein to central vein; this is known as **bridging necrosis.** Healing occurs by regeneration from surviving cells—usually without distortion of the normal architecture.

## Clinical Findings

The clinical picture of viral hepatitis is extremely variable, ranging from asymptomatic infection without jaundice (common in non-A, non-B posttransfusion hepatitis) to a fulminating disease and death in a few days.

**A. Symptoms:**

**1. Prodromal phase**–The speed of onset varies from abrupt to insidious, with general malaise, myalgia, arthralgia and occasionally arthritis, easy fatigability, upper respiratory symptoms (nasal discharge, pharyngitis), and severe anorexia out of proportion to the degree of illness. Nausea and vomiting are frequent, and diarrhea or constipation may occur. Fever is generally present but is rarely over 39.5 °C (103.1 °F). Defervescence often coincides with the onset of jaundice. Chills or chilliness may mark an acute onset.

Abdominal pain is usually mild and constant in the upper right quadrant or right epigastrium and is often aggravated by jarring or exertion. (On rare occasions, upper abdominal pain may be severe enough to simulate cholecystitis or cholelithiasis.) A distaste for smoking, paralleling anorexia, may occur early.

**2. Icteric phase**–Clinical jaundice occurs after 5–10 days but may appear at the same time as the initial symptomatology. Some patients never develop clinical icterus. With the onset of jaundice, there is often an intensification of the prodromal symptoms, followed by progressive clinical improvement.

**3. Convalescent phase**—There is an increasing sense of well-being, return of appetite, and disappearance of jaundice, abdominal pain and tenderness, and fatigability.

**4. Course and complications**—The acute illness usually subsides rapidly over a 2- to 3-week period with complete clinical and laboratory recovery by 8 weeks in the case of hepatitis A and by 16 weeks for hepatitis A and hepatitis non-A, non-B. In 5–10% of cases, the course may be more protracted, and less than 1–3% will have an acute fulminant course.

**B. Signs:** Hepatomegaly—rarely marked—is present in over half of cases. Liver tenderness is usually present. Splenomegaly is reported in 15% of patients, and soft, enlarged lymph nodes—especially in the cervical or epitrochlear areas—may occur. Signs of general toxemia vary from minimal to severe.

**C. Laboratory Findings:** The white cell count is normal to low, especially in the preicteric phase. Large atypical lymphocytes, such as are found in infectious mononucleosis, may occasionally be seen. Mild proteinuria is common, and bilirubinuria often precedes the appearance of jaundice. Acholic stools are often present during the initial icteric phase. Blood and urine studies tend to reflect hepatocellular damage, with abnormal SGOT (AST) or SGPT (ALT) values, increased gamma globulin, and urobilinogenuria. In the cholangiolitic variety, alkaline phosphatase is elevated. HBsAg is usually positive in hepatitis B.

## Differential Diagnosis

The differential diagnosis of viral hepatitis should include, in addition to viruses A, B, delta, and non-A, non-B, other viral diseases such as infectious mononucleosis and cytomegalic inclusion disease; spirochetal diseases such as leptospirosis and secondary syphilis; brucellosis; rickettsial diseases such as Q fever; and drug-induced liver disease.

The prodromal phase or the nonicteric form of the disease must be distinguished from other infectious diseases such as influenza, upper respiratory infections, and the prodromal stages of the exanthematous diseases. In the obstructive phase of viral hepatitis, it is necessary to rule out other obstructive lesions such as choledocholithiasis, chlorpromazine toxicity, and carcinoma of the head of the pancreas.

## Prevention

Strict isolation of patients is not necessary, but hand washing after bowel movements is required. Thorough hand washing by medical attendants who come into contact with contaminated utensils, bedding, or clothing is essential. Disinfection of feces is not necessary when waterborne sewage disposal is available. Hepatitis B is for the most part transmitted by the parenteral route, but the possibility of fecal-oral infection as well as sexual transmission must be considered. Screening by means of HBsAg and

SGOT (AST) determinations can remove potentially infectious individuals from blood donor lists. Unfortunately, there is increasing evidence that other viruses are responsible for similar clinical states. In blood donors, routine screening for HBsAg has reduced the incidence of posttransfusion hepatitis. In the USA, the avoidance of unnecessary transfusions and the exclusion of commercially obtained blood, along with clinical studies of the donor as well as the HBsAg and serum transaminase determinations, may be helpful in excluding potential sources of infectious blood. It may make possible the detection of one-third of infected donors. The use of disposable needles and syringes protects medical attendants as well as other patients.

**A. Gamma Globulin:** Gamma globulin should be routinely given to all close personal contacts of patients with hepatitis A. The recommended dose of 0.02 mL/kg body weight has been found to be protective for hepatitis A if administered during the incubation period. It is also desirable that individuals traveling to or residing in endemic regions receive gamma globulin within 2 weeks after arrival; if staying more than 2 months, the recommended dose is 5 mL for adults. In the event of prolonged residence, a second dose should be given after 5–6 months.

**B. Hepatitis B Hyperimmune Globulin:** Hepatitis B hyperimmune globulin may be protective if given in large doses within 7 days of exposure and again at 30 days (adult dose is 0.06 mL/kg body weight). At present, this preparation is recommended for individuals exposed to hepatitis B surface antigen-contaminated material via the mucous membranes or through breaks in the skin. Persons who have had sexual contact with patients with acute hepatitis B surface antigen-positive disease should also receive hepatitis B hyperimmune globulin. Hepatitis B hyperimmune globulin is also indicated for newborn infants of HBsAg-positive mothers; give 0.5 mL very soon after birth and at ages 3 and 6 months. Hepatitis B hyperimmune globulin does not seem to be indicated in the prevention of transfusion-associated hepatitis.

**C. Hepatitis B Vaccine:** Two vaccines for the prevention of hepatitis B have been developed, extensively tested, and found safe. They reduce the incidence of hepatitis B by approximately 92% in highly exposed persons. One vaccine consists of highly purified, formalin-activated HBsAg particles derived from plasma of chronic antigen carriers. The other is recombinant-derived. Recipients must have a negative serologic test for HBsAg and HBcAb. Potential candidates are persons at high risk, including renal dialysis patients and attending personnel, patients requiring repeated transfusions, spouses of HBsAg-positive individuals, male homosexuals, and newborns of HBsAg-positive mothers. Neither vaccine contains the AIDS virus. The dose for adults is 1 mL initially and 1 mL again at 1 and 6 months; the newborn and pediatric dose is one-half the adult dose.

## Treatment

**A. General Measures:** Bed rest should be at the patient's option during the acute initial phase of the disease, when symptoms are most severe. Bed rest beyond the most acute phase is not warranted. However, return to normal activity during the convalescent period should be gradual. If nausea and vomiting are significant problems, or if oral intake is substantially decreased, the intravenous administration of 10% glucose solution is indicated. If the patient shows signs of impending coma, protein should be temporarily interdicted and gradually reintroduced and increased as clinical improvement takes place. In general, dietary management consists of giving palatable meals as tolerated, without overfeeding. Patients with acute hepatitis should avoid strenuous physical exertion, alcohol, and hepatotoxic agents. While the administration of small doses of oxazepam is safe (not metabolized or excreted by the liver), it is recommended that morphine sulfate be avoided.

**B. Corticotropin and Corticosteroids:** Although these agents have been recommended by some authors for the treatment of fulminant hepatitis, controlled studies have demonstrated no benefit in patients with severe viral hepatitis treated relatively early in the course of the disease.

## Prognosis

The clinical course, morbidity, and mortality of viral hepatitis may vary considerably. In most cases of viral hepatitis, clinical recovery is complete in 3–16 weeks. Laboratory evidence of disturbed liver function may persist for a longer period, but most such patients go on to complete recovery. The overall mortality rate is less than 1%, but the rate is reportedly higher in older people (particularly post-menopausal women).

Hepatitis A does not progress to chronic liver disease, though persistent hepatitis with positive IgM has been seen for up to 1 year. The mortality rate is less than 0.2%. About 10% of hepatitis B patients and perhaps an even higher percentage of hepatitis non-A, non-B patients develop chronic liver disease (see below). The mortality rates quoted for hepatitis B and hepatitis non-A, non-B infections (0.1–15%) are higher than for hepatitis A infections, but these figures may reflect other factors (eg, age, associated illness).

Chronic hepatitis, as characterized by transaminasemia for more than 6 months, occurs in 5–10% of patients. Some of this latter group develop chronic active hepatitis with or without cirrhosis. Liver biopsy is necessary to make this distinction.

Hepatitis tends to be more severe and potentially has a poorer prognosis in the elderly or in those with other complicating illnesses. Posttransfusion hepatitis occurs as a complication in 0.25–3% of blood transfusions and as high as 12% of those receiving pooled blood products. The asymptomatic carrier state and persistent viremia after acute disease make control of contamination in donor blood extremely difficult.

Alter HJ, Holland PV: Indirect tests to detect the non-A, non-B hepatitis carrier state. (Editorial.) *Ann Intern Med* 1984;**101**:859.

Bonino F, Smedile A: Delta agent (type D) hepatitis. *Sem Liver Dis* 1986;**6**:28.

Bradley DW, Maynard JE: Etiology and natural history of post-transfusions and enterically transmitted non-A, non-B hepatitis. *Sem Liver Dis* 1986;**6**:56.

Centers for Disease Control: Recommendations for protection against viral hepatitis: Department of Health and Human Services. *MMWR* (June 7) 1985;**34**:313.

DeCock KM et al: Delta virus in the Los Angeles area: A report of 126 cases. *Ann Intern Med* 1986;**105**:108.

Dienstag JL, Alter HJ: Non-A, non-B hepatitis: Evolving epidemiologic and clinic perspective. *Sem Liver Dis* 1986;**6**:67.

Dienstag JL, Isselbacher KJ: Therapy for acute and chronic hepatitis. *Ann Intern Med* 1981;**141**:1419.

Gocke DJ: Hepatitis A revisited. *Ann Intern Med* 1986;**105**:960.

Jacobson IM, Dienstag JL: Viral hepatitis vaccines. *Annu Rev Med* 1985;**36**:241.

Mijch AM, Gust ID: Clinical, serological and epidemiological aspects of hepatitis A virus infection. *Sem Liver Dis* 1986;**6**:42.

Rosina F, Saracco G, Rizzetto M: Risk of posttransfusion infection with the hepatitis delta virus: A multicenter study. *N Engl J Med* 1985;**312**:1488.

Stevens CE et al: Hepatitis B virus antibody in blood donors and the occurrence of non-A, non-B hepatitis in transfusion recipients: An analysis of the Transfusion-Transmitted Viruses Study. *Ann Intern Med* 1984;**101**:733.

Tygstrup N, Ranek L: Assessment of prognosis in fulminant hepatic failure. *Semin Liver Dis* 1986;**6**:129.

## VARIANTS OF INFECTIOUS HEPATITIS

### Cholangiolitic Hepatitis

There is usually a cholestatic phase in the initial icteric phase of viral hepatitis, but in occasional cases, this is the dominant manifestation of the disease. The course tends to be more prolonged than that of ordinary hepatitis. The symptoms are often extremely mild, but jaundice is deeper, and pruritus is often present. Laboratory tests of liver function indicate cholestasis with hyperbilirubinemia, biliuria, and elevated alkaline phosphatase and cholesterol.

Differentiation of this type of hepatitis from extrahepatic obstruction may be difficult. Percutaneous transhepatic cholangiography or endoscopic retrograde cholangiography may be necessary to make the distinction.

### Fulminant Hepatitis

Hepatitis may take a rapidly progressive course terminating in less than 10 days. Up to 75% of those due to viral hepatitis are due to hepatitis B (with about half of these associated with the delta antigen). Most of the remainder are due to non-A, non-B hepatitis, but hepatitis A can also—rarely—induce fulminant hepatitis. Extensive necrosis of large areas of the liver gives the typical pathologic picture of acute liver atrophy. Toxemia and gastrointestinal symptoms are more severe, and hemorrhagic phenomena are common. Neurologic symptoms of hepatic coma develop (see Cirrhosis, p 408). Jaundice may be absent or minimal, but laboratory tests show extreme hepatocellular damage.

The treatment of fulminant hepatitis is directed toward those metabolic abnormalities associated with severe liver cell dysfunction. They include coagulation defects; disordered fluid, electrolyte, and acid-base balance; hypoglycemia; and nitrogenous intoxication. Careful monitoring of the patient, with vigorous correction of the deficits noted, provides the hope that some patients will survive who might otherwise succumb before liver regeneration can occur.

Adrenocorticosteroids, exchange transfusions, and perfusions through pig and baboon livers have not proved effective.

Zuckerman AJ: The enigma of fulminant viral hepatitis. *Hepatology* 1984;**4:**568.

## CHRONIC HEPATITIS

Chronic hepatitis is defined as a chronic inflammatory reaction of the liver of more than 6 months' duration, as demonstrated by persistently abnormal liver tests. For proper treatment, it is crucial to determine whether the disease will resolve, remain static, or progress to cirrhosis. The causes of chronic hepatitis are only partially defined. It may be a sequela of infection resulting from hepatitis B virus, as well as a sequela of non-A, non-B hepatitis. Hepatitis A virus has not yet been shown to lead to chronic hepatitis. Additionally, identical clinical entities may be associated with drug reactions, including oxyphenisatin, methyldopa, and isoniazid. Wilson's disease can also present as chronic liver disease, and $\alpha_1$-antitrypsin deficiency is also associated with chronic liver disease.

## 1. CHRONIC PERSISTENT HEPATITIS

This form of chronic hepatitis represents an essentially benign condition with a good prognosis. The diagnosis is confirmed by liver biopsy. The biopsy may show portal tract infiltration with primarily mononuclear cells and occasional areas of focal inflammation in the parenchyma. The boundary between portal tracts and parenchyma remains sharp, and there is little or no "piecemeal necrosis" (a process in which the liver cells are gradually destroyed and replaced by fibrous tissue septa). In essence, the architecture of the hepatic lobule remains intact. The symptomatology varies from the asymptomatic state to various vague manifestations including fatigability, anorexia, malaise, and lassitude. Physical examination is usually normal. Laboratory findings are those of intermittent or persistent transaminasemia, usually in the range of 2–3 times normal.

Liver biopsy helps establish the diagnosis of persistent hepatitis. The treatment is reassurance of the patient. Corticosteroids and immunosuppressive drugs should not be given. Dietary restrictions, excessive vitamin supplementation, and prolonged bed rest are not necessary. The prognosis is excellent. Rarely does the disease progress to chronic active hepatitis.

## 2. CHRONIC ACTIVE HEPATITIS (Chronic Aggressive Hepatitis, Lupoid Hepatitis)

This form of chronic hepatitis is usually characterized by progression to cirrhosis, although milder cases may resolve spontaneously. **Piecemeal necrosis** refers to this inflammatory process at the interface of the portal area and the liver lobule. In severe cases, piecemeal necrosis may be associated with considerable hepatic fibrosis and ultimately with cirrhosis. In very mild cases, it may be difficult to distinguish this entity from chronic persistent hepatitis. Liver biopsies repeated at varying intervals may be necessary to make the distinction as well as to monitor therapy.

### Clinical Findings
#### A. Symptoms and Signs:
**1. Chronic active hepatitis (lupoid type)**– This is generally a disease of young people, particularly young women. However, the disease can occur at any age. The onset is usually insidious, but about 25% of cases present as an acute attack of hepatitis. Although the serum bilirubin is usually increased, 20% of these patients have anicteric disease. Examination often reveals a healthy-appearing young woman with multiple spider nevi, cutaneous striae, acne, and hirsutism. Amenorrhea may be a feature of this disease. Multisystem involvement, including kidneys, joints, lungs, and bowel, and Coombs-positive hemolytic anemia are associated with this clinical entity. Markers for hepatitis B are absent.

**2. Chronic active hepatitis (HBsAg-positive type)**–This type of hepatitis clinically resembles the lupoid type of disease. The histologic pictures of these 2 types of chronic active hepatitis are indistinguishable. The HBsAg form of chronic active hepatitis appears to affect males predominantly. It may be noted as a continuum of acute hepatitis or may be manifested only by biochemical abnormalities of liver function.

**3. Delta agent in hepatitis B**–(See p 400.) Acute delta infection superimposed on chronic HBV infection may be subclinical and manifested only by a transient transaminase rise; in this setting, chronic delta infection ensues. Delta infection among HBsAg carriers is common and is associated with the presence of liver damage, characterized by chronic active hepatitis with or without cirrhosis.

**4. Chronic active hepatitis (non-A, non-B type)**–This type occurs in up to 5% of patients with posttransfusion hepatitis and in sporadic cases. It is clinically indistinguishable from chronic active hepatitis of other causes and may actually be the most common. The clinical setting, lack of hepatitis markers, absence of other potential causes (eg, drugs, Wilson's disease) and liver biopsy determine the category.

**B. Laboratory Findings:** The serum bilirubin is usually normal or only modestly increased (4.5–7 mg/dL); SGOT (AST), IgG, IgM, and gamma globulin levels are higher than normal. Late in the disease, serum albumin levels are usually decreased and prothrombin time may be significantly prolonged and will not respond to vitamin K therapy. Antinuclear and smooth muscle antibodies are positive 15–50% of the time but are nonspecific. Latex fixation tests for rheumatoid arthritis and anticytoplasmic and immunofluorescent antimitochondrial antibodies are positive in 28–50% of patients. Hepatitis B antigen is not found in the blood of patients with classic "lupoid" hepatitis.

The activity of chronic active hepatitis can be defined practically and accurately in terms of objective criteria. Thus, the magnitude of transaminase and gamma globulin elevations and the degree of hepatocellular necrosis are suitable means of defining activity and judging the response to treatment. Activity in chronic liver disease can be defined quantitatively quite readily by establishing arbitrary biochemical standards. For example, either a 10-fold increase in serum transaminase level or a 5-fold elevation of SGOT with a 2-fold increase in gamma globulin concentration constitutes "high-grade" activity.

## Differential Diagnosis

Chronic active hepatitis can be confused with 5 other chronic liver conditions: cholestatic viral hepatitis, chronic persistent hepatitis, subacute hepatic necrosis, postnecrotic cirrhosis, and Wilson's disease. Wilson's disease should be considered in any patient under the age of 30 who has chronic active hepatitis (see p 413). The differentiation is made on the basis of the clinical course, sequential laboratory testing, and liver biopsy.

## Treatment

Prolonged or enforced bed rest has not been shown to be beneficial. Activity should be modified according to the patient's symptoms. The diet should be well balanced, without specific limitations other than sodium or protein restrictions as dictated by water retention or encephalopathy.

Prednisone has been shown to decrease the serum bilirubin, SGOT (AST), and gamma globulin levels and reduce the piecemeal necrosis in patients with non-B chronic active hepatitis. Data from controlled clinical trials in patients with non-B chronic active hepatitis indicate that the mortality rate in patients treated with corticosteroids is significantly reduced. However, relapse after discontinuation of prednisone therapy occurs frequently. In assessing the necessity for corticosteroid therapy, the benefit of the therapy should outweigh its potential risk. For patients with chronic active hepatitis due to HBV infection, the risks of increasing viral replication and infectiousness with the use of corticosteroids are considerable and are a relative contraindication to their use. Patients with chronic active hepatitis who are symptomatic, those who are HBsAg-negative, and those who have severe histologic abnormalities appear at this time to be the most suitable candidates for corticosteroid therapy.

Prednisone or an equivalent drug is given initially in doses of 30 mg orally daily, with gradual reduction to the lowest maintenance level (usually 15–20 mg/d) that will control the symptomatology and reduce the abnormal liver function. If symptoms are not controlled, azathioprine (Imuran), 50–150 mg/d orally, is added, with the primary benefit being that doses of corticosteroids can be much lower. Azathioprine imposes a significant hazard of bone marrow depression, and complete blood counts should be obtained at least weekly for 6–8 weeks until the dose has been stabilized, and then at less frequent intervals as dictated by the maintenance dose and hematologic picture. In general, the combination of prednisone, 10–15 mg/d, and azathioprine, 50 mg/d, gives therapeutic efficacy with few significant side effects of both drugs.

## Prognosis

The course of chronic active hepatitis is variable and unpredictable. The sequelae of chronic active hepatitis secondary to hepatitis B include cirrhosis, liver cell failure, and hepatocellular carcinoma. It has been stated that 40–50% of patients with chronic active hepatitis die within 5 years of the onset of symptoms. Most patients die of hepatocellular failure and associated complications of portal hypertension.

Czaja AJ et al: Autoimmune features as determinants of prognosis in steroid-treated chronic active hepatitis of uncertain etiology. *Gastroenterology* 1983;**85:**713.

Czaja AJ et al: Complete resolution of inflammatory activity following corticosteroid treatment of HBsAg-negative chronic active hepatitis. *Hepatology* 1984;**4:**622.

Fattovich G: Clinical, virologic and histologic outcome following seroconversions from HBeAg to anti-HBe in chronic hepatitis type B. *Hepatology* 1986;**6:**167.

Redeker AG: Delta agent and hepatitis B. *Ann Intern Med* 1983;**98:**542.

Vyas GN, Blum HE: Hepatitis B virus infections: Current concepts of chronicity and immunity. *West J Med* 1984;**140:**754.

Weissberg JI et al: Survival in chronic hepatitis B: An analysis of 379 patients. *Ann Intern Med* 1984;**101:**613.

## ALCOHOLIC HEPATITIS

Alcoholic hepatitis is an acute or chronic inflammation of the liver that occurs as a result of parenchymal necrosis induced by alcohol abuse. Although a variety of terms were used in the past to describe this type of hepatitis in chronic alcoholics, the term alcoholic hepatitis is now regarded as the most appropriate one to describe this injury, which is currently accepted as the precursor of alcoholic cirrhosis.

While alcoholic hepatitis is often a reversible disease, it is the most common cause of cirrhosis in the USA. This is especially significant, since cirrhosis ranks among the most common causes of death of adults in this country. Alcoholic hepatitis does not develop in all chronic heavy drinkers; the exact prevalence and incidence are not known but have been estimated to be about one-third. Women appear to be more susceptible than men.

Alcoholic hepatitis usually occurs after years of excessive drinking. Although it may not develop in many patients even after several decades of alcohol abuse, it appears in a few individuals within a year of excessive drinking. Over 80% of patients with alcoholic hepatitis were drinking 5 years or more before developing any symptoms that could be attributed to liver disease. In general, the longer the duration of drinking (10–15 or more years) and the larger the alcoholic consumption (usually more than 120 g of alcohol per day, which is equal to 8 oz of 100-proof whiskey, 30 oz of wine, or 100 oz of beer [eight 12-oz cans]), the greater the probability of developing alcoholic hepatitis and cirrhosis. It is also important to realize that while drinking large amounts of alcoholic beverages is essential for the development of alcoholic hepatitis, drunkenness is not. In drinking individuals, the rate of ethanol metabolism can be sufficiently high to permit the consumption of large quantities of spirits without raising the blood alcohol level over 80 mg/dL, the concentration at which the conventional breath analyzer begins to detect ethanol.

The roles of proteins, vitamins, and calories in the development of alcoholic hepatitis or in the progression of this lesion to cirrhosis are not understood.

Only liver biopsy can establish the diagnosis with certainty, since any of the manifestations of alcoholic hepatitis can be seen in other types of alcoholic liver disease such as fatty liver or cirrhosis, as well as liver disease due to other causes.

## Clinical Findings

**A. Symptoms and Signs:** Alcoholic hepatitis is usually seen after a recent period of heavy drinking. That history in addition to complaints of anorexia and nausea and the objective demonstration of hepatomegaly and jaundice strongly suggest the diagnosis. Abdominal pain and tenderness, splenomegaly, ascites, fever, and encephalopathy support the diagnosis. The clinical presentation of alcoholic hepatitis can vary from an asymptomatic patient with an enlarged liver to a critically ill individual who dies quickly.

**B. Laboratory Findings:** Anemia is variable and usually macrocytic. Leukocytosis with shift to the left is common and is seen more frequently in patients with severe disease. Leukopenia is occasion-

ally seen and disappears after cessation of drinking. About 10% of patients have thrombocytopenia that appears related to a direct toxic effect of alcohol on megakaryocyte production.

SGOT (AST) is normal in 15–25% of patients; when increased, it is usually under 300 units/mL. SGPT (ALT) is almost invariably less than the SGOT, often by a factor of 2–5 or more. Serum alkaline phosphatase is generally elevated, but rarely more than 3 times the normal value. Serum bilirubin is increased in 60–90% of patients, and when levels greater than 6 mg/dL are demonstrated it can be assumed that the process is severe. The serum albumin is depressed, and the gamma globulin is elevated in 50–75% of individuals with alcoholic hepatitis even in the absence of cirrhosis.

Liver biopsy is diagnostic and may reveal both cirrhosis and alcoholic hepatitis.

**C. Special Procedures:** Scintiphotographic evaluation (liver scanning) using $^{99m}$Tc sulfur colloid will reveal patchy hepatic uptake of the isotope; marked bone marrow uptake, which is indicative of portal hypertension; and splenomegaly. Liver scanning is nonspecific and rarely indicated.

## Differential Diagnosis

Nausea, vomiting, abdominal pain, jaundice, fever, right upper abdominal tenderness, leukocytosis, and elevated serum alkaline phosphatase with concomitantly minimal to moderate elevation of SGOT (AST) occur in both alcoholic hepatitis and diseases of the hepatobiliary tree such as cholecystitis and cholelithiasis. A history of chronic insobriety and recent debauch is helpful but far from conclusive. Percutaneous liver biopsy, if there is no contraindication, is the only reliable means of differentiation.

## Complications

Clinical deterioration and worsening abdominal pain and tenderness may result in the unfortunate decision to perform laparotomy. The postoperative mortality rate of acutely ill patients with alcoholic hepatitis is far greater than that of those who are operated on for intra- or extrahepatic cholestasis.

## Treatment

**A. General Measures:** Discontinue all alcoholic beverages. During periods of anorexia, every effort should be made to provide sufficient amounts of carbohydrate and calories to reduce endogenous protein catabolism and gluconeogenesis and to prevent hypoglycemia. Although the clinical value of intravenous hyperalimentation has not been established, the judicious administration of parenteral fluids is most important. Caloric intake is gratifyingly improved by the use of palatable liquid formulas during the transition period between totally intravenous alimentation and normal feeding. The administration of vitamins, particularly folic acid, is an important part of treatment and is frequently associated with dramatic clinical improvement in patients with alcoholic liver disease.

**B. Steroids:** The use of corticosteroids in this disorder has been evaluated over a period of more than 20 years, with occasional reports of success. Anabolic steroids are not beneficial.

## Prognosis

**A. Short-Term:** The severity of liver injury, which can be ascertained clinically, biochemically, and histologically, enables valid speculation about prognosis. The presence of asterixis seems to be associated with an increased likelihood of death. Biochemically, it has been shown that when the prothrombin time is short enough to permit performance of liver biopsy without risk, the 1-year mortality rate is 7.1%, rising to 18% if there is progressive prolongation of that parameter during hospitalization. Individuals in whom the prothrombin time is so prolonged that liver biopsy cannot be attempted have a 42% mortality rate.

**B. Long-Term:** In the USA, the mortality rate over a 3-year period of persons who recover from acute alcoholic hepatitis is 10 times greater than that of average individuals of comparable age. The histologically severe form of the disease is associated with continued excessive mortality rates after 3 years, whereas the death rate is not increased after the same period in those whose liver biopsies show only mild alcoholic hepatitis.

The most important prognostic consideration is the indisputable fact that continued excessive drinking is associated with reduction of life expectancy in these individuals. The prognosis is indeed poor if the patient is unable to abstain from drinking.

Lieber CS: Alcohol and the liver: 1984 update. *Hepatology* 1984;**4**:1243.

Schenker S: Alcohol liver disease: Evaluation of natural history and prognostic factors. *Hepatology* 1984;**4**:365.

Zetterman RK, Sorrell MF: Immunologic aspects of alcoholic liver disease. *Gastroenterology* 1981;**81**:616.

## UNCOMMON HYPERBILIRUBINEMIA STATES

There are about a half-dozen hyperbilirubinemic states that must be distinguished from hemolytic disease, hepatitis, and surgical jaundice (Table 11–8). The disorders are benign, with the notable exception of the rare type I Crigler-Najjar syndrome, for which there is no known effective treatment. These hyperbilirubinemic states are very uncommon, with the exception of Gilbert's syndrome, which may occur in up to 5% of the population.

Wolkoff AW et al: Bilirubin metabolism and hyperbilirubinemia. *Semin Liver Dis* 1983;**8**:1.

## DRUG- & TOXIN-INDUCED LIVER DISEASE

The continuing synthesis, testing, and introduction of new drugs into clinical practice has resulted in

**Table 11–8.** Uncommon hyperbilirubinemic disorders.

| | Nature of Defect | Type of Hyper-bilirubinemia | Clinical and Pathologic Characteristics |
|---|---|---|---|
| Constitutional hepatic dysfunction (Gilbert's syndrome) | Glucuronyl transferase deficiency | Unconjugated (indirect) bilirubin | Benign, asymptomatic hereditary jaundice. Hyper-bilirubinemia increased by 24- to 36-hour fast. No treatment required. Prognosis excellent. |
| Crigler-Najjar syndrome | | | Severe, nonhemolytic hereditary jaundice of neonates. Type I cases sustain CNS damage (kernicterus). Milder cases (type II) may persist into adult life and may benefit from treatment with phenobarbital. |
| Familial chronic idio-pathic jaundice (Dubin-Johnson syn-drome) | Faulty excretory function of liver cells (hepatocytes) | Conjugated (direct) bilirubin | Benign, asymptomatic hereditary jaundice. BSP excretion impaired. Gallbladder does not visualize on oral cholecystography. Liver darkly pigmented on gross examination. Biopsy shows centrilobular brown pigment. Prognosis excellent. |
| Rotor's syndrome | | | Similar to Dubin-Johnson syndrome but liver is not pigmented and the gallbladder is visualized on oral cholecystography. Prognosis excellent. |
| Benign intermittent cholestasis | Cholestatic liver dysfunction | Unconjugated plus conjugated (total) bilirubin | Benign intermittent idiopathic jaundice, itching, and malaise. Onset in early life and may persist for lifetime. Alkaline phosphatase increased. Cholestasis found on liver biopsy. (Biopsy is normal during remission.) Prognosis excellent. |
| Recurrent jaundice of pregnancy | | | Benign cholestatic jaundice of unknown cause, usually occurring in the third trimester of pregnancy. Itching, gastrointestinal symptoms, and abnormal liver excretory function tests. Cholestasis noted on liver biopsy. Prognosis excellent, but recurrence with subsequent pregnancies or use of birth control pills is characteristic. |

an increase in toxic reactions of many types. Many widely used therapeutic agents may cause hepatic injury. The diagnosis of drug-induced liver injury is not always easy. Drug-induced liver disease can mimic viral hepatitis or biliary tract obstruction. The clinician must be aware of drug-induced liver disease and must question the patient carefully about the use of various drugs before dismissing this possibility.

## Direct Hepatotoxic Group

The liver lesion caused by this group of drugs is characterized by (1) dose-related severity, (2) reproducibility in experimental animals, (3) a latent period following exposure, and (4) susceptibility in all individuals:

| | |
|---|---|
| Acetaminophen | Phosphorus |
| Alcohol | Stilbamidine |
| Carbon tetrachloride | Tetracyclines |
| Chloroform | Valproic acid |
| Heavy metals | Vitamin A |
| Mercaptopurine | |

## Viral Hepatitis-Like Reactions

Reactions of this type are sporadic, suggesting host idiosyncrasy:

| | |
|---|---|
| Aspirin | Dantrolene |
| Chloramphenicol | Halothane |
| Chlortetracycline | Isoniazid |
| Cinchophen | Methoxyflurane |
| Methyldopa | Streptomycin |
| Oxacillin | Sulfamethoxypyridazine |
| Phenylbutazone | Zoxazolamine |
| Pyrazinamide | |

## Cholestatic Reactions

There are 2 general categories that differ in clinical presentation and histopathologic features. These reactions are dose-dependent, but marked differences in individual susceptibility exist:

**A. Noninflammatory:** Probable direct effect of agent on bile secretory mechanisms and on inflammatory reactions:

| | |
|---|---|
| Mestranol | Norethandrolone |
| Methyltestosterone | |

**B. Inflammatory:** Inflammation of portal areas, with allergic features, eg, eosinophilia:

| | |
|---|---|
| Chlorothiazide | Prochlorperazine |
| Chlorpromazine | Promazine |
| Chlorpropamide | Sulfadiazine |
| Erythromycin estolate | Thiouracils |

## Chronic Active Hepatitis

Clinically and histologically indistinguishable from postviral chronic active hepatitis:

| | |
|---|---|
| Acetaminophen | Isoniazid |
| Aspirin | Methyldopa |
| Chlorpromazine | Nitrofurantoin |
| Halothane | Oxyphenisatin |

## Miscellaneous Reactions

**A. Fatty Liver:**
Large fatty inclusions–Alcohol, corticosteroids
Small cytoplasmic droplets–Tetracyclines

**B. Granulomas:**
Allopurinol
Phenylbutazone
Phenytoin

**C. Cirrhosis:**
Methotrexate

**D. Peliosis Hepatis:**
Anabolic steroids (Halotestin)
Azathioprine
Oral contraceptive steroids

**E. Neoplasms:**
Oral contraceptive steroids

Black M: Acetaminophen hepatotoxicity. *Annu Rev Med* 1984;**35**:577.

Schiff ER: The liver and drugs: How to avoid reactions. *Mod Med* (Sept) 1984;**50**:66.

Timbrell JA: Drug hepatotoxicity. (Review.) *Br J Clin Pharmacol* 1983;**15**:3.

Zafrani ES, Pinaudeau Y, Dhumeaux D: Drug-induced vascular lesions of the liver. *Arch Intern Med* 1983;**143**:495.

## FATTY LIVER

It was formerly believed that malnutrition rather than ethanol was responsible for steatosis (fatty metamorphosis) of the liver in the alcoholic. More recently, it has come to be agreed that the role of deficient nutrition in such individuals has been overemphasized. However, it cannot be ignored that inadequate diets—specifically, those deficient in choline, methionine, and dietary protein—can produce fatty liver (kwashiorkor) in children.

Other nonalcoholic causes of steatosis are obesity (the commonest cause), starvation, diabetes mellitus, corticosteroids, poisons (carbon tetrachloride and yellow phosphorus), endocrinopathies such as Cushing's syndrome, tetracycline toxicity, Reye's syndrome, TPN, and, rarely, pregnancy.

Regardless of the cause, there are apparently at least 5 factors, acting in varying combinations, that are responsible for the accumulation of fat in the liver: (1) increased mobilization of fatty acids from peripheral adipose depots; (2) decreased utilization or oxidation of fatty acids by the liver; (3) increased hepatic fatty acid synthesis; (4) increased esterification of fatty acids into triglycerides; and (5) decreased secretion or liberation of fat from the liver.

Percutaneous liver biopsy is diagnostic.

Treatment consists of removing or modifying the offending factor.

Prognosis depends on the underlying condition.

Kaplan MM: Current concepts: Acute fatty liver of pregnancy. *N Engl J Med* 1985;**313**:367.

Sherlock S: Acute fatty liver of pregnancy and the microvesicular fat diseases. *Gut* 1983;**24**:265.

## CIRRHOSIS

The current concept of cirrhosis includes only those cases in which hepatocellular inj ̇ry leads to both fibrosis and nodular regeneration th. oughout the liver. These features delineate cirrhosis as a serious and irreversible disease—eighth leading cause of death in males, ninth in females in USA in 1981; rate of 12.3/100,000 per year; over 65% alcohol-related—that is characterized not only by variable degrees of hepatic cell dysfunction but also by portosystemic shunting and portal hypertension. Fibrosis alone, regardless of its severity, is excluded by the previous definition. Also excluded by definition are the early stages of chronic biliary obstruction, hemochromatosis, and primary biliary cirrhosis, none of which form regenerating nodules until late.

An important part of this concept is the realization that the type of cirrhosis changes with the passage of time in any one patient. Terms such as "portal" and "postnecrotic" refer not so much to separate disease states with different causes as to stages in the evolution of cirrhosis.

Attempts to classify cirrhosis on the basis of cause or pathogenesis are usually unsuccessful when applied to individual patients. Such persons often represent end-stage cirrhosis, enabling only speculation about the evolutionary process. The use of a purely anatomic and descriptive categorization facilitates easier and more practical classification. One such classification that is currently employed divides cirrhosis into micronodular, mixed, and macronodular forms. It is important, however, to remember that these are stages of development rather than separate diseases.

(1) Micronodular cirrhosis is the form in which the regenerating nodules are no larger than the original lobules, ie, approximately 1 mm in diameter or less. It has been suggested that this feature results from the persistence of the offending agent (alcohol), a substance that prevents regenerative growth.

(2) Macronodular cirrhosis is characterized by larger nodules, which can measure several centimeters in diameter. This form corresponds more or less to postnecrotic cirrhosis but does not necessarily follow episodes of massive necrosis and stromal collapse.

(3) Mixed macro- and micronodular cirrhosis points up the fact that the features of cirrhosis are highly variable and not always easy to classify. In any case, the configuration of the liver is determined by the mixture of liver cell death and regeneration as well as the deposition of fat, iron, and fibrosis.

Finally, it should be emphasized that there does exist a limited relationship between anatomic types and etiology as well as between anatomic types and prognosis. For example, alcoholics who continue to drink tend to have micronodular cirrhosis. The presence of fatty micronodular cirrhosis, although not an infallible criterion, is strongly suggestive of chronic alcoholism. On the other hand, there is a higher incidence of liver cell carcinoma in macronodular than in micronodular cirrhosis, although the latter is much more common in the USA because of the alcohol relationship. This propensity to malignancy is perhaps related either to the increased regeneration in macronodular cirrhosis or to the longer period required for the process to develop.

### Clinical Findings

**A. Symptoms and Signs:** Micronodular (Laennec's) cirrhosis may cause no symptoms for long periods, both at onset and later in the course (compensated phase). The onset of symptoms may be insidious or, less often, abrupt. Weakness, fatigability, and weight loss are common. In advanced cirrhosis, anorexia is usually present and may be extreme, with associated nausea and occasional vomiting. Abdominal pain may be present and is related either to hepatic enlargement and stretching of Glisson's capsule or to the presence of ascites. Menstrual abnormalities (usually amenorrhea), impotence, loss of libido, sterility, and painfully enlarged breasts in men (rare) may occur. Hematemesis is the presenting symptom in 15–25%.

In 70% of cases, the liver is enlarged, palpable, firm if not hard, has a blunt or nodular edge, and the left lobe may predominate. Skin manifestations consist of spider nevi (usually only on the upper half of the body), palmar erythema (mottled redness of the thenar and hypothenar eminences), telangiectases of exposed areas, and evidence of vitamin deficiencies (glossitis and cheilosis). Weight loss, wasting, and the appearance of chronic illness are present. Jaundice—usually not an initial sign—is mild at first, increasing in severity during the later stages of the disease. Ascites, pleural effusion, peripheral edema, and purpuric lesions are late findings. Precoma (sleep reversal, asterixis, tremor, dysarthrias, delirium, and drowsiness) and coma also occur very late except when precipitated by an acute hepatocellular insult or an episode of gastrointestinal bleeding. Fever may be present in 35% on presentation and usually reflects a complication such as alcoholic hepatitis, spontaneous bacterial peritonitis, cholangitis, or some other intercurrent event. Clinical splenomegaly is present in 35–50% of cases. The superficial veins of the abdomen and thorax are dilated and reflect the intrahepatic obstruction to portal blood flow.

**B. Laboratory Findings:** Laboratory abnormalities are either absent or minimal in latent or quiescent cirrhosis. Anemia, a frequent finding, is usually macrocytic and represents, in the heavy drinker, direct suppression of erythropoiesis by alcohol as well as folate deficiency, hemolysis, and insidious or overt blood loss from the gastrointestinal tract. The white cell count may be low, elevated, or normal, reflecting hypersplenism or infection. Coagulation abnormalities may be a result of failure of synthesis of clotting constituents in the liver. Proteinuria may be present. Oliguria is frequent in active or decompensated disease with ascites and is usually reflective of the secondary hyperaldosteronism state.

Blood chemical studies show primarily hepatocellular injury and dysfunction, reflected by elevations of SGOT (AST), alkaline phosphatase, and bilirubin. Serum albumin is low; gamma globulin is increased.

Liver biopsy shows cirrhosis.

**C. Imaging:** Plain films of the abdomen may reveal hepatic or splenic enlargement. Barium studies of the upper gastrointestinal tract may reveal the presence of esophageal or gastric varices. Splenoportography and arteriography are useful for evaluating the patency of the portal vein and splenic vein. Hepatic scanning using $^{99m}$Tc sulfur colloid may occasionally be helpful in documenting splenomegaly; however, this objective can be achieved at much less cost with a "flat plate" of the abdomen, and diffuse patchy uptake of the isotope in the liver makes the test useless in the evaluation of hepatoma.

**D. Special Examinations:** Esophagogastroscopy demonstrates or confirms the presence of varices and detects specific causes of bleeding in the esophagus, stomach, and proximal duodenum. Peritoneoscopy is helpful in judging the type of cirrhosis present.

## Differential Diagnosis

As previously noted, differentiation of one type of cirrhosis from another can be difficult. Actual visualization of the liver by peritoneoscopy, when correlated with biopsy results and the history, facilitates classification. Hemochromatosis may be associated with "bronzing" of the skin and diabetes mellitus; special staining of liver biopsies will be positive for increased iron deposition in the hepatic parenchyma. Primary biliary cirrhosis tends to occur more frequently in women and is associated with marked pruritus, significant elevation of alkaline phosphatase, and positive antimitochondrial antibodies.

## Complications

Upper gastrointestinal tract bleeding may occur from varices, hemorrhagic gastritis, or gastroduodenal ulcers. Hemorrhage may be massive, resulting in fatal exsanguination or portosystemic encephalopathy. Liver failure may also be precipitated by alcoholism, surgery, and infection. Carcinoma of the liver and portal vein thrombosis occur more frequently in patients with cirrhosis but are still uncommon. Lowered resistance often leads to serious infections, particularly of the lungs and peritoneum.

## Treatment

**A. General Measures:** The principles of treatment include abstinence from alcohol and adequate rest, especially during the acute phase. The diet should be palatable, with adequate calories and protein (75–100 g/d) and, in the stage of fluid retention, sodium and fluid restriction. In the presence of hepatic precoma or coma, protein intake should be reduced or excluded. Vitamin supplementation is desirable.

**B. Special Problems:**

**1. Ascites and edema due to sodium retention, hypoproteinemia, and portal hypertension–** Removal of ascites by paracentesis, for other than diagnostic purposes, is usually not indicated unless it is critically important to relieve respiratory distress or patient discomfort. Abdominal paracentesis is rarely associated with serious complications such as bleeding, infection, or bowel perforation.

In many patients, there is a rapid diminution of ascites on dietary sodium and fluid restriction alone. In individuals who pose more significant problems of fluid retention and who are considered to have "intractable" ascites, the urinary excretion of sodium is less than 10 meq/L. Mechanisms that have been postulated to explain sodium retention in cirrhosis include impaired liver inactivation of aldosterone and increased aldosterone secretion secondary to increased renin production, which is associated with decreased renal cortical blood flow of uncertain cause. If such persons are permitted unrestricted fluids, serum sodium progressively falls, representing dilution. With a 200-mg sodium diet and 500-mL allowance of oral fluids per day, ascites production ceases and the patient's abdominal discomfort abates; however, this regimen is unrealistic in most clinical situations.

**a. Restoration of plasma proteins–**This is dependent upon improving liver function and serves as a practical index of recovery. The use of albumin intravenously is of doubtful value except for maintaining intravascular volume during large-volume paracentesis.

**b. Diuretics–**Spironolactone should be used after documentation of secondary aldosteronism, as evidenced by markedly low urinary sodium. Starting with spironolactone, 50 mg twice daily, and monitoring the aldosterone antagonist effect, reflected by the urinary sodium concentration and the fact that sodium excretion exceeds sodium intake, the dose of spironolactone is increased 100 mg every 3 days (up to a daily dosage of 1000 mg) until the urinary sodium excretion exceeds 60 meq/L. Diuresis commonly occurs at this point and may be augmented by the addition of a potent agent such as furosemide. This potent diuretic, however, will maintain its effect even with a falling glomerular filtration rate, with resultant prerenal azotemia. The dose of furosemide ranges from 40 to 120 mg/d, and the drug should be administered with careful monitoring of serum electrolytes, especially potassium.

The goal of weight loss in the nonedematous ascitic patient should be no more than 1–1½ lb/d.

**c. Peritoneovenous shunts–**Peritoneovenous shunts have been advocated for use in patients with refractory ascites or hepatorenal syndrome. These shunts are frequently effective but carry a considerable complication rate: disseminated intravascular coagulation in 65% of patients (25% symptomatic; 5% total), bacterial infections in 4–8%, congestive heart failure in 2–4%, and variceal bleeding from sudden expansion of intravascular volume.

**2. Hepatic encephalopathy**–Hepatic encephalopathy is the result of biochemical abnormalities associated with hepatocellular deficit or hepatic bypass of portal vein blood into the systemic circulation. Although disturbed ammonia metabolism is inherent in the clinical entity of hepatic encephalopathy, it is clear that ammonia per se is not solely responsible for the disturbed mental status. The amount of ammonia produced is dependent upon the protein content, the bacterial flora, the pH, and the motility of the colon. Hepatic encephalopathy may be aggravated by sepsis. Bleeding into the intestinal tract may significantly increase the amount of protein in the bowel and may precipitate rapid development of liver coma. Other factors that may precipitate hepatic encephalopathy include alkalosis, potassium deficiency induced by diuretics, narcotics, hypnotics, and sedatives; medications containing ammonium or amino compounds; paracentesis with attendant hypovolemia; and hepatic or systemic infection.

Dietary protein should be curtailed or completely withheld during acute episodes. Parenteral or enteral nutrition is usually indicated.

Gastrointestinal bleeding should be controlled if possible and blood purged from the gastrointestinal tract. This can be accomplished with 120 mL of magnesium citrate by mouth or nasogastric tube every 3–4 hours until the stool is free of gross blood.

Lactulose (Cephulac), a nonabsorbable synthetic disaccharide, is digested by bacteria in the colon to short-chain fatty acids, resulting in acidification of colon contents. This acidification favors the ammonium ion in the $NH_4^+ \rightleftarrows NH_3$ equation; $NH_4^+$ is not absorbable, and it is the $NH_3$ that is absorbable and thought to be neurotoxic. When given orally, the initial dose of lactulose for acute hepatic encephalopathy is 30 mL 3 or 4 times daily, or a dose that will produce no more than 2–3 soft stools per day. When rectal use is indicated because of the patient's inability to take medicines orally, the dose is 300 mL of lactulose in 700 mL of saline or sorbitol as a retention enema for 30–60 minutes; it may be repeated every 4–6 hours. One liter of nonfat milk may be used instead, because there is no lactose in the colon and the bacteria reduce the lactose to short-chain fatty acids. The end result is the same as what can be achieved with lactulose for a fraction of the cost.

The intestinal flora may also be controlled with neomycin sulfate, 0.5–1 g orally every 6 hours for 5–7 days. Side effects of neomycin include diarrhea, malabsorption, superinfection, ototoxicity, and nephrotoxicity, usually only after prolonged use.

Treat shock as outlined in Chapter 1.

Treat infection with antibiotic agents chosen on the basis of culture and sensitivity studies. In some cases, broad-spectrum antimicrobials are indicated if the patient's condition is deteriorating.

If agitation is marked, give oxazepam, 10–30 mg orally or by nasogastric tube, cautiously as indicated. Avoid narcotics, tranquilizers, and sedatives excreted by the liver if possible.

**3. Anemia**–For hypochromic anemia, give ferrous sulfate, O.3-g enteric-coated tablets, one tablet 3 times daily after meals. Folic acid, 1 mg/d orally, is indicated in the treatment of macrocytic anemia associated with alcoholism.

**4. Hemorrhagic tendency**–A bleeding tendency due to hypoprothrombinemia may be treated with vitamin K preparations. This treatment is ineffective in the presence of severe hepatic disease when other coagulation factors are deficient. Transfusions with packed red blood cells may be necessary to replace blood loss. Increasing the prothrombin time in these situations requires large volumes of fresh-frozen plasma, and the effect is transient; for that reason, plasma infusions are not often indicated. Give menadione, 1–3 mg orally 3 times daily after meals.

**5. Hemorrhage from esophageal varices**–When active variceal bleeding is evident, attempts should be made to sclerose the bleeding varices transendoscopically if a physician with skill in the technique is available. If this procedure cannot be performed or is not successful, bleeding can often be controlled by use of the quadruple-lumen (Minnesota) tube. Unfortunately, there is a high incidence of recurrent variceal bleeding after balloon tamponade has been discontinued. Injection sclerotherapy has proved to be quite effective (80%) in stopping the acute episode of variceal bleeding. The advantages of this technique are simplicity and avoidance of a major surgical procedure in a poor-risk patient. Repeated injections may be necessary. If bleeding cannot be controlled by sclerotherapy, emergency surgical decompression of portal hypertension may be considered in selected patients. Morbidity and mortality rates are substantially lower when surgical shunting procedures are performed electively than when performed on an urgent basis. After the patient has been stabilized for 3–5 days, the beta-blocker propranolol can be given in an attempt to lower the portal pressure. The dosage is usually 20–80 mg twice daily, with the goal of reducing the pretreatment resting pulse by 25% but not below 60/min.

**6. Hemochromatosis**–See p 412.

**7. Spontaneous bacterial peritonitis**–This occurs in cirrhotic patients with ascites. Abdominal pain, increasing ascites, fever, and progressive encephalopathy suggest the possibility, although symptoms may be very mild. Liver function is grossly abnormal in these patients. Common organisms are pneumococci and *E coli*. The mortality rate is high.

## Prognosis

The prognosis in advanced cirrhosis has shown little change over the years. A major factor for survival is the patient's ability to discontinue the use of alcohol.

In established cases with severe hepatic dysfunction, only 50% survive 2 years and only about 35% survive 5 years. Hematemesis, jaundice, and ascites are unfavorable signs.

Many latent cases are discovered only at autopsy.

Benhamou JP, Lebrec D (editors): Non-cirrhotic intrahepatic portal hypertension in adults. *Clin Gastroenterol* 1985;**14:**1.

Crossley IR, Wardle EN, Williams R: Biochemical mechanisms of hepatic encephalopathy. *Clin Sci* 1983;**63:**247.

Epstein M: The sodium retention of cirrhosis: A reappraisal. *Hepatology* 1986;**6:**312.

Fogel MR et al: Continuous intravenous vasopressin in active upper gastrointestinal bleeding. *Ann Intern Med* 1982; **96:**565.

Fraser CL, Arieff AI: Hepatic encephalopathy. *N Engl J Med* 1985;**313:**865.

Gines P et al: Compensated cirrhosis: Natural history and prognostic factors. *Hepatology* 1987;**7:**122.

Groszmann RJ, Atterbury CE: The pharmacologic treatment of portal hypertension. *Annu Rev Med* 1985;**36:**81.

Harley HAJ et al: Results of a randomized trial of end-to-side portocaval shunt and distal splenorenal shunt in alcoholic liver disease and variceal bleeding. *Gastroenterology* 1986;**91:**802.

Lebrec D et al: A randomized controlled study of propranolol for prevention of recurrent gastrointestinal bleeding in patients with cirrhosis: A final report. *Hepatology* 1984;**4:**355.

LeVeen HH: The LeVeen shunt. *Annu Rev Med* 1985;**36:**453.

Pockros PJ, Reynolds TB: Rapid diuresis in patients with ascites from chronic liver disease: The importance of peripheral edema. *Gastroenterology* 1986;**90:**1827.

Sherlock S: Extrahepatic portal venous hypertension in adults. *Clin Gastroenterol* 1985;**14:**1.

Stassen WN, McCullough AS: Management of ascites. *Sem Liver Dis* 1985;**5:**291.

Terblanche J, Bornman PC, Kirsch RE: Sclerotherapy for bleeding esophageal varices. *Annu Rev Med* 1984;**35:**83.

Yang CH et al: White count, pH and lactate in ascites in the diagnosis of spontaneous bacterial peritonitis. *Hepatology* 1985;**5:**86.

# BILIARY CIRRHOSIS

## 1. PRIMARY BILIARY CIRRHOSIS

Primary biliary cirrhosis (chronic nonsuppurative destructive cholangitis) is a chronic disease of the liver manifested by cholestasis. It is insidious in onset, occurs usually in women age 40–60, and is often detected by chance finding of elevated alkaline phosphatase levels. The disease is progressive and complicated often by steatorrhea, xanthomatous neuropathy, osteomalacia, and portal hypertension.

### Clinical Findings

**A. Symptoms and Signs:** The onset is insidious and is heralded by pruritus. Jaundice usually occurs within 2 years of onset of pruritus. Physical examination reveals hepatosplenomegaly. Xanthomatous lesions may occur in the skin and tendons and around the eyelids.

**B. Laboratory Findings:** Hemograms are nor-

mal early in the disease. Serologic tests reflect cholestasis with elevation of alkaline phosphatase, cholesterol, and bilirubin. Mitochondrial antibodies are present in an incidence reported to be 83–98% in different series.

### Differential Diagnosis

The disease must be differentiated from chronic biliary tract obstruction (stone or stricture), carcinoma of the bile ducts, and cholestatic liver disease associated with inflammatory bowel disease.

### Treatment

Treatment is symptomatic. Cholestyramine may be beneficial for the pruritus. Vitamins A, K, and D should be administered parenterally if steatorrhea is present. Calcium supplementation may be helpful for osteomalacia. Penicillamine, corticosteroids, and azathioprine have proved to be of questionable benefit. Some successes with liver transplantation are being reported.

Cohen LB et al: Role of plasmapheresis in primary biliary cirrhosis. *Gut* 1985;**26:**291.

Cuervas-Mons V et al: Prognostic value of preoperatively obtained clinical and laboratory data in predicting survival following orthotopic liver transplantation. *Hepatology* 1986;**6:**922.

Dickson ER et al: Trial of penicillamine in advanced primary biliary cirrhosis. *N Engl J Med* 1985;**312:**1011.

Kaplan MM et al: A prospective trial of colchicine for primary biliary cirrhosis. *New England J Med* 1986;**315:**1448.

Roll J et al: The prognostic importance of clinical and histological features in asymptomatic and symptomatic primary biliary cirrhosis. *N Engl J Med* 1983;**308:**1.

Warnes TW: Treatment of primary biliary cirrhosis. *Sem Liver Dis* 1985;**5:**228.

Worner TM, Lieber CS: Perivenular fibrosis as precursor lesion of cirrhosis. *JAMA* 1985;**254:**627.

## 2. SECONDARY BILIARY CIRRHOSIS

Secondary biliary cirrhosis follows chronic obstruction to bile flow. Superimposed infection may hasten the process. Bile flow is most commonly impaired in an extrahepatic site by calculus, neoplasm, stricture, or biliary atresia.

### Clinical Findings

**A. Symptoms and Signs:** The clinical presentation is usually that of the underlying cause of the cholestasis (eg, carcinoma of the pancreas, choledocholithiasis, choledochal cysts).

**B. Laboratory Findings:** Hemograms are normal except insofar as they reflect the inciting lesion (eg, cholangitis associated with choledocholithiasis). Serologic tests reflect cholestasis with elevated alkaline phosphatase. The mitochondrial antibody is present in less than 1% of patients with secondary biliary cirrhosis.

**C. Imaging:** Ultrasound may reveal dilated ducts

(especially intrahepatic), hilar or pancreatic masses, and occasionally common duct stones. CT scan is more accurate than ultrasound for lesions of the pancreas.

The more definitive procedures are the invasive ones: endoscopic retrograde cholangiography (ERCP) and percutaneous transhepatic cholangiography. Selection of one or the other is dictated by the expertise available and the anticipated problem: For choledocholithiasis, ERCP is clearly the procedure of choice, since papillotomy with stone extraction can usually be accomplished and is therapeutic. Either method allows placement of stents. For balloon dilation of ductal strictures, ERCP is preferable.

Ferrucci JT et al: Advances in the radiology of jaundice: A symposium and review. *Am J Roentgenol* 1983;**141**:1.

## HEMOCHROMATOSIS

Primary or idiopathic hemochromatosis is considered to be a genetically determined disorder of iron metabolism characterized by increased accumulation of dietary iron. This iron is deposited as hemosiderin in the liver, pancreas, heart, adrenals, testes, pituitary, and kidneys. Eventually the patient may develop hepatic, pancreatic, and cardiac insufficiency. The disease usually occurs in males and is rarely recognized before the fifth decade.

### Clinical Findings

Clinical manifestations include arthropathy, hepatomegaly and evidence of hepatic insufficiency (late finding), occasional skin pigmentation (slate gray due to iron and brown due to melanin), cardiac enlargement with or without heart failure or conduction defects, diabetes mellitus with its complications, and impotence in the male. Bleeding from esophageal varices may occur, and in patients who develop cirrhosis, there is a 10% incidence of hepatic carcinoma.

Laboratory findings include elevated plasma iron, increased percentage saturation of transferrin, elevated serum ferritin, and the characteristic liver biopsy that stains positive for iron.

### Treatment

Early diagnosis and treatment in the precirrhotic phase of hemochromatosis is of great importance. Treatment consists initially of weekly phlebotomies of 500 mL of blood (about 250 mg of iron), perhaps continued for 2–3 years to achieve depletion of iron stores. This process is monitored by hematocrit and serum iron determinations. When iron store depletion is achieved, maintenance phlebotomies (every 2–4 months) are continued. The chelating agent, deferoxamine, administered intramuscularly to patients with hemochromatosis, has been shown to produce urinary excretion of up to 5–18 g of iron per year. This rate of urinary excretion compares favorably with the rate of 10–20 g of iron removed annually by weekly or biweekly phlebotomies. The treatment, however, is painful and not always practical. Active treatment of the complications of hemochromatosis— arthropathy, diabetes, heart and liver disease, and hypopituitarism—is important.

Although the long-term benefits of iron depletion therapy have not been completely established, available data indicate that the course of the disease may be favorably altered by chelation or bleeding. There appear to be fewer cardiac conduction defects and lower insulin requirements with these treatments.

Crosby WH: Hemochromatosis: Current concepts and management. *Hosp Pract* (Feb 15) 1987;**22**:173.

Tavill AS, Bacon BR: Hemochromatosis: How much iron is too much? *Hepatology* 1986;**6**:142.

Valberg LS, Ghent CN: Diagnosis and management of hereditary hemochromatosis. *Annu Rev Med* 1985;**36**:27.

## WILSON'S DISEASE

Wilson's disease (hepatolenticular degeneration) is a rare familial disorder that is inherited in an autosomally recessive manner and occurs in both males and females between the first and third decades. The condition is characterized by excessive deposition of copper in the liver and brain.

Awareness of the entity is important, since it may masquerade as chronic active hepatitis, psychiatric disorder, or neurologic disease. It is potentially reversible, and appropriate therapy will prevent neurologic and hepatic damage.

The major physiologic aberration in Wilson's disease is excessive absorption of copper from the small intestine and decreased excretion of copper by the liver, resulting in increased tissue deposition, especially in the liver, brain, cornea, and kidney. Ceruloplasmin, the plasma copper-carrying protein, is low. Urinary excretion of copper is high.

### Clinical Findings

Wilson's disease can present primarily as a neurologic abnormality, with liver involvement appearing later; or the reverse may be true, with hepatic disease being the initial manifestation. It may first be clinically recognized when jaundice appears in the first few years of life. The diagnosis should always be considered in any child with manifestations of atypical hepatitis, splenomegaly with hypersplenism, hemolytic anemia, portal hypertension, and neurologic or psychiatric abnormalities. Wilson's disease should also be considered in young adults (under 30 years of age) with chronic active hepatitis.

The neurologic manifestations are related to basal ganglia dysfunction and are characterized by rigidity or parkinsonian tremor. Hepatic involvement is evidenced by signs of cirrhosis, portal hypertension, and biochemical confirmation of hepatocellular insufficiency. The almost pathognomonic sign of the condition is the Kayser-Fleischer ring, which represents fine pigmented granular deposits in Descemet's membrane in the cornea close to the endothelial surface. Scattering and reflection of light by these deposits give rise to the typically brownish or gray-green appearance of the ring. The ring itself is not always complete and is usually most marked at the superior and inferior poles of the cornea. It can frequently be seen with the naked eye and almost invariably by slit lamp examination.

The diagnosis is based on demonstration of increased urinary copper excretion (> 100 $\mu$g/24 h) or low serum ceruloplasmin levels (< 20 mg/dL), elevated hepatic copper concentration (> 100 $\mu$g/g of dry liver). Histologically, the disease may present as an acute viral hepatitis. In other patients, it may present clinically and histologically as chronic active hepatitis. Cirrhosis ultimately occurs.

### Treatment

Early treatment is essential for removal of copper before it can produce neurologic or hepatic damage. Oral penicillamine (0.75–2 g/d in divided doses) is the drug of choice, making possible urinary excretion of chelated copper. Give supplemental pyridoxine, 50 mg per week, since penicillamine is an antimetabolite of this vitamin. If penicillamine treatment cannot be tolerated because of gastrointestinal, hypersensitivity or autoimmune reactions, consider the use of zinc therapy. Oral zinc acetate, 150 mg daily in divided doses, has been reported to produce a negative copper balance in patients with Wilson's disease, but its long-term effectiveness is not known. The use of copper restricted diets is of doubtful value.

Treatment should continue indefinitely. The prognosis is good in patients who are effectively treated before liver or brain damage has occurred.

McCullough AJ et al: Diagnosis of Wilson's disease presenting as fulminant hepatic failure. *Gastroenterology* 1983;**84**:161.
Sternlieb I: Wilson's disease: Indications to liver transplants. *Hepatology* 1984;**4**:155.

## HEPATIC VEIN OBSTRUCTION (Budd-Chiari Syndrome)

This uncommon disorder is due to occlusion of the hepatic veins from a variety of causes. Hepatovenous obstructions may be associated with caval webs, right-sided heart failure, polycythemia, use of birth control pills, pyrrolizidine alkaloids ("bush teas"), neoplasms causing hepatic vein occlusions, and pregnancy. Approximately 30% are idiopathic.

Clinical manifestations may include tender, painful hepatic enlargement; jaundice; splenomegaly; and ascites. With advanced disease, bleeding varices and hepatic coma may be evident. Isotopic liver scan may show prominent caudate lobes. Caval venogram can delineate caval webs and occluded hepatic veins. Percutaneous liver biopsy frequently shows a characteristic central lobular congestion.

Treatment consists of correcting the offending cause, when possible. Ascites should be treated with fluid and salt restriction and diuretics. Surgical decompression of the congested liver may be required. Mean survival is about 12–18 months, with a range of a few weeks to more than 20 years.

Friedman AC et al: Magnetic resonance imaging diagnosis of Budd-Chiari syndrome. *Gastroenterology* 1986;**91**:1289.
Mitchell MC et al: Budd-Chiari syndrome: Etiology, diagnosis and management. *Medicine* 1982;**61**:199.

## NONCIRRHOTIC PORTAL HYPERTENSION

Noncirrhotic portal hypertension must be considered in the differential diagnosis of splenomegaly or upper gastrointestinal bleeding due to esophageal or gastric varices. This syndrome may be due to portal vein obstruction, splenic vein obstruction (gastric varices without esophageal varices), schistosomiasis, noncirrhotic intrahepatic portal sclerosis, or arterial-portal vein fistula. Consideration of the diagnosis is most important. Angiography of the portal system is confirmatory, as is needle biopsy of the liver, particularly for schistosomiasis and noncirrhotic intrahepatic portal sclerosis. Other than for splenomegaly, the physical findings are not remarkable, and the endoscopic findings are those of esophageal gastric varices. The liver tests are usually normal, but there may be findings of hypersplenism.

Management consists of surgical decompression of the hypertension.

Benhamon JP, Lebrel D: Noncirrhotic intrahepatic portal hypertension in adults. *Clin Gastroenterol* 1985;**14**:21.
Sherlock S: Extrahepatic portal venous hypertension in adults. *Clin Gastroenterol* 1985;**14**:1.

## HEPATIC ABSCESS

### 1. PYOGENIC ABSCESS

Single or multiple local collections of pus in the liver that are large enough to be seen with the naked eye are presently quite rare, principally because of the use of antibiotics and improved methods of diagnosis of appendicitis, which was formerly the most common precursor of liver abscess. Although the actual clinical incidence cannot be determined because the condition is aborted or modified by antimicrobial treatment, hepatic abscess is still reported in 0.5–1.5% of autopsy specimens. It is equally distributed between men and women, usually in the sixth or seventh decade.

There are apparently 5 ways in which the liver can be invaded by bacteria: (1) by way of the portal vein; (2) by way of ascending cholangitis in the common duct; (3) by way of the hepatic artery, secondary to bacteremia; (4) by direct extension from an infectious process; and (5) by traumatic implantation of bacteria through the abdominal wall.

Despite the use of antimicrobial drugs, 10% of cases of liver abscess are secondary to appendicitis. Another 10% have no demonstrable cause and are classified as idiopathic. At present, ascending cholangitis is the most common cause of hepatic abscess in the USA. Bacterial infection of the hepatobiliary tree is more likely to accompany obstruction by stone than obstruction by carcinoma of the head of the pancreas and is probably attributable to dissemination of bacteria from an acutely inflamed gallbladder. The most frequently encountered organisms are *Escherichia coli, Proteus vulgaris, Enterobacter aerogenes,* and multiple anaerobic species.

## Clinical Findings

Clinically, fever is almost always present and may antedate other symptoms or signs. Pain is prominent and is localized to the right hypochondrium or epigastric area. Jaundice, tenderness in the right upper abdomen, and either steady or swinging fever are the chief physical findings.

Laboratory examination reveals leukocytosis with a shift to the left. Chest roentgenograms will usually reveal elevation of the diaphragm if the abscess is on the right side. Left-sided abscess does not produce significant diaphragmatic elevation. Liver scanning, using $^{99m}$Tc sulfur colloid, may reveal the presence of intrahepatic defects.

## Treatment

Treatment should consist of antimicrobial agents that are effective against coliform organisms. If adequate response to therapy is not rapid, needle or surgical drainage should be undertaken. Failure to recognize and treat the condition is attended by mortality rates of about 60% in patients with multiple abscesses.

Bertel CK, van Heerden JA, Sheedy PF II: Treatment of pyogenic abscesses: Surgical vs percutaneous drainage. *Arch Surg* 1986;**121**:554.
Greenstein AJ et al: Continuing changing patterns of disease in pyogenic liver abscess: A study of 38 patients. *Am J Gastroenterol* 1984;**79**:217.

## 2. AMEBIC LIVER ABSCESS

Amebic abscess is more common as a primary presentation than is pyogenic abscess. Usual symptoms and signs, which may have been present for 1–30 days, are right upper quadrant pain, often with associated fever, and right pleuritic chest pain. Associated dysentery is uncommon, but 20% of patients will have had a significant recent diarrheal episode. Usually there is a history of travel to endemic areas.

## Clinical Findings

Physical examination discloses fever in most cases, toxic appearance of varying degree, and a tender palpable liver with marked "punch" tenderness. Right lung base abnormalities and localized intercostal tenderness are common.

Laboratory findings usually consist of mild to moderate anemia, moderate leukocytosis with a shift to the left, and slightly abnormal liver tests. Serologic amebic gel diffusion test or indirect hemagglutination tests for *Entamoeba histolytica* are positive in 95% of patients but may be nondiagnostic on presentation, with a marked rise in titer over the subsequent 3–4 weeks.

An elevated right hemidiaphragm is frequently seen on chest radiograph. Ultrasonography, liver scan with $^{99m}$Tc sulfur colloid, or CT scan is helpful in delineating the location and number of abscesses. Most are in the right lobe.

## Treatment

Metronidazole, 750 mg 3 times per day orally for 5–10 days, is the drug of choice. Occasionally, a second course is necessary. In the acutely toxic patient, percutaneous needle aspiration and decompression of the abscess bring about a greater feeling of well-being and also allow for demonstration of the ameba in over 50% of cases. Following completion of treatment for the abscess, the patient needs to take iodoquinol (Yodoxin), 650 mg 3 times a day for 20 days (for adults), to eradicate the intestinal cyst phase of amebiasis.

Fever usually subsides rapidly once treatment is initiated. The hepatic defect may persist for as long as 6 months.

Complications include rupture of the abscess transcutaneously, into the peritoneal cavity, pleural space, lungs, or pericardium, with a significant associated mortality rate if undiagnosed. Rarely, distal embolization has been reported.

Kubitschek KR et al: Amebiasis presenting as pleuropulmonary disease. *West J Med* 1985;**142**:203.
Patterson M et al: The presentation of amebiasis. *Med Clin North Am* 1982;**66**:689.

## NEOPLASMS OF THE LIVER

Neoplasms of the liver arise either in the hepatic parenchymal cells or biliary ductules. A tumor that arises from parenchymal cells is called a hepatoma; one that originates in the ductular cells is called a cholangioma.

Although hepatoma was formerly thought to occur only in underdeveloped parts of the world where hepatitis B, malnutrition, and parasitism are prevalent, its incidence is now increasing in the USA. This neoplasm occurs in up to 20% of cases of macronodular cirrhosis. In the Orient, hepatitis B and *Clonorchis sinensis,* the liver fluke, are etiologically significant.

Histologically, the tumor may be made up of cords or sheets of cells that roughly resemble the hepatic parenchyma. In the case of a cholangioma, a fibrous stroma or tissue containing structures that simulate bile ducts will be seen. Blood vessels such as portal or hepatic veins are commonly involved by tumor.

## Clinical Findings

The presence of a hepatoma may be unsuspected until there is deterioration in the condition of a cirrhotic patient who was formerly stable. Cachexia, weakness, and weight loss are associated symptoms. The sudden appearance of ascites, which may be bloody, suggests portal or hepatic vein thrombosis by tumor or bleeding from the necrotic tumor.

Physical examination is positive for tender enlargement of the liver, with an occasionally palpable mass. Auscultation may reveal a bruit over the tumor, or a friction rub may be heard when the process has extended to the surface of the liver.

Laboratory tests may reveal leukocytosis, as opposed to the leukopenia that is frequently encountered in cirrhotic patients. Sudden and sustained elevation of the serum alkaline phosphatase in a patient who was formerly stable is a common finding. Hepatitis B surface antigen is present in more than 50% of cases. Alpha$_1$-fetoprotein—not usually found in adults—is demonstrable in 30–50% of patients with hepatoma. Cytologic study of ascitic fluid may reveal malignant cells.

Arteriography is frequently diagnostic, revealing a tumor "blush" that reflects the highly vascular nature of the tumor. Almost as helpful is the CT scan when done with and without intravenous contrast to characterize the location and vascularity of the tumor. Liver biopsy is diagnostic.

## Treatment

No therapy, including hepatic perfusion with cytotoxic agents, has proved effective. Attempts at surgical resection are usually fruitless because of the presence of cirrhosis and the frequent multifocal characteristics of the tumor. On rare occasions, surgical resection of "solitary" hepatomas has resulted in 5-year "cures."

## Liver Neoplasms in Women Taking Oral Contraceptives

Benign and malignant neoplasms have been encountered in women taking oral contraceptives. Two distinct entities with characteristic clinical, radiologic, and histopathologic features have been described. Focal nodular hyperplasia occurs at all ages. It is usually asymptomatic and hypervascular on CT scan. Microscopically, focal nodular hyperplasia consists of hyperplastic units of hepatocytes with centrally placed proliferating bile ducts. Liver cell adenoma occurs most commonly in the third and fourth decades of life; the clinical presentation is one of acute abdominal disease due to necrosis of the tumor with hemorrhage. The tumor is hypovascular and reveals a cold defect on liver scan. Grossly, the cut surface appears structureless. As seen microscopically, the liver cell ade-

noma consists of sheets of hepatocytes without portal tracts or central veins. The only physical finding in focal nodular hyperplasia or liver cell adenoma is a palpable abdominal mass in some cases. Liver function is usually normal. Treatment of focal nodular hyperplasia is resection in the symptomatic patient. The prognosis is excellent. Liver cell adenoma often undergoes necrosis and rupture; resection is advised. Regression of benign hepatic tumors may follow cessation of oral contraceptives.

Kew MC (editor): Hepatic tumors. *Semin Liver Dis* 1984;**4**:89.

Luna G, Florence L, Johansen K: Hepatocellular carcinoma: A 5-year institutional experience. *Am J Surg* 1985;**149**:591.

## CHOLELITHIASIS (Gallstones)

Gallstones are more common in women than in men and increase in incidence in both sexes and all races with aging. Data indicate that in the USA 10% of men and 20% of women between the ages of 55 and 65 have gallstones and that the total exceeds 15 million people. Although gallstones are less common in black people, cholelithiasis attributable to hemolysis has been encountered in over a third of individuals with sickle cell disease. American Indians have a high rate of cholesterol cholelithiasis. As many as 70% of Pima Indian women over age 25 have cholelithiasis. The incidence of gallstones is also high in individuals with certain diseases such as regional enteritis. Approximately one-third of individuals with inflammatory involvement of the terminal ileum have cholesterol gallstones due to disruption of bile salt resorption that results in decreased solubility of the bile. The incidence of cholelithiasis is also increased in patients with diabetes mellitus. Pregnancy as a significant association with gallstones has been over-emphasized.

## Classification of Gallstones

The simplest classification of gallstones is according to chemical composition: stones containing predominantly cholesterol and stones containing predominantly calcium bilirubinate. The latter comprise less than 5% of the stones found in Europe or the USA but 30–40% of stones found in Japan.

Three compounds comprise 80–95% of the total solids dissolved in bile: conjugated bile salts, lecithin, and cholesterol. Cholesterol is a neutral sterol; lecithin is a phospholipid; and both are almost completely insoluble in water. However, bile salts are able to form multimolecular aggregates (micelles) that solubilize lecithin and cholesterol in an aqueous solution. Bile salts alone are relatively inefficient in solubilizing cholesterol (approximately 50 molecules of bile salt are necessary to solubilize 1 molecule of cholesterol), but the solubilization of lecithin in bile salt solutions results in a mixed micelle that is 7 times more efficient in the solubilization of cholesterol. Precipitation of cholesterol microcrystals may come about through a simultaneous change in all 3 major components.

## Treatment

Cholelithiasis is frequently asymptomatic and is discovered fortuitously in the course of routine radiographic study, operation, or autopsy. Although there is disagreement about the desirability of cholecystectomy in patients with "silent" gallstones, it is generally agreed that diabetic patients should undergo gallbladder removal to avoid complications. Operation is usually indicated for symptomatic cholelithiasis.

Chenodeoxycholic acid (Chenix) is a bile salt that on oral administration is able to cause dissolution of some cholesterol stones. Although relatively safe, it may cause diarrhea or minor liver function test abnormalities. It is only effective in patients with a functioning gallbladder and an unobstructed biliary tract. Dissolution of gallstones may require 2 years or longer. Gallstones may recur when treatment stops. Obesity may induce resistance to therapy. Intermittent therapy is ineffective.

Allen MJ et al: Rapid dissolution of gallstones by methyl tert-butyl ether: Preliminary observations. *N Engl J Med* 1985;**312**:217.

Fromm H: Gallstone dissolution therapy: Current status and future prospects. *Gastroenterology* 1986;**91**:1560.

Heiss FW et al: Common bile duct calculi. 1. Surgical therapy. 2. Nonsurgical therapy. *Postgrad Med* (Feb 15) 1984;**75**:88, 109. [Special issue.]

Thistle JL et al: The natural history of cholelithiasis: The National Cooperative Gallstone Study. *Ann Intern Med* 1984;**101**:171.

## ACUTE CHOLECYSTITIS

### Essentials of Diagnosis

- Steady, severe pain and tenderness in the right hypochondrium or epigastrium.
- Nausea and vomiting.
- Jaundice.
- Fever and leukocytosis.

### General Considerations

Cholecystitis is associated with gallstones in over 90% of cases. It occurs when a calculus becomes impacted in the cystic duct and inflammation develops behind the obstruction. Vascular abnormalities of the bile duct or pancreatitis may rarely produce cholecystitis in the absence of gallstones. If the obstruction is not relieved, pressure builds up within the gallbladder as a result of continued secretion. Primarily as a result of ischemic changes secondary to distention, gangrene may develop, with resulting perforation. Although generalized peritonitis is possible, the leak usually remains localized and forms a chronic, well-circumscribed abscess cavity.

### Clinical Findings

**A. Symptoms and Signs:** The acute attack is often precipitated by a large or fatty meal and is characterized by the relatively sudden appearance of severe, minimally fluctuating pain which is localized to the epigastrium or right hypochondrium and which in the uncomplicated case may gradually subside over a period of 12–18 hours. Vomiting occurs in about 75% of patients and in half of instances affords variable relief. Right upper quadrant abdominal tenderness is almost always present and is usually associated with muscle guarding and rebound pain. A palpable gallbladder is present in about 15% of cases. Jaundice is present in about 25% of cases and, when persistent or severe, suggests the possibility of choledocholithiasis. Fever is usually present.

**B. Laboratory Findings:** The white count is usually high (12,000–15,000/$\mu$L). Total serum bilirubin values of 1–4 mg/dL may be reported even in the absence of common duct obstruction. Serum transaminase and alkaline phosphatase are often elevated—the former as high as 300 mU/mL and even higher when associated with ascending cholangitis. Serum amylase may also be moderately elevated.

**C. Imaging:** Films of the abdomen may show gallstones in 15% of cases. $^{99m}$Tc hepatobiliary imaging agents (iminodiacetic acid compounds), also known as HIDA scan, are useful in demonstrating an obstructed cystic duct, which is the cause of acute cholecystitis in most patients. This test is reliable if the bilirubin is under 5 mg/dL. Right upper quadrant abdominal ultrasound may show the presence of gallstones but is not specific for acute cholecystitis.

### Differential Diagnosis

The disorders most likely to be confused with acute cholecystitis are perforated peptic ulcer, acute pancreatitis, appendicitis in a high-lying appendix, perforated carcinoma or diverticulum of the hepatic flexure, liver abscess, hepatitis, and pneumonia with pleurisy on the right side. The definite localization of pain and tenderness in the right hypochondrium, with frequent radiation to the infrascapular area, strongly favors the diagnosis of acute cholecystitis.

### Complications

**A. Gangrene of the Gallbladder:** Continuation or progression of right upper quadrant abdominal pain, tenderness, muscle guarding, fever, and leukocytosis after 24–48 hours suggests severe inflammation and possible gangrene of the gallbladder. Necrosis may occasionally develop without definite signs in either the obese or the elderly.

**B. Cholangitis:** Intermittently high fever and chills strongly suggest choledocholithiasis.

### Treatment

Acute cholecystitis will usually subside on a conservative regimen (withholding of oral feedings, intravenous alimentation, analgesics and antibiotics if indicated). Cholecystectomy can be performed within

2–3 days after hospitalization or can be scheduled for 6–8 weeks later, depending on the surgeon's preference and the clinical aspects of the individual case. If, as occasionally happens, recurrent acute symptoms develop during this waiting period, cholecystectomy is indicated without delay. If nonsurgical treatment has been elected, the patient (especially if diabetic or elderly) should be watched carefully for evidence of gangrene of the gallbladder or cholangitis.

Operation is mandatory when there is evidence of gangrene or perforation. Operation during the first 24 hours can be justified as a means of reducing overall morbidity in good-risk patients in whom the diagnosis is unequivocal. It is usually best to defer surgery, if possible, in the presence of acute pancreatitis, unless choledocholithiasis is suspected.

**A. Medical Treatment:** During the acute period, the patient should be observed frequently, with careful abdominal examination and sequential determination of the white cell count several times a day. Analgesics such as pentazocine or meperidine are preferred for pain control. Morphine derivatives in effective doses are known to produce spasm of the sphincter of Oddi and may cause spurious elevations of serum amylase. Meperidine may have the same effects but to a much lesser degree. Anticholinergic agents are rarely indicated for these patients, in part because they may mask the development of paralytic ileus or prolong its duration. Appropriate antimicrobial agents should be employed in all but the most mild and rapidly subsiding cases.

**B. Surgical Treatment:** When surgery is elected for acute cholecystitis, cholecystectomy is the procedure of choice. Cholangiography should be performed at the time of operation to ascertain the need for common duct exploration. In the poor-risk patient or when technical difficulties preclude cholecystectomy, cholecystostomy can be performed under local anesthesia.

## Prognosis

Mild acute cholecystitis usually subsides, but recurrences are common. Symptomatic cholecystitis is a definite indication for surgery. Persistence of symptoms after removal of the gallbladder implies either mistaken diagnosis, functional bowel disorder, or technical error, since cholecystectomy is curative.

Dawson SL, Mueller PR: Nonoperative management of biliary obstruction. *Annu Rev Med* 1985;**36:**1.

Fajman WA: Acute right upper quadrant abdominal pain: Radionuclide approach. *JCU* 1983;**11:**193.

Fink-Bennett D et al: The sensitivity of hepatobiliary imaging and realtime ultrasonography in the detection of acute cholecystitis. *Arch Surg* 1985;**120:**904.

Fox MS et al: Acute acalculous cholecystitis. *Surg Gynecol Obstet* 1984;**159:**13.

Norrby S et al: Early or delayed cholecystectomy in acute cholecystitis: A clinical trial. *Br J Surg* 1983;**70:**163.

Ralls PW et al: Realtime sonography in suspected acute cholecystitis: Prospective evaluation of primary and secondary signs. *Radiology* 1985;**155:**767.

# CYSTIC DUCT SYNDROMES

## Precholecystectomy

A small group of patients (mostly women) has been reported in whom right upper quadrant abdominal pain occurred frequently following meals. Conventional radiographic study of the upper gastrointestinal tract and gallbladder—including intravenous cholangiography—was unremarkable. Using cholecystokinin (CCK) as a gallbladder stimulant, contraction and evacuation of the viscus did not take place, as usually occurs in the 3- to 5-minute period after injection of the hormone. However, the gallbladder assumed a "golf ball" configuration, and biliary type pain was reproduced. At the time of cholecystectomy, the gallbladders were found to be enlarged and could not be emptied by manual compression. Anatomic and histologic examination of the operative specimens revealed obstruction of the cystic ducts either because of fibrotic stenosis at their proximal ends or because of adhesions and kinking.

## Postcholecystectomy

Following cholecystectomy, a variable group of patients complain of continuing symptoms, ie, right upper quadrant pain, flatulence, and fatty food intolerance. The persistence of symptoms in this group of patients suggests the possibility of an incorrect diagnosis prior to cholecystectomy, eg, esophagitis, pancreatitis, radiculitis, or functional bowel disease. It is important to rule out the possibility of choledocholithiasis or common duct stricture as a cause for persistent symptoms in the postoperative period.

Pain has been associated with dilatation of the cystic duct remnant, neuroma formation in the ductal wall, foreign body granuloma, or traction on the common duct by a long cystic duct. The clinical presentation of colicky pain, chills, fever, or jaundice should suggest biliary tract disease. Liver tests for cholestasis, abdominal ultrasonography, or retrograde cholangiography may be necessary to rule out biliary tract disease. Surgery, with common duct exploration for stones and removal of the cystic duct remnant, may be necessary.

Alberti-Flor JJ et al: Mirizzi syndrome. *Am J Gastroenterol* 1985;**80:**822.

Bode WE, Aust JB: Isolated cystic dilatations of the cystic duct. *Am J Surg* 1983;**145:**828.

Jennings SA et al: Management of retained cystic duct stone. *Br J Surg* 1982;**69:**91.

# CHRONIC CHOLECYSTITIS

The most common disability that results from cholelithiasis is chronic cholecystitis. It is characterized pathologically by varying degrees of chronic inflammation on gross inspection or microscopic examination of the gallbladder. In about 4–5% of cases, the villi of the gallbladder undergo polypoid enlargement due to deposition of cholesterol that may be visible to the naked eye ("strawberry gallbladder," cholesterolosis). In other instances, adenomatous hyperplasia of all or part of the gallbladder wall may be so marked as to give the appearance of a myoma (pseudotumor). Calculi are usually present. The diagnosis is often erroneously applied to collections of symptoms that are only vaguely or indirectly related to gallbladder dysfunction.

## Clinical Findings

### A. Symptoms and Signs:

**1. Pain**—Chronic cholecystitis is associated with discrete bouts of right hypochondriac and epigastric pain that is either steady or intermittent. Discomfort is usually persistent, but, if intermittent, the height of pain may be separated by 15- to 60-minute intervals.

The onset of pain is usually abrupt, with maximum intensity and plateau reached within 15 minutes to 1 hour. Attacks of biliary colic may persist for as long as several hours or be as brief as 15–20 minutes, the average duration being about 1 hour. Pain referral to the interscapular area is occasionally noted.

**2. Chronic indigestion**—Chronic indigestion is considered by many to be commonly due to gallbladder disease. Fatty food intolerance, belching, flatulence, a sense of epigastric heaviness, upper abdominal pain of varying intensity, and pyrosis are some of the symptoms that have been erroneously considered to be suggestive of cholelithiasis and cholecystitis. Efforts have therefore been made to evaluate "dyspeptic" symptomatology in relationship to objective evidence of gallbladder disease. In one prospective study of 142 women who experienced "chronic indigestion," only 24 had either gallstones or nonvisualization of the gallbladder on oral cholecystograms. Sixty-three (53%) of the 118 who had normal cholecystograms complained of "dyspepsia." Accordingly, it can be assumed that the association of chronic indigestion and gallstones is fortuitous. If cholecystectomy is performed in patients with calculi who have complained of a constellation of "dyspeptic" symptoms, the results of operation may be unpredictable and unsatisfactory.

**3. Physical examination**—Physical examination is nonspecific, revealing abdominal tenderness which may be localized to the right hypochondrium and epigastric area but which may also be diffuse. Hydrops of the gallbladder results when subsidence of acute cholecystitis occurs but cystic duct obstruction persists, producing distention of the gallbladder with a clear mucoid fluid. The gallbladder in that circumstance is palpable in the right upper abdomen. The presence of jaundice obviously supports the diagnosis of cholecystitis with choledocholithiasis.

**B. Laboratory Findings:** Laboratory studies are usually not diagnostic.

**C. Imaging:** Films of the abdomen taken prior to oral cholecystography may reveal opacification of the gallbladder caused by high concentrations of calcium carbonate (limy bile) or radiopaque stones. Nonvisualization of the gallbladder implies cholecystitis (95% accuracy) provided there is radiologic evidence that the oral contrast material has been absorbed and excreted. It is important to remember the following technical reasons for nonvisualization: failure to ingest the dye, vomiting or diarrhea, gastric outlet obstruction or esophageal stricture, intestinal malabsorption, abnormal location of the gallbladder, liver disease (including preicteric hepatitis), Dubin-Johnson-Sprinz-Nelson syndrome, fat-free diet prior to cholecystography, and previous cholecystectomy.

Ultrasound examination of the gallbladder is a useful means of detecting stones. The accuracy of diagnosis of cholelithiasis (but not cholecystitis) in some centers is high (96%) and the incidence of false-positive results low (2%).

## Differential Diagnosis

When nonspecific symptoms are present, it is necessary to consider the possibilities of gastroduodenal ulcer disease, chronic relapsing pancreatitis, irritable colon syndrome, and malignant neoplasms of the stomach, pancreas, hepatic flexure, or gallbladder. Barium enema and upper gastrointestinal series complement cholecystography. Microscopic examination of bile obtained by biliary drainage is occasionally helpful in demonstrating calculous disease of the gallbladder. (The test is valid only in the absence of hepatic disease.)

## Complications

The presence of cholelithiasis with chronic cholecystitis can result in acute exacerbation of gallbladder inflammation, common duct stone, cholecystenteric fistulization, pancreatitis, and, rarely, carcinoma of the gallbladder. Calcified gallbladder has a high association with gallbladder carcinoma and is an indication for cholecystectomy.

## Treatment

Although documented cholelithiasis and cholecystitis ideally should be managed surgically, significant metabolic and cardiovascular disease or other factors may preclude operation. Nonspecific "dyspeptic" symptoms (eg, heartburn, belching, abdominal pain, bloating, flatulence, constipation) frequently are ameliorated by careful use of low-fat diets and weight reduction. Anticholinergics and sedatives, along with antacids and hydrophilic agents, may prove helpful.

Surgical treatment is the same as for acute cholecystitis, with operative cholangiography employed if there is a possibility of choledocholithiasis.

## Prognosis

The overall mortality rate of cholecystectomy is less than 1%, but hepatobiliary tract surgery is a more formidable procedure in the elderly and has a mortality rate of 5–10%. A technically successful surgical procedure in an appropriately selected patient is generally followed by complete cessation of symptoms.

Aranha GV et al: Cholecystectomy in cirrhotic patients: A formidable operation. *Am J Surg* 1982;**143**:55.

Escallon A Jr et al: Reliability of pre- and intraoperative tests for biliary lithiasis. *Ann Surg* 1985;**201**:640.

See also references on pp 398 and 417.

## CHOLEDOCHOLITHIASIS

### Essentials of Diagnosis
- Often a history of biliary colic or jaundice.
- Sudden onset of severe right upper quadrant or epigastric pain, which may radiate to the right scapula or shoulder.
- Nausea and vomiting.
- Fever, often followed by hypothermia and gram-negative shock.
- Jaundice.
- Leukocytosis.
- Abdominal films may reveal gallstones.

### General Considerations
About 15% of patients with gallstones have choledocholithiasis. The percentage rises with age, and the incidence in elderly people may be as high as 50%. Common duct stones usually originate in the gallbladder but may also form spontaneously in the common duct postcholecystectomy. The stones are frequently "silent," as no symptoms result unless there is obstruction.

### Clinical Findings
**A. Symptoms and Signs:** A history suggestive of biliary colic or prior jaundice can usually be obtained. The additional features that suggest the presence of a common duct stone are (1) frequently recurring attacks of right upper abdominal pain that is severe and persists for hours; (2) chills and fever associated with severe colic; and (3) a history of jaundice that was chronologically associated with abdominal pain. The combination of pain, fever (and chills), and jaundice represents Charcot's triad and denotes the classic picture of cholangitis. The presence of altered sensorium, lethargy, and septic shock connotes acute suppurative cholangitis accompanied by pus in the obstructed duct and represents a surgical emergency.

Biliary colic in choledocholithiasis is apparently caused by rapidly increasing biliary pressure that is secondary to sudden obstruction to the flow of bile. Radiation of pain into the interscapular area may be helpful in differentiating choledocholithiasis from cholecystolithiasis. Hepatomegaly may be present in calculous biliary obstruction, and tenderness is usually present in the right hypochondrium and epigastrium. Usually, there are no specific physical findings.

**B. Laboratory Findings:** Bilirubinuria and elevation of serum bilirubin are present if the common duct is obstructed. Serum alkaline phosphatase elevation is especially suggestive of obstructive jaundice. Not uncommonly, serum amylase elevations are present because of secondary pancreatitis. Because prolonged obstruction of the common duct results in hepatocellular dysfunction, SGOT (AST) will be abnormal. Prolongation of the prothrombin time occurs when there is disturbance of the normal enterohepatic circulation of bile, with its exclusion from the intestinal tract. When extrahepatic obstruction persists for more than a few weeks, differentiation of obstruction from primarily inflammatory disease becomes progressively more difficult.

**C. Imaging:** Although ultrasonography, CT scan, and radionuclide imaging may help to differentiate hepatocellular and obstructive jaundice, percutaneous transhepatic cholangiography or endoscopic retrograde cholangiography (ERCP) provides the most direct and accurate nonsurgical means of determining the cause, location, and extent of obstruction. If the obstruction is thought to be probably due to a stone, ERCP is the procedure of choice because of its therapeutic potential.

### Differential Diagnosis
The most common cause of obstructive jaundice is common duct stone. Next in frequency is carcinoma of the pancreas, ampulla of Vater, or common duct. Metastatic carcinoma (usually from the gastrointestinal tract) and direct extension of gallbladder cancer are other important causes of obstructive jaundice. Hepatocellular jaundice can usually be differentiated by the history, clinical findings, and liver tests, but liver biopsy is necessary on occasion.

### Complications
**A. Biliary Cirrhosis:** Common duct obstruction lasting longer than 30 days results in severe liver damage. Hepatic failure with portal hypertension occurs in untreated cases.

**B. Cholangitis:** If bacteria enter the duct proximal to the obstruction and inoculation of these organisms into the bloodstream occurs as the result of elevated biliary pressure in the ductal system, fever (and chills), jaundice, and pain will appear (Charcot's triad). Cholangitis may be nonsuppurative or suppurative. The former usually responds well to antimicrobial therapy, whereas the latter is a surgical emergency. Untreated cholangitis is the most common cause of multiple pyogenic hepatic abscesses, resulting in a progressively downhill course and septic death.

**C. Hypoprothrombinemia:** Patients with obstructive jaundice or liver disease may bleed excessively as a result of prolonged prothrombin times. If the hypoprothrombinemia is due to faulty vitamin K absorption, the following preparations are of value. When prothrombin response to parenteral versus oral administration of these agents is compared, the nature of the underlying lesion (hepatocellular versus obstructive) can be determined; obstructive jaundice will respond to parenteral vitamin K or water-soluble oral vitamin K.

For subcutaneous administration, phytonadione, 10 mg daily, is the preparation of choice. For oral administration, menadiol sodium diphosphate, 5 mg twice daily, is the preferred oral agent. It is water-soluble and is absorbed from the intestinal tract in the absence of bile.

## Treatment

Common duct stone is usually treated by cholecystectomy and choledochostomy. In the postcholecystectomy patient with choledocholithiasis, endoscopic papillotomy with stone extraction is preferable to transabdominal surgery.

**A. Preoperative Preparation:** Emergency operation is rarely necessary unless severe ascending cholangitis is present. A few days devoted to careful evaluation and preparation will be well spent.

Liver function should be evaluated thoroughly. Prothrombin time should be restored to normal by parenteral administration of vitamin K preparations (see above). Nutrition should be restored by a high-carbohydrate, high-protein diet and vitamin supplementation. Cholangitis, if present, should be controlled with antimicrobials, but may necessitate more urgent surgical decompression.

**B. Indications for Common Duct Exploration:** At every operation for cholelithiasis, the advisability of exploring the common duct must be considered. Operative cholangiography via the cystic duct is a very useful procedure for demonstrating common duct stone.

1. Preoperative findings suggestive of choledocholithiasis include a history (or the presence) of obstructive jaundice; frequent attacks of biliary colic; cholangitis; a history of pancreatitis; and a percutaneous transhepatic cholangiogram showing stone, obstruction, or dilatation of the duct.

2. Operative findings of choledocholithiasis are palpable stones in the common duct; dilatation or thickening of the wall of the common duct; gallbladder stones small enough to pass through the cystic duct; and pancreatitis.

3. For the patient with a T tube and a common duct stone, manipulation with various special instruments via the T tube or T tube sinus tract is often successful in extracting the stone.

**C. Postoperative Care:**

**1. Antibiotics**—Postoperative antibiotics are not administered routinely after biliary tract surgery. Cultures of the bile are always taken at operation. If biliary tract infection was present preoperatively or is apparent at operation, ampicillin or a cephalosporin is administered postoperatively until the results of sensitivity tests on culture specimens are available.

**2. Management of the T tube**—Following choledochostomy, a simple catheter or T tube is placed in the common duct for decompression. It must be attached securely to the skin or dressing because accidental removal of the tube may be disastrous. A prop-erly placed tube should drain bile at the operating table and continuously thereafter; otherwise, it should be considered blocked or dislocated. The volume of bile drainage varies from 100 to 1000 mL daily (average, 200–400 mL). Above-average drainage may be due to obstruction at the ampulla (usually by edema), increased bile output, low resistance or siphonage effect in the drainage system, or a combination of these factors.

**3. Cholangiography**–A cholangiogram should be taken through the T tube on about the seventh or eighth postoperative day. Under fluoroscopic control, a radiopaque medium is aseptically and gently injected until the duct system is outlined and the medium begins to enter the duodenum. The injection of air bubbles must be avoided, since on x-ray they resemble stones in the duct system. Spot films are always taken. If the cholangiogram shows no stones in the common duct and the opaque medium flows freely into the duodenum, the tube is clamped overnight and removed by simple traction on the following day. A small amount of bile frequently leaks from the tube site for a few days. A rubber tissue drain is usually placed alongside the T tube at operation. This drain is partially withdrawn on the fifth day and shortened daily until it is removed completely on about the seventh day.

In poor-risk patients with common duct stones, an endoscopic sphincterotomy should be considered if a skilled endoscopist is available.

Escourrou J et al: Early and late complications after endoscopic sphincterotomy for biliary lithiasis with and without the gallbladder "in situ." *Gut* 1984;**25**:598.

Hauer-Jensen M et al: Predictive ability of choledocholithiasis indicators: A prospective evaluation. *Ann Surg* 1985;**202**:64.

Kelly TR: Gallstone pancreatitis: Local predisposing factors. *Ann Surg* 1984;**200**:479.

Mitchell SE, Clark RA: A comparison of computed tomography and sonography in choledocholithiasis. *AJR* 1984;**142**:729.

## BILIARY STRICTURE

Benign biliary strictures are the result of surgical trauma in about 95% of cases. The remainder are caused by blunt external injury to the abdomen, pancreatitis, or erosion of the duct by a gallstone.

Signs of injury to the duct may or may not be recognized in the immediate postoperative period. If complete occlusion has occurred, jaundice will develop rapidly; but more often a tear has been accidentally made in the duct, and the earliest manifestation of injury may be excessive or prolonged loss of bile from the surgical drains. Bile leakage contributes to the production of localized infection, which in turn accentuates scar formation and the ultimate development of a fibrous stricture.

Cholangitis is the most common syndrome produced by stricture. Typically, the patient notices episodes of pain, fever, chills, and jaundice within a few weeks to months after cholecystectomy. With the exception of jaundice during an attack of cholangitis and right upper quadrant abdominal tenderness, physical findings are usually not significant.

Serum alkaline phosphatase is usually elevated. Hyperbilirubinemia is variable, fluctuating during exacerbations and usually remaining in the range of 5–10 mg/dL. Blood cultures may be positive during an episode of cholangitis. Percutaneous transhepatic cholangiography or endoscopic retrograde cholangiopancreatography can be valuable in demonstrating the stricture.

Differentiation from choledocholithiasis may require surgical exploration. Operative treatment of a stricture frequently necessitates performance of choledochojejunostomy or hepaticojejunostomy to reestablish bile flow into the intestine.

Biliary stricture is not a benign condition, since significant hepatocellular disease will inevitably occur if it is allowed to continue uncorrected. The death rate for untreated stricture ranges from 10 to 15%.

Bolton JS et al: Management of benign biliary stricture. *Surg Clin North Am* 1980;**60:**313.

## PRIMARY SCLEROSING CHOLANGITIS

Primary sclerosing cholangitis is a rare nonspecific inflammatory reaction of unknown cause involving both the intra- and extrahepatic biliary ducts. It is characterized by a diffuse inflammation of the biliary tract leading to fibrosis and strictures of the biliary system. The disease is closely associated with ulcerative colitis, which is present in approximately two-thirds of patients with primary sclerosing cholangitis. Primary sclerosing cholangitis appears to be often associated with increased HLA-B8 histocompatibility antigen. Primary sclerosing cholangitis may occur at any period of life and may initially simulate a slowly growing bile duct carcinoma. However, the chronicity of the process militates against neoplasm. The criteria for making the diagnosis of primary sclerosing cholangitis are as follows: (1) progressive obstructive jaundice; (2) absence of calculi in the gallbladder or biliary ducts; (3) absence of prior surgical injury to the biliary tract; (4) absence of diseases causing cholangitis; (5) absence of congenital biliary anomalies; (6) thickening and narrowing of the biliary ductal system, demonstrated by palpation at surgery, biopsy, or x-ray techniques; (7) absence of biliary cirrhosis; and (8) exclusion of cholangiocarcinoma by long-term follow-up and multiple liver biopsies. Endoscopic retrograde cholangiography is the best means of establishing the diagnosis of primary sclerosing cholangitis other than surgical exploration.

Clinically, the disease presents as progressively obstructive jaundice, frequently preceded by malaise, pruritus, anorexia, and indigestion. Treatment consists of surgical bypass such as cholecystoduodenostomy. Corticosteroids and broad-spectrum antimicrobial agents have been employed with rare success, but generally the results have been inconstant and unpredictable. The prognosis is regarded as poor, with few individuals living more than a few years after the appearance of symptoms.

Chapman RWG, Jewell DP: Primary sclerosing cholangitis: An immunologically mediated disease? *West J Med* 1985; **143:**193.

LaRusso NF et al: Primary sclerosing cholangitis. (Current concepts.) *N Engl J Med* 1984;**310:**899.

## CARCINOMA OF THE BILIARY TRACT

Carcinoma of the gallbladder occurs in approximately 2% of all people operated on for biliary tract disease. It is notoriously insidious, and the diagnosis is usually made unexpectedly at surgery. Spread of the cancer—by direct extension into the liver or to the peritoneal surface—may be the initial manifestation.

Carcinoma of the extrahepatic bile ducts accounts for 3% of all cancer deaths in the USA. It affects both sexes equally but is more prevalent in individuals age 50–70. There is a questionable increased incidence in patients with chronic nonspecific ulcerative colitis.

### Clinical Findings

Progressive jaundice is the most common and is usually the first sign of obstruction of the extrahepatic biliary system. Pain is usually present in the right upper abdomen and radiates into the back. Anorexia and weight loss are common and are frequently associated with fever and chills. Rarely, hematemesis may be a confusing presentation that results from erosion of tumor into a blood vessel. Fistula formation between the biliary system and adjacent organs may also occur. The course is usually one of rapid deterioration, with death occurring within a few months.

Physical examination will reveal profound jaundice. A palpable gallbladder with obstructive jaundice usually signifies malignant disease. Courvoisier's law states that the most frequent cause of obstructive jaundice distal to the cystic duct with a normal gallbladder wall is neoplasm. This clinical generalization has been proved to be accurate about 90% of the time. Hepatomegaly is usually present and is associated with liver tenderness. Ascites may occur with peritoneal implants. Pruritus and skin excoriations are common.

Laboratory examinations reveal hyperbilirubinemia, predominantly of the conjugated variety. Total serum bilirubin values range from 5 to 30 mg/dL. There is usually concomitant elevation of the alkaline phosphatase and serum cholesterol. SGOT (AST) is normal or minimally elevated.

The most helpful diagnostic studies before surgery are either percutaneous transhepatic or endoscopic retrograde cholangiography. One or both of these procedures may be required in order to define the pathologic anatomy of the ductal obstruction. Differentiation of benign strictures of the ductal system from progressive sclerosing cholangitis is suggested by a history of prior exploration of the hepatobiliary tree with resultant injury that was unrecognized at the time of the initial celiotomy.

## Treatment

Unless there are overwhelming contraindications, palliative surgery is indicated to decompress the hepatobiliary system and relieve jaundice. This can be accomplished by cholecystoduodenostomy or by T tube drainage of the common duct. The prognosis is poor, few patients surviving for more than 6 months after surgery.

Alexander F et al: Biliary carcinoma: A review of 109 cases. *Am J Surg* 1984;**147**:503.

# DISEASES OF THE PANCREAS

## ACUTE PANCREATITIS

### Essentials of Diagnosis

- Abrupt onset of dull epigastric pain, often with radiation to the back.
- Nausea, vomiting, sweating, weakness.
- Abdominal tenderness and distention, fever.
- Leukocytosis, elevated serum and urinary amylase, elevated serum lipase.
- History of previous episodes, often related to alcohol intake.

### General Considerations

Acute pancreatitis is often a severe intra-abdominal disease due to acute inflammation of the pancreas and associated "escape" of pancreatic enzymes from acinar cells into surrounding tissues. Most cases are related to biliary tract disease or heavy alcohol intake. Among the more than 80 other causes or associations are hypercalcemia, hyperlipidemias (types I, IV, and V), abdominal trauma (including surgery), drugs (including prednisone and thiazides), vasculitis, and viral infections. The exact pathogenesis is not known but may include edema or obstruction of the ampulla of Vater with resultant reflux of bile into pancreatic ducts, stenosis of the accessory pancreatic duct (duct of Santorini), and direct injury to the acinar cells.

Pathologic changes vary from acute edema and cellular infiltration to necrosis of the acinar cells, hemorrhage from necrotic blood vessels, and intra- and extrapancreatic fat necrosis. All or part of the pancreas may be involved.

## Clinical Findings

**A. Symptoms and Signs:** Epigastric abdominal pain, generally abrupt in onset, is steady and severe and is often made worse by walking and lying supine and better by sitting and leaning forward. The pain usually radiates into the back but may radiate to the right or left. Nausea and vomiting are usually present. Severe weakness, sweating, and anxiety are noted in severe attacks. There may be a history of alcohol intake or a heavy meal immediately preceding the attack, or a history of milder but otherwise similar episodes in the past, even suggestive of biliary colic.

The abdomen is tender mainly in the upper abdomen, most often without guarding, rigidity, or rebound. The abdomen may be distended, and bowel sounds may be absent in associated paralytic ileus. Fever of 38.4–39 °C (101.1–102.2 °F), tachycardia, hypotension (even true shock), pallor, and a cool clammy skin are often present. Mild jaundice is common. An upper abdominal mass may be present but is not characteristic. Acute renal failure may occur early in the course of acute pancreatitis, usually prerenal in character.

**B. Laboratory Findings:** Findings of leukocytosis (10,000–30,000/$\mu$L), proteinuria, casts (25% of cases), glycosuria (10–20% of cases), hyperglycemia, and elevated serum bilirubin may be present. Blood urea nitrogen and serum alkaline phosphatase may be elevated and coagulation tests abnormal. Decrease in serum calcium may reflect a decreased serum albumin (because fluids have collected in the third space) and correlates well with severity of disease; it is lowest on about the sixth day. Levels lower than 7 mg/dL are associated with tetany and an unfavorable prognosis.

Serum amylase and lipase are elevated within 24 hours in 90% of cases, and return to normal is variable depending on the severity of disease. Urine amylase may be very high and may remain elevated longer than serum amylase. In those who develop ascites or left pleural effusions, amylase content is high and is indicative of the cause of these fluid collections.

**C. Imaging:** A 2-way view of the abdomen may show gallstones, a "sentinel loop" (a segment of air-filled small intestine most commonly in the left upper quadrant), the "colon cutoff sign" (a gas-filled segment of transverse colon abruptly ending at the area of pancreatic inflammation), or linear focal atelectasis of the left lower lobe of the lungs with or without pleural effusion. These findings suggest acute pancreatitis but are not diagnostic. CT scan is useful in demonstrating an enlarged pancreas, in detecting pseudocysts, and in determining the extent of phlegmons. Ultrasonography is less reliable, because the echoes are deflected by the gas-distended small intestine frequently associated with acute pancreatitis.

**D. Electrocardiographic Findings:** ST–T wave changes may occur, but they usually differ from those of myocardial infarction. Abnormal Q waves do not occur as a result of pancreatitis.

## Differential Diagnosis

Acute pancreatitis may be difficult to differentiate from an acutely perforated duodenal ulcer. One must keep in mind that pancreatitis may be the presenting clinical picture of choledocholithiasis with or without cholangitis, as well as of a penetrating duodenal ulcer. It may occur owing to infection by mumps virus, post-ERCP, or postoperatively owing to surgical manipulation in the area of the pancreas. Serum amylase may also be elevated in high intestinal obstruction, in mumps not involving the pancreas (salivary amylase), in ectopic pregnancy, after administration of narcotics, and after abdominal surgery. Other conditions to be differentiated are acute cholecystitis, acute intestinal obstruction, dissecting aortic aneurysm, renal colic, and acute mesenteric vascular insufficiency or thrombosis.

## Complications

Intravascular volume depletion secondary to leakage of fluids in the pancreatic bed and ileus with fluid-filled loops of bowel may result in prerenal azotemia and even acute tubular necrosis without overt shock. This usually occurs within 24 hours of the onset of acute pancreatitis and lasts 8–9 days. Some patients require peritoneal dialysis or hemodialysis.

One of the most serious complications of acute pancreatitis is pulmonary edema with or without cardiac failure ("shock lung"). It usually occurs 3–7 days after the onset of pancreatitis in patients who have required large volumes of fluid and colloid to maintain blood pressure and urine output. Most require assisted respiration with positive end-expiratory pressure for 1–2 weeks.

Pancreatic abscess is a suppurative process in necrotic tissue, with rising fever, leukocytosis, and localized tenderness and epigastric mass. This may be associated with a left-sided pleural effusion or an enlarging spleen secondary to splenic vein thrombosis.

Pseudocysts, encapsulated fluid collections with high enzyme content, commonly appear in pancreatitis when CT scans are used to monitor the evolution of an acute attack. Although the natural history of pseudocysts is still not well delineated, it appears that those less than 6 cm in diameter are likely to resolve spontaneously. Pseudocysts most commonly are within or adjacent to the pancreas but can present most anywhere (eg, mediastinal, retrorectal), having extended along anatomic planes. Multiple pseudocysts occur in 14% of patients with pseudocysts. Pseudocysts may become secondarily infected, necessitating drainage as for an abscess. Erosion of the inflammatory process into a blood vessel can result in a major hemorrhage into the cyst.

Chronic pancreatitis develops in about 10% of cases.

Permanent diabetes mellitus and exocrine pancreatic insufficiency occur uncommonly after a single acute episode.

## Prevention

Potential causative factors should be removed or corrected, eg, biliary tract disease, alcohol intake, hypercalcemia, duodenal ulcer, or certain offending drugs. The patient should be warned not to eat large meals or foods that are high in fat content and not to drink alcohol. The most common precipitating factor in acute pancreatitis is alcohol intake.

## Treatment

**A. Management of Acute Disease:** The pancreatic rest program includes withholding food and liquids by mouth, bed rest, and in those with moderately severe pain or ileus, nasogastric suction. Pain is controlled with meperidine (Demerol), 100–150 mg intramuscularly every 3–4 hours as necessary. Other narcotics may be used if pain control is not achieved, but they may cause smooth muscle contractions (spasm of the ampulla of Vater). Atropine sulfate, 0.4–0.6 mg subcutaneously, may be given as an antispasmodic and to decrease pancreatic exocrine secretions but may complicate the picture in respect to possible ileus.

In more severe pancreatitis, there may be considerable leakage of fluids, necessitating more than the normal amount of intravenous fluids to maintain intravascular volume. Saline is chiefly used, but fresh-frozen plasma or serum albumin may be necessary. With colloid solutions, there may be an increased risk of developing adult respiratory distress syndrome. If shock persists after adequate volume replacement (including packed red cells), norepinephrine or dopamine may be required. For the severe pancreatitis patient requiring a large volume of parenteral fluids, central venous pressure and blood gases should be monitored at regular intervals.

Calcium gluconate must be given intravenously if there is evidence of hypocalcemia with tetany. Antibiotics should be reserved for specific infections. If fever exceeds 39 °C (102.2 °F) and blood, urine, sputum, and effusions (if present) have been obtained for culture, institution of antibiotic therapy has been recommended.

The patient with severe pancreatitis requires attention in an intensive care unit. Close follow-up of blood count, hematocrit, serum electrolytes, and creatinine is required.

**B. Follow-Up Care:** After the patient has recovered from shock (or if shock does not develop), it is necessary to choose between expectant medical management and exploratory surgery. Medical management is preferred. Observe the patient closely for evidence of continued inflammation of the pancreas or related structures. A surgeon should be consulted in all cases of suspected acute pancreatitis. If the diagnosis is in doubt and there is a strong possibility of a serious surgically correctable lesion (eg, perforated peptic ulcer, common duct stone), exploration is indicated.

Aggressive surgery and enteral or parenteral hyperalimentation may increase survival in patients with hemorrhagic or suppurative pancreatitis. Initially, enterostomy tubes and drainage are established. Subsequent surgery is performed to debride necrotic pancreas and surrounding tissue.

When acute pancreatitis is unexpectedly found on exploratory laparotomy, it is usually wise to close without intervention of any kind. If the pancreatitis appears mild and cholelithiasis is present, cholecystostomy or cholecystectomy may be justified. Patients with unsuspected pancreatitis who receive the least intra-abdominal manipulation have the lowest morbidity and mortality rates after laparotomy, except as noted above. Peritoneal lavage improves early survival in severe acute pancreatitis. Late septic complications are unaffected.

The development of a pancreatic abscess is an indication for prompt drainage, usually through the flank. If a pseudocyst develops and persists, surgical treatment may be required, although most subside over a period of 3–6 months. Pseudocysts may require drainage when infected or associated with persisting pain, pancreatitis, or common duct obstruction.

The patient should be examined frequently. Periodic blood counts, blood glucose determinations, and serum and urine enzyme determinations should be carried out as indicated. Antibiotic therapy should be reserved for patients with septic complications.

No fluid or foods should be given orally until the patient is largely free of pain and has bowel sounds. Clear liquids are then given, and a gradual progression to a regular low-fat diet is pursued, guided by the patient's tolerance and by the absence of pain. Pancreatitis complicated by prolonged ileus (24 hours or more), abdominal distention, or vomiting requires nasogastric suction until they subside, along with parenteral nutrition. Intravenous fluids are given as needed to replace lost fluids, electrolytes, and blood.

**C. Convalescent Care:** When clinical evidence of pancreatic inflammation has cleared, institute a low-fat diet.

## Prognosis

Recurrences are common. The mortality rate for acute hemorrhagic pancreatitis is high, especially when hepatic, cardiovascular, or renal impairment is present. Surgery is indicated only when the diagnosis is in doubt, when the patient is desperately ill despite conservative therapy, or in the presence of an associated disorder such as stones in the biliary tract.

Barkin JS et al: Diagnosis of pancreatic abscess via percutaneous aspiration. *Dig Dis Sci* 1982;**27**:1011.

Geokas MC et al: Acute pancreatitis. *Ann Intern Med* 1985;**103**:86.

Goulet RJ et al: Multiple pancreatic pseudocyst disease. *Ann Surg* 1984;**199**:6.

Heij HA et al: Timing of surgery for acute biliary pancreatitis. *Am J Surg* 1985;**149**:371.

Mallory A, Kern F Jr: Drug-induced pancreatitis: A critical review. *Gastroenterology* 1980;**78**:813.

Moossa AR: Current concepts: Diagnostic tests and procedures in acute pancreatitis. *N Engl J Med* 1984;**311**:639.

Pellegrini CA: The treatment of acute pancreatitis: A continuing challenge. (Editorial.) *N Engl J Med* 1985;**312**:436.

Rosseland AR, Solhaug JH: Early or delayed endoscopic papillotomy (EPT) in gallstone pancreatitis. *Ann Surg* 1984;**199**:165.

Steinberg WM et al: Diagnostic assays in acute pancreatitis: A study of sensitivity and specificity. *Ann Intern Med* 1985;**102**:576.

Wade JW: Twenty five year experience with pancreatic pseudocysts: Are we making progress? *Am J Surg* 1985;**149**:705.

## CHRONIC PANCREATITIS
## (Chronic Relapsing Pancreatitis)

Chronic pancreatitis occurs most often in patients with alcoholism, hereditary pancreatitis, hypercalcemia, and hyperlipoproteinemias (types I, IV, and V). Progressive fibrosis and destruction of functioning glandular tissue occur as a result. Pancreaticolithiasis and obstruction of the duodenal end of the pancreatic duct are often present. Pancreatitis recurring after cholecystectomy for cholelithiasis should raise the suspicion of a retained or newly developed common duct stone.

Differentiation of chronic from recurrent pancreatitis is important in that recurrent pancreatitis is initiated by a specific event (eg, alcoholic binge, passage of a stone), whereas chronic pancreatitis is a self-perpetuating disease characterized by pain and pancreatic exocrine or endocrine insufficiency.

### Clinical Findings

**A. Symptoms and Signs:** Persistent or recurrent episodes of epigastric and left upper quadrant pain with referral to the upper left lumbar region are typical. Anorexia, nausea, vomiting, constipation, flatulence, and weight loss are common. Abdominal signs during attacks consist chiefly of tenderness over the pancreas, mild muscle guarding, and paralytic ileus: Attacks may last only a few hours or as long as 2 weeks; pain may eventually be almost continuous. Steatorrhea (as indicated by bulky, foul, fatty stools) and other types of intestinal maldigestion may occur.

**B. Laboratory Findings:** Serum amylase and bilirubin may be elevated during acute attacks. Glycosuria may be present. Excess fecal fat may be demonstrated on chemical analysis of the stool.

**C. Imaging:** Plain films often show pancreaticolithiasis and mild ileus. A cholecystogram may reveal biliary tract disease, and upper gastrointestinal series may demonstrate a widened duodenal loop. Endoscopic retrograde cholangiopancreatography is a technique that has been widely used. It may show dilated ducts, intraductal stones, strictures, or tumor. Failure to cannulate the duct occurs in about 20% of cases.

### Complications

Narcotic addiction is common. Other frequent complications include diabetes mellitus, pancreatic pseudocyst or abscess, cholestatic liver disease with or without jaundice, steatorrhea, malnutrition, and peptic ulcer.

## Treatment

Correctable coexistent biliary tract disease should be treated surgically.

**A. Medical Measures:** A low-fat diet should be prescribed. Alcohol is forbidden because it frequently precipitates attacks. Mild sedatives or anticholinergics may be helpful. Narcotics should be avoided if possible. Steatorrhea is treated with pancreatic supplements that are selected on the basis of their lipase activity. Cotazym, Festal, Ilozyme, Ku-Zyme HP, Pancrease, and Viokase have high lipase activity. The usual dose is 2 capsules before, during, and after meals. Concurrent administration of $H_2$ receptor antagonists decreases the inactivation of lipase by acid and may thereby decrease steatorrhea further; however, the drugs are expensive. It is not necessary to reduce fat excretion to normal to have a good clinical response. Treat associated diabetes as for any other insulinopenic patient. Every effort is made to manage the disease medically.

**B. Surgical Treatment:** The only indication for surgery in chronic pancreatitis, other than internal drainage of persistent pseudocysts or to treat other complications, is to attempt to relieve pain. The objectives of surgical intervention are to eradicate biliary tract disease, ensure a free flow of bile into the duodenum, and eliminate obstruction of the pancreatic duct. When obstruction of the duodenal end of the duct can be demonstrated by endoscopic retrograde cholangiopancreatography, dilatation of the duct or resection of the tail of the pancreas with implantation of the distal end of the duct by pancreaticojejunostomy may be successful. Anastomosis between the longitudinally split duct and a defunctionalized limb of jejunum without pancreatectomy may be in order. In advanced cases it may be necessary, as a last resort, to do subtotal or total pancreatectomy.

## Prognosis

This is a serious disease and often leads to chronic invalidism. The prognosis is best when patients with acute pancreatitis are carefully investigated with their first attack and are found to have some remediable condition such as chronic cholecystitis and cholelithiasis, choledocholithiasis, stenosis of the sphincter of Oddi, or hyperparathyroidism. Medical management of the hyperlipidemias frequently associated with the condition may also prevent recurrent attacks. Surgical relief of these aggravating conditions may prevent recurrent pancreatic disease.

Ammann RW et al: Course and outcome of chronic pancreatitis: Longitudinal study of a mixed medical-surgical series of 245 patients. *Gastroenterology* 1984;**86**:820.

Creutzfeldt W (editor): The exocrine pancreas. *Clin Gastroenterol* 1984;**13**:655.

Dutta SK, Rubin J, Harvey J: Comparative evaluations of the therapeutic efficacy of a pH-sensitive enteric coated pancreatic enzyme preparation with conventional pancreatic enzyme therapy in the treatment of exocrine pancreatic insufficiency. *Gastroenterology* 1983;**84**:426.

Frey CF, Bodai BI: Surgery in chronic pancreatitis. *Clin Gastroenterol* 1984;**13**:913.

Niederau C, Grendell JH: Diagnosis of chronic pancreatitis. *Gastroenterology* 1985;**88**:1973.

Rossi RL, Heiss FW, Braasch JW: Surgical management of chronic pancreatitis. *Surg Clin North Am* 1985;**65**:79.

## CARCINOMA OF THE HEAD OF THE PANCREAS & THE PERIAMPULLARY AREA

### Essentials of Diagnosis

- Obstructive jaundice (may be painless).
- Enlarged gallbladder may be painful.
- Upper abdominal pain with radiation to back, weight loss, and thrombophlebitis are usually late manifestations.

### General Considerations

Carcinoma is the commonest neoplasm of the pancreas. About 75% are in the head and 25% in the body and tail of the organ. Carcinomas involving the head of the pancreas, the ampulla of Vater, the common bile duct, and the duodenum are considered together, because they are usually indistinguishable clinically. They comprise 3% of cancers and 5% of cancer deaths.

### Clinical Findings

**A. Symptoms and Signs:** Pain is present in over 70% of cases and is often vague, diffuse, and located in the epigastrium. Radiation of pain into the back is common and sometimes predominates. Sitting up and leaning forward may afford some relief, and this usually indicates that the lesion has spread beyond the pancreas and is inoperable. The pain is rarely confused with biliary colic. Diarrhea, as a relatively early symptom, is seen occasionally. Migratory thrombophlebitis is a rare sign. Jaundice and weight loss are common but late findings. An uncommon occurrence but a useful clinical rule (Courvoisier's law) is that jaundice associated with a palpable gallbladder is indicative of obstruction by neoplasm. In addition, a hard, fixed, occasionally tender mass may be present.

**B. Laboratory Findings:** There may be mild anemia. Glycosuria, hyperglycemia, and impaired glucose tolerance or true diabetes mellitus are found in 10–20% of cases. The serum amylase or lipase level is occasionally elevated. Liver function tests are those of obstructive jaundice. Steatorrhea in the absence of jaundice is uncommon. The secretin test of exocrine secretion usually has a low volume with normal bicarbonate concentration. In about 60% of cases, duodenal cytologic studies have shown malignant cells. Occult blood in the stool is suggestive of carcinoma of the ampulla of Vater. Carcinoembryonic antigen is elevated in most patients but is nonspecific.

**C. Imaging:** Radiographic examination is usually noncontributory in involvement of the body and tail of the pancreas, except when the splenic vein is involved. With obstruction of the splenic vein, splenomegaly or gastric varices are present, the latter delineated by an upper gastrointestinal series, endoscopy, or angiography. With carcinoma of the head of the pancreas, the gastrointestinal series may show a widening of the duodenal loop, mucosal abnormalities in the duodenum ranging from edema to invasion or ulceration, or spasm or compression. Hypotonic duodenography and selective celiac and superior mesenteric arteriography may be most helpful by demonstrating either the encroachment of the duodenum or abnormal vessels in the region of the pancreas. Endoscopic retrograde cholangiopancreatography may delineate the pancreatic duct system and suggest carcinoma. Data are not available on how often this procedure leads to a therapeutic decision. CT scan is most helpful in delineating the extent of the pancreatic mass and allows for percutaneous aspiration of the mass for cytologic studies.

## Treatment

Abdominal exploration is usually necessary when cytologic diagnosis cannot be made or if resection is to be attempted, which includes about 30% of patients. Radical pancreaticoduodenal resection is indicated for lesions strictly limited to the head of the pancreas, periampullary zone, and duodenum. When resection is not feasible, cholecystojejunostomy is performed to relieve the jaundice. A gastrojejunostomy is performed to relieve the jaundice. A gastrojejunostomy is also done if duodenal obstruction is expected to develop later. High-voltage irridation and combination drug chemotherapy should be considered.

## Prognosis

Carcinoma of the head of the pancreas has a very poor prognosis. Reported 5-year survival rates range from 2.3 to 5.2%. Lesions of the ampulla, common duct, and duodenum have a better prognosis, with reported 5-year survival rates of 20–40% after resection. The reported operative mortality rate of radical pancreaticoduodenectomy is 10–15%.

Nix GA et al: Carcinoma of the head of the pancreas: Therapeutic implications of endoscopic retrograde cholangiopancreatography findings. *Am J Surg* 1984;**87**:37.

## CARCINOMA OF THE BODY & TAIL OF THE PANCREAS

About 25% of pancreatic cancers arise in the body or tail. Islet cell tumors arise in the pancreas, as do the non-B cell gastrin-secreting tumors associated with Zollinger-Ellison syndrome. There are no charac-

teristic findings in the early stages. The initial symptoms are vague epigastric or left upper quadrant distress. Anorexia and weight loss usually occur. Later, pain becomes more severe and frequently radiates through to the left lumbar region. A mass in the mid or left epigastrium may be palpable. The spontaneous development of thrombophlebitis is suggestive. If suspected, the diagnosis can often be supported by CT scanning and confirmed by percutaneous aspiration of the mass for cytologic analysis. Sometimes, surgical exploration is necessary for diagnosis. Resection is rarely feasible, and cure is rarer still. The response to fluorouracil (5-FU) has been disappointing. Studies are under way to evaluate multiple-drug therapy.

Moossa AR: Pancreatic cancer: Approach to diagnosis, selection for surgery and choice of operation. *Cancer* 1982;**50**:2689.

Trede M: The surgical treatment of pancreatic carcinoma. *Surgery* 1985;**97**:28.

Van Dyke JA, Stanley RJ, Berland LL: Pancreatic imaging. *Ann Intern Med* 1985;**102**:212.

# ACUTE PERITONITIS

## Essentials of Diagnosis

- Abdominal pain, vomiting, fever, and prostration.
- Abdominal rigidity and diffuse or local tenderness (often rebound).
- Later, abdominal distention and paralytic ileus.
- Leukocytosis.

## General Considerations

Localized or generalized peritonitis is the most important complication of a wide variety of acute abdominal disorders. Peritonitis may be caused by infection or chemical irritation. Perforation or necrosis of the gastrointestinal tract is the usual source of infection. Chemical peritonitis occurs in acute pancreatitis and in the early stages of gastroduodenal perforation. Spontaneous bacterial peritonitis may occur in decompensated cirrhotic patients with ascites. Sclerosing peritonitis may be associated with neoplastic disease and certain drugs (eg, beta-blockers, methysergide).

## Clinical Findings

**A. Systemic Reaction:** Malaise, prostration, nausea, vomiting, septic fever, leukocytosis, and electrolyte imbalance are usually seen in proportion to the severity of the process. If infection is not controlled, toxemia is progressive, and septic shock may develop.

**B. Abdominal Signs:**

**1. Pain and tenderness**–Depending upon the extent of involvement, pain and tenderness may be localized or generalized. Abdominal pain on coughing, rebound tenderness referred to the area of peritonitis, and tenderness to light percussion over the inflamed peritoneum are characteristic. Pelvic peritonitis is associated with rectal and vaginal tenderness.

**2. Muscle rigidity**–The muscles overlying the area of inflammation usually become spastic. When peritonitis is generalized (eg, after perforation of a peptic ulcer), marked rigidity of the entire abdominal wall may develop immediately. Rigidity is frequently diminished or absent in the late stages of peritonitis, in severe toxemia, and when the abdominal wall is weak.

**3. Paralytic ileus**–Intestinal motility is markedly inhibited by peritoneal inflammation. Diminished to absent peristalsis and progressive abdominal distention are the cardinal signs. Vomiting occurs as a result of pooling of gastrointestinal secretions and gas, most of which is swallowed air.

**C. Imaging:** Abdominal films show gas and fluid collections in both large and small bowel, usually with generalized rather than localized dilatation. The bowel walls, when thrown into relief by the gas patterns, may appear to be thickened, indicating the presence of edema or peritoneal fluid. A gentle barium enema will determine whether large bowel obstruction is present or not.

**D. Diagnostic Abdominal Tap:** Recovery of ascitic fluid for amylase and protein measurements, culture and cytologic examination may be useful.

### Differential Diagnosis

Peritonitis, which may present a highly variable clinical picture, must be differentiated from acute intestinal obstruction, acute cholecystitis with or without choledocholithiasis, pancreatitis, renal colic, gastrointestinal hemorrhage, lower lobe pneumonias, porphyria, periodic fever, hysteria, black widow spider bite, and central nervous system disorders (eg, tabes dorsalis).

### Complications

The most frequent sequela of peritonitis is abscess formation in the pelvis, in the subphrenic space, between the leaves of the mesentery, or elsewhere in the abdomen. Antibiotic therapy may mask or delay the appearance of localizing signs of abscess. When fever, leukocytosis, toxemia, or ileus fails to respond to the general measures outlined for the management of peritonitis, a collection of pus should be suspected. This will usually require surgical drainage. Liver abscess and pylephlebitis are rare complications. Adhesions may cause early or, more frequently, late intestinal obstruction.

### Treatment

The measures employed in peritonitis as outlined below are generally applicable as supportive therapy in most acute abdominal disorders. The objectives are (1) to control infection, (2) to minimize the effects of paralytic ileus, and (3) to correct fluid, electrolyte, and nutritional disorders.

**A. Specific Measures:** Operative procedures to close perforations, to remove sources of infection such as gangrenous bowel or an inflamed appendix, or to drain abscesses are frequently required. The cause of the peritonitis should always be identified and treated promptly.

**B. General Measures:** No matter what specific operative procedures are employed, their ultimate success will often depend upon the care with which the following general measures are performed:

1. Bed rest in the medium Fowler (semi-sitting) position is preferred.

2. Nasogastric suction is started as soon as peritonitis is suspected, to prevent gastrointestinal distention. Suction is continued until peristaltic activity returns and the patient begins passing flatus. A self-tending sump tube should be used, but it must be checked frequently for patency. In persistent paralytic ileus, the intestinal tract may be more adequately decompressed by means of a long intestinal tube (eg, Miller-Abbott), although passage of such a tube into the small bowel is frequently difficult because of poor intestinal motility. In rare cases, combined gastric and long intestinal tube suction may be necessary to relieve or prevent distention.

3. Give nothing by mouth. Oral intake can be resumed slowly after nasogastric suction is discontinued.

4. Fluid and electrolyte therapy and parenteral feeding are required.

5. Narcotics and sedatives should be used liberally to ensure comfort and rest.

6. Antibiotic therapy–Initial antibiotic therapy should be broad spectrum, eg, cephalothin, clindamycin-gentamicin. When cultures are available, antibiotics are chosen according to sensitivity studies.

7. Blood transfusions are used as needed to control anemia.

8. Septic shock, if it develops, requires intensive treatment.

### Prognosis

If the cause of peritonitis can be corrected, the infection, accompanying ileus, and metabolic derangement can usually be managed successfully.

Clark C, Terris R: Sclerosing peritonitis associated with metoprolol. *Lancet* 1983;**1**:937.

Crossley IR, Williams R: Spontaneous bacterial peritonitis. *Gut* 1985;**26**:325.

Kerr CM et al: Fungal peritonitis in patients on continuous ambulatory peritoneal dialysis. *Ann Intern Med* 1983;**99**:334.

Levy M: Intraperitoneal drainage. *Am J Surg* 1984;**147**:309.

### PERIODIC DISEASE
### (Benign Paroxysmal Peritonitis, Familial Mediterranean Fever, Periodic Fever, Recurrent Polyserositis)

Periodic disease is a heredofamilial disorder of unknown pathogenesis, probably metabolic, characterized by recurrent episodes of abdominal or chest pain, fever, and leukocytosis. It is usually restricted to people of Mediterranean ancestry, primarily Armenians, Sephardic Jews, and Arabs and to some extent people of Egypto-Arabic origin living in Turkey, Greece, and Italy. The disease suggests surgical peritonitis, but the acute attacks are recurrent, self-limited, and not fatal. Amyloidosis of the primary type occurs in some cases, and death may result from renal or cardiac failure. Acute episodes may be precipitated by emotional upsets, alcohol, or dietary indiscretion. Treatment is symptomatic and supportive. A low-fat diet may reduce the number and severity of attacks. Daily administration of colchicine, 0.6–1.8 mg, strikingly reduces the number of attacks.

Pras M et al: Variable incidence of Mediterranean fever among different ethnic groups. *Johns Hopkins Med J* 1982;**150**:22.

# REFERENCES

Berk JE et al (editors): *Bockus Gastroenterology*, 4th ed. 7 vols. Saunders, 1985.

Dooley CP et al: Double-contrast barium meal and upper gastrointestinal endoscopy. *Ann Intern Med* 1984;**101**:538.

Gastroenterology Committee, American College of Physicians: Gastroenterology: An annotated bibliography of recent literature. *Ann Intern Med* 1982;**97**:287.

Haaga J, Reich NE: *Computed Tomography of Abdominal Abnormalities*, 2nd ed. Mosby, 1983.

Kirsner JB, Shorter RG: *Inflammatory Bowel Disease*, 2nd ed. Lea & Febiger, 1980.

Laws JW (editor): Non-invasive radiology. *Clin Gastroenterol* 1984;**13**:1.

Lennard-Jones JE: Current concepts: Functional gastrointestinal disorders. *N Engl J Med* 1983;**308**:431.

Margulis AR, Burhenne HJ: *Alimentary Tract Roentgenology*, 3rd ed. Vols 1 and 2, 1983; Vol 3, 1979. Mosby.

Schiff L: *Diseases of the Liver*, 6th ed. Lippincott, 1987.

Sherlock S: *Diseases of the Liver and Biliary System*, 7th ed. Lippincott/Blackwell, 1985.

Silen W: *Cope's Early Diagnosis of the Acute Abdomen*, 15th ed. Oxford Univ Press, 1983.

Sleisenger MH, Fordtran JS (editors): *Gastrointestinal Disease: Pathophysiology, Diagnosis, Management*, 3rd ed. Saunders, 1983.

Spiro HM: *Clinical Gastroenterology*, 3rd ed. Macmillan, 1983.

Taylor KB, Thomas HC: Gastrointestinal and liver diseases. Pages 520–543 in: *Basic & Clinical Immunology*, 5th ed. Stites DP et al (editors). Lange, 1984.

Welch CE, Malt RA: Abdominal surgery. (3 parts.) *N Engl J Med* 1983;**308**:624, 685, 753.

# Breast

# 12

*Armando E. Giuliano, MD*

## CARCINOMA OF THE FEMALE BREAST

### Essentials of Diagnosis

- Higher incidence in women who have delayed child bearing, those with a family history of breast cancer, and those with a personal history of breast cancer or some types of mammary dysplasia.
- Early findings: Single, nontender, firm to hard mass with ill-defined margins; mammographic abnormalities and no palpable mass.
- Later findings: Skin or nipple retraction; axillary lymphadenopathy; breast enlargement, redness, edema, pain, fixation of mass to skin or chest wall.
- Late findings: Ulceration; supraclavicular lymphadenopathy; edema of arm; bone, lung, liver, brain, or other distant metastases.

### General Considerations

The breast is the most common site of cancer in women, and cancer of the breast has been the leading cause of death from cancer among women in the USA. However, in 1986, lung cancer will account for more deaths in women than breast cancer. The probability of developing breast cancer increases throughout life. The mean and the median age of women with breast cancer is 60–61 years.

There were about 120,000 new cases of breast cancer and about 38,000 deaths from this disease in women in the USA in 1985. At the present rate of incidence, one of every 11 American women will develop breast cancer during her lifetime. Women whose mothers or sisters had breast cancer are more likely to develop the disease than controls. Risk is increased in patients whose mothers' or sisters' breast cancers occurred before menopause or was bilateral, or was present in 2 or more first-degree relatives. However, there is no history of breast cancer among female relatives in over 90% of patients with breast cancer. Nulliparous women and women whose first full-term pregnancy was after age 35 have a slightly higher incidence of breast cancer than multiparous women. Late menarche and artificial menopause are associated with a lower incidence of breast cancer, whereas early menarche (under age 12) and late natural menopause (after age 50) are associated with a slight increase in risk of developing breast cancer as is increased use of alcohol. Mammary dysplasia (fibrocystic disease of the breast), when accompanied

by proliferative changes, papillomatosis, or atypical epithelial hyperplasia, is associated with an increased incidence of cancer. A woman who has had cancer in one breast is at increased risk of developing cancer in the opposite breast. Women with cancer of the uterine corpus have a breast cancer risk significantly higher than that of the general population, and women with breast cancer have a comparably increased endometrial cancer risk. In the USA, breast cancer is more common in whites than in nonwhites. The incidence of the disease among nonwhites (mostly blacks), however, is increasing, especially in younger women. In general, rates reported from developing countries are low, whereas rates are high in developed countries, with the notable exception of Japan. Some of the variability may be due to underreporting in the developing countries, but a real difference probably exists. Dietary factors, particularly increased fat content, may account for some differences in incidence. There is some evidence that administration of estrogens to postmenopausal women may result in a slightly increased risk of breast cancer, but only with higher, long-term doses of estrogens.

Women who are at greater than normal risk of developing breast cancer (Table 12–1) should be identified by their physicians, taught the techniques of breast self-examination, and followed carefully. Screening programs involving periodic physical examination and mammography of asymptomatic high-risk women increase the detection rate of breast cancer and may improve the survival rate. Unfortunately, most women who develop breast cancer do not have significant identifiable risk factors, and analysis of

**Table 12–1.** Factors associated with increased risk of breast cancer.[*]

| | |
|---|---|
| Race | White |
| Age | Older |
| Family history | Breast cancer in mother or sister (especially bilateral or premenopausal) |
| Previous medical history | Endometrial cancer<br>Some forms of mammary dysplasia<br>Cancer in other breast |
| Menstrual history | Early menarche (under age 12)<br>Late menopause (after age 50) |
| Pregnancy | Late first pregnancy |

[*] Normal lifetime risk in white women = 1 in 11.

epidemiologic data has failed to identify women who are not at significant risk and would not benefit from screening. Therefore, virtually all women over about age 35 could possibly benefit from screening, although the cost-benefit ratio of screening programs to society as a whole is unclear. New, less expensive screening techniques, such as single-view mammography and the use of mobile vans, are being investigated in an attempt to reduce the cost of widespread screenings.

Growth potential of tumor and resistance of host vary over a wide range from patient to patient and may be altered during the course of the disease. The doubling time of breast cancer cells ranges from several weeks in a rapidly growing lesion to nearly a year in a slowly growing one. Assuming that the rate of doubling is constant and that the neoplasm originates in one cell, a carcinoma with a doubling time of 100 days may not reach clinically detectable size (1 cm) for about 8 years. On the other hand, rapidly growing cancers have a much shorter preclinical course and a greater tendency to metastasize to regional nodes or more distant sites by the time a breast mass is discovered.

The relatively long preclinical growth phase and the tendency of breast cancers to metastasize have led many clinicians to believe that breast cancer is a systemic disease at the time of diagnosis. Although it may be true that breast cancer cells are released from the tumor prior to diagnosis, variations in the host-tumor relationship may prohibit the growth of disseminated disease in many patients. For this reason, a pessimistic attitude concerning the management of localized breast cancer is not warranted, and many patients can be cured with proper treatment.

## Staging

The extent of disease evident from physical findings and special preoperative studies is used to determine the clinical stage of the lesion. Histologic staging is performed after examination of the axillary specimen. The results of clinical staging are used in designing the treatment plan (Table 12–2). Both clinical and histologic staging are of prognostic significance.

## Clinical Findings

The patient with breast cancer usually presents with a lump in the breast. Clinical evaluation should include assessment of the local lesion and a search for evidence of metastases in regional nodes or distant sites. After the diagnosis of breast cancer has been confirmed by biopsy, additional studies are often needed to complete the search for distant metastases or an occult primary in the other breast. Then, before any decision is made about treatment, all the available clinical data are used to determine the extent or "stage" of the patient's disease.

**A. Symptoms:** When the history is taken, special note should be made of menarche, pregnancies, parity, artificial or natural menopause, date of last menstrual period, previous breast lesions, and a family history of breast cancer. Back or other bone pain

**Table 12–2.** Clinical and histologic staging of breast carcinoma and relation to survival.

| Clinical Staging (American Joint Committee) | 5-Year Survival (%) |
|---|---|
| **Stage I** | 85 |
| Tumor <2 cm in diameter | |
| Nodes, if present, not felt to contain metastases | |
| Without distant metastases | |
| **Stage II** | 66 |
| Tumor <5 cm in diameter | |
| Nodes, if palpable, not fixed | |
| Without distant metastases | |
| **Stage III** | 41 |
| Tumor >5 cm or— | |
| Tumor any size with invasion of skin or attached to chest wall | |
| Nodes in supraclavicular area | |
| Without distant metastases | |
| **Stage IV** | 10 |
| With distant metastases | |

| | Survival (%) | |
|---|---|---|
| **Histologic Staging** | 5 Years | 10 Years |
| All patients | 63 | 46 |
| Negative axillary lymph nodes | 78 | 65 |
| Positive axillary lymph nodes | 46 | 25 |
| 1–3 positive axillary lymph nodes | 62 | 38 |
| >4 positive axillary lymph nodes | 32 | 13 |

may be the result of osseous metastases. Systemic complaints or weight loss should raise the question of metastases, which may involve any organ but most frequently the bones, liver, and lungs. The more advanced the cancer in terms of size of primary, local invasion and extent of regional node involvement, the higher the incidence of metastatic spread to distant sites.

The presenting complaint in about 70% of patients with breast cancer is a lump (usually painless) in the breast (Table 12–3). About 90% of breast masses are discovered by the patient herself. Less frequent symptoms are breast pain; nipple discharge; erosion, retraction, enlargement, or itching of the nipple; and redness, generalized hardness, enlargement, or shrinking of the breast. Rarely, an axillary mass, swelling of the arm, or bone pain (from metastases)

**Table 12–3.** Initial symptoms of mammary carcinoma.*

| Symptom | Percentage of All Cases |
|---|---|
| Painless breast mass | 66 |
| Painful breast mass | 11 |
| Nipple discharge | 9 |
| Local edema | 4 |
| Nipple retraction | 3 |
| Nipple crusting | 2 |
| Miscellaneous symptoms | 5 |

* Adapted from report of initial symptoms in 774 patients treated for breast cancer at Ellis Fischel State Cancer Hospital, Columbia, Missouri. Reproduced, with permission, from Spratt JS Jr, Donegan WL: *Cancer of the Breast*. Saunders, 1967.

may be the first symptom. Thirty-five to 50% of women involved in organized screening programs have cancers detected by mammography only and not physical examination.

**B. Signs:** The relative frequency of carcinoma in various anatomic sites in the breast is shown in Fig 12–1.

Inspection of the breast is the first step in physical examination and should be carried out with the patient sitting, arms at sides and then overhead. Abnormal variations in breast size and contour, minimal nipple retraction, and slight edema, redness, or retraction of the skin can be identified. Asymmetry of the breasts and retraction or dimpling of the skin can often be accentuated by having the patient raise her arms overhead or press her hands on her hips in order to contract the pectoralis muscles. Axillary and supraclavicular areas should be thoroughly palpated for enlarged nodes with the patient sitting (Fig 12–2). Palpation of the breast for masses or other changes should be performed with the patient both seated and supine with the arm abducted (Fig 12–3).

Breast cancer usually consists of a nontender, firm or hard lump with poorly delineated margins (caused by local infiltration). Slight skin or nipple retraction is an important sign. Minimal asymmetry of the breast may be noted. Very small (1–2 mm) erosions of the nipple epithelium may be the only manifestation of Paget's carcinoma. Watery, serous, or bloody discharge from the nipple is an occasional early sign but is more often associated with benign disease.

A lesion smaller than 1 cm in diameter may be difficult or impossible for the examiner to feel and yet may be discovered by the patient. She should always be asked to demonstrate the location of the mass; if the physician fails to confirm the patient's

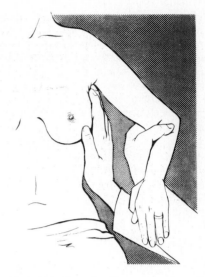

**Figure 12–2.** Palpation of axillary region for enlarged lymph nodes.

suspicions, the examination should be repeated in 1 month. During the premenstrual phase of the cycle, increased innocuous nodularity may suggest neoplasm or may obscure an underlying lesion. If there is any question regarding the nature of an abnormality under these circumstances, the patient should be asked to return after her period.

The following are characteristic of advanced carcinoma: edema, redness, nodularity, or ulceration of the skin; the presence of a large primary tumor; fixation to the chest wall; enlargement, shrinkage, or retraction of the breast; marked axillary lymphadenopathy; supraclavicular lymphadenopathy; edema of the ipsilateral arm; and distant metastases.

Metastases tend to involve regional lymph nodes, which may be clinically palpable. With regard to the axilla, one or 2 movable, nontender, not particu-

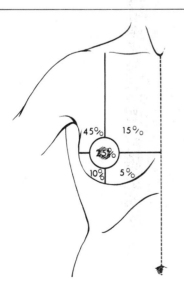

**Figure 12–1.** Frequency of breast carcinoma at various anatomic sites.

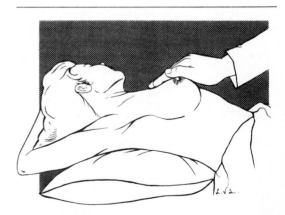

**Figure 12–3.** Palpation of breasts. Palpation is performed with the patient supine and arm abducted.

larly firm lymph nodes 5 mm or less in diameter are frequently present and are generally of no significance. Firm or hard nodes larger than 5 mm in diameter usually contain metastases. Axillary nodes that are matted or fixed to skin or deep structures indicate advanced disease (at least stage III). Histologic studies show that microscopic metastases are present in about 30% of patients with clinically negative nodes. On the other hand, if the examiner thinks that the axillary nodes are involved, this will prove on histologic section to be correct in about 85% of cases. The incidence of positive axillary nodes increases with the size of the primary tumor and with the local invasiveness of the neoplasm.

Usually no nodes are palpable in the supraclavicular fossa. Firm or hard nodes of any size in this location or just beneath the clavicle (infraclavicular nodes) are suggestive of metastatic cancer and should be biopsied. Ipsilateral supraclavicular or infraclavicular nodes containing cancer indicate that the patient is in an advanced stage of the disease (stage IV). Edema of the ipsilateral arm, commonly caused by metastatic infiltration of regional lymphatics, is also a sign of advanced (stage IV) cancer.

**C. Special Clinical Forms of Breast Carcinoma:**

**1. Paget's carcinoma**–The basic lesion is an infiltrating intraductal carcinoma, usually well differentiated and multicentric in the nipple and breast ducts. The nipple epithelium is infiltrated, but gross nipple changes are often minimal, and a tumor mass may not be palpable. The first symptom is often itching or burning of the nipple, with a superficial erosion or ulceration. The diagnosis is established by biopsy of the erosion.

Paget's carcinoma is not common (about 1% of all breast cancers), but it is important because it appears innocuous. It is frequently diagnosed and treated as dermatitis or bacterial infection, leading to unfortunate delay in detection. When the lesion consists of nipple changes only, the incidence of axillary metastases is about 5%, and the prognosis is excellent. When a breast tumor is also present, the incidence of axillary metastases rises, with an associated marked decrease in prospects for cure by surgical or other treatment.

**2. Inflammatory carcinoma**–This is the most malignant form of breast cancer and constitutes less than 3% of all cases. The clinical findings consist of a rapidly growing, sometimes painful mass that enlarges the breast. The overlying skin becomes erythematous, edematous, and warm. Often there is no distinct mass, since the tumor infiltrates the involved breast diffusely. The diagnosis should be made when the redness involves more than one-third of the skin over the breast and biopsy shows invasion of the subdermal lymphatics. The inflammatory changes, often mistaken for an infectious process, are caused by carcinomatous invasion of the dermal lymphatics, with resulting edema and hyperemia. If the physician suspects infection but the lesion does not respond rapidly (1–2 weeks) to antibiotics, a biopsy must be performed. Metastases tend to occur early and widely, and for this reason inflammatory carcinoma is rarely curable. Mastectomy is seldom, if ever, indicated. Radiation, hormone therapy, and anticancer chemotherapy are the measures most likely to be of value.

**3. Occurrence during pregnancy or lactation**–Only 1–2% of breast cancers occur during pregnancy or lactation. Breast cancer complicates approximately one in 3000 pregnancies. The diagnosis is frequently delayed, because physiologic changes in the breast may obscure the true nature of the lesion. This results in a tendency of both patients and physicians to misinterpret the findings and to procrastinate in deciding on biopsy. When the neoplasm is confined to the breast, the 5-year survival rate after mastectomy is about 70%. Axillary metastases are already present in 60–70% of patients, and for them the 5-year survival rate after mastectomy is only 30–40%. Pregnancy (or lactation) is not a contraindication to modified radical mastectomy, and treatment should be based on the stage of the disease as in the nonpregnant (or nonlactating) woman. Overall survival rates have improved as cancers are now diagnosed in pregnant women earlier than in the past.

**4. Bilateral breast cancer**–Clinically evident simultaneous bilateral breast cancer occurs in less than 1% of cases, but there is a 5–8% incidence of later occurrence of cancer in the second breast. Bilaterality occurs more often in women under age 50 and is more frequent when the tumor in the primary breast is of the lobular type. The incidence of second breast cancers increases directly with the length of time the patient is alive after her first cancer.

In patients with breast cancer, mammography should be performed before primary treatment and at regular intervals thereafter, to search for occult cancer in the opposite breast. Routine biopsy of the opposite breast is usually not warranted.

**D. Laboratory Findings:** A consistently elevated sedimentation rate may be the result of disseminated cancer. Liver or bone metastases may be associated with elevation of serum alkaline phosphatase. Hypercalcemia is an occasional important finding in advanced cancer of the breast. Carcinoembryonic antigen (CEA) may be used as a marker for recurrent breast cancer.

**E. Imaging:** Chest radiographs may show pulmonary metastases. CT scan of liver and brain is of value only when metastases are suspected in these areas. Bone scans utilizing technetium Tc 99m-labeled phosphates or phosphonates are more sensitive than skeletal x-rays in detecting metastatic breast cancer. Bone scanning has not proved to be of clinical value as a routine preoperative test in the absence of symptoms, physical findings, or abnormal alkaline phosphatase levels. The frequency of abnormal findings on bone scan parallels the status of the axillary lymph nodes on pathologic examination.

**F. Biopsy:** The diagnosis of breast cancer depends ultimately upon examination of tissue removed by biopsy. Treatment should never be undertaken without an unequivocal histologic diagnosis of cancer. The safest course is biopsy examination of all suspicious masses found on physical examination and, in the absence of a mass, of suspicious lesions demonstrated by mammography. About 30% of lesions thought to be definitely cancer prove on biopsy to be benign, and about 15% of lesions believed to be benign are found to be malignant. These findings demonstrate the fallibility of clinical judgment and the necessity for biopsy.

The simplest method is needle biopsy, either by aspiration of tumor cells (fine needle aspiration cytology) or by obtaining a small core of tissue with a Vim-Silverman or other special needle. A negative needle biopsy should be followed by open biopsy, because false-negative needle biopsies may occur in 15–20% of cancers.

The preferred method is open biopsy under local anesthesia as a separate procedure prior to deciding upon definitive treatment. The patient need not be admitted to the hospital. Decisions on additional workup for metastatic disease and on definitive therapy can be made and discussed with the patient after the histologic diagnosis of cancer has been established. This approach has the advantage of avoiding unnecessary hospitalization and diagnostic procedures in many patients, since cancer is found in the minority of patients who require biopsy for diagnosis of a breast lump. In addition, in situ cancers are not easily diagnosed cytologically.

As an alternative in patients for whom mastectomy is considered to be the treatment of choice in highly suspicious circumstances, the patient may be admitted directly to the hospital, where the diagnosis is made on frozen section of tissue obtained by open biopsy under general anesthesia. If the frozen section is positive, the surgeon could proceed immediately with mastectomy. This previously accepted one-step method should rarely be used today.

In general, the 2-step approach—that is, outpatient biopsy followed by definitive operation at a later date—is preferred in the diagnosis and treatment of breast cancer, because patients can be given time to adjust to the diagnosis of cancer, can carefully consider alternative forms of therapy, and can seek a second opinion should they feel it important. Studies have shown no adverse effect from the short (1–2 weeks) delay of the 2-step procedure, and this is the current recommendation of the National Cancer Institute.

At the time of the initial biopsy of breast cancer, it is important for the physician to preserve a portion of the specimen for determination of estrogen and progesterone receptors.

**G. Cytology:** Cytologic examination of nipple discharge or cyst fluid may be helpful on rare occasions. As a rule, mammography and breast biopsy are required when nipple discharge or cyst fluid is bloody or cytologically questionable.

**H. Mammography:** The 2 methods of mammography in common use are ordinary film radiography and xeroradiography. From the standpoint of diagnosing breast cancer, they give comparable results. It is now possible to perform a high-quality mammogram while delivering less than 1 rad to the mid breast.

Mammography is the only reliable means of detecting breast cancer before a mass can be palpated in the breast. Some breast cancers can be identified by mammography as long as 2 years before reaching a size detectable by palpation.

Although false-positive and false-negative results are occasionally obtained with mammography, the experienced radiologist can interpret mammograms correctly in about 90% of cases. Where mammography is employed proficiently, the yield of malignant lesions on biopsy remains around 35%. This is in spite of the fact that more biopsies are done.

Indications for mammography are as follows: (1) to evaluate each breast when a diagnosis of potentially curable breast cancer has been made, and at yearly intervals thereafter; (2) to evaluate a questionable or ill-defined breast mass or other suspicious change in the breast; (3) to search for an occult breast cancer in a woman with metastatic disease in axillary nodes or elsewhere from an unknown primary; (4) to screen women prior to cosmetic operations or prior to biopsy of a mass, to examine for an unsuspected cancer; and (5) to screen at regular intervals a selected group of women who are at high risk for developing breast cancer (see below).

Patients with a dominant or suspicious mass must undergo biopsy despite mammographic findings. The mammogram should be obtained prior to biopsy so that other suspicious areas can be noted and the contralateral breast can be checked. Mammography is never a substitute for biopsy, because it may not reveal clinical cancer in a very dense breast, as may be seen in young women with mammary dysplasia, and often does not reveal medullary type cancer. Breast ultrasonography can be used to differentiate a cystic from a solid mass.

### Early Detection

**A. Screening Programs:** A number of mass screening programs consisting of physical and mammographic examination of the breasts of asymptomatic women have been conducted. They are identifying more than 6 cancers per 1000 women. About 80% of these women have negative axillary lymph nodes at the time of surgery, whereas, by contrast, only 45% of patients found in the course of usual medical practice have uninvolved axillary nodes. Detecting breast cancer before it has spread to the axillary nodes greatly increases the chance of survival, and about 85% of such women will survive at least 5 years.

Both physical examination and mammography are necessary for maximum yield in screening programs, since about 40% of early breast cancers can be discovered only by mammography and another 40% can be detected only by palpation. Women 20–40 years of age should have a breast examination as part of routine medical care every 2–3 years. Women over age 40 should have yearly breast examinations.

The American College of Radiology and the American Cancer Society have recently revised their recommendations regarding use of mammography in asymptomatic women. A baseline mammogram should be performed on all women between ages 35 and 40 years. Women aged 40–49 years should have a mammogram every 1–2 years. Annual mammograms are indicated for women age 50 years or older. High-risk women—those whose mothers or sisters had bilateral or premenopausal breast cancer, those who have had cancer of one breast, and those with histologic abnormalities associated with subsequent cancer (eg, atypical epithelial hyperplasia, papillomatosis, lobular carcinoma in situ)—should have an annual mammogram and biannual examinations. The usefulness of screening mammography in young women without identifiable risk factors is not yet of proved value. However, in a recent large study of women under age 50, nearly half of all cancers were detected by mammography alone. Critics of screening question whether early detection actually improves survival sufficiently to justify its cost. Mammographic patterns are not a reliable predictor of the risk of developing breast cancer.

Other modalities of breast imagery have been investigated. Automated breast ultrasonography is very useful in distinguishing cystic from solid lesions but should be used only as a supplement to physical examination and mammography in screening for breast cancer. Diaphanography (transillumination of the breasts) and thermography are of no proved screening value.

**B. Self-Examination:** All women over age 20 should be advised to examine their breasts monthly. Premenopausal women should perform the examination 7–8 days after the menstrual period, and high-risk patients may be asked to perform a second examination in mid cycle. The breasts should be inspected initially while standing before a mirror with the hands at the sides, overhead, and pressed firmly on the hips to contract the pectoralis muscles. Masses, asymmetry of breasts, and slight dimpling of the skin may become apparent as a result of these maneuvers. Next, in a supine position, each breast should be carefully palpated with the fingers of the opposite hand. Physicians should instruct women in the technique of self-examination and advise them to report at once for medical evaluation if a mass or other abnormality is noted. Some women discover small breast lumps more readily when their skin is moist while bathing or showering. Most women do not practice self-examination, and its value is controversial. Clearly, however, it is not harmful and may be beneficial.

## Differential Diagnosis

The lesions most often to be considered in the differential diagnosis of breast cancer are the following, in order of frequency: mammary dysplasia (cystic disease of the breast), fibroadenoma, intraductal papilloma, and fat necrosis. The differential diagnosis of a breast lump should be established without delay by biopsy, by aspiration of a cyst, or by observing the patient until disappearance of the lump within a period of a few weeks.

## Pathologic Types

Numerous pathologic subtypes of breast cancer can be identified histologically (Table 12–4). These pathologic types are distinguished by the histologic appearance and growth pattern of the tumor. In general, breast cancer arises either from the epithelial lining of the large or intermediate-sized ducts (ductal) or from the epithelium of the terminal ducts of the lobules (lobular). The cancer may be invasive or in situ. Most breast cancers arise from the intermediate ducts and are invasive (invasive ductal, infiltrating ductal), and most histologic types are merely subtypes of invasive ductal cancer with unusual growth patterns (colloid, medullary, scirrhous, etc). Ductal carcinoma that has not invaded the extraductal tissue is intraductal or in situ ductal. Lobular carcinoma may be either invasive or in situ.

Except for the in situ cancers, the histologic subtypes have only a slight bearing on prognosis when outcomes are compared after accurate staging. Various histologic parameters, such as invasion of blood vessels, tumor differentiation, invasion of breast lymphatics, and tumor necrosis have been examined, but they too seem to have little prognostic value.

The noninvasive cancers by definition lack the ability to spread. However, in patients whose biopsies show noninvasive intraductal cancer, associated inva-

**Table 12–4.** Histologic types of breast cancer.

|  | Percent Occurrence |
|---|---|
| Infiltrating ductal (not otherwise specified) | 70–80 |
| Medullary | 5–8 |
| Colloid (mucinous) | 2–4 |
| Tubular | 1–2 |
| Papillary | 1–2 |
| Invasive lobular | 6–8 |
| Noninvasive | 4–6 |
| Intraductal | 2–3 |
| Lobular in situ | 2–3 |
| Rare cancers | <1 |
| Juvenile (secretory) | . . . |
| Adenoid cystic | . . . |
| Epidermoid | . . . |
| Sudiferous | . . . |

sive ductal cancers are present in about 1–3% of cases. Lobular carcinoma in situ is considered by some to be a premalignant lesion that by itself is not a true cancer. It lacks the ability to spread but is associated with the subsequent development of invasive cancer in at least 30% of cases.

## Hormone Receptor Sites

The presence or absence of estrogen and progesterone receptors in the cytoplasm of tumor cells is of paramount importance in managing patients with recurrent or metastatic disease. Up to 60% of patients with metastatic breast cancer will respond to hormonal manipulation if their tumors contain estrogen receptors. However, fewer than 10% of patients with metastatic, estrogen receptor–negative tumors can be successfully treated with hormonal manipulation.

Progesterone receptors may be an even more sensitive indicator than estrogen receptors of patients who may respond to hormonal manipulation. Up to 80% of patients with metastatic progesterone receptor–positive tumors seem to respond to hormonal manipulation. Receptors probably have no relationship to response to chemotherapy.

Some studies suggest that estrogen receptors are of prognostic significance. Patients whose primary tumors are receptor-positive have a more favorable course after mastectomy than those whose tumors are receptor-negative.

Receptor status is not only valuable for the management of metastatic disease but may help in the selection of patients for adjuvant therapy. Some studies suggest that hormonal therapy (tamoxifen) for patients with receptor-positive tumors treated by mastectomy may improve survival rates.

It is advisable to obtain an estrogen-receptor assay for every breast cancer at the time of initial diagnosis. Receptor status may change after hormonal therapy, radiotherapy, or chemotherapy. The specimen requires special handling, and the laboratory should be prepared to process the specimen correctly.

## Curative Treatment

Treatment may be curative or palliative. Curative treatment is advised for clinical stage I and II disease (see Table 12–2). Treatment can only be palliative for patients in stage IV and for previously treated patients who develop distant metastases or unresectable local recurrence.

**A. Therapeutic Options:** "Radical mastectomy involves en bloc removal of the breast, pectoral muscles, and axillary nodes and was the standard curative procedure for breast cancer from the turn of the century until about 10 years ago. Radical mastectomy removes the primary lesion and the axillary nodes with a wide margin of surrounding tissue, including the pectoral muscles. **Extended radical mastectomy** involves, in addition to standard radical mastectomy, removal of the internal mammary nodes. It has been recommended by a few surgeons for medially or centrally placed breast lesions and for tumors associated with positive axillary nodes, because of the known frequency of internal mammary node metastases under these circumstances. **Modified radical mastectomy** (total mastectomy plus axillary dissection) consists of en bloc removal of the breast with the underlying pectoralis major fascia (but not the muscle) and axillary lymph nodes. Some surgeons remove the pectoralis minor muscle. Others retract or transect the muscle to facilitate removal of the axillary lymph nodes. Modified radical mastectomy gives superior cosmetic and functional results compared with standard radical mastectomy. **Simple mastectomy** (total mastectomy) consists of removing the entire breast, leaving the axillary nodes intact. Limited procedures such as **segmental mastectomy** (lumpectomy, quadrant excision, partial mastectomy) are becoming more popular as definitive treatment. The proved efficacy of **irradiation** in sterilizing the primary lesion and the axillary and internal mammary nodes has made radiation therapy with segmental mastectomy a reasonable option for primary treatment of certain breast cancers.

**B. Choice of Primary Therapy:** The extent of disease and its biologic aggressiveness are the principal determinants of the outcome of primary therapy. Clinical and pathologic staging help in assessing extent of disease (Table 12–2), but each is to some extent imprecise. Since about two-thirds of patients eventually manifest distant disease regardless of the form of primary therapy, there is a tendency to think of breast carcinoma as being systemic in most patients at the time they first present for treatment.

There is a great deal of controversy regarding the optimal method of primary therapy of stage I, II, and III breast carcinoma, and opinions on this subject have changed considerably in the past decade. Legislation initiated in California and Massachusetts and now adopted in numerous states requires physicians to inform patients of alternative treatment methods in the management of breast cancer.

## Radical Mastectomy

For about three-quarters of a century, radical mastectomy was considered standard therapy for this disease. The procedure was designed to remove the primary lesion, the breast in which it arose, the underlying muscle, and, by dissection in continuity, the axillary lymph nodes that were thought to be the first site of spread beyond the breast. When radical mastectomy was introduced by Halsted, the average patient presented for treatment with advanced local disease (stage III), and a relatively extensive procedure was often necessary just to remove all gross cancer. This is no longer the case. Patients present now with much smaller, less locally advanced lesions. Most of the patients in Halsted's original series would now be considered incurable by surgery alone, since they had extensive involvement of the chest wall, skin, and supraclavicular regions.

Although radical mastectomy is extremely effective in controlling local disease, it has the disadvantage of being one of the most deforming of any of the available treatments for management of primary breast cancer. The surgeon and patient are both eager to find therapy that is less deforming but does not jeopardize the chance for cure. This operation is rarely performed now.

## Less Radical Surgery & Radiation Therapy

A number of clinical trials have been performed in the past decade in which the magnitude of the surgical procedure undertaken for removal of cancer in the breast and adjacent lymph nodes has been varied, with and without the use of local radiotherapy to the chest wall and node-bearing areas.

Radical mastectomy, modified radical mastectomy, and simple mastectomy have been compared in numerous clinical trials. In general, radical mastectomy has a slightly lower local recurrence rate than modified radical or simple mastectomy. Simple mastectomy has the highest regional recurrence rate, since the lymph nodes are not removed, and as many as 30% of patients with clinically negative nodes will have metastatic breast cancer within these nodes. At least half of these patients subsequently develop regional recurrences. Despite these differences in local and regional effect, no significant differences in survival have been consistently demonstrated among these 3 types of treatment. The addition of radiotherapy to mastectomy will also reduce the incidence of local recurrence, but in general, radiotherapy does not improve overall survival rates. Even the removal of occult cancer in axillary lymph nodes generally is not reflected in improvement in overall survival rates, although regional failures will be much lower.

The most significant recent advance in the management of primary breast cancer has been the realization that less than total mastectomy combined with radiotherapy may be as effective as more radical operations alone for certain patients with small primary tumors. Studies are still relatively recent, however, and long-term follow-up is necessary for definitive conclusions. Patients with large or stage III breast cancers may benefit from a combination of surgery, radiotherapy, and systemic chemotherapy.

Radiation therapy alone (without surgery) in the treatment of primary breast cancer fails to achieve local control in about 50% of cases. Small, nonrandomized studies have suggested that removal of the tumor by segmental mastectomy, or "lumpectomy" combined with postoperative irradiation, is as effective as mastectomy in achieving local control without diminishing long-term survival.

The results of the Milan trial and a large randomized trial conducted by the National Surgical Adjuvant Breast Project (NSABP) in the USA showed that disease-free survival rates were similar for patients treated by partial mastectomy plus axillary dissection followed by radiation therapy and for those treated by modified radical mastectomy (total mastectomy plus axillary dissection). All patients whose axillary nodes contained tumor received adjuvant chemotherapy.

In the NSABP trial, patients were randomized to 3 treatment types: (1) "lumpectomy" (removal of the tumor with *confirmed* tumor-free margins) plus whole breast irradiation, (2) lumpectomy alone, and (3) total mastectomy. All patients underwent axillary lymph node dissection. Some patients in this study had tumors as large as 4 cm with (or without) palpable axillary lymph nodes. Few local treatment failures were observed in any group. The lowest local recurrence rate was among patients treated with lumpectomy and postoperative irradiation; the highest was among patients treated with lumpectomy alone. However, no statistically significant differences were observed in overall or disease-free survival among the 3 treatment groups. This study shows that—at least in the early years postoperatively—lumpectomy and axillary dissection is as effective as modified radical mastectomy for the management of patients with stage I and stage II breast cancer. The high predicted local failure rate (nearly 30% at 5 years) for lumpectomy without radiation therapy makes this therapeutic alternative unacceptable in most cases.

In an earlier NSABP trial, patients were randomized to one of the following treatments: (1) radical mastectomy, (2) total mastectomy plus radiation therapy, and (3) total mastectomy followed by axillary dissection if clinically negative axillary nodes later became clinically positive. Among patients with clinically negative nodes, there were no differences in disease-free or overall survival rates with the 3 modes of treatment. Among those with clinically positive axillary nodes, there were no differences in outcome following radical mastectomy or total mastectomy plus radiation therapy.

The results of these and other trials have demonstrated that much less aggressive surgical treatment of the primary lesion than has previously been thought necessary gives equivalent results.

It is important to recognize that axillary dissection is valuable both in planning therapy and in staging of the cancer. Operation is extremely effective in preventing axillary recurrences. In addition, lymph nodes removed during the procedure can be pathologically assessed. This assessment is essential for the planning of adjuvant therapy, which is often recommended for patients with gross or occult involvement of axillary nodes.

## Current Recommendations

We believe that partial mastectomy plus axillary dissection and radiation therapy or total mastectomy plus axillary dissection (modified radical mastectomy) are the best initial treatments for most patients with potentially curable carcinoma of the breast. Premenopausal patients with involvement of axillary lymph nodes should receive adjuvant chemotherapy. Radical mastectomy may rarely if ever be required. Extended radical mastectomy would rarely be appropriate and could only be justified for patients with medial lesions and no signs of more distant spread.

Preoperatively, full discussion with the patient regarding the rationale for mastectomy and the manner of coping with the cosmetic and psychologic effects of the operation is essential. Patients often have questions about possible alternatives to standard or modified radical mastectomy—eg, local excision, simple mastectomy, and radiotherapy—and wish detailed explanations of the risks and benefits of the various procedures. Women with small tumors (< 4 cm) with or without axillary lymph node involvement should have the option of treatment by partial mastectomy (lumpectomy) plus axillary dissection and radiotherapy. Breast reconstruction should be discussed with the patient if this is a realistic possibility. Time spent preoperatively in educating the patient and her family is time well spent.

## Adjuvant Therapy

Chemotherapy is now being used as adjunctive treatment of patients with curable breast cancer and positive axillary nodes, since there is a great likelihood that these patients harbor occult metastases. Overall, about 75% of such patients eventually succumb within 10 years, even though the initial therapy, either surgery or irradiation, eradicated all neoplasm evident at that time. The objective of adjuvant chemotherapy is to eliminate the occult metastases responsible for late recurrences while they are microscopic and theoretically most vulnerable to anticancer agents.

Numerous clinical trials with various adjuvant chemotherapeutic regimens have been completed. The most extensive clinical experience to date is with the CMF regimen (cyclophosphamide, methotrexate, and fluorouracil). The regimen should be continued for 6 months in patients with axillary metastases. Follow-up studies at 8 years show that premenopausal women definitely benefit from receiving adjuvant chemotherapy, whereas postmenopausal women may not. The recurrence rate in premenopausal patients who received no adjuvant chemotherapy was more than 1½ times that of those who received therapy. No therapeutic effect with CMF has been shown in postmenopausal women, perhaps because therapy was modified so often in response to side effects that the total amount of drugs administered was less than planned. Other trials with different agents support the value of adjuvant chemotherapy; in some cases, postmenopausal women appear to benefit. Combinations of drugs are clearly superior to single drugs.

Adjuvant chemotherapy can be offered confidently to premenopausal women with metastases in axillary lymph nodes, but the use of adjuvant chemotherapy in postmenopausal women is more controversial. It is difficult to determine which regimen is appropriate for which subgroup of women with breast cancer. Some studies show a beneficial effect in premenopausal but not postmenopausal women, while other studies utilizing different combinations of agents show a beneficial effect in postmenopausal but not premeno-

pausal women. In addition, the estrogen receptor status of the tumor must be taken into consideration when chemotherapy is being planned. Some agents were shown to be effective in randomized studies, and others have been shown to be effective when compared to historical controls. In general, comparison with historical controls is less convincing proof of effect than are concurrent randomized prospective trials. For this reason, controversy remains regarding which agents are most beneficial for particular patients with breast cancer.

The addition of hormones may improve the results of adjuvant therapy. For example, tamoxifen has been shown to enhance the beneficial effects of melphalan and fluorouracil in women whose tumors are estrogen receptor-positive. Interestingly, in this study, improvement in disease-free survival rates was seen only in postmenopausal women. Tamoxifen has been used alone with some success as adjuvant treatment for postmenopausal women with estrogen receptor-positive tumors.

The length of time adjuvant therapy must be administered remains uncertain. Several studies suggest that shorter treatment periods may be as effective as longer ones. The Milan group has compared 6 versus 12 cycles of postoperative CMF and found 5-year disease-free survival rates to be comparable. One of the earliest adjuvant trials (Nissen-Meyer) used a 6-day perioperative regimen of intravenous cyclophosphamide alone; follow-up at 15 years shows a 15% improvement in disease-free survival rates for treated patients, suggesting that short-term therapy may be effective.

Patients with estrogen receptor-negative tumors, even without axillary lymph node involvement, may have a recurrence rate as high as 30% within the first 2 years after operation. For this reason, a number of clinical studies are investigating the value of adjuvant chemotherapy in women with estrogen receptor–negative tumors and no evidence of axillary lymph node involvement. Preliminary results suggest that these patients may benefit from adjuvant systemic chemotherapy; however, these studies are not yet conclusive, and we do not routinely employ adjuvant systemic therapy for patients without lymph node involvement.

A recent NIH Consensus Development Conference panel studied the results of adjuvant chemotherapy for breast cancer and concluded as follows: (1) Premenopausal women with positive nodes should be treated with adjuvant combination chemotherapy. (2) Premenopausal patients with negative nodes should not receive adjuvant chemotherapy—although certain high-risk patients (eg, those with estrogen receptor-negative tumors) could be considered for adjuvant chemotherapy. (3) Postmenopausal patients with positive nodes and positive hormone receptor tumors should receive adjuvant tamoxifen. (4) Postmenopausal women with positive nodes and negative hormone receptor tumors may be treated with adjuvant chemotherapy, but in general this practice is not recom-

**Table 12–5.** Summary of NIH Consensus Conference on adjuvant chemotherapy for premenopausal women.

| Nodal Involvement | Estrogen Receptors | Adjuvant Systemic Therapy |
|---|---|---|
| Yes | Positive | Combination chemotherapy |
| Yes | Negative | Combination chemotherapy |
| No | Positive | None |
| No | Negative | Perhaps; combination chemotherapy |

mended. (5) Postmenopausal women with negative nodes should not receive adjuvant chemotherapy regardless of the hormone receptor status of their tumors. (See Tables 12–5 and 12–6.)

Important questions remaining to be answered are the timing and duration of adjuvant chemotherapy; which chemotherapeutic agents should be applied for which subgroups of patients; how best to coordinate adjuvant chemotherapy with postoperative radiation therapy; the use of hormonal therapy; the use of combinations of hormonal and chemotherapy; and the value of adjuvant therapy for node-negative patients.

## Follow-Up Care

After primary therapy, patients with breast cancer should be followed for life for at least 2 reasons: to detect recurrences and to observe the opposite breast for a second primary carcinoma. Local and distant metastases occur most frequently within the first 3 years. During this period, the patient is examined every 3–4 months. Thereafter, examination is done every 6 months until 5 years postoperatively and then every 6–12 months. Special attention is given to the remaining breast, because of the increased risk of developing a second primary. The patient should examine her own breast monthly, and a mammogram should be obtained annually. In some cases, metastases are dormant for long periods and may appear up to 10–15 years or longer after removal of the primary tumor. Use of estrogen or progestational agents is probably inadvisable in patients free of disease after treatment of primary breast cancer, particularly those patients whose tumor was hormone receptor–positive. If topical estrogens are needed for senile

**Table 12–6.** Summary of NIH Consensus Conference on adjuvant chemotherapy for postmenopausal women.

| Nodal Involvement | Estrogen Receptors | Adjuvant Systemic Therapy |
|---|---|---|
| Yes | Positive | Tamoxifen |
| Yes | Negative | Perhaps; combination chemotherapy |
| No | Positive | None |
| No | Negative | None |

vaginitis or urinary incontinence, periodic use of a topical testosterone preparation will usually suffice.

**A. Local Recurrence:** The incidence of local recurrence correlates with tumor size, the presence and number of involved axillary nodes, the histologic type of tumor, and the presence of skin edema or skin and fascia fixation with the primary. About 15% of patients develop local recurrence after total mastectomy and axillary dissection. When the axillary nodes are not involved, the local recurrence rate is 5%, but the rate is as high as 25% when they are involved. A similar difference in local recurrence rate was noted between small and large tumors. Factors that affect the rate of local recurrence in patients who had partial mastectomies are not yet determined. However, early studies show that such things as multifocal cancer, in situ tumors, and positive resection margins are likely to be important.

Chest wall recurrences usually appear within the first 2 years, but may occur as late as 15 or more years after mastectomy. Suspect nodules should be biopsied. Local excision or localized radiotherapy may be feasible if an isolated nodule is present. If lesions are multiple or accompanied by evidence of regional involvement in the internal mammary or supraclavicular nodes, the disease is best managed by radiation treatment of the whole chest wall including the parasternal, supraclavicular, and axillary areas.

Local recurrence usually signals the presence of widespread disease and is an indication for bone and liver scans, posteroanterior and lateral chest x-rays, and other examinations as needed to search for evidence of metastases. When there is no evidence of metastases beyond the chest wall and regional nodes, radical irradiation for cure or complete local excision should be attempted. Most patients with locally recurrent tumor will develop distant metastases within 2 years. For this reason, many physicians use systemic therapy for treatment of patients with local recurrence. Although this seems reasonable, it should be pointed out that patients with local recurrence may be cured with local resection or radiation. Systemic chemotherapy or hormonal treatment should be used for patients who develop disseminated disease or those in whom local recurrence occurs following adequate local therapy.

**B. Edema of the Arm:** Significant edema of the arm occurs in 10–30% of patients after radical mastectomy and in about 5% after modified radical mastectomy. Edema of the arm is less frequent after modified radical mastectomy than after radical mastectomy and occurs more commonly if radiotherapy has been given or if there was postoperative infection. Early trials suggest that partial mastectomy with radiation to the axillary lymph nodes is followed by chronic edema of the arm in 10–20% of patients. To avoid this complication, many authorities advocate axillary lymph node sampling rather than complete axillary dissection. Judicious use of radiotherapy, with treatment fields carefully planned to spare the axilla as much as possible, can greatly diminish the incidence of edema. Since axillary dissection is a more accurate staging operation than axillary sampling, we recommend axillary dissection, with removal of at least level I and II lymph nodes, in combination with partial mastectomy.

Late or secondary edema of the arm may develop years after radical mastectomy, as a result of axillary recurrence or of infection in the hand or arm, with obliteration of lymphatic channels. There is usually no obvious cause of late arm swelling.

**C. Breast Reconstruction:** Breast reconstruction, with the implantation of a prosthesis, is usually feasible after standard or modified radical mastectomy. Reconstruction should probably be discussed with patients prior to mastectomy, because it offers an important psychologic focal point for recovery. However, most patients who are initially interested in reconstruction decide later that they no longer wish to undergo the procedure. Reconstruction is not an obstacle to the diagnosis of recurrent cancer.

**D. Risks of Pregnancy:** Data are insufficient to definitely determine whether interruption of pregnancy improves the prognosis of patients who are discovered during pregnancy to have potentially curable breast cancer and who receive definitive treatment. Theoretically, the increasingly high levels of estrogen produced by the placenta as the pregnancy progresses could be detrimental to the patient with occult metastases of hormone-sensitive breast cancer. Moreover, occult metastases are present in most patients with positive axillary nodes, and treatment by adjuvant chemotherapy would be potentially harmful to the fetus. Under these circumstances, interruption of early pregnancy seems reasonable, with progressively less rationale for the procedure as term approaches. Obviously, the decision must be highly individualized and will be affected by many factors, including the patient's desire to have the baby and the generally poor prognosis when axillary nodes are involved.

Equally problematic and important is the advice regarding future pregnancy (or abortion in case of pregnancy) to be given to women of child-bearing age who have had a mastectomy or other definitive treatment for breast cancer. Under these circumstances, one must assume that pregnancy will be harmful if occult metastases are present, although this has not been shown. Patients whose tumors are ER-negative probably would not be affected by pregnancy.

In patients with inoperable or metastatic cancer (stage IV disease), induced abortion is usually advisable, because of the possible adverse effects upon the fetus of hormonal treatment, radiotherapy, or chemotherapy.

## Prognosis

The stage of breast cancer is the single most reliable indicator of prognosis. Patients with disease localized to the breast and no evidence of regional spread after microscopic examination of the lymph nodes have by far the most favorable prognosis. Estrogen and progesterone receptors appear to be an important prognostic variable, because patients with hormone receptor–negative tumors and no evidence of metastases to the axillary lymph nodes have a much higher recurrence rate than do patients with hormone receptor–positive tumors and no regional metastases. The histologic subtype of breast cancer (eg, medullary, lobular, comedo) seems to have little, if any, significance in prognosis once these tumors are truly invasive.

As mentioned above, several different treatment regimens achieve approximately the same results when given to the appropriate patient. Localized disease can be controlled with local therapy—either surgery alone or limited surgery in combination with radiation therapy. However, the criteria for selection of patients to be treated with conservative resection and radiation therapy require further clarification.

Most patients who develop breast cancer will ultimately die of breast cancer. The mortality rate of breast cancer patients exceeds that of age-matched normal controls for nearly 20 years. Thereafter, the mortality rates are equal, although deaths that occur among the breast cancer patients are often directly the result of tumor. Five-year statistics do not accurately reflect the final outcome of therapy.

When cancer is localized to the breast, with no evidence of regional spread after pathologic examination, the clinical cure rate with most accepted methods of therapy is 75–90%. Exceptions to this may be related to the hormonal receptor content of the tumor, tumor size, host resistance, or associated illness. Patients with small estrogen and progesterone receptor–positive tumors and no evidence of axillary spread probably have a 5-year survival rate of nearly 90%. When the axillary lymph nodes are involved with tumor, the survival rate drops to 40–50% at 5 years and probably less than 25% at 10 years. In general, breast cancer appears to be somewhat more malignant in younger than older women, and this may be related to the fact that fewer younger women have estrogen receptor–positive tumors.

### General

Canellos GP, Hellman S, Veronesi U: The management of early breast cancer. *N Engl J Med* 1982;**306**:1430.

Council on Scientific Affairs, AMA: Early detection of breast cancer. *JAMA* 1984;**252**:3008.

Devitt JE: How breast cancer presents. *Can Med Assoc J* 1983;**129**:43.

Durand JC et al: Wide excision of the tumor, axillary dissection, and postoperative radiotherapy as treatment of small breast cancers. *Cancer* 1984;**53**:2439.

Fentiman IS, Rubens RD, Hayward JL: Control of pleural effusions in patients with breast cancers: A randomized trial. *Cancer* 1983;**52**:737.

Fisher B: Reappraisal of breast biopsy prompted by the use of lumpectomy. *JAMA* 1985;**253**:3585.

Fisher B: The revolution in breast cancer surgery: Science or anecdotalism? *World J Surg* 1985;**9**:655.

Fisher B, Wolmark N: Limited surgical management for primary breast cancer: A commentary on the NSABP reports. *World J Surg* 1985;**9**:682.

Fisher B et al: Five-year results of a randomized clinical

trial comparing total mastectomy and segmental mastectomy with or without radiation in the treatment of breast cancer. *N Engl J Med* 1985;**312**:665.

Fisher B et al: Relation of number of positive axillary nodes to the prognosis of patients with primary breast cancer: An NSABP update. *Cancer* 1983;**52**:1551.

Fisher B et al: Ten-year results of a randomized clinical trial comparing radical mastectomy and total mastectomy with or without radiation. *N Engl J Med* 1985;**312**:674.

Foster RS Jr, Costanza MC: Breast self-examination practices and breast cancer survival. *Cancer* 1984;**53**:999.

Greenberg ER et al: Breast cancer in mothers given diethylstilbestrol in pregnancy. *N Engl J Med* 1984;**311**:1393.

Hagelberg RS, Jolly PC, Anderson RP: Role of surgery in the treatment of inflammatory breast carcinoma. *Am J Surg* 1984;**148**:125.

Harris JR et al: Clinical-pathologic study of early breast cancer treated by primary radiation therapy. *J Clin Oncol* 1983;**1**:184.

Health and Public Policy Committee, American College of Physicians: The use of diagnostic tests for screening and evaluating breast lesions. *Ann Intern Med* 1985;**103**:143.

Israel L et al: Two years of high-dose cyclophosphamide and 5-fluorouracil followed by surgery after 3 months for acute inflammatory breast carcinomas. *Cancer* 1986;**57**:24.

Lagios MD et al: Paget's disease of the nipple: Alternative management in cases without or with minimal extent of underlying breast carcinoma. *Cancer* 1984;**54**:545.

Lipsztein R, Dalton JF, Bloomer WD: Sequelae of breast irradiation. *JAMA* 1985;**253**:3582.

Maddox WA et al: A randomized prospective trial of radical (Halsted) mastectomy versus modified radical mastectomy in 311 breast cancer patients. *Ann Surg* 1983; **198**:207.

Mansour EG et al: Tissue and plasma carcinoembryonic antigen in early breast cancer: A prognostic factor. *Cancer* 1983;**51**:1243.

Martinez A, Clarke D: Irradiation as an alternative to mastectomy for early breast cancer: An important consideration because of changes in laws. *West J Med* 1983;**138**:676.

Mushlin AI: Diagnostic decision: Diagnostic tests in breast cancer: Clinical strategies based on diagnostic probabilities. *Ann Intern Med* 1985;**103**:79.

O'Malley MS, Fletcher SW: Screening for breast cancer with breast self-examination. *JAMA* 1987;**257**:2197.

Pigott J et al: Metastases to the upper levels of the axillary nodes in carcinoma of the breast and its implications for nodal sampling procedures. *Surg Gynecol Obstet* 1984;**158**:255.

Seidman H, Stellman SD, Mushinski MH: A different perspective on breast cancer risk factors: Some implications of the nonattributable risks. *CA* 1982;**32**:301.

Skrabanek P: False premises and false promises of breast cancer screening. *Lancet* 1985;**2**:316.

Sunshine JA et al: Breast carcinoma in situ: A retrospective review of 112 cases with a minimum 10-year followup. *Am J Surg* 1985;**150**:44.

Veronesi R, Zucali R, Del Vecchio M: Conservative treatment of breast cancer with the QU.A.RT. technique. *World J Surg* 1985;**9**:676.

Willet WC: Moderate alcohol consumption and the risk of breast cancer. *New England J Med* 1987;**316**:1174.

## Mammography

Boyd NF et al: Mammographic signs as risk factors for breast cancer. *Br J Cancer* 1982;**45**:185.

Carlile T et al: Breast cancer prediction and the Wolfe classification of mammograms. *JAMA* 1985;**254**:1050.

Egan RL: Mammography: Current recommendations and their rationale. *Consultant* 1984;**28**:166.

Kopans DB, Meyer JE, Sadowsky N: Breast imaging. *N Engl J Med* 1984;**310**:960.

Lamas AM, Horwitz RI, Peck D: Usefulness of mammography in the diagnosis and management of breast disease in postmenopausal women. *JAMA* 1984;**252**:2999.

Mammography 1982: A statement of the American Cancer Society. *CA* 1982;**32**:226.

Mann BD et al: Delayed diagnosis of breast cancer as a result of negative mammogram. *Arch Surg* 1983; **118**:23.

Sickles EA et al: Mammography after needle aspiration of palpable breast masses. *Am J Surg* 1983;**145**:395.

## Hormone Receptors

Aamdal S et al: Estrogen receptors and long-term prognosis in breast cancer. *Cancer* 1984;**53**:2525.

Lesser ML et al: Estrogen and progesterone receptors in breast carcinoma: Correlations with epidemiology and pathology. *Cancer* 1981;**48**:299.

Manni A: Hormone receptors and breast cancer. *N Engl J Med* 1983;**309**:1383.

McCarty KS Jr et al: Relationship of age and menopausal status to estrogen receptor content in primary carcinoma of the breast. *Ann Surg* 1983;**197**:123.

Qazi R, Chuang JL, Drobyski W: Estrogen receptors and the patterns of relapse in breast cancer. *Arch Intern Med* 1984;**144**:2365.

Steroid receptors in breast cancer. *Cancer* 1980;**46** **(Suppl)**:2759. [Entire issue.]

## Adjuvant Chemotherapy

Bonadonna G, Valagussa P: Adjuvant systemic therapy for resectable breast cancer. *J Clin Oncol* 1985;**3**:259.

Bonadonna G, Valagussa P: Review: Adjuvant systemic therapy for breast cancer. *J Clin Oncol* 1985;**3**:259.

Cummings FJ et al: Adjuvant tamoxifen treatment of elderly women with stage II breast cancer: A double blind comparison with placebo. *Ann Intern Med* 1985;**103**: 324.

Fisher B et al: Influence of tumor estrogen and progesterone receptor levels on the response to tamoxifen and chemotherapy in primary breast cancer. *J Clin Oncol* 1983; **1**:227.

Henderson IC: Adjuvant chemotherapy of breast cancer: A promising experiment or standard practice. (Editorial.) *J Clin Oncol* 1985;**3**:140.

Ingle JN et al: Randomized trial of tamoxifen alone or combined with aminoglutethimide and hydrocortisone in women with metastatic breast cancer. *J Clin Oncol* 1986;**B4**:958.

National Institutes of Health Consensus Development Conference Statement: Adjuvant chemotherapy for breast cancer. Vol 5, No. 12, 1985.

Nissen-Meyer R: The Scandinavian clinical trials. *Experientia [Suppl]* 1982;**41**:571.

Planting AST et al: Tamoxifen therapy in premenopausal women with metastatic breast cancer. *Cancer Treatment Reports* 1985;**69**:363.

Rose C et al: Anti-estrogen treatment of postmenopausal breast cancer patients with high risk of recurrence: 72 months of life table analysis and steroid hormone receptor status. *World J Surg* 1985;**9**:765.

Tancini G et al: Adjuvant CMF in breast cancer: Comparative

5-year results of 12 versus 6 cycles. *J Clin Oncol* 1983;**1**:2.

Wolmark N, Fisher B: Adjuvant chemotherapy in stage II breast cancer: A brief overview of the NSABP clinical trials. *World J Surg* 1985;**9**:699.

## TREATMENT OF ADVANCED BREAST CANCER

This section covers palliative therapy of disseminated disease incurable by surgery (stage IV).

### Radiotherapy

Palliative radiotherapy may be advised for locally advanced cancers with distant metastases in order to control ulceration, pain, and other manifestations in the breast and regional nodes. Irradiation of the breast and chest wall and the axillary, internal mammary, and supraclavicular nodes should be undertaken in an attempt to cure locally advanced and inoperable lesions when there is no evidence of distant metastases. A small number of patients in this group are cured in spite of extensive breast and regional node involvement. Adjuvant chemotherapy should be considered for such patients.

Palliative irradiation is also of value in the treatment of certain bone or soft tissue metastases to control pain or avoid fracture. Radiotherapy is especially useful in the treatment of the isolated bony metastasis and chest wall recurrences.

### Hormone Therapy

Disseminated disease may respond to prolonged endocrine therapy such as administration of hormones; ablation of the ovaries, adrenals, or pituitary; or administration of drugs that block hormone receptor sites (eg, antiestrogens) or drugs that block the synthesis of hormones (eg, aminoglutethimide). Hormonal manipulation is usually more successful in postmenopausal women. If treatment is based on the presence of estrogen receptor protein in the primary tumor or metastases, however, the rate of response is nearly equal in premenopausal and postmenopausal women. A favorable response to hormonal manipulation occurs in about one-third of patients with metastatic breast cancer. Of those whose tumors contain estrogen receptors, the response is about 60% and perhaps as high as 80% for patients whose tumors contain progesterone receptors as well. Because only 5–10% of women whose tumors do not contain estrogen receptors respond, they should not receive hormonal therapy except in unusual circumstances.

Since the quality of life during a remission induced by endocrine manipulation is usually superior to a remission following cytotoxic chemotherapy, it is usually best to try endocrine manipulation first in cases where the estrogen receptor status of the tumor is unknown. However, if the estrogen receptor status is unknown but the disease is progressing rapidly or involves visceral organs, endocrine therapy is rarely successful, and introducing it may waste valuable time.

In general, only one type of systemic therapy should be given at a time, unless it is necessary to irradiate a destructive lesion of weight-bearing bone while the patient is on another regimen. The regimen should be changed only if the disease is clearly progressing but not if it appears to be stable. This is especially important for patients with destructive bone metastases, since minor changes in the status of these lesions are difficult to determine radiographically. A plan of therapy that would simultaneously minimize toxicity and maximize benefits is often best achieved by hormonal manipulation.

The choice of endocrine therapy depends on the menopausal status of the patient. Women within 1 year of their last menstrual period are considered to be premenopausal, while women whose menstruation ceased more than a year ago are postmenopausal. The initial choice of therapy is referred to as primary hormonal manipulation; subsequent endocrine treatment is called secondary or tertiary hormonal manipulation.

**A. The Premenopausal Patient:**

**1. Primary hormonal therapy**–Bilateral oophorectomy is usually the first choice for primary hormonal manipulation in premenopausal women. It can be achieved rapidly and safely by surgery or, if the patient is a poor operative risk, by irradiation to the ovaries. Ovarian radiation therapy should be avoided in otherwise healthy patients, however, because of the high rate of complications and longer time necessary to achieve results. Oophorectomy presumably works by eliminating estrogens, progestins, and androgens, which stimulate growth of the tumor. The average remission is about 12 months.

The potent antiestrogen tamoxifen has been tried as an alternative to oophorectomy in the premenopausal patient. In limited trials, the response rate to tamoxifen is similar to that of oophorectomy, leading some authorities to recommend tamoxifen as the primary hormonal treatment of metastatic breast cancer in premenopausal women with estrogen receptor–positive tumors. However, only a few premenopausal patients have received tamoxifen without prior oophorectomy, and the optimal dosage remains unclear. In a study in which 40–120 mg/d was given, serum levels of estrone and estradiol were markedly elevated, presumably due to an increased output of pituitary gonadotropins. Although 5 out of 11 women responded to tamoxifen, it appears that either escalating the drug dosage or oophorectomy plus tamoxifen may be necessary in premenopausal patients.

Tamoxifen may eventually become the preferred agent for primary hormonal manipulation in premenopausal women, but experience is presently insufficient to advocate tamoxifen in preference to oophorectomy. The operation is not associated with long-term endocrine dysfunction, as are adrenalectomy and hypophysectomy. Oophorectomy should not be abandoned yet. Randomized trials now being conducted comparing tamoxifen with oophorectomy should clarify this issue. In general, there appears to be no advantage to combining tamoxifen with other hormones simultaneously.

**2. Secondary or tertiary hormonal therapy**—Although patients who do not respond to oophorectomy should be treated with cytotoxic drugs, those who respond and then relapse may subsequently respond to another form of endocrine treatment. The initial choice for secondary endocrine manipulation has not been clearly defined. Adrenalectomy or hypophysectomy induces regression in approximately 30–50% of patients who have previously responded to oophorectomy.

Patients who respond initially to oophorectomy but subsequently relapse should receive tamoxifen. If this treatment fails, use of aminoglutethimide (Cytadren) should be considered. Aminoglutethimide is an inhibitor of adrenal hormone synthesis and, when combined with a corticosteroid, provides a therapeutically effective "medical adrenalectomy." Aminoglutethimide causes less morbidity and mortality than surgical adrenalectomy; can be discontinued once the patient improves; and is not associated with the many problems of postsurgical hypoadrenalism, so that patients who require chemotherapy are more easily managed.

**B. The Postmenopausal Patient:**

**1. Primary hormonal therapy**—Tamoxifen, 10 mg twice daily, is now the initial therapy of choice for postmenopausal women with metastatic breast cancer amenable to endocrine manipulation. It has fewer side effects than diethylstilbestrol, the former therapy of choice, and is just as effective. The main side effects of tamoxifen are nausea, vomiting, and skin rash. Rarely, it may induce hypercalcemia.

**2. Secondary or tertiary hormonal therapy**—Postmenopausal patients who do not respond to primary endocrine manipulation should be given cytotoxic drugs. Postmenopausal women who respond initially to tamoxifen but later manifest progressive disease could be given diethylstilbestrol. Some authorities use aminoglutethimide, but diethylstilbestrol is much easier to administer. Aminoglutethimide should be reserved for patients who respond initially to tamoxifen, progress, respond to diethylstilbestrol, and progress for a second time. An alternative treatment is use of progestins (eg, megestrol acetate). Androgens have many side effects and should rarely be used. In general, hypophysectomy or adrenalectomy is rarely necessary.

## Chemotherapy

Cytotoxic drugs should be considered for the treatment of metastatic breast cancer (1) if visceral metastases are present (especially brain or lymphangitic pulmonary); (2) if hormonal treatment is unsuccessful or the disease has progressed after an initial response to hormonal manipulation; or (3) if the tumor is estrogen receptor–negative. The most useful single chemotherapeutic agent to date is doxorubicin (Adriamycin), with a response rate of 40–50%. The remissions tend to be brief, and in general, experience with single-agent chemotherapy in patients with disseminated disease has not been encouraging.

Combination chemotherapy using multiple agents has proved to be more effective, with objectively observed favorable responses achieved in 60–80% of patients with stage IV disease. Various combinations of drugs have been used, and clinical trials are continuing in an effort to improve results and to reduce undesirable side effects. Doxorubicin and cyclophosphamide produced an objective response in 87% of 46 patients who had an adequate trial of therapy. Other chemotherapeutic regimens have consisted of various combinations of drugs, including cyclophosphamide, vincristine, methotrexate, and fluorouracil, with response rates ranging up to 60–70%. Prior adjuvant chemotherapy does not seem to alter response rates in patients who relapse. Few new drugs or combinations of drugs have been sufficiently effective in breast cancer to warrant wide acceptance.

## Malignant Pleural Effusion

This condition develops at some time in almost half of patients with breast cancer. When severe and persistent, the effusion is best controlled by closed tube drainage of the chest and intrapleural instillation of a sclerosing agent. An intercostal tube is inserted in a low interspace and placed on suction or water-seal drainage until as much fluid as possible has been removed, and 500 mg of tetracycline dissolved in 30 mL of saline is then injected into the pleural cavity through the tube, which is clamped for 6 hours. The patient's position is changed frequently to distribute the tetracycline within the pleural space. The tube is unclamped and continued on water-seal drainage until drainage has decreased to less than 60 mL in 24 hours. This will usually occur within 5–6 days if the sclerosing action of the tetracycline is effective in causing adherence of visceral to parietal pleura. Transient reaction to the tetracycline such as pleural pain or low-grade fever is treated symptomatically. Fluid reaccumulation is prevented in 50–75% of patients. The procedure may be repeated in a few weeks if fluid recurs. Tetracycline is preferable to various chemotherapeutic agents such as mechlorethamine and thiotepa that may cause bone marrow depression or nausea and vomiting.

Bitran JD et al: Response to secondary therapy in patients with adenocarcinoma of the breast previously treated with adjuvant chemotherapy. *Cancer* 1983;**51:**381.

Corle DK, Sears ME, Olson KB: Relationship of quantitative estrogen–receptor level and clinical response to cytotoxic chemotherapy in advanced breast cancer. *Cancer* 1984;**54:**1554.

Henderson IC: Chemotherapy of breast cancer: A general overview. *Cancer* 1983;**51:**2553.

Henderson IC: Less toxic treatment of advanced breast cancer. *N Engl J Med* 1981;**305:**575.

Hubay CA et al: Antiestrogen-cytotoxic chemotherapy and bacillus Calmette-Guérin vaccination in stage II breast cancer: Seventy-two-month follow-up. *Surgery* 1984;**96**:61.

Ingle JN: Integration of hormonal agents and chemotherapy for the treatment of women with advanced breast cancer. *Mayo Clin Proc* 1984;**59**:232.

Ingle JN et al: Randomized clinical trial of diethylstilbestrol versus tamoxifen in postmenopausal women with advanced breast cancer. *N Engl J Med* 1981;**304**:16.

Lipton A et al: A randomized trial of aminoglutethimide versus tamoxifen in metastatic breast cancer. *Cancer* 1982;**50**:2265.

Minton MJ et al: Corticosteroids for elderly patients with breast cancer. *Cancer* 1981;**48**:883.

Nemoto T et al: Tamoxifen (Nolvadex) versus adrenalectomy in metastatic breast cancer. *Cancer* 1984;**53**:1333.

Powles TJ et al: Failure of chemotherapy to prolong survival in a group of patients with metastatic breast cancer. *Lancet* 1980;**1**:580.

Powles TJ et al: Treatment of disseminated breast cancer with tamoxifen, aminoglutethimide, hydrocortisone, and danazol, used in combination or sequentially. *Lancet* 1984;**1**:1369.

Pritchard KI et al: Tamoxifen therapy in premenopausal patients with breast cancer. *Cancer Treat Rep* 1980;**64**:787.

Santen RJ et al: Aminoglutethimide as treatment of postmenopausal women with advanced breast carcinoma. *Ann Intern Med* 1982;**96**:94.

Santen RJ et al: A randomized trial comparing surgical adrenalectomy with aminoglutethimide plus hydrocortisone in women with advanced breast cancer. *N Engl J Med* 1981;**305**:545.

Schweitzer RJ: Oophorectomy/adrenalectomy. *Cancer* 1980; **46**:1061.

## CARCINOMA OF THE MALE BREAST

### Essentials of Diagnosis

- A painless lump beneath the areola in a man usually over 50 years of age.
- Nipple discharge, retraction, or ulceration may occur.

### General Considerations

Breast cancer in men is a rare disease; the incidence is only about 1% of that in women. The average age at occurrence is about 60—somewhat older than the commonest presenting age in women. The prognosis, even in stage I cases, is worse in men than in women. Blood-borne metastases are commonly present when the male patient appears for initial treatment. These metastases may be latent and may not become manifest for many years. As in women, hormonal influences are probably related to the development of male breast cancer. There is a high incidence of both breast cancer and gynecomastia in Bantu men, theoretically owing to failure of estrogen inactivation by a damaged liver associated with vitamin B deficiency.

### Clinical Findings

A painless lump, occasionally associated with nipple discharge, retraction, erosion, or ulceration, is the chief complaint. Examination usually shows a hard, ill-defined, nontender mass beneath the nipple or areola. Gynecomastia not uncommonly precedes or accompanies breast cancer in men. Nipple discharge is an uncommon presentation for breast cancer in men, as it is in women. However, nipple discharge in a man is an ominous finding associated with carcinoma in nearly 75% of cases.

Breast cancer staging is the same in men as in women. Gynecomastia and metastatic cancer from another site (eg, prostate) must be considered in the differential diagnosis of a breast lesion in a man. Biopsy settles the issue.

### Treatment

Treatment consists of modified radical mastectomy in operable patients, who should be chosen by the same criteria as women with the disease. Irradiation is the first step in treating localized metastases in the skin, lymph nodes, or skeleton that are causing symptoms.

Since breast cancer in men is frequently a disseminated disease, endocrine therapy is of considerable importance in its management. Castration in advanced breast cancer is the most successful palliative measure and more beneficial than the same procedure in women. Objective evidence of regression may be seen in 60–70% of men who are castrated—approximately twice the proportion in women. The average duration of tumor growth remission is about 30 months, and life is prolonged. Bone is the most frequent site of metastases from breast cancer in men (as in women), and castration relieves bone pain in most patients so treated. The longer the interval between mastectomy and recurrence, the longer the tumor growth remission following castration. As in women, there is no correlation between the histologic type of the tumor and the likelihood of remission following castration. In view of the marked benefits of castration in advanced disease, prophylactic castration has been suggested in stage II breast cancer in men, but there is no certainty that this approach is warranted, and this should probably not be done.

Bilateral adrenalectomy (or hypophysectomy) has been proposed as the procedure of choice when tumor has reactivated after castration. Aminoglutethimide therapy should replace adrenalectomy in men as it has in women. Corticosteroid therapy is considered by some to be efficacious but probably has no value when compared to major endocrine ablation.

Estrogen therapy—5 mg of diethylstilbestrol 3 times daily orally—may rarely be effective. Androgen therapy may exacerbate bone pain. Castration, bilateral adrenalectomy, and corticosteroids are the main lines of therapy for advanced breast cancer in men at present. Tamoxifen has been reported to be successful in several cases and is becoming increasingly popular and may replace castration as the initial therapy for metastatic disease. Chemotherapy should be administered for the same indications and using the same dose schedules as for women with metastatic disease.

Examination of the cancer for hormone receptor protein may in the future prove to be of value in predicting response to endocrine ablation. Adjuvant chemotherapy for the same indications as in breast cancer in women may be useful, but experience with this form of treatment is lacking at present.

## Prognosis

The prognosis of breast cancer is poorer in men than in women. The crude 5- and 10-year survival rates for clinical stage I breast cancer in men are about 58% and 38%, respectively. For clinical stage II disease, the 5- and 10-year survival rates are approximately 38% and 10%. The overall survival rates at 5 and 10 years are 36% and 17%.

Axelsson J, Andersson A: Cancer of the male breast. *World J Surg* 1983;**7**:281.

Kantarjian H et al: Hormonal therapy for metastatic male breast cancer. *Arch Intern Med* 1983;**143**:237.

Patel JK, Nemoto T, Dao TL: Metastatic breast cancer in males: Assessment of endocrine therapy. *Cancer* 1984;**53**:1344.

Yap HY et al: Chemotherapy for advanced male breast cancer. *JAMA* 1980;**243**:1739.

## MAMMARY DYSPLASIA
## (Fibrocystic Disease)

### Essentials of Diagnosis

- Painful, often multiple, usually bilateral masses in the breast.
- Rapid fluctuation in the size of the masses is common.
- Frequently, pain occurs or increases and size increases during premenstrual phase of cycle.
- Most common age is 30–50. Rare in postmenopausal women.

### General Considerations

This disorder, also known as fibrocystic disease or chronic cystic mastitis, is the most frequent lesion of the breast. It is common in women 30–50 years of age but rare in postmenopausal women; this suggests that it is related to ovarian activity. Estrogen hormone is considered a causative factor. The term "mammary dysplasia," or "fibrocystic disease," is imprecise and encompasses a wide variety of pathologic entities. These lesions are always associated with benign changes in the breast epithelium, some of which are found so commonly in normal breasts that they are probably variants of normal breast histology but have unfortunately been termed a "disease."

The microscopic findings of fibrocystic disease include cysts (gross and microscopic), papillomatosis, adenosis, fibrosis, and ductal epithelial hyperplasia. Although mammary dysplasia has been considered to increase the risk of subsequent breast cancer, it is probable that only the variants in which proliferation

of epithelial components is demonstrated represent true risk factors.

### Clinical Findings

Mammary dysplasia may produce an asymptomatic lump in the breast that is discovered by accident, but pain or tenderness often calls attention to the mass. There may be discharge from the nipple. In many cases, discomfort occurs or is increased during the premenstrual phase of the cycle, at which time the cysts tend to enlarge. Fluctuation in size and rapid appearance or disappearance of a breast tumor are common in cystic disease. Multiple or bilateral masses are common, and many patients will give a history of transient lump in the breast or cyclic breast pain.

### Differential Diagnosis

Pain, fluctuation in size, and multiplicity of lesions are the features most helpful in differentiation from carcinoma. However, if a dominant mass is present, the diagnosis of cancer should be assumed until disproved by biopsy. Final diagnosis often depends on biopsy. Mammography may be helpful, but the breast tissue in these young women is usually too radiodense to permit a worthwhile study. Sonography is useful in differentiating a cystic from a solid mass.

### Treatment

Because mammary dysplasia is frequently indistinguishable from carcinoma on the basis of clinical findings, it is advisable to perform biopsy examination of suspicious lesions, which is usually done under local anesthesia. Surgery should be conservative, since the primary objective is to exclude cancer. Simple mastectomy or extensive removal of breast tissue is rarely, if ever, indicated for mammary dysplasia.

When the diagnosis of mammary dysplasia has been established by previous biopsy or is practically certain, because the history is classic, aspiration of a discrete mass suggestive of a cyst is indicated. The patient is reexamined at intervals thereafter. If no fluid is obtained, or if fluid is bloody, if a mass persists after aspiration, or if at any time during follow-up a persistent lump is noted, biopsy should be performed.

Breast pain associated with generalized mammary dysplasia is best treated by avoiding trauma and by wearing (night and day) a brassiere that gives good support and protection. Hormone therapy is not advisable, because it does not cure the condition and has undesirable side effects. Recently, danazol, a synthetic androgen, has been used for patients with severe pain. This treatment suppresses pituitary gonadotropins and should be reserved for the unusual, severe case.

The role of caffeine consumption in the development and treatment of fibrocystic disease is controversial. Some studies suggest that eliminating caffeine from the diet is associated with improvement. Many patients are aware of these studies and report relief of symptoms after giving up coffee, tea, and chocolate. Similarly, many women find vitamin E helpful. However, these observations have been difficult to confirm.

### Prognosis

Exacerbations of pain, tenderness, and cyst formation may occur at any time until the menopause, when symptoms usually subside, except in patients receiving estrogens. The patient should be advised to examine her own breasts each month just after menstruation and to inform her physician if a mass appears. The risk of breast cancer in women with mammary dysplasia showing proliferative or atypical changes in the epithelium is higher than that of women in general. Follow-up examinations at regular intervals should therefore be arranged.

Dupont WD, Page DL: Risk factor for breast cancer in women with proliferative breast disease. *N Engl J Med* 1985; **312**:146.

Ernster VL et al: Effects of caffeine-free diet on benign breast disease: A randomized trial. *Surgery* 1982;**91**:263.

Humphrey LJ et al: Fibrocystic breast disease. *Contemp Surg* 1983;**23**:97.

Hutter RVP: Goodbye to "fibrocystic disease." (Editorial.) *N Engl J Med* 1985;**312**:179.

Minton JP et al: Response of fibrocystic disease to caffeine withdrawal and correlation of cyclic nucleotides with breast disease. *Am J Obstet Gynecol* 1979;**135**:157.

Wisbey JR et al: Natural history of breast pain. *Lancet* 1983;**2**:672.

## FIBROADENOMA OF THE BREAST

This common benign neoplasm occurs most frequently in young women, usually within 20 years after puberty. It is somewhat more frequent and tends to occur at an earlier age in black than in white women. Multiple tumors in one or both breasts are found in 10–15% of patients.

The typical fibroadenoma is a round, firm, discrete, relatively movable, nontender mass 1–5 cm in diameter. The tumor is usually discovered accidentally. Clinical diagnosis in young patients is generally not difficult. In women over 30, cystic disease of the breast and carcinoma of the breast must be considered. Cysts can be identified by aspiration. Fibroadenoma does not normally occur after the menopause, but postmenopausal women may occasionally develop fibroadenoma after administration of estrogenic hormone.

Treatment is by excision under local anesthesia as an outpatient procedure, with pathologic examination of the specimen.

**Cystosarcoma phyllodes** is a type of fibroadenoma with cellular stroma that tends to grow rapidly. This tumor may reach a large size and if inadequately excised will recur locally. The lesion is rarely malignant. Treatment is by local excision of the mass with a margin of surrounding breast tissue. The treatment

of malignant cystosarcoma phyllodes is more controversial. In general, complete removal of the tumor and a rim of normal tissue should avoid recurrence. Since these tumors tend to be large, simple mastectomy is often necessary to achieve complete control.

Briggs RM, Walters M, Rosenthal D: Cystosarcoma phyllodes in adolescent female patients. *Am J Surg* 1983;**146**:712.

Browder W, McQuitty JT, McDonald JC: Malignant cystosarcoma phyllodes: Treatment and prognosis. *Am J Surg* 1978;**136**:239.

Pietruszka M, Barnes L: Cystosarcoma phyllodes: A clinicopathologic analysis of 42 cases. *Cancer* 1978;**41**:1974.

## DIFFERENTIAL DIAGNOSIS OF NIPPLE DISCHARGE

In order of increasing frequency, the following are the commonest causes of nipple discharge in the nonlactating breast: carcinoma, intraductal papilloma, mammary dysplasia with ectasia of the ducts. The important characteristics of the discharge and some other factors to be evaluated by history and physical examination are as follows:

(1) Nature of discharge (serous, bloody, or other).

(2) Association with a mass or not.

(3) Unilateral or bilateral.

(4) Single duct or multiple duct discharge.

(5) Discharge is spontaneous (persistent or intermittent) or must be expressed.

(6) Discharge produced by pressure at a single site or by general pressure on the breast.

(7) Relation to menses.

(8) Premenopausal or postmenopausal.

(9) Patient taking contraceptive pills, or estrogen for postmenopausal symptoms.

Unilateral, spontaneous serous or serosanguineous discharge from a single duct is usually caused by an intraductal papilloma or, rarely, by an intraductal cancer. In either case, a mass may not be present. The involved duct may be identified by pressure at different sites around the nipple at the margin of the areola. Bloody discharge is more suggestive of cancer but is usually caused by a benign papilloma in the duct. Cytologic examination of the discharge should be accomplished and may identify malignant cells, but negative findings do not rule out cancer, which is more likely in women over age 50. In any case, the involved duct, and a mass if present, should be excised.

In premenopausal females, spontaneous multiple duct discharge, unilateral or bilateral, most marked just before menstruation, is often due to mammary dysplasia. Discharge may be green or brownish. Papillomatosis and ductal ectasia are usually seen on biopsy. If a mass is present, it should be removed.

Milky discharge from multiple ducts in the nonlactating breast may occur in certain syndromes (Chiari-Frommel syndrome, Argonz-Del Castillo [Forbes-Albright] syndrome), presumably as a result of increased secretion of pituitary prolactin. An endocrine workup may be indicated. Drugs of the chlorpromazine type and contraceptive pills may also cause milky discharge that ceases on discontinuance of the medication.

Oral contraceptive agents may cause clear, serous, or milky discharge from a single duct, but multiple duct discharge is more common. The discharge is more evident just before menstruation and disappears on stopping the medication. If it does not and is from a single duct, exploration should be considered.

Purulent discharge may originate in a subareolar abscess and require excision of the abscess and related lactiferous sinus.

When localization is not possible and no mass is palpable, the patient should be reexamined every week for 1 month. When unilateral discharge persists, even without definite localization or tumor, exploration must be considered. The alternative is careful follow-up at intervals of 1–3 months. Mammography should be done. Cytologic examination of nipple discharge for exfoliated cancer cells may be helpful in diagnosis.

Chronic unilateral nipple discharge, especially if bloody, is an indication for resection of the involved ducts.

Discharge from the nipple. (Editorial.) *Lancet* 1983;**2**:1405.

## FAT NECROSIS

Fat necrosis is a rare lesion of the breast but is of clinical importance, because it produces a mass, often accompanied by skin or nipple retraction, that is indistinguishable from carcinoma. Trauma is presumed to be the cause, although only about half of patients give a history of injury to the breast. Ecchymosis is occasionally seen near the tumor. Tenderness may or may not be present. If untreated, the mass associated with fat necrosis gradually disappears. As a rule, the safest course is to obtain a biopsy. The entire mass should be excised, primarily to rule out carcinoma. Fat necrosis is common after segmental resection and radiation therapy.

## BREAST ABSCESS

During nursing, an area of redness, tenderness, and induration not infrequently develops in the breast. In the early stages, the infection can often be reversed while continuing nursing with that breast and administering an antibiotic (see Puerperal Mastitis, p 495). If the lesion progresses to form a localized mass with local and systemic signs of infection, an abscess is present and should be drained, and nursing should be discontinued.

A subareolar abscess may develop (rarely) in young or middle-aged women who are not lactating. These infections tend to recur after incision and drainage unless the area is explored in a quiescent interval with excision of the involved lactiferous duct or ducts at the base of the nipple. Except for the subareolar type of abscess, infection in the breast is very rare unless the patient is lactating. Therefore, findings suggestive of abscess in the nonlactating breast require incision and biopsy of any indurated tissue.

## GYNECOMASTIA

Hypertrophy of the male breast may result from a variety of causes. Pubertal hypertrophy is very common during adolescence and is characterized by a tender discoid enlargement 2–3 cm in diameter beneath the areola with hypertrophy of the breast. The changes are usually bilateral and subside spontaneously within a year in the majority of cases.

Breast hypertrophy is common in men past the age of 65, particularly when there is associated weight gain.

Certain organic diseases may be associated with gynecomastia, eg, cirrhosis of the liver, hyperthyroidism, Addison's disease, testicular tumors, androgen insensitivity, hypogonadism, feminizing adrenal tumors, testicular tumors, and hepatomas. Gynecomastia may be observed in individuals who recover weight rapidly after prolonged illness or undernutrition.

Many drugs may cause gynecomastia, including estrogens, androgens, human chorionic gonadotropin, antihypertensive agents (reserpine, spironolactone, methyldopa), digitalis, cimetidine, isoniazid, phenothiazines, diazepam, tricyclic antidepressants, amphetamines, and antineoplastic drugs.

If there is uncertainty about the diagnosis of the breast lesion, especially when symptomatic or of recent onset, a biopsy should be done to rule out cancer. Otherwise, the treatment of gynecomastia is nonsurgical unless the patient insists on excision for cosmetic reasons or because of pain.

Bercovici JP et al: Hormonal profile of Leydig cell tumors with gynecomastia. *J Clin Endocrinol Metab* 1984;**59**:625.

Migeon CJ et al: A clinical syndrome of mild androgen insensitivity. *J Clin Endocrinol Metab* 1984;**59**:672.

Niewoehner CB, Nuttall FQ: Gynecomastia in a hospitalized male population. *Am J Med* 1984;**77**:633.

## REFERENCES

Bassett L: *Mammography, Thermography, and Ultrasound in Breast Cancer Detection.* Grune & Stratton, 1982.

Cooperman AM, Hermann RE (editors): Symposium on breast cancer. *Surg Clin North Am* 1984;**64**:1029. [Entire issue.]

Haagensen CD: *Diseases of the Breast,* 3rd ed. Saunders, 1985.

Haagensen CD, Bodian C, Haagensen DE Jr: *Breast Carcinoma: Risk and Detection.* Saunders, 1981.

Harris JR, Hellman S, Silen WP (editors): *Conservative Management of Breast Cancer.* Lippincott, 1983.

McDivitt RW: *The Breast.* Williams & Wilkins, 1984.

Najarian JS, Delaney JP (editors): *Advances in Breast and Endocrine Surgery.* Year Book, 1986.

# Gynecology & Obstetrics

# 13

*Alan J. Margolis, MD, & Sadja Greenwood, MD, MPH*

## GYNECOLOGY

### ABNORMAL PREMENOPAUSAL BLEEDING

**Normal menstrual bleeding** lasts an average of 4 days (range, 1–7 days), with a mean blood loss of 35 mL. Blood loss of over 80 mL per cycle is abnormal and frequently produces anemia. Excessive bleeding, often with the passage of clots, may occur at regular menstrual intervals **(menorrhagia)** or irregular intervals **(dysfunctional uterine bleeding).** When there are fewer than 21 days between the onset of bleeding episodes, the cycles are likely to be anovular. **Ovulation bleeding,** a single episode of spotting between regular menses, is quite common. Heavier or irregular intermenstrual bleeding warrants investigation.

### Clinical Findings

**A. Symptoms and Signs:** The diagnosis of the disorders underlying the bleeding usually depends upon (1) a careful description of the duration and amount of flow, related pain, and relationship to the last menstrual period (LMP); (2) a history of pertinent illnesses; (3) a history of all medications the patient has taken in the past month, so that possible inhibition of ovulation or endometrial stimulation can be assessed; and (4) a careful pelvic examination to look for pregnancy, uterine myomas, adnexal masses, infection, or evidence of endometriosis.

**B. Laboratory Studies:** Cervical smears should be obtained as needed for cytologic and culture studies. Blood studies should include measurements of hemoglobin, hematocrit, white blood cell count and differential, sedimentation rate, and platelet count. Urinalysis and measurement of blood sugar levels should be performed to rule out diabetes. A test for pregnancy and studies of thyroid function and blood clotting should be considered in the clinical evaluation. Tests for ovulation in cyclic menorrhagia include basal body temperature records, serum progesterone measured 1 week before the expected onset of menses, and analysis of an endometrial biopsy specimen for secretory activity.

**C. Imaging:** Pelvic ultrasound may be useful to diagnose intrauterine or ectopic pregnancy, subserous or intrauterine myomas, endometriosis, or adnexal masses that may be related to abnormal bleeding. Hysterosalpingography can outline endometrial polyps, submucous myomas, or uterine synechias. MRI can definitively diagnose submucous myomas and adenomyosis.

**D. Cervical Biopsy and Endometrial Curettage:** Biopsy, curettage, or aspiration of the endometrium and curettage of the endocervix are often necessary to diagnose the cause of bleeding. Polyps, tumors, and submucous myomas are commonly identified in this way. Obtain cultures for acid-fast bacilli if tuberculosis is suspected. If cancer of the cervix is a possibility, multiple quadrant biopsies (colposcopically directed if possible) and endocervical curettage are indicated as first steps.

**E. Hysteroscopy:** Hysteroscopy can visualize endometrial polyps, submucous myomas, and exophytic endometrial cancers. It is useful immediately before D&C.

### Treatment

**A. Emergency Measures:** For acute blood loss, employ the shock position and give sedation, intravenous fluids, and blood transfusions when necessary. Hemostasis may require surgical D&C. Definitive treatment depends on the underlying cause.

**B. Management of Dysfunctional Uterine Bleeding:** Premenopausal patients with abnormal uterine bleeding include those with early abortion, salpingitis, myomas, or pelvic neoplasms. The history, physical examination, and laboratory findings should identify such patients, who require definitive therapy depending upon the cause of the bleeding. A large group of patients without discernible causes of bleeding remains, most of whom have dysfunctional uterine bleeding.

Dysfunctional uterine bleeding is usually caused by overgrowth of endometrium due to estrogen stimulation without adequate progesterone to stabilize growth; this occurs in anovular cycles. Anovulation associated with high estrogen levels commonly occurs in teenagers, in women aged late 30s to late 40s, and in extremely obese women or those with polycystic ovaries. The use of synthetic estrogen without added progestin is another common cause. Prolonged low levels of unopposed estrogen can cause spotting; high levels can result in profuse or prolonged bleeding.

Such bleeding can usually be treated hormonally; progestins, which limit and stabilize endometrial growth, are generally effective. Routine D&C is usually not necessary. Medroxyprogesterone acetate, 10 mg/d, or norethindrone acetate, 5 mg/d, should be given for 10–14 days starting on day 15 of the cycle, following which withdrawal bleeding (so-called medical curettage) will occur. The treatment is repeated for several cycles; it can be reinstituted if amenorrhea or dysfunctional bleeding recurs. Alternatively in young women, oral contraceptives can be given 4 times daily for 5–7 days; after withdrawal bleeding occurs, pills are taken in the usual dosage for 3 cycles. In cases of intractable heavy bleeding, danazol in doses of 200 mg 4 times daily is sometimes used to create an atrophic endometrium. This drug generally stops bleeding and will allow the patient to build up her hemoglobin for a few months prior to definitive surgery.

If the abnormal bleeding is not controlled by hormonal treatment, a D&C is necessary to check for incomplete abortion, polyps, submucous myomas, or endometrial cancer. In women over age 40 with severe or persistent dysfunctional bleeding, a D&C or careful endometrial biopsy is generally indicated to rule out neoplasm before beginning hormonal therapy.

Endometrial ablation through the hysteroscope using laser photocoagulation is currently being tested; this technique is designed to reduce or prevent any future menstrual flow.

Use of iron supplements, investigation of clotting disorders, and evaluation of the causes of anovulation should be considered as appropriate.

Nonsteroidal anti-inflammatory drugs (ibuprofen, naproxen, mefenamic acid, etc) will often reduce blood loss in menorrhagia, even that associated with an IUD. Ibuprofen is now available without a prescription.

Prolonged use of a progestin, as in a minipill, in injectable contraceptives, or in the therapy of endometriosis, can also lead to intermittent bleeding, sometimes severe. In this instance, the endometrium is atrophic and fragile. If bleeding occurs, it should be treated with estrogen as follows: ethinyl estradiol, 20 μg, or conjugated estrogens, 1.25 mg/d for 7 days. In cases of heavy bleeding, intravenous conjugated estrogens, 25 mg every 4 hours for 3–4 doses, can be used, followed by oral estrogen for 1 week or a combination oral contraceptive. This will thicken the endometrium and control the bleeding.

It is useful for the patient and the physician to discuss stressful situations or life-styles that may contribute to anovulation and dysfunctional bleeding, such as prolonged emotional turmoil or excessive use of drugs or alcohol.

**C. Use of Thyroid Hormone:** Hypermenorrhea or metrorrhagia is often noted in hypothyroidism. Oligomenorrhea or amenorrhea accompanies hyperthyroidism if the periods are altered. Thyroid hormone will improve menstrual function if a deficiency in thyroid hormone production is the only problem. It should not be used for all patients with abnormal menstrual periods.

### Prognosis

In the absence of cancer, large tumors, and salpingitis, about 50% of patients with hypermenorrhea will resume normal menstrual periods after curettage alone. The prognosis is even better with the program of hormone therapy described above.

Loffer FD: Hysteroscopic endometrial ablation with the Nd:YAG laser using a nontouch technique. *Obstet Gynecol* 1987;**69:**679.

Mishell DR et al: Menorrhagia: A symposium. *J Reprod Med* 1984;**29:**763.

## POSTMENOPAUSAL VAGINAL BLEEDING

Vaginal bleeding that occurs 6 months or more following cessation of menstrual function should be investigated. The most common causes are endometrial hyperplasia or cancer, cervical cancer, and administration of estrogens in a noncyclic manner or without added progestin. Other causes include atrophic vaginitis, trauma, polyps, submucous myomas, trophic ulcers of the cervix associated with prolapse of the uterus, blood dyscrasias, and endogenous estrogen production by a feminizing ovarian tumor. Uterine bleeding is usually painless, but pain will be present if the cervix is stenotic, if bleeding is severe and rapid, or if infection or torsion or extrusion of a tumor is present. The patient may report a single episode of spotting or profuse bleeding for days or months.

### Diagnosis

The vulva and vagina should be carefully inspected for areas of bleeding, ulcers, or neoplasms. A cytologic smear of the cervix and vaginal pool should be taken; this may disclose exfoliated neoplastic cells. An unstained wet mount of vaginal fluid in saline and potassium hydroxide may reveal white blood cells, infective organisms, or free basal epithelial cells indicative of a low estrogen effect. Endocervical curettage and aspiration curettage of the endometrium should be performed next. These procedures often can be performed in the office with sedation and a paracervical block. A careful search for endometrial polyps should be made. The tissue obtained may reveal polyps, endometrial hyperplasia (with or without an atypical glandular pattern), or cancer.

### Treatment

Aspiration curettage (with polypectomy if indicated) will frequently be curative. If simple endometrial hyperplasia is found, give cyclic progestin therapy (medroxyprogesterone acetate, 10 mg/d, or norethindrone acetate, 5 mg/d) for 21 days of each month for 3 months. A repeat D&C can then be performed, and if tissues are normal and estrogen replacement therapy is reinstituted, a progestin should be prescribed (as above) for the last 10–14 days of each estrogen cycle, followed by 5 days with no hormone therapy, so that the uterine lining will be shed. If endometrial hyperplasia with atypical cells or carcinoma of the endometrium is found, hysterectomy is necessary.

Gambrell RD, Bagnell CA, Greenblatt RB: Role of estrogens and progesterone in the etiology and prevention of endometrial cancer: Review. *Am J Obstet Gynecol* 1983;**146**:696.

Gibbons WE et al: Biochemical and histologic effects of sequential estrogen/progestin therapy on the endometrium of postmenopausal women. *Am J Obstet Gynecol* 1986;**154**:456.

Grimes DA: Diagnostic dilation and curettage: A reappraisal. *Am J Obstet Gynecol* 1982;**142**:1.

## TOXIC SHOCK SYNDROME
### (See also Chapter 23.)

Toxic shock syndrome has occurred in menstruating women using tampons and occasionally in women with a retained vaginal foreign object (eg, contraceptive diaphragm or sponge), in postpartum or female postsurgical patients, in children, and in men with infected wounds. The disease is most common in women under age 30; it is possible that immunity may develop with older age. The disease may recur during subsequent menses. The probable cause is an exotoxin from certain strains of *Staphylococcus aureus* that enters the bloodstream through vaginal ulcerations produced by tampons or other foreign bodies.

### Clinical Findings & Treatment

Toxic shock syndrome is a severe multisystem illness with fever, hypotension, diffuse erythroderma, and later desquamation of the palms and soles. Intravenous fluids should be given immediately to maintain blood pressure and perfusion of vital organs. Tampons or other vaginal foreign bodies should be removed. Cultures should be made of tissues from focal lesions, tissues of all mucous membranes, and blood samples. A β-lactamase-resistant antibiotic (nafcillin or an appropriate cephalosporin) is used to prevent recurrence. Corticosteroids, renal dialysis, mechanical ventilation, and other intensive care treatments may be necessary.

### Prevention

Recommendations to women to reduce the risk of toxic shock syndrome include the following: (1) Avoid using tampons completely, or avoid using them continuously by alternating with menstrual pads. Avoid using tampons overnight. (2) If high fever, vomiting, diarrhea, or other symptoms develop during a menstrual period, stop using tampons. Seek immediate medical care. (3) Women who have had toxic shock syndrome should not use tampons. (4) A contraceptive diaphragm, cap, or sponge should not be left in the vagina for more than 12 hours. These devices should not be used during a menstrual period.

Tampons made with high-absorbency synthetic compounds (carboxymethylcellulose, polyester, polyacrylates, viscose rayon), which are believed to enhance the risk of toxic shock syndrome by encouraging the growth of *S aureus* and producing vaginal microulcerations. There has been a return to use of cotton or cotton and rayon fibers by tampon manufacturers in recent years in response to medical and consumer demands.

Lanes SF et al: Toxic shock syndrome, contraceptive methods, and vaginitis. *Am J Obstet Gynecol* 1986;**154**:989.

Wager GP: Toxic shock syndrome: A review. *Am J Obstet Gynecol* 1983;**146**:93.

## PREMENSTRUAL SYNDROME
### (Premenstrual Tension)

The premenstrual syndrome is a recurrent, variable cluster of troublesome, ill-defined symptoms and signs that develop during the 7–14 days before the onset of menses and subside when menstruation occurs. The syndrome affects about one-third of all premenopausal women, primarily those 25–40 years of age. In about 10% of these, the syndrome may be severe. Although not every woman experiences all the symptoms or signs at one time, many describe bloating, breast pain, ankle swelling, a sense of increased weight, skin disorders, irritability, aggressiveness, depression, inability to concentrate, libido change, lethargy, and food cravings. Depression may be the presenting symptom.

The pathogenesis of premenstrual syndrome is still uncertain. Theories include neuroendocrine changes and elevated or lowered levels of estrogen or progesterone. Suppression of ovarian function with GnRH has been shown to diminish all symptoms temporarily.

It is obvious that further investigation and well-controlled therapeutic studies of this heterogeneous syndrome will be necessary for rational treatment. Current treatment methods are mainly empiric. The physician should provide the best support possible for the patient's emotional and physical distress. This includes the following:

(1) Careful evaluation of the patient, with understanding, explanation, and reassurance, is of first importance.

(2) Advise the patient to keep a daily diary of all symptoms for 2–3 months, to help in evaluating the timing and characteristics of the syndrome. Psychotherapy may be important for some women or couples.

(3) Daily exercise and a diet emphasizing complex carbohydrates (whole grains, vegetables, and fruits) can be recommended. Foods high in sugar content and alcohol should be avoided to minimize reactive hypoglycemia. Salt intake should be restricted to re-

duce fluid retention. Use of caffeine should be minimized whenever tension and irritability predominate.

(4) A variety of vitamins and minerals in relatively high doses have been suggested for this syndrome, but none have proved useful in double-blind studies, and some have undesirable side effects. If a supplement is desired, use a single daily dose of a multivitamin-multimineral containing the RDA for these substances.

(5) Natural progesterone, 200–400 mg in vaginal or rectal suppositories daily for 10–14 days before the menstrual period, has been alleged to be of therapeutic value. These suppositories must be made up from natural progesterone powder by the pharmacist and are not widely available. Controlled studies have not validated the effectiveness of this treatment. Low-dose birth control pills may help some younger women by virtue of ovarian suppression.

Abplanalp JM: Psychologic components of the premenstrual syndrome: Evaluating the research and choosing the treatment. *J Reprod Med* 1983;**28**:517.

Keye WR, Hammond DC, Strong T: Medical and psychologic characteristics of women presenting with premenstrual symptoms. *Obstet Gynecol* 1986;**68**:634.

Rossignol AM: Caffeine-containing beverages and premenstrual syndrome in young women. *Am J Public Health* 1985;**75**:1335.

Woods NF, Most A, Dery GK: Prevalence of perimenstrual symptoms. *Am J Public Health* 1982;**72**:1257.

# DYSMENORRHEA

## 1. PRIMARY DYSMENORRHEA

Primary dysmenorrhea is menstrual pain associated with ovular cycles in the absence of pathologic findings. The pain usually begins within 1–2 years after the menarche and may become more severe with time. The frequency of cases increases up to age 20 and then decreases with age and markedly with parity. Thirty to 50% of women are affected at some time, and 5–10% have severe pain.

Primary dysmenorrhea is low, midline, wavelike, cramping pelvic pain often radiating to the back or upper thighs. Cramps may last for 1 or more days and may be associated with nausea, syncope, diarrhea, headache, and flushing. The pain is produced by uterine vasoconstriction, anoxia, and sustained contractions mediated by prostaglandins.

## Clinical Findings

The pelvic examination is normal between menses; examination during menses may produce more severe pain, but no pathologic findings are seen.

## Treatment

Nonsteroidal anti-inflammatory drugs (ibuprofen, mefenamic acid, naproxen) are generally helpful. Ibuprofen is now available without a prescription. Drugs should be given at the onset of bleeding to avoid inadvertent drug use during early pregnancy. Ovulation can be suppressed and dysmenorrhea usually prevented by oral contraceptives. Women with less severe dysmenorrhea often get relief with aspirin or acetaminophen. A high fluid intake and avoidance of exposure to extreme cold can be helpful. Acupuncture has been reported to be helpful by some investigators.

## 2. SECONDARY DYSMENORRHEA

Secondary dysmenorrhea is menstrual pain for which an organic cause exists. It usually begins well after menarche, sometimes even as late as the third or fourth decade of life.

## Clinical Findings

The history and physical examination commonly suggest endometriosis or pelvic inflammatory disease. Other causes may be submucous myoma, IUD use, cervical stenosis with obstruction, or blind uterine horn (rare).

## Diagnosis

Laparoscopy is often needed to differentiate endometriosis from pelvic inflammatory disease. Submucous myomas can be detected by passing a sound or curet over the uterine cavity during D&C or by hysterogram or hysteroscopy. Cervical stenosis may result from induced abortion, creating crampy pain at the time of expected menses with no blood flow; this is easily cured by passing a sound into the uterine cavity after administering a paracervical block.

## Treatment

**A. Specific Measures:** Periodic use of analgesics, including the nonsteroidal anti-inflammatory drugs given for primary dysmenorrhea, may be beneficial, and oral contraceptives may give relief, particularly in endometriosis and chronic salpingitis. Danazol is effective in the treatment of endometriosis (see p 458).

**B. Surgical Measures:** If disability is marked or prolonged, laparoscopy or exploratory laparotomy is usually warranted. Definitive surgery depends upon the degree of disability and the findings at operation.

Dawood MY: Dysmenorrhea. *J Reprod Med* 1985;**30**:154.

# VAGINITIS

Inflammation and infection of the vagina are common gynecologic problems, resulting from a variety of pathogens, allergic reactions to vaginal contraceptives or other products, or the friction of coitus. The normal vaginal pH is 4.5 or less, and *Lactobacillus* is the predominant organism. At the time of the midcycle estrogen surge, clear, elastic, mucoid secretions from the cervical os are often profuse. In the luteal phase and during pregnancy, vaginal secretions are thicker, white, and sometimes adherent to the vaginal walls. These normal secretions can be confused with vaginitis.

## Clinical Findings

When the patient complains of vaginal irritation, pain, or unusual discharge, a careful history should be taken, noting the onset of the menstrual period; recent sexual activity; use of contraceptives, tampons, or douches; and the presence of vaginal burning, pain, pruritus, or unusually profuse or malodorous discharge. The physical examination should include careful inspection of the vulva and speculum examination of the vagina and cervix. The cervix is cultured for gonococcus or *Chlamydia* if applicable (see pp 879 and 882). The vagina should be cultured for *S aureus* if toxic shock syndrome is suspected (see p 449) or for *Candida* if yeast forms are not demonstrated by wet mount but are strongly suspected. A specimen of vaginal discharge is examined under the microscope in a drop of saline solution to look for trichomonads, bacteria, white blood cells, and clue cells (stippled or granulated epithelial cells whose cell borders are obscured by bacteria; see Bacterial Vaginosis, below). Discharge from the vaginal walls should be inspected in a drop of 10–20% potassium hydroxide to search for *Candida*. The vaginal pH can be tested; it is frequently greater than 4.5 in infections due to trichomonads and anaerobic bacteria, including *Gardnerella*. A bimanual examination to look for evidence of pelvic infection should follow.

**A. Candida Albicans:** Pregnancy, diabetes, and use of broad-spectrum antibiotics or corticosteroids predispose to *Candida* infections. Heat, moisture, and occlusive clothing also contribute to the risk. Pruritus, vulvovaginal erythema, and a white curdlike discharge that is not malodorous are found. Microscopic examination with 10–20% potassium hydroxide reveals filaments and spores. Cultures with Nickerson's medium may be used if *Candida* is suspected but not demonstrated.

**B. Trichomonas Vaginalis:** This protozoan flagellate infects the vagina, Skene's ducts, and lower urinary tract in women and the lower genitourinary tract in men. It is transmitted through coitus. Pruritus and a malodorous discharge occur, along with diffuse vaginal redness with edematous papillae in severe cases. Motile organisms with flagella are seen by microscopic examination of a wet mount with saline solution. The organism can sometimes be found in a first-morning specimen of urine from an infected male.

**C. Bacterial Vaginosis:** (Formerly *Gardnerella, Haemophilus,* or bacterial vaginitis.) An overgrowth of *Gardnerella* and other anaerobes is often associated with increased malodorous discharge without obvious vulvitis or vaginitis. The discharge is grayish and sometimes frothy, with a pH of 5.0–5.5. An aminelike ''fishy'' odor is present if a drop

of discharge is alkalinized with 10–20% potassium hydroxide. On wet mount in saline, no trichomonads are found; epithelial cells are covered with bacteria to the extent that cell borders are obscured (clue cells).

**D. Atrophic Vaginitis:** In the absence of estrogen stimulation, the vulvar and vaginal tissues shrink, the vaginal walls become thin and dry, and rugal folds disappear. Tenderness and pruritus, with resulting dysuria and dyspareunia, may occur. Fissures and ulcerations of tissue with spotting or bleeding may result from coitus. The wet mount will reveal predominantly parabasal cells.

**E. Condylomata Acuminata (Genital Warts):** Warty growths on the vulva, perianal area, vaginal walls, or cervix are caused by the human papillomavirus. They are sexually transmitted. Pregnancy and immunosuppression favor growth. Cervical lesions may be visible only by colposcopy and are believed to be related to dysplasia and cervical cancer.

## Treatment

**A. Candida Albicans:** Treatment with butaconazole, clotrimazole, or miconazole nightly for 3–7 days is generally effective; nystatin suppositories, gentian violet solution (1–2%), or boric acid capsules (600 mg twice daily) have also been successful. In recurrent cases, prophylaxis may be attempted with use of these fungicides twice weekly or with oral nystatin, 500,000–1,000,000 units 3 times daily for 3 weeks. The sexual partner may be treated with fungicidal creams.

**B. Trichomonas Vaginalis:** Treatment of both partners simultaneously is necessary; metronidazole, 2 g for 1 day (8 tablets at once or 4 tablets in 2 doses) or 250 mg 3 times daily for 7 days, is usually used. In resistant cases, use 250 mg of metronidazole 3 times daily for 14 days, or 2 g daily for 5 days. Metronidazole should be avoided in the first trimester of pregnancy. Patients who refuse metronidazole (see p 899) may obtain relief with daily douches containing 4 tablespoons of vinegar and 4 drops of detergent shampoo in 1 quart of water. The male partner should use a condom during sexual intercourse. Clotrimazole vaginal cream is also said to be useful.

**C. Bacterial Vaginosis:** Treatment of both sexual partners with metronidazole, 500 mg twice daily for 7 days, is effective. However, the wisdom of using a potentially toxic drug for a mild condition that may disappear spontaneously is questionable. Either or both of the following treatments may be used alternatively: (1) ampicillin or amoxicillin, 500 mg 4 times a day for 7 days, or (2) douching with povidone-iodine solution (1 tablespoon per quart of water), vinegar (3–4 tablespoons per quart of water), or a milky suspension of yogurt to restore *Lactobacillus* levels, plus use of condoms by the sexual partner. The use of vaginal iodine solutions is not recommended in pregnancy.

**D. Atrophic Vaginitis:** Treatment consists of oral hormone replacement therapy or local applications of estrogen cream. Conjugated estrogen cream, one-eighth applicatorful (0.3 mg of conjugated estrogens), applied daily for 1 week and then every other day, will relieve most symptoms of dyspareunia with minimal systemic effects. Testosterone propionate cream 1% is helpful for individuals unable to use estrogen. For symptomatic relief, this treatment must be maintained indefinitely.

**E. Condylomata Acuminata:** Both partners should be treated for warts anywhere on their bodies. Treatment for small vulvar warts is with podophyllum resin 25% in tincture of benzoin (do not use during pregnancy or on bleeding lesions) or trichloroacetic acid, carefully applied to avoid the surrounding skin. Podophyllum resin must be washed off after 2–4 hours. Freezing with liquid nitrogen is also effective. Treatment of large warts (> 2 cm) and vaginal warts is with $CO_2$ laser or electrodesiccation and curettage of the base, following local or general anesthesia. Multiple vaginal warts may be treated with intravaginal applications of fluorouracil. Use one-half applicatorful of 5% fluorouracil cream nightly for 5 days. A tampon is inserted after cream insertion, and the introitus and vulva are further protected by application of zinc oxide ointment. In all cases, treat any other vaginal infections and sexually transmitted diseases.

Bump RC et al: The prevalence, six-month persistence, and predictive values of laboratory indicators of bacterial vaginosis (nonspecific vaginitis) in asymptomatic women. *Am J Obstet Gynecol* 1984;**150**:917.

Ferenczy A: Comparison of 5-fluorouracil and $CO_2$ laser for treatment of vaginal condylomata. *Obstet Gynecol* 1984;**64**:773.

Kaufman RH (editor): Vulvovaginal candidiasis: A symposium. *J Reprod Med* 1986;**31(Suppl 7)**:639.

Osborne NG, Grubin L, Pratson L: Vaginitis in sexually active women: Relationship to nine sexually transmitted organisms. *Am J Obstet Gynecol* 1982;**142**:962.

## CERVICITIS

Infection of the cervix must be distinguished from physiologic ectopy of columnar epithelium, which is common in young women. True cervicitis is characterized by a red edematous cervix with purulent, often blood-streaked discharge and tenderness on cervical motion. The infection may follow tears during delivery or abortion or may result from a sexually transmitted pathogen such as *Neisseria gonorrhoeae, Chlamydia,* or herpesvirus (which presents with vesicles and ulcers on the cervix during a primary herpetic infection).

The symptoms of cervicitis include leukorrhea, low back pain, dyspareunia, dysmenorrhea, dysuria, urinary frequency and urgency, and spotting or bleeding. Yellow mucopurulent endocervical secretions and the presence of 10 or more polymorphonuclear leukocytes per oil immersion field are suggestive of chlamydial infection.

Cultures should be taken from the cervical os, including cultures for *N gonorrhoeae* and *Chlamydia.*

Appropriate antibiotics should be given to the patient (and to her partner in cases of gonorrhea or chlamydial infection). See Chapter 23 for a more detailed discussion.

Brunham RC et al: Mucopurulent cervicitis: The ignored counterpart in women of urethritis in men. *N Engl J Med* 1984;**311**:1.

Paavonen J et al: Etiology of cervical inflammation. *Am J Obstet Gynecol* 1986;**154**:56.

## CYST & ABSCESS OF BARTHOLIN'S DUCT

Gonorrhea and other infections often involve Bartholin's duct, causing obstruction of the gland. Drainage of secretions is prevented, leading to pain, swelling, and abscess formation. The infections usually resolve and pain disappears, but stenosis of the duct outlet with distention often persists. Reinfection causes recurrent tenderness and further enlargement of the duct.

The principal symptoms are periodic painful swelling on either side of the introitus and dyspareunia. A fluctuant swelling 1–4 cm in diameter in the inferior portion of either labium minus is a sign of occlusion of Bartholin's duct. Tenderness is evidence of active infection.

Treat infections with broad-spectrum antibiotics and frequent warm soaks. If an abscess develops, aspiration or incision and drainage are the simplest forms of therapy, but the problem may recur. Marsupialization, incision and drainage with the insertion of an indwelling Word catheter, or laser treatment will establish a new duct opening. This can be done at the time of abscess formation or as an interval procedure.

Cheetham DR: Bartholin's cyst: Marsupialization or aspiration? *Am J Obstet Gynecol* 1985;**152**:569.

Davis GD: Management of Bartholin duct cysts with the carbon dioxide laser. *Obstet Gynecol* 1985;**65**:279.

## EFFECTS OF EXPOSURE TO DIETHYLSTILBESTROL IN UTERO

Between 1947 and 1971, diethylstilbestrol (DES) was widely used in the USA for diabetic women during pregnancy and to treat threatened abortion. It is estimated that 2–3 million fetuses were exposed. A relationship between fetal DES exposure and clear cell carcinoma of the vagina was later discovered, and a number of other related anomalies have since been noted. In one-third of all exposed women, there are changes in the vagina (adenosis, septa), cervix (deformities and hypoplasia of the vaginal portion of the cervix), or uterus (T-shaped cavity). In males exposed to DES in utero, testicular and epididymal abnormalities and an increase in oligospermia (although not carcinoma) have been reported.

At present, all exposed women are advised to have

an initial colposcopic examination to outline vaginal and cervical areas of abnormal epithelium, followed by cytologic examination of the vagina (all 4 quadrants of the upper half of the vagina) and cervix at 6-month intervals. Lugol's iodine stain of the vagina and cervix will also outline areas of metaplastic squamous epithelium.

Many women are not aware of having been exposed to DES. Therefore, in the age groups at risk, examiners should pay attention to structural changes of the vagina and cervix that may signal the possibility of DES exposure and indicate the need for follow-up.

The incidence of clear cell carcinoma is approximately one in 1000 exposed women, and the incidence of cervical intraepithelial neoplasia (dysplasia and carcinoma in situ) is also increased. DES daughters conceive with regularity but have an increased incidence of early abortion, ectopic pregnancy, and premature births. In addition, mothers treated with DES in pregnancy appear to have a small increase in the incidence of breast cancer, beginning 20 years after exposure.

Melnick S et al: Rates and risks of diethylstilbestrol-related clear-cell adenocarcinoma of the vagina and cervix. *New England J Med* 1987;**316**:514.

Report of the Recommendations of the 1985 DES Task Force of the US Department of Health and Human Services. *JAMA* 1986;**255**:1849.

Robboy SJ et al: Increased incidence of cervical and vaginal dysplasia in 3,980 diethylstilbestrol-exposed young women: Experience of the National Collaborative Diethylstilbestrol Adenosis Project. *JAMA* 1984;**252**:2979.

Stillman RJ: In utero exposure to diethylstilbestrol: Adverse effects on the reproductive tract and reproductive performance in male and female offspring. *Am J Obstet Gynecol* 1982;**142**:905.

## CERVICAL INTRAEPITHELIAL NEOPLASIA (CIN; Dysplasia of the Cervix)

The squamocolumnar junction of the uterine cervix represents an area of active squamous cell proliferation. In childhood, this junction is located on the exposed vaginal portion of the cervix. At puberty, because of hormonal influence and possibly because of changes in the vaginal pH, the squamous margin begins to encroach on the single-layered, mucus-secreting epithelium, creating an area of metaplasia (transformation zone). Factors associated with coitus (see Prevention, below) may lead to cellular abnormalities, which over a period of years can result in the development of squamous cell dysplasia or cancer. There are varying degrees of cervical intraepithelial dysplasia (Table 13–1), defined by the degree of cellular atypia; all types must be observed and treated if they persist or become more severe. At present, the malignant potential of a specific lesion cannot be predicted. Some lesions remain stable for long periods of time; some regress; and others advance.

**Table 13–1.** Classification systems for Papanicolaou smears.

| Classification | Dysplasia | Cervical Intraepithelial Neoplasia (CIN) |
|---|---|---|
| 1 | Benign | Benign |
| 2 | Benign with inflammation | Benign with inflammation |
| 3 | Mild dysplasia | CIN I |
| 3 | Moderate dysplasia | CIN II |
| 3 | Severe dysplasia | CIN III |
| 4 | Carcinoma in situ | CIN III |
| 5 | Invasive cancer | Invasive cancer |

### Clinical Findings

There are no specific signs or symptoms of cervical intraepithelial neoplasia. The diagnosis is made by cytologic screening of an asymptomatic population with no grossly visible cervical changes. All grossly abnormal cervical lesions should be biopsied.

### Diagnosis

**A. Cytologic Examination (Papanicolaou Smear):** All specimens can be spread on one slide and fixed. For optimal screening, specimens should be taken from the vaginal pool, the squamocolumnar junction, and the endocervical canal.

Cytologic reports from the laboratory may describe findings in one of several ways (see Table 13–1). Vaginal infection, cervicitis, and atrophy prevent adequate screening. Repeat smear is indicated after appropriate therapy.

**B. Colposcopy:** Viewing the cervix with 10–20 × magnification allows for assessment of the size and margins of an abnormal transformation zone and to see whether it extends into the endocervical canal. The application of 3% acetic acid dissolves mucus, and the acid's desiccating activity sharpens the contrast between normal and actively proliferating thickened squamous epithelium. Abnormal changes include white patches and vascular atypia, which indicate areas of greatest cellular activity. Paint the cervix with Lugol's solution (strong iodine solution [Schiller's test]). Normal squamous epithelium will take the stain; nonstaining squamous epithelum should be biopsied. (The single-layered, mucus-secreting endocervical tissue will not stain either but can readily be distinguished by its darker pink, shinier appearance.)

**C. Biopsy:** Colposcopically directed punch biopsy and endocervical curettage are office procedures. If colposcopic examination is not performed, the normal-appearing cervix shedding atypical cells can be evaluated by endocervical curettage and multiple punch biopsies of nonstaining squamous epithelium or tissue from each quadrant of the cervix.

Microscopic examination of biopsy specimens is a more exact way of diagnosing the degree of cellular atypia suggested by the cytologic examination. Endocervical curettage will confirm the presence of abnormalities in the endocervical canal. Data from both procedures are important in deciding on treatment.

## Prevention

Cervical dysplasia and cancer appear to be initiated by one or more sexually transmitted factors; human papillomavirus is currently suspected. Cervical cancer almost never occurs in virginal women; it is epidemiologically related to the number of sexual partners a woman has had and the number of other female partners a male partner has had. Use of the diaphragm or condom has been associated with a protective effect. Long-term oral contraceptive users develop more dysplasias and cancers of the cervix than users of other forms of birth control, and smokers are also more at risk. Preventive measures therefore include the following:

(1) Sexually active women should undergo regular cytologic screening to detect abnormalities.

(2) Women should limit the number of sexual partners.

(3) Use of a diaphragm by the woman or condom by the man will protect the cervix.

(4) Women should stop smoking.

(5) If a cytologic abnormality is found, the woman should stop using oral contraceptives or other contraceptive methods that leave the cervix exposed and should use a diaphragm or ask her male partner to use a condom.

(6) Prompt treatment of genital warts is advisable for men and women.

## Treatment

Treatment varies depending on the degree and extent of cervical intraepithelial neoplasia. Biopsies should always precede treatment.

**A. Cauterization or Cryosurgery:** The use of either hot cauterization or freezing (cryosurgery) is effective for noninvasive small visible lesions without endocervical extension.

**B. CO₂ Laser:** This well-controlled method minimizes tissue destruction. It is colposcopically directed and requires special training. It may be used with large visible lesions.

**C. Conization of the Cervix:** Conization allows for complete histopathologic assessment and generally results in excision of the lesion. It should be reserved for cases of severe dysplasia or cancer in situ (CIN III), particularly those with endocervical extension.

**D. Examination of Male Partners:** If the male partners of women with cervical dysplasia or cancer have genital warts, these should be removed. Thorough examination of men requires magnification with a hand lens or colposcope after application of 3% acetic acid.

**E. Follow-Up:** Because recurrence is possible, especially in the first 2 years after treatment, close follow-up is imperative. Repeat vaginal cytologic examinations at 6-month intervals. After 2 years, yearly examinations suffice.

Burk RD et al: Human papillomavirus infection of the cervix detected by cervicovaginal lavage and molecular hybridization: Correlation with biopsy results and Papanicolaou smear. *Am J Obstet Gynecol* 1986;**154**:982.

Sand PK et al: Evaluation of male consorts of women with genital human papilloma virus infection. *Obstet Gynecol* 1986;**68**:679.

## CARCINOMA OF THE UTERINE CERVIX

### Essentials of Diagnosis

- Abnormal uterine bleeding and vaginal discharge.
- Cervical lesion may be visible on inspection as a tumor or ulceration.
- Vaginal cytology usually positive; must be confirmed by biopsy.

### General Considerations

Cancer appears first in the intraepithelial layers (the preinvasive stage, or carcinoma in situ). Preinvasive cancer is a common diagnosis in women 25–40 years of age. Two to 10 years are required for carcinoma to penetrate the basement membrane and invade the tissues. After invasion, death usually occurs in 3–5 years in untreated or unresponsive patients.

### Clinical Findings

**A. Symptoms and Signs:** The most common signs are metrorrhagia, postcoital spotting, and cervical ulceration. Bloody or purulent, odorous, nonpruritic discharge appears after invasion. Bladder and rectal dysfunction or fistulas and pain are late symptoms. Anemia, anorexia, and weight loss are signs of advanced disease.

**B. Cervical Biopsy and Endocervical Curettage, or Cold Conization:** These procedures are necessary steps after a positive Papanicolaou smear to determine the extent and depth of invasion of the cancer. Even if the smear is positive, treatment is never justified until definitive diagnosis has been established through biopsy studies.

**C. "Staging," or Estimate of Gross Spread of Cancer of the Cervix:** The depth of penetration of the malignant cells beyond the basement membrane is a reliable clinical guide to the extent of primary cancer within the cervix and the likelihood of secondary to metastatic cancer. It is customary to stage cancers of the cervix under anesthesia as shown in Table 13–2. Further assessment may be carried out by abdominal and pelvic CT scanning or MRI.

### Complications

Metastases to regional lymph nodes occur with increasing frequency from stage I to stage IV. Paracervical extension occurs in all directions from the cervix. The ureters are often obstructed lateral to the cervix, causing hydroureter and hydronephrosis and consequently impaired kidney function. Almost two-thirds

**Table 13–2.** International classification of cancer of the cervix (1973).[*]

**Preinvasive carcinoma**

Stage 0      Carcinoma in situ, intraepithelial carcinoma.

**Invasive carcinoma**

Stage I      Carcinoma strictly confined to the cervix (extension to the corpus should be disregarded).

    Ia      Microinvasive carcinoma (early stromal invasion).

    Ib      All other cases of stage I. (Occult cancer should be labeled "occ.")

Stage II      Carcinoma extends beyond the cervix but has not extended onto the pelvic wall. The carcinoma involves the vagina, but not the lower third.

    IIa      No obvious parametrial involvement. The vagina has been invaded, but not the lower third.

    IIb      Obvious parametrial involvement.

Stage III      Carcinoma has extended onto the pelvic wall. On rectal examination, there is no cancer-free space between the tumor and the pelvic wall. The tumor involves the lower third of the vagina. All cases with hydronephrosis or nonfunctioning kidney.

    IIIa      No extension onto the pelvic wall. Vaginal involvement, but not the lower third.

    IIIb      Extension onto the pelvic wall and/or hydronephrosis or nonfunctioning kidney.

Stage IV      Carcinoma extended beyond the true pelvis or clinically involving the mucosa of the bladder or rectum. Do not allow a case of bullous edema as such to be allotted to stage IV.

    IVa      Spread of growth to adjacent organs (that is, rectum or bladder with positive biopsy from these organs).

    IVb      Spread of growth to distant organs.

[*] Approved by the International Federation of Gynecology and Obstetrics (FIGO). Adopted by American College of Obstetrics and Gynecology (1976).

of patients with carcinoma of the cervix die of uremia when ureteral obstruction is bilateral. Pain in the back and in the distribution of the lumbosacral plexus is often indicative of neurologic involvement. Gross edema of the legs may be indicative of vascular and lymphatic stasis due to tumor.

Pelvic infections may complicate cervical carcinoma. Vaginal fistulas to the rectum and urinary tract are severe late complications. Incontinence of urine and feces is a major late complication, particularly in debilitated individuals.

Hemorrhage is the cause of death in 10–20% of patients with extensive invasive carcinoma.

## Treatment

**A. Emergency Measures:** Vaginal hemorrhage originates from gross ulceration and cavitation in stage II–IV cervical carcinoma. Ligation and suturing of the cervix are usually not feasible, but ligation of the uterine or hypogastric arteries may be lifesaving when other measures fail. Styptics such as negatol (Negatan), Monsel's solution, or acetone are effective, although delayed sloughing may result in further bleeding. Wet vaginal packing is helpful. Irradiation usually controls bleeding.

**B. Specific Measures:**

**1. Noninvasive carcinoma (stage 0)**–In a woman over 40 with in situ carcinoma of the cervix, total hysterectomy is the surgical treatment of choice; rarely, irradiation may be used alternatively in women who are poor operative risks. In a younger woman who wishes to retain her uterus, conization of the cervix may be acceptable. This is a calculated risk and imposes the absolute necessity of cytologic examinations every 6 months for an indefinite time.

**2. Invasive carcinoma**–Irradiation is generally the best treatment for invasive squamous cell carcinoma or adenocarcinoma of the cervix. The objectives of irradiation are (1) the destruction of primary and secondary carcinoma within the pelvis and (2) the preservation of tissues not invaded. Gamma emissions derived from x-rays, $^{60}Co$, radium, the cyclotron, the linear accelerator, and comparable sources are employed. All stages of cancer may be treated by this method, and there are fewer medical contraindications to irradiation than to radical surgery. Selected stage I cases can be treated satisfactorily with radical surgical procedures by experienced pelvic surgeons.

## Prognosis

The overall 5-year arrest rate for squamous cell carcinoma or adenocarcinoma originating in the cervix is about 45% in the major clinics. Percentage arrest rates are inversely proportionate to the stage of cancer: stage 0, 99%; stage I, 77%; stage II, 65%; stage III, 25%; stage IV, about 5%.

Boyce J et al: Prognostic factors in stage I carcinoma of the cervix. *Gynecol Oncol* 1981;**12(2-Part 1)**:154.

Shingleton HM et al: Adenocarcinoma of the cervix. 1. Clinical evaluation and pathologic features. *Am J Obstet Gynecol* 1981;**139**:799.

## CARCINOMA OF THE ENDOMETRIUM (Corpus or Fundal Cancer)

Adenocarcinoma of the uterine corpus is the second most common cancer of the female genital tract. It occurs most often in women 50–70 years of age. Many patients with this problem will have taken unopposed estrogen in the past; their increased risk appears to persist for 10 or more years after stopping the drug. Obesity, nulliparity, diabetes, and polycystic ovaries with prolonged anovulation are also risk factors.

Abnormal bleeding is the presenting sign in 80% of cases. Pyometra or hematometra may be due to carcinoma of the endometrium. Pain occurs late in the disease, with metastases or infection.

Papanicolaou smears of the cervix occasionally show atypical endometrial cells but are an inconsistent diagnostic tool. Endocervical curettage and endometrial curettage or aspiration are the only reliable means of diagnosis. Adequate specimens of each can usually be obtained during an office procedure performed following local anesthesia (paracervical block) and sedation. General anesthesia may sometimes be necessary for a satisfactory examination and safe diagnostic procedure. Simultaneous hysteroscopy can be a valuable addition in order to find localized growth or polyps within the uterine cavity.

Pathologic assessment is important in identifying hyperplasias, which often can be treated with cyclic oral progestins.

### Prevention

Routine screening of all women by periodic pelvic examinations and cervical smears and prompt D&C for patients who report abnormal menstrual bleeding or postmenopausal uterine bleeding will reveal many incipient as well as clinical cases of endometrial cancer. Postmenopausal women taking estrogens or younger women with prolonged anovulation can be given oral progestins for 10 days at the end of each estrogen cycle in order to promote periodic shedding of the uterine lining; this has been associated with a decreased incidence of uterine adenocarcinoma.

### Staging

Examination under anesthesia, fractional D&C, chest x-ray, intravenous urography, cystoscopy, sigmoidoscopy, and MRI will help determine the extent of the disease and its appropriate treatment (Table 13–3).

### Treatment

Treatment consists of total hysterectomy and bilateral salpingo-oophorectomy. Preliminary external irradiation or intracavitary radium therapy is indicated if the cancer is poorly differentiated or if the uterus is definitely enlarged in the absence of myomas. If invasion deep into the myometrium has occurred or if sampled preaortic lymph nodes are positive for tumor, postoperative irradiation is indicated.

---

**Table 13–3.** Staging of endometrial adenocarcinoma.[*]

| |
|---|
| Stage I: The carcinoma is confined to the corpus. |
| Subdivision according to size of uterus: |
| Stage Ia: The uterine cavity sounds to 8 cm or less. |
| Stage Ib: The uterine cavity sounds to > 8 cm. |
| Subdivision according to histology: |
| $G_1$: Highly differentiated adenomatous carcinomas. |
| $G_2$: Differentiated adenomatous carcinomas with partly solid areas. |
| $G_3$: Predominantly solid or entirely undifferentiated carcinomas. |
| Stage II: The carcinoma has involved the corpus and the cervix. |
| Stage III: The carcinoma has extended outside the uterus but not outside the true pelvis. |
| Stage IV: The carcinoma has extended outside the true pelvis or has obviously involved the mucosa of the bladder or rectum. Bullous edema as such does not permit allotment of a case to stage IV. |

[*] Established by FIGO at the Sixth World Congress, 1970.

---

Palliation of advanced or metastatic endometrial adenocarcinoma may be accomplished with large doses of progestins, eg, medroxyprogesterone, 400 mg intramuscularly weekly, or megestrol acetate, 80–160 mg daily orally.

### Prognosis

With early diagnosis and treatment, the 5-year arrest rate is 80–85%.

Shapiro S et al: Risk of localized and widespread endometrial cancer in relation to recent and discontinued use of conjugated estrogens. *N Eng J Med* 1985;**313**:969.

## CERVICAL POLYPS

Cervical polyps commonly occur after the menarche and are occasionally noted in postmenopausal women. The cause is not known, but inflammation may play an etiologic role. The principal symptoms are discharge and abnormal vaginal bleeding. The polyps are visible in the cervical os on speculum examination.

Cervical polyps must be differentiated from polypoid neoplastic disease of the endometrium, small submucous pedunculated myomas, and endometrial polyps. Cervical polyps rarely contain malignant foci.

### Treatment

All cervical polyps should be removed; this can often be accomplished in the office by avulsion. All tissue recovered should be examined by a pathologist to rule out malignant change. If the cervix is soft, patulous, or definitely dilated and the polyp is large, surgical D&C is required (especially if the pedicle is not readily visible). Exploration of the cervical and uterine cavities with the polyp forceps and curet may reveal multiple polyps.

## MYOMA OF THE UTERUS
### (Fibroid Tumor, Fibromyoma)

### Essentials of Diagnosis

- Irregular enlargement of the uterus (may be asymptomatic).
- Heavy or irregular vaginal bleeding, dysmenorrhea.
- Acute and recurrent pelvic pain if the tumor becomes twisted on its pedicle or infarcted.
- Symptoms due to pressure on neighboring organs (large tumors).

### General Considerations

Myoma is the most common benign neoplasm of the female genital tract. It is a discrete, round, firm uterine tumor composed of smooth muscle and connective tissue. The most convenient classification is by anatomic location: (1) intramural, (2) submucous, (3) subserous, (4) intraligamentous, (5) parasitic (ie, deriving its blood supply from an organ to which it becomes attached), and (6) cervical. A submucous myoma may become pedunculated and descend through the cervix into the vagina.

## Clinical Findings

**A. Symptoms and Signs:** In nonpregnant women, myomas are frequently asymptomatic. However, they can cause urinary frequency, dysmenorrhea, heavy bleeding (often with anemia), or other complications due to the presence of an abdominal mass. Occasionally, degeneration occurs, causing intense pain. Infertility may be due to a myoma that obstructs the tubes or distorts the uterine cavity.

In pregnant women, myomas cause additional hazards: abortion, malpresentation, failure of engagement, premature labor, localized pain (from red degeneration or torsion), dystocia, ineffectual labor, and postpartum hemorrhage.

**B. Laboratory Findings:** Hemoglogin levels may be decreased as a result of blood loss, but in occasional cases polycythemia is present, presumably as a result of the production of erythropoietin by the myomas.

**C. Imaging:** Ultrasonography will confirm the presence of uterine myomas and can be used sequentially to monitor growth. When multiple subserous or pedunculated myomas are being followed, ultrasonography is important to exclude ovarian masses. MRI delineates intramural and submucous myomas very early. Hysterography or hysteroscopy can also confirm cervical or submucous myomas.

## Differential Diagnosis

Irregular myomatous enlargement of the uterus must be differentiated from the similar but symmetric enlargement that may occur with uterine pregnancy or adenomyosis. Subserous myomas must be distinguished from ovarian tumors. Malignant leiomyosarcoma is a very rare tumor; the average age at onset is 55 years.

## Treatment

**A. Emergency Measures:** Give blood transfusions if necessary. If the patient is markedly anemic as a result of long, heavy menstrual periods, preoperative treatment with depot medroxyprogesterone acetate or danazol will slow or stop bleeding, and medical treatment of anemia can be given prior to surgery. Emergency surgery is required for acute torsion of a pedunculated myoma. The only emergency indication for myomectomy during pregnancy is torsion; abortion is not an inevitable result.

**B. Specific Measures:**

**1. Nonpregnant women–**In women who are not pregnant, small asymptomatic myomas should be observed at 6-month intervals. Elective myomectomy can be done to preserve the uterus. Myomas do not urgently require surgery unless they cause significant pressure on the ureters, bladder, or bowel or severe bleeding leading to anemia or are undergoing

rapid growth. Cervical myomas larger than 3–4 cm in diameter or pedunculated myomas that protrude through the cervix must be removed.

GnRH analogs have been used to induce reversible hypogonadism, which occasionally reduces the size of myomas, suppresses further growth, and reduces surrounding vascularity. These effects are desirable before myomectomy or hysterectomy.

**2. Pregnant patients–**If the uterus is no larger than a 6-month pregnancy by the fourth month of gestation, an uncomplicated course may be anticipated. If the mass (especially a cervical tumor) is the size of a 5- or 6-month pregnancy by the second month, abortion will probably occur. If possible, defer myomectomy or hysterectomy until 6 months after delivery, at which time involution of the uterus and regression of the tumor will be complete.

**C. Surgical Measures:** The measures available for the treatment of myoma are myomectomy and total or subtotal abdominal or vaginal hysterectomy. Myomectomy is the treatment of choice during the childbearing years. The ovaries should be preserved if possible in women under age 50.

## Prognosis

Surgical therapy is curative. Future pregnancies are not endangered by myomectomy, although cesarean delivery may be necessary after wide dissection with entry into the uterine cavity. Careful hysterectomy with retention of normal ovaries does not hasten menopause.

Maheux R et al: Luteinizing hormone-releasing hormone agonist and uterine leiomyoma: A pilot study. *Am J Obstet Gynecol* 1985;**152:**1034.

## CARCINOMA OF THE VULVA

### Essentials of Diagnosis

- Occurs most often in the postmenopausal age group.
- History of prolonged vulvar irritation, with pruritus, local discomfort, or slight bloody discharge.
- Early lesions may suggest or include chronic vulvitis.
- Late lesions appear as a mass, an exophytic growth, or a firm, ulcerated area in the vulva.
- Biopsy is necessary to make the diagnosis.

### General Considerations

While cancer of the vulva is a disorder of unknown cause, numerous predisposing or contributing factors are recognized, such as chronic granulomatous disorders. The vast majority are squamous carcinomas. More than 50% of patients with this disorder are over age 50 years; the average age is 65 years.

### Differential Diagnosis

Biopsy is essential for the diagnosis of vulvar cancer and should be performed with any localized atypical vulvar lesion, including white patches. Multiple skin-punch specimens can be taken in the office under local anesthesia, with care to include tissue from the edges of each lesion sampled.

Benign vulvar disorders that must be excluded in the diagnosis of carcinoma of the vulva include chronic granulomatous lesions (eg, lymphogranuloma venereum, syphilis), vulvar nodulations, condylomas, hidradenoma, or neurofibroma. Kraurosis, lichen sclerosis et atrophicus, or other associated leukoplakic changes in the skin should be biopsied but usually are not malignant.

## Treatment

**A. General Measures:** Early diagnosis and treatment of irritative or other predisposing or contributing causes to carcinoma of the vulva should be pursued. Remove prominent or enlarging pigmented moles of the vulva before they become malignant.

**B. Surgical Measures:**

1. In situ squamous cell carcinoma of the vulva and small, invasive basal cell carcinoma of the vulva should be excised with a wide margin. If the squamous carcinoma in situ is extensive or multicentric, laser therapy or superficial removal of vulvar skin may be required. In this way, the clitoris and uninvolved portions of the vulva may be spared. Skin grafting is possible, and mutilating vulvectomy is avoided.

2. Invasive carcinoma confined to the vulva without evidence of spread to adjacent organs or to the regional lymph nodes will necessitate radical vulvectomy and inguinal lymphadenectomy if the patient is able to withstand surgery. Debilitated patients may be candidates for palliative irradiation only.

## Prognosis

Patients with vulvar carcinoma 3 cm in diameter or less without inguinal lymph node metastases who can sustain radical surgery have about a 90% chance of a 5-year arrest of the cancer. If the lesion is greater than 3 cm and has metastasized, the likelihood of 5-year survival is less than 25%.

Morley GW: Cancer of the vulva: A review. *Cancer* 1981;**48(2 Suppl)**:597.

## ENDOMETRIOSIS

Aberrant growth of endometrium outside the uterus, particularly in the dependent parts of the pelvis and in the ovaries, is a common cause of abnormal bleeding and secondary dysmenorrhea. This condition is known as endometriosis. Depending on the location of the endometrial implants, infertility, dyspareunia, or rectal pain with bleeding may result. Aching pain tends to be constant, beginning 2–7 days before the onset of menses to become increasingly severe until flow slackens. Pelvic examination may disclose tender indurated nodules in the cul-de-sac, especially if the examination is done at the onset of menstruation.

Endometriosis must be distinguished from pelvic inflammatory disease, ovarian neoplasms, and uterine myomas. In general, only in salpingitis and endometriosis are the symptoms aggravated by menstruation. Bowel invasion by endometrial tissue may produce clinical findings, including blood in the stool, that must be distinguished from bowel neoplasm. Differentiation in these instances depends upon proctosigmoidoscopy and biopsy.

The clinical diagnosis of endometriosis is presumptive and must be confirmed by laparoscopy or laparotomy. Ultrasound examination will often reveal complex fluid-filled masses that cannot be distinguished from neoplasms. Barium enema may delineate colonic involvement of endometriosis.

## Treatment

**A. Medical Treatment:** The goal of medical treatment is to preserve the fertility of women wanting future pregnancies, ameliorate symptoms, and simplify future surgery or make it unnecessary. Medications are designed to inhibit ovulation over 6–9 months and lower hormone levels, thus preventing cyclic stimulation of endometriotic implants and decreasing their size.

1. Danazol (Danocrine), 200–400 mg twice daily for 6–9 months, in the lowest dose necessary to suppress menstruation, is the current treatment of choice.

2. Combination estrogen-progestin oral contraceptives, one daily continuously for 6–9 months. Increase the dose only with the onset of breakthrough bleeding.

3. Medroxyprogesterone acetate (Depo-Provera), 100 mg intramuscularly every 2 weeks for 4 doses; then 100 mg every 4 weeks; add oral estrogen or estradiol valerate, 30 mg intramuscularly, for breakthrough bleeding. Use for 6–9 months.

4. GnRH analogs are currently being evaluated as treatment for endometriosis because of their ability to suppress ovulation with minimal side effects. Studies are under way to determine the optimal dose to avoid symptoms of hypoestrinism.

5. Low-dose oral contraceptives can be given for 21 days out of each 28; prolonged suppression of ovulation will often inhibit further stimulation of residual endometriosis, especially if taken after one of the therapies mentioned above.

6. Analgesics, with or without codeine, may be needed during menses. Nonsteroidal anti-inflammatory drugs may be helpful.

**B. Surgical Measures:** The surgical treatment of moderately extensive endometriosis depends upon the patient's age and symptoms and her desire to preserve reproductive function. If the patient is under 35, resect the lesions, free adhesions, and suspend the uterus. At least 20% of patients so treated can become pregnant, although some must undergo surgery again if the disease progresses. If the patient is over 35 years old, is disabled by pain, and has involvement of both ovaries, bilateral salpingo-oophorectomy and hysterectomy will probably be necessary.

Small foci of endometriosis can be treated at laparoscopy by bipolar coagulation or laser vaporization.

## Prognosis

The prognosis for reproductive function in early or moderately advanced endometriosis is good with conservative therapy. Bilateral ovariectomy is curative for patients with severe and extensive endometriosis with pain. Following hysterectomy and oophorectomy, estrogen replacement therapy is indicated.

Cramer DW et al: The relation of endometriosis to menstrual characterisitics, smoking, and exercise. *JAMA* 1986; **255**:1904.

Molgaard CA, Golbeck AL, Gresham L: Current concepts in endometriosis. *West J Med* 1985;**143**:42.

Schriock E et al: Treatment of endometriosis with a potent agonist of gonadotropin-releasing hormone (nafarelin). *Fertil Steril* 1985;**44**:583.

## VAGINAL HERNIAS
### (Cystocele, Rectocele, Enterocele)

Cystocele, rectocele, and enterocele are vaginal hernias commonly seen in multiparous women. Cystocele is a hernia of the bladder wall into the vagina, causing a soft anterior fullness. Cystocele may be accompanied by urethrocele, which is not a hernia but a sagging of the urethra following its detachment from the symphysis during childbirth. Rectocele is a herniation of the terminal rectum into the posterior vagina, causing a collapsible pouchlike fullness. Enterocele is a vaginal vault hernia containing small intestine, usually in the posterior vagina and resulting from a deepening of the pouch of Douglas. Enterocele may also accompany uterine prolapse or follow hysterectomy, when weakened vault supports or a deep unobliterated cul-de-sac containing intestine protrudes into the vagina. One or more of the 3 types of hernias often occur in combination.

Supportive measures include a high-fiber diet for constipation and care to empty the bladder completely. Weight reduction in obese patients and limitation of straining and lifting are helpful. Pessaries may reduce cystocele, rectocele, or enterocele temporarily and are helpful in women who do not wish surgery or are chronically ill.

The only cure for cystocele, rectocele, or enterocele is corrective surgery. The prognosis following an uncomplicated procedure is good. Hysterectomy without closure of a significant defect in the pelvic floor will be followed by enterocele.

## UTERINE PROLAPSE

Uterine prolapse most commonly occurs as a delayed result of childbirth injury to the pelvic floor (particularly the transverse cervical and uterosacral ligaments). Unrepaired obstetric lacerations of the levator musculature and perineal body augment the weakness. Attenuation of the pelvic structures with aging and congenital weakness can accelerate the development of prolapse.

In slight prolapse, the uterus descends only part way down the vagina; in moderate prolapse, the corpus descends to the introitus and the cervix protrudes slightly beyond; and in marked prolapse (procidentia), the entire cervix and uterus protrude beyond the introitus and the vagina is inverted. Inability to walk comfortably because of protrusion or discomfort from the presence of a vaginal mass is an indication that surgical treatment should be considered.

## Treatment

The type of surgery depends upon the extent of prolapse and the patient's age and her desire for menstruation, pregnancy, and coitus. The simplest, most effective procedure is vaginal hysterectomy with appropriate repair of the cystocele and rectocele. If the patient desires pregnancy, a partial resection of the cervix with plication of the cardinal ligaments can be attempted. For elderly women who do not desire coitus, partial obliteration of the vagina is surgically simple and effective. Abdominal uterine suspension or ventrofixation will fail in the treatment of prolapse.

A well-fitted vaginal pessary (eg, inflatable doughnut type, Gellhorn pessary) may give relief if surgery is refused or contraindicated.

## PELVIC INFLAMMATORY DISEASE
### (PID; Salpingitis, Endoparametritis)

### Essentials of Diagnosis

- Abdominal, cervical, and adnexal tenderness.
- One or more of the following:
    Temperature > 38 °C.
    White blood cell count > 10,000/$\mu$L.
    Purulent material on culdocentesis.
    Pelvic abscess or inflammatory mass on pelvic examination or ultrasound.
    Gonococci present in endocervix on culture or Gram stain.

### General Considerations

Pelvic inflammatory disease has increased in incidence in recent years owing to the rise in sexually transmitted disease. It is most common in young, nulliparous, sexually active women with multiple partners. Use of an IUD is associated with a 2-fold increase in risk; condoms, diaphragms, spermicides, and oral contraceptives provide significant protection. Endoparametritis can result from induced abortion or any other instrumentation of the uterus.

Pelvic inflammatory disease is a polymicrobial infection caused by a variety of aerobic and anaerobic bacteria, including *N gonorrhoeae, Peptostreptococ-*

*cus, Peptococcus, Bacteroides,* and *Chlamydia.* Organisms present in the endocervix may not be the same ones present in the uterine tubes and peritoneal cavity.

Tuberculous salpingitis is rare in the USA but more common in developing countries; it is characterized by pain and irregular pelvic masses not responsive to antibiotic therapy. Spread of disease is hematogenous from the primary lesion and is not acquired by sexual contact.

## Clinical Findings

**A. Symptoms and Signs:** Patients with pelvic inflammatory disease often have lower abdominal pain, chills and fever, menstrual disturbances, purulent cervical discharge, and cervical and adnexal tenderness. Right upper quadrant pain may indicate perihepatitis (Fitz-Hugh and Curtis syndrome), which is localized peritonitis involving the anterior surface of the liver and the adjacent peritoneum of the anterior abdominal wall. However, since these findings are not always present and are not specific to pelvic inflammatory disease, the criteria for diagnosis remain as stated above. In chronic pelvic inflammatory disease, dysmenorrhea, dyspareunia, infertility, recurrent low-grade fever, and tender pelvic masses are common.

**B. Laboratory Findings:** The white blood cell count and sedimentation rate are not consistently elevated. Gram stains and cultures of endocervical material and fluid obtained from culdocentesis (if available) are valuable guides to therapy. Gram stains of urethral material and cultures from the sexual partner, if available, are also useful.

**C. Ultrasonic Findings:** Pelvic ultrasound may help to distinguish the masses of pelvic infection from those of endometriosis, uterine myomas, ovarian cysts or tumors, and ectopic pregnancy.

## Differential Diagnosis

Appendicitis, ectopic pregnancy, septic abortion, hemorrhagic or ruptured ovarian cysts or tumors, twisted ovarian cyst, degeneration of a myoma, and acute enteritis must be considered. Pelvic inflammatory disease is more likely to occur when there is a history of pelvic inflammatory disease, recent sexual contact, recent onset of menses, or an IUD in place or if the partner has a sexually transmitted disease. Acute pelvic inflammatory disease is highly unlikely when recent intercourse has not taken place or an IUD is not being used. A sensitive serum pregnancy test should be obtained to rule out ectopic pregnancy. Culdocentesis will differentiate between causes of hemoperitoneum (ruptured ectopic pregnancy or hemorrhagic cyst) and pelvic sepsis (salpingitis, ruptured pelvic abscess, or ruptured appendix). Pelvic ultrasound is helpful in the differential diagnosis of ectopic pregnancy of over 6 weeks. Laparoscopy is often utilized to diagnosis pelvic inflammatory disease, and it is imperative if the diagnosis is not certain or if the patient has not responded to antibiotic therapy

after 48 hours. The appendix should be visualized at laparoscopy to rule out appendicitis. Cultures obtained at the time of laparoscopy are often specific and helpful.

## Treatment

**A. Hospitalization:** Patients with acute pelvic inflammatory disease should be hospitalized if there is fever higher than 38 °C or a possible pelvic abscess, if they are pregnant, if diagnosis is uncertain, or if oral antibiotics are not tolerated.

**B. Antibiotics:** Early treatment with appropriate antibiotics effective against *N gonorrhoeae, Chlamydia,* and anaerobes is essential to preserve fertility. Treatment of the sexual partner with tetracycline, 500 mg 4 times daily for 7 days, to eradicate *N gonorrhoeae* and *Chlamydia* should be given if possible.

Various treatment regimens for acute pelvic inflammatory disease are effective. Hospitalized patients can be given one of the following regimens: (1) Cefoxitin, 2 g intravenously every 6 hours, plus doxycycline, 100 mg intravenously twice daily. Continue intravenous administration for at least 48 hours after fever has abated. Continue tetracycline, 500 mg 4 times daily, or doxycycline, 100 mg twice daily, orally to complete 10–14 days of therapy. (2) Clindamycin, 600 mg intravenously every 6 hours, plus gentamicin or tobramycin, 2 mg/kg intravenously followed by 1.5 mg/kg intravenously every 8 hours. Continue intravenous administration for at least 48 hours after temperature is normal. Continue clindamycin, 450 mg 4 times daily orally to complete 10–14 days of therapy. (3) Metronidazole, 1 g intravenously every 12 hours, plus doxycycline, 100 mg intravenously every 12 hours. Continue intravenous administration for at least 48 hours after fever has abated. Then continue both drugs orally at the same dosage to complete 10–14 days of therapy.

Outpatients with milder cases of pelvic inflammatory disease should receive one of the following regimens: (1) ceftriaxone, 250 mg intramuscularly, followed by doxycycline, 100 mg twice daily orally, or tetracycline, 500 mg 4 times daily orally, for 10–14 days; or (2) amoxicillin, 3 g orally, or aqueous procaine penicillin G, 4.8 units intramuscularly, followed by doxycycline or tetracycline as above.

**C. General Measures:** Fluids, a nutritious diet, and bed rest are advisable. Pain is controlled with simple analgesics. Sexual intercourse should be delayed until recovery is complete, often 2–3 months. Subsequent use of oral contraceptives, condoms, or a diaphragm rather than the IUD will reduce the risk of reinfection. Women who have had pelvic inflammatory disease should ask new or promiscuous partners to use condoms and should avoid coitus during menses, when flare-ups are most common.

**D. Surgical Measures:** Tubo-ovarian abscesses may require surgical excision or transcutaneous or transvaginal aspiration. Unless rupture is suspected, institute high-dose antibiotic therapy in the hospital, and monitor therapy with ultrasound. In 70% of cases, antibiotics are effective; in 30%, there is inadequate response in 48–72 hours, and intervention is required. Unilateral adnexectomy in the presence of unilateral abscess is acceptable. Hysterectomy and bilateral salpingo-oophorectomy may be necessary for overwhelming infection or in cases of chronic disease with intractable pelvic pain.

## Prognosis

One-fourth of women with acute disease develop long-term sequelae, including repeated episodes of infection, chronic pelvic pain, dyspareunia, ectopic pregnancy, or infertility. The risk of infertility increases with repeated episodes of salpingitis: it is estimated at 11% after the first episode, 23% after a second episode, and 54% after a third episode.

Keith LG et al: On the causation of pelvic inflammatory disease. *Am J Obstet Gynecol* 1984;**149**:215.

Landers DV, Sweet RL: Current trends in the diagnosis and treatment of tuboovarian abscess. *Am J Obstet Gynecol* 1985;**151**:1098.

Wolner-Hanssen P et al: Treatment of pelvic inflammatory disease: Use doxycycline with an appropriate β-lactam while we wait for better data. *JAMA* 1986;**256**:3262.

## OVARIAN TUMORS

Ovarian tumors are common forms of neoplastic disease in women. Most are benign, but some are malignant. The wide range of types and patterns of ovarian tumors is due to the complexity of ovarian embryology and differences in tissue of origin. Most systems of classification utilize largely the tumor histogenesis, but there may be advantages to employing other criteria such as clinical behavior—functional and nonfunctional, cystic or solid—and always macroscopic or microscopic appearance (Table 13–4).

The history and physical examination may be supplemented with cervical cytologic studies, ultrasound, and laparoscopy. Upper gastrointestinal series, barium enema, and other studies may help to rule out metastatic origin from other primary sites. An intravenous urogram is important to determine distortion or obstruction of the ureters caused by the tumor.

## Treatment

The treatment of ovarian tumors must be individualized. Small unilocular tumors (as determined by ultrasound) in premenopausal women can be observed for a few months. A 2-month trial of suppression of ovulation with oral contraceptives usually causes functional cysts to disappear. If ultrasound suggests septation or solid components, a neoplasm is more likely, and surgical exploration should be prompt. If a plain film of the abdomen shows calcification, a benign teratoma is likely. Whenever possible in young women, ovarian cystectomy rather than total removal of the ovary is desirable. An enlarged ovary in a postmenopausal woman should be evaluated

promptly. If ultrasound study shows enlargement to twice the size of the contralateral ovary, surgery is indicated.

The initial surgery is the optimum time for a complete evaluation of the extent of the tumor and for its definitive treatment. Operations for suspected ovarian cancer should be performed at hospitals with facilities for performing frozen section biopsy and by personnel familiar with extended surgery, including bowel and bladder procedures.

Treatment for ovarian cancer is surgery (excision or debulking of any visible neoplasia, hysterectomy and bilateral oophorectomy, appendectomy, omentectomy, selective lymphadenectomy) and chemotherapy.

## Prognosis

The prognosis for benign ovarian tumors after surgical removal is excellent. The outlook for ovarian cancer, unless diagnosed in the earliest stages, is poor.

Richardson GS et al: Common epithelial cancer of the ovary. *N Engl J Med* 1985;**312**:415.

## PERSISTENT ANOVULATION
## (Polycystic Ovary Syndrome, Stein-Leventhal Syndrome)

### Essentials of Diagnosis

- Chronic anovulation.
- Infertility.
- Elevated plasma LH values and a reversed FSH/LH ratio.
- Hirsutism (in 70% of patients).

### General Considerations

These patients have a relatively steady state of high estrogen, androgen, and LH levels, rather than the fluctuating condition seen in ovulating women. The thecal and stromal tissues of the ovary secretes high amounts of androgens, and the peripheral conversion of androstenedione in body fat gives high estrone levels. Sex hormone-binding globulin levels are low, allowing for increased free circulating sex steroids. LH levels are higher than normal; FSH is low or low normal. New follicles in the ovary are continually stimulated but not to the point of ovulation; they may persist for months as follicle cysts. The polycystic ovary has a thickened, pearly white capsule.

### Clinical Findings

The patient is anovular, generally with amenorrhea and sometimes with irregular heavy bleeding. The ovaries may be enlarged, but this is not a consistent finding. Similarly, she may or may not be obese. Hirsutism occurs in about 70% of patients with this condition. These patients are generally infertile, although they may ovulate occasionally. They have an increased long-term risk of cancer of the breast

**Table 13–4.** Ovarian functional and neoplastic tumors.

| Tumor | Incidence | Size | Consistency | Menstrual Irregularities | Endocrine Effects | Potential For Malignancy | Special Remarks |
|---|---|---|---|---|---|---|---|
| Follicle cysts | Rare in childhood; frequent in menstrual years; never in postmenopausal years. | < 6 cm, often bilateral. | Moderate | Occasional | Occasional anovulation with persistently proliferative endometrium. | 0 | Often disappear after a 2-month regimen of oral contraceptives. |
| Corpus luteum cysts | Occasional, in menstrual years. | 4–6 cm, unilateral. | Moderate | Occasional delayed period | Prolonged secretory phase. | 0 | Functional cysts. Intraperitoneal bleeding occasionally. |
| Theca lutein cysts | Occurs with hydatidiform mole, choriocarcinoma; also with gonadotropin or clomiphene therapy. | To 4–5 cm, multiple, bilateral. (Ovaries may be ≥ 20 cm in diameter.) | Tense | Amenorrhea | hCG elevated as a result of trophoblastic proliferation. | 0 | Functional cysts. Hematoperitoneum or torsion of ovary may occur. Surgery to be avoided. |
| Inflammatory (tubo-ovarian abscess) | Concomitant with acute salpingitis. | To 15–20 cm, often bilateral. | Variable, painful | Menometrorrhagia | Anovulation usual. | 0 | Unilateral removal indicated if possible. |
| Endometriotic cysts | Never in preadolescent or postmenopausal years. Most common in women age 20–40 years. | To 10–12 cm, occasionally bilateral. | Moderate to softened | Rare | 0 | Very rare | Associated pelvic endometriosis. Medical treatment or conservative surgery recommended. |
| Teratoid tumors: Benign teratomas (dermoid cysts) | Childhood to postmenopause. | < 15 cm; 15% are bilateral. | Moderate to softened | 0 | 0 | Rare | Torsion can occur. Partial oophorectomy recommended. |
| Malignant teratomas | < 1% of ovarian tumors. Usually in infants and young adults. | > 20 cm, unilateral. | Irregularly firm | 0 | Occasionally, hCG elevated. | All | Unresponsive to any therapy. |
| Cystadenoma, cystadenocarcinoma | Common in reproductive years. | Serous: < 25 cm, often bilateral. Mucinous; up to 1 meter, occasionally bilateral. | Moderate to softened. Moderate to softened | 0 | 0 | > 50% for serous. About 5% for mucinous. | Peritoneal implants often occur with serous tumors, rarely occur with mucinous tumors. If mucinous tumor is ruptured, pseudomyxoma peritonei may occur. |
| Endometrioid carcinoma | 15% of ovarian carcinomas. | Moderate. | Firm | 0 | 0 | All | Adenocarcinoma of endometrium coexists in 15–30% of cases. |
| Fibroma | < 5% of ovarian tumors. | Usually < 15 cm. | Very firm | 0 | 0 | Rare | Ascites in 20% (rarely, pleural fluid). |
| Arrhenoblastoma | Rare. Average age 30 years or more. | Often small (< 10 cm), unilateral. | Firm to softened | Amenorrhea | Androgens elevated. | < 20% | Recurrences are moderately sensitive to irradiation. |
| Theca cell tumor (thecoma) | Uncommon. | < 10 cm, unilateral. | Firm | Occasionally irregular periods | Estrogens or androgens elevated. | < 1% | ... |
| Granulosa cell tumor | Uncommon. Usually in prepubertal girls or women older than 50 years. | May be very small. | Firm to softened | Menometrorrhagia | Estrogens elevated. | 15–20% | Recurrences are moderately sensitive to irradiation. |
| Dysgerminoma | About 1–2% of ovarian tumors. | < 30 cm, bilateral in one-third of cases. | Moderate to softened | 0 | ... | All | Very radiosensitive. |
| Brenner tumor | About 1% of ovarian tumors. | < 30 cm, unilateral. | Firm | 0 | ... | Very rare | > 50% occur in postmenopausal years. |
| Secondary ovarian tumors | 10% of fatal malignant disease in women. | Varies, often bilateral. | Firm to softened | Occasional | Very rare (thyroid, adrenocortical origin). | All | Bowel or breast metastases to ovary common. |

and endometrium because of unopposed estrogen secretion.

## Differential Diagnosis

Anovulation in the reproductive years may also be due to (1) premature menopause (high FSH and LH levels); (2) rapid weight loss or extreme physical exertion (normal FSH and LH levels for age); (3) discontinuation of oral contraceptives (anovulation for 6 months or more occasionally occurs); (4) pituitary adenoma with elevated prolactin (galactorrhea may or may not be present); (5) hyper- or hypothyroidism; (6) Cushing's syndrome or congenital adrenal hyperplasia. Always check FSH, LH, prolactin, and TSH levels when amenorrhea has persisted for 6 months or more without a diagnosis. A 10-day course of progestin (eg, medroxyprogesterone acetate, 10 mg/d) will cause withdrawal bleeding if estrogen levels are adequate; bleeding will not occur if estrogen levels are low. This will aid in the diagnosis and prevent endometrial hyperplasia. In long-term anovular patients over age 35, it is wise to search for an estrogen-stimulated cancer with mammography and endometrial aspiration.

## Treatment

If the patient wishes to become pregnant, clomiphene or other drugs can be employed for ovulatory stimulation. Wedge resection of the ovary is often successful in restoring ovulation and fertility, although this procedure is used less commonly now that medical treatments are available.

If the patient does not desire pregnancy, give medroxyprogesterone acetate, 10 mg/d for the first 10 days of each month. This will ensure regular shedding of the endometrium so that hyperplasia will not occur. If contraception is desired, a low-dose combination oral contraceptive can be used; this is also useful in controlling hirsutism, for which treatment must be continued for 6–12 months before results are seen.

Hirsutism may be managed with epilation and electrolysis. If hirsutism is severe, some patients will elect to have a hysterectomy and bilateral oophorectomy followed by estrogen replacement therapy. Spironolactone, an aldosterone antagonist, is also useful for hirsutism in doses of 25 mg 3 or 4 times daily. The benefits of this drug in reducing hair growth must be weighed against its potential side effects of hyperkalemia, menstrual abnormalities, sedation, headache, ataxia, etc.

Coney P: Polycystic ovarian disease: Current concepts of pathophysiology and therapy. *Fertil Steril* 1984;**42**:667.

## URINARY INCONTINENCE

Loss of urine under a variety of circumstances is a common gynecologic complaint. Urinary frequency, nocturia, and urgency are sometimes associated with incontinence. A careful history of drinking and voiding habits, amount of leakage and timing of leakage, and evidence of urinary tract infection will help in diagnosis. The normal bladder holds up to 500 mL, and voiding generally occurs every 2–3 hours while awake.

Women with stress incontinence following childbirth have urethras displaced downward from the normal position above the urogenital diaphragm. Sudden increases in intra-abdominal pressure are transmitted to the otherwise normally functioning bladder but not to the prolapsed urethra, and so urine tends to leak at that moment. Estrogen-deprived postmenopausal women have similar urine loss due to decreased urethral tone.

Abnormal bladder muscle (detrusor) function can also cause incontinence. A hypotonic (neurogenic) bladder will have a large capacity and will empty incompletely by overflow. A hypertonic bladder with a small capacity and variable levels of high detrusor tone will also cause urine loss.

Symptoms, history, physical examination, and routine laboratory tests sometimes are insufficient for diagnosis. When the type of incontinence is unclear or when there are multiple symptoms, cystometric study of the bladder may be needed. Cystometry measures pressures within the bladder and along the urethra during bladder filling and with the patient in different positions and with different stress mechanisms such as coughing.

## Treatment

Effective therapy for pure stress incontinence will increase the patient's ability to transmit intravesical pressure to the mid urethra but will not necessarily improve intraurethral pressure per se. A trial of medical treatment is always indicated before surgery is considered.

Medical disorders such as diabetes mellitus, extreme obesity, and chronic and recurrent urinary tract infections should be controlled if possible. Postmenopausal women should receive a trial of estrogen replacement (either cyclic oral medication or small doses of vaginal cream). Patients who do not have serious neurologic disorders and have not sustained severe physical injury can be taught to contract the pubococcygeus muscles repeatedly to help reestablish and increase control of the urogenital diaphragm and thus improve urinary function (Kegel isometric exercises). For maximum effect, sequences of exercises should be done 3–4 times a day for several months. Patients who fail to respond to exercises or medical treatment may be candidates for surgery, particularly when cystocele or prolapse of the bladder and uterus is present.

A study of bladder dynamics will identify abnormal detrusor activity as well as an unusually large or small bladder capacity. Measurement of closing pressures along the urethra will help in determining whether surgical procedures to lengthen and support the urethra will be successful. A voiding cystourethrogram will identify an excessively mobile prolapsing urethra. A useful surgical prognostic test is to elevate the anterior vaginal wall lateral to the urethra at the urethrovesical junction with a Smith-Hodge pessary. If loss of urine does not occur with cough, the surgical prognosis is good.

Medical therapy alone improves half of cases to some degree. The overall cure rate in patients who require operation is about 85%. The most successful procedure is retropubic suspension of the paravaginal tissues (Burch procedure). Other types of urethral suspension (Pereya operation) and vaginal urethral plication are occasional alternatives.

Patients with irritable bladders of decreased capacity who have annoying frequency and urge incontinence can be encouraged to retrain their bladders by scheduled voidings at increasing intervals. Initial improvement occurs within 2–4 weeks, and retraining should continue for 4–6 months. A variety of drugs with anticholinergic activity have also proved useful for frequency, nocturia, and urge incontinence. Among these are propantheline, 5 mg twice daily; dicyclomine, 10 mg daily or twice daily; oxybutinin, 5 mg twice daily; and flavoxate, 100 mg twice daily. Imipramine, 25 mg daily or twice daily, and amitriptyline, 25 mg daily or twice daily, can be used for their anticholinergic effects as well as their antidepressant activity. In older women, the risk of these drugs for precipitation of angle-closure glaucoma should be recognized. Indomethacin, 50 mg daily or twice daily, and nifedipine, 10 mg daily or twice daily, have also been tried.

Fantl JA: Urinary incontinence due to detrusor instability. *Clin Obstet Gynecol* 1984;**27**:474.

## PAINFUL INTERCOURSE
(Dyspareunia)

Painful intercourse may be caused by vulvovaginitis; vaginismus; an incompletely stretched hymen; insufficient lubrication of the vagina; or infection, tumors, or other pathologic conditions. Careful history taking and a thorough pelvic examination are essential. During the pelvic examination, the patient should be placed in a half-sitting position and given a hand-held mirror and then asked to point out the site of pain and describe the type of pain. The physician should be able to provide sex counseling and should allow adequate time for a discussion of problems related to sexuality, personal relationships, contraception, and fears of pregnancy.

### Etiology

**A. Vulvovaginitis:** Vulvovaginitis is inflammation or infection of the vagina. Areas of marked tenderness in the vulvar vestibule without visible inflammation occasionally show lesions resembling small condylomas on colposcopy. For a detailed discussion of vaginitis, see p 450.

**B. Vaginismus:** Vaginismus is voluntary or involuntary contraction of muscles around the introitus. It results from fear, pain, sexual trauma, or having learned negative attitudes toward sex during childhood.

**C. Remnants of the Hymen:** The hymen is usually adequately stretched during initial intercourse, so that pain does not occur subsequently. In some women, the pain of initial intercourse may produce vaginismus. In others, a thin or thickened rim or partial rim of hymen remains after several episodes of intercourse, causing pain.

**D. Insufficient Lubrication of the Vagina:** Insufficient vaginal lubrication may be due to inadequate time for sexual arousal or to low estrogen effect during lactation or following menopause. When estrogen levels are normal (as evidenced by the occurrence of menstrual periods or the presence of moist, healthy-appearing vaginal mucosa with rugal folds), dyspareunia is probably due to inadequate sexual arousal prior to coitus. Low estrogen levels are evidenced by decreased introital diameter, dry vaginal mucosa, fewer rugal folds, and thinned, reddened epithelium.

**E. Infection, Endometriosis, Tumors, or Other Pathologic Conditions:** Pain occurring with deep thrusting during coitus is usually due to acute or chronic infection of the cervix, uterus, or adnexa; endometriosis; adnexal tumors; or adhesions resulting from prior pelvic disease or operation. Careful history taking and a pelvic examination will generally help in the differential diagnosis.

**F. Dyspareunia Due to Unknown Cause:** Occasionally, no organic cause of pain can be found. These patients may have psychosexual conflicts or a history of childhood sexual abuse.

### Treatment

**A. Vulvovaginitis:** Infection or inflammation should be treated after careful diagnosis. The sexual partner should also be treated in recurrent cases. Irritation from spermicides may be a factor. The couple may be helped by a discussion of noncoital techniques to achieve orgasm until the infection subsides.

**B. Vaginismus:** Sexual counseling and education on anatomy and sexual functioning may be appropriate. The patient can be instructed in self-dilation, using a lubricated finger or test tubes of graduated sizes. Before coitus (with adequate lubrication) is attempted, the patient—and then her partner—should be able to easily and painlessly introduce 2 fingers into the vagina. Penetration should never be forced, and the woman should always be the one to control the depth of insertion during dilation or intercourse.

**C. Remnants of the Hymen:** In rare situations, manual dilation of a remaining hymen under general anesthesia is necessary. Surgery should be avoided.

**D. Insufficient Lubrication of the Vagina:** If inadequate sexual arousal is the cause, sexual counseling for the woman—and her partner if possible—is helpful. Lubricants may be used during sexual foreplay. For women with low plasma estrogen levels, use of a lubricant during coitus is sometimes sufficient.

If not, use conjugated estrogen cream, one-eighth applicatorful daily for 10 days and then every other day. Using the applicator or a finger, the patient can apply the cream directly to the most tender area, usually the hymenal ring. Testosterone cream 1–2% in a water-soluble base is also helpful.

**E. Infection, Endometriosis, Tumors, or Other Pathologic Conditions:** Medical treatment of acute cervicitis, endometritis, or salpingitis and temporary abstention from coitus usually relieves pain. Hormonal or surgical treatment of endometriosis may be helpful. Dyspareunia resulting from chronic pelvic inflammatory disease or any condition causing extensive adhesions or fixation of pelvic organs is difficult to treat without extirpative surgery. Couples can be advised to try coital positions that limit deep thrusting and to use manual and oral sexual techniques.

**F. Dyspareunia Due to Unknown Cause:** Colposcopy in discrete areas of pain without obvious lesions may be useful to rule out papilloma virus infections. Biopsies should be avoided if there is no identifiable lesion. Supportive, understanding discussion may be helpful. Small amounts of topical remedies such as 1% testosterone cream, estrogen cream, or topical lidocaine gel may relieve pain. Resolution of psychosexual problems or problems relating to traumatic sexual experiences may be necessary.

Lynch PJ: Vulvodynia: A syndrome of unexplained vulvar pain, psychologic disability, and sexual dysfunction. *J Reprod Med* 1986;**31**:773.

Reamy K: The treatment of vaginismus by the gynecologist: An eclectic approach. *Obstet Gynecol* 1982;**59**:58.

Steege JF: Dyspareunia and vaginismus. *Clin Obstet Gynecol* 1984;**27**:750.

## INFERTILITY

A couple is said to be infertile if pregnancy does not result after 1 year of normal sexual activity without contraceptives. About 10% of couples are infertile; the incidence of infertility increases with age. The male partner contributes to about 40% of cases of infertility. A combination of factors is common.

### Diagnostic Survey

A basic infertility study can be performed, usually within a 3-month period, although timing can vary depending on convenience and the desires of the couple. Both partners are evaluated.

During the initial interview, the physician can present an overview of infertility and discuss a plan of study. Separate private consultations are then conducted, allowing appraisal of psychosexual adjustment without embarrassment or criticism. Pertinent details (eg, sexually transmitted disease or prior pregnancies) must be obtained. A complete medical, surgical, occupational, and obstetric history must be taken. The ill effects of cigarettes, alcohol, and other recreational drugs on fertility in both men and women should be discussed. Prescription drugs that impair male potency should be noted. The gynecologic history should include queries regarding the menstrual pattern. The present history includes use and types of contraceptives, douches, libido, sex techniques, frequency and success of coitus, and correlation of intercourse with time of ovulation. Family history includes familial traits, illnesses, repeated abortions, and abnormal children.

General physical and genital examinations are performed on both partners. Basic laboratory studies include complete blood count, urinalysis, serologic test for syphilis, rubella antibody determination, and thyroid function tests. Tay-Sachs and sickle cell screening tests should be offered to appropriate couples. Screening mammography can also be offered to women over 35.

The woman is instructed to chart her basal body temperature orally daily on arising and to record on a graph episodes of coitus and days of menstruation. Self-performed urine tests for the midcycle LH surge can be used to enhance temperature observations relating to ovulation.

The man is instructed to bring a complete ejaculate for analysis. Sexual abstinence for at least 3 days before the semen is obtained is emphasized. A clean, dry, wide-mouthed bottle for collection is preferred. Condoms should not be employed, as the protective powder may be spermicidal. Semen should be examined within 1–2 hours after collection. Semen is considered normal with the following minimum values: volume, 3 mL; concentration, 20 million sperm per milliliter; motility, 50% after 2 hours; and normal forms, 60%.

**A. First Testing Cycle:** A postcoital test (Sims-Huhner test) is scheduled for just before ovulation (eg, day 12 or 13 in an expected 28-day cycle). The patient is examined within 6 hours after coitus. The cervical mucus should be clear, elastic, and copious owing to the influence of the preovular estrogen surge. (The mucus is scantier and more viscid before and after ovulation.) A good spinnbarkeit (stretching to a fine thread 4 cm or more in length) is desirable. A small drop of cervical mucus should be obtained from within the cervical os and examined under the microscope. The presence of 5 or more active sperm per high-power field constitutes a satisfactory postcoital test. If no spermatozoa are found, the test should be repeated (assuming that active spermatozoa were present in the semen analysis). Sperm agglutination and sperm immobilization tests should be considered if the sperm are immotile or show ineffective tail motility.

The presence of more than 3 white blood cells per high-power field in the postcoital test suggests cervicitis in the woman or prostatitis in the man. When estrogen levels are normal, the cervical mucus dried on the slide will form a fernlike pattern when viewed with a low-power microscope. This type of mucus is necessary for normal sperm transport.

The serum progesterone level should be measured at the midpoint of the secretory phase (21st day); a level of 10–20 ng/mL confirms adequate luteal function.

**B. Second Testing Cycle:** Hysterosalpingography is performed within 3 days following the menstrual period. This x-ray study will demonstrate uterine abnormalities (septa, polyps, submucous myomas) and tubal obstruction. A repeat x-ray film 24 hours later will confirm tubal patency if there is wide pelvic dispersion of the dye. This test has been associated with an increased pregnancy rate by some observers. If the woman has had prior pelvic inflammation, give tetracycline, 2 g/d, beginning immediately before and for 7 days after the x-ray study.

**C. Further Testing:**

1. Gross deficiencies of sperm (number, motility, or appearance) require repeat analysis. Zona-free hamster egg penetration tests are available to evaluate the ability of human sperm to fertilize the egg.

2. Obvious obstruction of the uterine tubes requires assessment for microsurgery or in vitro fertilization.

3. Absent or infrequent ovulation requires additional laboratory evaluation. Elevated FSH and LH levels indicate ovarian failure causing premature menopause (in women under age 30, karyotyping is indicated to rule out chromosomal abnormalities). Elevated LH levels in the presence of normal FSH levels confirm the presence of polycystic ovaries. Elevation of blood prolactin (PRL) levels suggests pituitary microadenoma.

**D. Laparoscopy:** Approximately 25% of women whose basic evaluation is normal will have findings on laparoscopy explaining their infertility (eg, peritubal adhesions, endometriotic implants).

## Treatment

**A. Medical Measures:** Fertility may be restored by appropriate treatment in many patients with endocrine imbalance, particularly those with hypo- or hyperthyroidism. Antibiotic treatment of cervicitis is of value. After 6 months of condom protection during intercourse, an antigen-antibody reaction will usually resolve, and sperm agglutination or immobilization should cease to be a problem.

Women who engage in vigorous athletic training often have low sex hormone levels; fertility improves with reduced exercise and some weight gain.

**B. Surgical Measures:** Excision of ovarian tumors or ovarian foci of endometriosis can improve fertility. Microsurgical relief of tubal obstruction due to salpingitis or tubal ligation will reestablish fertility in a significant number of cases. In special instances of cornual or fimbrial block, the prognosis with newer surgical techniques has become much better. Peritubal adhesions or endometriotic implants often can be treated via laparoscopy or via laparotomy immediately following laparoscopic examination if prior consent has been obtained.

With varicocele in the male, sperm characteristics are often improved following surgical treatment.

**C. Induction of Ovulation:**

**1. Clomiphene citrate (Clomid)–**Clomiphene citrate stimulates gonadotropin release, especially LH. Consequently, plasma estrone ($E_1$) and estradiol ($E_2$) also rise, reflecting ovarian follicle maturation. If $E_2$ rises sufficiently, an LH surge occurs to trigger ovulation.

After a normal menstrual period or induction of withdrawal bleeding with progestin, give 50 mg of clomiphene orally daily for 5 days. If ovulation does not occur, increase the dose to 100 mg orally daily for 5 days. If ovulation still does not occur, repeat the course with 150 and then 200 mg daily for 5 days and add chorionic gonadotropin, 10,000 units intramuscularly, 7 days after clomiphene.

The rate of ovulation following this treatment is 90% in the absence of other infertility factors. The pregnancy rate is high. Twinning occurs in 5% of these patients; an increased incidence of congenital anomalies has not been reported. Painful ovarian cyst formation occurs in 8% of patients and may warrant discontinuation of therapy.

In the presence of increased androgen production (DHEA-S > 200 $\mu$g/dL), the addition of dexamethasone, 0.5 mg at bedtime, improves the response to clomiphene. Dexamethasone should be discontinued after pregnancy is confirmed.

**2. Bromocriptine (Parlodel)–**Use only if PRL levels are elevated and there is no withdrawal bleeding following progesterone administration (otherwise use clomiphene). The usual dose is 2.5 mg twice daily. To minimize side effects (nausea, diarrhea, dizziness, headache, fatigue), bromocriptine should be taken with meals. Begin with 2.5 mg once daily and increase to 2–3 times daily in increments of 1.25 mg. The drug is discontinued once pregnancy has occurred.

**3. Human menopausal gonadotropins (hMG) (Pergonal)–**hMG is indicated in cases of hypogonadotropism and most other types of anovulation (exclusive of ovarian failure). Because of the complexities, laboratory tests, and expense associated with this treatment, patients who require hMG for the induction of ovulation should be referred to a specialist. Current reports suggest that hypothalamic amenorrhea unresponsive to clomiphene will be reliably and successfully treated with subcutaneous pulsatile gonadotropin-releasing hormone (GnRH). Use of this substance will avoid the dangerous ovarian complications and the 25% incidence of multiple pregnancy associated with hMG.

**4. Ovarian wedge resecton–**Wedge resection is indicated rarely and only when medical measures are not effective.

**D. Treatment of Endometriosis:** See p 458.

**E. Treatment of Low Midluteal Progesterone Levels:** Midluteal progesterone levels of less than 10 ng/mL can be treated with one of the following regimens:

1. Progesterone suppositories, 50 mg twice daily

on days 17–31 of the ovarian cycle. If the woman becomes pregnant, continue for 8 weeks.

2. Clomiphene (see above) can also be used for luteal phase insufficiency.

**F. Treatment of Inadequate Transport of Sperm:**

1. Cervical mucus will provide better transport following administration of 0.3 mg of conjugated equine estrogens from days 5 to 15 of the ovarian cycle (ovulation may be delayed).

2. Intrauterine insemination of concentrated washed sperm has been used to bypass a poor cervical environment. The sperm must be handled by sterile methods, washed in sterile saline or tissue culture solutions, and centrifuged. A small amount of fluid (0.5 mL) containing the sperm is then instilled into the uterus.

**G. Artificial Insemination in Azoospermia:** If azoospermia is present, artificial insemination by a donor usually results in pregnancy, assuming female function is normal. Both partners must consent to this method. The use of frozen sperm is currently preferable to fresh sperm because the frozen specimen can be held pending cultures and blood test results for sexually transmitted diseases, including AIDS.

**H. In Vitro Fertilization and Implantation of Embryos:** This technique is becoming a standard approach to fertility problems involving severe tubal disease and has also been used in cases of premature menopause, in couples with unexplained long-term infertility, and where the male is oligospermic. A highly organized team of specialists in reproductive function and sophisticated technology are required for successful results.

**Prognosis**

The prognosis for conception and normal pregnancy is good if minor (even multiple) disorders can be identified and treated; poor if the causes of infertility are severe, untreatable, or of prolonged duration (over 3 years).

It is important to remember that in the absence of severe causes of infertility (azoospermia, prolonged amenorrhea, or bilateral tubal obstruction), 30% of couples will achieve a pregnancy within 3 years. Most of these successes will be unrelated to therapy. Offering appropriately timed information about adoption is considered part of a complete infertility regimen.

Collins JA et al: Treatment-independent pregnancy among infertile couples. *N Engl J Med* 1983;**309**:1201.

Howe G et al: Effects of age, cigarette smoking, and other factors on fertility: Findings in a large prospective study. *Br Med J* 1985;**290**:1697.

Hurley DM et al: Induction of ovulation and fertility in amenorrheic women by pulsatile low-dose gonadotropin-releasing hormone. *N Engl J Med* 1984;**310**:1069.

# CONTRACEPTION

Voluntary control of childbearing benefits women, men, and the children born to them. Contraception should be available to all women and men of reproductive ages. Education about contraception and access to contraceptive pills or devices is especially important for sexually active teenagers and for women following childbirth or abortion.

Education about sexually transmitted disease, especially AIDS, should be given to all sexually active people, along with information that condoms with spermicide offer a high degree of protection (but not complete protection) to both sexes against sexually transmitted disease as well as pregnancy. The worldwide AIDS epidemic should cause a significant shift in the choice of contraception in the years to come.

## 1. ORAL CONTRACEPTIVES

### Combined Oral Contraceptives

**A. Efficacy and Methods of Use:** Oral contraceptives (birth control pills) have a failure rate of less than 0.5% if taken absolutely on schedule. Their primary mode of action is suppression of ovulation. The pills are initially started on the fifth day of the ovarian cycle and taken daily for 21 days, followed by 7 days of placebos or no medication, and this schedule is then continued for each cycle. The pills are often started on the first Sunday after the onset of menses, to help patients remember their starting day and to avoid menses on the weekend. If a pill is missed at any time, 2 pills should be taken the next day, and another method of contraception should be used for the rest of the cycle (eg, condoms or foam). A backup method should also be used during the first cycle if the pills are started later than the fifth day.

**B. Benefits of Oral Contraceptives:** Besides offering convenient, effective contraception, there are noncontraceptive advantages to oral contraceptives. Menstrual flow is lighter and resultant anemia is less common, and dysmenorrhea is relieved for most women. Functional ovarian cysts generally disappear with oral contraceptive use, and new cysts do not occur. Pain with ovulation and postovulatory aching are relieved. The risk of ovarian and endometrial cancer is decreased. The risk of salpingitis is diminished. Acne is usually improved.

**C. Selection of an Oral Contraceptive:** Most clinicians first prescribe 30–35 $\mu$g of estrogen combined with 1 mg or less of progestin. This low dose of estrogen provides highly effective contraception but is also associated with more spotting, breakthrough bleeding, and missed menstrual periods than higher doses, and the patient should be warned of these side effects. Patients taking pills containing more than 50 $\mu$g of estrogen should be switched to lower doses whenever possible, since many adverse side effects of the pill are dose-related. The progestins vary in potency and androgenicity. When hirsutism or acne is a problem, it is best to use ethynodiol diacetate or norethindrone. When breakthrough bleeding or dysfunctional bleeding occurs, many clinicians use a compound with norgestrel. Low-dose oral contraceptives currently used in the USA are shown in Table 13–5.

**D. Drug Interactions:** Several drugs interact with oral contraceptives to decrease their efficacy by causing induction of microsomal enzymes in the liver, by increasing sex hormone-binding globulin, and by other mechanisms. Some commonly prescribed drugs in this category are the anticonvulsants phenytoin, phenobarbital (and other barbiturates), primidone, and carbamazepine and the antituberculous drug rifampin. Women taking these drugs should use another means of contraception for maximum safety.

**E. Contraindications and Adverse Effects:** Oral contraceptives have been associated with many adverse effects; they are contraindicated in some situations and should be used with caution in others (Table 13–6).

**1. Myocardial infarction–**The risk of heart attack is higher with use of oral contraceptives. Age over 35 years; cigarette smoking; obesity; or the presence of hypertension, diabetes, or hypercholesterolemia increases the risk. Young nonsmoking women have minimal increased risk. Smokers over age 30–35 and women with other cardiovascular risk factors should use other methods of birth control.

**2. Thromboembolic disease–**An increased rate of fatal and nonfatal venous thromboembolism is found in oral contraceptive users. Women who develop thrombophlebitis should stop using this method, as should those at risk of thrombophlebitis because of surgery, fracture, serious injury, or immobilization.

**3. Cerebrovascular disease–**An increased risk of thrombotic and hemorrhagic stroke and subarachnoid hemorrhage has been found; smoking is associated with increased risk. Women who develop warning symptoms such as severe headache, blurred or lost vision, or other transient neurologic disorders should stop using oral contraceptives. Women with hypertensive disease should not use the pill.

**4. Carcinoma–**A relationship between long-term (3–4 years) oral contraceptive use and occurrence of cervical dysplasia and cancer has been suggested in various studies. No confirmed relationship has been

**Table 13–5.** Commonly used low-dose oral contraceptives.

| Name | Type | Progestin | Estrogen (Ethinyl Estradiol) |
|---|---|---|---|
| Lo/Ovral | Combination | 0.3 mg dl-norgestrel | 30 $\mu$g |
| Nordette and Levelen | Combination | 0.15 mg levonorgestrel | 30 $\mu$g |
| Norinyl 1/35 and Ortho-Novum 1/35 | Combination | 1 mg norethindrone | 35 $\mu$g |
| Loestrin 1.5/30 | Combination | 1.5 mg norethindrone acetate | 30 $\mu$g |
| Demulen 1/35 | Combination | 1 mg ethynodiol diacetate | 35 $\mu$g |
| Brevicon and Modicon | Combination | 0.5 mg norethindrone | 35 $\mu$g |
| Ovcon 35 | Combination | 0.4 mg norethindrone | 35 $\mu$g |
| Ortho-novum 10/11 | Biphasic | 0.5 mg norethindrone (days 1–10) 1 mg norethindrone (days 11–21) | 35 $\mu$g |
| Ortho-novum 777 | Triphasic | 0.5 mg norethindrone (days 1–7) 0.75 mg norethindrone (days 8–14) 1 mg norethindrone (days 15–21) | 35 $\mu$g |
| Tri-Norinyl | Triphasic | 0.5 mg norethindrone (days 1–7) 1 mg norethindrone (days 8–16) 0.5 mg norethindrone (days 17–21) | 35 $\mu$g |
| Triphasil and Trilevin | Triphasic | 0.05 mg levonorgestrel (days 1–6) 0.075 mg levonorgestrel (days 7–11) 0.125 mg levonorgestrel (days 12–21) | 30 $\mu$g 40 $\mu$g 30 $\mu$g |
| Micronor and Nor-QD | Progestin-only minipill | 0.35 mg norethindrone to be taken continuously | |
| Ovrette | Progestin-only minipill | 0.075 mg dl-norgestrel to be taken continuously | |

**Table 13–6.** Contraindications to use or oral contraceptives.

**Absolute contraindications**
 Pregnancy
 Thrombophlebitis or thromboembolic disorders (past or present)
 Stroke or coronary artery disease (past or present)
 Cancer of the breast (known or suspected)
 Undiagnosed abnormal vaginal bleeding
 Estrogen-dependent cancer (known or suspected)
 Benign or malignant tumor of the liver (past or present)
**Relative contraindications**
 Age over 35 years and heavy cigarette smoking (> 15 cigarettes daily)
 Age over 40–45 years
 Cervical intraepithelial neoplasia
 Migraine or recurrent persistent, severe headache
 Hypertension
 Cardiac or renal disease
 Diabetes
 Gallbladder disease
 Cholestasis during pregnancy
 Active hepatitis or infectious mononucleosis
 Sickle cell disease (S/S or S/C type)
 Surgery, fracture, or severe injury
 Lactation
 Significant psychologic depression

found between use of oral contraceptives and cancer of the breast. Birth control pills appear to protect against endometrial and ovarian cancer. Rarely, oral contraceptives have been associated with the development of benign or malignant hepatic tumors; this may lead to rupture of the liver, hemorrhage, and death. The risk increases with higher dosage, longer duration of use, and older age.

**5. Gallbladder disease**–There is an increased risk of gallbladder disease and subsequent cholecystectomy for cholesterol stones in pill users.

**6. Metabolic disorders**–A decrease in glucose tolerance and an increase in triglyceride levels is seen in pill takers, and women with diabetes should therefore rarely use this method.

**7. Hypertension**–Oral contraceptives may cause hypertension in some women; the risk is increased with longer duration of use and older age. Women who have or develop hypertension should use other contraceptive methods.

**8. Headache**–Migraine or other vascular headaches may occur or worsen with pill use. If severe or frequent, the pill should not be used.

**9. Amenorrhea**–Postpill amenorrhea lasting a year or longer occurs occasionally, sometimes with galactorrhea. PRL levels should be checked; if elevated, a pituitary prolactinoma may be present.

**10. Disorders of lactation**–Combined oral contraceptives can impair the quantity and quality of breast milk and should therefore not be given before the infant is weaned. Progestin-only minipills can be used during lactation.

**11. Other disorders**–Psychologic depression may occur or be worsened with oral contraceptive use. Fluid retention may lead to worsening of cardiac, renal, or convulsive problems. Asthma may be worsened. Patients who had cholestatic jaundice during pregnancy may develop jaundice while taking birth control pills. Contact lens use may become more difficult.

**F. Minor Side Effects:** Nausea and dizziness may occur in the first few months of pill use. A weight gain of 2–5 lb commonly occurs. Spotting or break-through bleeding between menstrual periods may occur, especially if a pill is skipped or taken late; this may be helped by switching to a pill of slightly greater potency (see ¶ C, above). Missed menstrual periods may occur, especially with low-dose pills. A pregnancy test should be performed if pills have been skipped or if 2 or more menstrual periods are missed. Depression, fatigue, and decreased libido can occur. Chloasma may occur, as in pregnancy, and is increased by exposure to sunlight.

**Progestin Minipill**

**A. Efficacy and Methods of Use:** Formulations containing 0.35 mg of norethindrone or 0.075 mg of norgestrel are available in the USA. Their efficacy is slightly lower than that of combined oral contraceptives, with failure rates of 1–4% being reported. The minipill is believed to prevent conception by causing thickening of the cervical mucus to make it hostile to sperm, alteration of ovum transport (which may account for the higher rate of ectopic pregnancy with these pills), and inhibition of implantation. Ovulation is inhibited inconsistently with this method. The minipill is begun on the first day of a menstrual cycle and then taken continuously for as long as contraception is desired.

**B. Advantages:** The low dose and absence of estrogen make the minipill safe during lactation; it may increase the flow of milk. It is often tried by women who want minimal doses of hormones and by patients who are over age 35. The minipill can be used by women with uterine myomas or sickle cell disease (S/S or S/C). Like the combined pill, the minipill decreases the likelihood of pelvic inflammatory disease by its effect on cervical mucus.

**C. Complications and Contraindications:** Minipill users often have bleeding irregularities (eg, prolonged flow, spotting, or amenorrhea); such patients may need monthly pregnancy tests. Ectopic pregnancies are more frequent, and complaints of abdominal pain should be investigated with this in mind. The absolute contraindications and many of the relative contraindications listed in Table 13–4 apply to the minipill. Exceptions are mentioned in ¶ B, above. Minor side effects of combination oral contraceptives such as weight gain and mild headache may also occur with the minipill.

Corson SL (editor): Oral contraceptives: Minimizing metabolic risk. *J Reprod Med* 1986;**31(Suppl 9):**839.

Rosenfield A (editor): Update on oral contraceptives. *J Reprod Med* 1984;**29:**501.

## 2. CONTRACEPTIVE INJECTIONS & IMPLANTS (Long-Acting Progestins)

Injections of long-acting progestins such as medroxyprogesterone acetate or norethindrone enanthate are widely used in many countries. They are not approved for contraception in the USA because of FDA concerns about animal studies showing an increased incidence of associated breast and genital tract cancer. Injections are given at 3- to 6-month intervals. Pregnancy rates are as low as those of combined oral contraceptives taken conscientiously. Uterine bleeding may be irregular at first, and amenorrhea eventually occurs. Ovulation after the last injection may be delayed. Absolute and relative contraindications are similar to those of the minipill.

Norplant, a new contraceptive implant containing levonorgestrel, is available in Finland, Sweden, England, Thailand, and some other countries. Thirty micrograms of levonorgestrel is released daily from 6 subcutaneously placed rods. The system is effective for 5 years. Contraceptive efficacy is very high, but some patients request removal of the implants because of irregular bleeding.

Lopez G et al: Two-year prospective study in Columbia of Norplant implants. *Obstet Gynecol* 1986;**68**:204.

## 3. INTRAUTERINE DEVICES (IUDs)

The only IUD currently manufactured in the USA is the Progestasert (which secretes progesterone into the uterus), but copper-bearing IUDs (Copper-7 and Copper-T) are widely used in other countries, and some all-plastic IUDs (Lippes Loop) are also still in use. Failure rates of most IUDs are 2–4%; the mechanism of action is thought to be prevention of implantation.

The all-plastic IUDs do not need to be replaced at a specific time, and some women use them for 10 years or more. The copper-bearing IUDs are more suitable for a smaller uterus; they must be replaced every 3–4 years for maximum efficacy. The progesterone-secreting IUDs must be replaced yearly but have the advantage of causing decreased cramping and menstrual flow.

The IUD is often an excellent contraceptive method for parous women with one sexual partner. It is less desirable for young nulliparas because of the greater threat of pelvic inflammatory disease in young women and the possible impairment of future fertility.

### Insertion

Insertion can be performed during or after the menses, at midcycle to prevent implantation, or later in the cycle if the patient has not become pregnant. Immediate postpartum insertion with IUDs designed to minimize expulsion has been successful in some studies; most clinicians wait until 8 weeks postpartum. When insertion is performed during lactation, there is greater risk of uterine perforation or embedding of the IUD. Insertion immediately following abortion is acceptable if there is no sepsis and if follow-up insertion a month later will not be possible; otherwise, it is wise to wait until 4 weeks postabortion.

### Contraindications & Complications

Contraindications to use of IUDs are outlined in Table 13–7.

**A. Pregnancy:** An IUD can be inserted within 5 days following a single episode of unprotected midcycle coitus as a postcoital contraceptive. An IUD should not be inserted into a pregnant uterus. If pregnancy occurs as an IUD failure, there is a greater chance of spontaneous abortion if the IUD is left in situ (50%) than if it is removed (25%). Spontaneous abortion with an IUD in place is associated with a high risk of severe sepsis, and death can occur rapidly. Women using an IUD who become pregnant should have the IUD removed if the string is visible. It can be removed at the time of abortion if this is desired. If the string is not visible and the patient wants to continue the pregnancy, she should be informed of the serious risk of sepsis and, occasionally, death with such pregnancies. She should be informed that any flulike symptoms such as fever, myalgia, headache, or nausea warrant immediate medical attention for possible septic abortion.

Since the ratio of ectopic to intrauterine pregnancies is increased among IUD wearers, clinicians should search for adnexal masses in early pregnancy and should always check the products of conception for placental tissue following abortion.

**B. Pelvic Inflammatory Disease:** IUD use is associated with double the normal risk of pelvic inflammatory disease, and therefore the IUD should rarely be used by teenagers, women desiring more children, women with multiple sexual partners, and women with a past history of pelvic inflammatory disease or ectopic pregnancy. The IUD should never

**Table 13–7.** Contraindications to IUD use.

**Absolute contraindications**
 Pregnancy
 Acute or subacute pelvic inflammatory disease or purulent cervicitis

**Relative contraindications**
 Past history of pelvic inflammatory disease or ectopic pregnancy
 Multiple sexual partners
 Nulliparous woman concerned about future fertility
 Lack of available follow-up care
 Menorrhagia or severe dysmenorrhea
 Cervical or uterine neoplasia
 Abnormal size or shape of uterus, including myomas distorting cavity
 Valvular heart disease
 Diabetes

be inserted in the presence of cervicitis, endometritis, or salpingitis.

If pelvic infection develops, the signs and symptoms may be minimal at first. When infection is strongly suspected, the IUD should be removed and antibiotic treatment begun (see p 459). With pelvic pain in IUD users, it is wise to consider ectopic pregnancy in the differential diagnosis.

IUDs without transcervical tails appear to cause less pelvic inflammatory disease; however, they are more difficult to check at follow-up and require uterine instrumentation at removal.

**C. Menorrhagia or Severe Dysmenorrhea:** The IUD can cause heavier menstrual periods, bleeding between periods, and more cramping, so it is generally not suitable for women who already suffer from these problems. However, progesterone-secreting IUDs can be tried in these cases, as they often cause decreased bleeding and cramping with menses. Nonsteroidal anti-inflammatory drugs are also helpful in decreasing bleeding and pain in IUD users.

**D. Complete or Partial Expulsion:** Spontaneous expulsion of the IUD occurs in 10–20% of cases during the first year of use. Remove any IUD if the body of the device can be seen or felt in the cervical os.

**E. Missing IUD Strings:** If the transcervical tail cannot be seen, this may signify unnoticed expulsion, perforation of the uterus with abdominal migration of the IUD, or simply retraction of the string into the cervical canal or uterus owing to movement of the IUD or uterine growth with pregnancy. Once pregnancy is ruled out, one should probe for the IUD with a sterile sound or forceps designed for IUD removal, after administering a paracervical block. If the IUD cannot be detected, pelvic ultrasound will demonstrate the IUD if it is in the uterus. Alternatively, obtain anteroposterior and lateral x-rays of the pelvis with another IUD or a sound in the uterus as a marker, to confirm an extrauterine IUD. If the IUD is in the abdominal cavity, it should generally be removed by laparoscopy or laparatomy. Open-looped all-plastic IUDs such as the Lippes Loop can be left in the pelvis without danger, but ring-shaped IUDs may strangulate a loop of bowel and copper-bearing IUDs may cause tissue reaction and adhesions.

Perforations of the uterus are less likely if insertion is performed slowly, with meticulous care taken to follow directions applicable to each type of IUD.

Cramer DW et al: Tubal infertility and the intrauterine device. *N Engl J Med* 1985;**312**:941.

Tatum HG: Connell EB: A decade of intrauterine contraception: 1976–1986. *Fertil Steril* 1986;**46**:173.

## 4. DIAPHRAGM & CERVICAL CAP

The diaphragm (with contraceptive jelly) is a safe and effective contraceptive method with features that make it acceptable to some women and not others. Failure rates range from 2 to 20%, depending on the motivation of the woman and the care with which the diaphragm is used. The advantages of this method are that it has no systemic side effects and gives significant protection against pelvic infection and cervical dysplasia as well as pregnancy. The disadvantages are that it must be inserted near the time of coitus and that pressure from the rim predisposes some women to cystitis after intercourse.

The cervical cap (with contraceptive jelly) is similar to the diaphragm but fits snugly over the cervix only (the diaphragm stretches from behind the cervix to behind the pubic symphysis). The cervical cap is more difficult to insert and remove than the diaphragm and is associated with a higher failure rate. The main advantages are that it can be used by women who cannot be fitted for a diaphragm because of a relaxed anterior vaginal wall or by women who have discomfort or develop repeated bladder infections with the diaphragm.

Because of the small risk of toxic shock syndrome, a cervical cap or diaphragm should not be left in the vagina for over 12–18 hours, nor should these devices be used during the menstrual period (see above).

Koch JP: The Prentif contraceptive cervical cap: A contemporary study of its clinical safety and effectiveness. *Contraception* 1982;**25**:135.

## 5. CONTRACEPTIVE SPONGE, FOAM, CREAM, JELLY, & SUPPOSITORY

These products are available without prescription, are easy to use, and are fairly effective, with reported failure rates of 2–29%. All contain the spermicides nonoxynol 9 or octoxynol 9, which also have some virucidal and bactericidal activity. The contraceptive sponge is inserted before intercourse and can be used for repeated acts of intercourse but should not be left in the vagina for longer than 12–18 hours, because of the risk of toxic shock syndrome (see above). The sponge is considerably more effective in nulliparous women than in parous women. Foams, creams, jellies, and suppositories also have the advantages of being simple to use and easily available. Their disadvantage is a slightly higher failure rate than with the diaphragm or condom. Teratogenesis due to spermicides used at the time of conception has been studied, but no correlation has been proved.

McIntyre SL, Higgins JE: Parity and use effectiveness with the contraceptive sponge. *Am J Obstet Gynec* 1986;**155**:796.

## 6. CONDOM

The male sheath of rubber or animal membrane affords good protection against pregnancy—equivalent to that of a diaphragm and spermicidal jelly; it also offers protection against sexually transmitted disease and cervical dysplasia. Men and women seeking protection against AIDS transmission are advised to use a condom along with spermicide during vaginal or rectal intercourse. When a spermicide such as vaginal foam is used with the condom, the failure rate approaches that of oral contraceptives. Condoms coated with spermicide are now available in the USA. The disadvantages are dulling of sensation and sperm loss due to tearing, slipping, or leakage with detumescence of the penis.

## 7. CONTRACEPTION BASED ON AWARENESS OF FERTILE PERIODS

There is renewed interest in methods to identify times of ovulation and avoidance of unprotected intercourse at that time as a means of family planning. These methods are most effective when the couple restricts intercourse to the postovular phase of the cycle or uses a barrier method at other times. Women benefit from learning to identify their fertile periods. Well-instructed, motivated couples may achieve low pregnancy rates with fertility awareness, but in many field trials, the pregnancy rates were as high as 20%.

### "Symptothermal" Natural Family Planning

The basis for this approach is patient-observed increase in clear elastic cervical mucus, brief abdominal midcycle discomfort ("mittelschmerz"), and a sustained rise of the basal body temperature about 2 weeks after onset of menstruation. Unprotected intercourse is avoided from shortly after the menstrual period, when fertile mucus is first identified, until 48 hours after ovulation, as identified by a sustained rise in temperature and the disappearance of clear elastic mucus.

### Calendar Method

After the length of the menstrual cycle has been observed for at least 8 months, the following calculations are made: (1) The first fertile day is determined by subtracting 18 days from the shortest cycle; (2) the last fertile day is determined by subtracting 11 days from the longest cycle. For example, if the observed cycles run from 24 to 28 days, the fertile period would extend from the sixth day of the cycle (24 minus 18) through the 17th day (28 minus 11).

### Basal Body Temperature Method

This method indicates the safe time after ovulation has passed. The temperature must be taken immediately upon awakening, before any activity. A slight drop in temperature often occurs 1–1½ days before ovulation, and a rise of about 0.4 °C (0.7 °F) occurs 1–2 days after ovulation. The elevated temperature continues throughout the remainder of the cycle. The

second day after the rise marks the end of the fertile period.

Periodic abstinence: How well do new approaches work? Population Information Program, Johns Hopkins Univ (Sept) 1981;9:33.

## 8. POSTCOITAL CONTRACEPTION

If unprotected intercourse occurs in midcycle and the woman is certain she has not inadvertently become pregnant earlier in the cycle, the following regimens are effective in preventing implantation. The failure rate is less than 1.5%. These methods should be started within 72 hours after coitus. (1) Ethinyl estradiol, 2.5 mg twice daily for 5 days. (2) Ovral (50 $\mu$g of ethinyl estradiol with 0.5 mg of norgestrel), 2 tablets at once followed by 2 tablets 12 hours later. Antinausea medication may be necessary with these regimens. Bleeding should occur within 3–4 weeks. If pregnancy occurs, abortion is advisable because of fetal exposure to possibly teratogenic doses of sex steroids.

IUD insertion within 5 days after one episode of unprotected midcycle coitus will also prevent pregnancy; copper-bearing IUDs have been tested for this purpose. The disadvantage of this method is possible infection, especially in rape cases; the advantage is ongoing contraceptive protection if this is desired in a patient for whom the IUD is a suitable choice.

Yuzpe AA, Smith RP, Rademaker AW: A multicenter clinical investigation employing ethinyl estradiol combined with dlnorgestrel as a postcoital contraceptive agent. *Fertil Steril* 1982;37:508.

## 9. ABORTION

Since the legalization of abortion in the USA in 1973, the related maternal mortality rate has fallen markedly, because illegal and self-induced abortions have been replaced by safer medical procedures. Abortions in the first trimester of pregnancy are performed by vacuum aspiration under local anesthesia. A similar technique, dilatation and evacuation, is often used in the second trimester, with general or local anesthesia. Techniques utilizing intra-amniotic instillation of hypertonic saline solution or prostaglandins are also used after 15 weeks from the LMP. Abortions are rarely performed after 20 weeks from the LMP. It is currently believed that fetal viability begins at about 24 weeks. Legal abortion has a mortality rate of 1:100,000. Rates of morbidity and mortality rise with length of gestation. Currently in the USA, 90% of abortions are performed before 12 weeks' gestation and only 3–4% after 17 weeks. Every effort should be made to continue the trend toward earlier abortion.

Complications resulting from abortion include retained products of conception (often associated with infection and heavy bleeding) and unrecognized ectopic pregnancy. Immediate analysis of the removed tissue for placenta can exclude or corroborate the diagnosis of ectopic pregnancy. Women presenting with fever, bleeding, or abdominal pain after abortion should be examined; use of broad-spectrum antibiotics and reaspiration of the uterus are frequently necessary. Hospitalization is advisable if acute salpingitis requires intravenous administration of antibiotics (see p 460). Complications following illegal abortion often need emergency care for hemorrhage, septic shock, or uterine perforation.

Rh immune globulin should be given to all Rh-negative women following abortion. Contraception should be thoroughly discussed and contraceptive supplies or pills provided at the time of abortion.

Long-term sequelae of repeated induced abortions have been studied, but as yet there is no consensus on whether there are increased rates of fetal loss or premature labor. It is felt that such adverse sequelae can be minimized by performing early abortion with minimal cervical dilatation or by the use of *Laminaria* to induce gradual cervical dilatation.

Cates W: Legal abortion: The public health record. *Science* 1982;**215**:1586.

## 10. STERILIZATION

In the USA, sterilization is the most popular method of birth control for couples who want no more children. Although sterilization is reversible in some instances, reversal surgery in both men and women is costly, complicated, and not always successful. Therefore, patients should be counseled carefully before sterilization and should view the procedure as final.

Vasectomy is a safe, simple procedure in which the vas deferens is severed and sealed through a scrotal incision under local anesthesia. Long-term follow-up studies on vasectomized men show no excess risk of heart disease, cancer, or immune system problems.

Female sterilization is currently performed via laparoscopic bipolar electrocoagulation or plastic ring application of the uterine tubes or via minilaparotomy with Pomeroy tubal resection. The advantages of laparoscopy are minimal postoperative pain, small incisions, and rapid recovery. The advantages of minilaparotomy are that it can be performed with standard surgical instruments under local or general anesthesia. However, there is more postoperative pain and a longer recovery period. Failure rates after tubal sterilization are approximately 0.5%; this fact should be discussed with women preoperatively. There are recent reports that menstrual irregularities may increase after sterilization by unipolar tubal coagulation, but probably not after other techniques.

DeStefano F et al: Long-term risk of menstrual disturbances after tubal sterilization. *Am J Obstet Gynecol* 1985;**152**:835.

Petitti DB et al: Vasectomy and the incidence of hospitalized illness. *J Urol* 1983;**129**:760.

## RAPE

Rape, or sexual assault, is legally defined in different ways in various jurisdictions. Physicians and emergency room personnel who deal with rape victims should be familiar with the laws pertaining to sexual assault in their own state. From a medical and psychologic viewpoint, it is essential that persons treating rape victims recognize the nonconsensual and violent nature of the crime. About 95% of reported rape victims are women. Penetration may be vaginal, anal, or oral and may be by the penis, hand, or a foreign object. The absence of genital injury does not imply consent by the victim.

"Unlawful sexual intercourse," or statutory rape, is intercourse with a female before the age of majority even with her consent.

Rape represents an expression of anger, power, and sexuality on the part of the rapist. The rapist is usually a hostile man who uses sexual intercourse to terrorize and humiliate a woman. Women neither secretly want to be raped, nor do they expect, encourage, or enjoy rape.

Rape involves severe physical injury in 5–10% of cases and is always a terrifying experience in which most victims fear for their lives. Consequently, all victims suffer some psychologic aftermath. Moreover, some may acquire sexually transmissible disease or become pregnant.

Because rape is a personal crisis, each patient will react differently. The rape-trauma syndrome comprises 2 principal phases:

(1) Immediate or acute–Shaking, sobbing, and restless activity may last from a few days to a few weeks. The patient may experience anger, guilt, shame, and fear of revenge or may repress these emotions. Reactions vary depending on the victim's personality and the circumstances of the attack.

(2) Late or chronic–Problems related to the attack may develop weeks or months later. The life-style and work patterns of the individual may change. Sleep disorders or phobias often develop. Loss of self-esteem can rarely lead to suicide.

Physicians and emergency room personnel who deal with rape victims should work with community rape crisis centers whenever possible to provide ongoing supportive, skilled counseling.

### General Office Procedures

The physician who first sees the alleged rape victim should be empathetic. Begin with a statement such as, "This is a terrible thing that has happened to you. I want to help."

(1) Secure written consent from the patient, guardian, or next of kin for gynecologic examination; for photographs if they are likely to be useful as evidence; and for notification of police. If police are to be

notified, do so, and obtain advice on the transfer of evidence.

(2) Obtain and record the history in the patient's own words. The sequence of events, ie, the time, place, and circumstances, must be included. Note the date of the LMP, whether or not the woman is pregnant, and the time of the most recent coitus prior to the sexual assault. Note the details of the assault such as body cavities penetrated, use of foreign objects, and number of assailants.

Note whether the alleged victim is calm, agitated, or confused (drugs or alcohol may be involved). Record whether the patient came directly to the hospital or whether she bathed or changed her clothing. Record findings but do not issue even a tentative diagnosis lest it be erroneous or incomplete. Do not use the word "rape" in the recorded history.

(3) Have the patient disrobe while standing on a white sheet. Hair, dirt, and leaves; underclothing; and any torn or stained clothing should be kept as evidence. Scrape material from beneath fingernails and comb pubic hair for evidence. Place all evidence in separate clean paper bags or envelopes and label carefully.

(4) Examine the patient, noting any traumatized areas that should be photographed. Examine the body and genitals with a Wood light to identify semen, which fluoresces; positive areas should be swabbed with a premoistened swab and air-dried in order to identify acid phosphatase from prostatic secretions.

(5) Perform a pelvic examination, explaining all procedures and obtaining the patient's consent before proceeding gently with the examination. (In children, general anesthesia may be necessary during the pelvic examination or for repair of vaginal lacerations.) Use a narrow speculum lubricated with water only. Collect material with sterile cotton swabs from the vaginal walls and cervix and make 2 air-dried smears on clean glass slides. Swab the mouth (around molars and cheeks) and anus in the same way, if appropriate. Label all slides carefully. Collect secretions from the vagina, anus, or mouth with a premoistened cotton swab, place at once on a slide with a drop of saline, and cover with a coverslip. Look for motile or nonmotile sperm under high, dry magnification, and record the percentage of motile forms.

(6) Perform appropriate laboratory tests as follows. Culture the vagina, anus, or mouth (as appropriate) for *N gonorrhoeae* and *Chlamydia*. Perform a Papanicolaou smear of the cervix, a baseline pregnancy test, and VDRL test. Repeat the pregnancy test if the next menses is missed, and repeat the VDRL test in 6 weeks. Obtain blood (10 mL without anticoagulant) and urine (100 mL) specimens if there is a history of forced ingestion or injection of drugs or alcohol.

(7) Transfer clearly labeled evidence, eg, laboratory specimens, directly to the clinical pathologist in charge or to the responsible laboratory technician, in the presence of witnesses (never via messenger), so that the rules of evidence will not be breached.

## Treatment

(1) Give analgesics or tranquilizers if indicated.

(2) Administer tetanus toxoid if deep lacerations contain soil or dirt particles.

(3) Give prophylactic probenecid, 1 g orally, and 30 minutes later aqueous penicillin G, 4.8 million units intramuscularly, to prevent syphilis and gonorrhea. In addition, give tetracycline, 500 mg 4 times daily for 7 days, or doxycycline, 100 mg twice daily for 7 days, to increase the efficacy of treatment against penicillin-resistant gonococci and to treat chlamydial infection.

(4) Prevent pregnancy by using one of the methods discussed under Postcoital Contraception, if necessary (see above).

(5) Make sure the patient and her family and friends have a source of ongoing psychologic support.

Glaser JB, Hammerschlag MR, McCormack WM: Sexually transmitted diseases in victims of sexual assault. *New England J Med* 1986;**313**:625.

Hicks DJ: Rape: Sexual assault. *Am J Obstet Gynecol* 1980;**137**:931.

# MENOPAUSAL SYNDROME

## Essentials of Diagnosis

- Cessation of menses due to aging or to bilateral oophorectomy.
- Elevation of FSH and LH levels.
- Hot flushes and night sweats (in 80% of women).
- Decreased vaginal lubrication; thinned vaginal mucosa with or without dyspareunia.

## General Considerations

The term "menopause" refers to the final cessation of menstruation, either as a normal part of aging or as the result of surgical removal of both ovaries. In a broader sense, as the term is commonly used, it denotes a 1- to 3-year period during which a woman adjusts to a diminishing and then absent menstrual flow and the physiologic changes that may be associated—hot flushes, night sweats, and vaginal dryness or soreness with coitus.

The average age at menopause in Western societies today is 51 years. Premature menopause is defined as ovarian failure and menstrual cessation before age 40; this often has a genetic or autoimmune basis. Surgical menopause due to bilateral oophorectomy is common and can cause more severe symptoms owing to the sudden rapid drop in sex hormone levels.

There is no objective evidence that cessation of ovarian function is associated with increased emotional disturbance or personality changes. However, the time of menopause often coincides with other major life changes, such as departure of children from home, a midlife identity crisis, or divorce. These events, coupled with a sense of the loss of youth, may exacerbate the symptoms of menopause and cause psychologic distress.

## Clinical Findings

### A. Symptoms and Signs:

**1. Cessation of menstruation**–Menstrual cycles generally become irregular as menopause approaches. Anovular cycles occur more often, with irregular cycle length and occasional menorrhagia. Menstrual flow usually diminishes in amount owing to decreased estrogen secretion, resulting in less abundant endometrial growth. Finally, cycles become longer, with missed periods or episodes of spotting only. When no bleeding has occurred for one year, the menopausal transition can be said to have occurred. Any bleeding after this time warrants investigation by endometrial curettage or aspiration to rule out endometrial cancer.

**2. Hot flushes**–Hot flushes (feelings of intense heat over the trunk and face, with flushing of the skin and sweating) occur in 80% of women as a result of the sudden decrease in ovarian hormones. An increase in pulsatile release of gonadotropin-releasing hormone from the hypothalamus is believed to trigger the hot flushes by affecting the adjacent temperature-regulating area of the brain. Hot flushes are more severe in women who undergo surgical menopause. Flushing is more pronounced late in the day, during hot weather, after ingestion of hot foods or drinks, or during periods of tension. Occurring at night, they often cause sweating and insomnia and result in fatigue on the following day.

**3. Dyspareunia**–With decreased estrogen secretion, thinning of the vaginal mucosa and decreased vaginal lubrication occur and may lead to dyspareunia. The introitus decreases in diameter. Pelvic examination reveals pale, smooth vaginal mucosa and a small cervix and uterus. The ovaries are not normally palpable after the menopause. Continued sexual activity will help prevent tissue shrinkage; use of lubricants, estrogen or testosterone cream, or oral estrogen therapy can prevent or relieve pain.

**4. Osteoporosis**–Osteoporosis may occur as a late sequela of menopause, with about 25% of women eventually developing fractures or loss of height and back pain due to vertebral compression. Hip and vertebral fractures with ensuing complications are significant causes of morbidity in elderly women. Risk factors for osteoporosis are listed in Table 13–8. Osteoporosis can be prevented or halted by hormone replacement therapy; exercise, calcium therapy, and other changes in life-style also play a role in prevention and treatment.

### B. Laboratory Findings:
Vaginal cytologic examination will show a low estrogen effect with predominantly parabasal cells. Serum FSH and LH levels are elevated.

## Treatment

### A. Natural Menopause:
Education and support from health providers, midlife discussion groups, and reading material will help most women having difficulty adjusting to the menopause. Physiologic symptoms can be treated as follows:

**Table 13–8.** Risk factors for osteoporosis.

| Genetic or Medical Factors | Life-style Factors |
|---|---|
| All races except blacks | High alcohol use |
| Previous fractures not due to major trauma | Smoking |
| Female relatives with osteoporosis | Lack of exercise |
| Thin body habitus | Low dietary intake of calcium |
| Early menopause (before age 40) | Lack of vitamin D |
| Inflammatory bowel disease; bowel resection | High-protein or high-salt diet (promotes calciuria) |
| Prolonged use of corticosteroids, phenytoin, aluminum-containing antacids, or high doses of thyroid | High caffeine use (more than 5 cups of coffee daily) |
| Chronic renal failure | |

**1. Vasomotor symptoms**–Give conjugated estrogens, 0.3 mg or 0.625 mg (or ethinyl estradiol, 0.02 mg; estradiol, 1 mg; or estrone sulfate 0.625 mg) from day 1 to day 25 of each calendar month. Alternatively, estradiol can be given transdermally as skin patches that are changed twice weekly and secrete 0.05–0.1 mg of hormone daily (Estraderm). Use from day 1 to day 25 of the calendar month. When either form of estrogen is used, add a progestin (medroxyprogesterone acetate, 10 mg, or norethindrone acetate, 2.5–5 mg) on days 16–25, to prevent endometrial hyperplasia or cancer. Withhold hormones from day 26 until the end of the month, when the endometrium will be shed, producing a light, generally painless monthly period. If the patient has had a hysterectomy, a progestin need not be used. Explain to the patient that hot flushes will probably return if the hormone is discontinued. When women wish to stop hormone therapy, the dose should be tapered.

Clonidine, an α-adrenergic agonist, has been found to be effective in reducing hot flashes when given orally in doses of 100–150 μg daily. Side effects include dry mouth, drowsiness, and blood pressure decrease, but the effects are usually mild at these low dosages. Transdermal clonidine may soon be available.

**2. Dyspareunia**–This problem can be treated with hormone therapy as outlined above. Alternatively, topical use of hormone creams in small doses will often relieve pain with minimal systemic absorption. Use conjugated estrogen vaginal cream, one-eighth applicatorful (0.3 mg of conjugated estrogen) nightly for 7–10 nights. Thereafter, use every other night or twice weekly. Dienestrol cream can also be used. Testosterone propionate 1–2% in a vanishing cream base used in the same manner is also effective if estrogen is contraindicated. A bland lubricant such as unscented cold cream or water-soluble gel can be helpful at the time of coitus.

**3. Osteoporosis**–Women should ingest at least 800 mg of calcium daily throughout life. In addition, 1 g of elemental calcium (as calcium carbonate) should be taken as a daily supplement at the time of the menopause and thereafter. Vitamin D, 400 IU/d from food, sunlight, or supplements is necessary to enhance calcium absorption. A daily program of energetic

**Table 13–9.** Contraindications to estrogen therapy.

| |
|---|
| Cancer of the breast or uterus |
| Estrogen-dependent ovarian cancer |
| History of thromboembolic disease |
| Diabetes |
| Hepatic adenoma or other significant liver disease |
| Gallstones or gallbladder disease |
| Large uterine myomas |

walking or other physical exercise helps maintain bone mass. CT scans and photon absorptiometry will detect demineralization of the vertebral bodies and cortical bone, but both tests are expensive. At present, factors indicated in Table 13–8 are generally used to identify patients most in need of hormone therapy. Dosage is usually the same as for treatment of vasomotor symptoms. Regular follow-up is needed with ongoing treatment.

**B. Surgical Menopause:** The abrupt hormonal decrease resulting from oophorectomy generally results in severe vasomotor symptoms and rapid onset of dyspareunia and osteoporosis unless treated. Estrogen replacement is generally started immediately after surgery. Conjugated estrogen, 1.25 mg (or ethinyl estradiol 0.05 mg, or estrone sulfate, 1.25 mg), is given for 25 days of each month. After age 45–50 years, this dose can be tapered to 0.625 mg of conjugated estrogen or equivalent.

**C. Contraindications to Estrogen Therapy:** Women with conditions listed in Table 13–9 should generally not use estrogen. Progestins can be substituted in some cases but are not advisable for patients with diabetes or circulatory disease. At present, there is little evidence that postmenopausal estrogens are associated with breast cancer development. Estrogens must be given with progestins as outlined above in women who have a uterus, to avoid endometrial cancer. Most authorities believe that estrogen in low doses will retard atherosclerosis by raising high-density lipoprotein levels, but progestins have the opposite effect. Since estrogen doubles the risk of gallbladder disease necessitating cholecystectomy, its use in women with gallstones or a history of cholecystitis

is unwise. Estrogen causes growth of uterine myomas, which otherwise shrink after the menopause.

Deutsch S, Ossowski R, Benjamin I: Comparison between degree of systemic absorption of vaginally and orally administered estrogens at different dose levels in postmenopausal women. *Am J Obstet Gynecol* 1981;**139:**967.

Ettinger B, Genant HK, Cann CE: Postmenopausal bone loss is prevented by treatment with low-dosage estrogen with calcium. *Ann Intern Med* 1987;**106:**40.

Padwick ML, Endacott J, Whitehead MI: Efficacy, acceptability, and metabolic effects of transdermal estradiol in the management of postmenopausal women. *Am J Obstet Gynecol* 1985;**152:**1085.

# OBSTETRICS

## DIAGNOSIS & DIFFERENTIAL DIAGNOSIS OF PREGNANCY

It is advantageous to diagnose pregnancy as promptly as possible when a sexually active woman misses a menstrual period or has symptoms suggestive of pregnancy. In the event of a wanted pregnancy, she can begin prenatal care early and discontinue use of recreational drugs (eg, alcohol, tobacco, marihuana) or potentially teratogenic medication in the critical weeks of embryogenesis in the first trimester. In the event of an unwanted pregnancy, she can consider termination of the pregnancy at an early stage.

### Pregnancy Tests

Currently available tests (Table 13–10) permit very early diagnosis of pregnancy, sometimes even before the time of the missed menses. All urine or blood tests rely on the detection of hCG produced by the placenta. hCG levels increase shortly after implantation, double approximately every 48 hours, reach a peak at 50–75 days, and fall to lower levels in the second and third trimesters. The older slide tests for

**Table 13–10.** Selected diagnostic tests for pregnancy.

| Test | Sensitivity (in mIU of hCG/mL) | Comments |
|---|---|---|
| Slide test with urine | 1000–3000 | Hemagglutination (or agglutination) inhibition tests to detect hCG. Convenient for office use. Quick and inexpensive. Accurate 4 weeks after conception. May cross-react with LH. Proteinuria, opiates, and psychotropic drugs may give false-positive results. |
| Tube test with urine | 175–250 | As above. May be accurate 2–4 weeks after conception. May cross-react with LH. |
| Monoclonal antibody test with urine | 20–50 | Colorimetric test. Some designed for home use. Accurate 2–4 weeks after conception. Specific for hCG. |
| Radioimmunoassay (RIA) | 5 | Some tests accurate 1 week after conception. Specific for hCG. Also used for quantitative assays in abnormal pregnancies (molar, ectopic, threatened abortion.) |

pregnancy, which are of lower sensitivity, become accurate 7–10 days after the missed period. Most laboratories (and newer home pregnancy tests) now use monoclonal antibodies specific for hCG; these tests are performed on urine or serum and are accurate at the time of the missed period or shortly after it, depending on their sensitivity.

Compared with intrauterine pregnancies, ectopic pregnancies may show lower levels of hCG, which level off or fall in serial determinations. Quantitative assays of hCG repeated at 48- to 72-hour intervals are used in the diagnosis of ectopic pregnancy, as well as in cases of molar pregnancy, threatened abortion, and missed abortion. Comparison of hCG levels between laboratories may be misleading in a given patient because different international standards produce results that vary by a factor or two.

## Manifestations of Pregnancy

The following symptoms and signs are usually due to pregnancy, but none are diagnostic. A record or history of time and frequency of coitus may be of considerable value.

**A. Symptoms:** Amenorrhea, nausea and vomiting, breast tenderness and tingling, urinary frequency and urgency, "quickening" (may be noted at about the 18th week), weight gain.

**B. Signs (in Weeks From LMP):** Breast changes (enlargement, vascular engorgement, colostrum), abdominal enlargement, cyanosis of vagina and cervical portio (about the seventh week), softening of the cervix (seventh week), softening of the cervicouterine junction (eighth week), generalized enlargement and diffuse softening of the corpus (after eighth week).

By 14–15 weeks from the LMP, the uterine fundus is palpable above the pubic symphysis, and by 20–22 weeks, it has reached the umbilicus. By 28 weeks it is usually halfway between the umbilicus and the xiphoid process, and by 38 weeks it has reached the xiphoid process. The fetal heart can be heard at the end of the first trimester with an ultrasonic stethoscope and by 20 weeks with an ordinary fetoscope.

## Differential Diagnosis

The nonpregnant uterus enlarged by myomas can be confused with the gravid uterus, but it is usually very firm and irregular. An ovarian tumor may be found midline, displacing the nonpregnant uterus to the side or posteriorly. Ultrasonography and a pregnancy test will help make an accurate diagnosis in these circumstances.

## ESSENTIALS OF PRENATAL CARE

The first prenatal visit, occurring as early as possible after the diagnosis of pregnancy, should include the following:

## History

Age, ethnic background, occupation. Onset of LMP and its normality, possible conception dates, bleeding after LMP, medical history, all prior pregnancies (duration, outcome, and complications), symptoms of present pregnancy. Use of drugs, alcohol, tobacco, caffeine, nutritional habits. Family history of congenital anomalies and heritable diseases.

## Physical Examination

Height, weight, blood pressure, general physical examination. Abdominal and pelvic examination: (1) estimate uterine size or measure fundal height; (2) evaluate bony pelvis for symmetry and adequacy; (3) evaluate cervix for infection, effacement, dilatation; (4) detect fetal heart sounds with Doppler device (or ultrasound) after 10 weeks from LMP if fetal demise is suspected because of uterine bleeding or inadequate uterine growth.

## Laboratory Tests

Urinalysis, complete blood count with red cell indices, serologic test for syphilis; rubella antibody titer, blood group, Rh type, and atypical antibody screening. If indicated clinically, cervical cultures for *Neisseria gonorrhoeae* and *Chlamydia;* Papanicolaou smear of the cervix, culture for herpes simplex if suspicious lesions seen. Hemoglobin electrophoresis for anemic black (Hgb S, C, F) and Asian women (Hgb $A_2$); HBsAg and HBeAg for women from Asia and Africa. Women at high risk of carrying the AIDS virus should be offered confidential HIV antibody studies (intravenous drug users, prostitutes, partners of AIDS-ARC patients, women from Haiti or Africa, recipients of transfusions from 1978 to 1985). Tuberculosis skin tests when indicated. Chorionic villus sampling at 9–12 weeks or amniocentesis at 16 weeks from LMP if patient is over 35 or has had prior offspring with chromosomal abnormality; Tay-Sachs blood screening for Jewish women with Jewish partners.

## Advice to Patients

A. Take no medications unless prescribed by a doctor or a registered midwife.

B. Avoid x-rays unless they are essential; inform the dentist or radiologist of pregnancy.

C. Avoid all street drugs, alcohol, and tobacco.

D. Decrease caffeine to 0–1 cup of coffee or tea daily.

E. Avoid eating raw or rare meat. Wash hands after handling raw meat.

F. Pay attention to good nutrition and take prenatal vitamins with iron and folate as directed. Do not diet to lose weight. Plan to gain about 11kg during pregnancy.

G. Get adequate daily rest; avoid exhausting work.

H. Do not work where there are chemical or radiation hazards.

I. Avoid excessive heat in saunas or hot tubs.

J. Perform mild to moderate exercises daily; avoid exhausting or hazardous exercise or new athletic training programs.

K. Enroll with your partner in a class on preparation for childbirth.

## Schedule of Prenatal Visits for Normal Pregnancy

Up to 28 weeks: every 4 weeks.
Up to 36 weeks: every 2 weeks.
36 weeks to delivery: weekly.

## Tests & Procedures in Second & Third Trimesters

**A. Each Visit:** Weight, blood pressure, fundal height, fetal heart rate, urine specimen for protein and sugar. Fetal position. Review of patient's concerns about pregnancy; health and nutritional advice.

**B. 15–18 Weeks:** Genetic amniocentesis for women over 35; or with family history of congenital anomalies; or with previous child with chromosomal abnormality, errors of metabolism, or neural tube defect; or with history of repeated spontaneous abortions.

**C. 16–18 Weeks:** Alpha-fetoprotein (AFP) determination on maternal blood in patients with history of fetuses with neural tube defects and in diabetics. In some states, this test may become mandatory for all women.

**D. 14–26 Weeks:** Ultrasound examination (if needed) for determining pregnancy duration (most accurate in second trimester).

**E. 24–28 Weeks:** Oral glucose tolerance test with 50 g glucose and 1-hour blood sugar (< 140mg/dL is normal) to screen for gestational diabetes.

**F. 28 Weeks:** Rh immunoglobulin for unsensitized Rh-negative patients.

**G. 28 Weeks On:** Ultrasound examination for suspected intrauterine growth retardation (most accurate after 28 weeks); repeat every 3–4 weeks to assess changes. Ultrasound examination near term or postterm may be used for suspected macrosomia.

**H. 28–32 Weeks:** Repeat complete blood count.

**I. 36 Weeks to Delivery:** Careful assessment of the presenting part to diagnose breech presentations so that external version with the aid of tocolytic drugs can be accomplished after labor. Weekly vaginal examination to determine cervical ripeness and descent of presenting part. Weekly speculum examination to culture for genital herpes infection if active infection is suspected. At 38 weeks, culture the cervix for group B β-hemolytic streptococci; if positive, treat mother in labor.

**J. Postterm to Beyond 41 Weeks:** Review dates and milestones of pregnancy. Evaluate cervical status. Perform nonstress tests twice weekly and obtain ultrasound profile for fetal weight, breathing, and limb movements; fetal position and body tone; and amniotic fluid volume (biophysical profile). Perform ultrasound-directed amniocentesis for lung maturity tests and the presence of meconium. Consider

**Table 13–11.** Common drugs that are teratogenic or fetotoxic.*

| | |
|---|---|
| Alcohol | Antidiabetics |
| Amebicides | Oral hypoglycemics |
| Carbarsone | Antihypertensives |
| Analgesics and antipyretics | Diazoxide, thiazide diuretics, reserpine |
| Aspirin and other salicylates (in third trimester); narcotics (prolonged use) | Antineoplastics |
| | All agents |
| | Antithyroid drugs |
| Antibiotics | Radioiodine, propylthiouracil, methimazole |
| Kanamycin, streptomycin, tetracyclines, trimethoprim, sulfonamides (in third trimester) | Disulfiram (Antabuse) |
| | Hormones |
| Anticoagulants | Estrogens, diethylstilbestrol, progestins, androgens |
| Warfarin, dicumarol and other coumarin derivatives | Isotretinoin (Accutane) |
| | Nonsteroidal anti-inflammatory drugs in third trimester |
| Anticonvulsants | Psychoactive drugs |
| Aminoglutethimide, ethotoin, phenytoin, paramethadione, trimethadione, valproic acid | Lithium, benzodiazepines, amitriptyline |
| | Tobacco smoking |

* Additional drugs may also be contraindicated during pregnancy. Evaluate any drug for its need and its potential adverse effects.

induction of labor during confirmed 42nd week of gestation.

Guinan ME, Hardy A: Epidemiology of AIDS in women in the United States. *JAMA* 1987;**257**:2039.
Manning FA et al: Fetal biophysical profile score and the non-stress test: A comparative trial. *Obstet Gynecol* 1984;**64**:326.
Stillman RJ et al: Smoking and reproduction. *Fertil Steril* 1986;**46**:545.

## NUTRITION IN PREGNANCY

Nutrition in pregnancy significantly affects maternal health and infant size and well-being. Pregnant women should have nutrition counseling early in prenatal care and access to supplementary food programs if they lack funds for adequate nutrition. Counseling should stress abstention from alcohol, smoking, and drugs. Caffeine and artificial sweeteners should be used only in small amounts. "Empty calories" should be avoided, and the diet should contain the following foods: protein foods of animal and vegetable origin; milk and milk products; whole-grain cereals and breads; and fruits and vegetables, especially green leafy vegetables.

Weight gain in pregnancy should be at least 11kg, which includes the added weight of the fetus, placenta, and amniotic fluid and of maternal reproductive tissues, fluid, blood, increased fat stores, and increased lean body mass. Maternal fat stores are a caloric reserve for pregnancy and lactation; weight restriction in pregnancy to avoid developing such fat stores may affect the development of other fetal and maternal tissues and is not advisable. Obese women can have adequate-sized infants with less weight gain but should be encouraged to eat high-quality foods. Normally, a pregnant woman gains 1–2 kg in the first trimester and slightly less than 0.5 kg/wk thereafter. She needs approximately an extra 200–300 kcal/d (depending on energy output) and 30 g/d of additional protein, for a total protein intake of about 75 g/d. Appropriate caloric intake in pregnancy helps prevent infants of low birth weight.

Rigid salt restriction is not necessary. While the consumption of highly salted snack foods and prepared foods is not desirable, 2–3 g/d of sodium is permissible. The increased calcium needs of pregnancy (1200 mg/d) can be met with milk, milk products, green vegetables, soybean products, corn tortillas, and calcium carbonate supplements.

The increased need for iron and folic acid should be met from foods as well as vitamin and mineral supplements. (See section on anemia in pregnancy.) Megavitamins should not be taken in pregnancy, as they may result in fetal malformation or disturbed metabolism. However, a balanced prenatal supplement containing 30–60 mg of elemental iron, 0.5–0.8 mg of folate, and the recommended daily allowances of various vitamins and minerals is widely used in the USA and is probably beneficial to many women with marginal diets. There is some evidence that periconceptional vitamin supplements decrease the risk of neural tube defects in the fetus. Lactovegetarians and ovolactovegetarians do well in pregnancy; vegetarian women who eat neither eggs nor milk products should have their diets assessed for adequate calories and protein and should take oral vitamin $B_{12}$ supplements during pregnancy and lactation.

Abrams BF, Laros RK: Prepregnancy weight, weight gain, and birth weight. *Am J Obstet Gynecol* 1986;**154**:503.
Susser M: Prenatal nutrition, birth weight, and psychological development: An overview of experiments, quasi experiments and natural experiments in the past decade. *Am J Clin Nutr* 1981;**34**:784.

## VOMITING OF PREGNANCY
(Morning Sickness)
## & HYPEREMESIS GRAVIDARUM
(Pernicious Vomiting of Pregnancy)

Morning or evening nausea and vomiting usually begin soon after the first missed period and cease after the fourth to fifth months of gestation. At least half of women, most of them primiparas, complain of nausea and vomiting during early pregnancy. This problem exerts no adverse effects on the pregnancy and does not presage other complications, though it is common with multiple pregnancy and hydatidiform mole. Persistent severe vomiting during pregnancy—hyperemesis gravidarum—can be disabling and require hospitalization. Dehydration, acidosis, and nutritional deficiencies may develop with protracted vomiting.

The cause of vomiting during pregnancy is believed to be high estrogen levels.

### Treatment
**A. Mild Nausea and Vomiting of Pregnancy:** Reassurance and dietary advice are all that is required in most instances. Frequent small meals of nutritious, easily digested low-fat foods should be suggested. Begin prenatal vitamin and mineral supplements as soon as tolerated.

Because of possible teratogenicity, drugs used during the first half of pregnancy should be restricted to those of major importance to life and health. Antiemetics, antihistamines, and antispasmodics are generally unnecessary to treat nausea of pregnancy. Vitamin $B_6$ (pyridoxine), 50–100 mg/d orally, is nontoxic and may be helpful in some patients.

**B. Hyperemesis Gravidarum:** Hospitalize the patient in a private room at bed rest. Give nothing by mouth for 48 hours, and maintain hydration and electrolyte balance by giving appropriate parenteral fluids and vitamin supplements as indicated. Rarely, total parenteral nutrition may become necessary. As soon as possible, place the patient on a dry diet consisting of 6 small feedings daily with clear liquids 1 hour after eating. Prochlorperazine rectal suppositories may be useful, and psychosocial consultation is advisable. After stabilization in the hospital, the patient can be maintained at home even if she requires intravenous fluids in addition to her oral intake.

## SPONTANEOUS ABORTION

### Essentials of Diagnosis

- Vaginal bleeding in a pregnant woman before the 20th week of gestation.
- Uterine cramping.
- Disappearance of symptoms and signs of pregnancy.
- Negative or equivocal pregnancy tests.
- The products of conception may or may not be expelled.

### General Considerations

Abortion is defined as termination of gestation before the 20th week of pregnancy. About three-fourths of spontaneous abortions occur before the 16th week of gestation; of these, three-fourths occur before the eighth week. About 15% of all clinically recognized pregnancies terminate in spontaneous abortion.

More than 60% of spontaneous abortions result from ovular defects due to maternal or paternal factors; about 15% are caused by maternal trauma, infections, dietary deficiencies, diabetes mellitus, hypothyroidism, or anatomic malformations. There is no reliable evidence that abortion may be induced by psychic stimuli such as severe fright, grief, anger, or anxiety. In about one-fourth of cases, the cause of abortion cannot be determined.

It is important to identify those cases of late abortion (after 16 weeks) that result from cervical incompetence, since this is treatable. Often these women will have a history of late abortions associated with spontaneous rupture of the membranes and minimal labor. Some will have a history of wide cervical dilatation during D&C. In the nonpregnant state, an incompetent cervix will easily admit a dilator 8 mm in diameter.

### Clinical Findings

**A. Symptoms and Signs:**

**1. Threatened abortion**–Bleeding or cramping occurs, but the pregnancy continues.

**2. Inevitable abortion**–The passage of some or all of the products of conception is impending. Bleeding and cramping persist, and the cervix is effaced and dilated.

**3. Complete abortion**–All of the conceptus is expelled. The fetus and the placenta may be expelled separately. When the entire conceptus has been expelled, pain ceases but spotting persists.

**4. Incomplete abortion**–A significant portion of the pregnancy (usually a placental fragment) remains in the uterus. Only mild cramps are reported, but bleeding is persistent and often excessive.

**5. Missed abortion**–The pregnancy has ceased to develop for at least 1 month, but the conceptus has not been expelled. Symptoms of pregnancy disappear. There is a brownish vaginal discharge but no free bleeding. Pain does not develop. The cervix is semifirm and slightly patulous; the uterus becomes smaller and irregularly softened; the adnexa are normal.

**B. Laboratory Findings:** Pregnancy tests show low or falling levels of hCG. A complete blood count should be obtained if bleeding is heavy. Determine Rh type, and give Rh immune globulin if the type is Rh-negative. All tissue recovered should be assessed by a pathologist.

**C. Ultrasonographic Findings:** An expert ultrasonographer can identify a gestational sac at 6 weeks from the LMP and a fetal pole at 7 weeks. Serial observations are often required to evaluate changes in size. A small, irregular sac without a fetal pole is diagnostic of a failing pregnancy.

### Differential Diagnosis

The bleeding that occurs in abortion of a uterine pregnancy must be differentiated from the abnormal bleeding of an ectopic pregnancy and anovular bleeding in a nonpregnant woman. The passage of hydropic villi in the bloody discharge is diagnostic of the abortion of a hydatidiform mole.

### Complications

Hemorrhage in abortion is a major cause of maternal death. Infection is common after illegally induced abortion or spontaneous abortion associated with an IUD.

### Treatment

**A. General Measures:**

1. Threatened abortion requires 24–48 hours of bed rest followed by gradual resumption of usual activities, with abstinence from coitus and douching. Hormonal treatment is contraindicated. Antibiotics should be used only if there are signs of infection.

2. Missed abortion requires counseling regarding the fate of the pregnancy and planning for its elective termination at a time chosen by the patient and physician. Insertion of *Laminaria* stems to dilate the cervix followed by aspiration is the method of choice. Prostaglandin vaginal suppositories are an effective alternative.

**B. Emergency Measures:**

1. Incomplete abortion requires prompt removal of any products of conception remaining within the uterus. Analgesia and a paracervical block are useful, followed by uterine exploration with ovum forceps or uterine aspiration.

2. If shock is present, intravenous fluids or blood may be necessary, as well as other intensive care measures.

3. Uterine contraction to expel clots and tissue may be stimulated by oxytocin infusion (40 units in 1000 mL of intravenous fluid). If the uterus is empty,

0.2 mg of methylergonovine maleate (Methergine) may be used to induce uterine spasm.

**C. Surgical Measures:** In the second trimester of pregnancy, an incompetent cervix can be closed by cerclage using a 5-mm woven Dacron strip (Shirodkar method) or circumsuture with braided silk (McDonald method).

## RECURRENT (HABITUAL) ABORTION

Recurrent, or habitual, abortion has been defined for years as the loss of 3 or more previable (< 500 g) pregnancies in succession. Recurrent or chronic abortion occurs in about 0.4–0.8% of all pregnancies. Abnormalities related to repeated abortion can be identified in approximately half of the couples. If a woman has lost 3 previous pregnancies without identifiable cause, she still has a 70–80% chance of carrying a fetus to viability. If she has aborted 4 or 5 times, the likelihood of a successful pregnancy is 65–70%.

Recurrent abortion is a clinical rather than pathologic diagnosis. The clinical findings are similar to those observed in other types of abortion (see above).

### Treatment

**A. Preconception Therapy:** Preconception therapy is aimed at detection of maternal or paternal defects that may contribute to abortion. A thorough general and gynecologic examination is essential. Cervical cultures for *Chlamydia,* herpesvirus, and cytomegalovirus and endometrial cultures for *Ureaplasma urealyticum* and *Toxoplasma gondii* should be taken. A random blood glucose test, thyroid function studies, and an antinuclear antibody test are indicated. Endometrial tissue should be examined in the postovulation stage of the cycle to determine the adequacy of the response of the endometrium to hormones. The competency of the cervix must be determined and hysteroscopy or hysterography used to exclude submucous myomas and congenital anomalies. Chromosomal (karyotype) analysis of both partners rules out balanced translocations. Every attempt should be made to restore and maintain good physical and emotional health.

Recent experiments have focused on the major histocompatibility complex (MHC) of chromosome 6, which carries HLA loci and other genes that may influence reproductive success. Many couples who experience habitual abortion share a significant number of HLA antigens, and some women demonstrate a lack of maternal antibody response to paternal lymphocytes, which is customarily found in normal women after successful childbearing. Centers where HLA typing can be performed will identify couples whose unusual gene sharing may play a role in habitual abortion. The immunologic approach of enhancing maternal antibody response to paternal lymphocytes is still experimental.

**B. Postconception Therapy:** Provide early prenatal care and schedule frequent office visits. Complete bed rest is justified only for bleeding or pain. Empiric steroid sex hormone therapy is contraindicated.

### Prognosis

The prognosis is excellent if the cause of abortion can be corrected.

Menge AC, Beer AE: The significance of human leukocyte antigen profiles in human infertility, recurrent abortion, and pregnancy disorders. *Fertil Steril* 1985;**43**:693.

Stray-Pedersen B, Stray-Pedersen S: Etiologic factors and subsequent reproductive performance in 195 couples with a prior history of habitual abortion. *Am J Obstet Gynecol* 1984;**148**:140.

## ECTOPIC PREGNANCY

### Essentials of Diagnosis

- Abnormal vaginal bleeding with symptoms suggestive of pregnancy.
- Cramping pains in the lower abdomen.
- A tender mass palpable outside the uterus.
- Pelvic ultrasound finding of empty uterus after seventh week from LMP.
- Failure to recover placental tissue at the time of induced abortion.

### General Considerations

Any pregnancy arising from implantation of the ovum outside the cavity of the uterus is ectopic. Ectopic implantation occurs in about one out of 150 live births. About 98% of ectopic pregnancies are tubal. Other sites of ectopic implantation are the peritoneum or abdominal viscera, the ovary, and the cervix. Peritonitis, salpingitis, abdominal surgery, and pelvic tumors may predispose to abnormally situated pregnancy. Combined intra- and extrauterine pregnancy (heterotopic) may occur rarely. In the USA, ectopic pregnancy is currently the most common cause of maternal death in pregnancies with abortive outcomes.

### Clinical Findings

**A. Symptoms and Signs:** The cardinal symptoms and signs of tubal pregnancy are (1) amenorrhea or irregular bleeding and spotting, followed by (2) pelvic pain, and (3) pelvic (adnexal) mass formation. They may be acute or chronic.

**1. Acute (about 40% of tubal ectopic pregnancies)**—Severe lower quadrant pain occurs in almost every case. It is sudden in onset, lancinating, intermittent, and does not radiate. Backache is present during attacks. Collapse and shock occur in about 10%, often after pelvic examination. At least two-thirds of patients give a history of abnormal menstruation; many have been infertile.

**2. Chronic (about 60% of tubal ectopic pregnancies)**—Blood leaks from the tubal ampulla over a period of days, and considerable blood may accumulate in the peritoneum. Slight but persistent vaginal spotting is reported, and a pelvic mass can be palpated. Abdominal distention and mild paralytic ileus are often present.

**B. Laboratory Findings:** Blood studies show anemia and slight leukocytosis. Quantitative serum pregnancy tests will show levels generally lower than expected for normal pregnancies of the same duration. If pregnancy tests are followed over a few days, there may be a slow rise or a plateau rather than the doubling every 2 days associated with early intrauterine pregnancy or the falling levels that occur with spontaneous abortion.

**C. Imaging:** Ultrasonography can reliably demonstrate a gestational sac 6 weeks from the LMP and a fetal pole at 7 weeks if located in the uterus. An empty uterine cavity raises a strong suspicion of extrauterine pregnancy, which can occasionally (but not reliably) be revealed by ultrasound.

**D. Special Examinations:** Aspiration of the pouch of Douglas (culdocentesis) with an 18-gauge spinal needle will confirm hemoperitoneum. Laparoscopy to confirm an ectopic pregnancy is of great value prior to laparotomy.

### Differential Diagnosis

Clinical and laboratory findings suggestive or diagnostic of pregnancy will distinguish ectopic pregnancy from many acute abdominal illnesses such as acute appendicitis, acute pelvic inflammatory disease, ruptured corpus luteum cyst or ovarian follicle, and urinary calculi. Uterine enlargement with clinical findings similar to those found in ectopic pregnancy is also characteristic of an aborting uterine pregnancy or hydatidiform mole.

### Treatment

Hospitalize the patient if there is a reasonable likelihood of ectopic pregnancy. Type and cross-match blood. Ideally, diagnosis and operative treatment should precede frank rupture of the tube and intra-abdominal hemorrhage.

Surgical treatment is imperative. Generally, salpingectomy will be required if the tube has ruptured. If the condition of the patient permits, assessment of the other tube is important at the time of laparotomy. Patency of the contralateral tube can be established by the injection of indigo carmine into the uterus, with appropriate compression of the lower uterine segment. Under certain circumstances, a conservative operation may be indicated (removing an unruptured ectopic pregnancy by salpingostomy or via the laparoscope, simple excision of the ectopic pregnancy, leaving portions of the tube for later microsurgery).

Iron therapy for anemia may be necessary during convalescence. Give $Rh_o$ (D) immune globulin to Rh-negative patients.

### Prognosis

Repeat tubal pregnancy occurs in about 12% of cases. This should not be regarded as a contraindication to future pregnancy, but the patient requires careful observation and early ultrasound confirmation of an intrauterine pregnancy.

Loffer FD (editor): Current concepts in the management of ectopic pregnancies: A symposium. *J Reprod Med* 1986;**31**:73.

## PREGNANCY-INDUCED HYPERTENSION (Preeclampsia-Eclampsia)

### Essentials of Diagnosis

- Onset of symptoms in the third trimester of pregnancy.
- Blood pressure > 140/90 mm Hg, or a rise of 30 mm Hg systolic or 15 mm Hg diastolic, noted on 2 occasions 6 hours apart, associated with the following:

  Significant proteinuria (500 mg/dL/24 h).

  Generalized edema, headache, visual disturbances, and epigastric pain.

  Increasing symptoms and signs preceding convulsions.

### General Considerations

Preeclampsia-eclampsia usually occurs in the last trimester of pregnancy. It is often first observed during labor or in the first 24 hours after delivery. The term preeclampsia denotes the nonconvulsive form; with the development of convulsions and coma, the disorder is termed eclampsia. About 5% of pregnant women in the USA develop preeclampsia. Primiparas are most commonly affected. The incidence of preeclampsia is increased with multiple pregnancies, essential hypertension, diabetes mellitus, chronic renal disease, collagen disorders, and hydatidiform mole. Uncontrolled eclampsia is a significant cause of maternal death. Five percent of cases of preeclampsia progress to eclampsia. Perinatal survival is very low when severe preeclampsia develops before the 28th week of pregnancy.

The cause is not known. Before the syndrome is clinically manifested, there is generalized vasospasm apparently initiated by the presence of chorionic tissue. The longer vasospasm continues, the greater the likelihood of associated pathologic changes in maternal organs, including the placenta; this indirectly affects the fetus.

None of the interventions recommended to reduce the incidence or severity of the process have proved to be of significant value when studied objectively, including diuretics, dietary restriction or enhancement, sodium restriction, and vitamin-mineral supplements. The only cure is termination of the pregnancy at a time as favorable as possible for fetal survival in the light of the medical condition of the mother.

### Clinical Findings

**A. Preeclampsia:**

**1. Mild**–Symptoms are absent. Diastolic blood

pressure is elevated to 90–100 mm Hg. There is minimal proteinuria and no evidence of intrauterine growth retardation.

**2. Severe**–Headache, visual changes, and upper abdominal pain are present, as is oliguria. Intrauterine growth retardation is present. Blood pressure exceeds 160/110 mm Hg. Ophthalmoscopic examination reveals arteriolar spasm, occasional edema of the optic disks, and cotton-wool exudates. Laboratory findings include proteinuria ($>$ 2000 mg/dL/24 h), evidence of azotemia (increased serum creatinine, uric acid, or urea nitrogen), disseminated intravascular coagulation (thrombocytopenia, decreased fibrinogen, and increased fibrin split products), and hepatocellular damage, including hyperbilirubinemia.

**B. Eclampsia:** The symptoms of eclampsia usually are engrafted on those of severe preeclampsia and include the following: (1) generalized tonic-clonic convulsions; (2) coma followed by amnesia and confusion; (3) 3–4+ proteinuria; (4) marked hypertension preceding a convulsion, and hypotension thereafter (during coma or vascular collapse); and (5) oliguria or anuria.

## Differential Diagnosis

The combination of renal, neurologic, and hypertensive findings in a previously normal pregnant woman distinguishes preeclampsia-eclampsia from primary hypertensive, renal, or neurologic disease.

## Treatment

**A. Preeclampsia:** This condition should be recognized as early as possible by meticulous prenatal care. The objectives of treatment are (1) to prevent eclampsia, abruptio placentae, hepatic rupture, and ocular or vascular accidents; and (2) to deliver a normal baby that will survive. Place the patient at bed rest and give small doses of a benzodiazepine if necessary to make bed rest more acceptable. Delivery should be delayed, if possible, until the disease is under control and the fetus is mature.

**1. Home management**–Most patients can be managed at home (at bed rest) under alert supervision, including frequent blood pressure readings, daily urine protein determinations, and careful recording of fluid intake and output. Mild sodium restriction ($<$ 3 g of salt per day) is advisable. If improvement does not occur in 48 hours, transfer the patient to a hospital.

**2. Hospital care**–Determine blood pressure, serum electrolytes, and urine protein at frequent intervals. Examine the ocular fundi every day, noting particularly arteriolar spasm, edema, hemorrhages, and exudates. The diet should be high in calcium, low in fat, high in complex carbohydrate, and moderate in protein content. Sedatives to promote quiet rest are indicated. Intravenous hydralazine is the antihypertensive of choice if diastolic blood pressure goes above 110 mm Hg. When labor ensues, parenteral magnesium sulfate is required to prevent seizures.

**3. Observation of the fetus**–With stabilization of preeclampsia, an optimal time for delivery minimizes perinatal illness and death. Deliver the fetus after 37 weeks by appropriate induction of labor, with cesarean section reserved for obstetric indications. Earlier in the third trimester, the status of the fetus can be followed with nonstress tests and oxytocin challenge tests done at 48-hour intervals. Regular maternal observations of fetal movements ("kick counts") are also useful. Estriol and human placental lactogen determinations are not necessary.

**B. Eclampsia:**

**1. Emergency care**–If the patient is convulsing, turn her on her side to prevent aspiration of vomitus and mucus and to prevent the caval syndrome. Insert a padded tongue blade or plastic airway between the teeth to prevent biting of the tongue and to maintain respiratory exchange. Aspirate fluid and food from the glottis or trachea. Give oxygen by nasal prongs. Give magnesium sulfate, 4 g (20 mL of a 20% solution) intravenously over a 4-minute period. At the same time, give 10 g of magnesium sulfate (20 mL of a 50% solution), one-half (10 mL) deep in each buttock (1 mL of 2% lidocaine may be added to each syringe to minimize pain). Thereafter, every 4 hours give 5 g of magnesium sulfate (10 mL of a 50% solution) in alternate buttocks as long as (1) knee jerk is present, (2) respirations are regular in rate (not $<$ 16/min), and (3) urine output was at least 100 mL in the previous 4 hours. In cases of overdosage, give calcium gluconate (or equivalent), 20 mL of a 10% aqueous solution intravenously slowly, and repeat every hour until urinary, respiratory, and neurologic depression have cleared.

**2. General care**–Hospitalize the patient in a darkened, quiet room at absolute bed rest, lying on her side, with side rails for protection during convulsions. Allow no visitors. Do not disturb the patient for unnecessary procedures (eg, baths, enemas), and leave the blood pressure cuff on her arm. Typed and cross-matched blood must be available for immediate use, because patients with eclampsia often develop premature separation of the placenta with hemorrhage and are susceptible to shock.

**3. Laboratory evaluation**–Insert a retention catheter for accurate measurement of the quantity of urine passed. Determine the protein content of each 24-hour specimen until the fourth or fifth postpartum day. Blood tests to evaluate clotting factors, liver function, and electrolytes should be obtained as often as the severity and progression of the disease indicate.

**4. Physical examination**–Check blood pressure frequently during the acute phase and every 2–4 hours thereafter. Monitor the fetal heart constantly, if possible. Perform ophthalmoscopic examination once a day. Examine the face, extremities, and especially the sacrum (which becomes dependent when the patient is in bed) for edema.

**5. Diet and fluids**–If the patient is convulsing, give nothing by mouth. Record fluid intake and output for each 24-hour period. If she can eat and drink, give a high-carbohydrate, moderate-protein, low-fat diet. If the urine output exceeds 700 mL/d, replace the output plus visible fluid loss with isotonic fluid. If the output is less than 700 mL/d, allow no more than 2000 mL of fluid per day (including parenteral fluid).

**6. Diuretics**–Because maternal hypovolemia is the rule in patients with preeclampsia-eclampsia, diuretics should be avoided. Hypertonic solutions are also unnecessary. Furosemide may be used in cases of pulmonary edema.

**7. Sedatives**–Use these agents sparingly if at all.

**8. Antihypertensives**–Hydralazine given in 5- to 10-mg increments intravenously every 20 minutes is used whenever the diastolic pressure is above 110 mm Hg. A satisfactory response is a decrease to 90 – 100 mm Hg. Further lowering may impair placental perfusion.

**9. Delivery**–Because severe hypertensive disease, renal disease, and preeclampsia-eclampsia are usually aggravated by continuing pregnancy, the best method of treatment of any of these disorders is termination of pregnancy, preferably after definite fetal viability. Control eclampsia before attempting induction of labor or delivery. Vaginal delivery is preferred. Induce labor, preferably by amniotomy alone, when the patient's condition permits. Use oxytocin to stimulate labor if necessary. Monitor the fetus carefully. Regional anesthesia is the technique of choice. Nitrous oxide (70%) and oxygen (30%) may be given with contractions, but 100% oxygen should be administered between contractions during the second stage.

Elective cesarean section may be considered if the patient is not at term or if labor is not inducible. Convulsions or coma must be absent for 12 or more hours before cesarean section is performed.

## Prognosis

The maternal mortality rate in eclampsia is 10 – 15%. Most patients improve strikingly in 24 – 48 hours with appropriate therapy, but early termination of pregnancy is usually required.

Although babies of mothers with preeclampsia-eclampsia are usually small for gestational age (probably because of placental malfunction), they fare better than preterm babies of the same weight born of women who do not develop preeclampsia-eclampsia.

Pritchard JA, Cunningham FG, Pritchard SA: The Parkland Memorial Hospital Protocol for Treatment of Eclampsia: Evaluation of 245 cases. *Am J Obstet Gynecol* 1984;**148**:951.

Wheeler AS, Harris BA: Anesthesia for pregnancy-induced hypertension. *Clin Perinatol* 1982;**9**:95.

## GESTATIONAL TROPHOBLASTIC NEOPLASIA (Hydatidiform Mole & Choriocarcinoma)

### Essentials of Diagnosis

- Uterus sometimes larger than expected for duration of pregnancy.
- Excessively elevated levels of hCG.
- Vesicles passed from vagina.
- Ultrasound findings characteristic of mole.
- Uterine bleeding in pregnancy.

### General Considerations

Gestational trophoblastic neoplasia is a spectrum of disease that includes hydatidiform mole, invasive mole, and choriocarcinoma. Cytogenetics has demonstrated that true moles are almost always euploid and sex chromatin-positive, 46,XX with all genetic material of paternal origin. Partial moles are usually triploid, with a maternal set of 23 chromosomes and added chromosomal material from paternal origins. Partial moles generally show evidence of an embryo or gestational sac, are slower growing and less symptomatic, and are often present clinically as a missed abortion. Recent investigations suggest that partial moles tend to follow a benign course, while true moles have a greater tendency to become choriocarcinomas.

The highest rates of gestation trophoblastic neoplasia occur in some developing countries, with rates of 1:125 pregnancies in certain areas of the Orient. In the USA, the frequency is 1:1500 pregnancies. Risk factors include low socioeconomic status, a history of mole, and age below 18 or above 40. Approximately 10% of women require further treatment after evacuation of the mole; 5% develop choriocarcinoma.

### Clinical Findings

**A. Symptoms and Signs:** Excessive nausea and vomiting occur in over one-third of patients with hydatidiform mole. Uterine bleeding, beginning at 6 –8 weeks, is observed in virtually all instances and is indicative of threatened or incomplete abortion. In about one-fifth of cases, the uterus is larger than would be expected in a normal pregnancy of the same duration. Intact or collapsed vesicles may be passed through the vagina. These grapelike clusters of enlarged villi are diagnostic. Bilaterally enlarged cystic ovaries are sometimes palpable. They are the result of ovarian hyperstimulation due to excess hCG.

Preeclampsia-eclampsia, frequently of the fulminating type, may develop during the second trimester of pregnancy, but this is unusual.

Choriocarcinoma may be manifested by continued or recurrent uterine bleeding after evacuation of a mole or following a delivery, abortion, or ectopic pregnancy. The presence of an ulcerative vaginal tumor, pelvic mass, or evidence of distant metastatic tumor may be the presenting observation. The diagnosis is established by pathologic examination of curettings or by biopsy.

**B. Laboratory Findings:** A serum hCG beta-subunit value above 40,000 mIU/mL or a urinary hCG value in excess of 100,000 IU/24 h increases the likelihood of hydatidiform mole, although such values are occasionally seen with a normal pregnancy (eg, in multiple gestation).

**C. Ultrasonography:** Ultrasound has virtually replaced all other means of preoperative diagnosis of hydatidiform mole. The multiple echoes indicating edematous villi within the enlarged uterus and the absence of a fetus and placenta are pathognomonic.

**D. Imaging:** A preoperative chest film is indicated to rule out pulmonary metastases of trophoblast.

## Treatment

**A. Specific (Surgical) Measures:** Empty the uterus as soon as the diagnosis of hydatidiform mole is established, preferably by suction. Do not resect ovarian cysts or remove the ovaries; spontaneous regression of theca lutein cysts will occur with elimination of the mole.

If malignant tissue is discovered at surgery or during the follow-up examination, chemotherapy is indicated.

Thyrotoxicosis indistinguishable clinically from that of primary thyroid or pituitary origin may occur. Surgical removal of the mole promptly corrects the thyroid overactivity.

**B. Follow-up Measures:** Effective contraception (preferably birth control pills) should be prescribed. Weekly quantitative hCG level measurements are initially required. Moles show a progressive decline in hCG. After 2 negative weekly tests ($< 5$ mIU/mL), the interval may be increased to monthly for 6 months and then to every 2 months for a year. If levels plateau or begin to rise, the patient should be evaluated by repeat chest film and D&C before the initiation of chemotherapy.

**C. Antitumor Chemotherapy:** For low-risk patients with a good prognosis, give methotrexate, 0.4 mg/kg intramuscularly over a 5-day period, or dactinomycin, 10–12 $\mu$g/kg/d intravenously over a 5-day period (see pp 1067 and 1068). Refer patients with a poor prognosis to a tumor center, where multiple-agent chemotherapy probably will be given. The side effects—anorexia, nausea and vomiting, stomatitis, rash, diarrhea, and bone marrow depression—usually are reversible in about 3 weeks. They can be ameliorated by the administration of folic acid. Death occurs occasionally from agranulocytosis or toxic hepatitis. Repeated courses of methotrexate 2 weeks apart generally are required to destroy the trophoblast and maintain a zero chorionic gonadotropin titer, as indicated by hCG $\beta$-subunit determination.

**D. Supportive Measures:** Replace blood, give iron, and encourage good nutrition. If infection is suspected, give broad-spectrum antibiotics for 24 hours before and 3–4 days after surgery. Prescribe oral contraceptives (if acceptable) or another reliable birth control method to avoid the hazard and confusion of elevated hCG from a new pregnancy. hCG levels should be negative for a year before pregnancy is again attempted. In the pregnancy following a mole, the hCG level should be checked 6 weeks postpartum.

## Prognosis

A 5-year arrest after courses of chemotherapy, even when metastases have been demonstrated, can be expected in at least 85% of cases of choriocarcinoma. The risk of chronic abortion or fetal anomaly is not greater in women who have had hydatidiform mole.

Grimes DA: Epidemiology of gestational trophoblastic disease. *Am J Obstet Gynecol* 1984;**150:**309.

Szulman AE: Syndromes of hydatidiform moles: Partial vs. complete. *J Reprod Med* 1984;**29:**788.

## THIRD-TRIMESTER BLEEDING

Five to 10% of women have vaginal bleeding in late pregnancy. Multiparas are more commonly affected. The physician must distinguish between placental causes of obstetric bleeding (placenta previa, premature separation of the placenta) and nonplacental causes (systemic disease or disorders of the lower genital tract).

The approach to the problem of bleeding in late pregnancy should be conservative and expectant.

The patient should be hospitalized at once and placed at complete bed rest. Perform a gentle abdominal examination. Significant degrees of premature separation of the placenta (abruptio placentae) cause uterine tetany and tenderness, whereas placenta previa is associated with painless bleeding, abnormal fetal position (breech, transverse lie), and a high presenting part. Inspect the vagina and cervix with a speculum for cancer or infection. Avoid digital rectal or vaginal examination, which may result in excessive bleeding. Typed and cross-matched blood should be ready in case of need during the examination. Ultrasonography is accurate in detecting placental location. Over 90% of patients with third-trimester bleeding will stop bleeding in 24 hours with bed rest alone, although the bleeding may recur at a later time. If bleeding is profuse and persistent, and especially if there are persistent uterine contractions, vaginal examination is indicated after preparation for cesarean section and blood replacement.

If the patient is less than 36 weeks pregnant, it may be necessary to keep her in the hospital or at home at bed rest until the chances of delivering a viable infant improve and amniotic fluid tests confirm lung maturity.

Gillieson MS, Winer-Muram HT, Muram D: Low-lying placenta. *Radiology* 1982;**144:**577.

# MEDICAL CONDITIONS COMPLICATING PREGNANCY

## Anemia

Plasma volume increases approximately 50% during pregnancy, while red cell volume increases 25%, causing hemodilution with lowered hemoglobin and hematocrit values. True anemia in pregnancy is often defined as a hemoglobin measurement below 11 g/dL or hematocrit below 33%. Anemia is very common in pregnancy, causing fatigue, anorexia, dyspnea, and edema. Prevention through optimal nutrition and iron and folic acid supplementation is desirable.

**A. Iron Deficiency Anemia:** Many women enter pregnancy with low iron stores resulting from heavy menstrual periods, previous pregnancies, or poor nutrition. It is difficult to meet the increased requirement for iron through diet, so that anemia often develops unless iron supplements are given. Red cells may not become hypochromic and microcytic until the hematocrit has fallen far below normal levels. The reticulocyte count is low. A serum iron level below 40 $\mu$g/dL and a transferrin saturation less than 16% suggest iron deficiency anemia. Treatment consists of a diet containing iron-rich foods and 60 mg of elemental iron (eg, 300 mg of ferrous sulfate) 3 times a day with meals. Iron is best absorbed if taken with a source of vitamin C (raw fruits and vegetables, lightly cooked greens). For prevention of anemia, all pregnant women should take daily iron supplements containing 60 mg of elemental iron.

**B. Folic Acid Deficiency Anemia:** Folic acid deficiency anemia is the main cause of macrocytic anemia in pregnancy, since vitamin $B_{12}$ deficiency anemia is rare in the childbearing years. The daily folate requirement doubles from 400 $\mu$g to 800 $\mu$g in pregnancy. Twin pregnancies, acute infections, malabsorption syndromes, and use of anticonvulsant drugs such as phenytoin can precipitate folic acid deficiency. The anemia may first be seen in the puerperium owing to the increased need for folate during lactation.

The diagnosis is made by finding macrocytic red cells and hypersegmented neutrophils in a blood smear. However, blood smears in pregnancy may be difficult to interpret, since they frequently show iron deficiency changes as well. Because the deficiency is hard to diagnose and folate intake is inadequate in some socioeconomic groups, 0.8–1 mg of folic acid is routinely given as a supplement in pregnancy. Treat an established deficiency with 1–5 mg/d. Good sources of folate in food are leafy green vegetables, orange juice, peanuts, and beans. Cooking and storage of food destroy folic acid. Strict vegetarians who eat no eggs or milk products should take vitamin $B_{12}$ supplements during pregnancy and lactation.

**C. Sickle Cell Anemia:** Women with sickle cell anemia are subject to serious complications in pregnancy. The anemia becomes more severe, and crises may occur more frequently. Complications include infections, bone pain, pulmonary infarction, congestive heart failure, and preeclampsia. There is an increased rate of spontaneous abortion and higher maternal and perinatal mortality rates. Newer methods of intensive medical treatment have improved the outcome for mother and fetus. Frequent transfusions of packed cells or leukocyte-poor washed red cells are used to lower the level of hemoglobin S and elevate the level of hemoglobin A; this minimizes the severity of anemia and sickle cell crises. Folic acid supplements should be given, and analgesics and adequate hydration are important.

Parents with sickle cell disease or sickle cell trait may wish to undergo first-trimester chorionic villus biopsy or second-trimester amniocentesis to determine whether sickle cell anemia has been passed on to the fetus. Genetic counseling should be available before pregnancy and postpartum for all patients with hemoglobinopathies and their partners. Elective sterilization and therapeutic abortion should be available if desired. IUDs and oral contraceptives are contraindicated for these patients, but progestin-only contraceptives may be used.

Women with sickle cell trait alone generally have an uncomplicated gestation. Sickle cell-hemoglobin C disease in pregnancy is similar to sickle cell anemia and is treated similarly.

## Asthma

The effect of pregnancy on asthma is unpredictable. About 50% of patients have no change, 25% improve, and 25% get worse. For acute attacks of bronchospasm, subcutaneous epinephrine is the treatment of choice. For mild episodes, theophylline or ephedrine can be used; cromolyn for prevention is also considered safe. For severe cases, 5–7 days of prednisone (30–50 mg/d) can be helpful, with inhaled beclomethasone dipropionate being used to permit a gradual decrease in oral corticosteroids.

Greenberger PA, Patterson R: Current concepts: Management of asthma during pregnancy. N Engl J Med 1985;312:897.

## Diabetes Mellitus

During pregnancy there is increased tissue resistance to insulin with resultant increased levels of blood insulin as well as glucose and triglycerides. These changes result from secretion of human placental lactogen and increasing levels of estrogen and progesterone. The prevention of common hazards of diabetes, such as hypoglycemia, ketosis, and diabetic coma, requires great effort and attention to detail on the part of both the physician and the patient. Although pregnancy does not appear to alter the ultimate severity of diabetes, retinopathy and nephropathy may appear or become worse during pregnancy. Over the years, the White classification of diabetes during pregnancy (Table 13–12) has allowed for uniform description and comparison of diabetic pregnant women.

Even in carefully managed diabetics, the incidence of obstetric complications such as hydramnios, pre-

**Table 13–12.** Classification of diabetes during pregnancy (Priscilla White).[*]

| Class | Characteristics | Implications |
|---|---|---|
| Gestational diabetes | Abnormal glucose tolerance during pregnancy; postprandial hyperglycemia during pregnancy. | Diagnosis before 30 weeks' gestation important to prevent macrosomia. Treat with diet adequate in calories to prevent maternal weight loss. Goal is postprandial blood glucose < 130 mg/dL at 1 hour, or < 105 mg/dL at 2 hours. If insulin is necessary, manage as in classes B, C, and D. |
| A | Chemical diabetes diagnosed before pregnancy; managed by diet alone; any age at onset. | Management as for gestational diabetes. |
| B | Insulin treatment used before pregnancy; onset at age 20 or older; duration < 10 years. | Some endogenous insulin secretion may persist. Fetal and neonatal risks same as in classes C and D, as is management. |
| C | Onset at age 10–20, or duration 10–20 years. | Insulin-deficient diabetes of juvenile onset. |
| D | Onset before age 10, or duration > 20 years, or chronic hypertension (not preeclampsia), or background retinopathy (tiny hemorrhages). | Fetal macrosomia or intrauterine growth retardation possible. Retinal microaneurysms, dot hemorrhages, and exudates may progress during pregnancy, then regress after delivery. |
| F | Diabetic nephropathy with proteinuria. | Anemia and hypertension common; proteinuria increases in third trimester, declines after delivery. Fetal intrauterine growth retardation common; perinatal survival about 85% under optimal conditions; bed rest necessary. |
| H | Coronary artery disease. | Serious maternal risk. |
| R | Proliferative retinopathy. | Neovascularization, with risk of vitreous hemorrhage or retinal detachment; laser photocoagulation useful; abortion usually not necessary. With active process of neovascularization, prevent bearing-down efforts. |

[*] Reproduced, with permission, from Benson RC (editor): *Current Obstetric & Gynecologic Diagnosis & Treatment*, 5th ed. Lange, 1984.

eclampsia-eclampsia, infections, and prematurity is increased. The infants are larger than those of nondiabetic women. There is an increase in the number of unexplained fetal deaths in the last few weeks of pregnancy as well as a high rate of neonatal deaths.

The maintenance of euglycemia is improved by patient-performed blood sugar monitoring at home 4 times daily with added postmeal observations once or twice a week. Attempts are under way to decrease the number of congenital anomalies associated with diabetic pregnancies. Prepregnancy evaluation and adjustment of insulin control based on glycosylated hemoglobin ($A_{1c}$) will maintain strict euglycemia in early pregnancy when organogenesis is occurring. The use of a continuous insulin pump is under study for its effect in lowering the frequency of anomalies. Time of delivery is dictated by deterioration of diabetic control, the onset of preeclampsia, decreased fetal reactivity as judged by nonstress or oxytocin challenge tests, or confirmation of lung maturity at or about 38 weeks of pregnancy. Cesarean sections are performed for obstetric indications.

Because 50% of gestational diabetics go on to develop overt diabetes mellitus and because the infants of gestational diabetics suffer risks similar to those borne by infants of diabetic mothers, screening of all pregnant women for glucose intolerance has been recommended between the 24th and 28th weeks of pregnancy (Table 13–13). Nutritional advice, blood glucose monitoring, and obstetric surveillance should be meticulous.

Gestational diabetes should be evaluated 6–8 weeks postpartum by a 2-hour oral glucose tolerance test (75 g glucose load).

Freinkel N, Dooley SL, Metzger BE: Current concepts: Case of the pregnant woman with insulin-dependent diabetes mellitus. *N Engl J Med* 1985;**313**:96.
Gabbe SG: Definition, detection and management of gestational diabetes. *Obstet Gynecol* 1986;**67**:121.

**Table 13–13.** Screening and diagnostic criteria for gestational diabetes mellitus.

**Screening for gestational diabetes**
1. Glucose measurement in blood.
2. 50-g oral glucose load, administered between the 24th and 28th weeks, without regard to time of day or time of last meal, to all pregnant women who have not been identified as having glucose intolerance before the 24th week.
3. Venous plasma glucose measured 1 hour later.
4. Value of 140 mg/dL (7.8 mmol/L) or above in venous plasma indicates the need for a full diagnostic glucose tolerance test.

**Diagnosis of gestational diabetes mellitus**
1. 100-g oral glucose load, administered in the morning after overnight fast lasting at least 8 hours but not more than 14 hours, and following at least 3 days of unrestricted diet (> 150 g carbohydrate) and physical activity.
2. Venous plasma glucose is measured fasting and at 1, 2, and 3 hours. Subject should remain seated and not smoke throughout the test.
3. Two or more of the following venous plasma concentrations must be equaled or exceeded for positive diagnosis: fasting, 105 mg/dL (5.8 mmol/L); 1 hour, 190 mg/dL (10.6 mmol/L); 2 hours, 165 mg/dL (9.2 mmol/L); 3 hours, 145 mg/dL (8.1 mmol/L).

## Heart Disease

Most cases of heart disease complicating pregnancy in the USA now are of congenital origin. About 5% of maternal deaths are due to heart disease. Pregnancy causes a significant increase in pulse rate, an increase of cardiac output of more than 30%, and a rise in plasma volume greater than red cell mass with relative hemodilution. Both vital capacity and oxygen consumption rise only slightly.

For practical purposes, the functional capacity of the heart is the best single measurement of cardiopulmonary status.

Class I: Ordinary physical activity causes no discomfort (perinatal mortality rate about 5%).

Class II: Ordinary activity causes discomfort and slight disability (perinatal mortality rate 10–15%).

Class III: Less than ordinary activity causes discomfort or disability; patient is barely compensated (perinatal mortality rate about 35%).

Class IV: Patient decompensated; any physical activity causes acute distress (perinatal mortality rate over 50%).

In general, patients with class I or class II functional disability (80% of pregnant women with heart disease) do well obstetrically. Over 80% of maternal deaths due to heart disease occur in women with class III or IV cardiac disability. Congestive failure is the usual cause of death. Three-fourths of these deaths occur in the early puerperium. Pregnancy is contraindicated in Eisenmenger's complex; in severe mitral stenosis if there is pulmonary hypertension; in Marfan's syndrome, in which the aorta is prone to rupture; and in primary pulmonary hypertension. In addition, pregnancy is poorly tolerated in patients with aortic stenosis (uncorrected), aortic coarctation, tetralogy of Fallot, active rheumatic carditis, and any other lesion with class III or class IV symptoms.

Therapeutic abortion and elective sterilization should be offered to patients with significant cardiac disease. Cesarean section should be performed only upon obstetric indications. Appropriate antibiotic prophylaxis against infective endocarditis is indicated after delivery or termination of pregnancy.

McAnulty JH, Metcalfe J, Ueland K: General guidelines in the management of cardiac disease during pregnancy. *Clin Obstet Gynecol* 1981;**24**:773.

Sullivan JM, Ramanathan KB: Current concepts: Management of medical problems of pregnancy: Severe cardiac disease. *N Engl J Med* 1985;**313**:304.

## Herpes Genitalis
## (See also Chapters 4 and 21.)

Infection of the lower genital tract by herpes simplex virus type 2 (HSV-2) is a common sexually transmitted disease of potential seriousness to pregnant women and their newborn infants.

Cesarean section is indicated at the time of labor if there are definite prodromal symptoms, active genital lesions, or a positive cervical culture obtained within the past week. Abdominal delivery is protective to the baby even several hours after rupture of the membranes.

Women who have had primary herpes infection late in pregnancy are at high risk of shedding virus at delivery. They should be screened by means of weekly cultures during the last month of pregnancy.

Women with a history of recurrent genital herpes should be followed by clinical observation and culture of any suspicious lesions. Since asymptomatic viral shedding is not predictable by antepartum cultures, current recommendations do not include routine cultures in individuals with a past history of herpes but with no active disease. However, when labor begins, vulvar and cervical cultures should be taken. Prompt treatment of a potentially infected newborn after a positive maternal herpes culture should permit successful management of the baby.

For treatment, see Chapter 28. The safety of acyclovir in pregnancy has not been established.

Arvin AM et al: Failure of antepartum maternal cultures to predict the infant's risk of exposure to herpes simplex virus infections. *New Engl J Med* 1986;**315**:796.

Prober CG et al: Low risk of herpes simplex virus infections in neonates exposed to the virus at the time of vaginal delivery to mothers with recurrent genital herpes simplex virus infections. *New Engl J Med* 1987;**316**:240.

## Hypertensive Disease

Hypertensive disease in women of childbearing age is usually essential hypertension. Other less common but important causes should be looked for: coarctation of the aorta, pheochromocytoma, aldosteronism, and renovascular and renal hypertension.

Preeclampsia is superimposed on 20% of pregnancies in women with hypertensive disease, and in such patients it appears earlier, is more severe, and is more often associated with intrauterine growth retardation. It may be difficult to determine whether or not hypertension in a pregnant woman precedes or derives from the pregnancy if she is not examined until after the 20th week and there is no reliable medical history. When in doubt, treat for preeclampsia. The hypertension of preeclampsia usually recedes 6 weeks after delivery. If it persists for 3 months postpartum, it is probably essential hypertension.

Pregnant women with probable hypertensive disease require antihypertensive drugs only if the diastolic pressure is sustained at or above 110 mm Hg. One should strive to keep the diastolic pressure between 90 and 100 mm Hg. However, if the pressure is over 110 mm Hg, do not attempt to lower it quickly by more than 25%.

If a hypertensive woman is being managed successfully by medical treatment when she registers for antenatal care, one may generally continue the antihypertensive medication. Diuretics can be continued in pregnancy; propranolol is best replaced by a more selective β-adrenergic antagonist that is less lipid-soluble (eg, metoprolol). For initiation of treatment, one may begin with hydralazine, 25 mg orally daily, and increase the dosage as indicated. If the response is unsatisfactory or if the patient is not near term, give methyldopa, 250 mg orally twice daily, again building in divided doses as needed to as much as 2 g daily.

The incidence or severity of preeclampsia and the increased perinatal mortality rate associated with hypertensive syndromes are reduced slightly by long-term drug therapy.

Therapeutic abortion may be indicated in cases of severe hypertension during pregnancy. If pregnancy is allowed to continue, the risk to the fetus must be assessed periodically in anticipation of early delivery. An early second-trimester ultrasound examination will confirm the duration of pregnancy, and follow-up examinations after 28 weeks will evaluate intrauterine growth retardation.

## Maternal Hepatitis B Carrier State

There are an estimated 200 million chronic carriers of hepatitis B virus worldwide. Among these people there is an increased incidence of chronic active hepatitis, cirrhosis, and hepatocellular carcinoma. The frequency of the hepatitis B carrier state varies from 1% in the USA and Western Europe to 35% in parts of Africa and Asia. Pregnant women in high-risk groups should be screened. The mother who will transmit the virus to her baby after delivery can be recognized by positive blood tests for hepatitis B surface antigen (HBsAg) and hepatitis B e antigen (HBeAg). Vertical transmission can be blocked by the immediate postdelivery administration to the newborn of 0.5 mL of hepatitis B immunoglobulin and 10 μg of hepatitis B vaccine intramuscularly. The vaccine dose is repeated at 1 and 6 months of age.

For further discussion of viral hepatitis, see p 398.

Stevens CE et al: Perinatal hepatitis B virus transmission in the United States: Prevention by passive-active immunization. *JAMA* 1985;**253**:1740.

## Seizure Disorders

Women contemplating pregnancy who have not had a seizure for 5 years should consider a prepregnancy trial of withdrawal from seizure medication. Those with recurrent epilepsy should use a single drug with blood level monitoring. Trimethadione and valproic acid are contraindicated during pregnancy; phenytoin is also considered teratogenic and should not be used unless absolutely necessary. Phenobarbital is considered the drug of choice in pregnancy. Anticonvulsant serum levels should be measured at least monthly and dosage adjustments made to keep serum levels in the low normal therapeutic range.

Newborns of mothers taking phenobarbital or phenytoin are at risk of bleeding tendencies due to decreased levels of vitamin K-dependent clotting factors. Such infants should receive an injection of vitamin $K_1$, 1 mg given subcutaneously immediately after delivery, and should have clotting studies 2–4 hours later.

Dalessio DJ: Current concepts: Seizure disorders and pregnancy. *N Engl J Med* 1985;**312**:559.

## Syphilis, Gonorrhea, & *Chlamydia trachomatis* Infection (See also Chapters 23 and 24.)

These sexually transmitted diseases have significant consequences for mother and child. Untreated syphilis in pregnancy will cause late abortion or transplacental infection with congenital syphilis. Gonorrhea will produce large-joint arthritis by hematogenous spread as well as newborn eye damage. Maternal chlamydial infections are largely asymptomatic but are manifested in the newborn by inclusion conjunctivitis and, at age 2–4 months, by pneumonia. The diagnosis of each can be reliably made by appropriate laboratory tests, which should be included in all prenatal care. The sexual partners of women with sexually transmitted diseases should be identified and treated also if that can be done.

Mascola L et al: Congenital syphilis: Why is it still occurring? *JAMA* 1984;**252**:1719.

## Thyrotoxicosis

Thyrotoxicosis during pregnancy may result in fetal anomalies, late abortion, or preterm labor and fetal hyperthyroidism with goiter. Thyroid storm in late pregnancy or labor is a life-threatening emergency.

Radioactive isotope therapy must never be given during pregnancy. The thyroid inhibitor of choice is propylthiouracil, which acts to prevent further thyroxine formation by blocking iodination of tyrosine. There is a 2- to 3-week delay before the pretreatment hormone level begins to fall. The initial dose of propylthiouracil is 100–150 mg 3 times a day; the dose is lowered as the euthyroid state is approached. It is desirable to keep thyroxine ($T_4$) in the high normal range during pregnancy. A maintenance dose of 100 mg/d minimizes the chance of fetal hypothyroidism and goiter. Elective thyroidectomy is recommended by some in preference to medical management during and even after pregnancy (see Chapter 18).

Recurrent postpartum thyroiditis is a newly recognized entity occurring 3–6 months after delivery. A hyperthyroid state of 1–3 months' duration is followed by hypothyroidism, sometimes misdiagnosed as depression. Microsomal thyroid antibodies and thyroglobulin antibodies are present. Recovery is spontaneous in over 90% of cases after 3–6 months.

Burrow GN: Current concepts: The management of thyrotoxicosis in pregnancy. *N Engl J Med* 1985;**313**:562.

## Tuberculosis

The diagnosis of tuberculosis in pregnancy is made by history taking, physical examination, and skin testing, with special attention to women from ethnic groups with a high prevalence of the disease (such as women from southeast Asia). Chest films should not be obtained as a routine screening measure in pregnancy but should be used only in patients with a skin test that has converted from negative to positive or with suggestive findings in the history and physical examination. Use abdominal shielding if a chest film is obtained.

If adequately treated, tuberculosis in pregnancy has an excellent prognosis. There is no increase in spontaneous abortion, fetal problems, or congenital anomalies in patients receiving antitubercular chemotherapy.

Treatment is with isoniazid and ethambutol or isoniazid and rifampin, in a short course (9–12 months) or standard course (18–24 months). Because isoniazid therapy may result in vitamin $B_6$ deficiency, a supplement of 50 mg/d of vitamin $B_6$ should be given simultaneously. Streptomycin, ethionamide, and most other antituberculous drugs should be avoided in pregnancy.

Snider DE Jr et al: Treatment of tuberculosis during pregnancy. *Am Rev Respir Dis* 1980;**122**:65.

## Urinary Tract Infection

The urinary tract is especially vulnerable to infections during pregnancy because the altered secretions of steroid sex hormones and the pressure exerted by the gravid uterus upon the ureters and bladder cause hypotonia and congestion and predispose to urinary stasis. Labor and delivery and urinary retention postpartum also may initiate or aggravate infection. *Escherichia coli* is the offending organism in over two-thirds of cases.

From 2 to 8% of pregnant women have asymptomatic bacteriuria, which some believe to be associated with increased risk of prematurity. It is estimated that 20–40% of these women will develop pyelonephritis during pregnancy.

A first-trimester urine culture is indicated in women with a history of recurrent or recent episodes of urinary tract infection. If the culture is positive, treatment should be initiated as a prophylactic measure. Sulfisoxazole, nitrofurantoin, penicillins, and cephalosporins are acceptable medications for 7–10 days. Sulfonamides should not be given in the third trimester. If bacteriuria returns, suppressive medication (one daily dose of an appropriate antibiotic) for the remainder of the pregnancy is indicated. Acute pyelonephritis requires hospitalization for intravenous administration of antibiotics until the patient is afebrile; this is followed by a full course of oral antibiotics.

Gilstrap LC III, Cunningham FG, Whalley PJ: Acute pyelonephritis in pregnancy: An anterospective study. *Obstet Gynecol* 1981;**57**:409.

## SURGICAL COMPLICATIONS DURING PREGNANCY

Elective major surgery should be avoided during pregnancy. However, normal, uncomplicated pregnancy has no debilitating effect and does not alter operative risk except as it may interfere with the diagnosis of abdominal disorders and increase the technical problems of intra-abdominal surgery. Abortion is not a serious hazard after operation unless peritoneal sepsis or other significant complication occurs.

During the first trimester, congenital anomalies may be induced in the developing fetus by hypoxia. Avoid surgical intervention during this period; if surgery does become necessary, the greatest precautions must be taken to prevent hypotension and hypoxia.

The second trimester is usually the optimal time for elective operative procedures.

### Appendicitis

Appendicitis occurs in about one of 5000 pregnancies. Diagnosis is more difficult than when the disease occurs in nonpregnant persons, since the appendix is carried high and to the right, away from McBurney's point, and localization of pain and infection does not usually occur. Nausea, vomiting, fever, and leukocytosis occur regularly. Any right-sided pain associated with these symptoms should raise a suspicion of appendicitis. In at least 20% of obstetric patients, the diagnosis of appendicitis is not made until the appendix has ruptured and peritonitis has become established. Such a delay may lead to premature labor or abortion. With early diagnosis and appendectomy, the prognosis is good for mother and baby.

Horowitz MD et al: Acute appendicitis during pregnancy: Diagnosis and management. *Arch Surg* 1985;**120**:1362.

### Carcinoma of the Breast

Cancer of the breast (see also Chapter 12) is diagnosed approximately once in 3500 pregnancies. Pregnancy may accelerate the growth of cancer of the breast; however, delay in diagnosis affects the outcome of treatment more significantly. Inflammatory carcinoma is an extremely virulent type of breast cancer that occurs most commonly during lactation. Prepregnancy mammography should be encouraged for women over age 35 who are anticipating a pregnancy.

Breast enlargement obscures parenchymal masses, and breast tissue hyperplasia decreases the accuracy of mammography. Any perceived discrete mass should be promptly evaluated by aspiration to verify cystic structure and then by fine-needle biopsy if it is solid. A definitive diagnosis may require excisional biopsy under local anesthesia. If breast biopsy confirms the diagnosis of cancer, surgery should be done regardless of the stage of the pregnancy. If spread to the regional glands has occurred, irradiation or chemotherapy should be considered. Under these circumstances, termination of an early pregnancy or delay of therapy for fetal maturation is indicated.

Sahni K et al: Carcinoma of breast associated with pregnancy and lactation. *J Surg Oncol* 1981;**16:**167.

## Choledocholithiasis, Cholecystitis, & Idiopathic Cholestasis of Pregnancy

Severe choledocholithiasis and cholecystitis are not common during pregnancy despite the fact that women tend to form gallstones. When they do occur, it is usually in late pregnancy or in the puerperium. About 90% of patients with cholecystitis have gallstones; 90% of stones will be visualized by ultrasonography.

Symptomatic relief may be all that is required.

Gallbladder surgery in pregnant women should be attempted only in extreme cases (eg, obstruction), because it increases the perinatal mortality rate to about 15%. Cholecystostomy and lithotomy may be all that is feasible during advanced pregnancy, cholecystectomy being deferred until after delivery. On the other hand, withholding surgery when it is definitely needed may result in necrosis and perforation of the gallbladder and peritonitis. Cholangitis due to impacted common duct stone requires surgical removal of gallstones and establishment of biliary drainage.

Idiopathic cholestasis of pregnancy is due to a hereditary metabolic (hepatic) deficiency aggravated by the high estrogen levels of pregnancy. It causes intrahepatic biliary obstruction of varying degrees. The rise in bile acids is sufficient in the third trimester to cause severe, intractable, generalized itching and sometimes clinical jaundice. There may be mild elevations in blood bilirubin and alkaline phosphatase levels. The fetus is generally unaffected, although an increased prematurity rate has been reported. Resins such as cholestyramine (4 g 3 times a day) absorb bile acids in the large bowel and relieve pruritus but are difficult to take and may cause constipation. Their use requires vitamin K supplementation. The disorder is relieved once the infant has been delivered, but it recurs in subsequent pregnancies and sometimes with the use of oral contraceptives.

Douwas SG et al: Liver disease and pregnancy. *Obstet Gynecol Surv* 1983;**38:**531.

## Ovarian Tumors

The most common adnexal mass in early pregnancy is the corpus luteum, which may become cystic and enlarge to 6 cm in diameter. Any persistent mass over 5 cm should be evaluated by ultrasound examination; unilocular cysts are likely to be corpus luteum cysts, whereas septated or semisolid tumors are likely to be neoplasms. Ovarian tumors may undergo torsion and cause abdominal pain and nausea and vomiting and must be differentiated from appendicitis, other bowel disease, and ectopic pregnancy. Patients with suspected ovarian cancer should be referred to a gynecologic oncologist to determine whether the pregnancy can progress to fetal viability or whether treatment should be instituted without delay.

## PREVENTION OF HEMOLYTIC DISEASE OF THE NEWBORN (Erythroblastosis Fetalis)

The antibody anti-$Rh_o$ (D) is responsible for most severe instances of hemolytic disease of the newborn (erythroblastosis fetalis). About 15% of whites and much lower proportions of blacks and Asians are $Rh_o$ (D)-negative. If an $Rh_o$ (D)-negative woman carries an $Rh_o$ (D)-positive fetus, she may develop antibodies against $Rh_o$ (D) when fetal red cells enter her circulation at delivery (or during abortion, ectopic pregnancy, abruptio placentae, or other antepartum bleeding problems). This antibody, once produced, remains in the woman's circulation and poses a serious threat of hemolytic disease for subsequent Rh-positive fetuses.

Passive immunization against hemolytic disease of the newborn now is possible with $Rh_o$ (D) immune globulin, a purified concentrate of antibodies against $Rh_o$ (D) antigen. To be maximally effective, the $Rh_o$ (D) immune globulin should be given within 72 hours after delivery (or spontaneous or induced abortion or ectopic pregnancy). The antibodies in the immune globulin destroy fetal Rh-positive cells so that the mother will not produce anti-$Rh_o$ (D). During her next Rh-positive gestation, erythroblastosis will be prevented.

The usual dose of $Rh_o$ (D) immune globulin for prevention of isoimmunization is 1 vial (300 $\mu$g) intramuscularly.

It has recently been demonstrated that a rare Rh-negative woman will become sensitized by small fetomaternal bleeding episodes in the early third trimester. An additional safety measure is the administration of the immune globulin at the 28th week of pregnancy. The antibody molecules are too large to pass through the placenta and affect an Rh-positive fetus. The maternal clearance of the globulin is slow enough that protection will continue for 12 weeks.

Mild to moderate degrees of hemolytic disease continue to occur in association with Rh subgroups (C, c, or E) or the Kell (k) factor. Therefore, atypical antibodies should be checked in the third trimester of all pregnancies.

Bowman JM: Controversies in Rh prophylaxis: Who needs Rh immune globulin and when should it be given? *Am J Obstet Gynecol* 1985;**151:**289.

## PREVENTION OF PRETERM (PREMATURE) LABOR

Preterm (premature) labor is labor that begins before the 37th week of pregnancy; it is responsible for 85% of neonatal illnesses and deaths. The onset of labor is a result of a complex sequence of biologic events involving regulatory factors that are still poorly understood. It is theorized that the delicate balance of hormones and other agents which maintain pregnancy may be upset by maternal changes such as alteration in estrogen-progesterone-prostaglandin production or by fetal factors such as increases in fetal ACTH and cortisol. If these events occur too early, preterm labor may ensue. The most significant risk factors for the onset of preterm labor are a past history of preterm delivery, premature rupture of the membranes, urinary tract infection, or exposure to diethylstilbestrol. In the current pregnancy, multiple gestation and abdominal or cervical surgery are especially important. To estimate the clinical risk, see Table 13–14.

Low rates of preterm delivery are associated with success in educating patients to identify regular, frequent uterine contractions and in alerting medical and nursing staff to evaluate these patients early and initiate treatment if cervical changes can be identified. Cessation of work or physical activities that seem related to increased uterine activity is mandatory. Resting at home will often suffice to slow contractions. In more acute situations, sedation with opiates and hydration with oral or intravenous fluids, if given before uterine contractions have changed the cervix appreciably, will often avert the need for specific drug therapy. Intravenous magnesium sulfate in doses similar to those used for the treatment of preeclampsia is an effective tocolytic and can be used before intravenous beta-adrenergic drugs are initiated.

Uterine smooth muscle is largely under sympathetic nervous system control, and stimulation of $\beta_2$ receptors relaxes the myometrium. Consequently, inhibition of uterine contractility often can be accomplished by the administration of $\beta$-adrenergic drugs such as ritodrine (Yutopar).

Ritodrine may be administered by intravenous infusions of 0.05–0.3 mg/min to decrease the frequency

**Table 13–14.** Risk of preterm delivery.*

| Score† | Socioeconomic Status | Past History | Daily Habits | Current Pregnancy | |
| --- | --- | --- | --- | --- | --- |
| | | | | Mother | Fetus |
| 1 | 2 children at home. Low socioeconomic status. | One first trimester abortion. Less than 1 year since last birth. | Work outside home. | Unusual fatigue. | . . . |
| 2 | Under 20 years of age. Over 40 years of age. Single parent. | Two first trimester abortions. | More than 10 cigarettes per day. | Less than 12 lb weight gain by 32 weeks. Albuminuria. Hypertension. Bacteriuria. | . . . |
| 3 | Very low socioeconomic status. Malnourished. Shorter than 150 cm (5 ft). Weighs less than 45 cm (100 lb). | Three first trimester abortions. | Unusual anxiety. Heavy work. Long, tiring travel. Long commute distance. | Weight loss of 2 kg. Febrile illness. Leiomyomas. | Head engaged before 34 weeks. |
| 4 | Under 18 years of age. | Pyelonephritis. | . . . | Uterine bleeding after 12 weeks. Effacement or dilation of cervix before 36 weeks. Uterine irritability. | . . . |
| 5 | . . . | Uterine anomaly. Second trimester abortion. Cone biopsy. | . . . | Placenta previa. Hydramnios. | . . . |
| 10 | . . . | Premature delivery. DES exposure. Repeated second trimester abortion. | . . . | Abdominal surgery. Cervical surgery. | Twins. Small-for-dates fetus. |

* Modified and reproduced, with permission, from Zuspan FK, Quilligan EJ (editors): *Practical Manual of Obstetric Care.* Mosby, 1982. (Modified from Creasy R: Personal communication.)
† Score is computed by addition of the number of points given any item. 0–5 = minimal risk; 6–9 = moderate risk; 10 or more = high risk.

and intensity of uterine contractions. Within several hours after cessation of contractions, ritodrine infusion may be scaled back by 0.05 mg every 15 minutes until a minimum effective dose is established. Oral therapy is started 30 minutes before stopping intravenous ritodrine and is continued in a dose of 10–20 mg every 4–6 hours. A dose-related elevation of heart rate of 20–40 beats/min may occur. An increase of systolic blood pressure up to 10 mm Hg is likely, and the diastolic pressure may fall 10–15 mm Hg during the infusion. Nonetheless, cardiac output increases considerably. Transient elevation of blood glucose, insulin, and fatty acids together with slight reduction of serum potassium have been reported. Fetal tachycardia may be slight or absent. No drug-caused perinatal deaths have been reported. Maternal side effects requiring dose limitation are tachycardia ($\geq$ 140 beats/min), palpitations, and nervousness. Fluids should be limited to 2500 mL/24 h. Serious side effects (pulmonary edema, chest pain with or without electrocardiographic changes) are often idiosyncratic, not dose-related, and warrant termination of therapy.

One must identify cases in which untimely delivery is the sole threat to the life or health of the infant. An effort should be made to eliminate (1) maternal conditions that compromise the intrauterine environment and make premature birth the lesser risk, eg, preeclampsia-eclampsia; (2) fetal conditions that either are helped by early delivery or render attempts to stop premature labor meaningless, eg, severe erythroblastosis fetalis; and (3) clinical situations in which it is likely that an attempt to stop labor will be futile, eg, ruptured membranes, cervix fully effaced and dilated more than 3 cm, strong labor in progress.

In pregnancies of less than 34 weeks' duration, betamethasone (12 mg intramuscularly repeated in 24 hours) is administered to hasten fetal lung maturation and permit delivery 48 hours after initial treatment when prolongation of pregnancy is contraindicated.

Herron M, Katz M, Creasy RK: Evaluation of a preterm birth prevention program. *Obstet Gynecol* 1982;**59:**452.

Katz M, Robertson PA, Creasy RK: Cardiovascular complications associated with terbutaline treatment of preterm labor. *Am J Obstet Gynecol* 1981;**139:**605.

## LACTATION

Breast feeding should be encouraged by educative measures throughout pregnancy and the puerperium. Mothers should be told the benefits of breast feeding—it is emotionally satisfying, promotes mother-infant bonding, is economical, and gives significant immunity to the infant. If the mother must return to work, even a brief period of nursing is beneficial.

Transfer of immunoglobulins in colostrum and breast milk protects the infant against many systemic and enteric infections. Macrophages and lymphocytes transferred to the infant from breast milk play an immunoprotective role. The intestinal flora of breast-fed infants inhibits the growth of pathogens. Breast-fed infants have fewer bacterial and viral infections, less severe diarrhea, fewer allergy problems, and less subsequent obesity than bottle-fed infants.

Frequent breast feeding on an infant demand schedule enhances milk flow and successful breast feeding. Mothers breast-feeding for the first time need help and encouragement from physicians, nurses, and other nursing mothers or lay groups such as the La Leche League. Milk supply can be increased by increased suckling and increased rest.

Nursing mothers should have a fluid intake of over 2 L/d. WHO suggests 24 g of extra protein (over the 41 g/d baseline for an adult woman) and 550 extra kcal/d in the first 6 months of nursing. Calcium intake should be 1200–1500 mg/d. Continuation of a prenatal vitamin and mineral supplement is wise. Strict vegetarians who eschew both milk and eggs should always take vitamin $B_{12}$ supplements during pregnancy and lactation.

### Effects of Drugs in a Nursing Mother

Drugs taken by a nursing mother may accumulate in milk and be transmitted to the infant. The amount of a drug entering the milk depends on the drug's lipid solubility, mechanism of transport, and degree of ionization (Table 13–15).

### Suppression of Lactation

**A. Mechanical Suppression:** The simplest and safest method of suppressing lactation after it has started is to gradually transfer the baby to a bottle or a cup over a 3-week period. Milk supply will decrease with decreased demand, and minimal discomfort ensues. If nursing must be stopped abruptly, the mother should avoid nipple stimulation, refrain from expressing milk, and use a snug brassiere. Ice packs and analgesics can be helpful. If suppression is desired before nursing has begun, use this same technique. Engorgement will gradually recede over a 2- to 3-day period.

**B. Hormonal Suppression:** Oral and long-acting injections of hormonal preparations are available to suppress lactation. They are all effective if begun at the time of delivery but have occasional side effects—increased thromboembolic episodes (estrogens), hair growth (androgens), changes in blood pressure and temporary emotional changes (bromocriptine).

**1. Suppression with estrogens**—Ethinyl estradiol, 0.05 mg, is administered as follows:

a. Four tablets (0.2 mg) twice daily on first postpartum day.

b. Three tablets (0.15 mg) twice daily on second day.

c. Two tablets (0.1 mg) twice daily on third day.

d. One tablet (0.05 mg) twice daily on fourth to seventh days.

**2. Suppression with estrogen and andro-**

**Table 13–15.** Drugs or substances to be used cautiously or not at all by nursing mother.[*]

| Drugs or Substances | Effect on Nursing Infant |
|---|---|
| Alcohol | No harmful effects unless taken in excess, when it can be associated with decreased linear growth and sedation. |
| Antibiotics<br>  Aminoglycosides | Not advised; will alter infant's bowel flora. |
|   Nitrofurantoin | May cause hemolytic anemia in infant with glucose-6-phosphate dehydrogenase (G6PD) deficiency. |
|   Tetracycline | Effects are dose-related; amount infant receives from milk is too small to cause discoloration of teeth. Safe. |
|   Chloramphenicol[†] | Neonate may be unable to conjugate the drug; potential harm to bone marrow, leading to anemia, shock, and death. |
|   Sulfonamides[†] | May cause jaundice in the neonatal period; may cause hemolytic anemia in infant with glucose-6-phosphate dehydrogenase (G6PD) deficiency. |
|   Metronidazole | Nursing may be resumed 48 hours after last dose. |
| Anticoagulants<br>  Phenindione | Can use heparin or warfarin instead. |
| Antihistamines | Not appreciably excreted in milk, but large doses may affect milk supply. |
| Antineoplastics[†] | Suspend nursing if these drugs are taken. |
| Antithyroids<br>  Thiouracil;[†] methimazole[†] | Contraindicated; may cause goiter or agranulocytosis. |
|   Propylthiouracil | Considered safe. |
| Cardiac drugs<br>  Quinidine[†] | Contraindicated; may cause arrhythmia in infant. |
| Cimetidine[†] | Concentrated in breast milk; may suppress gastric acidity and cause central nervous system stimulation. |
| Ergot alkaloids<br>  Ergotamine (in doses to treat migraine)[†] | Causes vomiting, diarrhea, convulsions. May suppress lactation. |
|   Bromocriptine[†] | Suppresses lactation. |
| Gold salts[†] | Contraindicated. |
| Hormones<br>  Oral contraceptives[†] | Contraindicated; may cause reduction of milk supply. |
| Laxatives<br>  Cascara, senna | Can cause diarrhea in infant. |
| Lithium carbonate[†] | Contraindicated because of toxicity. |
| Nicotine | Increased respiratory disease in infants exposed to smoke. |
| Radioactive materials for testing[†]<br>  $^{67}$Ga | Insignificant amount excreted in milk; no nursing for 2 weeks.. |
|   $^{125}$I | Discontinue nursing for 48 hours. |
|   $^{131}$I | After a test dose, nursing may be resumed after 24–36 hours; after a treatment dose, nursing may be resumed after 2–3 weeks. |
|   $^{99m}$Tc | Discontinue nursing for 72 hours (half-life, 6 hours) |
| Sedatives and tranquilizers | Can cause sedation in infant. Benzodiazepines should be avoided. |
| Other drugs<br>  Caffeine | Irritability, poor sleep pattern with large amounts. |
|   Cannabis;[†] cocaine;[†] polyhalogenated biphenyls[†] (eg, PCB$_5$, PBB$_5$); D-lysergic acid[†] (LSD) | Contraindicated; may interfere with mother's caretaking abilities and nutrition. |

[*] Modified and reproduced, with permission, from Sahu S: Drugs and the nursing mother. *Am Fam Physician* (Dec) 1981;**24**:137.
[†] Absolutely contraindicated.

**gens**–Testosterone enanthate, 180 mg/mL, and estradiol valerate, 8 mg/mL, 2 mL injected intramuscularly immediately after delivery, is very effective.

**3. Suppression with bromocriptine**–Bromocriptine (Parlodel), 2.5 mg orally twice daily with meals for 10–14 days, will suppress lactation in women who do not wish to nurse their infants or after stillbirth or abortion. The drug should not be started until 4 hours postpartum, when vital signs are stable. Postural hypotension, nausea, headache, dizziness, nasal congestion, and mild constipation have been noted as side effects. These symptoms can be allayed by reducing the dose of the drug temporarily. Hypertension, seizures, and stroke have also been reported in a small number of women.

Committee on Drugs: The transfer of drugs and other chemicals into human breast milk. *Pediatrics* 1983;**72**:375.

## PUERPERAL MASTITIS
### (See also Chapter 12)

Postpartum mastitis occurs sporadically in nursing mothers shortly after they return home, or it may occur in epidemic form in the hospital. Hemolytic *Staphylococcus aureus* is usually the causative agent. Inflammation is generally unilateral, and women nursing for the first time are more often affected.

Mastitis frequently begins within 3 months after delivery and may start with a sore or fissured nipple. There is obvious cellulitis in an area of breast tissue, with redness, tenderness, local warmth, and fever. Treatment consists of antibiotics effective against penicillin-resistant organisms (dicloxacillin or a cephalosporin) and regular emptying of the breast by nursing followed by expression of any remaining milk by hand or with a mechanical suction device.

If the mother begins antibiotic therapy before suppuration begins, infection can usually be controlled in 24 hours. If delay is permitted, breast abscess can result. Incision and drainage are required for abscess formation. Despite puerperal mastitis, the baby usually thrives without prophylactic antimicrobial therapy.

Thomsen AC, Espersen T, Maigaard S: Course and treatment of milk stasis, noninfectious inflammation of the breast, and infectious mastitis in nursing women. *Am J Obstet Gynecol* 1984;**149**:492.

## REFERENCES

Benson RC (editor): *Current Obstetric & Gynecologic Diagnosis & Treatment,* 5th ed. Lange, 1984.

Briggs GG et al: *Drugs in Pregnancy and Lactation.* Williams & Wilkins, 1983.

Callen P: *Ultrasonography in Obstetrics and Gynecology.* Saunders, 1983.

Creasy RK, Resnik R: *Maternal-Fetal Medicine: Principles and Practice.* Saunders, 1984.

Cutler WB, Garcia CR: *The Medical Management of Menopause and Premenopause.* Lippincott, 1984.

Danforth DM, Scott JR (editors): *Obstetrics and Gynecology,* 5th ed. Lippincott, 1986.

Ellis J, Beckman C (editors): *Clinical Manual of Obstetrics.* Appleton-Century-Crofts, 1983.

Hatcher RA et al: *Contraceptive Technology 1986–1987.* Irvington, 1986.

Jones HW Jr, Jones GS: *Novak's Textbook of Gynecology,* 10th ed. Williams & Wilkins, 1981.

Kaplan HS: *The New Sex Therapy.* Brunner/Mazel, 1974.

Pritchard JA, MacDonald PC, Gant NF: *Williams Obstetrics,* 17th ed. Appleton-Century-Crofts, 1985.

Speroff L, Glass R, Kase N: *Clinical Gynecologic Endocrinology and Infertility,* 3rd ed. Williams & Wilkins, 1983.

Worthington-Roberts BS, Vermeersch J, Williams SL: *Nutrition in Pregnancy and Lactation,* 2nd ed. Mosby, 1985.

# 14 Arthritis & Musculoskeletal Disorders

*Martin A. Shearn, MD*

## Examination of the Patient

The diagnosis of a rheumatic disease can often be made at the bedside or in the office by history and physical examination; special attention is paid to signs of articular inflammation (eg, heat, soft tissue swelling, effusion) and the functional status of the joints (eg, range of motion, deformity). Laboratory procedures complete the study, most commonly including sedimentation rate, tests for rheumatoid factor and antinuclear or other antibodies, synovianalysis, and x-rays of affected joints. These studies are important for diagnosis and as a baseline for judging the results of therapy.

## Examination of Joint Fluid

Synovial fluid examination (Table 14–1) may provide specific diagnostic information in joint disease.

When performed, the following studies should be included:

**(1) Gross examination:** If fluid is green or purulent, a Gram's stain is indicated. If grossly bloody, consider a bleeding disorder, trauma, or "traumatic tap." Note if the fluid is xanthochromic.

**(2) Microscopic examination:**

**(a) Cytology:** Collect 2–5 mL in a heparinized tube. The red and white cells are counted, using the same equipment and technique as for a standard white count. The diluent, however, should be normal saline solution, since the usual acidified diluent causes the fluid to clot in the pipette. One drop of methylene blue added to the diluent makes the cells distinguishable. Differential counts are performed on thin smears with Wright's stain.

**(b) Crystals:** Compensated polarized light microscopy identifies the existence and type of crystals. The demonstration of urate or calcium pyrophosphate crystals is most important diagnostically.

**(3) Culture:** Collect 1 mL of fluid in a sterile culture tube and perform routine bacterial cultures as well as special studies for gonococci, tubercle bacilli, or fungi when indicated.

**(4) Glucose:** Collect 2–3 mL of fluid in a fluoride tube. The patient should be in a fasting state and the blood glucose determined at the time of joint aspiration.

**Interpretation.** (See Table 14–2). Synovial fluid studies are not diagnostic unless a specific organism is identified in the culture or urate crystals of gout or calcium pyrophosphate crystals of pseudogout are demonstrated. There is considerable overlap in the cytologic and biochemical values obtained in different diseases. These studies do make possible, however, a differentiation according to severity of inflammation. Thus, joint fluids in inflammatory diseases such as infections and rheumatoid arthritis are often turbid, with an elevated white count (usually well above 3000 cells/µL, with over 50% polynucleated forms) and a synovial fluid sugar content that is considerably lower than the blood glucose. In diseases characterized by relatively mild articular inflammation, such as degenerative joint disease or traumatic arthritis, the synovial fluid is usually clear, with a low white

**Table 14–1.** Examination of joint fluid.

| Measure | Normal | Group I (Noninflammatory) | Group II (Inflammatory) | Group III (Septic) |
|---|---|---|---|---|
| Volume (mL) (knee) | < 3.5 | Often > 3.5 | Often > 3.5 | Often > 3.5 |
| Clarity | Transparent | Transparent | Translucent-opaque | Opaque |
| Color | Clear | Yellow | Yellow to opalescent | Yellow to green |
| WBC (per µL) | < 200 | 200–3000 | 3000–100,000 | > 100,000* |
| Polymorphonuclear leukocytes (%) | < 25% | < 25% | 50% or more | 75% or more* |
| Culture | Negative | Negative | Negative | Usually positive |
| Glucose (mg/dL) | Nearly equal to serum | Nearly equal to serum | > 25, lower than serum | < 25, much lower than serum |

* Counts are lower with infections caused by organisms of low virulence or if antibiotic therapy as been started.

**Table 14–2.** Differential diagnosis by joint fluid groups.[*]

| Group I (Noninflammatory) | Group II (Inflammatory) | Group III (Septic) | Hemorrhagic |
|---|---|---|---|
| Degenerative joint disease<br>Trauma[†]<br>Osteochondritis dissecans<br>Osteochondromatosis<br>Neuropathic arthropathy[†]<br>Subsiding or early inflammation<br>Hypertrophic osteoarthropathy[‡]<br>Pigmented villonodular synovitis[†] | Rheumatoid arthritis<br>Acute crystal-induced synovitis (gout and pseudogout)<br>Reiter's syndrome<br>Ankylosing spondylitis<br>Psoriatic arthritis<br>Arthritis accompanying ulcerative colitis and regional enteritis<br>Rheumatic fever[‡]<br>Systemic lupus erythematosus[‡]<br>Progressive systemic sclerosis (scleroderma)[‡] | Bacterial infections | Hemophilia or other hemorrhagic diathesis<br>Trauma with or without fracture<br>Neuropathic arthropathy<br>Pigmented villonodular synovitis<br>Synovioma<br>Hemangioma and other benign neoplasm |

[*] Reproduced from Rodnan GP (editor): Primer on the rheumatic diseases, 7th ed. *JAMA* 1973;**244(Suppl):**662.
[†] May be hemorrhagic.
[‡] Groups I or II.

cell count (usually below 3000/μL), and the synovial fluid and blood glucose levels are within 10 mg/dL of each other.

# AUTOIMMUNE DISEASES (Collagen Diseases, Connective Tissue Diseases

The autoimmune disorders are a protean group of acquired diseases in which genetic factors appear to play a role. They have in common widespread immunologic and inflammatory alterations of connective tissue.

These illnesses share certain clinical features, and differentiation among them is often difficult because of this. Common findings include synovitis, pleuritis, myocarditis, endocarditis, pericarditis, peritonitis, vasculitis, myositis, skin rash, alterations of connective tissues, and nephritis. Laboratory tests may reveal Coombs-positive hemolytic anemia, thrombocytopenia, leukopenia, immunoglobulin excesses or deficiencies, antinuclear antibodies (which include antibodies to many nuclear constituents, including DNA and extractable nuclear antigen), rheumatoid factors, cryoglobulins, false-positive serologic tests for syphilis, elevated muscle enzymes, and alterations in serum complement.

Although the autoimmune disorders are regarded as acquired diseases, their causes cannot be determined in most instances. Heredity, environmental antigens, immunoglobulin deficiency, inappropriate T lymphocyte function, immune complexes, anaphylaxis, cytolysis, or some combination of all of these factors appear to play causative and pathogenic roles. The causative role of viruses is also being investigated.

Some of the laboratory alterations that occur in this group of diseases (eg, false-positive serologic tests for syphilis, rheumatoid factor) occur in asymptomatic individuals. These changes may also be demonstrated in certain asymptomatic relatives of patients with connective tissue diseases, in older persons, in patients using certain drugs, and in patients with chronic infectious diseases.

# RHEUMATOID ARTHRITIS

## Essentials of Diagnosis

- Prodromal systemic symptoms of malaise, fever, weight loss, and morning stiffness.
- Onset usually insidious and in small joints; progression is centripetal and symmetric; deformities common.
- Radiographic findings: juxta-articular osteoporosis, joint erosions, and narrowing of the joint spaces.
- Rheumatoid factor usually present.
- Extra-articular manifestations: subcutaneous nodules, pleural effusion, pericarditis, lymphadenopathy, splenomegaly with leukopenia, and vasculitis.

## General Considerations

Rheumatoid arthritis is a chronic systemic inflammatory disease of unknown cause, chiefly affecting synovial membranes of multiple joints. The disease has a wide clinical spectrum with considerable variability in joint and extra-articular manifestations. The prevalence in the general population is 1–2%; female patients outnumber males almost 3:1. The usual age at onset is 20–40 years, although rheumatoid arthritis may begin at any age.

The pathologic findings in the joint include chronic synovitis with pannus formation. The pannus erodes cartilage, bone, ligaments, and tendons. In the acute phase, effusion and other manifestations of inflammation are common. In the late stage, organization may result in fibrous ankylosis; true bony ankylosis is rare. In both acute and chronic phases, inflammation of soft tissues around the joints may be prominent and is a significant factor in joint damage.

The microscopic findings most characteristic of rheumatoid arthritis are those of the subcutaneous nodule. This is a granuloma with a central zone of fibrinoid necrosis, a surrounding palisade of radially arranged elongated connective tissue cells, and a periphery of chronic granulation tissue. Pathologic alterations indistinguishable from those of the subcutaneous nodule are occasionally seen in the myocardium, pericardium, endocardium, heart valves, visceral pleura, lungs, sclera, dura mater, spleen, and larynx as well as in the synovial membrane, periarticular tissues, and tendons. Nonspecific pericarditis and pleuritis are found in 25–40% of patients at autopsy. Additional nonspecific lesions associated with rheumatoid arthritis include inflammation of small arteries, pulmonary fibrosis, round cell infiltration of skeletal muscle and perineurium, and hyperplasia of lymph nodes. Secondary amyloidosis may also be present.

## Clinical Findings

**A. Symptoms and Signs:** The clinical manifestations of rheumatoid disease are highly variable. The onset of articular signs of inflammation is usually insidious, with prodromal symptoms of malaise, weight loss, vasomotor disturbances (eg, paresthesias, Raynaud's phenomenon), and vague periarticular pain or stiffness. Less often, the onset is acute, apparently triggered by a stressful situation such as infection, surgery, trauma, emotional strain, or the postpartum period. There is characteristically symmetric joint swelling with associated stiffness, warmth, tenderness, and pain. Stiffness is prominent in the morning and subsides during the day; its duration is a useful indicator of activity of disease. Stiffness may recur after daytime inactivity and may be much more severe after strenuous activity. Although any joint may be affected in rheumatoid arthritis, the proximal interphalangeal and metacarpophalangeal joints of the fingers as well as the wrists, knees, ankles, and toes are most often involved. Monarticular disease is occasionally seen early. Synovial cysts and rupture of tendons may occur. Entrapment syndromes are not unusual—particularly entrapment of the median nerve at the carpal tunnel of the wrist. Palmar erythema is noted occasionally, as are tiny hemorrhagic infarcts in the nail folds or finger pulps, which are signs of vasculitis. Twenty percent of patients have subcutaneous nodules, most commonly situated over bony prominences but also observed in the bursas and tendon sheaths. A small number of patients have splenomegaly and lymph node enlargement. Low-grade fever, anorexia, weight loss, fatigue, and weakness often persist; chills are rare. After months or years, thickening of the periarticular tissue, flexion deformities, subluxation, fibrosis, and ankylosis may occur. Atrophy of skin or muscle is common. Dryness of the eyes, mouth, and other mucous membranes, is found especially in advanced disease (see Sjögren's Syndrome). Other ocular manifestations include episcleritis and scleromalacia, often due to scleral nodules. Pericarditis and pleural disease, when present, are frequently silent clinically.

**B. Laboratory Findings:** Serum protein abnormalities are often present. Rheumatoid factor, an IGM antibody directed against other globulins, is present in the sera of 75% of patients. High titers of rheumatoid factor are commonly associated with severe rheumatoid disease. Titers may also be significantly elevated in a number of diverse conditions, including syphilis, sarcoidosis, infective endocarditis, tuberculosis, leprosy, and parasitic infections; in advanced age; and in asymptomatic relatives of patients with autoimmune diseases. Antinuclear antibodies are often demonstrable, although their titers are lower in rheumatoid arthritis than in systemic lupus erythematosus.

During both the acute and chronic phases, the erythrocyte sedimentation rate and the gamma globulins (most commonly IgM and IgG) are typically elevated. A moderate hypochromic normocytic anemia is common. The white cell count is normal or slightly elevated, but leukopenia may occur, often in the presence of splenomegaly (eg, Felty's syndrome). Joint fluid examination is valuable, reflecting abnormalities that are associated with varying degrees of inflammation. (See Tables 14–1 and 14–2.) Low synovial complement values are found in severe forms of rheumatoid arthritis.

**C. Imaging:** Early radiographic signs are soft tissue swelling, osteoporosis around the involved joint, and erosion of the peripheral "bare space" of bone surface that is not covered by cartilage. Later, extensive erosion of cartilage causes joint space narrowing. Bony cysts result from invasion by granulation tissue. Rheumatoid synovium may invade the joint capsule, ligaments, and tendons, and it may add to joint instability induced by destruction of cartilage and bone. After some years, the degenerative changes of secondary osteoarthritis may be superimposed. Special attention should be directed to the upper cervical spine and especially to C1–2, where subluxation may result in the development of serious neurologic complications. This most commonly occurs after several years of active disease, though neck pain without x-ray findings occurs early in the course.

## Differential Diagnosis

The differentiation of rheumatoid arthritis from other diseases of connective tissue can be difficult. However, certain clinical features are helpful. Rheumatic fever is characterized by the migratory nature of the arthritis, the more common occurrence of carditis, and an elevated antistreptolysin titer. Butterfly rash, discoid lupus erythematosus, photosensitivity, alopecia, high titer to anti-DNA, renal disease, and central nervous system abnormalities point to the diagnosis of systemic lupus erythematosus. Degenerative joint disease (osteoarthritis) is not associated with constitutional manifestations, and the joint pain is characteristically relieved by rest, in contrast to the morning stiffness of rheumatoid arthritis. Signs of articular inflammation, prominent in rheumatoid arthritis, are usually minimal in degenerative joint disease. Gouty arthritis may be confused with rheumatoid arthritis, but acute onset in one joint, the identification of urate crystals in the joint fluid, the presence of tophi in chronic disease, and the response to colchicine indicate gout. Pyogenic arthritis can be distinguished by chills and fever, the demonstration of the causative organism in the joint fluid, and the frequent presence of a primary focus elsewhere, eg, gonococcal urethritis.

## Treatment

**A. Basic Program (Conservative Management):** Evidence indicates that conservative management offers a long-term prognosis that may be as good as that of more aggressive and potentially more toxic regimens. Since no measures are curative, a conservative approach should be initiated first.

The primary objectives of treatment of rheumatoid arthritis are reduction of inflammation and pain, preservation of function, and prevention of deformity. A regimen consisting of rest, physical therapy, and nonsteroidal anti-inflammatory agents is a worthwhile means of rehabilitating the patient. These measures constitute the basic program of treatment to which other treatment may be added.

**1. Systemic rest–** The amount of rest required depends upon the severity of the disease. Complete bed rest may be desirable in patients with profound systemic and articular involvement. In mild disease, 2 hours of rest each day may suffice. In general, rest should be continued until significant improvement is sustained for at least 2 weeks; thereafter, the program may be liberalized. However, the increase of physical activity must proceed gradually and with appropriate support for any involved weight-bearing joints.

**2. Emotional factors–**The importance of emotional factors in rheumatoid arthritis and the need for psychologic support cannot be overemphasized. This depends in part upon rapport between the patient and the doctor and involves a support system at home. Patients need help in dealing with fear, disability, loss, and helplessness.

**3. Articular rest–**Decrease of articular inflammation may be expedited by articular rest. Relaxation and stretching of the hip and knee muscles, to prevent flexion contractures, can be accomplished by having the patient lie in the prone position for 15 minutes several times daily in addition to nighttime rest. Sitting in a flexed position for prolonged periods is a poor form of joint rest. Appropriate adjustable supports provide rest for inflamed weight-bearing joints, relieve spasm, and may reduce deformities, soft tissue contracture, or instability of the ligaments. The supports must be removable to permit daily range of motion and exercise of the affected extremities (see below). When ambulation is started, care must be taken to avoid weight bearing, which may aggravate

flexion deformities. This is accomplished with the aid of crutches or braces until the tendency toward contracture has subsided.

**4. Exercise–**This is the most important measure in the physical therapy of rheumatoid arthritis. The management of rheumatoid arthritis is based on the concomitant use of rest and therapeutic exercise in proper balance. Therapeutic exercises are designed to preserve joint motion, muscular strength, and endurance. Most effective are exercises of the active-assistive type, which should be performed, within the limits of pain tolerance, from the outset of management. As tolerance for exercise increases and the activity of the disease subsides, progressive resistance exercises may be introduced.

**5. Heat and cold–**These are used primarily for their muscle-relaxing and analgesic effect. Radiant or moist heat is generally most satisfactory. The ambulatory patient will find warm tub baths convenient. Paraffin baths for the hands are inexpensive and help many patients to reduce morning stiffness. Exercise may be better performed after exposure to heat. Some patients derive more relief of joint pain from local application of cold.

**6. Nonsteroidal anti-inflammatory drugs–**

**a. Aspirin–**Aspirin is an effective anti-inflammatory antipyretic agent and the least expensive of the various drugs available to treat rheumatoid arthritis. It is usually the first drug employed unless there is some contraindication to its use. The proper dose is the amount that provides optimal relief of symptoms without causing toxic reactions. Most adults can tolerate daily doses of 4–6 g, which result in therapeutic serum salicylate levels of 20–30 mg/dL. After 1 week, the salicylate half-life increases to 15 hours; therefore, the patient need not be given aspirin every 4 hours, as is often recommended. If tinnitus—an early manifestation of toxicity—occurs, the daily dose should be lowered by decrements of 0.6 or 0.9 g until this symptom disappears. Symptoms of gastric irritation may be lessened by the ingestion of salicylates with meals and antacid. The use of enteric-coated tablets may also reduce gastric irritation. Salicylates should not be used by patients with a history of allergy to aspirin or related products. Nearly all patients receiving high doses of salicylates test positively for occult blood in the stool; however, more significant hemorrhage may also occur, with or without gastrointestinal symptoms.

**b. Other nonsteroidal anti-inflammatory drugs–**If aspirin proves ineffective or if intolerable gastrointestinal effects occur, a trial of the newer anti-inflammatory analgesic agents is indicated. Because of a simpler dosage schedule for most of these agents, compliance may be better. A number of nonsteroidal anti-inflammatory analgesic drugs are available, including ibuprofen (Motrin), fenoprofen (Nalfon), naproxen (Naprosyn), tolmetin (Tolectin), sulindac (Clinoril), meclofenamate sodium (Meclomen), and piroxicam (Feldene). Other drugs of this class are also available, some only outside the USA.

The new drugs themselves are not free of gastroduodenal and other side effects (particularly renal) but tend to cause less gastrointestinal discomfort than does aspirin in full dosage. Renal toxicity may occur, including interstitial nephritis; nephrotic syndrome reversible renal failure may be associated. Hyperkalemia due to hyporeninemic hypoaldosteronism may also be seen. While more expensive, none of the drugs is superior to salicylates in efficacy. Each of them, however, may be effective in patients who fail to respond to salicylate therapy. Drug toxicity also varies from individual to individual.

Indomethacin is probably no more effective than the salicylates in rheumatoid arthritis, and its untoward effects are far greater. Phenylbutazone is not advised for chronic therapy because of its toxicity.

**7. Physical therapy**–See p 530.

**B. Other anti-inflammatory drugs:**

**1. Antimalarials**–Hydroxychloroquine sulfate (Plaquenil), the agent most often used in this group, has antirheumatic properties. A dosage of 200–400 mg/d minimizes the likelihood of toxic reactions. The most important reaction, pigmentary retinitis causing visual loss, is fortunately rare when the dosage is kept low. Periodic ophthalmologic examinations are suggested when this drug is employed for long-term therapy. Other reactions include neuropathies and myopathies of both skeletal and cardiac muscle, which usually improve when the drug is withdrawn.

**2. Gold salts (chrysotherapy)**–Gold salts in the treatment of rheumatoid arthritis have gained increased popularity in recent years. There is evidence that these agents may retard the bone erosions of rheumatoid arthritis. About 60% of patients may be expected to benefit from gold therapy, although complete remissions are uncommon. Their mode of action is not known.

**a. Indications**–Disease responding unfavorably to conservative management; erosive disease.

**b. Contraindications**–Previous gold toxicity; significant renal, hepatic, or hematopoietic dysfunction.

**c. Preparations of choice**–Intramuscular gold sodium thiomalate or aurothioglucose; oral auranofin.

**d. Dosage**–The intramuscular dose is 50 mg weekly until toxic reactions appear or there is a clinical response. If there is no response after 800 mg have been administered, the drug should be discontinued. If the response is good, a total dose of 1 g should be given, followed by a regimen of 50 mg every 2 weeks and, with continued improvement, every 3 and then every 4 weeks for an indefinite period. Recent studies suggest that smaller doses may be effective. The oral dose of auranofin is 3 mg twice daily until benefit or toxicity occurs.

**e. Toxic reactions**–About 32% of patients (range in various series: 4–55%) experience toxic reactions to gold therapy; the mortality rate is less than 0.4%. The manifestations of toxicity are similar to those of poisoning by other heavy metals (notably arsenic) and include dermatitis (mild to exfoliative,

and pruritic), stomatitis, neutropenia, nephritis, and nitritoid reactions (especially to gold thiomalate and presumably due to its vehicle). Auranofin causes side effects less frequently than gold, though diarrhea is common. In order to prevent or reduce the severity of toxic reactions, gold should not be given to patients with any of the contraindicating disorders listed above. Periodic urinalyses and complete blood counts should be obtained.

If signs of toxicity appear, the drug should be withdrawn immediately. Severe toxicity may require corticosteroids for control, and failure to respond might then be an indication for the cautious use of penicillamine or dimercaprol (BAL) as chelating agents for the gold. Worsening of articular symptoms after the initial dose is often temporary and is not an indication for withdrawal of the drug. Patients so affected may ultimately respond favorably if treatment is continued.

**3. Corticosteroids**–Although corticosteroids usually produce an immediate and dramatic anti-inflammatory effect in rheumatoid arthritis, they do not alter the natural progression of the disease; furthermore, clinical manifestations of active disease commonly reappear when the drug is discontinued. The serious problem of untoward reactions resulting from prolonged corticosteroid therapy greatly limits its long-term use. Another disadvantage that might stem from the use of steroids lies in the tendency of the patient and the physician to neglect the less spectacular but proved benefits derived from general supportive treatment, physical therapy, and orthopedic measures.

The corticosteroids may be used on a short-term basis to tide patients over acute disabling episodes, to facilitate other treatment measures (eg, physical therapy), or to manage serious extra-articular manifestations (eg, pericarditis, perforating eye lesions). Corticosteroids may also be indicated for active and progressive disease that does not respond favorably to conservative management and when there are contraindications to or therapeutic failure of gold salts and penicillamine.

The least amount of steroid that will achieve the desired clinical effect should be given, but not more than 10 mg of prednisone or equivalent per day is appropriate for articular disease. Many patients do reasonably well on 5–7.5 mg daily. (The use of 1-mg tablets is to be encouraged.) When the steroids are to be discontinued, they should be phased out gradually on a planned schedule appropriate to the duration of treatment.

Intra-articular corticosteroids may be helpful if one or 2 joints are the chief source of difficulty. Intra-articular hydrocortisone, 25–50 mg, may be given for symptomatic relief, but no more often than 4 times a year.

**4. Penicillamine**–This agent may be used in patients with severe rheumatoid arthritis who have continuing rheumatic activity in spite of therapy with the agents discussed above. Penicillamine may prove effective in a number of such patients, although toxicity is substantial. The mechanism of action is not understood. Up to one-half of patients experience some side effects such as oral ulcers, loss of taste, fever, rash, thrombocytopenia, leukopenia, and aplastic anemia. Proteinuria and nephrotic syndrome may occur. Immune complex diseases (eg, myasthenia gravis, systemic lupus erythematosus, polymyositis, Goodpasture's syndrome) appear to be induced by the drug. It should not be used during pregnancy.

If penicillamine is employed, one should start with small doses: 250 mg daily, increasing by 125 mg every 2–3 months up to a maximum of 750 mg–1 g/d. Penicillamine is given between meals to enhance absorption. Careful monitoring for toxicity is essential.

**C. Experimental Cytotoxic Drugs:** Cyclophosphamide, methotrexate, azathioprine, and chlorambucil have been used in patients with severe rheumatoid arthritis. Response to treatment is not invariably correlated with laboratory parameters of rheumatoid activity. The toxicity of these drugs and their potential teratogenic and oncogenic capacities are such that they should not be employed except by a physician thoroughly conversant with their use. At this time, only azathioprine has been approved by the FDA for the treatment of rheumatoid arthritis.

**D. Surgical Measures:** See p 531.

## Prognosis

The course of rheumatoid arthritis is totally unpredictable, although spontaneous remissions and relapses are common early in the disease. Occasionally, in well-established cases, permanent spontaneous remission occurs, with either return to normal function of the involved joints (if involvement is early and minimal) or some decrease in the degree of disability (if of longer duration). Although the disease is commonly progressive—and although some degree of permanent deformity may result—it must be emphasized that after 10 years most patients are capable of self-care and fully employable.

Maksymowych W, Russell AS: Antimalarials in rheumatology: Efficacy and safety. *Semin Arthritis Rheum* 1987;**16**:206.
Million R et al: Long-term study of management of rheumatoid arthritis. *Lancet* 1984;**1**:812.
O'Brien WM, Bagby GF: Rare adverse reactions to nonsteroidal antiinflammatory drugs. *J Rheumatol* 1985;**12**:1.

## JUVENILE CHRONIC ARTHRITIS

Rheumatoidlike disease with onset before age 17 is referred to as juvenile chronic arthritis. Synovitis that persists for at least 6 weeks is an essential criterion of diagnosis. Various expressions of the disease have been described, including (1) a form with systemic onset often called Still's disease; (2) pauciarticular arthritis, often with iritis; (3) polyarticular arthritis, including both seronegative and seropositive types, resembling adult disease; and (4) a peripheral arthritis

of few or many joints in older boys, who later develop ankylosing spondylitis. In systemic-onset disease, there is a characteristic evanescent, salmon-colored morbilliform rash, a high spiking fever that may antedate the arthritis by months, and common occurrence of hepatosplenomegaly, lymphadenopathy, and pleuropericarditis. Iritis may be asymptomatic and detected only by slit lamp examination; it occurs commonly in patients with mild arthritis. A clinical presentation with features identical to those of juvenile chronic arthritis may recur in adulthood after an episode before age 17 or may even appear for the first time in adult life.

In many children with polyarticular chronic arthritis, the apophyseal joints of the cervical spine, especially C2–3, are affected. Abnormalities of bony growth and development are related to active disease and may be transient and reversible or, with chronic disease activity, may be irreversible and result in premature closure of epiphyses or ossification centers; micrognathia is one consequence.

The differential diagnosis of juvenile chronic arthritis includes idiopathic ankylosing spondylitis, leukemia or lymphoma, and chronic infectious disease. Joint fluid examination, culture, and synovial biopsy may be useful in diagnosis. Antinuclear antibody is often found in the subgroup that develops iritis. Rheumatoid factor is positive only in the small subset of patients whose disease resembles adult rheumatoid arthritis. HLA-B27 positivity is common in patients without rheumatoid factor but is of little use diagnostically because of its cost and the high incidence of false-positives.

The treatment of juvenile chronic arthritis must be individualized; in general, the approach to therapy is similar to that for adult rheumatoid arthritis.

Kredich DW: Chronic arthritis in childhood. *Med Clin North Am* 1986;**70**:305.
Wouters JMGW, van de Putte LBA: Adult-onset Still's disease: Clinical and laboratory features, treatment and progress of 45 cases. *Quart J Med* 1986;**61**:1055.

## SYSTEMIC LUPUS ERYTHEMATOSUS

### Essentials of Diagnosis

- Occurs mainly in young women.
- Rash over areas exposed to sunlight.
- Joint symptoms in 90% of patients.
- Multiple system involvement.
- Depression of hemoglobin, white blood cells, platelets.
- Serologic findings: antinuclear antibody with high titer to native DNA.

### General Considerations

Systemic lupus erythematosus is an inflammatory autoimmune disorder that may affect multiple organ systems. Its clinical manifestations are thought to be secondary to the trapping of antigen-antibody complexes in capillaries of visceral structures. The clinical course may vary from a mild episodic disorder to a rapidly fulminating fatal illness.

Systemic lupus erythematosus is not uncommon. Figures from a large representative urban community population indicate a prevalence exceeding one in 2000 persons. About 85% of patients are women. Although the disease may occur at any age, most patients are between ages 10 and 50, with greatest clustering between 20 and 40. Blacks are affected more often than members of other races.

Before making a diagnosis of spontaneous systemic lupus erythematosus, it is imperative to ascertain that the condition has not been induced by a drug. Approximately 25 pharmacologic agents have been implicated as causing a lupuslike syndrome, but only a few cause the disorder with appreciable frequency. Procainamide and hydralazine are the most important and best studied of these drugs. While antinuclear antibody tests and other serologic findings become positive in many persons receiving these agents, in only a few do clinical manifestations occur.

Four features of drug-induced lupus separate it from spontaneously occurring disease: (1) the sex ratio is nearly equal; (2) nephritis and central nervous system features are not ordinarily present; (3) depressed serum complement and antibodies to native DNA are absent; and (4) the clinical features and most laboratory abnormalities must often revert toward normal when the offending drug is withdrawn.

The familial occurrence of systemic lupus erythematosus has been repeatedly documented, and the disorder has involved identical twins in a number of instances. Aggregation of serologic features (positive antinuclear antibody, antibodies to DNA, hypergammaglobulinemia) is seen in asymptomatic family members, and the prevalence of other rheumatic diseases is increased among close relatives of patients. There is increased incidence of HLA-DR2 and -DR3 in lupus. A current hypothesis suggests that there is an underlying genetically determined abnormality in immunologic regulation, related to defective T lymphocyte suppressor function, resulting in overactivity of B cells. This leads to production of multiple autoantibodies, which causes tissue damage through the mechanism of immune complex deposition.

Viruses are thought to play a role in the induction of this disorder in a genetically disposed host. The New Zealand mouse, in which a clinical syndrome develops that is remarkably similar to idiopathic lupus in humans, harbors the murine leukemia virus. Patients with systemic lupus have increased antibody titers to various viral antigens, including those of measles, rubella, and parainfluenza. Electron micrographs of capillary endothelial cells in renal biopsy tissue and of circulating lymphocytes have shown tubular reticular structures thought to be virus-related.

The diagnosis of systemic lupus erythematosus should be suspected in patients having a multisystem disease with serologic positivity (eg, antinuclear antibody, serologic test for syphilis). Differential diagnosis includes diseases that may present in a similar manner, such as rheumatoid arthritis, scleroderma, chronic active hepatitis, acute drug reactions, polyarteritis, and drug-induced lupus.

The American Rheumatism Association has proposed that the diagnosis of systemic lupus erythematosus can be made with reasonable probability if 4 of the 11 following criteria are present, serially or simultaneously, during any interval of observation: malar rash; discoid rash; photosensitivity; oral ulcers; nonerosive arthritis; serositis; renal disorder; neurologic disorder; hematologic abnormality (hemolytic anemia, leukopenia, lymphopenia, or thrombocytopenia); immune dysfunction (positive LE preparation, antinative DNA, anti-Sm, false-positive syphilis serologic tests for more than 6 months); and positive antinuclear antibody.

## Clinical Findings

**A. Symptoms and Signs:** The systemic features include fever, anorexia, malaise, and weight loss. Most patients have skin lesions at some time; the characteristic "butterfly" rash affects fewer than half of patients. Other cutaneous manifestations are discoid lupus, typical fingertip lesions, periungual erythema, nail fold infarcts, and splinter hemorrhages. Alopecia is common. Mucous membrane lesions tend to occur during periods of exacerbation. Raynaud's phenomenon, present in about 20% of patients, often antedates other features of the disease.

Joint symptoms, with or without active synovitis, occur in over 90% of patients and are often the earliest manifestation. The arthritis is rarely deforming; erosive changes are almost never noted on x-ray study. Subcutaneous nodules are rare.

Ocular manifestations include conjunctivitis, photophobia, transient blindness, and blurring of vision. Cotton-wool spots on the retina (cytoid bodies) represent degeneration of nerve fibers due to occlusion of retinal blood vessels.

Pleurisy, pleural effusion, bronchopneumonia, and pneumonitis are frequent. Restrictive lung disease is often demonstrated.

The pericardium is affected in the majority of patients. Cardiac failure may result from myocarditis and hypertension. Cardiac arrhythmias are common. Atypical verrucous endocarditis of Libman-Sacks, occasionally seen at autopsy, rarely alters cardiac dynamics during life.

Abdominal pains, ileus, and peritonitis may result from vasculitis; the right colon is especially susceptible. Nonspecific reactive hepatitis or that induced by salicylates may alter liver function.

Neurologic complications of systemic lupus erythematosus are usually observed in patients who have highly active disease. Severe depression and psychosis are sometimes heightened by the administration of large doses of corticosteroids. Convulsive disorders, peripheral and cranial neuropathies, transverse myelitis, cerebrovascular accidents, and Guillain-Barré syndrome may be seen.

Several forms of renal disease are encountered. Proliferative glomerulonephritis, which may be associated with nephrotic syndrome and renal insufficiency, is the major threat to life in systemic lupus erythematosus. Mesangial nephritis is usually benign but occasionally may progress. A third type, membranous glomerulonephritis, is associated with profuse proteinuria, and tends to be very slowly progressive. With appropriate therapy, the survival rate even for patients with serious renal disease (proliferative glomerulonephritis) is favorable.

Other clinical features include lymphadenopathy, splenomegaly, Hashimoto's thyroiditis, hemolytic anemia, and thrombocytopenic purpura.

**B. Laboratory Findings:** The LE cell is neither sensitive nor specific for systemic lupus erythematosus. Antinuclear antibody is detected in more than 95% of cases. Serum elevations of antibodies to double-stranded DNA and Sm have a greater specificity than does that of antinuclear antibody, but they are less sensitive. Depressed serum complement—a finding suggestive of disease activity—often returns toward normal in remission. Anti-DNA antibody levels also correlate with disease activity; anti-Sm levels do not. Hypergammaglobulinemia, a positive Coombs test reaction, and rheumatoid factor may be demonstrable in the serum. Biologically false-positive serologic tests for syphilis occur in about 20% of patients. The fluorescent treponemal antibody absorption test may also be falsely positive, though much less often; a beaded pattern of immunofluorescence may serve to distinguish it from a true positive reaction. Antibody titers to a wide variety of other cellular tissues and organ tissues may be observed.

There is often mild normocytic, normochromic anemia and occasionally autoimmune hemolytic anemia. The sedimentation rate is almost always elevated when the disease is active. Leukopenia and lymphopenia are common; thrombocytopenia occasionally may be severe, resulting in purpura or bleeding. A lupus anticoagulant results in elevation of the partial thromboplastin time but not in clinical bleeding.

Liver function tests are often mildly abnormal. Abnormality of urinary sediment is almost always found in association with renal lesions. Showers of red blood cells, with or without casts, and mild proteinuria are frequent during exacerbation of the disease; these usually abate with remission.

## Treatment

Many patients with systemic lupus erythematosus have a benign form of the disease requiring only supportive care and need little or no medication. Patients with photosensitivity should be cautioned against sun exposure and should apply a protective lotion to the skin while out of doors. Skin lesions often respond to the local administration of corticosteroids. Joint symptoms can usually be alleviated by rest and full salicylate dosage. Every drug that may have precipitated the condition should be withdrawn if possible.

Antimalarials (hydroxychloroquine) may be helpful in treating the joint and skin features. When these are used, the dose should generally not exceed 200 mg/d, and periodic monitoring for retinal changes is necessary. Drug-induced neuropathy and myopathy may be erroneously ascribed to the underlying disease (see p 499). Corticosteroids are required for the control of certain serious complications. These include thrombocytopenic purpura, hemolytic anemia, myocarditis, pericarditis, convulsions, and nephritis. Forty to 60 mg of prednisone are often needed initially; however, the lowest dose of corticosteroid that controls the condition should be employed. Central nervous system lupus may require higher doses of corticosteroids than are usually given; however, steroid psychosis may mimic lupus cerebritis, in which case reduced doses are appropriate. In lupus nephritis, sequential studies of serum complement and antibodies to DNA often permit early detection of disease exacerbation and thus prompt increase in corticosteroid therapy. Such studies also allow for lowering the dosage of the drugs and withdrawing them when they are no longer needed. Immunosuppressive agents such as cyclophosphamide, chlorambucil, and azathioprine are used in cases resistant to corticosteroids. Patients with proliferative glomerulonephritis may do better when an immunosuppressive agent is added to steroid therapy. Very close follow-up is needed to watch for potential side effects when immunosuppressants are employed; these agents should be given by those experienced in their use. Systemic steroids are not usually given for arthritis, skin rash, leukopenia, or the anemia associated with chronic disease. Positive serologic findings in asymptomatic patients are not an indication for treatment.

## Course & Prognosis

The prognosis for patients with systemic lupus appears to be considerably better than older reports implied. From both community settings and university centers, 10-year survival rates exceeding 85% are routine. In most patients, the illness pursues a mild chronic course, occasionally interrupted by disease activity. With time, the number and intensity of exacerbations decrease and the probability of major insult to visceral structures declines. After 5 years of disease, abnormal laboratory findings such as raised sedimentation rates and anti-DNA titers tend to become normal in many patients. However, there are some in whom the disease pursues a virulent course, leading to serious impairment of vital structures such as lung, heart, brain, or kidneys, and the disease may lead to death. Although such manifestations are more likely to be seen in the early phases of the illness, one must be alert to the possibility of their occurrence at any time. The most frequently observed serious complication is progressive renal disease followed by central nervous system involvement. Another important cause of sickness and death is infection, related in part to the use of corticosteroids. With careful management, however, the outlook for most patients with systemic lupus erythematosus is increasingly favorable.

Balow JE et al: Lupus nephritis. *Ann Intern Med* 1987;**106**:79.
Branch DW et al: Obstetric complications associated with the lupus anticoagulant. *N Engl J Med* 1985;**313**:1322.
Hochberg MC et al: Systemic lupus erythematosus: A review of clinico-laboratory features and immunogenetic markers in 150 patients with emphasis on demographic subsets. *Medicine* 1985;**64**:285.
Nived O et al: Systmic lupus erythematosus and infection: A controlled and prospective study including an epidemiological group. *Quart J Med* 1985;**55**:271.

## PROGRESSIVE SYSTEMIC SCLEROSIS (Scleroderma)

### Essentials of Diagnosis

- Diffuse thickening of skin, with telangiectasia and areas of increased pigmentation and depigmentation.
- Raynaud's phenomenon in 90% of patients.
- Systemic features of dysphagia, hypomotility of gastrointestinal tract, pulmonary fibrosis, and cardiac and renal involvement.

### General Considerations

Progressive systemic sclerosis is a chronic disorder characterized by diffuse fibrosis of the skin and internal organs. Its cause is unknown, although abnormal serologic features have suggested the importance of an altered immune status. Symptoms usually appear in the third to fifth decades, and women are affected 2–3 times as frequently as men.

Scleroderma may appear in any of several forms. A localized form of scleroderma (morphea) is benign and unassociated with visceral disease. Eosinophilic fasciitis, which may be a variant of scleroderma, is a rare disorder presenting with skin changes like those of scleroderma. Biopsy of involved tissue shows fasciitis with eosinophilia. Visceral features are generally absent, although aplastic anemia has been an associated feature.

Another group of patients have a relatively benign, slowly progressive disorder characterized by calcinosis cutis, Raynaud's phenomenon, esophageal involvement, sclerodactyly, and telangiectasia (CREST syndrome). Still others have an overlapping syndrome called mixed connective tissue disease that consists of myositis, certain features of systemic lupus erythematosus, and a high titer of extractable nuclear antigen (ENA); this disorder tends to respond to relatively small doses of corticosteroids, usually less than 20 mg of prednisone daily. Finally, in occasional individuals, systemic sclerosis may take a rapidly progressive course in which the function of major viscera is compromised, leading to death within a few years.

## Clinical Findings

**A. Symptoms and Signs:** Most frequently, the disease makes its appearance in the skin, although visceral involvement may precede cutaneous alteration. Polyarthralgia and Raynaud's phenomenon (present in 90% of patients) are early manifestations. Subcutaneous edema, fever, and malaise are common. With time the skin becomes thickened and hidebound, with loss of normal folds. Telangiectasia, pigmentation, and depigmentation are characteristic. Ulceration about the fingertips and subcutaneous calcification are seen. Dysphagia due to esophageal dysfunction, which occurs in 90% of patients, results from abnormalities in motility and later from fibrosis. Fibrosis and atrophy of the gastrointestinal tract cause hypomotility, and malabsorption results from bacterial overgrowth. Large-mouthed diverticula occur in the jejunum, ileum, and colon. Diffuse pulmonary fibrosis and pulmonary vascular disease are reflected in low diffusing capacity and decreased lung compliance. Cardiac abnormalities include pericarditis, heart block, myocardial fibrosis, and right heart failure secondary to pulmonary hypertension. Hypertensive-uremic syndrome, resulting from obstruction to smaller renal blood vessels, indicates a grave prognosis.

**B. Laboratory Findings:** Mild anemia is often present, and it is occasionally hemolytic because of mechanical damage to red cells from diseased small vessels. Elevation of the sedimentation rate and hypergammaglobulinemia are also common. Proteinuria and cylindruria appear in association with renal involvement. Antinuclear antibody tests are frequently positive, often with a speckled or nucleolar pattern. Rheumatoid factor and a positive LE preparation may be found. The scleroderma antibody (SCL-70) is found in about 35% of patients with systemic sclerosis and is rare in the CREST syndrome; an anticentromere antibody is seen in 60% of those with CREST syndrome and in 5% of individuals with systemic sclerosis. Though these tests may be useful and of academic interest, their lack of sensitivity and (usually) specificity precludes cost-effective application in diagnosis.

## Treatment

Treatment is symptomatic and supportive. Broad-spectrum antibiotics are useful when intestinal malabsorption occurs. Claims of efficacy of various specific therapeutic modalities are largely unfounded. The prognosis tends to be worse in blacks, in males, and in older patients. In most cases, death results from renal, cardiac, or pulmonary failure.

Rocco VK, Hurt ER: Scleroderma and scleroderma-like disorders. *Semin Arthritis Rheum* 1986;**16**:22.
Shuck JW, Oetgen WJ, Tesar JT: Pulmonary vascular response during Raynaud's phenomenon in progressive systemic sclerosis. *Am J Med* 1985;**78**:221.

# POLYMYOSITIS-DERMATOMYOSITIS

## Essentials of Diagnosis

- Bilateral proximal muscle weakness (all cases).
- Heliotrope suffusion of upper eyelids, characteristic rash, papules over knuckles (many cases).
- Diagnostic tests: elevated CPK and other muscle enzymes, muscle biopsy, electromyogram.
- Increased incidence of malignancy, especially when rash is present and with late age at onset.

## General Considerations

Polymyositis is a systemic disorder of unknown cause whose principal manifestation is muscle weakness. It is the most frequent primary myopathy in adults. When skin manifestations are associated with it, the entity is designated dermatomyositis. The true incidence is not known, since milder cases are frequently not diagnosed. The disease may affect persons of any age group, but the peak incidence is in the fifth and sixth decades of life. Women are affected twice as commonly as men.

## Clinical Findings

**A. Symptoms and Signs:** Polymyositis may begin abruptly, although often it is gradual and progressive. The characteristic rash is dusky red and may be seen over the butterfly area of the face, neck, shoulders, and upper chest and back. Periorbital edema and a purplish (heliotrope) suffusion over the upper eyelids are typical signs. Subungual erythema, cuticular telangiectases, and scaly patches over the dorsum of the proximal interphalangeal and metacarpophalangeal joints (Gottron's sign) are highly suggestive. Muscle weakness chiefly involves proximal groups, especially of the extremities. Neck flexor weakness occurs in two-thirds of cases. Pain and tenderness of affected muscles are frequent but not universal, and Raynaud's phenomenon and joint symptoms may be associated. Atrophy and contractures occur late. Associated myocarditis is uncommon. Interstitial pulmonary disease, usually mild, is sometimes associated, and calcinosis may be observed, especially in children. Association with malignant neoplasms, particularly in older patients, is well recognized, but the frequency in several large series appears to be less than 20%; however, a search for a visceral cancer is unwarranted unless symptoms and signs suggest its presence. Polymyositis may occur in association with Sjögren's syndrome. It may also be a prominent feature of mixed connective tissue disease.

**B. Laboratory Findings:** Measurement of serum levels of muscle enzymes, especially creatine phosphokinase and aldolase, is most useful in diagnosis and in assessment of disease activity. Anemia is uncommon. The sedimentation rate is not appreciably elevated. Rheumatoid factor is found in a minority of patients. Electromyographic abnormalities consisting of polyphasic potentials, fibrillations, and high-frequency action potentials are helpful in establishing the diagnosis. None of the studies are specific.

**C. Muscle Biopsy:** Biopsy of clinically involved muscle, usually proximal, is the only specific diagnostic study. Findings include necrosis of muscle fibers associated with inflammatory cells, sometimes located near blood vessels. The muscle biopsy may, however, reveal little change in spite of significant muscle weakness owing to the patchy distribution of pathologic abnormalities.

## Treatment

Most patients respond to corticosteroids. Often a daily dose of 40–60 mg or more of prednisone is required initially. The dose is then adjusted downward according to the response of sequentially observed serum levels of muscle enzymes. Long-term use of steroids is often needed, and the disease may recur or reemerge when they are withdrawn. Patients with an associated neoplasm have a poor prognosis, although remission may follow treatment of the tumor; steroids may or may not be effective in these patients. In patients resistant or intolerant to corticosteroids, therapy with methotrexate or azathioprine has been advised, but these agents should be used with caution in view of their adverse effects.

Hochberg MC et al: Adult onset polymyositis/dermatomyositis: An analysis of clinical and laboratory features and survival in 76 patients with a review of the literature. *Semin Arthritis Rheum* 1986;**15**:168.

Lakhanpal S et al: Polymyositis-dermatomyositis and malignant lesions: Does an association exist? *Mayo Clin Proc* 1986;**61**:645.

# MIXED CONNECTIVE TISSUE DISEASE

Mixed connective tissue disease (MCTD) is a clinical syndrome in which overlapping features of systemic lupus erythematosus, scleroderma, and myositis are present in conjunction with high titers of an extractable nuclear antigen (ENA). The antigen contains ribonucleoprotein and is associated with a speckled pattern on the antinuclear antibody (ANA). Patients with MCTD usually have nondeforming arthritis, swollen hands with taut and thickened skin, Raynaud's phenomenon, and myositis. Abnormal esophageal motility and interstitial pulmonary disease are also common. Renal disease is characterized by mesangial or membranous changes but is uncommon. Laboratory findings often show exceedingly high titers of ENA of the ribonucleoprotein type, speckled ANA, absent or low anti-DNA titers, and normal complement.

In a multicenter study of MCTD with a mean duration of 6 years, 4% of patients died. Longer-term follow-up has shown that many patients subsequently developed scleroderma. The prognosis of this disorder is generally good if pulmonary involvement and renal involvement are not severe. Treatment of

MCTD is similar to that of systemic lupus erythematosus, although MCTD tends to be milder, with less serious renal and central nervous system disease; patients respond to lower doses of corticosteroids. Mild disease is often controlled with nonsteroidal anti-inflammatory drugs.

Sullivan WD et al: A prospective evaluation emphasizing pulmonary involvement in mixed connective tissue disease. *Medicine* 1984;**63**:92.

## SJÖGREN'S SYNDROME

### Essentials of Diagnosis

- 90% of patients are women; the average age is 50 years.
- Dryness of eyes and dry mouth (sicca components) are the most common features; they occur alone or in association with rheumatoid arthritis or other connective tissue disease.
- Rheumatoid factor and other autoantibodies common.
- Increased incidence of lymphoma.

### General Considerations

Sjögren's syndrome, an autoimmune disorder, is the result of chronic dysfunction of exocrine glands in many areas of the body. It is characterized by dryness of the eyes, mouth, and other areas covered by mucous membrane and is frequently associated with a rheumatic disease, most often rheumatoid arthritis. The disorder is predominantly a disease of women, in a ratio of 9:1, with greatest incidence between age 40 and 60 years.

Disorders with which Sjögren's syndrome is frequently associated include rheumatoid arthritis, systemic lupus erythematosus, primary biliary cirrhosis, scleroderma, polymyositis, Hashimoto's thyroiditis, polyarteritis, and interstitial pulmonary fibrosis. When Sjögren's syndrome occurs without rheumatoid arthritis, HLA-DR2 and -DR3 antigens are present with increased frequency.

### Clinical Findings

**A. Symptoms and Signs:** Keratoconjunctivitis sicca results from inadequate tear production caused by lymphocyte and plasma cell infiltration of the lacrimal glands. Symptoms include burning, itching, ropy secretions, and impaired tear production during crying. Parotid enlargement, which may be chronic or relapsing, develops in one-third of patients. Dryness of the mouth (xerostomia) leads to difficulty in speaking and swallowing and to severe dental caries. There may be loss of taste and smell. Desiccation may involve the nose, throat, larynx, bronchi, vagina, and skin.

Systemic manifestations include dysphagia, pancreatitis, pleuritis, neuropsychiatric dysfunction, and vasculitis; they may be related to the associated diseases noted above. Renal tubular acidosis (type I,

distal) occurs in 20% of patients. Chronic interstitial nephritis, which may result in impaired renal function, may be seen. A glomerular lesion is rarely observed but may occur secondary to associated cryoglobulinemia.

A spectrum of lymphoproliferation ranging from benign to malignant may be found. Malignant lymphomas and Waldenström's macroglobulinemia occur with greater frequency than could be explained by chance alone.

**B. Laboratory Findings:** Laboratory findings include mild anemia, leukopenia, and eosinophilia. Rheumatoid factor is found in 70% of patients. Heightened levels of gamma globulin, antinuclear antibodies, and antibodies against RNA, salivary gland, lacrimal duct, and thyroid may be noted. Antibodies against cytoplasmic antigens SS-A and SS-B are found predominantly in Sjögren's syndrome alone, whereas antibodies against salivary ducts and the RANA antigen are found in Sjögren's syndrome in association with rheumatoid arthritis. When SS-A antibodies are present, extraglandular manifestations of Sjögren's syndrome are far more common.

Useful ocular diagnostic tests include the Schirmer test, which measures the quantity of tears secreted. The salivary gland may be evaluated by radionuclide scanning. Labial biopsy, a simple procedure, is the only specific diagnostic technique and has minimal risk; if lymphoid foci are seen, the diagnosis is confirmed. Biopsy of the parotid gland should be reserved for patients with atypical presentations such as unilateral gland enlargement.

### Treatment & Prognosis

Treatment is symptomatic and supportive. Artificial tears applied frequently will relieve ocular symptoms and avert further desiccation. The mouth should be kept well lubricated. Atropine drugs and decongestants decrease salivary secretions and should be avoided. A program of oral hygiene is essential in order to preserve dentition. If there is an associated rheumatic disease, its treatment is not altered by the presence of Sjögren's syndrome.

The disease is usually benign and may be consistent with a normal life span; it is influenced mainly by the nature of the associated disease.

Daniels TE: Labial salivary gland biopsy in Sjögren's syndrome: Assessment as a diagnostic criterion in 362 suspected cases. *Arthritis Rheum* 1984;**27**:147.

Fox RI et al: Sjögren's syndrome. Proposed criteria for classification. *Arthritis Rheum* 1986;**29**:577.

## VASCULITIC SYNDROMES

The vasculitic syndromes are a heterogenous group of disorders characterized by the pathologic features of inflammation and necrosis of blood vessels. In most disorders characterized as vasculitides, no cause has been found. Hepatitis B is clearly the cause of one form, and other infections have been implicated, as in the vasculitis that occurs in bacterial endocarditis. No common pathogenic link has been identified for these disorders, although the deposition of immune complexes in the vascular system occurs in many.

Although vasculitis is seen in multiple disorders, only the major vasculitides will be discussed here.

## POLYARTERITIS NODOSA

### Essentials of Diagnosis

- Clinical findings depend on arteries involved.
- Affects kidneys, muscles, joints, nerves, heart, gastrointestinal tract in most patients; cutaneous and pulmonary involvement unusual but possible.
- Manifestations of fever, hypertension, abdominal pain, livedo reticularis, mononeuritis multiplex, anemia, hematuria, elevated sedimentation rate.
- Diagnostic confirmation by biopsy or angiogram.

### General Considerations

Polyarteritis is characterized by focal or segmental lesions of blood vessels, especially arteries of small to medium size, resulting in a variety of clinical presentations depending upon the specific site of the blood vessel involved. The pathologic hallmark of the disease is acute necrotizing inflammation of the arterial media, with fibrinoid necrosis and extensive inflammatory cell infiltration of all coats of the vessel and surrounding tissue. Aneurysmal dilatations occur; hemorrhage, thrombosis, and fibrosis may lead to occlusion of the lumen. Arterial lesions may be seen in all stages—acute, healing, and healed. Such vascular lesions may involve virtually every organ of the body but are especially prominent in the kidney, heart, liver, gastrointestinal tract, muscle, and testes.

The cause of polyarteritis is unknown. The disease occurs in drug abusers and may be induced by allopurinol, sulfonamides, and other drugs; hepatitis B surface antigen is found in the serum of over a third of patients. It affects chiefly young adults but may appear at any age. Men are affected 3 times as frequently as women. It should be suspected in any polysystemic illness of obscure cause.

### Clinical Findings

**A. Symptoms and Signs:** The clinical onset may be abrupt, often accompanied by fever, chills, and tachycardia. Arthralgia and myositis with muscle tenderness are prominent. A wide variety of cutaneous abnormalities develop. Livedo reticularis is most common; vasculitic involvement causing skin ulcers is less common. Occlusion of retinal vessels results in cotton-wool spots (cytoid bodies). Hypertension occurs in half of patients and renal involvement in more than 80%. The renal lesion is a segmental necrotizing glomerulonephritis with extracapillary proliferation, often with localized intravascular coagulation. Abdominal pain and nausea and vomiting are common. Infarction due to the arteritis compromises the function of major viscera and may lead to cholecystitis, appendicitis, and intestinal obstruction. Cardiac involvement is manifested by pericarditis, myocarditis, and arrhythmias; myocardial infarction secondary to coronary vasculitis also occurs. Multiple asymmetric neuropathies occur as a result of vasculitis of the vasa vasorum. Polyarteritis is an occasional cause of fever of unknown origin.

**B. Laboratory Findings:** Laboratory findings include proteinuria, hematuria, and cylindruria. Most patients manifest anemia and leukocytosis. Eosinophilia is more frequently encountered in association with pulmonary lesions, which may represent a different disease process (Churg-Strauss vasculitis), though overlap is not universal. The sedimentation rate is almost always elevated. Rheumatoid factor, antinuclear antibody, positive serologic test for syphilis, and increased serum concentration of gamma globulin are neither sensitive nor specific. Serum complement is often normal or elevated.

**C. Biopsy and Angiography:** Diagnosis may be difficult and should be confirmed, if possible, by histologic evidence of a typical arteritic lesion. Visceral angiography demonstrating aneurysmal dilatation of renal, mesenteric, and hepatic arteries is useful; it is positive in about 50% of cases.

### Treatment

Corticosteroids in high doses (up to 60 mg of prednisone daily) may control fever and constitutional symptoms and heal vascular lesions. Immunosuppressive agents, especially cyclophosphamide, significantly improve the survival of patients when given with steroids. These drugs may be required for long periods, and relapses are not infrequent when they are withdrawn.

### Prognosis

The course is variable and unpredictable. Spontaneous remission may occur, but the disease usually runs a fulminant course, with death occurring in months to years.

Savage COS et al: Microscopic polyarteritis: Presentation, pathology and prognosis. *Quart J Med* 1985;**56**:467.

## POLYMYALGIA RHEUMATICA & GIANT CELL ARTERITIS

Polymyalgia rheumatica, a disorder affecting middle-aged or elderly persons, is rare before age 50. The disease often develops abruptly, with pain and stiffness of the pelvis and shoulder girdle in association with fever, malaise, and weight loss. Anemia and a markedly elevated sedimentation rate are almost always present. The course is generally limited to 1–2 years.

Polymyalgia rheumatica bears a close relationship to giant cell arteritis. The 2 conditions often coexist, but each may occur independently; when they coexist, the clinical manifestations of polymyalgia rheumatica almost always precede those of giant cell arteritis. The importance of diagnosing arteritis lies in the risk of blindness due to obstruction of the ophthalmic arteries; this may occur unless treatment is given. Suggestive symptoms include unilateral throbbing headache, scalp sensitivity, visual symptoms, and jaw claudication, but arteritis may be present without local symptoms. Biopsy of the temporal artery should be performed whenever the clinical picture is suggestive and will usually reveal inflammation of the vessel, often with giant cells. Some clinicians recommend empiric temporal artery biopsy in patients with polymyalgia rheumatica alone; arteritis may be found in a minority of such individuals, despite the absence of local symptoms. An adequate biopsy specimen (5 cm in length) is essential because the disease tends to be segmental; bilateral biopsies add 15–20% to the yield. Ten to 15% of patients have vasculitis of other major arteries.

In the presence of headache and other symptoms suggestive of cranial arteritis and following confirmation by biopsy, corticosteroids should be administered immediately (eg, prednisone, 60 mg daily) and continued for several months before tapering. Where there is polymyalgia without local cranial symptoms, smaller doses of prednisone (10–15 mg daily) bring almost immediate relief. If such a response does not occur, the diagnosis should be questioned. In adjusting the dosage of steroid, the erythrocyte sedimentation rate (ESR) is a useful guide to disease activity. One should administer the smallest dose of corticosteroid that normalizes the ESR. Blindness rarely occurs when the ESR has reached the normal range. The drug may be discontinued when disease activity ceases, although the disorder may recur and in some patients remains active for years. Chronic infectious disease such as bacterial endocarditis, which have systemic symptoms similar to those of polymyalgia rheumatica, should always be excluded before corticosteroids are started.

Ayoub WT, Franklin CM, Torretti D: Polymyalgia rheumatica: Duration of therapy and long term outcome. *Am J Med* 1985;**79**:309.
Olhagen B: Polymyalgia rheumatica. *Clin Rheum Dis* 1986;**12**:33.
Shearn MA, Kang IY: Effect of age and sex on the erythrocyte sedimentation rate. *J Rheumatol* 1986;**13**:297.

## WEGENER'S GRANULOMATOSIS

Wegener's granulomatosis is a rare disorder characterized by vasculitis, necrotizing granulomatous lesions of both upper and lower respiratory tract, and glomerulonephritis. Without treatment it is invariably fatal, most patients surviving less than a year after diagnosis. It occurs most commonly in the fourth and fifth decades of life and affects men and women with equal frequency.

### Clinical Findings

The disorder presents as a febrile illness with weakness, malaise, and weight loss. Symptoms include those of purulent sinusitis and rhinitis; polyarthralgia may also be present. Dyspnea, cough, chest pain, and hemoptysis may dominate the clinical picture. Ulcerations of the nasal septum are noted on physical examination. X-ray of the chest often reveals nodular pulmonary lesions, frequently cavitating; histologic examination of the lesions shows necrotizing vasculitis with granuloma formation. Although limited forms of Wegener's granulomatosis have been described in which the kidney is spared, severe progressive renal disease usually ensues and results in rapid deterioration of renal function. In such cases the urinary sediment invariably contains red cells, with or without white cells, and red cell casts. Renal biopsy discloses a segmental necrotizing glomerulonephritis with multiple crescents; this is characteristic but not diagnostic. Granulomas are observed in 10%.

Laboratory studies show anemia (occasionally microangiopathic), leukocytosis, and a rapid sedimentation rate. Immunologic findings are variable but not specific.

### Treatment

It is essential that the diagnosis be made early, since treatment may be lifesaving; lung tissue is preferred, as findings are more often specific than in tissue from nasal mucosal biopsy. Remissions have been induced in up to 90% of patients treated with cyclophosphamide. Corticosteroids are usually of limited value.

Fauci AS et al: Wegener's granulomatosis: Prospective clinical and therapeutic experience with 85 patients for 21 years. *Ann Intern Med* 1983;**98**:76.

## HENOCH-SCHÖNLEIN PURPURA

This is a form of purpura of unknown cause; the underlying pathologic feature is vasculitis, which principally affects small blood vessels. Although the disease is predominantly seen in children, adults are also affected. Hypersensitivity to aspirin and food and drug additives has been reported. The purpuric skin lesions are typically located on the lower extremities but may also be seen on the hands, arms, and trunk. Localized areas of edema, especially common on the dorsal surfaces of the hands, are frequently observed. Joint symptoms are present in the vast majority of patients, the knees and ankles being most commonly involved. Abdominal pain secondary to vasculitis of the intestinal tract is often associated with gastrointestinal bleeding. Hematuria signals the presence of a renal lesion that is usually reversible, although it occasionally may progress to renal insufficiency. Biopsy of the kidney reveals segmental glomerulonephritis with crescents and mesangial deposition of IgA and, sometimes, IgG. Aside from an elevated sedimentation rate, most laboratory findings are noncontributory; the platelet count is normal or elevated.

The disease is usually self-limited, lasting 1–6 weeks, and subsides without sequelae if renal involvement is not severe. There is no effective treatment, although immunosuppressive drugs have met with some success in the nephropathy of this disorder.

Roth DA et al: Schönlein-Henoch syndrome in adults. *Quart J Med* 1985;**55**:145.

# SERONEGATIVE ARTHROPATHIES

## ANKYLOSING SPONDYLITIS

### Essentials of Diagnosis
- Chronic low backache in young adults.
- Progressive limitation of back motion and of chest expansion.
- Transient (50%) or permanent (25%) peripheral arthritis.
- Diagnostic x-ray changes in sacroiliac joints.
- Uveitis in 20–25%.
- Accelerated erythrocyte sedimentation rate and negative serologic tests for rheumatoid factor.
- HLA-B27 usually positive.

### General Considerations
Ankylosing spondylitis is a chronic inflammatory disease of the joints of the axial skeleton, manifested clinically by pain and progressive stiffening of the spine. The age at onset is usually in the late teens or early 20s. The incidence is about the same in both sexes, but symptoms are more prominent in men, and ascending involvement of the spine is more likely to occur.

### Clinical Findings
**A. Symptoms and Signs:** The onset is usually gradual, with intermittent bouts of back pain that may radiate down the thighs. As the disease advances, symptoms progress in a cephalad direction and back motion becomes limited, with the normal lumbar curve flattened and the thoracic curvature exaggerated. Atrophy of the trunk muscles is common. Chest expansion is often limited as a consequence of costovertebral joint involvement. Radicular symptoms due to the cauda equina syndrome may occur years after onset of the disease. In advanced cases, the entire spine becomes fused, allowing no motion in any direction. Transient acute arthritis of the peripheral joints occurs in about 50% of cases, and permanent changes

in the peripheral joints—most commonly the hips, shoulders, and knees—are seen in about 25%.

Spondylitic heart disease, characterized chiefly by atrioventricular conduction defects and aortic insufficiency, occurs in 3–5% of patients with long-standing severe disease. Nongranulomatous anterior uveitis is associated in as many as 25% of cases and may be a presenting feature. Pulmonary fibrosis of the upper lobes, with progression to cavitation and bronchiectasis mimicking tuberculosis, may occur, characteristically long after the onset of skeletal symptoms. Constitutional symptoms similar to those of rheumatoid arthritis are absent in most patients.

**B. Laboratory Findings:** The erythrocyte sedimentation rate is elevated in 85% of cases, but serologic tests for rheumatoid factor are characteristically negative. There may be leukocytosis and anemia.

HLA-B27 is found in 90% of patients with ankylosing spondylitis, as opposed to 6–8% among normal individuals. These figures are lower in blacks. HLA-B27 is found with greater than normal frequency in some other rheumatic diseases such as Reiter's syndrome, psoriasis, and inflammatory bowel disease. The incidence of B27 positivity is highest in ankylosing spondylitis. Because of the noted incidence of this antigen in the normal population, it is not used as a diagnostic aid.

Persons with other rheumatic diseases such as rheumatoid arthritis, degenerative joint disease (osteoarthritis), and gout do not show a higher than normal incidence of HLA-B27.

**C. Imaging:** Early in the course of ankylosing spondylitis, radiographs of the sacroiliac joints may be normal; erosion and sclerosis of these joints soon develop, however. Later, involvement of the apophyseal joints of the spine, ossification of the annulus fibrosus, calcification of the anterior and lateral spinal ligaments, and squaring and generalized demineralization of the vertebral bodies may occur. The term "bamboo spine" has been used to describe the late radiographic changes.

Additional x-ray findings include periosteal new bone formation on the iliac crest, ischial tuberosities and calcanei, and alterations of the symphysis pubica and sternomanubrial joint similar to those of the sacroiliacs. Radiologic changes in peripheral joints, when present, tend to be asymmetric and lack the demineralization and erosions seen in rheumatoid arthritis.

### Differential Diagnosis
Although rheumatoid arthritis may ultimately involve the spine, it does so characteristically in the cervical region, usually sparing the sacroiliac joints. Other features that differentiate ankylosing spondylitis from rheumatoid arthritis are the rare involvement of the small joints of the hands and feet, the absence of subcutaneous nodules, and the negative serologic tests for rheumatoid factor in spondylitis. The history and physical findings of ankylosing spondylitis serve to distinguish this disorder from other causes of low

back pain such as disk disease and often low back pain, osteoporosis, soft tissue trauma, and tumors. The single most valuable distinguishing radiologic sign of ankylosing spondylitis is the appearance of the sacroiliac joints, although a similar pattern may be seen in Reiter's syndrome and in the arthritis associated with inflammatory intestinal diseases and psoriasis. In ankylosing hyperostosis (diffuse idiopathic skeletal hyperostosis [DISH], Forestier's disease), there is exuberant osteophyte formation. The osteophytes are thicker and more anterior than the syndesmophytes of ankylosing spondylitis, and the sacroiliac joints are not affected. The x-ray appearance of the sacroiliac joints in spondylitis should be distinguished from that in osteitis condensans ilii. In some geographic areas and in persons with appropriate occupations, brucellosis and fluoride poisoning may be important in the differential diagnosis.

## Treatment

**A. Basic Program:** In general, treatment is similar to that of rheumatoid arthritis. The importance of postural and breathing exercises should be stressed.

**B. Drug Therapy:** The nonsteroidal anti-inflammatory agents are employed in the treatment of this disorder. Of these, indomethacin appears to be the most effective, though it is not unreasonable to begin therapy with aspirin. The dosage of indomethacin is usually 25–50 mg 3 times a day, but the least amount should be used that will provide symptomatic improvement. Agents such as naproxen, fenoprofen, tolmetin, sulindac, and piroxicam are valuable alternatives and may even be used as primary therapy. Indomethacin may produce a variety of untoward reactions, including headache, giddiness, nausea and vomiting, peptic ulcer, depression, and psychosis.

**C. Physical Therapy:** See p 530.

## Prognosis

Spontaneous remissions and relapses are common and may occur at any stage. Occasionally, the disease progresses to ankylosis of the entire spine. In general, the functional prognosis is good unless the hips are seriously involved and consequently ankylosed.

van der Linden S, Valkenburg HA, Cats A: Evaluation of diagnostic criteria for ankylosing spondylitis: A proposal for modification of the New York criteria. *Arthritis Rheum* 1984;**27**:361.

## PSORIATIC ARTHRITIS

### Essentials of Diagnosis

- Psoriasis precedes onset of arthritis in 80% of cases.
- Arthritis usually asymmetrical, with "sausage" appearance of fingers and toes; resembles rheumatoid arthritis; rheumatoid factor is absent from serum.
- Sacroiliac joint involvement common; ankylosing spondylitis may be associated.

- X-ray findings: osteolysis; pencil-in-cup deformity; relative lack of osteoporosis; bony ankylosis; asymmetrical sacroiliitis and atypical syndesmophytes.

### General Considerations

In 15–20% of patients with psoriasis, arthritis coexists. The patterns or subsets of arthritis that may accompany psoriasis include the following:

(1) Joint disease that resembles rheumatoid arthritis in which polyarthritis is symmetric. Usually, fewer joints are involved than in rheumatoid arthritis, and rheumatoid factor is absent from the serum.

(2) An oligoarticular form that may lead to considerable destruction of the affected joints.

(3) A pattern of disease in which the distal interphalangeal joints are primarily affected. Early, this may be monarticular, and often the joint involvement is asymmetric. Pitting of the nails and onycholysis are frequently associated.

(4) A severe deforming arthritis (arthritis mutilans) in which osteolysis is severe.

(5) A spondylitic form with sacroiliitis and spinal involvement predominating; 45% of these patients are HLA-B27 positive.

### Clinical Findings

**A. Symptoms and Signs:** Although psoriasis usually precedes the onset of arthritis, in 20–25% of patients the arthritis precedes the skin disease. Arthritis is at least 5 times more common in patients with severe skin disease than in those with only mild skin findings. Occasionally, though, patients may have a single patch of psoriasis and are unaware of it. Thus, a detailed search for cutaneous lesions is essential in patients with arthritis of new onset. Also, the psoriatic lesions may have cleared when arthritis appears—in such cases, the history is most useful. Nail pitting, a residue of previous psoriasis, is sometimes the only clue.

**B. Laboratory Findings:** Laboratory studies show an elevation of the sedimentation rate, but rheumatoid factor is not present. Uric acid levels may be high, reflecting the active turnover of skin affected by psoriasis. There is a correlation between the extent of psoriatic involvement and the level of uric acid, but gout is no more common than in patients without psoriasis. Desquamation of the skin may also reduce iron stores.

**C. Imaging:** Radiographic findings are most helpful in distinguishing the disease from other forms of arthritis. There are marginal erosions of bone and irregular destruction of joint and bone, which, in the phalanx, may give the appearance of a sharpened pencil. Fluffy periosteal new bone may be marked, especially at the insertion of muscles and ligaments into bone. Such changes will also be seen along the shafts of metacarpals, metatarsals, and phalanges. Paravertebral ossification occurs, which may be distinguished from ankylosing spondylitis by the absence of ossification in the anterior aspect of the spine.

## Treatment

Treatment regimens are symptomatic. Nonsteroidal anti-inflammatory drugs are useful. Antimalarials may exacerbate the psoriasis. Gold therapy is often effective. In resistant cases, methotrexate has been used with some success, but it should be employed only by those fully conversant with its use. Successful treatment of the skin lesions commonly—though not invariably—is accompanied by an improvement in peripheral articular symptoms.

Bird HA et al: Psoriatic arthritis. *Clin Rheum Dis* 1983;**9:**675.
Willkens RF et al: Randomized, double-blind, placebo controlled trial of low-dose pulse methotrexate in psoriatic arthritis. *Arthritis Rheum* 1984;**27:**376.

## REITER'S SYNDROME

Reiter's syndrome is a clinical tetrad of unknown cause consisting of urethritis, conjunctivitis (or, less commonly, uveitis), mucocutaneous lesions, and arthritis. It occurs most commonly in young men. It may follow (within days or weeks) infection with *Chlamydia, Campylobacter, Salmonella,* or *Yersinia* and is usually accompanied by a systemic reaction, including fever. The arthritis is most commonly asymmetric and frequently involves the large weight-bearing joints (chiefly the knee and ankle); sacroiliitis or ankylosing spondylitis is observed in at least 20% of patients, especially after frequent recurrences. The mucocutaneous lesions may include balanitis, stomatitis, and keratoderma blenorrhagicum, resembling pustular psoriasis with involvement of the skin and nails. Carditis and aortic regurgitation may occur. While most signs of the disease disappear within days or weeks, the arthritis may persist for several months or even years. The test for HLA-B27 is positive in 80% of white patients, but these percentages are 20–30% lower in blacks. (See p 505 for further discussion of HLA-B27.) Characteristically, the initial attack is self-limited and terminates spontaneously.

Recurrences involving any combination of the clinical manifestations are common and are sometimes followed by permanent sequelae, especially in the joints. X-ray signs of permanent or progressive joint disease may be seen in the sacroiliac as well as the peripheral joints.

Reiter's syndrome must be distinguished from gonococcal arthritis, especially when conjunctivitis has been mild or overlooked. Rheumatoid arthritis, idiopathic ankylosing spondylitis, and psoriatic arthritis must also be considered.

Treatment is symptomatic. Antibiotics are ineffective. As in psoriatic arthritis, the most useful agents are the nonsteroidal anti-inflammatory agents.

Marks JS, Holt PJL: The natural history of Reiter's disease: 21 years of observations. *Quart J Med* 1986;**60:**685.

## ARTHRITIS & INFLAMMATORY INTESTINAL DISEASES

Arthritis is a common complication of ulcerative colitis, regional enteritis, and Whipple's disease. Occasionally, such joint disease is indistinguishable from rheumatoid arthritis and may represent a coincidence of the 2 disorders. More commonly, however, intestinal arthritis is asymmetric, affects large joints, parallels the course of the bowel disease, and rarely results in residual deformity. Articular symptoms may be prominent enough to cause the patient to overlook intestinal spasm. Ankylosing spondylitis, which may accompany inflammatory bowel disease, is indistinguishable from idiopathic ankylosing spondylitis and usually runs a course separate from bowel disease activity.

The synovitis is pathologically nonspecific. Rheumatoid factor is usually negative and HLA-B27 is often positive, and its presence may predispose to the development of spondylitis. Treatment of intestinal arthritis involves control of intestinal inflammation and use of supportive anti-inflammatory drugs; that of ankylosing spondylitis is the same as for idiopathic ankylosing spondylitis.

About 15% of patients who have jejunoileal bypass surgery for morbid obesity develop an inflammatory symmetric polyarticular disorder. The arthritis is usually acute in onset and nonmigratory and may affect the small as well as the large joints. The sedimentation rate is elevated, and antinuclear antibody and rheumatoid factor tests may be positive. Nonsteroidal anti-inflammatory agents are often effective, although some patients require prednisone.

Jorizzi JL: Bowel-associated dermatosis-arthritis syndrome. *Arch Intern Med* 1984;**144:**738.

## BEHÇET'S SYNDROME

Named after the Turkish dermatologist who first described it, this disease of unknown cause is characterized by recurrent oral and genital ulcers, uveitis, seronegative arthritis, and central nervous system abnormalities. Other features include ulcerative skin lesions, erythema nodosum, thrombophlebitis, and vasculitis. Arthritis occurs in about two-thirds of patients, most commonly affecting the knees and ankles. Keratitis, uveitis—often with hypopyon—and optic neuritis are observed. The ocular involvement is often fulminant and may result in blindness. Involvement of the central nervous system often results in serious disability or death. Findings include cranial nerve palsies, convulsions, encephalitis, mental disturbances, and spinal cord lesions. Leukocytosis and a rapid sedimentation rate are common.

The clinical course may be chronic but is often characterized by remissions and exacerbations. Corticosteroids and immunomodulating drugs have been used with beneficial results.

Benezra D et al: Treatment and visual prognosis in Behçet's disease. *Br J Ophthalmol* 1986;**70:**589.

•    •    •

## RELAPSING POLYCHONDRITIS

This is a rare disease of unknown cause characterized by inflammatory destructive lesions of cartilaginous structures, principally the ears, nose, trachea, and larynx. It may be associated with other immunologic disorders such as systemic lupus erythematosus, rheumatoid arthritis, or Hashimoto's thyroiditis. The disease, which is usually episodic, affects males and females equally. The cartilage is painful, swollen, and tender during an attack and subsequently becomes atrophic, resulting in permanent deformity. Biopsy of the involved cartilage shows inflammation, loss of basophilia, and chondrolysis. Noncartilaginous manifestations of the disease include fever, episcleritis, uveitis, deafness, aortic insufficiency, and rarely immune complex-mediated renal disease. In 85% of patients, an arthropathy is seen that tends to be migratory, asymmetric, and seronegative, affecting both large and small joints and the parasternal articulation.

Corticosteroid therapy is often effective. Involvement of the tracheobronchial tree, leading to its collapse, may cause death if tracheostomy is not done promptly.

Michet CT et al: Relapsing polychondritis: Survival and predictive role of early disease manifestations. *Ann Int Med* 1986;**104:**74.

## PALINDROMIC RHEUMATISM

Palindromic rheumatism is a disease of unknown cause characterized by frequent recurring attacks (at irregular intervals) of acutely inflamed joints. Periarticular pain with swelling and transient subcutaneous nodules may also occur. The attacks cease within several hours to several days. The knee and finger joints are most commonly affected, but any peripheral joint may be involved. Systemic manifestations do not occur. Although hundreds of attacks may take place over a period of years, there is no permanent articular damage. Laboratory findings are usually normal. Palindromic rheumatism must be distinguished from acute gouty arthritis and an atypical, acute onset of rheumatoid arthritis.

Symptomatic treatment is usually all that is required during the attacks. Chrysotherapy may be of value in preventing recurrences.

## DEGENERATIVE JOINT DISEASE (Osteoarthritis)

### Essentials of Diagnosis

- A degenerative disorder without systemic manifestations.
- Pain relieved by rest; morning stiffness brief.
- Articular inflammation minimal.
- X-ray findings: narrowed joint space, osteophytes, increased density of subchondral bone, bony cysts.
- Commonly secondary to other articular disease.

### General Considerations

Osteoarthritis is the most common form of joint disease, sparing no age, race, or geographic area. At least 20 million adults in the USA suffer from the effects of this condition at any one time, and 90% of all people will have radiographic features of osteoarthritis in weight-bearing joints by age 40. Symptomatic disease also increases with age.

This arthropathy is characterized by degeneration of cartilage and by hypertrophy of bone at the articular margins. Inflammation is usually minimal. Hereditary and mechanical factors may be variably involved in the pathogenesis.

Degenerative joint disease is traditionally divided into 2 types: (1) primary, which most commonly affects the terminal interphalangeal joints (Heberden's nodes) and less commonly the proximal interphalangeal joints (Bouchard's nodes), the metacarpophalangeal and carpometacarpal joints of the thumb, the hip, the knee, the metatarsophalangeal joint of the big toe, and the cervical and lumbar spine; and (2) secondary, which may occur in any joint as a sequela to articular injury resulting from either intra-articular (including rheumatoid arthritis) or extra-articular causes. The injury may be acute, as in a fracture; or chronic, as that due to occupational overuse of a joint, metabolic disease (eg, hyperparathyroidism, hemochromatosis, ochronosis), or neurologic disorders (tabes dorsalis; see below).

Pathologically, the articular cartilage is first roughened and finally worn away, and spur formation and lipping occur at the edge of the joint surface. The synovial membrane becomes thickened, with hypertrophy of the villous processes; the joint cavity, however, never becomes totally obliterated, and the synovial membrane does not form adhesions. Inflammation is prominent only in occasional patients with acute interphalangeal joint involvement (Heberden's nodes).

### Clinical Findings

**A. Symptoms and Signs:** The onset is insidious. Initially, there is articular stiffness, seldom lasting more than 15 minutes; this develops later into pain on motion of the affected joint and is made worse by prolonged activity and relieved by rest.

Deformity may be absent or minimal; however, bony enlargement is occasionally prominent, and flexion contracture or valgus or varus deformity of the knee is not unusual. There is no ankylosis, but limitation of motion of the affected joint or joints is common. Coarse crepitus may often be felt in the joint. Joint effusion and other articular signs of inflammation are mild. There are no systemic manifestations.

**B. Laboratory Findings:** Elevated sedimentation rate and other laboratory signs of inflammation are not present.

**C. Imaging:** Radiographs may reveal narrowing of the joint space, sharpened articular margins, osteophyte formation and lipping of marginal bone, and thickened, dense subchondral bone. Bone cysts may also be present.

### Differential Diagnosis

Because articular inflammation is minimal and systemic manifestations are absent, degenerative joint disease should seldom be confused with other arthritides. The appearance of the hands in degenerative joint disease may mimic that in rheumatoid arthritis. Bony rather than soft tissue swelling and lack of involvement of the metacarpophalangeal joints are helpful indications in diagnosis. Neurogenic arthropathy is easily distinguished by physical examination. Degenerative joint disease may coexist with any other type of joint disease. Furthermore, one must be cautious in attributing all skeletal symptoms to degenerative changes in joints, especially in the spine, where metastatic neoplasia, osteoporosis, multiple myeloma, or other bone disease may coexist.

### Treatment

**A. General Measures:**

**1. Rest**–Occupational or recreational overuse of an affected joint must be prevented. If weight-bearing joints are involved, activities such as climbing stairs, walking, or prolonged standing should be minimized. Most patients are aware of these limitations by the time they consult a physician.

**2. Diet**–Diet should be adjusted to meet the patient's needs. In obese patients, weight reduction may help diminish stress on the joints.

**3. Local heat**–Local heat in any form and other forms of physical therapy are often of symptomatic value.

**B. Analgesic and Anti-inflammatory Drugs:** Salicylates or other nonsteroidal anti-inflammatory drugs (see Chapter 1) are indicated for the relief of pain. High doses of salicylates, as used in more inflammatory arthritides, are unnecessary.

**C. Orthopedic Measures:** Orthopedic measures to correct developmental anomalies, deformities, disparity in leg length, and severely damaged joint surfaces may be required (see p 530).

**D. Surgical Measures:** Total hip replacement provides excellent symptomatic and functional improvement when that joint is seriously afflicted. Knee replacement is also an option, though the results are less impressive.

### Prognosis

Marked disability is less common than in rheumatoid arthritis, but symptoms may be quite severe and limit activity considerably (especially with involvement of the hips, knees, and cervical spine). Proper treatment may relieve symptoms and improve function.

Bellamy N: The clinical evaluation of osteoarthritis in the elderly. *Clin Rheum Dis* 1986;**12**:131.

## NEUROGENIC ARTHROPATHY (Charcot's Joint)

Neurogenic arthropathy is joint destruction resulting from loss or diminution of proprioception, pain, and temperature perception. Although traditionally associated with tabes dorsalis, it is more frequently seen in diabetic neuropathy, syringomyelia, spinal cord injury, pernicious anemia, leprosy, and peripheral nerve injury. Prolonged administration of hydrocortisone by the intra-articular route may also cause Charcot's joint. As normal muscle tone and protective reflexes are lost, a marked secondary degenerative joint disease ensues; this results in an enlarged, boggy, painless joint with extensive erosion of cartilage, osteophyte formation, and multiple loose joint bodies. X-ray changes may be degenerative or hypertrophic in the same patient.

Treatment is directed against the primary disease; mechanical devices are used to assist in weight bearing and prevention of further trauma. In some instances, amputation becomes unavoidable.

## ACUTE BACTERIAL (SEPTIC) ARTHRITIS

### Essentials of Diagnosis

- Sudden onset of acute arthritis, usually monarticular, most often in large weight-bearing joints and wrists, frequently preceded by migratory arthralgia.
- Chills and fever.
- Joint fluid findings often diagnostic.
- Dramatic therapeutic response to appropriate antibiotic.
- Infection with causative organisms commonly found elsewhere in body.

### General Considerations

The pyogenic cocci (gonococcus, meningococcus, *Staphylococcus*, *Streptococcus pneumoniae*, and other streptococci), *Haemophilus influenzae*, and gram-negative bacilli are the usual causes of this form of arthritis. The organisms may enter the joints directly, as in local trauma or needling, by extension from adjacent bone, or, more commonly, by hematogenous spread. The synovium is highly vascular and has no limiting basement membrane, and various blood-borne substances can therefore enter the synovial cavity. In recent years this type of disease has been seen more commonly as a result of the increasing therapeutic use of intra-articular injections, intravenous drug abuse, and the increasing survival rate of premature infants, in whom the incidence of septic arthritis is relatively high. Septic arthritis is more apt to localize in previously diseased joints (eg, gouty arthritis, rheumatoid arthritis). The widespread use of arthroscopy and prosthetic joint surgery has also increased the frequency of septic arthritis. In the latter conditions, *S epidermidis* is the usual offending organism. The worldwide increase of gonococcal infections, particularly with antibiotic-resistant gonococci, has posed a special problem. Pathologic changes include varying degrees of acute inflammation, with synovitis, effusion, abscess formation in synovial or subchondral tissues, and, if treatment is not adequate, articular destruction.

## Clinical Findings

**A. Symptoms and Signs:** The onset is usually sudden; the joint becomes acutely painful, hot, and swollen; and chills and fever are often present. The large weight-bearing joints and the wrists are most frequently affected.

Disseminated infection is not uncommon in individuals whose anogenital or throat infection is asymptomatic. Dissemination in women usually occurs during pregnancy or menstruation. The initial bacteremic stage may persist for days and is characterized by migratory arthralgias, tenosynovitis, and typical skin lesions. The latter are violaceous papules or petechiae that may disappear or progress through transient vesicular, pustular, and bullous stages. The organism is rarely recovered from these lesions. Frank arthritis develops after these premonitory symptoms and is often confined to one joint. Less common systemic complications are liver function abnormalities, myocarditis, pericarditis, meningitis, and endocarditis.

**B. Laboratory Findings:** The leukocyte count of the synovial fluid may be greater than 100,000/μL, with 90% or more polymorphonuclear cells. Synovial fluid sugar is usually low. The organisms are occasionally demonstrated by smear. However, there is increasing evidence that articular infection starts in the periarticular tissues and that organisms do not appear in synovial fluid unless the infective focus ulcerates into the joint cavity. In gonococcal arthritis, for example, the gonococcus is recovered from joint fluid in less than half of cases. Throat and anorectal cultures for gonococci as well as blood and genital cultures are required whenever infection with this organism is suspected.

**C. Imaging:** Radiographs are usually normal early in the disease, but evidence of demineralization may be present within days of onset. Bony erosions and narrowing of the joint space followed by osteomyelitis and periostitis may be seen within 2 weeks.

## Differential Diagnosis

The septic course with chills and fever, the acute systemic reaction, the joint fluid findings, evidence of infection elsewhere in the body, and the dramatic response to appropriate antibiotics are diagnostic of bacterial arthritis. Gout and pseudogout are excluded by the failure to find crystals on synovial fluid analysis. Acute rheumatic fever and rheumatoid arthritis commonly involve many joints; Still's disease may mimic septic arthritis, but laboratory evidence of infection is absent. Pyogenic arthritis may be superimposed on other types of joint disease, notably rheumatoid arthritis, and must be excluded (by joint fluid examination) in any apparent acute relapse of the primary disease, particularly when a joint has been needled or one is more strikingly inflamed than the others.

## Treatment

Prompt systemic antibiotic therapy of any septic arthritis should be based on the best clinical judgment of the causative organism and the results of smear and culture of joint fluid, blood, urine, or other specific sites of potential infection. If the organism cannot be determined clinically, treatment should be started with bactericidal antibiotics effective against staphylococci, pneumococci, gonococci, and gram-negative organisms.

Frequent (even daily) local aspiration is indicated when synovial fluid rapidly reaccumulates and causes symptoms. Surgical drainage is reserved for septic arthritis of the hip, because of its inaccessibility to repeated aspiration. Pain can be relieved with local hot compresses and by immobilizing the joint with a splint or traction. Rest, immobilization, and elevation are used at the onset of treatment. Early active motion exercises within the limits of tolerance will hasten recovery.

## Prognosis

With prompt antibiotic therapy, functional recovery is usually complete. Bony ankylosis and articular destruction commonly occur if treatment is inadequate.

Bacterial arthritis. (Editorial) *Lancet* 1986;**2**:721.

Goldenberg DL, Reed JI: Bacterial arthritis. *N Engl J Med* 1985;**312**:764.

## OTHER INFECTIOUS ARTHROPATHIES

### Lyme Disease

This disease is named after Lyme, Connecticut, the site where the first recognized case occurred, but it is now recognized to be widespread. Lyme arthritis is caused by *Borrelia burgdorferi*, a spirochete transmitted by a tick (*Ixodes dammini* or related species) that harbors the organism. The common animal hosts are mice and deer. Clinical manifestations start with a characteristic skin lesion at the site of the tick bite (erythema chronicum migrans), fever, chills, and headache. Oligoarticular arthritis is common, but polyarticular disease occurs also, often with large effusions. Involvement of the heart (eg, arrhythmias, myocarditis) and nervous system (eg, neuropathies, meningoencephalitis) occurs in immunologically predisposed individuals, as a high incidence of HLA-DR2 is observed in this group. In these patients, the arthritis is more common and often recurrent and may develop into a proliferative erosive synovitis. Penicillin is the preferred treatment. It should be given intravenously in established cases. The condition also responds to tetracycline, cephalosporins, and doxycycline.

### Viral Arthritis

Arthritis may be a manifestation of many viral infections. It is generally mild and of short duration, and it terminates spontaneously without lasting ill effects. Mumps arthritis may occur in the absence of parotitis. Rubella arthritis, which occurs more commonly in adults than in children, may appear immediately before, during, or soon after the disappearance of the rash. Its usual polyarticular and symmetric distribution mimics that of rheumatoid arthritis. However, the seronegative tests for rheumatoid factor and the rising rubella titers in convalescent serum help to confirm the diagnosis. Postrubella vaccination arthritis may have its onset as long as 6 weeks following vaccination and occurs in all age groups.

Polyarthritis may be associated with type B hepatitis and typically occurs before the onset of jaundice; it may occur in anicteric hepatitis as well. Urticaria or other types of skin rash may be present. Indeed, the clinical picture may be indistinguishable from that of serum sickness. Serum transaminase levels are elevated, and hepatitis B surface antigen is most often present. Serum complement levels are usually low during active arthritis and become normal after remission of arthritis. False-positive tests for rheumatoid factor, when present, disappear within several weeks. The arthritis is mild; it rarely lasts more than a few weeks and is self-limiting and without deformity.

Sergent JS: Extrahepatic manifestations of hepatitis B infection. *Bull Rheum Dis* 1983;**33**:1.
Steere AC et al: Successful parenteral penicillin therapy of established Lyme arthritis. *N Engl J Med* 1985;**312**:869.

# INFECTIONS OF BONES

Direct microbial contamination of bones results from open fracture, surgical procedures, gunshot wounds, diagnostic needle aspirations, and therapeutic or self-administered drug injections.

Indirect or secondary infections are first noticed in other areas of the body and extend to bones by hematogenous routes.

## ACUTE PYOGENIC OSTEOMYELITIS

### Essentials of Diagnosis

- Fever and chills associated with pain and tenderness of involved bone.
- Aspiration of involved bone is usually diagnostic.
- Culture of blood or lesion tissue is essential for precise diagnosis.
- Radiographs early in the course are typically negative.

### General Considerations

Initial bone infections are indirectly seeded by a single strain of pyogenic bacteria about 95% of the time. About 75% of hematogenous acute infections of bone are due to staphylococci; group A hemolytic streptococci are the next most common pathogens. Vertebral osteomyelitis, due to more indolent organisms, is being encountered with increasing frequency in elderly patients. Infections of bone due to trauma are often polymicrobial.

Salmonellae cause many cases of bacteremia associated with sickle cell disease. Among patients with hemoglobinopathies, osteomyelitis is caused by salmonellae almost 10 times as often as by other pyogenic bacteria. In otherwise healthy patients with salmonellosis, bone lesions are likely to be solitary. In typhoid fever, however, infections of bones occur as a complication in less than 1% of cases. (See Salmonellosis, p 865.)

Bone infection is an uncommon complication of brucellosis, but the clinical picture when it does occur is characteristic. Bone lesions most commonly occur in the lumbar spine or sacroiliac joints.

### Clinical Findings

**A. Symptoms and Signs:** The onset of acute osteomyelitis in adults is less likely to be striking than the sudden and alarming presentation often seen in children. Generalized toxic symptoms of bacteremia may be absent, and vague or evanescent local pain may be the earliest manifestation. Tenderness may be present or absent, depending upon the extent and duration of bone involvement.

**B. Laboratory Findings:** Aspiration of bone and periosteum to recover organisms for culture is necessary for accurate diagnosis. Blood cultures are frequently positive, particularly when systemic symptoms are prominent, in which case the white count and sedimentation rate are often elevated.

With infections due to *Salmonella* or *Brucella*, significant rising serologic agglutination titers support a tentative diagnosis during the acute stage. Culture of material from the osteoid focus is specific.

**C. Imaging:** Early findings may include soft tissue swelling, loss of tissue planes, and periarticular demineralization of bone. About 2 weeks after onset of symptoms, erosion of bone and alteration of cancellous bone appear, followed by periostitis. Xeroradiography and radionuclide imaging may localize occult lesions several days before conventional radiographic studies are suggestive. When osteomyelitis involves the vertebrae, it commonly traverses the disk space— a finding that is not observed in tumor.

### Differential Diagnosis

Acute hematogenous osteomyelitis should be distinguished from suppurative arthritis, rheumatic fever, and cellulitis. More subacute forms must be differentiated from tuberculous or mycotic infections of bone and Ewing's sarcoma or from metastatic tumor (vertebral osteomyelitis).

### Complications

Inadequate treatment of bone infections results in chronicity of infection, and this possibility is increased by delay in diagnosis and treatment. Extension to adjacent bone or joints may complicate acute osteomyelitis. Recurrence of bone infections often results in anemia, weight loss, weakness, and rarely amyloidosis. Pseudoepitheliomatous hyperplasia, squamous cell carcinoma, or fibrosarcoma may occasionally arise in persistently infected tissues.

### Treatment

Cultures and antibiotic sensitivity studies should determine the choice of antibiotic agents; the initial selection of drug is based on clinical assessment of the most probable cause. Open or closed drainage of the local lesion is important when prompt clinical response to initial treatment does not occur. Parenteral antibiotic therapy should be continued for a total of 6 weeks. Analgesics, rest, immobilization, and elevation of the part should be used from the beginning of treatment.

### Prognosis

If sterility of the lesion is achieved within 2–4 days, a good result can be expected in most cases if there is no compromise of the patient's immune system. However, progression of the disease to a chronic form may occur. It is especially common in the lower extremities and in patients in whom circulation is impaired (eg, diabetics). Surgical saucerization, excision of bone, and debridement of healthy tissues are often necessary.

Blockey NJ: Chronic osteomyelitis. *J Bone Joint Surg [Br]* 1983;**65**:120.

Kern RZ, Houpt JB: Pyogenic vertebral osteomyelitis: Diagnosis and management. *Can Med Assoc J* 1984;**130**:1025.

## OTHER INFECTIONS OF BONES & JOINTS

### 1. MYCOTIC INFECTIONS OF BONES & JOINTS

Fungal infections of the skeletal system are usually secondary to a primary infection in another organ, frequently the lungs (see Chapter 27). Although skeletal lesions have a predilection for the cancellous extremities of long bones and the bodies of vertebrae, the predominant lesion—a granuloma with varying degrees of necrosis and abscess formation—does not produce a characteristic clinical picture.

Differentiation from other chronic focal infections depends upon culture studies of synovial fluid or tissue obtained from the local lesion. Serologic tests and skin tests provide presumptive support of the diagnosis.

### Coccidioidomycosis

Coccidioidomycosis of bones and joints is usually secondary to primary pulmonary infection (see p 955). Early arthralgia with periarticular swelling, especially in the knees and ankles, should be differentiated from organic bone and joint involvement. Osseous lesions commonly occur in cancellous bone of the vertebrae or near the ends of long bones. These lesions are initially osteolytic and thus may mimic metastatic tumor or myeloma.

The precise diagnosis depends upon recovery of *Coccidioides immitis* from the lesion or histologic examination of tissue obtained by open biopsy. Rising titers of IgA complement-fixing antibodies provide further evidence of the disseminated nature of the disease.

Systemic treatment with amphotericin B should be tried for bone and joint infections (see p 956). Treatment with miconazole may be effective, but the results remain unproved. Chronic infection may require operative excision of infected bone and soft tissue; amputation may be the only solution for stubbornly progressive infections. Immobilization of joints by plaster casts and avoidance of weight bearing provide benefit. Synovectomy, joint debridement, and arthrodesis are reserved for more advanced joint infections.

### Histoplasmosis

Focal skeletal or joint involvement in histoplasmosis is rare and generally represents dissemination from a primary focus in the lungs (see p 956). Skeletal lesions may be single or multiple and are not characteristic.

### 2. TUBERCULOSIS OF BONES & JOINTS

Most tuberculous infections in the USA are caused by the human strain of *Mycobacterium tuberculosis* (see Chapter 7). Infection of the musculoskeletal system is caused by hematogenous spread from a primary lesion of the respiratory tract; it may occur shortly after primary infection or may be seen years later as a reactivation disease. Tuberculosis of the thoracic or lumbar spine (Pott's disease) may be associated with an active lesion of the genitourinary tract or may occur as an isolated finding. It is usually a disease of childhood, occurring most commonly before puberty; adult infection is uncommon. Tuberculous osteomyelitis secondary to cutaneous inoculation has been reported.

## Clinical Findings

**A. Symptoms and Signs:** The onset of symptoms is generally insidious and not accompanied by general manifestations of fever, sweating, toxicity, or prostration. Pain may be mild at onset, is usually worse at night, and may be accompanied by stiffness. As the disease process progresses, limitation of joint motion becomes prominent because of muscle contractures and destruction of the joint. The knee is the most commonly involved peripheral joint. Symptoms of pulmonary tuberculosis may also be present.

Local findings during the early stages may be limited to tenderness, soft tissue swelling, joint effusion, and increase in skin temperature about the involved area. As the disease progresses without treatment, muscle atrophy and deformity become apparent. Abscess formation with spontaneous drainage externally leads to sinus formation. Progressive destruction of bone in the spine may cause a gibbus, especially in the thoracolumbar region.

**B. Laboratory Findings:** The precise diagnosis rests upon recovery of the acid-fast organism from joint fluid, pus, or tissue specimens. Biopsy of the bony lesion, synovium, or a regional lymph node may demonstrate the characteristic histopathologic picture of caseating necrosis and giant cells.

**C. Imaging:** There is a latent period between the onset of symptoms and the initial positive radiographic finding. The earliest changes of tuberculous arthritis are those of soft tissue swelling and distention of the capsule by effusion. Subsequently, bone atrophy causes thinning of the trabecular pattern, narrowing of the cortex, and enlargement of the medullary canal. As joint disease progresses, destruction of cartilage, both in the spine and in peripheral joints, is manifested by narrowing of the joint cleft and focal erosion of the articular surface, especially at the margins. Extensive destruction of joint surfaces causes deformity. As healing takes place, osteosclerosis becomes apparent around areas of necrosis and sequestration. Where the lesion is limited to bone, especially in the cancellous portion of the metaphysis, the x-ray picture may be that of single or multilocular cysts surrounded by sclerotic bone. As intraosseous foci expand toward the limiting cortex and erode it, subperiosteal new bone formation takes place. When bony tuberculosis is suspected, a chest film may be helpful in revealing characteristic pulmonary abnormalities even in the absence of symptoms.

## Differential Diagnosis

Tuberculosis of the musculoskeletal system must be differentiated from all subacute and chronic infections, rheumatoid arthritis, gout, and, occasionally, osseous dysplasia. In the spine, metastatic tumor may be suggested.

## Complications

Destruction of bones or joints may occur in a few weeks or months if adequate treatment is not provided. Deformity due to joint destruction, abscess formation with spread into adjacent soft tissues, and sinus formation are common. Paraplegia is the most serious complication of spinal tuberculosis. As healing of severe joint lesions takes place, spontaneous fibrous or bony ankylosis follows.

## Treatment
## (See also Chapter 7.)

**A. General Measures:** General care is especially important when prolonged recumbency is necessary; skillful nursing care must be provided.

**B. Chemotherapy:** Combinations of antituberculosis agents are recommended. Cure without need for surgical intervention may be effected in most cases, even with extensive disease.

**C. Surgical Measures:** In acute infections where synovitis is the predominant feature, treatment can be conservative, at least initially: Immobilization by splint or plaster, aspiration, and chemotherapy may suffice to control the infection. This treatment is especially desirable for the management of infections of large joints of the lower extremities in children during the early stage of the infection. Synovectomy may be valuable for less acute hypertrophic lesions that involve tendon sheaths, bursae, or joints.

Halsey JP et al: A decade of skeletal tuberculosis. *Ann Rheum Dis* 1982;**41**:7.

Versfeld GA, Solomon A: A diagnostic approach to tuberculosis of bones and joints. *J Bone Joint Surg [Br] 1982;***64**:446.

## OSTEOGENESIS IMPERFECTA
## (Fragilitas Ossium, Brittle Bones)

### Essentials of Diagnosis

- Fragility of bone manifested by repeated pathologic fracture.
- Clearness or blue coloration of scleras.
- Deafness.
- Positive family history.
- Ligamentous laxity.
- Dental defects.

### General Considerations

Osteogenesis imperfecta is a heritable disorder of connective tissue usually transmitted as an autosomal dominant, although some cases may be autosomal recessive. Two recognized clinical types may occur: osteogenesis imperfecta congenita (fetal type), in which fractures occur in utero and skeletal deformities are apparent at birth; and osteogenesis imperfecta tarda, in which fractures and deformities occur after birth.

### Clinical Findings

**A. Symptoms and Signs:** Fragility of bones is the single most obvious diagnostic criterion. Repeated long-bone fractures in childhood should suggest the underlying disorder. Clearness or blue coloration of the scleras, conductive deafness, and spinal deformities (scoliosis and kyphosis) are often present.

Defective dentin formation (dentinogenesis imperfecta), joint hypermobility, hernias, and hyperelasticity of the skin suggest a soft tissue dysplasia.

The milder cases of the late form may simulate idiopathic juvenile or menopausal osteoporosis.

**B. Imaging:** The cortices of the major long bones in the congenita type are thin, and the marrow cavities are broad. In the late type, the bones may be "slender," with narrow shafts, reduced marrow cavities, and bell-shaped widening of the epiphyses. Callus formation after fracture may be meager or luxuriant. Hyperplastic callus formation may occur with or without apparent fracture.

### Treatment

There is no treatment for the inadequate formation of osteoid. Calcitonin may be of some value in the tarda group.

Most fractures require immobilization for the relief of pain and prevention of malhealing. Extensive deformities of the diaphysis of a major long bone require more elaborate surgical treatment (eg, multiple osteotomies and internal fixation). Surgical treatment of kyphoscoliosis may have to be delayed until late adolescence, when skeletal structures are stronger.

### Prognosis

Because of the protean manifestations of this disease, the course and prognosis are variable. Transmission of the more severe traits is probably prevented by death before puberty or by prevention of reproduction of invalids. The incidence of fracture and the extent of ligamentous laxity are likely to decrease after puberty, and this favorable turn tends to continue through adolescence into later life. However, menopause-associated osteoporosis may worsen the picture in women.

Molecular genetics and osteogenesis imperfecta. (Editorial.) *Lancet* 1986;**2**:496.

# PAIN SYNDROMES

## CERVICOBRACHIAL PAIN SYNDROMES

A large group of articular and extra-articular disorders is characterized by pain that may involve simultaneously the neck, shoulder girdle, and upper extremity. Diagnostic differentiation is often difficult. Some of these entities and clinical syndromes represent primary disorders of the cervicobrachial region; others are local manifestations of systemic disease. The clinical picture is further complicated when 2 or more of these conditions occur coincidentally.

### Clinical Findings

**A. Symptoms and Signs:** Neck pain may be limited to the posterior neck region or, depending upon the level of the symptomatic joint, may radiate segmentally to the occiput, anterior chest, shoulder girdle, arm, forearm, and hand. It may be intensified by active or passive neck motions. The general distribution of pain and paresthesias corresponds roughly to the involved dermatome in the upper extremity. Radiating pain in the upper extremity is often intensified by hyperextension of the neck and deviation of the head to the involved side. Limitation of cervical movements is the most common objective finding. Neurologic signs depend upon the extent of compression of nerve roots or the spinal cord. Compression of the spinal cord may cause long-tract involvement resulting in paraparesis or paraplegia.

**B. Imaging:** The radiographic findings depend on the cause of the pain; many are completely normal. An early finding is loss of the normal anterior convexity of the cervical curve (loss of cervical lordosis). Comparative reduction in height of the involved disk space is a frequent finding. The most common late x-ray finding is osteophyte formation anteriorly, adjacent to the disk; other late changes occur around the apophyseal joint clefts, chiefly in the lower cervical spine. Computer-assisted myelography is a valuable radiographic means of demonstrating nerve root or spinal cord compression; MRI may be preferable but is less apt to be available.

### Differential Diagnosis & Treatment

The causes of neck pain include acute and chronic cervical strain or sprains, herniated nucleus pulposus, osteoarthritis, ankylosing spondylitis, rheumatoid arthritis, osteomyelitis, neoplasms, spinal stenosis, compression fractures, and functional disorders.

**A. Acute or Chronic Cervical Musculotendinous Strain:** Cervical strain is generally caused by mechanical postural disorders, overexertion, or injury (eg, whiplash). Acute episodes are associated with pain, decreased cervical spine motion, and paraspinal muscle spasm, resulting in stiffness of the neck and loss of motion. Muscle trigger points can often be localized. Management includes neck and head immobilization by traction, a cervical collar, and administration of analgesics. Gradual return to full activity is encouraged.

Patients with chronic symptoms often have few objective findings. Mechanical stress due to work or recreational activities is often implicated. Chronic pain, especially that radiating into the upper extremity, may require additional treatment such as bracing.

**B. Herniated Nucleus Pulposus:** Rupture or prolapse of the nucleus pulposus of the cervical disks into the spinal canal causes pain that radiates to the arms at the level of C6–7. When intra-abdominal pressure is increased by coughing, sneezing, or other movements, symptoms are aggravated, and cervical muscle spasm may often occur. Neurologic abnormalities may include decreased reflexes of the deep tendons of the biceps and triceps and decreased sensation and muscle atrophy or weakness in the forearm or hand. Cervical traction, bed rest, and other conservative measures are usually successful. Myelography or electromyography help delineate lesions that may require surgical treatment (laminectomy, fusion). Chemonucleolysis is not a useful treatment alternative in cervical disk disease.

**C. Arthritic Disorders:** Cervical spondylosis (degenerative arthritis) is a collective term describing degenerative changes that occur in the apophyseal joints and intervertebral disk joints, with or without neurologic signs. Osteoarthritis of the articular facets is characterized by progressive thinning of the cartilage, subchondral osteoporosis, and osteophytic proliferation around the joint margins. Degeneration of cervical disks and joints may occur in adolescents but is more common after age 40. Degeneration is progressive and is marked by gradual narrowing of the disk space, as demonstrated by x-ray. Osteocartilaginous proliferation occurs around the margin of the vertebral body and gives rise to osteophytic ridges that may encroach upon the intervertebral foramens and spinal canal, causing compression of the neurovascular contents. A large anterior osteophyte may occasionally cause dysphagia.

Ankylosing spondylitis is discussed on pp 509 and 521. Rheumatoid arthritis can mimic ankylosing spondylitis, with intervertebral disk and connective tissue involvement. Atlantoaxial subluxation may occur in patients with rheumatoid arthritis, regardless of the severity of disease. Inflammation of the synovial structures resulting from erosion and laxity of the transverse ligament can lead to neurologic signs of spinal cord compression. Treatment may vary from use of a cervical collar or more rigid bracing to operative treatment, depending on the degree of subluxation and neurologic progression. Surgical treatment may involve stabilization of the cervical spine.

**D. Other Disorders:** Osteomyelitis is discussed on pp 515 and 520; neoplasms on p 521; compression fractures and osteoporosis on p 521; and functional disorders on p 522.

Hirsh LF: Cervical degenerative arthritis: Possible cause of neck and arm pain. *Postgrad Med* (July) 1983;**74:**123.

## LOW BACK PAIN SYNDROME

Low back pain is one of the most ubiquitous of ailments. About 80% of people are so afflicted at some time during their lives, and of these, 1–2% become chronically impaired. Low back pain may be associated with a variety of causes. These patients are subjected to a large number of diagnostic procedures with ambiguous or unrevealing results. This reflects inadequate clinical evaluation and a failure to utilize information obtained from properly conducted history and physical examination.

### Clinical Findings

A history of the patient's illness should include occupation, injuries, onset of symptoms, pattern of pain and relationship to physical activity, aggravating and relieving factors, emotional status, loss of time from work, and possible litigation.

Inspection and palpation of the painful area are important. Since pain from nerve roots or nerves is commonly referred toward the periphery, the physician should explore the entire nerve lengths leading from the painful area and should note the presence of any masses or tenderness and, where possible, the size and consistency of nerves.

Muscle spasm and tenderness to percussion and deep pressure may give evidence suggesting radicular irritation, particularly when associated with local deformity or restriction of spinal motion. Lumbar paraspinal muscle spasm frequently is noted with local radiculitis, which is due to many causes, including herniated lumbar intervertebral disk.

Psoas muscle spasm usually indicates disease of the psoas muscle or of the lumbar vertebrae and soft tissue adjacent to this muscle. It may be tested with the patient prone and the pelvis firmly pressed against the table with one hand by the examiner. With the other hand grasping the ankle, the leg is moved to the vertical position with the knee flexed at a right angle. The hip is passively hyperextended by lifting up on the ankle. Limitation of motion is produced by involuntary psoas muscle spasm.

Limitation of passive lumbar flexion and resulting pain often accompany disease of the lumbar or lumbosacral articulations. With the patient supine, the examiner grasps one lower extremity with both hands, moves the thigh to a position of maximal flexion, and then presses firmly downward toward the table and upward toward the patient's head, passively flexing the lumbar spinal column.

The range of motion of joints and the effect of movement on the pain should be determined, since pain from areas such as the hip may be referred distally.

The regional blood vessels and those of the extremity should be checked for adequacy of pulsation and aneurysmal dilatation. Rectal and vaginal examination rule out local lesions and involvement of accessible lumbodorsal plexuses.

Sciatic stretch tests (eg, the straight leg-raising test and Lasègue's sign) should be elicited. With the patient supine, the relaxed, extended lower extremity is gently lifted from the bed or table. A test is positive if back pain and radicular radiation are duplicated. It is suggestive but not diagnostic of herniated nucleus pulposus.

Patrick's sign helps to differentiate sciatic from hip joint disease. The patient lies supine, and the heel of the lower extremity being tested is passively placed on the opposite knee. The knee on the side being tested is then pressed laterally and downward as far as it will go. The test is positive if motion is involuntarily restricted; pain frequently accompanies limitation of motion. The test is positive in hip joint disease and negative in sciatica.

## Low Back Pain Without Characteristic Radiographic Changes

Disorders of the spine that may present without characteristic radiographic changes causing back pain include musculotendinous strain of the thoracic and lumbar spine, herniated nucleus pulposus, ankylosing spondylitis, osteomyelitis, and primary and metastatic bone tumors.

**A. Musculotendinous Strain:** Strain is generally related to postural or mechanical causes. Acute episodes of pain are severe and usually limited in duration, with decreased back motion and paraspinal muscle spasm, resulting in a list and loss of lordosis. Muscle trigger points can often be localized. Management includes bed rest, local heat, a firm sleeping surface, and analgesics. After 24 hours of pain-free recumbency without medication, walking activity is tried, with progression to full activity if symptoms do not recur. Patients with chronic symptoms present few objective findings, and stress is often implicated. Predisposing factors may include poor posture, obesity, poor abdominal muscle tone, and pregnancy. Ongoing management may include daily exercises or sport activities appropriate for age, a firm mattress, and a weight reduction program if needed.

**B. Herniated Nucleus Pulposus:** This is the most common radicular syndrome manifested in the lumbosacral region and occurs principally in young adult males. Backache, exacerbated by increased intra-abdominal pressure due to coughing, sneezing, and movement, usually antedates the sciatic syndrome. The latter is noted by a positive Lasègue and a negative Patrick sign. Intervertebral disks L4–5 and L5–S1 are most commonly affected, causing weakness or atrophy of the thigh or calf, decreased sensation in a radicular pattern, and hyporeflexia.

Except for an occasional narrowed intervertebral space, x-rays are not generally helpful. Pain from a herniated nucleus pulposus is almost always relieved by bed rest in recumbency, analgesics, sedation, and a firm sleeping surface. The duration of bed rest to be recommended is controversial; there is no evidence that more than 48–72 hours is beneficial, though some clinicians feel otherwise. The patient who does not respond to conservative treatment in 14–21 days or who demonstrates progression of neurologic deficits should undergo contrast myelography with CT scanning. Based upon these findings, operation may be indicated. Extradural corticosteroid injections are helpful in some cases, especially for the short term. **Chemonucleolysis** is a useful but controversial alternative to surgical diskectomy but should not preclude conservative treatment. Patients who are good candidates for surgical disk excision may benefit from this special technique.

**C. Inflammatory Disorders:** Ankylosing spondylitis (see p 509) occurs principally in men. Few significant radiographic changes are noted during the first 1–2 years following onset of symptoms. The disorder is progressive and leads to calcification of the anterior longitudinal ligaments.

Rheumatoid arthritis can cause severe low back pain from intervertebral disk degeneration.

**D. Osteomyelitis:** (See p 515.) Osteomyelitis of the spine produces destructive lesions with localized pain and sensitivity to percussion. Indeed, the combination of both pain and fever should be considered to signify infection until some other cause is identified. In young patients, there is often a history of respiratory tract (staphylococcal or streptococcal) infection; in older patients, manipulation of the genitourinary tract (gram-negative bacilli) may be the precipitating event. Radiographs may show localized decalcification of the vertebrae and subperiosteal calcification 10–14 days after an acute pyogenic episode. Postoperative infections following diskectomy may develop in 1–8 weeks. Management by immobilization of the back usually alleviates the pain. If antibiotic therapy does not control the infection, surgical debridement and drainage with or without bone grafting of the defect are required. Chronic pyogenic osteomyelitis resulting from bacteria is more common in areas where narcotic addiction is frequent. Brucellosis, coccidioidomycosis, and mycobacterial infection may follow an ill-defined or insidious course with low-grade fever; radiographic changes are evident even later than the symptoms. Back pain, constitutional symptoms, weight loss, and a list develop. Hyperemic osteoporosis of cancellous bone may result in vertebral collapse, producing neurologic symptoms. When abscesses form, they may dissect along fascial planes, affecting the psoas muscle and the gluteal and paravertebral areas. Management is similar to that of acute pyogenic infection. Abscess drainage may be needed. Occasionally, spinal fusion may be necessary for instability or progressive deformity causing neurologic deficit.

**E. Neoplasms:** Benign or malignant neoplasms may affect the spinal cord or the osseous vertebrae at any level. The patient who complains of constant night pain and worsening sleep difficulties due to pain should be suspected of having a tumor. The most common primary tumor in patients over 40 is multiple myeloma; secondary neoplasms are metastatic carcinoma from the breast, prostate, kidney, or lung. Neck or back pain may be the initial complaint, and x-rays of the spine may be normal until 30% of the bone has been destroyed. Tumors may be bone-producing or bone-destroying, depending upon the origin of the lesion. Serum alkaline phosphatase (elevated in bone-producing tumors), calcium, and phosphorus may help; and bone scanning is more sensitive than plain films for bone-producing tumors. Management includes symptomatic treatment, needle or open biopsy, and computer-assisted myelography or MRI. Radiotherapy is the initial treatment of choice for metastatic tumors compressing the spinal cord. Surgery is reserved for radiation failures or for cases in which the diagnosis has not been established. Prognosis is best if therapy is initiated before neurologic signs of cord compression develop.

## Low Back Pain With Characteristic Radiographic Changes

These include osteoarthritis, spondylolisthesis, spinal stenosis, facet tropism, transitional vertebra, untreated scoliosis, and osteoporosis.

**A. Degenerative Changes:** Degenerative changes of the intervertebral disks (spondylosis) and the posterior articulating facets (osteoarthritis) and spinal stenosis are often interrelated and may affect the entire spine. They occur chiefly in patients of middle age or older. Early morning stiffness and pain aggravated by prolonged sitting and standing and improved by walking (except for spinal stenosis, which worsens with exertion), are often relieved by recumbency. Sciatic radiation may occur. Fatigue, obesity, and muscle tension or spasm aggravate the problem. Musculotendinous strain may be superimposed. The formation of osteophytes around the periphery of the vertebral body and facet joints may lead to entrapment of the lateral spinal nerve roots. Early radiographic findings show osteophyte formation lateral and anterior (traction spur) to the vertebral body, with later narrowing of the disk and facet joints and foraminal encroachment. CT scan with myelography is confirmatory. Management includes analgesics, antiinflammatory agents, weight loss, modification of activities, and decompressive surgery.

**B. Spondylolysis and Spondylolisthesis:** A defect in the pars interarticularis (spondylolysis) and a bilateral defect with vertebral slippage (spondylolisthesis) are believed in most cases to be acquired disorders resulting from stress fractures. Although often asymptomatic, they may cause low back pain with or without sciatic radiation. Involvement of L5 is most common, followed by L4. A depression above

the sacrum is seen on physical examination. Radiographs (particularly oblique views) are necessary to confirm the diagnosis. Management of acute symptoms remains conservative, with bed rest and analgesics. Recurrent and increasingly severe symptoms with or without neurologic involvement and continuing radiographic evidence of slippage warrant surgical decompression or fusion.

**C. Facet Tropism and Transitional Vertebra:** Normally, the facets are symmetrically aligned at each vertebral level. Facet tropism occurs with asymmetry, adding rotational stresses to the joint. Asymmetric stress resulting from unilateral transitional vertebra (Bertolotti's syndrome) often causes a herniated nucleus pulposus one level above the sacralized or lumbarized segment. Both are diagnosed by radiography. When conservative measures fail, spinal fusion with or without decompression may be of benefit.

**D. Compression Fractures:** Compression fractures often result from trauma and are diagnosed by radiographic examination. The level and degree of injury determine the degree of neurologic involvement and the necessity for thorough and repeated neurologic examinations. The possibility of cancer or osteoporosis should be considered in patients with a history of fractures resulting from trivial trauma. Stable injuries respond to bed rest and conservative care; unstable ones require longer periods of bed rest and orthotic or surgical treatment (or both).

**E. Untreated Scoliosis:** Uncorrected scoliosis in adults can cause back pain. After skeletal maturity has been achieved, spinal curves can progress up to 2 degrees per year and up to 8 degrees per pregnancy or period of exogenous hormone use. Degenerative changes develop more rapidly. Symptomatic treatment may be helpful. Adult patients with progressive symptoms of pain in the area of the deformity may get relief from operative treatment.

**F. Osteoporosis:** Osteoporosis is the most common metabolic disorder causing back pain. It affects postmenopausal women more commonly than older men. Radiographs reveal a marked decrease in vertebral bone density and decreased height, with thoracic kyphosis or lumbar lordosis. The intervertebral disks often bulge into the vertebral end plate, and compression fractures may be noted. Laboratory values are normal; metastatic tumor and multiple myeloma must be ruled out. Treatment is directed toward the cause, as noted on p 719. Activity strengthens bone and favors increased deposition of all bony elements. Orthotic support may be useful. In advanced cases, surgical measures must be considered to minimize neurologic symptoms.

## Miscellaneous Causes of Low Back Pain

Other causes of back pain not accompanied by radiographic abnormalities include aneurysms, visceral disorders, and functional problems.

**A. Aneurysms:** Atherosclerosis of the aorta, resulting in abdominal aneurysm of the terminal aorta, gives rise to back pain similar to that of herniated nucleus pulposus or neoplasm. Deep, boring pain in the lumbar or pelvic region and a pulsating abdominal mass suggest the diagnosis. Thrombotic occlusion of the terminal aorta, with or without associated aneurysm, may produce pain in the buttocks, thighs, or legs, with fatigue, weakness, or muscle atrophy along with male impotence; persistent peripheral pulses may still be present. Vascular surgery may provide symptomatic relief.

**B. Visceral Disorders:** Gastrointestinal and genitourinary disease may be a source of back pain. Pancreatic disease and duodenal ulcer may give rise to left thoracolumbar and midback pain. Flank pain can be caused by renal disease. Lumbosacral pain can be due to prostatitis, gynecologic disorders (pelvic inflammatory disease, uterine fibroids, and endometriosis), and retrocolic processes.

**C. Functional Disorders:** Complaints of a tired and weak back with pain (not necessarily severe) and no objective findings may suggest a psychologic problem. Hysterical back pain may be severe and dramatically exaggerated. A history of domestic or work-related problems and observation of a flat affect with a bizarre reaction to treatment will further suggest the disorder. Treatment may include reassurance and judicious use of mild analgesics and sedatives. Chronicity of complaints is common, and psychiatric referral may be necessary.

The patient with compensatory back or neck pain may be interested in monetary gain, whereas the malingerer seeks a conscious real or imagined secondary gain. Subjective complaints in both types of patients are out of proportion to objective findings. The experienced clinician can often identify the malingerer or the patient with compensatory back or neck pain. These diagnostic impressions should not be conveyed to the patient. It is best to state simply that no organic disorder can be found that explains the patient's symptoms.

Fredrickson BE et al: The natural history of spondylolysis and spondylolisthesis. *J Bone Joint Surg* [*Am*] *1984;***66:**699.

Hall S et al: Lumbar spinal stenosis: Clinical features, diagnostic procedures and results of surgical treatment in 68 patients. *Ann Intern Med* 1985;**103:**271.

Mooney V: Evaluation and guidelines for nonoperative care of the low back. In: *Instructional Course Lectures.* Stauffer ES (editor). Mosby, 1985.

Reuler JB: Low back pain. *West J Med* 1985;**143:**259.

# THORACIC OUTLET SYNDROMES

Thoracic outlet syndromes include those disorders that result in compression of the neurovascular structures supplying the upper extremity. Among them are cervical rib syndrome, costoclavicular syndrome, scalenus anticus and scalenus medius syndromes, pectoralis minor syndrome, "effort thrombosis" of the axillary and subclavian veins, and the subclavian steal syndrome. Patients often have a history of trauma to the head and neck areas.

Symptoms and signs may arise from intermittent or continuous pressure on elements of the brachial plexus and the subclavian or axillary vessels by a variety of anatomic structures of the shoulder girdle region. The neurovascular bundle can be compressed between the anterior or middle scalene muscles and a normal first thoracic rib or a cervical rib. Descent of the shoulder girdle may continue during adulthood and cause compression. Faulty posture, chronic illness, and occupation may be other predisposing factors. The components of the median nerve that encircle the axillary artery may cause compression and vascular symptoms. Sudden or repetitive strenuous physical activity may initiate "effort thrombosis" of the axillary or subclavian vein.

Pain may radiate from the point of compression to the base of the neck, the axilla, the shoulder girdle region, arm, forearm, and hand. Paresthesias are frequently present and are commonly distributed to the volar aspect of the fourth and fifth digits. Sensory symptoms may be aggravated at night or by prolonged use of the extremities. Weakness and muscle atrophy are the principal motor abnormalities. Vascular symptoms consist of arterial ischemia characterized by pallor of the fingers on elevation of the extremity, sensitivity to cold, and, rarely, gangrene of the digits or venous obstruction marked by edema, cyanosis, and engorgement.

Deep reflexes are usually not altered. When the site of compression is between the upper rib and clavicle, partial obliteration of subclavian artery pulsation may be demonstrated by abduction of the arm to a right angle with the elbow simultaneously flexed and rotated externally at the shoulder so that the entire extremity lies in the coronal plane. Neck or arm position has no effect on the diminished pulse, which remains constant in the subclavian steal syndrome.

Radiographic examination is helpful in differential diagnosis. Plethysmography as an objective method of recording brachial arterial pulsations has been emphasized. When venous or arterial obstruction is intravascular, venography or arteriography demonstrates the location of the occlusion. Determinations of the conduction velocities of the ulnar and other peripheral nerves of the upper extremity may help to localize the site of their compression.

Thoracic outlet syndrome must be differentiated from symptomatic osteoarthritis of the cervical spine, tumors of the cervical spinal cord or nerve roots, periarthritis of the shoulder, and other cervicobrachial pain syndromes.

Conservative treatment is directed toward relief of compression of the neurovascular bundle. The patient is instructed to avoid physical activities likely to precipitate or aggravate symptoms. Overhead pulley exercises are useful to improve posture. Shoulder bracing, although uncomfortable, provides a constant stimulus to improve posture. When lying down, the shoulder girdle should be bolstered by arranging pillows in an inverted "V" position.

Symptoms may disappear spontaneously or may be relieved by conservative treatment. Operative treatment is more likely to relieve the neurologic rather than the vascular component that causes symptoms.

Coccia MR, Satiani B: Thoracic outlet syndrome. *Am Fam Physician* (Feb) 1984;**29:**121.

## SCAPULOHUMERAL CALCAREOUS TENDINITIS

Calcareous tendinitis of the shoulder joint is an acute or chronic inflammatory disorder of the capsulotendinous cuff (especially the supraspinatus portion) characterized by deposits of calcium salts among tendon fibers. It is a common cause of acute pain near the lateral aspect of the shoulder joint in men over age 30. The calcium deposit may be restricted to the tendon substance or may rupture into the overlying bursa.

Symptoms consist of pain (at times severe), tenderness to pressure, and restriction of shoulder joint motion.

Radiographic examination confirms the diagnosis and demonstrates the site of the lesion.

Calcareous tendinitis must be differentiated from other cervicobrachial pain syndromes, pyogenic arthritis, osteoarthritis, gout, and tears of the rotator cuff.

The aim of treatment is to relieve pain and restore shoulder joint function. Pain is best treated by injection of the lesion with a local anesthetic with corticosteroid. After treatment, early recovery of shoulder joint function should be fostered by supervised exercises. Acute symptoms occasionally subside after spontaneous rupture of the calcium deposit into the subacromial bursa. Chronic symptoms may be treated by analgesics, exercises, and injection of local anesthetics with corticosteroids. Rarely, calcific deposits may require surgical evacuation.

When x-ray examination shows that a deposit has disappeared, recurrence of that deposit is rare. Symptoms of periarthritis may persist if shoulder joint motion is not completely regained.

Post M (editor): The painful shoulder. (Symposium.) *Clin Orthop* (March) 1983;**173:**1.

## SCAPULOHUMERAL PERIARTHRITIS (Adhesive Capsulitis, Frozen Shoulder)

Periarthritis of the shoulder joint is an inflammatory disorder primarily involving the soft tissues. The condition may be divided into a primary type, in which no obvious cause can be identified, and a secondary type associated with an organic lesion (eg, rheumatoid arthritis, osteoarthritis, fracture or dislo-

cation). The primary type is most common in the minor shoulder among women after the fourth decade. It may be manifested as inflammation of the articular synovia, the tendons around the joint, the intrinsic ligamentous capsular bands, the paratendinous bursae (especially the subacromial), or the bicipital tendon sheath. Calcareous tendinitis and attritional disease of the rotator cuff, with or without tears, are incidental lesions.

The onset of pain, which is aggravated by extremes of shoulder joint motion, may be acute or insidious. Pain may be most annoying at night and may be intensified by pressure on the involved extremity when the patient sleeps in the lateral decubitus position. Tenderness upon palpation is often noted near the tendinous insertions into the greater tuberosity or over the bicipital groove. Although a sensation of stiffness may be noted only at onset, restriction of shoulder joint motion soon becomes apparent and is likely to progress unless effective treatment is instituted.

Pain can usually be controlled with nonsteroidal anti-inflammatory agents. Passive exercise of the shoulder by an overhead pulley mechanism should be repeated slowly for about 2 minutes 4 times daily. Forceful manipulation of the shoulder joint during this exercise should be avoided. Injection of tender areas with corticosteroids gives transitory relief. Operative treatment should be reserved for the occasional refractory case.

White RH, Paull DM, Fleming KW: Rotator cuff tendonitis: Comparison of subacromial injection of a long-acting corticosteroid versus oral indomethacin therapy. *J Rheumatol* 1986;**13:**3.

## EPICONDYLITIS (Tennis Elbow, Epicondylalgia)

Epicondylitis is a pain syndrome affecting the mid portion of the upper extremity; no single causative lesion has been identified. It has been postulated that chronic strain of the forearm muscles due to repetitive grasping or rotatory motions of the forearm causes microscopic tears and subsequent chronic inflammation of the common extensor or common flexor tendon at or near their respective osseous origins from the epicondyles.

Epicondylitis occurs most frequently in the dominant extremity during middle life. Pain is predominantly on the medial or lateral aspect of the elbow region, may be aggravated by grasping, and may radiate proximally into the arm or distally into the forearm. The point of maximal tenderness to pressure is 1–2 cm distal to the epicondyle but may also be present in the muscle bellies more distally. Resisted dorsiflexion or volar flexion of the wrist may accentuate the pain. X-ray examination generally reveals no significant change.

Treatment is directed toward relief of pain. Most symptoms can be relieved by rest and mild analgesics.

An elastic bandage applied about the proximal forearm may ameliorate discomfort when the patient is grasping forcefully. Infiltration of "trigger points" by local anesthetic solutions with corticosteroids may be helpful. Operative treatment is reserved for severe, refractory cases.

Berson BL, McGinniss GH: Common tennis injuries. *Hosp Med* (April) 1983;**19**:122.

## FIBROSITIS
## (Fibromyalgia)

Fibrositis is a relatively common form of nonarticular rheumatism. The condition is characterized by diffuse musculoskeletal aching associated with multiple tender points in soft tissues. It affects chiefly women in the fourth through sixth decades of life. Associated symptoms include morning stiffness, fatigue, headache, neck pain, and sleep disturbances. Laboratory tests are noncontributory. Fibrositis usually occurs in the absence of any other disease, and it may be mimicked by polymyalgia rheumatica or rheumatoid arthritis. Attention to the sleep disorder may lead to improvement in the symptom complex; tricyclic antidepressants in low doses may help. Cardiovascular fitness training may also be of value.

Bennett RM (editor): The fibrositis/fibromyalgia syndrome: Current issues and perspectives. *Am J Med* 1986;**81**:1. [Entire issue.]
Campbell SM et al: Clinical characteristics of fibrositis. 1. A "blinded," controlled study of symptoms and tender points. *Arthritis Rheum* 1983;**26**:817.

## CARPAL TUNNEL SYNDROME

Carpal tunnel syndrome is a common painful disorder caused by compression of the median nerve between the carpal ligament and other structures within the carpal tunnel (entrapment neuropathy). The volume of the contents of the tunnel can be increased by organic lesions such as synovitis of the tendon sheaths or carpal joints, recent or malhealed fractures, tumors, and occasionally congenital anomalies. Even though no anatomic lesion is apparent, flattening or even circumferential constriction of the median nerve may be observed during operative section of the ligament. The disorder may occur in pregnancy and is seen in individuals with a history of repetitive use of the hands, and it may follow injuries of the wrists. A familial type of carpal tunnel syndrome has been reported in which no etiologic factor can be identified.

Carpal tunnel syndrome can also be a feature of many systemic diseases: rheumatoid arthritis and other rheumatic disorders (inflammatory tenosynovitis); myxedema, amyloidosis, sarcoidosis, and leukemia (tissue infiltration); acromegaly; hyperparathyroidism, hypocalcemia, and diabetes mellitus.

### Clinical Findings

Pain in the distribution of the median nerve, which may be burning and tingling (acroparesthesia), is the initial symptom. Aching pain may radiate proximally into the forearm and occasionally proximally to the shoulder, neck, and chest. Pain is exacerbated by manual activity, particularly by extremes of volar flexion or dorsiflexion of the wrist. It may be most bothersome at night. Impairment of sensation in the median nerve distribution may not be apparent. Subtle disparity between the affected and opposite sides can be demonstrated by requiring the patient to identify different textures of cloth by rubbing them between the tips of the thumb and the index finger. Tinel's sign (tingling or shocklike pain on volar wrist percussion) may be positive. Muscle weakness or atrophy, especially of the abductor pollicis brevis, appears later than sensory disturbances. Useful special examinations include electromyography and determinations of segmental sensory and motor conduction delay. Distal median sensory conduction delay may be evident before motor delay.

### Differential Diagnosis

This syndrome should be differentiated from other cervicobrachial pain syndromes and from compression syndromes of the median nerve in the forearm or arm. When left-sided, it may be confused with angina pectoris.

### Treatment

Treatment is directed toward relief of pressure on the median nerve. Conservative treatment usually relieves mild symptoms of recent onset. When a primary lesion is discovered, specific treatment should be given. When soft tissue swelling is a cause, elevation of the extremity may relieve symptoms. Splinting of the hand and forearm at night may be beneficial. When nonspecific inflammation of the ulnar bursa is thought to be a cause, injection of corticosteroids into the carpal tunnel may be helpful.

Operative division of the volar carpal ligament gives lasting relief from pain, which usually subsides within a few days. Muscle strength returns gradually, but complete recovery cannot be expected when atrophy is pronounced.

Golding DN et al: Clinical tests for carpal tunnel syndrome: An evaluation. *Br J Rheumatol* 1986;**25**:388.

## DUPUYTREN'S CONTRACTURE

This relatively common disorder is characterized by hyperplasia of the palmar fascia and related structures, with nodule formation and contracture of the palmar fascia. The cause is unknown, but the condition has a genetic predisposition and occurs primarily in white men over 50 years of age. The incidence of Dupuytren's contracture is higher among alcoholics and patients with chronic systemic disorders (eg, cirrhosis, diabetes, epilepsy, tuberculosis). The onset may be acute, but slowly progressive chronic disease is more common.

Dupuytren's contracture manifests itself by nodular or cordlike thickening of one or both hands, with the fourth and fifth fingers most commonly affected. The patient may complain of tightness of the involved digits, with inability to satisfactorily extend the fingers, and on occasion there is tenderness. The resulting functional and cosmetic problems may be extremely disabling. Fasciitis involving other areas of the body may lead to plantar fibromatosis (10% of patients) or Peyronie's disease (1–2%).

Periodic examination of patients in early stages of disease is recommended. If the palmar nodule is growing rapidly, injections of triamcinolone into the nodule may be of benefit. Surgical intervention is indicated in patients with significant flexion contractures, depending on the location, but recurrence is not uncommon.

Bradlow A, Mowat AG: Dupuytren's contracture and alcohol. *Ann Rheum Dis* 1986;**45**:304.

## REFLEX SYMPATHETIC DYSTROPHY

Reflex sympathetic dystrophy (shoulder-hand syndrome) is a complex of symptoms and signs arising from various painful disorders of the shoulder joint and hand of the same extremity. The syndrome is essentially a combination of scapulohumeral periarthritis and Sudeck's atrophy of the hand and wrist, and occurs with increasing frequency during the middle years of life. Pain and restricted motion of the shoulder may precede or follow the ipsilateral painful hand involvement. The elbow joint is usually spared; when the elbow is involved, there is painful restriction of motion. Osteoporosis of the bones of the involved hand is common and prominent.

This syndrome should be differentiated from other cervicobrachial pain syndromes, rheumatoid arthritis, polymyositis, scleroderma, and gout.

In addition to specific treatment of the underlying disorder, treatment is directed toward restoration of function. Therapy described for scapulohumeral periarthritis (see above) and Sudeck's atrophy is given simultaneously. The prognosis depends in part upon the stage in which the lesions of the shoulder joint and hand are encountered and the extent and severity of associated organic disease. Early treatment offers the best prognosis for recovery.

Schutzer SF, Gossling HR: The treatment of reflex sympathetic dystrophy syndrome. *J Bone Joint Surg [Am] 1984;***66**:625.

## BURSITIS

Inflammation of the synoviumlike cellular membrane overlying bony prominences may be secondary to trauma, infection, or arthritic conditions. The most common locations are the subdeltoid, olecranon, ischial, and prepatellar bursae. Clinically and anatomically, this syndrome can be differentiated from adjacent inflammatory disorders of tendons, and the attacks may suggest an arthritic process. On occasion, calcific deposits are noted on x-rays of the involved bursae.

Various methods of treatment have been used, including local heat, immobilization, analgesics, nonsteroidal anti-inflammatory agents, and local steroid injections. Infected bursae usually require surgical drainage or aspiration and antibiotic therapy.

## CRYSTAL DEPOSITION ARTHRITIS

### 1. GOUTY ARTHRITIS

#### Essentials of Diagnosis

- Acute onset, usually monarticular, often involving the first metatarsophalangeal joint.
- Postinflammatory desquamation and pruritus.
- Hyperuricemia.
- Identification of urate crystals in joint fluid or tophi.
- Asymptomatic periods between acute attacks.
- With chronicity, urate deposits in subcutaneous tissue, bone, cartilage, joints, and other tissues.
- Dramatic therapeutic response to colchicine and nonsteroidal anti-inflammatory agents.

#### General Considerations

Gout is a metabolic disease of heterogeneous nature, often familial, associated with abnormal amounts of urates in the body and characterized early by a recurring acute arthritis, usually monarticular, and later by chronic deforming arthritis.

Primary gout is a heritable metabolic disease in which hyperuricemia is usually due to overproduction or underexcretion of uric acid—sometimes both. It is rarely due to a specifically determined genetic aberration (eg, Lesch-Nyhan syndrome). Secondary gout, which may have some latent heritable component, is related to acquired causes of hyperuricemia, eg, myeloproliferative disorders, multiple myeloma, hemoglobinopathies, chronic renal disease, and lead poisoning.

About 90% of patients with primary gout are men, usually over 30 years of age. In women the onset is usually postmenopausal. The characteristic histologic lesion is the tophus, a nodular deposit of monosodium urate monohydrate crystals, and an associated foreign body reaction. These may be found in cartilage, subcutaneous and periarticular tissues, tendon, bone, the kidneys, and elsewhere. Urates have been demonstrated in the synovial tissues (and fluid) during acute arthritis; indeed, the acute inflammation of gout is believed to be activated by the phagocytosis by polymorphonuclear cells of urate crystals with the ensuing release from the nucleated neutrophils of chemotactic and other substances capable of mediating inflammation. The precise relationship of hyperuricemia to acute gouty arthritis is still obscure, since chronic hyperuricemia is a frequent finding in people who never develop gout or uric acid stones (Table 14–3). Rapid fluctuations in serum urate levels, either increasing or decreasing, are important factors in precipitating acute gout. The mechanism of the late, chronic stage of gouty arthritis is better understood. This is characterized pathologically by tophaceous invasion of the articular and periarticular tissues, with structural derangement and secondary degeneration (osteoarthritis).

Uric acid kidney stones are present in 10–20% of patients with gouty arthritis. The term gouty nephropathy (or ''gouty nephritis'') refers to kidney disease due to sodium urate deposition in the renal interstitium. Uric acid stones are not related to its pathogenesis, and a relationship to renal insufficiency has not been established.

Unless there is a rapid breakdown of cellular nucleic acid following aggressive treatment of leukemia or lymphoma, uric acid-lowering drugs need not be instituted until arthritis, renal calculi, or tophi become apparent. Psoriasis, sarcoidosis, and diuretic drugs are commonly overlooked causes of hyperuricemia and may precipitate attacks in patients with gout. Asymptomatic hyperuricemia need not be treated.

## Clinical Findings

**A. Symptoms and Signs:** The acute arthritis is characterized by its sudden onset, frequently nocturnal, either without apparent precipitating cause or following rapid fluctuations in serum urate levels from food and alcohol excess, surgery, infection, diuretics,

**Table 14–3.** Origin of hyperuricemia.[*]

**Primary Hyperuricemia**
A. Increased production of purine:
   1. Idiopathic.
   2. Specific enzyme defects (eg, Lesch-Nyhan syndrome, glycogen storage disease).
B. Decreased renal clearance of uric acid (idiopathic).
**Secondary Hyperuricemia**
A. Increased catabolism and turnover of purine:
   1. Myeloproliferative disorders.
   2. Lymphoproliferative disorders.
   3. Carcinoma and sarcoma (disseminated).
   4. Chronic hemolytic anemias.
   5. Cytotoxic drugs.
   6. Psoriasis.
B. Decreased renal clearance of uric acid:
   1. Intrinsic kideny disease.
   2. Functional impairment of tubular transport:
      a. Drug-induced (eg, thiazides, probenecid).
      b. Hyperlacticemia (eg, lactic acidosis, alcoholism).
      c. Hyperketoacidemia (eg, diabetic ketoacidosis, starvation).
      d. Diabetes insipidus (vasopressin-resistant).
      c. Bartter's syndrome.

[*] Modified from Rodnan GP: Gout and other crystalline forms of arthritis. *Postgrad Med* (Oct) 1975;**58:**6.

chemicals (eg, meglumine diatrizoate, Urografin), or uricosuric drugs. The metatarsophalangeal joint of the great toe is the most susceptible joint, although others, especially those of the feet, ankles, and knees, are commonly affected. Hips and shoulders are rarely involved in gouty arthritis. More than one joint may occasionally be affected during the same attack; in such cases, the distribution of the arthritis is usually asymmetric. As the attack progresses, the pain becomes intense. The involved joints are swollen and exquisitely tender and the overlying skin tense, warm, and dusky red. Fever is common and may reach 39 °C. Local desquamation and pruritus during recovery from the acute arthritis are characteristic of gout but are not always present. Tophi may be found in the external ears, hands, feet, olecranon, and prepatellar bursas. They are usually seen only after several attacks of acute arthritis.

Asymptomatic periods of months or years commonly follow the initial acute attack. Later, gouty arthritis may become chronic, with symptoms of progressive functional loss and disability. Gross deformities, due usually to tophaceous invasion, are seen. Signs of inflammation may be absent or superimposed.

**B. Laboratory Findings:** The serum uric acid is practically always elevated (> 7.5 mg/dL) unless uricopenic drugs are being given. During an acute attack, the erythrocyte sedimentation rate and white cell count are usually elevated. Examination of the material aspirated from a tophus shows the typical crystals of sodium urate and confirms the diagnosis. Further confirmation is obtained by identification of sodium urate crystals by compensated polariscopic examination of wet smears prepared from joint fluid aspirates. Such crystals are negatively birefringent and needlelike and may be found free or in neutrophils.

**C. Imaging:** Early in the disease, radiographs show no changes. Later, punched-out areas in the bone (radiolucent urate tophi) are seen. When these are adjacent to a soft tissue tophus, they are diagnostic of gout.

## Differential Diagnosis

Once the diagnosis of acute gouty arthritis is suspected, it is confirmed by the presence of hyperuricemia, dramatic response to colchicine, local desquamation and pruritus as the edema subsides, and polariscopic examination of joint fluid. Acute gout is often confused with cellulitis. Appropriate bacteriologic studies should exclude acute pyogenic arthritis. Acute chondrocalcinosis (pseudogout) may be distinguished by the identification of calcium pyrophosphate crystals in the joint fluid, usually normal serum uric acid, the x-ray appearance of chondrocalcinosis, and the relative therapeutic ineffectiveness of colchicine.

Chronic tophaceous arthritis may rarely mimic chronic rheumatoid arthritis. In such cases, the diagnosis of gout is established by the demonstration of urate crystals in the contents of a suspected tophus.

Biopsy may be necessary to distinguish tophi from rheumatoid nodules. An x-ray appearance similar to that of gout may be found in rheumatoid arthritis, sarcoidosis, multiple myeloma, hyperparathyroidism, or Hand-Schüller-Christian disease. Chronic lead intoxication may result in attacks of gouty arthritis and renal insufficiency.

## Treatment

### A. Acute Attack:

**1. Colchicine,** which may inhibit the chemotactic property of leukocytosis and thus interfere with the inflammatory response to urate crystals, is the traditional drug; it is used diagnostically as well as therapeutically. It should be given as early as possible in the acute attack or during the prodrome to obtain maximum benefit, since 75% of patients with acute gouty arthritis respond to colchicine, and failure of relief in the remainder may be related to a delay in the initiation of treatment. Trial with colchicine should not replace joint aspiration for diagnosis when an aspirable joint is readily accessible, since 80% of patients receiving colchicine have significant abdominal cramping, diarrhea, nausea, or vomiting. The dose is 0.5 or 0.6 mg every hour or 1 mg every 2 hours until pain is relieved or until nausea or diarrhea appears, and then stop the drug. The usual total dose required is 4–8 mg. The pain and swelling will subside in 24–72 hours. Once the patient knows how much will produce toxic symptoms, the drug should be given in a dose of about 1 mg less than the toxic dose. Colchicine-induced diarrhea is controlled with diphenoxylate with atropine (Lomotil) or with loperamide (Imodium). The incidence of gastrointestinal side effects of colchicine can be reduced by intravenous administration in an initial dose of 1–3 mg in 10–20 mL of saline solution. This may be repeated in a few hours, but no more than 4 mg should be given intravenously within a period of 24 hours for a single attack. Colchicine may cause local pain and tissue damage from extravasation during injection. This route of administration is rarely necessary and is inadvisable if the oral route can be used. Administration of usual doses of colchicine to patients with significant renal or hepatic disease may result in serious toxicity. Oral colchicine should not be used in patients with inflammatory bowel disease.

**2. Indomethacin** is as effective as colchicine in acute gout and is the drug of choice if the attack has lasted more than a few hours before therapy is instituted. The dose is 50 mg every 6 hours until a response occurs; dosage is then reduced to 25 mg 3–4 times daily for 4–5 days. Active peptic ulcer is a contraindication.

**3. Newer nonsteroidal anti-inflammatory agents** have been shown to be effective and may be used instead of indomethacin.

**4. Corticotropin (ACTH) and the corticosteroids** often give dramatic symptomatic relief in acute episodes of gout and, if given for a sufficient length of time, will control most acute attacks. However, when corticotropin and corticosteroids are discontinued shortly after termination of attacks, many patients promptly undergo relapse unless colchicine is given. Since colchicine and nonsteroidal anti-inflammatory agents are so effective, these agents are preferred unless they are poorly tolerated by the patient.

**5. Analgesics**–At times the pain of an acute attack may be so severe that analgesia is necessary before a more specific drug becomes effective. In these cases, codeine or meperidine may be given. Low to moderate doses of aspirin increase the serum uric acid and are not indicated.

**6. Bed rest** is important in the management of the acute attack and should be continued for about 24 hours after the acute attack has subsided. Early ambulation may precipitate a recurrence. **Physical therapy** is of little value during the acute attack, although hot or cold compresses to or elevation of the affected joints makes some patients more comfortable.

**B. Management Between Attacks:** Treatment during symptom-free periods is intended to minimize urate deposition in tissues, which causes chronic tophaceous arthritis, and to reduce the frequency and severity of recurrences.

**1. Diet**–From a dietary standpoint, it is important to avoid obesity, fasting, and dehydration. Rigid diets fail to influence the hyperuricemia or the course of gouty arthritis. Since dietary sources of purines contribute very little to the causation of the disease, restriction of foods high in purine (eg, kidney, liver, sweetbreads, sardines, anchovies, meat extracts) cannot be expected to contribute significantly to the management of the disease. Specific foods or alcoholic beverages that precipitate attacks should be avoided. However, there is little evidence that alcohol in moderation will precipitate attacks or is otherwise harmful in patients with gout. A high liquid intake and, more importantly, a daily urinary output of 2 L or more will aid urate excretion and minimize urate precipitation in the urinary tract.

**2. Colchicine**–The daily administration of colchicine in a dose of 0.5 mg 3 times daily should be started simultaneously with uricosuric drugs or allopurinol in order to suppress the acute attack that may be precipitated by these drugs. After several weeks of such treatment, it is usually possible to lower the daily dose of colchicine to 0.5 mg. There is some suggestion that colchicine, even in this small dosage, has preventive value and should be continued indefinitely.

**3. Reduction of serum uric acid**–Indications include frequent acute arthritis not controlled by colchicine prophylaxis, tophaceous deposits, or renal damage. It is emphasized that hyperuricemia which is either asymptomatic or associated only with infrequent attacks of arthritis may not require treatment.

Two classes of agents may be used to lower the serum uric acid—the uricosuric drugs and allopurinol (neither is of value in the treatment of acute gout).

**a. Uricosuric drugs**–These drugs, by blocking

tubular reabsorption of filtered urate and reducing the metabolic pool of urates, prevent the formation of new tophi and reduce the size of those already present. Furthermore, when administered concomitantly with colchicine, they may lessen the frequency of recurrences of acute gout. The indication for uricosuric treatment is the increasing frequency or severity of acute attacks.

The following uricosuric drugs may be employed:

(1) Probenecid 0.5 g daily initially with gradual increase to 1–2 g daily.

(2) Sulfinpyrazone, 100 mg daily initially with gradual increase to 200–400 mg daily. The maintenance dose is determined by observation of the serum uric acid response and the urinary uric acid response. Ideally, one attempts to maintain a normal serum urate level.

Hypersensitivity to either uricosuric drug in the form of fever and rash occurs in 5% of cases; gastrointestinal complaints occur in 10%.

**Precautions with uricosuric drugs.** It is important to maintain a daily urinary output of 2000 mL or more in order to minimize the precipitation of uric acid in the urinary tract. This can be further prevented by giving alkalinizing agents to maintain a urine pH of above 6.0. If a significant uricosuric effect is not obtained in the presence of overt renal dysfunction, do not increase the dose of the drug beyond the limits stated above. Uricosuric drugs are best avoided in patients with a history of uric acid lithiasis. Avoid using salicylates, since they antagonize the action of uricosuric agents.

**b. Allopurinol–**The xanthine oxidase inhibitor allopurinol (Zyloprim) promptly lowers plasma urate and urinary uric acid concentrations and facilitates tophus mobilization. The drug is of special value in uric acid overproducers (as defined by urinary excretion of uric acid in excess of 800 mg/d while on a purine-free diet); in tophaceous gout; in patients unresponsive to the uricosuric regimen; and in gouty patients with uric acid renal stones. It should be used cautiously in patients with renal insufficiency and is not indicated in asymptomatic hyperuricemia. The most frequent adverse effect is the precipitation of an acute gouty attack. However, the commonest sign of hypersensitivity to allopurinol (occurring in 5% of cases) is a pruritic rash that may progress to toxic epidermal necrolysis, a potentially fatal complication. Vasculitis is a related complication.

The daily dose is determined by the serum uric acid response. A normal serum uric acid level is often obtained with a daily dose of 200–300 mg. Occasionally (and in selected cases) it may be helpful to continue the use of allopurinol with a uricosuric drug. Neither of these drugs is useful in acute gout.

**C. Chronic Tophaceous Arthritis:** Tophaceous deposits can be made to shrink in size and disappear altogether with allopurinol therapy. The treatment is essentially the same as that outlined for the intervals between acute attacks. Surgical excision of large tophi

offers immediate mechanical improvement in selected deformities but is rarely required.

## Prognosis

Without treatment, the acute attack may last from a few days to several weeks, but proper treatment quickly terminates the attack. The intervals between acute attacks vary up to years, but the asymptomatic periods often become shorter if the disease progresses. Chronic tophaceous arthritis occurs after repeated attacks of acute gout, but only after inadequate treatment. Although the deformities may be marked, only a small percentage of patients become bedridden. The younger the patient at the onset of disease, the greater the tendency to a progressive course. Destructive arthropathy is rarely seen in patients whose first attack is after age 50.

Patients with gout have an increased incidence of hypertension, renal disease (eg, nephrosclerosis, tophi, pyelonephritis), diabetes mellitus, hypertriglyceridemia, and atherosclerosis, although these relationships are not well understood.

Lalley EV et al: The clinical spectrum of gouty arthritis in women. *Arch Intern Med* 1986;**146:**2221.

Lo B: Hyperuricemia and gout. (Topics in Primary Care Medicine.) *West J Med* 1985;**142:**104.

## 2. CHONDROCALCINOSIS & PSEUDOGOUT (Calcium Pyrophosphate Dehydrate [CPPD] Deposition Disease)

The term chondrocalcinosis refers to the presence of calcium-containing salts in articular cartilage. It is most often first diagnosed radiologically. It may be familial and is commonly associated with a wide variety of metabolic disorders, eg, hemochromatosis, hyperparathyroidism, ochronosis, diabetes mellitus, hypothyroidism, Wilson's disease, and true gout. Pseudogout, most often seen in persons age 60 or older, is characterized by acute, recurrent and rarely chronic arthritis that usually involves large joints (principally the knees) and is almost always accompanied by chondrocalcinosis of the affected joints. Identification of calcium pyrophosphate crystals in joint aspirates is diagnostic of pseudogout. Like the intraarticular urate crystals of gouty synovitis, calcium pyrophosphate crystals are believed to induce the synovitis of pseudogout. They may be seen with the ordinary light microscope but are best visualized under polarized light, in which they exhibit a positive birefringence; like gouty crystals, they may be intracellular or extracellular. X-ray examination shows not only calcification (usually symmetric) of cartilaginous structures but also signs of degenerative joint disease (osteoarthritis). Unlike gout, pseudogout is usually associated with normal serum urate levels and is not dramatically improved by colchicine.

Treatment of chondrocalcinosis is directed at the primary disease, if present. Some of the nonsteroidal anti-inflammatory agents (salicylates, indomethacin, naproxen, and other drugs) are helpful in the treatment of acute episodes of pseudogout. Colchicine may be of benefit. Aspiration of the inflamed joint and intraarticular injection of a hydrocortisone ester is also of value in resistant cases.

McCarty DJ: Arthritis associated with crystals containing calcium. *Med Clin North Am* 1986;**70**:437.

## ARTHRITIS IN SARCOIDOSIS

The frequency of arthritis among patients with sarcoidosis is variously reported between 10% and 35%. It is usually acute in onset, but articular symptoms may appear insidiously and often antedate other manifestations of the disease. Knees and ankles are most commonly involved, but any joint may be affected. Distribution of joint involvement is usually polyarticular and symmetric. The arthritis is commonly self-limiting after several weeks or months; infrequently, the arthritis is recurrent or chronic. Despite its occasional chronicity, the arthritis is rarely associated with joint destruction or significant deformity. Although sarcoid arthritis is often associated with erythema nodosum, the diagnosis is contingent upon the demonstration of other extra-articular manifestations of sarcoidosis and, notably, biopsy evidence of noncaseating granulomas. In chronic arthritis, x-ray shows rather typical changes in the bones of the extremities with intact cortex and cystic changes.

Treatment of arthritis in sarcoidosis is usually symptomatic and supportive. Colchicine may be of value. A short course of corticosteroids may be effective in patients with severe and progressive joint disease.

## JOGGING INJURIES

The beneficial effects on cardiovascular function and the sense of well-being associated with aerobic activity have led to considerable enthusiasm for jogging and running. This has resulted in a large number of musculoskeletal injuries, which are estimated to occur in about 75% of runners. In addition, osteoporosis, hematuria, heat stroke, exercise-induced ectopy, and even death have occurred as consequences of running.

Many of the deleterious effects can be prevented by appropriate precautions, such as stretching exercises, proper footwear, avoidance of overexertion, and prompt attention to injuries. After an injury has healed, a graduated schedule for returning to training is necessary to avoid recurrence. Since injuries occur frequently in long-distance runners, it is most important that these individuals avoid overexertion, and, when early signs of injury appear, reduce the amount of distance run. The psychologic effects of complete inactivation in athletes whose identity is intimately tied to their sport should be recognized and addressed, since severe depression may develop in such circumstances.

Temple C: Sports injuries: Hazards of jogging and marathon running. *Br J Hosp Med* 1983;**3**:237.

## TUMORS & TUMORLIKE LESIONS OF BONE

### Essentials of Diagnosis
- Persistent pain, swelling, or tenderness of a skeletal part.
- Pathologic ("spontaneous") fractures.
- Suspicious areas of bony enlargement, deformity, radiodensity, or radiolucency on x-ray.
- Histologic evidence of bone neoplasm on biopsy specimen.

### General Considerations
Primary tumors of bone are relatively uncommon in comparison with secondary or metastatic neoplasms. They are, however, of great clinical significance because of the possibility of cancer and because some of them grow rapidly and metastasize widely.

Although tumors of bone have been categorized classically as primary or secondary, there is some disagreement about which tumors are primary to the skeleton. Tumors of mesenchymal origin that reflect skeletal tissues (eg, bone, cartilage, and connective tissue) and tumors developing in bones that are of hematopoietic, nerve, vascular, fat cell, and notochordal origin should be differentiated from secondary malignant tumors that involve bone by direct extension or hematogenous spread. Because of the great variety of bone tumors, it is difficult to establish a satisfactory simple classification of bone neoplasms.

### Clinical Findings
Persistent skeletal pain and swelling, with or without limitation of motion of adjacent joints or spontaneous fracture, are indications for prompt clinical, x-ray, laboratory, and possibly biopsy examination. X-rays may reveal the location and extent of the lesion and certain characteristics that may suggest the specific diagnosis. The so-called classic x-ray findings of certain tumors (eg, punched-out areas of the skull in multiple myeloma, "sun ray" appearance of osteogenic sarcoma, and "onion peel" effect of Ewing's sarcoma), although suggestive, are not pathognomonic. Even histologic characteristics of the tumor, when taken alone, cannot provide infallible information about the nature of the process. The age of the patient, the duration of complaints, the site of involvement and the number of bones involved, and the presence or absence of associated systemic disease—

as well as the histologic characteristics—must be considered collectively for proper management.

The possibility of benign developmental skeletal abnormalities, metastatic neoplastic disease, or infections (eg, osteomyelitis), posttraumatic bone lesions, or metabolic disease of bone must always be kept in mind. If bone tumors occur in or near the joints, they may be confused with the various types of arthritis, especially monarticular arthritis.

### Specific Bone Tumors

Tumors arising from osteoblastic connective tissue include osteoid osteoma and osteogenic sarcoma. Osteoid osteomas are benign tumors of children and adolescents that should be surgically removed. Osteogenic sarcomas usually involve the knees or long bones and are treated by resection and chemotherapy, with improving survival in recent years. Fibrosarcomas, which are derived from nonosteoblastic connective tissue, have an outlook similar to that of the osteogenic sarcomas. Tumors derived from cartilage include enchondromas, chondromyxoid fibromas, and chondrosarcomas. Histologic examination is confirmatory in this group, and the outlook with appropriate curettement or surgery is generally good.

Other bone tumors include giant cell tumors (osteoclastomas), chondroblastomas, and Ewing's sarcoma. Of these, chondroblastomas are almost always benign. About 50% of giant cell tumors are benign, while the rest may be frankly malignant or recur after excision. Ewing's sarcoma, which affects children, adolescents, and young adults, has a 50% mortality rate in spite of chemotherapy, irradiation, and surgery.

### Treatment

Although prompt action is essential for optimal treatment of certain bone tumors, accurate diagnosis is required because of the great potential for harm that may result either from temporization or from radical or ablative operations or unnecessary irradiation.

Brown KT et al: Computed tomography analysis of bone tumors: Patterns of cortical destruction and soft tissue extension. *Skeletal Radiol* 1986;**15**:448.

Sim FH et al: Osteosarcoma: State of the art. *Minn Med* 1986;**69**:42.

# OTHER DISORDERS OF BONES & JOINTS

## FAT EMBOLIZATION SYNDROME

Fat embolization syndrome is a life-threatening form of acute respiratory failure that may occur following severe trauma, especially long-bone fractures.

The pathophysiology is not completely understood, but it is thought that embolic fat released from injured tissues is deposited within the pulmonary capillaries. Release and local accumulation of free fatty acids cause alveolocapillary damage leading to respiratory failure, changes in blood coagulation, and central nervous system dysfunction. Apparently, all degrees of embolization syndrome occur, ranging from minor symptoms to frank respiratory failure and death.

The syndrome may not become clinically apparent until 12 hours to 3 or 4 days after the injury occurs. Symptoms and signs include tachypnea, tachycardia, fever, skin petechiae, changes in mental status (ranging from restlessness to stupor or coma), and convulsions. Hypoxemia, often clinically inapparent initially, usually occurs early and before the development of other signs and symptoms. Other laboratory findings may include anemia, thrombocytopenia, and lipuria. Chest x-rays are not characteristic but may show diffuse, fluffy infiltrates in both lung fields.

Prompt immobilization of long-bone fractures is considered to be an important factor in prevention of the syndrome. Successful treatment of fat embolization syndrome requires early detection, management of respiratory failure (see Adult Respiratory Distress Syndrome, p 182), restoration of blood volume, and other supportive measures. Corticosteroids may be useful for prophylaxis of fat embolism, particularly in high-risk patients. The prognosis for fat embolization syndrome is usually good if the disorder can be detected early and proper treatment given promptly.

Serota M: Fat embolism syndrome. *West J Med* 1984;**141**:501.

# GENERAL PRINCIPLES IN THE PHYSICAL MANAGEMENT OF ARTHRITIC JOINTS

Proper physical management of arthritic joints can improve patient comfort and help preserve joint and muscle function and total well-being. In order to obtain optimal results, as well as to conserve financial resources and time, it is important for the physician to be as specific as possible in instructions to the patient or to the occupational and physical therapists conducting treatment.

### Exercise

**A. Passive Range of Motion:** Since someone other than the patient puts the joints through the range of motion once or twice daily, the patient is not directly involved and maintenance of muscle tone is not assisted. Passive exercises should be ordered infrequently and only for specific purposes.

**B. Active Range of Motion:** This type of exercise requires the patient to actively contract the muscles in order to put joints through the range of motion. The prescribed motions should be repeated 3–10 times once or twice daily. Such active exercise should be encouraged, since it involves the patient, costs no money, protects joint motion, and assists in maintaining muscle tone.

**C. Isometric Exercise:** With this type of exercise the muscle is contracted but not shortened, while the joint is minimally moved, for 3–10 repetitions several times daily. This maintains or even increases muscle strength and tone; the patient is involved; joint use is minimal; and the cost is nil. Isometric exercise should be used to supplement passive or active range-of-motion exercises.

**D. Isotonic Exercise:** In isotonic exercise, the muscle is contracted and shortened and the joint is maximally moved and stressed. This type of exercise should seldom be used (see below).

**E. Hydrotherapy:** The buoyancy of water permits maximum isotonic and isometric exercise with no more stress on joints than active range-of-motion exercises. Although ideal for arthritic patients, its cost often precludes use and it is generally prescribed only for specific short-term goals.

**F. Active-Assistive Exercise:** The therapist provides direct supervision, physical support, and exercise guidance. Although this is ideal for arthritic patients, cost again often precludes its use except for specific short-term goals. A member of the family may be taught to assist the patient in exercises on a long-term basis.

*Note:* Any exercise in the arthritic patient may be associated with some pain, but pain lasting for hours after exercise is an indication for a change in the duration or type of exercise.

### Heat, Cold, & Massage

**A. Heat:** Most patients with chronic arthritis find that some form of heat gives temporary muscle relaxation and relief of pain. Generally, moist heat is more effective than electric pads or heat lamps. Tub baths may require bar supports for ease of entry and exit. Paraffin dips may spare the patient the "dishpan hands" caused by water.

**B. Cold:** Some patients with particularly acute arthritis or acutely injured arthritic joints find that cold (ice pack or bag) relieves pain more effectively than does heat.

**C. Massage:** While massage is helpful in relaxing muscles and giving psychologic support, it provides only temporary relief, and its cost is usually high.

### Splints

Splints may provide joint rest, reduce pain, and prevent contracture, but certain principles should be adhered to.

(1) Night splints of the hands or wrists (or both) should maintain the extremity in the position of optimum function. The elbow and shoulder lose motion

so rapidly that other local measures and corticosteroid injections are usually preferable to splints.

(2) The best "splint" for the hip is prone-lying for several hours a day on a firm bed. For the knee, prone-lying may suffice, but splints in maximum tolerated extension are frequently needed. Ankle splints are of the simple right-angle type.

(3) Splints should be applied for the shortest period needed, should be made of lightweight materials for comfort, and should be easily removable for range-of-motion exercises once or twice daily to prevent loss of motion.

(4) Corrective splints, such as those for overcoming knee flexion contractures, should be used under the guidance of a physician familiar with their proper use.

*Note:* Avoidance of prolonged sitting or knee pillows may decrease the need for splints.

### Braces

Unstable joints—particularly the knee and wrist—can be supported, and the pain of weight bearing may be relieved by appropriately prescribed braces.

### Assistive Devices

Patient-oriented publications, physical therapists, occupational therapists, and home health nurses can help the patient to obtain appropriate gripping bars, raised toilet seats, long-handled reachers, and other devices to help in coping with daily living.

### Referral of the Patient for Surgical Opinion by an Orthopedist

**A. Synovectomy:** This procedure has been used for over 50 years to attempt to retard joint destruction by invasive synovial pannus of rheumatoid arthritis. However, its prophylactic effect has not been documented, and inflammation of regenerated synovial membrane occurs. Thus, the only indication for synovectomy is intractable pain in an isolated joint, most commonly the knee.

**B. Joint Replacement:** (See also Total Joint Arthroplasty, below.) Total hip replacement by methylmethacrylate has been highly successful. Infection, the major complication, is uncommon. The long-term effects of replacement of the knee—and more recently the ankle, shoulder, and other joints—have not been fully determined.

**C. Arthroplasty:** Realignment and reconstruction of the knee, wrist, and small joints of the hand are feasible in a small number of selected patients.

**D. Tendon Rupture:** This is a fairly common complication in rheumatoid arthritis and requires immediate orthopedic referral. The most common sites are the finger flexors and extensors, the patellar tendon, and the Achilles tendon.

**E. Arthrodesis:** Arthrodesis (fusion) is being used less now than formerly, but a chronically infected, painful joint may be an indication for this surgical procedure.

## Joint Protection Program

Physical and occupational therapists can instruct patients in changing their daily habits and their occupational and recreational activities to lessen damage to joints, maintain range of motion, and lessen pain and muscle atrophy.

Delisa JA: Practical use of therapeutic physical modalities. *Am Fam Physician* (May) 1983;**27**:129.

## TOTAL JOINT ARTHROPLASTY

In the last 2 decades, remarkable progress has been made in the replacement of severely damaged joints with prosthetic materials. At present, artificial joint replacement is primarily indicated to relieve pain and only secondarily to restore function. Many patients who have minimal pain, therefore, even with marked destruction of the joint on radiographic examination, are not suitable candidates for joint replacement.

Success of the replacement depends upon the amount of physical stress to which the prosthetic components are subjected. Vigorous impact activity, even with the most advanced biomaterials and design, will result in failure of the prosthesis with time. Revision operations are technically more difficult, and the results may not be as good as with the primary procedure. The patient, therefore, must understand the limitations of joint replacement and the consequences of unrestrained joint usage.

### Total Hip Arthroplasty

Hip replacement was originally designed for use in patients over 65 years of age with severe osteoarthritis. In these patients—usually less active physically—the prosthesis not only functioned well but outlasted the patients. Severe arthritis that fails to respond to conservative measures (see p 513) remains the principal indication for hip arthroplasty. Hip arthroplasty may also be indicated in younger patients severely disabled by painful hip disease (eg, rheumatoid arthritis), since in such cases it can be assumed that stress on the prosthetic joint will not be great. Contraindications to the operation include active infection and neurotrophic joint disease. Serious complications may occur in about 1% of patients and include thrombophlebitis, pulmonary embolization, sepsis, and dislocation of the joint. Extensive experience has now been accumulated, and the results are generally successful in properly selected patients.

### Total Knee Arthroplasty

The indications and contraindications for total knee arthroplasty are similar to those for hip arthroplasty, but experience with the artificial knee is not as extensive. Results are slightly better in osteoarthritis patients than in those with rheumatoid arthritis. Knee arthroplasty is probably not advisable in younger individuals. Complications are similar to those with hip arthroplasty. The failure rate of knee arthroplasty is slightly higher than that of hip arthroplasty.

### Total Arthroplasty

Prostheses are now available for total arthroplasty of every major joint of the extremities, but experience with joints other than the hip and the knee has been limited.

Cornell CN et al: Survivorship analysis of total hip replacements: Results in a series of active patients who were less than fifty-five years old. *J Bone Joint Surg [Am]* 1986;**68**:1430.

Scott WN (editor): Symposium on total knee arthroplasty. *Orthop Clin North Am* 1982;**13**:1.

## REFERENCES

Blechman WJ et al (editors): The state of the art in arthritis therapy. *Postgrad Med* (May) 1983. [Special report.]

Coles LS et al: From experiment to experience: Side effects of nonsteroidal anti-inflammatory drugs. *Am J Med* 1983;**74**:820.

Kelley W et al: *Textbook of Rheumatology,* 2nd ed. Saunders, 1985.

Shearn MA: Nonsteroidal anti-inflammatory agents; nonopiate analgesics; drugs used in gout. Chapter 34 in: *Basic & Clinical Pharmacology,* 3rd ed. Katzung B (editor). Appleton-Lange, 1987.

Stites DP, Stobo JD, Wells JV (editors): *Basic & Clinical Immunology,* 6th ed. Appleton-Lange, 1987.

Turek SL: *Orthopaedics,* 4th ed. Lippincott, 1984.

# Genitourinary Tract

**15**

*Marcus A. Krupp, MD*

## NONSPECIFIC MANIFESTATIONS OF DISEASE OR DISORDERS

### Pain

The localization, pattern of referral, and type of pain are important clues to the diagnosis of genitourinary tract disease.

**(1) Pain caused by renal disease** is usually felt as a dull ache in the "flanks" or costovertebral angle, often extending along the rib margin toward the umbilicus. Because many renal diseases do not produce sudden distention of the capsules of the kidney, there is often no pain.

**(2) Ureteral pain** is related to obstruction and is usually acute in onset, severe, and colicky and radiates from the costovertebral angle down the course of the ureter into the scrotum or vulva and the inner thigh. The radiation of the pain may be a clue to the site of obstruction. High ureteral pain is usually referred to the testicle or vulva; midureteral pain to the lower quadrants of the abdomen; and low ureteral pain to the bladder.

**(3) Bladder pain** accompanies overdistention of the bladder in acute urinary retention and distention of a bladder wall altered by tuberculosis or interstitial cystitis. Relief comes with emptying the bladder. Pain due to bladder infection is usually referred to the distal urethra and accompanies micturition. Pain caused by chronic bladder disease is uncommon.

**(4) Acute prostatic inflammation** may produce perineal or low mid back pain.

**(5) Pain caused by testicular inflammation or trauma** is acute and severe and is occasionally referred to the costovertebral angle. Pain associated with infection of the epididymis is similar to that associated with testicular inflammation.

### Urinary Symptoms

Infection, inflammation, and obstruction produce symptoms associated with urination.

**(1) Frequency, urgency, and nocturia** are common when inflammation of the urinary tract is present. Severe infection produces a constant desire to urinate even though the bladder contains only a few milliliters of urine. Frequency and nocturia occur when bladder capacity is diminished by disease or when the bladder cannot be emptied completely, leaving a large volume of residual urine. Nocturia associated with a large urine volume may occur with heart failure, renal insufficiency, mobilization of edema due to any cause, diabetes insipidus, hyperaldosteronism, hypercalcemia, and ingestion of large amounts of fluid late in the evening.

**(2) Dysuria and burning pain in the urethra on urination** are associated with infection of the bladder and prostate.

**(3) Enuresis** may be due to urinary tract disease but is most often caused by functional disorders.

**(4) Urinary incontinence** may be due to anatomic abnormality, physical stress, the urgency associated with infection or nervous system disease, or the dribbling associated with an overdistended flaccid bladder.

### Characteristics of Urine

**Urinalysis,** an essential part of the examination of all patients, is critical in the study of patients who may have renal disease. Some organic and inorganic materials in solution in the urine are diagnostic of metabolic disease (inherited or acquired) and of renal disease.

**(1) Proteinuria (albuminuria):** Normally, up to 150 mg of protein is excreted daily in urine. Exercise, febrile illness, or severe dehydration may produce increased proteinuria in persons without renal disease. Rarely, a normal person may have significant proteinuria when in an upright position but none while recumbent (postural or orthostatic proteinuria). Proteinuria in excess of 200–500 mg/d is almost always indicative of renal disease. In most cases of significant proteinuria, increased filtration of protein occurs because of reduction in the density of anionic charges in the glomerular capillary wall, not because of altered epithelial pore size. The "dipstick" test for albumin will usually not detect light-chain globulins (eg, Bence Jones protein) and will be false-positive with highly alkaline urine. Tests with sulfosalicylic acid will be false-positive with sulfisoxazole metabolites, tolbutamide metabolites, acetazolamide, some penicillins (nafcillin, ampicillin, piperacillin), some cephalosporins, levodopa, and tolmetin and with radiographic contrast media.

**(2) Urinary sediment** provides evidence of renal disease that is not available from other sources, and some elements are characteristic of the type and extent of renal disease. The physician should examine the sediment if renal disease may be present.

**(3) Cloudy urine** is most frequently due to the urates or phosphates that precipitate out as urine collects in the bladder and is usually of no significance.

**(4) Hematuria** nearly always means structural genitourinary disease. It may be due to glomerular disease, neoplasms, vascular accidents, infections, anomalies, stones, coagulation defects, or trauma to the urinary tract. When blood appears only during the initial period of voiding, the most likely source is the anterior urethra or prostate. When blood appears during the terminal period of voiding, the most likely source is the posterior urethra, vesical neck, or trigone. Blood mixed in with the total urine volume is from the kidneys, ureters, or bladder. Red blood cells that have come from the glomerulus may be dysmorphic and show a variety of distorted forms and swollen forms. Red cells from elsewhere in the urinary tract are not distorted.

The causes of hematuria can be summarized as follows:

**A. Localized:**

1. Urethra–Trauma, infection.

2. Bladder–Infection, stone, neoplasm, varices (especially of bladder neck with prostatic enlargement), drug reaction (cyclophosphamide), radiation injury, parasite infection (*Schistosoma haematobium*).

3. Ureter–Infection, stone, tumor.

4. Kidney–Glomerular disease, infection, stone, anatomic anomalies (including polycystic disease, arteriovenous malformations), renal vein or artery thrombosis, neoplasms, trauma (including renal biopsy).

**B. Systemic:**

1. Anticoagulant therapy.

2. Bleeding diathesis–Hemophilia, thrombocytopenia, disseminated intravascular coagulation.

3. Hemolytic disease–Hemoglobinurias, hemolytic-uremic syndrome.

4. Sickle cell disease.

5. Anaphylactoid purpura with renal involvement.

## RENAL FUNCTION TESTS

Diagnosis of renal diseases and evaluation of renal function depend on laboratory determinations. As renal function becomes impaired, laboratory observations provide reliable indices of the capacity of the kidney to meet the demands of excretion, reabsorption, and secretion and to fulfill its role in maintaining homeostasis. Useful tests may be categorized according to the physiologic function measured:

**(1) Glomerular filtration rate (GFR):** Inulin clearance is the reference method for measuring GFR. After a single intravenous injection of $^{51}$Cr edetate, $^{99m}$technetium diethylenetriamine penta-acetate, or $^{131}$I iothalamate, the slope of decreasing concentration in plasma can be determined to give a precise measure of GFR. For routine clinical use, the less precise endogenous creatinine clearance is adequate. Plasma creatinine or urea levels reflect GFR, rising as the

filtration rate diminishes. GFR may be estimated from the serum creatinine by the following formula:

$$\text{GFR (mL/min)} = \frac{(140 - \text{Age}) \times \text{Weight (kg)}}{72 \times \text{Serum creatinine (mg/dL)}}$$

The result is for men; for women, decrease by 15%.

Concentrations of serum urea nitrogen and creatinine are used as indicators of adequacy of renal function. Urea nitrogen concentration will vary directly with the quantity of protein in the diet and will increase with increased catabolism following trauma or stressful disease or with decreased renal blood flow (decreased filtration and increased reabsorption). The combination of a high protein load and decreased renal blood flow consequent to bleeding into the upper gastrointestinal tract will result in a transient elevation of serum urea nitrogen. Creatinine is produced at a relatively constant rate independently of diet. It is excreted at a fairly constant rate by glomerular filtration; for clinical purposes, tubular secretion is of little consequence except when renal failure is well advanced and tubular secretion becomes a significant portion of the total creatinine excreted. Creatinine clearance in the presence of chronic renal failure yields higher values than does inulin clearance. The concentration of serum creatinine increases as renal impairment advances; the concentration exceeds the normal level when creatinine clearance reaches about 50% of normal. The ratio of concentration of serum or blood urea nitrogen to creatinine is normally about 10:1. Ratios greater than 15:1 occur with prerenal azotemia, postrenal azotemia due to acute obstructive uropathy, and upper gastrointestinal hemorrhage.

**(2) Tubular function:** Clinical means of assessing tubular function include the ability to produce urine that is more concentrated or less concentrated than the osmolality of plasma and the ability to acidify the urine.

## RENAL BIOPSY

Renal biopsy is useful to confirm the diagnosis in instances in which choice of therapy depends on tissue diagnosis. Tissue should be prepared for light and electron microscopy and for immunofluorescent stains. Percutaneous renal biopsy is used to distinguish by structural characteristics the causes of nephrotic syndrome, to determine the presence of generalized disease (amyloidosis, autoimmune diseases), to define the lesion of rapidly progressive glomerulonephritis, and to identify other causes of hematuria and proteinuria. Biopsy is also used to assess rejection response in a transplanted kidney. Absolute contraindications include anatomic presence of only one kidney; severe malfunction of one kidney even though function is adequate in the other; bleeding diathesis; the presence of hemangioma, tumor, or large cysts; perinephric abscess or renal infection; hydronephrosis; and an uncooperative patient. Relative contraindications are the presence of serious hypertension, end-stage chronic renal failure, severe arteriosclerosis, and unusual difficulty in doing a biopsy owing to obesity, anasarca, or inability of the patient to lie flat.

## RADIOGRAPHIC EXAMINATION & ULTRASOUND

### Renal Radiography

Radiography is an essential resource for the diagnosis and evaluation of renal disease amenable to medical as well as surgical treatment. Kidney size, shape, and position may be critical elements of information. Routine films, tomography, urography, angiography, and CT and MRI scans are sources of anatomic and physiologic data that often are definitive, revealing details of circulation, structure, and calcification available by no other means. Collaboration with the radiologist provides the greatest opportunity for properly performed and interpreted examinations. Radiographic contrast agents are hazardous in the presence of severe dehydration, renal disease, diabetic nephropathy, liver failure, and multiple myeloma.

### Scanning With Radionuclides

Use of appropriate radioisotope-tagged compounds (iodohippurate sodium I 131, chlormerodrin Hg 203, technetium $^{99m}$Tc), sensitive detectors, and scintillation cameras provides ready assessment of renal blood flow and clearance of the compound, as well as visualization of the size and shape of the kidneys, the site of ureteral obstruction, and the presence of dilated ureters and urinary bladder. The 2 kidneys can be compared as a means of identifying unilateral disease.

### Ultrasound (Sonography)

Ultrasound is a noninvasive technique that is free of hazard. Devices utilizing high-frequency sound waves are capable of delineating solid or fluid-filled organs or masses. Kidney size and shape can often be distinguished clearly enough to identify tumors or cysts and anomalies such as horseshoe kidney. Calcification within the kidney and urinary tract can sometimes be best demonstrated in this way. It is a useful guide in performing renal biopsy. Dilated renal calices, the renal pelvis, and the ureters and bladder can be identified. Bladder and prostatic neoplasms can often be demonstrated.

Abuels JG: Proteinuria: Diagnostic principles and procedures. *Ann Intern Med* 1983;**98**:186.

Fairley KF, Birch DF: Hematuria: A simple method for detecting glomerular bleeding. *Kidney Int* 1982;**21**:105.

Hanglustaine D et al: Detection of glomerular bleeding using a simple staining method for light microscopy. *Lancet* 1982;**2**:761.

Morrin PAF: Urinary sediment in the interpretation of proteinuria. (Editorial.) *Ann Intern Med* 1983;**98**:254.

Schwab SJ et al: Quantitation of proteinuria by the use of protein-to-creatinine ratios in single urine samples. *Arch Intern Med* 1987;**147**:943.

Stamey T, Kindrachuk RW: *Urinary Sediment and Urinalysis: A Practical Guide for the Health Professional.* Saunders, 1985.

## DISORDERS OF THE KIDNEYS

### GLOMERULONEPHRITIS

Information obtained from experimentally induced glomerular disease in animals and from correlations with evidence derived by modern methods of examination of tissue obtained by biopsy and at necropsy has provided a new concept of glomerulonephritis.

The clinical manifestations of renal disease are apt to consist only of varying degrees of microscopic hematuria, excretion of characteristic formed elements in the urine, proteinuria, and renal insufficiency and its complications. Alterations in glomerular architecture as observed in tissue examined by light microscopy are also apt to be minimal and difficult to interpret.

Immunologic techniques for demonstrating a variety of antigens, antibodies, and complement fractions have helped toward understanding the origins and pathogenesis of glomerular disease. Electron microscopy has complemented the immunologic methods. Information gleaned from use of these methods has provided a satisfactory basis for diagnosis, treatment, and prognosis.

Briefly, glomerular disease resulting from immunologic reactions may be divided into 2 groups:

**(1) Immune complex disease,** in which soluble antigen-antibody complexes in the circulation are trapped in the glomeruli. The antigens are not derived from glomerular components; they may be exogenous (bacterial, viral, chemical, including antibiotics and other drugs) or endogenous (circulating native DNA, tumor antigens, thyroglobulin). Factors in the pathogenic potential of the antigen include its origin, quantity, and route of entry and the host's duration of exposure to it. The immune response varies with the capacity of the host to react to antigens.

In the presence of antigen excess and, in some cases, antibody excess, antigen-antibody complexes form in the circulation and are trapped in the glomeruli as they are filtered through capillary walls rendered permeable by the action of vasoactive amines. The antigen-antibody complexes bind components of complement, particularly C3. Activated complement provides factors that attract leukocytes whose lysosomal enzymes incite the injury to the glomerulus.

Light microscopy will show reduced or occluded capillary lumens from proliferating mesangial and endothelial cells and infiltration with polymorphonuclear leukocytes, monocytes, and eosinophils in the mesangium. Bowman's space may be occupied by crescents of accumulated epithelial cells and monocytes. By immunofluorescence methods and by electron microscopy, these complexes appear as lumpy deposits between the epithelial cells and the glomerular basement membrane and in the mesangium. IgG, IgM, occasionally IgA, and C3 have been identified.

**(2) Anti-glomerular basement membrane disease,** in which antibodies are generated against the glomerular basement membrane of the kidney and often against lung basement membrane, which appears to be antigenically similar to glomerular basement membrane. The autoantibodies may be stimulated by autologous glomerular basement membrane altered in some way or combined with an exogenous agent. The reaction of antibody with glomerular basement membrane is accompanied by activation of complement, the attraction of leukocytes, and the release of lysosomal enzymes. The presence of thrombi in glomerular capillaries is often accompanied by leakage of fibrinogen and precipitation of fibrin in Bowman's space, with subsequent development of epithelial "crescents" in the space.

Immunofluorescence techniques and electron microscopy show the anti-glomerular basement membrane complexes as linear deposits outlining the membrane. IgG and C3 are usually demonstrable.

## Classification of Glomerulonephritis

A current classification of glomerulonephritis is based on the immunologic concepts described above. However, the discussions in the following pages are organized according to traditional clinical categories.

### I. Immunologic Mechanisms Likely
#### A. Immune Complex Disease:
Glomerulonephritis clearly poststreptococcal
Glomerulonephritis associated with infectious
    agents, including staphylococci, pneumo-
    cocci, infective endocarditis, secondary
    syphilis, leprosy, malaria, toxoplasmosis,
    schistosomiasis, viruses of hepatitis
    (HBAg), measles, and varicella
Glomerulonephritis associated with other sys-
    temic (autoimmune?) disease such as sys-
    temic lupus erythematosus, polyarteritis
    nodosa, scleroderma, anaphylactoid pur-
    pura, idiopathic cryoglobulinemia, and tu-
    mor antigens (eg, tumors of the colon,
    bronchus, kidney; melanoma)
Membranous glomerulonephritis, cause un-
    known
Membranoproliferative glomerulonephritis,
    cause unknown
Focal glomerulonephritis
Rapidly progressive glomerulonephritis (some
    cases)
#### B. Anti-Glomerular Basement Membrane Disease:
Goodpasture's syndrome

Rapidly progressive glomerulonephritis (some cases)

### II. Immunologic Mechanisms Not Clearly Shown
Lipoid nephrosis (minimal lesion)
Focal glomerulonephritis (some cases)
Focal glomerulosclerosis
Diabetic glomerulosclerosis
Amyloidosis
Hemolytic-uremic syndrome and thrombotic
    thrombocytopenic purpura
Wegener's granulomatosis
Alport's syndrome
Sickle cell disease

## 1. ACUTE GLOMERULONEPHRITIS

Acute nephritis is often related to an antecedent infection with a group A hemolytic streptococcus or, less frequently, to a variety of other infectious agents. The clinical syndrome of acute nephritis occurs with other renal diseases, including systemic lupus erythematosus, idiopathic mesangiocapillary proliferative (membranoproliferative) glomerulonephritis, Henoch-Schönlein purpura, acute interstitial nephritis, and mixed cryoglobulinemia.

The following description of the clinical presentation of poststreptococcal glomerulonephritis applies in whole or in part to the syndrome of acute glomerulonephritis due to any other cause.

### Essentials of Diagnosis
- History of preceding streptococcal or, rarely, other infection.
- Concurrent systemic vasculitis or hypersensitivity reaction.
- Malaise, headache, anorexia, low-grade fever.
- Mild generalized edema, mild hypertension, retinal hemorrhages.
- Gross hematuria; protein, red cell casts, granular and hyaline casts, white cells, and renal epithelial cells in urine.
- Evidence of impaired renal function, especially nitrogen retention.

### General Considerations
Glomerulonephritis is a disease affecting both kidneys. In most cases, recovery from the acute stage is complete; however, progressive involvement may destroy renal tissue, in which case renal insufficiency results. Poststreptococcal acute glomerulonephritis is most common in children 3–10 years of age, although 5% or more of initial attacks occur in adults over age 50. By far the most common cause is an antecedent infection of the pharynx and tonsils or of the skin with group A β-hemolytic streptococci, certain strains of which are nephritogenic. In children under age 6, pyoderma (impetigo) is the most common antecedent; in older children and young adults, pharyngitis

is a common antecedent and skin infection a rare one. Rarely, nephritis may follow other infections (see above) and exposure to some drugs, including penicillins, sulfonamides, phenytoin, aminosalicylic acid, and aminoglycoside antibiotics. *Rhus* dermatitis and reactions to venom or chemical agents may be associated with renal disease clinically indistinguishable from glomerulonephritis.

The pathogenesis of the glomerular lesion has been further elucidated by the use of immunologic techniques (immunofluorescence) and electron microscopy. A likely sequela to infection by nephritogenic strains of β-hemolytic streptococci is injury to the mesangial cells in the intercapillary space. The glomerulus may then become more easily damaged by antigen-antibody complexes developing from the immune response to the streptococcal infection. The C3 component of complement is deposited in association with IgG (rarely IgA or IgM) or alone in a granular pattern on the epithelial side of the basement membrane and occasionally in subendothelial sites as well. Similar immune complex deposits in the glomeruli can often be demonstrated when the origin is other than streptococcal.

Gross examination of the involved kidney shows only punctate hemorrhages throughout the cortex. Microscopically, the primary alteration is in the glomeruli, which show proliferation and swelling of the mesangial and endothelial cells of the capillary tuft. The proliferation of capsular epithelium produces a thickened crescent about the tuft, and in the space between the capsule and the tuft there are collections of leukocytes, red cells, and exudate. Edema of the interstitial tissue and cloudy swelling of the tubule epithelium are common. Immune complexes are demonstrable by means of immunofluorescence techniques. Electron microscopy reveals the dense immune complex deposits as well as altered glomerular structures. As the disease progresses, the kidneys may enlarge. The typical histologic findings in glomerulitis are enlarging crescents that become hyalinized and converted into scar tissue and obstruct the circulation through the glomerulus. Degenerative changes occur in the tubules, with fatty degeneration and necrosis and ultimate scarring of the nephron. Arteriolar thickening and obliteration become prominent.

## Clinical Findings

**A. Symptoms and Signs:** Nephritis begins about 2 weeks after the streptococcal infection or exposure to a drug or other inciting agent. Often the disease is very mild, and there may be no reason to suspect renal involvement unless the urine is examined. In severe cases, the patient develops malaise, headache, mild fever, flank pain, and oliguria. The urine is noted as "bloody," "coffee-colored," or "smoky." Salt and water retention result from the diminished GFR and relatively increased tubular reabsorption. Edema appears in the periorbital areas and may include the extremities and pleural and peritoneal spaces. Increased blood volume is accompanied by increased cardiac output and some increase in arterial peripheral resistance with consequent arterial hypertension. Pulmonary vascular congestion occurs frequently and produces shortness of breath. Frank pulmonary edema may ensue.

**B. Laboratory Findings:** The diagnosis is confirmed by examination of the urine, which may be grossly bloody or coffee-colored (acid hematin) or may show only microscopic hematuria. Red cell morphology provides a clue as to whether the origin of the red cell is glomerular or nonglomerular. Red cells of glomerular origin are dysmorphic and show a variety of distorted forms and swollen forms; red cells of nonglomerular origin are not distorted. Examine the sediment with phase microscopy or with oil immersion in light microscopy after using one of the commercially available sediment stains. The urine contains protein (1–3+) and casts. Hyaline and granular casts are commonly found in large numbers, but the diagnostic sign of glomerulitis, the erythrocyte cast (blood cast), may be rare and require careful search of a centrifuged urinary sediment. The erythrocyte cast resembles a blood clot formed in the lumen of a renal tubule; it is usually of small caliber, intensely orange or red, and under high power with proper lighting may show the mosaic pattern of the packed red cells held together by the clot of fibrin and plasma protein.

With the impairment of renal function and with oliguria, plasma or serum urea nitrogen and creatinine become elevated, the levels varying with the severity of the renal lesion. The sedimentation rate is rapid. Infection of the throat with nephritogenic streptococci is frequently followed by increasing antistreptolysin O (ASO) titers in the serum, whereas high titers are usually not demonstrable following skin infections. Production of antibody against streptococcal deoxyribonuclease B (anti-DNase B) is more regularly observed following both throat and skin infections. Serum complement levels are usually low.

These studies are unnecessary in the diagnosis of the typical case. Confirmation is made by examination of the urine, although the history and clinical findings in typical cases leave little doubt. The finding of erythrocytes that are dysmorphic or contained in a cast is proof of their glomerular origin.

## Differential Diagnosis

Although considered to be the hallmark of poststreptococcal glomerulonephritis, erythrocyte casts also occur along with other abnormal elements in any disease in which glomerular inflammation is present, ie, polyarteritis nodosa, disseminated lupus erythematosus, dermatomyositis, sarcoidosis, subacute infective endocarditis, "focal" nephritis, Goodpasture's syndrome, Henoch's purpura.

## Complications

In severe cases, signs compatible with cardiac failure appear as a result of salt and water retention;

they include cardiac enlargement, tachycardia, $S_3$ gallop, pulmonary passive congestion, pleural fluid, and peripheral edema. Hypertension may be severe and may contribute to left ventricular failure.

Hypertensive encephalopathy may be striking: severe headache, drowsiness, muscle twitchings and convulsions, vomiting, and at times papilledema and retinal hemorrhage.

## Treatment

**A. Specific Measures:** There is no specific treatment. Eradication of β-hemolytic streptococci with penicillin or other antibiotic is desirable. Adrenocorticosteroids are of no value and may be contraindicated because they increase protein catabolism, sodium retention, and hypertension. Immunosuppressive and cytotoxic drugs have been ineffective in this form of nephritis. (See Nephrotic Syndrome, below.)

**B. General Measures:** In uncomplicated cases, treatment is symptomatic and designed to prevent overhydration and hypertension. Hospitalization is indicated if oliguria, nitrogen retention, and hypertension are present. Bed rest is of great importance and should be continued until clinical signs abate. Excretion of protein and formed elements in the urine will increase with resumption of activity, but such increases should not be great. Erythrocytes may be excreted in large numbers for months, and the rate of excretion is not a good criterion for evaluating convalescence.

In the presence of elevated blood urea nitrogen and oliguria, dietary protein restriction is indicated. If severe oliguria is present, no more than 20 g of protein should be given. If no nitrogen retention is apparent, the diet may contain 0.5 g of protein per kilogram of ideal weight. Carbohydrates should be given liberally to provide calories and to reduce the catabolism of protein and prevent starvation ketosis. With severe oliguria, hyperkalemia may occur, requiring dialysis.

The degree of oliguria and fluid retention and the severity of circulatory congestion and edema dictate the degree of restriction of salt and water. Loop diuretics are useful in reduction of fluid overload and of accompanying hypertension. Hemodialysis is performed as indicated by the severity of the acute renal insufficiency and for volume overload unresponsive to conservative measures.

If anemia becomes severe (hematocrit < 30%), give transfusions of packed red cells.

**C. Treatment of Complications:**

**1. Hypertensive encephalopathy** should be treated vigorously. Drowsiness and confusion accompanied by severe headache, nausea, blurred vision, and twitching progress to stupor and coma. A greatly elevated blood pressure (often > 250/150 mm Hg) and evidence of retinal arteriolar spasm with or without papilledema and hemorrhages are characteristic. The goal of therapy is to reduce blood pressure to near normal levels without further impairing renal function. The first-line drugs include nitroprusside, diazoxide, hydralazine, labetalol, and nifedipine.

Treatment for hypertensive crisis requires close monitoring.

a. Sodium nitroprusside by intravenous infusion pump at 2–50 μg/kg/min acts promptly but is of brief duration. Observation in an intensive care unit with intra-arterial blood pressure monitoring is required.

b. Nifedipine, 10–20 mg sublingually, may be used initially for rapid control under close monitoring.

c. Hydralazine, 5–10 mg intravenously every 15 minutes or 30–50 mg intravenously every 4–6 hours, is slower to act. Propranolol, 1–5 mg intravenously, may be required to reduce tachycardia.

d. Labetalol, an alpha- and beta-adrenergic blocking agent, is given intravenously at a rate of 2 mg/min up to a total of 20 mg. Its effects begin after 5 minutes and last for 3–6 hours. Subsequent infusions of 20–80 mg up to a total of 300 mg may be given. Both this agent and propranolol (as noted above) should be used with caution if at all if cardiac dysfunction is present.

e. Diazoxide, 150–300 mg, may be given rapidly as a bolus and 150 mg repeated as needed every 5–10 minutes. A continuous infusion of 300 mg/min may be substituted. Close monitoring is essential. Diazoxide produces sodium retention, which should be corrected by intravenous furosemide.

f. Clonidine, minoxidil, or prazosin may be useful for maintenance therapy.

g. Phenytoin may be of value in controlling seizures.

**2. Heart failure** should be treated as any case of left ventricular failure, ie, with severe restriction of fluid and sodium intake and the use of agents that reduce peripheral resistance (afterload) and venous return (preload) (see Chapter 8). Oxygen helps relieve respiratory distress. If digitalis is used, its effects must be monitored closely. Dialysis may be dramatic in relieving symptoms.

## Prognosis

Most patients with acute disease recover completely within 1–2 years; 5–20% show progressive renal damage. If oliguria, heart failure, or hypertensive encephalopathy is severe, death may occur during the acute attack.

See references under Chronic Glomerulonephritis, below.

## 2. CHRONIC GLOMERULONEPHRITIS

If acute glomerulonephritis does not heal within 1–2 years, the vascular and glomerular lesions continue to progress, and tubular changes occur. In the presence of smoldering active nephritis, the patient is usually asymptomatic, and the only evidence of disease is the excretion of abnormal urinary elements.

The urinary excretion of protein, red cells, white cells, epithelial cells, and casts (including erythrocyte casts, granular casts, and hyaline and waxy casts) continues at levels above normal. As renal impairment progresses, signs of renal insufficiency appear (see below).

## Treatment

Treat intercurrent infections promptly and vigorously as indicated. Avoid unnecessary vaccinations.

Exacerbations are treated as for the acute attack. A protein intake of 0.5–1 g/kg is permissible as long as renal function is adequate to maintain a normal blood urea nitrogen. A liberal fluid intake is desirable.

Strenuous exercise may be harmful; otherwise, normal activity is permitted.

## Prognosis

Worsening of the urinary findings may occur with infection, trauma, or fatigue. Exacerbations may resemble the acute attack or may be typical of the nephrotic syndrome (see below). Death in uremia is the usual outcome, but the course is variable, and the patient may live a reasonably normal life for 20–30 years.

Baldwin DS: Chronic glomerulonephritis: Nonimmunologic mechanisms of progressive glomerular damage. *Kidney Int* 1982;**21**:109.

Couser WG: Mesangial IgA nephropathies: Steady progress. *West J Med* 1984;**140**:89.

Couser WG: What are circulating immune complexes doing in glomerulonephritis? *N Engl J Med* 1981;**304**:1230.

Culpepper RM, Andreoli TE: The pathophysiology of the glomerulopathies. *Adv Intern Med* 1983;**28**:161.

Hood SA et al: IgA-IgG nephropathy: Predictive indices of progressive disease. *Clin Nephrol* 1981;**16**:55.

## 3. NEPHROTIC SYNDROME

### Essentials of Diagnosis

- Massive edema.
- Proteinuria more than 3.5 g/d.
- Hypoalbuminemia less than 3 g/dL.
- Hyperlipidemia with cholesterol more than 300 mg/dL.
- Free fat, oval fat bodies, fatty casts in urinary sediment.

### General Considerations

Because treatment and prognosis vary with the cause of nephrotic syndrome (nephrosis), renal biopsy and appropriate examination of an adequate tissue specimen are important. Light microscopy, electron microscopy, and immunofluorescence identification of immune mechanisms provide critical information for identification of most of the causes of nephrosis.

Glomerular diseases associated with nephrotic syndrome include the following: (See Table 15–1.)

(1) Minimal glomerular lesions: Lipoid nephrosis accounts for about 20% of cases of nephrotic syndrome in adults.

(2) Membranous glomerulonephritis: About 30% of cases.

(3) Mesangial proliferative glomerulonephritis: About 5% of cases.

(4) Focal glomerular sclerosis: About 10% of cases.

(5) Membranoproliferative glomerulonephritis: About 7% of cases.

(6) Miscellaneous diseases: These include diabetic glomerulopathy, systemic lupus erythematosus, polyarteritis, Wegener's granulomatosis, amyloidosis, multiple myeloma, neoplasms (including lymphomas and carcinomas), hepatitis B, syphilis, reaction to toxins (bee venom, *Rhus* antigen), reaction to drugs, and exposure to heavy metals.

### Clinical Findings

**A. Symptoms and Signs:** Edema may appear insidiously and increase slowly; often it appears suddenly and accumulates rapidly. As fluid collects in the serous cavities, the abdomen becomes protuberant, and the patient may complain of anorexia and become short of breath. Symptoms other than those related to the mechanical effects of edema and serous sac fluid accumulation are not remarkable.

On physical examination, massive edema is apparent. Signs of hydrothorax and ascites are common. Pallor is often accentuated by the edema, and striae commonly appear in the stretched skin of the extremities. Hypertension, changes in the retina and retinal vessels, and cardiac and cerebral manifestations of hypertension may be demonstrated more often when autoimmune disease, diabetes mellitus, or renal insufficiency is present.

**B. Laboratory Findings:** The urine contains large amounts of protein, 4–10 g/24 h or more. The sediment contains casts, including the characteristic fatty and waxy varieties; renal tubule cells, some of which contain lipid droplets (oval fat bodies); and variable numbers of erythrocytes. A mild normochromic anemia is common, but anemia may be more severe if renal damage is great. Nitrogen retention varies with the severity of impairment of renal function. The plasma is often lipemic, and cholesterol and triglycerides are usually elevated. Plasma protein is greatly reduced. The albumin fraction is typically decreased to less than 3 g/dL. Some reduction of gamma globulin occurs in most types of nephrosis, but in inflammatory disease such as systemic lupus erythematosus the protein of the gamma fraction may be greatly elevated. Serum complement may be low in active disease. The serum electrolyte concentrations are often normal, although the serum sodium may be slightly low; total serum calcium may be low, in keeping with the degree of hypoalbuminemia and decrease in the protein-bound calcium moiety. During edema-forming periods, urinary sodium excretion is very low and urinary aldosterone excretion elevated. If renal insufficiency (see above) is present, the blood and urine findings are usually altered accordingly.

**Table 15–1.** Morphologic characteristics of selected glomerulopathies.

| | Light Microscopy | Electron Microscopy | Immunofluorescence* | IgG | IgA | IgM | C3 | FRA |
|---|---|---|---|---|---|---|---|---|
| **Primary glomerulonephritis** | | | | | | | | |
| Diffuse proliferative, including poststreptococcal | Proliferation of mesangial cells, endothelial cells, and/or epithelial cells. | Subepithelial GBM† deposits. Mesangial cells and matrix increased. | Variable and irregular granular deposits along capillary walls and in mesangium. | ++ | v | v | + | v |
| Focal proliferative | Focal proliferative changes plus increased mesangial cellularity. | Mesangial deposits. | Segmental granular GBM and mesangial deposits. | ++ | + | + | ++ | v |
| Proliferative with crescent formation | Crescent formation from proliferation of epithelial cells filling Bowman's space. | Subendothelial deposits along GBM with increased mesangial matrix; proliferating epithelial cells. | Diffuse granular or linear deposits involving peripheral capillary loops. | ++ | + | + | + | + |
| Mesangiocapillary (membranoproliferative) | Proliferation of mesangial cells, increased mesangial matrix, thickening of capillary walls. | I. Deposits in mesangium; endothelial cells separated from endothelial cells by mesangial matrix. II. Confluent intra-GBM deposit. | I. Granular deposit along GBM. C3 alone in mesangium. II. Intramembranous deposit in GBM and TBM.† | ++ | v | ++ | +++ | v |
| Membranous | Thickening of capillary wall. Subepithelial spikes (silver stain). | Dense subepithelial deposits. | Coarse granular deposits along capillary wall. | ++ | v | v | ++ | v |
| Focal sclerosing | Segmental sclerosis with hyaline deposits in subendothelial areas of affected loops, especially of juxtamedullary cortex. | Subendothelial and mesangial dense deposits. Diffuse or segmental alteration of foot processes. | Irregular granular or nodular deposits at site of focal lesions. | + | ± | ++ | ++ | − |
| Chronic, end stage | Hyalinization of glomerular tufts, loss of tubules, interstitial fibrosis. | Fibrosis, hyaline deposits, advanced alterations characteristic of primary disease. | Granular deposits in scarred and partially intact glomeruli and in interstitial areas. | ± | ± | ± | + | ± |
| **Systemic disease** | | | | | | | | |
| Systemic lupus erythematosus | Variable patterns of minimal changes, mesangial proliferative, focal proliferative, membranous and subepithelial deposits; wire loop lesions. Hematoxylin bodies in capillary loops. | Characteristic massive subendothelial, intramembranous and subepithelial deposits; wire loop lesions. Microtubules in endothelial cells and leukocytes. | Variable. Granular deposits corresponding to type and location of altered glomeruli. | ++ | + | ++ | ++ | + |
| **Disease of uncertain immunologic cause** | | | | | | | | |
| Lipoid nephrosis | No alteration, or minimal lesion of proliferative type. | Abnormalities of epithelial cells with smudging of foot processes and obliteration of slit pore membrane. | Minimal irregular clumps in mesangial areas. | ± | − | ± | ± | − |
| Berger's IgA nephropathy | Segmental to diffuse mesangial proliferation and increase in mesangial matrix. | Deposits in mesangium. | Granular deposits in mesangium. | + | ++ | ++ | ++ | + |
| Henoch-Schönlein purpura | Focal and diffuse proliferative lesions and mesangial lesions. | Same as focal and diffuse proliferative types with increased mesangial deposits. | Diffuse glomerular deposits, largely in mesangium. | + | ++ | − | ++ | + |
| Wegener's granulomatosis | Proliferative and crescent-forming lesions. | Dense GBM deposits. | Variable scattered granular deposits. | + | + | + | + | + |

* FRA = Fibrin/fibrinogen-related antigen; v = variable.
† GBM = Glomerular basement membrane; TBM = tubular basement membrane.

Renal biopsy is essential to confirm the type of lesion, to indicate prognosis, and to guide therapy.

## Differential Diagnosis

Constrictive pericarditis may present with a clinical picture resembling nephrosis. Renal vein thrombosis is associated with nephrotic syndrome; it is likely that renal vein thrombosis is secondary to nephrosis rather than a cause of it.

## Treatment

There is no specific treatment except for syphilis or for heavy metal poisoning. Bed rest is indicated for patients with severe edema or those who have infections. Hospitalization may be desirable when corticosteroid therapy is initiated. The diet should provide a normal protein ration (0.75–1 g/kg/d), with adequate calories. Sodium intake should be restricted to 0.5–1 g/d. Potassium need not be restricted. If edema, ascites, or pleural effusion becomes disabling, a cautious trial of diuretics is warranted; the physician should watch for reduction of an already diminished plasma volume (postural hypotension, prerenal azotemia, shock).

Adrenocorticosteroids are useful for treatment of the nephrotic syndrome in children and in adults when the underlying disease is the minimal glomerular lesion (lipoid nephrosis), systemic lupus erythematosus, proliferative glomerulonephritis, or idiosyncrasy to toxin or venom. In the adult with minimal glomerular lesion, a trial of corticosteroid therapy is justified, although the advantage over no treatment is uncertain and complications of therapy are more frequent. Prednisone, 1 mg/kg/d orally or 2 mg/kg orally as a single morning dose on alternate days for 4–8 weeks, is an adequate trial. Diuresis and diminishing proteinuria are evidence of response to therapy. The dose of prednisone may then be reduced slowly over a period of a month or more. Failure to respond indicates that the cause is probably not minimal lesion disease.

For treatment of patients with membranous glomerular lesions, the alternate-day prednisone program (120 mg on alternate mornings) may be employed for up to 8 weeks.

Focal glomerulosclerosis, mesangiocapillary (membranoproliferative) glomerulonephritis, and proliferative glomerulonephritis do not respond to steroid alone or to steroid plus immunosuppressive therapy. Treatment is solely symptomatic.

Diuretics are often ineffective, though loop diuretics, thiazides, chlorthalidone, and others may be employed. Spironolactone may be helpful when employed concurrently with other diuretics. Salt-free albumin, dextran, and other oncotic agents are of little help, and their effects are transient.

*Caution:* Elevation of serum potassium, development of hypertension, and sudden severe increase in edema contraindicate continuation of corticosteroid therapy. Such complications usually arise during the first 2 weeks of continuous therapy.

Immunosuppressive drugs, including alkylating agents, cyclophosphamide, mercaptopurine, azathioprine, and others, have been employed in the treatment of the nephrotic syndrome. The use of corticosteroids plus immunosuppressive agents is similar to that employed in reversing rejection of homotransplants in humans. Encouraging results have been reported in children and adults with membranous lesions and with systemic lupus erythematosus. Those with minimal lesions refractory to corticosteroid therapy do no better when immunosuppressive agents are added.

Serious side effects related both to corticosteroids and to the cytotoxic agents are common. This form of therapy should be employed only by those experienced in treating the nephrotic syndrome in patients who have proved refractory to well-established treatment regimens.

For renal vein thrombosis, the treatment is directed against progress of thrombus formation and consists of heparin or thrombolytic agents and long-term use of coumarin drugs.

## Prognosis

The course and prognosis depend upon the cause of the nephrotic syndrome. In more than half of cases of childhood nephrosis, the disease appears to run a rather benign course when properly treated and to leave insignificant sequelae. Of the others, most develop chronic renal insufficiency. Adults with nephrosis fare less well, particularly when the associated disorder is glomerulonephritis, systemic lupus erythematosus, amyloidosis, or diabetic nephropathy. In those with minimal lesions, remissions, either spontaneous or following corticosteroid therapy, are common. Treatment is more often unsuccessful or only ameliorative when the other glomerular lesions are present.

Cogan MG: Nephrotic syndrome. *West J Med* 1982;**136**:411.

Glassock RJ et al: The nephrotic syndrome. Page 955 in: *The Kidney,* 3rd ed. Brenner BM, Rector FC (editors). Saunders, 1986.

Harrington JT: Thrombolytic therapy in renal vein thrombosis. (Editorial.) *Arch Intern Med* 1984;**144**:33.

Llach F, Papper S, Massry SG: The clinical spectrum of renal vein thrombosis: Acute and chronic. *Am J Med* 1980;**69**:819.

Ponticelli C et al: Controlled trial of methylprednisolone and chlorambucil in idiopathic membranous nephropathy. *N Engl J Med* 1984;**310**:946.

Wagoner RD et al: Renal vein thrombosis in idiopathic membranous glomerulopathy and nephrotic syndrome: Incidence and significance. *Kidney Int* 1983;**23**:368.

## 4. IgA NEPHROPATHY (Idiopathic Benign Hematuria)

The entity of primary hematuria (idiopathic benign and recurrent hematuria, or Berger's disease) is now included among the immune complex glomerulopathies in which deposition of IgA with C3 and fibrin-related antigens occurs in a granular pattern in the mesangium of the glomerulus.

Recurrent macroscopic and microscopic hematuria and mild proteinuria are characteristically the only manifestations of renal disease. Prospective studies have shown progression of renal disease, with destruction of glomeruli and loss of renal function, often with hypertension. Exacerbations have been observed with upper respiratory tract disease. Progression is usually slow, extending over 2–3 decades.

Berger's nephropathy has appeared in siblings and identical twins. HLA-DR4 antigen occurs in 49% of patients, an incidence 2.5 times that of the control population.

Diagnosis is made by renal biopsy and demonstration of the mesangial deposits of IgA often accompanied by C3 and by small amounts of IgG. IgA may be deposited in skin capillaries as well. Similar deposits may be seen in Henoch-Schönlein purpura, disseminated lupus erythematosus, eclampsia, membranous glomerulonephritis, acute postinfectious glomerulonephritis, and other rare causes of glomerulopathy. The urine sediment resembles that of any latent glomerulonephritis, with protein, red cells, and casts, including erythrocyte casts. The paucity of clinical manifestations and slow progress may be determining factors in the diagnosis.

No specific treatment has been advocated for this indolent disease.

## 5. ANTI-GLOMERULAR BASEMENT MEMBRANE NEPHRITIS (Goodpasture's Syndrome)

The patient usually gives a history of recent hemoptysis and often of malaise, anorexia, and headache. The clinical syndrome is that of severe acute glomerulonephritis accompanied by diffuse hemorrhagic inflammation of the lungs. Occasionally, acute renal disease with a similar clinical and immunologic pattern may occur without associated lung disease (see next section). The urine shows gross or microscopic hematuria, and laboratory findings of severely suppressed renal function are usually evident. Biopsy shows glomerular crescents, glomerular adhesions, and inflammatory infiltration interstitially. Electron microscopic examination shows an increase in basement membrane material and deposition of fibrin beneath the capillary endothelium. In some cases, circulating antibody against glomerular basement membrane can be identified. IgG and C3 complement can be demonstrated as linear deposits on the basement membranes of the glomeruli and the lung. Antiglomerular basement membrane antibody also reacts with lung basement membrane.

Only rare cases of survival have been documented. Large doses of corticosteroids in combination with immunosuppressive agents are indicated. In addition, plasmapheresis may be employed to remove circulating antibody. Hemodialysis and nephrectomy with renal transplantation may offer the only hope for rescue. Transplantation should be delayed until circulating antiglomerular antibodies have disappeared.

Briggs WA et al: Anti-glomerular basement membrane antibody-mediated glomerulonephritis and Goodpasture's syndrome. *Medicine* 1979;**58**:348.

Johnson JP et al: Therapy of anti-glomerular basement membrane antibody disease: Analysis of prognostic significance of clinical, pathologic, and treatment factors. *Medicine* 1985;**64**:219.

## 6. RAPIDLY PROGRESSIVE GLOMERULONEPHRITIS

Rapid deterioration of renal function in the course of a few weeks to a few months is characteristic of fulminant anti-glomerular basement membrane glomerulonephritis. Other glomerular disorders that can follow the same clinical course include poststreptococcal glomerulonephritis, mesangiocapillary (membranoproliferative) glomerulonephritis, Wegener's granulomatosis, systemic lupus erythematosus, polyarteritis, Henoch-Schönlein purpura, hemolyticuremic syndrome, thrombotic thrombocytopenic purpura, mixed cryoglobulinemia, and ventriculovenous shunt nephritis. Scleroderma may produce a similar picture.

Oliguria, hematuria and proteinuria, and mild hypertension may be the only signs. Abdominal pain and nausea and vomiting may be prominent.

Exuberant proliferation of epithelial cells of Bowman's capsule with crescent formation is the main feature of renal biopsy. Immunofluorescent stains show either fine linear deposits of IgG and segmental deposits of C3 related to anti-glomerular basement membrane antibody or granular deposits of IgG and IgM accompanied by C3 related to immune complex disease.

Treatment with corticosteroids and immunosuppressive drugs has not been successful. Plasmapheresis may be helpful. Dialysis and transplantation may be necessary.

Spontaneous recovery is rare. Progression of renal failure is the rule.

Oredugba O et al: Pulse methylprednisolone therapy in idiopathic rapidly progressive glomerulonephritis. *Ann Intern Med* 1980;**92**:504.

## CHRONIC RENAL INSUFFICIENCY

### Essentials of Diagnosis

- Weakness and easy fatigability, headaches, anorexia, nausea and vomiting, pruritus, polyuria, nocturia.
- Hypertension with secondary encephalopathy, retinal damage, heart failure.
- Anemia, azotemia, and acidosis, with elevated

serum potassium, phosphate, and sulfate and decreased serum calcium and protein.

- Urine specific gravity low and fixed; mild to moderate proteinuria; few red cells, white cells, and broad renal failure casts.

## General Considerations

Chronic renal insufficiency may be a consequence of a variety of diseases involving the kidney parenchyma or obstruction of the excretory tract. Causes of chronic renal failure include the following: (1) primary glomerular disease (immune complex glomerulonephritis), (2) renal vascular disease, (3) chronic pyelonephritis, (4) metabolic diseases with renal involvement, (5) nephrotoxins, (6) infection, (7) chronic radiation nephritis, (8) interstitial nephritis, (9) chronic obstructive uropathy, (10) congenital anomalies of both kidneys, (11) embolization of glomeruli by cholesterol crystals incident to aortic catheterization for angiography, and (12) nephropathy of particular geographic distribution.

The pathologic picture varies with the cause of the damage to the kidney. Extensive scarring with decrease in kidney size, hyalinization of glomeruli, and obliteration of some tubules and hypertrophy and dilatation of others produce great distortion of renal architecture. The vascular changes are due to the effects of scar formation and of prolonged hypertension, with thickening of the media, fragmentation of elastic fibers, intimal thickening, and obliteration of the lumens in some areas. In diabetic nephropathy, the typical glomerular lesions of intercapillary sclerosis are often distinct. The vascular lesions of periarteritis or of systemic lupus erythematosus often serve to establish these diagnoses. Obstructive uropathy presents the classic picture of hydronephrosis with compression and destruction of the renal parenchyma. Polycystic disease, multiple myeloma, amyloid disease, persistent hypercalcemia, and other causes of renal failure usually can be identified by characteristic lesions.

## Pathophysiology of Uremia

The clinical findings of the uremic syndrome result from loss of nephrons and decreased renal blood flow and glomerular filtration.

With the loss of nephrons, the burden of solute excretion falls on fewer functional units, with subsequent impaired ability of the kidney to maintain body water, osmolality of body fluids, and electrolyte and acid-base balance. The consequences of nephron loss are, briefly, as follows.

**A. Water:** Increased solute load per nephron produces an osmotic diuresis with associated impaired ability to excrete concentrated or dilute urine. Dehydration is common and hazardous; water intoxication may occur if fluid intake is excessive.

**B. Electrolyte:**

1. Both excretion and conservation of electrolyte are inadequate. Reduced filtration and excretion of phosphate, sulfate, and organic acid end products of metabolism result in increased concentration of these anions in body fluids, with displacement of bicarbonate. Furthermore, decreased ability to produce $H^+$ and $NH_4^+$ for excretion with anion in the urine contributes to acidosis.

2. Sodium loss due to the impaired reabsorption that accompanies osmotic diuresis contributes to a decrease in extracellular fluid volume. With reduction of plasma volume, renal perfusion declines, with worsening renal failure. Since the kidney cannot respond appropriately, a sudden increase in sodium intake cannot be excreted readily, and edema will usually ensue.

3. Potassium regulation is usually not impaired until oliguria is severe or acidosis becomes prominent.

4. Metabolism of calcium and phosphate is seriously disturbed as a consequence of reduction of glomerular filtration and tubule function, impairment of 1-hydroxylation of the vitamin D metabolite 25-hydroxycholecalciferol to 1,25-dihydroxycholecalciferol, and reduced effect of parathyroid hormone on the skeleton. The ensuing hyperphosphatemia and hypocalcemia elicit the development of secondary hyperparathyroidism. The combination of hyperparathyroidism and impaired vitamin D metabolism results in bone disease (renal osteodystrophy) characterized by osteitis fibrosa, osteomalacia, osteoporosis, osteosclerosis, and, in children, impaired growth. Calcification in soft tissue may occur. Rarely, parathyroid secretion cannot be influenced by therapy, a condition termed tertiary hyperparathyroidism. Pertinent laboratory findings include hyperphosphatemia, hypocalcemia (even when corrected for hypoalbuminemia), hypermagnesemia, and elevated parathyroid hormone levels.

**C. Nitrogen Retention:** High urea, creatinine, and urate levels are manifestations of reduced clearance. Urea load is related to protein metabolism, while creatinine load is related to muscle mass and is independent of protein intake.

**D. Anemia:** Depression of red cell production probably results from reduced secretion of erythropoietin by the kidney. Survival time of red cells is shorter than normal. Size and hemoglobin content of red cells are usually normal.

**E. Hypertension:** With renal ischemia and increasing destruction of the renal parenchyma, hypertension may become evident, with further deterioration of kidney function. The coincidence of malignant hypertension and uremia is particularly ominous.

## Clinical Findings

**A. Symptoms and Signs:** Progressive weakness, easy fatigability, and lethargy are often prominent. Thirst, weight loss, anorexia, gastrointestinal irritability, diarrhea, hiccup, and itching are common complaints. Occasionally, a persistent bad or metallic taste annoys the patient. Symptoms of nervous system involvement include paresthesias and burning sensations associated with peripheral neuropathy, myoclonic jerking, and seizures. Headache, visual difficulties, and symptoms of left heart failure result from hypertension. Cerebral hemorrhage, pulmonary edema, and heart failure are usually late occurrences. Purpura and bleeding from the nose and gastrointestinal tract may be severe. Bone pain and, in children, retarded growth reflect osteodystrophy.

The history should include a review of familial disease and questions regarding previous renal disease, drug ingestion, and symptoms of lower urinary tract obstruction.

Physical examination of the patient reveals pallor, hyperpnea, uremic breath, dehydration, excoriated skin, and purpura. Hypertension with retinopathy is usually present. Cardiac enlargement, pulmonary edema, and pericarditis may be evident. Evidence of peripheral neuropathy should be sought. Bone deformity and awkwardness of gait are evidence of osteodystrophy.

**B. Laboratory Findings:** Anemia, azotemia, and acidosis are the principal findings. The anemia is usually normochromic and normocytic, with hemoglobin in the range of 6–9 g/dL. Prolonged bleeding time is attributed to defective platelet function. The urine is usually dilute and contains small amounts of protein; few red, white, and epithelial cells; and a few granular and waxy casts, some of which are large (broad renal failure casts). Serum concentrations of urea nitrogen, creatinine, and often uric acid are greatly elevated. Serum sodium may be slightly lower than normal and serum potassium slightly to markedly elevated; serum calcium is decreased; with bone disease, alkaline phosphatase activity in the serum is increased, and circulating parathyroid hormone is often elevated. Serum magnesium may be elevated. With retention of phosphate, sulfate, and, frequently, chloride, plasma bicarbonate concentration is decreased. (Phosphate and sulfate participate in the "anion gap" of uremia.) Both retention of organic acids and impaired tubular secretion of hydrogen ion plus loss of sodium and bicarbonate buffer are accompanied by a decrease in blood pH.

**C. Imaging:** Chest radiographs may show evidence of cardiac enlargement, midzone interstitial edema of the lung, frank pulmonary congestion, or pulmonary edema. The size of the kidneys should be determined by ultrasonography, which also may demonstrate evidence of obstructed ureter and bladder outlet. Radiologic evidence of bone disease (osteomalacia and osteitis fibrosa) is common long before overt symptoms and clinical signs appear.

**D. Other Findings:** Echocardiography is useful in confirming the presence of pericardial effusion. The ECG reflects left ventricular strain or hypertrophy and changes due to potassium toxicity.

## Differential Diagnosis

Chronic renal insufficiency presents symptoms and signs related to the functional disability resulting from a reduction in the number of functioning nephrons rather than to the cause of the renal damage. It is often impossible to distinguish the cause. The presence of large kidneys characteristic of polycystic disease should serve to identify this cause of renal failure. The physician must identify remediable causes of renal insufficiency such as obstruction, infection, persistent hypercalcemia, gout, myeloma, and drug toxicity. Bilaterally small kidneys and the presence of bone disease imply irreversible damage to renal function.

## Treatment

Hypertension or heart failure should be treated as indicated with agents that sustain renal function and coronary artery blood flow (see below).

**A. Diet and Fluids:** Limitation of protein of high biologic value to 0.5 g/kg/d helps to reduce azotemia, acidosis, and hyperkalemia. Trials of mixtures of essential amino acids or of amino acid precursors such as $\alpha$-keto and $\alpha$-hydroxy acid analogs are promising approaches to protein replacement.

The diet should include adequate calories and a multivitamin product plus folic acid, 1 mg daily, particularly when protein is severely restricted. Sodium intake need not be restricted and should be tailored to urine losses, which tend to be fixed in amount. Fluid intake should be sufficient to maintain an adequate urine volume, but no attempt should be made to force diuresis. Obligatory water loss may be quite high because of the large solute load (eg, sodium and urea) that must be excreted by a reduced number of nephrons. Intake of up to 2–3 L may be required when creatinine clearance is reduced to 10–20 mL/min. With decreasing clearance, urine volume decreases. Intake must be sufficient to maintain renal function without causing excessive diuresis or water retention. If edema is present, a cautious trial of furosemide or ethacrynic acid is indicated, with careful monitoring of serum electrolytes. *Caution:* Water restriction for laboratory examination, tests of renal function, or any other reason may lead to serious volume depletion.

**B. Electrolyte Replacement:**

1. Sodium supplements may be required to restore sodium losses resulting from failure of the kidney to provide $NH_4^+$ and $H^+$ for sodium conservation. A mixture of NaCl and $NaHCO_3$ in equal parts, 1–2 g 2–3 times daily with meals, may be required in addition to dietary sources. Weight loss and a decreasing urine volume indicate a need for additional sodium. Hypertension and edema are signs that a trial of sodium restriction is in order.

2. Potassium intake may have to be restricted or supplemented. In severe hyperkalemia, active measures to remove potassium may be required (see discussion in Chapter 3). Measurement of the serum potassium concentration will provide indications.

3. Serum phosphate levels may be lowered and secondary hyperparathyroidism ameliorated by reducing absorption of phosphate in the gastrointestinal tract with administration of aluminum hydroxide gel, 30 mL, or (as tablets) 4–5 g 3–4 times daily.

4. Calcium lactate, 4 g 2–3 times daily, may be given to relieve hypocalcemic tetany. Intravenous administration of calcium salts may be required at times.

**C. Bone Disease (Renal Osteodystrophy):** In the presence of bone disease, phosphate binders and supplemental calcium are employed as above. In addition, cholecalciferol (vitamin $D_3$) or, more effectively, its metabolites—ie, calcifediol (25-hydroxycholecalciferol) and calcitriol (1,25-dihydroxycholecalciferol)—are useful in correcting osteomalacia and osteitis fibrosa, with some amelioration of myopathy. *Caution:* Close observation is mandatory to prevent hypercalcemia and soft tissue calcification, which may ensue if the dosage is too great. Thorough knowledge of indications and hazards must be obtained before using these potent agents.

Parathyroidectomy may be required if "tertiary" hyperparathyroidism is present.

**D. Anemia; Hemostasis:** Iron is of little value unless iron deficit exists. With evidence that transfusion is responsible for improved acceptance of renal allografts, there should be no hesitation in giving blood transfusions to patients whose anemia is symptomatic or if the hematocrit falls to the low 20s. Prolonged bleeding time and difficulty with hemostasis can be corrected transiently with cryoprecipitate. Desmopressin acetate (1-deamino-8-D-arginine vasopressin; DDAVP), 0.3 μg/kg body weight diluted in 50–100 mL of saline solution, may be infused intravenously over 30 minutes to shorten the bleeding time for about 4 hours. DDAVP is sometimes used to prevent bleeding during minor surgical procedures.

**E. General Measures:** Nausea and vomiting may be alleviated with chlorpromazine, 15–25 mg orally or 10–20 mg intramuscularly (or equivalent amounts of related compounds). The barbiturate drugs may be used for sedation as required.

Hypertension is a common manifestation of uremia. An expanded extracellular fluid volume is often responsible for hypertension, and the circumstances can be ameliorated by reduction of extracellular fluid volume by a trial of furosemide or by hemodialysis. Combinations of hydralazine and propranolol may be effective; nifedipine, minoxidil, metoprolol, clonidine, and prazosin are useful drugs. Angiotensin-converting enzyme inhibitors are enjoying increasing applications. Very rarely, bilateral nephrectomy may be necessary to rescue the patient from persistent hypertension. (See references for details of management of hypertension in the presence of renal failure.)

**F. Approach to Drug Therapy:** Because the half-life of many drugs is prolonged in patients with renal failure, the physician must monitor the effects of drugs closely. The dosage of drugs must often be reduced and guided by blood levels (see references).

**G. Chronic Dialysis and Kidney Transplants:** These approaches to the treatment of renal insufficiency due to any cause have been under investigation for many years, and encouraging experience has prompted expansion of facilities for scheduled, repeated extracorporeal dialysis. Successful renal transplantation has extended life for patients with chronic renal failure.

Amelioration of complications such as neuropathy, hyperparathyroidism, and anemia can be frequently achieved by dialysis or transplantation.

1. Simplified mechanisms for dialysis with the artificial kidney and ingenious cannulas and arteriovenous fistulas permit periodic dialysis with a minimum of professional supervision in hospital centers and in the patient's home. Patients with creatinine clearances of 0–2 mL/min have been kept alive for 6–10 years in reasonable health and activity by dialysis once or twice a week. The criteria for selection of patients are now clear. Centers have been established for the treatment of chronic renal insufficiency, and home units are generally available, although considerable skill is required to operate the devices. A recent survey indicates a 1-year survival rate on dialysis of 87%, a 2-year survival rate of 73%, and, in the 20- to 45-year age group, a 6-year survival rate of 60%.

Peritoneal dialysis can be used for temporary or long-term therapy. Chronic ambulatory peritoneal dialysis provides less effective clearance of small molecules (urea, creatinine) than does hemodialysis, but because it is continuous, it is adequate to relieve symptoms of uremia and provides excellent treatment. One to 2 L of dialysate modified to meet the needs of the patient can be exchanged 3–5 times daily. With good technique, the risk of peritonitis is reduced; it can usually be treated successfully with appropriate antibiotics.

Hemofiltration, a variant of dialysis in which a highly permeable membrane is employed, may prove a useful alternative to conventional dialysis.

2. Transplantation of kidneys from one human to another has been technically feasible for many years. Survival of such grafts has been limited by rejection of the foreign organ by the recipient except when donor and recipient were identical twins. Blood typing and leukocyte typing for histocompatibility antigens have improved the matching of donor and recipient, with an encouraging decrease in the rejection rate. The enhanced survival of cadaver renal grafts in patients who have had 5 or more blood transfusions compared to those who have had none is clear (1-year graft survival > 60% versus 42%). Further experience with immunosuppressive drugs (azathioprine or cyclophosphamide) and adrenal corticosteroids has improved protection of the homologous transplant from rejection for extended periods. The use of cyclosporine (cyclosporin A) to suppress immunity has been impressively effective. The high incidence of nephrotoxicity is a serious complication requiring close monitoring of renal function and reduction of dosage for long-term use. Total lymphoid irradiation (TLI) has resulted in improved tolerance for the graft, permitting reduced dosage of prednisone. The goal with cyclosporine and with TLI is to effect

tolerance for the graft in the absence of immunosuppressive drugs.

Survival data since January 1970 are much improved over prior experience. When the donor is a parent or an HLA-matched sibling, recipient survival with the first transplant still functional at 2 years is 80% or greater and at 3 years 70%. Cyclosporine has extended survival of the recipient and the transplanted cadaveric kidney, with some reduction of acute rejection episodes. One study showed that the 4-year survival rate for patients receiving cyclosporine was 86%, while the rate for those receiving azathioprine and corticosteroids was 76%.

Adequate dialysis. (Editorial.) *Lancet* 1982;**1**:147.

Anemia of chronic renal failure. (Editorial.) *Lancet* 1983;**1**:965.

Bennett WM et al: Drug prescribing in renal failure: Dosing guidelines for adults. *Am J Kidney Dis* 1983;**3**:155.

Brenner BM, Meyer TW, Hostetter TH: Dietary protein intake and the progressive nature of kidney disease. *N Engl J Med* 1982;**307**:652.

Carpenter CB, Strom TB: Transplantation: Immunogenetic and clinical aspects. (Part 1.) *Hosp Pract* (Dec) 1982;**17**:125.

Carvalho A: Bleeding in uremia: A clinical challenge. (Editorial.) *N Engl J Med* 1983;**308**:38.

Cohen DJ et al: Cyclosporine: A new immunosuppressive agent for organ transplantation. *Ann Intern Med* 1984;**101**:667.

Hosfeffer TH: Diabetic nephropathy. *N Engl J Med* 1985;**312**:642.

Kurtzman NA: Chronic renal failure: Metabolic and clinical consequences. *Hosp Pract* (Aug) 1982;**17**:107.

Levey AS, Harrington JT: Continuous peritoneal dialysis for chronic renal failure. *Medicine* 1982;**61**:330.

Levin B et al: Treatment of cadaveric renal transplant recipients with total lymphoid irradiation, anti-thymocyte globulin and low dose prednisone. *Lancet* 1985;**2**:1321.

Mannucci PM et al: Deamino-8-D-arginine vasopressin shortens the bleeding time in uremia. *N Engl J Med* 1983;**308**:8.

Merion RM et al: Cyclosporine: Five years' experience in cadaveric renal transplantation. *N Engl J Med* 1984;**310**:148.

Mooradian AD, Morley JE: Endocrine dysfunction in chronic renal failure. *Arch Intern Med* 1984;**144**:351.

Murray BM: Cyclosporine nephrotoxicity. *The Kidney* 1986;**19**:5.

Quarles LD: The renal dystrophies: Therapeutic principles. *The Kidney* 1985;**18**:11.

Rosanski SJ, Sugimoto T: An analysis of the United States renal transplant patient population and organ survival characteristics: 1977 to 1980. *Kidney Int* 1982;**22**:685.

Rosman JB et al: Prospective randomised trial of early dietary protein restriction in chronic renal failure. *Lancet* 1984;**2**:1291.

Strom TB, Carpenter CB: Transplantation: Immunogenetic and clinical aspects. (Part 2.) *Hosp Pract* (Jan) 1983;**18**:135.

Symposium on continuous ambulatory peritoneal dialysis. *Kidney Int* 1983;**23**:2. [Entire issue.]

Walser M: Nutritional support in renal failure: Future directions. *Lancet* 1983;**1**:340.

## HEMOLYTIC-UREMIC SYNDROME

This syndrome, though still uncommon, is being recognized with increasing frequency. Many features are similar to thrombotic thrombocytopenic purpura.

The essential features include renal microangiopathy (with decreased glomerular filtration, proteinuria, and hematuria), microangiopathic hemolytic anemia, and thrombocytopenia. Endothelial damage involves renal arterioles and glomerular capillaries, with rare extension to other organs. Ischemic necrosis in the renal cortex may occur with obstruction from intravascular coagulation. Acute renal insufficiency is the major threat to life.

Two types of the syndrome have been described. Sporadic cases may be idiopathic or secondary to infections with *Shigella, Salmonella, E coli* strain O157:H7, or viral agents. This form is more common in children, and the mortality rate is low (under 5%). The syndrome may occur in pregnant women, in women taking oral contraceptives, or as a complication of malignant hypertension or renal transplantation.

A familial, or hereditary, type has been identified in which members of a family may have recurrent episodes over several years. The mortality rate is 30%.

Postpartum renal failure has many characteristics of the hemolytic uremic syndrome or thrombotic thrombocytopenic purpura. It occurs within a few days to a few months after normal pregnancy and delivery. The characteristics are those of the hemolytic uremic syndrome, and therapy is just as unrewarding.

Initial treatment is the conservative management of acute renal failure. Persistent thrombocytopenia and microangiopathic hemolytic anemia and worsening renal disease with serious hypertension are indications for more radical treatment as for thrombotic thrombocytopenic purpura. Heparin, antiplatelet drugs (dipyridamole, aspirin), and corticosteroids (prednisone) have been employed with some success. Plasmapheresis, prednisone, antiplatelet agents, and vincristine have also been tried.

The disease in adults has a high mortality rate. Relapses are common. Chronic renal failure is a frequent outcome.

Campos A et al: The hemolytic-uremic syndrome. *The Kidney* 1981;**14**:23.

Hayslett JP: Postpartum renal failure. *N Engl J Med* 1985;**312**:1556.

Ponticelli C et al: Hemolytic uremic syndrome in adults. *Arch Intern Med* 1980;**140**:353.

Shumak KH, Rock GA: Therapeutic plasma exchange. *N Engl J Med* 1984;**310**:762.

## DISEASES OF THE RENAL TUBULES & INTERSTITIUM

### 1. ACUTE RENAL FAILURE

#### Essentials of Diagnosis

- Sudden onset of oliguria; urine volume 20–200 mL/d. (Oliguria may not occur.)

- Proteinuria and hematuria; isosthenuria with a specific gravity of 1.010–1.016.
- Anorexia, nausea and vomiting, lethargy, elevation of blood pressure. Signs of uremia.
- Progressive increase in serum urea nitrogen, creatinine, potassium, phosphate, sulfate; decrease in sodium, calcium, bicarbonate.
- Spontaneous recovery in a few days to 6 weeks.

## General Considerations

Acute renal failure is a term applied to a state of sudden cessation of renal function following a variety of insults to normal kidneys. Emphasis has recently been placed on vasomotor constriction of afferent arterioles as the initial lesion—hence the term vasomotor nephropathy. Among the causes of acute renal failure are the following: (1) Toxic agents, eg, carbon tetrachloride, methoxyflurane, sulfonamides, aminoglycoside antibiotics, amphotericin B, mercury bichloride, arsenic, diethylene glycol, and mushroom poisoning. X-ray contrast materials are hazardous in patients with dehydration, renal disease, diabetic nephropathy, liver failure, or multiple myeloma. (2) Traumatic shock due to severe injury, surgical shock, or myocardial infarction, and ischemia associated with surgery on the abdominal aorta (vasomotor nephropathy). (3) Tissue destruction due to crushing injury, rhabdomyolysis, burns, intravascular hemolysis (transurethral resection of the prostate, incompatible blood transfusion). (4) Infectious diseases, eg, leptospirosis, hemorrhagic fever, gram-negative bacteremia with shock, toxic shock syndrome, peritonitis. (5) Disseminated intravascular coagulation. (6) Complications of pregnancy, eg, bilateral cortical necrosis. (7) Immunologic mechanisms induced by methicillin, penicillin, phenytoin, and other drugs.

Return of renal function can be expected, but even with the best treatment the mortality rate is high.

Renal tubular necrosis is the characteristic pathologic finding. In some instances, after exposure to a specific toxin, the proximal tubule may be primarily damaged; and renal tubule cell disintegration and desquamation with collection of debris in the lumens of the tubules are found uniformly throughout both kidneys. In other cases, tubule cell destruction and basement membrane disruption are scattered throughout both kidneys. In cases due to hemolysis or crushing injury, heme or myoglobin casts may be present, but it is unlikely that such casts produce tubule cell destruction. The spotty distribution of the damage caused by ischemic necrosis is consistent with a great reduction in cortical blood flow in addition to a moderate to marked decrease in total renal blood flow. In bilateral cortical necrosis, ischemic infarcts are distributed throughout both kidneys.

## Clinical Findings

The history is critical in identification of the cause. The cardinal sign of acute renal failure is acute reduction of urine output following injury, surgery, a transfusion reaction, or other causes listed above. The daily volume of urine may be reduced to 20–30 mL/d or may be as high as 400–500 mL/d. In some cases, urine volume may always be greater than 600 mL/d. After a few days to 6 weeks of oliguria, the daily urine volume slowly increases. Anorexia, nausea, and lethargy are common symptoms. Other symptoms and signs are related to the causative agent or event.

The course of the disease may be divided into the oliguric and diuretic phases.

**A. Oliguric Phase:** During the oliguric phase, the urine excretion is greatly reduced. The urine contains protein, red cells, epithelial cells, and characteristic "dirty" brown granular casts; and the specific gravity of the urine is usually 1.010–1.016. The rate of catabolism of protein determines the rate of increase of metabolic end products in body fluids. In the presence of injury, rhabdomyolysis, or fever, the blood urea nitrogen and the serum creatinine, potassium, phosphate, sulfate, and organic acids increase rapidly. Typically, because of dilution and intracellular shifts, the serum sodium concentration drops to 120–130 meq/L. As organic acids and phosphate accumulate, serum bicarbonate concentration decreases. Normochromic anemia is common. With prolonged oliguria, signs of uremia appear, with nausea, vomiting, diarrhea, neuromuscular irritability, convulsions, somnolence, and coma. Hypertension frequently develops and may be associated with retinopathy, left heart failure, and encephalopathy. During this phase of the disease, therapy modifies the clinical picture significantly. Overhydration produces signs of water intoxication, with convulsions, edema, and the serious complication of pulmonary edema. Excess saline administration may produce edema and congestive failure. Failure to restrict potassium intake or to employ agents to remove potassium at the proper time may result in hyperkalemia manifested by neuromuscular depression that progresses to paralysis and interference with the cardiac conduction system, resulting in arrhythmias; death may follow respiratory muscle paralysis or cardiac arrest (see p 36). With proper treatment, potassium intoxication is almost always reversible, and death should not occur because of it.

**B. Diuretic Phase:** After a few days to 6 weeks of oliguria, the diuretic phase begins, signifying that the nephrons have recovered to the point that urine excretion is possible. The urine volume usually increases in increments of a few milliliters to 100 mL/d until 300–500 mL/d is excreted, after which the rate of increase in flow is usually more rapid. Rarely, the urine volume increases rapidly during the first day or so of diuresis. Diuresis may be the result of impaired nephron function, with loss of water and electrolytes; but this is uncommon, and true deficits of water, sodium, and potassium seldom occur. More often, diuresis represents an unloading of excess extracellular fluid that has accumulated during the oliguric phase as a result of either overhydration during therapy or unusual metabolic production of water.

Diuresis usually occurs when the total nephron function is still insufficient to excrete nitrogenous metabolic products, potassium, and phosphate, and the concentration of these constituents in the serum may continue to rise for several days after urine volumes exceed 1 L/d. Renal function returns slowly toward normal, and blood chemical findings usually become normal.

## Differential Diagnosis

Because acute glomerulonephritis, collagen disease, acute interstitial nephritis, uric acid nephropathy, myeloma, hepatorenal syndrome, Reye's syndrome, ureteral obstruction due to edema at the ureterovesical junction following ureteral catheterization, ureteral obstruction by neoplasm, bilateral renal artery occlusion due to embolism or aortic dissection, and, rarely, a ruptured bladder may present with symptoms and signs indistinguishable from those of tubular necrosis, appropriate diagnostic procedures (ultrasound examination of kidneys and bladder, radiograph of abdomen, etc) should be employed as suggested by the history and by physical examination. Functional or prerenal azotemia consequent to shock, severe volume depletion, congestive heart failure, pressor agents, or diuretics must be distinguished to assure appropriate immediate therapy.

In the differentiation between acute renal failure and prerenal azotemia, the ability to excrete creatinine and urea and to conserve sodium are useful criteria (Table 15–2).

The loss of normal capacity to excrete creatinine and to conserve sodium indicates acute renal failure. The clinical setting must be carefully assessed, for in chronic renal insufficiency the ability to conserve sodium is lost, and after administration of diuretics sodium excretion is elevated.

## Treatment

**A. Specific Measures:** Immediate treatment of the cause of oliguria is essential.

**1. Decreased renal perfusion**–Diminished circulating blood volume resulting in decreased renal perfusion (prerenal failure) can be ruled out by infusion of 500–1000 mL of 0.9% NaC1 solution and use of a loop diuretic. Treatment in the very early period of acute renal shutdown with mannitol, loop diuretics, or dopamine is controversial.

**2. Shock**–Vigorous measures to restore normal blood pressure levels are mandatory in order to overcome renal ischemia. *Caution:* When it is apparent that tubular necrosis has occurred, fluid volume must be sharply curtailed.

**3. Transfusion reaction**–See Chapter 10.

**4. Obstruction of ureters**–Cystoscopy and catheterization of ureters may be necessary.

**5. Heavy metal poisoning**–Dimercaprol (BAL) may be of use in mercury or arsenic poisoning, although by the time the renal lesion is apparent it may be too late.

**B. General Measures:** Conservative medical management often serves adequately for the uncomplicated case. **Indications for dialysis** include rapidly increasing blood urea nitrogen, serum creatinine, and potassium, and metabolic acidosis often consequent to severe trauma or infection. Overhydration, usually from too vigorous treatment with intravenous solutions, and oliguria lasting 4–5 days are also indications for dialysis. Hemodialysis is more effective, but peritoneal dialysis may be adequate in instances where hemodialysis is not immediately accessible. Aggressive supportive therapy (combating infection, use of hyperalimentation, etc) should accompany treatment by dialysis. Conservative management is summarized below.

**1. Oliguric phase**–The objectives of therapy are to maintain normal body fluid volume and electrolyte concentration, reduce tissue catabolism to a minimum, and prevent infection until healing occurs.

**a. Bed rest**–"Reverse isolation" is indicated to protect the patient from exposure to hospital infections.

**b. Fluids**–Restrict fluids to a basic ration of 400 mL/d for the average adult. Additional fluid may be given to replace unusual losses due to vomiting, diarrhea, sweating, etc. The metabolism of fat, carbohydrate, and protein provides water of combustion; and catabolism of tissues provides intracellular water. These sources must be included in calculations of water balance, thus leaving only a small ration to be provided as "intake" (see ¶ e, below).

**c. Diet**–In order to limit sources of nitrogen, potassium, phosphate, and sulfate, no protein should be given. Glucose, 100–200 g/d, should be given to prevent ketosis and to reduce protein catabolism. Although fat may be given as butter or emulsion orally or intravenously, it is usually better if the patient fulfills caloric needs from existing fat deposits.

The fluid and glucose may be given orally or intravenously. When administered intravenously as a 20–50% glucose solution, the 400 mL of fluid should be given continuously throughout the 24-hour period through an intravenous catheter threaded into a large

**Table 15–2.** Acute renal failure versus prerenal azotemia.

|  | Acute Renal Failure | Prerenal Azotemia |
|---|---|---|
| Urine osmolality (mosm/L) | <350 | >500 |
| Urine/plasma urea | <10 | >20 |
| Urine/plasma creatinine | <20 | >40 |
| Urine Na (meq/L) | >40 | <20 |
| Renal failure index = $\dfrac{U_{Na}}{U/P_{Cr}}$ | >1 | <1 |
| * FENa = $\dfrac{U/P_{Na}}{U/P_{Cr}} \times 100$ | >1 | <1 |

* Excreted fraction of filtered sodium. See Espinel CH: The FENa test: Use in the differential diagnosis of acute renal failure. *JAMA* 1976;**236**:579; and Miller TR et al: Urinary diagnostic indices in acute renal failure: A prospective study. *Ann Intern Med* 1978;**89**:47.

vein to reduce the likelihood of thrombosis. Vitamin B complex and vitamin C should be provided.

For patients on dialysis, parenteral hyperalimentation with a mixture of essential amino acids and nonessential amino acids (particularly those partially synthesized in the kidney) supplemented by glucose and lipid for calories prevents excessive catabolism of tissue and enhances recovery.

**d. Electrolyte replacement**–Electrolyte therapy is not necessary unless it is required to repair clear-cut losses, as in vomiting, diarrhea, etc. *Note:* Potassium must not be administered unless proved deficits exist, and then only with caution.

**e. Observations**–Daily records of fluid intake and output are essential; avoid an indwelling catheter if at all possible. Weight should be recorded daily whenever possible. Because the patient's own tissues are being consumed, weight loss should be about 0.5 kg/d. If weight loss does not occur, too much fluid is being given. Frequent (often daily) measurements of serum electrolytes (especially potassium) and creatinine are essential.

**f. Infection**–Treat vigorously with appropriate antibiotics in doses commensurate with renal failure.

**g. Congestive heart failure**–See discussion in Chapter 8.

**h. Anemia**–A hematocrit of less than 30% is an indication for cautious transfusion with a small volume of packed fresh red blood cells.

**i. Hyperkalemia**–See discussion in Chapter 3.

**j. Uremia**–Hemodialysis and peritoneal dialysis are effective, but they require expert management in a well-equipped hospital. With appropriate facilities, dialysis has proved to be of great value if employed "prophylactically" before serum creatinine reaches 7–8 mg/dL.

**k. Convulsions and encephalopathy**–Seizures are treated as medical emergencies. (See treatment of tonic-clonic seizures, p 575). Hemodialysis may be instituted if the seizure activity is clearly a result of the renal failure or of treatment (eg, overhydration, administration of bicarbonate).

**2. Diuretic phase**–Unless water and electrolyte deficits clearly exist, no attempt should be made to "keep up" with the diuresis; collections of excess water and electrolyte are usually being excreted. Fluid and diet intake can be liberalized as diuresis progresses until a normal daily intake is reached. Protein restriction should be continued until blood urea nitrogen and serum creatinine levels are declining. Infection is still a hazard. Diuresis is occasionally accompanied by sodium retention, hypernatremia, and hyperchloremia associated with confusion, neuromuscular irritability, and coma. When this happens, water and glucose must be given in sufficient quantities to correct hypernatremia. Serum electrolytes and blood urea nitrogen or serum creatinine should be measured frequently.

**Prognosis**

If severe complications of trauma and infection are not present, skillful treatment often will tide the patient over the period of oliguria until spontaneous healing occurs. Death may occur as a result of water intoxication, congestive heart failure, acute pulmonary edema, potassium intoxication, and encephalopathy. With recovery, there often is little residual impairment of renal function.

Miller TR et al: Urinary diagnostic indices in acute renal failure: A prospective study. *Ann Intern Med* 1978;**89**:47.

Schrier RW: Acute renal failure: Pathogenesis, diagnosis, and management. *Hosp Pract* (March) 1981;**16**:93.

Smolens P, Stein JH: Pathophysiology of acute renal failure. *Am J Med* 1981;**70**:479.

## 2. INTERSTITIAL NEPHRITIS

Acute interstitial nephritis may be due to systemic infections from bacteria, viruses, and spirochetes and sensitivity to drugs, including antibiotics (penicillins, cephalosporins, sulfonamides, rifampin, vancomycin), diuretics (thiazides, furosemide), nonsteroidal anti-inflammatory agents, phenindione, allopurinol, cimetidine, and others. Some patients will show other signs of hypersensitivity such as rash, arthralgia, fever, and eosinophilia. Hematuria, proteinuria, and enlargement of the kidneys are commonly demonstrable. Occasionally, acute renal failure may occur. Recovery may be complete.

Chronic interstitial nephritis is characterized by focal or diffuse interstitial fibrosis accompanied by infiltration with inflammatory cells ultimately associated with extensive atrophy of renal tubules. It represents a nonspecific reaction to a variety of causes: analgesic abuse, lead and cadmium toxicity, nephrocalcinosis, urate nephropathy, radiation nephritis, sarcoidosis, Balkan nephritis, and some instances of obstructive uropathy. There are cases in which antitubule basement membrane antibodies have been identified by means of immunofluorescence linear staining of IgG and C3. Most patients with anti-glomerular basement membrane disease (Goodpasture's syndrome) and some with other forms of rapidly progressive glomerulonephritis will have anti-tubular basement membrane disease as well.

Linton AL, Lindsay RM: Drug-induced acute interstitial nephritis. *The Kidney* 1982;**15**:1.

Pusey CD et al: Drug-associated acute interstitial nephritis: Clinical and pathological features and the response to high-dose steroid therapy. *Q J Med* 1983;**52**:194.

## 3. DISORDERS OF PROSTAGLANDIN SYNTHESIS

The roles of prostaglandins $PGE_2$, $PGF_2\alpha$, and $PGI_2$ (prostacyclin) and of $TXA_2$ (thromboxane), all of which have been isolated from the kidney, are only partially understood. There is evidence that prostaglandin biosynthesis is influenced by bradykinin, angiotensin II, catecholamines, glucocorticoids, and nonsteroidal anti-inflammatory drugs. Prostaglandins modify salt and water excretion by their influence on glomerular filtration rate, proximal tubule fluid reabsorption, gradients in concentration of medullary solute, and reabsorption of water and electrolyte in the distal nephron. Prostaglandins mediate release of renin in response to depletion of intravascular volume. Altered prostaglandin metabolism is seen with hypertension, obstructive uropathy, Bartter's syndrome, and disorders of water reabsorption. Nonsteroidal analgesics can produce acute renal failure, nephrotic syndrome, and interstitial nephritis, all of which may be in part the result of inhibition of prostaglandin synthesis.

Levenson DJ, Simmons CE Jr, Brenner BM: Arachidonic acid metabolism, prostaglandins and the kidney. *Am J Med* 1982;**72**:354.

## 4. DISORDERS RELATED TO NONSTEROIDAL ANTI-INFLAMMATORY DRUGS

The kidney can be adversely affected by nonsteroidal anti-inflammatory drugs (NSAIDs). Renal damage may be structural or functional. Structural changes may produce acute or chronic renal failure, nephrotic syndrome, interstitial nephritis, and renal papillary necrosis. Functional changes include abnormal metabolism of water, sodium, and potassium.

Diminished prostaglandin synthesis induced by NSAIDs is the likely cause of the associated kidney disease. The offending drugs include salicylates (acetylated and nonacetylated), oxicams, and the derivatives of indoleacetic acid, propionic acid, anthranilic acid, and pyrazolone.

NSAIDs are particularly dangerous in conditions in which blood volume or effective arterial volume is reduced: congestive heart failure, nephrotic syndrome, diuretic use, and salt depletion. Patients with chronic renal disease may suffer further decrease of kidney function, which may not be reversible.

Papillary necrosis with interstitial nephritis is a serious complication of NSAID use. Associated urinary tract infection, particularly in patients with diabetes mellitus, probably plays a role in the setting of long-term intake of large doses of analgesic drugs.

Water metabolism is regulated in part by renal prostaglandins. NSAIDs inhibit prostaglandin synthesis and thereby reduce excretion of free water, and this may lead to hyponatremia (see Chapter 3). Simultaneous use of thiazides may exaggerate this effect.

Sodium retention is a common side effect of treatment with NSAIDs. Mild to massive edema may occur. Potassium excretion is often reduced; when this occurs in the setting of mild renal insufficiency, hyperkalemia can result. NSAIDs can blunt renin activity and ultimately reduce aldosterone production, which will in turn enhance potassium retention.

Blackshear JL, Davidman M, Stillman MT: Identification of risk for renal insufficiency from nonsteroidal anti-inflammatory drugs. *Arch Intern Med* 1983;**143**:1130.

Carmichael J, Shankel SW: Effects of nonsteroidal anti-inflammatory drugs on prostaglandins and renal function. *Am J Med* 1985;**78**:992.

Clive DM, Stoff JS: Renal syndromes associated with nonsteroidal antiinflammatory drugs. *N Engl J Med* 1984;**310**:563.

Dunn MJ: Clinical effects of prostaglandins in renal disease. *Hosp Pract* (March) 1984;**19**:99.

Eknoyan G et al: Renal papillary necrosis: An update. *Medicine* 1982;**61**:55.

Garella S, Matarese RA: Renal effects of prostaglandins and clinical adverse effects of nonsteroidal anti-inflammatory agents. *Medicine* 1984;**63**:165.

Hartman GW et al: Analgesia-associated nephropathy. *JAMA* 1984;**251**:1734.

Nanra RS: Renal effects of antipyretic analgesics: Proceedings of a symposium on antipyretic analgesic therapy. *Am J Med* 1983;**75**:70.

## 5. URIC ACID NEPHROPATHY

See section on gout, above.

Crystals of urate produce an interstitial inflammatory reaction. Urate may precipitate out in acid urine in the calices or distally in the ureters to form uric acid stones. Patients with myeloproliferative disease under treatment may develop hyperuricemia and are subject to occlusion of the upper urinary tract by uric acid crystals. Alkalinization of the urine and a liberal fluid intake will help prevent crystal formation. Allopurinol is a useful drug to prevent hyperuricemia and hyperuricosuria.

## 6. MYELOMATOSIS

Features of myelomatosis that contribute to renal disease include proteinuria (including filtrable Bence Jones protein and κ and λ chains), with precipitation in the tubules leading to accumulation of abnormal proteins in the tubule cells; amyloidosis; hypercalcemia; and, occasionally, increase in viscosity of the blood associated with macroglobulinemia. A Fanconi-like syndrome may develop.

Plugging of tubules, giant cell reaction around tubules, tubular atrophy, and, occasionally, the accumulation of amyloid are evident on examination of renal tissue.

Renal failure may occur acutely or may develop slowly depending on the cause. Hemodialysis may rescue the patient during efforts to control the myeloma with chemical agents.

Cohen DJ et al: Acute renal failure in patients with multiple myeloma. *Am J Med* 1984;**76**:247.

## HEREDITARY RENAL DISEASES

The importance of inheritance and the familial incidence of disease warrants inclusion of the classification of hereditary renal diseases suggested by Perkoff. Although relatively uncommon in the population at large, hereditary disease must be recognized to permit early diagnosis and treatment in other family members and to prepare the way for genetic counseling.

Many of the renal diseases that can occur as heritable abnormalities are listed in Table 31–1. Selected diseases are discussed briefly below.

## 1. HEREDITARY CHRONIC NEPHRITIS

Evidence of the disease usually appears in childhood, with episodes of hematuria often following an upper respiratory infection. Renal insufficiency commonly develops in males but only rarely in females. Survival beyond age 40 is rare.

In many families, deafness and abnormalities of the eyes accompany the renal disease (Alport's syndrome). Another form of the disease is accompanied by polyneuropathy. Infection of the urinary tract is a common complication.

The anatomic features in some cases resemble proliferative glomerulonephritis; in others, there is thickening of the glomerular basement membrane or podocyte proliferation and thickening of Bowman's capsule. In a few cases, there are fat-filled cells (foam cells) in the interstitial tissue or in the glomeruli.

Laboratory findings are commensurate with existing renal function.

Treatment is symptomatic.

## 2. CYSTIC DISEASES OF THE KIDNEY

Congenital structural anomalies of the kidney must always be considered in any patient with hypertension, pyelonephritis, or renal insufficiency. The manifestations of structural renal abnormalities are related to the superimposed disease, but management and prognosis are modified by the structural anomaly.

### Polycystic Kidneys

Polycystic kidney disease is familial (autosomal dominant) and often involves not only the kidney but the liver and pancreas as well.

The formation of cysts in the cortex of the kidney is thought to result from failure of union of the collecting tubules and convoluted tubules of some nephrons. New cysts do not form, but those present enlarge and, by pressure, cause destruction of adjacent tissue. Cysts may be found in the liver and pancreas. The incidence of cerebral vessel ("berry") aneurysms is higher than normal.

Cases of polycystic disease are discovered during the investigation of hypertension, by diagnostic study in patients presenting with pyelonephritis or hematuria, or by investigating the families of patients with polycystic disease. At times, flank pain due to hemorrhage into a cyst will call attention to a kidney disor-

der. Otherwise, the symptoms and signs are those commonly seen in hypertension or renal insufficiency. On physical examination the enlarged, irregular kidneys are easily palpable.

The urine may contain leukocytes and red cells. With bleeding into the cysts, there may also be bleeding into the urinary tract. The blood chemical findings reflect the degree of renal insufficiency. Examination by echography or x-ray shows the enlarged kidneys, and urography demonstrates the classic elongated calices and renal pelves stretched over the surface of the cysts.

No specific therapy is available, and surgical interference is contraindicated unless ureteral obstruction is produced by an adjacent cyst. Hypertension, infection, and uremia are treated in the conventional manner.

Because persons with polycystic kidneys may live in reasonable comfort with slowly advancing uremia, it is difficult to determine when renal transplantation is in order. Hemodialysis can extend the life of the patient, but recurrent bleeding and continuous pain indicate the need for a transplant, which carries an excellent prognosis.

Although the disease may become symptomatic in childhood or early adult life, it usually is discovered in the fourth or fifth decades. Unless fatal complications of hypertension or urinary tract infections are present, uremia develops very slowly, and patients live longer than with other causes of renal insufficiency.

### Cystic Disease of the Renal Medulla

Two syndromes have become more frequent as their diagnostic features have become better known.

**Medullary cystic disease** is a familial disease (either autosomal dominant or recessive) that may become symptomatic during adolescence. Anemia is usually the initial manifestation, but azotemia, acidosis, and hyperphosphatemia soon become evident. Hypertension may develop. The urine is not remarkable, although there is often an inability to produce a concentrated urine. Many small cysts are scattered through the renal medulla. Renal transplantation is indicated by the usual criteria for the operation.

**Sponge kidney** is asymptomatic and is discovered by the characteristic appearance of the urogram. Enlargement of the papillae and calices and small cavities within the pyramids are demonstrated by the contrast media in the excretory urogram. Many small calculi often occupy the cysts, and infection may be troublesome. Life expectancy is not affected, and only symptomatic therapy for ureteral impaction of a stone or for infection is required.

Gardner KD Jr (editor): *Cystic Diseases of the Kidney*. Wiley, 1976.

## 3. ANOMALIES OF FUNCTION OF THE PROXIMAL TUBULE

### Defects of Amino Acid Reabsorption

**A. Congenital Cystinuria:** Increased excretion of cystine results in the formation of cystine calculi in the urinary tract. Ornithine, arginine, and lysine are also excreted in abnormally large quantities. There is also a defect in absorption of these amino acids in the jejunum. Nonopaque stones should be examined chemically to provide a specific diagnosis.

Maintain a high urine volume by giving a large fluid intake. Maintain the urine pH above 7 by giving sodium bicarbonate and sodium citrate plus acetazolamide (Diamox) at bedtime to ensure an alkaline night urine. In refractory cases, a low-methionine (cystine precursor) diet may be necessary. Penicillamine has proved useful in some cases.

**B. Aminoaciduria:** Hereditary defects of renal tubule function or defects of amino acid metabolism are manifested by loss of a variety of amino acids. Failure to thrive and the presence of other tubular deficits suggest the diagnosis.

There is no treatment.

**C. Hepatolenticular Degeneration (Wilson's Disease):** In this congenital familial disease, aminoaciduria is associated with cirrhosis of the liver and neurologic manifestations.

### Multiple Defects of Tubular Function

**A. De Toni-Fanconi-Debré Syndrome:** Aminoaciduria, phosphaturia, glycosuria, and a variable degree of renal tubular acidosis characterize this syndrome. Osteomalacia is a prominent clinical feature; other clinical and laboratory manifestations are associated with specific tubular defects described above.

The proximal segment of the renal tubule is replaced by a thin tubular structure constituting the swan-neck deformity. The proximal segment also is shortened to less than half the normal length.

Treatment consists of replacing cation deficits (especially potassium), correcting acidosis with bicarbonate or citrate, replacing phosphate loss with isotonic neutral phosphate (mono- and disodium salts) solution, and a liberal calcium intake. Vitamin D is usually helpful, but the dose used must be controlled by monitoring serum calcium and phosphate.

**B. Acquired Fanconi Syndrome:** Defects in tubular reabsorption resembling those of the Fanconi syndrome can be induced by heavy metal poisoning (cadmium, lead, copper, uranium, mercury), by a degradation product of tetracycline, by cresol poisoning, by galactosemia, by renal tubule damage in myeloma and by tubulointerstitial disease.

Treatment is directed at the primary cause and at correction of electrolyte abnormalities.

### Defects of Phosphorus & Calcium Absorption

**A. Vitamin D-Resistant Rickets:** Excessive loss of phosphorus and calcium results in rickets or osteomalacia poorly responsive to vitamin D therapy. Treatment consists of giving large doses of vitamin D and dietary phosphorus and calcium supplementation.

**B. Pseudohypoparathyroidism:** See Chapter 18.

### Defects of Glucose Absorption (Renal Glycosuria)

Relative inability to reabsorb glucose means that glycosuria is present when blood glucose levels are normal. Ketosis is not present. The glucose tolerance test response is usually normal. In some instances, renal glycosuria may precede the onset of true diabetes mellitus.

There is no treatment for renal glycosuria.

### Defects of Glucose & Phosphate Absorption (Glycosuric Rickets)

The symptoms and signs are those of rickets or osteomalacia, with weakness, pain, or discomfort of the legs and spine, and tetany. The bones become deformed, with bowing of the weight-bearing long bones, kyphoscoliosis, and, in children, signs of rickets. Radiography shows markedly decreased density of the bone, with pseudofracture lines and other deformities. Nephrocalcinosis may occur with excessive phosphaturia, and renal insufficiency may follow. Urinary calcium and phosphorus are increased, and glycosuria is present. Serum glucose is normal, serum calcium normal or low, serum phosphorus low, and serum alkaline phosphatase elevated.

Treatment consists of giving large doses of vitamin D and dietary phosphorus and calcium supplementation.

## 4. RENAL TUBULAR ACIDOSIS

Both the proximal tubule and the distal tubule can secrete hydrogen ion ($H^+$) and reclaim bicarbonate ($HCO_3^-$) from the luminal fluid. Normally, the preponderance of filtered $HCO_3^-$ is reclaimed in the proximal tubule, leaving a smaller demand on the distal segment of the nephron to provide hydrogen for reabsorption of a small amount of $HCO_3^-$ and excretion of metabolic acids.

### Proximal Renal Tubular Acidosis (Type II)

The defect in $H^+$ secretion in the proximal tubule results in a decrease in absorption of filtered bicarbonate, loss of bicarbonate in the urine, and decreased concentration of bicarbonate in extracellular fluid. Secretion of $H^+$ in the distal tubule is unimpaired.

As plasma bicarbonate concentration diminishes, less bicarbonate is filtered, and ultimately an equilibrium is reached. This sets a limit on bicarbonate loss, and the resultant acidosis is only moderate. Accompanying the limitation of hydrogen ion secretion are increased potassium secretion into the urine and retrieval of $Cl^-$ instead of $HCO_3^-$. The acidosis is therefore associated with hypokalemia and hyperchloremia. Because $Cl^-$ replaces $HCO_3^-$ in the extracellular fluid, there is no anion gap. Hypercalciuria is moderate, and stone formation is uncommon. Transport of glucose, amino acids, phosphate, and urate may be deficient as well and may result in the Fanconi syndrome (see above).

Proximal renal tubular acidosis may be genetic in origin. It is transiently seen with acetazolamide therapy, use of outdated tetracycline, and exposure to some heavy metals (eg, lead). Proximal renal tubular acidosis may occur when the kidney is involved with medullary cystic disease or multiple myeloma. (See also de Toni-Fanconi-Debré Syndrome, above.)

The pH of the urine is high except if acidosis becomes severe when bicarbonate disappears from the urine and the pH drops to a lower limit of 5.5–5.4.

When treatment is required for the acidosis, it consists of replacement with large amounts of $HCO_3^-$ and replacement of wasted $K^+$. Bicarbonate in doses of 6–15 mmol/kg/d may be required; some of this should be $KHCO_3$. Shohl's solution, a mixture of sodium citrate and citric acid (1 mL = 1 mmol $HCO_3^-$), in doses of 20–50 mL 3 times a day, may be substituted for part of the $HCO_3^-$ requirement. A combination of hydrochlorothiazide, to produce slight volume depletion with resultant increased $HCO_3^-$ reabsorption, plus spironolactone, to reduce $K^+$ excretion, has been employed to ameliorate proximal renal tubular acidosis.

## Distal Renal Tubular Acidosis (Type I)

The distal tubule cells, like those of the proximal tubule, generate carbonic acid from $CO_2$ and $H_2O$ and retrieve the bicarbonate by secreting $H^+$ to exchange for $Na^+$ in the tubular fluid. $H^+$ is excreted with acid anion and buffers in the urine and is also combined with $NH_3$ to form $NH_4^+$, an additional cation that accompanies acid anion in the excreted urine.

The defect in distal renal tubular acidosis is either a defect in secretion of $H^+$ or an inability to transport $H^+$ against a steep concentration gradient between extracellular fluid and urine in the terminal segments of the nephron (eg, plasma pH 7.4 = $4 \times 10^{-8}$ molar $[H^+]$ versus urine pH 4.5 = $32 \times 10^{-6}$ molar $[H^+]$) or both of these. The defect persists no matter how severe the acidosis, and diagnosis depends on the observation that in the presence of acidosis, the urine pH remains greater than 5.5. Potassium excretion is heightened by failure of $H^+$ secretion and by activation of the secretion of aldosterone; hypokalemia is often apparent clinically. Hypercalciuria with renal stone and nephrocalcinosis and metabolic bone disease are seen in severe and long-standing cases. There is an incomplete form of distal renal tubular acidosis that is revealed only when it is necessary to excrete a large acid load. To prove that this incomplete form of renal tubular acidosis exists, 0.1 g of $NH_4Cl$ per kilogram is administered orally. Within

6–8 hours, arterial blood pH should be less than 7.35, plasma bicarbonate should be less than 20 mmol/L, and the urine pH should remain greater than 5.5.

Distal renal tubular acidosis may be genetically transmitted. It can occur in association with sickle cell anemia, a variety of autoimmune diseases, chronic interstitial nephritis and urolithiasis, cirrhosis of the liver, diseases in which nephrocalcinosis occurs, and therapy with amphotericin B or analgesics.

Treatment of the acute emergency of severe metabolic acidosis includes vigorous bicarbonate replacement supplemented with adequate $K^+$. The chronic case requires lifelong therapy with enough $NaHCO_3$ or Shohl's solution to neutralize the metabolic acids that must be excreted (50 mmol/d or more) and to correct hypercalciuria. Potassium loss will usually diminish enough so that $K^+$ replacement is not required, but in some cases, potassium intake may have to be increased.

Appropriate therapy will protect against development of nephrocalcinosis, azotemia, and metabolic bone disease.

## Type IV Renal Tubular Acidosis

Recognition of type IV renal tubular acidosis is increasingly common as the clinical manifestations become known. It occurs with hyporeninemic hypoaldosteronism when moderate renal insufficiency is associated with diabetes mellitus; with chronic renal insufficiency from many causes; or as an adverse effect of drugs such as spironolactone (especially with cirrhosis) and nonsteroidal anti-inflammatory agents. It also occurs with normal aldosterone activity when there is chronic renal insufficiency (rarely) or urinary obstruction. The characteristics of type IV renal tubular acidosis include impairment of renal acidification accompanied by reduced renal clearance of potassium, which results in hyperkalemia and acidosis. The disorder is related to lack of aldosterone or inability of aldosterone to stimulate $H^+$ secretion at the cation exchange portion of the distal tubule.

Treatment with fludrocortisone in doses that do not induce hypervolemia and hypertension (0.1–0.3 mg/d) may correct acidosis and hyperkalemia. Alternatively, reducing potassium intake, use of potassium-binding resins, and use of loop diuretics may correct the hyperkalemia. Acidosis may be corrected by small doses of sodium bicarbonate (2 meq/kg/d).

## 5. ANOMALIES OF THE DISTAL TUBULE

### Excess Potassium Secretion (Potassium "Wastage" Syndrome)

Excessive renal secretion or loss of potassium may occur in 4 situations: (1) chronic renal insufficiency with diminished $H^+$ secretion; (2) renal tubular acidosis and de Toni-Fanconi syndrome, with cation loss resulting from diminished $H^+$ and $NH_4^+$ secretion; (3) aldosteronism and hyperadrenocorticism; and (4) excessive tubular secretion of potassium, the cause of which is unknown. Hypokalemia indicates that the deficit is severe. Muscle weakness, metabolic alkalosis, and polyuria with dilute urine are signs of hypokalemia (see Chapter 3).

## Defects of Water Absorption (Renal Diabetes Insipidus)

Nephrogenic diabetes insipidus occurs more frequently in males. Unresponsiveness to antidiuretic hormone is the key to differentiation from pituitary diabetes insipidus.

In addition to congenital refractoriness to antidiuretic hormone, obstructive uropathy, lithium, methoxyflurane, and demeclocycline may also render the tubule refractory. Impaired water reabsorption may be present with sickle cell anemia, medullary cystic disease, hypokalemia, and hypercalcemia.

Symptoms are related to an inability to reabsorb water, with resultant polyuria and polydipsia. The daily urine volume approaches 12 L, and osmolality and specific gravity are low. Atonic bladder and hydronephrosis occur frequently.

Treatment consists primarily of an adequate water intake. Chlorothiazide may ameliorate the diabetes; the mechanism of action is unknown, but the drug may act by increasing isosmotic reabsorption in the proximal segment of the tubule secondary to volume contraction.

## 6. UNSPECIFIED RENAL TUBULAR ABNORMALITIES

In idiopathic hypercalciuria, decreased reabsorption of calcium predisposes to the formation of renal calculi. Serum calcium and phosphorus are normal. Urine calcium excretion is high; urine phosphorus excretion is low.

Hruska KA, Ban D: Renal tubular acidosis. *Arch Intern Med* 1982;**142**:1909.
Mattern WD: Renal tubular acidosis. *The Kidney* 1982;**15**:11.

## 7. CONGENITAL ANOMALIES

### Renal Agenesis

Occasionally, one kidney (usually the left) is congenitally absent. The remaining kidney is hypertrophied. Before performing a nephrectomy for any reason, it is mandatory to prove the patient has a second kidney.

### Horseshoe Kidney

A band of renal tissue or of fibrous tissue may join the 2 kidneys. Associated abnormalities of the ureterocaliceal system predispose to pyelonephritis, as does hydronephrosis resulting from ureteral obstruction by aberrant vessels.

### Ectopic Kidney

The kidney may occupy a site in the pelvis, and the ureter may be shorter than normal. Infection is common in ectopic kidneys compromised by ureteral obstruction or urinary reflux.

### Nephroptosis

Unusual mobility of the kidney permits it to move from its normal position to a lower one. The incidence of ureteral occlusion due to movement of a kidney is extremely low.

### Megaloureter & Hydronephrosis

These anatomic abnormalities may occur congenitally but are more commonly the result of vesicoureteral urinary reflux.

Kissane JM: Congenital malformations. Page 83 in: *Pathology of the Kidney*, 3rd ed. Heptinstall RH (editor). Little, Brown, 1983.

## 8. RENAL DISEASE INCIDENT TO OTHER DISEASES

Abnormalities of renal function occur with other diseases and may be of therapeutic and prognostic importance. In sickle cell anemia, circulatory changes resulting from sickling and aggregation of red cells contribute to decreased concentrating ability, a defect in acidification of urine, hematuria, renal infarction, glomerulopathy, papillary necrosis, and renal failure. With acute pancreatitis, acute renal failure may occur in the absence of shock. In hepatorenal syndrome, severe renal failure may appear with cirrhosis of the liver and ascites or with severe jaundice of either parenchymatous or obstructive origin. Limited space precludes an adequate discussion. Acute renal failure in pregnancy occurs with toxemia, intrauterine hemorrhage, and complications of abortion and in the immediate postpartum period (hemolytic-uremic syndrome).

Brenner BM, Rector FC Jr: *The Kidney*, 3rd ed. Saunders, 1986.
Wong PY et al: The hepatorenal syndrome. (Clinical Conference.) *Gastroenterology* 1979;**77**:1326.

# INFECTIONS OF THE URINARY TRACT

*Ernest Jawetz, MD, PhD*

The term urinary tract infection denotes a wide variety of clinical entities in which the common denominator is the presence of a significantly large number of microorganisms in any portion of the urinary tract. Microorganisms may be evident only in the urine (bacteriuria), or there may be evidence of infection of an organ, eg, urethritis, prostatitis, cystitis, pyelonephritis. At any given time, any one of these organs may be asymptomatic or symptomatic. Infection in any part of the urinary tract may spread to any other part of the tract.

Symptomatic urinary tract infection may be acute or chronic. The term relapse implies recurrence of infection with the same organism; the term reinfection implies infection with another organism.

## Pathogenesis

Urine secreted by normal kidneys is sterile until it reaches the distal urethra. Bacteria can reach the urinary tract by the ascending route or by hematogenous spread. The latter occurs during bacteremia (eg, with staphylococci) and results in abscess formation in the cortex or the perirenal fat. Far commoner is ascending infection, where bacteria are introduced into the urethra (from fecal flora on the perineum or the vaginal vestibule, or by instrumentation) and travel up the urinary tract to reach the bladder, ureter, or renal pelvis. The most important factor in aiding or perpetuating ascending infection is anatomic or functional obstruction to free urine flow. Free flow, large urine volume, complete emptying of the bladder, and acid pH are important antibacterial defenses.

## Age & Sex Distribution of Urinary Tract Infection

In infants, urinary tract infection occurs more frequently in boys than in girls, in keeping with a higher incidence of obstructive anomalies of the urinary tract. After the first year of life, urinary tract infection is more frequent in girls because the female urethra is short and because the vaginal vestibule can become contaminated with fecal flora. In surveys of schoolchildren, only 0.05% of boys have bacteriuria, whereas at least 2% of girls do. In later life, urinary tract infection is rare among men until the age of prostatic hypertrophy (over 40), but there is a regular increase in incidence among women until age 70, when about 10% of women have urinary tract infection. There is some correlation of the incidence of urinary tract infection with sexual activity in women, as well as with parity.

## Infecting Microorganisms

Virtually any microorganism introduced into the urinary tract may cause urinary tract infection. However, the vast majority of cases of urinary tract infection are caused by aerobic members of the fecal flora, especially *Escherichia* (*E coli* O serotypes 4, 6, and 75 are especially common), *Enterobacter, Klebsiella,* enterococci, *Pseudomonas,* and *Proteus.* Other organisms (eg, *Staphylococcus saprophyticus*) occasionally appear in spontaneous urinary tract infection, but their significance must be assessed as described below. Infections with strict anaerobes are very rare. Viruses may cause immune complex nephritis but—except for adenovirus type 11 in hemorrhagic cystitis of children—do not cause urinary tract infections. Chlamydiae, mycoplasmas, and other organisms causing urethritis, vaginitis, and other genital tract disorders are listed below.

## Significant Bacteriuria

The concept of significant bacteriuria is basic to the proper interpretation of urine cultures. Urine secreted by the normal kidney is sterile and remains so while it travels to the bladder. However, the normal urethra has a microbial flora, and any voided urine in normal persons may therefore contain thousands of bacteria per milliliter derived from this normal flora. To differentiate this smaller number of microorganisms from the larger number commonly found in infections of the urinary tract, it is essential to count the number of bacteria in fresh, properly collected specimens by appropriate methods (quantitative culture). In general, active urinary tract infections are characterized by more than 100,000 bacteria per milliliter. If such numbers are found in 2 consecutive specimens and if the bacteria are of a single type, there is more than a 95% chance that an active infection is present. On the other hand, a significant proportion of acutely dysuric women have pyuria with only $10^3–10^5$ bacteria per milliliter at times but respond promptly to antibacterial treatment. In persons who chronically show low-grade bacteriuria, suprapubic aspiration may help in diagnosis.

## Pathology

Acute urinary tract infection shows inflammation of any part of the tract and sometimes intense hyperemia or even bleeding of the mucous membranes. The prominent lesion in the kidney is acute inflammation of the interstitial tissue, which may progress to frank suppuration and patchy necrosis. Papillary necrosis (eg, in diabetics) may lead to slough of papillae and ureteral obstruction. Recurrent urinary tract infection may cause only minimal changes or progressively more severe scarring in any part of the tract. Chronic pyelonephritis may lead to widespread fibrosis and scarring of functional cortical and medullary tissue, resulting in renal insufficiency; it appears unlikely that repeated urinary tract infection causes renal insufficiency unless there is concomitant obstruction. Chronic interstitial nephritis may result from bacterial infection or from other causes (eg, hypersensitivity, vasculitis, use of analgesics).

## Collection of Urine for Culture

**A. Voided Midstream Specimen:** This is the optimal method, involving no risk to the patient. The urethral meatus or vaginal vestibule is cleansed, the labia are spread, and the first part of the stream is discarded. The mid part of the stream is aseptically collected in a sterile container.

**B. Specimen Obtained by Catheterization:** Each urethral catheter insertion carries a 1–2% risk of introducing microorganisms into the bladder and thus initiating urinary tract infection. Results of quantitative culture from a single catheterized urine specimen yielding more than 100,000 bacteria of a single species per milliliter of urine indicate that active urinary tract infection is present. In persons with indwelling urethral catheters, specimens must be obtained by aseptic needle aspiration of urine through the catheter wall, *not* by disconnecting the closed system.

**C. Specimen Obtained by Suprapubic Aspiration:** While the bladder is distended, the suprapubic skin is aseptically prepared, and a sterile needle is then thrust into the bladder. This permits aspiration of bladder urine free from urethral contamination. It is especially useful in infants (from whom satisfactory specimens for culture may be difficult to obtain) and in patients with equivocal counts on several occasions. However, this procedure is technically more difficult in adults; it should rarely be necessary.

## Examination of Urine

Urine must be cultured or examined microscopically within 1 hour of collection or after no more than 18 hours of refrigeration. Urine is a good culture medium for many microorganisms, and growth can occur at room temperature.

**A. Microscopic Examination:** A drop of fresh urine or a drop of resuspended sediment from centrifuged fresh urine is placed on a microscope slide, covered with a cover glass, and examined with the high-dry objective under reduced illumination. The prevalence of leukocytes is noted. The presence of more than 10 bacteria (often motile) per field in the unstained specimen suggests a bacteria count of more than 100,000/mL of urine. Smears may also be made from fresh urine, stained with Gram's stain, and examined under the oil immersion objective. Three bacteria or more per field in such stains suggest infection. By immunofluorescence, bacteria in urine are coated with immunoglobulin if they are derived from tissue infection (especially pyelonephritis, prostatitis) but usually are not so coated if the infection is limited to the outflow system (cystitis, urethritis). This procedure is expensive, however, and rarely used in routine cases.

**B. Urine Culture:** With a calibrated loop, undiluted urine and urine diluted 1:100 are spread on eosin-methylene blue and blood agar plates. After incubation, numbers of colonies are estimated and multiplied by the dilution factor to yield the bacterial count per milliliter. A number of simplified semiquantitative culture methods are available that are readily performed in the physician's office at nominal cost. The dip-slide method and its several variations involve dipping an agar-coated slide or similar device into fresh urine, incubating it, and then comparing the resultant growth with optical density standards.

**C. Chemical Tests of Urine:** The presence and number of bacteria can also be estimated by various chemical tests that rely on the enzymatic activity of viable bacteria, eg, the reduction of nitrate. These indirect tests are much less reliable than tests employing quantitative estimates of bacterial growth.

**D. Identification of Microorganisms:** In most cases of acute urinary tract infection, detailed identification of the etiologic organism may not be required. However, in chronic or recurrent urinary tract infection, identification of the organism by standard microbiologic methods is desirable. Antimicrobial drug susceptibility tests are not needed in the first attack of urinary tract infection. Most of these infections are due to coliform organisms and are often treated with sulfonamide, ampicillin, or amoxicillin. In chronic or recurrent urinary tract infection, antimicrobial drug susceptibility tests are needed. It must be kept in mind that many drugs appear in the urine in very high concentration, whereas "standard" disk tests indicate susceptibility only to levels achieved in blood.

## ACUTE URINARY TRACT INFECTION (Urethritis, Cystitis, Pyelonephritis)

### Clinical Findings

**A. Lower Tract Involvement (Urethritis, Cystitis):**

**1. Symptoms and signs**–Manifestations include burning pain on urination, often with turbid, foul-smelling, or dark urine, frequency, and suprapubic or lower abdominal discomfort. There are usually no positive physical findings unless the upper tract is involved also.

**2. Laboratory findings**–Microscopic examination of a properly collected urine specimen usually shows significant bacteriuria and pyuria and occasionally hematuria. Bacteriuria may be confirmed by dipslide or similar test.

**B. Upper Tract Involvement (Pyelonephritis):**

**1. Symptoms and signs**–Findings include headache, malaise, vomiting, chills and fever, costovertebral angle pain and tenderness, and abdominal pain. The absence of upper tract signs does not exclude bacterial invasion of the upper tract, however.

**2. Laboratory findings**–Significant bacteriuria is often accompanied by proteinuria and pyuria. The bacteria in the urine are often coated with immunoglobulin, as revealed by immunofluorescence. Leukocytosis is common, with a marked shift to the left. Blood culture is only rarely positive.

### Differential Diagnosis

Acute urinary tract infection may occasionally present as an "acute abdomen," acute pancreatitis, or pneumonia. In all of these circumstances, the presence of significant bacteriuria usually establishes the diagnosis. On the other hand, dysuria, frequency, nocturia, and lower abdominal pain may be due to traumatic cystitis, the "urethral" or "bladder" syndrome, especially in sexually active women. It may also represent vaginitis ("vaginosis"); urethritis; cervicitis attributable to *Trichomonas, Gardnerella, mixed anaerobes, Chlamydia, Neisseria,* or *Ureaplasma.*

## Prevention

Certain women have a high rate of urinary reinfection, sometimes related to sexual activity. In the latter situation, one or two doses of an effective antimicrobial (eg, trimethoprim-sulfamethoxazole, ampicillin) taken after intercourse tend to prevent establishment of infection. In other women, recurrences can be greatly reduced if the patient takes trimethoprim-sulfamethoxazole, one tablet 3 times weekly or one-half tablet daily at bedtime for months.

In patients who must have an indwelling catheter postoperatively and in whom closed sterile drainage is established, the onset of bacteriuria is delayed if suitable antimicrobial drugs are given during the first 3 days after insertion. Thereafter, there is no benefit.

## Treatment

### A. Specific Measures:

**1. First attack of urinary tract infection–**For uncomplicated acute symptomatic cystitis in nonpregnant women, previously untreated, a single dose of sulfisoxazole, 1 g, or of amoxicillin, 500 mg—or 2 tablets of trimethoprim 80 mg plus sulfamethoxazole 400 twice in 1 day— is effective treatment in 80–90% of cases. Alternatively, the administration of sulfisoxazole, 4 g/d, ampicillin, 2–4 g/d, cephalexin, 2–4 g/d, or trimethoprim-sulfamethoxazole, 2–4 tablets daily for 1–3 days, may be effective. Acute infection in men or infections suggestive of upper tract involvement should be treated with similar drugs for 7–10 days. If symptoms have not improved and the urine has not cleared as shown by microscopy on day 4 of treatment, reexamine the urine for possible resistant microorganisms. Follow-up at 2 and 6 weeks after treatment is stopped should show absence of bacteriuria; otherwise, retreat. All men with urinary tract infections should be investigated for obstructive uropathy.

**2. Recurrence of urinary tract infection–**In this situation, an antimicrobial drug is selected on the basis of antimicrobial susceptibility tests of cultured organisms. The drug is administered for 10–14 days in doses sufficient to maintain high urine levels. Reexamine the urine 2 and 6 weeks after treatment is stopped.

**3. Second recurrence, or failure of bacteriuria to be suppressed–**Women should be investigated for possible obstruction, reflux, and localization of infection in the upper or lower tract. Men with recurrent urinary tract infection and no obstruction are likely to have a prostatic focus, and a 12- to 20-week trial of trimethoprim-sulfamethoxazole or ampicillin is indicated.

**B. General Measures:** Forcing fluids may relieve signs and symptoms. Analgesics may be required briefly.

## Prognosis

Initial attacks of acute urinary tract infection, in the absence of obstruction, tend to subside with treatment or spontaneously. The symptoms and bacteriuria often disappear. This is not true in recurrent or chronic urinary tract infection. About 20% of pregnant women with asymptomatic bacteriuria in the first trimester develop symptomatic pyelonephritis later in pregnancy.

## CHRONIC URINARY TRACT INFECTION (Cystitis, Pyelonephritis)

### Essentials of Diagnosis

- Recurrent episodes of lower or upper tract involvement.
- Absence of symptoms or signs referable to the urinary tract, but persistent asymptomatic bacteriuria.
- Obstruction or other anatomic abnormality in the urinary tract is consistently found in men, occasionally in women.
- Impairment of renal function rare unless obstruction is present.

### General Considerations

Chronic or recurrent episodes of urinary tract infection usually produce no permanent harm unless obstruction is present. In these patients, chronic bacterial pyelonephritis may progress to inflammation of interstitial tissue, scarring, atrophy, and, rarely, progressive renal failure. In most patients with these pathologic findings, ''chronic pyelonephritis'' is in fact not caused by infection but instead represents interstitial nephritis of immunologic or toxic cause. Occasionally, chronic infection is due to a unilateral structural abnormality (eg, ureteral stricture), and nephrectomy may be curative. With bilateral nephritis, chronic suppression of infection may stabilize renal function. Some women have chronic bacteremia which is asymptomatic; in the absence of anatomic abnormalities, the prognosis for preservation of renal function appears to be good.

### Clinical Findings

**A. Symptoms and Signs:** There are often no positive clinical findings in chronic urinary tract infection except significant bacteriuria. There may be episodes of recurrent acute urinary tract infection with symptoms referable to the lower or to the upper urinary tract. Hypertension and anemia appear only in the late stages of chronic pyelonephritis.

Whenever chronic bacteriuria is discovered, it is mandatory to perform a complete urologic study, including excretory urograms or renal ultrasonography, cystograms, and voiding cystourethrograms, followed by procedures to localize the source of bacteriuria to one or both sides and to the lower or upper tract. Surgical correction of any abnormality (reflux, obstruction, etc) found in these studies must be considered while chronic suppression of bacteriuria is undertaken.

**B. Laboratory Findings:** The white blood count is usually normal, but significant anemia may be present in early renal failure. Blood urea and serum creatinine are elevated, and creatinine clearance may be reduced. Repeated and meticulous urine culture is the crucial laboratory procedure that is a guide to medical treatment. In addition, methods such as "bladder washout" may be used to distinguish infection of the lower from that of the upper tract. When significant chronic bacteriuria is discovered, an attempt may be made to eradicate or suppress it (see below). If no significant bacteriuria is found in the presence of unexplained hematuria and pyuria, infection by tubercle bacilli, anaerobic bacteria, or fungi must be considered.

Immunofluorescence staining usually shows that bacteria derived from tissue infection are coated with immunoglobulin, eg, in pyelonephritis and prostatitis. Bacteria from the ureter or bladder are not usually stained by this technique.

## Treatment

**A. Specific Measures:** Specific treatment may consist of surgical correction of functional or anatomic abnormalities by the urologist, or it may consist of antimicrobial treatment. The latter usually involves attempts to eradicate the infectious agent by short-term treatment and, if bacteriuria recurs, long-term suppression of the bacteria by administration of urinary antiseptics.

1. If the same organism is isolated from at least 2 sequential urine cultures, antimicrobial drug sensitivity tests should be performed. From the group of drugs to which the organism is susceptible in vitro, the least toxic and least expensive agent is selected (for choice of drugs, see Chapter 28) and administered daily in full systemic doses orally for 4 weeks. The urine is checked after 3 days of treatment and then at weekly intervals to make certain that bacteriuria is suppressed and that a new infection with another organism has not occurred. At the end of treatment, all drug administration is stopped and, 2 and 6 weeks later, the urine is checked again. If bacteriuria is not found, it may be assumed that the particular organism has been eradicated. Repeated examinations for bacteriuria are necessary to confirm absence of recurrent infection.

2. If the foregoing measures fail to eradicate the infection, chronic suppression of bacteriuria is attempted by daily dosage with a urinary antiseptic, eg, nitrofurantoin, methenamine mandelate or hippurate, nalidixic acid, or acidifying agents (see Chapter 28). Urinary pH must be adjusted to the optimum for the drug selected and usually should be held below pH 6.0. The patient can monitor urine pH with indicator paper once a day. After 1 week of treatment and monthly thereafter, the urine must be examined for bacteria. Chronic suppression is continued for 6 months or even longer if the patient can tolerate the drug and superinfection does not occur. If the latter should occur, a specific antimicrobial drug may be selected, by laboratory test, for a 14-day course of treatment, and suppression with another urinary anti-

septic may then be continued. At the end of 1 year of suppressive treatment, renal function and bacteriuria are reevaluated.

**B. General Measures:** Water diuresis may often provide relief from minor discomfort of lower urinary tract symptoms. Water and electrolyte balance must be maintained and renal failure managed as described above. Prevention of infection is all-important, particularly by avoidance of catheterization and instrumentation and by practicing good hygiene. In some women, prophylactic administration of nitrofurantoin, 50–100 mg daily, or trimethoprim-sulfamethoxazole, 2 tablets every other day, may prevent recurrences of infection.

Prolonged drug administration should be avoided in patients with neurogenic bladder or long-term indwelling catheter. Removal of the catheter takes priority over drug treatment.

## Prognosis

Probably 10% or fewer of asymptomatic bacteriuria patients develop renal failure attributable to the infection; hypertension is even more rare. Chronic urinary tract infection is eradicated by short-term therapy (2–6 weeks) in about 25–35% of patients. Some of the others have relapses caused by the same organism; some have reinfection caused by other organisms.

Long-term suppression (> 6 months) with urinary antiseptics eradicates bacteriuria in about two-thirds of patients, but some may become reinfected later. Many elderly patients tolerate recurrent urinary tract infection well, and therapy of their asymptomatic bacteriuria is inappropriate. Antimicrobial drugs should be limited to the relief of symptomatic exacerbations.

Komaroff AL: Acute dysuria in women. *N Engl J Med* 1984;**310**:368.

Kunin CM: Duration of treatment of urinary tract infections. *Am J Med* 1981;**71**:849.

Nicolle LE et al: Bacteriuria in elderly institutionalized men. *N Engl J Med* 1983;**309**:1420.

Sheehan G, Harding GKM, Ronald AR: Advances in treatment of urinary tract infection. *Am J Med* 1984;**76**:141.

Souney P, Polk BF: Single-dose therapy for urinary tract infections in women. *Rev Infect Dis* 1982;**4**:29.

Stamm WE: Prevention of urinary tract infections. *Am J Med* 1984;**76**:148.

Stamm WE et al: Diagnosis of coliform infection in acutely dysuric women. *N Engl J Med* 1982;**307**:463.

## TUBERCULOSIS OF THE GENITOURINARY TRACT

### Essentials of Diagnosis

- Fever, easy fatigability, night sweats, or other signs of systemic infection.
- Symptoms or signs of upper or lower urinary tract infection.
- Urine may contain leukocytes and erythrocytes but no visible bacteria. Routine urine culture is negative.

- Special culture of urine for mycobacteria reveals *Mycobacterium tuberculosis.*
- Excretory urogram may show deformed or "moth-eaten" calices and varying types of kidney tissue destruction.
- Cystoscopy may reveal ulcers or granulomas of bladder wall.

## General Considerations

Reactivation of foci originating from hematogenous dissemination of tubercle bacilli after primary pulmonary infection is the usual source of tuberculosis of the kidney; rarely does the infection originate in the genital tract. The genital organs may become similarly infected by hematogenous spread or secondary to kidney infection. The prostate, seminal vesicles, epididymides, and, rarely, the testes may be infected. The oviducts are more frequently involved than the ovaries and uterus.

The kidney and ureter may show little gross change. However, caseous nodules in the renal parenchyma and abscess formation with destruction of tissue and fibrosis often produce extensive damage. Calcification in the lesions is common. The ureter and calices are thickened, and stenosis may occur, with total destruction of functioning renal tissue above. The bladder shows mucosal inflammation and submucosal tubercles that become necrotic and form ulcers. Fibrosis of the bladder wall occurs late or upon healing. Tubercles with caseous necrosis and calcification are found in the genital organs. Microscopically, typical tubercles are found, and demonstration of the tubercle bacilli in the lesions is usually easily accomplished.

A search must be made for tuberculosis elsewhere in the body whenever urinary tract tuberculosis is found.

## Clinical Findings

**A. Symptoms and Signs:** Symptoms are not characteristic or specific. Manifestations of chronic infection, with malaise, fever, fatigability, and night sweats, may be present. Tuberculous kidney and ureter infection is usually silent, but bladder infection produces frequency, burning on urination, nocturia, and, occasionally, tenesmus. If bleeding occurs with clot formation, ureteral or vesical colic may occur. Gross hematuria is fairly common. There may be nodular induration of the testes, epididymides, or prostate and thickened seminal vesicles. Occasionally, pain and tenderness occur in the costovertebral angle. A draining sinus may form from any of these sites.

**B. Laboratory Findings:** The urine contains "pus without bacteria," red cells, and, usually, protein; occasionally, culture for routine bacterial pathogens may also be positive. Culture for tubercle bacilli confirms the diagnosis. If renal damage is extensive, blood urea nitrogen and creatinine are elevated. A mild anemia usually is present, and the sedimentation rate is rapid.

**C. Imaging and Cystoscopic Findings:** Excretory urograms reveal the moth-eaten appearance of the involved calices or the obliteration of calices, stenosis of calices, abscess cavities, ureteral thickening and stenosis, and the nonfunctioning kidney (autonephrectomy). Calcification of involved tissues is common. Cystoscopic examination is required to determine the extent of bladder wall infection and to provide biopsy material if needed.

## Differential Diagnosis

The "sterile" pyuria of chronic interstitial nephritis, chronic nonspecific urethritis, and cystitis may mimic tuberculous infection. If hematuria is prominent, urinary calculi or bladder carcinoma may be suspected.

## Treatment

Intensive and prolonged antituberculosis therapy is indicated, employing 2 or 3 drugs simultaneously for 9–18 months (see Chapter 28). In 1988, the drugs of choice are isoniazid, 5–8 mg/kg/d (usually 300 mg/d orally); ethambutol, 15 mg/kg/d as a single oral dose; and rifampin, 10–20 mg/kg/d (usually 600 mg as a single oral dose). Alternative drugs are listed in Chapter 28.

Pyridoxine, 100 mg/d orally, is usually given simultaneously with isoniazid to prevent neurotoxic reactions. Surgical procedures are generally limited to situations in which extensive destruction of one kidney makes it unlikely that infection can be eradicated and useful function restored (nephrectomy), obstruction in the tract interferes with proper function, or erosion of a vessel leads to severe bleeding.

## Prognosis

The outlook depends largely on the degree of destruction of renal tissue and impairment of renal function. If urinary tract tuberculosis is detected early, prolonged drug treatment can suppress and arrest the infectious process successfully. Structural defects resulting from infection or fibrosis require surgical correction.

Alvarez S, McCabe WR: Extrapulmonary tuberculosis revisited. *Medicine* 1984;**63**:25.
American Thoracic Society: Treatment of tuberculosis and other mycobacterial diseases. *Am Rev Respir Dis* 1983;**127**:790.
Dutt AK et al: Short-course chemotherapy for extrapulmonary tuberculosis. *Ann Intern Med* 1986;**104**:7.

## PROSTATITIS

Bacteria may reach the prostate from the bloodstream (eg, tuberculosis) or from the urethra. Prostatitis is thus commonly associated with urethritis (eg, gonococcal, chlamydial, mycoplasmal) or with active bacterial infection of the lower urinary tract. Perineal pain, lumbosacral backache, fever, dysuria, and frequency may be symptoms of acute prostatic bacterial infection.

Prostatitis is more commonly chronic. In this instance, symptoms are less impressive, and specific bacterial pathogens are seldom isolated from prostatic secretions.

## Clinical Findings

**A. Symptoms and Signs:** These include perineal pain, fever, dysuria, frequency, and urethral discharge. In acute prostatitis, the prostate feels enlarged, boggy, and very tender; fluctuation occurs only if an abscess has formed. Even gentle palpation of the prostate results in expression of copious purulent discharge.

In chronic prostatitis there may be dull lumbosacral and perineal pain, mild dysuria and frequency, and scanty urethral discharge. Palpation reveals a symmetrically enlarged, boggy, and slightly tender prostate.

**B. Laboratory Findings:** With acute febrile prostatitis, there is often leukocytosis. The expressed prostatic fluid shows pus cells and bacteria on microscopy and culture. During the acute phase, prostatic palpation may express frank pus. In acute and chronic prostatitis, the first glass of urine contains a far larger number of white cells than do subsequent urine samples.

## Differential Diagnosis

Prostatitis should be differentiated from lower urinary tract infection, although it may form part of it. In the latter case, the infected prostate may serve as a source of recurrent lower urinary tract infections. Perirectal infections may be considered, as well as epididymitis, gonococcal infection, and tuberculosis.

## Complications

Epididymitis and cystitis as well as urethritis commonly accompany acute prostatitis. Chronic prostatitis commonly predisposes to recurrent urinary tract infection and occasionally to urethral obstruction and acute urinary retention.

## Treatment

**A. Specific Measures:** For acute prostatitis, initial treatment may consist of sulfamethoxazole, 400 mg, plus trimethoprim, 80 mg, 6–8 tablets daily; tetracycline, 2 g daily by mouth; or ampicillin, 250 mg 6 times daily, until culture of prostatic fluid and susceptibility tests indicate the drug of choice. Treatment for 2 weeks usually abates the acute inflammation, but chronic prostatitis may continue.

Eradication of bacteria in chronically infected prostatic tissue is exceedingly difficult. Antimicrobial drugs diffusing best into prostatic acini must be lipid-soluble and basic (eg, trimethoprim-sulfamethoxazole). Erythromycins are quite active in the prostate but effective mainly against gram-positive organisms, which are rare in urinary tract infections and prostatitis. Conversely, most drugs that are active against gram-negative coliform bacteria (the commonest cause of prostatitis) fail to reach the prostatic acini.

**B. General Measures:** During the acute phase, the patient should be kept at rest, with good hydration, and kept comfortable by means of analgesics, stool softeners, and sitz baths. Urethral instrumentation and prostatic massage must be avoided. Surgical drainage of an abscess is mandatory.

Chronic prostatitis should be treated by prolonged antimicrobial therapy accompanied by vigorous prostatic massage once weekly to promote drainage. Transurethral prostatectomy offers uncertain benefits.

## Prognosis

Although the symptoms of acute prostatitis will usually subside with treatment, the prospects for the eventual elimination of chronic prostatitis are often discouraging.

Krieger JN: Prostatitis syndromes: Pathophysiology, differential diagnosis, and treatment. *Sex Transm Dis* 1984;**11**:100.

# URINARY STONES

Urinary stones and calcification in the kidney may be associated with metabolic disease; may be secondary to infection in the urinary tract; may occur in sponge kidney, tuberculosis of the kidney, or papillary necrosis; or may be idiopathic. The incidence of urinary tract calculus is higher in men.

## NEPHROCALCINOSIS

Chronic hypercalciuria and hyperphosphaturia may result in precipitation of calcium salts in the renal parenchyma (nephrocalcinosis). The commonest causes are hyperparathyroidism, hypervitaminosis D (particularly with associated high calcium intake), and excess calcium and alkali intake. Chronic interstitial nephritis predisposes to nephrocalcinosis. Other causes include acute osteoporosis following immobilization, sarcoidosis, renal tubular acidosis, the de Toni-Fanconi syndrome, and destruction of bone by metastatic carcinoma.

The symptoms, signs, and laboratory findings are those of the primary disease. The diagnosis is usually established by x-ray demonstration of calcium deposits in the kidney, which appear as minute calcific densities with linear streaks in the region of the renal papillae. True renal stones may be present as well in these patients.

Specific treatment is directed at the primary disorder. Particular attention is directed to treatment of urinary tract infection and renal insufficiency. When renal tubular acidosis or the de Toni-Fanconi defect is present, it is essential to maintain a high fluid intake, to replace cation deficit, and to alkalinize the urine with sodium bicarbonate. See Renal Tubular Acidosis, above.

## RENAL STONE

### Essentials of Diagnosis
- Often asymptomatic.
- Symptoms of obstruction of calix or ureteropelvic junction, with flank pain and colic.
- Nausea, vomiting, abdominal distention.
- Hematuria.
- Chills and fever and bladder irritability if infection is present.

### Etiology
**A. Excessive Excretion of Relatively Insoluble Urinary Constituents:**
  **1. Calcium–**
   a. Hypercalciuria with normocalcemia.
      (1) Idiopathic hypercalciuria (30–40% of stone formers).
      (2) Renal tubular acidosis, type I; distal tubule deficit (see p 553).
   b. Hypercalciuria with hypercalcemia or normocalcemia.
      (1) Primary hyperparathyroidism (see Chapter 18). (Five to 7% of stone formers.)
      (2) High vitamin D intake.
      (3) Renal tubular acidosis, type I.
      (4) Excessive intake of milk and alkali.
      (5) Destructive bone disease due to neoplasm or of metabolic origin (corticosteroid excess, thyrotoxicosis).
      (6) Sarcoidosis.
      (7) Prolonged immobilization.
  **2. Oxalate–**Over half of urinary stones are composed of calcium oxalate or calcium oxalate mixed with phosphate.
   a. Congenital or familial oxaluria (rare).
   b. Ileal disease; ileal resection or bypass.
   c. High oxalate intake (tea, cocoa, spinach, beets, rhubarb, parsley, nuts). Vitamin C is an oxalate precursor.
   d. Methoxyflurane anesthesia.
  **3. Uric acid–**
   a. Gout–Stones may form spontaneously or as a result of treatment with uricosuric agents.
   b. Hyperuricosuria with or without hyperuricemia. Idiopathic or secondary to high purine intake (see C, below).
   c. Anticancer therapy with agents that cause rapid destruction of cells, resulting in increased excretion of uric acid.
   d. Myeloproliferative disease (leukemia, lymphoma, myeloid metaplasia, etc).
  **4. Cystine–**Hereditary cystinuria.
**B. Physical Changes in the Urine:**
  1. Increased concentration of urine solute as a consequence of low intake of fluid and low urine volume.
  2. Urinary pH–
   a. Low pH–Organic substances less soluble (uric acid, cystine).
   b. High pH–Inorganic salts usually less soluble (calcium phosphate and mixed calcium phosphate-calcium oxalate stones).
   c. High pH associated with urinary tract infection with organisms containing urease (especially *Proteus*). Hydrolysis of urea yields ammonia, which produces an increase in pH. $Mg + NH_4 + PO_4^{3-}$ precipitates as magnesium ammonium phosphate (struvite) to form stones.
**C. Nucleus (Nidus) for Stone Formation:**
  1. Uricosuria–Crystals of uric acid or sodium hydrogen urate may initiate precipitation of calcium oxalate from solution.
  2. Bits of necrotic tissue, blood clots, and clumps of bacteria, particularly in the presence of stasis or infection, may serve as a nucleus for stone formation.
**D. Congenital or Acquired Deformities of the Kidneys:**
  1. Sponge kidney.
  2. Horseshoe kidney.
  3. Local caliceal obstruction or defect.

### General Considerations
The location and size of the stone and the presence or absence of obstruction determine the changes that occur in the kidney and caliceal system. The pathologic changes may be modified by ischemia due to pressure or by infection.

### Clinical Findings
**A. Symptoms and Signs:** Often a stone trapped in a calix or in the renal pelvis is asymptomatic. If a stone produces obstruction in a calix or at the ureteropelvic junction, dull flank pain or even colic may occur. Hematuria and symptoms of accompanying infection may be present. Nausea and vomiting may suggest enteric disease. Flank tenderness and abdominal distention may be the only findings.

**B. Laboratory Findings:** Urinalysis is the most important laboratory test. In addition to gross or microscopic hematuria, the presence of pyuria suggests associated urinary tract infection. Crystals may provide a lead to the composition of the stone and the underlying metabolic disorder (hypercalciuria, gout, cystinuria, renal tubular acidosis, oxaluria). Chemical analysis of serum with a broad biochemical profile will assist in confirming the metabolic disorder. Always obtain a stone for analysis.

**C. Imaging:** A plain abdominal radiograph (kidney, ureter, and bladder) will assist in discovering symptomatic and asymptomatic radiopaque stones and related bone lesions (eg, hyperparathyroidism). If the stone has not passed within a day or 2 after the acute onset of symptoms, radionuclide renography may reveal the presence of persistent obstruction. Ultrasonography will usually define renal size and caliceal and ureteral dilatation above the site of obstruction. Excretory and retrograde urograms help to delineate the site and degree of obstruction and to confirm the presence of nonopaque stones (uric acid).

## Differential Diagnosis

Renal stone may be confused with acute pyelonephritis, renal tumor, renal tuberculosis, and infarction of the kidney. In occasional cases, the symptoms may mimic those of acute abdomen.

## Complications

Infection and hydronephrosis may destroy renal tissue.

## Prevention of Further
## Stone Formation

(1) Obtain a stone for analysis whenever possible. It is useful for diagnosis and therapy.

(2) Review the family history to identify metabolic causes (cystinuria, gout, hypercalcemia, renal tubular acidosis, hyperoxaluria).

(3) Treat predisposing diseases such as hyperparathyroidism, gout, cystinuria, renal tubular acidosis, infection, sarcoidosis, hypercortisolism, and hyperoxaluria and anatomic defects of the urinary tract.

(4) Instruct the patient to maintain a high fluid intake to produce a dilute urine, ie, urine volume of more than 2000 mL/d with a specific gravity less than 1.015.

(5) Maintain urine pH at a suitable level: (a) Above pH 6.5 for uric acid stones; above 7.5 for cystine stones: Use Shohl's solution (see p 553), 10–30 mL 5 times a day, ie, after each meal, at bedtime, and during the night. (b) Below pH 6.5 for struvite stones: There is no practical long-term therapy that will not produce metabolic acidosis. For a brief trial, one may use ascorbic acid, 3 g/d or more, or methionine, 8–12 g/d.

(6) If hyperuricosuria is present in those who form calcium stones, allopurinol, 100 mg twice a day, plus restriction of intake of purine-containing foods will often reduce stone formation.

(7) If idiopathic hypercalciuria is present, the patient should reduce calcium intake by avoiding milk and milk products, calcium-containing medications, and vitamin D-fortified foods. A high fluid intake is essential. Chronic use of thiazide diuretics in modest doses (hydrochlorothiazides, 50 mg twice daily, or equivalent) plus modest restriction of salt intake will reduce calcium excretion and may enhance excretion of magnesium, which has an inhibitory effect on stone formation. Thiazides reduce excretion of citrate in the urine. Citrate inhibits calcium stone formation by complexing with calcium, thus reducing its concentration, and by directly inhibiting crystal growth. The addition of potassium citrate, 10–20 meq 3 times daily by mouth, appears to be effective. Inorganic orthophosphate has proved beneficial when used alone or with thiazides. Combinations of dibasic and monobasic phosphate salts of sodium and potassium provide a mix of neutral pH. Most formulations provide 250 mg of phosphorus per capsule or tablet. Give in divided doses 3 or 4 times a day to provide a total of 1250–1500 mg of phosphorus per day. Cellulose phosphate chelates cations and may be used to reduce intestinal absorption of calcium. When used, it should be accompanied by a low-calcium diet and magnesium supplementation.

(8) Magnesium inhibits calcium stone formation. It may be supplied as magnesium oxide in doses that will not produce diarrhea. If stones consist of calcium oxalate, a reduction of oxalate intake is in order. Cocoa, tea, rhubarb, spinach, Swiss chard, beets, parsley, nuts, and excess vitamin C should be avoided.

(9) Treat patients who are "idiopathic calcium stone formers" according to paragraphs 7 and 8 above.

(10) In the presence of urinary tract infection with urease-containing organisms, suppression of struvite stone formation is difficult. Infection must be eradicated or reduced with appropriate antibiotics.

(11) Prevention of uric acid stones by inhibiting the formation of uric acid is now possible by blocking the conversion of xanthine to uric acid with the xanthine oxidase inhibitor allopurinol. The usual adult dose of allopurinol is 600 mg/d (300 mg every 12 hours). This will reduce elevated serum uric acid to normal levels and markedly reduce the excretion of uric acid. It is effective even in the presence of renal failure associated with gouty nephropathy. The drug is well tolerated and apparently produces no alteration of renal function. Allopurinol may be used in association with antileukemia and anticancer agents. While the allopurinol effect is developing, treatment should include a high fluid intake and alkalinization of the urine with sodium bicarbonate, 10–12 g/d in divided doses, or Shohl's solution, 50–150 mL/d.

(12) Cystine stone formation can be reduced by forcing fluids to produce a urine output of 3–4 L daily and alkalinizing the urine with sodium bicarbonate or sodium citrate and acetazolamide at bedtime. Urine pH should be maintained at 7.5 or higher, at which levels cystine solubility is greatly increased. A low-methionine diet may help, but protein deprivation must be avoided. Patients with severe cystinuria may require penicillamine, which complexes cystine and reduces the total excretion of cystine. There are many side effects of penicillamine that appear to be dose-related.

## Treatment

Small stones may be passed. They do no harm if infection is not present. Larger stones may be removed by percutaneous nephrostomy plus mechanical, ultrasonic, or electrohydraulic disintegration of the stone to permit easy removal of the debris. Surgical removal may be required. Nephrectomy may be necessary.

## Prognosis

If obstruction can be prevented and infection eradicated, the prognosis is good.

## URETERAL STONE

### Essentials of Diagnosis

- Obstruction of ureter produces severe colic with radiation of pain to regions determined by the position of the stone in the ureter.
- Gastrointestinal symptoms common.
- Urine usually contains fresh red cells.
- May be asymptomatic.
- Exacerbations of infection when obstruction occurs.

### General Considerations

Ureteral stones are formed in the kidney but produce symptoms as they pass down the ureter.

### Clinical Findings

**A. Symptoms and Signs:** The pain of ureteral colic is intense. The patient may be in mild shock, with cold, moist skin. There is marked tenderness in the costovertebral angle. Abdominal and back muscle spasm may be present. Referred areas of hyperesthesia may be demonstrated.

**B. Laboratory Findings:** As for renal stone.

**C. Imaging and Instrumental Examination:** Radiographs may show the stone lodged in the ureter or at the ureterovesical junction. Nonopaque stones can be demonstrated by radionuclide renography, ultrasonography, or excretory urograms, which reveal the site of obstruction and the dilated ureteropelvic system above it. Because of the danger of infection, cystoscopy and ureteral catheterization should be avoided unless retrograde urography is essential.

### Differential Diagnosis

Ureteral stones require differentiation from clots due to hemorrhage, from tumor, and from acute pyelonephritis as well as acute cholecystitis and other causes of acute surgical abdomen.

### Prevention

Proceed as for renal stone. Every effort should be made to obtain a stone for analysis.

### Treatment

**A. Specific Measures:** Most stones will pass spontaneously if spasm of the ureter is relieved and fluids are forced. By a cystoscopic or percutaneous approach, removal of stones may be accomplished with baskets or by ultrasound lithotripsy. Surgical ureterolithotomy may be necessary.

**B. General Measures:** Morphine or other opiates should be given in doses adequate to control pain. Morphine sulfate, 8 mg (or equivalent dosage of other drugs), may be given intravenously and repeated in 5–10 minutes if necessary. Thereafter, subcutaneous administration is usually adequate. Atropine sulfate, 0.8 mg subcutaneously, or methantheline bromide, 0.1 g intravenously, may be used as an antispasmodic.

### Prognosis

If obstruction and infection can be treated successfully, the outlook is excellent.

## VESICAL STONE

### Essentials of Diagnosis

- Bladder irritability, with dysuria, urgency, and frequency.
- Interruption of urinary stream as stone occludes urethra.
- Hematuria and pyuria.
- Benign prostatic hypertrophy is occasionally present in men.

### General Considerations

Vesical stones occur most commonly when there is residual urine infected with urea-splitting organisms (eg, *Proteus,* staphylococci). Thus, bladder stones are associated with urinary stasis due to bladder neck or urethral obstruction, diverticula, neurogenic bladder, and cystocele. Foreign bodies in the bladder act as foci for stone formation. Ulceration and bladder inflammation predispose to stone formation.

Most vesical stones are composed of calcium phosphate, calcium oxalate, or magnesium ammonium phosphate. Uric acid stones are common in the presence of an enlarged prostate and uninfected urine.

### Clinical Findings

**A. Symptoms and Signs:** Symptoms of chronic urinary obstruction or stasis and infection are usually present. Dysuria, frequency and urgency, and interruption of the urinary stream (causing pain in the penis) when the stone occludes the urethra are common complaints. Physical findings include prostatic enlargement, evidence of distended (neurogenic) bladder, and cystocele. The stone may be palpable.

**B. Laboratory Findings:** The urine usually shows signs of infection and contains red cells.

**C. Imaging and Cystoscopic Examination:** Radiographic examination shows the calcified stone, and urograms show the bladder abnormalities and upper urinary tract dilatation due to long-standing back pressure. Direct cystoscopic examination may be necessary.

### Treatment & Prognosis

Stones can be removed by fragmentation using ultrasound, mechanical, or electrohydraulic lithotripsy. Surgical lithotomy may be necessary.

Urethral obstruction, cystocele, and other contributing anatomic factors must be eliminated by appropriate surgery.

Give analgesics as required, and treat infection with appropriate antibiotics.

The prognosis is excellent.

Coe FL: Prevention of kidney stones. *Am J Med* 1981;**71**:514.

Health and Public Policy Committee of the American College of Physicians: Lithotripsy. *Ann Intern Med* 1985;**103**:626.

Smith DR: *General Urology,* 11th ed. Lange, 1984.

Pak CYC et al: Correction of hypocitraturia and prevention of stone formation by combined thiazide and potassium citrate therapy in thiazide-unresponsive hypercalciuric nephrolithiasis. *Am J Med* 1985;**99**:284.

Smith LH: Medical treatment of idiopathic calcium urolithiasis. *The Kidney* 1983;**16**:9.

Symposium on surgery of stone disease. *Urol Clin North Am* 1983;**10**:583. [Entire issue.]

•   •   •

## OBSTRUCTIVE UROPATHY

Obstruction of the urinary tract can result in serious damage to the kidneys; early detection and treatment are required to prevent irreversible function and anatomic damage. The site and degree of obstruction, the duration of obstruction, and the complication of urinary tract infection determine the presenting manifestations.

### Etiology & Pathogenesis

Obstructive uropathy is the result of (1) congenital anatomic abnormalities (eg, ureteropelvic, ureterovesical, or urethral stricture); (2) stone, tumor, or clot that obstructs a ureter or the bladder neck; (3) extrinsic tumors, bands, or fibrosis; or (4) neuromuscular disorder related to the spinal cord or peripheral nerve lesions.

Complete obstruction to the flow of urine produces increase in pressure in the ureters and in the renal pelvis, which then become dilated. Renal papillae become flattened, the renal tubules dilate, and glomerular filtration is impeded. Functional impairment of tubule function affects the excretion of solute, the reabsorption of sodium, and the secretion of hydrogen ion. Renal blood flow is reduced. Destruction of the kidney results within a few weeks. Partial obstruction produces lesser impairment of renal function.

### Clinical Findings

**A. Symptoms and Signs:** The site of obstruction and rapidity of onset determine the presentation. Chronic or low-grade obstruction is usually asymptomatic. Acute and complete obstruction of a ureter will produce pain in the flank or groin associated with distention of the renal capsule or ureteral colic. Acute obstruction of the urethra by an enlarged prostate, postoperative bladder dysfunction, or stone will produce painful distention of the bladder. (See below for discussion of prostatic hyperplasia.) Chronic urethral obstruction may result in a distended bladder with "overflow" dribbling. If a neurologic lesion is the cause of bladder dysfunction, there may be overflow dribbling from a distended bladder, involuntary voiding, and frequency with incomplete emptying of the bladder.

The history and physical examination should be directed at excluding circulatory or intrinsic renal disease as causes of oliguria. The history should focus on recurrent urinary tract infection, symptoms of incomplete lower urinary tract obstruction (nocturia, hesitancy, urgency, incontinence), evidence of diabetes mellitus, use of anticholinergic drugs, stone disease, and neurologic disease. In some patients, the only symptoms may be those of renal failure. The presence of extrinsic tumor, an enlarged prostate, or neurologic disease should be evident on examination.

**B. Laboratory Findings:** Bacteriuria and leukocytes in the urine signify accompanying infection. Lower urinary tract obstruction results in elevated BUN and creatinine and, if renal impairment is severe, increased serum $K^+$, phosphate, and uric acid.

**C. Special Examinations:** Ultrasound imaging will reveal dilatation of the renal pelvis, ureters, and bladder and help to distinguish unilateral ureteral obstruction from lower tract obstruction. Cystoscopy and retrograde urography may be indicated.

### Treatment

Relief of obstruction is urgent. Urethral obstruction can be relieved by catheterization. An indwelling urethral or suprapubic catheter may be required. Operation may be necessary to relieve ureteral obstruction, remove a stone, place nephrostomy tubes or ureteral stents, and relieve urethral obstruction (prostatic resection). Vigorous treatment of infection is imperative. Urologic or surgical consultation should be sought as needed. Treatment of neurogenic bladder is a complex subject beyond the scope of this chapter.

Postobstructive diuresis is usually limited, but losses may continue beyond elimination of retained fluid and require aggressive replacement of water and electrolyte.

Klahr S: Pathophysiology of obstructive nephropathy. *Kidney Int* 1983;**23**:414.

## URETERAL OBSTRUCTION

Obstruction of one or both ureters may be due to a variety of acquired diseases, including injury to ureters during pelvic surgery; postirradiation fibrosis; compression by extrinsic neoplastic disease; occlusion of the ureterovesical junction by cancer of the bladder, prostate, uterine cervix, or rectum; endometriosis; chronic infections of the urinary tract; retroperitoneal fibrosis; ureteral stone; chronic vesical outlet obstruction from prostatic hyperplasia or cancer, urethral stricture, or vesical stone.

Although rare, retroperitoneal fibrosis warrants

further discussion. Chronic inflammatory disease of retroperitoneal tissues over the lower lumbar vertebrae may compress one or both ureters, with consequent dilatation of the ureter and renal pelvis proximal to the site of obstruction. The vena cava and, occasionally, the aorta or other major arteries in the area may be occluded. Rarely, extension upward may extend to the mediastinum, with occlusion of retroperitoneal viscera.

The reaction occurs in some patients taking methysergide for migraine or beta-blocker drugs (propranolol, atenolol, oxprenolol) for the usual indications. Retroperitoneal fibrosis may accompany sclerosing Hodgkin's disease. Lymphomas and spread of metastatic tumor retroperitoneally may simulate the disease by occluding the ureters and great vessels.

Symptoms and signs include low back pain, abdominal pain, anorexia, weight loss, fever, urinary frequency, and, depending on the degree of renal insufficiency, polyuria or anuria. Occlusion of arteries trapped in the fibrotic reaction can produce claudication and weakness of the legs and impotence. A mass is often palpable over the promontory of the sacrum.

Laboratory findings are those of impaired renal function secondary to chronic obstruction, with elevated blood urea nitrogen and serum creatinine, metabolic acidosis, and anemia (see Chronic Renal Insufficiency). Excretory urograms show medial deviation of the ureters and dilatation of the excretory tract proximal to the obstruction.

Therapy includes abstaining from the offending drug and a trial of corticosteroid. Give prednisone, 30–60 mg/d orally, until evidence of improvement permits reduction to a maintenance dose of 5–15 mg/d. Operation may be required to relieve ureteral obstruction.

## URINARY INCONTINENCE

Urinary incontinence occurs in many clinical settings. In adults, there are 7 circumstances in which incontinence occurs. Elderly people are more likely to be affected. Urology texts should be consulted for diagnosis and treatment.

(1) Congenital defects of the bladder or urethra often result in incontinence.

(2) Urinary tract infection—especially severe cystitis—may lead to bladder detrusor muscle spasm, frequency, and involuntary loss of urine.

(3) Diminished bladder capacity from intrinsic disease of the bladder wall (eg, scarring from infection or stone, carcinoma of the bladder) results in frequency and incontinence.

(4) Urethral obstruction by stricture or tumor may produce urinary retention and "overflow" incontinence.

(5) Central nervous system disease—especially strokes, brain stem and spinal cord damage, and autonomic neuropathy—may result in urinary retention with overflow incontinence, involuntary micturition, reflex incontinence, and detrusor-sphincter asynergy.

(6) Drugs whose effects can produce incontinence include diuretics, long-acting sedatives, anticholinergic agents, and calcium channel blockers as well as others.

(7) Stress incontinence (discussed below).

Stress incontinence is common in elderly women as a result of urethral hypermobility referable to a lax pelvic floor musculature and sphincter incompetence and inadequate detrusor muscle control, permitting involuntary escape of urine with coughing, laughing, or increased intra-abdominal pressure due to other causes. Treatment consists of correction of cystocele (if present), pelvic floor muscle exercises, and correction of atrophic vaginitis by use of topical or oral estrogen. Urologic consultation should be sought as needed.

Resnick NM, Yalla SV: Management of urinary incontinence in the elderly. *N Engl J Med* 1985;**313**:800.

Urinary continence in elderly patients. (Editorial.) *Lancet* 1986;**2**:1316.

## TESTICULAR DISEASE

### 1. EPIDIDYMITIS

Acute epididymitis is caused by bacterial infection ascending from the urethra or prostate. In older men, it usually follows urinary tract obstruction and infection or instrumentation of the lower genitourinary tract.

Sudden pain in the scrotum, rapid unilateral scrotal enlargement, and marked tenderness of the testes, spermatic cord, and groin are the characteristic manifestations. Secondary orchitis with a swollen, painful testicle may occur. Elevation of the scrotum provides some relief.

Laboratory findings include leukocytosis, pyuria, and bacteriuria. Urine culture will usually demonstrate the organism—frequently *E coli* in men over age 35. A sterile urine culture strongly suggests chlamydial infection. Ultrasound examination often can differentiate a swollen epididymis from testicular tumor.

Bed rest and elevation and support of the scrotum provide symptomatic relief. Nonsteroidal analgesics may be useful. If chlamydial infection is the likely cause, give tetracycline. Appropriate antibiotics should be used for identified bacteria. Trimethoprim-sulfamethoxazole, ampicillin, or a cephalosporin may be employed for men over 35 years of age, in whom *E coli* is the most frequent organism.

Berger RE: Urethritis and epididymitis. *Semin Urol* 1983;**1**:139.

## 2. ORCHITIS

Acute orchitis is usually due to mumps and occurs during the years just following adolescence. It is most often unilateral but may be bilateral. Mumps may produce acute oophoritis as well.

Chronic orchitis may be due to syphilis, tuberculosis, leprosy, filariasis, and schistosomiasis haematobia. Destruction of the testis usually leaves some hormonal cell function.

Meares EM Jr: Nonspecific infections of the urinary tract. In: Smith DR (editor): *General Urology,* 11th ed. Lange, 1984.

## 3. TESTICULAR TORSION

Testicular torsion (torsion of the spermatic cord) is most common in adolescent males and young men under age 25. An anomaly of the tunica vaginalis or of the relationship of the epididymis to the testis is usually present.

The characteristic presentation is with a sudden onset of unabating pain in the scrotum, groin, or lower abdomen, made worse by elevation of the scrotum. The testis is swollen, tender, and retracted.

Testicular torsion must be differentiated from epididymitis, orchitis, and trauma to the testis. A technetium 99m Tc pertechnetate scan will demonstrate decreased blood flow with torsion and increased blood flow with epididymitis. Ultrasound examination of the testes may be helpful.

Treatment consists of immediate surgery to remove the infarcted testis. Orchiopexy of the other testis is desirable because of the high incidence of the bilateral anatomic abnormality associated with torsion.

Lee LM, Wright JE, McLoughlin MG: Testicular torsion in the adult. *J Urol* 1983;**130:**93.

# TUMORS OF THE GENITOURINARY TRACT

## ADENOCARCINOMA OF KIDNEY (Renal Cell Carcinoma, Hypernephroma)

### Essentials of Diagnosis
- Gross hematuria with or without flank pain.
- Fever.
- Enlarged kidney may be palpable.

### General Considerations
The commonest malignant tumor of the kidney is adenocarcinoma, which occurs more frequently in men. It rarely occurs before age 35 and more commonly after age 50. This tumor metastasizes early to the lungs, liver, and long bones.

Adenocarcinoma of the kidney apparently arises from renal tubule cells or adenomas. It invades blood vessels early. On microscopic examination, the cells resemble renal tubule cells arranged in cords and varying patterns.

### Clinical Findings
**A. Symptoms and Signs:** Gross hematuria is the most frequent sign. Fever is often the only symptom. A flank mass may be palpable. Pain of renal or ureteral origin may occur with bleeding into the tumor or renal pelvis. Vena caval occlusion may produce characteristic patterns of collateral circulation and edema of the legs.

A hypernephroma may not produce classic symptoms of renal tumor. It may produce symptoms and signs suggesting a wide variety of diseases: fever of obscure origin, leukemoid reaction, refractory anemia, erythrocytosis, hypercalcemia, hypoglycemia, peripheral neuropathy, and increased production of gonadotropins and prostaglandins.

**B. Laboratory Findings:** Polycythemia occasionally develops as a result of increased secretion of erythropoietin by the tumor. Anemia is more commonly found. Hematuria is almost always present. Alkaline phosphatase may be elevated in the absence of hepatic metastases. Urinary cytologic examination may aid in diagnosis. The erythrocyte sedimentation rate is rapid.

**C. Imaging:** Ultrasound imaging can define the size and contour of the kidneys. Cysts can often be differentiated from solid tumors. The presence of tumor in the renal vein and vena cava can often be demonstrated. With visualization by real-time ultrasound scan, an experienced operator may perform "thin-needle" biopsy of the renal mass.

Radiographic examination may show an enlarged kidney. Metastatic lesions of bone and lung may be revealed. Excretory or retrograde urograms, as well as angiograms, may be necessary to establish the presence of a renal tumor. CT scans with contrast medium may help differentiate renal cyst or anomaly from tumor, define tumor size and consistency, and document any extension of tumor into the renal vein and vena cava. MRI may prove to be the diagnostic test of choice.

### Differential Diagnosis
The differential diagnosis includes hydronephrosis, polycystic kidneys, renal tuberculosis, renal calculi, and renal infarction. The most challenging problem is to distinguish benign renal cyst from carcinoma; aspiration of the lesion may be necessary.

### Treatment
Nephrectomy is indicated if no metastases are present. Even when metastases are present, nephrectomy may be indicated for intractable bleeding or pain.

X-ray irradiation of metastases may be of value,

although the lesions are usually fairly radioresistant. Isolated single pulmonary metastases can occasionally be removed surgically. At present, chemotherapy is ineffective. Palliation may be achieved with medroxyprogesterone. Therapy with interleukin-II is under investigation.

## Prognosis

The course is variable. Some patients may not develop metastases for 10–15 years after removal of the primary tumor. About 35% of patients live more than 5 years.

Garnick MB, Richie JP: Renal neoplasia. Page 1533 in: *The Kidney,* 3rd ed. Brenner B, Rector F (editors). Saunders, 1986.

McDonald MW: Current therapy for renal cell carcinoma. *J Urol* 1982;**127**:211.

## TUMORS OF THE RENAL PELVIS & URETER

Epithelial tumors of the renal pelvis and ureter are relatively rare. They are usually papillary and tend to metastasize along the urinary tract. Epidermoid tumors are highly malignant and metastasize early. Transitional cell tumors have occurred in cases of interstitial nephritis and papillary necrosis due to phenacetin abuse.

Painless hematuria is the most common complaint. Colic occurs with obstruction due to blood clot or tumor. Tenderness in the flank may be found. Anemia due to blood loss occurs. The urine contains red cells and clots; white cells and bacteria are present when infection is superimposed. Urography should reveal the filling defect in the pelvis or show obstruction and dilatation of the ureter. At cystoscopy, the bleeding from the involved ureter may be seen and satellite tumors identified. Exfoliative cytologic studies should be done.

Radical removal of the kidney, the involved ureter, and the periureteral portion of the bladder should be done unless metastases are extensive.

Irradiation of metastases is usually of little value.

The prognosis depends upon the type of tumor. With anaplastic neoplasms, death usually occurs within 5 years.

## TUMORS OF THE BLADDER

### Essentials of Diagnosis

- Hematuria, gross or microscopic.
- Malignant cells by urine cytology.
- Suprapubic pain and bladder symptoms associated with infection.
- Visualization of tumor at cystoscopy.

### General Considerations

Bladder tumors are the second most common urinary tract tumors. At least 75% of bladder tumors occur in men over age 50. Tumors usually arise at the base of the bladder and involve ureteral orifices and the bladder neck. The common tumor is transitional cell carcinoma, which is often of low-grade malignancy; epidermoid tumors, adenocarcinomas, and sarcomas are rare. Metastases involve regional lymph nodes, bone, liver, and lungs.

### Clinical Findings

**A. Symptoms and Signs:** Hematuria is the commonest symptom and may occur early in the course. Cystitis with frequency, urgency, and dysuria is a frequent complication. With encroachment of the tumor on the bladder neck, the urinary stream is diminished. Suprapubic pain occurs as the tumor extends beyond the bladder. Obstruction of the ureters produces hydronephrosis, frequently accompanied by renal infection, in which case the signs of urinary tract infection may be present. Physical examination is not notable. The bladder tumor may be palpable on bimanual (abdominorectal or abdominovaginal) examination.

**B. Laboratory Findings:** Anemia is common. The urine contains red cells, white cells, and bacteria. Exfoliative cytology is often confirmatory.

**C. Imaging and Instrumental Examination:** Excretory urography may reveal ureteral obstruction. Cystograms usually show the tumor. Cystoscopy and biopsy confirm the diagnosis. Ultrasonography and CT scanning are helpful in diagnosis and staging.

### Differential Diagnosis

Hematuria and pain can be produced by other tumors of the urinary tract, urinary calculi, renal tuberculosis, acute cystitis, or acute nephritis.

### Treatment

**A. Specific Measures:** Tumor staging is required to serve as a guide to selection of treatment. Endoscopic transurethral resection of superficial and submucosal tumors can provide a cure in many cases. Cystectomy with ureterosigmoidostomy or another urinary diversion procedure is required for invasive tumors. Radiation therapy may be useful for more anaplastic tumors. Thiotepa or mitomycin C instillations may be effective in eradicating superficial and papillary bladder epithelial tumors. For metastatic disease, cyclophosphamide, cisplatin, and doxorubicin may be effective.

**B. General Measures:** Urinary tract infection should be controlled with appropriate antibiotics. Anastomosis of ureters to an isolated loop of ileum or sigmoid colon, one end of which is brought to the skin to act as a conduit, is relatively free of renal complications and of alteration of body fluid electrolytes. An isolated loop of ileum or sigmoid colon can be used as a urinary conduit when anastomosed to the ureters.

### Prognosis

There is a tendency toward recurrence and increasing malignancy. With infiltrating carcinomas the outlook is poor even with radical resection.

Grossman HB: Current therapy of bladder carcinoma. *J Urol* 1979;**121**:1.

Soloway MS: Rationale for intensive intravesical chemotherapy for superficial bladder cancer. *J Urol* 1980;**123**:461.

## BENIGN PROSTATIC HYPERPLASIA

### Essentials of Diagnosis

- Prostatism: hesitancy and straining to initiate micturition, reduced force and caliber of the urinary stream, nocturia.
- Acute urinary retention.
- Enlarged prostate.
- Uremia follows prolonged obstruction.

### General Considerations

Hyperplasia of the prostatic lateral and subcervical lobes that are invaded by periurethral glands results in enlargement of the prostate and urethral obstruction.

### Clinical Findings

**A. Symptoms and Signs:** The symptoms of prostatism increase in severity as the degree of urethral obstruction increases. Symptoms may be overlooked or not reported when the progression of obstruction is slow. On rectal examination, the prostate is usually found to be enlarged. The bladder may be seen and palpated as retention of urine increases. Infection commonly occurs with stasis and retention of "residual urine." Hematuria may occur. Uremia may result from prolonged back pressure and severe bilateral hydronephrosis. Determination of blood urea nitrogen may provide the only clue to slowly advancing and relatively asymptomatic obstructive disease. Residual urine can be measured by postvoiding catheterization or estimated by ultrasonography. In the presence of prostatism, ganglionic blocking agents and parasympatholytic drugs used in the treatment of hypertension, as well as tranquilizers, weaken the power of detrusor contraction, thus causing symptoms simulating vesical neck obstruction and in some cases urinary retention.

**B. Imaging and Cystoscopic Examination:** Excretory urograms reveal the complications of back pressure: ureteral dilatation, hydronephrosis, and postvoiding urinary retention. Cystoscopy will reveal enlargement of the prostate and secondary bladder wall changes such as trabeculation, diverticula, inflammation due to infection, and vesical stone.

### Differential Diagnosis

Other causes of urethral obstruction include urethral stricture, vesical stone, bladder tumor, neurogenic bladder, and carcinoma of the prostate.

### Treatment

**A. Specific Measures:** Conservative (nonsurgical) management should be undertaken only in collaboration with a urologist. Acute urinary retention is relieved by catheterization, and catheter drainage is maintained if the degree of obstruction is severe. Surgery is usually necessary. There are various indications for each of the 4 approaches: treatment by transurethral resection or by suprapubic, retropubic, or perineal prostatectomy. Occasionally, partial obstruction may be ameliorated by empirical therapy with trimethoprim-sulfamethoxazole, which relieves the commonly associated chronic prostatitis.

**B. General Measures:** Treat infection of the urinary tract with appropriate antibiotics. The patient who develops postobstructive diuresis must be sustained with appropriate water and electrolyte replacement.

### Prognosis

Surgical resection will relieve symptoms. The surgical mortality rate is low.

## CARCINOMA OF THE PROSTATE

### Essentials of Diagnosis

- Prostatism.
- Hard consistency of the prostate.
- Metastases to bone produce pain, particularly in the low back.
- Elevated serum acid phosphatase in 85% of patients with extension of the cancer beyond the prostatic capsule.

### General Considerations

Cancer of the prostate is rare before age 60. It metastasizes early to the bones of the pelvis and locally may produce urethral obstruction with subsequent renal damage. The growth of the tumor is increased by androgens and inhibited by estrogens. The prostatic tissue is rich in acid phosphatase, and when cancer has extended beyond the prostate to the periprostatic tissue or to bone, the serum acid phosphatase is increased. The serum acid phosphatase concentration thus provides a good index of extension and growth of the tumor.

### Clinical Findings

**A. Symptoms and Signs:** Obstructive symptoms similar to those of benign prostatic hyperplasia are common. Rectal examination reveals a stone-hard prostate that is often nodular and fixed. Low back pain occurs with metastases to the bones of the pelvis and spine. Pathologic fractures may occur at the sites of metastases. Obstruction may produce renal damage and the symptoms and signs of renal insufficiency. An enlarged nodular liver and an enlarged supraclavicular sentinel lymph node are late signs of metastatic disease.

**B. Laboratory Findings:** Anemia may be extreme if bone marrow is replaced by tumor. The urine may show evidence of infection. Serum prostatic acid phosphatase is increased when metastases have occurred, and serum alkaline phosphatase may be elevated as new bone is formed at the site of metastases. Hypercalcemia is a serious complication of metastatic disease. Biopsy by transurethral resection or by needle aspiration through the perineum establishes the diagnosis.

**C. Imaging:** MRI is a sensitive indicator of the presence of cancer within the prostate. Ultrasonography with a rectal probe transducer can often identify the presence of carcinoma. Radiographic examination of the bones of the pelvis, spine, ribs, and skull will reveal the typical osteoblastic metastases; radionuclide bone scan is more sensitive. Excretory urograms delineate changes secondary to urethral obstruction and the back pressure of urine retention. Lymphangiography may demonstrate metastases to pelvic nodes.

### Differential Diagnosis

Differentiation from benign prostatic hyperplasia, urethral stricture, vesical stone, bladder tumor, and neurogenic bladder is necessary.

### Treatment

Every effort must be made to ascertain the stage of disease by anatomic extent and histologic characteristics in order to apply appropriate therapy. Before metastasis has occurred, cure may be obtained by radical resection of the prostate, including the seminal vesicles and a portion of the bladder neck, with or without lymph node dissection. Newer surgical techniques have resulted in a lower incidence of impotence after the procedure. Palliative therapy includes transurethral resection to relieve obstruction. Interstitial implantation of radioactive iodine ($^{125}$I) has proved useful in selected cases of localized cancer. Radiotherapy of the primary tumor with the linear accelerator or radioactive cobalt has provided good remission. Irradiation of bone metastases may afford relief. In late stages (stage D), antiandrogen therapy slows the rate of growth and extension of the cancer. Orchiectomy or estrogen therapy alone (1 mg diethylstilbestrol daily) is often effective in reducing symptoms and extending survival. Blocking testosterone production with leuteinizing hormone-releasing hormone (LHRH) analogs that inhibit gonadotropin release from the pituitary has proved effective and may replace castration and estrogen therapy. Treatment of metastatic disease should not be instituted unless the patient is symptomatic. Chemotherapy is of little use.

The effectiveness of therapy can be judged by clinical response and by periodic measurements of the serum acid and alkaline phosphatase.

### Prognosis

Palliative therapy is often not effective for long. Most patients die within 3 years; a few survive for 5–10 years. Since the tumor affects older men, many patients die of unrelated conditions.

Glide LM: Gonadotropin-releasing hormone analogues and other new hormonal treatments of prostatic cancer. Page 105 in: *Genitourinary Cancer: Contemporary Issues in Clinical Oncology,* Vol 5. Garnick MB (editor). Churchill Livingstone, 1985.

The Leuprolide Study Group: Leuprolide versus diethylstilbestrol for metastatic prostate cancer. *N Engl J Med* 1984;**311**:1281.

## TUMORS OF THE TESTIS
### (See also Chapter 18.)

### Essentials of Diagnosis
- Painless enlargement of the testis.
- Mass does not transilluminate.
- Evidence of metastases.

### General Considerations

The incidence of testicular tumors is about 0.5% of all types of cancer in males. Tumors occur most frequently between ages 18 and 35 and are often malignant. Classification of tumors of the testes is based upon their origin from germinal components or from nongerminal cells. The most common are the germinal tumors: seminomas; embryonal tumors, including embryoma, choriocarcinoma, embryonal carcinoma, teratocarcinoma, and adult teratoma; and the gonadoblastomas of intersexes. Nongerminal tumors include those of interstitial cell, Sertoli cell, and stromal origin. Rarely, lymphomas, leukemias, plasmacytomas, and metastatic carcinoma may involve the testis.

Seminomas, the most common testicular tumors, tend to spread slowly via the lymphatics to the iliac and periaortic nodes and disseminate late. Embryonal tumors invade the spermatic cord and metastasize early, particularly to the lungs. Seminomas are usually radiosensitive; embryonal tumors are usually radioresistant. Chemotherapy may be helpful in choriocarcinoma.

Secretion of gonadotropic hormones occurs with only about 10% of tumors. The literature on tumor-hormonal relationships is limited and confusing, but gonadotropin secretion is usually indicative of a carcinomatous tumor.

Gynecomastia may be associated with testicular tumors. Interstitial cell tumors, which occur at any age and are rarely malignant, are occasionally associated with gynecomastia and with sexual precocity and virilization.

### Clinical Findings

**A. Symptoms and Signs:** Painless enlargement of the testes is typical. The enlarged testis may produce a dragging inguinal pain. The tumor is usually symmetric and firm, and pressure does not produce the typical testicular pain. The tumors do not transilluminate. Attachment to the scrotal skin is rare. Gynecomastia may be present. Virilization may occur in preadolescent boys with Leydig cell tumors. Hydrocele may develop.

Metastases commonly go to regional lymph nodes and then to those of the mediastinum and supraclavicular region. The lungs and the liver are often sites of metastases.

**B. Laboratory Findings:** Gonadotropins may be present in high concentrations in urine and plasma in cases of choriocarcinoma, and pregnancy tests are positive. Radioimmunoassay for the beta unit of human chorionic gonadotropin is the test of choice for diagnosis and follow-up assessment. Urinary 17-ketosteroids are normal or low in Leydig cell tumors. Estrogens may be elaborated in both Sertoli cell and Leydig cell tumors. Alpha-fetoprotein is a useful tumor marker for diagnosis and assessment of the tumor burden of teratocarcinoma and embryonal carcinoma (derivatives of the extraembryonic primitive yolk sac).

**C. Imaging:** Pulmonary metastases are demonstrated by chest radiographs. Lymphangiography will reveal enlarged iliac and periaortic nodes. Displacement of ureters by enlarged lymph nodes can be demonstrated by use of urography or venacavograms. Tumors of the testicle are easily discerned with ultrasonography.

## Differential Diagnosis

Tuberculosis, syphilitic orchitis (gumma of the testicle), hydrocele, spermatocele, and tumors or granulomas of the epididymis may produce similar local manifestations.

## Treatment

The testicle should be removed and the lumbar and inguinal nodes examined. Radical resection of iliac and lumbar nodes is usually indicated except for seminoma, which is radiosensitive. Radiation therapy is the treatment of choice following removal of the testis bearing a seminoma. Radiation therapy is employed following radical surgery for other malignant tumors. Chemotherapy is effective against chorionic tumors (choriocarcinoma). Metastatic disease may be curable with combination chemotherapy, including cisplatin, vinblastine, and bleomycin. Other drugs that may be effective in various combinations include vincristine, dactinomycin, doxorubicin, and cyclophosphamide.

## Prognosis

The presence of metastases or high gonadotropin secretion indicates a less favorable prognosis. Seminomas are least malignant, with 90% 5-year cures. With modern chemotherapeutic regimens, other cell types are increasingly effectively treated, resulting in cures of even widespread metastatic disease.

Drasga RE, Einhorn LH, Williams SD: The chemotherapy of testicular cancer. *CA* 1982;**32:**66.

Einhorn LH: Cancer of the testis: A new paradigm. *Hosp Pract* (April 15) 1986;**21:**165.

Fraley EE, Lange PH, Kennedy BJ: Germ-cell testicular cancer in adults. (2 parts.) *N Engl J Med* 1979;**301:**1370, 1420.

Hainsworth JD, Greco FA: Testicular germ cell neoplasms. *Am J Med* 1983;**75:**817.

# REFERENCES

Brenner BM, Rector FC Jr: *The Kidney,* 3rd ed. Saunders, 1986.

Heptinstall RH: *Pathology of the Kidney,* 3rd ed. Little, Brown, 1983.

Klahr S: Pathophysiology of obstructive nephropathy. *Kidney Int* 1983;**23:**414.

Massry SG, Glassock RJ (editors): *Textbook of Nephrology.* Williams & Wilkins, 1983.

Maxwell MH, Kleeman CR, Narins RG (editors): *Clinical Disorders of Fluid and Electrolyte Metabolism,* 4th ed. McGraw-Hill, 1987.

Schrier RW (editor): *Renal and Electrolyte Disorders,* 2nd ed. Little, Brown, 1980.

Stanbury JB et al (editors): *The Metabolic Basis of Inherited Disease,* 5th ed. McGraw-Hill, 1983.

Tanagho EA, McAninch JW: *Smith's General Urology,* 12th ed. Appleton & Lange, 1987.

Tanagho EA, Williams RD: Urology. Pages 823–883 in: *Current Surgical Diagnosis & Treatment.* Way LW (editor). Lange, 1985.

# Nervous System

*Michael J. Aminoff, MD, FRCP*

## HEADACHE

Headache is such a common complaint and can occur for so many different reasons that its proper evaluation may be difficult. Although underlying structural lesions are not present in most patients presenting with headache, it is nevertheless important to bear this possibility in mind. About one-third of patients with brain tumors, for example, present with a primary complaint of headache.

The intensity, quality, and site of pain—and especially the duration of the headache and the presence of associated neurologic symptoms—may provide clues to the underlying cause. The onset of severe headache in a previously well patient is more likely than chronic headache to relate to an intracranial disorder such as subarachnoid hemorrhage or meningitis. Headaches that disturb sleep, exertional headaches, and late-onset paroxysmal headaches are also more suggestive of an underlying structural lesion, as are headaches accompanied by neurologic symptoms such as drowsiness, visual or limb problems, seizures, or altered mental status. Chronic headaches are commonly due to migraine, tension, or depression, but they may be related to intracranial lesions, head injury, cervical spondylosis, dental or ocular disease, temporomandibular joint dysfunction, sinusitis, hypertension, and a wide variety of general medical disorders. Depending on the initial clinical impression, the need for such investigations as CT scan of the head, electroencephalography, and lumbar puncture must be assessed on an individual basis. The diagnosis and treatment of primary neurologic disorders associated with headache are considered separately under these disorders.

### Tension Headache

Patients frequently complain of poor concentration and other vague nonspecific symptoms, in addition to constant daily headaches that are often viselike or tight in quality and may be exacerbated by emotional stress, fatigue, noise, or glare. The headaches are usually generalized, may be most intense about the neck or back of the head, and are not associated with focal neurologic symptoms.

When treatment with simple analgesics is not effective, a trial of antimigrainous agents (see Migraine, below) is worthwhile. Techniques to induce relaxation are also useful and include massage, hot baths, and biofeedback. Exploration of underlying causes of chronic anxiety is often rewarding.

### Depression Headache

Depression headaches are frequently worse on arising in the morning and may be accompanied by other symptoms of depression. Headaches are occasionally the focus of a somatic delusional system (eg, fear that the brain is "rotting"). Tricyclic antidepressant drugs are often helpful, as may be psychiatric consultation.

### Migraine

Classic migrainous headache is a lateralized throbbing headache that occurs episodically following its onset in adolescence or early adult life. In many cases, however, the headaches do not conform to this pattern, although their associated features and response to antimigrainous preparations nevertheless suggest that they have a similar basis. In this broader sense, migrainous headaches may be lateralized or generalized, may be dull or throbbing, and are sometimes associated with anorexia, nausea, vomiting, photophobia, and blurring of vision (so-called sick headaches). They usually build up gradually and may last for several hours or longer. They have been related to dilatation and excessive pulsation of branches of the external carotid artery. Focal disturbances of neurologic function may precede or accompany the headaches and have been attributed to constriction of branches of the internal carotid artery. Visual disturbances occur quite commonly and may consist of field defects; of luminous visual hallucinations such as stars, sparks, unformed light flashes (photopsia), geometric patterns, or zigzags of light; or of some combination of field defects and luminous hallucinations (scintillating scotomas). Other focal disturbances such as aphasia or numbness, tingling, clumsiness, or weakness in a circumscribed distribution may also occur.

Patients often give a family history of migraine. Attacks may be triggered by emotional or physical stress, lack or excess of sleep, missed meals, specific foods (eg, chocolate), alcoholic beverages, menstruation, or use of oral contraceptives.

An uncommon variant is so-called basilar artery migraine, in which blindness or visual disturbances throughout both visual fields are initially accompanied or followed by dysarthria, dysequilibrium, tinnitus, and perioral and distal paresthesias and are sometimes followed by transient loss or impairment of consciousness or by a confusional state. This, in turn, is followed by a throbbing (usually occipital) headache, often with nausea and vomiting.

In ophthalmoplegic migraine, lateralized pain—often about the eye—is accompanied by nausea, vomiting, and diplopia due to transient external ophthalmoplegia. The ophthalmoplegia is due to third nerve palsy, sometimes with accompanying sixth nerve involvement, and may outlast the orbital pain by several days or even weeks. The ophthalmic division of the fifth nerve has also been affected in some patients. Ophthalmoplegic migraine is rare; more common causes of a painful ophthalmoplegia are internal carotid artery aneurysms and diabetes.

In rare instances, the neurologic or somatic disturbance accompanying typical migrainous headaches becomes the sole manifestation of an attack (''migraine equivalent''). On other occasions, the patient may be left with a permanent neurologic deficit following a migrainous attack, presumably because of irreversible cerebral ischemic damage.

Management of migraine consists of avoidance of any precipitating factors, together with prophylactic or symptomatic pharmacologic treatment if necessary.

During acute attacks, many patients find it helpful to rest in a quiet, darkened room until symptoms subside. A simple analgesic (eg, aspirin) taken right away often provides relief, but treatment with extracranial vasoconstrictors or other drugs is sometimes necessary. Cafergot, a combination of ergotamine tartrate and caffeine, is often particularly helpful; 1–4 tablets are taken at the onset of headache or warning symptoms, and more are taken after about 20 minutes if symptoms have not begun to subside. Ergonovine maleate, up to 5 tablets (1 mg) taken at the onset of symptoms, may also provide relief. Because of impaired absorption or vomiting during acute attacks, oral medication sometimes fails to help. Cafergot given rectally as suppositories, ergotamine tartrate given intramuscularly (0.25–0.5 mg), or dihydroergotamine mesylate given either intramuscularly or intravenously (0.5–1 mg) may be useful in such cases. Ergotamine-containing preparations may affect the gravid uterus and thus should be avoided during pregnancy. Mefenamic acid may also help if taken (with food) at the onset of an acute migraine attack.

Prophylactic treatment may be necessary if migrainous headaches occur frequently. Some of the more common drugs used for this purpose are listed in Table 16–1. Drugs that are least likely to produce severe or disabling side effects should be tried first. Several drugs may have to be tried in turn, however, before the headaches are brought under control. Once a drug has been found to help, it should be continued for several months. If the patient remains headache-free, the dose can then be tapered and the drug eventually withdrawn. Many patients have spontaneous remission, so that medication can be discontinued, at least for a while.

## Cluster Headache
## (Migrainous Neuralgia)

Cluster headache affects predominantly middle-aged men. There is often no family history of headache or migraine. Episodes of severe unilateral periorbital pain occur daily for several weeks and are often accompanied by one or more of the following: ipsilateral nasal congestion, rhinorrhea, lacrimation, redness of the eye, and Horner's syndrome. Episodes usually occur at night, awaken the patient from sleep, and last for less than 2 hours. Spontaneous remission then occurs, and the patient remains well for weeks or months before another bout of closely spaced attacks occurs. During a bout, many patients report that alcohol triggers an attack; others report that stress, glare, or ingestion of specific foods occasionally precipitates attacks. In experimental studies, sublingual nitroglycerin or subcutaneous histamine was found to provoke attacks in some patients.

In occasional patients, typical attacks of pain and associated symptoms recur at intervals without remission. This variant has been referred to as chronic cluster headache.

Clinical examination reveals no abnormality apart from Horner's syndrome that either occurs transiently

**Table 16–1.** Prophylactic treatment of migraine.*

| Drug | Usual Adult Daily Dose (mg) | Common Side Effects |
|---|---|---|
| Propranolol | 80–240 | Fatigue, lassitude, depression, insomnia, nausea, vomiting, constipation. |
| Amitriptyline | 10–150 | Sedation, dry mouth, constipation, weight gain, blurred vision, edema, hypotension, urinary retention. |
| Ergonovine maleate | 0.6–2 | Nausea, abdominal pain, diarrhea. |
| Cyproheptadine | 12–20 | Sedation, dry mouth, epigastric discomfort, gastrointestinal disturbances. |
| Clonidine | 0.2–0.6 | Dry mouth, drowsiness, sedation, headache, constipation. |
| Methysergide | 4–8 | Nausea, vomiting, diarrhea, abdominal pain, cramps, weight gain, insomnia, edema, peripheral vasoconstriction. Retroperitoneal and pleuropulmonary fibrosis and fibrous thickening of cardiac valves may occur; patients must be closely supervised. |

* Reproduced, with permission, from Aminoff MJ: Neurologic disorders. In: *Handbook of Medical Treatment,* 17th ed. Watts HD (editor). Jones, 1983.

during an attack or, in long-standing cases, remains as a residual deficit between attacks.

Treatment of an individual attack with oral drugs is generally unsatisfactory, but use of ergotamine tartrate aerosol or inhalation of 100% oxygen (7 L/min for 15 minutes) is often effective. Drugs should be given to prevent further attacks until the ongoing bout is over. Ergotamine tartrate is an effective prophylactic and can be given as rectal suppositories (0.5–1 mg at night or twice daily), by mouth (2 mg daily), or by subcutaneous injection (0.25 mg 3 times daily for 5 days per week). Various prophylactic agents that have been found to be effective in individual patients are propranolol, amitriptyline, cyproheptadine, lithium carbonate (monitored by plasma lithium determination), prednisone (20–40 mg daily or on alternate days for 2 weeks, followed by gradual withdrawal), and methysergide (4–6 mg daily).

## Giant Cell (Temporal or Cranial) Arteritis

The superficial temporal, vertebral, ophthalmic, and posterior ciliary arteries are often the most severely affected pathologically. The major symptom is headache, often associated with or preceded by myalgia, malaise, anorexia, weight loss, and other nonspecific complaints. Loss of vision is the most feared manifestation and occurs quite commonly. Clinical examination often reveals tenderness of the scalp and over the temporal arteries, which may become thrombosed. Further details, including approaches to treatment, are given in Chapter 14.

## Posttraumatic Headache

A variety of nonspecific symptoms may follow a closed head injury, regardless of whether or not consciousness is lost. Headache is often a conspicuous feature. Some authorities believe that psychologic factors bear on the development of the syndrome, because its development does not correlate with the severity of the injury and neurologic signs are lacking.

The headache itself usually appears within a day or so following injury, may worsen over the ensuing weeks, and then gradually subsides. It is usually a constant dull ache, with superimposed throbbing that may be localized, lateralized, or generalized. It is sometimes accompanied by nausea, vomiting, or scintillating scotomas.

Dysequilibrium, sometimes with a rotatory component, may also occur in the posttraumatic syndrome and is often enhanced by postural change or head movement. Impaired memory, poor concentration, emotional instability, and increased irritability are other common complaints and occasionally are the sole manifestations of the syndrome. The duration of symptoms relates in part to the severity of the original injury, but even trivial injuries are sometimes followed by symptoms that persist for months.

Special investigations are usually not helpful. The electroencephalogram may show minor nonspecific changes, while the electronystagmogram sometimes suggests either peripheral or central vestibulopathy. CT scans of the head usually show no abnormal findings.

Treatment is difficult, but optimistic encouragement and graduated rehabilitation, depending upon the occupational circumstances, are advised. Headaches often respond to simple analgesics, but severe headaches may necessitate treatment with amitriptyline, propranolol, or ergot derivatives.

## Cough Headache

Severe head pain may be produced by coughing (and by straining, sneezing, and laughing) but, fortunately, usually lasts for only a few minutes or less. The pathophysiologic basis of the complaint is not known, and often there is no underlying structural lesion. However, intracranial lesions, usually in the posterior fossa (eg, Arnold-Chiari malformation, basilar impression), are present in about 10% of cases, and brain tumors or other space-occupying lesions may certainly present in this way. Accordingly, CT scanning should be undertaken in all patients and repeated annually, since a small structural lesion may not show up initially.

The disorder is usually self-limited, although it may persist for several years. For unknown reasons, symptoms sometimes clear completely after lumbar puncture. Indomethacin may provide relief.

## Headache Due to Other Neurologic Causes

Intracranial mass lesions of all types may cause headache owing to displacement of vascular structures. Posterior fossa tumors often cause occipital pain, and supratentorial lesions lead to bifrontal headache, but such findings are too inconsistent to be of value in attempts at localizing a pathologic process. The headaches are nonspecific in character and may vary in severity from mild to severe. They may be worsened by exertion or postural change and may be associated with nausea and vomiting, but this is true of migraine also. Headaches are also a feature of pseudotumor cerebri (see below). Signs of focal or diffuse cerebral dysfunction or of increased intracranial pressure will indicate the need for further investigation. Similarly, a progressive headache disorder or the new onset of headaches in middle or later life merits investigation if no cause is apparent.

Cerebrovascular disease may be associated with headache, but the mechanism is unclear. Headache may occur with internal carotid artery occlusion or carotid dissection and after carotid endarterectomy. Diagnosis is facilitated by the clinical accompaniments and the circumstances in which the headache developed.

Acute severe headache accompanies subarachnoid hemorrhage and meningeal infections, but the accompanying signs of meningeal irritation and the frequent impairment of consciousness then indicate the need for further investigations. A dramatically severe headache may also occur in association with paroxysmal hypertension in patients with pheochromocytoma.

Dull or throbbing headache is a frequent sequela of lumbar puncture and may last for several days. It is aggravated by the erect posture and alleviated by recumbency. The exact mechanism is unclear, but it is commonly attributed to leakage of cerebrospinal fluid through the dural puncture site.

Caviness VS, O'Brien P: Headache. *N Engl J Med* 1980;**302**:446.

Diamond S, Dalessio DJ: *The Practicing Physician's Approach to Headache*, 3rd ed. Williams & Wilkins, 1982.

Kudrow L: *Cluster Headache: Mechanisms and Management*. Oxford Univ Press, 1980.

Lance JW: Headache. *Ann Neurol* 1981;**10**:1.

Raskin NH, Appenzeller O: *Headache*. Vol 19 of: *Major Problems in Internal Medicine*. Saunders, 1980.

## FACIAL PAIN

### Trigeminal Neuralgia

Trigeminal neuralgia may begin at any age but is most common in middle and later life. It affects women more frequently than men. The disorder is characterized by momentary episodes of sudden lancinating facial pain that commonly arises near one side of the mouth and then shoots toward the ear, eye, or nostril on that side. The pain may be triggered or precipitated by such factors as touch, movement, drafts, and eating. Indeed, in order to lessen the likelihood of triggering further attacks, many patients try to hold the face still while talking. Spontaneous remissions for several months or longer may occur. As the disorder progresses, however, the episodes of pain become more frequent, remissions become shorter and less common, and a dull ache may persist between the episodes of stabbing pain. Symptoms remain confined to the distribution of the trigeminal nerve (usually the second or third division) on one side only.

The characteristic features of the pain in trigeminal neuralgia usually distinguish it without difficulty from other causes of facial pain. In general, neurologic examination shows no abnormality except in a few patients in whom trigeminal neuralgia is symptomatic of some underlying lesion, such as multiple sclerosis or a brain stem neoplasm, in which case the finding will depend on the nature and site of the lesion. Similarly, CT scans and radiologic contrast studies are normal in patients with classic trigeminal neuralgia. In a young patient presenting with trigeminal neuralgia, multiple sclerosis must be suspected even if there are no other neurologic signs. In such circumstances, findings on evoked potential testing and examination of cerebrospinal fluid may be corroborative. When the facial pain is due to a posterior fossa tumor, CT scanning and arteriography generally reveal the lesion, which should then be surgically removed if possible.

The drug most helpful for treatment of trigeminal neuralgia is carbamazepine, given in a dose of up to 1200 mg/d, with monitoring by serial blood counts and liver function tests. If carbamazepine is ineffective or cannot be tolerated by the patient, phenytoin should be tried. (Doses and side effects of these drugs are shown in Table 16–2.) Baclofen may also be helpful, either alone or in combination with carbamazepine or phenytoin.

In the past, various surgical and other means of providing symptomatic relief (eg, alcohol injection of the affected nerve, rhizotomy, or tractotomy) were recommended if pharmacologic treatment was unsuccessful. More recently, however, posterior fossa exploration has frequently revealed some structural cause for the neuralgia (despite normal findings on CT scans or arteriograms), such as an anomalous artery or vein impinging on the trigeminal nerve root. In such cases, simple decompression and separation of the anomalous vessel from the nerve root produce lasting relief of symptoms. In elderly patients with a limited life expectancy, radiofrequency rhizotomy is sometimes preferred because it is easy to perform, has few complications, and provides symptomatic relief for a period of time. Surgical exploration generally reveals no abnormality and is inappropriate in patients with trigeminal neuralgia due to multiple sclerosis.

### Atypical Facial Pain

Facial pain without the typical features of trigeminal neuralgia is generally a constant, often burning pain that may have a restricted distribution at its onset but soon spreads to the rest of the face on the affected side and sometimes involves the other side, the neck, or the back of the head as well. The disorder is especially common in middle-aged women, many of them emotionally depressed, but it is not clear whether depression is the cause of or a reaction to the pain. Most forms of treatment either are unhelpful or provide benefit for only a limited period. Simple analgesics should be given a trial, as should tricyclic antidepressants, carbamazepine, and phenytoin. Opiate analgesics should be avoided, since addiction is a very real danger in patients with this disorder. Attempts at surgical treatment are not indicated.

### Glossopharyngeal Neuralgia

Glossopharyngeal neuralgia is an uncommon disorder in which pain similar in quality to that in trigeminal neuralgia occurs in the throat, about the tonsillar fossa, and sometimes deep in the ear and at the back of the tongue. The pain may be precipitated by swallowing, chewing, talking, or yawning and is sometimes accompanied by syncope. In most instances, no underlying structural abnormality is present. Carbamazepine is the treatment of choice and should be tried before any surgical procedures are considered.

### Postherpetic Neuralgia

About 10% of patients who develop shingles suffer from postherpetic neuralgia. This complication seems

**Table 16–2.** Drug treatment for seizures.*

| | Usual Adult Daily Dose (mg/kg) | Usual Adult Daily Dose (mg) | Minimum Number of Daily Doses | Time to Steady-State Drug Levels (days) | Optimal Blood Level (per mL) | Selected Side Effects and Idiosyncratic Reactions |
|---|---|---|---|---|---|---|
| **Generalized tonic-colonic (grand mal) or partial (focal) seizures** | | | | | | |
| Phenytoin | 4–8 | 200–400 | 1 | 5–10 | 10–20 µg | Nystagmus, ataxia, dysarthria, sedation, confusion, gingival hyperplasia, hirsutism, megaloblastic anemia, blood dyscrasias, skin rashes, fever, systemic lupus erythematosus, lymphadenopathy, peripheral neuropathy, dyskinesias. |
| Carbamazepine | 5–25 | 600–1200 | 2 | 3–4 | 4–8 µg | Nystagmus, dysarthria, diplopia, ataxia, drowsiness, nausea, blood dyscrasias, hepatotoxicity. |
| Phenobarbital | 2–5 | 100–200 | 1 | 14–21 | 10–40 µg | Drowsiness, nystagmus, ataxia, skin rashes, learning difficulties, hyperactivity. |
| Primidone | 5–20 | 750–1500 | 3 | 4–7 | 5–15 µg | Sedation, nystagmus, ataxia, vertigo, nausea, skin rashes, megaloblastic anemia, irritability. |
| Valproic acid | 10–60 | | 3 | 2–4 | 50–100 µg | Nausea, vomiting, diarrhea, drowsiness, alopecia, weight gain, hepatotoxicity, thrombocytopenia, tremor. |
| **Absence (petit mal) seizures** | | | | | | |
| Ethosuximide | 20–35 | 100–1500 | 2 | 5–10 | 40–100 µg | Nausea, vomiting, anorexia, headache, lethargy, unsteadiness, blood dyscrasias, systemic lupus erythematosus, urticaria, pruritus. |
| Valproic acid | 10–60 | | 3 | 2–4 | 50–100 µg | See above. |
| Clonazepam | 0.05–0.2 | | 2 | ? | 20–80 ng | Drowsiness, ataxia, irritability, behavioral changes, exacerbation of tonic-clonic seizures. |
| **Myoclonic seizures** | | | | | | |
| Valproic acid | 10–60 | | 3 | 2–4 | 50–100 µg | See above. |
| Clonazepam | 0.05–0.2 | | 2 | ? | 20–80 ng | See above. |

* Reproduced, with permission, from Aminoff MJ: Neurologic disorders. In: *Handbook of Medical Treatment,* 17th ed. Watts HD (editor). Jones, 1983.

especially likely to occur in the elderly and when the first division of the trigeminal nerve is affected. A history of shingles and the presence of cutaneous scarring resulting from shingles aid in the diagnosis. Severe pain with shingles correlates with the intensity of postherpetic symptoms.

The incidence of postherpetic neuralgia may be reduced by the treatment of shingles with steroids. Management of the established complication is essentially medical. If simple analgesics fail to help, a trial of a tricyclic drug (eg, amitriptyline, up to 100–150 mg/d) in conjunction with a phenothiazine (eg, perphenazine, 2–8 mg/d) is often effective. Many patients derive benefit from using a vibrator on the affected area and gradually increasing the frequency of application and the intensity of vibration with time, as tolerance increases.

## Facial Pain Due to Other Causes

Facial pain may be caused by temporomandibular joint dysfunction in patients with malocclusion, abnormal bite, or faulty dentures. There may be tenderness of the masticatory muscles, and an association between pain onset and jaw movement is sometimes noted. Treatment consists of correction of the underlying problem.

A relationship of facial pain to chewing or temperature changes may suggest a dental disturbance. Facial swelling and trismus, when present, help to establish the diagnosis. Nevertheless, the cause is sometimes not obvious, and diagnosis requires careful dental examination and x-rays.

Sinusitis and ear infections causing facial pain are usually recognized by the history of respiratory tract infection and fever and, in some instances, aural discharge. There may be localized tenderness. Radiologic evidence of sinus infection or mastoiditis is confirmatory.

Glaucoma is an important ocular cause of facial pain, usually localized to the periorbital region. The underlying cause should be treated.

On occasion, pain in the jaw may be the principal manifestation of angina pectoris. Precipitation by exertion and radiation to more typical areas help to establish the cardiac origin of pain.

Facial pain may also be due to cluster headache or to preeruptive herpes zoster (see above).

Sweet WH: The treatment of trigeminal neuralgia (tic douloureux). *New Engl J Med* 1986;**315**:174.

Zorman G, Wilson CB: Outcome following microvascular decompression or partial sensory rhizotomy in 125 cases of trigeminal neuralgia. *Neurology* 1984;**34**:1362.

# EPILEPSY

## Essentials of Diagnosis

- Recurrent seizures.
- Characteristic electroencephalographic changes accompany seizures.
- Mental status abnormalities or focal neurologic symptoms may persist for hours postictally.

## General Considerations

The term epilepsy denotes any disorder characterized by recurrent seizures. A seizure is a transient disturbance of cerebral function due to an abnormal paroxysmal neuronal discharge in the brain. Epilepsy is common, affecting approximately 0.5% of the population in the USA.

## Etiology

Epilepsy has several causes. Its most likely cause in individual patients relates to the age of onset.

**A. Idiopathic or Constitutional Epilepsy:** Seizures usually begin between 5 and 20 years of age but may start later in life. No specific cause can be identified, and there is no other neurologic abnormality.

**B. Symptomatic Epilepsy:** There are many causes for recurrent seizures.

**1. Congenital abnormalities and perinatal injuries** may result in seizures presenting in infancy or childhood.

**2. Metabolic disorders** such as hypocalcemia, hypoglycemia, pyridoxine deficiency, and phenylketonuria are major treatable causes of seizures in newborns or infants. In adults, withdrawal from alcohol or drugs is a common cause of recurrent seizures, and other metabolic disorders such as renal failure and diabetes may also be responsible.

**3. Trauma** is an important cause of seizures at any age, but especially in young adults. Posttraumatic epilepsy is more likely to develop if the dura mater was penetrated and generally becomes manifest within 2 years following the injury. However, seizures developing in the first week after head injury do not necessarily imply that future attacks will occur. There is suggestive evidence that prophylactic anticonvulsant drug treatment reduces the incidence of posttraumatic epilepsy.

**4. Tumors and other space-occupying lesions** may lead to seizures at any age, but they are an especially important cause of seizures in middle and later life, when the incidence of neoplastic disease increases. The seizures are commonly the initial symptoms of the tumor and often are partial (focal) in character. They are most likely to occur with structural lesions involving the frontal, parietal, or temporal regions. Tumors must be excluded by appropriate laboratory studies in all patients with onset of seizures after 30 years of age, focal seizures or signs, or a progressive seizure disorder.

**5. Vascular diseases** become increasingly frequent causes of seizures with advancing age and are the most common cause of seizures with onset at age 60 years or older.

**6. Degenerative disorders** are a cause of seizures in later life.

**7. Infectious diseases** must be considered in all age groups as potentially reversible causes of seizures. Seizures may occur with an acute infective or inflammatory illness, such as bacterial meningitis or herpes encephalitis, or in patients with more longstanding or chronic disorders such as neurosyphilis or cerebral cysticercosis. Seizures are a common sequela of supratentorial brain abscess, developing most frequently in the first year after treatment.

## Classification of Seizures

Seizures can be categorized in various ways, but the descriptive classification proposed by the International League Against Epilepsy is clinically the most useful. Seizures are divided into those that are generalized and those affecting only part of the brain (partial seizures).

**A. Partial Seizures:** The initial clinical and electroencephalographic manifestations of partial seizures indicate that only a restricted part of one cerebral hemisphere has been activated. The ictal manifestations depend upon the area of the brain involved. Partial seizures are subdivided into simple seizures, in which consciousness is preserved, and complex seizures, in which it is impaired. Partial seizures of either type sometimes become secondarily generalized, leading to a tonic, clonic, or tonic-clonic attack.

**1. Simple partial seizures**–Simple seizures may be manifested by focal motor symptoms (convulsive jerking) or somatosensory symptoms (eg, paresthesias or tingling) that spread (or "march") to different parts of the limb or body depending upon their cortical representation. In other instances, special sensory symptoms (eg, light flashes or buzzing) indicate involvement of visual, auditory, olfactory, or gustatory regions of the brain, or there may be autonomic symptoms or signs (eg, abnormal epigastric sensations, sweating, flushing, pupillary dilation). When psychic symptoms occur, they are usually accompanied by impairment of consciousness, but the sole manifestations of some seizures are phenomena such as dysphasia, dysmnesic symptoms (eg, *déjà vu, jamais vu*), affective disturbances, illusions, or structured hallucinations.

**2. Complex partial seizures**–Impaired consciousness may be preceded, accompanied, or followed by the psychic symptoms mentioned above, and automatisms may occur. Such seizures may also begin with some of the other simple symptoms mentioned above.

**B. Generalized Seizures:** There are several different varieties of generalized seizures, as outlined below. In some circumstances, seizures cannot be classified because of incomplete information or because they do not fit into any category.

**1. Absence (petit mal) seizures**–These are characterized by impairment of consciousness, sometimes with mild clonic, tonic, or atonic components (ie, reduction or loss of postural tone), autonomic components (eg, enuresis), or accompanying automatisms. Onset and termination of attacks are abrupt. If attacks occur during conversation, the patient may miss a few words or may break off in mid sentence for a few seconds. The impairment of external awareness is so brief that the patient is unaware of it. Absence seizures almost always begin in childhood and frequently cease by the age of 20 years, although occasionally they are then replaced by other forms of generalized seizure. Electroencephalographically, such attacks are associated with bursts of bilaterally synchronous and symmetric 3-Hz spike-and-wave activity. A normal background in the electroencephalogram and normal or above-normal intelligence imply a good prognosis for the ultimate cessation of these seizures.

**2. Atypical absences**–There may be more marked changes in tone, or attacks may have a more gradual onset and termination than in typical absences.

**3. Myoclonic seizures**–Myoclonic seizures consist of single or multiple myoclonic jerks.

**4. Tonic-clonic (grand mal) seizures**–In these seizures, which are characterized by sudden loss of consciousness, the patient becomes rigid and falls to the ground, and respiration is arrested. This tonic phase, which usually lasts for less than a minute, is followed by a clonic phase in which there is jerking of the body musculature that may last for 2 or 3 minutes and is then followed by a stage of flaccid coma. During the seizure, the tongue or lips may be bitten, urinary or fecal incontinence may occur, and the patient may be injured. Immediately after the seizure, the patient may either recover consciousness, drift into sleep, have a further convulsion without recovery of consciousness between the attacks (**status epilepticus**), or after recovering consciousness have a further convulsion (**serial seizures**). In other cases, patients will behave in an abnormal fashion in the immediate postictal period, without subsequent awareness or memory of events (**postepileptic automatism**). Headache, disorientation, confusion, drowsiness, nausea, soreness of the muscles, or some combination of these symptoms commonly occurs postictally.

**5. Tonic, clonic, or atonic seizures**–Loss of consciousness may occur with either the tonic or clonic accompaniments described above, especially in children. Atonic seizures (**epileptic drop attacks**) have also been described.

## Clinical Findings

**A. Symptoms and Signs:** Nonspecific changes such as headache, mood alterations, lethargy, and myoclonic jerking alert some patients to an impending seizure hours before it occurs. These prodromal symptoms are distinct from the aura which may precede a generalized seizure by a few seconds or minutes and which is itself a part of the attack, arising locally from a restricted region of the brain.

In most patients, seizures occur unpredictably at any time and without any relationship to posture or ongoing activities. Occasionally, however, they occur at a particular time (eg, during sleep) or in relation to external precipitants such as lack of sleep, missed meals, emotional stress, menstruation, alcohol ingestion (or alcohol withdrawal; see below), or use of certain drugs. Fever and nonspecific infections may also precipitate seizures in known epileptics; in infants and young children, it may be hard to distinguish such attacks from febrile seizures. In a few patients, seizures are provoked by specific stimuli such as flashing lights or a flickering television set (**photosensitive epilepsy**), music, or reading.

Clinical examination between seizures shows no abnormality in patients with idiopathic epilepsy, but in the immediate postictal period, extensor plantar responses may be seen. The presence of lateralized or focal signs postictally suggests that seizures may have a focal origin. In patients with symptomatic epilepsy, the findings on examination will reflect the underlying cause.

**B. Imaging:** CT or MRI scan is indicated in all patients with focal neurologic symptoms or signs, focal seizures, or electroencephalographic findings of a focal disturbance. It should also be performed in patients with clinical evidence of a progressive disorder and in those presenting with seizures after the age of 30 years, because of the possibility of an underlying neoplasm. A chest radiograph should also be obtained in such patients, since the lungs are a common site for primary or secondary neoplasms.

**C. Laboratory and Other Studies:** In patients older than 10 years, initial investigations should always include a full blood count, blood glucose determination, liver and renal function tests. The hematologic and biochemical screening tests are important both in excluding various causes of seizures and in providing a baseline for subsequent monitoring of long-term effects of treatment.

Electroencephalography should be performed. The findings may support the clinical diagnosis of epilepsy (by demonstrating paroxysmal abnormalities containing spikes or sharp waves), may provide a guide to prognosis, and may help classify the seizure disorder. Classification of the disorder is important for determining the most appropriate anticonvulsant drug with which to start treatment. For example, absence (petit mal) and complex partial seizures may be difficult to distinguish clinically, but the electroencephalographic findings and treatment of choice differ in these 2 conditions. Finally, the electroencephalographic findings are important in evaluating candidates for surgical treatment.

## Differential Diagnosis

The distinction between the various disorders likely to be confused with generalized seizures is usually made on the basis of the history. The importance of obtaining an eyewitness account of the attacks cannot be overemphasized.

**A. Differential Diagnosis of Partial Seizures:**

**1. Transient ischemic attacks**–These attacks are distinguished from seizures by their longer duration, lack of spread, and symptomatology. There is a loss of motor or sensory function (eg, weakness or numbness) with transient ischemic attacks, whereas positive symptomatology (eg, convulsive jerking or paresthesias) characterizes seizures.

**2. Rage attacks**–Rage attacks are usually situational and lead to goal-directed aggressive behavior.

**3. Panic attacks**–These may be hard to distinguish from simple or complex partial seizures unless there is evidence of psychopathologic disturbances between attacks and the attacks have a clear relationship to external circumstances.

**B. Differential Diagnosis of Generalized Seizures:**

**1. Syncope**–Episodes of syncope usually occur while the patient is standing or after a sudden change in posture to the erect position, especially in patients with autonomic insufficiency. Syncope may occur in healthy individuals in hot weather, after pain or blood loss, during intense emotional stimulation, and following prolonged coughing or straining (which impedes venous return to the heart). Premonitory symptoms such as nausea, sweating, unsteadiness, yawning, and graying of vision are followed by loss of consciousness during which the patient is pale, sweaty, and flaccid and may experience one or 2 convulsive jerks. Injury is rare. Incontinence may occur and does not reliably distinguish seizures from syncope. Recovery is rapid once the patient is recumbent, but residual headache, nausea, sweatiness, and unsteadiness are common. If the patient is unable to fall into the recumbent position but is maintained upright (for example, by room fixtures and fittings), more conspicuous convulsive movements will occur.

**2. Cardiac dysrhythmias**–Cerebral hypoperfusion due to a disturbance of cardiac rhythm should be suspected in patients with known cardiac or vascular disease or in elderly patients who present with episodic loss of consciousness. A relationship of attacks to physical activity is suggestive of aortic stenosis. Repeated Holter monitoring may be necessary to establish the diagnosis; monitoring initiated by the patient ("event monitor") may be valuable if the disturbances of consciousness are rare.

**3. Brain stem ischemia**–Loss of consciousness is preceded or accompanied by other brain stem signs. Basilar artery migraine is discussed on p 572 and vertebrobasilar vascular disease on p 583.

**4. Pseudoseizures**–The term pseudoseizures is used to denote both hysterical conversion reactions and attacks due to malingering when these simulate epileptic seizures. Many patients with pseudoseizures also have true seizures or a family history of epilepsy. Although pseudoseizures tend to occur at times of emotional stress, this may also be the case with true seizures.

Clinically, the attacks superficially resemble tonic-clonic seizures, but there may be obvious preparation before pseudoseizures occur. Moreover, there is usually no tonic phase; instead, there is a wild and asynchronous thrashing about of the limbs, which increases if restraints are imposed and which rarely leads to injury or incontinence. Consciousness may be normal or "lost," but in the latter context the occurrence of goal-directed behavior or of shouting, swearing, etc, indicates that loss of consciousness is feigned. Postictally, there are no changes in behavior or neurologic findings, and the patient may vaguely recall some incident that occurred while consciousness was supposedly lost.

There are no electrocerebral changes during pseudoseizures. The serum level of prolactin has been found to increase dramatically between 15 and 30 minutes after a tonic-clonic convulsion in most patients, whereas it is unchanged after a pseudoseizure; similarly, temporary metabolic acidosis accompanies true generalized seizures.

## Treatment

**A. General Measures:** For patients with recurrent seizures, drug treatment is prescribed with the goal of preventing further attacks and is usually continued until there have been no seizures for at least 4 years. Epileptic patients should be advised to avoid situations that could be dangerous or life-threatening if further seizures should occur. State legislation may require physicians to report to the authorities any patients with seizures or other episodic disturbances of consciousness.

**1. Choice of medication**–The drug with which treatment is best initiated depends upon the type of seizures to be treated (Table 16–2). The dose of the selected drug is gradually increased until seizures are controlled, blood levels reach the upper limit of the optimal therapeutic range, or side effects prevent further increases. If seizures continue despite treatment at the maximal tolerated dose, a second drug is added and the dose increased until its blood levels are in the therapeutic range; the first drug is then gradually withdrawn. In treatment of partial and secondarily generalized tonic-clonic seizures, the success rate is higher with carbamazepine or phenytoin than with phenobarbital or primidone. In most patients with seizures of a single type, satisfactory control can be achieved with a single anticonvulsant drug. Treatment with 2 drugs may further reduce seizure frequency or severity, but usually only at the cost of greater toxicity. Treatment with more than 2 drugs is almost always unhelpful unless the patient is having seizures of different types. If the drugs shown in Table 16–2 are ineffective, a number of second-line anticonvulsant drugs can be tried, but these have more frequent and troublesome side effects, which limit their use.

**2. Monitoring**–Monitoring plasma drug levels has led to major advances in the management of seizure disorders. The same daily dose of a particular drug leads to markedly different blood concentrations in different patients, and this will affect the therapeutic response. Steady-state drug levels in the blood should therefore be measured after treatment is initiated, dosage is changed, or another drug is added to the therapeutic regimen and when seizures are poorly controlled. Dose adjustments are then guided by the laboratory findings. The most common cause of a lower concentration of drug than expected for the prescribed dose is poor patient compliance. Compliance can be improved by limiting to a minimum the number of daily doses. Recurrent seizures or status epilepticus may result if drugs are taken erratically, and in some circumstances noncompliant patients may be better off without any medication.

All anticonvulsant drugs have side effects, and some of these are shown in Table 16–2. A complete blood count should be performed at least annually in all patients, because of the risk of anemia or blood dyscrasia. Treatment with certain drugs may require more frequent monitoring or use of additional screening tests. For example, periodic tests of hepatic function are necessary if valproic acid or carbamazepine is used, and serial blood counts are important with carbamazepine or ethosuximide.

**3. Discontinuation of medication**–Only when patients have been seizure-free for several (at least 4) years should withdrawal of medication be considered. Unfortunately, there is no way of predicting which patients can be managed successfully without treatment, although seizure recurrence is more likely in patients who initially failed to respond to therapy, those with seizures having focal features or of multiple types, and those with continuing electroencephalographic abnormalities. Dose reduction should be gradual over a period of weeks or months, and drugs should be withdrawn one at a time. If seizures recur, treatment is reinstituted with the same drugs used previously. Seizures are no more difficult to control after a recurrence than before.

**B. Special Circumstances:**

**1. Solitary seizures**–In patients who have had only one seizure, investigation should exclude an underlying cause requiring specific treatment. Prophylactic anticonvulsant drug treatment is generally not required unless further attacks occur. The risk of seizure recurrence varies in different series, but in one recent survey it was only 27% over 3 years, with none occurring thereafter. Epilepsy should not be diagnosed on the basis of a solitary seizure, since the diagnosis of epilepsy is based on a history of repeated attacks in a patient expected to have further attacks. Similarly, if seizures occur only in the context of a transient, nonrecurrent systemic disorder, such as acute cerebral anoxia, the diagnosis of epilepsy

should be avoided, and long-term prophylactic anticonvulsant drug treatment is unnecessary.

**2. Alcohol withdrawal seizures**–One or a few generalized tonic-clonic seizures may occur within 48 hours or so of withdrawal from alcohol after a period of high or chronic intake. If the seizures have consistently focal features, the possibility of an associated structural abnormality, often traumatic in origin, must be considered. Treatment with anticonvulsant drugs is generally not required for alcohol withdrawal seizures, since they are self-limited. Status epilepticus may rarely follow alcohol withdrawal and is managed along conventional lines (see below). Long-term prophylactic anticonvulsant drug treatment is unnecessary and may even be hazardous if the patient complies poorly. Further attacks will not occur if the patient abstains from alcohol.

**3. Tonic-clonic status epilepticus**–Poor compliance with the anticonvulsant drug regimen is the most common cause of tonic-clonic status epilepticus. Other causes include alcohol withdrawal, intracranial infection or neoplasms, metabolic disorders, and drug overdose. The mortality rate may be as high as 20%, and among survivors the incidence of neurologic and mental sequelae may be high. The prognosis relates to the length of time between onset of status epilepticus and the start of effective treatment.

*Status epilepticus is a medical emergency.* Management includes maintenance of the airway to ensure adequate pulmonary ventilation. In adults, unless the cause of the seizures is obvious, 50% dextrose (25–50 mL) is routinely given intravenously in case hypoglycemia is responsible. If seizures continue, 10 mg of diazepam is given intravenously over the course of 2 minutes, and the dose is repeated after 10 minutes if necessary. This is usually effective in halting seizures for a brief period, but a long-acting anticonvulsant must also be given to provide continuing control. Regardless of the response to diazepam, therefore, phenytoin (15 mg/kg) is given intravenously at a rate of 50 mg/min, which permits therapeutic levels to be reached in the brain within a few minutes. The drug is best injected directly but can also be given in saline; it precipitates, however, if injected into glucose-containing solutions. Because cardiac arrhythmias may develop during rapid administration of large doses of phenytoin, electrocardiographic monitoring during administration is indicated.

If seizures continue, phenobarbital is then given in a loading dose of 10–15 mg/kg intravenously by slow or intermittent injection. Equipment for assisted respiration should be available for immediate use if required, since respiratory depression and hypotension are common complications. In refractory cases, one or more of the following may be necessary: lidocaine, 50–100 mg intravenously; paraldehyde, 5–10 mL intravenously (as a 4% solution in normal saline), by deep intramuscular injection, or rectally (in mineral oil); and amobarbital, 200–1000 mg by infusion. Since paraldehyde will dissolve plastic syringes and nasogastric tubes, they should not be used for its administration.

If these measures fail, general anesthesia with ventilatory assistance and neuromuscular junction blockade may be required.

Intravenous diazepam sometimes leads to respiratory depression and hypotension, and these complications become more probable as additional drugs are given. It is therefore important to monitor vital signs frequently during the course of treatment. Other benzodiazepines have also been used in the immediate management of status epilepticus. Lorazepam given intravenously is effective and has more prolonged clinical effects than diazepam. It is unclear whether lorazepam is as safe and as rapidly effective as diazepam, but ongoing comparative studies may clarify the issue.

After status epilepticus is controlled, an oral drug program for the long-term management of seizures is started, and investigations into the cause of the disorder are pursued.

**4. Nonconvulsive status epilepticus**–Absence (petit mal) and complex partial status epilepticus are characterized by fluctuating abnormal mental status, confusion, impaired responsiveness, and automatism. Electroencephalography is helpful both in establishing the diagnosis and in distinguishing the 2 varieties. Initial treatment with intravenous diazepam is usually helpful regardless of the type of status epilepticus, but phenytoin, phenobarbital, carbamazepine, and other drugs may also be needed to obtain and maintain control in complex partial status epilepticus.

Aminoff MJ, Simon RP: Status epilepticus: Causes, clinical features and consequences in 98 patients. *Am J Med* 1980;**69**:657.

Bleck TP: Therapy for status epilepticus. *Clin Neuropharmacol* 1983;**6**:255.

Berkovic SF et al: Progressive myoclonus epilepsies: Specific causes and diagnosis. *N Engl J Med* 1986;**315**:296.

Bruni J, Albright PS: The clinical pharmacology of antiepileptic drugs. *Clin Neuropharmacol* 1984;**7**:1.

Delgado-Escueta AV, Treiman DM, Walsh GO: The treatable epilepsies. (2 parts.) *N Engl J Med* 1983;**308**:1508, 1576.

Delgado-Escueta AV et al: Current concepts in neurology: Management of status epilepticus. *N Engl J Med* 1982;**306**:1337.

Mattson RH et al: Comparison of carbamazepine, phenobarbital, phenytoin, and primidone in partial and secondarily generalized tonic-clonic seizures. *N Engl J Med* 1985;**313**:145.

## TRANSIENT ISCHEMIC ATTACKS

### Essentials of Diagnosis

- Risk factors for vascular disease often present.
- Focal neurologic deficit of acute onset.
- Clinical deficit resolves completely within 24 hours.

### General Considerations

Transient ischemic attacks are characterized by focal ischemic cerebral neurologic deficits that last for less than 24 hours (usually less than 1–2 hours). Patients with recent onset of attacks are at high risk for cerebral infarction, myocardial infarction, or death. About 30% of patients with stroke have a past history of transient ischemic attacks, and proper treatment of the attacks is an important means of preventing strokes. The incidence of stroke does not relate to either the number or the duration of individual attacks but is increased in patients with hypertension or diabetes.

### Etiology

An important cause of transient cerebral ischemia is embolization. In many patients with these attacks, a source of embolization is readily apparent in the heart or a major extracranial artery to the head, and emboli sometimes are visible in the retinal arteries. Moreover, an embolic phenomenon explains why separate attacks may affect different parts of the territory supplied by the same major vessel. Cardiac causes of embolic ischemic attacks include rheumatic heart disease, mitral valve disease, cardiac dysrhythmia, infective endocarditis, atrial myxoma, and mural thrombi complicating myocardial infarction. In patients with stenosis or ulceration of a major artery to the brain, a mural thrombus may form and serve as a source of emboli. In the anterior circulation, atherosclerotic changes occur most commonly in the region of the carotid bifurcation extracranially, and these changes may cause a bruit. In some patients with transient ischemic attacks or strokes, an acute or recent hemorrhage is found to have occurred into this atherosclerotic plaque, and this finding may have pathologic significance.

Other (less common) abnormalities of blood vessels that may cause transient ischemic attacks include fibromuscular dysplasia, which affects particularly the cervical internal carotid artery; inflammatory arterial disorders such as giant cell arteritis, systemic lupus erythematosus, polyarteritis, and granulomatous angiitis; and meningovascular syphilis. Transient severe hypotension (eg, due to blood loss, cardiac dysrhythmia, or postural change) may cause a reduction of cerebral blood flow if a major extracranial artery to the brain is markedly stenosed, but this is a rare cause of transient ischemic attack.

Hematologic causes of ischemic attacks include polycythemia, sickle cell disease, and hyperviscosity syndromes. Severe anemia may also lead to transient focal neurologic deficits in patients with preexisting cerebral arterial disease.

The **subclavian steal syndrome** may lead to transient vertebrobasilar ischemia. Symptoms develop when there is localized stenosis or occlusion of one subclavian artery proximal to the source of the vertebral artery, so that blood is "stolen" from this artery. A bruit in the supraclavicular fossa, unequal radial pulses, and a difference of 20 mm Hg or more between the systolic blood pressures in the arms should suggest the diagnosis in patients with vertebrobasilar transient ischemic attacks.

## Clinical Findings

**A. Symptoms and Signs:** The symptoms of transient ischemic attacks vary markedly among patients; however, the symptoms in a given individual tend to be constant in type. Onset is abrupt and without warning, and recovery usually occurs rapidly, often within a few minutes.

If the ischemia is in the carotid territory, common symptoms are weakness and heaviness of the contralateral arm, leg, or face, singly or in any combination. Numbness or paresthesias may also occur either as the sole manifestation of the attack or in combination with the motor deficit. There may be slowness of movement, dysphasia, or monocular visual loss in the eye contralateral to affected limbs. During an attack, examination may reveal flaccid weakness with pyramidal distribution, sensory changes, hyperreflexia or an extensor plantar response on the affected side, dysphasia, or any combination of these findings. Subsequently, examination reveals no neurologic abnormality, but the presence of a carotid bruit or cardiac abnormality may provide a clue to the cause of symptoms.

Vertebrobasilar ischemic attacks may be characterized by vertigo, ataxia, diplopia, dysarthria, dimness or blurring of vision, perioral numbness and paresthesias, and weakness or sensory complaints on one, both, or alternating sides of the body. These symptoms may occur singly or in any combination. Drop attacks due to bilateral leg weakness, without headache or loss of consciousness, may occur, sometimes in relation to head movements.

The natural history of attacks is variable. Some patients will have a major stroke after only a few attacks, whereas others may have frequent attacks for weeks or months without having a stroke. Attacks may occur intermittently over a long period of time, or they may stop spontaneously. In general, carotid ischemic attacks are more liable than vertebrobasilar ischemic attacks to be followed by stroke.

**B. Imaging:** CT scan of the head will exclude the possibility of a small cerebral hemorrhage or a cerebral tumor masquerading as a transient ischemic attack. A number of noninvasive techniques, such as ultrasonography, have been developed for studying the cerebral circulation and imaging the major vessels to the head, but they have not replaced arteriography as a means of demonstrating the status of the cerebrovascular system. Accordingly, if findings on CT scan are normal, if there is no cardiac source of embolization, and if age and general condition indicate that the patient is a good operative risk, bilateral carotid arteriography should be undertaken in the further evaluation of carotid ischemic attacks.

**C. Laboratory and Other Studies:** Clinical and laboratory evaluation must include assessment for hypertension, heart disease, and diffuse vascular disease. It should include complete blood count, blood glucose determination, serologic tests for syphilis, and an ECG and chest x-ray. Echocardiography is performed in patients with heart murmurs, and blood cultures are undertaken if endocarditis is suspected. Holter monitoring is indicated if a transient, paroxysmal disturbance of cardiac rhythm is suspected.

## Differential Diagnosis

Focal seizures must be distinguished. They usually cause abnormal motor or sensory phenomena such as clonic limb movements, paresthesias, or tingling, rather than weakness or loss of feeling. Symptoms generally spread (''march'') up the limb and may lead to a generalized tonic-clonic seizure. The electroencephalogram may help in detecting the epileptogenic source.

Classic migraine is easily recognized by the visual premonitory symptoms, followed by nausea, headache, and photophobia, but less typical cases may be hard to distinguish. The patient's age and medical history (including family history) may be helpful in this regard. Patients with migraine commonly have a history of episodes since adolescence and report that other family members have a similar disorder.

Focal neurologic deficits may occur during periods of hypoglycemia in diabetic patients receiving treatment, and the lack of general hypoglycemic symptoms does not exclude this possibility.

## Treatment

When arteriography reveals a surgically accessible lesion on the side appropriate to carotid ischemic attacks and there is relatively little atherosclerosis elsewhere in the cerebrovascular system, operative treatment (carotid thromboendarterectomy) may be appropriate, especially when transient ischemic attacks are of recent onset ($< 2$ months). When more extensive atherosclerotic disease is angiographically evident in the cerebral circulation, the benefits of surgery are less clear and the operative risks greater. Studies to compare the results of surgery with those of medical treatment alone are currently in progress.

In patients with carotid ischemic attacks who are poor operative candidates (and thus have not undergone arteriography) or who are found to have extensive vascular disease, medical treatment should be instituted. Similarly, patients with vertebrobasilar ischemic attacks are treated medically and are not subjected to arteriography unless there is clinical evidence of stenosis or occlusion in the carotid or subclavian arteries.

Medical treatment is aimed at preventing further attacks and stroke. Cigarette smoking should be stopped, and cardiac sources of embolization, hypertension, diabetes, arteritis, or hematologic disorders should be treated appropriately. If anticoagulants are indicated for the treatment of embolism from the heart, they should be started immediately, provided there is no contraindication to their use. There is no advantage in delay, and the common fear of causing hemorrhage into a previously infarcted area is misplaced, since there is a far greater risk of further embolism to the cerebral circulation if treatment is withheld.

Treatment is initiated with intravenous heparin while warfarin sodium is introduced.

In patients with presumed or angiographically verified atherosclerotic changes in the extracranial or intracranial cerebrovascular circulation, antithrombotic medication is prescribed. The treatment selected will depend upon the patient's age, the likelihood of compliance in taking the drug, and the ready availability of medical and laboratory services. Some physicians use anticoagulant drugs (eg, warfarin, with temporary heparinization until the dose of warfarin is adequate) unless they are medically contraindicated, continuing them for 3–6 months before they are tapered and ultimately replaced with aspirin or, in women, dipyridamole, which is continued for another year. However, there is no convincing evidence that anticoagulant drugs are of value in this context. Other physicians therefore prefer aspirin, dipyridamole, or both, from the onset.

The evidence supporting a therapeutic role for aspirin and other agents that suppress platelet aggregation is increasing. Platelets adhere to and aggregate around an atherosclerotic plaque and release various substances including thromboxane $A_2$. In a double-blind prospective study performed in Canada, it was found that treatment with aspirin significantly reduced the frequency of transient ischemic attacks and the incidence of stroke or death in men. A number of other studies in which different doses of aspirin were used similarly suggest a beneficial effect and suggest also that men and women respond differently to treatment. Nevertheless, several studies have demonstrated therapeutic responses in patients of either sex. The optimal daily dose remains to be established, but four 325-mg aspirin tablets is currently recommended. Studies of low-dose aspirin therapy (325 mg or less daily) are in progress. Dipyridamole added to aspirin does not offer any advantage over aspirin alone for stroke prevention, but it may itself have some effect in preventing vascular disease, perhaps by enhancing the production of prostacyclin (which has antithrombotic activities) in the vessel wall.

In recent years, many patients with transient ischemic attacks associated with stenotic lesions of the distal internal carotid or the proximal middle cerebral arteries have undergone surgical extracranial-intracranial arterial anastomosis. Most commonly, a connection is made between the superficial temporal and middle cerebral arteries, and the operative mortality rate is generally low. The indications for such surgery are unclear, and no benefit of surgical treatment could be demonstrated in a recently published large controlled prospective study.

Dyken ML: Anticoagulant and platelet-antiaggregating therapy in stroke and threatened stroke. *Neurol Clin* 1983;**1**:223.

EC/IC Bypass Study Group: Failure of extracranial-intracranial arterial bypass to reduce the risk of ischemic stroke: Results of an international randomized trial. *N Engl J Med* 1985;**313**:1191.

Yatsu FM, Mohr JP: Anticoagulation therapy for cardiogenic emboli to brain. *Neurology* 1982;**32**:274.

## STROKE

### Essentials of Diagnosis

- Sudden onset of characteristic neurologic deficit.
- Patient often has history of hypertension, valvular heart disease, or atherosclerosis.
- Distinctive neurologic signs reflect the region of the brain involved.

### General Considerations

In the USA, stroke remains the third leading cause of death, despite a general decline in the incidence of stroke in the last 30 years. The precise reasons for this decline are uncertain, but increased awareness of risk factors (hypertension, diabetes, hyperlipidemia, cigarette smoking, cardiac abnormalities, heavy alcohol consumption, family history of stroke) and improved prophylactic measures and surveillance of those at increased risk have been contributory. A previous stroke makes individual patients more susceptible to further strokes.

For years, strokes have been subdivided pathologically into infarcts (thrombotic or embolic) and hemorrhages, and clinical criteria for distinguishing between these possibilities have been emphasized. However, in one autopsy study of 1000 cases of stroke, a clinical diagnosis of cerebral hemorrhage was confirmed in only 65% of cases and that of cerebral infarction in only 58%. Similar findings have been reported in other studies. These findings indicate the difficulty in determining on clinical grounds the pathologic basis of stroke.

### 1. LACUNAR INFARCTION

Lacunar infarcts are among the most common cerebral vascular lesions. They are small infarcts (usually < 5 mm in diameter) that occur in the distribution of short penetrating arterioles in the basal ganglia, pons, cerebellum, anterior limb of the internal capsule, and, less commonly, the deep cerebral white matter. Lacunar infarcts may be associated with hypertension or diabetes and have been found in conjunction with several clinical syndromes, including contralateral pure motor or pure sensory deficit, ipsilateral ataxia with crural paresis, and dysarthria with clumsiness of the hand. The neurologic deficit may progress over 24–36 hours before stabilizing.

Lacunar infarcts are sometimes visible on CT scans as small, punched-out, hypodense areas, but in other patients no abnormality is seen. In some instances, patients with a clinical syndrome suggestive of lacunar infarction are found on CT scanning to have a severe hemispheric infarct.

The prognosis for recovery from the deficit produced by a lacunar infarct is usually good, with partial or complete resolution occurring over the following 4–6 weeks in many instances.

Mohr MP: Lacunes. *Neurol Clin* 1983;**1**:201.

## 2. CEREBRAL INFARCTION

Thrombotic or embolic occlusion of a major vessel leads to cerebral infarction. Causes include the disorders predisposing to transient ischemic attacks (see above) and atherosclerotic degeneration of cerebral arteries. The resulting deficit depends upon the particular vessel involved and the extent of any collateral circulation.

### Clinical Findings

**A. Symptoms and Signs:** Onset is usually abrupt, and there may then be very little progression except that due to brain swelling. Clinical evaluation always includes examination of the heart and auscultation over the subclavian and carotid vessels to determine whether there are any bruits.

**1. Obstruction of carotid circulation**—Occlusion of the ophthalmic artery is probably symptomless in most cases because of the rich orbital collaterals, but its transient embolic obstruction leads to amaurosis fugax—sudden and brief loss of vision in one eye.

Occlusion of the anterior cerebral artery distal to its junction with the anterior communicating artery causes weakness and cortical sensory loss in the contralateral leg and sometimes mild weakness of the arm, especially proximally. There may be a contralateral grasp reflex, paratonic rigidity, and abulia or frank confusion. Urinary incontinence is not uncommon, particularly if behavioral disturbances are conspicuous. Bilateral anterior cerebral infarction is especially likely to cause marked behavioral changes and memory disturbances. Unilateral anterior cerebral artery occlusion proximal to the junction with the anterior communicating artery is generally well tolerated because of the collateral supply from the other side.

Middle cerebral artery occlusion leads to contralateral hemiplegia, hemisensory loss, and homonymous hemianopia, with the eyes deviated to the side of the lesion. If the dominant hemisphere is involved, global aphasia is also present. It may be impossible to distinguish this clinically from occlusion of the internal carotid artery. With occlusion of either of these arteries, there may also be considerable swelling of the hemisphere, leading to drowsiness, stupor, and coma in extreme cases. Occlusions of different branches of the middle cerebral artery cause more limited findings. For example, involvement of the anterior main division leads to a predominantly expressive dysphasia and to contralateral paralysis and loss of sensations in the arm, the face, and to a lesser extent, the leg. Posterior branch occlusion produces a receptive (Wernicke's) aphasia and a homonymous visual field defect. With involvement of the nondominant hemisphere, speech and comprehension are preserved, but there may be a confusional state, dressing apraxia, and constructional and spatial deficits.

**2. Obstruction of vertebrobasilar circulation**—Occlusion of the posterior cerebral artery may lead to a thalamic syndrome in which contralateral hemisensory disturbance occurs, followed by the development of spontaneous pain and hyperpathia. There is often a macular-sparing homonymous hemianopia and sometimes a mild, usually temporary, hemiparesis. Depending on the site of the lesion and the collateral circulation, the severity of these deficits varies and other deficits may also occur, including involuntary movements and alexia. Occlusion of the main artery beyond the origin of its penetrating branches may lead solely to a macular-sparing hemianopia.

Vertebral artery occlusion distally, below the origin of the anterior spinal and posterior inferior cerebellar arteries, may be clinically silent because the circulation is maintained by the other vertebral artery. If the remaining vertebral artery is congenitally small or severely atherosclerotic, however, a deficit similar to that of basilar artery occlusion is seen unless there is good collateral circulation from the anterior circulation through the circle of Willis. When the small paramedian arteries arising from the vertebral artery are occluded, contralateral hemiplegia and sensory deficit occur in association with an ipsilateral cranial nerve palsy at the level of the lesion. An obstruction of the posterior inferior cerebellar artery or an obstruction of the vertebral artery just before it branches to this vessel leads ipsilaterally to spinothalamic sensory loss involving the face, ninth and tenth cranial nerve lesions, limb ataxia and numbness, and Horner's syndrome, combined with contralateral spinothalamic sensory loss involving the limbs.

Occlusion of both vertebral arteries or the basilar artery leads to coma with pinpoint pupils, flaccid quadriplegia and sensory loss, and variable cranial nerve abnormalities. With partial basilar artery occlusion, there may be diplopia, visual loss, vertigo, dysarthria, ataxia, weakness or sensory disturbances in some or all of the limbs, and discrete cranial nerve palsies. In patients with hemiplegia of pontine origin, the eyes are often deviated to the paralyzed side, whereas in patients with a hemispheric lesion, the eyes commonly deviate from the hemiplegic side.

Occlusion of any of the major cerebellar arteries produces vertigo, nausea, vomiting, nystagmus, ipsilateral limb ataxia, and contralateral spinothalamic sensory loss in the limbs. If the superior cerebellar artery is involved, the contralateral spinothalamic loss also involves the face; with occlusion of the anterior inferior cerebellar artery, there is ipsilateral spinothalamic sensory loss involving the face, usually in conjunction with ipsilateral facial weakness and deafness. Massive cerebellar infarction may lead to coma, tonsillar herniation, and death.

**3. Coma**—Infarction in either the carotid or vertebrobasilar territory may lead to loss of consciousness. For example, an infarct involving one cerebral hemisphere may lead to such swelling that the function of the other hemisphere or the rostral brain stem is disturbed and coma results. Similarly, coma occurs with bilateral brain stem infarction when this involves the reticular formation, and it occurs with brain stem compression after cerebellar infarction.

**B. Imaging:** Radiography of the chest may reveal cardiomegaly or valvular calcification; the presence of a neoplasm would suggest that the neurologic deficit is due to metastasis rather than stroke. A CT scan of the head is important in excluding cerebral hemorrhage, but it may not permit distinction between a cerebral infarct and tumor.

**C. Laboratory and Other Studies:** Investigations should include a complete blood count, sedimentation rate, blood glucose determination, and serologic tests for syphilis. Electrocardiography will help exclude a cardiac dysrhythmia or recent myocardial infarction that might be serving as a source of embolization. Blood cultures should be performed if endocarditis is suspected, echocardiography if heart murmur is present, and Holter monitoring if paroxysmal cardiac dysrhythmia requires exclusion. Examination of the cerebrospinal fluid is not always necessary but may be helpful if there is diagnostic uncertainty; it should be delayed until after CT scanning.

## Treatment

The patient must be examined in detail, and if the neurologic deficit progresses over the following minutes or hours, heparinization may be of value in limiting or arresting further deterioration. Since the signs of progressing stroke may be simulated by an intracerebral hematoma, the latter must be excluded by immediate CT scanning or angiography before the patient is heparinized.

Early management of a completed stroke consists of attention to general supportive measures. During the acute stage, there may be marked brain swelling and edema, with symptoms and signs of increasing intracranial pressure, an increasing neurologic deficit, or herniation syndrome. Corticosteroids have been prescribed in an attempt to reduce vasogenic cerebral edema. Prednisone (up to 100 mg/d) or dexamethasone (16 mg/d) has been used, but the evidence that corticosteroids are of any benefit is conflicting. Dehydrating hyperosmolar agents have also been prescribed in efforts to reduce brain swelling, but there is little evidence of any lasting benefit.

There is no convincing evidence of clinical benefit from treatment with vasodilators such as papaverine. Similarly, neither hypercapnia nor hypocapnia has been shown to have any benefit. Barbiturates are known to decrease neuronal metabolism and energy requirements and have been reported to improve functional recovery in experimental stroke models; their use in humans, however, is experimental and premature at present. Attempts to lower the blood pressure of hypertensive patients during the acute phase of a stroke should be avoided, since there is loss of cerebral autoregulation and since lowering the blood pressure may further compromise ischemic areas.

Anticoagulant drugs have no role in the management of patients with a completed stroke, except when there is a cardiac source of embolization. Treatment is then started with intravenous heparin while warfarin is introduced. If the CT scan shows no evidence of hemorrhage and the cerebrospinal fluid is clear, anticoagulant treatment may be started without delay. Many physicians, however, prefer to wait for about 5–7 days (to reduce any risk of cerebral hemorrhage) before initiating anticoagulant treatment. There are insufficient data to indicate which of these alternatives is preferable.

Physical therapy has an important role in the management of patients with impaired motor function. Passive movements at an early stage will help prevent contractures. As cooperation increases and some recovery begins, active movements will improve strength and coordination. In all cases, early mobilization and active rehabilitation are important. Occupational therapy may improve morale and motor skills, while speech therapy may be beneficial in patients with expressive dysphasia or dysarthria. When there is a severe and persisting motor deficit, a device such as a leg brace, toe spring, frame, or cane may help the patient move about, and the provision of other aids to daily living may improve the quality of life.

## Prognosis

The prognosis for survival after cerebral infarction is better than after cerebral or subarachnoid hemorrhage. Loss of consciousness after a cerebral infarct implies a poorer prognosis than otherwise. The extent of the infarct governs the potential for rehabilitation. Patients who have had a cerebral infarct are at risk for further strokes and for myocardial infarcts.

Barnett HJM: Heart in ischemic stroke: A changing emphasis. *Neurol Clin* 1983;**1**:291.

Buonanno F, Toole JF: Management of patients with established ("completed") cerebral infarction. *Stroke* 1981;**12**:7.

Wolf PA, Kannel WB, Verter J: Current status of risk factors for stroke. *Neurol Clin* 1983;**1**:317.

## 3. INTRACEREBRAL HEMORRHAGE

Spontaneous intracerebral hemorrhage in patients with no angiographic evidence of an associated vascular anomaly (eg, aneurysm or angioma) is usually due to hypertension. The pathologic basis for hemorrhage is probably the presence of microaneurysms that are now known to develop on perforating vessels of 100–300 μm in diameter in hypertensive patients. Hypertensive intracerebral hemorrhage occurs most frequently in the basal ganglia and less commonly in the pons, thalamus, cerebellum, and cerebral white matter. Hemorrhage may extend into the ventricular system or subarachnoid space, and signs of meningeal irritation are then found. Hemorrhages usually occur suddenly and without warning, often during activity.

In addition to its association with hypertension, nontraumatic intracerebral hemorrhage may occur with hematologic and bleeding disorders (eg, leukemia, thrombocytopenia, hemophilia, or disseminated intravascular coagulation), anticoagulant therapy, liver disease, cerebral amyloid angiopathy, and primary or secondary brain tumors. Bleeding is primarily into the subarachnoid space when it occurs from an intracranial aneurysm or arteriovenous malformation (see below), but it may be partly intracerebral as well. In some cases, no specific cause for cerebral hemorrhage can be identified.

## Clinical Findings

**A. Symptoms and Signs:** With hemorrhage into the cerebral hemisphere, consciousness is initially lost or impaired in about one-half of patients. Vomiting occurs very frequently at the onset of bleeding, and headache is sometimes present. Focal symptoms and signs then develop, depending on the site of the hemorrhage. With hypertensive hemorrhage, there is generally a rapidly evolving neurologic deficit with hemiplegia or hemiparesis. A hemisensory disturbance is also present with more deeply placed lesions. With lesions of the putamen, loss of conjugate lateral gaze may be conspicuous. With thalamic hemorrhage, there may be a loss of upward gaze, downward or skew deviation of the eyes, lateral gaze palsies, and pupillary inequalities.

Cerebellar hemorrhage may present with sudden onset of nausea and vomiting, disequilibrium, headache, and loss of consciousness that may terminate fatally within 48 hours. Less commonly, the onset is gradual and the course episodic or slowly progressive—clinical features suggesting an expanding cerebellar lesion. In yet other cases, however, the onset and course are intermediate, and examination shows lateral conjugate gaze palsies to the side of the lesion; small reactive pupils; contralateral hemiplegia; peripheral facial weakness; ataxia of gait, limbs, or trunk; periodic respiration; or some combination of these findings.

**B. Imaging:** CT scanning is important not only in confirming that hemorrhage has occurred but also in determining the size and site of the hematoma. If the patient's condition permits further intervention, cerebral angiography may be undertaken thereafter to determine if an aneurysm or arteriorvenous malformation is present (see below).

**C. Laboratory and Other Studies:** A complete blood count, platelet count, bleeding time, prothrombin and partial thromboplastin times, and liver function tests may reveal a predisposing cause for the hemorrhage. Lumbar puncture may precipitate a herniation syndrome in patients with a large hematoma, and CT scanning is far superior.

## Treatment

Neurologic management is generally conservative and supportive, regardless of whether the patient has a profound deficit with associated brain stem compression, in which case the prognosis is grim, or a more localized deficit not causing increased intracranial pressure or brain stem involvement. Attention is directed to maintaining fluid and electrolyte balance and ensuring adequate ventilation. In patients with cerebellar hemorrhage, however, prompt surgical evacuation of the hematoma is appropriate, because spontaneous unpredictable deterioration may otherwise lead to a fatal outcome and because operative treatment may lead to complete resolution of the clinical deficit.

Drury I, Whisnant JP, Garraway WM: Primary intracerebral hemorrhage: Impact of CT on incidence. *Neurology* 1984;**34**:653.

## 4. SUBARACHNOID HEMORRHAGE

Between 5 and 10% of strokes are due to subarachnoid hemorrhage. Although hemorrhage is usually from rupture of an aneurysm or arteriovenous malformation, no specific cause can be found in 20% of cases.

## Clinical Findings

**A. Symptoms and Signs:** Subarachnoid hemorrhage has a characteristic clinical picture. Its onset is with sudden headache of a severity never experienced previously by the patient. This may be followed by nausea and vomiting and by a loss or impairment of consciousness that can either be transient or progress inexorably to deepening coma and death. If consciousness is regained, the patient is often confused and irritable and may show other symptoms of an altered mental status. Neurologic examination generally reveals nuchal rigidity and other signs of meningeal irritation, except in deeply comatose patients. A focal neurologic deficit is occasionally present and may suggest the site of the underlying lesion.

**B. Imaging:** A CT scan should be performed immediately to confirm that hemorrhage has occurred and to search for clues regarding its source. Findings sometimes are normal in patients with suspected hemorrhage, and the cerebrospinal fluid must then be examined before the possibility of subarachnoid hemorrhage is discounted.

Cerebral arteriography may be undertaken to determine the source of bleeding; it is not performed unless or until the patient's condition has stabilized and is good enough so that operative treatment is feasible. In deeply comatose patients, for example, arteriography should usually not be performed. In general, bilateral carotid and vertebral arteriography are necessary because aneurysms are often multiple, while arteriovenous malformations may be supplied from several sources.

## Treatment

The medical management of patients is important. The measures outlined on p 604 must be applied to comatose patients. Conscious patients are confined to bed, advised against any exertion or straining, treated symptomatically for headache and anxiety, and given laxatives or stool softeners to prevent straining. If there is severe hypertension, the blood pressure can be lowered gradually, but not below a diastolic level of 100 mm Hg. Phenytoin or phenobarbital is generally prescribed routinely to prevent seizures. Further comment concerning the specific operative management of arteriovenous malformations and aneurysms follows.

## 5. INTRACRANIAL ANEURYSM

Saccular aneurysms (''berry'' aneurysms) tend to occur at arterial bifurcations, are considerably more common in adults than in children, are frequently multiple (20% of cases), and are usually asymptomatic. They may be associated with polycystic kidney disease and coarctation of the aorta. Most aneurysms are located on the anterior part of the circle of Willis—particularly on the anterior or posterior communicating arteries, at the bifurcation of the middle cerebral artery, and at the bifurcation of the internal carotid artery.

### Clinical Findings

**A. Symptoms and Signs:** Aneurysms may cause a focal neurologic deficit by compressing adjacent structures. However, most are asymptomatic or produce only nonspecific symptoms until they rupture, at which time subarachnoid hemorrhage results. There is often a paucity of focal neurologic signs in patients with subarachnoid hemorrhage, but when present, such signs may relate either to a focal hematoma or to ischemia in the territory of the vessel with the ruptured aneurysm. Hemiplegia or other focal deficit sometimes occurs after a delay of 4–14 days and is due to focal arterial spasm in the vicinity of the ruptured aneurysm. This spasm is of uncertain, probably multifactorial, cause, but it sometimes leads to significant cerebral ischemia or infarction, and it may further aggravate any existing increase in intracranial pressure. Subacute hydrocephalus due to interference with the flow of cerebrospinal fluid may occur after 2 or more weeks, and this leads to a delayed clinical deterioration that is relieved by shunting.

In some patients, ''warning leaks'' of a small amount of blood from the aneurysm precede the major hemorrhage by a few hours or days. They lead to headaches, sometimes accompanied by nausea and neck stiffness, but the true cause of these symptoms is often not appreciated until massive hemorrhage occurs.

**B. Imaging:** The CT scan generally confirms that subarachnoid hemorrhage has occurred, but occasionally it is normal. Angiography (bilateral carotid and vertebral studies) generally indicates the size and site of the lesion, sometimes reveals multiple aneurysms, and may show arterial spasm. If arteriograms show no abnormality, the examination should be repeated after 2 weeks, because vasospasm may have prevented detection of an aneurysm during the initial study.

**C. Laboratory and Other Studies:** The cerebrospinal fluid is bloodstained. The electroencephalogram sometimes indicates the side or site of hemorrhage but frequently shows only a diffuse abnormality. Diffuse deep T wave inversions on the ECG have been well described and are of uncertain origin. Peripheral leukocytosis and transient glycosuria are also common findings.

### Treatment

The major aim of treatment is to prevent further hemorrhages. Definitive treatment requires a surgical approach to the aneurysm and ideally consists of clipping of the aneurysmal base. If surgery is not feasible, medical management as outlined above for subarachnoid hemorrhage is continued for about 6 weeks and is followed by gradual mobilization.

The optimal time for surgery depends upon the clinical status of the patient. Although some surgeons now favor early operation, others have shown that the operative morbidity and mortality rates are decreased by delaying surgery for at least 10 days after the hemorrhage. (The optimal timing of surgery is currently being investigated in a multicenter study that is nearing completion.) Unfortunately, the risk of further hemorrhage is greatest within a few days of the first hemorrhage; approximately 20% of patients will have further bleeding within 2 weeks and 40% within 6 months. Accordingly, attempts have been made to reduce this risk pharmacologically. Since antifibrinolytic drugs prevent lysis of any blood clot that has formed near the site of rupture, aminocaproic acid (Amicar) is often given for the first 2 weeks or so, or until surgery, to reduce the incidence of early recurrence of bleeding. The daily dose is 24–36 g (5 g initially, followed by 1–1.25 g hourly) given intravenously for the first week and then orally, while the streptokinase clot lysis time is monitored. Outside of the USA, use of tranexamic acid is preferred. Potential complications include venous thrombosis, pulmonary embolism, and ischemic focal neurologic deficits. Recent studies indicate that aminocaproic acid and tranexamic acid do indeed lower the incidence of recurrent bleeding, but their use is associated with such an increase in cerebral ischemic complications that the mortality rate and the degree of disability among survivors are unchanged.

There is currently no specific treatment for cerebral vasospasm, but calcium channel-blocking agents have helped to reduce or reverse experimental vasospasm, and results of a clinical study in which nimodipine was given orally to neurologically normal patients after subarachnoid hemorrhage indicate that it significantly reduced the incidence of ischemic deficits from arterial spasm without producing any side effects. The initial dose of nimodipine was 0.7 mg/kg, followed by 0.35 mg/kg every 4 hours for 21 days.

With regard to unruptured aneurysms, those that are symptomatic merit prompt surgical treatment, whereas small asymptomatic ones discovered incidentally are often followed arteriographically and corrected surgically only if they increase in size to over 5 mm. The natural history of unruptured aneurysms is not clearly defined, however, and the age and condition of the patient and experience of the surgeon will clearly bear on any therapeutic decisions.

Allen GS et al: Cerebral arterial spasm: A controlled trial of nimodipine in patients with subarachnoid hemorrhage. *N Engl J Med* 1983;**308:**619.

Kassell NF, Drake CG. Review of the management of saccular aneurysms. *Neurol Clin* 1983;**1:**73.

Vermeulen M et al: Antifibrinolytic treatment in subarachnoid hemorrhage. *N Engl J Med* 1984;**311:**432.

Weibers DO, Whisnant JP, O'Fallon WM: The natural history of unruptured intracranial aneurysms. *N Engl J Med* 1981;**304:**696.

## 6. ARTERIOVENOUS MALFORMATIONS

Arteriovenous malformations are congenital vascular malformations that result from a localized maldevelopment of part of the primitive vascular plexus and consist of abnormal arteriovenous communications without intervening capillaries. They vary in size, ranging from massive lesions that are fed by multiple vessels and involve a large part of the brain to lesions so small that they are hard to identify at arteriography, surgery, or autopsy. In approximately 10% of cases, there is an associated arterial aneurysm, while 1–2% of patients presenting with aneurysms have associated arteriovenous malformations. Clinical presentation may relate to hemorrhage from the malformation or an associated aneurysm or may relate to cerebral ischemia due to diversion of blood by the anomalous arteriovenous shunt or due to venous stagnation. Regional maldevelopment of the brain, compression or distortion of adjacent cerebral tissue by enlarged anomalous vessels, and progressive gliosis due to mechanical and ischemic factors may also be contributory. In addition, communicating or obstructive hydrocephalus may occur and lead to symptoms.

### Clinical Findings

#### A. Symptoms and Signs:

**1. Supratentorial lesions–**Most cerebral arteriovenous malformations are supratentorial, usually lying in the territory of the middle cerebral artery. Initial symptoms consist of hemorrhage in 30–60% of cases, epilepsy in 20–40%, headache in 5–25%, and miscellaneous complaints (including focal deficits) in 10–15%. Up to 70% of arteriovenous malformations bleed at some point in their natural history, most commonly before the patient reaches the age of 40 years. This tendency to bleed is unrelated to the lesion site or to the patient's sex, but small arteriovenous malformations are more likely to bleed than large ones. Arteriovenous malformations that have bled once are more likely to bleed again. Hemorrhage is commonly intracerebral as well as into the subarachnoid space, and it has a fatal outcome in about 10% of cases. Focal or generalized seizures may accompany or follow hemorrhage, or they may be the initial presentation, especially with frontal or parietal arteriovenous malformations. Headaches are especially likely when the external carotid arteries are involved in the malformation. These sometimes simulate migraine but more commonly are nonspecific in character, with nothing about them to suggest an underlying structural lesion.

In patients presenting with subarachnoid hemorrhage, examination may reveal an abnormal mental status and signs of meningeal irritation. Additional findings may help to localize the lesion and sometimes indicate that intracranial pressure is increased. A cranial bruit always suggests the possibility of a cerebral arteriovenous malformation, but bruits may also be found with aneurysms, meningiomas, acquired arteriovenous fistulas, and arteriovenous malformations involving the scalp, calvarium, or orbit. Bruits are best heard over the ipsilateral eye or mastoid region and are of some help in lateralization but not in localization. Absence of a bruit in no way excludes the possibility of arteriovenous malformation.

**2. Infratentorial lesions–**Brain stem arteriovenous malformations are often clinically silent, but they may hemorrhage, cause obstructive hydrocephalus, or lead to progressive or relapsing brain stem deficits. Cerebellar arteriovenous malformations may also be clinically inconspicuous but sometimes lead to cerebellar hemorrhage.

**B. Imaging:** In patients presenting with suspected hemorrhage, CT scanning indicates whether subarachnoid or intracerebral bleeding has recently occurred, helps to localize its source, and may reveal the arteriovenous malformation. If the CT scan shows no evidence of bleeding but subarachnoid hemorrhage is diagnosed clinically, the cerebrospinal fluid should be examined.

When intracranial hemorrhage is confirmed but the source of hemorrhage is not evident on the CT scan, arteriography is necessary to exclude aneurysm or arteriovenous malformation. Even if the findings on CT scan suggest arteriovenous malformation, arteriography is required to establish the nature of the lesion with certainty and to determine its anatomic features, so that treatment can be planned. The examination must generally include bilateral opacification of the internal and external carotid arteries and the vertebral arteries. Arteriovenous malformations typically appear as a tangled vascular mass with distended tortuous afferent and efferent vessels, a rapid circulation time, and arteriovenous shunting. Findings on plain radiographs of the skull are often normal unless an intracerebral hematoma is present.

**C. Laboratory and Other Studies:** Electroencephalography is usually indicated in patients presenting with seizures and may show consistently focal or lateralized abnormalities resulting from the underlying cerebral arteriovenous malformation. This should be followed by CT scanning.

### Treatment

Surgical treatment to prevent further hemorrhage

is justified in patients with arteriovenous malformations that have bled, provided that the lesion is accessible and the patient has a reasonable life expectancy. Surgical treatment is also appropriate if intracranial pressure is increased or if there is cardiac decompensation, as occurs in children, and to prevent further progression of a focal neurologic deficit. In patients presenting solely with seizures, anticonvulsant drug treatment is usually sufficient and operative treatment unnecessary unless there are further developments.

Definitive operative treatment consists of excision of the arteriovenous malformation if it is surgically accessible and is not in a critical location. Arteriovenous malformations that are inoperable because of their location are sometimes treated solely by embolization; although the risk of hemorrhage is not reduced, neurologic deficits may be stabilized or even reversed by this procedure. Two other new techniques for the treatment of intracerebral arteriovenous malformations are injection of a vascular occlusive polymer through a flow-guided microcatheter and permanent occlusion of feeding vessels by positioning detachable balloon catheters in the desired sites and then inflating them with quickly solidifying contrast material. Proton beam therapy may also be useful in the management of inoperable cerebral arteriovenous malformations.

Aminoff MJ: Angiomas and fistulae involving the nervous system. In: *Vascular Disease of the Central Nervous System.* Ross Russell RW (editor). Churchill Livingstone, 1983.
Drake CG: Arteriovenous malformations of the brain: The options for management. *N Engl J Med* 1983;**309**:308.

## 7. INTRACRANIAL VENOUS THROMBOSIS

Intracranial venous thrombosis may occur in association with intracranial or maxillofacial infections, hypercoagulable states, polycythemia, sickle cell disease, and cyanotic congenital heart disease and in pregnancy or during the puerperium. It is characterized by headache, focal or generalized convulsions, drowsiness, confusion, increased intracranial pressure, and focal neurologic deficits—and sometimes by evidence of meningeal irritation. The cerebrospinal fluid may be under increased pressure. The diagnosis is confirmed by CT scanning and angiography.

Treatment includes anticonvulsant drugs if seizures have occurred and antiedema agents (eg, dexamethasone) to reduce intracranial pressure. The use of anticoagulant drugs is controversial.

## 8. SPINAL CORD VASCULAR DISEASES

### Infarction of the Spinal Cord

Infarction of the spinal cord is rare. It occurs only in the territory of the anterior spinal artery because this vessel, which supplies the anterior two-thirds

of the cord, is itself supplied by only a limited number of feeders. Infarction usually results from interrupted flow in one or more of these feeders, eg, with aortic dissection, aortography, polyarteritis, or severe hypotension, or after surgical resection of the thoracic aorta. The paired posterior spinal arteries, by contrast, are supplied by numerous arteries at different levels of the cord.

Since the anterior spinal artery receives numerous feeders in the cervical region, infarcts almost always occur more caudally. Clinical presentation is characterized by acute onset of flaccid, areflexive paraplegia that evolves after a few days or weeks into a spastic paraplegia with extensor plantar responses. There is an accompanying dissociated sensory loss, with impairment of appreciation of pain and temperature but preservation of sensations of vibration and position. Treatment is symptomatic.

### Epidural or Subdural Hemorrhage

Epidural or subdural hemorrhage may lead to sudden severe back pain followed by an acute compressive myelopathy necessitating urgent myelography and surgical evacuation. It may occur in patients with bleeding disorders or those who are taking anticoagulant drugs, sometimes following trauma or lumbar puncture. Epidural hemorrhage may also be related to a vascular malformation or tumor deposit.

### Arteriovenous Malformation of the Spinal Cord

Arteriovenous malformations of the cord are congenital lesions that present with spinal subarachnoid hemorrhage or myeloradiculopathy. Since most of these malformations are located in the thoracolumbar region, they lead to motor and sensory disturbances in the legs and to sphincter disorders. Pain in the legs or back is often severe. Examination reveals an upper, lower, or mixed motor deficit in the legs; sensory deficits are also present and are usually extensive, although occasionally they are confined to radicular distribution. Cervical arteriovenous malformations lead also to symptoms and signs in the arms. In general, the diagnosis is suggested at myelography (performed with the patient prone and supine) when serpiginous filling defects due to enlarged vessels are found. Selective spinal arteriography confirms the diagnosis. Most lesions are extramedullary, are posterior to the cord (lying either intra- or extradurally), and can easily be treated by ligation of feeding vessels and excision of the fistulous anomaly.

Aminoff MJ: *Spinal Angiomas.* Blackwell, 1976.
Henson RA, Parson M: Ischaemic lesions of the spinal cord: An illustrated review. *Q J Med* 1967;**36**:205.

# INTRACRANIAL & SPINAL SPACE-OCCUPYING LESIONS

## 1. PRIMARY INTRACRANIAL TUMORS

### Essentials of Diagnosis
- Generalized or focal disturbance of cerebral function, or both.
- Increased intracranial pressure in some patients.
- Neuroradiologic evidence of space-occupying lesion.

### General Considerations
Approximately half of all primary intracranial neoplasms (Table 16–3) are gliomas, and the remainder are meningiomas, pituitary adenomas, neurofibromas, and other tumors. Certain tumors, especially neurofibromas, hemangioblastomas, and retinoblastomas, may have a familial basis, and congenital factors bear on the development of craniopharyngiomas. Tumors may occur at any age, but certain gliomas show particular age predilections (Table 16–3).

### Clinical Findings
**A. Symptoms and Signs:** Intracranial tumors may lead to a generalized disturbance of cerebral function and to symptoms and signs of increased intracranial pressure. In consequence, there may be personality changes, intellectual decline, emotional lability, seizures, headaches, nausea, and malaise. If the pressure is increased in a particular cranial compartment, brain tissue may herniate into a compartment with lower pressure. The most familiar syndrome is herniation of the temporal lobe uncus through the tentorial hiatus, which causes compression of the third cranial nerve, midbrain, and posterior cerebral artery. The earliest sign of this is ipsilateral pupillary dilatation, followed by stupor, coma, decerebrate posturing, and respiratory arrest. Another important herniation syndrome consists of displacement of the cerebellar tonsils through the foramen magnum, which causes medullary compression leading to apnea, circulatory collapse, and death. Other herniation syndromes are less common and of less clear clinical importance.

Intracranial tumors also lead to focal deficits depending on their location.

**1. Frontal lobe lesions**–Tumors of the frontal lobe often lead to progressive intellectual decline, slowing of mental activity, personality changes, and contralateral grasp reflexes. They may lead to expressive aphasia if the posterior part of the left inferior frontal gyrus is involved. Anosmia may also occur as a consequence of pressure on the olfactory nerve. Precentral lesions may cause focal motor seizures or contralateral pyramidal deficits.

**2. Temporal lobe lesions**–These lesions may produce a variety of disturbances. Tumors of the uncinate region may be manifested by seizures with olfactory or gustatory hallucinations, motor phenomena

such as licking or smacking of the lips, and some impairment of external awareness without actual loss of consciousness. Temporal lobe lesions also lead to depersonalization, emotional changes, behavioral disturbances, sensations of *déjà vu* or *jamais vu,* micropsia or macropsia, visual field defects (crossed upper quadrantanopia), and auditory illusions or hallucinations. Left-sided lesions may lead to dysnomia and receptive aphasia, while right-sided involvement sometimes disturbs the perception of musical notes and melodies.

**3. Parietal lobe lesions**–Tumors in this location characteristically cause contralateral disturbances of sensation and may cause sensory seizures, sensory loss or inattention, or some combination of these symptoms. The sensory loss is cortical in type and involves postural sensibility and tactile discrimination, so that the appreciation of shape, size, weight, and texture is impaired. Objects placed in the hand may not be recognized (astereognosis). Extensive parietal lobe lesions may produce contralateral hyperpathia and spontaneous pain (thalamic syndrome). Involvement of the optic radiation leads to a contralateral homonymous field defect that sometimes consists solely of lower quadrantanopia. Lesions of the left angular gyrus cause Gerstmann's syndrome (a combination of alexia, agraphia, acalculia, right-left confusion, and finger agnosia), whereas involvement of the left submarginal gyrus causes ideational apraxia. Anosognosia (the denial, neglect, or rejection of a paralyzed limb) is seen in patients with lesions of the nondominant (right) hemisphere. Constructional apraxia and dressing apraxia may also occur with right-sided lesions.

**4. Occipital lobe lesions**–Tumors of the occipital lobe characteristically produce crossed homonymous hemianopia or a partial field defect. With left-sided or bilateral lesions, there may be visual agnosia both for objects and for colors, while irritative lesions on either side can cause unformed visual hallucinations. Bilateral occipital lobe involvement causes cortical blindness in which there is preservation of pupillary responses to light and lack of awareness of the defect by the patient. There may also be loss of color perception, prosopagnosia (inability to identify a familiar face), simultagnosia (inability to integrate and interpret a composite scene as opposed to its individual elements), and Balint's syndrome (failure to turn the eyes to a particular point in space, despite preservation of spontaneous and reflex eye movements). The denial of blindness or a field defect constitutes Anton's syndrome.

**5. Brain stem and cerebellar lesions**–Brain stem lesions lead to cranial nerve palsies, ataxia, incoordination, nystagmus, and pyramidal and sensory deficits in the limbs on one or both sides. Intrinsic brain stem tumors, such as gliomas, tend to produce an increase in intracranial pressure only late in their course. Cerebellar tumors produce marked ataxia of the trunk if the vermis cerebelli is involved and produce ipsilateral appendicular deficits (ataxia, incoordi-

**Table 16–3.** Primary intracranial tumors.

| Tumor | Clinical Features | Treatment and Prognosis |
|---|---|---|
| Glioblastoma multiforme | Presents commonly with nonspecific complaints and increased intracranial pressure. As it grows, focal deficits develop. | Course is rapidly progressive, with poor prognosis. Total surgical removal is usually not possible, and response to radiation therapy is poor. |
| Astrocytoma | Presentation similar to glioblastoma multiforme but course more protracted, often over several years. Cerebellar astrocytoma, especially in children, may have a more benign course. | Prognosis is variable. By the time of diagnosis, total excision is usually impossible; tumor often is not radiosensitive. In cerebellar astrocytoma, total surgical removal is often possible. |
| Medulloblastoma | Seen most frequently in children. Generally arises from roof of fourth ventricle and leads to increased intracranial pressure accompanied by brain stem and cerebellar signs. May seed in subarachnoid space. | Treatment consists of surgery combined with radiation therapy and chemotherapy. |
| Ependymoma | Glioma arising from the ependyma of a ventricle, especially the fourth ventricle; leads early to signs of increased intracranial pressure. Arises also from central canal of cord. | Tumor is not radiosensitive and is best treated surgically if possible. |
| Oligodendroglioma | Slow-growing. Usually arises in cerebral hemisphere in adults. Calcification may be visible on skull x-ray. | Treatment is surgical, which is usually successful. |
| Brain stem glioma | Presents during childhood with cranial nerve palsies and then with long-tract signs in the limbs. Signs of increased intracranial pressure occur late. | Tumor is inoperable; treatment is by irradiation and shunt for increased intracranial pressure. |
| Cerebellar hemangioblastoma | Presents with disequilibrium, ataxia of trunk or limbs, and signs of increased intracranial pressure. Sometimes familial. May be associated with retinal and spinal vascular lesions, polycythemia, and hypernephromas. | Treatment is surgical. |
| Pineal tumor | Presents with increased intracranial pressure, sometimes associated with impaired upward gaze (Parinaud's syndrome) and other deficits indicative of midbrain lesion. | Ventricular decompression by shunting is followed by surgical approach to tumor; irradiation is indicated if tumor is malignant. Prognosis depends on histopathologic findings and extent of tumor. |
| Craniopharyngioma | Originates from remnants of Rathke's pouch above the sella, depressing the optic chiasm. May present at any age but usually in childhood, with endocrine dysfunction and bitemporal field defects. | Treatment is surgical, but total removal may not be possible. |
| Acoustic neurinoma | Ipsilateral hearing loss is most common initial symptom. Subsequent symptoms may include tinnitus, headache, vertigo, facial weakness or numbness, and long-tract signs. (May be familial and bilateral when related to neurofibromatosis.) Most sensitive screening test is brain stem auditory evoked potential. | Treatment is excision by translabyrinthine surgery, craniectomy, or a combined approach. Outcome is usually good. |
| Meningioma | Originates from the dura mater or arachnoid; compresses rather than invades adjacent neural structures. Increasingly common with advancing age. Tumor size varies greatly. Symptoms vary with tumor site—eg, unilateral exophthalmos (sphenoidal ridge); anosmia and optic nerve compression (olfactory groove). Tumor is usually benign and readily detected by CT scanning; may lead to calcification and bone erosion visible on plain x-rays of skull. | Treatment is surgical. Tumor may recur if removal is incomplete. |

nation, and hypotonia of the limbs) if the cerebellar hemispheres are affected.

**6. False localizing signs**–Tumors may lead to neurologic signs other than by direct compression or infiltration, thereby leading to errors of clinical localization. These false localizing signs include third or sixth nerve palsy produced by herniation syndromes, bilateral extensor plantar responses, and an extensor plantar response occurring ipsilateral to a hemispheric tumor as a result of compression of the opposite cerebral peduncle against the tentorium.

**B. Imaging:** CT scanning detects the lesion and may also define its location, shape, and size; the extent to which normal anatomy is distorted; and the degree of any associated cerebral edema or mass effect. CT scanning is not so helpful in the posterior fossa, but MRI is of particular value in this regard. The characteristic appearance of meningiomas on CT scanning is virtually diagnostic; ie, a lesion in a typical site (parasagittal and sylvian regions, olfactory groove, sphenoidal ridge, tuberculum sellae) that appears as a homogeneous area of increased density in noncontrast CT scans and enhances uniformly with contrast.

Arteriography may show stretching or displacement of normal cerebral vessels by the tumor and the presence of tumor vascularity. The presence of an avascular mass is a nonspecific finding that could be due to tumor, hematoma, abscess, or any space-occupying lesion. In patients with normal hormone levels and an intrasellar mass, angiography is necessary to distinguish with confidence between a pituitary adenoma and an arterial aneurysm.

MRI scans may be diagnostic when a clinically suspected tumor is not detected by CT scanning.

**C. Laboratory and Other Studies:** The ECG provides supporting information concerning cerebral function and may show either a focal disturbance due to the neoplasm or a more diffuse change reflecting altered mental status. The findings on CT scan dispose of the need for lumbar puncture; in any case, findings are seldom diagnostic.

## Treatment

Treatment depends on the type and site of the tumor (Table 16–3) and the condition of the patient. Complete surgical removal may be possible if the tumor is extra-axial (eg, meningioma, acoustic neuroma) or is not in a critical or inaccessible region of the brain (eg, cerebellar hemangioblastoma). Surgery also permits the diagnosis to be verified and may be beneficial in reducing intracranial pressure and relieving symptoms even if the neoplasm cannot be completely removed. Clinical deficits are sometimes due in part to obstructive hydrocephalus, in which case simple surgical shunting procedures often produce dramatic benefit. In patients with malignant gliomas, radiation therapy increases median survival rates regardless of any preceding surgery, and its combination with chemotherapy provides additional benefit. Indications for irradiation in the treatment of patients with other primary intracranial neoplasms depend upon tumor type and accessibility, and the feasibility of complete surgical removal. Corticosteroids help reduce cerebral edema and are usually started before surgery. Herniation is treated with intravenous dexamethasone and intravenous mannitol (20%). Anticonvulsants are also commonly administered.

Baker HL, Houser OW, Campbell JK: National Cancer Institute Study: Evaluation of computed tomography in the diagnosis of intracranial neoplasms. *Radiology* 1980;**136:**91.

Wilson CB: Current concepts in cancer: Brain tumors. *N Engl J Med* 1979;**300:**1469.

Wilson CB, Fulton DS, Seager ML: Supportive management of the patient with malignant brain tumor. *JAMA* 1980;**244:**1249.

## 2. METASTATIC INTRACRANIAL TUMORS

### Cerebral Metastases

Metastatic brain tumors present in the same way as other cerebral neoplasms, ie, with increased intracranial pressure, with focal or diffuse disturbance of cerebral function, or with both of these manifestations. Indeed, in patients with a single cerebral lesion, the metastatic nature of the lesion may only become evident on histopathologic examination. In other patients, there is evidence of widespread metastatic disease, or an isolated cerebral metastasis develops during treatment of the primary neoplasm.

The most common source of intracranial metastasis is carcinoma of the lung; other common sources are neoplasms of the breast, kidney, and gastrointestinal tract. Most cerebral metastases are located supratentorially. The laboratory and radiologic studies used to evaluate patients with metastases are similar to those described in the preceding section on primary neoplasms. CT scanning should be performed both with and without contrast material. Lumbar puncture is necessary only in patients with suspected carcinomatous meningitis (see below). In patients with verified cerebral metastasis from an unknown primary, investigation should be guided by symptoms and signs. In women, mammography is regularly indicated; in men, attention should be paid to a possible germ cell origin. Both have therapeutic implications.

In patients with only a single cerebral metastasis who are otherwise well, it may be possible to remove the lesion, and then treat with irradiation. Alternatively, irradiation may be selected as the sole means of treatment. In patients with multiple metastases or widespread systemic disease, the long-term outlook is gloomy, and treatment by radiation therapy or chemotherapy is palliative.

### Leptomeningeal Metastases (Carcinomatous Meningitis)

The neoplasms metastasizing most commonly to the leptomeninges are carcinoma of the breast, lymphomas, and leukemia. Leptomeningeal metastases lead to multifocal neurologic deficits, which may be associated with infiltration of cranial and spinal nerve roots, direct invasion of the brain or spinal cord, obstructive hydrocephalus, or some combination of these factors.

The diagnosis is confirmed by examination of the cerebrospinal fluid. Findings may include elevated cerebrospinal fluid pressure, pleocytosis, increased protein concentration, and decreased glucose concentration. Cytologic studies may indicate that malignant cells are present; if not, spinal tap should be repeated at least twice to obtain further samples for analysis.

CT scans showing contrast enhancement in the basal cisterns or showing hydrocephalus without any evidence of a mass lesion support the diagnosis. Myelography may show deposits on multiple nerve roots.

Treatment is by irradiation to symptomatic areas, combined with intrathecal methotrexate. The long-term prognosis is poor—only about 10% of patients survive for a year.

Henson RA, Urich H: *Cancer and the Nervous System.* Blackwell, 1982.

### 3. PRIMARY & METASTATIC SPINAL TUMORS

Approximately 10% of spinal tumors are intramedullary. Ependymoma is the most common type of intramedullary tumor; the remainder are other types of glioma. Extramedullary tumors may be extradural or intradural in location. Among the primary extramedullary tumors, neurofibromas and meningiomas are relatively common, are benign, and may be intra- or extradural. Carcinomatous metastases, lymphomatous or leukemic deposits, and myeloma are usually extradural; in the case of metastases, the prostate, breast, lung, and kidney are common primary sites.

Tumors may lead to spinal cord dysfunction by direct compression, by ischemia secondary to arterial or venous obstruction, and, in the case of intramedullary lesions, by invasive infiltration.

### Clinical Findings

**A. Symptoms and Signs:** Symptoms usually develop insidiously. Pain is often conspicuous with extradural lesions; is characteristically aggravated by coughing or straining; may be radicular, localized to the back, or felt diffusely in an extremity; and may be accompanied by motor deficits, paresthesias, or numbness, especially in the legs. When sphincter disturbances occur, they are usually particularly disabling. Pain, however, often precedes specific neurologic symptoms from epidural metastases.

Examination may reveal localized spinal tenderness. A segmental lower motor neuron deficit or dermatomal sensory changes (or both) are sometimes found at the level of the lesion, while an upper motor neuron deficit and sensory disturbance are found below it.

**B. Imaging:** Findings on plain radiography of the spine may be normal but are commonly abnormal when there are metastatic deposits. Myelography, CT scanning with metrizamide, or both, may be necessary to identify and localize the site of cord compression. The combination of known tumor elsewhere in the body, back pain, and either abnormal plain films of the spine or neurologic signs of cord compression is an indication to perform these studies on an urgent basis. Some clinicians proceed to myelography based solely on new back pain in a cancer patient. If a complete block is present at lumbar myelography, a cisternal myelogram is performed to determine the upper level of the block and to investigate the possibility of block higher in the cord.

MRI scanning provides images in 3 planes, requires no contrast, and visualizes the whole spinal column. With increasing availability, MRI will probably become the imaging procedure of choice in the investigation of spinal tumors.

**C. Laboratory Findings:** The cerebrospinal fluid removed at myelography is often xanthochromic and contains a greatly increased protein concentration with normal cell content and glucose concentration.

### Treatment

Intramedullary tumors are treated by decompression and surgical excision (when feasible), and irradiation. The prognosis depends upon the cause and severity of cord compression before it is relieved.

Treatment of epidural spinal metastases consists of irradiation, irrespective of cell type. Dexamethasone is also given in a high dosage (eg, 25 mg 4 times daily for 3 days, followed by rapid tapering of the dosage, depending on response) to reduce cord swelling and relieve pain. Surgical decompression is reserved for patients with tumors that are unresponsive to irradiation or have previously been irradiated and for cases in which there is some uncertainty about the diagnosis. The long-term outlook is poor, but radiation treatment may at least delay the onset of major disability. Analgesics are given as necessary.

### 4. BRAIN ABSCESS

Infectious disorders are considered elsewhere in this book, but brief comment will be made here concerning cerebral abscess, which presents as an intracranial space-occupying lesion. Brain abscess may arise as a sequela of disease of the ear or nose, may be a metastatic complication of infection elsewhere in the body, or may result from infection introduced intracranially by trauma or surgical procedures. The most common infective organisms are streptococci and staphylococci. Headache, drowsiness, inattention, confusion, and seizures are early symptoms, followed by signs of increasing intracranial pressure and then a focal neurologic deficit. There may be little or no evidence of systemic infection.

A CT scan of the head characteristically shows an area of increased contrast surrounding a low-density core. Similar abnormalities may, however, be found in patients with metastatic neoplasms. Arteriography indicates the presence of a space-occupying lesion, which appears as an avascular mass with displacement of normal cerebral vessels, but this procedure provides no clue to the nature of the lesion.

Treatment consists of intravenous antibiotics, combined with surgical drainage (aspiration or excision) if necessary to reduce the mass effect, or sometimes to establish the diagnosis. Abscesses smaller than 2 cm can often be cured medically; the regimen should include drugs with activity against gram-positive organisms and anaerobes (eg, chloramphenicol).

### NONMETASTATIC NEUROLOGIC COMPLICATIONS OF MALIGNANT DISEASE

A variety of nonmetastatic neurologic complications of malignant disease can be recognized:

(1) Metabolic encephalopathy due to electrolyte abnormalities, infections, drug overdose, or the fail-

ure of some vital organ may be reflected by drowsiness, lethargy, restlessness, insomnia, agitation, confusion, stupor, or coma. The mental changes are usually associated with tremor, asterixis, and multifocal myoclonus. The electroencephalogram is generally diffusely slowed. Laboratory studies are necessary to detect the cause of the encephalopathy, which must then be treated appropriately.

(2) Immune suppression resulting from either the malignant disease or its treatment (eg, by chemotherapy) predisposes patients to brain abscess, progressive multifocal leukoencephalopathy, meningitis, herpes zoster infection, and other infectious diseases. Moreover, an overt or occult cerebrospinal fluid fistula, as occurs with some tumors, may also increase the risk of infection. CT scanning aids in the early recognition of a brain abscess, but metastatic brain tumors may have a similar appearance. Examination of the cerebrospinal fluid is essential in the evaluation of patients with meningitis but is of no help in the diagnosis of brain abscess. Treatment should be specific for the infective organism.

(3) Cerebrovascular disorders that cause neurologic complications in patients with systemic cancer include nonbacterial thrombotic endocarditis and septic embolization. Cerebral, subarachnoid, or subdural hemorrhages may occur in patients with myelogenous leukemia and may be found in association with metastatic tumors, especially malignant melanoma. Spinal subdural hemorrhage sometimes occurs after lumbar puncture in patients with marked thrombocytopenia.

Disseminated intravascular coagulation occurs most commonly in patients with acute promyelocytic leukemia or with some adenocarcinomas and is characterized by a fluctuating encephalopathy, often with associated seizures, that frequently progresses to coma or death. There may be few accompanying neurologic signs.

Venous sinus thrombosis, which usually presents with convulsions and headaches, may also occur in patients with leukemia or lymphoma. Examination commonly reveals papilledema and focal or diffuse neurologic signs. Treatment is with anticonvulsants and drugs to lower the intracranial pressure. The role of anticoagulants is controversial.

(4) Subacute cerebellar degeneration occurs most commonly in association with carcinoma of the lung. Symptoms may precede those due to the neoplasm itself, which may be undetected for several months or even longer. Typically, there is a pancerebellar syndrome causing dysarthria, nystagmus, and ataxia of the trunk and limbs. Treatment is of the underlying malignant disease.

(5) Malignant disease is more commonly associated with sensorimotor polyneuropathy than with pure sensory neuropathy (ie, dorsal root ganglionitis) or autonomic neuropathy.

(6) Dermatomyositis or a myasthenic syndrome may be seen in patients with underlying carcinoma (see Chapter 14 and p 612).

## PSEUDOTUMOR CEREBRI
### (Benign Intracranial Hypertension)

Symptoms of pseudotumor cerebri consist of headache, diplopia, and other visual disturbances due to papilledema and abducens nerve dysfunction. Examination reveals the papilledema and some enlargement of the blind spots, but patients otherwise look well. Investigations reveal no evidence of a space-occupying lesion, and the CT scan shows small or normal ventricles. Lumbar puncture confirms the presence of intracranial hypertension, but the cerebrospinal fluid is normal.

There are many causes of pseudotumor cerebri. Thrombosis of the transverse venous sinus as a noninfectious complication of otitis media or chronic mastoiditis is an important cause, and sagittal sinus thrombosis may lead to a clinically similar picture. Other causes include chronic pulmonary disease, endocrine disturbances such as hypoparathyroidism or Addison's disease, vitamin A toxicity, and the use of nalidixic acid, tetracycline, or oral contraceptives. Cases have also followed withdrawal of corticosteroids after long-term use. In many instances, however, no specific cause can be found, and the disorder remits spontaneously after several months. This idiopathic variety is said to be especially common in overweight young women.

Untreated pseudotumor cerebri leads to secondary optic atrophy and permanent visual loss. Repeated lumbar puncture to lower the intracranial pressure by removal of cerebrospinal fluid is effective, but pharmacologic approaches to treatment are now more satisfactory. Acetazolamide reduces formation of cerebrospinal fluid and can be used to start treatment; furosemide serves the same function and can be added to the treatment regimen if necessary. Oral corticosteroids have also been used. Obese patients should be advised to lose weight. Treatment is monitored by checking visual acuity, funduscopic appearance, and pressure of the cerebrospinal fluid.

If medical treatment fails to control the intracranial pressure, surgical placement of a lumboperitoneal or other shunt should be undertaken to preserve vision.

In addition to the above measures, any specific cause of pseudotumor cerebri requires appropriate treatment. Thus, hormone therapy should be initiated if there is an underlying endocrine disturbance. Discontinuing the use of nalidixic acid, tetracycline, oral contraceptives, or vitamin A will allow for resolution of pseudotumor cerebri due to these agents. If corticosteroid withdrawal is responsible, the medication should be reintroduced and then tapered more gradually.

Rush JA: Pseudotumor cerebri. *Br J Hosp Med* 1983;**29**:320.

## SELECTED NEUROCUTANEOUS DISEASES

### Tuberous Sclerosis

Tuberous sclerosis may occur sporadically or on a familial basis with autosomal dominant inheritance. Its pathogenesis is unknown. Neurologic presentation is with seizures and progressive psychomotor retardation beginning in early childhood. The cutaneous abnormality, adenoma sebaceum, becomes manifest usually between 5 and 10 years of age and typically consists of reddened nodules on the face (cheeks, nasolabial folds, sides of the nose, and chin) and sometimes on the forehead and neck. Other typical cutaneous lesions include subungual fibromas, shagreen patches, and leaf-shaped hypopigmented spots. Associated abnormalities include retinal lesions and tumors, benign rhabdomyomas of the heart, lung cysts, benign tumors in the viscera, and bone cysts.

The disease is slowly progressive and leads to increasing mental deterioration. There is no specific treatment, but anticonvulsant drugs may help in controlling seizures.

### Neurofibromatosis (Recklinghausen's Disease)

Neurofibromatosis may occur either sporadically or on a familial basis with autosomal dominant inheritance. Neurologic presentation is usually with symptoms and signs of tumor. Multiple neurofibromas characteristically are present and may involve spinal or cranial nerves, especially the eighth cranial nerve. Examination of the superficial cutaneous nerves usually reveals palpable mobile nodules. In some cases, there is an associated marked overgrowth of subcutaneous tissues (plexiform neuromas), sometimes with an underlying bony abnormality. Associated cutaneous lesions include axillary freckling and patches of cutaneous pigmentation (café au lait spots). Malignant degeneration of neurofibromas occasionally occurs and may lead to peripheral sarcomas. Meningiomas, gliomas (especially optic nerve gliomas), bone cysts, pheochromocytomas, scoliosis, and obstructive hydrocephalus may also occur.

It may be possible to correct disfigurement by plastic surgery. Intraspinal or intracranial tumors and tumors of peripheral nerves should be treated surgically if they are producing symptoms.

### Sturge-Weber Syndrome

Sturge-Weber syndrome consists of a congenital, usually unilateral, cutaneous capillary angioma involving the upper face, leptomeningeal angiomatosis, and, in many patients, choroidal angioma. It has no sex predilection and usually occurs sporadically. The cutaneous angioma sometimes has a more extensive distribution over the head and neck and is often quite disfiguring, especially if there is associated overgrowth of connective tissue. Focal or generalized seizures are the usual neurologic presentation and may commence at any age. There may be contralateral homonymous hemianopia, hemiparesis and hemisensory disturbance, ipsilateral glaucoma or buphthalmos, and mental subnormality. Skull x-rays taken after the first 2 years of life usually reveal gyriform ("tramline") intracranial calcification, especially in the parieto-occipital region, due to mineral deposition in the cortex beneath the intracranial angioma.

Treatment is aimed at controlling seizures pharmacologically. Ophthalmologic advice should be sought concerning the management of choroidal angioma and of increased intraocular pressure.

Riccardi VM: Von Recklinghausen neurofibromatosis. *N Engl J Med* 1981;**305**:1617.

## MOVEMENT DISORDERS

### 1. BENIGN ESSENTIAL (FAMILIAL) TREMOR

The cause of benign essential tremor is uncertain, but it is sometimes inherited in an autosomal dominant manner. Tremor may begin at any age and is enhanced by emotional stress. The tremor usually involves one or both hands, the head, or the hands and head, while the legs tend to be spared. Examination reveals no other abnormalities. A small quantity of alcohol commonly provides remarkable but short-lived relief by an unknown mechanism.

Although the tremor may become more conspicuous with time, it generally leads to little disability other than cosmetic and social embarrassment, and treatment is often therefore unnecessary. Occasionally, however, it interferes with manual skills and leads to impairment of handwriting. Speech may also be affected if the laryngeal muscles are involved. In such circumstances, propranolol may be helpful but will need to be continued indefinitely in daily doses of 60–240 mg. It is not clear whether the response to propranolol depends on central or peripheral mechanisms. Primidone may be helpful when propranolol is ineffective, but patients with essential tremor are often very sensitive to it. They are therefore started on 50 mg daily, and the daily dose is increased by 50 mg every 2 weeks depending on the response; a maintenance dose of 125 mg 3 times daily is commonly effective.

Larsen TA, Calne DB: Essential tremor. *Clin Neuropharmacol* 1983;**6**:185.

### 2. PARKINSONISM

### Essentials of Diagnosis

- Any combination of tremor, rigidity, bradykinesia, progressive postural instability.
- Seborrhea of skin quite common.
- Mild intellectual deterioration is common.

## General Considerations

Parkinsonism is a relatively common disorder that occurs in all ethnic groups, with an approximately equal sex distribution. The most common variety, idiopathic Parkinson's disease (paralysis agitans), begins most often between 45 and 65 years of age.

## Etiology

Postencephalitic parkinsonism is becoming increasingly rare. Exposure to certain toxins (eg, manganese dust, carbon disulfide) and severe carbon monoxide poisoning may lead to parkinsonism. Recently, typical parkinsonism was reported in a group of individuals who had attempted to make a narcotic drug related to meperidine but actually synthesized and then took 1-methyl-4-phenyl-1,2,5,6-tetrahydropyridine (MPTP). This compound selectively destroys dopaminergic neurons in the substantia nigra. Reversible parkinsonism may develop in patients receiving neuroleptic drugs (see Chapter 17) and has also been caused by reserpine and metoclopramide. Only rarely is hemiparkinsonism the presenting feature of a brain tumor or some other progressive space-occupying lesion.

In idiopathic parkinsonism, dopamine depletion due to degeneration of the dopaminergic nigrostriatal system leads to an imbalance of dopamine and acetylcholine, which are neurotransmitters normally present in the corpus striatum. Treatment is directed at redressing this imbalance by blocking the effect of acetylcholine with anticholinergic drugs or by the administration of levodopa, the precursor of dopamine.

## Clinical Findings

Tremor, rigidity, bradykinesia, and postural instability are the cardinal features of parkinsonism and may be present in any combination. There may also be a mild decline in intellectual function. The tremor of about 4–6 cycles per second is most conspicuous at rest, is enhanced by emotional stress, and is often less severe during voluntary activity. Although it may ultimately be present in all limbs, the tremor is commonly confined to one limb or to the limbs on one side for months or years before it becomes more generalized. In some patients, tremor is absent.

Rigidity (an increase in resistance to passive movement) is responsible for the characteristically flexed posture seen in many patients, but the most disabling symptoms of parkinsonism are due to bradykinesia, manifested as a slowness of voluntary movement and a reduction in automatic movements such as swinging of the arms while walking. Curiously, however, effective voluntary activity may briefly be regained during an emergency (eg, the patient is able to leap aside to avoid an oncoming motor vehicle).

Clinical diagnosis of the well-developed syndrome is usually simple. The patient has a relatively immobile face with widened palpebral fissures, infrequent blinking, and a certain fixity of facial expression. Seborrhea of the scalp and face is common. There is often mild blepharoclonus, and a tremor may be present about the mouth and lips. Repetitive tapping (about twice per second) over the bridge of the nose produces a sustained blink response (Myerson's sign). Other findings may include saliva drooling from the mouth, perhaps due to impairment of swallowing; soft and poorly modulated voice; a variable rest tremor and rigidity in some or all of the limbs; slowness of voluntary movements; impairment of fine or rapidly alternating movements; and micrographia. There is typically no muscle weakness (provided that sufficient time is allowed for power to be developed) and no alteration in the tendon reflexes or plantar responses. It is difficult for the patient to arise from a sitting position and begin walking. The gait itself is characterized by small shuffling steps and a loss of the normal automatic arm swing; there may be unsteadiness on turning and difficulty in stopping.

## Differential Diagnosis

Diagnostic problems may occur in mild cases, especially if tremor is minimal or absent. For example, mild hypokinesia or slight tremor is commonly attributed to old age. Depression, with its associated expressionless face, poorly modulated voice, and reduction in voluntary activity, can be difficult to distinguish from mild parkinsonism, especially since the 2 disorders may coexist; in some cases, a trial of antidepressant drug therapy may be necessary. The family history, the character of the tremor, and lack of other neurologic signs should distinguish essential tremor from parkinsonism. Wilson's disease can be distinguished by its early age at onset, the presence of other abnormal movements, Kayser-Fleischer rings, chronic hepatitis, and increased concentrations of copper in the tissues. Huntington's disease presenting with rigidity and bradykinesia may be mistaken for parkinsonism unless the family history and accompanying dementia are recognized. In Shy-Drager syndrome, the clinical features of parkinsonism are accompanied by autonomic insufficiency (leading to postural hypotension, anhidrosis, disturbances of sphincter control, impotence, etc) and more widespread neurologic deficits (pyramidal, lower motor neuron, or cerebellar signs). In progressive supranuclear palsy, bradykinesia and rigidity are accompanied by a supranuclear disorder of eye movements, pseudobulbar palsy, and axial dystonia. Creutzfeldt-Jakob disease may be accompanied by features of parkinsonism, but dementia is usual, myoclonic jerking is common, ataxia and pyramidal signs may be conspicuous, and the electroencephalographic findings are usually characteristic. Hypothyroidism may also resemble parkinsonism, as may advanced ankylosing spondylitis.

## Treatment

**A. Medical Measures:** Drug treatment is not required early in the course of parkinsonism, but the nature of the disorder and the availability of medical treatment for use when necessary should be discussed with the patient.

**1. Amantadine**–Patients with mild symptoms but no disability may be helped by treatment with amantadine. This drug improves all of the clinical features of parkinsonism, but its mode of action is unclear. Side effects include restlessness, confusion, depression, skin rashes, edema, nausea, constipation, anorexia, postural hypotension, and disturbances of cardiac rhythm. However, these are relatively uncommon with the usual dose (100 mg 2 times daily).

**2. Anticholinergic drugs**–Anticholinergics are more helpful in alleviating tremor and rigidity than bradykinesia. Treatment is started with a small dose of one preparation (Table 16–4), and the dose is gradually increased until benefit occurs or side effects limit further increments. If treatment is ineffective, the drug is gradually withdrawn and another preparation then tried. Ethopropazine is probably the most helpful drug in this group for the relief of tremor.

Common side effects include dryness of the mouth, nausea, constipation, palpitations, cardiac arrhythmias, urinary retention, confusion, agitation, restlessness, drowsiness, mydriasis, increased intraocular pressure, and defective accommodation.

Anticholinergic drugs are contraindicated in patients with prostatic hypertrophy, closed-angle glaucoma, or obstructive gastrointestinal disease.

**3. Levodopa**–Levodopa, which is converted in the body to dopamine, improves all of the major features of parkinsonism, including bradykinesia. Long-term levodopa therapy does not stop progression of the disorder; moreover, its effectiveness may decline after 2 or 3 years, and certain complications or adverse reactions to it may develop with time. Levodopa is therefore best reserved for patients with definite disability. The commonest early side effects of levodopa are nausea, vomiting, and hypotension, but cardiac irregularities may also occur. Dyskinesias, restlessness, confusion, and other behavioral changes tend to occur somewhat later and become more com-

mon with time. Levodopa-induced dyskinesias may take any conceivable form, including chorea, athetosis, dystonia, tremor, tics, and myoclonus. An even later complication is the "on-off phenomenon," in which abrupt but transient fluctuations in the severity of parkinsonism occur unpredictably but frequently during the day. The "off" period of marked bradykinesia has been shown to relate in some instances to falling plasma levels of levodopa. During the "on" phase, dyskinesias are often conspicuous but mobility is increased.

Carbidopa, which inhibits the enzyme responsible for the breakdown of levodopa to dopamine, does not cross the blood-brain barrier. When levodopa is given in combination with carbidopa, the extracerebral breakdown of levodopa is largely prevented. This reduces the amount of levodopa required daily for beneficial effects, and it lowers the incidence of nausea, vomiting, hypotension, and cardiac irregularities. Such a combination does not prevent the development of the "on-off phenomenon," and the incidence of other side effects (dyskinesias or psychiatric complications) may actually be increased.

Sinemet, a commercially available preparation that contains carbidopa and levodopa in a fixed ratio (1:10 or 1:4), is generally used. Treatment is started with a small dose—eg, one tablet of Sinemet 25/100 (containing 25 mg of carbidopa and 100 mg of levodopa) 3 times daily—and gradually increased depending on the response.

The dyskinesias and behavioral side effects of levodopa are dose-related, but reduction in dose may eliminate any therapeutic benefit. In such circumstances, a drug holiday may be helpful. Levodopa medication is gradually withdrawn over several days and not reinstated for 1–2 weeks. When it is reintroduced, up to two-thirds of patients show improved responsiveness and so derive benefit at a lower daily dose than previously required. The "on-off phenomenon" may also be improved by a drug holiday, but any benefit in this regard is usually short-lived. Unfortunately, there is no way of predicting which patients will benefit from a drug holiday, and it is a distressing and difficult experience that may necessitate hospitalization. Complications of a drug holiday include depression, decubitus ulcers, aspiration pneumonia, and thromboembolism.

Levodopa therapy is contraindicated in patients with psychotic illness or closed-angle glaucoma. It should not be given to patients taking monoamine oxidase A inhibitors or within 2 weeks of their withdrawal, because hypertensive crises may result. Levodopa should be avoided in patients with suspected malignant melanomas, which may be activated, and in patients with active peptic ulcers, which may bleed.

**4. Bromocriptine**–This ergot derivative acts directly on dopamine receptors and has been used as adjunctive therapy in parkinsonism. Bromocriptine may have a role as a first-line drug, because there is some suggestive evidence that its use in parkinsonism is associated with a lower incidence of the side

**Table 16–4.** Some anticholinergic antiparkinsonian drugs.*

| Drug | Usual Daily Dose (mg) |
| --- | --- |
| Benztropine mesylate (Cogentin) | 1–6 |
| Biperiden (Akineton) | 2–12 |
| Chlorphenoxamine (Phenoxene) | 150–400 |
| Cycrimine (Pagitane) | 5–20 |
| Ethopropazine (Parsidol) | 150–300 |
| Orphenadrine (Disipal, Norflex) | 150–400 |
| Procyclidine (Kemadrin) | 7.5–30 |
| Trihexyphenidyl (Artane) | 6–20 |

* Reproduced, with permission, from Aminoff MJ: Pharmacologic management of parkinsonism and other movement disorders. In: *Basic & Clinical Pharmacology*, 3rd ed. Katzung BG (editor). Appleton-Lange, 1987.

effects that occur with long-term levodopa therapy. It is often reserved for patients who have either become refractory to levodopa or developed the "on-off phenomenon." Patients who have never responded to levodopa generally fail to respond to bromocriptine as well. The initial dosage of bromocriptine is 1.25 mg twice daily; this is increased by 2.5 mg at 2-week intervals until benefit occurs or side effects limit further increments. The usual daily maintenance dose in patients with parkinsonism is between 10 and 30 mg.

Side effects include anorexia, nausea, vomiting, constipation, postural hypotension, digital vasospasm, cardiac arrhythmias, various dyskinesias and mental disturbances, headache, nasal congestion, erythromelalgia, and pulmonary infiltrates.

Bromocriptine is contraindicated in patients with a history of mental illness or recent myocardial infarction and is probably best avoided in those with peripheral vascular disease or peptic ulcers (bleeding from peptic ulcers has been reported).

**5. Other drugs**–A number of other dopamine agonists, including lisuride and pergolide, have been used to treat parkinsonism, but these are still under study.

**B. General Measures:** Physical therapy or speech therapy helps many patients. The quality of life can often be improved by the provision of simple aids to daily living, eg, rails or banisters placed strategically about the home, special table cutlery with large handles, nonslip rubber table mats, and devices to amplify the voice.

**C. Surgical Measures:** Surgical treatment (thalamotomy) is generally reserved for the patient who is relatively young, has predominantly unilateral tremor and rigidity that have failed to respond to medication, and has no evidence of diffuse vascular disease.

Current concepts and controversies in Parkinson's disease. *Can J Neurol Sci* 1984;**11(Suppl)**. [Entire issue.]

Langston JW et al: Chronic parkinsonism in humans due to a product of meperidine-analog synthesis. *Science* 1983; **219:**979.

## 3. HUNTINGTON'S DISEASE

### Essentials of Diagnosis

- Gradual onset and progression of chorea and dementia
- Family history of the disorder.

### General Considerations

Huntington's disease is characterized by chorea and dementia. It is inherited in an autosomal dominant manner and occurs throughout the world, in all ethnic groups, with a prevalence rate of about 5 per 100,000. The gene responsible for the disease has been located on the short arm of chromosome No. 4. Symptoms do not usually develop until after 30 years of age.

Thus, by the time of diagnosis the patient has usually had children, and so the disease continues from one generation to the next. The cause of Huntington's disease is unknown.

### Clinical Findings

Clinical onset is usually between 30 and 50 years of age. The disease is progressive and usually leads to a fatal outcome within 15–20 years. The initial symptoms may consist of either abnormal movements or intellectual changes, but ultimately both occur. The earliest mental changes are often behavioral, with irritability, moodiness, antisocial behavior, or a psychiatric disturbance, but a more obvious dementia subsequently develops. The dyskinesia may initially be no more than an apparent fidgetiness or restlessness, but eventually choreiform movements and some dystonic posturing occur. Progressive rigidity and akinesia (rather than chorea) sometimes occur in association with dementia, especially in cases with childhood onset. CT scanning usually demonstrates cerebral atrophy and atrophy of the caudate nucleus in established cases. MRI spectroscopy and positron emission tomography (PET) have shown reduced glucose utilization in an anatomically normal caudate nucleus.

Chorea developing with no family history of choreoathetosis should not be attributed to Huntington's disease, at least until other causes of chorea have been excluded clinically and by appropriate laboratory studies. In younger patients, self-limiting Sydenham's chorea develops after group A streptococcal infections on rare occasions. If a patient presents solely with progressive intellectual failure, it may not be possible to distinguish Huntington's disease from other causes of dementia unless there is a characteristic family history or a dyskinesia develops.

### Treatment

There is no cure for Huntington's disease, progression cannot be halted, and treatment is purely symptomatic. The reported biochemical changes suggest a relative underactivity of neurons containing gamma-aminobutyric acid (GABA) and acetylcholine or a relative overactivity of dopaminergic neurons. Treatment with drugs blocking dopamine receptors, such as phenothiazines or haloperidol, may control the dyskinesia and any behavioral disturbances. Haloperidol treatment is usually begun with a dose of 1 mg once or twice daily, which is then increased every 3 or 4 days depending on the response. Tetrabenazine, a drug that depletes central monoamines, is widely used in Europe to treat dyskinesia but is not yet available in the USA. Reserpine is similar in its actions to tetrabenazine and may be helpful; the daily dose is built up gradually to between 2 and 5 mg, depending on the response. Attempts to compensate for the relative GABA deficiency by enhancing central GABA activity or to compensate for the relative cholinergic underactivity by giving choline chloride have not been therapeutically helpful. High levels of somatostatin (a neuropeptide) have recently been reported in certain areas of the brain in patients with Huntington's disease, and the therapeutic response to cysteamine (a selective depleter of somatostatin in the brain) is currently under study.

Offspring should be offered genetic counseling. There is no certain way of determining whether asymptomatic offspring have inherited the disease.

Martin JB, Gusella JF: Huntington's disease: Pathogenesis and management. *New England J Med* 1986;**315:**1267.
Martindale B, Yale R: Huntington's chorea: Neglected opportunities for preventive medicine. *Lancet* 1983;**1:**634.

### 4. IDIOPATHIC TORSION DYSTONIA

#### Essentials of Diagnosis

- Dystonic movements and postures.
- Normal birth and developmental history.
- No other neurologic signs.
- Investigations (including CT scan) reveal no cause of dystonia.

#### General Considerations

Idiopathic torsion dystonia may occur sporadically or on a hereditary basis, with autosomal dominant, autosomal recessive, and X-linked recessive modes of transmission. It may begin in childhood or later and persists throughout life.

#### Clinical Findings

The disorder is characterized by the onset of abnormal movements and postures in a patient with a normal birth and developmental history, no relevant past medical illness, and no other neurologic signs. Investigations (including CT scan) reveal no cause for the abnormal movements. Dystonic movements of the head and neck may take the form of torticollis, blepharospasm, facial grimacing, or forced opening or closing of the mouth. The limbs may also adopt abnormal but characteristic postures. The age at onset influences both the clinical findings and the prognosis. With onset in childhood, there is usually a family history of the disorder, symptoms commonly commence in the legs, and progression is likely until there is severe disability from generalized dystonia. In contrast, when onset is later, a positive family history is unlikely, initial symptoms are often in the arms or axial structures, and severe disability does not usually occur, although generalized dystonia may ultimately develop in some patients. If all cases are considered together, about one-third of patients eventually become so severely disabled that they are confined to chair or bed, while another one-third are affected only mildly.

Before a diagnosis of idiopathic torsion dystonia is made, it is imperative to exclude other causes of dystonia. For example, perinatal anoxia, birth trauma, and kernicterus are common causes of dystonia, but abnormal movements usually then develop before the age of 5, the early development of the patient is usually abnormal, and a history of seizures is not unusual. Moreover, examination may reveal signs of mental retardation or pyramidal deficit in addition to the movement disorder. Dystonic posturing may also occur in Wilson's disease, Huntington's disease, or parkinsonism; as a sequela of encephalitis lethargica or previous neuroleptic drug therapy; and in certain other disorders. In these cases, diagnosis is based on the history and accompanying clinical manifestations.

#### Treatment

Idiopathic torsion dystonia usually responds poorly to drugs. Diazepam, baclofen, carbamazepine, amantadine, or anticholinergic medication (in high dosage) is occasionally helpful; if not, a trial of treatment with phenothiazines, haloperidol, or tetrabenazine (not available in USA) may be worthwhile. However, the doses of these latter drugs that are required for benefit lead usually to mild parkinsonism. Stereotactic thalamotomy is sometimes helpful in patients with predominantly unilateral dystonia, especially when this involves the limbs.

Fahn S: High dosage anticholinergic therapy in dystonia. *Neurology* 1983;**33:**1255.

### 5. FOCAL TORSION DYSTONIA

A number of the dystonic manifestations that occur in idiopathic torsion dystonia may also occur as isolated phenomena. They are best regarded as focal dystonias that either occur as formes frustes of idiopathic torsion dystonia in patients with a positive family history or represent a focal manifestation of the adult-onset form of that disorder when there is no family history. Medical treatment is generally unsatisfactory. A trial of the drugs used in idiopathic torsion dystonia is worthwhile, however, since a few patients do show some response. In addition, with restricted dystonias such as blepharospasm or torticollis, local injection of botulinum A toxin into the overactive muscles may produce benefit for several weeks or months and can be repeated as needed.

Both **blepharospasm** and **oromandibular dystonia** may occur as an isolated focal dystonia. The former is characterized by spontaneous involuntary forced closure of the eyelids for a variable interval. Oromandibular dystonia is manifested by involuntary contraction of the muscles about the mouth causing, for example, involuntary opening or closing of the mouth, roving or protruding tongue movements, and retraction of the platysma.

**Spasmodic torticollis,** usually with onset between 25 and 50 years of age, is characterized by a tendency for the neck to twist to one side. This initially occurs episodically, but eventually the neck is held to the side. Spontaneous resolution may occur in the first year or so. The disorder is otherwise usually lifelong.

Selective section of the spinal accessory nerve and the upper cervical nerve roots is sometimes helpful if medical treatment is unsuccessful. Local injection of botulinum A toxin may provide benefit in some cases.

**Writer's cramp** is characterized by dystonic posturing of the hand and forearm when the hand is used for writing and sometimes when it is used for other tasks, eg, playing the piano, using a screwdriver or eating utensils. Drug treatment is usually unrewarding, and patients are often best advised to learn to use the other hand for activities requiring manual dexterity.

Jankovic J, Havins WE, Wilkins RB: Blinking and blepharospasm: Mechanism, diagnosis, and management. *JAMA* 1982;**248**:3160.
Scott AB et al: Botulinum A toxin injection as a treatment for blepharospasm. *Arch Ophthalmol* 1985;**103**:347.

## 6. MYOCLONUS

Occasional myoclonic jerks may occur in anyone, especially when drifting into sleep. General or multifocal myoclonus is common in patients with idiopathic epilepsy and is especially prominent in certain hereditary disorders characterized by seizures and progressive intellectual decline, such as the lipid storage diseases and Lafora's disease. It is also a feature of various rare degenerative disorders, notably Ramsay Hunt syndrome, and is common in subacute sclerosing panencephalitis and Creutzfeldt-Jakob disease. Generalized myoclonic jerking may accompany uremic and other metabolic encephalopathies, result from levodopa therapy, occur in alcohol or drug withdrawal states, or follow anoxic brain damage. It also occurs on a hereditary or sporadic basis as an isolated phenomenon in otherwise healthy subjects.

Segmental myoclonus is a rare manifestation of a focal spinal cord lesion. It may also be the clinical expression of **epilepsia partialis continua,** a disorder in which a repetitive focal epileptic discharge arises in the contralateral sensorimotor cortex, sometimes from an underlying structural lesion. An electroencephalogram is often helpful in clarifying the epileptic nature of the disorder, and CT or MRI scan may reveal the causal lesion. An interesting segmental form is diaphragmatic myoclonus, which clinically resembles hiccup but occurs at a faster rate and is more apt to be associated with the causes of general myoclonus.

Myoclonus may respond to certain anticonvulsant drugs, especially valproic acid, or to one of the benzodiazepines, particularly clonazepam. Myoclonus following anoxic brain damage is often responsive to 5-hydroxytryptophan, the precursor of 5-hydroxytryptamine, and sometimes to clonazepam. In patients with segmental myoclonus, a localized lesion should be searched for and treated appropriately.

Berkovic SF et al: Progressive myoclonus epilepsies: Specific causes and diagnosis. *N Engl J Med* 1986;**315**:296.
Kelly JJ, Sharbrough FW, Daube JR: A clinical and electrophysiological evaluation of myoclonus. *Neurology* 1981; **31**:581.

## 7. WILSON'S DISEASE

In this metabolic disorder, abnormal movements and postures of all sorts may occur with or without coexisting signs of liver involvement. It is discussed in detail in Chapter 11.

## 8. DRUG-INDUCED ABNORMAL MOVEMENTS

Phenothiazines and butyrophenones may produce a wide variety of abnormal movements, including parkinsonism, akathisia, acute dystonia, chorea, and tardive dyskinesia. These complications are discussed in Chapter 17. Chorea may also develop in patients receiving levodopa, bromocriptine, anticholinergic drugs, phenytoin, carbamazepine, lithium, amphetamines, or oral contraceptives, and it resolves with withdrawal of the offending substance. Similarly, dystonia may be produced by levodopa, bromocriptine, lithium, metoclopramide, or carbamazepine; and parkinsonism by reserpine, tetrabenazine, and metoclopramide. Postural tremor may occur with a variety of drugs, including epinephrine, isoproterenol, theophylline, caffeine, lithium, thyroid hormone, tricyclic antidepressants, and valproic acid.

## 9. GILLES DE LA TOURETTE'S SYNDROME

### Essentials of Diagnosis
- Multiple motor and phonic tics.
- Symptoms begin before age 15 years.
- Chronic lifelong disorder with relapses and remissions.

### Clinical Findings
Motor tics are the initial manifestation in 80% of cases and most commonly involve the face, whereas in the remaining 20%, the initial symptoms are phonic tics; all patients ultimately develop a combination of different motor and phonic tics. These are noted first in childhood, generally between the ages of 2 and 15. Motor tics occur especially about the face, head, and shoulders (eg, sniffing, blinking, frowning, shoulder shrugging, head thrusting, etc). Phonic tics commonly consist of grunts, barks, hisses, throat-clearing, coughs, etc, but sometimes also of verbal utterances including coprolalia. There may also be echolalia, echopraxia, and palilalia. Some tics may be self-mutilating in nature, such as severe nail-biting, hair-pulling, or biting of the lips or tongue. The disorder is chronic, but the course may be punctuated by relapses and remissions.

Examination usually reveals no abnormalities other than the multiple tics. Psychiatric disturbances may occur, however, because of the cosmetic and social embarrassment produced. Investigations are unrevealing except that the electroencephalogram may show minor nonspecific abnormalities of no diagnostic relevance.

The diagnosis of the disorder is often delayed for years, the tics being interpreted as psychiatric illness or some other form of abnormal movement. Patients are thus often subjected to unnecessary and expensive treatments before the true nature of the disorder is recognized. The ticlike character of the abnormal movements and the absence of other neurologic signs should differentiate this disorder from other movement disorders presenting in childhood. Wilson's disease, however, can simulate the condition and should be excluded.

## Treatment

Treatment is symptomatic and may need to be continued indefinitely. Haloperidol is generally regarded as the drug of choice. It is started in a low daily dose (0.25 mg) that is gradually increased (by 0.25 mg every 4 or 5 days) until there is maximum benefit with a minimum of side effects, or until side effects limit further increments. A total daily dose of between 2 and 8 mg is usually optimal, but higher doses are sometimes necessary. Treatment with clonazepam or clonidine may also be helpful, and it seems sensible to begin with one of these drugs in order to avoid some of the long-term extrapyramidal side effects of haloperidol. Phenothiazines, such as fluphenazine, have been used, but patients unresponsive to haloperidol are usually unresponsive to these as well.

Pimozide, an oral dopamine-blocking drug related to haloperidol, may be helpful in patients who cannot tolerate or have not responded to haloperidol. Treatment is started with 1 mg daily and the daily dose increased by 1–2 mg every 10 days; the average dose is between 7 and 16 mg daily. The long-term safety of the drug is unclear.

Lees AJ et al: A clinical study of Gilles de la Tourette syndrome in the United Kingdom. *J Neurol Neurosurg Psychiatry* 1984;**47**:1.

## DEMENTIA

Dementia, the symptom complex of progressive global impairment of intellectual function, is a major medical, social, and economic problem that is worsening as the number of elderly people in the general population increases. In the USA, more than 20 million people were more than 65 years old in 1970; 10% of these were mildly demented and another 5% so severely demented that they could not cope with the tasks of independent daily life. By the turn of the century, a 50% increase in the number of demented

elderly persons has been projected. Nevertheless, the clinical features of dementia are often not recognized at an early stage, so that investigations are delayed and treatment is withheld.

It is clinically important to distinguish dementia from other disturbances of cognitive function.

(1) It is sometimes difficult to distinguish between dementia and a confusional state. In general, however, a **confusional state,** which represents the mildest level of a disturbance in consciousness, has an acute or subacute onset and fluctuating course, is frequently reversible, and is characterized by short attention span and variable degrees of disorientation; if there is excessive agitation, the term **delirium** is often used. In dementia, by contrast, there is no alteration in the level of consciousness, and the course is usually chronic and progressive, although it may be possible to arrest or reverse it in some cases.

(2) The global cognitive impairment in dementia clearly distinguishes it from disorders characterized by focal, circumscribed deficits of higher cortical function. Nevertheless, **aphasia,** and especially the fluent, articulate, but meaningless speech (jargon aphasia) that occurs with lesions in Wernicke's area, is often mistaken for dementia. Similarly, patients with memory disturbances may be held to be demented until it is recognized that their difficulties result from a selective **amnestic syndrome.**

(3) Psychiatric disorders may masquerade as dementia. **Depression** is especially likely to cause a so-called pseudodementia, because it leads to retardation, withdrawal, lack of spontaneity, and paucity of ideas. However, such a pseudodementia generally has a more abrupt onset and rapid progression and is accompanied by a variety of somatic complaints (eg, anorexia, insomnia, headaches, constipation, weight loss) in addition to a depressed affect; moreover, patients make little attempt to respond to tests of intellectual function, and there may be a history of depressive illness. **Schizophrenic disturbances** generally begin before the age of 40 years and are considered in detail in Chapter 17.

(4) **Mental retardation** is distinguished by the age and history, since it represents a failure of development rather than a deterioration from a previous level of intellectual functioning.

Reversible or treatable causes of dementia include normal pressure hydrocephalus, intracranial mass lesions, vascular disease (multi-infarct dementia), hypothyroidism, vitamin $B_{12}$ deficiency, Wilson's disease, drug toxicity, hepatic or renal failure, and any of the chronic meningitides, including neurosyphilis. Investigations in all patients should be undertaken with this in mind.

The clinical findings, laboratory investigation, and management of Alzheimer's disease and other disorders presenting with dementia are discussed in Chapters 2 and 17.

# VERTIGO

Dysfunction of the vestibular system leads to vertigo, a feeling of rotatory disequilibrium. The vertigo that results from peripheral vestibulopathy is usually of sudden onset, may be so severe that the patient is unable to walk or stand, and is frequently accompanied by nausea and vomiting. Tinnitus and deafness may be associated and provide strong support for a peripheral origin. Nystagmus is found on examination and is usually horizontal with a rotatory component, the fast phase being toward the intact side. Visual fixation tends to inhibit both the nystagmus and the complaint of vertigo.

With central nervous system lesions, vertigo may develop gradually and then become progressively more severe. Nystagmus is not always present, can occur in any direction, and may be dissociated in the 2 eyes; vertical nystagmus always indicates a central lesion.

Episodic vertigo can occur in patients with diplopia from external ophthalmoplegia and is maximal when the patient looks in the direction where the separation of images is greatest. Cerebral lesions involving the temporal cortex may also produce vertigo, which is sometimes the initial symptom of a seizure. Finally, vertigo may be a feature of a number of systemic disorders and can occur as a side effect of certain anticonvulsant, antibiotic, hypnotic, analgesic, and tranquilizing drugs and alcohol.

## Syndromes Characterized by Vertigo

### A. Vertigo Due to Peripheral Lesions:

**1. Benign positional vertigo—**This form of vertigo is usually peripheral in origin, although it occasionally occurs with central lesions. Vertigo and nystagmus occur as posture-dependent phenomena and are especially likely to occur when the patient is lying down or the head is tilted backward. Typically with peripheral lesions, there is a latency period of up to about 45 seconds before they develop, and after another 10–60 seconds they subside and then cease; they habituate with constant repetition of the positional change that induces them. In central lesions, there is no latent period, fatigability, or habituation of the symptoms and signs.

**2. Meniere's disease—**Meniere's disease is characterized by vertiginous episodes lasting up to several hours and occurring on a background of increasing hearing loss, tinnitus, and vertigo. Caloric testing commonly reveals loss or impairment of thermally induced nystagmus on the involved side. The disorder and its treatment are discussed in detail in Chapter 6.

**3. Vestibular neuronitis—**In vestibular neuronitis, a paroxysmal, usually single attack of vertigo occurs without accompanying impairment of auditory function and may persist for several weeks before clearing. Examination reveals nystagmus and absent responses to caloric stimulation on one or both sides.

The cause of the disorder is unclear. Treatment is symptomatic.

**4. Labyrinthitis—**Acute or chronic labyrinthitis is accompanied by severe vertigo, as discussed in Chapter 6.

**5. Acoustic neuromas—**These tumors may produce vertigo but usually not as an initial manifestation of the lesion. They are considered further in Table 16–3.

**B. Vertigo Due to Central Nervous System Lesions:** Central nervous system causes of vertigo include brain stem vascular disease, arteriovenous malformations or tumors, multiple sclerosis, and vertebrobasilar migraine. There are usually other signs of brain stem dysfunction (eg, cranial nerve palsies; motor, sensory, or cerebellar deficits in the limbs) or of increased intracranial pressure. Auditory function is generally spared. The underlying cause should be treated.

## Treatment

Investigations such as audiologic evaluation, caloric stimulation, electronystagmography, CT scan, and brain stem auditory evoked potential studies will help to distinguish between central and peripheral lesions and to identify causes requiring specific therapy. Medical treatment is otherwise symptomatic. Bed rest may reduce the severity of vertigo, and treatment with antihistamines such as meclizine, cyclizine, or dimenhydrate (25–50 mg 4 times daily) is sometimes helpful. If these fail, scopolamine, ephedrine, or diazepam is worthy of trial. A combination of drugs sometimes helps when the response to one drug is disappointing.

Snow JB: Positional vertigo. *N Engl J Med* 1984;**310:**1740.

# MULTIPLE SCLEROSIS

## Essentials of Diagnosis

- Episodic symptoms that may include sensory abnormalities, blurred vision, sphincter disturbances, and weakness with or without spasticity.
- Patient usually under 55 years of age at onset.
- Single pathologic lesion cannot explain clinical findings.
- Multiple foci best demonstrated radiographically by MRI.

## General Considerations

This common neurologic disorder of unknown cause has its greatest incidence in young adults. Epidemiologic studies indicate that multiple sclerosis is much more common in persons of western European lineage who live in temperate zones. No population with a high risk for multiple sclerosis exists between latitudes 40 °N and 40 °S. Genetic, dietary, and climatic factors cannot account for these differences. There may be a familial incidence of the disease, since affected relatives are sometimes reported. The strong association between multiple sclerosis and specific HLA antigens (HLA-DR2) provides support for a theory of genetic predisposition. Many believe that the disease has an immunologic basis, but verification of this is awaited. Pathologically, focal—often perivenular—areas of demyelination with reactive gliosis are found scattered in the white matter of brain and spinal cord and in the optic nerves.

## Clinical Findings

**A. Symptoms and Signs:** The common initial presentation is weakness, numbness, tingling, or unsteadiness in a limb; spastic paraparesis; retrobulbar neuritis; diplopia; disequilibrium; or a sphincter disturbance such as urinary urgency or hesitancy. Symptoms may disappear after a few days or weeks, although examination often reveals a residual deficit.

In most patients, there is an interval of months or years after the initial episode before new symptoms develop or the original ones recur. Eventually, however, relapses and usually incomplete remissions lead to increasing disability, with weakness, spasticity, and ataxia of the limbs, impaired vision, and urinary incontinence. The findings on examination at this stage commonly include optic atrophy, nystagmus, dysarthria, and pyramidal, sensory, or cerebellar deficits in some or all of the limbs.

Less commonly, symptoms are steadily progressive from their onset, and disability develops at a relatively early stage. The diagnosis cannot be made with confidence unless the total clinical picture indicates involvement of different parts of the central nervous system at different times.

A number of factors (eg, infection, trauma) may precipitate or trigger exacerbations. Relapses are also more likely during the 2 or 3 months following pregnancy, possibly because of the increased demands and stresses that occur in the postpartum period.

**B. Imaging:** CT scanning, especially with high doses of contrast medium and delayed scanning techniques, is sometimes helpful in demonstrating the presence of a multiplicity of lesions. Magnetic resonance imaging can detect a multiplicity of lesions even when CT scans are normal.

In patients presenting with myelopathy alone and in whom there is no clinical or laboratory evidence of more widespread disease, myelography may be necessary to exclude a congenital or acquired surgically treatable lesion. The foramen magnum region must be visualized to exclude the possibility of Arnold-Chiari malformation, in which part of the cerebellum and the lower brain stem are displaced into the cervical canal and produce mixed pyramidal and cerebellar deficits in the limbs.

**C. Laboratory and Other Studies:** Investigations may help to support the clinical diagnosis and exclude other disorders, but a definitive diagnosis can never be based solely on the laboratory findings. If there is clinical evidence of only a single lesion in the central nervous system, multiple sclerosis cannot properly be diagnosed unless it can be shown that other regions are affected subclinically. The electrocerebral responses evoked in the clinical neurophysiology laboratory by monocular visual stimulation with a checkerboard pattern stimulus, by monaural click stimulation, and by electrical stimulation of a sensory or mixed peripheral nerve have been used to detect subclinical involvement of the visual, brain stem auditory, and somatosensory pathways, respectively.

There may be mild lymphocytosis or a slightly increased protein concentration in the cerebrospinal fluid, especially soon after an acute relapse. Of more help in diagnosis is the fact that the IgG level in cerebrospinal fluid may be increased, and protein electrophoresis characteristically shows the presence of discrete bands of IgG, called oligoclonal bands, in many patients. The presence of such bands is not specific, however, since they have been found in a variety of inflammatory neurologic disorders and occasionally in patients with vascular or neoplastic disorders of the nervous system.

## Treatment

At least partial recovery from acute exacerbations can reasonably be expected, but further relapses may occur without warning, and there is no means of preventing progression of the disorder. Some disability is likely to result eventually, but about half of all patients are without significant disability even 10 years after onset of symptoms.

Recovery from acute relapses may be hastened by treatment with corticosteroids, but the extent of recovery is unchanged. A high dose (eg, prednisone, 60 or 80 mg) is given daily for a week, after which medication is tapered over the following 2 or 3 weeks. Long-term treatment with steroids provides no benefit and does not prevent further relapses.

Several recent studies have suggested that intensive immunosuppressive therapy with cyclophosphamide given intravenously in high doses may help to arrest the course of chronic progressive active multiple sclerosis. Further clinical trials are in progress. There is some evidence that plasmapheresis may enhance any beneficial effects of immunosuppression in some patients with chronic progressive multiple sclerosis, at least for a time, but its role in the management of the various clinical forms of multiple sclerosis is uncertain. The findings in a recent trial of systemic interferon therapy suggested some benefit in patients whose disease was characterized by relapses and remissions rather than by steady progression, further studies to evaluate this form of treatment in selected patients are planned.

Treatment for spasticity (see below) and for neurogenic bladder may be needed in advanced cases. In all cases, care of the general health is important. Excessive fatigue must be avoided, and patients should rest during periods of acute relapse.

Hauser SL et al: Intensive immunosuppression in progressive multiple sclerosis: A randomized, three-arm study of high-dose intravenous cyclophosphamide, plasma exchange, and ACTH. *N Engl J Med* 1983;**308**:173.

Khatri BO et al: Chronic progressive multiple sclerosis: Double-blind controlled study of plasmapheresis in patients taking immunosuppressive drugs. *Neurology* 1985;**35**:312.

Knobler RL et al: Systemic alpha-interferon therapy of multiple sclerosis. *Neurology* 1984;**34**:1273.

Lukes SA et al: Nuclear magnetic resonance imaging in multiple sclerosis. *Ann Neurol* 1983;**13**:592.

Symposium on multiple sclerosis. *Neurol Clin* 1983;**1–Part 3**.[Entire issue.]

## SPASTICITY

The term ''spasticity'' is commonly used for an upper motor neuron deficit, but it properly refers to a velocity-dependent increase in resistance to passive movement that affects different muscles to a different extent, is not uniform in degree throughout the range of a particular movement, and is commonly associated with other features of pyramidal deficit. It is often a major complication of stroke, cerebral or spinal injury, and multiple sclerosis.

Spasticity should be treated when it interferes with daily activities or causes distress or disability. Treatment may increase functional disability when increased extensor tone is providing additional support for patients with weak legs.

Physical therapy with appropriate stretching programs is important during rehabilitation after the development of an upper motor neuron lesion and in subsequent management of the patient. The aim is to prevent joint and muscle contractures and, perhaps, to modulate spasticity.

Drug management is important in reducing spasticity that interferes with function or causes distress. Dantrolene weakens muscle contraction by interfering with the role of calcium. It may be helpful in the treatment of spasticity but is best avoided in patients with poor respiratory function or severe myocardial disease. Treatment is begun with 25 mg once daily, and the daily dose is built up by 25-mg increments every 3 days, depending on tolerance, to a maximum of 100 mg 4 times daily. The drug should be withdrawn if no benefit has occurred after treatment with the maximum tolerated dose for about 2 weeks. Side effects include diarrhea, nausea, weakness, hepatic dysfunction (that may rarely be fatal, especially in women older than 35), drowsiness, lightheadedness, and hallucinations.

Baclofen seems to be the most effective drug for treating spasticity of spinal origin. It is particularly helpful in relieving painful flexor (or extensor) spasms. The maximum recommended daily dose is 80 mg; treatment is started with a dose of 5 or 10 mg twice daily and then built up gradually. Side effects include gastrointestinal disturbances, lassitude, fatigue, sedation, unsteadiness, confusion, and hallucinations. Diazepam may modify spasticity by its action on spinal interneurons and perhaps also by influencing supraspinal centers.

Motor-point blocks by intramuscular phenol have been used to reduce spasticity selectively in one or a few important muscles and may permit return of function in patients with incomplete myelopathies. Intrathecal injection of phenol or absolute alcohol may be helpful in more severe cases, but greater selectivity can be achieved by nerve root or peripheral nerve neurolysis. These procedures should not be undertaken until the spasticity syndrome is fully evolved, ie, only after about 1 year or so, and only if long-term drug treatment either has been unhelpful or carries a significant risk to the patient.

A number of surgical procedures, eg, adductor or heel cord tenotomy, may help in the management of spasticity. Neurectomy may also facilitate patient management. For example, obturator neurectomy is helpful in patients with marked adductor spasms that interfere with personal hygiene or cause gait disturbances. Posterior rhizotomy reduces spasticity, but its effect may be short-lived, whereas anterior rhizotomy produces permanent wasting and weakness in the muscles that are denervated.

Spasticity may be exacerbated by decubitus ulcers, urinary or other infections, and nociceptive stimuli, which must therefore be prevented.

## SUBACUTE COMBINED DEGENERATION OF THE SPINAL CORD

Subacute combined degeneration of the spinal cord is due to vitamin $B_{12}$ deficiency, such as occurs in pernicious anemia. It is characterized by myelopathy with predominant pyramidal and posterior column deficits, sometimes in association with polyneuropathy, mental changes, or optic neuropathy. Megaloblastic anemia may also occur, but this does not parallel the neurologic disorder, and the former may be obscured if folic acid supplements have been taken. Treatment is with vitamin $B_{12}$.

## WERNICKE'S ENCEPHALOPATHY

Wernicke's encephalopathy is characterized by confusion, ataxia, and nystagmus leading to ophthalmoplegia (lateral rectus muscle weakness, conjugate gaze palsies); peripheral neuropathy may also be present. It is due to thiamine deficiency and in the USA occurs most commonly in alcoholics. In suspected cases, thiamine (50 mg) is given intravenously immediately and then intramuscularly on a daily basis until a satisfactory diet can be ensured. Intravenous glucose given before thiamine may precipitate the syndrome or worsen the symptoms. The diagnosis is confirmed by the response to treatment.

## STUPOR & COMA

The patient who is stuporous is unresponsive except when subjected to repeated vigorous stimuli, while the comatose patient is unrousable and unable to respond to external events or inner needs, although reflex movements and posturing may be present.

Coma is a major complication of serious central nervous system disorders. It can result from seizures, hypothermia, metabolic disturbances, or structural lesions causing bilateral cerebral hemispheric dysfunction or a disturbance of the brain stem reticular activating system. A mass lesion involving one cerebral hemisphere may cause coma by compression of the brain stem.

## Assessment & Emergency Measures

The diagnostic workup of the comatose patient must proceed concomitantly with management. In particular, immediate steps must be taken to evaluate and maintain vital functions, with supportive therapy for respiration or blood pressure being initiated if necessary. This is especially true in coma due to hypothermia, where all vital signs may be absent; all such patients should be rewarmed before the prognosis is assessed.

The patient can be positioned on one side with the neck partly extended, dentures removed, and secretions cleared by suction; if necessary, the patency of the airways is maintained with an oropharyngeal airway. In order to determine the cause of the coma, blood is then drawn for determination of serum glucose, electrolyte, and calcium levels; arterial blood gases; liver and renal function tests; and toxicologic studies if necessary. Dextrose 50% (25 g), naloxone (0.4–1.2 mg), and thiamine (50 mg) to counteract possible hypoglycemia, opiate overdosage, or thiamine deficiency should be given intravenously without delay. The intravenous line is left in place to facilitate further access to the circulation.

After these initial measures, further details are obtained from attendants of the patient's medical history, the circumstances surrounding the onset of coma, and the time course of subsequent events. Abrupt onset of coma suggests subarachnoid hemorrhage, brain stem stroke, or intracerebral hemorrhage, whereas a slower onset and progression occur with other structural or mass lesions. A metabolic cause is suggested by a preceding intoxicated state or agitated delirium. A detailed general and neurologic examination is undertaken, with particular attention to the behavioral response to painful stimuli, the pupils and their response to light, the position of the eyes and their movement in response to passive movement of the head and ice-water caloric stimulation, and the respiratory pattern.

**A. Response to Painful Stimuli:** Purposive limb withdrawal from painful stimuli implies that sensory pathways from and motor pathways to the stimulated limb are functionally intact, at least in part. Unilateral absence of responses despite application of stimuli to both sides of the body in turn implies a corticospinal lesion; bilateral absence of responsiveness suggests brain stem involvement, bilateral pyra-

midal tract lesions, or psychogenic unresponsiveness. Inappropriate responses may also occur. Decorticate posturing may occur with lesions of the internal capsule and rostral cerebral peduncle, decerebrate posturing with dysfunction or destruction of the midbrain and rostral pons, and decerebrate posturing in the arms accompanied by flaccidity or slight flexor responses in the legs in patients with extensive brain stem damage extending down to the pons at the trigeminal level.

**B. Ocular Findings:**

**1. Pupils**–Hypothalamic disease processes may lead to unilateral Horner's syndrome, while bilateral diencephalic involvement or destructive pontine lesions may lead to small but reactive pupils. Ipsilateral pupillary dilation with no direct or consensual response to light occurs with compression of the third cranial nerve, eg, with uncal herniation. The pupils are slightly smaller than normal but responsive to light in many metabolic encephalopathies; however, they may be fixed and dilated following overdosage with atropine, scopolamine, or glutethimide, and pinpoint (but responsive) with opiates. Pupillary dilatation for several hours following cardiopulmonary arrest implies a poor prognosis.

**2. Eye movements**–Conjugate deviation of the eyes to the side suggests the presence of an ipsilateral hemispheric lesion or a contralateral pontine lesion. A mesencephalic lesion is suggested by downward conjugate deviation. Dysconjugate ocular deviation in coma suggests a structural brain stem lesion unless there was preexisting strabismus.

The oculomotor responses to passive head turning and to caloric stimulation relate to each other and provide complementary information. In response to brisk rotation of the head from side to side and to flexion and extension of the head, normally conscious patients with open eyes do not exhibit contraversive conjugate eye deviation (doll's-head eye response) unless there is voluntary visual fixation or bilateral frontal pathology. With cortical depression in lightly comatose patients, a brisk doll's-head eye response is seen. With brain stem lesions, this oculocephalic reflex becomes impaired or lost, depending on the site of the lesion.

The oculovestibular reflex is tested by caloric stimulation using irrigation with ice water. In normal subjects, jerk nystagmus is elicited for about 2 or 3 minutes, with the slow component toward the irrigated ear. In unconscious patients with an intact brain stem, the fast component of the nystagmus disappears, so that the eyes tonically deviate toward the irrigated side for 2–3 minutes before returning to their original position. With impairment of brain stem function, the response becomes perverted and finally disappears. In metabolic coma, oculocephalic and oculovestibular reflex responses are preserved, at least initially.

**C. Respiratory Patterns:** Diseases causing coma may lead to respiratory abnormalities. Cheyne-Stokes respiration may occur with bihemispheric or diencephalic disease or in metabolic disorders. Central neurogenic hyperventilation occurs with lesions of the brain stem tegmentum; apneustic breathing suggests damage at the pontine level (eg, due to basilar artery occlusion); and atactic breathing (a completely irregular pattern of breathing with deep and shallow breaths occurring randomly) is associated with lesions of the lower pontine tegmentum and medulla.

## Continuing Care

The continuing care of patients with impaired consciousness includes maintenance of a clear airway and removal of secretions by suction as necessary. Patients are kept on their side and turned regularly, and pressure is avoided on bony prominences such as the heels. Bladder function is controlled by catheterization and bowel function by nursing care. Fluid and nutrients can be given intravenously or by nasogastric tube depending on the duration of the disorder, and metabolic parameters are monitored. The prognosis depends on the underlying disorder.

Plum F, Posner JB: *The Diagnosis of Stupor and Coma,* 3rd ed. Davis, 1980.

## 1. STUPOR & COMA DUE TO STRUCTURAL LESIONS

Supratentorial mass lesions tend to affect brain function in an orderly way. There may initially be signs of hemispheric dysfunction, such as hemiparesis. As coma develops and deepens, cerebral function becomes progressively disturbed, producing a predictable progression of neurologic signs that suggest rostrocaudal deterioration.

Thus, as a supratentorial mass lesion begins to impair the diencephalon, the patient becomes drowsy, then stuporous, and finally comatose. There may be Cheyne-Stokes respiration; small but reactive pupils; doll's-head eye responses with side-to-side head movements, but sometimes an impairment of reflex upward gaze with brisk flexion of the head; tonic ipsilateral deviation of the eyes in response to vestibular stimulation with cold water; and initially a positive response to pain but subsequently only decorticate posturing. With further progression, midbrain failure occurs. Motor dysfunction progresses from decorticate to bilateral decerebrate posturing in response to painful stimuli, Cheyne-Stokes respiration is gradually replaced by sustained central hyperventilation; the pupils become middle-sized and fixed; and the oculocephalic and oculovestibular reflex responses become impaired, perverted, or lost. As the pons and then the medulla fail, the pupils remain unresponsive; oculovestibular responses are unobtainable; respiration is rapid and shallow; and painful stimuli may lead only to flexor responses in the legs. Finally, respiration becomes irregular and stops, the pupils often then dilating widely.

In contrast, a subtentorial (ie, brain stem) lesion

may lead to an early, sometimes abrupt disturbance of consciousness without any orderly rostrocaudal progression of neurologic signs. Compressive lesions of the brain stem, especially cerebellar hemorrhage, may be clinically indistinguishable from intraparenchymal processes.

A structural lesion should always be suspected if the findings suggest dysfunction at a particular level of the nervous system. In such circumstances, a CT scan or cerebral angiogram should be performed before, or instead of, a lumbar puncture in order to avoid any risk of cerebral herniation. Further management is of the causal lesion and is considered separately under the individual disorders.

## 2. STUPOR & COMA DUE TO METABOLIC DISTURBANCES

Patients with a metabolic cause of coma generally have signs of patchy, diffuse, and symmetric neurologic involvement that cannot be explained by loss of function at any single level or in a sequential manner, although focal or lateralized deficits may occur in hypoglycemia. Moreover, pupillary reactivity is usually preserved, while other brain stem functions are often grossly impaired. Comatose patients with meningitis, encephalitis, or subarachnoid hemorrhage may also have little in the way of focal neurologic signs, however, and clinical evidence of meningeal irritation is sometimes very subtle in comatose patients. Examination of the cerebrospinal fluid in such patients is essential to establish the correct diagnosis.

In patients with coma due to cerebral ischemia and hypoxia suggests that absence of pupillary light reflexes at the time of initial examination indicates that there is little chance of regaining independence; by contrast, preserved pupillary light responses, the development of spontaneous eye movements (roving, conjugate, or better), and extensor, flexor, or withdrawal responses to pain at this early stage imply a relatively good prognosis.

Treatment of metabolic encephalopathy is of the underlying disturbance and is considered in other chapters. If the cause of the encephalopathy is obscure, all drugs except essential ones may have to be withdrawn in case they are responsible for the altered mental status.

Levy DE et al: Predicting outcome from hypoxic-ischemic coma. *JAMA* 1985;**253**:1420.

## 3. BRAIN DEATH

The definition of brain death is controversial, and diagnostic criteria have been published by many different professional organizations. In order to establish brain death, the irreversibly comatose patient must be shown to have lost all brain stem reflex responses, including the pupillary, corneal, oculovestibular, oculocephalic, oropharyngeal, and respiratory reflexes, and should have been in this condition for at least 6 hours. Spinal reflex movements do not exclude the diagnosis, but ongoing seizure activity or decerebrate or decorticate posturing is not consistent with brain death. The apnea test (presence or absence of spontaneous respiratory activity at a $P_{aCO2}$ of at least 60 mm Hg) serves to determine whether or not the patient is capable of respiratory activity.

Reversible coma simulating brain death may be seen with hypothermia (temperature < 32 °C), and overdosage with central nervous system depressant drugs, and these conditions must be excluded. Certain ancillary tests may assist the determination of brain death but are not essential. An isoelectric electroencephalogram, when the recording is made according to the recommendations of the American Electroencephalographic Society, is especially helpful in confirming the diagnosis. Alternatively, the demonstration of an absent cerebral circulation by angiography of the 4 major vessels to the brain can be confirmatory.

Black PM: Brain death. (2 parts.) *N Engl J Med* 1978;**299**:338, 393.
Chatrian GE: Electrophysiologic evaluation of brain death: A critical appraisal. In: *Electrodiagnosis in Clinical Neurology,* Aminoff MJ (editor). 2nd ed. Churchill Livingstone, 1986.

## 4. PERSISTENT VEGETATIVE STATE

Patients with severe bilateral hemispheric disease may show some improvement from an initially comatose state, so that, after a variable interval, they appear to be awake but lie motionless and without evidence of awareness or higher mental activity. This persistent vegetative state has been variously referred to as akinetic mutism, apallic state, or coma vigil. Most patients in this persistent vegetative state will die in months or years, but partial recovery has occasionally occurred and in rare instances has been sufficient to permit communication or even independent living.

## 5. LOCKED-IN SYNDROME (De-efferented State)

Acute destructive lesions (eg, infarction, hemorrhage, demyelination, encephalitis) involving the ventral pons and sparing the tegmentum may lead to a mute, quadriparetic but conscious state in which the patient is capable of blinking and of voluntary eye movement in the vertical plane, with preserved pupillary responses to light. Such a patient can mistakenly be regarded as comatose. Physicians should recognize that "locked-in" individuals are fully aware of their surroundings. Prognosis is variable, but recovery has occasionally been reported, in some cases including resumption of independent daily life, though this may take up to 2 or 3 years.

## HEAD INJURY

Trauma is the most common cause of death in young people, and head injury accounts for almost half of these trauma-related deaths. The prognosis following head injury depends upon the site and severity of brain damage. Some guide to prognosis is provided by the mental status, since loss of consciousness for more than 1 or 2 minutes implies a worse prognosis than otherwise. Similarly, the degree of retrograde and posttraumatic amnesia provides an indication of the severity of injury and thus of the prognosis. Absence of skull fracture does not exclude the possibility of severe head injury. During the physical examination, special attention should be given to the level of consciousness and extent of any brain stem dysfunction.

*Note:* In general, patients who have lost consciousness for 2 minutes or more following head injury should be admitted to the hospital for observation, as should patients with focal neurologic deficits, lethargy, or skull fractures. If patients are not to be detained, responsible family members should be given clear instructions about the need for, and manner of, checking on them at regular (hourly) intervals and for obtaining additional medical help if necessary. Deterioration is an indication for further investigation.

Skull radiographs may provide evidence of fractures. An air-fluid level in the frontal or sphenoidal sinuses suggests the possibility of basilar fractures. Because injury to the spine may have accompanied head trauma, cervical spine radiographs (especially in the lateral projection) should always be obtained in comatose patients and in patients with severe neck pain or a deficit possibly related to cord compression. CT scanning has an important role in demonstrating intracranial hemorrhage and may also provide evidence of cerebral edema and displacement of midline structures.

### Cerebral Injuries

These are summarized in Table 16–5, where treatment is also indicated.

### Scalp Injuries & Skull Fractures

Scalp lacerations and depressed or compound depressed skull fractures should be treated surgically as appropriate. Simple skull fractures require no specific treatment.

The clinical signs of basilar skull fracture include bruising about the orbit (raccoon sign), blood in the external auditory meatus (Battle's sign), and leakage of cerebrospinal fluid (which can be identified by its glucose content) from the ear or nose. Cranial nerve palsies (involving especially the first, second, third, fourth, fifth, seventh, and eighth nerves in any combination) may also occur. Prophylactic antibiotics should be given if there is any leakage of cerebrospinal fluid. Conservative treatment, with elevation of the head, restriction of fluids, and administration of aceta-

**Table 16–5.** Acute cerebral sequelae of head injury.

| Sequelae | Clinical Features | Pathology |
|---|---|---|
| Concussion | Transient loss of consciousness with bradycardia, hypotension, and respiratory arrest for a few seconds followed by retrograde and posttraumatic amnesia. Occasionally followed by transient neurologic deficit. | Bruising on side of impact (coup injury) or contralaterally (contrecoup injury). |
| Cerebral contusion/ laceration | Loss of consciousness longer than with concussion. May lead to death or severe residual neurologic deficit. | Cerebral contusion, edema, hemorrhage, and necrosis. May have subarachnoid bleeding. |
| Acute epidural hemorrhage | Headache, confusion, somnolence, seizures, and focal deficits occur several hours after injury and lead to coma, respiratory depression, and death unless treated by surgical evacuation. | Tear in meningeal artery, vein, or dural sinus, leading to hematoma visible on CT scan. |
| Acute subdural hemorrhage | Similar to epidural hemorrhage, but interval before onset of symptoms is longer. Treatment is by surgical evacuation. | Hematoma from tear in veins from cortex to superior sagittal sinus or from cerebral laceration, visible on CT scan. |
| Cerebral hemorrhage | Generally develops immediately after injury. Clinically resembles hypertensive hemorrhage. Surgical evacuation is sometimes helpful. | Hematoma, visible on CT scan. |

zolamide (250 mg 4 times daily), is often helpful; but if the leak continues for more than a few days, lumbar subarachnoid drainage may be necessary. Only very occasional patients require intracranial repair of the dural defect because of persistence of the leak or recurrent meningitis.

## Late Complications of Head Injury

The relationship of **chronic subdural hemorrhage** to head injury is not always clear. In many elderly persons there is no history of trauma, but in other cases a head injury, often trivial, precedes the onset of symptoms by several weeks. The clinical presentation is usually with mental changes such as slowness, drowsiness, headache, confusion, memory disturbances, personality change, or even dementia. Focal neurologic deficits such as hemiparesis or hemisensory disturbance may also occur but are less common. CT scan is an important means of detecting the hematoma, which is sometimes bilateral. Treatment is by surgical evacuation to prevent cerebral compression and tentorial herniation.

**Normal-pressure hydrocephalus** may follow head injury, subarachnoid hemorrhage, or meningoencephalitis, but in many instances there are no specific antecedents. Hydrocephalus occurs because flow and absorption of cerebrospinal fluid are interrupted. The resulting clinical syndrome is characterized by intellectual deterioration, urinary incontinence, and an apraxic gait. CT scan reveals enlarged ventricles without evidence of cortical atrophy. Radionuclide cisternography helps to confirm the diagnosis by demonstrating the obstruction to flow of cerebrospinal fluid. Surgical shunting procedures may be of clinical benefit, especially in the presence of the full clinical triad and typical appearance on CT scan; it is most effective if a cause (eg, recent injury, hemorrhage, or infection) can be identified.

Other late complications of head injury include posttraumatic seizure disorder (see p 576) and posttraumatic headache (see p 573).

Seelig JM et al: Traumatic acute subdural hematoma: Major mortality reduction in comatose patients treated within four hours. *N Engl J Med* 1981;**304**:1511.

## SPINAL TRAUMA

While spinal cord damage may result from whiplash injury, severe injury usually relates to fracture-dislocation causing compression or angular deformity of the cord either cervically or in the lower thoracic and upper lumbar region. Extreme hypotension following injury may also lead to cord infarction.

Total cord transection results in immediate flaccid paralysis and loss of sensation below the level of the lesion. Reflex activity is lost for a variable period, and there is urinary and fecal retention. As reflex function returns over the following days and weeks, spastic paraplegia or quadriplegia develops, with hyperreflexia and extensor plantar responses, but a flaccid atrophic (lower motor neuron) paralysis may be found depending on the segments of the cord that are affected. The bladder and bowels also regain some reflex function, permitting urine and feces to be expelled at intervals. As spasticity increases, flexor or extensor spasms (or both) of the legs become troublesome, especially if the patient develops bed sores or a urinary tract infection. Paraplegia with the legs in flexion or extension may eventually result.

With lesser degrees of injury, patients may be left with mild limb weakness, distal sensory disturbance, or both. Sphincter function may also be impaired, urinary urgency and urgency incontinence being especially common. More particularly, a unilateral cord lesion leads to an ipsilateral motor disturbance with accompanying impairment of proprioception and contralateral loss of pain and temperature appreciation below the lesion (Brown-Séquard syndrome). A central cord syndrome may lead to a lower motor neuron deficit and loss of pain and temperature appreciation, with sparing of posterior column functions. A radicular deficit may occur at the level of the injury—or, if the cauda equina is involved, there may be evidence of disturbed function in several lumbosacral roots.

Treatment of the injury consists of immobilization and—if there is cord compression—decompressive laminectomy and fusion. Anatomic realignment of the spinal cord by traction and other orthopedic procedures is also important. Subsequent care of the residual neurologic deficit—paraplegia or quadriplegia—requires treatment of spasticity and care of the skin, bladder, and bowels.

## SYRINGOMYELIA

Destruction or degeneration of gray and white matter adjacent to the central canal of the cervical spinal cord leads to cavitation and accumulation of fluid within the spinal cord. The precise pathogenesis is unclear, but many cases are associated with Arnold-Chiari malformation, in which there is displacement of the cerebellar tonsils, medulla, and fourth ventricle into the spinal canal, sometimes with accompanying meningomyelocele. In such circumstances, the cord cavity connects with and may merely represent a dilated central canal. In other cases, the cause of cavitation is less clear. There is a characteristic clinical picture, with segmental atrophy and areflexia and loss of pain and temperature appreciation in a ''cape'' distribution owing to the destruction of fibers crossing in front of the central canal. Thoracic kyphoscoliosis is usually present. With progression, involvement of the long motor and sensory tracts occurs as well, so that a pyramidal and sensory deficit develops in the legs. Upward extension of the cavitation (syringobulbia) leads to dysfunction of the lower brain stem and thus to bulbar palsy, nystagmus, and sensory impairment over one or both sides of the face.

Syringomyelia, ie, cord cavitation, may also occur in association with an intramedullary tumor or following severe cord injury, and the cavity then does not communicate with the central canal.

In patients with Arnold-Chiari malformation, there are commonly abnormalities on plain x-rays of the skull and cervical spine. CT scans show caudal displacement of the fourth ventricle. Positive contrast myelography may demonstrate Arnold-Chiari malformation, whereas with gas myelography the cord cavity may vary in size depending on the position of the patient. Focal cord enlargement is found at myelography in patients with cavitation related to past injury or intramedullary neoplasms.

Treatment of Arnold-Chiari malformation with associated syringomyelia is by suboccipital craniectomy and upper cervical laminectomy, with the aim of decompressing the malformation at the foramen magnum. The cord cavity should be drained, and if necessary an outlet for the fourth ventricle can be made. In cavitation associated with intramedullary tumor, treatment is surgical, but radiation therapy may be necessary if complete removal is not possible. Posttraumatic syringomyelia is also treated surgically if it leads to increasing neurologic deficits or to intolerable pain.

## MOTOR NEURON DISEASES

This group of disorders is characterized clinically by weakness and variable wasting of affected muscles, without accompanying sensory changes. Certain of these disorders, such as Werdnig-Hoffman disease and Kugelberg-Welander syndrome, occur in infants or children and are not considered further here.

Motor neuron disease in adults generally commences between 30 and 60 years of age. There is degeneration of the anterior horn cells in the spinal cord, the motor nuclei of the lower cranial nerves, and the corticospinal and corticobulbar pathways. The disorder is usually sporadic, but familial cases may occur.

### Classification

Five varieties have been distinguished on clinical grounds.

**A. Progressive Bulbar Palsy:** Bulbar involvement predominates owing to disease processes affecting primarily the motor nuclei of the cranial nerves.

**B. Pseudobulbar Palsy:** Bulbar involvement predominates in this variety also, but it is due to bilateral corticobulbar disease and thus reflects upper motor neuron dysfunction.

**C. Progressive Spinal Muscular Atrophy:** This is characterized primarily by a lower motor neuron deficit in the limbs due to degeneration of the anterior horn cells in the spinal cord.

**D. Primary Lateral Sclerosis:** There is a purely upper motor neuron deficit in the limbs.

**E. Amyotrophic Lateral Sclerosis:** A mixed upper and lower motor neuron deficit is found in the limbs. This disorder is sometimes associated with dementia, parkinsonism, and other neurologic diseases.

### Clinical Findings

**A. Symptoms and Signs:** Difficulty in swallowing, chewing, coughing, breathing, and talking (dysarthria) occur with bulbar involvement. In progressive bulbar palsy, there is drooping of the palate, a depressed gag reflex, pooling of saliva in the pharynx, a weak cough, and a wasted, fasciculating tongue. In pseudobulbar palsy, the tongue is contracted and spastic and cannot be moved rapidly from side to side. Limb involvement is characterized by motor disturbances (weakness, stiffness, wasting, fasciculations) reflecting lower or upper motor neuron dysfunction; there are no objective changes on sensory examination, though there may be vague sensory complaints. The sphincters are generally spared.

The disorder is progressive and usually fatal within 3–5 years; death usually results from pulmonary infections. Patients with bulbar involvement generally have the poorest prognosis.

**B. Laboratory and Other Studies:** Electromyography may show changes of chronic partial denervation, with abnormal spontaneous activity in the resting muscle and a reduction in the number of motor units under voluntary control. Motor conduction velocity is usually normal but may be slightly reduced, and sensory conduction studies are also normal. Biopsy of a wasted muscle shows the histologic changes of denervation. The serum creatine phosphokinase may be slightly elevated but never reaches the extremely high values seen in some of the muscular dystrophies. The cerebrospinal fluid is normal.

There have been recent reports of juvenile spinal muscular atrophy due to hexosaminidase deficiency, with abnormal findings on rectal biopsy and reduced hexosaminidase A in serum and leukocytes. Pure motor syndromes resembling motor neuron disease may also occur in association with monoclonal gammopathy.

## Treatment

There is no specific treatment except in patients with gammopathy, in whom plasmapheresis and immunosuppression may lead to improvement. Symptomatic and supportive measures may include prescription of anticholinergic drugs (such as trihexyphenidyl, amitriptyline, or atropine) if drooling is troublesome, braces or a walker to improve mobility, and physical therapy to prevent contractures. Spasticity may be helped by baclofen or diazepam. A semiliquid diet or nasogastric tube feeding may be needed if dysphagia is severe. Gastrostomy or cricopharyngomyotomy is sometimes resorted to in extreme cases of predominant bulbar involvement, and tracheostomy may be necessary if respiratory muscles are severely affected; however, in the terminal stages of these disorders, the aim of treatment should be to keep patients as comfortable as possible.

Parry GJ et al: Gammopathy with proximal motor axonopathy simulating motor neuron disease. *Neurology* 1986;**36**:273.
Rowland LP (editor): *Human Motor Neuron Diseases.* Vol 36 of: *Advances in Neurology.* Raven Press, 1982.

## PERIPHERAL NEUROPATHIES

Peripheral neuropathies can be categorized on the basis of the structure primarily affected. The predominant pathologic feature may be axonal degeneration (axonal or neuronal neuropathies) or paranodal or segmental demyelination. The distinction may be possible on the basis of neurophysiologic findings. Motor and sensory conduction velocity can be measured in accessible segments of peripheral nerves. In axonal

neuropathies, conduction velocity is normal or reduced only mildly and needle electromyography provides evidence of denervation in affected muscles. In demyelinating neuropathies, conduction may be slowed considerably in affected fibers, and in more severe cases, conduction is blocked completely, without accompanying electromyographic signs of denervation.

Peripheral neuropathies may also occur as a result of disorders affecting the connective tissues of the nerves or the blood vessels supplying the nerves, but these are much less common than the preceding varieties.

Nerves may be injured or compressed by neighboring anatomic structures at any point along their course. Common **mononeuropathies** of this sort are considered on p 613. They lead to a sensory, motor, or mixed deficit that is restricted to the territory of the affected nerve. A similar clinical disturbance is produced by peripheral nerve tumors, but these are rare except in patients with Recklinghausen's disease. Multiple mononeuropathies suggest a patchy multifocal disease process such as vasculopathy (eg, diabetes, arteritis), an infiltrative process (eg, leprosy, sarcoidosis), radiation damage, or an immunologic disorder (eg, brachial plexopathy). Diffuse **polyneuropathies** lead to a symmetric sensory, motor, or mixed deficit, often most marked distally. They include the hereditary, metabolic, and toxic disorders; idiopathic inflammatory polyneuropathy (Guillain-Barré syndrome); and the peripheral neuropathies that may occur as a nonmetastatic complication of malignant diseases. Involvement of motor fibers leads to flaccid weakness that is most marked distally; dysfunction of sensory fibers causes impaired sensory perception. Tendon reflexes are depressed or absent. Paresthesias, pain, and muscle tenderness may also occur.

## 1. POLYNEUROPATHIES & MONONEURITIS MULTIPLEX

The cause of polyneuropathy or mononeuritis multiplex is suggested by the history, mode of onset, and predominant clinical manifestations. Laboratory workup includes a complete blood count and sedimentation rate, serum protein electrophoresis, determination of plasma urea and electrolytes, liver and thyroid function tests, tests for rheumatoid factor and antinuclear antibody, a serologic test for syphilis, fasting blood glucose level, urinary heavy metal levels, cerebrospinal fluid examination, and chest radiography. These tests should be ordered selectively, as guided by symptoms and signs. Measurement of nerve conduction velocity is important in confirming the peripheral nerve origin of symptoms and providing a means of following clinical changes, as well as indicating the likely disease process (ie, axonal or demyelinating neuropathy). Cutaneous nerve biopsy may help establish a precise diagnosis. In about half of cases, no specific cause can be established; of these, slightly less than half are heredofamilial.

Treatment is of the underlying cause, when feasible, and is discussed below under the individual disorders. Symptomatic and general measures are also important, especially in advanced cases. Physical therapy helps prevent contractures, and splints can maintain a weak extremity in a position of useful function. Anesthetic extremities must be protected from injury. To guard against burns, patients should check the temperature of water and hot surfaces with a portion of skin having normal sensation, measure water temperature with a thermometer, and use cold water for washing or lower the temperature setting of their hot-water heaters. Shoes should be examined frequently during the day for grit or foreign objects in order to prevent pressure lesions.

Patients with polyneuropathies or mononeuritis multiplex are subject to additional nerve injury at pressure points and should therefore avoid such behavior as leaning on elbows or sitting with crossed legs for lengthy periods.

Neuropathic pain is sometimes troublesome and may respond to simple analgesics such as aspirin. Narcotics or narcotic substitutes may be necessary for severe hyperpathia or pain induced by minimal stimuli, but their use should be avoided as far as possible. The use of a frame or cradle to reduce contact with bedclothes may be helpful. Many patients experience episodic stabbing pains, which may respond to phenytoin, carbamazepine, or tricyclic antidepressants.

Symptoms of autonomic dysfunction are occasionally troublesome. Postural hypotension is often helped by wearing waist-high elastic stockings and sleeping in a semierect position at night. Fludrocortisone reduces postural hypotension, but doses as high as 1 mg/d are sometimes necessary in diabetics and may lead to recumbent hypertension. Indomethacin is sometimes helpful. Impotence and diarrhea are difficult to treat; a flaccid neuropathic bladder may respond to parasympathomimetic drugs such as bethanechol chloride, 10–50 mg 3 or 4 times daily.

### Inherited Neuropathies

**A. Charcot-Marie-Tooth Disease:** Several distinct varieties of Charcot-Marie-Tooth disease can be recognized. There is usually an autosomal dominant mode of inheritance, but occasional cases occur on a sporadic, recessive, or X-linked basis. Clinical presentation may be with foot deformities or gait disturbances in childhood or early adult life. Slow progression leads to the typical features of polyneuropathy, with distal weakness and wasting that begin in the legs, a variable amount of distal sensory loss, and depressed or absent tendon reflexes. Tremor is a conspicuous feature in some instances. Pathologic examination reveals segmental demyelination and remyelination of peripheral nerves, an increase in their transverse fascicular area, and hyperplasia of Schwann cells. Electrodiagnostic studies show a marked reduction in motor and sensory conduction velocity (hereditary motor and sensory neuropathy [HMSN] type I).

In other instances (HMSN type II), motor conduction velocity is normal or only slightly reduced, sensory nerve action potentials may be absent, and signs of chronic partial denervation are found in affected muscles electromyographically. The predominant pathologic change is axonal loss rather than segmental demyelination.

A similar disorder may occur in patients with progressive spinal muscular atrophy, but there is no sensory loss; electrophysiologic investigation reveals that motor conduction velocity is normal or only slightly reduced, and nerve action potentials are normal.

**B. Dejerine-Sottas Disease (HMSN Type III):** Both recessive and dominantly inherited forms of this disorder have been described. The recessive form has its onset in infancy or childhood and leads to a progressive motor and sensory polyneuropathy with weakness, ataxia, sensory loss, and depressed or absent tendon reflexes. The peripheral nerves may be palpably enlarged and are characterized pathologically by segmental demyelination, Schwann cell hyperplasia, and thin myelin sheaths. Electrophysiologically, there is slowing of conduction, and sensory action potentials may be unrecordable. Cases with a dominant mode of inheritance are best classified with neuropathies of the Charcot-Marie-Tooth type.

**C. Friedreich's Ataxia:** Patients generally present in childhood or early adult life with this autosomal recessive disorder. The gait becomes atactic, the hands become clumsy, and other signs of cerebellar dysfunction develop accompanied by weakness of the legs and extensor plantar responses. Involvement of peripheral sensory fibers leads to sensory disturbances in the limbs and depressed tendon reflexes. There is bilateral pes cavus. Pathologically, there is a marked loss of cells in the posterior root ganglia and degeneration of peripheral sensory fibers. In the central nervous system, changes are conspicuous in the posterior and lateral columns of the cord. Electrophysiologically, conduction velocity in motor fibers is normal or only mildly reduced, but sensory action potentials are small or absent.

**D. Refsum's Disease (HMSN Type IV):** This autosomal recessive disorder is due to a disturbance in phytanic acid metabolism. Clinically, pigmentary retinal degeneration is accompanied by progressive sensorimotor polyneuropathy and cerebellar signs. Auditory dysfunction, cardiomyopathy, and cutaneous manifestations may also occur. The cerebrospinal fluid contains increased protein but normal cell content. Motor and sensory conduction velocity is reduced, often markedly, and there may be electromyographic evidence of denervation in affected muscles. Dietary restriction of phytanic acid and its precursors may be helpful therapeutically.

**E. Porphyria:** Peripheral nerve involvement may occur during acute attacks in both variegate porphyria and acute intermittent porphyria. The general clinical features of these disorders are discussed in Chapter 31. Motor symptoms usually occur first, and weakness is often most marked proximally and in the upper limbs rather than the lower. Sensory symptoms and signs may be proximal or distal in distribution. Autonomic involvement is sometimes pronounced. The electrophysiologic findings are in keeping with the results of neuropathologic studies suggesting that the neuropathy is axonal in type. A high-carbohydrate diet and, in severe cases, intravenous glucose or levulose may be helpful in treatment. Propranolol may also be beneficial in acute attacks.

## Neuropathies Associated With Systemic & Metabolic Disorders

**A. Diabetes Mellitus:** In this disorder, involvement of the peripheral nervous system may lead to symmetric sensory or mixed polyneuropathy, asymmetric motor neuropathy (diabetic amyotrophy), thoracoabdominal radiculopathy, autonomic neuropathy, or isolated lesions of individual nerves. These may occur singly or in any combination.

Sensory polyneuropathy, the most common manifestation, may lead to no more than depressed tendon reflexes and impaired appreciation of vibration in the legs. When symptomatic, there may be pain, paresthesias, or numbness in the legs, but in severe cases distal sensory loss occurs in all limbs. Diabetic amyotrophy is characterized by asymmetric weakness and wasting involving predominantly the proximal muscles of the legs, accompanied by local pain. Thoracoabdominal radiculopathy leads to pain over the trunk. In patients with autonomic neuropathy, postural hypotension, postgustatory hyperhidrosis, constipation, flatulence, diarrhea, impotence, urinary retention, and incontinence may occur, and there may be abnormal pupillary responses. Isolated lesions of individual peripheral nerves are common and in the limbs tend to occur at sites of compression or entrapment. Treatment is symptomatic. Entrapment neuropathies may be helped by surgical decompression. Treatment of neuropathic pain is discussed on p 609.

**B. Uremia:** Uremia may lead to a symmetric sensorimotor polyneuropathy that tends to affect the lower limbs more than the upper limbs and is more marked distally than proximally. The diagnosis can be confirmed electrophysiologically, for motor and sensory conduction velocity is moderately reduced. The neuropathy improves both clinically and electrophysiologically with prolonged dialysis or renal transplantation and to a lesser extent with chronic dialysis.

**C. Alcoholism and Nutritional Deficiency:** Many alcoholics have an axonal distal sensorimotor polyneuropathy that is frequently accompanied by painful cramps, muscle tenderness, and painful paresthesias and is often more marked in the legs than in the arms. Symptoms of autonomic dysfunction may also be conspicuous. Motor and sensory conduction velocity may be slightly reduced, even in subclinical cases, but gross slowing of conduction is uncom-

mon. A similar distal sensorimotor polyneuropathy is a well-recognized feature of beriberi. In vitamin $B_{12}$ deficiency, distal sensory polyneuropathy may develop but is usually overshadowed by central nervous system manifestations (eg, myelopathy, optic neuropathy, or intellectual changes).

**D. Paraproteinemias:** A symmetric sensorimotor polyneuropathy that is gradual in onset, progressive in course, and often accompanied by pain and dysesthesias in the limbs may occur in patients (especially men) with multiple myeloma. The neuropathy is of the axonal type in classic lytic myeloma, but segmental demyelination (primary or secondary) and axonal loss occur in sclerotic myeloma and lead to predominantly motor clinical manifestations. Both demyelinating and axonal neuropathies are also observed in patients with paraproteinemias without myeloma. A small fraction will develop myeloma if serially followed. The demyelinating neuropathy in these patients may be due to the monoclonal protein's reacting to a component of the nerve myelin. The neuropathy of classic multiple myeloma is poorly responsive to therapy. The polyneuropathy of benign monoclonal gammopathy may respond to plasmapheresis.

Polyneuropathy may also occur in association with macroglobulinemia and cryoglobulinemia and sometimes responds to plasmapheresis. Entrapment neuropathy, such as carpal tunnel syndrome, is more common than polyneuropathy in patients with primary amyloidosis or in amyloidosis associated with multiple myeloma. With polyneuropathy due to amyloidosis, sensory and autonomic symptoms are especially conspicuous, whereas distal wasting and weakness occur later; there is no specific treatment.

## Neuropathies Associated With Infectious & Inflammatory Diseases

**A. Leprosy:** Leprosy is an important cause of peripheral neuropathy in certain parts of the world. Sensory disturbances are mainly due to involvement of intracutaneous nerves. In tuberculoid leprosy, they develop at the same time and in the same distribution as the skin lesion but may be more extensive if nerve trunks lying beneath the lesion are also involved. In lepromatous leprosy, there is more extensive sensory loss, and this develops earlier and to a greater extent in the coolest regions of the body, such as the dorsal surfaces of the hands and feet, where the bacilli proliferate most actively. Motor deficits result from involvement of superficial nerves where their temperature is lowest, eg, the ulnar nerve in the region proximal to the olecranon groove, the median nerve as it emerges from beneath the forearm flexor muscle to run toward the carpal tunnel, the peroneal nerve at the head of the fibula, and the posterior tibial nerve in the lower part of the leg; patchy facial muscular weakness may also occur owing to involvement of the superficial branches of the seventh cranial nerve.

Motor disturbances in leprosy are suggestive of multiple mononeuropathy, whereas sensory changes resemble those of distal polyneuropathy. Careful examination, however, relates the distribution of sensory deficits to the temperature of the tissues; in the legs, for example, sparing frequently occurs between the toes and in the popliteal fossae, where the temperature is higher. Treatment is with antileprotic agents.

**B. Sarcoidosis:** Sarcoidosis may affect the central nervous system. In addition, cranial nerve palsies (especially facial palsy), multiple mononeuropathy, and, less commonly, symmetric polyneuropathy may all occur, the latter sometimes preferentially affecting either motor or sensory fibers. Improvement may occur with use of corticosteroids.

**C. Polyarteritis:** Involvement of the vasa nervorum by the vasculitic process may result in infarction of the nerve. Clinically, one encounters an asymmetric sensorimotor polyneuropathy (mononeuritis multiplex) that pursues a waxing and waning course. Steroids and cytotoxic agents—especially cyclophosphamide—may be of benefit in severe cases.

**D. Rheumatoid Arthritis:** Compressive or entrapment neuropathies, ischemic neuropathies, mild distal sensory polyneuropathy, and severe progressive sensorimotor polyneuropathy can occur in rheumatoid arthritis.

## Toxic Neuropathies

Axonal polyneuropathy may follow exposure to industrial agents or pesticides such as acrylamide, organophosphorus compounds, hexacarbon solvents, methyl bromide, and carbon disulfide; metals such as arsenic, thallium, mercury, and lead; and drugs such as phenytoin, perhexiline, isoniazid, nitrofurantoin, vincristine, and pyridoxine in high doses. Detailed occupational, environmental, and medical histories and recognition of clusters of cases are important in suggesting the diagnosis. Treatment is by preventing further exposure to the causal agent. Isoniazid neuropathy is prevented by pyridoxine supplementation.

Diphtheritic neuropathy results from a neurotoxin released by the causative organism and is common in many areas. Palatal weakness may develop 2–4 weeks after infection of the throat, and infection of the skin may similarly be followed by focal weakness of neighboring muscles. Disturbances of accommodation may occur about 4–5 weeks after infection and distal sensorimotor demyelinating polyneuropathy after 1–3 months.

## Neuropathies Associated With Malignant Diseases

Both a sensorimotor and a purely sensory polyneuropathy may occur as a nonmetastatic complication of malignant diseases. The sensorimotor polyneuropathy may be mild and occur in the course of known malignant disease; or it may have an acute or subacute onset, lead to severe disability, and occur before there is any clinical evidence of the cancer, occasionally following a remitting course.

## Acute Idiopathic Polyneuropathy (Guillain-Barré Syndrome)

This acute or subacute polyradiculoneuropathy sometimes follows infective illness, inoculations, or surgical procedures but often occurs in a previously well person. It probably has an immunologic basis, but the precise mechanism is unclear. The main complaint is of weakness that varies widely in severity in different patients and often has a proximal emphasis and symmetric distribution. It usually begins in the legs, spreading to a variable extent but frequently involving the arms and often one or both sides of the face. The muscles of respiration or deglutition may also be affected. Sensory symptoms are usually less conspicuous than motor ones, but distal paresthesias and dysesthesias are common, and neuropathic or radicular pain is present in many patients. Autonomic disturbances are also common, may be severe, and are sometimes life-threatening; they include tachycardia, cardiac irregularities, hypotension or hypertension, facial flushing, abnormalities of sweating, pulmonary dysfunction, and impaired sphincter control.

The cerebrospinal fluid characteristically contains a high protein concentration with a normal cell content, but these changes may take 2 or 3 weeks to develop. Electrophysiologic studies may reveal marked abnormalities, which do not necessarily parallel the clinical disorder in their temporal course. Pathologic examination has shown that primary demyelination occurs in regions infiltrated with inflammatory cells, and it seems probable that myelin disruption has an autoimmune basis.

When the diagnosis is made, the history and appropriate laboratory studies should exclude the possibility of porphyric, diphtheritic, or toxic (heavy metal, hexacarbon, organophosphate) neuropathies. Poliomyelitis, botulism, and tick paralysis must also be considered. The presence of pyramidal signs, a markedly asymmetric motor deficit, a sharp sensory level, or early sphincter involvement should suggest a focal cord lesion.

Most patients eventually make a good recovery, but this may take many months, and 10–20% patients are left with persisting disability. Treatment is controversial. Corticosteroids were often prescribed in the past, but a prospective randomized trial has now shown that early treatment with prednisone is ineffective and may actually affect the outcome adversely by prolonging recovery time. Plasmapheresis is of value; it is best performed within the first few days of illness and is best reserved for clinically severe cases. Severely affected patients are best managed in intensive care units where respiratory and circulatory function can be monitored and respiration assisted if necessary. Patients should be admitted to such units if they are continuing to deteriorate and their forced vital capacity is declining, and intubation should be considered if the forced vital capacity reaches 15 mL/kg, dyspnea becomes evident, or the blood oxygen saturation declines. Careful respiratory toilet and chest physical therapy help prevent bronchial obstruction and atelectasis. Marked hypotension may respond to volume replacement or pressor agents. Frequent turning of the patient helps prevent decubitus ulcers, and physical therapy helps prevent contractures. Low-dose heparin to prevent pulmonary embolism should be considered.

Approximately 3% of patients with acute idiopathic polyneuropathy have one or more relapses, sometimes several years after the initial illness. Relapses are clinically similar to the original illness. Plasma exchange therapy may produce improvement in chronic and relapsing inflammatory polyneuropathy.

## Chronic Inflammatory Polyneuropathy

Chronic inflammatory polyneuropathy, an acquired immunologically mediated disorder, is clinically similar to Guillain-Barré syndrome except that it has a relapsing or steadily progressive course over months or years. In the relapsing form, partial recovery may occur after some relapses, but in other instances there is no recovery between exacerbations. Although remission may occur spontaneously with time, the disorder frequently follows a progressive downhill course leading to severe functional disability.

Electrodiagnostic studies show marked slowing of motor and sensory conduction, and focal conduction block. Signs of partial denervation may also be present owing to secondary axonal degeneration. Nerve biopsy may show chronic perivascular inflammatory infiltrates in the endoneurium and epineurium, without accompanying evidence of vasculitis. However, a normal nerve biopsy result or the presence of nonspecific abnormalities does not exclude the diagnosis.

Corticosteroids may be effective in arresting or reversing the downhill course. Treatment is usually begun with prednisone, 60 mg daily, continued for 2–3 months or until a definite response has occurred. If no response has occurred despite 3 months of treatment, a higher dose may be tried. In responsive cases, the dose is gradually tapered, but most patients become corticosteroid-dependent, often requiring prednisone, 20 mg daily on alternate days, on a long-term basis. Patients unresponsive to corticosteroids may benefit instead from treatment with a cytotoxic drug such as azathioprine. There are increasing anecdotal reports of benefit with plasmapheresis.

Dowling PC, Cook SD, Prineas JW (editors): Guillain-Barré syndrome: Proceedings of a conference sponsored by the Kroc Foundation. *Ann Neurol* 1981;**9(Suppl)**. [Entire issue.]

Ewing DJ, Campbell IW, Clarke BF: The natural history of diabetic autonomic neuropathy. *Q J Med* 1980;**49**:95.

Hallett M, Tandon D, Berardelli A: Treatment of peripheral neuropathies. *J Neurol Neurosurg Psychiatry* 1985;**48**:1193.

Kelly JJ et al: The spectrum of peripheral neuropathy in myeloma. *Neurology* 1981;**31**:24.

Lotti M et al: Occupational peripheral neuropathies. *West J Med* 1982;**137**:493.

Sabin TD, Swift TR: Leprosy. In: *Peripheral Neuropathy:* Dyck PJ et al (editors). Saunders, 1984.

## 2. MONONEUROPATHIES

An individual nerve may be injured along its course, or compressed, angulated, or stretched by neighboring anatomic structures, especially at a point where it passes through a narrow space (entrapment neuropathy). The relative contributions of mechanical factors and ischemia to the local damage are not clear. With involvement of a sensory or mixed nerve, pain is commonly felt distal to the lesion. Symptoms never develop with some entrapment neuropathies, resolve rapidly and spontaneously in others, and become progressively more disabling and distressing in yet other cases. The precise neurologic deficit depends on the nerve involved. Percussion of the nerve at the site of the lesion may lead to paresthesias in its distal distribution.

Entrapment neuropathy may be the sole manifestation of subclinical polyneuropathy, and this must be borne in mind and excluded by nerve conduction studies. Such studies are also indispensable for the accurate localization of the focal lesion.

In patients with acute compression neuropathy such as Saturday night palsy, no treatment is necessary. Complete recovery generally occurs, usually within 2 months, presumably because the underlying pathology is demyelination. However, axonal degeneration can occur in severe cases, and recovery then takes longer and may never be complete.

In chronic compressive or entrapment neuropathies, local infiltration of the region about the nerve with corticosteroids may be of value; in addition, surgical decompression may help if there is a progressively increasing neurologic deficit or if electrodiagnostic studies show evidence of partial denervation in weak muscles.

Peripheral nerve tumors are uncommon, except in Recklinghausen's disease, but also give rise to mononeuropathy. This may be distinguishable from entrapment neuropathy only by noting the presence of a mass along the course of the nerve and by demonstrating the precise site of the lesion with appropriate electrophysiologic studies. Treatment of symptomatic lesions is by surgical removal if possible.

### Carpal Tunnel Syndrome

See p 524.

### Pronator Teres or Anterior Interosseous Syndrome

The median nerve gives off its motor branch, the anterior interosseous nerve, below the elbow as it descends between the 2 heads of the pronator teres muscle. A lesion of either nerve may occur in this region, sometimes after trauma or owing to compression from, for example, a fibrous band. With anterior interosseous nerve involvement, there is no sensory loss, and weakness is confined to the pronator quadratus, flexor pollicis longus, and the flexor digitorum profundus to the second and third digits. Weakness is more widespread and sensory changes occur in an appropriate distribution when the median nerve itself is affected. The prognosis is variable. If improvement does not occur spontaneously, decompressive surgery may be helpful.

## Ulnar Nerve Lesions

Ulnar nerve lesions are likely to occur in the elbow region as the nerve runs behind the medial epicondyle and descends into the cubital tunnel. In the condylar groove, the ulnar nerve is exposed to pressure or trauma. Moreover, any increase in the carrying angle of the elbow, whether congenital, degenerative, or traumatic, may cause excessive stretching of the nerve when the elbow is flexed. Ulnar nerve lesions may also result from thickening or distortion of the anatomic structures forming the cubital tunnel, and the resulting symptoms may also be aggravated by flexion of the elbow, because the tunnel is then narrowed by tightening of its roof or inward bulging of its floor. A severe lesion at either site causes sensory changes in the medial 1½ digits and along the medial border of the hand. There is weakness of the ulnar-innervated muscles in the forearm and hand. With a cubital tunnel lesion, however, there may be relative sparing of the flexor carpi ulnaris muscle. Electrophysiologic evaluation using nerve stimulation techniques allows more precise localization of the lesion.

If conservative measures (eg, avoidance of factors liable to cause compression or stretch of the nerve) are unsuccessful in relieving symptoms and preventing further progression, surgical treatment may be necessary. This consists of nerve transposition if the lesion is in the condylar groove, or a release procedure if it is in the cubital tunnel.

Ulnar nerve lesions may also develop at the wrist or in the palm of the hand, usually owing to repetitive trauma or to compression from ganglia or benign tumors. They can be subdivided depending upon their presumed site. Compressive lesions are treated surgically. If repetitive mechanical trauma is responsible, this is avoided by occupational adjustment or job retraining.

## Radial Nerve Lesions

The radial nerve is particularly liable to compression or injury in the axilla (eg, by crutches or by pressure when the arm hangs over the back of a chair). This leads to weakness or paralysis of all the muscles supplied by the nerve, including the triceps. Sensory changes may also occur but are often surprisingly inconspicuous, being marked only in a small area on the back of the hand between the thumb and index finger. Injuries to the radial nerve in the spiral groove occur characteristically during deep sleep, as in intoxicated individuals (Saturday night palsy), and there

is then sparing of the triceps muscle, which is supplied more proximally. The nerve may also be injured at or above the elbow; its purely motor posterior interosseous branch, supplying the extensors of the wrist and fingers, may be involved immediately below the elbow, but then there is sparing of the extensor carpi radialis longus, so that the wrist can still be extended. The superficial radial nerve may be compressed by handcuffs or a tight watch strap.

## Femoral Neuropathy

The clinical features of femoral nerve palsy consist of weakness and wasting of the quadriceps muscle, with sensory impairment over the anteromedian aspect of the thigh and sometimes also of the leg to the medial malleolus, and a depressed or absent knee jerk. Isolated femoral neuropathy may occur in diabetics or from compression by retroperitoneal neoplasms or hematomas (eg, expanding aortic aneurysm). Femoral neuropathy may also result from pressure from the inguinal ligament when the thighs are markedly flexed and abducted, as in the lithotomy position.

## Meralgia Paresthetica

The lateral femoral cutaneous nerve, a sensory nerve arising from the L2 and L3 roots, may be compressed or stretched in obese or diabetic patients and during pregnancy. The nerve usually runs under the outer portion of the inguinal ligament to reach the thigh, but the ligament sometimes splits to enclose it. Hyperextension of the hip or increased lumbar lordosis—such as occurs during pregnancy—leads to nerve compression by the posterior fascicle of the ligament. However, entrapment of the nerve at any point along its course may cause similar symptoms, and several other anatomic variations predispose the nerve to damage when it is stretched. Pain, paresthesia, or numbness occurs about the outer aspect of the thigh, usually unilaterally, and is sometimes relieved by sitting. Examination shows no abnormalities except in severe cases when cutaneous sensation is impaired in the affected area. Symptoms are usually mild and commonly settle spontaneously, so patients can be reassured about the benign nature of the disorder. Hydrocortisone injections about the nerve where it lies medial to the anterosuperior iliac spine often relieve symptoms temporarily, while nerve decompression by transposition may provide more lasting relief.

## Sciatic & Common Peroneal Nerve Palsies

Misplaced deep intramuscular injections are probably still the most common cause of sciatic nerve palsy. Trauma to the buttock, hip, or thigh may also be responsible. The resulting clinical deficit depends on whether the whole nerve has been affected or only certain fibers. In general, the peroneal fibers of the sciatic nerve are more susceptible to damage than those destined for the tibial nerve. A sciatic nerve lesion may therefore be difficult to distinguish from peroneal neuropathy unless there is electromyographic evidence of involvement of the short head of the biceps femoris muscle. The common peroneal nerve itself may be compressed or injured in the region of the head and neck of the fibula. There is weakness of dorsiflexion and eversion of the foot, accompanied by numbness or blunted sensation of the anterolateral aspect of the calf and dorsum of the foot.

### Tarsal Tunnel Syndrome

The tibial nerve, the other branch of the sciatic, supplies several muscles in the lower extremity, gives origin to the sural nerve, and then continues as the posterior tibial nerve to supply the plantar flexors of the foot and toes. It passes through the tarsal tunnel behind and below the medial malleolus, giving off calcaneal branches and the medial and lateral plantar nerves that supply small muscles of the foot and the skin on the plantar aspect of the foot and toes. Compression of the posterior tibial nerve or its branches between the bony floor and ligamentous roof of the tarsal tunnel leads to pain, paresthesias, and numbness over the bottom of the foot, especially at night, with sparing of the heel. Muscle weakness may be hard to recognize clinically. Compressive lesions of the individual plantar nerves may also occur more distally, with similar clinical features to those of the tarsal tunnel syndrome. Treatment is surgical decompression.

Dawson DM, Hallett M, Millender LH: *Entrapment Neuropathies*. Little, Brown, 1983.

### 3. BELL'S PALSY

Bell's palsy is an idiopathic facial paresis of lower motor neuron type that has been attributed to an inflammatory reaction involving the facial nerve near the stylomastoid foramen or in the bony facial canal. A relationship of Bell's palsy to reactivation of herpes simplex virus has recently been suggested, but there is little evidence to support this.

The clinical features of Bell's palsy are characteristic. The facial paresis generally comes on abruptly, but it may worsen over the following day or so. Pain about the ear precedes or accompanies the weakness in many cases but usually lasts for only a few days. The face itself feels stiff and pulled to one side. There may be ipsilateral restriction of eye closure, and difficulty with eating and fine facial movements. A disturbance of taste is common, owing to involvement of chorda tympani fibers, and hyperacusis due to involvement of fibers to the stapedius occurs occasionally.

The management of Bell's palsy is controversial. Approximately 60% of cases recover completely without treatment, presumably because the lesion is so mild that it leads merely to conduction block. Considerable improvement occurs in most other cases, and only about 10% of all patients are seriously dissatisfied

with the final outcome because of permanent disfigurement or other long-term sequelae. Treatment is unnecessary in most cases but is indicated for patients in whom an unsatisfactory outcome can be predicted. The best clinical guide to progress is the severity of the palsy during the first few days after presentation. Patients with clinically complete palsy when first seen are less likely to make a full recovery than those with an incomplete one. A poor prognosis for recovery is also associated with advancing age, hyperacusis, and severe initial pain. Electromyography and nerve excitability or conduction studies provide a guide to prognosis but not early enough to aid in the selection of patients for treatment.

The only medical treatment that may influence the outcome is administration of corticosteroids, but studies supporting this concept have been criticized on methodologic grounds, and controlled trials have shown no convincing benefit. Many physicians nevertheless routinely prescribe corticosteroids for patients with Bell's palsy seen within 5 days of onset. The author prescribes them only when the palsy is clinically complete or there is severe pain. Treatment with prednisone, 60 or 80 mg daily in divided doses for 4 or 5 days, followed by tapering of dose over the next 7–10 days, is a satisfactory regimen. It is helpful to protect the eye with a patch if eye closure is not possible. There is no evidence that surgical procedures to decompress the facial nerve are of benefit.

Adour KK: Current concepts in neurology: Diagnosis and management of facial paralysis. *N Engl J Med* 1982;**307**:348.

## NECK & BACK PAIN
### (See also Chapter 14.)

### 1. BACK PAIN

Spinal disease may lead to local pain, root pain, or both. It may also lead to pain that is referred to other parts of the involved dermatomes. Local pain may lead to protective reflex muscle spasm, which in turn causes further pain and may result in abnormal posture and limitation of movement. Radicular pain arises from compression, stretch, or irritation of nerve roots and usually radiates from the back to the territory of the affected root, being exacerbated by coughing, straining, or stretching of the nerve fibers, eg, by straight leg raising. Root disturbances may also lead to paresthesias and numbness in dermatomal distribution and to weakness in segmental distribution; reflex changes may accompany involvement of motor or sensory fibers.

Localized back pain at rest (eg, at night) is common with vertebral involvement due to neoplasm, infection, or primary bone disease. The presence of fever suggests that back pain has an infective basis.

## Selected Causes of Low Back Pain

**A. Acute lumbar intervertebral disk prolapse** generally involves the L4–5 or the L5–S1 disk and leads to back and radicular (L5 or S1) pain. The L4 root is occasionally affected, but involvement of a higher lumbar root should arouse suspicion of other causes of root compression. There may be accompanying numbness and paresthesias in dermatomal distribution or segmental motor deficit. An L5 radiculopathy causes weakness of dorsiflexion of the foot and toes. With an S1 root lesion, there is weakness of eversion and plantar flexion of the foot and a depressed ankle jerk. A centrally prolapsed disk may lead to bilateral limb disturbances and sphincter involvement. Pelvic and rectal examination and plain x-rays of the spine help to exclude other disorders such as local primary cancers or metastatic deposits. Symptoms are often relieved with simple analgesics, diazepam, and bed rest on a firm mattress. Persisting pain, an increasing neurologic deficit, or any evidence of sphincter dysfunction calls for investigation by CT scanning with myelography or MRI followed by surgical treatment.

**B. Neoplastic disease** involving the spine may lead to localized, diffuse, or radicular pain, as discussed on p 521.

**C. Infections of the vertebral column** may cause progressive, unremitting local pain and tenderness, sometimes without systemic signs of infection. The peripheral white cell count and sedimentation rate may not be elevated. Radiographs may show disk space narrowing and a soft tissue mass but are frequently normal in the early stages. Osteomyelitis may be pyogenic or tuberculous and requires long-term antimicrobial therapy; surgical debridement and drainage may also be necessary. Spinal epidural abscess similarly presents with localized pain and tenderness, but flaccid paraplegia then develops rapidly; myelography is undertaken urgently and is followed by operative treatment.

**D. Nonspecific chronic bank pain** that occurs without objective clinical signs or obvious cause despite detailed investigations poses a difficult management problem. In some cases it may have a postural basis, while in others it may be a somatic manifestation of some psychiatric disorder. In yet other cases, pain that has arisen on an organic basis is enhanced or perpetuated by nonorganic factors and leads to disability out of proportion to symptoms. Treatment with tricyclic antidepressant drugs is sometimes helpful, and psychiatric evaluation may be worthwhile. Nonessential surgical procedures must be avoided.

## 2. NECK PAIN

A variety of congenital abnormalities may involve the cervical spine and lead to neck pain; these include hemivertebrae, fused vertebrae, basilar impression, and instability of the atlantoaxial joint. The traumatic, infective, and neoplastic disorders that cause back pain may also lead to pain in the neck. When rheumatoid arthritis involves the spine, it tends to affect especially the cervical region, leading to pain, stiffness, and reduced mobility; displacement of vertebrae or atlantoaxial subluxation may lead to cord compression that can be life-threatening if not treated by fixation.

## Selected Causes of Neck Pain

**A. Acute cervical disk protrusion:** Acute cervical disk protrusion leads to pain in the neck and radicularly in the arm, exacerbated by head movement. With lateral herniation of the disk, motor, sensory, or reflex changes may be found in a radicular (usually C6 or C7) distribution on the affected side; with more centrally directed herniations, the spinal cord may also be involved, leading to spastic paraparesis and sensory disturbances in the legs, sometimes accompanied by impaired sphincter function. The diagnosis is confirmed by myelography and CT scanning. In mild cases, bed rest or intermittent neck traction may help, followed by immobilization of the neck in a collar for several weeks. If these measures are unsuccessful or the patient has a significant neurologic deficit, surgical removal of the protruding disk may be necessary.

**B. Cervical Spondylosis:** Cervical spondylosis results from chronic cervical disk degeneration, with herniation of disk material, secondary calcification, and associated osteophytic outgrowths. One or more of the cervical nerve roots may be compressed, stretched, or angulated; and myelopathy may also develop as a result of compression, vascular insufficiency, or recurrent minor trauma to the cord. Patients present with neck pain and restricted head movement, occipital headaches, radicular pain and other sensory disturbances in the arms, weakness of the arms or legs, or some combination of these symptoms. Examination generally reveals that lateral flexion and rotation of the neck are limited. A segmental pattern of weakness or dermatomal sensory loss (or both) may be found unilaterally or bilaterally in the upper limbs, and tendon reflexes mediated by the affected root or roots are depressed. The C5 and C6 nerve roots are most commonly involved, and examination frequently then reveals weakness of muscles supplied by these roots (eg, deltoids, supra- and infraspinous, biceps, brachioradialis), pain or sensory loss about the shoulder and outer border of the arm and forearm, and depressed biceps and brachioradialis reflexes. Spastic paraparesis may also be present if there is an associated myelopathy, sometimes accompanied by posterior column or spinothalamic sensory deficits in the legs.

Plain radiographs of the cervical spine show osteophyte formation, narrowing of disk spaces, and encroachment on the intervertebral foramens, but such changes are common in middle-aged persons and may be unrelated to the presenting complaint. Myelography helps to confirm the diagnosis and exclude other structural causes of the myelopathy.

Restriction of neck movements by a cervical collar may relieve pain. Operative treatment may be necessary to prevent further progression if there is a significant neurologic deficit or if root pain is severe, persistent, and unresponsive to conservative measures.

Management of cervical spondylotic myelopathy. (Editorial.) *Lancet* 1984;**1**:1058.

## BRACHIAL PLEXUS LESIONS

### Brachial Plexus Neuropathy

Brachial plexus neuropathy may be idiopathic, sometimes occurring in relationship to a number of different nonspecific illnesses or factors. In other instances, brachial plexus lesions follow trauma or result from congenital anomalies, neoplastic involvement, or injury by various physical agents. In rare instances, the disorder occurs on a familial basis.

Idiopathic brachial plexus neuropathy (neuralgic amyotrophy) characteristically begins with severe pain about the shoulder, followed within a few days by weakness, reflex changes, and sensory disturbances involving especially the C5 and C6 segments. Symptoms and signs are usually unilateral but may be bilateral. Wasting of affected muscles is sometimes profound. The disorder relates to disturbed function of cervical roots or part of the brachial plexus, but its precise cause is unknown. Recovery occurs over the ensuing months but may be incomplete. Treatment is purely symptomatic.

### Cervical Rib Syndrome

Compression of the C8 and T1 roots or the lower trunk of the brachial plexus by a cervical rib or band arising from the seventh cervical vertebra leads to weakness and wasting of intrinsic hand muscles, especially those in the thenar eminence, accompanied by pain and numbness in the medial 2 fingers and the ulnar border of the hand and forearm. The subclavian artery may also be compressed, and this forms the basis of Adson's test for diagnosing the disorder; the radial pulse is diminished or obliterated on the affected side when the seated patient inhales deeply and turns the head to one side or the other. Electromyography, nerve conduction studies, and somatosensory evoked potential studies may help confirm the diagnosis. X-rays sometimes show the cervical rib or a large transverse process of the seventh cervical vertebra, but normal findings do not exclude the possibility of a cervical band. Treatment of the disorder is by surgical excision of the rib or band.

### Lumbosacral Plexus Lesions

A lumbosacral plexus lesion usually develops in association with diseases such as diabetes, cancer, or bleeding disorders or in relation to injury. It occasionally occurs as an isolated phenomenon similar to idiopathic brachial plexopathy, and pain and weakness then tend to be more conspicuous than sensory symptoms. The distribution of symptoms and signs depends on the level and pattern of neurologic involvement.

Gilliatt RW et al: Peripheral nerve conduction in patients with cervical rib and band. *Ann Neurol* 1978;**4**:124.
Kori SH, Foley KM, Posner JB: Brachial plexus lesions in patients with cancer: 100 cases. *Neurology* 1981;**31**:45.
Lascelles RG et al: The thoracic outlet syndrome. *Brain* 1977;**100**:601.

## DISORDERS OF NEUROMUSCULAR TRANSMISSION

### 1. MYASTHENIA GRAVIS

#### Essentials of Diagnosis

- Fluctuating weakness of commonly used voluntary muscles, producing symptoms such as diplopia, ptosis, and difficulty in swallowing.
- Activity increases weakness of affected muscles.
- Short-acting anticholinesterases transiently improve the weakness.

#### General Considerations

Myasthenia gravis occurs at all ages, sometimes in association with a thymic tumor or thyrotoxicosis, as well as with rheumatoid arthritis and lupus erythematosus. It is commonest in young women with HLA-DR3; if thymoma is associated, older men are more commonly affected. Onset is usually insidious, but the disorder is sometimes unmasked by a coincidental infection that leads to exacerbation of symptoms. Exacerbations may also occur before the menstrual period or during or shortly after pregnancy. Symptoms are due to a variable degree of block of neuromuscular transmission. This probably has an immunologic basis, and autoantibodies binding to acetylcholine receptors are found in most patients with the disease. These antibodies have a primary role in reducing the number of functioning acetylcholine receptors. Additionally, cellular immune activity against the receptor is found. Clinically, this leads to weakness; initially powerful movements fatigue readily. The external ocular muscles and certain other cranial muscles, including the masticatory, facial, and pharyngeal muscles, are especially likely to be affected, and the respiratory and limb muscles may also be involved.

#### Clinical Findings

**A. Symptoms and Signs:** Patients present with ptosis, diplopia, difficulty in chewing or swallowing, respiratory difficulties, limb weakness, or some combination of these problems. Weakness may remain localized to a few muscle groups, especially the ocular muscles, or may become generalized. Symptoms often fluctuate in intensity during the day, and this diurnal variation is superimposed on a tendency to longer-term spontaneous relapses and remissions that may last for weeks. Nevertheless, the disorder follows a slowly progressive course and may have a fatal outcome owing to respiratory complications such as aspiration pneumonia.

Clinical examination confirms the weakness and fatigability of affected muscles. In most cases, the extraocular muscles are involved, and this leads to ocular palsies and ptosis, which are commonly asymmetric. Pupillary responses are normal. The bulbar and limb muscles are often weak, but the pattern of involvement is variable. Sustained activity of affected muscles increases the weakness, which improves after a brief rest. Sensation is normal, and there are usually no reflex changes.

The diagnosis can generally be confirmed by the response to a short-acting anticholinesterase. Edrophonium (Tensilon) can be given intravenously in a dose of 10 mg (1 mL), 2 mg being given initially and the remaining 8 mg about 30 seconds later if the test dose is well tolerated; in myasthenic patients, there is an obvious improvement in strength of weak muscles lasting for about 5 minutes. Alternatively, 1.5 mg of neostigmine can be given intramuscularly, and the response then lasts for about 2 hours; atropine sulfate (0.6 mg) should be available to reverse muscarinic side effects.

**B. Imaging:** Lateral and anteroposterior x-rays of the chest and CT scans should be obtained to demonstrate a coexisting thymoma, but normal studies do not exclude this possibility.

**C. Laboratory and Other Studies:** Electrophysiologic demonstration of a decrementing muscle response to repetitive 2- or 3-Hz stimulation of motor nerves indicates a disturbance of neuromuscular transmission. Such an abnormality may even be detected in clinically strong muscles with certain provocative procedures. Needle electromyography of affected muscles shows a marked variation in configuration and size of individual motor unit potentials, and single-fiber electromyography reveals an increased jitter, or variability in the time interval between 2 muscle fiber action potentials from the same motor unit.

Assay of serum for elevated levels of circulating acetylcholine receptor antibodies is another approach—increasingly used—to the laboratory diagnosis of myasthenia gravis.

**Treatment**

Anticholinesterase drugs provide symptomatic benefit without influencing the course of the disease. Neostigmine, pyridostigmine, or both can be used, the dose being determined on an individual basis. Overmedication may temporarily increase weakness, which is then unaffected or enhanced by intravenous edrophonium.

Thymectomy usually leads to symptomatic benefit or remission and should be undertaken in patients younger than age 60, unless weakness is restricted to the extraocular muscles. If the disease is of recent onset and only slowly progressive, operation is sometimes delayed for a year or so, in the hope that spontaneous remission will occur.

Treatment with corticosteroids is indicated for patients who have responded poorly to anticholinesterase drugs and have already undergone thymectomy. It is introduced with the patient in the hospital, since weakness may initially be aggravated. Once weakness has stabilized after 2–3 weeks or any improvement is sustained, further management can be on an outpatient basis. Alternate-day treatment is usually well tolerated, but if weakness is enhanced on the nontreatment day it may be necessary for medication to be taken daily. The dose of corticosteroids is determined on an individual basis, but an initial high daily dose can gradually be tapered to a relatively low maintenance level as improvement occurs; total withdrawal is difficult, however. Treatment with azathioprine may also be effective, and the relative merit of this approach is currently under investigation.

In patients with major disability in whom conventional treatment is either unhelpful or contraindicated, plasmapheresis may be beneficial.

Seybold ME: Myasthenia gravis: A clinical and basic science review. *JAMA* 1983;**250**:2516.

## 2. MYASTHENIC SYNDROME (Eaton-Lambert Syndrome)

Myasthenic syndrome may be associated with small cell carcinoma, underlying carcinoma, sometimes developing before the tumor is diagnosed, and occasionally occurs with certain autoimmune diseases. There is defective release of acetylcholine in response to a nerve impulse, and this leads to weakness especially of the proximal muscles of the limbs. Unlike myasthenia gravis, however, power steadily increases with sustained contraction. The diagnosis can be confirmed electrophysiologically, because the muscle response to stimulation of its motor nerve increases remarkably if the nerve is stimulated repetitively at high rates, even in muscles that are not clinically weak.

Treatment with plasmapheresis and immunosuppressive drug therapy (prednisone and azathioprine) may lead to clinical and electrophysiologic improvement, in addition to therapy aimed at tumor when present. Guanidine hydrochloride (25–50 mg/kg/d in divided doses) is occasionally helpful in seriously disabled patients, but adverse effects of the drug include marrow suppression. The response to treatment with anticholinesterase drugs such as pyridostigmine or neostigmine, either alone or in combination with guanidine, is variable.

Dau PC, Denys EH: Plasmapheresis and immunosuppressive drug therapy in the Eaton-Lambert syndrome. *Ann Neurol* 1982;**11**:570.

## 3. BOTULISM

The toxin of *Clostridium botulinum* prevents the release of acetylcholine at neuromuscular junctions and autonomic synapses. Botulism occurs most commonly following the ingestion of contaminated home-canned food and should be suggested by the development of sudden, fluctuating, severe weakness in a previously healthy person. Symptoms begin within 72 hours following ingestion of the toxin and may progress for several days. Typically, there is diplopia, ptosis, facial weakness, dysphagia, and nasal speech, followed by respiratory difficulty and finally by weakness that appears last in the limbs. Blurring of vision (with unreactive dilated pupils) is characteristic, and there may be dryness of the mouth, constipation (paralytic ileus), and postural hypotension. Sensation is preserved, and the tendon reflexes are not affected unless the involved muscles are very weak. If the diagnosis is suspected, the local health authority should be notified and a sample of serum and contaminated food (if available) sent to be assayed for toxin. Support for the diagnosis may be obtained by electrophysiologic studies; with repetitive stimulation of motor nerves at fast rates, the muscle response increases in size progressively.

Patients should be hospitalized in case respiratory assistance becomes necessary. Treatment is with trivalent antitoxin, once it is established that the patient is not allergic to horse serum. Guanidine hydrochloride (25–50 mg/kg/d in divided doses) to facilitate release of acetylcholine from nerve endings sometimes helps to increase muscle strength. Anticholinesterase drugs are of no value. Respiratory assistance and other supportive measures should be provided as necessary.

## 4. DISORDERS ASSOCIATED WITH USE OF AMINOGLYCOSIDES

Aminoglycoside antibiotics, eg, gentamicin, may produce a clinical disturbance similar to botulism by preventing the release of acetylcholine from nerve endings, but symptoms subside rapidly as the responsible drug is eliminated from the body. These antibiotics are particularly dangerous in patients with preexisting disturbances of neuromuscular transmission and are therefore best avoided in patients with myasthenia gravis.

## MYOPATHIC DISORDERS

### Muscular Dystrophies

These inherited myopathic disorders are characterized by progressive muscle weakness and wasting. They are subdivided by mode of inheritance, age at onset, and clinical features, as shown in Table 16–6. In the Duchenne type, pseudohypertrophy of muscles frequently occurs at some stage; intellectual retardation is common; and there may be skeletal deformities, muscle contractures, and cardiac involvement. The serum creatine phosphokinase level is increased, especially in the Duchenne and Becker varieties, and mildly increased also in limb-girdle dystrophy. Electromyography may help to confirm that weakness is myopathic rather than neurogenic. Similarly, histopathologic examination of a muscle biopsy specimen may help to confirm that weakness is due to a primary disorder of muscle and to distinguish between various muscle diseases.

There is no specific treatment, but it is important to encourage patients to lead as normal lives as possi-

**Table 16–6.** The muscular dystrophies.

| Disorder | Inheritance | Age at Onset (years) | Distribution | Prognosis |
|---|---|---|---|---|
| Duchenne type | X-linked recessive | 1–5 | Pelvic, then shoulder girdle; later, limb and respiratory muscles. | Rapid progression. Death within about 15 years after onset. |
| Becker's | X-linked recessive | 5–25 | Pelvic, then shoulder girdle. | Slow progression. May have normal life span. |
| Limb-girdle (Erb's) | Autosomal recessive (may be sporadic or dominant) | 10–30 | Pelvic or shoulder girdle initially, with later spread to the other. | Variable severity and rate of progression. Possible severe disability in middle life. |
| Facioscapulo-humeral | Autosomal dominant | Any age | Face and shoulder girdle initially; later, pelvic girdle and legs. | Slow progression. Minor disability. Usually normal life span. |
| Distal | Autosomal dominant | 40–60 | Onset distally in extremities; proximal involvement later. | Slow progression. |
| Ocular | Autosomal dominant | Any age | External ocular muscles. May also be mild weakness of face, neck, and arms. | |
| Oculopharyngeal | Autosomal dominant | Any age | As the ocular form, but with dysphagia. | |

ble. Prolonged bed rest must be avoided, as inactivity often leads to worsening of the underlying muscle disease. Physical therapy and orthopedic procedures may help to counteract deformities or contractures.

## Myotonic Dystrophy

Myotonic dystrophy, a slowly progressive, dominantly inherited disorder, usually manifests itself in the third or fourth decade but occasionally appears early in childhood. Myotonia leads to complaints of muscle stiffness and is evidenced by the marked delay that occurs before affected muscles can relax after a contraction. This can often be demonstrated clinically by delayed relaxation of the hand after sustained grip or by percussion of the belly of a muscle. In addition, there is weakness and wasting of the facial, sternocleidomastoid, and distal limb muscles. Associated clinical features include cataracts, frontal baldness, testicular atrophy, diabetes mellitus, cardiac abnormalities, and intellectual changes. Electromyographic sampling of affected muscles reveals myotonic discharges in addition to changes suggestive of myopathy.

Myotonia can be treated with quinine sulfate (300–400 mg 3 times daily), procainamide (0.5–1 g 4 times daily), or phenytoin (100 mg 3 times daily). In myotonic dystrophy, phenytoin is preferred, since the other drugs may have undesirable effects on cardiac conduction. Neither the weakness nor the course of the disorder is influenced by treatment.

## Myotonia Congenita

Myotonia congenita is commonly inherited as a dominant trait. Generalized myotonia without weakness is usually present from birth, but symptoms may not appear until early childhood. Patients complain of muscle stiffness that is enhanced by cold and inactivity and relieved by exercise. Muscle hypertrophy, at times pronounced, is also a feature. A recessive form with later onset is associated with slight weakness and atrophy of distal muscles. Treatment with quinine sulfate, procainamide, or phenytoin may help the myotonia, as in myotonic dystrophy.

## Polymyositis & Dermatomyositis

See Chapter 14.

## Myopathies Associated With Other Disorders

Myopathy may occur in association with chronic hypokalemia, hyper- or hypothyroidism, hyper- or hypoparathyroidism, hyper- or hypoadrenalism, hypopituitarism, and acromegaly and in patients taking corticosteroids, chloroquine, colchicine, bretylium tosylate, or drugs causing potassium depletion. Treatment is of the underlying cause. Myopathy also occurs with chronic alcoholism, whereas acute reversible muscle necrosis may occur shortly after acute alcohol intoxication.

# PERIODIC PARALYSIS SYNDROME

Periodic paralysis may have a familial (dominant inheritance) basis. Episodes of flaccid weakness or paralysis occur, sometimes in association with abnormalities of the plasma potassium level. Strength is normal between attacks. The **hypokalemic** variety is characterized by attacks that tend to occur on awakening, after exercise, or after a heavy meal and may last for several days. Patients should avoid excessive exertion. A low-carbohydrate and low-salt diet may help prevent attacks, as may acetazolamide, 250–750 mg/d. An ongoing attack may be aborted by potassium chloride given orally or by intravenous drip, provided the ECG can be monitored and renal function is satisfactory. It is sometimes associated with hyperthyroidism, and treatment of the endocrine disorder may then prevent recurrences. In **hyperkalemic** periodic paralysis, attacks also tend to occur after exercise but usually last for less than an hour. Severe attacks may be terminated by intravenous calcium gluconate (1–2 g) or by intravenous diuretics (furosemide, 20–40 mg), glucose, or glucose and insulin; daily acetazolamide or chlorothiazide may prevent recurrences. In **normokalemic** periodic paralysis, the patient may be unable to move his or her limbs in severe attacks; fortunately, respiration and swallowing are rarely affected, because treatment with acetazolamide is not always helpful.

# REFERENCES

Adams RD, Victor M: *Principles of Neurology,* 3rd ed. McGraw-Hill, 1985.

Aminoff MJ (editor): *Electrodiagnosis in Clinical Neurology,* 2nd ed. Churchill Livingstone, 1986.

Baraitser M: *The Genetics of Neurological Disorders.* Oxford, 1982.

Dyck PJ et al (editors): *Peripheral Neuropathy,* 2nd ed. Saunders, 1984.

Fishman RA: *Cerebrospinal Fluid in Diseases of the Nervous System.* Saunders, 1980.

Rowland LP (editor): *Merritt's Textbook of Neurology,* 7th ed. Lea & Febiger, 1984.

Walton JN (editor): *Brain's Diseases of the Nervous System,* 9th ed. Oxford, 1985.

Walton JN (editor): *Disorders of Voluntary Muscle,* 4th ed. Churchill Livingstone, 1981.

# Psychiatric Disorders

# 17

*James J. Brophy, MD*

Psychiatric disorders may result from disturbance of one or more of the following interrelated factors: (1) biologic function, (2) psychodynamic adaptation, (3) learned behavior, and (4) social and environmental conditions. Although the clinical situation at a given time determines which area of dysfunction will be emphasized, proper patient care requires an approach that simultaneously encompasses all factors.

**(1) Biologic function.** Psychiatric disorders of biologic origin may be secondary to identifiable physical illness or caused by as yet unexplained biochemical disturbances of the brain. A wide variety of psychiatric disorders (eg, psychosis, depression, delirium, anxiety), as well as nonspecific symptoms frequently considered to be of psychogenic origin, may be caused by organic brain disease or by derangement of cerebral metabolism resulting from illness, nutritional deficiencies, or toxic agents.

Research in biopsychiatry, utilizing techniques such as radioimmunoassay, magnetic resonance imaging (MRI), and positron emission tomography (PET), is now providing information about the localization, concentration, and chemical characteristics of the neuroactive transmitters and modulators in the living human brain. PET studies may be helpful in the subtle distinctions between unipolar and bipolar disorders. Serotoninergic mechanisms are intimately involved in affective disorders, autism, and the anxiety disorders. Studies of the physiologic interactions that take place along the hypothalamic-pituitary-adrenocortical axis has resulted in a recognized association between depression and thyroid dysfunction. Research in this area is also fundamental to the investigation of psychoimmunologic interactions and biochemical markers in psychiatric disorders. The isolation of a protein (amyloid precursor) and the investigations of a gene (chromosome 21) associated with Alzheimer's disease hold promise for earlier diagnosis and further clarification of this disorder. Of both heuristic and clinical interest is the increasing utilization of anticonvulsant drugs in the treatment of affective disorders and panic attacks. The calcium channel-blocking agents will probably also be of value in the treatment of some affective disorders.

**(2) Psychodynamic maladaptation** involves intrapsychic aberrations and is usually treated by a psychotherapeutic approach. There are over 100 alleged forms of psychotherapy, excluding behavioral approaches. Depending on the therapist's approach, psychotherapy can be classified as supportive, interpretive, cognitive, persuasive, educative, or some combination of these. Depth, duration, intensity, and frequency of sessions may vary. Various theoretic frameworks may be employed—freudian, jungian, adlerian, sullivanian, kleinian, etc. The "dynamic" approaches have their roots in classic freudian psychoanalytic theory, whereas "experiential" psychotherapy is of more recent origin, including many tenuous offshoots currently popular but of dubious long-term significance.

**(3) Learned behavior** is part of the pathogenetic mechanism in all psychiatric disorders. Although a biochemical abnormality may be the matrix of a schizophrenic process, the content of the psychotic material is to a great degree learned and socially relevant. Paranoid delusions reflect current concerns (eg, radar, electronic eavesdropping). In the case of anxiety disorders, many behavioral scientists feel that learned behavior alone is the major consideration. Appropriate parenting or training consists in great part of utilizing proper behavioral practices, rewarding correct behavior, and punishing delinquent behavior. Personality disorders are examples of failure to learn and incorporate patterns of behavior acceptable in societal surroundings.

**(4) Social and environmental conditions** have always been considered vital factors in the mental balance of the individual. Without the encounter with the environment, there can be no socially recognized illness: the exigencies of everyday life contribute both to the development of a stable personality and to the deviations from the norm. There is a constantly changing cultural influence that determines which types of behavior will be tolerated or considered deviant. The principal vehicle for modeling and learning in our social structure is the family unit, which has shifted from an extended group with numerous relatives to a smaller nuclear group consisting of one or both parents and their children. This changes when remarriage and perhaps the presence of children of previous unions result in a loose, fluid family unit with variable degrees of bonding. Changes in the family unit have coincided with changes in work patterns of parents and in schooling and work patterns of young adults. The changes are complex and generally have lengthened the period of dependency and increased stresses in the family unit; this, in turn, affects the underlying social fabric, with consequences for each individual.

Barnes DM: Biological issues in schizophrenia. *Science* 1987;**235**:430.

Gur RE et al: Regional brain function in schizophrenia: A positron emission tomography study. *Arch Gen Psychiat* 1987;**44**:119.

Pardes H: Future relationship of neuroscience and psychiatry. *Am J Psychiat* 1986;**143**:1205.

## PSYCHIATRIC ASSESSMENT

Psychiatric diagnosis rests upon the established principles of a thorough history and examination. All of the forces contributing to the individual's life situation must be identified, and this can only be done if the examination includes the history; mental status; medical conditions; and pertinent social, cultural, and environmental factors impinging on the individual.

### Interview

The appearance and behavior of the interviewer influences the interviewee. Lateness, obesity, smoking, and use of the patient's first name may all create a negative ambience. The manner in which the history is taken is important not only because it affects success in eliciting pertinent data but also because it may be of therapeutic value in itself. The setting should be quiet, with an appropriate degree of professional decorum at all times, and patients should initially be allowed to talk about their problems in an unstructured way without interruption. The interviewer should minimize writing, unnecessary direct questioning, and interpretive comments. Long, rambling discussions may be controlled by subtly interjecting questions relevant to the topic, although the patient's digressions sometimes provide important clues to his or her mental status. The first few minutes are often the most important part of the interview.

The interviewer should be alert for key words or phrases that can be used to help the patient develop the theme of the main difficulty. For example, if the patient says, "Doctor, I hurt, and when we have marital problems, things just get worse"—the words "hurt" and "marital problems" are important clues that need amplification when the physician makes another comment. Nonverbal clues may be as important as words, and one should notice gestures, tones of voice, and facial expressions. Obvious omissions, shying away from painful subjects, and sudden shifts of subject matter give important clues to unconscious as well as conscious sources of difficulty.

Every psychiatric history should cover the following points: (1) complaint, from the patient's viewpoint; (2) the present illness, or the evolution of the complaints; (3) previous disorders and the nature and extent of treatment; (4) the family history—important for genetic aspects and family influences; (5) personal history—childhood development, adolescent adjustment, level of education, and adult coping patterns; (6) sexual history; (7) current life functioning, with attention to vocational, social, educational, and avocational areas; and (8) current medications or other drugs.

It is often essential to obtain additional information from the family. Observing interactions of significant other people with the patient in the context of a family interview may give significant diagnostic information and may even underscore the nature of the problem and suggest a therapeutic approach.

### The Mental Status Examination

Observation of the patient and the content of the remarks made during the interview constitute the informal part of the mental status examination, ie, that which is obtained indirectly. The remainder of the information comes from direct questioning, which really is intended only to fill in the gaps.

The mental status examination includes the following: (1) Appearance: Note unusual modes of dress, makeup, etc. (2) Activity and behavior: Gait, gestures, coordination of bodily movements, etc. (3) Affect: Outward manifestation of emotions such as depression, anger, elation, fear, resentment, or lack of emotional response. (4) Mood: Inward feelings, sum of statements, and observable emotional manifestations. (5) Speech: Coherence, spontaneity, articulation, hesitancy in answering, and duration of response. (6) Content of thought: Associations, preoccupations, obsessions, depersonalization, delusions, hallucinations, paranoid ideation, anger, fear, or unusual experiences. (7) Sensorium: (a) orientation to person, place, time, and circumstances; (b) remote and recent memory and recall; (c) calculations, digit retention (forward and backward), serial 7s and 3s; (d) general fund of knowledge (presidents, states, distances, events); (e) abstracting ability, often tested with common proverbs or with analogies and differences (eg, how are a lie and a mistake the same, and how are they different?); (f) ability to identify by naming, reading, and writing specified test names and objects; (g) ideomotor function, which combines understanding and the ability to perform a task (eg, "Show me how to throw a ball"); (h) ability to reproduce geometric constructions (eg, parallelogram, intersecting squares); and (i) right-left differentiation. (8) Judgment regarding commonsense problems such as what to do when one runs out of medicine. (9) Insight into the nature and extent of the current difficulty and its ramifications in the patient's daily life.

The mental status examination is important in establishing a diagnosis and must be *recorded clearly and completely in the chart*.

### Medical Examination

*The examination of a psychiatric patient must include a complete medical history and physical examination as well as all necessary laboratory and other special studies.* Physical illness may frequently present as psychiatric disease, and vice versa. It is hazardous to assign a "functional" cause to symptoms simply because they arose during an emotional crisis.

## Special Diagnostic Aids

Many tests and evaluation procedures are available that can be used to support and clarify initial diagnostic impressions.

**A. Psychologic Testing:** Psychologic testing by a trained psychologist may measure intelligence and cognitive functioning; provide information about personality, feelings, psychodynamics, and psychopathology; and differentiate psychic problems from organic ones. The place of such tests is similar to that of other tests in medicine—helpful in diagnostic problems but a useless expense when not needed.

**1. Objective tests**–These tests provide quantitative evaluation compared to standard norms.

**a. Intelligence tests**–The test most frequently used is the Wechsler Adult Intelligence Scale—Revised (WAIS-R). Intelligence tests often reveal more than IQ. The results, given expert interpretation, can lend objective support to the ultimate psychiatric diagnosis. They provide information regarding different aspects of cognitive functioning, eg, short-term memory, abstract reasoning skills, and judgment.

**b. Minnesota Multiphasic Personality Inventory (MMPI)**–The MMPI is an empirically based test of personality assessment. The patient's scores are interpreted in comparison with data about others with the same response pattern to assess psychopathologic changes.

**c. Bender Gestalt Test**–This test is used to elicit evidence of psychomotor dysfunction in persons with organic disorders.

**d. Vocational aptitude and interest tests**–Several are available and may be used as a source of advice regarding vocational plans.

**2. Projective tests**–These tests are unstructured, so that the subject is forced to respond in ways that reflect fantasies and individual modes of adaptation. Conscious and unconscious attitudes (particularly disordered thinking) may be deduced from the subject's responses.

**a. Rorschach Psychodiagnostics**–This test utilizes 10 inkblots. It requires expert interpretation but can provide important information on psychodynamic themes and aberrations.

**b. Thematic Apperception Test (TAT)**–This test uses 20 pictures of people in different situations. Interpretation is based on psychoanalytic theory concerning defenses against feelings of anxiety and reflects areas of interpersonal conflicts.

**c. Sentence completion tests, draw-a-person tests, etc**–These tests are most useful in providing information about the patient's present concerns and conflicts.

**3. Miscellaneous tests**–Other tests designed for specific purposes include aphasia screening tests, inventories of depression, tests of different types of memory, and neurologic, behavior, and anxiety screening tests.

**B. Neurologic Evaluation:** Consultation is often necessary and may include specialized tests such as electroencephalography, echoencephalography, brain scanning, CT scanning, positron emission tomography (PET), and magnetic resonance imaging (MRI).

**C. Amobarbital Interviews:** The success of any of the sedative agents in eliciting clinically useful information is quite limited. The suggestive force of giving substances by injection is helpful, as judged from a comparison of amobarbital and saline interviews. The procedure can be helpful in differentiating psychosis from delirium; the former improves with amobarbital, whereas the latter worsens. Some cases of conversion disorders or dissociative disorders respond to this approach. Hypnosis can provide similar relief in selected subjects.

**D. Biologic Markers:** The dexamethasone suppression test (DST) and the thyrotropin-releasing hormone (TRH) test have been used as aids in the diagnosis, treatment, and follow-up of patients with depressive illness. Clinical usefulness of the tests is limited, but they represent progress in the search for reliable biologic markers.

## Formulation of the Diagnosis

A psychiatric diagnosis must be based upon positive evidence accumulated by the above techniques. It must not be based simply on the exclusion of organic findings.

A thorough psychiatric evaluation has therapeutic as well as diagnostic value and should be expressed in ways best understood by the patient, family, and other physicians. The problem-oriented medical record is applicable to psychiatric disorders.

Asaad G, Shapiro B: Hallucinations: Theoretical and clinical overview. *Am J Psychiat* 1986;**143**:1088.

Bech P, Kastrup M, Rafaelson OJ: Mini-compendium of rating scales of anxiety, depression, mania, schizophrenia, with corresponding DSM-III syndromes. *Acta Psychiatr Scand* 1986;**73(Suppl. 326)**:1.

Roca RP: Bedside cognitive examination. *Psychosomatics* 1987;**28**:73.

# TREATMENT APPROACHES

The approaches to treatment of psychiatric patients are, in a broad sense, similar to those in other branches of medicine. For example, the internist treating a patient with heart disease uses not only **medical** measures such as digitalis and pacemakers but also **psychologic** techniques to change attitudes and behaviors, **social** and **environmental** manipulation to mitigate deleterious influences, and **behavioral** techniques to change behavior patterns.

The psychiatrist may utilize the same general therapeutic approaches (conceptual models). The **medical** approaches used by the psychiatrist include, for example, medications and electroconvulsive therapy. The **psychologic** techniques include individual, group, and family therapies. **Social** interventions relate to the patient's environment by means of milieu therapy, halfway house placement, mutual aid support groups, or alteration in job or living situation. **Behavioral** therapy is directed toward identifying specific behavior patterns, factors determining such behavior, and ways of modifying it.

Regardless of the methods employed, treatment must be directed toward an objective, ie, **goal-oriented.** This usually involves (1) obtaining active cooperation on the part of the patient; (2) establishing reasonable goals and modifying the goal downward if failure occurs; (3) emphasizing positive behavior (goals) instead of symptom behavior (problems); (4) delineating the method; and (5) setting a time frame (which can be modified later).

The physician must resist pressures for prescribed treatment and instantaneous results, on the part of either the patient or relatives or close friends. The physician should be flexible and find ways to modify and work around patient resistance. Beware of unrealistic demands by the patient or the patient's family for a speedy resolution to a complex psychiatric problem. In almost all cases, psychiatric treatment involves the *active participation* of the significant people in the patient's life. It takes time to unravel the complex interrelationships between the psyche, the soma, and the sociocultural milieu of the patient. Time must be spent with the patient, but the frequency and duration of appointments are highly variable and should be adjusted to meet both the patient's psychologic needs and financial restrictions. Compliance (collaboration) is the end product of many factors, the most important being clear communication, attention to cost, and simple dosage regimens when drugs are prescribed. *The physician can unwittingly promote chronic illness by prescribing inappropriate medication.* The patient may come to believe that problems respond only to medication, and the more drugs prescribed, the stronger the misconception becomes.

### Psychiatric Referrals

All physicians have always treated most psychiatric problems and are in an excellent position to meet their patients' emotional needs in an organized and competent way, referring to psychiatrists for consultation *or* treatment those patients who represent particularly complex problems. The most pressing problems involve evaluation of suicidal or assaultive potential and diagnostic differentiation in affective disorders and psychoses. The psychiatric problems associated with unusual psychopharmacologic therapy and with medications used in other branches of medicine may require expert pharmacologic consultation. When a psychiatric referral is made, it should be conducted like any other referral: in an open manner, with full explanation of the problem to the patient and the referral appointment made while the patient is still in the office.

Schwartz MA, Wiggins OP: Systems and the structuring of meaning: Contributions to a biopsychosocial medicine. *Am J Psychiat* 1986;**143**:1213.
Wallen J et al: Psychiatric consultations in short-term general hospitals. *Arch Gen Psychiat* 1987;**44**:163.

## MEDICAL APPROACHES

### 1. ANTIPSYCHOTIC DRUGS (Neuroleptics, "Major Tranquilizers")

This group of drugs includes **phenothiazines** and **thioxanthenes** (both similar in structure), **butyrophenones, dihydroindolones,** and **dibenzoxazepines.** Table 17–1 lists the drugs in order of increasing milligram potency and decreasing side effects (with the exception of extrapyramidal symptoms). Thus, chlorpromazine has lower milligram potency and causes more severe side effects and fewer extrapyramidal complications than fluphenazine.

The phenothiazines comprise the bulk of the currently used neuroleptic drugs. The only butyrophenone commonly used in the USA is haloperidol, which

**Table 17–1.** Commonly used antipsychotics.

| | Chlor-proma-zine Ratio | Usual Daily Oral Dose | Usual Daily Maximum Dose* |
|---|---|---|---|
| **Phenothiazines** | | | |
| Chlorpromazine (Thorazine and other trade names) | 1:1 | 100–400 mg | 1 g |
| Thioridazine (Mellaril) | 1:1 | 100–400 mg | 600 mg |
| Mesoridazine (Serentil) | 1:2 | 50–200 mg | 400 mg |
| Perphenazine (Trilafon)† | 1:10 | 16–32 mg | 64 mg |
| Trifluoperazine (Stelazine)† | 1:20 | 5–15 mg | 60 mg |
| Fluphenazine (Permitil, Prolixin)† | 1:50 | 2–10 mg | 60 mg |
| **Thioxanthenes** | | | |
| Chlorprothixene (Taractan) | 1:1 | 100–400 mg | 600 mg |
| Thiothixene† (Navane) | 1:20 | 5–10 mg | 80 mg |
| **Butyrophenone** | | | |
| Haloperidol (Haldol) | 1:50 | 2–5 mg | 80 mg |
| **Dihydroindolone** | | | |
| Molindone (Moban) | 1:12 | 30–100 mg | 225 mg |
| **Dibenzoxazepine** | | | |
| Loxapine (Loxitane) | 1:10 | 20–60 mg | 200 mg |

* Can be higher in some cases.
† Indicates piperazine structure.

is totally different in structure but very similar in action and extrapyramidal side effects to the piperazine phenothiazines such as fluphenazine, perphenazine, and trifluoperazine. Haloperidol has a paucity of autonomic side effects, markedly lowers hyperactivity and psychotic ideation, and is particularly effective in movement disorders such as those seen in Gilles de la Tourette's syndrome. Molindone and loxapine are similar in action, side effects, and safety to the piperazine phenothiazines.

None of the antipsychotics produce true physical dependency, and they have a wide safety margin between therapeutic and toxic effects. All are efficacious in ameliorating psychotic symptoms. Previous response and experience with the drug and its side effects dictate the choice of a drug.

## Clinical Indications

The antipsychotics are used to treat the **schizophrenias** and **psychotic ideation in organic brain psychoses, psychotic depression, mania,** and **other psychoses.** They are effective in drug-induced psychoses such as psychedelic abuse and stimulant psychosis. They quickly lower the arousal (activity) level and, perhaps indirectly, gradually improve socialization and thinking.

Symptoms that are ameliorated by these drugs include hyperactivity, hostility, delusions, hallucinations, irritability, and poor sleep. Individuals with acute psychosis and good premorbid function respond quite well. The most common cause of failure in the treatment of acute psychosis is inadequate dosage, and the most common cause of relapse is noncompliance. *A simple regimen, preferably one dose given at bedtime, is usually the most effective plan.*

## Dosage Forms & Patterns

The dosage range is quite broad. For example, haloperidol, 1 mg orally at bedtime, may be sufficient for the elderly person with a mild organic brain syndrome, whereas 60 mg/d may be used in a young schizophrenic patient. For this reason, it is misleading to depend on static dosage levels. Haloperidol, 10 mg intramuscularly, is quite effective in the very active patient, particularly in mania, acute delirium, or acute schizophrenic disorder. Psychomotor agitation, racing thoughts, and auditory hallucinations are the symptoms most responsive to this initial treatment. Intramuscular medication is absorbed rapidly and uniformly. It achieves an initial 10-fold plasma level advantage over equal oral doses. This advantage levels off after 24 hours of haloperidol administration, and oral doses are then usually quite effective. Observe the response, and repeat the dose every 2–3 hours until the patient is under control. Most patients will not require more than 50 mg in a 24-hour period. The use of a benzodiazepine to diminish agitation may permit lower doses of neuroleptics. The potency of intramuscular administration is 1½ times that of the oral form. The onset of action occurs in 30 minutes.

The philosophy of administration of these drugs is similar to that which governs the use of insulin in acute diabetic coma. Insulin is given until the glucose level approaches normal. In the acute psychotic patient, the antipsychotic drug is given until behavior becomes as near normal as possible. After the acute diabetic situation is resolved, insulin is titrated to maintain a reasonable glucose level, and patients vary widely in their required dosage. After the acute psychiatric situation is resolved, the psychiatric patient will require *only enough medication* to help maintain reasonable behavior. In the case of the chronic schizophrenic patient—like the brittle diabetic patient—the drugs may be required indefinitely and on a varying dosage schedule related to the patient's needs. Plasma drug levels are not of major clinical assistance at this time.

The principal side effects are extrapyramidal reactions. Antiparkinsonism drugs usually need not be used prophylactically, particularly with the low-potency antipsychotic drugs. Most patients taking *depot* neuroleptic drugs will require ongoing treatment with antiparkinsonism agents.

Loxapine may have some advantage for schizophrenic patients who are also severely depressed, since it is metabolized partially to amoxapine (an antidepressant drug).

In most cases, oral medications are adequate. The concentrate is best absorbed, the tablet next best. Various factors play a role in the absorption of oral medications. Of particular importance are previous gastrointestinal surgery and concomitant administration of other drugs, eg, antacids (Table 17–2). There are racial differences in metabolizing these drugs— eg, many Asians require only about half the usual dosage. Bioavailability is influenced by other factors such as microsomal stimulation with alcohol or barbiturates and enzyme-altering drugs such as carbamazepine or methylphenidate.

Divided daily doses are not necessary after a main-

**Table 17–2.** Antipsychotic drug interactions with other drugs.

| Drug | Effects |
|------|---------|
| Antacids | Decreased absorption of antipsychotic drugs. |
| All anticholinergics | Increased anticholinergic effects. |
| Barbiturates | Central nervous system depression and decreased antipsychotic drug levels. |
| Carbamazepine | Decreased haloperidol levels. |
| Cyclic antidepressants | Increased antidepressant blood levels. |
| Guanadrel | Increased hypotensive effect. |
| Guanethidine | Decreased hypotensive effect. |
| Indomethacin | Severe drowsiness (with haloperidol). |
| Levodopa | Decreased antiparkinson effect. |
| Methyldopa | Decreased hypotensive effect. |
| Phenytoin | Increased phenytoin levels. |
| Propranolol | Increased thioridazine levels. |
| Thiazide diuretics | Increased hypotensive effect. |
| Trihexyphenidyl | Decreased antipsychotic levels. |

tenance dose has been established, and most patients can then be maintained on a single daily dose, usually taken at bedtime. This is particularly appropriate in a case where the sedative effect of the drug is desired for nighttime sleep, and undesirable sedative effects can be avoided during the day. Costs of medication, nursing time, and patient unreliability are reduced when either a single daily dose or a large bedtime/smaller morning dose schedule is utilized.

Psychiatric patients—particularly paranoid individuals—often neglect to take their medication. In these cases, the enanthate and decanoate (the latter is slightly longer lasting and has fewer extrapyramidal side effects) forms of fluphenazine or the decanoate form of haloperidol may be given subcutaneously or intramuscularly to achieve an effect that will usually last 7–28 days. A patient who cannot be depended on to take oral medication (or who overdoses on minimal provocation) will generally agree to come to the physician's office for a "shot." The usual dose of the fluphenazine long-acting preparations is 25 mg (1 mL) every 2 weeks. Dosage and frequency of administration vary from about 100 mg weekly to 12.5 mg monthly. Use the smallest amount as infrequently as possible. A biweekly injection of 25 mg of fluphenazine decanoate is equivalent to about 15–20 mg of oral fluphenazine daily.

Intravenous use of haloperidol (the only neuroleptic used in this manner) is reserved for special situations (eg, severely burned patients, postsurgical agitation).

## Side Effects

The side effects *decrease* as one goes from the sedating, lower milligram potency drugs such as chlorpromazine to those of higher milligram potency such as fluphenazine and haloperidol (Table 17–1). However, the extrapyramidal effects *increase* as one goes down the list (consider chlorprothixene as similar to chlorpromazine).

The most common side effects occur with use of low-potency drugs. Anticholinergic effects include dry mouth, blurred vision, urinary retention (particularly in elderly men with enlarged prostates), delayed gastric emptying, ileus, and precipitation of acute glaucoma in patients with narrow anterior chamber angles. Other autonomic effects include orthostatic hypotension, impotence, and inhibition of ejaculation. Cardiac arrhythmias may occur frequently as electrocardiographic findings and less frequently as clinical conditions, usually in the elderly. Thioridazine, which has the fewest extrapyramidal side effects, has the most cardiac effects. One should avoid the concomitant use of thioridazine and sympathomimetic drugs. The most frequently seen electrocardiographic changes include diminution of the T wave amplitude, appearance of prominent U waves, depression of the ST segment, and prolongation of the QT interval. These electrocardiographic findings do not alter treatment.

Metabolic and endocrine effects include weight gain, hyperglycemia, infrequent temperature irregularities (particularly in hot weather), and water intoxication that may be due to inappropriate antidiuretic hormone function. Lactation and menstrual irregularities are common, as are problems in achieving erection, ejaculation (including retrograde ejaculation), and orgasm in males (approximately 50% of cases) and orgasm in females (approximately 30%). Delay in achieving orgasm is sometimes a factor in medication noncompliance. Both antipsychotic and antidepressant drugs inhibit sperm motility. Bone marrow depression and cholestatic jaundice occur rarely; these are sensitivity reactions, and they usually appear in the first 2 months of treatment. They subside on discontinuance of the drug. There is cross-sensitivity among all of the phenothiazines, and a drug from a different group must be used when allergic reactions occur.

Photosensitivity (including retinal effects) is commonly related to chlorpromazine use. Retinopathy and hyperpigmentation are associated with use of fairly high dosages of chlorpromazine and thioridazine. The appearance of particulate melanin deposits in the lens of the eye is related to the total dose given, and patients on long-term medication should have periodic eye examinations. Teratogenicity has not been causally related to these drugs, but prudence is indicated in the first trimester of pregnancy. The seizure threshold is lowered, particularly in older patients taking higher dosages. It is safe to use these medications in epileptics controlled by anticonvulsants.

The **neuroleptic malignant syndrome** of extrapyramidal signs, blood pressure changes, altered consciousness, and hyperpyrexia is an uncommon but serious complication of neuroleptic treatment. Rigidity, involuntary movements, confusion, dysarthria, and dysphagia are accompanied by pallor, cardiovascular instability, fever, pulmonary congestion, and diaphoresis and may result in stupor, coma, and death. The cause may be related to a number of factors, including poor dosage control of neuroleptic medication and increased sensitivity of dopamine receptor sites. It may occur very rapidly and with small doses of neuroleptic drugs. Dantrolene, 50 mg every 12 hours, has been of some value in the treatment of this condition. Bromocriptine mesylate, 2.5–15 mg 3 times a day, has been reported to be effective over a 10-day period, as has amantadine, 100 mg orally twice daily. None of the treatments are wholly satisfactory.

**Extrapyramidal symptoms. Akathisia** is the most common (about 20%) so-called extrapyramidal symptom. It occurs early in treatment (but may persist after neuroleptics are discontinued) and is frequently mistaken for anxiety or exacerbation of psychosis. It is characterized by a subjective desire to be in constant motion followed by an inability or sit or stand still and consequent pacing. It may include feelings of fright, rage, terror, or sexual torment. Insomnia is often present. In all cases, reevaluate the dosage requirement of the neuroleptic drug. Antiparkinsonism drugs such as trihexyphenidyl, 2–5 mg orally 3 times daily, or benztropine mesylate, 1–2 mg twice daily, may be helpful. There are increasing reports of the abuse of the antiparkinsonism agents (see Substance Use Disorders, below). In resistant cases, propranolol, 30–80 mg orally daily, diazepam, 5 mg 3 times daily, or amantadine, 100 mg orally 3 times daily, may alleviate the symptoms. Patients whose behavioral symptoms worsen with use of antipsychotic drugs may have an undiagnosed organic condition.

**Acute dystonias** are often of sudden onset early in treatment and most commonly produce bizarre muscle spasms of the head, neck, and tongue. Frequently present are torticollis, oculogyric crises, swallowing difficulties, and masseter spasms. The back, arm, or leg muscles are occasionally affected. Diphenhydramine, 50 mg intramuscularly, is effective for the acute crisis; then give benztropine mesylate, 2 mg twice daily, or biperiden, 2 mg 3 times daily, for several weeks; then discontinue gradually, since few of the extrapyramidal symptoms require long-term use of the antiparkinsonism drugs (all of which are about equally efficacious), although trihexyphenidyl tends to be mildly stimulating and benztropine mildly sedating. Neuroleptic-induced catatonia is similar to catatonic stupor with rigidity, drooling, urinary incontinence, and cogwheeling. It usually responds slowly to withdrawal of the offending medication and use of antiparkinsonism agents.

**Drug-induced parkinsonism** is indistinguishable from idiopathic parkinsonism, but it occurs later in treatment than the preceding extrapyramidal symptoms. The condition includes the typical signs of apathy and reduction of facial and arm movements (akinesia, which can mimic depression), festinating gait, rigidity, loss of postural reflexes, and the pill-rolling tremor. This extrapyramidal symptom also responds to the aforementioned antiparkinsonism drugs in the same dosages. After 4–6 weeks, these drugs can often be discontinued with no recurrent symptoms. In any of the extrapyramidal symptoms, amantadine, 100–400 mg daily, may be used instead of the antiparkinsonism drugs if anticholinergic effects are a problem. Anticholinergic toxicity is characterized by impaired attention and short-term memory, disorientation, anxiety, visual and auditory hallucinations, and other psychotic ideation. Physostigmine, 2–4 mg intramuscularly, can reverse this central anticholinergic organic mental state.

**Tardive dyskinesia** is a syndrome of abnormal involuntary stereotyped movements of the face, mouth, tongue, trunk, and limbs that may occur after months or (usually) years of treatment with neuroleptic agents. The syndrome affects 15–20% of patients who have undergone long-term neuroleptic therapy.

Early manifestations include fine wormlike movements of the tongue at rest, difficulty in sticking out the tongue, facial tics, increased blink frequency, or jaw movements of recent onset. Later manifestations may include bucco-linguo-masticatory movements, lip smacking, chewing motions, mouth opening and closing, disturbed gag reflex, puffing of the cheeks, disrupted speech, respiratory distress, or choreoathetoid movements of the extremities (the last being more prevalent in younger patients).

Early signs of dyskinesia must be differentiated from those reversible signs produced by ill-fitting dentures or nonneuroleptic drugs such as levodopa, tricyclic antidepressants, antiparkinsonism agents, anticonvulsants, and antihistamines. Other neurologic conditions such as Huntington's chorea can be differentiated by history and examination.

The incidence of tardive dyskinesia increases with age (3 times more common in patients over 40). Brain damage is said to be predisposing, although conclusive studies are lacking. It is estimated that approximately 25% of neuroleptic-treated patients with an abnormal movement disorder develop the disorder owing to reasons other than drug therapy. There may be other predisposing factors (eg, nicotine exposure) not proved at this time. Such factors may explain why some patients develop the dyskinesia after only a few months of medication while others never do. There may also be subgroups of dyskinesias that are not yet well defined.

The dyskinesias do not occur during sleep and can be voluntarily suppressed for short periods. Stress and movements in other parts of the body will often aggravate the condition. Tardive dyskinesia is not alleviated by antiparkinsonism agents and may be worsened by them. There is concern that the chronic use of antiparkinsonism drugs may contribute to the development of the dyskinesia, either by masking early signs or by altering neurochemical balance, but this has not been proved. *There is no known difference among any of the antipsychotic drugs in the development of this syndrome.* There is a correlation between the incidence of tardive dyskinesia and interruption of drug therapy; thus, the concept of drug holidays as a beneficial treatment plan is in doubt.

At present, the emphasis is on prevention. When the tardive dyskinesic syndrome is first noted, stop all anticholinergic drugs and gradually discontinue all neuroleptic drugs if possible. In about one-third of cases, symptoms will gradually disappear over several months. In cases that do not improve with discontinuation of the antipsychotic drugs and those in which psychotic symptoms necessitate the use of neuroleptics, a rauwolfia derivative such as reserpine can be given instead. This is an effective antipsychotic agent and does not produce the dyskinetic symptoms, although the depressive and gastrointestinal side effects limit usage. There is evidence that the benzodiazepines may alleviate the syndrome through their action on the GABA neurotransmitter system. Pure lecithin, lithium, propranolol, clonidine, and sodium valproate have been helpful only in a limited number of cases. In some cases, one must weigh the advantages against the side effects, and—with the consent of the patient—continue the antipsychotic drug therapy at the lowest therapeutic dosage that produces stabilization or remission of the dyskinesia.

Guze BH, Baxter LR Jr: Current concepts: Neuroleptic malignant syndrome. *N Engl J Med* 1985;**313**:163.

Lake CR (editor): Symposium on clinical pharmacology. (2 parts.) *Psychiatr Clin North Am* 1984;**7**:409, 655. [Two entire issues.]

Ortiz A, Gershon S: The future of neuroleptic psychopharmacology. *J Clin Psychiatry* 1986;**47(5–Suppl)**:3.

Simpson GM, Pi EH, Stramek JJ: An update on tardive dyskinesia. *Hosp Commun Psychiat* 1986;**37**:362.

Yassa R et al: Nicotine exposure and tardive dyskinesia. *Biol Psychiat* 1987;**22**:67.

## 2. LITHIUM

The use of lithium over the last 4 decades has dramatically affected both diagnosis and treatment in psychiatry. The discovery of lithium's effectiveness in affective disorders has shown that many of these patients were erroneously diagnosed as having a schizophrenic disorder. It has also become evident that some alcohol-dependent individuals have affective disorders and can be successfully treated with lithium. This has led to further research on a number of poorly defined and treated conditions, including aggressive states, movement disorders, drug dependencies, and organic brain syndromes.

### Clinical Indications

As a prophylactic drug for bipolar affective disorder, lithium significantly decreases the frequency and severity of both manic and depressive attacks in about 80% of patients. A positive response is more predictable if the patient has a low frequency of episodes (no more than 2 per year with intervals free of psychopathology). A positive response occurs more frequently in individuals who have blood relatives with a diagnosis of manic or hypomanic attacks. Patients who swing rapidly back and forth between manic and depressive attacks (at least 4 cycles per year) usually respond poorly to lithium prophylaxis initially, but some improve with continued long-term treatment. Carbamazepine has been used with some success in this group.

Acute manic or hypomanic symptoms will respond to lithium therapy, but it is common to use neuroleptic drugs to treat the excited or psychotic manic stage (as outlined in the treatment of the psychoses) and then make a decision with the patient and family about the feasibility of long-term prophylactic lithium therapy. The decision is usually based on the severity of the condition. Schizoaffective disorders and some cases of schizophrenia are probably atypical bipolar affective disorder, for which lithium treatment may be effective.

Lithium alone and combined with cyclic antidepressants in the acute phases is useful in the prophylaxis of some recurrent unipolar depressions (perhaps undiagnosed bipolar disorder). Its use in the treatment of acute depression is not warranted except in depressions occurring in a bipolar patient who has previously responded to the drug and in cases that have not responded to antidepressant drugs. Lithium is compatible with other commonly used psychotherapeutic drugs, although the concomitant use of an antipsychotic drug may worsen lithium toxicity. Lithium is not effective in primary alcoholism, sedative abuse, hyperkinesis, or obsessive compulsive neurosis unless there is an underlying primary affective disorder. Most patients with bipolar disease can be managed with lithium alone, though some will require continued or intermittent use of a neuroleptic or antidepressant medication.

### Dosage Forms & Patterns

Lithium carbonate (Eskalith, Lithane, Lithobid, Lithonate, Lithotabs) is available in the USA in 300-mg capsules. Although lithium citrate liquid is available, capsules are usually preferred because they are associated with less nausea and less metallic taste. Tablets (Lithotabs), which can be broken, are used in patients requiring a more exact dosage than a multiple of 300 mg. Side effects can be mitigated by taking the drug with food or by use of Lithobid (slow release). Lithium citrate is available as a syrup for patients in whom compliance is a problem. The dosage is that required to maintain blood levels in the therapeutic range. For acute attacks this ranges from 1 to 1.6 meq/L, whereas the prophylactic dose is usually 0.4–1 meq/L. Maintenance levels should be kept as low as clinically feasible. The dose required to meet this need will vary in individuals and should be determined by giving a test dose of 600 mg of lithium carbonate after the clinical workup, which should include a medical history and physical examination; complete blood count; $T_4$, TSH, blood urea nitrogen, creatinine, and electrolyte determinations; urinalysis; and ECG. Twenty-four hours after the administration of the test dose, a blood sample is drawn for lithium determination. (See Table 17–3 for dosage requirements based on a test dose.) The usual practice is to administer lithium in the most convenient way, with a minimum of side effects. There is no evidence that once-a-day dosage is deleterious, but some patients have less nausea when they take the drug in divided doses with meals.

**Table 17–3.** Predicted lithium daily dosage necessary to produce therapeutic levels. (Based on 600-mg test dose.)

| 24-h Lithium Level (meq/L) | Total Daily Dose (mg) |
|---|---|
| <0.05 | 3600 |
| 0.05–0.09 | 2700 |
| 0.10–0.14 | 1800 |
| 0.15–0.19 | 1200 |
| 0.20–0.23 | 900 |
| 0.24–0.30 | 600 |
| >0.30 | 300 |

Lithium is readily absorbed, with peak serum levels occurring within 1–3 hours and complete absorption in 8 hours. Half of the total body lithium is excreted in 18–24 hours (95% in the urine). *The blood for the lithium levels should be drawn 12 hours after the last dose.* Serum levels should be measured every 1–3 weeks in the early maintenance stage and thereafter when clinically indicated, particularly when there is any condition that may lower sodium levels (eg, diarrhea; dehydration; use of diuretics). Patients receiving lithium should use diuretics with caution and only under close medical supervision. The thiazide diuretics cause increased lithium reabsorption from the proximal renal tubules, resulting in increased serum lithium levels (Table 17–4), and adjustment of lithium intake must be made to compensate for this. Reduce lithium dosage by 25–40% when the patient is receiving 50 mg of hydrochlorothiazide daily. Potassium-sparing diuretics (spironolactone, amiloride, triamterene) may also cause increased serum lithium levels and require careful monitoring of lithium levels. Loop diuretics (furosemide, ethacrynic acid, bumetanide) appear not to alter serum lithium levels.

### Side Effects

**A. Early Side Effects:** Mild gastrointestinal symptoms (take lithium with food), fine tremors (treat with propranolol, 20–60 mg/d orally, only if persistent), slight muscle weakness, and some degree of somnolence are early side effects that are usually transient. Moderate polyuria (reduced renal responsiveness to antidiuretic hormone) and polydipsia (associated with increased plasma renin concentration) are occasionally present. Weight gain (often a result of calories in fluids taken for polydipsia) and leukocytosis are fairly common.

**B. Lithium Toxicity:** Frank toxicity usually occurs at blood levels above 2 meq/L. This is often a result of sodium loss or kidney disease, since sodium and lithium are reabsorbed at the same loci in the proximal renal tubules. Any sodium loss such as that which occurs with diarrhea, use of diuretics, or excessive perspiration results in increased lithium levels.

**Table 17–4.** Lithium interactions with other drugs.

| Drug | Effects |
|---|---|
| Ibuprofen | Increased lithium levels. |
| Indomethacin | Increased lithium levels. |
| Iodine | Enhanced goitrogenic effect. |
| Methyldopa | Rigidity, mutism, fascicular twitching. |
| Osmotic diuretics (urea, mannitol) | Increased lithium excretion. |
| Phenylbutazone | Increased lithium levels. |
| Potassium-sparing diuretics (spironolactone, amiloride, triamterene) | Increased lithium levels. |
| Sodium bicarbonate | Increased lithium excretion. |
| Succinylcholine | Increased succinylcholine duration of action. |
| Theophylline, aminophylline | Increased lithium excretion. |
| Thiazide diuretics | Increased lithium levels. |

Symptoms and signs include vomiting and diarrhea, the latter exacerbating the problem since more sodium is lost. Other signs and symptoms include tremors, marked muscle weakness, confusion, dysarthria, vertigo, ataxia, hyperreflexia, rigidity, seizures, opisthotonos, and coma. Toxicity is higher in the elderly, who should be maintained on slightly lower serum levels. Lithium overdosage may be accidental or intentional or may occur as a result of poor monitoring. Compliance with lithium therapy is adversely affected by the loss of some hypomanic experiences valued by the patient. These include social extroversion and a sense of heightened enjoyment in many activities such as sex and business dealings, often with increased productivity in the latter.

**C. Other Side Effects:** These include weight gain, goiter (3%; often euthyroid), occasionally hypothyroidism (5%; concomitant administration of lithium and iodide enhances the hypothyroid and goitrogenic effect of either drug), changes in the glucose tolerance test toward a diabeticlike curve, nephrogenic diabetes intipiders, edema, pseudotumor cerebri (do funduscopy if there are complaints of headache or blurred vision), and leukocytosis. Thyroid and kidney function should be checked at 3- to 6-month intervals. Most of these side effects subside when lithium is discontinued; when residual side effects exist, they are usually not serious. Most clinicians treat lithium-induced hypothyroidism (more common in women) with thyroid hormone while continuing lithium therapy. Hypercalcemia and elevated parathyroid hormone levels occur in some patients. Electrocardiographic abnormalities (principally T wave flattening or inversion) may occur during lithium administration but are not of major clinical significance. Sinoatrial block may occur, particularly in the elderly. It is important that other drugs which prolong intraventricular conduction, such as tricyclic antidepressants, be used with caution in conjunction with lithium. Lithium impairs ventilatory function in patients with airway obstruction. Lithium may precipitate or exacerbate psoriasis in some patients. Patients receiving long-term lithium therapy may have cogwheel rigidity and, occasionally, other extrapyramidal signs. Lithium potentiates the parkinsonian effects of haloperidol. A wide variety of neurologic sequelae have been reported; most remit quickly when lithium therapy is discontinued.

The long-term use of lithium has adverse effects on renal function (with interstitial fibrosis, tubular atrophy, and glomerulosclerosis) in some patients that are not always completely reversible. A rise in serum creatinine levels is an indication for indepth evaluation of renal function. Incontinence has been reported in women, apparently related to changes in bladder cholinergic-adrenergic balance. Lithium increases parathyroid hormone levels, with increased serum calcium and decreased serum phosphate. Long-term lithium therapy has also been associated with a relative lowering of the level of memory and perceptual processing (affecting compliance in some cases). Some impairment of attention and emotional reactivity has also been noted. Lithium-induced delirium with therapeutic lithium levels is an infrequent complication and often persists for several days after serum levels have become negligible. Encephalopathy has occurred in patients on combined lithium/neuroleptic therapy.

Lithium exposure in early pregnancy increases the frequency of congenital anomalies, with a marked shift toward major cardiovascular anomalies. *It is advisable for women using lithium either to avoid pregnancy or to not use lithium at all during a planned pregnancy, particularly during the first trimester.* If there has been exposure in the first trimester, especially between the eighth and twelfth weeks, the possibility of teratogenic defect is highest. Bottle-feeding should be considered in mothers using lithium, since concentration in breast milk is one-third to one-half that in serum.

Patients with massive ingestions of lithium or levels above 3 meq/L should be treated with induced emesis and gastric lavage. In normal renal function, osmotic and saline diuresis increases renal lithium clearance. Urinary alkalinization is also helpful, since sodium bicarbonate decreases lithium reabsorption in the proximal tubule, as does acetazolamide also. Aminophylline potentiates the diuretic effect by increasing the glomerular filtration rate of lithium. Drugs affecting the distal loop have no effect on lithium reabsorption. In exceptional cases, hemodialysis and peritoneal dialysis decrease plasma concentration; this gradually shortens recovery time.

Mander AJ: Is lithium justified after one manic episode? *Acta Psychiatr Scand* 1986;**73**:60.

Swartz CM: Correction of lithium levels for dose and blood sampling times. *J Clin Psychiat* 1987;**48**:60.

## 3. ANTIDEPRESSANT DRUGS
### (Table 17–5)

The antidepressant drugs are classified into 3 groups: (1) the tricyclic antidepressants—the mainstay of therapy for over 20 years; (2) the monoamine oxidase (MAO) inhibitors, which have become less popular in recent years because their use imposes certain dietary restrictions; and (3) the cyclic—so-called new-generation—antidepressants, which are achieving widespread use mainly because they cause fewer anticholinergic side effects.

### Clinical Indications

Antidepressant drugs are indicated for severe depression of any type, but particularly the major affective disorders. Some of the drugs—especially the tricyclics—are effective in enuresis, catalepsy, chronic pain syndromes, attention deficit disorders, and peptic disease. Certain symptoms of depression signify a positive response to drug therapy—ie, vegetative signs of sleep disturbances, anorexia and weight loss, and ruminations and feelings of hopelessness and guilt.

Drug selection depends on specific symptoms and side effects. If there is no dominant symptom (such as sleeplessness, calling for a sedating drug such as amitriptyline), a tricyclic such as desipramine is a reasonable choice. If the dominant symptom is anxiety or if unpleasant anticholinergic side effects must be

**Table 17–5.** Commonly used antidepressants.

| | Usual Daily Oral Dose (mg) | Usual Daily Maximum Dose (mg) | Sedative Effects* | Anticholinergic Effects* | Serotonin Uptake* | Norepinephrine Uptake* |
|---|---|---|---|---|---|---|
| **Tricyclic compounds** | | | | | | |
| Amitriptyline | 150–200 | 300 | 4 | 4 | 4 | 0 |
| Amoxapine | 150–200 | 400 | 2 | 2 | 1 | 4 |
| Desipramine | 150–200 | 300 | 1 | 1 | 0 | 4 |
| Doxepin | 150–200 | 300 | 4 | 3 | 1 | 1 |
| Imipramine | 150–200 | 300 | 3 | 3 | 3 | 2 |
| Nortriptyline | 100–150 | 200 | 2 | 3 | 2 | 2 |
| Protriptyline | 15–40 | 60 | 1 | 2 | — | — |
| Trimipramine | 75–150 | 200 | 4 | 4 | — | — |
| **Monoamine oxidase inhibitors** | | | | | | |
| Isocarboxazid | 10–20 | 50 | — | — | — | — |
| Phenelzine | 45–60 | 90 | — | — | — | — |
| Tranylcypromine | 20 | 50 | — | — | — | — |
| **New cyclic compounds** | | | | | | |
| Maprotiline | 150–200 | 300 | 4 | 1 | 0 | 4 |
| Trazodone | 200–400 | 600 | 4 | 1 | 4 | 1 |

* 4 = strong effect; 1 = weak effect; 0 = no effect.

avoided, trazodone, one of the MAO inhibitors, or alprazolam can be used. For patients with atypical depression characterized by excessive sleepiness and voracious appetite but little agitation and marked signs of social withdrawal, an MAO inhibitor may be the initial drug of choice.

There has been an attempt to relate subgroups of depression to variations in neurotransmitter metabolism, but it is not yet clinically feasible to select antidepressant drugs on this basis.

If, after an adequate trial (see below), the patient does not respond to a given drug, one must consider switching to a drug with a different neurotransmitter effect (Table 17–5). One may rapidly decrease the dosage of the ineffective drug (eg, desipramine) while giving the new drug (eg, amitriptyline) in increasing doses and then continuing for an adequate trial period. If this does not work, one should consider the use of an MAO inhibitor. (It is common practice to stop the tricyclic drug and wait for a week before starting the MAO inhibitor. Combined therapy with both drugs is used by some physicians experienced in the technique when the patient can be closely monitored.)

Alprazolam has been used successfully in some cases of depression, particularly in patients with severe anxiety or those (eg, elderly patients) unable to tolerate the side effects of the tricylics.

Although lithium is used chiefly in bipolar disorder, a number of reports have been published claiming success with lithium in treating major depression without mania. In cases of depression unresponsive to other drugs, lithium alone or in combination with an antidepressant drug may be effective (see Affective Disorders, below).

## Dosage Forms & Patterns

The tricyclic antidepressants are characterized more by their similarities than by their differences. Side effects and neurotransmitter activity of these drugs are outlined in Table 17–5. The dosages tend to be quite similar, except for protriptyline and trazodone. The newer cyclic antidepressants are generally about as effective as the tricyclic drugs; side effects and time of onset of action may differ. Side effects dictate the choice of drug.

The lag in clinical response may be as much as several weeks; however, the side effects of these drugs limit the clinician's ability to increase the dosage rapidly. One can use perphenazine in small doses (4–8 mg daily) to block hydroxylation and boost antidepressant blood levels more rapidly than by increasing dosage alone. The lag time is apparently related to delays in achieving therapeutic blood levels and the interval required to affect neurotransmitter systems. Even though they receive similar dosages, individuals vary considerably (up to 30-fold) in concentration of the drug in plasma. Plasma level determinations of the antidepressant drugs can be clinically useful. There is a consistent relationship between clinical response and plasma levels in some of the antidepressants studied. For example, nortriptyline is most

effective if the plasma levels are between 50 and 150 ng/mL. Imipramine has the best clinical response if plasma levels are about 200–250 ng/mL. Desipramine shows maximal response at about 125 ng/mL. The indications for the test in most cases would be nonresponse to therapeutic doses and high-risk medical patients in whom dosages should be kept as low as possible. Adsorption plays a role in the blood level of these drugs, and patients who have had gastrointestinal surgery often have lower levels. Early responses include relief of both anxiety and insomnia. Even though the patient may state that the depression has not lifted, there is usually increased energy and less preoccupation with somatic concerns in the first several weeks of therapy. Mood depression and sexual dysfunction, which are side effects of the drugs, are often the last problems to be relieved.

The 2 most common reasons for clinical failure in the treatment of depression are (1) poor selection of treatable depressions and (2) inadequate trial of medication (including noncompliance, which is frequently related to poor instruction about side effects). *An adequate trial includes adequate dosages over an appropriate period of time.* Usually, treatment starts with a moderate dose (eg, desipramine, 100 mg at bedtime) that is increased by 25–50 mg every several days depending on the side effects and the clinical response to maximum doses. (See Table 17–5.) The drug should be tried for several weeks at maximum doses (300 mg/d) before it is considered a failure. The elderly require small doses. Many patients respond when the dosage is in the range of 150–200 mg. Once clinical relief of symptoms is achieved, the dosage is maintained for several months, and thereafter the drug is given in the lowest effective dose for as long as the depression continues. This involves a gradual downward adjustment of the dosage until the patient requires no medication—a process that usually takes 6 or more months from the start of the depression. Sudden withdrawal of the medication may result in gastrointestinal symptoms or sleep disturbances with vivid dreams; movement disorders and hyperactivity rarely occur on withdrawal. *Some patients will require medication for considerably longer periods.* Patients with bipolar affective disorders respond best to lithium, whereas the recurrent major depressive disorders respond better to antidepressants. Patients with bipolar disorders are at higher risk for precipitation of the manic phase when taking a tricyclic antidepressant; the manic phase usually occurs within 12 weeks of the onset of therapy. Bipolar patients also tend to cycle more rapidly when treated with tricyclic antidepressants. Either of these occurrences should alert the physician to possible bipolar illness, and the patient should be evaluated for lithium treatment. Maintenance dosages of tricyclic antidepressants are usually one-half to one-third the amount needed by the individual for treatment of an acute episode.

Except for some early adjustments, it is not necessary to use divided doses of antidepressants: a single dose at bedtime is adequate (particularly when the clinician takes advantage of the sedative side effects to help treat associated insomnia). Trazodone, amitriptyline, and doxepin are the most sedating of the antidepressants. The bedtime dose helps achieve compliance, since people tend to take drugs at bedtime and not during the day. Frightening dreams can be alleviated by using divided doses.

Essentially the same procedures apply to the use of the monoamine oxidase inhibitors. There is less lag time and a narrower range of dosages, so that therapeutic levels are more quickly achieved. With these drugs it is vital to instruct patients about dietary restrictions (see Side Effects, below). Combined antipsychotic-antidepressant drug therapy is needed only in unusual cases, and in those instances, the fixed dosage of the commercial combinations is a disadvantage. Amoxapine, which has a relatively rapid onset of action, has some neuroleptic action and may be useful when mild psychotic symptoms are present. Triiodothyronine, 25–50 $\mu$g/d orally, is sometimes used to increase responsiveness to tricyclic antidepressants.

## Side Effects

The tricyclic and newer cyclic antidepressants have **anticholinergic effects** (highest in amitriptyline, lowest in trazodone), commonly including dry mouth (the most persistent side effect), blurred vision, constipation, and urinary retention to varying degrees, the worst occurring in men with prostatic hypertrophy. The anticholinergic effects predispose to other medical problems such as heat stroke or dental problems (xerostomia). Orthostatic hypotension occasionally occurs and may not remit with continued use of a drug (nortriptyline and desipramine produce less hypotension than most of the tricyclics). **Cardiac effects** of the tricyclic drugs include altered rate, rhythm, and contractility. The cardiac abnormality is a function of the anticholinergic effect, direct myocardial depression (quinidine effect), and interference with adrenergic neurons. As one might expect, the incidence of clinical abnormalities secondary to these drugs is significantly greater in patients with preexisting disease. Electrocardiographic changes range from benign ST segment and T wave changes and sinus tachycardia to a variety of complex and serious arrhythmias, the latter requiring a change in medication. The seizure threshold is lowered (particularly with maprotiline), and a patient will occasionally become psychotic. Loss of libido and decreased orgasm occur. Erectile and ejaculatory disturbances are fairly common. Anticholinergic side effects ameliorate with time. If intervention is warranted, a 1% solution of pilocarpine applied locally 3–4 times a day helps promote salivation if sugarless gum or candy is inadequate. Bethanechol, 10–30 mg orally 3 times a day, may help the urinary hesitation, and neostigimine, 7.5–15 mg orally 30 minutes prior to sexual activity, may help libido and retarded ejaculation. Photosensitivity is infrequent. Delirium, severe agitation, and mania are infrequent complications (occurring in about 10% of patients with bipolar disorder), as are extrapyramidal reactions similar to those caused by the phenothiazines (particularly amoxapine).

Monoamine oxidase inhibitor therapy can cause **sympathomimetic symptoms** of tachycardia, sweating, and tremor. The monoamine oxidase inhibitors frequently cause orthostatic hypotension. One advantage is the relative lack of anticholinergic effects, but nausea, insomnia, and sexual dysfunction are common. Weight gain is a common problem associated with the use of these drugs and is often related to a craving for sweets. **Central nervous system side effects** include agitation and toxic psychoses. Great care must be taken to avoid the ingestion of sympathomimetic amines, since the reduction of effective monoamine oxidase leaves the individual vulnerable to the effects of exogenous amines, including those foods containing tyramine, eg, liver of all types, sausage and bologna, aged cheeses (cream, cottage, and ricotta cheeses are permissible), pickled herring, concentrated yeast extract, Chinese pea pods, and English bean pods. Beer, ale, wines (particularly red wine and sherry), sardines, and anchovies contain varying amounts of tyramine. Avocados and overripe fruits are to be avoided. All stimulants should be avoided, including both prescribed and over-the-counter decongestants, most of which contain phenylpropanolamine. (See Table 17–6.) Treatment of a hypertensive crisis is the same as that for pheochromocytoma (see Chapter 18); give phentolamine, 1.2 mg intravenously every 5 minutes as needed to lower blood pressure.

Severe depression involves a high risk of suicide, and these groups of drugs have a narrow margin of safety in overdoses. Since most people who commit suicide with drugs take what is at hand, it is important that the amount of medication dispensed be less than the lethal dose, ie, less than a week's supply. Since the clinician will see the severely depressed patient frequently, the medication can be given at each visit, and the reasons for this can be discussed with the patient. Rather than being annoyed at this supposed lack of trust, most suicidal patients are relieved that the physician cares.

Overdoses of antidepressants are dangerous and must be considered a medical emergency. Major complications include coma with shock, respiratory depression, seizures, hyperpyrexia, smooth muscle paralysis, delirium, and severe cardiac arrhythmias. The drug should be removed from the gastrointestinal tract as soon as possible after insertion of a cuffed endotracheal tube if the patient is comatose. Ventilatory support should be provided. Shock is treated with fluids and hyperpyrexia by cooling techniques. Arterial blood gases and pH must be monitored for early correction of any abnormalities, particularly since these contribute to cardiac complications. Seizures should be treated with intravenous anticonvulsants. Cardiac complications are treated on the basis of electrocardiographic findings. Lidocaine is considered initial therapy for immediate control of ventricular arrhythmias due to tricyclic antidepressant overdose.

APA Symposium Proceedings: Beyond depression: New uses of antidepressants. *Psychosomatics* 1986;**27(11)**:[Entire issue.]

Frommer DA et al: Tricyclic antidepressant overdose: A review. *JAMA* 1987;**257**:521.

Pollack MH, Rosenbaum JF: Management of antidepressant-induced side effects: A practical guide for the clinician. *J Clin Psychiat* 1987;**48**:3.

Zisook S: A clinical overview of monoamine oxidase inhibitors. *Psychosomatics* 1985;**26**:240.

## 4. SEDATIVE-HYPNOTIC & OTHER ANTIANXIETY DRUGS
### (Anxiolytic Agents, "Minor Tranquilizers")

The sedatives are a heterogeneous group of drugs that differ in chemical structure but have quite similar pharmacologic and behavioral effects. They are often marketed as "minor tranquilizers" or "antianxiety agents," and all have hypnotic properties when given in adequate dosage. Ethanol is the most commonly used antianxiety drug. The various sedatives differ mainly in milligram potency, dose-response curves, and onset and duration of action. All are general depressants of brain function and decrease anxiety, producing disinhibition and a lowering of passive avoidance in sufficient dosage. To varying degrees, all have the potential for dependency with tolerance and severe withdrawal symptoms. Short-acting drugs may present a greater risk of withdrawal reactions than longer-acting agents. They are additive and have cross tolerance and cross dependence. Some have anticonvulsant and muscle relaxant properties, although muscle relaxation usually occurs in the ataxic dosage range.

The highly addicting drugs with a narrow margin of safety such as glutethimide, methaqualone, ethchlorvynol, methyprylon, meprobamate, and the barbiturates (with the exception of phenobarbital) should be avoided. Phenobarbital, in addition to its anticonvulsant properties, is a reasonably safe and very cheap sedative but has the disadvantage of enzyme stimulation (not the case with benzodiazepines), which markedly reduces its usefulness if any other medications are being used by the patient. Although its effect on dicumarol is the most widely known, it increases the catabolism of practically all other drugs, including antipsychotics and antidepressants.

The benzodiazepines are the latest in a long line of sedatives that were initially regarded as safe, effective, and not likely to cause dependency. However, like its predecessors, the benzodiazepine group has potential for abuse and complex metabolic actions. When ingested by themselves, these agents are safer than other drugs used in suicide attempts. Despite the fact that the "safer" benzodiazepines are replacing barbiturates for purposes of sedation, there has been no significant reduction in suicides caused by drugs.

**Table 17–6.** Antidepressant drug interactions with other drugs.

| Drug | Effects |
|---|---|
| **Tricyclic and cyclic antidepressants** | |
| Antacids | Decreased absorption of antidepressants. |
| Anticoagulants | Increased hypoprothrombinemic effect. |
| Cimetidine | Increased antidepressant blood levels. |
| Clonidine | Decreased antihypertensive effect. |
| Digitalis | Increased incidence of heart block. |
| Guanadrel | Decreased antihypertensive effect. |
| Guanethidine | Decreased antihypertensive effect. |
| Insulin | Decreased blood sugar. |
| Methyldopa | Decreased antihypertensive effect. |
| Other anticholinergic drugs | Marked anticholinergic responses. |
| Phenytoin | Increased blood levels. |
| Procainamide | Decreased ventricular conduction. |
| Procarbazine | Hypertensive crisis. |
| Propranolol | Increased hypotension. |
| Quinidine | Decreased ventricular conduction. |
| Rauwolfia derivatives | Increased stimulation. |
| Sedatives | Increased sedation. |
| Sympathomimetic drugs | Increased pressor effect. |
| **Monoamine oxidase inhibitors** | |
| Antihistamines | Increased sedation. |
| Belladonnalike drugs | Increased blood pressure. |
| Guanadrel | Increased blood pressure. |
| Guanethidine | Decreased blood pressure. |
| Insulin | Decreased blood sugar. |
| Levodopa | Increased blood pressure. |
| Meperidine | Increased mood lability, agitation, seizures. |
| Methyldopa | Decreased blood pressure. |
| Reserpine | Increased blood pressure and temperature. |
| Succinylcholine | Increased neuromuscular blockade. |
| Sulfonylureas | Decreased blood sugar. |
| Sympathomimetic drugs | Increased blood pressure. |

Furthermore, many attempted suicides involve not only multiple drug use but also alcohol. It is clear that carelessly dispensing drugs for obscure complaints and persistent patient demands is a part of the problem.

Onset of action varies, with diazepam and clorazepate being the most rapidly absorbed. This characteristic, along with high lipid solubility, may explain the popularity of diazepam. Halazepam and prazepam are the least rapidly absorbed. The length of action of the benzodiazepines varies as a function of the active metabolites they produce. Short-acting benzodiazepines, which do not produce active metabolites, have half-lives of 5–20 hours, and ultra–short-acting ones have half-lives of less than 5 hours. The other benzodiazepines produce active metabolites and have half-lives of 1–8 days. The long-acting sedatives are poorly absorbed when given intramuscularly, while the short-acting benzodiazepines are rapidly absorbed by this route. The antihistamines hydroxyzine and diphenhydramine are often prescribed for their sedative properties even though the effect is limited.

Buspirone is the only anxiolytic drug that is not a sedative. It is not believed to produce depressant effects or dependence. Abuse potential is thought to be low. Thus, it differs from the sedatives in that motor skills are not impaired and it does not potentiate the effects of alcohol or cause a withdrawal syndrome. Efficacy is apparently slightly less than that of the benzodiazepines.

## Clinical Indications

The sedatives are used clinically for the treatment of anxiety, which may be the result of many factors, eg, transient situational problems, acute and chronic stresses of life, chronic medical problems, intractable pain exacerbated by apprehension and depression, and problems that people cannot or will not resolve (unhappy marriages, unsatisfactory jobs, etc). In higher doses these drugs act as hypnotics. Whether the indications are anxiety or insomnia, the drugs should be used judiciously. There are no indications for sedatives that cannot be met by one of the benzodiazepines.

Clonazepam (Klonopin), approved in the USA as an oral benzodiazepine antiepileptic agent, has been found to be effective in a variety of other conditions. It is not used as a sedative (although it has sedative properties) but has been shown to be effective as an antimanic drug and in the treatment of panic attacks.

In the treatment of panic attacks, both alprazolam and clonazepam are effective. The other benzodiazepines are *not* considered adequate treatment for this disorder.

## Dosage Forms & Patterns
## (Table 17–7)

All of the sedatives may be given orally, and several are available in parenteral form. There is evidence that chlordiazepoxide, diazepam, and other long-acting benzodiazepines are slowly and erratically absorbed when given intramuscularly, but intravenous use produces rapid clinical results. Short-acting benzodiazepines are absorbed rapidly when given intramuscularly. Antacids significantly alter the absorption of chlorazepate and prazepam; this is an important consideration, since many anxious individuals suffer from gastrointestinal disturbances and use both types of drugs concomitantly. Food also modifies the absorption of diazepam (and possibly the other benzodiazepines), initially slowing absorption but resulting in higher levels over many hours. In the average case of anxiety, diazepam, 5–10 mg orally every 4–6 hours as needed, is a reasonable starting regimen. Since people vary widely in their response and since the drugs are long-lasting, one must individualize the dosage. Once this is established, an *adequate*

**Table 17–7.** Commonly used antianxiety agents.

| | Usual Oral Anxiolytic Dose (mg) | Usual Oral Hypnotic Dose (mg) | Usual Maximum Daily Oral Dose (mg) |
|---|---|---|---|
| **Benzodiazepines** | | | |
| Alprazolam* (Xanax) | 0.5 | | 4 |
| Chlordiazepoxide (Librium) | 5–30 | 50–100 | 75–100 |
| Clorazepate (Tranxene) | 3.25–15 | 30 | 60 |
| Diazepam (Valium) | 2–10 | 20–30 | 40 |
| Flurazepam (Dalmane) | | 15 | 60 |
| Halazepam (Paxipam) | 20 | 40–60 | 160 |
| Lorazepam* (Ativan) | 2 | | |
| Oxazepam* (Serax) | 10–30 | 30–60 | 90 |
| Prazepam (Centrax) | 10 | | 60 |
| Temazepam* (Restoril) | | 15 | 30 |
| Triazolam† (Halcion) | | 0.5–1 | 1.5 |
| **Miscellaneous** | | | |
| Buspirone | 5–10 | | 60 |
| Chloral hydrate (Noctec)* | 250 | 500–1000 | 2000 |
| Hydroxyzine pamoate (Vistaril) | 25–50 | 100 | 300 |
| Phenobarbital | 15–30 | 90 | 300 |

* Shorter-acting sedatives.
† Ultra-short-acting sedatives.

dose early in the course of symptom development will obviate the need for "pill-popping," which contributes to dependency problems. Flurazepam and temazepam are both marketed for management of sleep problems. The latter has a somewhat shorter duration of action but a delayed onset of action in the range of 1–3 hours. Triazolam has achieved popularity as a hypnotic drug because of its very short duration of action.

## Side Effects

The side effects are mainly behavioral and depend on patient reaction and dosage. As the dosage exceeds the levels necessary for sedation, the side effects include disinhibition, ataxia, dysarthria, nystagmus, errors of commission (machinery should not be operated until the patient is well stabilized), and excessive sedation, with sleep followed by coma and death if large doses are taken. Elderly or debilitated patients usually require much smaller doses for sedation. Use the shortest-acting drugs, eg, triazolam, in the elderly. Bradycardia, hypotension, phlebitis, and respiratory arrest have occurred after the intravenous use of diazepam, but this has usually happened in patients with preexisting cardiopulmonary diseases and is also thought to be related to the propylene glycol solvent.

A serious side effect of chronic excessive dosage is drug dependency, which may involve tolerance, and physiologic dependency with withdrawal symptoms similar in morbidity and mortality to alcohol withdrawal (withdrawal effects must be distinguished from reemergent anxiety). Abrupt withdrawal of sedative drugs may cause serious and even fatal convulsive seizures. Both duration of action and duration of exposure are major factors; withdrawal symptoms are more severe when the individual has been using the drug for more than 8 months. The symptoms are similar to those of barbiturate dependency. They are more gradual in onset in the case of the longer-acting benzodiazepines. They include perceptual distortions, anxiety, faintness, some cardiovascular lability, nightmares, insomnia, and hyperreactivity to external stimuli, with seizures as late as the twelfth day of withdrawal. In the case of the benzodiazepines, several months of overusage have usually preceded the development of dependency; in the case of the less safe drugs, such as the barbiturates, overusage for a period of weeks may result in a dependent state requiring planned withdrawal. Taper dosages every several days for gradual withdrawal (eg, 1 mg every 3 days for alprazolam and 5–10 mg every 3 days for diazepam).

The sedatives produce **cumulative** clinical effects with repeated dosage (especially if the patient has not had time to metabolize the previous dose); **additive** effects when given with other classes of sedatives or alcohol (many "accidental" deaths are the result of concomitant use of sedatives and alcohol); and **residual** effects after termination of treatment (particularly in the case of drugs that undergo slow biotransformation). Other side effects are rare, although inhibition of orgasm and hypomania have been reported with the use of alprazolam.

Benzodiazepine interactions with other drugs are listed in Table 17–8.

Busto U et al: Withdrawal reaction after long-term therapeutic use of benzodiazepines. *N Engl J Med* 1986;**315:**854.

Chouinard G: Neurologic and psychiatric aspects of clonazepam: An update. *Psychosomatics* 1985;**26(12-Suppl).** [Entire issue.]

Ray WA et al: Reducing long-term diazepam prescribing in office practise: A controlled trial of educational visits. *JAMA* 1986;**256:**2536.

## 5. OTHER ORGANIC THERAPIES

**Electroconvulsive therapy (ECT)** causes a central nervous system seizure (peripheral convulsion is not necessary) by means of electric current. The key objective is to exceed the seizure threshold, which can be accomplished by a variety of means. Electrical stimulation is more reliable and simpler than the use of chemical convulsants such as hexafluorodiethyl ether (flurothyl). The mechanism of action is not known, but it is thought to involve major neurotransmitter responses at the cell membrane. Current insufficient to cause a seizure produces no therapeutic benefit and causes more postictal confusion.

Electroconvulsive therapy is the most effective (about 70%) treatment of severe depression, particularly with delusions and agitation commonly seen in the involutional period. It is indicated when medical conditions preclude the use of antidepressants or in cases of nonresponsiveness to these medications. Comparative controlled studies of electroconvulsive therapy in severe depression show that it is more effective than chemotherapy. It is also effective in the manic disorders and psychoses during pregnancy (when drugs may be contraindicated). It has not been shown to be helpful in chronic schizophrenic disorders, and it is generally not used in acute schizophrenic episodes unless drugs are not effective and it is urgent that the psychosis be controlled (eg, a catatonic stupor complicating an acute medical condition).

Before electroconvulsive therapy is administered, a history and physical examination are performed, along with indicated laboratory tests. Lateral spine films and an electroencephalogram (EEG) are frequently done, particularly in elderly patients. Occasionally, the EEG will reveal a clinically silent intracranial lesion that may be a factor in the depression and is a contraindication to electroconvulsive therapy. The patient should not eat or drink for at least 8 hours before treatment. Medications that heighten the seizure threshold (eg, sedatives, clonidine) should be discontinued several days prior to electroconvulsive therapy. Lithium may aggravate the central nervous system side effects, including memory loss. Dentures are removed prior to electroconvulsive therapy. An empty bladder is desirable because of incontinence resulting from the seizure. Atropine sulfate, 0.6–1 mg intramuscularly, is given for its vagolytic effect. A short-acting barbiturate such as methohexital, 40–70 mg, is given carefully intravenously (extravasation is very irritating to tissues) to cause unconsciousness. Succinylcholine, 30–60 mg intravenously, will produce a flaccid paralysis, and the anesthesiologist can then ventilate the patient with 100% oxygen from the onset of unconsciousness until spontaneous respiration resumes. Succinylcholine is contraindicated if the patient is using echothiophate iodide for glaucoma, since the latter is absorbed in amounts sufficient to interfere with the hydrolysis of succinylcholine and can thus precipitate prolonged apnea. Chronic renal dialysis, excessive supported ventilation, and congenital pseudocholinesterase deficiency may also result in prolonged apnea.

Placement of electrodes may be bitemporal or unilateral on the nondominant side. The latter is considered to produce less impairment of memory, although it may be slightly less effective and require more

**Table 17–8.** Benzodiazepine interactions with other drugs.

| Drug | Effects |
|------|---------|
| Antacids | Decreased absorption of benzodiazepines. |
| Cimetidine | Increased half-life of flurazepam, alprazolam. |
| Contraceptives | Increased levels of diazepam and triazolam. |
| Dicumarol | Decreased prothrombin time. |
| Digoxin | Alprazolam and diazepam raise digoxin level. |
| Disulfiram | Increased duration of action of sedatives. |
| Isoniazid | Increased plasma diazepam. |
| Levodopa | Inhibition of antiparkinsonism effect. |
| Rifampin | Decreased plasma diazepam. |

than the usual 9–12 treatments. Patients with a history of manic symptoms respond better to bitemporal electroconvulsive therapy. Electroconvulsive therapy may be performed every few days (3 per week is usual), or all of the treatments may be given in 1–3 sessions under electrocardiographic monitoring of seizure activity (multiple-monitored electroconvulsive therapy).

A seizure usually lasts 5–20 seconds, with a brief postictal state. The patient can resume activity in about an hour. The most common side effects are memory disturbance and headache. Memory loss or confusion is usually related to number and frequency of electroconvulsive therapy treatments and proper oxygenation during treatment. Some memory loss is occasionally permanent, but most memory faculties return to full capacity within several weeks. There have been reports that lithium administration concurrent with electroconvulsive therapy resulted in greater memory loss. Before anesthesia was used, spinal compression fractures and severe anticipatory anxiety were common.

Increased intracranial pressure is a positive contraindication. Other problems such as cardiac disorders, aneurysms, bronchopulmonary disease, and venous thrombosis, are relative contraindications and must be evaluated in light of the severity of the medical problem versus the need for electroconvulsive therapy. Serious complications arising from electroconvulsive therapy occur in less than one in a thousand cases. Most of these problems are cardiovascular or respiratory in nature (eg, aspiration of gastric contents). Patient education and acceptance of the technique and public opinion are the biggest obstacles to the use of electroconvulsive therapy.

**Psychosurgery** has a limited place in selected cases of severe, unremitting anxiety and depression, obsessional neuroses, and, to a lesser degree, some of the schizophrenias. The stereotactic techniques now being used, including modified bifrontal tractotomy, are great improvements over the crude methods of the past. In the controversial area of **megavitamin treatment** for the schizophrenic patient, the overall therapeutic efficacy of nicotinic acid or nicotinamide as the sole or adjuvant medication is no better than that of an inactive placebo. **Acupuncture** and **electrosleep,** while currently of interest, are of unproved usefulness for any psychiatric conditions.

Consensus conference: Electroconvulsive therapy. *JAMA* 1985;**254**:2103.

Fink M: Update on ECT. *Psychiatr Ann* 1987;**17**:47.

Hansen H et al: Stereotactic psychosurgery: A psychiatric and psychological investigation of the effects and side effects of the interventions. *Acta Psychiatr Scand [Suppl]* 1982;**301**:1.

## 6. HOSPITALIZATION

The need for hospital care may range from admission to a medical bed in a general hospital for an acute situational stress reaction to admission to a psychiatric ward when the patient is in acute psychosis. The trend over recent years has been to admit patients to general hospitals in the community, treat patients aggressively, and discharge them promptly to the next appropriate level of treatment—day hospital, halfway house, outpatient therapy, etc. Involuntary hospitalization should be objectively determined on the basis of patient and society welfare. Sixty percent of admissions are readmissions. The total "in residence" population (hospital plus residential) is the same as the hospital total of 20 years ago.

Hospital care may be indicated when patients are too sick to care for themselves or when they present serious threats to themselves or others; when observation and diagnostic procedures are necessary; or when specific kinds of treatment such as electroconvulsive therapy, complex medication trials, or hospital environment (milieu) are required. Symptoms correlating best with hospitalization are self-neglect, violent or bizarre behavior, paranoid ideation or delusions, marked intellectual impairment, and poor judgment.

The disadvantages of psychiatric hospitalization include decreased self-confidence as a result of needing hospitalization; the stigma of being a "psychiatric patient"; possible increased dependency and regression; and the expense. Generally, there is no advantage to prolonged hospital stays for most psychiatric disorders.

Lieberman PB, Strauss JS: Brief psychiatric hospitalization: What are its effects? *Am J Psychiat* 1986;**143**:1557.

Spiegel D, Wissler T: Family environment as a predictor of psychiatric rehospitalization. *Am J Psychiatry* 1986;**143**:56.

## PSYCHOLOGIC APPROACHES

Psychotherapy is a process whereby a socially sanctioned healer seeks to help people overcome or ameliorate psychologic distress and disability by a systematic treatment method based on a theory of the origin and nature of the patient's problems. There are over 100 different types of psychotherapy, but all of them with one exception fall into 2 broad categories—dynamic or experiential—and all are reported to give similar results. Harm as well as good can be done by psychotherapy. Bad results can usually be shown to be due to the inexperience, poor judgment, or inflexibility of the therapist.

The exception referred to in the preceding paragraph is behavioral therapy, which professes no interest in the origins of psychologic distress but only in modification of its symptoms.

**Dynamic psychotherapy.** The basic concepts of dynamic psychotherapy rest in the role of the unconscious with libidinal drives and conflicts that remain out of awareness and in the importance of determinism, which emphasizes that each psychic event is determined by the ones that preceded it. The ideologic framework is not a critical factor. The variables that correlate highly with improvement are support by the therapist and identification with the therapist (both being functions of the patient-therapist relationship), improved self-esteem, and appropriate use of defense mechanisms.

The defense mechanisms of particular importance are **repression** (purposeful forgetting), **reaction formation** (substituting a pleasant thought for a painful one), **isolation** (separating original memory from affective response), **denial** (refusing to deal with obvious reality issues), **projection** (attributing a wish or impulse to some other person), **rationalization** (substituting acceptable reason for unacceptable reason), and **undoing** (neutralizing objectionable thoughts).

The focus is rooted in the subjective past, and the mode of change is to make the unconscious conscious, ie, to achieve insight with an understanding of the early past and its connection with conflicts. To achieve reduction of the conflicts, the therapist in a dyadic relationship uses free associations, interpretations, and analysis of both resistance and transference of feelings (a repetition of the past that is inappropriate to the present) onto the therapist. The process is long-term (in classic psychoanalysis, daily sessions; in later modifications, weekly to thrice-weekly meetings) and is set in a doctor-patient relationship with the expectation of a major reorganization of the psyche.

**Experiential psychotherapy.** This includes gestalt therapy, client-centered psychotherapy, cognitive therapy, existential analysis, and structural analysis. Experiential therapy evolved from the concepts of fragmentation of the self, existential despair, and the lack of unity with one's own experiences. The focus of therapy is on the present. The mode of change is in the immediate experiencing of one's emotions. The past is not significant in the therapeutic process. The therapist uses intense interactions in a comfortable setting that stimulates self-expression. The sharing is an important element in the encounter to ameliorate the feelings of isolation and alienation and emphasize the possibility of unlimited psychic growth. The goals in this short-term process (weekly meetings for weeks or months) are self-determination; integration of new perceptions, thinking patterns, and self-awareness; rational thinking; creativity; and self-affirmation within a setting of adult, humanistic, peer-oriented relationships.

**Supportive psychotherapy** is a commonly used approach. While it has its theoretical roots in psychoanalytic theory, it usually denotes a positive relationship with the patient, strengthening of existing defenses, enhancing self-esteem (remoralization), and an emphasis on the here and now. The goals are primarily alleviation of symptoms and termination of therapy when this has been accomplished. There is little effort to make substantial changes in the personality structure. Emphasis is on maintaining morale and hope in the future, recognizing responses to stress, and identifying and practicing new ways of coping with stress. Success in all forms of disorders (medical

and psychiatric) has been correlated with assumption of responsibility by the patient, a positive approach with a will to live, confidence in the treating professional, and supportive family and friends. Termination should occur within the framework of therapist availability in the event of future needs.

**Group therapy.** The decision for group versus individual therapy is usually based on the patient's need to improve interpersonal relationships, and the group setting may provide the "laboratory" for improvisation and practice of new behaviors that can then be generalized to everyday activities. Therapy groups are usually composed of individuals who have no outside connection with one another, but groups may be made up of couples or families.

The various schools of therapy often purport to be unique, more effective, or of more lasting value than others. In reality, they have many similarities and common derivations, with about the same results. The attitude of the patient and the skill of the therapist rather than the ideology are usually the major factors in producing change.

Foulks EF, Persons JB, Merkel RL: The effect of patients' beliefs about their illnesses on compliance in psychotherapy. *Am J Psychiatry* 1986;**143**:340.

Ursano RJ, Hales RE: A review of brief individual psychotherapies. *Am J Psychiat* 1986;**143**:1507.

## SOCIAL APPROACHES

In contrast to psychologic techniques, which deal principally with intrapsychic phenomena and interpersonal problems, the social approaches to psychiatric treatment attempt to modify attitudes and behavior by altering the **environmental** factors contributing to the patient's maladaptation. The scope of the attempt may range from provision of a therapeutic milieu—eg, in a day hospital or residential community—to minor alterations in school procedures or daily family activities. The family, friends, and neighbors provide the major social support in the large majority of cases. Various psychologic and behavioral techniques are used within social approaches.

### Part-Time Hospitalization

The patient either participates in the hospital milieu during the day (day hospitals—going home at night), or stays the night (night hospitals—going to work or school during the day), or spends several hours a day in the hospital for up to 5 or 6 days a week. This is a cost-effective alternative to full hospitalization.

### Self-Help Communities

These are usually sponsored by nongovernmental agencies for the purpose of helping people with a particular type of difficulty. The individual lives-in full time for varying periods and usually continues to be affiliated with the group after leaving. Examples of self-help communities include halfway houses, residences for alcoholics, Salvation Army, and church-sponsored agencies. They are often a bridge between hospitalization and independent living.

## Substitute Homes

Substitute homes provide shelter and treatment-related programs for longer periods of time. Examples of "substitute" homes are foster homes, usually for children; board and care homes, primarily for people who are disabled and unlikely to return to productive function; residential treatment centers, taking a number of children and offering fairly intensive treatment programs; and shelters for young people—often in the process of withdrawing from drugs.

## Nonresidential Self-Help Organizations

The following are examples of organizations usually administered by people who have survived similar problems and have banded together to help others cope with the same problem: Alcoholics Anonymous (and Al-Anon, to help families of alcoholics); Recovery Inc., organized and run by people who have had an emotional problem that required hospitalization; Schizophrenics Anonymous; Gamblers Anonymous; Overeaters Anonymous; colostomy clubs; mastectomy clubs; the Epilepsy Society; the Alzheimer's Disease and Related Disorders Association; the American Heart Association's Stroke Clubs of America; burn recovery groups; other groups organized to help people deal with practical and psychologic problems of a particular illness; and friendship centers that assist people in their efforts to find specific kinds of help. At times, the best support for a patient is contact with another patient who has conquered a similar problem.

A national self-help clearinghouse at the City University of New York, 33 West 42nd St., New York, NY 10036, maintains up-to-date listings of mutual aid organizations in the USA.

## Special Professional & Paraprofessional Organizations

Examples of special organizations of this type are Homemaker Service, made up of individuals who come into the home to help the partially disabled maintain the household; Visiting Nurse Associations, which usually provide more than medical assistance; adult protective services for the elderly; genetic counseling services; family service agencies, for marriage counseling and family problems; crisis centers, eg, "free clinics" and county-sponsored satellite clinics; and church-sponsored agencies. Religion (personal beliefs) and churches (organized groups) play major roles in psychosocial adjustment. Medication groups exist, in which physicians, nurses, and pharmacists provide education regarding drugs and help patients to accept the need for long-term medication.

## Stress Reduction Techniques

Social and environmental factors are major aids in lowering stress and should be part of the activities of daily living. Both active recreation (sports, physical exercise, participant hobbies) and passive pursuits (reading, music, painting) are necessary for a balanced life and alleviation of stress. Although they are major factors in causing stress, job pressures and uncertainty about vocational goals are frequently ignored. Family structure and dynamics must be evaluated, and there will be occasions (eg, adult children living at home, presence of in-laws) when a social restructuring is in order.

Johnson HA: Stroke clubs: Undervalued and underused. *JAMA* 1984;**251**:1881.

Mollice RF, Milic M: Social class and psychiatric practice: A revision of the Hollingshead and Redlich model. *Am J Psychiatry* 1986;**143**:12.

## BEHAVIORAL APPROACHES

Behavior therapy has its foundations in theories of the learning process. The role of the behavior therapist is that of a teacher who attempts to bring about change in the patient's maladaptation. The specific problem (target behavior) and the factors that play a role in precipitating or perpetuating the problem must first be identified. An attempt can then be made to alter those factors that perpetuate unwanted behavior.

The emphasis of behavior therapy is on "here and now" and *direct* change. The goal is to "unlearn" those destructive or unproductive types of behavior that result from faulty learning and to enhance the individual's repertoire of useful social and adaptive skills. Great emphasis is placed on identifying and then ablating whatever is maintaining the maladaptive behavior.

Whereas **conditioning** is understood by some to be synonymous with a specific type of learning (eg, Pavlov's dogs), behavior therapy is much broader. It includes the relationship with the therapist, utilizes verbal techniques, although to a lesser degree than other therapies, and interprets "behavior" in a broad sense that includes thoughts and feelings.

Many of the techniques of behavior therapy require a cooperative effort on the part of a number of people who must all understand and be *consistent* in their responses to specified behaviors. Thus, a cooperative social setting such as a milieu ward or the patient's own home and family is important in implementing many of the following techniques.

## Techniques of Behavior Therapy

**A. Modeling:** Much learning occurs by imitation. From the earliest years of childhood, the individual's behavior is modeled after parents, teachers, peers, employers, public personalities, historical figures, etc ("significant others"). The therapist makes a conscious effort to serve as a model of particular kinds of behavior that are significant to and attainable by the patient. This device is particularly useful in treating patients with low self-esteem.

**B. Operant Conditioning:** Operant conditioning is the deliberate implementation of a system of rewards to encourage repetition of specific desired behaviors. A voluntary behavior is singled out for a specific reward every time the behavior is used. The objective is to develop a habit in the use of that behavior. Like modeling, operant conditioning is a common procedure in families, and the child soon learns that "good" behavior is rewarded. "Token economies" (tokens are given for acceptable behavior, and these tokens can be redeemed for foods, outings, etc) in centers for retarded or autistic patients and those with behavioral problems are effective, particularly where verbal techniques have little impact.

**C. Aversive Conditioning:** Aversive conditioning is the opposite of operant conditioning but is a less potent shaper of behavior. Undesirable behavior (eg, alcohol ingestion) is paired with an unpleasant consequence (eg, vomiting induced by apomorphine, mild electric or sound shock), whereas satisfactory alternative responses are operantly encouraged. The most common conditions treated by this technique have been enuresis, smoking, alcoholism, and homosexuality. The results have been varied, but some successes have been reported, particularly in enuresis.

**D. Extinction:** Extinction is the process of refusing to reinforce behavior on the theory that behavior cannot be sustained without some sort of reinforcement. Temper tantrums and noxious behavior, usually contrived to gain attention of any sort, are "extinguished" in this way.

**E. Desensitization:** Familiarity lessens anxiety and reduces the tendency to avoid exposure to the feared object, person, or situation. The subject is repeatedly exposed to the feared stimulus (eg, looking at a picture of an elevator when the fear has been riding in elevators) at such a low level of intensity that the fear response is minimal. Exposures are then gradually increased (eg, walking past a real elevator) until the subject is able to tolerate the real experience with markedly reduced fear. This technique has been most effective in the treatment of phobias and a variety of situations (such as frigidity or impotence) that engender fears of failure, disapproval, and embarrassment.

**F. Emotive Imagery:** Deliberate evocation of mental images that arouse certain feelings can be used as a way of warding off painful emotions resulting from stress-inducing circumstances. Noxious imagery can be used in aversive conditioning and "pleasant thoughts" in operant training. In "mental imagery" desensitization, the phobic or sensitive situation is reproduced in graded quantities and the patient learns to handle minor upsetting imagined situations

without anxiety before proceeding to the more difficult ones.

**G. Flooding:** Flooding (implosion) consists of overwhelming the individual, in a safe setting, with anxiety-producing stimuli. The anxiety responses gradually lessen (law of diminishing returns) until extinction occurs. In some ways, flooding is a desensitization technique without the graded approach. It has been used in treatment of obsessive compulsive patients and those with such behavior problems as compulsive hoarding.

**H. Role Playing:** In the role-playing technique, patients can practice various types of behaviors in anxiety-producing but "safe" situations. For example, the therapist may assume the role of an angry friend and the patient uses different ways of handling the situation. Role reversal—where the therapist and the patient change roles—then gives the patient a chance to experience the other's feelings and attitudes. Assertiveness training for inhibited individuals is a variant to help people learn to be more spontaneous.

**I. Relaxation Techniques:** These include muscle relaxation, self-hypnosis, and biofeedback procedures. The names are descriptive. Biofeedback requires some equipment to measure and signal physiologic change. It is particularly helpful in such somatic disorders as migraine headache and hyperactive bowel syndome (see Somatoform Disorders). Relaxation techniques may be used concomitantly with other therapeutic approaches.

Gorsman RM: The psychodynamics of prescribing in behavior therapy. *Am J Psychiatry* 1985;**142**:675.

---

# COMMON PSYCHIATRIC DISORDERS

---

## STRESS & ADJUSTMENT DISORDERS
### (Situational Disorders)

Stress exists when the adaptive capacity of the individual is overwhelmed by events. The event may be an insignificant one objectively considered, and even favorable changes (eg, promotion and transfer) requiring adaptive behavior can produce stress. For each individual, stress is subjectively defined, and the response to stress is a function of each person's personality and physiologic endowment.

### Classification & Clinical Findings

Opinion differs about what events are most apt to produce stress reactions. The Holmes/Rahe studies of psychosocial factors provide some insights into the stress-inducing potential of marriage, family relationships, work and social relationships, financial problems, illness and injury, etc. The causes of stress are different at different ages—eg, in young adulthood, the sources of stress are found in the marriage or parent-child relationship, the employment relationship, and the struggle to achieve financial stability; in the middle years, the focus shifts to changing spousal relationships, problems with aging parents, and problems associated with having young adult offspring who themselves are encountering stressful situations; in old age, the principal concerns are apt to be retirement, loss of physical capacity, major personal losses, and thoughts of death.

An individual may react to stress by becoming anxious or depressed, by developing a physical symptom, by running away, by having a drink or starting an affair, or in limitless other ways. Common subjective responses are fear (of repetition of the stress-inducing event), rage (at frustration), guilt (over aggressive impulses), and shame (over helplessness). Acute stress may be manifested by restlessness, irritability, fatigue, increased startle reaction, and a feeling of tension. Inability to concentrate, sleep disturbances (insomnia, bad dreams), and somatic preoccupations often lead to self-medication, most commonly with alcohol or other central nervous system depressants. Maladaptive behavior to stress is called adjustment disorder, with the major symptom specified (eg, "adjustment disorder with depressed mood").

**Posttraumatic stress disorder** (eg, the so-called post-Vietnam syndrome) is a syndrome with symptoms of reexperiencing the traumatic event (eg, rape, military combat), along with decreased responsiveness to current events, startle reactions, intrusive thoughts, illusions, overgeneralized associations, sleep problems, nightmares, difficulties in concentration, and hyperalertness. The symptoms may be precipitated or exacerbated by distant events that are a reminder of the original stress. Symptoms frequently arise after a long latency period. The sooner the symptoms arise after the initial trauma and the sooner therapy is initiated, the better the prognosis. The therapeutic approach is to facilitate the normal recovery that was blocked at the time of the trauma. Therapy at that time should be brief, simple (catharsis and working through of the traumatic experience), and expectant (of quick recovery and a rapid return to work).

## Differential Diagnosis

Adjustment disorders must be distinguished from anxiety disorders, affective disorders, and personality disorders exacerbated by stress and from structural somatic disorders with psychic overlay.

## Treatment

**A. Behavioral:** Stress reduction techniques include immediate symptom reduction (eg, rebreathing in a bag for hyperventilation) or early recognition and removal from a stress source before full-blown symptoms appear. It is often helpful for the patient to keep a daily log of stress precipitators, responses, and alleviators. Relaxation and exercise techniques are also helpful in reducing the reaction to stressful events. Specific behavioral techniques such as desensitization are indirectly helpful in anxiety reduction of stress reactions. For example, alleviation of a phobia can lead to a general reduction of tension and thus raise the response threshold to stress stimuli.

**B. Medical:** Judicious use of sedatives (eg, lorazepam, 1–2 mg orally daily) for a limited time and as a part of an overall treatment plan can provide relief from acute anxiety symptoms. Problems arise when the situation becomes chronic through inappropriate treatment or when the treatment approach supports the development of chronicity (see Sedative-Hypnotic Drugs, above).

**C. Psychologic:** Prolonged depth psychotherapy is seldom necessary in cases of isolated stress response or adjustment disorder. Supportive psychotherapy (see above) with an emphasis on the here and now and strengthening of existing defenses, is a helpful approach while time and the patient's own resiliency allow a restoration to the previous level of function. A more prolonged psychotherapeutic approach is helpful in revising poor coping patterns, repetitive symptom patterns, and marked susceptibility to life's vicissitudes. Posttraumatic stress syndromes respond to catharsis and dynamic psychotherapy oriented toward acceptance of the event. Marital problems are a major area of concern, and it is important that the physician have available a dependable referral source when marriage counseling is indicated.

**D. Social:** The stress reactions of life crisis problems are, more than any other category, a function of psychosocial upheaval, and it is patients responding to these problems who so frequently present with somatic symptoms. While it is not easy for the patient to make necessary changes (or they would have been made long ago), it is important for the physician to establish the framework of the problem, since the patient's denial system may obscure the issues. Clarifying the problem allows the patient to begin viewing it within the proper context and facilitates the sometimes very difficult decisions the patient eventually must make (eg, change of job or relocation of adult dependent offspring). It is important that the physician *not dictate what changes must be made.*

## Prognosis

Return to satisfactory function after a short period is part of the clinical picture of this syndrome. Resolution may be delayed if others' responses to the patient's difficulties are thoughtlessly harmful or if the secondary gains outweigh the advantages of recovery.

Mellion MB: Exercise therapy for anxiety and depression. 1. Does the evidence justify its recommendation? *Postgrad Med* (Feb) 1985;**77**:59.

Modlin HC: Posttraumatic stress disorder no longer just for war veterans. *Postgrad Med* 1986;**79**:26.

## ANXIETY DISORDERS & DISSOCIATIVE DISORDERS (Neuroses)

### Essentials of Diagnosis

- Overt anxiety or an overt manifestation of a defense mechanism (such as a phobia) or both.
- Not limited to an adjustment disorder.
- Somatic symptoms referable to the autonomic nervous system or to a specific organ system (eg, dyspnea, palpitations, paresthesias).
- Not a result of physical disorders, psychiatric conditions (eg, schizophrenia), or drugs (eg, caffeine).

### General Considerations

Anxiety is a reaction to real or imagined danger. It is ubiquitous and can be a transient symptom or a chronic debilitated state. Anxiety disorders may reflect the result of a maladaptive attempt to resolve internal conflicts. These conflicts usually include unresolved childhood problems such as dependency, insecurity, hostility, excessive need for affection, concerns about intimacy, and overly strong drives for power and control.

Principal components of anxiety are **psychologic** (tension, fears, difficulty in concentration, apprehension) and **somatic** (tachycardia, hyperventilation, palpitations, tremor, sweating). Other organ systems (eg, gastrointestinal) may be involved in multiple-system complaints. Fatigue and sleep disturbances are common. Sympathomimetic symptoms of anxiety are both a response to a central nervous system state and a reinforcement of further anxiety. Anxiety can become self-generating, since the symptoms reinforce the reaction, causing it to spiral.

The resultant anxiety is handled in different ways. Anxiety may be free-floating, resulting in acute anxiety attacks, occasionally becoming chronic. When one or several defense mechanisms (see above) are functioning, the consequences are well-known problems such as phobias, conversion reactions, dissociative states, obsessions, and compulsions. *Lack of structure is frequently a contributing factor,* as noted in those people who have ''Sunday neuroses.'' They do well during the week with a planned work schedule but cannot tolerate the unstructured weekend. Planned-time activities tend to bind anxiety, and many people have increased difficulties when this is lost, as in retirement.

Some believe that various manifestations of anxiety are not a result of unconscious conflicts but are ''habits''—persistent patterns of nonadaptive behavior acquired by learning. The ''habits,'' being nonadaptive, are unsatisfactory ways of dealing with life problems—hence the resultant anxiety. Help is sought only when the anxiety becomes too painful. *Exogenous factors such as stimulants (eg, caffeine) must be considered as causative or contributing factors.*

The treatment approach adopted in the management of the neuroses tends to reflect the philosophic bias of the therapist. Results do not differ significantly among various treatment methods.

### Clinical Findings

**A. Generalized Anxiety Disorder:** This is the most common of the clinically significant anxiety disorders and occurs with equal frequency in both sexes. The disabling anxiety symptoms of apprehension, worry, irritability, hypervigilance, and somatic complaints are long-lasting and persist for at least 1 month. Symptoms include cardiac (eg, tachycardia, increased blood pressure), gastrointestinal (eg, increased acidity, epigastric pain), and neurologic (eg, headache, syncope) systems. Some of the origins or exacerbating causes of the anxiety may be identified in life situations.

**B. Panic Disorder:** This is characterized by short-lived, recurrent, unpredictable episodes of intense anxiety accompanied by marked physiologic manifestations. Distressing symptoms such as dyspnea, tachycardia, palpitations, headaches, dizziness, paresthesias, nausea, and bloating are associated with feelings of impending doom. Although panic attacks usually arise spontaneously, caffeine may be a precipitating factor. Panic disorder tends to be familial, with onset under age 25, and there is a 2:1 prevalence in women. Patients frequently undergo emergency medical evaluations (eg, for ''heart attacks'' or ''hypoglycemia'') before the correct diagnosis is made. Mitral valve prolapse may be present but is not necessarily a significant factor. ''Air hunger'' and tetany due to **hyperventilation syndrome** are promptly relieved when rebreathing is induced by placing an airtight bag over the patient's nose and mouth. Patients with recurrent panic disorder often become **demoralized, agoraphobic and depressed.** Alcohol abuse results from self-treatment and is not infrequently combined with dependence on sedatives.

**C. Phobic Disorder:** Phobic ideation can be considered a mechanism of ''displacement'' in which the patient transfers feelings of anxiety from their true object to one that can be avoided so as not to feel anxiety. However, since phobias are ineffective defense mechanisms, there tends to be an increase in the scope, intensity, and number of phobias. Agoraphobia (fear of open places and public areas) is frequently associated with severe panic attacks. Patients often develop the syndrome in early adult life, making a normal life-style difficult.

**D. Obsessive Compulsive Disorder:** In the obsessive compulsive reaction, the irrational idea or the impulse persistently intrudes into awareness. Obsessions (constantly recurring thoughts such as fears of hitting somebody) and compulsions (repetitive actions such as washing hands many times prior to peeling a potato) are recognized by the individual as absurd and are resisted, but anxiety is alleviated only by ritualistic performance or mechanical impulse or entertainment of the idea. The primary underlying concern of the patient is to not lose control. These patients are usually predictable, orderly, conscientious, and intelligent, traits that are seen in many compulsive behaviors such as anorexia and compulsive running. Under extreme stress, these patients sometimes exhibit paranoid and delusional behaviors, often associated with depression.

**E. Dissociative Disorder:** Fugue, amnesia, somnambulism, and multiple personality are the usual dissociative states. The reaction is precipitated by emotional crisis, and although the primary gain is anxiety reduction, the secondary gain is a temporary solution of the crisis. Mechanisms include repression and isolation as well as particularly limited concentration such as seen in hypnotic states. This condition is similar in many ways to symptoms seen in patients with temporal lobe dysfunction.

### Treatment

**A. Psychologic:** Psychotherapy is still a customary way of treating these disorders. Irrespective of the therapist's philosophic orientation, the relationship with the therapist in individual therapy is anxiety-reducing and effective when the therapy deals with the conflict producing the anxiety. The therapist who can help the patient delineate specific problems and goals is helping the patient find specific alternatives to unproductive or harmful ways of dealing with problems. When economically feasible, psychoanalysis can be helpful, particularly when the patient is motivated to deal with the past events that have laid the groundwork for the present problem. Other individual approaches such as reality therapy or transactional analysis are particularly helpful when interpersonal relationships are a major factor. Group therapy is the treatment of choice when the anxiety is clearly a function of the patient's difficulties in dealing with others, and if these other people are part of the family it is appropriate to include them and initiate family or couples therapy.

**B. Behavioral:** Behavioral approaches are widely used in various anxiety disorders. Any of the behavioral techniques (see above) can be used beneficially in altering the contingencies (precipitating factors or rewards) supporting any anxiety-provoking behavior. Relaxation techniques can sometimes be helpful in reducing anxiety. Desensitization, by exposing the patient to graded doses of a phobic object or situation, is an effective technique and one that the patient can practice outside of the therapy session. Emotive imagery, wherein the patient imagines the anxiety-provoking situation while at the same time learning to relax, helps to decrease the anxiety when the patient faces the real life situation. Some compulsions are treated by "flooding," ie, saturating the person with the anxiety-producing situation or phobic object. This changes the relationship of the compulsion to the anxiety, and the compulsion is given up, since it no longer serves to ward off anxiety.

**C. Medical:** In all cases, underlying medical disorders must be ruled out (eg, thyroid disease, partial complex seizures). Benzodiazepines are the sedatives of choice in most cases of generalized anxiety. Other classes of drugs, such as antipsychotics, and the older sedatives, such as the barbiturates, have no advantages

over the benzodiazepines and have numerous disadvantages (diverse side effects and more dependency problems, respectively). Beta blockers such as propranolol may be helpful in the reduction of peripheral somatic symptoms. Ethanol is the most frequently self-administered drug, but it has no role in the treatment of anxiety.

Panic attacks may be treated in several ways. Tricyclic antidepressants and MAO inhibitors (imipramine, 100–300 mg/d orally, or phenelzine, 30–60 mg/d orally) are effective against the panic attacks but less so in blocking phobic-avoidant behavior. Norepinephrine reuptake blockers have been more effective than serotonin reuptake blockers. Alprazolam (0.5–8 mg/d orally) and clonazepam (1–8 mg/d orally) are exceptions because of their unique structures. They have been used in conjuction with propranolol (40–160 mg/d orally) in resistant cases. Phobic disorder may be part of the panic disorder and are treated within that framework. Benzodiazepine sedatives lower anticipatory anxiety and may be used in conjunction with desensitization procedures for a wide range of phobic behaviors.

Obsessive compulsive disorders show a variable response to medications. Clomipramine has been the most useful drug, but it is not generally available. Imipramine (150–300 mg/d orally) is better than placebo but not as effective as clomipramine. L-Tryptophan in dosages of 1.5–2 g/d orally has been beneficial in some cases.

**D. Social:** Social modification may require measures such as family counseling to aid acceptance of the patient's symptoms. Any help in maintaining the social structure is anxiety-alleviating, and work, school, and social activities should be maintained. School and vocational counseling may be provided by professionals, who often need help from the physician in defining the patient's limitations.

### Prognosis

Anxiety disorders are usually of long standing and may be quite difficult to treat. Some, such as obsessions and compulsions, tend to be most resistant. All can be relieved to varying degrees with psychotherapy and behavioral techniques. The prognosis is much better if one can break the commonly observed anxiety-panic-phobia-depression cycle with the medication resources discussed above.

Anderson RW, Lev-Ran A: Hypoglycemia: The standard and the fiction. *Psychosomatics* 1985;**26**:38.

Barlow DA et al: Generalized anxiety and generalized anxiety disorders: Description and reconceptualization. *Am J Psychiatry* 1986;**143**:40.

Hayes PE, Dommisse CS: Current concepts in clinical therapeutics: Anxiety disorders. (Part 1.) *Clin Pharmacol* 1987;**6**:140.

Insel TR, Akiskal HS: Obsessive-compulsive disorder with psychotic features: A phenomenologic analysis. *Am J Psychiat* 1986;**143**:1527.

Noyes R Jr et al: Relationship between panic disorders and agoraphobia. *Arch Gen Psychiatry* 1986;**43**:227.

Smith CW: Hyperventilation: A much overlooked disorder. *Postgrad Med* 1985;**78**:40.

## SOMATOFORM DISORDERS
### (Psychophysiologic Disorders, Psychosomatic Disorders)

### Essentials of Diagnosis

- Symptoms may involve one or more organ systems.
- Subjective complaints exceed objective findings.
- Correlations of symptom development and psychosocial stresses.
- Matrix of biogenetic and developmental patterns.

### General Considerations

A major source of diagnostic confusion in medicine has been to assume cause-and-effect relationships when parallel events have been observed. This post hoc ergo propter hoc reasoning has been particularly vexing in many situations where the individual exhibits psychosocial distress that could well be secondary to a chronic illness but has been assumed to be primary and causative. An example is the person with a chronic bowel disease who becomes querulous and demanding. Is this a result of problems of coping with a chronic disease, or is it a personality pattern that causes the gastrointestinal problem?

People react differently to illness. Emotional stress often exacerbates or precipitates an acute illness. Vulnerability in one or more organ systems and exposure to family members with somatization problems play a major role in the development of particular symptoms, and the "functional" versus "organic" dichotomy is a hindrance to good treatment.

In any patient presenting with a condition judged to be somatoform, depression must be considered in the diagnosis.

### Clinical Findings

**A. Conversion Disorder:** "Conversion" of psychic conflict into physical symptoms in parts of the body innervated by the sensorimotor system (eg, paralysis, aphonia) is a disorder that is more common in unsophisticated individuals and certain cultures. The term "hysterical conversion" was previously used to describe this condition. The defense mechanisms utilized in this condition are repression (a barring from consciousness) and isolation (a splitting of the affect from the idea). The somatic manifestation that takes the place of anxiety is typically paralysis, and in some instances the organ dysfunction may have symbolic meaning (eg, arm paralysis in marked anger). Hysterical seizures ("pseudoseizures") are usually difficult to differentiate from intoxication states or panic attacks. Retention of consciousness, random flailing with asynchronous movements of the right and left sides, and resistance to having the nose and mouth pinched closed during the attack all point toward a hysterical event. Electroencephalography

*during the attack* is the most helpful diagnostic aid in excluding seizure states. Serum prolactin levels rise abruptly in the postictal state but not in pseudoseizures. There is usually a past history of other conversion situations. The conversion may temporarily "solve the problem." La belle indifférence is not a significant characteristic (as commonly believed). Important criteria in diagnosis include a history of conversion or somatization disorder, modeling, a serious precipitating emotional event, associated psychopathology (eg, schizophrenia, personality disorders), a temporal correlation between the precipitating event and the symptom, and a temporary "solving of the problem" by the conversion. *It is important to consider physical disorders with unusual presentations (eg, multiple sclerosis).*

**B. Somatization Disorder (Briquet's Syndrome, Hysteria):** This is characterized by multiple physical complaints referable to several organ systems. It usually occurs before age 30 and is more common in women. Polysurgery is often a feature of the history. Preoccupation with medical and surgical therapy becomes a life-style that excludes most other activities. The symptoms are a reflection of adaptive patterns, coping techniques, and reactivity of the particular organ system. There is often evidence of long-standing somatic symptoms (particularly dysmenorrhea, a lump in the throat, vomiting, shortness of breath, burning in the sex organs, painful extremities, and amnesia), often with a history of similar organ system involvement in other family members. Multiple symptoms that constantly change and inability of more than 3 doctors to make a diagnosis are strong clues to the problem.

**C. Psychogenic Pain Disorder:** This involves a long history of complaints of severe pain not consonant with anatomic and clinical signs. This diagnosis should be made only after extended evaluation has established a clear correlation of psychogenic factors with exacerbations and remissions of complaints. Furthermore, there should be evidence that the pain confers some secondary gain. This diagnosis must not be made by exclusion but must be supported by positive psychologic factors.

**D. Hypochondriasis:** This is a fear of disease and preoccupation with the body, with perceptual amplification and heightened responsiveness. A process of social learning is usually involved, frequently with a role model who was a member of the family and may be a part of the underlying psychodynamic etiology.

**E. Factitious Disorders:** These are characterized by self-induced symptoms or false physical and laboratory findings for the purpose of deceiving physicians or other hospital personnel. The deceptions may involve self-mutilation, fever, hemorrhage, hypoglycemia, seizures, and an almost endless variety of manifestations—often presented in an exaggerated and dramatic fashion (Munchausen's syndrome). The duplicity may be either simple or extremely complex and difficult to recognize. The patients are frequently connected in some way with the health professions, they are often migratory, and their motivation in complex cases is usually unclear.

## Complications

A poor doctor-patient relationship, with iatrogenic disorders and "doctor shopping," are the principal problems. Sedative and analgesic dependency is the most common iatrogenic complication.

## Treatment

**A. Medical:** Medical support with careful attention to building a therapeutic doctor-patient relationship is the mainstay of treatment. *It must be accepted that the patient's distress is real. Every problem not found to have an organic basis is not necessarily a mental disease.* Diligent attempts should be made to relate symptoms to adverse developments in the patient's life. It may be useful to have the patient keep a meticulous diary, paying particular attention to various pertinent factors evident in the history. Regular, frequent, short appointments may be helpful. Drugs should not be prescribed to replace appointments. One doctor should be the primary physician, and consultants should be used mainly for evaluation. An emphatic, realistic, optimistic approach must be maintained in the face of the expected ups and downs.

**B. Psychologic:** Psychologic approaches can be used by the primary physician when it is clear that the patient is ready to make some changes in lifestyle in order to achieve symptomatic relief. This is often best approached on a here-and-now basis and oriented toward pragmatic changes rather than an exploration of early experiences that the patient frequently fails to relate to current distress. Individual group therapy with others who have similar problems is sometimes of value to improve coping, allow ventilation, and focus on interpersonal adjustment. Hypnosis and amobarbital interviews used early are helpful in resolving conversion disorders. If the primary physician has been working with the patient on psychologic problems related to the physical illness, the groundwork is often laid for successful psychiatric referral.

**C. Behavioral:** Behavioral therapy is probably best exemplified by the current efforts in biofeedback techniques. In biofeedback, the particular abnormality (eg, increased peristalsis) must be recognized and monitored by the patient and therapist (eg, by an electronic stethoscope to amplify the sounds). This is immediate feedback, and after learning to recognize it the patient can then learn to identify any change thus produced (eg, a decrease in bowel sounds) and so become a conscious originator of the feedback instead of a passive recipient. Relief of the symptom operantly conditions the patient to utilize the maneuver that relieves symptoms (eg, relaxation causing a decrease in bowel sounds). With emphasis on this type of learning, the patient is able to identify symptoms early and initiate the countermaneuvers, thus

decreasing the symptomatic problem. Migraine and tension headaches have been particularly responsive to biofeedback methods.

**D. Social:** Social endeavors include family, work, and other interpersonal activity. Family members should come for some appointments with the patient so that they can learn how best to live with the patient. This is particularly important in treatment of the somatization and psychogenic pain disorders. Ileostomy clubs and similar mutual aid groups provide a climate for encouraging the patient to accept and live with the problem. Ongoing communication with the employer may be necessary to encourage long-term continued interest in the employee. Employers can become just as discouraged as physicians in dealing with employees who have chronic problems.

## Prognosis

The prognosis is much better if the primary physician is able to intervene early before the situation has deteriorated. After the problem has crystallized into chronicity, it is very difficult to effect change.

Ford CV: The somatizing disorders. *Psychosomatics* 1986;**27**:327.

Ford CV, Folks DG: Conversion disorders: An overview. *Psychosomatics* 1985;**26**:371.

Lesser RP: Psychogenic seizures. *Psychosomatics* 1986;**27**:823.

Othmer E, DeSouza C: A screening test for somatization disorder (hysteria). *Am J Psychiatry* 1985;**142**:1146.

Smith GR, Mouson RA; Psychiatric consultation in somatization disorder: A randomized controlled study. *N Engl J Med* 1986;**314**:1407.

## CHRONIC PAIN DISORDERS

### Essentials of Diagnosis

- Chronic complaints of pain.
- Symptoms frequently exceed signs.
- Minimal relief with standard treatment.
- History of many physicians.
- Frequent use of many nonspecific medications.

### General Considerations

A problem in the management of pain is the lack of distinction between acute and chronic pain syndromes. Most physicians are adept at dealing with acute pain problems but have difficulty handling the patient with chronic pain. This type of patient frequently takes too many medications, stays in bed a great deal, has had many physicians, has lost skills, and experiences little joy in either work or play. All relationships suffer (including those with physicians), and life becomes a constant search for succor. The search results in complex physician-patient relationships that usually include many drug trials, particularly sedatives. Treatment failures provoke angry responses and depression from both the physician and the patient, and the pain syndrome is exacerbated.

When frustration becomes too great, a new physician is found, and the cycle is repeated. The longer the existence of the pain, the more important the psychologic factors of anxiety and depression, which are often a consequence rather than a cause of chronic pain. As with all other conditions, it is counterproductive to speculate about whether the pain is "real." It is real to the patient, and acceptance of the problem underlines a mutual endeavor to alleviate the disturbance.

## Clinical Findings

Components of the chronic pain syndrome include anatomic changes, chronic anxiety and depression, and changed life-style. Usually, the anatomic problem is irreversible, since it has already been subjected to many interventions with increasingly unsatisfactory results.

Chronic anxiety and depression produce heightened irritability and overreaction to stimuli. A marked decrease in pain threshold is apparent. This pattern develops into a hypochondriacal preoccupation with the body and a constant need for reassurance. The pressure on the doctor becomes wearing and often leads to covert rejection devices, such as not being available or making referrals to other physicians. This is perceived by the patient, who then intensifies the effort to get help, and the typical cycle is under way. Anxiety and depression are seldom discussed, almost as if there is a tacit agreement not to deal with these issues.

Changes in life-style involve some of the so-called pain games. These usually take the form of a family script in which the patient accepts the role of being sick, and this role then becomes the focus of most family interactions and may become important in maintaining the family, so that neither the patient nor the family wants the patient's role to change. Demands for attention and efforts to control the behavior of others revolve around the central issue of control of other people (including physicians). Cultural factors frequently play a role in the behavior of the patient and how the significant people around the patient cope with the problem. Some cultures encourage demonstrative behavior, while others value the stoic role. The physician's recognition of this fact is important, since overt dramatization of the discomfort is sometimes helpful in alleviating the problem.

Another secondary gain that frequently maintains the patient in the sick role is financial compensation or other benefits ("green poultice"). Frequently, such systems are structured so that they reinforce the maintenance of sickness and discourage any attempts to give up the role. Physicians unwittingly reinforce this role because of the very nature of the practice of medicine, which is to respond to complaints of illness. Helpful suggestions are often met with responses like "Yes, but. . . ." Medications then become the principal approach, and drug dependency problems may develop.

## Treatment

**A. Behavioral:** The cornerstone of a unified approach to chronic pain syndromes is a comprehensive behavioral program. This is necessary to identify and eliminate pain reinforcers, to decrease drug use, and to use effectively those positive reinforcers that shift the focus from the pain. *It is critical that the patient be made a partner in the effort to alleviate pain.* (Avoid the concept of cure.) The patient should agree to discuss the pain only with the physician and not with family members; this tends to stabilize the patient's personal life, since the family is usually tired of the subject. At the beginning of treatment, the patient should be assigned self-help tasks graded up to maximal activity, as a means of positive reinforcement. The tasks should not exceed capability. The patient can also be asked to keep a self-rating chart to log accomplishments, so that progress can be measured and remembered. Instruct the patient to record degrees of pain on a self-rating scale in relation to various situations and mental attitudes so that similar circumstances can be avoided or modified.

Avoid negative reinforcers such as sympathy and attention to pain. Emphasize a positive response to productive activities, which remove the focus of attention from the pain. Activity is also desensitizing, since the patient learns to tolerate increasing activity levels.

Biofeedback techniques (see Somatoform Disorders, above) and hypnosis have been successful in ameliorating some pain syndromes. Hypnosis tends to be most effective in those patients with a high level of denial, who are more responsive to suggestion. Hypnosis can be used to lessen anxiety, alter perception of the length of time that pain is experienced, and encourage relaxation.

**B. Medical:** A *single physician* in charge of the multiple treatment approach is the highest priority. Consultations as indicated and technical procedures done by others are appropriate, but the care of the patient should remain in the hands of the primary physician. Referrals should not be allowed to raise the patient's hopes unrealistically or to become a way for the physician to reject the case. The attitude of the doctor should be one of honesty, interest, and hopefulness—not for a cure but for alleviation of symptoms and continuing improvement.

Medications, nerve stimulation, and surgery should be used appropriately, not out of desperation (see Chapter 1). Physical means of relief (heat, cold) should be part of the daily routine; this tends to encourage compliance. Neither analgesics nor sedatives should be given on an "as needed" schedule. A fixed schedule lessens the conditioning effects of these drugs. Tricyclic antidepressants in doses smaller than those used in depression may be helpful by blocking central nervous system pain interpretation and promoting sleep.

**C. Social:** *Involvement of family members and other significant persons in the patient's life should* *be an early priority*. The best efforts of both patient and therapists can be unwittingly sabotaged by other persons who may feel that they are "helping" the patient. They frequently tend to reinforce the negative aspects of the pain syndrome. The patient becomes more dependent and less active, and the pain syndrome becomes an immutable way of life. The more destructive "pain games" described by many experts in chronic pain syndromes are results of well-meaning but misguided efforts of family members. Ongoing therapy with the family can be helpful in the early identification and elimination of these behavior patterns.

Alteration of behavior in others (including employers and friends) requires repetition of instructions and fairly frequent contact. The tendency is to slip back into behavior patterns that impede progress. Group instruction by a nurse or physician's assistant is valuable and is enhanced by interchanges of people in the group. Repetition and group interaction tend to fix the instructions.

**D. Psychologic:** In addition to group therapy with family members and others, groups of patients can be helpful if properly led. The major goal, whether of individual or group therapy, is to gain patient *involvement*. A group can be a powerful instrument for achieving this goal, with the development of group loyalties and cooperation. People will frequently make efforts with group encouragement that they would never make alone. Individual therapy should be directed toward strengthening existing defenses and improving self-esteem. The rapport between patient and physician, as in all psychotherapeutic efforts, is the major factor in therapeutic success.

Kanner R: Pain management. *JAMA* 1986;**256**:2112.

Katon W, Egan K, Miller D: Chronic pain: Lifetime psychiatric diagnoses and family history. *Am J Psychiatry* 1985;**142**:1156.

## PSYCHOSEXUAL DISORDERS

The stages of sexual activity include **excitement** (arousal), **plateau, orgasm,** and **resolution.** The precipitating excitement or arousal is psychologically determined. Arousal response leading to plateau is a physiologic and psychologic phenomenon of vasocongestion, a parasympathetic reaction causing erection in the male and labial/clitoral congestion in the female. The orgasmic response includes emission in the male and clonic contractions of the analogous striated perineal muscles of both male and female. Resolution is a gradual return to normal physiologic status.

While the arousal stimuli—vasocongestive and orgasmic responses—constitute a single response in a well-adjusted person, they can be considered as separate stages that can produce different syndromes responding to different treatment procedures.

## Clinical Findings

There are 3 major groups of sexual disorders.

**A. Paraphilias (Sexual Arousal Disorders):** In these conditions, formerly called "deviations" or "variations," the excitement stage of sexual activity is associated with sexual objects or orientations different from those usually associated with adult heterosexual stimulation. The stimulus may be a woman's shoe, a child, the genitalia of persons of the same sex, animals, instruments of torture, or incidents of aggression. The pattern of sexual stimulation is usually one that has early psychologic roots. Poor experiences with heterosexual activity frequently reinforce this pattern over time.

**Exhibitionism** is the impulsive behavior of exposing the genitalia in order to achieve sexual excitation. It is a childhood sexual behavior carried into adult life, and it is limited as a clinical condition to males.

**Transvestism** is the wearing of clothes and the enactment of a role of the opposite sex for the purpose of sexual excitation. Such fetishistic cross-dressing can be part of masturbation foreplay in heterosexual men who in all other respects behave in a masculine way. Transvestism in homosexuality and transsexualism is not done to cause sexual excitement but is a function of the gender disorder.

**Voyeurism** involves the achievement of sexual arousal by secretly watching the activities of women, usually in various stages of undress or sexual activity. In both exhibitionism and voyeurism, excitation leads to masturbation as a *replacement* for heterosexual activity.

**Pedophilia** is the use of a child of either sex to achieve sexual arousal and, in many cases, gratification. Contact is frequently oral, with either participant being dominant, but pedophilia includes intercourse of any type. Adults of both sexes engage in this behavior, but because of social and cultural factors it is more commonly identified with males. The pedophile has difficulty in adult sexual relationships, and males who perform this act are frequently impotent.

**Incest** involves a sexual relationship with a person in the immediate family, most frequently a child. In many ways it is similar to pedophilia (intrafamilial pedophilia). Incestuous feelings are fairly common, but cultural mores are usually sufficiently strong to act as a barrier to the expression of sexual feelings.

**Bestiality** is the attainment of sexual gratification by intercourse with an animal. The intercourse may involve penetration or simply contact with the human genitalia by the tongue of the animal. The practice is more common in rural or isolated areas and is frequently a substitute for human sexual contact rather than an expression of preference.

**Sadism** is the attainment of sexual arousal by inflicting pain upon the sexual object, and **masochism** is the attainment of sexual excitation by enduring pain. Much sexual activity has aggressive components (eg, biting, scratching). Forced sexual acquiescence (eg, rape) is considered to be primarily an act of aggression.

**Bondage** is the achievement of erotic pleasure by being humiliated, enslaved, physically bound, and restrained. It is life-threatening, since neck binding or partial asphyxiation usually forms part of the ritual.

**Necrophilia** is sexual intercourse with a dead body or the use of parts of a dead body for sexual excitation, often with masturbation.

**B. Gender Identity Variations:** *Core gender identity* reflects a biologic self-image—the conviction that "I am a male" or "I am a female." While this is a fixed self-image, *gender role identity* is a dynamic, changing self-representation. Variances of core gender identity are rare, while those of gender role identity are common. The major gender variation is transsexualism.

**Transsexualism** (a core gender identity problem) is an attempt to deny and reverse biologic sex by maintaining sexual identity with the opposite gender. Transsexuals do not alternate between gender roles; rather, they assume a fixed role of attitudes, feelings, fantasies, and choices consonant with those of the opposite sex, all of which clearly date back to early development. For example, male transsexuals in early childhood behave, talk, and fantasize as if they were girls. They do not grow out of feminine patterns, they do not work in professions traditionally considered to be masculine, and they have no interest in their own penises either as evidence of maleness or as organs for erotic behavior. The desire for sex change starts early and may culminate in assumption of a feminine life-style, hormonal treatment, and use of surgical procedures, including castration and vaginoplasty.

**Homosexuality** is no longer considered to be a classifiable sexual disorder. Problems arise in this group when the individual has difficulty accepting the sexual orientation or is under stress in a society that is intolerant.

**C. Psychosexual Dysfunction:** This category includes a large group of vasocongestive and orgasmic disorders. Often, they involve problems of sexual adaptation, education, and technique that are often initially discussed with, diagnosed by, and treated by the family physician.

There are 2 conditions common in the male: impotence and ejaculation disturbances.

**Impotence** (erectile dysfunction) is the inability to attain or maintain an erection firm enough for satisfactory intercourse. Causes for this vasocongestive disorder can be psychologic, physiologic, or both. After the onset of the problem, a history of repeated erections (particularly nocturnal penile tumescence, which may be evaluated in a sleep laboratory) is evidence that the dysfunction is psychologic in origin. Psychologic impotence is caused by either interpersonal or intrapsychic factors (eg, marital disharmony, depression). Organic factors include diabetes mellitus, drug abuse (alcohol, narcotics, stimulants), pharmacologic agents (anticholinergic drugs, antihyper-

tensive medication, disulfiram, all psychotherapeutic drugs, narcotics, estrogens), organ system failure (circulatory, cardiorespiratory, renal), surgical complications (prostatectomy, vascular and back surgery), trauma (disk and spinal cord injuries), endocrine disturbances (pituitary, thyroid, adrenal), zinc deficiency, neurologic disorders (multiple sclerosis, tumors, peripheral neuropathies, pernicious anemia, syphilis), urologic problems (phimosis, Peyronie's disease, priapism), and congenital abnormalities (Klinefelter's syndrome).

**Ejaculation disturbances** include premature ejaculation, inability to ejaculate, and retrograde ejaculation. (One may ejaculate even though impotent.) Ejaculation is usually connected with orgasm, and ejaculatory control is an acquired behavior that is minimal in adolescence and increases with experience. Pathogenic factors are those that interfere with learning control, most frequently sexual ignorance. Intrapsychic factors (anxiety, guilt, depression) and interpersonal maladaptation (marital problems, unresponsiveness of mate, power struggles) are also common. Organic causes include interference with sympathetic nerve distribution (often due to surgery or trauma) and the effects of pharmacologic agents on sympathetic tone. Postcoital cephalalgia is common and may be a variant of migraine.

In females, the 2 most common forms of sexual dysfunction are vaginismus and frigidity.

**Vaginismus** is a conditioned response in which a spasm of the perineal muscles occurs if there is any stimulation of the area. The desire is to avoid penetration. Sexual responsiveness and vasocongestion may be present, and orgasm from clitoral stimulation is common.

**Frigidity** is a complex condition in which there is a general lack of sexual responsiveness. The woman has difficulty in experiencing erotic sensation and does not have the vasocongestive response. Sexual activity varies from active avoidance of sex to an occasional orgasm. Orgasmic dysfunction—in which a woman has a vasocongestive response but varying degrees of difficulty in reaching orgasm—is sometimes differentiated from frigidity. Causes for the dysfunctions include poor sexual techniques, early traumatic sexual experiences, interpersonal disharmony (marital struggles, use of sex as a means of control), and intrapsychic problems (anxiety, fear, guilt). Organic causes include any conditions that might cause pain in intercourse, pelvic pathology, mechanical obstruction, and neurologic deficits.

**Disorders of sexual desire** refer to reduction or absence of sexual desire in either sex and may be a function of organic or psychologic difficulties. Any chronic illness can sap desire, but cerebral problems such as partial complex seizures, panhypopituitarism, Cushing's syndrome, and parkinsonism frequently cause a decrease in sexual drive. Hormonal variations, including use of antiandrogen compounds such as cyproterone acetate, and chronic renal failure contribute to deterioration in sexual activity. Alcohol, sedatives, narcotics, marihuana, and some medications may affect sexual drive.

### Treatment

#### A. Paraphilias and Gender Identity Disorders:

**1. Psychologic**–Sexual arousal disorders involving variant sexual activity (paraphilia), particularly those of a more superficial nature (eg, voyeurism) and those of recent onset, are responsive to psychotherapy in a moderate percentage of cases. The prognosis is much better if the motivation comes from the individual rather than the legal system; unfortunately, however, court intervention is frequently the only stimulus to treatment, because the condition persists and is reinforced until conflict with the law occurs. Therapies frequently focus on barriers to normal arousal response; the expectation is that the variant behavior will decrease as normal behavior increases.

**2. Behavioral**–Aversive and operant conditioning techniques have been tried frequently in gender role disorders but have been only occasionally successful. In some cases, the sexual arousal disorders improve with modeling, role-playing, and conditioning procedures. Emotive imagery is occasionally helpful in lessening anxiety in fetish problems.

**3. Social**–Although they do not produce a change in sexual arousal patterns or gender role, self-help groups have facilitated adjustment to an often hostile society. Attention to the family is particularly important in helping persons in such groups to accept their situation and alleviate their guilt about the role they think they had in creating the problem.

**4. Medical**–After careful evaluation, some transsexuals are treated with hormones and genital surgery. The surgical procedures include penectomy in the male, with preservation of the invaginated penile skin for vaginoplasty. The meatus is occasionally partially preserved as a cervix substitute, and the scrotal skin is used in the construction of labia. Surgical procedures—particularly the construction of a penis—are more complicated in female-to-male conversion.

#### B. Psychosexual Dysfunction:

**1. Medical**–Identification of a contributory reversible cause is most important. Even if the condition is not reversible, identification of the specific cause helps the patient to accept the condition. Marital disharmony, with its exacerbating effects, may thus be avoided. Of all the sexual dysfunctions, impotence is the condition most likely to have an organic basis. When the condition is irreversible, penile implants may be considered. One type is an inserted pump device that offers the patient a choice of flaccidity or erection, but this is costly, complex, and subject to mechanical problems. Another type of implant results in permanent erection but is simple and relatively trouble-free. Revascularization surgery has been done in patients with impotence due to circulatory problems.

**2. Behavioral**–Syndromes resulting from conditioned responses have been treated by conditioning techniques, with excellent results. Vaginismus responds well to desensitization with graduated Hegar dilators along with relaxation techniques. Masters and Johnson have used behavioral approaches in all of the sexual dysfunctions, with concomitant supportive psychotherapy and with improvement of the communication patterns of the couple.

**3. Psychologic**–The use of psychotherapy by itself is best suited for those cases in which interpersonal difficulties or intrapsychic problems predominate. Anxiety and guilt about parental injunctions against sex constitute the most frequent psychopathology contributing to sexual dysfunction. Even in these cases, however, a combined behavioral-psychologic approach usually produces results most quickly.

**4. Social**–The proximity of other people (eg, a mother-in-law) in a household is frequently an inhibiting factor in sexual relationships. In such cases, some social engineering may alleviate the problem.

The physician's guide to sexual counseling. (Special issue.) *Med Aspects Hum Sex* (March) 1986;**20**. [Entire issue.]

Verhulst JM, Heiman JR: Sexual dysfunction: A guide to evaluation and intervention. *Postgrad Med* (March) 1985;**77**:295.

## PERSONALITY DISORDERS

### Essentials of Diagnosis

- Long history dating back to childhood.
- Recurrent maladaptive behavior.
- Low self-esteem and lack of confidence.
- Minimal introspective ability.
- Major difficulties with interpersonal relationships or society.
- Depression with anxiety when maladaptive behavior fails.

### General Considerations

Personality—a hypothetical construct—is the result of the prolonged interaction of an individual with personal drives and with outside influences, the sum being the enduring and unique patterns of behavior which are adopted in order to cope with the environment and which characterize one as an individual. Obviously, the more satisfactory the early development of a person, the stronger the personality development. The personality structure, or character, is an integral part of self-image and is important to one's sense of identity. People who fail to integrate satisfactory early experiences tend to have personality structures that manifest more primitive responses.

Lack of a self-identity is characteristic and is manifested by marked dependence on others and a tendency to imitate someone who may be important at a given time. There are repeated attempts to move toward another person, often in this dependent fashion, followed by the inevitable rejections that elicit the overreactive response.

The ambiguity of the term is one of the principal characteristics that perpetuates its use. It implies a developmental maladaption from an early age, with subsequent problems of behavior that are repetitive, personally handicapping, and annoying to others. The individual does not learn from bad experiences and feels little anxiety unless the pathologic coping pattern fails.

The classification of subtypes depends upon the predominant symptoms and their severity. The most severe disorders—those that bring the patient into greatest conflict with society—tend to be classified as antisocial (psychopathic) or borderline.

## Classification & Clinical Findings

**Paranoid:** Defensive, oversensitive, secretive, suspicious, hyperalert, with limited emotional response. **Schizoid:** Shy, introverted, withdrawn, avoids close relationships. **Compulsive:** Perfectionist, egocentric, indecisive, with rigid thought patterns and need for control. **Histrionic (hysterical):** Dependent, immature, seductive, histrionic, egocentric, vain, emotionally labile (a mnemonic device describing these traits is *dishevel*). **Schizotypal:** Superstitious, socially isolated, suspicious, with limited interpersonal ability and odd speech. **Narcissistic:** Exhibitionist, grandiose, preoccupied with power, lacks interest in others, with excessive demands for attention. **Avoidant:** Fears rejection, hyperreacts to rejection and failure, with poor social endeavors and low self-esteem. **Dependent:** Passive, overaccepting, unable to make decisions, lacks confidence, with poor self-esteem. **Passive-aggressive:** Stubborn, procrastinating, argumentative, sulking, helpless, clinging, negative to authority figures. **Antisocial:** Selfish, callous, promiscuous, impulsive, unable to learn from experience, has legal problems. **Borderline:** Impulsive, has unstable and intense interpersonal relationships, lacks self-control and self-fulfillment, has identity problems, affective instability, suicidal and aggressive behavior, feelings of emptiness, and occasional psychotic decompensation.

## Differential Diagnosis

Patients with personality disorders tend to show anxiety and depression when pathologic techniques fail, and their symptoms can be similar to those occurring with anxiety disorders. Occasionally, the more severe cases may decompensate into psychosis under stress and mimic other psychotic disorders.

## Treatment

**A. Social:** Social and therapeutic environments such as day hospitals, halfway houses, and self-help communities utilize peer pressures to modify the self-destructive behavior. The patient with a personality disorder often has failed to profit from experience, and difficulties with authority impair the learning experience. The use of peer relationships and the repetition possible in a structured setting of a helpful community enhances the educational opportunities and increases learning. When one's companions note

every flaw in one's character and insist that it be corrected immediately, a powerful learning environment is being created. When problems are detected early, both the school and the home can serve as foci of intensified social pressure to change the behavior, particularly with the use of behavioral techniques.

**B. Behavioral:** The behavioral techniques used are principally operant and aversive conditioning. The former simply emphasizes the recognition of acceptable behavior and reinforcement of this with praise or other tangible rewards. Aversive responses usually mean punishment, although this can range from a mild rebuke to some specific punitive responses such as verbal abuse or deprivation of privileges. Extinction plays a role in that an attempt is made not to respond to inappropriate behavior, and the lack of response eventually causes the person to abandon that type of behavior. Pouting and tantrums, for example, diminish quickly when such behavior elicits no reaction.

**C. Psychologic:** Psychologic intervention is most usefully accomplished in group settings. Group therapy is helpful when specific interpersonal behavior needs to be improved (eg, schizoid and inadequate types, where involvement with people is markedly impaired). This mode of treatment also has a place with so-called acting-out patients, ie, those who frequently act in an impulsive and inappropriate way. The peer pressure in the group tends to impose restraints on rash behavior. The group also quickly identifies the patient's types of behavior and helps to improve the validity of the patient's self-assessment, so that the antecedents of the unacceptable behavior can be effectively handled, thus decreasing its frequency. Individual therapy is of limited usefulness even in motivated patients.

**D. Medical:** Hospitalization is rarely indicated. In most cases, treatment can be accomplished in the day treatment center or self-help community. Antipsychotics may be required for short periods in conditions that have temporarily decompensated into transient psychoses (eg, haloperidol, 2–5 mg orally every 3–4 hours until the patient has quieted down and is regaining contact with reality). In most cases, these drugs are required only for several days and can be discontinued after the patient has regained a previously established level of adjustment. Sedatives (eg, diazepam, 5–10 mg orally several times a day) can be used when a decrease of passive avoidance is desired to allow the patient to learn and practice new kinds of behavior in a therapeutic setting (eg, in the very fearful schizoid patient who passively avoids people and is attempting to learn to interact in a group therapy setting).

## Prognosis

Antisocial and borderline categories generally have a poor prognosis, whereas persons with mild schizoid or passive-aggressive tendencies have a good prognosis with appropriate treatment.

Akiskal HS et al: Borderline: An adjective in search of a noun. *J Clin Psychiatry* 1985;**46:**41.

Livesley WJ: The classification of personality disorder. 1. The choice of category concept. *Can J Psychiatry* 1985;**30:**353.

Livesley WJ: Trait and behavioral prototypes of personality disorder. *Am J Psychiat* 1986;**143:**728.

# SCHIZOPHRENIC & OTHER PSYCHOTIC DISORDERS

## Essentials of Diagnosis (Schizophrenia)

- Social withdrawal, usually slowly progressive, often with deterioration in personal care.
- Loss of ego boundaries, with inability to perceive oneself as a separate entity.
- Loose thought associations, often with slowed thinking or overinclusive and rapid shifting from topic to topic.
- Autism with absorption in inner thoughts and frequent sexual or religious preoccupations.
- Auditory hallucinations, often of a derogatory nature.
- Delusions, frequently of a grandiose or persecutory nature.
- Symptoms of at least 6 months' duration.

*Frequent additional signs:*

- Flat affect and rapidly alternating mood shifts irrespective of circumstances.
- Hypersensitivity to environmental stimuli, with a feeling of enhanced sensory awareness.
- Variability or changeable behavior incongruent with the external environment.
- Concrete thinking with inability to abstract; inappropriate symbolism.
- Impaired concentration worsened by hallucinations and delusions.
- Depersonalization, wherein one behaves like a detached observer of one's own actions.

## General Considerations

The schizophrenic disorders are a group of syndromes manifested by massive disruption of thinking, mood, and overall behavior. According to *DSM-III* criteria, the onset of illness occurs before age 45; signs must be continuous for at least 6 months; the illness is not preceded by a full depressive or manic syndrome; and symptoms are not due to mental retardation or organic mental disorder. The characterization and nomenclature of the disorders are quite arbitrary and are influenced by sociocultural factors and schools of psychiatric thought.

It is currently believed that the schizophrenic disorders are of multifactorial cause, with genetic, environmental, neuroendocrine, and pathophysiologic components. At present, there is no laboratory method to confirm the diagnosis of schizophrenia. There may or may not be a history of a major disruption in the individual's life (failures, losses, physical illness) be-fore gross psychotic deterioration is evident. History obtained from others may indicate a long-standing "strange" premorbid personality.

"Other psychotic disorders" are conditions that are similar to schizophrenic illness in their acute symptoms but have a less pervasive influence over the long term. The individual usually attains higher levels of functioning. The acute psychotic episodes tend to be less disruptive of the person's life-style, with a fairly quick return to previous levels of functioning.

## Classifications

**A. Schizophrenic Disorders:** Schizophrenic disorders are subdivided on the basis of certain prominent phenomena that are frequently present. **Disorganized (hebephrenic) schizophrenia** is characterized by marked incoherence and an incongruous or silly affect. **Catatonic schizophrenia** is distinguished by a marked psychomotor disturbance of either excitement (purposeless and stereotyped) or rigidity with mutism. Infrequently, there may be rapid alternation between excitement and stupor (see under catatonic syndrome, below). **Paranoid schizophrenia** includes marked persecutory or grandiose delusions often consonant with hallucinations of similar content. **Undifferentiated schizophrenia** denotes a category in which symptoms are not specific enough to warrant inclusion of the illness in the other subtypes. **Residual schizophrenia** is a classification that includes persons who have clearly had an episode warranting a diagnosis of schizophrenia but who at present have no overt psychotic symptoms, although they show milder signs such as social withdrawal, flat affect, and eccentric behaviors.

**B. Paranoid (Delusional) Disorders:** Paranoid disorders are psychoses in which the predominant symptoms are persistent persecutory delusions, with minimal impairment in daily function (the schizophrenic disorders show significant impairment). Intellectual and occupational activities are little affected, whereas social and marital functioning tend to be markedly involved. Hallucinations are not usually present. Many of these patients are misdiagnosed as paranoid schizophrenics. The category includes such states as paranoia, shared paranoid disorder (folie à deux), and paranoid state, the last being characterized by its transitory nature, whereas the others are more chronic.

**C. Schizoaffective Disorders:** Schizoaffective disorders are those cases that fail to fit comfortably either in the schizophrenic or in the affective categories. They are usually cases with affective symptoms that precede or develop concurrently with psychotic manifestations. They were formerly included under the heading of schizoaffective schizophrenia and more recently have been labeled by some as atypical bipolar affective disorders.

**D. Schizophreniform Disorders:** Schizophreniform disorders are similar in their symptoms to the schizophrenic disorders except that the duration of the illness is less than 6 months but more than 1 week.

**E. Brief Reactive Psychotic Disorders:** These disorders last less than 1 week. They are the result of psychologic stress. The shorter duration is significant and correlates with a more acute onset and resolution as well as a much better prognosis.

## Clinical Findings (Schizophrenia)

The signs and symptoms vary markedly among individuals as well as in the same person at different times. **Appearance** may be bizarre, although the usual finding is a mild to moderate unkempt blandness. **Motor activity** is generally reduced, although extremes ranging from catatonic stupor to frenzied excitement occur. **Social behavior** is characterized by marked withdrawal, coupled with disturbed interpersonal relationships and a reduced ability to experience pleasure. Dependency and a poor self-image are common. **Verbal utterances** are variable, the language being concrete yet symbolic, with unassociated rambling statements (at times interspersed with mutism) during an acute episode. Neologisms (made-up words or phrases), echolalia (repetition of words spoken by others), and verbigeration (repetition of senseless words or phrases) are occasionally present. **Affect** is usually flattened and shallow, with occasional inappropriateness. **Depression** is ubiquitous but may be less apparent during the acute psychotic episode and become more obvious during recovery. It is not usually necessary to give antidepressant medication. Depression is sometimes confused with akinetic side effects of antipsychotic drugs.

**Thought content** may vary from a paucity of ideas to a rich complex of delusional fantasy with archaic thinking. One frequently notes after a period of conversation that little if any information has actually been conveyed. Incoming stimuli produce varied responses. In some cases a simple question may trigger explosive outbursts, whereas at other times there may be no overt response whatsoever (catatonia). When paranoid ideation is present, the patient is often irritable and less cooperative. Delusions (false beliefs) are characteristic of paranoid thinking, and they usually take the form of a preoccupation with the supposedly threatening behavior exhibited by other individuals. This ideation may cause the patient to adopt active countermeasures such as locking doors and windows, taking up weapons, covering the ceiling with aluminum foil to counteract radar waves, and other bizarre efforts. Somatic delusions revolve around issues of bodily decay or infestation. **Perceptual distortions** usually include auditory hallucinations—visual hallucinations are more commonly associated with organic mental states—and may include illusions (distortions of reality) such as figures changing in size or lights varying in intensity. Cenesthetic hallucinations (eg, burning sensation in the brain, feeling blood flowing in blood vessels) are fairly common. Lack of humor, feelings of dread, depersonaliza-

tion (a feeling of being apart from the self), and fears of annihilation may be present. Any of the above symptoms generates higher anxiety levels, with heightened arousal and occasional panic, as the individual fails to cope.

Ventricular enlargement in the brain, as seen on the CT scan, has been correlated with a chronic course, severe cognitive impairment, and nonresponsiveness to neuroleptic medications.

The development of the acute episode in schizophrenia frequently is the end product of a gradual decompensation. Frustration and anxiety appear early, followed by depression and alienation, along with decreased effectiveness in day-to-day coping. This often leads to feelings of panic and increasing disorganization, with loss of the ability to test and evaluate the reality of perceptions. The stage of so-called psychotic resolution includes delusions, autistic preoccupations, and psychotic insight, with acceptance of the decompensated state. The schizophrenic process is frequently complicated by the use of alcohol and other recreational drugs. Polydipsia with hyponatremia occasionally occurs in these patients. It may be related to the disorder, antipsychotic drugs (dosage and type not a factor), or cigarette smoking (which is very common in this population).

## Differential Diagnosis

*First and foremost should be a reconsideration of the diagnosis of schizophrenia in any person who has been so diagnosed in the past, particularly when the clinical course has been atypical.* A number of these patients have been found to actually have atypical episodic affective disorders that have responded well to lithium. Manic episodes often mimic schizophrenia. Also, many individuals have been diagnosed as schizophrenic because of inadequacies in psychiatric nomenclature. Thus, persons with brief reactive psychoses, paranoid disorders, and schizophreniform disorders were often inappropriately diagnosed as having schizophrenia. Toxic reactions to drugs have also been incorrectly diagnosed as schizophrenia in many instances.

Psychotic depressions, psychotic organic mental states, and any illness with psychotic ideation tend to be confused with schizophrenia, partly because of the regrettable tendency to use the terms interchangeably. Adolescent phases of growth and counterculture behaviors constitute another area of diagnostic confusion. It is particularly important to avoid a misdiagnosis in these groups, because of the long-term implications arising from having such a serious diagnosis made in a formative stage of life.

**Medical disorders** such as thyroid dysfunction, adrenal and pituitary disorders, and practically all of the organic mental states in the early stages must be ruled out. **Complex partial seizures,** especially when psychosensory phenomena are present, are an important differential consideration. Toxic drug states arising from prescription, over-the-counter, and street drugs may mimic all of the psychotic disorders. The chronic use of amphetamines, cocaine, and other stimulants frequently produces a psychosis that is almost identical to the acute paranoid schizophrenic episode. Stimulants (including caffeine) and marihuana (antagonizes neuroleptics) may precipitate acute psychiatric symptoms in the schizophrenic. The presence of formication and stereotypy suggests the possibility of stimulant abuse. Phencyclidine (see below) has become a very common street drug, and in many cases an adverse reaction to it is difficult to distinguish from other psychotic disorders. Cerebellar signs, excessive salivation, dilated pupils, and increased deep tendon reflexes should alert the physician to the possibility of a toxic psychosis. Industrial chemicals (both organic and metallic), degenerative disorders, and metabolic deficiencies must be considered in the differential diagnosis.

**Catatonic syndrome,** frequently assumed to exist solely as a component of schizophrenic disorders, is actually the end product of a number of illnesses, including various organic conditions. Neoplasms, viral encephalopathies, central nervous system hemorrhage, metabolic derangements such as diabetic ketoacidosis, sedative withdrawal, and hepatic and renal malfunction have all been implicated. It is particularly important to realize that drug toxicity (eg, overdoses of antipsychotic medications such as fluphenazine or haloperidol can cause catatonic syndrome, which may be misdiagnosed as a catatonic schizophrenic disorder and inappropriately treated with more antipsychotic medication.

### Treatment

**A. Medical:** Hospitalization is often necessary, particularly when the patient's behavior shows gross disorganization. The presence of competent family members lessens the need for hospitalization, and each case should be judged individually. The major considerations are to prevent self-inflicted harm or harm to others and to provide the patient's basic needs. CT scanning should be considered in first episodes of schizophreniform disorder and other psychotic episodes of unknown cause.

**Antipsychotic medications** (see Antidepressant Drugs, p. 630) are the treatment of choice. The relapse rate can be reduced by 50% with proper maintenance neuroleptic therapy. The so-called **positive symptoms** such as hallucinations and delusions respond best, while **negative symptoms** such as withdrawal, psychomotor retardation, and poor interpersonal relationships may show little improvement. The addition of a benzodiazepine drug to the neuroleptic regimen may prove helpful in treating the agitated psychotic patient who has not responded to neuroleptics alone; the benzodiazepine may make possible maintenance with a lower neuroleptic dose (perhaps reducing the risk of tardive dyskinesia).

**B. Social:** Environmental considerations are most important in the individual with a chronic illness, who usually has a history of repeated hospitalizations, a continued low level of functioning, and symptoms that never completely remit. This type of patient has usually never lived up to basic potential and frequently has been rejected by family members. The work record has frequently been poor, with a disability pension being the usual means of financial support. In these cases, board and care homes experienced in caring for psychiatric patients are most important. There is frequently an inverse relationship between stability of the living situation and the amounts of required antipsychotic drugs.

Nonresidential self-help groups such as Recovery, Inc. should be utilized whenever possible. They provide a setting for sharing, learning, and mutual support and are frequently the only social involvement with which this type of patient is comfortable. Work agencies (eg, Goodwill Industries, Inc.) and vocational rehabilitation departments provide assessment, training, and job opportunities at a level commensurate with the person's clinical condition.

**C. Psychologic:** The need for psychotherapy varies markedly depending on the patient's current status and past history. Patients with a long history of chronic disability do not benefit appreciably from the usual verbal, insight-oriented therapies. A person with a single psychotic episode and a previously good level of adjustment may do very well with psychologic therapy after the acute phase has been resolved with medication and the passage of time. Supportive psychotherapy may be helpful in assisting the patient to reintegrate the experience, gain some insight into antecedent problems, and become a more self-observant individual who can recognize early signs of stress. Insight-oriented psychotherapy is often counterproductive in this type of disorder. More importantly, family therapy should be given concomitantly to help alleviate the patient's stress and to assist relatives in coping with the patient.

**D. Behavioral:** Behavioral techniques (see above) are most frequently used in therapeutic settings such as day treatment centers, but there is no reason why they cannot be incorporated into family situations or any therapeutic setting. Many behavioral techniques are used unwittingly (eg, positive reinforcement—whether it be a word of praise or an approving nod—after some positive behavior), and with some careful thought, this approach can be a most powerful instrument for helping a person learn behaviors that will facilitate social acceptance. The family or board and care situation is the most important place for practice of such techniques, since so much of the patient's time is spent in such settings.

Cloninger CR et al: Diagnosis and prognosis in schizophrenia. *Arch Gen Psychiatry* 1985;**42**:15.

Johnstone EC et al: The relative stability of positive and negative factors in chronic schizophrenia. *Br J Psychiat* 1987; **150**:60.

Jos CJ, Evenson RC, Mallya AR: Self-induced water intoxication: A comparison of 34 cases with matched controls. *J Clin Psychiat* 1986;**47**:368.

Mann SC: Lathal catatonia. *Am J Psychiat* 1986;**143**:1374.

Solovay MR, Shenton ME, Holzman PS: Comparative studies

of thought disorders: 1. Mania and schizophrenia. *Arch Gen Psychiat* 1987;**44**:13.

# MOOD DISORDERS
## (Depression & Mania)

## Essentials of Diagnosis

*Present in most depressions:*

- Lowered mood, varying from mild sadness to intense feelings of guilt, worthlessness, and hopelessness.
- Difficulty in thinking, including inability to concentrate and lack of decisiveness.
- Loss of interest, with diminished involvement in work and recreation.
- Somatic complaints such as headache; disrupted, lessened, or excessive sleep; loss of energy; change in appetite; decreased sexual drive.
- Anxiety.

*Present in some severe depressions:*

- Psychomotor retardation or agitation.
- Delusions of a hypochondriacal or persecutory nature.
- Withdrawal from activities.
- Physical symptoms of major severity, eg, anorexia, insomnia, reduced sexual drive, weight loss, and various somatic complaints.
- Suicidal ideation.

## General Considerations

Depression, like anxiety, is ubiquitous and is a reality of everyday life. It may be the final expression of (1) genetic factors (neurotransmitter dysfunction), (2) developmental problems (personality defects, childhood events), or (3) psychosocial stresses (divorce, job loss). It frequently presents in the form of somatic complaints with negative medical workup. It can be a normal reaction to a wide variety of events and must be evaluated as such. When the depression is appropriate to a life event and is not of major magnitude, specific treatment is not necessary. In many cases the patient comes to the physician to find out if the depression is abnormal, and in a significant number of cases all that is needed is reassurance. Not every depression requires treatment, and the inappropriate use of antidepressant medications is a direct result of the physician's failure to appreciate this.

The whole issue of depression is further confused by the fact that the word is used as an expression of a mood, a symptom, a syndrome, or a disease. Furthermore, the classifications are totally different and do not necessarily relate to each other.

## Clinical Findings

In general, there are 3 major groups of depressions, with similar symptoms in each group.

**A. Reactive to Psychosocial Factors:** Depression may occur in reaction to some outside (exogenous) adverse life situation, usually loss of a person by death, divorce, etc; financial reversal; or loss of an established role, such as being needed. Anger and aggression or repression are frequently associated with the loss, and this in turn often produces a feeling of guilt. The loss, anger, and guilt are readily apparent as the patient discusses the depression with the physician, who should be particularly alert to these components. Adjectives such as reactive and neurotic (implying anxiety, which is often present in these depressions) are often used in this group of depressions. The symptoms range from mild sadness, anxiety, irritability, worry, lack of concentration, discouragement, and somatic complaints to the more severe symptoms of the next group.

**B. Depressive Disorders:** The subclassifications include major depressive episodes and dysthymia.

**1. A major depressive episode** (endogenous unipolar disorder, involutional melancholia) is a period of serious mood depression that occurs relatively independently of the patient's life situations or events. Many consider a physiologic or metabolic aberration to be causative. Complaints vary widely but most frequently include a loss of interest and pleasure (anhedonia), withdrawal from activities, and feelings of guilt. Also included are inability to concentrate, some cognitive function, anxiety, chronic fatigue, feelings of worthlessness, somatic complaints (unidentifiable somatic complaints frequently indicate depression), and loss of sexual drive. Diurnal variation with improvement as the day progresses is common. Vegetative signs that frequently occur are insomnia (particularly early morning awakening), anorexia with weight loss, and constipation and loss of sexual drive. Occasionally, severe agitation and psychotic ideation (paranoid thinking, somatic delusions) are present. Paranoid symptoms may range from general suspiciousness to ideas of reference with delusions. The somatic delusions frequently revolve around feelings of impending annihilation or hypochondriacal beliefs (eg, that the body is rotting away with cancer). Hallucinations are uncommon. Major depressive disorders may occur at any time from childhood through adult life. The incidence is somewhat higher in women, and there is a greater chance of occurrence during the involutional period with symptoms of severe agitation, somatic complaints, insomnia, and feelings of guilt. Puerperal psychosis may be linked to the major affective disorders, as is seasonal affective depression (SAD), which occurs more commonly in the winter because of decreased exposure to light.

Atypical depression is a subtype that is characterized by hypersomnia, overeating, lethargy, and rejection sensitivity. Patients with atypical depression may respond better to treatment with a monoamine oxidase inhibitor.

**2. Dysthymic disorder** is a chronic depressive disturbance. Sadness, loss of interest, and withdrawal from activities over a period of 2 or more years with a relatively persistent course is necessary for this diagnosis. Generally, the symptoms are milder and longer-lasting than those in a major depressive episode.

**C. Bipolar Disorders:** Bipolar disorders (manic *and* depressive episodes) and individual manic episodes usually occur earlier (late teens or early adult life) than major depressive episodes.

**1. A manic episode** is a mood change characterized by elation with hyperactivity, overinvolvement in life activities, low irritability threshold, flight of ideas, easy distractibility, and little need for sleep. The overenthusiastic quality of the mood and the expansive behavior initially attract others, but the irritability, mood lability, aggressive behavior, and grandiosity usually lead to marked interpersonal difficulties. Activities may occur that are later regretted, eg, excessive spending, resignation from a job, a hasty marriage, sexual acting out, and exhibitionistic behavior, with alienation of friends and acquaintances. Atypical manic episodes can include gross delusions, paranoid ideation of severe proportions, and auditory hallucinations usually related to some grandiose perception. The episodes begin abruptly (sometimes precipitated by life stresses) and may last from several days to months. Generally, the manic episodes are of shorter duration than the depressive episodes. In almost all cases, the manic episode is part of a broader bipolar (manic-depressive) disorder. Some causes of maniclike symptoms include drugs such as levodopa and steroids. Partial complex seizures, head injury, and a wide variety of medical conditions may cause agitation and restlessness that may mimic mania (see Delusions, below). Manic patients differ from schizophrenics in that the former use more effective interpersonal maneuvers, are more sensitive to the social maneuvers of others, and are more able to utilize weakness and vulnerability in others to their own advantage. Catatonia may be a feature of bipolar disorder. Schizophrenics are more withdrawn, less sensitive to nuances, and less flexible; unlike the manic, they seldom if ever function on an efficient interpersonal level.

**2. Cyclothymic disorders** are chronic mood disturbances with episodes of depression and hypomania. The symptoms must have at least a 2-year duration and are milder than those in a depressive or manic episode. Occasionally, the symptoms will escalate into a full-blown manic or depressive episode, in which case it would be classified as a bipolar disorder.

**D. Secondary to Illness and Drugs:** Any illness, severe or mild, can cause significant depression. Conditions such as rheumatoid arthritis, multiple sclerosis, and chronic heart disease are particularly likely to be associated with depression, as are all other chronic illnesses. Hormonal variations clearly play a role in some depressions. Varying degrees of depression occur at various times in schizophrenic disorders and organic mental states. **Alcohol dependency** frequently coexists with serious depression. Any patient overusing alcohol should be evaluated for an affective disorder. Conversely, any patient with symptoms of depression should be questioned carefully for problems of alcohol abuse (or abuse of any other sedative drug).

The classic model of drug-induced depression (which is diagnosed as organic mood disorders) occurs with the use of reserpine, both in a clinical and a neurochemical sense. Corticosteroids and oral contraceptives are commonly associated with affective changes. Antihypertensive medications such as methyldopa, guanethidine, clonidine, and propranolol have been associated with the development of depressive syndromes. Infrequently, disulfiram and anticholinesterase drugs may be associated with symptoms of depression. The appetite-suppressing drugs, while initially stimulating, often result in a depressive syndrome when the drug is withdrawn (as does all stimulant abuse). Alcohol, sedatives, opiates, and most of the psychedelic drugs are depressants and, paradoxically, are often used in self-treatment of depression. They inevitably worsen the problem; the suicide rate is highest with the use of these drugs.

## Differential Diagnosis

Since depression may be a part of any illness—either reactively or as a secondary symptom—careful attention must be given to personal life adjustment problems, the role of medications (eg, reserpine), schizophrenia, and brain syndromes. Eating disorders are often associated with affective problems. Psychomotor symptoms (eg, olfactory hallucinations, metamorphopsia [visual distortion]) may occur in bipolar disorders and must be differentiated from partial complex seizures. Subtle thyroid dysfunction must be ruled out (check antithyroid antibodies).

## Complications

The longer the depression continues, the more crystallized it becomes, particularly when there is an element of secondary reinforcement. The most important complication is **suicide,** which always includes some elements of aggression. There are 4 major groups of people who make suicide attempts:

(1) Those who are overwhelmed by problems in living. By far the greatest number fall into this category. There is often great ambivalence; they don't really want to die, but they don't want to go on as before either.

(2) Those who are clearly attempting to control others. This is the blatant attempt in the presence of a significant other person in order to hurt or control that person.

(3) Those with severe depressions (*high-risk group*). This group includes both exogenous and endogenous conditions. It also includes those who may not be diagnosed as having depression but who are overwhelmed by a serious transient situation (eg, the man charged with child molestation who hangs himself in his cell). A patient may seem to make a dramatic improvement, but the lifting of depression may be due to the patient's decision to commit suicide. Hopelessness and guilt tend to be the 2 major symptom determinants.

(4) Those with psychotic illness (*high-risk group*). These individuals tend not to verbalize their concerns, are unpredictable, and are often successful but comprise a small percentage of the total.

The immediate goal of psychiatric evaluation is to assess the current suicidal risk and the need for hospitalization versus outpatient management. The intent is less likely to be truly suicidal, for example, if small amounts of poison were ingested or scratching of wrists was superficial; if the act was performed in the presence of others or with early notification of others; or if the attempt was arranged so that early detection would be anticipated. There is a significant correlation between suicide and delusional thoughts. Other risk factors are previous suicide attempts, male sex, older age, contemplation of violent methods, drug and alcohol use, severe depression, and psychosis.

The patient's current mood status is best evaluated by direct evaluation of plans and concerns about the future, personal reactions to the attempt, and thoughts about the reactions of others. The patient's immediate resources should be assessed—people who can be significantly involved (most important), family support, job situation, financial resources, etc.

If hospitalization is not indicated, the physician must formulate and institute a treatment plan or make an adequate referral. Medication should be dispensed in small amounts to at-risk patients. Guns and drugs should be removed from the patient's household. Driving should be interdicted until the patient improves. The problem is often worsened by the long-term complications of the suicidal attempt, eg, brain damage due to hypoxia; peripheral neuropathies caused by staying for long periods in one position, causing nerve compressions; and uncorrectable medical or surgical problems such as esophageal strictures and tendon dysfunctions.

The reasons for self mutilation, most commonly wrist cutting (but also autocastration, autoamputation, and autoenucleation, which are associated with psychoses), may be very different from the reasons for a suicide attempt. The initial treatment plan, however, should presume suicidal ideation, and conservative treatment should be initiated as for attempted suicide.

**Sleep disturbances** in the depressions are discussed below.

## Treatment

**A. Medical:** Depression associated with reactive disorders usually does not call for drug therapy and can be managed by psychotherapy and the passage of time. In severe cases—particularly when vegetative signs are present or impending—antidepressant drug therapy (see Antidepressant Drugs, p. 630) may prevent deepening of depression and provide symptomatic relief. Drugs should be given in sufficient dosage over a long enough period of time to constitute an adequate trial before being withdrawn or replaced with another drug.

If psychotic ideation is present—usually paranoia or somatic delusions—antipsychotic drugs should be given initially (eg, trifluoperazine, 10–20 mg/d orally) and the dosage increased every 2–3 days until symptoms abate. If depression persists as the psychosis comes under control, it may be necessary to add an antidepressant drug later. Loxapine may logically be the first antipsychotic drug considered, since it is metabolized to amoxapine, an antidepressant.

Hospitalization is called for if suicide is a realistic possibility or if symptoms are incapacitating. Suicide precautions should be instituted as necessary. In patients who do not respond to medications—particularly those with involutional melancholia or those who are considered at risk of suicide—hospitalization is mandatory and should not be withheld out of concern for cost to the family or the presumed social stigma of psychiatric detention.

Electroconvulsive therapy has consistently been more effective than the antidepressant groups of drugs, particularly for involutional depressions (see Other Organic Therapies, above). Convenience, expense, and public opinion have been major limiting factors in the use of electroconvulsive therapy. It should be considered in those who are at risk of suicide and in those who fail to respond to adequate trials of medication. Stimulants have little, if any, place in the treatment of depression. Their uses are in the treatment of apathy in geriatric cases, depression in severe medical illness when antidepressants or electroconvulsive therapy is not feasible, childhood hyperkinesis, and narcolepsy.

**Manic episodes** are treated with haloperidol, 5–10 mg orally or intramuscularly every 2–3 hours until symptoms subside. A decision must then be made about the need for long-term lithium maintenance. The dosage of haloperidol is gradually reduced after lithium is started (see Lithium, above).

If lithium alone does not control symptoms, a neuroleptic may be added. The addition of L-tryptophan or clonazepam may obviate the need for a neuroleptic. If lithium is contraindicated or if problems develop with lithium (eg, kidney dysfunction), clonazepam alone (2–8 mg/d orally) may be effective. Carbamazepine, 800–1600 mg/d orally, is also an effective substitute, particularly in rapid-cycling bipolar patients, but it has caused hepatic and hematologic toxicity in some patients.

Full-spectrum light therapy for 1–2 hours daily in the morning has been successful in depression related to seasonal affective disorder (SAD).

**B. Psychologic:** It is seldom possible to engage an individual in penetrating psychotherapeutic endeavors during the acute stage of a severe depression. While medications may be taking effect, a supportive approach to strengthen existing defenses and appropriate consideration of the patient's continuing need to function at work, to engage in recreational activities, etc, are necessary as the severity of the depression lessens. If the patient is not seriously depressed, it is often quite appropriate to initiate intensive psychotherapeutic efforts, since flux periods are a good time to effect change. A catharsis of repressed anger and guilt may be beneficial. Therapy during or just after the acute stage may focus on coping techniques, with some practice of alternative choices. When lack of self-confidence and identity problems are factors in the depression, individual psychotherapy can be oriented to ways of improving self-esteem, increasing assertiveness, and lessening dependency. It is usually helpful to involve the spouse or other significant family members early in treatment. Timing is important—the particular therapeutic approach should be initiated when the patient is ready. Inflexible dedication to any particular treatment modality can be counterproductive. Good clinical judgment may dictate early psychotherapy in a patient with mild to moderate depression, whereas in another patient the initial approach might be medical.

**C. Social:** Flexible use of appropriate social services can be of major importance in the treatment of depression. Since alcohol is often associated with depression, early involvement in alcohol treatment programs such as Alcoholics Anonymous can be important to future success (see Alcohol Dependency and Abuse, below). The *structuring* of daily activities during severe depression is often quite difficult for the patient. The help of family, employer, or friends is often necessary to mobilize the patient who experiences no joy in daily activities and tends to remain uninvolved and to deteriorate. Insistence on sharing activities will help involve the patient in simple but important daily functions. In some severe cases, the use of day treatment centers or support groups of a specific type (eg, mastectomy groups) is indicated. It is not unusual for a patient to have multiple legal, financial, and vocational problems. As the depression lifts, support agencies that provide legal aid and vocational rehabilitation can be of great assistance.

**D. Behavioral:** When depression is a function of self-defeating coping techniques such as passivity, the role-playing approach can be useful. Behavioral techniques, including desensitization, may be used in problems such as phobias where depression is a by-product. When depression is a regularly used interpersonal style, behavioral counseling to family members or others can help in extinguishing the behavior in the patient.

### Prognosis

Reactive depressions are usually time-limited, and the prognosis with treatment is good if suicide or a pathologic pattern of adjustment does not intervene. Major affective disorders frequently respond well to effective drug treatment given early and in adequate amounts for a reasonable period of time.

Bick PA: Seasonal major affective disorder. *Am J Psychiatry* 1986;**143**:90.

Consensus Development Panel, NIMH: Mood disorders: Pharmacologic prevention of recurrences. *Am J Psychiatry* 1985;**142**:469.

Michel K: Suicide risk factors: A comparison of suicide attempts with suicide complications. *Br J Psychiat* 1987;**150**:78.

Othmer E (ed): Atypical bipolar disorders. *Psychiatr Ann* 1987;**17(1)**: [Entire issue.]

Placidi GF et al: The comparative efficacy and safety of carbamazepine versus lithium: A randomized double-blind 3-year trial in 83 patients. *J Clin Psychiat* 1986;**47**:490.

Simons AD et al: Cognitive therapy and pharmacotherapy for depression. *Arch Gen Psychiatry* 1086;**43**:43.

## SLEEP DISORDERS

Sleep consists of 2 distinct states as shown by electroencephalographic studies: REM (rapid eye movement) sleep, also called dream sleep, D state sleep, paradoxic sleep; and NREM (non-REM) sleep, also called slow (delta) wave sleep or S state sleep, which is divided into stages 1, 2, 3, and 4 recognizable by different electroencephalographic patterns. Dreaming occurs mostly in REM and to a lesser extent in NREM sleep.

Sleep is a cyclic phenomenon, with 4–5 REM periods during the night accounting for about one-fourth of the total night's sleep (1½–2 hours). The first REM period occurs about 80–120 minutes after onset of sleep and lasts about 10 minutes. Later REM periods are longer (15–40 minutes) and occur mostly in the last several hours of sleep. Most stage 4 (deepest) sleep occurs in the first several hours.

Age-realted changes in normal sleep include a steady increase in REM sleep and less stage 3 and stage 4 sleep, with an increase in wakeful periods during the night. These normal changes and daytime naps play a role in the increased complaints of insomnia in older people. Variations in sleep patterns may be due to circumstances (eg, "jet lag") or to idiosyncratic patterns ("night owls") in persons who perhaps because of different "biologic rhythms" habitually go to bed late and sleep late in the morning. There are also rare individuals who have chronic difficulty in adapting to a 24-hour sleep-wake cycle (desynchronization sleep disorder).

The 3 major sleep disorders are discussed below.

### Disorders of Initiating & Maintaining Sleep (Insomnia)

Insomnia is the traditional term, though "dyssomnia" would be a more accurate one. Transient episodes are common and of no significance. Persistent insomnia (for longer than 3 weeks) is most common in elderly people for the reasons mentioned above. Patients may complain of difficulty getting to sleep or staying asleep, intermittent wakefulness during the night, early morning awakening, or combinations of any of these.

**A. Clinical Conditions:** Psychiatric disorders are often associated with persistent insomnia. **Depression** is usually associated with fragmented sleep or early morning awakening, with diminished extent and altered distribution of NREM sleep, earlier onset of REM sleep, and a shift of REM activity to the first half of the night. In atypical cases, depression may be associated with hypersomnia (see below). In **manic disorders,** sleeplessness is a cardinal feature and an important early sign of impending mania in bipolar cases.

**Drug abuse** is frequently associated with insomnia. Abuse of alcohol may cause or be secondary to the sleep disturbance. There is a tendency to use alcohol as a means of getting to sleep without realizing that it disrupts the normal sleep cycle. Chronic alcohol abuse increases stage 1 and decreases REM sleep, with symptoms persisting for many months after the individual has stopped drinking. Acute alcohol withdrawal causes delayed onset of sleep and REM rebound with intermittent awakening during the night.

Heavy smoking (more than a pack a day) causes difficulty falling asleep—apparently independently of the often associated increase in coffee drinking. Excess intake near bedtime of caffeine and other stimulants (eg, over-the-counter cold remedies) causes decreased total sleep time—mostly NREM sleep—with some increased sleep latency.

**Sedative-hypnotics**—specifically, the benzodiazepines, which are the prescription drugs of choice to promote sleep—tend to increase total sleep time, decrease sleep latency, and decrease nocturnal awakening, with variable effects on NREM sleep. Withdrawal causes just the opposite effects—and that is the problem with chronic use of sedatives. After a while (usually 30–60 days of nightly use), continued use of the drug is for the purpose of preventing withdrawal symptoms. Various psychotherapeutic medications (eg, trazodone, thioridazine) have sedative side effects and may be selected—in those conditions for which they are indicated—because of this property. Some over-the-counter preparations (eg, antihistamines, stimulants) are marketed for their sleep-altering side effects. Antidepressants decrease REM sleep (with marked rebound on withdrawal in the form of nightmares) and have varying effects on NREM sleep. The effect on REM sleep correlates with reports that REM sleep deprivation parallels improvement in some depressions.

Persistent insomnias are also related to a wide variety of medical conditions, particularly pain and respiratory distress syndromes. Adequate analgesia and proper treatment of medical disorders will reduce symptoms and decrease the need for sedatives.

Other conditions associated with insomnia include nocturnal myoclonus, which involves repetitive leg movements in sleep (every 20–40 seconds) due to contraction of the anterior tibialis muscle. Intermittent awakening may occur, but the patient is usually unaware of the problem. Daytime sleepiness may result.

**B. Treatment:** In transient insomnias, deemphasis and reassurance are sufficient treatment. The patient should be given common-sense advice about room temperature (cool is best), late snacks (a small amount of food or liquid), daily exercise, avoidance of noxious habits (too much coffee, alcohol, cigarettes), and daytime naps (including dozing at the

TV set). Patients in acute distress because of sleepless nights may require a short course of benzodiazepine (eg, temazepam, 15 mg at bedtime). Antihistamines such as diphenhydramine or hydroxyzine are acceptable milder substitutes for benzodiazepines or chloral hydrate. The use of antipsychotic drugs or antidepressants just for sleep problems is not good practice.

## Disorders of Excessive Sleepiness (Sleep Apnea, Narcolepsy)

These disorders—also called hypersomnias—are a more severe problem than insomnia.

**A. Clinical Conditions:**

**1. Sleep apnea—** This disorder is characterized by cessation of breathing for at least 30 episodes (each lasting 10 seconds) during the night. There are 2 types: obstructive and central. The obstructive type is discussed in Chapter 7. Central sleep apnea is due to failure during sleep of the respiratory drive mechanism. Obese middle-aged and older men with hypertension are most often affected. Both types may occur simultaneously. Symptoms include snoring, restless sleep, and exessive daytime sleepiness, which may be associated with headaches and depression. Cardiac arrhythmias (particularly bradycardia) and blood gas irregularities occur during episodes. The patients tend to have poor judgment and a history of work-related problems. Definitive diagnostic evaluation may include otolaryngologic examination; polysomnography in the hospital to record sleep, heart rate, and respiratory movement; and oxygen saturation studies.

**2. Narcolepsy—** Narcolepsy consists of a tetrad of symptoms: (1) Sudden, brief (about 15 minutes) sleep attacks that may occur during any type of activity; (2) cataplexy—sudden loss of muscle tone involving specific small muscle groups or generalized muscle weakness that may cause the person to slump to the floor, unable to move; (3) sleep paralysis—a generalized flaccidity of muscles with full consciousness in the transition zone between sleep and waking; and (4) hypnagogic hallucinations, visual or auditory, which may precede sleep or occur during the sleep attack. The attacks are characterized by an abrupt transition into REM sleep—a necessary criterion for diagnosis. The disorder begins in early adult life, affects both sexes equally, and usually levels off in severity at about 30 years of age.

**3. Kleine-Levin syndrome—** This syndrome is characterized by hypersomnic attacks 3–4 times a year lasting up to 2 days, with confusion on awakening.

**B. Treatment:** Treatment of sleep attacks may include medical measures such as weight reduction, administration during sleep of low-flow oxygen by nasal prongs, and tongue restraining devices. Surgical treatment is discussed in Chapter 7. Diaphragmatic pacing has been helpful for central sleep apnea. Trials with protriptyline have improved daytime somnolence and nocturnal oxygenation, with no significant change, however, in the number of apneic episodes.

Narcolepsy is managed by daily administration of a stimulant such as amphetamine sulfate, 10 mg in the morning, with increased dosage as necessary. Imipramine, 75–100 mg daily, has been effective in treatment of cataplexy but not narcolepsy.

There is no treatment for Kleine-Levin syndrome.

## Parasomnias (Abnormal Behaviors During Sleep)

These disorders are fairly common in children and less so in adults.

**A. Clinical Presentations: Sleep terror (pavor nocturnus)** is an abrupt, terrifying arousal from sleep, usually in preadolescent boys. Symptoms are fear, sweating, tachycardia, and confusion for several minutes, with amnesia for the event. **Nightmares** occur during REM sleep; sleep terrors in stage 3 or stage 4 sleep. **Sleepwalking (somnambulism)** includes ambulation or other intricate behaviors while still asleep, with amnesia for the event. It affects mostly children aged 6–12 years, and episodes occur during stage 3 or stage 4 sleep in the first third of the night. Sleepwalking in elderly people is a feature of organic brain syndrome. Idiosyncratic reactions to drugs (eg, marihuana, alcohol) and medical conditions (eg, partial complex seizures) may be causative factors in adults.

**Enuresis** is involuntary micturition during sleep in a person who usually has voluntary control. Like other parasomnias, it is more common in children, usually in the 3–4 hours after bedtime, but is not limited to a specific stage of sleep. Confusion during the episode and amnesia for the event are common.

**B. Treatment:** Treatment for sleep terrors is with benzodiazepines (eg, diazepam, 5–20 mg at bedtime), since it will suppress stage 3 and stage 4 sleep. Somnambulism responds to the same treatment for the same reason, but simple safety measures should not be neglected. Enuresis may respond to imipramine, 50–100 mg at bedtime. Behavioral approaches (eg, bells that ring when the pad gets wet) have also been successful.

Hartmann E et al: Who has nightmares: The personality of the lifelong nightmare sufferer. *Arch Gen Psychiat* 1987;**44**:59.

Kales A, Soldatos CR, Kales JD: Sleep disorders: Night terrors, nightmares, and enuresis. *Ann Intern Med* 1987;**106**:582.

Kales A, Vela-Bueno A, Kales JD: Sleep disorders: Sleep apnea and narcolepsy. *Ann Intern Med* 1987;**106**:434.

Karnovsky ML: Progress in sleep. *New England J Med* 1986;**315**:1027.

Kwentus J et al: Sleep apnea: A review. *Psychosomatics* 1985;**26**:713.

## DISORDERS OF AGGRESSION

Acts performed with the deliberate intent of causing physical harm to persons or property have a wide variety of causative factors. Aggression and violence are symptoms rather than diseases, and most frequently they are *not* associated with an underlying medical condition. In terms of demographic characteristics, the perpetrator of an act of aggression is often a male under age 25, a member of a minority group, a person in socially and economically deprived circumstances, and a resident of an inner-city area.

Those who commit acts of aggression fall into 2 general personality types. The more common is a person with a pattern of physically aggressive behavior from an early age, with a poor capacity for peer relationships; truancy; and a family member (usually the father) who has a history of brutality, psychosis, or antisocial behavior. The less common type is the overcontrolled, chronically frustrated person who seethes inside until some event precipitates a violent overreaction. Some clues to the dangerous patient include statements that they feel powerless, feel humiliated, have headaches, or feel that they are ''going to explode'' or have ''something terribly wrong with my body.'' Depression (and suicide) may be associated with aggression, particularly when it is precipitated by sexual infidelity (real or imagined). *In both types, disinhibiting drugs (most commonly alcohol) play a role in the aggressive outburst.*

In the USA, 50% of all violent deaths are alcohol-related. The ingestion of even small amounts of alcohol can result in pathologic intoxication that resembles an acute organic mental condition. Amphetamines or other stimulants are frequently associated with aggressive behavior. Barbiturates and, increasingly, the benzodiazepines (both of which are often combined with alcohol) are frequent factors in the outburst. Phencyclidine is a drug commonly associated with violent behavior that is occasionally of a bizarre nature. Treatment of the acute situation is the same as for any instance of substance abuse (see Substance Use Disorders, p 660). Psychotherapy is not successful in modifying the underlying personality problems. It has long been known that this type of individual does better with strong external controls to replace the lack of inner controls. Close probationary supervision and court-mandated restrictions can be most helpful. There should be a major effort to help the individual avoid drug usage (eg, help from Alcoholics Anonymous).

**Episodic dyscontrol syndrome** is a descriptive term for a cluster of behaviors that may or may not warrant the use of the term ''syndrome.'' The disorder is characterized by physical abuse, usually of wife or children, pathologic intoxication, impulsive sexual activities, and automobile misuse.

Wife-beating and rape (see Chapter 13) are much more widespread than heretofore recognized. Awareness of the problem is to some degree due to increasing recognition of the rights of women and the understanding by women that they do not have to accept abuse. Women frequently have remained in violent home situations because of financial, legal, and cultural restraints. Acceptance of this kind of aggression inevitably leads to more, with the ultimate aggression being murder—20–50% of murders in the USA occur within the family. Police are involved in more domestic disputes than *all other criminal incidents combined.* The woman is by far the most frequent victim of intrafamily strife—3:1 in the case of family homicide. Such violent behavior is clearly more prevalent in succeeding generations of families who have indulged in it. Paternal violence (often associated with alcohol abuse) toward a daughter who marries during the teens to escape the home (often accompanied by premarital pregnancy) and acceptance of violence from the new husband set the stage for replication of violent behavior by the next generation. Extreme jealousy in men, often exacerbated by alcohol, is frequently used as an excuse for aggression. This jealousy may lead to attempts to limit the wife's activities outside the home, thus furthering her financial dependency. Interspersed periods of ''sobriety'' encourage the wife's hope for change and delay any efforts she might make to break the cycle. Children who are a part of such relationships inevitably become victims. The majority of abused children come from this type of household.

Presenting symptoms of victims frequently are depression, anxiety, and somatic complaints, and it is often only after overcoming the patient's great reluctance by means of gentle questioning that one is able to elicit the truth. The physician should be suspicious about the origin of any injuries not fully explained, particularly if such incidents recur. Any history of alcohol excess warrants further careful questioning. If depression seems related to suppressed aggression, it is important to discuss the reasons for such feelings. Feelings of powerlessness often contribute to depression and acceptance of further violence.

Attempts to correlate brain dysrhythmias with episodic dyscontrol syndrome have not been successful. Clinicians are unable to predict dangerous behavior beyond the level of chance.

Major mental disorders such as affective disorders, schizophrenic disorders, and organic mental states are not major causes of violent behavior. However, young paranoid schizophrenics are the most dangerous of mentally disordered persons. When violence does occur in this group, it is frequently associated with attempts to control a person who is in the throes of an acute psychotic state.

### Treatment

**A. Psychologic:** Management of any violent individual includes appropriate psychologic maneuvers. Move slowly, talk slowly with clarity and reassurance, and evaluate the situation. Strive to create a setting that is minimally disturbing and eliminate people or things threatening to the violent individual. Do not threaten or abuse and do not touch or crowd the person. Proximity to a door is comforting to both the patient and the examiner. For purposes of negotiation, use an individual whom the violent person can relate to most comfortably. Honesty is important. Make no false promises, and continue to engage the subject verbally until the situation is under control.

**B. Pharmacologic:** Pharmacologic means are often necessary whether or not psychologic approaches have been successful. This is particularly true in the agitated or psychotic patient. The drug of choice in psychotic aggressive states is haloperidol, 10 mg intramuscularly every hour until symptoms are alleviated. Droperidol is another butyrophenone that acts very rapidly and can be given intramuscularly or intravenously (eg, 5–10 mg hourly to a maximum of 45 mg in 24 hours). Benzodiazepine sedatives (eg, diazepam, 5 mg orally or intravenously every several hours) can be used for mild to moderate agitation, but an antipsychotic drug is preferred for management of the seriously violent and psychotic patient. Chronic aggressive states, particularly in retardation and brain damage, have been successfully ameliorated with propranolol, 40–240 mg/d orally.

**C. Physical:** Physical management is necessary if psychologic and pharmacologic means are not sufficient. It requires the active and visible presence of an adequate number of personnel to reinforce the idea that the situation is under control despite the patient's lack of inner controls. Such an approach often precludes the need for actual physical restraint. If it becomes necessary, however, 2 people shielded by a mattress (single-bed size) can usually corner and subdue the patient without injury to anyone. Seclusion rooms and restraints should be used only when necessary, and the patient must then be observed at *frequent* intervals. Design of corridors and seclusion rooms is important. Narrow corridors, small spaces, and crowded areas exacerbate the potential for violence in an anxious patient.

**D. Other:** The treatment of beaten wives is a frustrating experience, chiefly because of the woman's reluctance to leave the situation. Reasons for staying vary, but common themes include the fear of more violence because of leaving; the hope that the situation may ameliorate (in spite of steady worsening); and the financial aspects of the situation, which are seldom to the woman's advantage. An early step is to get the woman into a therapeutic situation that provides the support of others in similar straits. Al-Anon is frequently a valuable asset and quite appropriate when alcohol is one of the factors in the abuse of the woman. The group can support the victim while she gathers strength to consider alternatives without being paralyzed by fear. Many cities now offer temporary emergency centers and counseling. ''Rescue'' attempts by physicians and other well-meaning individuals are often unsuccessful and discourage the would-be helper from ever again dealing with such problems. *Use the available resources,* attend to any medical or psychiatric problems, and maintain a compassionate interest.

Greendyke RM et al: Propranolol treatment of assaultive patients with organic brain disease. *J Nerv Ment Dis* 1986;**174:**290.

Holinger PC, Offer D, Ostrov E: Suicide and homicide in the

United States: An epidemiologic study of violent death population changes and the potential for prediction. *Am J Psychiat* 1987;**144**:215.

# SUBSTANCE USE DISORDERS
## (Drug Dependency, Drug Abuse)

The term "drug dependency" is used in a broad sense here to include both addictions and habituations. It involves the triad of compulsive drug use referred to as drug addiction, which includes (1) a **psychologic craving** or dependence, and the behavior included in the procurement of the drug ("hustle"); (2) **physiologic dependence,** with withdrawal symptoms on discontinuance of the drug; and (3) **tolerance,** ie, the need to increase the dose to obtain the desired effects. Drug dependency is a function of the amount of drug used and the duration of usage. The amount needed to produce dependency varies with the nature of the drug and the idiosyncratic nature of the user. The frequency of use is usually daily, and the duration is inevitably greater than 2–3 weeks. Dependency increases with increased amount and duration of drug usage. Polydrug abuse is very common. Transgenerational continuity of drug abuse is also common. A large percentage of drug abusers present themselves for something other than treatment (eg, avoiding legal consequences, obtaining more drugs).

The physician faces 3 problems with substance abuse: (1) the prescribing of substances such as sedatives, stimulants, or narcotics that might produce dependency, (2) the treatment of individuals who have already abused drugs, most commonly alcohol; and (3) the detection of illicit drug use in patients presenting with psychiatric symptoms. The usefulness of urinalysis for detection of drugs varies markedly with different drugs and under different circumstances (pharmacokinetics is a major factor). Water-soluble drugs (eg, alcohol, stimulants, opioids) are eliminated in a day or so. Lipophilic substances (eg, phencyclidine, tetrahydrocannabinol) appear in the urine over longer periods of time: several days in most cases, a month or 2 months in chronic marihuana users. Sedative drug determinations are quite variable, amount of drug and duration of use being important determinants. False-positives can be a problem related to ingestion of some legitimate drugs (eg, phenytoin for barbiturates, phenylpropanolamine for amphetamines, chlorpromazine for opiates) and some foods (eg, poppy seeds for opiates, coca leaf tea for cocaine). Manipulations can alter the legitimacy of the testing. Dilution, either in vivo or in vitro, can be detected by checking urine specific gravity. Addition of ammonia, vinegar, or salt may invalidate the test, but odor and pH determinatins are simple. Hair analysis can determine drug use over longer periods.

# ALCOHOL DEPENDENCY & ABUSE
## (Alcoholism)

### Essentials of Diagnosis
*Major criteria:*
- Physiologic dependence as manifested by evidence of withdrawal when intake is interrupted.
- Tolerance to the effects of alcohol.
- Evidence of alcohol-associated illnesses, such as alcoholic liver disease, cerebellar degeneration.
- Continued drinking despite strong medical and social contraindications and life disruptions.
- Impairment in social and occupational functioning.
- Depression.
- Blackouts.

*Other signs:*
- Alcohol stigmas: Alcohol odor on breath, alcoholic facies, flushed face, tremor, ecchymoses, peripheral neuropathy.
- Surreptitious drinking.
- Unexplained work absences.
- Frequent accidents, falls, or injuries of vague origin; in smokers, cigarette burns on hands or chest.

### General Considerations
Alcoholism is a syndrome consisting of 2 phases: problem drinking and alcohol addiction. Problem drinking is the repetitive use of alcohol, often to alleviate tension or solve other emotional problems. Alcohol addiction is a true addiction similar to that which occurs following the repeated use of barbiturates or similar drugs. Concurrent dependence on sedative-hypnotics is very common. It may occur in an attempt to control the anxiety generated by heavy alcohol abuse or in the mistaken belief that control by other pharmacologic agents will stop the alcohol abuse. Adoption and twin studies indicate some genetic influence, particularly in male alcoholics. *Depression is often present and should be evaluated carefully.* The majority of suicides and intrafamily homicides involve alcohol usage.

### Clinical Findings
**A. Acute Intoxication:** The signs of alcoholic intoxication are the same as those of overdosage with any other central nervous system depressant: drowsiness, errors of commission, disinhibition, dysarthria, ataxia, and nystagmus. For a 70-kg person, an ounce of whiskey, a glass of wine, or a 12-oz bottle of beer raises the level of alcohol in the blood by 25 mg/dL. Blood levels below 50 mg/dL rarely cause significant motor dysfunction. Intoxication as manifested by ataxia, dysarthria, and nausea and vomiting indicates a blood level above 150 mg/dL, and lethal blood levels range from 350 to 900 mg/dL. In severe cases, overdosage is marked by respiratory depression, stupor, shock syndrome, coma, and death. Serious overdoses are frequently due to a combination of alcohol with other sedatives.

**B. Withdrawal:** There is a wide spectrum of manifestations of alcoholic withdrawal, ranging from anxiety, decreased cognition, and tremulousness through increasing irritability and hyperreactivity to full-blown **delirium tremens.** The latter is an acute organic psychosis that is usually manifest within 24–72 hours after the last drink (but may occur up to 7–10 days later). It is characterized by mental confusion, tremor, sensory hyperacuity, visual hallucinations (often of snakes, bugs, etc), autonomic hyperactivity, diaphoresis, dehydration, electrolyte disturbances (hypokalemia, hypomagnesemia), seizures, and cardiovascular abnormalities. The acute withdrawal syndrome is often completely unexpected and occurs when the patient has been hospitalized for some unrelated problem and presents as a diagnostic problem. *Suspect alcohol withdrawal in every unexplained delirium.* Seizures occur early (the first 24 hours) and are more prevalent in persons who have a history of withdrawal syndromes. The mortality rate from delirium tremens is significant.

**C. Alcoholic (Organic) Hallucinosis:** This syndrome occurs either during heavy drinking or on withdrawal and is characterized by a paranoid psychosis without the tremulousness, confusion, and clouded sensorium seen in withdrawal syndromes. The patient appears normal except for the auditory hallucinations, which are frequently persecutory and may cause the patient to behave aggressively.

**D. Chronic Alcoholic Brain Syndromes:** These encephalopathies are characterized by increasing erratic behavior, memory and recall problems, and emotional instability—the usual signs of organic brain syndrome due to any cause (see Organic Mental Disorders, below). Early recognition and treatment of Wernicke's encephalopathy with intravenous thiamine and parenteral B complex vitamins can minimize damage.

### Differential Diagnosis

The differential diagnosis of problem drinking is essentially between primary alcoholism (when no other major psychiatric diagnosis exists) and secondary alcoholism, when alcohol is used as self-medication for major underlying psychiatric problems such as schizophrenia or affective disorder. The differentiation is important, since the latter group requires treatment for the specific psychiatric problem.

The differential diagnosis of alcoholic withdrawal includes other sedative abuse. Acute alcoholic hallucinosis must be differentiated from other acute paranoid states such as amphetamine psychosis or acute paranoid schizophrenia. An accurate history is the most important differentiating factor. The history is also the most important feature in differentiating chronic organic brain syndromes due to alcohol from those due to other causes. The form of the brain syndrome is of little help—eg, chronic brain syndromes from lupus erythematosus may be associated with confabulation similar to that resulting from long-standing alcoholism.

### Complications

The medical and psychosocial problems of alcoholism are staggering. The central and peripheral nervous system complications include chronic brain syndromes, cerebellar degeneration, cardiovascular disorders, and peripheral neuropathies. The effects on the liver result not only in cirrhosis with its direct complications such as liver failure and esophageal varicosities but also in the systemic effects of altered metabolism, protein abnormalities, and coagulation defects.

**Fetal alcohol syndrome** includes one or more of the following developmental defects in the offspring of alcoholic women: (1) low birth weight and small size with failure to catch up in size or weight; (2) mental retardation, with an average IQ in the 60s; and (3) a variety of birth defects, with a large percentage of cardiac abnormalities. The fetuses are very quiet in utero, and there is an increased frequency of breech presentations. There is a higher incidence of delayed postnatal growth and behavior development. The risk factors are appreciably higher when more than 6 drinks are ingested each day. With lesser amounts, the risk is not precisely established. Cigarette and marihuana smoking can also produce these effects on the fetus.

### Treatment of Problem Drinking

**A. Psychologic:** The most important consideration for the physician is to suspect the problem early and take a nonjudgmental attitude, though this does not mean a passive one. There must be an emphasis on the things that can be done. This approach emphasizes the fact that the physician cares and strikes a positive and hopeful note early in treatment.

Valuable time should not be wasted trying to find out why the patient drinks; come to grips early with the immediate problem of *how to stop the drinking.* Total abstinence (not "controlled drinking") should be the primary goal. This often means early involvement of the spouse and elucidation of specific ways in which he or she can be helpful in stopping the drinking. In fact, if there is a spouse or family, the prognosis is much better, and working with both of the marriage partners—alone or together—should be started immediately.

**B. Social:** Get the patient into Alcoholics Anonymous (AA) and the spouse into Al-Anon. Success is usually proportionate to the utilization of AA, other social agencies, religious counseling, and other resources. The patient should be seen frequently for short periods and charged an appropriate fee.

Do not underestimate the importance of religion, particularly since the alcoholic is often a dependent person who needs a great deal of support. Early enlistment of the help of a concerned religious adviser can often provide the turning point for a personal conversion to sobriety.

One of the most important considerations is the job; it is usually lost or in jeopardy. In the latter case, some specific recommendations to employers can be offered: (1) Avoid placement in jobs where the alcoholic must be alone, eg, traveling buyer or sales executive. (2) Use supervision but not surveillance. (3) Keep competition with others to a minimum. (4) Avoid positions that require quick decision making on important matters (high stress situations).

**C. Medical:** Hospitalization is not usually necessary or even desirable at this stage, which is not an acute one. It is sometimes used to dramatize a situation and force the patient to face the problem of alcoholism, but generally it should be used only on medical indications.

Because of the many medical complications of alcoholism, a complete physical examination with appropriate laboratory tests is mandatory, with special attention to the liver and nervous system. *Use of sedatives as a replacement for alcohol is not desirable.* Usually the result is a concomitant use of sedatives *and* alcohol and a worsening of the problem.

The medical deterrent drug disulfiram can be of critical importance in helping the alcoholic to make the essential decision to *stop drinking.* There should be nothing surreptitious about the use of disulfiram (no slipping the drug into the coffee by the spouse, etc). It should be discussed with the patient, with full disclosure of its side effects, mode of action, and dangers (organic brain syndrome is an infrequent complication). The initial dosage schedule of disulfiram (after a minimum of 12 hours' abstention from alcohol) is 500 mg/d in a single dose in the morning. This can be decreased to a maintenance dose of 250 mg/d, continued indefinitely. Reports of liver damage due to disulfiram warrant baseline hepatic studies and monitoring. (Impotence is an important side effect.) Any sedative or narcotic should be used cautiously when there is concomitant disulfiram administration. Disulfiram impairs elimination of caffeine. A disulfiram regimen need not interfere with other treatment approaches such as AA.

**D. Behavioral:** Conditioning approaches have been used in many settings in the treatment of alcoholism, most commonly as a type of aversion therapy. For example, the patient is given a drink of whisky and then a shot of apomorphine, and proceeds to vomit. In this way a strong association is built up between the vomiting and the drinking. Although this kind of treatment has been successful in some cases, many people do not retain the learned aversive response.

## Treatment of Withdrawal & Hallucinosis

### A. Medical:

**1. Alcoholic hallucinosis**–Alcoholic hallucinosis, which can occur either during or on cessation of a prolonged drinking period, is not a typical withdrawal syndrome and is handled differently. Since the symptoms are primarily those of a psychosis in the presence of a clear sensorium, they are handled like any other psychosis: hospitalization (when indi-

cated) and adequate amounts of antipsychotic drugs. Haloperidol, 5 mg orally twice a day for the first day or so, usually ameliorates symptoms quickly, and the drug can be decreased and discontinued over several days as the patient improves. It then becomes necessary to deal with the chronic alcohol abuse, which has been discussed.

**2. Withdrawal symptoms**–Withdrawal symptoms, ranging from a mild syndrome to the severe state usually called **delirium tremens,** are a medical problem with a significant morbidity and mortality rate. They usually occur when an intake of at least 7–8 pints of beer or 1 pint of spirits daily for several months has been stopped. The patient should be hospitalized and given adequate central nervous system depressants to counteract the excitability resulting from the sudden cessation of alcohol. Monitoring of vital signs and fluids and electrolyte levels is essential for the severely ill patient. Antipsychotic drugs such as chlorpromazine should *not* be used. The choice of the specific sedative is less important than using *adequate* doses to bring the patient to a level of moderate sedation, and this will vary from person to person. Mild to moderate dependency requires "drying out"—a short course of oral benzodiazepines on an outpatient basis with *no alcohol intake.* In severe withdrawal, hospitalize and use diazepam, 10 mg intravenously initially and then 5 mg intravenously every 5 minutes until the patient is calm. Then give the drug orally in a dosage of 5–10 mg every 1–4 hours depending on the clinical need. After stabilization, the amount of diazepam required to maintain a sedated state may be given orally every 8–12 hours. If restlessness, tremulousness, and other signs of withdrawal persist, the dosage is increased until moderate sedation occurs. The dosage is then gradually reduced until withdrawal is complete. This usually requires a week or so of treatment. Clonidine, 5 $\mu$g/kg orally every 2 hours, suppresses cardiovascular signs of withdrawal and also has some anxiolytic effect.

Meticulous examination for other medical problems is necessary. Alcoholics commonly have liver disease and associated clotting problems and are also prone to injury—and the combination all too frequently leads to undiagnosed subdural hematoma.

Anticonvulsant drugs are not needed unless there is a history of seizures. In these situations, phenytoin can be given in a loading dose—500 mg orally and, several hours later, another 500 mg orally (ie, 1 g over 4–6 hours). This drug is then continued in a dosage of 300 mg daily, which is checked by serum drug level.

A general diet should be given, and vitamins in high doses: thiamine, 100 mg 3 times a day; pyridoxine, 100 mg/d; folic acid, 5 mg 3 times a day; and ascorbic acid, 100 mg twice a day. Intravenous glucose solutions should not be given prior to the vitamins. Concurrent administration is satisfactory, and hydration should be meticulously assessed on an ongoing basis. Magnesium levels often decline, and replacement by magnesium sulfate solution intravenously several times a day for several days is desirable.

Chronic brain syndromes secondary to a long history of alcohol intake are not responsive to any specific measures. Attention to the social and environmental care of this type of patient is paramount.

**B. Psychologic and Behavioral:** The comments in the section on problem drinking apply here also; these methods of treatment become the primary consideration after the successful treatment of withdrawal or alcoholic hallucinosis. Psychologic and social measures should be initiated in the hospital shortly before discharge. This increases the possibility of continued posthospitalization treatment.

Fuller RK et al: Disulfiram treatment of alcohol: A Veterans Administration cooperative study. *JAMA* 1986;**256:**1449.

Helzer JE et al: The extent of long-term moderate drinking among alcoholics discharged from medical and psychiatric facilities. *N Engl J Med* 1985;**312:**1678.

Kamerow DB, Pincus HA, Macdonald DI: Alcohol abuse, other drug abuse, and mental disorders in medical practice. *JAMA* 1986;**255:**2054.

Pattison EM: Clinical approaches to the alcoholic patient. *Psychosomatics* 1986;**27:**762.

Schuckit MA: Genetic and clinical implications of alcoholism and affective disorder. *Am J Psychiatry* 1986;**143:**140.

## OTHER DRUG & SUBSTANCE DEPENDENCIES

### Opiates

The terms "opiates" and "narcotics" are used interchangeably and include a group of drugs with actions that mimic those of morphine. The group includes natural derivatives of opium, synthetic surrogates, and a number of polypeptides, some of which have been discovered to be natural neurotransmitters. The principal narcotic of abuse is heroin (metabolized to morphine), which is not used as a legitimate medication. A large percentage of heroin addicts have AIDS antibodies. The other common narcotics are prescription drugs and differ in milligram potency, duration of action, and agonist and antagonist capabilities (see Chapter 1). All of the narcotic analgesics can be reversed by the narcotic antagonist naloxone.

The clinical signs of mild narcotic intoxication include needle tracks; changes in mood, with feelings of euphoria; drowsiness; nausea with occasional emesis; and miosis. The incidence of snorting and inhaling heroin is increasing, particularly among cocaine users. This coincides with a decrease in the availability of methaqualone (no longer on the market) and other sedatives used to temper the cocaine "high." Overdosage causes respiratory depression, peripheral vasodilatation, pinpoint pupils, pulmonary edema, coma, and death.

Dependency is a major concern when continued use of narcotics occurs, although withdrawal causes only moderate morbidity (about the severity of a bout with the "flu"). Addicts sometimes consider themselves more addicted than they really are and may not require a withdrawal program. Grades of withdrawal are categorized from 0–4: grade 0 includes craving and anxiety; grade 1, yawning, lacrimation, rhinorrhea, and perspiration; grade 2, previous symptoms plus mydriasis, piloerection, anorexia, tremors, and hot and cold flashes with generalized aching; grades 3 and 4, increased intensity of previous symptoms and signs, with increased temperature, blood pressure, pulse, and respiratory rate and depth. In withdrawal from the most severe addiction, vomiting, diarrhea, weight loss, hemoconcentration, and spontaneous ejaculation or orgasm commonly occur.

Treatment for overdosage (or suspected overdosage) is naloxone (Narcan), 0.4 mg intravenously. If an overdose has been taken, the results are dramatic and occur within 2 minutes. Effects of naloxone are quickly dissipated, and administration of the drug can be repeated at 5- to 10-minute intervals. Since the length of action of naloxone is much shorter than that of the narcotics, the patient must be under close observation. Hospitalization, supportive care, naloxone administration, and observation for withdrawal from other drugs should be maintained for as long as necessary. Complications include infections (eg, pneumonia, septic emboli, hepatitis), traumatic insults (eg, arterial spasm due to drug injection, gangrene), and pulmonary edema (50% of patients).

Treatment for withdrawal begins if grade 2 signs develop. If a withdrawal program is necessary, use methadone, 10 mg orally (use parenteral administration if the patient is vomiting), and observe. If signs (piloerection, mydriasis, cardiovascular changes) persist for more than 4–6 hours, give another 10 mg; continue to administer methadone at 4- to 6-hour intervals until signs are not present (rarely more than 40 mg of methadone in 24 hours). Divide the total amount of drug required over the first 24-hour period by 2 and give this dose every 12 hours. Each day, reduce the total 24-hour dose by 5–10 mg. Thus, a moderately addicted patient initially requiring 30–40 mg of methadone could be withdrawn over a 4- to 8-day period. Clonidine, 0.1 mg in several divided doses over a 10- to 14-day period, is an excellent and faster alternative to methadone detoxification; it is not necessary to taper the dose. Clonidine is helpful in alleviating cardiovascular symptoms but does not significantly relieve anxiety, insomnia, or generalized aching.

Methadone maintenance programs are of some value in chronic recidivism. Under carefully controlled supervision, the narcotic addict is maintained on fairly high doses of methadone (40–120 mg/d) that satisfy craving and block the effects of heroin to a great degree. Methadyl acetate is longer lasting and is replacing methadone in some programs. Abrupt withdrawal from methadyl acetate does not result in more severe withdrawal problems than gradual withdrawal. Narcotic antagonists (eg, naltrexone) can be used successfully for treatment of the patient free of opioids for 7–10 days. Naltrexone blocks the narcotic "high" of heroin when 50 mg is given orally every 24 hours initially for several days and then 100 mg is given every 48–72 hours. Liver disorders are a major contraindication. Compliance tends to be poor, partly because of the dysphoria that can persist long after opioid discontinuance.

## Sedatives (Anxiolytics)

This group includes all of the so-called minor tranquilizers, antianxiety drugs, and sleeping medications (see Sedative-Hypnotic Drugs, above). They can all produce dependency and resemble alcohol in their behavioral manifestations. They are all additive (mixed usage along with alcohol is common), with cross dependency. Thus, selective sedatives may be used to withdraw a patient from other sedative addiction.

Acute intoxication states are manifested by drowsiness, errors of commission (which may result in accidents), slowed speech and thinking, impaired memory, disinhibition, nystagmus, ataxia, dysarthria, and sleep.

Overdosage is characterized by respiratory depression, severe hypotension, decreased gastrointestinal activity, stupor, shock syndrome, coma, and death.

Manifestations of withdrawal vary, depending on the nature of the sedative and the degree of dependency (the latter a function of dosage and length of dependency). The signs and symptoms range from mild restlessness to death. Manifestations include restlessness, tremor, anxiety (12–16 hours), intolerance to loud noise and bright lights, seizures, muscular weakness, gastrointestinal symptoms, palpitations, and orthostatic hypotension (16–36 hours). Delirium is occasionally present, accompanied by visual hallucinations, disorientation, and paranoid ideation; this may last up to 1 week. The longer-acting sedatives have a longer withdrawal pattern, and the symptoms tend to be milder.

Complications of sedative abuse include pneumonia, septicemia with injected drugs, bullous cutaneous lesions with barbiturates, renal failure secondary to muscle necrosis in overdoses, peripheral neuropathies related to extended time in pressure positions during coma, and the results of associated trauma.

Treatment of overdoses (see p 1022) and with drawal states are medical emergencies. *Unlike withdrawal from narcotics, which is relatively benign, sedative withdrawal is as dangerous as alcohol withdrawal and is treated in the same manner.* Treatment of sedative dependency is also handled in much the same way as treatment of alcohol dependency. Recognition of the problem and use of supporting treatment organizations are most important.

## Psychedelics

About 6000 species of plants have psychoactive properties. All of the common psychedelics (LSD, mescaline, psilocybin, dimethyltryptamine, and other derivatives of phenylalanine and tryptophan) produce similar behavioral and physiologic effects. An initial feeling of tension is followed by emotional release such as crying or laughing (1–2 hours). Later, perceptual distortions occur, with visual illusions and hallucinations, and occasionally there is fear of ego disintegration (2–3 hours). Major changes in time sense and mood lability then occur (3–4 hours). A feeling of detachment and a sense of destiny and control occur (4–6 hours). Of course, reactions vary among individuals, and some of the current street drugs produce markedly different time frames. Occasionally, the acute episode is terrifying (a "bad trip") and may not remit for long periods of time. The attitude of the user and the setting where the drug is used affect the experience. Most of the street drugs peddled as mescaline, LSD, and THC are really phencyclidine, the use of which has reached epidemic proportions (see below). Psychedelic usage in women during the first trimester of pregnancy is connected with an increased incidence of spontaneous abortion and congenital defects.

Treatment of the acute episode primarily involves protection of the individual from erratic behavior that may lead to injury or death. A structured environment is usually sufficient until the drug is metabolized. In severe cases, antipsychotic drugs with minimal side effects (eg, haloperidol, 5 mg intramuscularly) may be given every several hours until the individual has regained control. In cases where "flashbacks" occur (mental imagery from a "bad trip" that is later triggered by mild stimuli such as marihuana, alcohol, or psychic trauma), a short course of an antipsychotic drug (eg, trifluoperazine, 5 mg orally) for several days is sufficient. An occasional patient may have "flashbacks" for much longer periods and require small doses of neuroleptic drugs over the longer term.

## Phencyclidine

Phencyclidine (PCP, angel dust, peace pill, hog), developed as an anesthetic agent, first appeared as a street drug deceptively sold as tetrahydrocannabinol (THC). Because it is simple to produce and mimics to some degree the traditional psychedelic drugs, it has become a common deceptive substitute for LSD and mescaline. It is available in crystals, capsules, and tablets to be inhaled, injected, swallowed, or smoked (it is commonly sprinkled on marihuana).

Absorption after smoking is rapid, with onset of symptoms in several minutes and peak symptoms in 15–30 minutes. Mild intoxication produces a euphoria accompanied by a feeling of numbness. Moderate intoxication (5–10 mg) results in disorientation, detachment from surroundings, distortion of body image, combativeness, unusual feats of strength, and loss of ability to integrate sensory input, especially touch and proprioception. Physical symptoms include dizziness, ataxia, dysarthria, nystagmus, hyperreflexia, and tachycardia. There are increases in blood pressure, respiration, muscle tone, and urine production. Severe intoxication (20 mg or more) produces an increase in degree of moderate symptoms, with the addition of seizures, deepening coma, hypertensive crisis, and severe psychotic ideation. The drug is particularly long lasting (several days to several weeks) owing to high lipid solubility, gastroenteric recycling, and the production of active metabolites. Overdosage may be directly fatal, with the major causes of death being hypertensive crisis, respiratory arrest, and convulsions. Acute rhabdomyolysis has been reported and can result in myoglobinuric renal failure.

Differential diagnosis involves the whole spectrum of street drugs, since in some ways phencyclidine mimics sedatives, psychedelics, and marihuana in its effects. Blood and urine testing can detect the acute problem.

Treatment is discussed on p 1029.

## Marihuana

*Cannabis sativa,* a hemp plant, is the source of marihuana. The parts of the plant vary in potency. The resinous exudate of the flowering tops of the female plant (hashish, charas) is the most potent, followed by the dried leaves and flowering shoots of the female plant (bhang) and the resinous mass from small leaves of inflorescence (ganja). The least potent parts are the lower branches and the leaves of the female plant and all parts of the male plant. The drug is usually inhaled by smoking. Effects occur in 10–20 minutes and last 2–3 hours. "Joints" of good quality contain about 500 mg of marihuana (which contains approximately 5–15 mg of tetrahydrocannabinol with a half-life of 7 days). Marihuana soaked in formaldehyde and dried ("AMP") has produced unusual effects, including autonomic discharge and severe, transient cognitive impairment. The user and the setting, as in psychedelic use, are important factors in the effect of the drug.

With moderate dosage, marihuana produces 2 phases: mild euphoria followed by sleepiness. In the acute state, the user has an altered time perception, less inhibited emotions, impaired immediate memory, and conjunctival injection. High doses produce transient psychotomimetic effects. No specific treatment is necessary except in the case of the occasional "bad trip," in which case the person is treated in the same way as for psychedelic usage. Marihuana frequently aggravates existing mental illness and slows the learning process in children.

Studies of long-term effects have conclusively shown abnormalities in the pulmonary tree. Laryngitis and rhinitis are related to prolonged use, along with chronic obstructive pulmonary disease. Electrocardiographic abnormalities are common, but no long-term cardiac disease has been linked to marihuana use. Chronic usage has resulted in depression of plasma testosterone levels and reduced sperm counts. Abnormal menstruation and failure to ovulate have occurred in some female users. Sudden withdrawal produces insomnia, nausea, myalgia, and irritability. Psychologic effects of chronic marihuana usage are still unclear. Urine testing is reliable if samples are carefully collected and tested. Detection periods span 4–6 days in acute users and 20–30 days in chronic users.

## Stimulants

The abuse of stimulants has increased markedly since World War II, partly because of the proliferation of drugs marketed for weight reduction. The **amphetamines,** including methedrine ("speed"), methylphenidate, and phenmetrazine, are being placed under control, but street availability remains high. Moderate usage of any of the stimulants produces hyperactivity, a sense of enhanced physical and mental capacity, and sympathomimetic effects. The clinical picture of acute stimulant intoxication includes sweating, tachycardia, elevated blood pressure, mydriasis, hyperactivity, and an acute brain syndrome with confusion and disorientation. Tolerance develops quickly and, as the dosage is increased, paranoid ideation (with delusions of parasitosis), stereotypy, bruxism, and full-blown psychoses occur. Stimulant withdrawal is characterized by depression with symptoms of hyperphagia and hypersomnia.

People who have used stimulants chronically (eg, anorexigenics) occasionally become sensitized to future use of stimulants. In these individuals, even small amounts of mild stimulants such as caffeine can cause symptoms of paranoia and auditory hallucinations.

**Cocaine** is a stimulant, not a narcotic. It is a product of the coca plant. The derivatives include seeds, leaves, coca paste, cocaine HCl, and the free base of cocaine. Coca paste is a crude extract that contains 40–80% cocaine sulfate and other impurities. Cocaine HCl is the salt and the most commonly used form. Free base, a purer (and stronger) derivative called "crack" is prepared by simple extraction from cocaine HCl. The drug is powerfully addictive and extremely dangerous.

The use of cocaine has been steadily increasing in recent years. Higher purity has resulted in increased problems. Cocaine may be snorted (complications include septal ulceration), and the free base form can be "smoked" (the drug is vaporized and inhaled). Both forms can be injected intravenously. The latter 2 routes produce marked euphoria ("rush") but increased toxicity. Parenteral use also creates the many problems associated with injection of any street drug of questionable purity.

Cocaine produces powerful euphoria, excitement, and increased energy ("high") that lasts for several minutes. It creates a strong dependency and craving with tolerance and causes wide mood swings, erratic behavior, insomnia, paranoia (often severe), and hallucinations. Chronic use leads to increasing paranoia, delusions of parasitosis, and miniaturized visual perceptions (micropsia). Sedatives, alcohol, marihuana, and opiates are often used concomitantly to dampen some of the unpleasant stimulant effects. An injectable mixture of cocaine and heroin is called a "speedball." Some users now smoke a combination of freebase cocaine and Persian heroin. Overdoses may cause cardiac arrest, fatal hyperpyrexia, or exacerbation of symptoms of angina. Lung damage can result from vasoconstriction. Some individuals have become vitamin B and C deficient secondary to high ATP generation, and the rare person with pseudocholinesterase deficiency is particularly susceptible to small doses of cocaine. Cocaine use in pregnancy is associated with an increased incidence of congenital malformations and perinatal morbidity.

Physicians should be alert to cocaine use in patients presenting with unexplained nasal bleeding, headaches, fatigue, insomnia, anxiety, depression, and chronic hoarseness. Sudden withdrawal of the drug is not life-threatening but usually produces sleep disturbances, hyperphagia, lassitude, and severe depression (sometimes with suicidal ideation) lasting several days to several weeks. Infrequently, an abstinence syndrome consisting of delirium, sleeplessness, and increased motor activity develops 3–10 days after cessation of the drug. A short course of moderate doses of antipsychotic drugs is effective in treating this syndrome and any paranoid ideation resulting from cocaine use.

Successful treatment for behavioral or physiologic reactions arising from cocaine use may require hospitalization. A dopamine agonist such as bromocriptine, 1 mg 3 times a day orally, may alleviate craving and withdrawal symptoms. The patient with habituation must be followed in a comprehensive, structured treatment program which include cocaine recovery groups such as Cocaine Anonymous. There is a strong tendency to relapse, and pursuit of a different lifestyle is vital to recovery.

## Caffeine

The most popular mind-affecting drugs are caffeine, nicotine, and alcohol. Some 10 billion pounds of coffee (the richest source of caffeine) are consumed yearly throughout the world. Tea, cocoa, and cola drinks also contribute to an intake of caffeine that is often astoundingly high in a large number of people. The content of caffeine in a (180-mL) cup of beverage is as follows: brewed coffee, 80–140 mg; instant coffee, 60–100 mg; decaffeinated coffee, 1–6 mg; leaf tea, 30–80 mg; tea bags, 25–75 mg; instant tea, 30–60 mg; cocoa, 10–50 mg; and 12-oz cola drinks, 30–65 mg. A 1-oz chocolate candy bar has about 20 mg. Caffeine-containing analgesics usually contain approximately 30 mg per unit. Symptoms of caffeinism include anxiety, agitation, restlessness, insomnia, a feeling of being "wired," and somatic symptoms referable to the heart and gastrointestinal tract. *It is common for a case of caffeinism to present as an anxiety disorder.* It is also common for caffeine and other stimulants to precipitate severe symptoms in compensated schizophrenic and manic-depressive patients. Chronically depressed patients often use caffeine drinks as self-medication. This diagnostic clue may help distinguish some major affective disorders. Withdrawal from caffeine (more than 500 mg/d) can produce headaches, irritability, and occasional nausea.

## Miscellaneous Drugs & Solvents

The principal over-the-counter drugs (OTC) of concern are phenylpropanolamine and an assortment of antihistaminic agents. Frequently, these drugs are sold in combination as cold remedies (eg, Dristan, Triaminic). Not infrequently, a mild analgesic is added to the preparation. Most appetite suppressant drugs are combinations of phenylpropanolamine and caffeine (fenfluramine is an exception); these drugs are also heavily marketed as "stay-awake" drugs. Practically all of the so-called sleep aids are now antihistamines. Scopolamine and bromides have generally been removed from the over-the-counter market.

The major problem in the use of all these drugs relates to phenylpropanolamine, which has all the side effects of any stimulant, including precipitation of anxiety states, auditory and visual hallucinations, paranoid ideation, and, occasionally, delirium. Aggressiveness and some loss of impulse control have been reported. Sleep disturbances are common even with reasonably small doses.

Nicotine dependency is usually a function of cigarette smoking. It is a major causative or contributing factor in a number of medical illnesses. The 2 principal drugs of abuse in the USA are nicotine and alcohol.

Antihistamines usually produce some central nervous system depression—thus their use as over-the-counter sedatives. Drowsiness may be a problem. Antihistamine intoxication can produce excitement. The mixture of antihistamines with alcohol usually exacerbates the central nervous system effects.

The abuse of laxatives sometimes can lead to electrolyte disturbances that may contribute to the manifestations of an organic brain syndrome. The greatest use of laxatives tends to be in the elderly, who are most vulnerable to physiologic changes.

Amyl nitrite, a drug useful in angina pectoris, has been used in recent years as an "orgasm expander." The changes in time perception caused by the drug prompted its nonmedical use, and popular lore concerning the effects of inhalation just prior to orgasm has led to increased use. Tolerance develops readily, but there are no known withdrawal symptoms. Abstinence for several days reestablishes the previous level of responsiveness. Long-term effects are unknown.

Sniffing of solvents and inhaling of gases (including aerosols) produce a form of inebriation similar to that of the volatile anesthetics. Agents include gasoline, toluene, petroleum ether, lighter fluids, cleaning fluids, paint thinners, and nail polish. Typical intoxication states include euphoria, slurred speech, and confusion, and with high doses, acute manifestations are unconsciousness and cardiorespiratory depression or failure; chronic exposure produces a variety of symptoms related to the liver, kidney, or bone marrow. Lead encephalopathy can be associated with sniffing leaded gasoline. In addition, studies of workers chronically exposed to jet fuel showed significant increases in neurasthenic symptoms, including fatigue, anxiety, mood changes, memory difficulties, and somatic complaints. These same problems have been noted in long-term solvent abuse.

The so-called designer drugs are synthetic substitutes for commonly used recreational drugs and are produced in small, clandestine laboratories. The most common designer drugs have been methyl analogs of fentanyl and have been used as heroin substitutes. MDMA, an amphetamine derivative sometimes called "ecstasy," is also a designer drug with high abuse potential. Manufacture and use of these substances are a vexing problem for law enforcement, since the newest drugs have not yet reached an illegal status and there are no tests developed for detection. Furthermore, they present problems for physicians faced with symptoms from a totally unknown cause.

Charney DS, Heninger GR, Kleber HD: The combined use of clonidine and naltrexone as a rapid, safe, and effective treatment of abrupt withdrawal from methadone. *Am J Psychiat* 1986;**143**:831.

Dowling GP, McDonough ET III, Bost RO: "Eve" and "Ecstasy": A report of five deaths associated with the use of MDEA and MDMA. *JAMA* 1987;**257**:1615.

Dupon RL: Substance abuxe. *JAMA* 1986;**256**:2214.

Gavin FH, Kleber HD: Abstinence symptomatology and psychiatric diagnoses in cocaine abusers. *Arch Gen Psychiatry* 1986;**43**:107.

Gold MS (editor): Marijuana update. *Psychiatr Ann* 1986;**26(Apr).** [Entire issue.]

Hughes JR, Hatsukami D: Signs and symptoms of tobacco withdrawal. *Arch Gen Psychiatry* 1986;**43**:289.

Isner JM et al: Acute cardiac events temporally related to cocaine abuse. *New England J Med* 1986;**315**:1438.

## ORGANIC MENTAL DISORDERS
## (Organic Brain Syndrome [OBS])

### Essentials of Diagnosis

- Cognitive impairment: disorientation, defective sensation and perception, impairment of capacity for recall and recent memory, impaired thinking and logical reasoning.
- Emotional disturbances: affect, depression, shame, anxiety, irritability.
- Behavioral disturbances: decreased impulse control, exhibitionism, sexual acting-out, aggression.
- History or findings to indicate one or more of the etiologic factors listed below.

### General Considerations

The organic problem may be a primary brain disease or a secondary manifestation of some general disorder. All of the brain syndromes show some degree of cognitive impairment depending on the site of involvement, the rate of onset and progression, and the duration of the underlying brain lesion. Emotional disturbances are often inversely proportionate to the severity of the cognitive disorder. The behavioral disturbances tend to be more common with chronicity, more directly related to the underlying personality,

and not necessarily correlated with cognitive dysfunction.

### Etiology

**A. Intoxication:** Alcohol, sedatives, bromides, anticholinergic drugs, antidepressants, analgesics (eg, pentazocine), pollutants, psychedelic drugs, salicylates (chronic use), solvents, a wide variety of over-the-counter and prescribed drugs, and household, agricultural, and industrial chemicals.

**B. Drug Withdrawal:** Withdrawal from alcohol, sedative-hypnotics, corticosteroids.

**C. Long-Term Effects of Alcohol:** Wernicke-Korsakoff syndrome.

**D. Infections:** Septicemia; meningitis and encephalitis due to bacterial, viral, fungal, parasitic or tuberculous organisms or to central nervous system syphilis; acute and chronic infections due to the entire range of microbiologic pathogens.

**E. Endocrine Disorders:** Thyrotoxicosis, hypothyroidism, adrenocortical dysfunction (including Addison's disease and Cushing's syndrome), pheochromocytoma, insulinoma, hypoglycemia from insulin overdose, hyperparathyroidism, hypoparathyroidism, panhypopituitarism.

**F. Respiratory Disorders:** Hypoxia, hypocapnia, any imbalance in respiratory exchange.

**G. Metabolic Disturbances:** Fluid and electrolyte disturbances, acid-base disorders, hepatic disease (hepatic encephalopathy, Wilson's disease), renal failure, porphyria.

**H. Nutritional Deficiencies:** Deficiency of vitamin $B_1$ (beriberi), vitamin $B_{12}$ (pernicious anemia), nicotinic acid (pellagra); protein-calorie malnutrition.

**I. Trauma:** Subdural hematoma, subarachnoid hemorrhage, intracerebral bleeding, concussion syndrome.

**J. Cardiovascular Disorders:** Cardiac infarctions, arrhythmias, cerebrovascular spasms, hemorrhages, embolisms, occlusions.

**K. Neoplasms:** Primary or metastatic lesions of the central nervous system, cancer-induced hypercalcemia.

**L. Idiopathic Epilepsy:** Grand mal and postictal temporal lobe dysfunction.

**M. Collagen and Immunologic Disorders:** Systemic lupus erythematosus, acquired immunodeficiency syndrome (AIDS).

**N. Degenerative Diseases:** Alzheimer's disease, Pick's disease, multiple sclerosis, parkinsonism, Huntington's chorea, amyotrophic lateral sclerosis, normal pressure hydrocephalus.

**O. Miscellaneous:** Tourette's syndrome.

### Clinical Findings

The manifestations are many and varied and include problems with orientation, short or fluctuating attention span, loss of recent memory and recall, impaired judgment, emotional lability, lack of initiative, impaired impulse control, inability to reason through problems, depression (worse in mild to moderate types), confabulation (not limited to alcohol organic brain syndrome), constriction of intellectual functions, visual hallucinations, and delusions. Physical findings will naturally vary according to the cause. The EEG is often abnormal.

**A. Delirium:** Delirium is a disorder of attention, with clouding of consciousness. Onset is usually rapid. The mental status fluctuates (impairment is usually least in the morning), with varying inability to concentrate, maintain attention, and sustain purposeful behavior. (''Sundowning''—mild to moderate delirium at night—is more common in patients with preexisting dementia and may be precipitated by drugs and sensory deprivation.) There is a marked deficit of short-term memory and recall. Amnesia is retrograde (impaired recall of past memories) and anterograde (inability to recall events after the onset of the delirium). Orientation problems follow the inability to retain information. Perceptual disturbances (often visual hallucinations) and psychomotor restlessness with insomnia are common. Autonomic changes include tachycardia, dilated pupils, and sweating. The average duration is about 1 week, with full recovery in most cases. Physical illness or drug toxicity is usually present. Delirium can coexist with dementia.

**B. Dementia:** (See also Chapter 2.) Dementia is characterized by chronicity and deterioration of all mental functions. Onset is insidious in most cases. Dementia is usually progressive, more common in the elderly (although not an inevitable consequence of aging), and rarely reversible even if underlying disease can be corrected. Dementia can be classified as cortical or subcortical. The former (eg, Alzheimer's disease) is characterized by initial short-term memory loss (amnesia), gradual loss of expressive and comprehensive language (aphasia), and higher-order associative functions (visuospatial disturbance) with normal motor function. Subcortical forms include degeneration of subcortical structures (eg, parkinsonism, HIV infection) and are less likely to be associated with aphasia, agnosia, or loss of higher associative functions but more likely to produce apathy and movement disorders (eg, chorea, tremor, rididity). Loss of intellectual abilities and impairment of abstract thinking, along with personality disintegration, tend to markedly impair social and occupational function. Emotional lability is common—often associated with depression in the early stages. Loss of impulse control (sexual and language) is common. Paranoia and other psychotic symptoms are often present. The tenuous level of function makes the individual most susceptible to minor physical and psychologic stresses. The course depends on the underlying cause, and the general trend is steady deterioration.

There are 3 types of cortical dementia: (1) primary degenerative dementia, accounting for about 50–60% of cases; (2) atherosclerotic dementia, 15–20% of cases; and (3) mixtures of the first 2 types or due to miscellaneous causes, 15–20% of cases (see also

Chapter 2). Examples of primary degenerative dementia are Alzheimer's dementia (most common) and Pick, Parkinson, Creutzfeldt-Jacob, and Huntington dementias (less common). Alzheimer's dementia has a slow onset and tends to occur after 40 years of age. It is associated with a relative cholinergic deficiency, principally of choline acetyltransferase. The diagnosis can be established clinically only by exclusion of other known organic causes of dementia. The presence of Alzheimer's disorder in other family members ranges from 30 to 70% and shows a genetic transmission related to Down's syndrome. At present, the definitive diagnosis can be established only on the basis of characteristic pathologic findings on brain biopsy or postmortem examination.

**Pseudodementia** is a term applied to depressed patients who appear to be demented. It is occasionally used to include other reversible conditions that mimic dementia (eg, mass lesions, effects of medication). Depression should be considered in every apparent case of dementia. (See Table 17–9.)

**C. Amnestic Syndrome:** This is a memory disturbance without delirium or dementia. It is usually associated with thiamine deficiency and chronic alcohol use (eg, Korsakoff's syndrome). It impairs selective areas of cognitive functioning. The onset is usually sudden, but the course is usually chronic.

**D. Organic Hallucinosis:** This condition is characterized by persistent or recurrent hallucinations (usually auditory) without the other symptoms usually found in delirium or dementia. Alcohol or hallucinogens are often the cause, and some people seem to be particularly susceptible to stimulants. There does not have to be any other mental disorder, and there may be complete spontaneous resolution.

**E. Organic Personality Syndrome:** This syndrome is characterized by emotional lability and loss of impulse control along with a general change in personality. Cognitive functions are preserved. Social

**Table 17–9.** Differentiation of pseudodementia (depression) and dementia.

| Pseudodementia | Dementia |
|---|---|
| Rapid onset | Slow onset |
| Rapid progress | Usually slow course |
| Early loss of social skills | Social skills retained for a long time |
| Patient emphasizes disability | Patient conceals disability |
| Complaints of memory loss | Few complaints |
| Recent and remote memory equally affected | Loss of recent memory |
| More often previous psychiatric history | No previous psychiatric history |
| Vegetative symptoms common | Fewer vegetative symptoms |
| Inconsistency on examination | Consistent manifest deficiencies |
| Same problems night and day | Worse at night |

inappropriateness is common. Loss of interest and lack of concern with the consequences of one's actions are often present. The course depends on the underlying cause (eg, frontal lobe contusion may resolve completely).

## Differential Diagnosis

Patients with nonorganic ("functional") psychoses usually remain oriented; the onset is usually gradual; hallucinations are usually auditory rather than visual; and intellectual functions are relatively intact, with good memory and a normal EEG and no demonstrable organic disease.

## Complications

Chronicity is sometimes a function of early nonreversal, eg, subdural hematoma, low-pressure hydrocephalus. Prompt correction of reversible causes improves recovery of mental function. Accidents secondary to impulsive behavior and poor judgment are a major consideration. Secondary depression and impulsive behavior not infrequently lead to suicide attempts. Drugs, particularly sedatives, may worsen thinking abilities and contribute to the overall problems.

## Treatment

**A. Medical:** Provide a pleasant, comfortable, nonthreatening, and physically safe environment with adequate nursing or attendant services. *Establish the diagnosis and correct underlying medical problems.* Do not overlook any possibility of reversible organic disease. Avoid analgesic drugs. Give antipsychotics in small doses at first (eg, haloperidol, 2 mg orally at bedtime) and increase according to the need to reduce psychotic ideation or excessive irritability. Bedtime administration obviates the need for sedatives, which often worsen organic brain syndrome. Aggressiveness and rage states in central nervous system lesions can be reduced with propranolol, 40–240 mg/d. Emotional lability in some cases responds to small doses of imipramine, 25 mg 3 times daily.

Cerebral vasodilators were originally used on the assumption that cerebral arteriosclerosis and ischemia were the principal causes of the dementias. Although there is a slight reduction of blood flow in primary degenerative dementia (probably as a result of the basic disorder), there is no evidence that this is a major factor in this group of disorders or that vasodilators are of value. Ergotoxine alkaloids (Hydergine) have been studied, with mixed results; improvement in ambulatory self-care and depressed mood has been noted, but there has been no improvement of cognitive functioning on any standardized tests. Hyperbaric oxygen treatment has not produced significant improvement. Drugs having a stimulatory effect, such as methylphenidate, may cause affective improvement without a change in cognitive function. The affective improvement can benefit the patient and family by providing some improvement in the quality of life.

Numerous investigational drugs have been used, but there is no clear-cut evidence of benefit.

Failing sensory functions should be supported as necessary, with hearing aids, cataract surgery, etc.

**B. Social:** Substitute home care, board care, or convalescent home care may be most useful when the family is unable to care for the patient. The setting should include familiar people and objects, lights at night, and a simple schedule. Family counseling may help the family to cope with problems that may occur and may help keep the patient at home as long as possible. Volunteer services, including homemakers, visiting nurses, and adult protective services may be required if the patient is left at home.

**C. Behavioral:** Behavioral techniques include operant responses that can be used to induce positive behaviors, eg, paying attention to the patient who is trying to communicate appropriately, and extinction by ignoring inappropriate responses.

**D. Psychologic:** Formal psychologic therapies are not usually helpful and may make things worse by taxing the patient's limited cognitive resources.

## Prognosis

The prognosis is good in acute (reversible) cases, fair in moderate cases, and poor in deteriorated states.

Council on Scientific Affairs: Dementia. *JAMA* 1986;**256**:2234.

Cummings JL: Multi-infarct dementia: Diagnosis and management. *Psychosomatics* 1987;**28**:117.

Jenike MA: Alzheimer's disease: Clinical care and management. *Psychosomatics* 1986;**27**:407.

Navin BA, Jordan BD, Price RW: The AIDS dementia complex: 1. Clinical features. *Ann Neurol* 1986;**19**:517.

# GERIATRIC PSYCHIATRIC DISORDERS
## (See also Chapter 2.)

### Essentials of Diagnosis

- Some degree of organic brain syndrome often present.
- Depression, paranoid ideation, and easy irritability are common.
- High frequency of medical problems.
- Patient is frequently worsened by a wide variety of medications.
- Loneliness and fear of death are often factors.

### General Considerations

There are 3 basic factors in the process of aging: biologic, sociologic, and psychologic.

The complex **biologic** changes depend on inherited characteristics (the best guarantee of long life is to have long-lived parents), nutrition, declining sensory functions such as hearing or vision, disease, trauma, and life-style. A definite correlation between hearing loss and paranoid ideation exists in the elderly. (See Organic Brain Syndrome, above.) As a person ages, the central nervous system becomes less hardy, and relatively minor disorders or combinations of disorders may cause deficits in cognition and affective response. Hypochondriasis is frequently a mechanism of compensating for decreased function.

The **sociologic** factors derive from stresses connected with occupation, family, and community. Any or all of these areas may be disrupted in a general phenomenon of "disengagement" that older people experience as friends die, the children move away, and the surroundings become less familiar. Retirement commonly precipitates a major disruption in a well-established life structure. This is particularly stressful in the person whose compulsive devotion to a job has precluded other interests, so that sudden loss of this outlet leaves a void that is not easily filled.

The **psychologic** withdrawal of the elderly person is frequently related to a loss of self-esteem, which is based on the economic insecurity of older age with its congruent loss of independence, the realization of decreasing physical and mental ability, and the fear of approaching death. The process of aging is often poorly accepted, and the real or imagined loss of physical attractiveness may have a traumatic impact that the plastic surgeon can only soften for a time. In a culture that stresses physical and sexual attractiveness, it is difficult for most people to accept the change.

## Clinical Findings & Complications

The most common psychiatric syndrome in the elderly is organic brain syndrome of varying degree (see Chapter 2). Psychotic ideation (usually paranoid) may coexist with the organic brain syndrome. Frequently, in the milder cases, the individual is aware of the deficiency in sensorium and becomes depressed about actual or threatened loss of function. Depression becomes the most obvious symptom. Unless the examination is done with great care, the organic brain syndrome is missed and the patient is treated for the secondary symptom of depression without evaluation of the organic problem. Anxiety is often associated with organic illness. In organic brain syndrome, anxiety heightens preexisting confusion.

Abuse of the elderly—both physical neglect and physical injury—demands early recognition. Bruises, welts, fractures, and debilitation should alert the physician.

Depression may herald a mild or moderate organic brain syndrome. Depression in the absence of a brain syndrome is frequently manifested in the elderly as a somatic complaint without the overt signs of depression (see Affective Disorders, above). Night awakenings are common in depression in the elderly person. This is often diagnosed as hypochondriasis, which is also more frequent in older people (eg, preoccupation with bowel function). Polypharmacy (with both prescription and over-the-counter drugs) is a major cause of accidents and illness in the elderly. The increased and varied complaints are often an attempt to compensate and divert attention from decreased mental function. The triad of motor weakness, headache, and mental changes may be due to brain tumor. Overt depression is often related to life exigencies (80% of people over age 65 have some kind of medical problem). Alcoholism is present in approximately 15% of older patients presenting with psychiatric symptoms. The incidence of suicide is higher in elderly people—loneliness, age, and medical problems being directly related to the higher number of successful suicides. Because of somatic complaints hiding a "masked depression," it is necessary to be alert to suicidal ideation in this group. Direct questioning about suicidal intent is always warranted when any suspicion exists.

## Treatment

**A. Social:** Socialization, a structured schedule of activities, familiar surroundings, continued achievement, and avoidance of loneliness (probably the most important factor) are some of the major considerations in prevention and amelioration of the psychiatric problems of older age. Whenever possible, the patient should remain in a familiar setting or return to one for as long as possible. An inexorable downhill trend frequently follows dislocation, with the accompanying disengagement from adaptable activities. The patient can be supported in the primary environment by various agencies that can help avoid a premature change of habits. For patients with disabilities that make it difficult to cope with the problems of living alone, homemaker services can assist in continuing the day-to-day activities of the household; visiting nurses can administer medications and monitor the physical condition of the patient; and geriatric social groups can help maintain socialization and human contacts. In the hospital or nursing home, attention to the kinds of people placed in the same room is most important. All too often, the 4-bed ward is peopled by 4 withdrawn, nonfunctioning people who provide no stimulation for each other, and the resultant isolation increases the degree of depression; occasionally, a florid psychosis develops. Attention to the proper mixture of active and inactive people can help relieve the loneliness that so often pervades such placement.

**B. Medical:** Treatment of any reversible components of an organic brain syndrome is obviously the major medical consideration. One commonly overlooked factor is self-medication, frequently with over-the-counter drugs that further impair the patient's already precarious functioning. Frequent culprits are antihistamines and anticholinergic drugs.

Any signs of psychosis, such as paranoid ideation and delusions, respond very well to *small amounts* of antipsychotics. Trifluoperazine, 2–5 mg orally once a day, or fluphenazine, 1–2 mg orally daily, will usually decrease psychotic ideation markedly. Associated agitation is usually ameliorated. The use of long-acting fluphenazine for acute paranoid ideation or agitation is appropriate if it is used initially in low dosage (12.5 mg) every 2–3 weeks with close attention to the possibility of extrapyramidal side effects, which are more frequent in the geriatric population.

Judicious use of the antipsychotics can often maintain the older person in the home environment and delay the traumatic dislocation that usually worsens the patient's condition. Do not use drugs that cause significant orthostatic hypotension (resulting in dizziness, falls, fractures). Because of sensitivity to anticholinergic effects, avoid nonpiperazine phenothiazines and unnecessary antiparkinsonism drugs. Sedatives frequently have a worsening effect and should generally be avoided. All psychoactive drugs have a higher incidence of side effects and are metabolized and excreted more slowly in the elderly.

Antidepressants (in one-half to one-third the doses given to young adults) are used when indicated for depression. Low doses of amitriptyline have been effective in pathologic laughing and weeping, which occur in neurologic conditions such as multiple sclerosis. Infrequently, a stimulant in small doses (eg, methylphenidate, 5–10 mg orally daily) can be used to treat apathy. The stimulant may help increase the patient's energy for social involvement and help the patient to maintain life activities. Lithium is helpful in the treatment of severe mood swings but has a narrow margin of neurotoxicity in the elderly.

When sedatives are to be used, consider triazolam or lorazepam, since they have no active metabolites and thus have a shorter half-life. Sedatives can worsen memory and confusional states in people who are already impaired. The appropriate use of wine and beer for mild sedative effects is quite rewarding in the hospital and other care facilities as well as at home.

**C. Behavioral:** The impaired cognitive abilities of the geriatric patient necessitate simple behavioral techniques. Positive responses to appropriate behavior encourage the patient to repeat desirable kinds of behavior, and frequent repetition offsets to some degree the defects in recent memory and recall. It also results in participation—a most important element, since there is a tendency in the older population to withdraw, thus increasing isolation and functional decline.

One must be careful not to reinforce and encourage obstreperous behavior by responding to it; in this way, extinction or at least gradual reduction of inappropriate behavior will occur. At the same time, the obstreperous behavior often represents a nondirective response to frustration and inability to function, and a structured program of activity is necessary.

**D. Psychologic:** Patients may require help in adjusting to changing roles and commitments and in finding new goals and viewpoints. The older person steadily loses an important commodity—the future— and may attempt to compensate for this by preoccupation with the past. Involvement with the present and psychotherapy on a here-and-now basis can help make the adjustment easier.

Chairello RJ, Cole JO: The use of psychostimulants in general psychiatry: A reconsideration. *Arch Gen Psychiat* 1987;**44**:286.

Eslinger PJ et al: Neuropsychologic detection of abnormal mental decline in older persons. *JAMA* 1985;**253**:670.

Reding M, Haycox J, Blass J: Depression in patients referred to a dementia clinic. *Arch Neurol* 1985;**42**:894.

Thompson TL, Moran MG, Nies AS: Psychotropic drug use in the elderly. (2 parts.) *N Engl J Med* 1983;**308**:134, 194.

## DEATH & DYING

As Thomas Browne said, ''The long habit of living indisposeth us for dying.'' It is only when death comes close to us that we really begin to respond to the possibility of our own death.

Death means different things to different people. For some it may represent an escape from unbearable suffering or other difficulties; for others, entrance into a new transcendental life. Death may come as a narcissistic attempt to find lasting fame or importance in martyrdom or heroic adventure, or it may be an atonement for real or imagined guilt or a means of extorting from others posthumously the affection that was not forthcoming during life.

Often the process is more shattering to those whose charge it is to maintain life, and there is a good deal of question about the so-called agony of death. Some observers, including Sir William Osler, take the view that there is no such thing, and the experiences of people who have been resuscitated from cardiac standstill seem to substantiate his view. They describe a sensation of detachment, a final peaceful ''letting go''; and one is at times impressed with the fact that the dying patient resents any interference with the process by physicians and nurses.

How each individual responds to imminent death is a function not only of what death means to that person but also of the mechanisms used to deal with problems—and these are usually the same as those used throughout life. Patients frequently worry more about *how* they will die than about death itself. Responses frequently seen in the dying patient include denial, anger, bargaining, depression, and acceptance—stages that are seen in many people as they go through any significant flux or loss. Seldom are these stages seen in isolation, and the complexity of the process contributes to the juxtaposition of the stages and the noted lability of mood and attitude in the dying patient.

An ill person may at first deny any concern with dying and then later admit to a fear of going to sleep because of the possibility of not waking up. This is often demonstrated by a need to keep the light on and to call frequently during the night with minor complaints. Some find it necessary to deny impending death to the end. Their families and doctors will often join in the conspiracy of denial, either out of sympathy or for their own reasons. It is important not to force the patient to realize the truth but to allow the opportunity, *when the patient is ready,* to discuss and deal with the problem of impending death. Frank discussion can mitigate the terror some patients feel. For many it is a comfort to be actively involved in the process of dying, sharing in the anticipation of death, and making whatever plans may be important. Alleviation of pain is a primary concern of many patients. The physician should not be concerned about addiction to narcotics when treating a dying patient.

The reactions of the family are often a combination of pain, anger, sadness, and depression. They react to each other and to the personnel caring for the patient. The problem to be resolved with the survivors is the guilt feelings they may have—that they continue to exist while the other person has died. Also to be reconciled are the vague sense of being responsible for the death and the subconscious refusal to believe that the person is really dead. The staff must be careful not to alienate the family, because this can result in less than optimum care. Some emotional investment in the patient by the staff is proper and inevitable, but it must be handled with insight and professional restraint. An insecure staff member may respond to a patient's death as if it were a professional failure. If the emotional investment is too little, the staff member may seem to be aloof and insensitive, while over-concern may lead to depression and despair, further impairing the person's capacity to serve as a source of support for the family in a time of distress.

The physician and staff must be aware of their own anxieties; maintain an appropriate level of involvement (a change of physicians may be necessary when this is impossible); allow for free and ongoing communication between patient, physician, and family; and share as a group—staff and family—the impending and unavoidable loss.

Bayer R et al: The care of the terminally ill: Mortality and economics. *N Engl J Med* 1983;**309:**1490.

Brown JH et al: Is it normal for terminally ill patients to desire death? *Am J Psychiatry* 1986;**143:**208.

# PSYCHIATRIC PROBLEMS ASSOCIATED WITH MEDICAL & SURGICAL DISORDERS

## Essentials of Diagnosis

*Acute problems:*

- Psychotic organic brain syndrome secondary to the medical or surgical problem, or compounded by effect of the environment (eg, intensive care unit).
- Acute anxiety, often related to ignorance and fear of the immediate problem as well as uncertainty about the future.
- Anxiety as an intrinsic aspect of the medical problem (eg, hyperthyroidism).

*Intermediate problems:*

- Depression as a function of the illness or accep-

tance of the illness, often associated with realistic or fantasied hopelessness about the future.
- Behavioral problems, often related to denial of illness and, in extreme cases, causing the patient to leave the hospital against medical advice.

*Recuperative problems:*

- Decreasing cooperation as the patient sees improvement and is not compelled to follow orders closely.
- Readjustment problems with family, job, and society.

## General Considerations

### A. Acute Problems:

**1. "Intensive care unit psychosis"** is a type of delirium that is frequently accompanied by psychotic ideation. It is an expression of organic (frequently including a preexisting organic brain syndrome), psychologic, and environmental factors. Some factors include sleep deprivation, sedative and analgesic medications, alcohol withdrawal, metabolic fluctuations (particularly hypoxemia and hyponatremia), fear, and overstimulation. It is important to consider and recognize the problem early when it is more easily corrected. (See Organic Mental Disorders, above.)

**2. Pre- and postsurgical anxiety states** are common—and commonly ignored. Presurgical anxiety is ubiquitous and is principally a fear of death (note the high number of surgical patients who make out their wills). Patients may be fearful of anesthesia (improved by the preoperative anesthesia interview), the mysterious operating room, and the disease processes that might be uncovered by the surgeon. Such fears frequently cause people to delay examinations that might result in earlier surgery and a greater incidence of cure.

The opposite of this is **surgery proneness,** the quest for surgery to escape from overwhelming life stresses. Polysurgery patients are not easily categorized. Dynamic motivations include unconscious guilt, a masochistic need to suffer, an attempt to deal with another family member's illness, and psychogenic pain. More apparent reasons may include an attempt to get relief from pain and a life-style that has become almost exclusively medically oriented, with all of the risks entailed in such an endeavor.

**Postsurgical anxiety states** are usually related to pain, procedures, and loss of body image. Acute pain problems are quite different from chronic pain disorders (see Chronic Pain Disorders, above); the former are readily handled with *adequate* analgesic medication. Problems usually are due to inadequate dosage and overly long time intervals between administration, eg, meperidine is commonly administered every 4 hours even though the duration of action is closer to 3 hours. Anxiety about procedures can be eased by actually introducing the patient to the procedures *before* surgery, in effect desensitizing the patient to the forthcoming trauma. The alteration in body image is particularly difficult for mastectomy patients.

Any procedure that results in a stoma has the attendant ramifications of odor, excretion bag, and concern about intimate relationships with others.

**3. Iatrogenic problems** usually pertain to medications, complications of diagnostic and treatment procedures, and impersonal and unsympathetic staff behavior. Polypharmacy is often a factor. Patients with unsolved diagnostic problems are at higher risk. They are desirous of relief, and the quest engenders more diagnostic procedures with a higher incidence of complications. The upset patient and family may be very demanding. Negative responses or a lack of attention by the staff to excessive demands may result in complications that escape the attention of the staff. Experience teaches medical personnel to appreciate that obstreperous behavior or excessive demands usually result from anxiety. Such behavior is best handled with calm and measured responses.

**B. Intermediate Problems:**

**1. Prolonged hospitalization** presents unique problems in certain hospital services, eg, burn units, orthopedic services, and tuberculosis wards. The acute problems of the severely burned patient are discussed in Chapter 29. The problems often are behavioral difficulties related to length of hospitalization and necessary procedures. For example, in burn units, pain is a major problem in addition to anxiety about procedures. Debridement and grafting seem never-ending to the patient, who is angry about and becoming resistant to immobilization and apparent lack of progress. This is especially true for people who have led an unencumbered life-style. Disputes with staff are common and often concern pain medication or ward privileges. Some patients regress to infantile behavior and dependency. Staff members must agree about their approach to the patient in order to ensure the smooth functioning of the unit.

**2. Depression** frequently intervenes during this period. It can contribute to irritability and overt anger. Severe depression can lead to anorexia, which further complicates healing and metabolic balance. It is during this period that the issue of disfigurement arises. Relief at survival gives way to concern about future function and appearance.

**C. Recuperative Problems:**

**1. Anxiety** about return to the outside world can cause regression to a dependent position. Complications increase, and staff forbearance again is tested. Anxiety at this stage usually is handled more easily than previous behavior problems.

**2. Posthospital adjustment** is related to the severity of the deficits and the use of outpatient facilities (eg, physical therapy, rehabilitation programs, psychiatric outpatient treatment). In a broad sense, the issue of ''survivorship''—attention to the quality of life in somebody who had or has a major illness. Lack of appropriate follow-up can contribute to depression in the patient, who may feel that he or she is making poor progress and may have thoughts of ''giving up.'' Reintegration into work, educational, and social endeavors may be painfully slow. Life is

simply much more difficult when one is disfigured, disabled, or disfranchised.

### Clinical Findings

The symptoms that occur in these patients are similar to those discussed in previous sections of this chapter, eg, organic brain syndrome, anxiety, and depression. Behavior problems may include lack of cooperation, increased complaints, demands for medication, sexual approaches to nurses, threats to leave the hospital, and actual signing out against medical recommendations. The underlying personality structure of the individual is a major factor in coping styles (eg, compulsive increases indecision, hysterical increases dramatic behavior).

### Differential Diagnosis

Organic brain syndrome must always be ruled out, since it often presents with symptoms resembling anxiety, depression, or psychosis. The schizophrenias may present with any of the above complaints. Personality disorders existing prior to hospitalization often underlie the various behavior problems, but particularly the management problems.

### Complications

Prolongation of hospitalization causes increased expense, deterioration of patient-staff relationships, and increased probabilities of iatrogenic and legal problems. The possibility of increasing posthospital treatment problems is enhanced.

### Treatment

**A. Medical:** The most important consideration by far is to have *one* physician in charge, a physician whom the patient trusts and who is able to oversee multiple treatment approaches (see Somatoform Disorders, above). In the acute problems, attention must be paid to metabolic imbalance, alcohol withdrawal, and previous drug use—prescribed, recreational, or over-the-counter. Adequate sleep and analgesia are important in the prevention of delirium.

Most physicians are attuned to the early detection of the surgery-prone patient. Plastic and orthopedic surgeons are at particular risk. Appropriate consultations may help detect some problems and mitigate future ones.

Postsurgical anxiety states can be alleviated by personal attention from the surgeon. Anxiety is not so effectively lessened by ancillary medical personnel, whom the patient perceives as lesser authorities, until after the physician has reassured the patient. Inappropriate use of ''as needed'' analgesia places an unfair burden on the nurse.

Depression should be recognized early. If severe, it may be treated by antidepressant medications (see Antidepressant Drugs, above). In the majority of cases, early consideration leads to early diagnosis and treatment by psychotherapeutic measures without the need for medication. Unnecessary medications tend to reinforce the patient's impression that there must be a serious illness or medication would not be required.

**B. Psychologic:** Prepare the patient for what is to come. This includes the types of units where the patient will be quartered, the procedures that will be performed, and any disfigurements that will result from surgery. Often because of anxiety, a great number of patients do not really listen to these explanations and are greatly surprised after surgery. Explanations with other family members present *on several occasions* may be necessary. The nursing staff can be helpful, since patients frequently confide a lack of understanding to a nurse but are reluctant to do so to the physician.

Time taken to elicit and discuss the patient's fears goes far in reducing the normal anxiety experienced by most patients. Repetition gives the patient time to digest information and ask further questions. Valid concerns and distorted understandings often relate to the death of a relative.

Denial of illness is frequently a block to acceptance of treatment. This, too, should be handled with family members present (to help the patient face the reality of the situation) in a series of short interviews (for reinforcement). Dependency problems resulting from long hospitalization are best handled by focusing on the changes to come as the patient makes the transition to the outside world. Key figures are teachers, vocational counselors, and physical therapists. Challenges should be realistic and practical and handled in small steps.

Depression is usually related to the loss of familiar hospital supports, and the outpatient therapists and counselors help to lessen the impact of the loss. The effect of depression on the family can delay resolution. Some of the impact can be alleviated by anticipating, with the patient and family, the signal features of the common depression to help prevent the patient from assuming a permanent sick role (invalidism).

Communication with the patient must be done with tact and under the best possible conditions. Suicide is always a concern when a patient is faced with despair. Be honest and compassionate, and make it clear by your actions that you are on the patient's side. Do not give unrealistic reassurances. Try to see the situation from the patient's position. Help the patient maintain hope, and nurture your relationship.

**C. Behavioral:** Prior desensitization can significantly allay anxiety about medical procedures. A "dry run" can be done to reinforce the oral description. Cooperation during acute problem periods can be enhanced by the use of appropriate reinforcers such as a favorite nurse or *helpful* family member. People who are positive reinforcers are even more helpful during the intermediate phases when the patient becomes resistant to the seemingly endless procedures (eg, debridement of burned areas). Other small pleasures such as wine or beer with hospital meals or after procedures can improve cooperation. Analgesic

medications should be used effectively (see Chronic Pain Disorders, above).

Specific situations (eg, psychologic dependency on the respirator) can be corrected by weaning with appropriate reinforcers (eg, a loved one allowed in the room whenever the patient is disconnected from the respirator). Behavioral approaches should be done in a positive and optimistic way for maximal reinforcement.

**D. Social:** A change in environment requires adaptation. Because of the illness, admission and hospitalization may be more easily handled than discharge. Reintegration into society can be difficult. In some cases, the family is a negative influence. A predischarge evaluation must be made to determine whether the family will be able to cope with the physical or mental changes in the patient. Working with the family while the patient is in the acute stage may presage a successful transition later on.

A positive work situation is critical to the restoration of self-esteem. In many cases, the previous form of employment is no longer available. Vocational counseling can provide new career directions. It should be started in the hospital as early as possible and may include the occupational therapists.

Development of a new social life can be facilitated by various self-help organizations (eg, the stoma club). Sharing problems with others in similar circumstances eases the return to a social life which may be quite different from that prior to the illness.

## Prognosis

The prognosis is good in all patients who have reversible medical and surgical conditions. It is guarded when there is serious functional loss that impairs vocational, educational, or societal possibilities—especially in the case of progressive and ultimately life-threatening illness.

Boehnert CE, Popkin MK: Psychological issues in treatment of severely noncompliant diabetics. *Psychosomatics* 1986;**27:**11.

Case RB, Heller SS, Case NB: Type A behavior and survival after acute myocardial infarction. *N Engl J Med* 1985; **312:**737.

Dilley JW, Shelp EE, Batki SL: Psychiatric and ethical issues in the care of patients with AIDS. *Psychosomatics* 1986;**27:**562.

Geringer ES, Stern TA: Coping with medical illness: The impact of personality types. *Psychosomatics* 1986;**27:**251.

Kwentus JA et al: Psychiatric complications of closed head trauma. *Psychosomatics* 1985;**26:**8.

Robinson RG, Lipsey JR, Price TR: Diagnosis and clinical management of post-stroke depression. *Psychosomatics* 1985;**26:**769.

Rodin G, Voshart K: Depression in the medically ill: An overview. *Am J Psychiat* 1986;**143:**696.

Rogers MP; Rheumatoid arthritis: Psychiatric aspects and use of psychotropics. *Psychosomatics* 1985;**26:**915.

## REFERENCES

Bassuk EL, Birk AW (editors): *Emergency Psychiatry: Concepts, Methods, and Practices.* Plenum Press, 1984.

Extein IL (editor): *Medical Mimics of Psychiatric Disorders.* APA Press, 1986.

Goldman HH (editor): *Review of General Psychiatry.* Lange, 1984.

Horowitz MJ: *Stress Response Syndromes,* 2nd ed. Jason Aronson, 1986.

Kandel ER, Schwartz JH (eds): *Principles of Neural Science,* 2nd ed. Elsevier, 1985.

Kellner R: *Somatization and Hypochondriasis.* Praeger, 1986.

Raj PP: *Practical Management of Pain.* Year Book, 1986.

Schatzberg AF, Cole JO: *Manual of Clinical Psychopharmacology.* APA Press, 1986.

Vaillant GE: *The Natural History of Alcoholism.* Harvard Univ Press, 1983.

# 18

# Endocrine Disorders

*Carlos A. Camargo, MD, & Felix O. Kolb, MD*

Our concepts of the endocrine system, the mechanisms of action of hormones, the complex interrelationships among hormones in maintaining our internal milieu, and the diagnosis and therapy of disorders of the endocrine glands have all undergone radical changes during the last decade. The line separating a hormone from other information-carrying molecules is becoming a tenuous one. This chapter, however, deals with the classically accepted hormonal systems.

It is now clear that all hormones regulate intracellular mechanisms responsible for the production of cellular proteins and that the induction or activation of these proteins is responsible for the effects of the hormones. The process whereby these new proteins are formed is quite complex. We have learned that many hormones have predecessors without biologic activity and that these "prohormones" must be transformed into active moieties. These changes may take place inside the endocrine gland itself (eg, many pituitary hormones), in other tissues peripheral in location such as liver or kidney (eg, vitamin D transformations), or inside the target organ cell (eg, testosterone-dihydrotestosterone transformation in prostatic cells). It is also possible for a hormone to exert most of its actions via a mediator formed in another organ (growth hormone-somatomedin).

Hormones attach to cells via specific receptors found either in the surface of the cells (most peptide hormones) or inside the cellular cytoplasm (steroid and thyroid hormones). The importance of these receptors in modern concepts of endocrine function cannot be overemphasized. Our understanding of disease processes in endocrinology is currently being greatly enhanced by knowledge of the dynamic aspects of hormone receptors, their modulation and control, and endocrine abnormalities.

## The Challenges of Diagnosis of Endocrine Diseases

The diagnosis of endocrine disorders is complicated by the following factors:

**A. Interrelationships of the Endocrine Glands:** Because the endocrine glands are so closely interrelated, the presenting symptoms and signs of any endocrine disorder may represent a secondary disturbance in another gland or even in more than one gland. The diagnostic clue may therefore be in an organ that is secondarily affected by hypofunction or hyperfunction of the gland in question. For example, amenorrhea may be due to an abnormality of the pituitary or adrenal gland rather than to a primary ovarian lesion.

**B. Homeostatic (Compensatory) Mechanisms:** A well-balanced system of homeostasis often disguises the existence of a functional change in an endocrine gland, eg, partial pituitary suppression by cortisol administration. Special stress tests may be required to clarify the diagnosis.

**C. Complexity of Hormone Deficiencies:** A functional hormonal deficiency results not only from decreased production and concentration of a hormone but may also occur with a decreased number or decreased affinity of tissue receptors for the hormone, postreceptor defects of hormone action, antagonism to hormone effect by another hormone or drug, and other conditions. Functional insufficiency may occur in the presence of normal or even *high* hormone levels.

**D. Size of Lesion Versus Magnitude of Effect:** The metabolic effect of an endocrine disturbance is not necessarily proportionate to the size of the lesion. A small tumor may cause extensive disturbance, whereas a striking enlargement may have only modest pathologic significance.

**E. Physiologic Versus Pathologic States:** The line between a physiologic aberration and a pathologic state may be quite tenuous. For example, when does the delay in appearance of signs of puberty become pathologic? Family background, judicious use of statistical data, and evaluation of nonendocrine problems such as state of nutrition and general health often help suggest when a search for an endocrine abnormality should be started.

**F. Neurologic Integration:** Many of the endocrine glands are regulated by neuroendocrine factors elaborated in the hypothalamus that control the secretion of the pituitary hormones. The structure of many of these hypothalamic hormones has been elucidated. Some of the hormones have proved to be of diagnostic value, and others (and their synthetic analogs) are likely to become useful therapeutic agents in the near future.

**G. Endocrine Versus Paracrine Hormonal Control:** Although hormones are secreted into the blood stream and exert their effects at a distance from another organ or tissue (classic *endocrine* control), it has become increasingly clear that a hormone can also diffuse locally and exert an effect upon neighboring cells (*paracrine* control). Thus, testosterone produced by the Leydig cell locally influences seminiferous tubular function.

**H. Multiple and Nonendocrine Involvement:** The increasing number of recognized syndromes of multiple endocrine tumors and autoimmune deficiencies (often familial) and the endocrinopathies associated with nonendocrine gland tumors has complicated the problems of diagnosis. A patient may present with renal stone as the main complaint and be found to have not only hypercalcemia due to hyperparathyroidism but also an enlarged sella turcica due to a prolactin-secreting tumor (multiple endocrine neoplasia type I). Conversely, failure of multiple endocrine glands may be due to poorly understood autoimmune mechanisms (eg, simultaneous primary thyroid and adrenal insufficiencies [Schmidt's syndrome]).

A tumor of a nonendocrine organ may also produce, at the same time, several "ectopic" hormones (eg, oat cell carcinoma of the lung secreting ACTH and vasopressin simultaneously).

**I. Difficulties of Laboratory Diagnosis:** Direct chemical and radioimmunoassays of many hormones in blood, urine, saliva, and other biologic fluids have been developed. The concentration of hormones in these fluids, however, often varies from subject to subject and from hour to hour, making interpretation of data difficult on occasion. Bedside observation and sensitive indirect procedures are still required to establish the diagnosis of many endocrine disorders.

Clayton RN (editor): Receptors in health and disease. *Clin Endocrinol Metab* 1983;**12**:1. [Entire issue.]

Franchimont P (editor): Paracrine control. *Clin Endocr Metab* 1986;**15**:No. 1. [Entire issue.]

Krieger DT: Brain peptides: What, where and why? *Science* 1983;**222**:975.

Pollet RJ, Levey GS: Principles of membrane receptor physiology and their application to clinical medicine. *Ann Intern Med* 1980;**92**:663.

# COMMON PRESENTING COMPLAINTS

## Delayed Growth

Normal growth is a complex process resulting from the interplay of multiple hormonal, metabolic, nutritional, genetic, and environmental factors. Normal growth requires, among other things, a normal chromosomal complement; normal cardiovascular, renal, and gastrointestinal systems; adequate diet and exercise; and the absence of harmful drugs or toxins. The possible causes of growth failure are multiple, and determination of the cause requires careful, comprehensive evaluation of the entire patient, not just of the endocrine status.

Rule out bone diseases and nutritional, metabolic, emotional, and chronic cardiorespiratory, gastrointestinal, hematologic, or renal disorders that may delay growth. A common cause of short stature in girls is Turner's syndrome. Look for sexual infantilism, webbing of the neck, and other signs of this chromosomal disorder.

Hormonal abnormalities to be considered include the following:

**A. Juvenile Hypothyroidism:** The thyroid deficiency may be subtle and difficult to recognize clinically. It should be suspected whenever a growth chart shows arrest in a previously normally growing child. The most common cause is Hashimoto's thyroiditis. Skeletal maturation is delayed. Low serum thyroxine and elevated TSH levels make the diagnosis.

**B. Glucocorticoid Excess:** Cushing's syndrome, whether naturally occurring or due to exogenous glucocorticoid administration, in childhood or adolescence is always associated with growth retardation. Look for red or violaceous striae, centripetal obesity, and easy bruisability. If the diagnosis is in doubt, perform a screening test such as the overnight dexamethasone suppression test. If the results reveal an abnormality, a complete evaluation is indicated.

**C. Gonadal Steroid Excess:** Precocious puberty and pseudoprecocious puberty, of whatever origin, are associated with early rapid growth and premature epiphyseal closure, resulting in short final stature. Look for signs of masculinization or feminization. If gonadal steroid excess is suspected, a complete workup is indicated.

**D. Hypopituitarism:** Any disease of the hypothalamus or the pituitary, with the exception of pituitary growth hormone-secreting tumors, is capable of impairing growth. Ask in detail about a history of headaches, visual disturbances, or polyuria. Remember that craniopharyngiomas are common in this age group. Modern imaging techniques (CT scan, magnetic resonance imaging [MRI]) will detect pituitary and hypothalamic disease in the early stages. If pituitary disease is suspected, a complete endocrine evaluation is in order.

**E. Monotropic Lack of Growth Hormone:** This syndrome is a common cause of dwarfism. It is often "idiopathic" in that no specific cause such as neoplasia, infection, vascular disease, or anatomic abnormality is ever found. A hypothalamic defect is often found. Many of these patients are able to synthesize growth hormone when growth hormone-releasing factor is administered. It is often difficult to clinically separate true growth hormone deficiency from "constitutional delay" of growth in cases where both growth and puberty are delayed but will eventually occur without therapy. Dynamic tests with growth hormone stimulation are often helpful, but borderline cases occur. A rare cause of functional growth hormone deficiency is **Laron dwarfism,** a familial autosomal recessive disorder, in which there is normal or increased growth hormone secretion but no secretion of somatomedin, the mediator of growth hormone action.

**F. Other Syndromes Affecting Growth:** In addition to the disorders mentioned, there are a myriad of rare syndromes, most of them heritable, in which deficient growth is one feature. These include genetic syndromes causing deafness or facial or limb anomalies, mental retardation, or retinitis pigmentosa. (See McKusik reference under General References.)

## Excessive Growth

Excessive growth may be a familial or racial characteristic or a physiologic event (eg, the growth spurt of puberty) as well as a sign of endocrine disease. If precocious genital development occurs, consider true precocity due to pituitary or hypothalamic disorders, or pseudoprecocious puberty due to excess of adrenal, ovarian, or testicular hormones (often due to tumors). These patients, if not treated rapidly, will eventually be of short stature as a result of premature closure of their epiphyses. The administration of a synthetic luteinizing hormone-releasing hormone (LHRH) analog has recently been shown to be effective in suppressing gonadotropin secretion in cases of true precocious puberty. Pituitary tumors secreting excess growth hormone cause gigantism if present before puberty and acromegaly if growth hormone excess takes place after closure of the epiphyseal plates of long bones. A few cases of nonpituitary "cerebral gigantism" have been described. Marfan's syndrome should also be considered. Purely hypogonadal individuals tend to grow taller, with eunuchoid proportions (span exceeds height; excessive length of floor-to-pubis segment of body).

## Obesity

Although obesity is a common presenting "endocrine" complaint, the overwhelming majority of cases are due to excessive food intake or physical inactivity, or both. There is some experimental evidence favoring the concept that there are different rates of thermogenesis in obese and nonobese individuals, but the matter remains controversial. It is clear, however, that obesity is *always* the result of a positive energy balance and will not occur if "excess" calories are not ingested. This is true for *all* types of obesity.

Endocrine causes of obesity are extremely uncommon. A rapid onset of massive obesity associated with lethargy or polyuria suggests a hypothalamic lesion (rare). Some cases of extreme obesity are associated with delayed puberty. Hypothyroidism is usually *not* associated with marked obesity. In Cushing's disease or syndrome, there is roundness of the face with a characteristic "buffalo hump" and trunk obesity with thin extremities. Striae are common with any type of obesity. They are wider (over 10 mm) and more violaceous in Cushing's syndrome. Amenorrhea, hypertension, and glycosuria or a diabetic glucose tolerance curve are commonly associated with obesity and often improve after adequate weight loss. Insulin-secreting adenomas are often associated with weight gain, but these are quite rare. In most instances, the obese patient requires increased activity and reduction in caloric intake, and all such patients

require sympathetic understanding and reinforcement of motivation.

## Wasting & Weakness

Contrary to old beliefs, hypopituitarism is only rarely associated with cachexia. Always rule out nonendocrine causes and consider anorexia nervosa and dietary fanaticism before looking for endocrine disturbances. Consider diabetes mellitus, thyrotoxicosis, pheochromocytoma, and Addison's disease if weight loss is progressive. Occult cancer and depressive reactions should also be ruled out.

## Abnormal Skin Pigmentation or Color

First consider normal individual, familial, and racial variations. Hyperpigmentation may coexist with depigmentation (vitiligo) in Addison's disease, which must be ruled out by standard tests. Search carefully for pigmentary spots on mucous membranes, gums, and nipples. Differentiate Addison's disease from sprue, hemochromatosis, and argyria. Severe malnutrition is often associated with hyperpigmentation. It may be confined to skin areas exposed to sunlight, as in pellagra. Pregnancy and thyrotoxicosis are at times associated with spotty brown pigmentation, especially over the face (chloasma). A similar type of pigmentation has been seen occasionally with oral contraceptive administration. Other drugs (eg, diethylstilbestrol) will cause localized brown-black pigmentation over the nipples. Generalized hyperpigmentation can also occasionally be found after prolonged administration of busulfan or chlorpromazine. Brown pigment spots with a ragged border are typical of McCune-Albright syndrome (associated with fibrous dysplasia and precocious sexual development in the female); smooth pigmented (café au lait) spots are seen in neurofibromatosis. Acanthosis nigricans may be associated with acromegaly and other endocrine tumors but is also often seen in patients with severe obesity. Patients with Cushing's disease usually have a ruddy complexion. Hyperpigmentation, especially after adrenalectomy, suggests a pituitary tumor or, more rarely, an extra-adrenal cancer. Carotenemia with yellowish skin is characteristic of primary myxedema. Sudden flushing and skin discoloration suggest the carcinoid syndrome. Vitiligo is often associated with autoimmune endocrinopathies.

## Hirsutism & Hypertrichosis

Hirsutism and hypertrichosis are disorders involving increased growth of body hair. It is important to distinguish between the two.

**A. Hypertrichosis:** Hypertrichosis is a disorder in which there is a generalized increase in body hair, including areas that are *not* androgen-sensitive, such as the arms and legs, the forehead, and the eyebrows. The disorder occurs in both men and women. Hypertrichosis is seen rarely in patients with porphyria cutanea tarda, sometimes in patients with anorexia nervosa, and in patients taking phenytoin, diazoxide, or the new antihypertensive agent minoxidil. There is no known endocrine abnormality underlying hypertrichosis in these cases.

**B. Hirsutism:** In hirsutism, excess androgen causes **vellus hair** follicles, which produce fine, short, nonpigmented hairs, to become **terminal hair** follicles, which produce coarse, long, pigmented hairs. This occurs only in areas of the body sensitive to the effects of androgens (mainly testosterone), eg, the face, chest, and lower abdomen. This disorder occurs only in women. In diagnosing hirsutism, it is important to remember that there are wide variations in the ''normal'' amount of hair present in these areas. Racial, familial, and individual differences must be taken into account (eg, Native American women have much less body hair than southern European or eastern Mediterranean women). Concepts of ''normal'' are often based on images presented in the media and not on statistical standards for various ethnic or racial groups. A careful history and physical examination are important and will often indicate that the underlying pathology will not be found. If the increased hair growth began at puberty and is not progressing, if there are no signs of virilization, and if menstruation is regular, the process is probably benign.

**1. Idiopathic and familial hirsutism**—These are the most common forms of hirsutism. In the idiopathic form (hirsutism for which no metabolic cause can be found), there may be increased skin sensitivity to androgens. Familial or genetic hirsutism is evident in certain family or ethnic groups in which women tend to have a greater proportion of terminal facial or body hair (eg, eastern Mediterranean peoples). Localized treatment such as electrolysis, depilatory agents, bleaching compounds, and shaving are usually effective. Adrenal or ovarian hormonal suppression is potentially dangerous in these patients and should be avoided.

**2. True hirsutism**—True hirsutism is always caused by a relative or absolute excess of androgen, which may be of adrenal or ovarian origin, or both. This excess cannot always be demonstrated by laboratory tests; the free, non-protein-bound fraction of plasma testosterone is the most sensitive test. Adrenal disorders such as Cushing's syndrome are easily ruled out on the basis of the history and physical examination. Late-onset congenital adrenal hyperplasia (deficiency of 21-hydroxylase or 11-hydroxylase) can be diagnosed by measuring the steroid precursors immediately before the enzymatic block (17-hydroxyprogesterone and 11-deoxycortisol, respectively). ACTH stimulation is sometimes necessary to demonstrate the defect. Obesity may cause a previously asymptomatic defect to become apparent. 11-Hydroxylase deficiency is often associated with hypertension and hypokalemia. Satisfactory results are obtained with adrenal suppression (dexamethasone, 0.5–0.75 mg/d at bedtime).

Other systemic agents used for symptomatic therapy of hirsutism are androgen antagonists such as cimetidine, spironolactone, and, in Europe, cyproterone acetate. Results are variable and experience inconclusive.

**3. Ovarian abnormalities**—Other common causes of hirsutism are ovarian abnormalities such as polycystic ovary syndrome. This syndrome is accompanied by menstrual irregularities or amenorrhea, increased free plasma testosterone, decreased sex steroid-binding globulin, a high LH to FSH ratio (> 2), and multiple ovarian cysts. The hirsutism often responds to chronic ovarian suppression with an oral contraceptive agent. This therapy is not without problems and should not be used indiscriminately.

**4. Ovarian and adrenal tumors**—Ovarian and adrenal tumors are rare causes of hirsutism, but the possibility should always be taken into account. A sudden onset of hirsutism is suggestive, as well as signs of increased muscle mass, frontal balding, deepening of the voice, enlargement of the clitoris, and androgen excess. The plasma testosterone is usually markedly elevated (> 150 ng/dL). Urinary 17-ketosteroids are usually also markedly elevated in adrenal tumors causing hirsutism. CT scan and ovarian ultrasound often localize the tumor. Surgical removal of the neoplasm is often curative, but the patient should be warned that it may be years before the hair pattern returns to normal.

**5. Hyperprolactinemia**—A rare cause of hirsutism is hyperprolactinemia, which can result in excessive production of adrenal androgens. If a prolactinoma is demonstrated, surgical resection or bromocriptine therapy is in order.

## Change in Appetite

Polyphagia (associated with polydipsia and polyuria) is classically found in uncontrolled diabetes mellitus. However, excessive eating is usually not an endocrine problem but a compulsive personality trait. Only rarely is it due to a hypothalamic lesion, in which case it is associated with somnolence and other signs of the hypothalamic disease, eg, hypogonadism and also congenital abnormalities. Excessive appetite with weight loss is observed in thyrotoxicosis; polyphagia with weight gain may rarely indicate acromegaly or hypoglycemia due to an insulin-secreting islet cell adenoma.

Anorexia and nausea associated with weight loss and diarrhea may occur at the onset of addisonian crisis or uncontrolled diabetic acidosis. Weight loss due to anorexia plus increased metabolic rate is often seen in patients with pheochromocytoma. Anorexia and nausea with constipation are found with any state of hypercalcemia, eg, hyperparathyroidism, and may be indistinguishable from the same symptoms occurring in peptic ulcer (which may coexist with hyperparathyroidism). Recurrent peptic ulceration with high gastrin levels is diagnostic of pancreatic gastrinoma (Zollinger-Ellison syndrome).

## Polyuria & Polydipsia

Polyuria, commonly associated with polydipsia,

is usually of nonendocrine etiology, due to a habit of drinking excessive water (psychogenic). However, if it is severe and of sudden onset, it suggests diabetes mellitus or diabetes insipidus. Diabetes insipidus may develop insidiously or may appear suddenly after head trauma or brain surgery. Always attempt to rule out an organic lesion in or about the posterior pituitary-supraoptic tract. In children, the physician must consider nephrogenic diabetes insipidus and eosinophilic granuloma. Lithium and demeclocycline may induce polyuria by interfering with the renal action of ADH.

Polyuria and polydipsia are frequently seen in any state of hypercalcemia, such as hyperparathyroidism, and are also part of the syndrome of hypokalemic nephropathy, such as can occur in disorders of mineralocorticoid excess. Polyuria may occur in renal tubular disorders, such as renal tubular acidosis and Fanconi's syndrome, as well as in a multitude of renal diseases associated with damage to the medullary interstitium that is responsible for establishing the osmotic gradient required for concentration of urine.

## Gynecomastia

Gynecomastia, or breast enlargement in men, is fairly common. It is a physiologic phenomenon during puberty, when at least half of males experience enlargement of one or both breasts. It is also common among elderly men, although the exact incidence in men who are not suffering from hepatic, renal, or cardiac disease or are not taking drugs causing breast enlargement has not been ascertained. Gynecomastia can be the first sign of a serious disorder such as a testicular tumor, and medical evaluation is always indicated when breast enlargement occurs. Carcinoma of the male breast is an extremely rare cause of gynecomastia. It is more common, however, in patients with Klinefelter's syndrome.

The causes of gynecomastia are multiple and diverse (Table 18–1). A search for a common mechanism has not been successful. A number of researchers believe that in many cases (but not all), an altered androgen/estrogen ratio causes changes in cellular elements in breast tissue. This could be due to the following mechanisms: (1) A decrease in production of androgen (all cases of male hypogonadism; see Table 18–14). (2) An increase in estrogen formation (adrenal or testicular tumors, excessive gonadotropin secretion, hyperthyroidism, hepatic disease). (3) A decrease in sensitivity of breast tissue to androgens (hereditary states of androgen resistance such as Reifenstein's syndrome, complications of drugs such as cimetidine or spironolactone).

It is theoretically possible that increased tissue sensitivity to estrogens may also cause gynecomastia. This mechanism has been postulated by some to account for idiopathic gynecomastia, a condition for which no specific cause is found (most cases in almost all published series).

Many drugs induce gynecomastia by a variety of mechanisms. Estrogens or drugs having estrogenic effects (diethylstilbestrol, marihuana, digitalis, possi-

**Table 18–1.** Causes of gynecomastia.

| Physiologic causes | Drugs (cont'd) |
|---|---|
| Neonatal period | Methyldopa |
| Puberty | Metoclopramide |
| Aging | Penicillamine |
| **Drugs** | Phenothiazines |
| Alcohol | Reserpine |
| Alkylating agents | Spironolactone |
| Amphetamines | Testosterone |
| Busulfan | Tricyclic antidepressants |
| Chorionic gonadotropin | **Endocrine diseases** |
| Cimetidine | Male hypogonadism |
| Clomiphene | Hyperthyrodism |
| Cyclophosphamide | Androgen resistance syn- |
| Diazepam | dromes |
| Diethylstilbestrol | **Systemic diseases** |
| Digitalis | Chronic liver disease |
| Estrogens | Chronic renal disease |
| Ethionamide | Refeeding after starvation |
| Heroin | **Neoplasias** |
| Hydroxyzine | Testicular tumors |
| Isoniazid | Adrenal tumors |
| Ketoconazole | Bronchogenic carcinoma |
| Marihuana | Carcinoma of the breast |
| Meprobamate | **Idiopathic** |
| Methadone | |

bly heroin) are one group. Other drugs cause liver damage, which in turn can result in hyperestrogenemia (alcohol, isoniazid). A few drugs cause damage to the testicle or block the synthesis of testosterone by Leydig cells, with resulting hypotestosteronemia (cyclophosphamide, spironolactone, ketoconazole). Others (phenothiazines) induce hyperprolactinemia, with a resulting decrease in gonadotropin and testosterone secretion. It is paradoxic that testosterone itself can produce gynecomastia when given parenterally as testosterone esters over the long term. This is due to increased peripheral conversion of testosterone by aromatases to estradiol. Undoubtedly, some drugs produce gynecomastia by a combination of mechanisms. The mechanism of action has not yet been found in some drugs (busulfan, penicillamine, diazepam).

A careful history and physical examination will often clarify the cause of gynecomastia. An adolescent with slight gynecomastia or a patient with prostatic carcinoma taking diethylstilbestrol need not have further diagnostic workups. Careful examination of the testes is mandatory to look for a testicular tumor. The small, firm testes of Klinefelter's syndrome are characteristic. Look for eunuchoid features, signs of liver disease, and the enlarged thyroid of Graves' disease.

Laboratory investigation of unclear cases should include the following:

(1) A chest x-ray to search for metastatic or primary lung tumors.

(2) Measurements of plasma levels of the beta subunit of human chorionic gonadotropin (hCG). High levels may lead to finding a choriocarcinoma or other hCG-secreting tumors.

(3) Measurements of plasma testosterone and lu-

teinizing hormone (LH) are valuable in the diagnosis of primary or secondary hypogonadism. A high testosterone level may be seen in hyperthyroidism (due to increased sex steroid-binding protein). High testosterone levels *plus* high LH levels should alert the physician to the possibility of androgen resistance.

(4) Serum estradiol is often measured but is usually normal. Many estrogens and substances with estrogen activity are *not* detected by the estradiol radioimmunoassay. Other laboratory tests such as serum prolactin, thyroid function, and chromosomal analysis should not be performed indiscriminately but can be valuable when clinically indicated.

The treatment of gynecomastia should always take into account the underlying condition. Remove the cause if possible. The breast enlargement per se is not often responsive to medical therapy. It can be surgically corrected if aesthetic or psychologic considerations so indicate.

### Abnormal Lactation

Lactation is a physiologic phenomenon when seen in the newborn (''witch's milk''); it may occur before menstruation or may persist for prolonged periods after recent delivery and is part of the syndrome of pseudocyesis. It is frequently present in acromegaly and, more rarely, in thyrotoxicosis and myxedema. A common cause of the galactorrhea-amenorrhea syndrome is a prolactin-secreting tumor of the pituitary gland. The level of serum prolactin is usually above 100 ng/mL in these patients (see Clinical Disorders of Prolactin Secretion, p 688). CT scan allows visualization of small pituitary adenomas. Galactorrhea may also occur after pituitary stalk section. It can occur after thoracotomy or other injuries to the chest wall as well as after breast surgery. Abnormal lactation occurs rarely with estrogen-secreting adrenal tumors and quite rarely with corpus luteum cysts and choriocarcinoma. Many drugs (phenothiazines, antihypertensive agents such as reserpine and methyldopa, estrogen-containing medications such as oral contraceptives, etc) may produce lactation. Serum prolactin levels are high in many patients with galactorrhea, and they can be used to evaluate the response to therapy.

If the serum prolactin is normal, the condition is usually benign (idiopathic galactorrhea); it is interesting to note that galactorrhea ceases in many of these patients with bromocriptine therapy.

### Precocious Puberty (in Both Sexes)

Precocious puberty is often a normal variant or a familial trait, but it may indicate serious organic disease. One must differentiate true precocity (caused by release of pituitary gonadotropins) from pseudoprecocity. At times there is only premature breast development (''thelarche'') or only premature appearance of pubic and axillary hair (''adrenarche'') with normal subsequent menarche. Hypothalamic lesions, encephalitis, hydrocephalus, and certain tumors (eg,

hamartoma of the tuber cinereum, pineal tumors) may cause true sexual precocity. Precocious puberty also occurs in girls who have associated fibrous dysplasia of bone and pigment spots (McCune-Albright syndrome). Adrenal hyperplasia or tumor and gonadal tumors usually cause pseudoprecocious puberty with virilization or feminization. Hepatomas may rarely cause isosexual precocity. Reversible precocity with lactation and pituitary enlargement may be seen in juvenile hypothyroidism. The cause must be detected early, since all children with precocious puberty will eventually be short or even dwarfed as a result of premature closure of the epiphyses, and because many of the tumors responsible for precocious puberty are potentially malignant.

### Sexual Infantilism & Delayed Puberty

It is often difficult to differentiate between simple functional delay of puberty (often a familial trait) and organic causes for such delays. Any type of gonadal or genetic defect may manifest itself primarily by failure of normal sexual development (see Diseases of the Testes, p 736, and Diseases of the Ovaries, p 739). Many patients grow to eunuchoid proportions, with span exceeding height. Consider hypothalamic lesions, especially if familial and associated with loss of sense of smell (Kallmann's syndrome), craniopharyngioma, pituitary tumors, and defective testes or ovaries, and look for associated stigmas (webbed neck of Turner's syndrome, gynecomastia of Klinefelter's syndrome). The serum gonadotropins are very helpful in determining the site of disease. If high, they point to the gonad as the defective organ. Chromosomal disorders should be ruled out by chromosomal analysis. Buccal smear for chromatin sex pattern is less expensive but does not exclude mosaicism.

### Impotence & Lack of Libido in Males

Erectile impotence is a frequent, complex problem. Recent studies indicate that purely psychogenic factors are less important in causing impotence than formerly believed and that endocrine, vascular, and neurologic abnormalities are more important. Hypogonadism of whatever origin (see Table 18–14) is associated with lack of libido and consequent erectile dysfunction. These can also be the first clinical manifestations of a hyperprolactinemic disorder (see Table 18–4). Other endocrine causes of impotence include hyperthyroidism, Addison's disease, and acromegaly. Diabetes mellitus is a very common cause; as many as 50% of males seen in outpatient diabetic clinics suffer from erectile dysfunction. In the past, this was thought to be due to autonomic neuropathy. Arteriosclerotic disease leading to decrease of penile blood flow is a more frequent cause. Vascular disease is also a frequent factor in impotence in elderly men. Any debilitating systemic disorder (eg, heart failure, renal insufficiency, infections, cancer) can cause impotence at any age.

A careful history of drug use is extremely important. Many pharmacologic agents are known to cause impotence through a variety of mechanisms; some interfere directly with the neural erectile reflex, and a few induce hyperprolactinemia or interfere with testosterone action (Table 18–2). For many drugs, the mechanism is not known. All drugs are variable in effect, with some patients developing severe impotence with a given dose and others retaining normal erectile function with double that dose. The reasons for this are not known. If the effect is in doubt, the suspected offending agent should be discontinued and the patient's response evaluated.

Techniques such as monitoring of nocturnal penile tumescence, Doppler penile blood flow analysis, and bulbocavernosus reflex timing have been helpful in distinguishing "organic" from "psychogenic" impotence. Overlap does occur, however, and organic impotence can cause psychologic problems (fear of failure, performance anxiety) that persist even after the underlying disorder has been treated.

Treatment will vary with the cause. Testosterone administration is helpful in hypogonadal states. Bromocriptine is useful in hyperprolactinemic syndromes. Revascularization procedures can be effective in selected cases when performed by expert technicians. A variety of penile prostheses are now available for surgical implantation in patients not responsive to medical or psychologic therapy. Several psychologic therapeutic approaches can be tried for patients found to have no evidence of organic disease. A few new pharmacologic agents are being actively investigated.

## Cryptorchidism

Failure of descent of the testes is a common but poorly understood phenomenon. Not infrequently, spontaneous descent takes place at the time of puberty. Cryptorchid testes may be intra-abdominal or located anywhere in the inguinal canal. Cryptorchidism may be an isolated defect or associated with other congenital anomalies. More than 35 congenital syndromes associated with cryptorchidism have been recognized.

There is no agreement about when hormonal therapy should be instituted. If the testes are present, gonadotropic hormone will bring them down unless a hernia or blockage of the passageway prevents their descent. hCG, 1000 units 3 times per week for 3

weeks, is usually sufficient. If this fails, surgical orchiopexy is indicated. Early surgical repair is advisable because intra-abdominal testes may later fail to produce sperm normally and because the incidence of malignancy in intra-abdominal testes is high.

A new approach to cryptorchidism is therapy with gonadorelin (gonadotropin-releasing hormone). The use of synthetic gonadorelin in a nasal spray for 4 weeks has resulted in successful descent of the testes in a significant proportion of cases.

## Bone & Joint Pains & Pathologic Fractures

If the onset is at an early age and if there is a family history of similar disorders, consider osteogenesis imperfecta (look for blue scleras). Bowing of the bone and pseudofractures suggest rickets or osteomalacia, due either to intestinal or, more commonly, renal tubular disorders. Always consider hyperparathyroidism, specifically if bone pain, bone cysts, and fractures are associated with renal stones. Back pain with involvement of the spine suggests osteoporosis, especially when it occurs after the menopause. In cases of osteopenia of unknown cause, hyperthyroidism and Cushing's syndrome should always be considered and ruled out by appropriate tests. Aches and pains in the extremities are suggestive of rickets or osteomalacia. Rule out metastatic tumors, multiple myeloma, and Paget's disease in elderly patients by scintiscan and other tests. In doubtful cases, bone biopsy is indicated. Bone densitometry measurements are more accurate than x-ray in determining mineral losses from the skeleton.

## Renal Colic; Gravel & Stone Formation

A metabolic cause must be sought for recurrent stone formation and for kidney stones in children. If there is a family history, cystinuria and uric acid stones must be considered, or renal tubular acidosis with nephrocalcinosis. About 5% of stones are due to hyperparathyroidism, which must be ruled out in every instance of calcium stones. Look for bone disease, especially subperiosteal resorption of the bones of the fingers, and obtain a parathyroid hormone assay if the serum calcium is elevated. Look also for signs of osteomalacia associated with excessive renal loss of calcium. Vitamin D intoxication, sarcoidosis, and excessive intake of milk and alkali must be considered. Any rapid bone breakdown may give rise to renal calcium stones, eg, in Cushing's syndrome. Uric acid stones may occur in patients with gouty arthritis, but often they occur simply because the urinary pH is very acid; they occur also after any type of intensive therapy for leukemia or polycythemia. Idiopathic hypercalciuria is the most common metabolic cause of recurrent calcium stones in males. Primary hyperoxaluria is a rare cause of severe renal calcification and may be associated with deposition of oxalate in soft tissues (oxalosis). Oxalate stones are seen frequently in patients with intestinal disorders

**Table 18–2.** Drugs causing impotence.

| | |
|---|---|
| Alcohol | Methadone |
| Atropine | Methyldopa |
| Barbiturates | Monoamine oxidase inhibitors |
| Chlordiazepoxide | Phenothiazines |
| Cimetidine | Phenoxybenzamine |
| Clonidine | Propranolol |
| Diazepam | Reserpine |
| Ethionamide | Spironolactone |
| Guanethidine | Thiazides |
| Marihuana | Tricyclic antidepressants |

(eg, ileitis, shunt procedures for obesity). At times, stones form in a structurally abnormal kidney (eg, medullary sponge kidney). Metabolic causes of renal stones must be corrected early before renal damage due to infection and obstruction occurs, since this may not be reversed upon removal of the initiating factor. The keys to proper diagnosis are careful stone analysis and chemical tests in blood and urine for calcium, phosphate, and uric acid.

### Tetany & Muscle Cramps

Mild tetany with paresthesias and muscle cramps is usually due to hyperventilation with alkalosis resulting from an anxiety state. If tetany occurs in children, rule out idiopathic hypoparathyroidism or pseudohypoparathyroidism. Look for calcification in the lens, poor teeth, and x-ray evidence of basal ganglia calcification. Consider latent hypoparathyroidism in the postthyroidectomy patient. Tetany may be the presenting complaint of osteomalacia or rickets or of acute pancreatitis. Neonatal tetany is probably due to the high phosphate content of milk and relative hypoparathyroidism. A similar mechanism has been considered responsible for leg cramps during pregnancy. Neonatal tetany may rarely indicate maternal hyperparathyroidism. Severe hypocalcemic tetany will occasionally produce convulsions and must be differentiated from "idiopathic" epilepsy. Classic signs of tetany are Chvostek's sign and Trousseau's phenomenon. If tetany is associated with hypertension, hypokalemia, and polyuria, consider primary hyperaldosteronism. Leg cramps may occur in some diabetic patients. Magnesium deficiency must be considered in tetany unresponsive to calcium.

### Mental Changes

Disturbances of mentation are often subtle and may be difficult to recognize, but they may be important indications of underlying endocrine disorders. Nervousness, flushing, and excitability are characteristic of the menopause, hyperthyroidism, and anxiety states. Prolonged hypocalcemia from untreated hypoparathyroidism may be associated with intellectual deterioration. Convulsions with abnormal electroencephalographic findings may occur in hypocalcemic tetany or in hypoglycemia, either spontaneously or induced by insulin. Islet cell tumors may cause confusion, abnormal speech, and behavior or personality changes as well as sudden loss of consciousness, somnolence and prolonged lethary, or coma. Frank psychosis can occur but is rare. Diabetic acidosis may progress gradually into coma. Hypercalcemia leads to somnolence and lethargy, with marked weakness. Mental confusion may occur in hypopituitarism or Addison's disease or in long-standing myxedema. Severe depression can also occur in hypothyroidism. Confusion, lethargy, and nausea may be the presenting symptoms of water intoxication due to inappropriate or excessive secretion of antidiuretic hormone. Mental deterioration is the rule in long-standing and untreated hypoparathyroidism and hypothyroidism

(cretinism). Insomnia, mood changes, anxiety, and even frank psychosis can be associated with Cushing's syndrome, glucocorticoid status (either a sudden increase or a sudden decrease) may be associated with acute psychosis. Mental deficiency may be associated with abnormal excretion of amino acids in the urine (eg, phenylketonuria) and with chromosomal abnormalities.

# DISEASES OF THE HYPOTHALAMUS & OF THE PITUITARY GLAND

The function of the pituitary gland is controlled by regulating hormones (factors) produced by the hypothalamus. These releasing and release-inhibiting hormones are, for the most part, relatively simple polypeptides, many of which have been identified and synthesized (Table 18–3). Corticotropin-releasing factor has been recently isolated and characterized as a 41-amino acid peptide. A clinical disorder may be due to lack or excess of a pituitary hormone or, more commonly, to lack of releasing or inhibiting factor of the hypothalamus. Isolated or multiple defects may occur. Accurate radioimmunoassays and stimulation tests have made it possible to classify accurately the location of the defect. The exciting work of Guillemin and Schally in isolating and synthesizing these hypothalamic factors is proving of

**Table 18–3.** The pituitary hormones and their hypothalamic regulatory factors (hormones).*

| Hormones | Regulatory Factors (Hormones) |
|---|---|
| Growth hormone (somatotropin, STH) | Somatotropin-releasing factor (SRF, GH-RH, GH-RF); somatotropin release-inhibiting hormone (SIF, somatostatin)† |
| Corticotropin (ACTH) | Corticotropin-releasing factor (CRF or CRH)† |
| Thyrotropin (TSH) | Thyrotropin-releasing hormone (TRF, TRH)† |
| Follicle-stimulating hormone (FSH) | FSH and LH share a common hypothalamic peptide, gonadotropin-releasing hormone or gonadorelin (FSH-RH, LH-RH, LH-RF, LRH, GnRH)† |
| Luteinizing hormone (LH) | |
| Prolactin | Prolactin-releasing factor (PRF, PRH); prolactin release-inhibiting factor‡ (PIF) |
| Melanocyte-stimulating hormone | MSH-releasing factor (MRH, MRF); MSH release-inhibiting factor (MRIH, MIF) |

* Modified from Schally AV et al: Hypothalamic regulatory hormones. *Science* 1973;**179**:341.
† Presently fully identified and synthesized.
‡ One of which is certainly dopamine.

great value in the control of pituitary functional disorders. Clinical use of synthetic hypothalamic factors and their agonist or antagonist analogs is a new and promising development (eg, use of GnRH and analogs in cryptorchidism, delayed puberty, induction of ovulation, management of precocious puberty). A fascinating feature of at least one of the hypothalamic peptides (GnRH) is the opposite effects produced when it is given by constant infusion versus pulsatile administration; the latter mode stimulates and the former inhibits gonadotropin secretion. Tumors of the pituitary gland are recognized with increased frequency thanks to new methods of visualization of soft structures within the sella turcica (CT scans and MRI). Some are hormonally inactive. Others have been found to secrete excessive ACTH, growth hormone, prolactin, thyrotropin, LH, and FSH. A certain degree of overlap in function has been noted, eg, pituitary enlargement and lactation in juvenile myxedema reversed by the administration of thyroid hormone. Prolactin assays may be most important for the early diagnosis of pituitary lesions.

Cutler GB et al: Therapeutic applications of luteinizing hormone-releasing hormone and its analog. *Ann Intern Med* 1985;**102**:643.

Gillies G, Grossman A: The CRFs and their control: Chemistry, physiology and clinical implications. *Clin Endocrinol Metab* 1985;**14**:821.

Givens JR (editor): *The Hypothalamus.* Year Book, 1984.

Jordan RM, Kohler PO: Recent advances in diagnosis and treatment of pituitary tumors. *Adv Intern Med* 1987;**32**:299.

Krieger DT: Brain peptides: What, where and why? *Science* 1983;**222**:975.

Sanforo N et al: Hypogonadotropic disorders in men and women: Diagnosis and therapy with pulsatile gonadotropin-releasing hormone. *Endocr Rev* 1986;**7**:11.

Scanlon MF: Neuroendocrinology. *Clin Endocrinol Metab* 1983;**12**:3. [Entire issue.]

## PANHYPOPITUITARISM

### Essentials of Diagnosis

- Sexual dysfunction; weakness; easy fatigability; lack of resistance to stress, cold, and fasting; axillary and pubic hair loss.
- Low blood pressure; may have visual field defects.
- All low: $T_4$, $^{123}I$ uptake, FSH, LH, TSH, urinary 17-ketosteroids and hydroxycorticosteroids, growth hormone. Prolactin level may be elevated.
- X-ray may reveal sellar lesion.

### General Considerations

Hypopituitarism is a relatively rare disorder in which inactivity of the pituitary gland leads to insufficiency in the target organs. All or several of the tropic hormones may be involved. Isolated defects, eg, of the gonadotropins, are not rare. There is also great variation in the severity of the lesions, from those merely involving pathways (hypothalamic lesions) to almost complete destruction of the gland

itself. The pathogenesis of this disorder includes circulatory collapse due to hemorrhage following delivery and subsequent pituitary necrosis (Sheehan's syndrome), granulomas, hemochromatosis, cysts and tumors (chromophobe adenomas and craniopharyngiomas are most common), surgical hypophysectomy, external irradiation to the skull, trauma, metastatic disease, and aneurysms involving the sella turcica.

The pituitary tumor may be part of the syndrome of multiple endocrine adenomatosis (type I), with concomitant involvement of the parathyroid glands and pancreatic islets. Isolated or partial deficiencies of anterior pituitary hormones (eg, FSH, LH, TSH) or their releasing factors may occur and may be detected by refined techniques.

### Clinical Findings

These vary with the degree of pituitary destruction, and are related to the lack of hormones from the "target" endocrine glands.

**A. Symptoms and Signs:** Weakness; lack of resistance to cold, to infections, and to fasting; and sexual dysfunction (lack of development of primary and secondary sex characteristics, or regression of function) are the most common symptoms. In expanding lesions of the sella, interference with the visual tracts may produce loss of temporal vision, whereas a craniopharyngioma may cause blindness. Short stature is the rule if the onset is during the growth period. Amenorrhea and galactorrhea may be the first indications of a pituitary tumor. In men, impotence is usually an early complaint.

In both sexes there is sparseness or loss of axillary and pubic hair, and there may be thinning of the eyebrows and of the head hair, which is often silky.

The skin is often dry, with lack of sweating, and the patient appears pale. Pigmentation is lacking even after exposure to sunlight. Fine wrinkles are seen, and the facies presents a "sleepy" appearance.

The heart is small and the blood pressure low. Orthostatic hypotension is often present. Cerebrovascular symptoms may occur.

**B. Laboratory Findings:** The fasting blood glucose may be low. Dilutional hyponatremia is often present. Hyperkalemia does not occur, since aldosterone production, which is mainly controlled by the renin-angiotensin system, is not affected. Mild anemia may be present. Systematic analysis of pituitary hormones should be done: Serum growth hormone, measured by radioimmunoassay, is low and does not increase in response to insulin hypoglycemia, arginine infusion, or levodopa. The insulin tolerance test (use only 0.05 unit/kg intravenously) shows marked insulin sensitivity and is dangerous in these patients, since severe hypoglycemia reactions may occur. The $T_4$ level is low, and the TSH is not elevated (as in primary myxedema). Urinary 170-ketosteroids and 17-hydroxycorticosteroids and plasma cortisol are low but rise slowly after corticotropin administration. Corticotropin may have to be given for several days to demonstrate an adrenal response. Serum ACTH is low. The metyrapone (Metopirone) test has been used to demonstrate limited pituitary ACTH reserve. Plasma levels of sex steroids (testosterone and estradiol) are low, and so are the urinary and serum gonadotropins. TSH response to repeated intravenous infusions of thyrotropin-releasing hormone (TRH) may be of help in differentiating hypothalamic from pituitary lesions. Elevated prolactin levels are found in patients with prolactinomas and in cases of hypothalamic disease.

The demonstration of a low level of a hormone secreted by a target gland in the presence of a low level of a trophic hormone is strongly suggestive of hypothalamic or pituitary disease (low plasma cortisol *and* ACTH, $T_4$ *and* TSH, estradiol or testosterone *and* LH).

**C. Imaging:** Radiographs of the skull may show a lesion in or above the sella. Craniopharyngiomas are often calcified and may be seen in a plain film. CT scan is helpful in ascertaining the degree of suprasellar extension of a tumor, the presence of cysts, "empty sella," etc. Magnetic resonance imaging (MRI) provides even better detail.

**D. Eye Examination:** Visual field defects (bitemporal hemianopia) may be present.

### Differential Diagnosis

Anorexia nervosa may occasionally simulate hypopituitarism. In fact, severe malnutrition may give rise to functional hypopituitarism. By and large, cachexia is far more common in anorexia nervosa, and loss of axillary and pubic hair is rare; at times mild facial and body hirsutism is seen in anorexia nervosa. The 17-ketosteroids are low normal or not as low as in hypopituitarism; plasma and urinary cortisol may be high and may respond rapidly to corticotropin stimulation; and the gonadotropins are usually present at low levels. Thyroid function tests are not abnormal in anorexia nervosa except for low $T_3$. Pituitary growth hormone assays show high levels in anorexia nervosa and very low levels in hypopituitarism.

Primary Addison's disease and primary myxedema are at times difficult to differentiate from pituitary insufficiency, but the response to corticotropin and TSH often helps. Direct radioimmunoassays of ACTH and TSH are more accurate diagnostic methods, since they are invariably elevated in primary insufficiency of the adrenal or thyroid glands.

Enlargement of the sella may require CT scans or MRI to rule out "empty sella syndrome," where minimal endocrine abnormalities are present and radiation or surgery is not indicated.

The severe hypoglycemia after fasting may cause confusion with hyperinsulinism.

The mental changes of hypopituitarism may be mistaken for a primary psychosis.

### Complications

In addition to those of the primary lesion (eg, tumor), complications may develop at any time as a result of the patient's inability to cope with minor stressful situations. This may lead to high fever, shock, coma, and death. Sensitivity to thyroid may precipitate an adrenal crisis when thyroid is administered. Rarely, acute hemorrhage may occur in large pituitary tumors with rapid loss of vision, headache, and evidence of acute pituitary failure (pituitary apoplexy) requiring emergency decompression of the sella.

### Treatment

The pituitary lesion, if a tumor, is treated by surgical removal, x-ray irradiation, or both. Removal is usually via a transsphenoidal approach, which in expert hands is an effective and safe surgical procedure. Craniotomy is rarely necessary. Endocrine substitution therapy must be used before, during, and often permanently after such procedures.

Recently, new therapeutic vistas have been provided by the development of purified pituitary hormones and of hypothalamic releasing factor or their analogs. Some of these materials, however, are not extensively available yet. The mainstay of substitution therapy for pituitary insufficiency remains the replacement of the end-organ deficiencies (adrenal, thyroid, and gonad). This must be continued throughout life. Almost complete replacement therapy can be carried out with corticosteroids, thyroid hormone, and sex steroids.

**A. Corticosteroids:** Give hydrocortisone tablets, 15–25 mg/d orally in divided doses. Most patients do well with 15 mg in the morning and 5–10 mg in the late afternoon. A mineralocorticoid is rarely needed, since the adrenal conserves the capacity to secrete aldosterone. Additional amounts of rapid-acting corticosteroids must be given during states of stress, eg, during infection, trauma, or surgical procedures.

**B. Thyroid:** Thyroid (and insulin) should rarely, if ever, be used in panhypopituitarism unless the patient is receiving corticosteroids. Because of lack of adrenal function, patients may be exceedingly sensitive to these drugs. For this reason one should exercise special care in differentiating primary myxedema from hypopituitarism.

Levothyroxine is the drug of choice. The usual maintenance dose is 0.125 mg daily (range, 0.1–0.175 mg daily).

**C. Sex Hormones:**

1. If gonadal failure is present, appropriate sex steroid replacement should be instituted. For males, testosterone enanthate, cypionate, or any other long-acting ester is given intramuscularly every 3–4 weeks (200–400 mg/dose). Because of hepatic complications, the long-term use of oral androgens is not recommended.

2. Estrogens are extremely important in the female to prevent osteoporosis and to maintain secondary sex characteristics. The most frequently used oral agents are conjugated equine substances (eg, Premarin) and ethinyl estradiol. Give 0.625–1.25 mg of Premarin daily or 0.02–0.05 mg of ethinyl estradiol.

Three weeks of estrogen therapy are usually followed by 5 days of a progestational agent such as medroxyprogesterone acetate, 10 mg daily. If the patient is unwilling to take 2 different kinds of pills every month, a "low-dose" (30 μg of ethinyl estradiol) combination estrogen-progestin oral contraceptive preparation may be used. (See Table 13–5.)

3. Chorionic gonadotropic hormone (hCG) in combination with human pituitary FSH or postmenopausal urinary gonadotropin may be used in an attempt to produce fertility.

4. Clomiphene citrate and LH-releasing factor are sometimes useful in hypothalamic hypogonadism.

*Note:* Sex hormones, especially estrogens, should be employed cautiously in young patients with panhypopituitarism, or the epiphyses will close before maximum growth is achieved. Most androgens also share this property—especially when given in large doses.

**D. Human Growth Hormone:** This hormone is by far the most effective agent for increasing height. Previously used preparations were obtained from human pituitary glands collected at autopsy. They have been withdrawn from the market because of demonstrated transmission of Creutzfeldt-Jakob disease to recipients. New methods of production of hGH (human growth hormone) using recombinant DNA techniques have ensured increased availability and safety of this hormone. It has been used to increase the stature of some children who do *not* have clear-cut growth hormone deficiency. (See Rudman reference, below.) A better understanding of growth hormone-releasing factors may offer alternative forms of treatment in the future.

**E. Other Drugs:** Bromocriptine has been used successfully in the treatment of pituitary lesions producing lactation and amenorrhea, especially in prolactinomas. It is given orally in divided doses. Most patients respond very well to 5–10 mg daily. This treatment often induces marked regression in tumor size in addition to dramatic decreases of serum prolactin levels, with resumption of menses and ovulation. Unfortunately, cessation of therapy is almost always associated with regrowth of tumor. (See Disorders of Prolactin Secretion, p 688.)

## Prognosis

This depends on the primary cause. If it is due to postpartum necrosis (Sheehan's syndrome), partial or even complete recovery may occur. Functional hypopituitarism due to starvation and similar causes may also be corrected. The recent observation that some patients with hypopituitarism may suffer from failure of hypothalamic releasing factor offers hope for simpler therapy in the near future.

If the gland has been destroyed, the problem is to replace target hormones, since chronic replacement with pituitary tropic hormones is not yet feasible. With appropriate therapy, a patient with hypopituitarism can expect a normal life span. Major improvements in pituitary surgical techniques in the last decade have resulted in safe and satisfactory removal of many pituitary tumors.

Brook CED et al: Clinical features and investigation of growth hormone deficiency. *Clin Endocrinol Metab* 1986;**15**:479.

Ciric I: Pituitary tumors. *Neurol Clin* 1986;**3**:751.

Hickstein D, Chandler WF, Marshall JC: The spectrum of pituitary adenoma hemorrhage. *West J Med* 1986;**144**:435.

Preece MA: Diagnosis and treatment of children with growth hormone deficiency. *Clin Endocrinol Metab* 1982;**11**:1.

Rudman D et al: Children with normal variant short stature: Treatment with human growth hormone for six months. *N Engl J Med* 1981;**305**:123.

Veldhuis JD, Hammond JM: Endocrine function after spontaneous infarct of the anterior pituitary: Report, review and reappraisal. *Endocr Rev* 1980;**1**:100.

Wass JAH, Besser GM: The medical management of hormone-secreting tumors of the pituitary. *Annu Rev Med* 1983;**34**:283.

# ACROMEGALY & GIGANTISM

## Essentials of Diagnosis

- Excessive growth of hands (increased glove size), feet (increased shoe size), jaw (protrusion of lower jaw), and internal organs; or gigantism before closure of epiphyses.
- Amenorrhea, headaches, visual field loss, sweating, weakness.
- Elevated serum inorganic phosphorus; $T_4$ normal; glycosuria.
- Elevated serum growth hormone with failure to suppress after glucose. Elevated serum somatomedin.
- Imaging: Sellar enlargement and terminal phalangeal "tufting" on radiographs. Increased heel pad. CT or MRI demonstration of pituitary tumor.

## General Considerations

Growth hormone seems to exert its peripheral effects through the release of several somatomedins produced in the liver.

An excessive amount of growth hormone is most often produced by a benign pituitary adenoma. Rarely, it could be due to ectopic secretion of growth hormone by nonpituitary tissue (see Melmed reference, below). The disease may be associated with adenomas elsewhere, such as in the parathyroids or pancreas (multiple endocrine neoplasia type I). Acromegaly may also rarely occur as a result of secretion of ectopic growth hormone-releasing factor (GHRF) by tumors such as bronchial and intestinal carcinoids, hypothalamic gangliocytomas, pancreatic islet cell adenomas, and lung carcinomas. If the onset is before closure of the epiphyses, gigantism will result. If the epiphyses have already closed at onset, only overgrowth of soft tissues and terminal skeletal structures (acromegaly) results. At times the disease is transient ("fugitive acromegaly") and followed by pituitary insufficiency.

## Clinical Findings

**A. Symptoms and Signs:** Crowding of other hormone-producing cells, especially those concerned with gonadotropic hormones, causes amenorrhea and loss of libido. Production of excessive growth hormone causes doughy enlargement of the hands with spadelike fingers, large feet, jaw, face, tongue, and internal organs, wide spacing of the teeth, and an oily, tough, "furrowed" skin and scalp with multiple fleshy tumors (mollusca). Hoarse voice is common. Sleep apnea may occur. At times, acanthosis nigricans is present. Pressure of the pituitary tumor causes headache, bitemporal hemianopia, lethargy, and diplopia. In long-standing cases, secondary hormonal changes take place, including diabetes mellitus, goiter, and abnormal lactation. Less commonly, these may be the presenting picture in acromegaly. Excessive sweating may be the most reliable clinical sign of activity of the disease.

**B. Laboratory Findings:** Serum inorganic phosphorus is often elevated (over 4.5 mg/dL) during the active phase of acromegaly. Serum gonadotropins are normal or low. Glycosuria and hyperglycemia may be present, and there is resistance to the administration of insulin. Hypercalciuria is common. The $T_4$ is normal or low. 17-Ketosteroids and hydroxycorticosteroids may be high or low, depending upon the stage of the disease. In the active phase of the disease, serum levels of growth hormone are elevated above 7 ng/mL. Administration of glucose fails to suppress the serum level (as it does in normal individuals). Intravenous infusion of TRH or LRH often results in stimulation of growth hormone secretion, whereas in normal individuals there is no such effect. The plasma levels of immunoreactive somatomedin C have been reported to correlate closely with disease activity. Serum prolactin is often elevated. This may be due to simultaneous secretion of prolactin by the growth hormone-secreting tumor, to the presence of a small prolactinoma, or to interference with delivery of hypothalamic prolactin inhibitory factor (PIF) to the normal prolactin-secreting cells of the anterior pituitary.

**C. Imaging:** Radiography of the skull may show a large sella with destroyed clinoids, but a sella of usual size does not rule out the diagnosis. The frontal sinuses may be large. One may also demonstrate thickening of the skull and long bones, with typical overgrowth of vertebral bodies and severe spur formation. Dorsal kyphosis is common. Typical "tufting" of the terminal phalanges of the fingers and toes may be demonstrated, with increase in size of the sesamoid bone. A lateral view of the feet demonstrates increased thickness of the heel pad. Modern techniques of CT and MRI scanning can demonstrate even small pituitary tumors.

**D. Eye Examination:** Visual field examination may show bitemporal hemianopia.

## Differential Diagnosis

Growth hormone excess is to be considered if there is rapid growth or resumption of growth once stopped (eg, change in shoe size or ring size). Consider the diagnosis also in unexplained amenorrhea, insulin-resistant diabetes mellitus, or goiter with elevated basal metabolic rate that does not respond to antithyroid drugs. Physiologic spurts of growth and increase in tissue size from exercise, weight gain, or certain occupations enter into the differential diagnosis. The syndrome of cerebral gigantism with mental retardation and ventricular dilatation but normal growth hormone levels resembles acromegalic gigantism. Myxedema and, rarely, pachydermoperiostosis may resemble acromegaly. Serial photographs are of help in differentiating familial nonendocrine gigantism and facial enlargement. Other conditions causing visceromegaly must be considered.

## Complications

Complications include pressure of the tumor on surrounding structures, rupture of the tumor into the brain or sinuses, the complications of diabetes, cardiac enlargement, and cardiac failure. The carpal tunnel syndrome, due to compression of the median nerve at the wrist, may cause disability of the hand. Cord compression due to large intervertebral disks may be seen. Weakness due to myopathy often affects the limbs.

## Treatment

Pituitary surgery is the treatment of choice. Transsphenoidal microsurgery has removed the hyperfunctioning tissue while preserving anterior pituitary function in most patients. Pituitary irradiation is useful if surgical therapy fails to return the elevated growth hormone levels to normal. Periodic reassessment of pituitary function after these procedures is advisable. In the "burnt out" case, hormonal replacement as for hypopituitarism may be required. Medical treatment of active acromegaly with progesterone and chlorpromazine has been disappointing. Reports of medical treatment with bromocriptine have been disappointing. Large doses are often necessary (30–40 mg/d), and normalization of growth hormone secretion is not often achieved. A somatostatin analog has been described as effective in lowering growth hormone concentration in a small series of patients with acromegaly.

## Prognosis

Prognosis depends upon the age at onset and, more particularly, the age at which therapy is begun. Menstrual function may be restored. Severe headaches may persist even after treatment. Secondary tissue and skeletal changes do not respond completely to removal of the tumor. The diabetes may be permanent in spite of adequate pituitary ablation. The patient may succumb to the cardiovascular complications. The tumor may "burn out," causing symptoms of hypopituitarism, or it may appear as an "empty" sella.

Daughaday DW: A new treatment for an old disease. (Editorial.) *N Engl J Med* 1985;**313**:1604.

Melmed S et al: Acromegaly due to secretion of growth hormone by an ectopic pancreatic islet-cell tumor. *N Engl J Med* 1985;**312**:9.

Melmed S et al: Pituitary tumors secreting growth hormone and prolactin. *Ann Intern Med* 1986;**105**:238.

Schuster LD et al: Acromegaly: Reassessment of the long-term therapeutic effectiveness of transsphenoidal pituitary surgery. *Ann Intern Med* 1981;**95**:172.

Wass JAH et al: The treatment of acromegaly. *Clin Endocr Metab* 1986;**15**:683.

## CLINICAL DISORDERS OF PROLACTIN SECRETION

### Essentials of Diagnosis

- Women: Menstrual cycle disturbances (oligomenorrhea, amenorrhea).
- Men: Decreased libido and erectile impotence.
- Elevated serum prolactin.
- CT scan or MRI often demonstrates pituitary adenoma.

### Normal Physiology

Although the existence of prolactin has been known for over 40 years, it was only in the 1970s that a significant amount of knowledge accumulated concerning clinical disorders associated with this hormone. Prolactin is a peptide hormone with a molecular weight of 21,000 which is secreted by the pituitary and in the mammalian species has as its main role that of inducing lactation. The hormone is hypersecreted during pregnancy, and the levels in plasma increasingly rise until the time of delivery. Under the combined effect of prolactin, increased estrogen, and progesterone, further breast development takes place, with eventual formation of milk in the acini. After parturition, the sudden withdrawal of estrogen caused by the expulsion of the placenta results in the onset of lactation. Estrogens play a synergistic role along with prolactin to promote the differentiation and development of the breast, but they antagonize prolactin in inhibiting the actual secretion of milk. The presence of prolactin is absolutely essential for lactation. During the puerperal period, the act of suckling constitutes a powerful stimulus for the continued production of prolactin. Lactation will cease if prolactin secretion is interrupted by prolactin-lowering drugs or by pituitary destruction. Prolactin is an unusual hormone in terms of control of secretion in that it is under a predominantly inhibitory control. Thus, section of the pituitary stalk will result in marked increases in prolactin secretion. Also, a pituitary transplanted to another anatomic site will abundantly secrete prolactin. There is mounting evidence that the prolactin inhibitory factor (PIF) is dopamine and that the control of prolactin secretion is primarily modulated by secretion of PIF. A prolactin-stimulating factor also exists, but its physiologic role is less clear. Prolactin, like other peptide hormones, is secreted episodically, and its concentration in blood is not stable (0–20 ng/mL).

Elevated serum prolactin is found in association with multiple physiologic and pathologic causes (see Table 18–4). Estrogens increase serum prolactin levels slowly by increasing the number of prolactin-secreting cells in the anterior pituitary gland. Many drugs inhibit prolactin inhibitory factor, thereby raising the production of prolactin.

### Clinical Consequences of Prolactin Excess

In women, prolactin excess produces (1) disturbances of pituitary ovarian function with anovulatory cycles, oligomenorrhea, or (frequently) amenorrhea; (2) galactorrhea (less common); and (3) hirsutism (rare). (See p 739.)

In men, excess prolactin is associated with (1) impotence and decreased libido (very common), (2) hypogonadism (less common), and (3) galactorrhea (very rare). (See p 681.)

Of all patients with secondary amenorrhea, as many as 28% may have elevated prolactin levels. In men, increased prolactin concentrations are usually not associated with galactorrhea, because the male breast tissue has not been primed by estrogens and progesterone.

Most women with hyperprolactinemia have amenorrhea or manifestations of a short luteal phase. Several syndromes are characterized in part by clinical associations of galactorrhea-amenorrhea: Argonz-del Castillo syndrome (galactorrhea-amenorrhea in nulliparous women), Chiari-Frommel syndrome (galactorrhea-amenorrhea following normal parturition), and Forbes-Albright syndrome (galactorrhea-amenorrhea accompanied by pituitary enlargement). It is now clear that these syndromes are not different clinical entities and may represent transitional phases of the same basic problem. Recent studies indicate that amenorrhea is much more common than galactorrhea. Hyperprolactinemic women also tend to have decreased bone density and are therefore at increased risk to develop clinical osteoporosis if left untreated.

The most important cause of high serum prolactin

**Table 18–4.** Causes of hyperprolactinemia.

| Physiologic Causes | Pharmacologic Causes | Pathologic Causes |
|---|---|---|
| Sleep (REM phase) | Phenothiazines | Pituitary stalk section |
| Exercise | Tricyclic antidepressants | Hypothalamic disease |
| Stress (trauma, surgery) | Reserpine | Prolactin-secreting tumors |
| Pregnancy | Methyldopa | Nelson's syndrome |
| Puerperium | Amphetamines | Acromegaly |
| Suckling | Anesthetic agents | Hypothyroidism |
|  | Estrogens | Renal failure |
|  | Metoclopramide | Chronic chest wall stimulation (postthoracotomy; postmastectomy; herpes zoster, etc) |

is a pituitary tumor. As many as 65% of all pituitary tumors may be associated with hyperprolactinemia. The tumors may be small (microadenomas) or produce clear-cut enlargement of the sella (macroadenomas). A great number of tests have been devised in the last few years to separate a prolactin-secreting tumor from other causes of hyperprolactinemia. Most of them are unreliable. A possible exception may be the response of serum prolactin to the administration of thyrotropin-releasing hormone (TRH). In normal individuals, there is a significant increase in serum prolactin following the intravenous administration of 400 $\mu$g of TRH. In most patients with prolactin-secreting tumors, this increase in prolactin levels does not occur. More useful, however, is the actual level of circulating prolactin. In patients with proved pituitary tumors, plasma levels of prolactin are usually over 100 ng/mL. Macroadenomas tend to cause higher levels of serum prolactin than microadenomas and are more frequently associated with decreased secretion of gonadotropins (LH and FSH). Tomograms of the sella have been helpful in diagnosing small prolactin-secreting tumors that may produce subtle bony deformities. CT scan of the pituitary may also demonstrate small prolactinomas. Differentiation from normal variants, however, is not always possible. Magnetic resonance imaging (MRI) may prove superior to CT scan for evaluation of pituitary disease.

## Treatment

The treatment of a hyperprolactinemic state obviously depends upon the cause. If the problem is due to administration of exogenous estrogens, discontinuation of these drugs will produce improvement after a period of several months. Discontinuation of psychotropic agents usually results in a much faster recovery and resumption of menses. Most prolactin-secreting tumors are not responsive to radiation therapy, and surgical removal via the transsphenoidal route is the treatment of choice. In expert hands, surgical removal results in complete disappearance of the symptoms (amenorrhea-galactorrhea and hypogonadism, or impotence and decreased libido in the male). A follow-up period of several years, however, is necessary to determine if a ''cure'' has been achieved, since some patients show a tendency toward relapse of increased prolactin secretion. If hyperprolactinemia is due to hypothyroidism, administration of thyroid hormone will rapidly correct the situation. Bromocriptine, a drug that binds to the pituitary dopamine receptor, thus inhibiting both spontaneous as well as TRH-provoked secretion from the gland, is useful in the medical therapy of hyperprolactinemic syndromes. In doses of 2.5–10 mg/d, it promptly reduces the levels of circulating prolactin, with rapid resumption of menses and cessation of galactorrhea. Always start with a small dose (eg, 2.5 mg/d) given at bedtime to minimize problems of nausea, dizziness, and orthostatic hypotension. Gradually increase the dose as necessary to bring prolactin levels down to normal. The exact role of bromocriptine in the treatment of prolactin-secreting pituitary tumors is debatable at present, but the drug is certainly helpful where surgery fails to correct the problem. Dramatic reductions in size of prolactinomas can occur during bromocriptine administration. Unfortunately, discontinuation of therapy usually results in reappearance of hyperprolactinemia and galactorrhea-amenorrhea. Since the patient's fertility is usually promptly restored with bromocriptine therapy, many pregnancies have resulted, with no clear evidence that the drug is teratogenic. Pregnancy, however, with its concomitant hypersecretion of estrogens, may result in marked increase in pituitary tumor size, with danger of sudden development of visual disturbances. Close supervision of these patients is imperative.

Koppelman MCS et al: Hyperprolactinemia, amenorrhea and galactorrhea. *Ann Intern Med* 1984;**100**:115.

March CM et al: Longitudinal evaluation of patients with untreated prolactin-secreting pituitary adenomas. *Am J Obstet Gynecol* 1981;**139**:835.

Melmed S et al: Pituitary tumors secreting growth hormone and prolactin. *Ann Intern Med* 1986;**105**:238.

Molitch ME: Pregnancy and the hyperprolactinemic woman. *N Engl J Med* 1985;**312**:1364.

Molitch ME et al: Bromocriptine as primary therapy for prolactin-secreting macroadenomas: Results of a prospective multicenter study. *J Clin Endocr Metab* 1985;**60**:698.

Spark RF et al: Hyperprolactinaemia in males with and without pituitary macroadenomas. *Lancet* 1982;**2**:129.

Tucker H St G et al: Galactorrhea-amenorrhea syndrome: Follow-up of forty-five patients after pituitary tumor removal. *Ann Intern Med* 1981;**94**:302.

Vance ML et al: Bromocriptine. *Ann Intern Med* 1984;**100**:78.

Wass JAH, Besser JM: The medical management of hormone-secreting tumors of the pituitary. *Annu Rev Med* 1983;**34**:283.

Wollesen F, Bendsen BB: Effect rates of different modalities for treatment of prolactin adenomas. *Am J Med* 1985;**78**:114.

# DIABETES INSIPIDUS

## Essentials of Diagnosis

- Polydipsia (4–20 L/d); excessive polyuria.
- Urine specific gravity < 1.006.
- Inability to concentrate urine on fluid restriction.
- Hyperosmolality of plasma.
- Vasopressin reduces urine output (except in nephrogenic diabetes insipidus).

## General Considerations

Diabetes insipidus is an uncommon disease characterized by an increase in thirst and the passage of large quantities of urine of a low specific gravity. The urine is otherwise normal. The disease may occur acutely, eg, after head trauma or surgical procedures near the pituitary region, or may be chronic and insidious in onset. It is due to decreased or absent vasopressin secretion or, more rarely, unresponsiveness of the kidney to vasopressin (nephrogenic diabetes insipidus).

The causes may be classified as follows:

**A. Due to Deficiency of Vasopressin:**

1. Primary diabetes insipidus, due to a defect inherent in the gland itself (no organic lesion), may be familial, occurring as a dominant trait; or, more commonly, sporadic or "idiopathic."

2. Secondary diabetes insipidus is due to destruction of the functional unit by surgical or accidental trauma, infection (eg, encephalitis, tuberculosis, syphilis), primary tumor or metastatic tumors from the breast or lung (common), vascular accidents (rare), and xanthomatosis (eosinophilic granuloma or Hand-Schüller-Christian disease).

**B. "Nephrogenic" Diabetes Insipidus:** This disorder is due to a defect in the kidney tubules that interferes with water reabsorption and occurs as an X-linked recessive trait. The polyuria is unresponsive to vasopressin. In fact, these patients have normal secretion of vasopressin. Serum levels of ADH are normal or high. Adults with familial nephrogenic diabetes insipidus often have hyperuricemia. Acquired forms of vasopressin-resistant diabetes insipidus are seen in some patients with pyelonephritis, renal amyloidosis, potassium depletion, or chronic hypercalcemia. Certain drugs (eg, demeclocycline, lithium) may induce nephrogenic diabetes insipidus.

## Clinical Findings

**A. Symptoms and Signs:** The outstanding signs and symptoms of the disease are intense thirst, especially with a craving for ice water, and polyuria, the volume of ingested fluid varying from 4 to 20 L daily, with correspondingly large urine volumes. Restriction of fluids causes marked weight loss, dehydration, headache, irritability, fatigue, muscular pains, hypothermia, tachycardia, and shock.

**B. Laboratory Findings:** Polyuria of over 6 L daily with a specific gravity below 1.006 is highly suggestive of diabetes insipidus. Simple water deprivation with measurement of urine osmolality may be diagnostic. Special tests have been devised to distinguish true diabetes insipidus from psychogenic polydipsia. The latter will often respond (with reduction in urine flow and increase in urinary specific gravity) to administration of hypertonic (3%) saline solution; true diabetes insipidus does not. Hypertonic saline infusions may be dangerous to patients with abnormal cardiovascular status. Although a positive response tends to rule out true diabetes insipidus, a negative result must be followed by careful prolonged dehydration and measurement of both urine and plasma osmolality and body weight under hospital conditions. Plasma osmolality is normally maintained in the range of 285–290 mosm/kg associated with ADH concentrations of 1–3 $\mu$U/mL in plasma and 11–30 $\mu$U/h in urine. Impaired ability to either synthesize or release ADH results in diminished ability of the kidney to conserve water. Patients with severe diabetes insipidus minimally concentrate urine following dehydration. After administration of 5 units of vasopressin, urine osmolality promptly rises. Patients with milder degrees may fail to release ADH in response to hyper-

tonicity but retain the ability to release hormone following nonosmotic stimuli. Some patients respond to an osmotic stimulus only when the plasma osmolality exceeds normal levels ("high set osmoreceptor"). The presence of intact thirst perception results in polydipsia and polyuria. Failure to respond to vasopressin (Pitressin) indicates "nephrogenic" diabetes insipidus if the serum calcium and potassium levels are normal. A recently developed radioimmunoassay for arginine vasopressin will facilitate the differential diagnosis of diabetes insipidus and psychogenic polydipsia. The high levels of plasma vasopressin in nephrogenic diabetes insipidus are diagnostic.

If true primary diabetes insipidus seems likely on the basis of these tests, search for a possible brain lesion with x-rays of the skull, visual field tests, and CT scan of the pituitary hypothalamic area. Search also for associated bone lesions of xanthomatosis and obtain biopsy for confirmation. Look for a primary tumor in the lung or breast. In nephrogenic diabetes insipidus, rule out pyelonephritis or hydronephrosis and demeclocycline and lithium administration.

## Differential Diagnosis

The most important differentiation is from the "psychogenic" water-drinking habit (see above). This may be difficult, since patients with long-standing polydipsia develop a true defect in renal concentrating ability. The baseline serum osmolality is helpful, since subjects with psychogenic polydipsia have low values, whereas the serum osmolality is normal or high in patients with diabetes insipidus. Polydipsia and polyuria may also be seen in diabetes mellitus, chronic nephritis, hypokalemia (eg, in primary hyperaldosteronism), and in hypercalcemic states such as hyperparathyroidism. The low fixed specific gravity of the urine in chronic nephritis does not rise after administration of vasopressin. On the other hand, in spite of the inability of patients with diabetes insipidus to concentrate urine, other tests of renal function yield essentially normal results.

## Complications

If water is not readily available, the excessive output of urine will lead to severe dehydration, which rarely proceeds to a state of shock. Insomnia and dysphagia may occur. All the complications of the primary disease may eventually become evident. In patients who also have a disturbed thirst mechanism and who are receiving effective antidiuretic therapy, there is a danger of induced water intoxication. In untreated subjects, the passage of large volumes of urine for many years may be associated with dilatation of the ureters and urinary bladder.

## Treatment

**A. Specific Measures:** Aqueous vasopressin injection is rarely used in continuous treatment because of its short duration of action (1–4 hours). A synthetic analog of arginine vasopressin (desmopressin acetate [DDAVP]) is longer-acting and has become the treatment of choice. It is given intranasally in a dose of 5–10 µg once or twice daily. Vasopressin tannate (Pitressin Tannate) suspension in oil (warn the patient to shake the vial well before filling the syringe), 0.5–1 mL intramuscularly, has been the standard treatment for many years. It is effective for 24–72 hours. It is usually best to administer the drug in the evening so that maximal results can be obtained during sleep. Patients learn to administer the drug themselves, and the dosage is adjusted as necessary.

**B. Other Measures:** Mild cases require no treatment other than adequate fluid intake. Hydrochlorothiazide (Hydrodiuril), 50–100 mg/d (with potassium chloride), is of some help in reducing the urine volume of true or nephrogenic diabetes insipidus. Chlorpropamide (Diabinese) has been found to enhance the activity of ADH upon the renal tubule and is useful in patients with partial diabetes insipidus, who still maintain a residual secretion of vasopressin. It has no effect in the nephrogenic type. After an initial dose of 250 mg twice daily, many patients can be maintained on 125–250 mg daily. Side effects include nausea, skin allergy, hypoglycemia, and a disulfiram-like reaction to alcohol.

Other drugs with andidiuretic activity are clofibrate and carbamazepine. They induce release of ADH and may be used in combination with chlorpropamide for selected patients with partial vasopressin deficiency. They have no effect on nephrogenic diabetes insipidus.

Solute restriction (low-sodium, no-excess-protein diet) may be of additional help. Psychotherapy is required for most patients with compulsive water drinking.

**C. X-Ray Therapy:** This may be used in the treatment of some cases due to tumor (eg, eosinophilic granuloma).

## Prognosis

Diabetes insipidus may be latent, especially if there is associated lack of anterior pituitary function; and may be transient, eg, following head trauma. In most patients, the condition is permanent. With adequate therapy, all symptoms disappear and the patient can live a normal life. The ultimate prognosis is essentially that of the underlying disorder. In cases associated with organic brain disease, the prognosis is often poor. Surgical correction of the primary brain lesion rarely alters the diabetes insipidus.

If the disease is due to an eosinophilic granuloma of the skull, temporary amelioration or even complete cure may be effected with x-ray therapy.

The prognosis of the ''nephrogenic'' type is only fair, since intercurrent infections are common, especially in infants affected with the disease. The acquired forms of this type may be reversible—eg, if urinary tract infection or obstruction is alleviated.

Kimmel DW, O'Neill BP: Systemic cancer presenting as diabetes insipidus. *Cancer* 1983;**52**:2355.
Moses AM, Notman DD: Diabetes insipidus and syndrome of inappropriate antidiuretic hormone secretion (SIADH). *Adv Intern Med* 1982;**27**:73.
Richardson DW, Robinson AG: Drugs twenty years later: Desmopressin. *Ann Intern Med* 1985;**103**:228.

## INAPPROPRIATE SECRETION OF ANTIDIURETIC HORMONE

This syndrome, which is essentially water intoxication, may be mild and may only be manifested as asymptomatic hyponatremia, or it may be accompanied by irritability, lethargy, confusion, and seizures. It may lead to coma and death if not recognized. Laboratory findings include hyponatremia (which usually suggests the diagnosis) and hypo-osmolarity of the serum, continued renal excretion of sodium, formation of hyperosmolar urine, and expanded fluid volume. Adrenal and renal function are normal. Plasma arginine vasopressin levels are elevated or high normal but are inappropriate for plasma osmolality.

The disorder is most commonly caused by oat cell bronchogenic carcinoma, but it may also be present in patients with malignant tumors of the pancreas, prostate, and other organs. It is also seen in pulmonary tuberculosis, porphyria, acute leukemia, acute myocardial infarction, myxedema, and central nervous system disorders. It may be induced by chlorpropamide, vincristine, cyclophosphamide, and potassium-depleting diuretics.

Treatment is best accomplished by water restriction, which succeeds if the syndrome is recognized early. In severe cases of hyponatremia, when rapid correction is required, the use of furosemide diuresis with electrolyte replacement may be tried. Lithium carbonate has been found to be effective in this syndrome, but lithium intoxication may occur. Demeclocycline may be a safer drug to correct antidiuresis. Urea may be a safe and effective drug. A search for the primary cause of the disorder must also be undertaken (see Chapter 3).

Cooke CR et al: The syndrome of inappropriate antidiuretic hormone secretion (SIADH): Pathophysiologic mechanisms in solute and volume regulation. *Medicine* 1979;**58**:240.
Newsome HH: Vasopressin: Deficiency, excess and the syndrome of antidiuretic hormone secretion. *Nephron* 1979;**23**:125.

## DISEASES OF THE THYROID GLAND

Thyroid hormone affects cellular oxidative processes throughout the body. It is normally elaborated within the follicles of the gland by a combination of inorganic iodine, which is trapped by the gland under the influence of pituitary TSH, and tyrosine, forming monoiodotyrosine and diiodotyrosine, which further combine to form thyroxine ($T_4$) and triiodothyronine ($T_3$), the principal hormones of the gland. The "storage" form of the hormone is thyroglobulin, a combination of thyroxine and thyroid globulin, and it is in this colloidal form that the hormone is found within the follicles.

Under the influence of TSH, the active hormones are released from the gland as the need arises. Most of the circulating $T_3$, however, results from extra thyroidal metabolism of $T_4$. Circulating thyroxine is bound to plasma proteins, primarily thyroxine-binding globulins, and prealbumin. High levels of estrogen (eg, in pregnancy or in women taking oral contraceptives) increase the thyroxine-binding globulin levels and thus also the total level of $T_4$. The binding can be inhibited by certain compounds, eg, phenytoin and high doses of aspirin, which lower the $T_4$. The free (unbound) levels of circulating hormones regulate TSH release. The physiologic importance of triiodothyronine in clinical disorders is now well established. The availability of synthetic TSH-releasing hormone has been helpful in the evaluation of pituitary reserve and in the diagnosis of both hyper- and hypothyroidism.

The requirements for iodine are minimal (about 50–200 $\mu$g/d), but if a true deficiency arises or if the demand for iodine is increased (eg, during puberty), hormone production will be insufficient and circulating levels will be low. This leads to increase in pituitary TSH output, and thyroid hyperplasia follows.

The peripheral metabolism of the thyroid hormones, especially by the liver, and its alteration in disease states are significant. Most circulating $T_3$ derives from peripheral conversion of $T_4$, which is also metabolized to a biologically inactive compound, reverse $T_3$. In many acute and chronic nonthyroidal illnesses, starvation, etc, the proportion of $T_3$ formed decreases and that of reverse $T_3$ increases. Serum concentrations of free $T_4$ are usually normal, less frequently low (patients with more serious disease), and rarely elevated. Euthyroid hyperthyroxinemia is especially common in acute psychiatric illness and in hyperemesis gravidarum; the mechanisms are unclear.

Thyroid disorders may occur with or without diffuse or nodular enlargement of the gland (goiter). Symptoms may be due to pressure alone or to hyperfunction or hypofunction. A strong genetic predisposition to thyroid disease is being recognized.

Since thyroid hormone affects all vital processes of the body, the time of onset of a deficiency state is most important in mental and physical development. Prolonged insufficiency that is present since infancy (cretinism) causes irreversible changes. Milder degrees of hypofunction, especially in adults, may go unrecognized or may masquerade as symptoms of disease of another system, eg, menorrhagia. Diagnosis will then depend to a large extent upon laboratory aids, especially the finding of an elevated TSH level.

In any age group, whenever an isolated thyroid nodule is felt that is not associated with hyperfunction—and especially if there is any change in size of the nodule—the possibility of neoplasm must be considered.

Chopra IJ et al: Thyroid function in nonthyroidal illnesses. *Ann Intern Med* 1983;**98**:946.

Greenspan FS, Forsham PH (editors): *Basic & Clinical Endocrinology.* 2nd ed. Lange, 1986.

Kaplan MM, Larsen PR (editors): Thyroid disease. (Symposium.) *Med Clin North Am* 1985;**69(5)**:September. [Entire issue.]

Oppenheimer JH: Thyroid hormone action at the nuclear level. *Ann Intern Med* 1985;**102**:374.

Van der Spuy ZM, Jacobs HS: Management of endocrine disorders in pregnancy. 1. Thyroid and parathyroid disease. *Postgrad Med J* 1984;**60**:245.

## TESTS OF THYROID FUNCTION

The tests most widely used in clinical practice are $T_4$ and "free" $T_4$ radioimmunoassays. When the latter is not available, the resin uptake of $T_3$ and determination of free thyroxine index (FTI) are useful. The TSH (RIA) assay has been of great help in diagnosis.

### 1. THYROID HORMONES IN SERUM

**$T_4$ (RIA)**

Normal: 5–13 $\mu$g/dL.

This test measures thyroxine by radioimmunoassay. It is affected by states of altered thyroxine binding.

### "Free" Thyroxine Determination (FT$_4$)

Normal: 0.8–2.3 ng/dL.

This test measures the metabolically effective fraction of circulating $T_4$. If properly performed, it is the best measurement of thyroid hormones, since it is not affected by binding problems, chronic illness, etc. It is not yet generally available.

### Radioactive $T_3$ Uptake of Resin

Normal (varies with methods): 25–35%.

This test is not dependent upon exogenous organic or inorganic iodides. It is an indirect measure of thyroxine-binding protein and is of value in certain patients, eg, in pregnancy when the $T_4$ is high due to increased thyroxine-binding while $T_3$ uptake is low. In general, $T_3$ uptake parallels the $T_4$ except in the rare euthyroid patient with deficient thyroxine-binding protein, where the $T_4$ is low but the $T_3$ uptake normal or high. A test for $T_4$ should be done at the same time.

### Free Thyroxine Index (FTI)

The normal range varies in different laboratories.

The product of $T_4$ and resin $T_3$ uptake ($T_4 \times T_3$ uptake) usually (not always) corrects for abnormalities of thyroxine binding. If a free $T_4$ determination is available, this calculation is unnecessary.

### Thyroxine-Binding Globulin (TBG-RIA)

Normal: 2–4.8 mg/dL.

This is a direct and specific test for abnormal thyroxine binding and is not affected by alterations in other serum proteins.

### $T_3$ by Radioimmunoassay

Normal: 80–200 ng/mL.

This test is of value in the diagnosis of thyrotoxicosis with normal $T_4$ values ($T_3$ thyrotoxicosis) and in some cases of toxic nodular goiter. It decreases rapidly in states of malnutrition, chronic illnesses, weight reduction diets, etc.

### 2. IN VIVO UPTAKE OF THYROID GLAND

### Radioiodine ($^{123}$I) Uptake of Thyroid Gland

Normal: 5–35% in 24 hours. The normal range has been markedly lowered in the USA because of increase of dietary intake of iodine (primarily due to the addition of sodium iodate to bread).

**A. Elevated:** Thyrotoxicosis, hypofunctioning large goiter, iodine lack; at times, chronic thyroiditis.

**B. Low:** Administration of iodides, $T_4$, antithyroid drugs, thyroiditis, hypothyroidism.

A scintiscan over the gland outlines areas of increased and decreased activity. If the uptake of $^{123}$I is blocked, technetium ($^{99m}$Tc) may be used to obtain a scintiscan. Suppression of uptake after administration of 100 $\mu$g of $T_3$ daily for several days will determine if the area in the gland is autonomous or TSH-dependent.

### 3. MISCELLANEOUS TESTS OF THYROID FUNCTION

### Serum Cholesterol

Normal: 150–250 mg/dL. This test is nonspecific, since many factors influence cholesterol levels, including age, sex, genetic makeup, and dietary intake. The absolute level is less significant than the change after institution of therapy. A relatively high level occurs in hypothyroidism. A relatively low level may be seen in thyrotoxicosis.

### Achilles Tendon Reflex

The relaxation time is often prolonged in hypothyroidism but also in diabetes, old age, peripheral vascular disease, etc. It is rapid in hyperthyroidism. Although it lacks specificity for diagnosis, this test may be of value in following response to therapy.

### Thyrotropin Immunoassay & Response to TRF

Normal: TSH-RIA less than 8 $\mu$U/mL (varies with laboratory); TRF response: doubling of TSH within 40 minutes after administration of 400 $\mu$g intravenously.

Radioimmunoassay of serum TSH is the most sensitive test for the early detection of primary hypothyroidism. TSH elevations may occur in subclinical hypothyroidism (eg, after destructive thyroid treatment), in iodine deficiency goiter, and in some dyshormonogenic goiters. It may also be elevated in rare cases of thyroid hormone resistance (Refetoff syndrome). After adequate $T_4$ replacement, patients with myxedema should have undetectable or low TSH levels. A normal TSH response to TRF rules out pituitary hypothyroidism. A prolonged and exaggerated rise in TSH after administration of thyrotropin-releasing factor (TRF) in patients with borderline elevations of TSH may provide further evidence of primary thyroid failure. Patients with hyperthyroidism fail to respond to TRF, and a normal response virtually excludes hyperthyroidism.

"Ultrasensitive" assays for TSH have been developed that separate the normal range from the "suppressed" values found in hyperthyroidism. These may be of help in the diagnosis of mild hyperthyroidism and will render obsolete the use of TRF stimulation tests for this purpose. These new assays may provide the best cost-effective screening test for thyroid dysfunction (hypo- or hyperthyroidism).

### Thyroid Antibodies

Antibodies against several thyroid constituents (antithyroglobulin and antimicrosomal) are most commonly found in Hashimoto's thyroiditis but are also found in most patients with Graves' disease, a few patients with goiters or thyroid carcinomas, and in about 5–10% of normal subjects. In the latter, the titers tend to be low, and they increase with age. Thyroid-specific stimulating autoantibodies such as LATS (long-acting thyroid stimulator) and LATS protector (which is probably identical with human-specific thyroid stimulator [HSTS]) are found in Graves' disease. A generic test for these and other thyroid-stimulating immunoglobulins (TSI) measures their displacement of TSH in thyroid cell membranes. TSI titers are elevated in approximately 80% of patients with Graves' disease. These titers—and those of antithyroglobulin and antimicrosomal antibodies—often decrease during pregnancy and during treatment of Graves' disease with propylthiouracil. Other antibodies include thyroid growth-promoting antibodies, blocking antibodies, etc. Most of these factors can be measured only in research laboratories.

### Serum Thyroglobulin

The level of serum thyroglobulin rises in autoimmune thyroid disease, thyroid injury or inflammation, and thyroid cancer. Levels are of little value in diagnosing or distinguishing among these conditions, but

**Table 18–5.** Typical results of some blood thyroid function tests in various conditions.*
(N = Normal range. ↑ = Elevated. ↓ = Decreased. V = Variable.)

*Note:* The more direct tests are subject to technical variables. They should be used when the more standard tests do not give decisive information, since many drugs cause interference with these thyroid tests.

| | $T_4$ (RIA) | $T_3$ Resin | Free $T_4$ Index | $T_3$ Serum | RAI ($^{123}$I) Uptake | Other Useful Tests and Comments |
|---|---|---|---|---|---|---|
| Hyperthyroidism | ↑ | ↑ | ↑ | ↑ | ↑ | TSH ↓ |
| Hypothyroidism | ↓ | ↓ | ↓ | ↓ | ↓ | TSH ↑ in primary myxedema, ↓ in pituitary myxedema |
| Euthyroid, or hypothyroid therapy with: $T_4$ | N | N | N | V | ↓ | TSH ↓ with 0.1–0.2 mg $T_4$ |
| $T_3$ (1) | ↓ | ↓ | ↓ | | ↓ | TSH ↓ with 50 $\mu$g $T_3$ |
| Desiccated thyroid (2) | N | N | N | | ↓ | TSH ↓ with 120–200 mg |
| Euthyroid following (3) Radiographic contrast dyes | N | N | N or ↑ | N | ↓ | Effects may persist for 2 weeks to years |
| Pregnancy Hyperthyroid | ↑ | N or ↑ | ↑ | ↑ | ↑ | Effects persist for 6–10 weeks after termination |
| Euthyroid | ↑ | ↓ | N | ↑ | ↑ | |
| Hypothyroid | N or ↓ | ↓ | ↓ | ↓ | ↓ | |
| Birth control pills | ↑ | ↓ | N | ↑ | N | TSH normal |
| Nephrotic syndrome (4) | ↓ | ↑ | N | N | N | Low TP and TBG |
| Phenytoin, high doses of salicylates, testosterone | ↓ | ↑ | N | ↓ | N | TSH normal |
| Iodine deficiency | N | N | N | N | ↑ | $^{123}$I ↓ by $T_4$ or $T_3$ |
| Iodide ingestion | N | N | N | N | ↓ | |

* Modified and reproduced, with permission, from Leeper RD: *Current Concepts* 1972;1:1. Courtesy of the Upjohn Co., Kalamazoo, Mich.
(1) $T_3$ causes decreased measurements of serum thyroxine because $T_4$ secretion is depressed or absent. $T_3$ resin uptake is decreased because of decreased saturation of TBG with $T_4$.
(2) Assuming normal $T_3$:$T_4$ ratio. Different batches of thyroid extract may vary.
(3) Free $T_4$ index may be increased if measurement for serum $T_4$ is elevated by contamination.
(4) TBG is lost in this disease, which accounts for decreased serum thyroxine.

they provide a useful marker in thyroid cancer to indicate recurrence of disease and the need for further studies and therapy.

## Echo Scan (Ultrasound)

This simple technique has been used to determine if thyroid lesions are solid or cystic. Cysts are less likely to be malignant, since thyroid carcinomas rarely undergo cystic degeneration. One should remember, however, that most solid lesions are benign. The test has poor discriminating value.

## Fine-Needle Aspiration

Aspiration of thyroid tissue with a fine-gauge (21–26) needle has been shown to be helpful in the diagnosis of thyroid disorders, especially nodular lesions. Reading by an experienced cytopathologist is mandatory.

## Calcitonin Assay

Elevated in medullary carcinoma.

Borst GC et al: Euthyroid hyperthyroxinemia. *Ann Intern Med* 1983;**98**:366.

Chopra IJ et al: Thyroid function in nonthyroidal illness. *Ann Intern Med* 1983;**98**:946.
Frable WJ: *Fine Needle Aspiration Biopsy.* Saunders, 1983.
Kolesnick RN et al: Thyrotropin-releasing hormone and the pituitary. Am J Med 1985;**79**:729.
Melmed S et al: A comparison of methods for assessing thyroid function in nonthyroidal illness. *J Clin Endocrinol Metab* 1982;**54**:300.
Ollis CA et al: Thyroid stimulating immunoglobulins: Measurement and clinical use. *Clin Sci* 1985;**69**:113.
Ross DS: New sensitive immunoradiometric assays for thyrotropin. (Editorial.) *Ann Intern Med* 1986;**104**:718.

## SIMPLE & NODULAR GOITER

### Essentials of Diagnosis

- Enlarged thyroid gland in a patient living in an endemic area.
- No symptoms except those associated with compression by large gland.
- $T_4$ and serum cholesterol normal; radioactive iodine uptake normal or elevated.
- TSH may be elevated.

**Table 18–6.** Appropriate use of thyroid tests.

| Purpose | Test | Comment |
|---------|------|---------|
| For screening | Free-$T_4$ | Best test if available. |
| | $T_4$ (RIA) | Varies with TBG. |
| | $T_3$ resin uptake | Varies with TBG. |
| | Free thyroxine index | Useful combination. |
| For hypo-thyroidism | Serum TSH | Primary vs secondary hypothyroidism. "Feedback" with $T_4$ and $T_3$. |
| | TRH stimulation | Differentiates pituitary and hypothalamic disorders. |
| | Antithyroglobulin and antimicrosomal antibodies | Elevated in Hashimoto's thyroiditis. |
| For hyper-thyroidism | Serum TSH | Usually suppressed. |
| | $T_3$ (RIA) | Elevated. |
| | $^{123}$I uptake and scan | Increased diffuse vs "hot" areas. |
| | Suppression test (100 $\mu$g $T_3$ for 7 days) | Autonomy. For atypical Graves' disease with normal uptake. |
| | TRH stimulation | No response; safer than suppression test. |
| | Antithyroglobulin and antimicrosomal | Elevated in Graves' disease. |
| | TSH displacing immunoglobulin (TD) | Positive in Graves' disease (not always) |
| For nodules | $^{123}$I uptake and scan | "Warm" vs "cold." |
| | $^{99m}$Tc scan | Vascular vs avascular. |
| | Echo scan | Solid vs cystic. Pure cysts are not malignant. |
| | Thyroglobulin (TG) | High in metastatic, papillary, or follicular carcinomas. |
| | Calcitonin | High in medullary carcinoma. |
| | Thin-needle aspiration | Best diagnostic method for thyroid cancer. |

## General Considerations

Simple goiter in many parts of the world is due to iodine lack and occurs in endemic areas away from the seacoast. Deficiency of iodine leads to functional overactivity and hyperplasia of the gland, which becomes filled with colloid poor in iodine. If the deficiency is corrected, the enlargement may subside. In long-standing cases, the goiter persists and is often nodular. In the USA, the ingestion of iodine is now so high (due to iodates in bread and other iodine sources in the diet) that iodine deficiency due to lack of ingestion is extremely rare. Iodine excess can also cause goiter (excessive chronic ingestion of seaweed in Hokkaido, Japan; chronic treatment with saturated solution of potassium iodide or Lugol's solution). Unknown factors other than iodine lack play a role in the genesis of goiter. Simple goiter may occur transiently when there is greater demand for thyroid hormone, eg, with the onset of puberty or during pregnancy. Rarely, goiter may occur in spite of adequate iodine intake when there is interference with formation of thyroid hormones, eg, due to excess intake of certain goitrogenic vegetables (rutabagas, turnips), exposure to thiocyanate, or congenital lack of certain enzyme systems. Goitrogens occurring in contaminated water supplies have been described. Thyroid growth-stimulating immunoglobulins have been demonstrated in the serum of patients with goiters previously thought to be autoimmune. Goiter is more easily prevented than cured; it is rarer since the introduction of iodized salt. Simple goiters may show chronic thyroiditis on biopsy.

## Clinical Findings

**A. Symptoms and Signs:** The gland is visibly enlarged and palpable. There may be no symptoms, or symptoms may occur as a result of compression of the structures in the neck or chest: wheezing, dysphagia, respiratory embarrassment. (*Note:* Recurrent laryngeal compression is rare.) There may be associated congenital deafness (Pendred's syndrome) and disorders of taste.

**B. Laboratory Findings:** The $T_4$ and serum cholesterol are usually normal. The radioiodine uptake of the gland may be normal or high. The uptake over nodules shows them to be low in activity (in contrast to toxic nodular goiters).

With special techniques it is possible to demonstrate enzymatic defects in thyroid hormone production or abnormal circulating compounds in a number of patients with goiters, especially the familial types. The TSH levels may be elevated. Antimicrosomal and antithyroglobulin antibody titers are usually not elevated.

**C. Ultrasound Examination:** Echography provides information about the structure of the thyroid rapidly and safely: presence of single or multiple nodules, intrathoracic extension of goiters, etc. It should be remembered that demonstration of the cystic nature of a mass does not rule out malignancy.

## Differential Diagnosis

It may be difficult, by examination alone, to differentiate simple goiter from toxic diffuse or nodular goiter, especially in a patient with a great many nervous symptoms. A history of residence in an endemic area, a family history of goiter, or onset during stressful periods of life (eg, puberty or pregnancy) will often help. Thyroid function tests are usually normal in simple goiter. High titers of antithyroid antibodies point to the presence of autoimmune thyroid disease (Hashimoto's thyroiditis or Graves' disease). If the lesion is nodular, and especially if only a single nodule is present, neoplasm must be considered. Fine needle aspiration of the nodule is the most useful technique to distinguish neoplasia from other causes of nodule formation.

## Prevention

With a dietary intake of 100–200 μg of iodine daily, simple goiter due to iodine deficiency should not occur. During times of stress (puberty, pregnancy, and lactation), the upper limits of this dose may be necessary. This amount is provided in 1–2 g of iodized salt daily. Iodinated oil has been introduced in certain areas of the world as a prophylactic agent for goiter.

## Treatment

### A. Specific Measures:

**1. Thyroid**–Levothyroxine, 0.1 mg or more, is of value in most cases. The goiter will stop growing and often will decrease in size. As a guide to therapy, $T_4$ should be maintained in the high normal range. TSH levels should be suppressed by adequate replacement therapy. Since long-standing simple goiters may contain autonomous nodules, it is prudent to watch the patient carefully for possible hyperthyroidism.

**2. Iodine therapy**–If the enlargement is discovered early and is due to iodine deficiency, it may disappear completely with adequate iodine administration. Five drops daily of saturated solution of potassium iodide or strong iodine solution (Lugol's solution) in one-half glass of water is sufficient. Continue therapy until the gland returns to normal size, and then place the patient on a maintenance dosage or use iodized table salt.

### B. Indications for Surgery:

**1. Signs of pressure**–If signs of local pressure are present that are not helped by medical treatment, the gland should be removed surgically.

**2. Potential cancer**–Surgery should be considered for any thyroid gland with a single "cold" (low $^{123}$I or $^{99m}$Tc uptake) noncystic nodule, for the chances of a single nodule being malignant are high. This is particularly true in younger people and in any case when there is no decrease in size or abnormal growth in spite of thyroid therapy after a period of 3–6 months. Nodules can be aspirated for cytopathologic study.

## Prognosis

Simple goiter may disappear spontaneously or may become large, causing compression of vital structures. Multinodular goiters of long standing, especially in people over 50 years of age, may become toxic. This often happens after ingestion of large amounts of iodine (jodbasedow phenomenon). Whether they ever become malignant is not established.

Botazzo GF, Doniach D: Autoimmune thyroid disease. *Annu Rev Med* 1986;**37**:353.

Lever EG et al: Inherited disorders of thyroid metabolism. *Endocr Rev* 1983;**4**:213.

Studer H, Ramelli F: Simple goiter and its variants: Euthyroid and hyperthyroid multinodular goiters. *Endocr Rev* 1982;**3**:40.

## HYPOTHYROIDISM

In view of the profound influence exerted on all tissues of the body by thyroid hormone, lack of the hormone may affect virtually all body functions. The degree of severity ranges from mild and unrecognized hypothyroid states to striking myxedema.

A state of hypothyroidism may be due to primary disease of the thyroid gland itself, or lack of pituitary TSH or hypothalamic TRF. A true end-organ insensitivity to normal amounts of circulating hormone has been rarely observed. Although gross forms of hypothyroidism, ie, myxedema and cretinism, are readily recognized on clinical grounds alone, the far more common mild forms often escape detection without adequate laboratory facilities.

## 1. CRETINISM & JUVENILE HYPOTHYROIDISM

### Essentials of Diagnosis

- Dwarfism; mental retardation; dry, yellow, cold skin; "pot belly" with umbilical hernia.
- $T_4$ low; serum cholesterol elevated. Delayed bone age; "stippling" of epiphyses.
- TSH elevated.

### General Considerations

The causes of cretinism and juvenile hypothyroidism are as follows:

**A. Congenital (Cretinism):**

1. Thyroid gland absent or rudimentary (embryonic defect; most cases of sporadic cretinism).

2. Thyroid gland present but defective in hormone secretion, goitrous, or secondarily atrophied. Due to extrinsic factor (deficient iodine, goitrogenic substances, in most cases of endemic cretinism); or due to maternal factors (some cases of congenital goiter). Many cases are familial, and enzymatic defects in thyroid hormone synthesis may be demonstrated.

**B. Acquired (Juvenile Hypothyroidism):** Atrophy of the gland or defective function may be due to unknown causes, thyroiditis, or operative removal (lingual thyroid or toxic goiter), or secondary to pituitary deficiency.

### Clinical Findings

**A. Symptoms and Signs:** All degrees of dwarfism may be seen, with delayed skeletal maturation; apathy; physical and mental torpor; dry skin with coarse, dry, brittle hair; constipation; slow teething; poor appetite; large tongue; "pot belly" with umbilical hernia; deep voice; cold extremities and cold sensitivity; and true myxedema of subcutaneous and other tissues. A yellow skin due to carotenemia is not infrequent. The thyroid gland is usually not palpable, but a large goiter may be present that may be diffusely enlarged or nodular. Sexual development is retarded but maturation eventually occurs. Menometrorrhagia or amenorrhea may be seen in older girls. Rarely, sexual precocity and galactorrhea with pituitary enlargement may occur. Deafness is occasionally associated with goiters. Nephrocalcinosis is a rare finding in cretinism.

**B. Laboratory Findings:** Total serum $T_4$ and free $T_4$ are markedly decreased. Serum cholesterol is frequently elevated. Radioactive iodine uptake is very low in athyroid individuals, but it may be high in some goitrous cretins where the iodine is not bound in the gland and is released. By special techniques, abnormal circulating iodine compounds and enzymatic defects in thyroid hormone production and release are demonstrable in some patients. Others show circulating autoantibodies to thyroid constituents. TSH by radioimmunoassay is invariably elevated; this may be the best screening test if readily available, especially in newborns.

**C. Imaging:** Delayed skeletal maturation is a constant finding, often with "stippling" of the epiphyses (especially of the femoral head), with flattening; widening of the cortices of the long bones, absence of the cranial sinuses, and delayed dentition may also be noted.

## Differential Diagnosis

It is of practical interest to differentiate primary hypothyroidism from pituitary failure because in the latter instance a search for a pituitary lesion must be undertaken. TSH assay will help greatly in the differentiation of primary hypothyroidism from pituitary hypothyroidism. Treatment with thyroid hormone must be instituted cautiously when hypothyroidism is secondary to pituitary failure, since it may occasionally precipitate adrenal crisis. Cretinism is sometimes confused with Down's syndrome, although retarded skeletal development is rare in mongoloid infants. Macroglossia may be due to tumor, eg, lymphangioma. The dry skin of ichthyosis may be misleading. In children and adolescents, any unexplained decrease in the rate of growth should alert the physician to the possibility of early hypothyroidism. All causes of stunted growth and skeletal development (see above) must be considered as well.

## Treatment

See Myxedema, below.

## Prognosis

The progress and outcome of the disease depend largely upon the duration of thyroid deficiency and the adequacy and persistence of treatment. Since mental development is at stake, it is of utmost importance to start treatment early.

The prognosis for full mental and physical maturation is much better if the onset of disease occurs later in life. Congenital cretins often have variable degrees of intellectual impairment. With implementation of large-scale thyroid screening programs at birth, appropriate therapy is being instituted much earlier than before, and it is expected that most cretins will have a reasonably normal mental development.

By and large, the response to thyroid therapy is gratifying, but therapy usually must be maintained throughout life.

Dussault JH: Congenital hypothyroidism. In: *The Thyroid: A Fundamental and Clinical Text*, 5th ed. Ingbar SH, Braverman LE (editors). Lippincott, 1986.

Lever EG, Medeiros-Neto GA, DeGroot LJ: Inherited disorders of thyroid metabolism. *Endocr Rev* 1983;**4**:213.

Postellon DC: Diagnosis and treatment of congenital hypothyroidism. *Compr Ther* 1983;**9**:41.

Stanbury JB, Dumont JE: Familial goiter and related disorders. Chapter 11 in: *The Metabolic Basis of Inherited Disease*, 5th ed. Stanbury JB et al (editors). McGraw-Hill, 1983.

## 2. ADULT HYPOTHYROIDISM & MYXEDEMA

### Essentials of Diagnosis

- Weakness, fatigue, cold intolerance, constipation, menorrhagia, hoarseness.
- Dry, cold, yellow, puffy skin; scant eyebrows; thick tongue; bradycardia; delayed return of deep tendon reflexes.
- Anemia (often macrocytic).
- $T_4$ and radioiodine uptake low.
- TSH elevated in primary myxedema.

### General Considerations

Primary thyroid deficiency is much more common than secondary hypofunction due to pituitary insufficiency. Primary myxedema occurs after thyroidectomy, eradication of thyroid by radioactive iodine, ingestion of goitrogens (eg, thiocyanates, rutabagas, lithium carbonate), or chronic thyroiditis. The widely used antiarrhythmic agent amiodarone has induced goiter or hypothyroidism (or both) in a significant proportion of patients receiving it. Thyroid deficiency can also occur after external x-ray irradiation of the neck (as in patients with lymphoma). Most cases, however, are due to atrophy of the gland from unknown causes, probably due to an autoimmune mechanism. This may also involve other endocrine glands, eg, adrenals, in the same patient (Schmidt's syndrome).

Secondary hypothyroidism may follow destructive lesions of the pituitary gland, eg, chromophobe adenoma or postpartum necrosis (Sheehan's syndrome). It is usually manifested by associated disorders of the adrenals and gonads. Since thyroid hormone is necessary for all glandular functions, primary myxedema may lead to secondary hypofunction of the pituitary, adrenals, and other glands, making diagnosis difficult.

### Clinical Findings

These may vary from the rather rare full-blown myxedema to mild states of hypothyroidism, which are far more common and may escape detection unless a high index of suspicion is maintained.

**A. Symptoms and Signs:**

**1. Early**–The principal symptoms are weakness,

fatigue, cold intolerance, lethargy, dryness of skin, headache, and menorrhagia. Nervousness is a common finding. Physical findings may be few or absent. Outstanding are thin, brittle nails; thinning of hair, which may be coarse; and pallor, with poor turgor of the mucosa. Delayed return of deep tendon reflexes is often found.

**2. Late**—The principal symptoms are slow speech, absence of sweating, modest weight gain, constipation, peripheral edema, pallor, hoarseness, decreased sense of taste and smell, muscle cramps, aches and pains, dyspnea, anginal pain, and deafness. Some women have amenorrhea; others have menorrhagia. Galactorrhea may also be present. Physical findings include puffiness of the face and eyelids, typical carotenemic skin color and occasional purpura, thinning of the outer halves of the eyebrows, thickening of the tongue, hard pitting edema, and effusions into the pleural, peritoneal, and pericardial cavities, as well as into joints. Cardiac enlargement ("myxedema heart") is often due to pericardial effusion. The heart rate is slow; the blood pressure is more often normal than low, and even hypertension that reverses with treatment may be found. Pituitary enlargement due to hyperplasia of TSH-secreting cells, which may be reversible following thyroid therapy, may be seen in long-standing hypothyroidism. (**Note:** Obesity is not common in hypothyroidism.)

**B. Laboratory Findings:** The $T_4$ is under 3.5 $\mu$g/dL; the free $T_4$ is less than 0.8 ng/dL. Radioiodine uptake is decreased (below 10% in 24 hours), but this test is not always reliable. The radioactive $T_3$ resin uptake is usually low. Plasma cholesterol is elevated in primary and, less commonly, in secondary hypothyroidism (decrease on thyroid therapy is a sensitive index). Anemia is often present; it may be macrocytic, owing to associated pernicious anemia, or hypochromic microcytic, owing to iron deficiency in women with menorrhagia. Serum creatine phosphokinase (CPK) is often elevated. Plasma cortisol is normal unless the patient has associated autoimmune Addison's disease or the hypothyroidism is secondary to pituitary disease with associated adrenal insufficiency. Serum prolactin is elevated in some patients with primary hypothyroidism, presumably due to hypersecretion of hypothalamic thyrotropin-releasing hormone (TRH). The radioimmunoassay of TSH is a most useful test, since it is consistently elevated in primary hypothyroidism and low in pituitary hypothyroidism. Antithyroid antibody titers (antimicrosomal and antithyroglobulin) are high in patients with Hashimoto's thyroiditis and idiopathic primary myxedema.

### Differential Diagnosis

Mild hypothyroidism must be considered in many states of neurasthenia, menstrual disorders without grossly demonstrable pelvic disease, unexplained weight gain, and anemia. Myxedema enters into the differential diagnosis of unexplained heart failure that does not respond to digitalis or diuretics, "idiopathic"

hyperlipemia, and unexplained ascites. The protein content of myxedematous effusions is high. The thick tongue may be confused with that seen in primary amyloidosis. Pernicious anemia may be suggested by the pallor and the macrocytic type of anemia seen in myxedema. Some cases of primary psychosis and cerebral arteriosclerosis or even brain tumors must be differentiated from profound myxedema. (**Note:** The cerebrospinal fluid proteins may be elevated in myxedema.)

### Complications

Complications are mostly cardiac in nature, occurring as a result of advanced coronary artery disease and congestive failure, which may be precipitated by too vigorous thyroid therapy. There is an increased susceptibility to infection. Megacolon has been described in long-standing hypothyroidism. Organic psychoses with paranoid delusions may occur ("myxedema madness"). Rarely, adrenal crisis may be precipitated by thyroid therapy of pituitary myxedema. Hypothyroidism is a rare cause of infertility, which may respond to thyroid medication. Sellar enlargement and even well-defined TSH-secreting tumors may develop in untreated cases. These tumors decrease in size after replacement therapy is instituted.

A rare complication of severe hypothyroidism is deep stupor, at times progressing to **myxedema coma,** with severe hypothermia, hypoventilation, hypoxia, hypercapnia, and hypotension. Water intoxication and severe hyponatremia are common. Convulsions and abnormal central nervous system signs may occur. Myxedema coma is often induced by an underlying infection; cardiac, respiratory, or central nervous system illness; cold exposure; or drug use. It is most often seen in elderly women. The mortality rate is high.

*Caution:* Myxedematous patients are unusually sensitive to opiates and may die from average doses.

Refractory hyponatremia is often seen in severe myxedema, possibly due to inappropriate secretion of antidiuretic hormone; however, a defect in distal tubular reabsorption of sodium and water has been demonstrated in this disorder.

### Treatment

**A. Specific Therapy:** Thyroid or a synthetic preparation is used. The initial dosage varies with the severity of the hypothyroidism (Table 18–7).

**1.** *Caution*—When treating patients with severe myxedema or myxedema heart disease, or elderly patients with hypothyroidism with other associated heart disease, begin with small doses of levothyroxine, 25–50 $\mu$g daily for 1 week, and increase the dose every week by 25 $\mu$g daily up to a total of 100–150 $\mu$g daily. This dosage should be continued until signs of hypothyroidism have vanished or mild toxic symptoms appear, and the dosage then stabilized to maintain the $T_4$ at normal levels. Thyroxine tablets may vary in biologic potency and actual thyroxine content.

**Table 18–7.** Equivalency of thyroid preparations.

| Desiccated Thyroid | Approximate Equivalent In | | |
|---|---|---|---|
| | Levothyroxine Sodium (Levothroid, Synthroid, Etc) | Liothyronine Sodium (T₃, Cytomel) | Liotrix (Euthroid, Thyrolar) |
| 60 mg | 0.05 mg | 12.5 $\mu$g | Code: ½ |
| 65 mg | 0.1 mg | 25 $\mu$g | 1 |
| 130 mg | 0.2 mg | 50 $\mu$g | 2 |
| 200 mg | 0.3 mg | 75 $\mu$g | 3 |

2. Patients with early hypothyroidism may be started with larger doses, 50–100 $\mu$g daily, increasing by 25 $\mu$g every week to the limit of tolerance.

3. Maintenance–Each patient's dose must be adjusted to obtain the optimal effect. Most patients require 100–150 $\mu$g daily for maintenance. Optimal dosage can be estimated by following the free $T_4$ and TSH levels, but clinical judgment is often the best guide.

4. Desiccated thyroid may be used for replacement therapy, although it is not as well standardized or as predictable as crystalline levothyroxine. One grain (65 mg) of desiccated thyroid is equivalent to 100 $\mu$g of levothyroxine or 25 $\mu$g of triiodothyronine.

5. When a rapid response is necessary, sodium liothyronine ($T_3$ [Cytomel]) may be employed. Begin with very low doses because of the speed of action of this agent. Begin with 5 $\mu$g and increase slowly. *Note:* Serum $T_4$ cannot be used as a guide to $T_3$ therapy.

6. Mixtures of $T_4$ and $T_3$ in a ratio of 4:1—liotrix (Euthroid, Thyrolar)—have been introduced as "complete" replacement therapy. Since $T_4$ is normally converted to $T_3$ in extrathyroidal tissues, there is no need for this preparation.

7. **Myxedema coma** is a medical emergency with a high mortality rate. Triiodothyronine, 10–25 $\mu$g or more given by stomach tube every 8 hours, or, preferably, levothyroxine sodium, 200–400 $\mu$g intravenously as a single injection and repeated once in a dose of 100–200 $\mu$g in 12 hours, with the addition of hydrocortisone, 100 mg every 8 hours, may be lifesaving. The patient must not be warmed, adequate pulmonary ventilation must be provided, and fluid and electrolyte replacement must be carefully monitored. Infection is often present and must be vigorously treated.

8. Suppression of serum TSH has become a useful test of adequate replacement therapy in hypothyroidism.

**B. Needless Use of Thyroid:** The use of thyroid medication as nonspecific stimulating therapy is mentioned only to be condemned. It has been shown that the doses usually employed merely suppress the activity of the patient's own gland.

"Metabolic insufficiency" is a questionable entity. The use of thyroid in cases of amenorrhea or infertility warrants consideration only if the patient is likely to be hypothyroid.

**Prognosis**

The patient may succumb to the complications of the disease if treatment is withheld too long, eg, myxedema coma. With early treatment, striking transformations take place both in appearance and mental function. Return to a normal state is usually the rule, but relapses will occur if treatment is interrupted. On the whole, response to thyroid treatment is most satisfactory. Chronic maintenance therapy with unduly large doses of thyroid hormone may lead to subtle but important side effects (eg, bone demineralization).

Becker C: Hypothyroidism and atherosclerotic heart disease: Pathogenesis, medical management, and the role of coronary artery bypass surgery. *Endocr Rev* 1985;**6**:432.

Caldwell G et al: A new strategy for thyroid function testing. *Lancet* 1985;**1**:1117.

Klein I, Levey GS: Unusual manifestations of hypothyroidism. *Arch Intern Med* 1984;**144**:123.

Levine HD: Compromise therapy in the patient with angina pectoris and hypothyroidism: A clinical assessment. *Am J Med* 1980;**69**:411.

Martino E et al: Environmental iodine intake and thyroid dysfunction during chronic amiodarone therapy. *Ann Intern Med* 1984;**101**:28.

Sawin CT et al: Oral thyroxine: Variations in biologic action and tablet content. *Ann Intern Med* 1984;**100**:641.

Tachman MI, Guthrie GP: Hypothyroidism: Diversity of presentation. *Endocr Rev* 1984;**5**:456.

Wartofsky L: Myxedema coma. In: *The Thyroid: A Fundamental and Clinical Text*, 5th ed. Ingbar SH, Braverman LE (editors). Lippincott, 1986.

## HYPERTHYROIDISM (Thyrotoxicosis)

### Essentials of Diagnosis

- Weakness, sweating, weight loss, nervousness, loose stools, heat intolerance.
- Tachycardia; warm, thin, soft, moist skin; exophthalmos; stare; tremor.
- Goiter, bruit.
- $T_4$, radio-$T_3$ resin uptake, and radioiodine uptake elevated. Failure of suppression by $T_3$ administration.

### General Considerations

The term "thyrotoxicosis" denotes a series of clinical disorders associated with increased circulating levels of free thyroxine or triiodothyronine. By far the most common form of thyrotoxicosis is that associated with diffuse enlargement of the thyroid, hyperactivity of the gland, and the presence of antibodies against different fractions of the thyroid gland. This autoimmune thyroid disorder is called **Graves' disease** (or Basedow's disease in Europe and Latin America). It is much more common in women than in men (8:1), and its onset is usually between the ages of 20 and 40. It may be accompanied by a poorly understood infiltrative ophthalmopathy (Graves' exophthalmos) and, less commonly, by infiltrative dermopathy (pretibial myxedema). It may also be associated with other systemic autoimmune disorders such as pernicious anemia, myasthenia gravis, diabetes mellitus, etc. It has a familial tendency, and histocompatibility studies have shown an association with group HLA-B8 and DW3 (DRW3) in white subjects. Current thinking about the pathogenesis of the hyperthyroidism of Graves' disease involves the formation of autoantibodies that bind to the TSH receptor in thyroid cell membranes and stimulate the gland to hyperfunction. These thyroid-stimulating immunoglobulins (TSI) are demonstrable by special techniques in the plasma of most (but not all) patients with Graves' disease. Recent studies suggest that many other antibodies are generated in Graves' disease and even in some forms of thyrotoxicosis that have been traditionally thought to be nonautoimmune.

Other causes of hyperthyroidism include the following: **(1) Plummer's disease,** or autonomous toxic adenoma of the thyroid, which may be single or multiple. This is probably not an autoimmune disease and is not accompanied by infiltrative ophthalmopathy or dermopathy. Antithyroid antibodies are usually not present in the plasma, and tests for TSI are negative. **(2) Jodbasedow disease,** or iodine-induced hyperthyroidism, which may occur in patients with multinodular goiters after ingestion of large amounts of iodine. **(3) Thyrotoxicosis factitia,** which is due to ingestion of excessive amounts of exogenous thyroid hormone. **(4) Struma ovarii** or **hydatidiform mole,** which causes rare cases of clinical hyperthyroidism, although asymptomatic elevation of $T_4$ may be seen in chorionic tumors, presumably due to ectopic production of a TSH-like material. **(5) TSH-secreting tumor** of the pituitary, which is an extremely rare cause of hyperthyroidism. Much more commonly, these tumors are the consequence of long-standing **hypothyroidism. (6) Thyroiditis,** which may be associated with transient hyperthyroidism during the initial phase.

## Clinical Findings

**A. Symptoms and Signs:** Restlessness, nervousness, irritability; easy fatigability, especially toward the latter part of the day; and unexplained weight loss in spite of ravenous appetite are often the early features. There is usually excessive sweating and heat intolerance, and quick movements with incoordination varying from fine tremulousness to gross tremor. Less commonly, patients' primary complaints are difficulty in focusing their eyes, pressure from the goiter, diarrhea, or rapid, irregular heart action.

The patient is quick in all motions, including speech. The skin is warm and moist and the hands tremble. A diffuse or nodular goiter may be seen or felt with a thrill or bruit over it. The eyes appear bright, there may be a stare, at times periorbital edema, and commonly lid lag, lack of accomodation, exophthalmos, and even diplopia. The hair and skin are thin and of silky texture. At times there is increased pigmentation of the skin, but vitiligo may also occur. Spider angiomas and gynecomastia are common. Cardiovascular manifestations vary from tachycardia, especially during sleep, to paroxysmal atrial fibrillation and congestive failure of the "high-output" type. Mitral valve prolapse occurs much more frequently than in the general population. At times, a harsh pulmonary systolic murmur is heard (Means' murmur). Lymphadenopathy and splenomegaly may be present. Wasting of muscle and bone (osteoporosis) are common features, especially in long-standing thyrotoxicosis. Rarely, one finds nausea, vomiting, and even fever and jaundice (in which case the prognosis is poor). Mental changes are common, varying from mild exhilaration to delirium and exhaustion progressing to severe depression.

Associated with severe or malignant exophthalmos is at times a localized, bilateral, hard, nonpitting, symmetric swelling ("pretibial myxedema") over the tibia and dorsum of the feet (infiltrative dermopathy). At times there is clubbing and swelling of the fingers (acropachy). It often subsides spontaneously.

Thyroid **"storm,"** rarely seen today, is an extreme form of thyrotoxicosis that may occur after stress, thyroid surgery, or radioactive iodine administration and is manifested by marked delirium, severe tachycardia, vomiting, diarrhea, dehydration, and in many cases, very high fever. The mortality rate is high.

**B. Laboratory Findings:** The $T_4$ level and radioiodine and $T_3$ resin uptakes are increased. On rare occasions, the $T_4$ level may be normal but the serum $T_3$ elevated ("$T_3$ thyrotoxicosis"). The radioiodine uptake is elevated and cannot be suppressed by $T_3$ administration (see p 692). In toxic nodular goiter, a high radioiodine uptake in the nodule may be diagnostic if combined with elevated $T_4$ or $T_3$ and low TSH levels. Serum cholesterol levels are low (variable). Postprandial glycosuria is occasionally found. Urinary creatine is increased. Lymphocytosis is common. Urinary and, at times, serum calcium and phosphate are elevated. Serum alkaline phosphatase is often elevated. In patients with Graves' disease, thyroid-stimulating immunoglobulins (TSI) are often present in serum and tests for antithyroid antibodies (antimicrosomal and antithyroglobulin) are also positive. TSH is low and fails to rise after TRF administration.

**C. Imaging:** Skeletal changes include diffuse

demineralization or, at times, resorptive changes (osteitis). Hypertrophic osteoarthropathy with proliferation of periosteal bone may be present, especially in the hands (acropachy). CT or MRI scans of the orbit shows swelling of the extraocular muscles in cases of Graves' ophthalmopathy.

**D. Electrocardiographic Findings:** Electrocardiography may show tachycardia, atrial fibrillation, and P and T wave changes.

## Differential Diagnosis

A difficult differentiation is between hyperthyroidism and anxiety neurosis, especially in the menopause. Subacute thyroiditis may present with toxic symptoms, and the gland is usually quite tender. The thyroid antibody tests may be positive; $T_4$ may be elevated, but radioiodine uptake is very low. Exogenous thyroid administration will present the same laboratory features as thyroiditis. A rare pituitary tumor may produce the picture of thyrotoxicosis with high levels of TSH.

A hypermetabolic state due mainly to overproduction of $T_3$ has been described (''$T_3$ thyrotoxicosis''). The $T_4$ is normal or low and the radioiodine uptake is normal or moderately elevated but fails to be suppressed by $T_3$ administration. Serum $T_3$ is elevated.

Some states of hypermetabolism without thyrotoxicosis, notably severe anemia, leukemia, polycythemia, and cancer, rarely cause confusion. Pheochromocytoma and acromegaly, however, may be associated with hypermetabolism, enlargement of the thyroid, and profuse sweating. Appropriate laboratory tests will easily distinguish these entities.

Cardiac disease (eg, atrial fibrillation, failure) refractory to treatment with digitalis, quinidine, or diuretics suggests the possibility of underlying hyperthyroidism. Other causes of ophthalmoplegia (eg, myasthenia gravis) and exophthalmos (eg, orbital tumor) must be considered. Thyrotoxicosis must also be considered in the differential diagnosis of muscle wasting diseases and diffuse bone atrophy. Hypercalciuria and bone demineralization may resemble hyperparathyroidism. The 2 diseases may be present in the same patient. Diabetes mellitus and Addison's disease may coexist with thyrotoxicosis.

## Complications

The ocular and cardiac complications of longstanding thyrotoxicosis are most serious. Severe malnutrition and wasting with cachexia may become irreversible. If jaundice is present, the mortality rate increases. Episodes of periodic paralysis induced by exercise or heavy carbohydrate ingestion and accompanied by hypokalemia may complicate thyrotoxicosis in Orientals. Thyroid ''storm'' (see above) is rarely seen but may be fatal. Hypercalcemia and nephrocalcinosis may occur. Decreased libido, impotence, decreased sperm count, and gynecomastia are often found in men with Graves' disease. Complications of treatment for goiter include drug reactions following iodine and thiouracil treatment, hypoparathyroidism and laryn-

geal palsy after surgical treatment, and progressive exophthalmos. The exophthalmos may progress, despite adequate therapy, to the point of corneal ulceration and destruction of the globe unless orbital decompression is done.

## Treatment

Treatment is aimed at halting excessive secretion of the thyroid hormone. Several methods are available; the method of choice is still being debated and varies with different patients. The most widely accepted method in the past has been subtotal thyroidectomy after adequate preparation. There is a greater tendency toward trying long-term medical treatment with antithyroid drugs to achieve remission of the disease and to use radioactive iodine therapy rather than surgical thyroidectomy for thyroid ablation except for large multinodular glands. The age of the patient and reproductive history and wishes are important considerations. Children and young adults who have not yet had children are better treated with antithyroid drugs rather than with radioactive iodine. If medical therapy fails or the gland is very large, subtotal thyroidectomy should be strongly considered, subject to the availability of a skilled and experienced thyroid surgeon. It should be pointed out that even among experts, there is wide divergence of opinion as to the ''definitive'' treatment of Graves' disease, especially in the young.

**A. Subtotal Thyroidectomy:** Adequate preparation is of the utmost importance. One or 2 drugs are generally necessary for adequate preparation: one of the thiouracil group of drugs alone, or, preferably, a thiouracil plus iodine. The sympatholytic agent propranolol has been used successfully as the sole agent before surgery. This drug, however, does not return the patient to a normal metabolic rate, and most experts prefer to render the patient euthyroid prior to surgery.

**1. Preoperative use of thiouracil and similar drugs**–Several thiouracil drugs are available: propylthiouracil, methimazole, and carbimazole. The modes of action are probably identical. These agents block the intrathyroidal synthesis of hormone. Propylthiouracil has also been shown to impede the peripheral conversion of $T_4$ to $T_3$, and carbimazole has been recently described as decreasing autoimmune response in Graves' disease.

**Propylthiouracil** has been most widely used and appears to be the least toxic. It is the thiouracil preparation of choice. The $T_4$ invariably falls, the rate of fall depending upon the total quantity of previously manufactured hormone available from the gland. (More hormone is present if iodine has been given previously.) The average time required for the $T_4$ to return to normal is about 4–6 weeks. If the drug dose is not tapered, the $T_4$ will continue to fall until the patient becomes myxedematous.

Preparation is usually continued and surgery deferred until the $T_4$ and $T_3$ uptake are normal. There is no need to rush surgery and no danger of ''escape'' as with iodine. In severe cases, 100–200 mg 4 times daily (spaced as close to every 6 hours as possible) is generally adequate. Larger doses (eg, for patients with very large glands) are occasionally necessary. In milder cases, 100 mg 3 times daily is sufficient.

Propylthiouracil appears to be an ideal drug to prepare the patient for thyroidectomy except for 2 disadvantages: the danger of toxic reactions (especially agranulocytosis) and interference with surgery. Toxic reactions to propylthiouracil are rare, however. In practice, patients are instructed to watch for fever, sore throat, or rash and to notify their physicians immediately if any of these occurs, so that blood count and examination can be performed. If the white count falls below 3000/$\mu$L or if less than 45% granulocytes are present, therapy should be discontinued. Other rare reactions are drug fever, rash, and jaundice. The second objection is of a technical nature; since the gland may remain hyperplastic and vascular, surgical removal is more difficult. For this reason, combined therapy, using propylthiouracil and iodine, is the method of choice in preparing patients for thyroidectomy (see below).

**Methimazole (Tapazole)** has a mode of action similar to that of the thiouracils. The average dose is 10–15 mg every 8 hours. The smaller dosage is no guarantee against toxic reactions, especially skin rash, which are more common with this drug than with the thiouracils.

**Carbimazole** (not available in the USA but commonly used in Europe) is rapidly converted to methimazole and is similar in action. The average dose is 10–15 mg every 8 hours. Toxic side effects are slightly more common with this drug.

**2. Preoperative use of iodine–**Iodine is given in daily dosages of 5–10 drops of strong iodine solution (Lugol's solution) or saturated solution of potassium iodide with nonspecific therapy (see below) until the $T_4$ has dropped toward normal, the signs and symptoms have become less marked, and the patient has begun to gain weight. The disadvantages of preparation with iodine are that (1) a few patients may not respond, especially those who have received iodine recently; (2) sensitivity to iodides may be present; (3) if there is too long a wait before surgery, the gland may "escape" and the patient may develop a more severe hyperthyroidism than before; and (4) it is generally impossible to reduce the $T_4$ to normal with iodine alone.

**3. Combined propylthiouracil-iodine therapy–**The advantage of this method is that one obtains the complete inhibition of thyroid secretion with the involuting effect of iodine. This can be done in one of 2 ways:

**Propylthiouracil followed by iodine** appears at present to be the preoperative method of choice. Begin therapy with propylthiouracil; about 10–21 days before surgery is contemplated (when all thyroid tests have returned to normal or low normal range), begin the iodine and *continue* for 1 week after surgery.

**Concomitant administration** of the 2 drugs from the start in dosages as for the individual drugs, ie, propylthiouracil, 100–200 mg 4 times daily, and strong iodine solution, 10–15 drops daily. This method is less commonly used and less desirable than sequential administration (outlined above).

Patients who fail to be euthyroid after subtotal thyroidectomy can be re-treated with propylthiouracil or with radioiodine.

**4. Propranolol–**This drug may be used alone for the preoperative preparation of the patient in doses of 80–240 mg daily. It is the most rapid way of reversing some of the seemingly catecholamine-mediated toxic manifestations of the disease, and less time is necessary to prepare the patient for thyroidectomy. It has been suggested as the treatment of choice for thyrotoxicosis in pregnancy. Since it does not reverse the hypermetabolic state itself, escape and even thyroid storm may occur in patients so prepared. It should not be used in patients with bronchial asthma, and it should be employed with extreme caution if congestive heart failure seems likely to develop.

**B. Continuous Propylthiouracil Therapy (Medical Treatment):** Control of hyperthyroidism with propylthiouracil alone is often the treatment of choice, especially in young people, who are not good candidates for $^{131}$I therapy. The advantage is that it avoids the risks and postoperative complications of surgery, eg, laryngeal palsy, hypoparathyroidism. The disadvantage is the remote possibility of toxic reactions plus the necessity of watching the patient carefully for signs of hypothyroidism. Since the advent of propylthiouracil, it appears that the incidence of toxic reactions is slight. It had been thought that some patients were "resistant" to the effects of propylthiouracil, but the problem is one of compliance in taking the medication.

Begin with 100–200 mg every 6–8 hours and continue until the $T_4$ and $T_3$ uptake are normal and all signs and symptoms of the disease have subsided; then place the patient on a maintenance dose of 50–150 mg daily, observing the thyroid function tests periodically to avoid hypothyroidism.

An alternative method is to continue with doses of 50–200 mg every 6–8 hours until the patient becomes hypothyroid and then maintain the $T_4$ at normal levels with thyroid hormone.

The optimal duration of therapy and the recurrence rate with medical therapy have not been completely worked out. At present it would seem that of the patients kept on propylthiouracil between 18 and 24 months (the dosage slowly decreased), about 30–50% will have no recurrence. Patients with large thyroid glands that fail to decrease in size with medical therapy have a greater chance of recurrence of thyrotoxicosis after cessation of therapy. In some laboratories, the levels of thyroid-stimulating immunoglobulins (TSI) have been helpful in predicting outcome of medical therapy. Those having recurrences after cessation of treatment may be treated again with propylthiouracil, with radioiodine, or with surgery. Many patients remaining euthyroid after discontinuation of therapy may develop hypothyroidism spontaneously in subsequent decades. They should all have reevaluation of thyroid status at regular intervals.

**C. Radioactive Iodine ($^{131}$I):** The administration of radioiodine has proved to be an excellent method for destruction of overfunctioning thyroid tissue (either diffuse or toxic nodular goiter). The rationale of treatment is that the radioiodine, being concentrated in the thyroid, will destroy the cells that concentrate it. The only objections to date to radioiodine therapy are the possibility of carcinogenesis and the possibility of damage to the genetic pool of the individual treated. Studies to date have failed to show evidence of these effects. Nevertheless, the use of radioiodine is generally limited to older age groups (30 or above); however, the age level is not absolute, and some children may be best treated with radioiodine. *Do not use this drug in pregnant women.* There is a high incidence of hypothyroidism several years after this form of treatment, even when small doses are given (see Sridama reference, below). Prolonged follow-up, preferably with $T_4$ and TSH measurements, is therefore mandatory. There is a greater tendency toward higher-dosage radioiodine ablation of the toxic gland, with subsequent permanent replacement therapy with thyroid hormone. If smaller doses are used initially, retreatment may be required and myxedema may still occur several years later.

**D. General Measures:**

1. The patient with hyperthyroidism should not engage in strenuous activities. In severe cases, bed rest may be necessary. Mild cases may be treated with propylthiouracil or radioiodine on an ambulatory basis.

2. Diet should be high in calories, proteins, and vitamins. Hyperthyroid patients consume great quantities of food, are generally in negative nitrogen and calcium balance, and need the excess foods and vitamins because of their increased metabolic needs. Supplemental vitamin B complex should be given.

3. Sedation–When first seen, these patients are often very nervous. Sedation is sometimes necessary, eg, phenobarbital, 30 mg 3–6 times daily.

4. Since many signs resemble the effects of catecholamines, sympathetic blocking agents (reserpine, guanethidine, propranolol) have been recommended. Propranolol is especially useful in rapidly controlling tachycardia and cardiac irregularities, but it must be used cautiously in incipient or frank failure. It is especially effective in patients with neuromuscular signs, eg, periodic paralysis or upper motor neuron signs.

**E. Treatment of Complications:**

**1. Exophthalmos**–The exact cause of exophthalmos in Graves' disease is still not known. It has been shown that exophthalmos is due to edema and cellular infiltration of the orbital muscles, possibly because of an autoimmune reaction that may be facilitated by lymphatic channel communication between the thyroid gland and the ocular orbits. The onset and severity of this ocular complication bears no relationship to the hypermetabolic state. Removing the thyroid secretion (extirpation or administration of propylthiouracil) does not necessarily help this condition and may possibly even aggravate it, leading to malignant exophthalmos. It has been suggested that this is because the thyroid secretion exerts an inhibitory effect on the anterior pituitary, and removal of the gland allows the anterior pituitary to secrete more hormones and aggravate the condition. However, since the pituitary TSH levels are *always* low in thyrotoxicosis due to Graves' disease, it is questionable whether thyroid therapy is of use unless the patient is becoming hypothyroid.

a. Dark glasses, protection from dust, eye shields, tarsorrhaphy, and other measures may be necessary to protect the eyes. Elevation of the head of the bed at night, diuretics, and local use of methylcellulose solution (1%) to prevent drying of the protruding eyes are helpful. Ophthalmologic consultation should be requested.

b. Corticotropin (ACTH) or corticosteroids in large doses (60–100 mg of prednisone daily) have proved helpful in some cases. They act by reducing the inflammatory reaction in the periorbital tissues. They may also reduce the level of autoimmune activity. Unfortunately, relapse occurs frequently when the drug is discontinued, and the severe side effects of high-dose glucocorticoid therapy preclude prolonged therapy.

c. Surgery for malignant exophthalmos–Every patient with exophthalmos should be measured periodically with an exophthalmometer; do not rely upon clinical judgment to determine whether or not exophthalmos is present or progressing. In severe progressive cases, where corneal edema or ulceration, limitation of extraocular muscle movements, and failing vision occur, orbital decompression may be necessary to save the eyesight.

d. Orbital irradiation may be helpful and should be considered in severe cases. Immunosuppressive therapy has also been suggested, but the evidence in its favor is scanty and inconclusive.

**2. Cardiac complications**–A number of cardiac complications are at times associated with hyperthyroidism.

a. Some degree of tachycardia is almost always found if normal rhythm is present in thyrotoxicosis. This requires only the treatment of the thyrotoxicosis. Severe tachycardia responds promptly to propranolol therapy.

b. Congestive failure tends to occur in longstanding thyrotoxicosis, especially in the older age groups. Treatment is the same as for congestive failure due to any cause.

c. Atrial fibrillation may occur in association with thyrotoxicosis. Treat as any other atrial fibrillation, but do not try to convert the atrial fibrillation in a toxic patient. Most cases will revert to normal rhythm soon after toxicity is removed. However, if fibrillation remains for 2 weeks after surgery or for 2–4 weeks after $T_4$ or other thyroid function tests have returned to normal with propylthiouracil therapy, and if no contraindications are present, one should consider conversion to a normal rhythm.

**3. "Crisis" or "storm"**–Fortunately, this condition is rare with modern therapy. It occurs now mainly in patients inadequately prepared with propylthiouracil and iodine, those with complicating infection, immediately after subtotal thyroidectomy, or, rarely, after [131]I therapy. It can occur spontaneously or after stress such as trauma, infection, or parturition in an untreated patient with thyrotoxicosis. It is characterized by high fever, tachycardia, central nervous system irritability, and delirium. The cause is uncertain, though factors such as tissue hypoxia, hyperactivity of the adrenergic system, and decreased binding of thyroid hormones in blood have been postulated. It has also occurred after exposure of the thyrotoxic patient to iodinated materials, with rapid increase of thyroid hormone synthesis.

Therapy of thyroid storm is multifactorial. Treat aggressively any precipitating illness (infection, ketoacidosis, etc). Give large doses of antithyroid drugs, by nasogastric tube if necessary. Propylthiouracil, 1000–1500 mg daily in divided doses, is of crucial importance. Administer iodine to block release of thyroid hormone from glandular stores. Give large doses of $\beta$-adrenergic blocking agents, eg, propranolol (60–120 mg every 6 hours) to block adrenergic-mediated effects of thyroid hormone and to decrease synthesis of $T_3$ from $T_4$. Intravenous propranolol may be necessary, with careful monitoring of cardiac rhythm and function. Large doses of glucocorticoids (hydrocortisone hemisuccinate, 300–500 mg/d) have traditionally been used in these patients, who are at risk of developing adrenal insufficiency. Glucocorticoids may inhibit the peripheral transformation of $T_4$ to $T_3$ and should be of help.

Plasmapheresis has been used in cases not responsive to the above measures. Cholestyramine, which binds thyroid hormone in the gut, is an alternative drug. General measures consist of oxygen, cold packs, sedation, glucose infusions, multivitamins, and careful monitoring of the state of hydration, electrolyte balance, etc. Therapy is best carried out in an intensive care unit.

**4. Dermopathy**–Severe pretibial myxedema, an uncommon complication of Graves' disease, responds well to local glucocorticoid therapy.

## Prognosis

Graves' disease is a cyclic entity and may subside spontaneously and may even result in spontaneous hypothyroidism. More commonly, however, it progresses, especially with recurrent psychic trauma and other types of stress. The ocular, cardiac, and psychic complications often are more serious than the chronic wasting of tissues and may become irreversible even after treatment. Progressive exophthalmos is perhaps more common after surgical than after medical treatment. Permanent hypoparathyroidism and vocal cord palsy are risks of surgical thyroidectomy. With any form of therapy, unless radical thyroidectomy or large dosage [131]I therapy is used, recurrences are common. With adequate treatment and long-term follow-up, the results are good. It is perhaps wiser to speak of induced remission rather than cure. Posttreatment hypothyroidism is common. It may occur several years after radioactive iodine therapy or subtotal thyroidectomy. Use of [131]I to treat Graves' disease has not resulted in any demonstrable increase of thyroid cancer, leukemia, or other cancers.

Patients with jaundice and fever have a less favorable prognosis. Thyrotoxic periodic paralysis with hypokalemia—to which males of Oriental background are predisposed—may alter the prognosis. Periorbital swelling and chemosis often precede serious and progressive malignant exophthalmos leading to blindness, and they must be watched for carefully.

Thyroid storm (rare) has the worst prognosis. It is best avoided by careful preoperative preparation of the patient rather than treated once it appears.

Becker DV: Choice of therapy for Graves' hyperthyroidism. (Editorial.) *N Engl J Med* 1984;**311**:464.

Burrow GN: The management of thyrotoxicosis in pregnancy. (Current Concepts.) *N Engl J Med* 1985;**313**:562.

Cooper DS: Antithyroid drugs. *N Engl J Med* 1984;**311**:1353.

Dunn JT: Choice of therapy in young adults with hyperthyroidism of Graves' disease. *Ann Intern Med* 1984;**100**:891.

Fradkin JE, Wolff J: Iodide-induced thyrotoxicosis. *Medicine* 1983;**62**:1.

Gruebeck-Loebenstein B et al: Immunological features of non-immunogenic hyperthyroidism. *J Clin Endocrinol Metab* 1985;**60**:150.

Himsworth RL: Hyperthyroidism with a low iodine uptake. *Clin Endocrinol Metab* 1985;**14**:397.

Jacobson DH, Gorman CA: Endocrine ophthalmopathy: Current ideas concerning etiology, pathogenesis and treatment. *Endocr Rev* 1984;**5**:200.

Kriss JP, McDougall IR, Donaldson SS: Graves' ophthalmopathy. In: *Current Therapy in Endocrinology 1983–1984.* Krieger DT, Bardin CW (editors). Mosby, 1983.

Smallridge RC et al: Hyperthyroidism due to TSH-secreting pituitary tumors. *Arch Intern Med* 1983;**143**:503.

Smith LH, Rapoport B: The ophthalmopathy of Graves' disease. *West J Med* 1985;**142**:532.

Toft AD (editor): Hyperthyroidism. (Symposium.) *Clin Endocrinol Metab* 1985;**14(2)**:May. [Entire issue.]

Wartofsky L: Thyrotoxic storm. In: *The Thyroid: A Fundamental and Clinical Text,* 5th ed. Ingbar SH, Braverman LE (editors). Lippincott, 1986.

Weetman AP, McGregor AM: Autoimmune thyroid disease: Developments in our understanding. *Endocr Rev* 1984;**5**:309.

## THYROID NODULES & THYROID CANCER

### Essentials of Diagnosis

- Painless swelling in region of thyroid, or thyroid nodule not responding to suppression. Normal thyroid function tests.
- Past history of irradiation to neck, goiter, or thyroiditis.
- Positive thyroid needle aspiration.

## General Considerations
## (Table 18–8)

Although carcinoma of the thyroid is rarely associated with functional abnormalities, it enters into the differential diagnosis of all types of thyroid lesions. It is common in all age groups, but especially in patients who have received radiation therapy in childhood or infancy to the neck structures (eg, thymus gland). The cell type determines to a large extent the type of therapy required and the prognosis for survival. The most common varieties are papillary and follicular carcinomas, which are usually associated with prolonged survival. The anaplastic tumor is rare and carries a very bad prognosis. Finally, the medullary carcinoma of the thyroid originates in the parafollicular cells derived from the last branchial pouch, contains amyloid deposits, and secretes calcitonin. It is familial and often associated with pheochromocytomas (multiple endocrine neoplasia type II) and with the syndrome of multiple mucosal neuromas (multiple endocrine neoplasia type III). Other tumors of the thyroid, much less common than those mentioned above, include lymphomas, primary sarcomas, and teratomas.

## Clinical Findings

**A. Symptoms and Signs:** The principal signs of thyroid cancer are a painless nodule, a hard nodule in an enlarged thyroid gland, so-called lateral aberrant thyroid tissue, or palpable lymph nodes with thyroid enlargement. Signs of pressure or invasion of the neck structures are present in anaplastic or long-standing tumors.

**B. Laboratory Findings:** With very few exceptions, all thyroid function tests are normal unless the disease is associated with thyroiditis. The scintiscan usually shows a "cold" nodule. Serum thyroid autoantibodies are sometimes found. Thyroglobulin levels are high in metastatic papillary and follicular tumors. In medullary carcinoma, the calcitonin levels are elevated, especially after a calcium infusion. Calcitonin assay is a reliable clue to silent medullary carcinoma, especially in the familial syndrome, although an occasional extrathyroidal tumor (eg, lung) may also produce calcitonin. An excellent technique for determining the nature of a thyroid nodule is fine-needle aspiration biopsy. It requires the services of an experienced cytopathologist.

**C. Imaging:** Extensive bone and soft tissue metastases (some of which may take up radioiodine) may be demonstrable on radiographs. Calcified areas may be seen in medullary carcinoma (primary tumor or metastases).

## Differential Diagnosis
## (Table 18–9)

Since nonmalignant enlargements of the thyroid gland are far more common than carcinoma, it is at times most difficult to establish the diagnosis except by biopsy (which may be an open biopsy or a needle biopsy). Echography may be helpful in differentiating cystic and solid nodules. Purely cystic lesions are very frequently benign. The incidence of malignancy is much greater in single than in multinodular lesions, and far greater in nonfunctioning than in functioning nodules. The differentiation from chronic thyroiditis is at times most difficult, and the 2 lesions may occur together. Any nonfunctioning lesion in the region of the thyroid that does not decrease in size on thyroid therapy or increases rapidly must be considered carcinoma until proved otherwise. Percutaneous needle aspiration biopsy has been very useful in diagnosis.

## Complications

The complications vary with the type of carcinoma. Papillary tumors invade local structures, such as lymph nodes; follicular tumors metastasize through the bloodstream; anaplastic carcinomas invade local structures, causing constriction and nerve palsies, as well as leading to widespread metastases. Medullary carcinomas may be complicated by the coexistence of pheochromocytomas. The complications of radical

**Table 18–8.** Some characteristics of thyroid cancer.

|  | Papillary | Follicular | Medullary | Anaplastic |
|---|---|---|---|---|
| Incidence* (%) | 61 | 18 | 6 | 15 |
| Average age* | 42 | 50 | 50 | 57 |
| Females* (%) | 70 | 72 | 56 | 56 |
| Deaths due to thyroid cancer*† (%) | 6 | 24 | 33 | 98 |
| Invasion: Juxtanodal | +++++ | + | ++++++ | +++ |
|     Blood vessels | + | +++ | +++ | +++++ |
|     Distant sites | + | +++ | ++ | ++++ |
| Resemblance to normal thyroid | + | +++ | + | ± |
| $^{123}$I uptake | + | ++++ | 0 | 0 |
| Degree of malignancy | + | ++ to +++ | +++ | ++++++++ |

\* Data based upon 885 cases analyzed by Woolner et al; figures have been rounded to the nearest digit. (After Woolner.)
† Some patients have been followed up to 32 years after diagnosis.

**Table 18–9.** Differential diagnosis of thyroid nodules.*

| Clinical Evidence | Low Index of Suspicion | High Index of Suspicion |
|---|---|---|
| History | Familial history of goiter<br>Residence in area of endemic goiter | Previous therapeutic irradiation of head, neck, or chest<br>Hoarseness |
| Physical characteristics | Older women<br>Soft nodule<br>Multinodular goiter | Children, young adults; men<br>Solitary, firm, dominant nodule<br>Vocal cord paralysis<br>Enlarged lymph nodes<br>Distant metastatic lesions |
| Serum factors | High titer of antithyroid antibody | Elevated serum calcitonin |
| Scanning techniques<br>Uptake of $^{123}$I<br>Echo scan<br>Thermography<br>Roentgenogram<br><br>Technetium flow | "Hot" nodule<br>Cystic lesion<br>Cold<br>Shell-like calcification<br>Avascular | "Cold" nodule<br>Solid lesion<br>Warm<br>Punctate calcification<br>Vascular |
| Thyroxine therapy | Regression after 0.2 mg/d for 3 months or more | No regression |

* Reproduced, with permission, from Greenspan FS: Thyroid nodules and thyroid cancer. *West J Med* 1974;**121**:359.

neck surgery often include permanent hypoparathyroidism, vocal cord palsy, and myxedema.

## Treatment

Surgical removal is the treatment of choice for most thyroid carcinomas. The appropriate extent of surgical removal is debatable. In recent years, conservative surgery has been shown to be as effective as radical neck dissection, with a much lower incidence of complications. $^{131}$I has been used by most as an adjunct to surgical therapy, but there is no agreement among experts about the clear-cut indications, timing, or dosage. The protracted course of most thyroid cancers, with or without therapy, has made it difficult to establish a consensus for optimal therapy. Thyroxine administration to suppress TSH to undetectable levels is also useful as adjunct therapy for papillary and follicular cancers. External irradiation may be useful for local as well as distant metastases. Postoperative hypoparathyroidism must be treated in the usual manner.

Reports of chemotherapy of inoperable tumors with doxorubicin are encouraging, but the drug is fairly toxic.

## Prognosis

The prognosis is directly related to the cell type. The anaplastic carcinomas advance rapidly in spite of early diagnosis and treatment, while papillary tumors—in spite of frequent bouts of recurrence—are almost never fatal. Early detection and removal of medullary carcinomas by finding elevated calcitonin levels may lead to a better prognosis. In general, the prognosis is less favorable in elderly patients.

Bell RM: Thyroid carcinoma. *Surg Clin North Am* 1986;**66**:13.

Blum M: The diagnosis of the thyroid nodule using aspiration biopsy and cytology. (Editorial.) *Arch Intern Med* 1984;**144**:1140.

Crile G et al: The advantages of subtotal thyroidectomy and suppression of TSH in the primary treatment of papillary carcinoma of the thyroid. *Cancer* 1985;**55**:2691.

Frable WJ: *Fine Needle Aspiration Biopsy.* Saunders, 1983.

Mazzaferri EI, Young RL: Papillary thyroid carcinoma: A 10-year follow-up report of the impact of therapy in 576 patients. *Am J Med* 1981;**70**:511.

Molitch ME et al: The cold thyroid nodule: An analysis of diagnostic and therapeutic options. *Endocr Rev* 1984;**5**:185.

Rojeski MT, Gharib H: Nodular thyroid disease: Evaluation and management. *N Engl J Med* 1985;**313**:428.

Saad MF et al: Medullary carcinoma of the thyroid: A study of the clinical features and prognosis factors in 161 patients. *Medicine* 1984;**63**:319.

## THYROIDITIS

### Essentials of Diagnosis

- Swelling of thyroid gland, causing pressure symptoms in acute and subacute forms; painless enlargement in chronic form.
- Thyroid function tests variable; discrepancy in $T_4$ and radioiodine uptake common.
- Serologic autoantibody tests often positive.

### General Considerations

Thyroiditis has been more frequently diagnosed in recent years, since special serologic tests for thyroid autoantibodies became available. This heterogeneous group can be divided into 2 groups: (1) due to a specific cause (usually infection), and (2) due to unknown, often autoimmune factors. The second is the more common form.

### Clinical Findings

**A. Symptoms and Signs:**

**1. Thyroiditis due to specific causes (pyogenic infections, tuberculosis, syphilis)—**A rare disorder causing severe pain, tenderness, redness, and fluctuation in the region of the thyroid gland.

**2. Nonspecific (?autoimmune) thyroiditis—**

**a. Acute or subacute nonsuppurative thyroiditis** (de Quervain's thyroiditis, granulomatous thyroiditis, giant cell thyroiditis, giant follicular thyroiditis)—An acute, usually painful enlargement of the thyroid gland, with dysphagia. The pain radiates into the ears. The manifestations may persist for several weeks and may be associated with signs of thyrotoxicosis and malaise. Middle-aged women are most commonly affected. Viral infection has been suggested as the cause. Transient irradiation thyroiditis may be seen after radioactive iodine therapy.

**b. Lymphocytic subacute thyroiditis** (lymphocytic thyroiditis with hyperthyroidism, atypical subacute thyroiditis)—This form of thyroiditis, characterized by a silent (painless) swelling of the thyroid and associated with symptoms and signs of hyperthyroidism, is being increasingly recognized in the USA. The clinical manifestations are similar to those of moderate Graves' disease, and the differential diagnosis is not simple. Both may present with symmetric, painless, modest enlargement of the thyroid, tremor, weight loss, stare, lid lag, etc, as well as elevated levels of serum $T_4$. Antibody titers (antithyroglobulin and antithyroid microsomal) are higher in Graves' disease. The $^{123}$I uptake is *low* in this form of thyroiditis and *high* in Graves' disease. The hyperthyroid symptoms abate spontaneously, and normalcy is restored within a few months. The transient hyperthyroid state is due to leakage of preformed thyroid hormone from the inflamed gland and not to hyperactivity of the thyroid cells. These patients, therefore, should *not* receive propylthiouracil. Propranolol is useful for symptomatic control of the hyperthyroid phase. The etiology of this entity is unknown.

**c. Postpartum thyroiditis** is a form of autoimmune thyroiditis occurring soon after parturition and accompanied by transient hyperthyroidism followed by hypothyroidism. It has been described in women with thyroid autoimmune disease who had suppression of antibody titers during pregnancy and a rebound of immune activity after delivery.

**d. Hashimoto's thyroiditis** (struma lymphomatosa, lymphadenoid goiter, chronic lymphocytic thyroiditis)—The most common form of thyroiditis and probably the most common thyroid disorder. Evidence for an autoimmune cause is uniformly present. Onset of enlargement of the thyroid gland is insidious, with few pressure symptoms. The gland is firm, symmetrically enlarged, lobulated, and nontender to palpation. Signs of thyroid dysfunction seldom appear, but rarely the disease may progress to myxedema or even present as thyrotoxicosis ("hashitoxicosis"), which may be transient.

**e. Riedel's thyroiditis** (chronic fibrous thyroiditis, Riedel's struma, woody thyroiditis, ligneous thyroiditis, invasive thyroiditis)—This is the rarest form of thyroiditis and is found only in middle-aged women. Enlargement is often asymmetric; the gland is stony hard and adherent to the neck structures, causing signs of compression and invasion, including dysphagia, dyspnea, and hoarseness.

**B. Laboratory Findings:** The $T_4$ and $T_3$ resin uptake are usually markedly elevated in acute and subacute thyroiditis and normal or low in the chronic forms. Radioiodine uptake is characteristically very low in subacute thyroiditis; it may be high with an uneven scan in chronic thyroiditis with enlargement of the gland, and low in Riedel's struma. The TSH stimulation test shows lack of response in most forms of thyroiditis. Leukocytosis, elevation of the sedimentation rate, and increase in serum globulins are common in acute and subacute forms. Thyroid autoantibodies are most commonly demonstrable in Hashimoto's thyroiditis but are also found in the other types. The serum TSH level is elevated if inadequate amounts of biologically active thyroid hormones are elaborated by the thyroid gland.

## Complications

In the suppurative forms of thyroiditis, any of the complications of infection may occur; the subacute and chronic forms of the disease are complicated by the effects of pressure on the neck structures: dyspnea and, in Riedel's struma, vocal cord palsy. Hashimoto's thyroiditis often leads to hypothyroidism. Carcinoma or lymphoma may be associated with chronic thyroiditis and must be considered in the diagnosis of uneven painless enlargements that continue in spite of treatment. Hashimoto's thyroiditis may be associated with Addison's disease (Schmidt's syndrome), hypoparathyroidism, diabetes, pernicious anemia, various collagen diseases, biliary cirrhosis, vitiligo, and other autoimmune conditions. Mitral valve prolapse is also much more frequent in patients, with Hashimoto's thyroiditis than in normal persons. The reason for this is unknown.

## Differential Diagnosis

Thyroiditis must be considered in the differential diagnosis of all types of goiters, especially if enlargement is rapid. In the acute or subacute stages it may simulate thyrotoxicosis, and only a careful evaluation of several of the laboratory findings will point to the correct diagnosis. The very low radioiodine uptake in subacute thyroiditis with elevated $T_4$ and $T_3$ uptake and a rapid sedimentation rate is of the greatest help. Chronic thyroiditis, especially if the enlargement is uneven and if there is pressure on surrounding structures, may resemble carcinoma, and both disorders may be present in the same gland. The subacute and suppurative forms of thyroiditis may resemble any infectious process in or near the neck structures; and the presence of malaise, leukocytosis, and a high sedimentation rate is confusing. The thyroid autoantibody tests have been of help in the diagnosis of chronic thyroiditis, but the tests are not specific and may also be positive in patients with goiters, carcinoma, and thyrotoxicosis. Biopsy may be required for diagnosis.

## Treatment

**A. Suppurative Thyroiditis:** Antibiotics, and surgical drainage when fluctuation is marked.

**B. Subacute Thyroiditis:**

**1. De Quervain's thyroiditis**—All treatment is empiric and must be maintained for several weeks, since the recurrence rate is high. The drug of choice is aspirin, which relieves pain and inflammation. Severe cases may require a brief course of prednisone therapy: 10 mg 3 times a day for 1 or 2 weeks is effective, but symptoms and signs may recur after the drug is tapered off. Levothyroxine, propylthiouracil, and external x-ray neck irradiation have been used in the past, but there are no convincing data to justify their use.

**2. Lymphocytic thyroiditis** with hyperthyroidism does not require the use of anti-inflammatory agents. The symptoms of hyperthyroidism may be treated with propranolol. If hypothyroidism develops later, thyroid replacement therapy is indicated.

**C. Hashimoto's Thyroiditis:** Levothyroxine should be given in the usual doses (0.1–0.15 mg daily) if hypothyroidism or large goiter is present. If the thyroid gland is only minimally enlarged and the patient is euthyroid (with *normal* TSH levels), regular observation is in order, since approximately 10–15% of patients will develop hypothyroidism in future years.

**D. Riedel's Struma:** Partial thyroidectomy is often required to relieve pressure; adhesions to surrounding structures make this a difficult operation.

### Prognosis

The course of this group of diseases is quite variable. Spontaneous remissions and exacerbations are common in the subacute form, and therapy is nonspecific. The disease process may smolder for months. Thyrotoxicosis may occur. Hashimoto's thyroiditis may be associated with other autoimmune disorders (diabetes mellitus, Addison's disease, etc), with all the complications of those diseases. In general, however, patients with Hashimoto's thyroiditis have an excellent prognosis, since the condition either remains stable for years or progresses to hypothyroidism, which is easily treated. Rarely, lymphoma of the thyroid may complicate Hashimoto's thyroiditis.

Hamburger JI: The various presentations of thyroiditis: Diagnostic considerations. *Ann Intern Med* 1986;**104**:219.

Klein I et al: Silent thyrotoxic thyroiditis. *Ann Intern Med* 1982;**96**:242.

Marks AD et al: Chronic thyroiditis and mitral valve prolapse. *Ann Intern Med* 1985;**102**:479.

# THE PARATHYROIDS

## HYPOPARATHYROIDISM & PSEUDOHYPOPARATHYROIDISM

### Essentials of Diagnosis

- Tetany, carpopedal spasms, stridor and wheezing, muscle and abdominal cramps, urinary frequency, personality changes, mental torpor.
- Positive Chvostek's sign and Trousseau's phenomenon; defective nails and teeth; cataracts.
- Serum calcium low; serum phosphate high; alkaline phosphatase normal; urine calcium excretion reduced.
- Basal ganglia calcification on x-ray of skull.

### General Considerations

**Hypoparathyroidism** is most commonly seen following thyroidectomy or, more rarely, following surgery for parathyroid tumor. Very rarely it follows x-ray irradiation to the neck or massive radioactive iodine administration for cancer of the thyroid. Partial hypoparathyroidism occurs in a significant number of patients after thyroidectomy. It is rarely associated with hemochromatosis or metastatic cancer.

Transient hypoparathyroidism may be seen in the neonatal period, presumably due to a relative underactivity of the parathyroids, to magnesium deficiency, or to extraordinary demands on the parathyroids by the intake of cow's milk containing a great deal of phosphate. A similar mechanism may operate in the tetany of pregnancy. Hypomagnesemia may cause failure of release of parathyroid hormone and also resistance to hormonal action on bone, resulting in hypocalcemia reversible by magnesium repletion.

Neonatal tetany may be a manifestation of maternal hyperparathyroidism.

Idiopathic hypoparathyroidism, often associated with candidiasis, may be familial and may be associated with Addison's disease and thyroiditis due to an autoimmune disorder (multiple endocrine deficiency, autoimmune, candidiasis [MEDAC] syndrome).

**Pseudohypoparathyroidism** is a genetic defect associated with short stature, round face, obesity, short metacarpals, hypertension, and ectopic bone formation. The parathyroids are present and often hyperplastic, but the renal tubules do not respond to the hormone. This resistance, probably due to a receptor protein defect, may be incomplete and may disappear spontaneously or after restoration of serum calcium to normal. Recent evidence suggests a selective lack of 1,25-dihydroxyvitamin D in pseudohypoparathyroidism. Some investigators have found a biologically abnormal hormone in this disorder or an antagonist to parathyroid hormone. Various unusual syndromes have been described that have some features of Albright's original report (Albright's osteodystrophy) but lack others (pseudopseudohypoparathyroidism, pseudohypoparathyroidism type II, pseudoidiopathic hypoparathyroidism). In some patients, high levels of parathyroid hormone lead to osteitis fibrosa (''pseudohypo-hyperparathyroidism''), which is reversible with treatment with vitamin D. Resistance to other hormones (TSH, gonadotropins, glucagon) may be present in patients with pseudohypoparathyroidism.

### Clinical Findings
### (Table 18–10)

**A. Symptoms and Signs:** Acute hypoparathyroidism causes tetany, with muscle cramps, irritability, carpopedal spasm, and convulsions; stridor,

**Table 18–10.** Principal findings in the various parathyroid syndromes.*

| Syndrome | Low Serum Ca With High Serum P | Serum Alkaline Phosphatase | Cataracts; Calcification of Basal Ganglia | Micro-dactylia; Ectopic Bone | Sub-periosteal Resorption (Osteitis) | Para-thyroid Hyper-plasia | Responds to PTH | PTH Assay |
|---|---|---|---|---|---|---|---|---|
| Hypoparathyroidism | + | Normal | + | 0 | 0 | 0 | + | 0 |
| Pseudohypoparathyroidism | + | Normal | + | + | 0 | + | 0 | Normal or ↑ |
| Pseudopseudohypoparathyroidism | 0 | Normal | 0 | + | 0 | 0 | + | Normal |
| Secondary (renal) hyperparathyroidism | + (NPN ↑) | ↑ | 0 | 0 | + | + | ± | ↑ |
| Pseudohypoparathyroidism with secondary hyperparathyroidism | + (NPN normal) | ↑ | ± | + | + | + | 0 | ↑ |

\* Modified and reproduced, with permission, from Kolb FO, Steinbach HL: Pseudohypoparathyroidism with secondary hyperparathyroidism and osteitis fibrosa. *J Clin Endocrinol Metab* 1962;**22**:68.

wheezing, dyspnea; photophobia and diplopia; abdominal cramps; and urinary frequency. Symptoms of the chronic disease are lethargy, personality changes, anxiety state, blurring of vision due to cataracts, and mental retardation.

Chvostek's sign (facial muscle contraction on tapping the facial nerve near the angle of the jaw) is positive, and Trousseau's phenomenon (carpal spasm after application of a cuff) is present. Cataracts may occur; the nails may be thin and brittle; the skin dry and scaly, at times with fungus infection (candidiasis) and loss of hair (eyebrows); and deep reflexes may be hyperactive. Choreoathetosis may be found in an occasional patient but is reversible with adequate therapy. Choking of the optic disks is rarely found. Teeth may be defective if the onset of the disease occurs in childhood. Branchial anomalies (eg, cleft palate) may be found. In pseudohypoparathyroidism, the fingers and toes are short, with absence of the knuckles of the fourth and fifth fingers on making a fist; ectopic soft tissue calcification may be seen and felt.

**B. Laboratory Findings:** Serum calcium is low, serum phosphate high, urinary phosphate low (tubular reabsorption of phosphate above 95%), urinary calcium low to absent, and alkaline phosphatase normal. Alkaline phosphatase may be elevated in pseudohypoparathyroidism. Creatinine clearance is normal. Parathyroid hormone levels are low or absent in idiopathic or postsurgical hypoparathyroidism but normal or even markedly elevated in pseudohypoparathyroidism.

**C. Imaging:** Radiographs or CT scans of the skull may show basal ganglia calcifications; the bones may be denser than normal. In pseudohypoparathyroidism, short metacarpals and ectopic bone may be seen and bones may be demineralized.

**D. Other Examinations:** Slit lamp examination may show early posterior lenticular cataract formation. The ECG shows generalized dysrhythmia (par-

tially reversible) and may show prolonged QT intervals.

## Complications

Acute tetany with stridor, especially if associated with vocal cord palsy, may lead to respiratory obstruction requiring tracheostomy. Severe hypocalcemia may lead to cardiac dilatation and failure and cardiac irregularities resistant to digitalis. The complications of chronic hypoparathyroidism depend largely upon the duration of the disease and the age at onset. If it starts early in childhood, there may be stunting of growth, malformation of the teeth, and retardation of mental development. There may be associated sprue syndrome, pernicious anemia, and Addison's disease, probably on the basis of an autoimmune mechanism. In pseudohypoparathyroidism, hypothyroidism is often found. In long-standing cases, cataract formation and calcification of the basal ganglia are seen. Ossification of the paravertebral ligaments may occur with nerve root compression; surgical decompression may be required (see Okazaki reference, below). Permanent brain damage with convulsions or psychosis may lead to admission to mental institutions. There may be complications of overtreatment with calcium and vitamin D, with renal impairment and calcinosis.

## Differential Diagnosis

The symptoms of hypocalcemic tetany are most commonly confused with or mistaken for tetany due to metabolic or respiratory alkalosis, in which the serum calcium is normal. Symptoms of anxiety are common in both instances, and fainting is not uncommon in the hyperventilation syndrome. The typical blood and urine findings should differentiate the 2 disorders. With less common causes of hypocalcemic tetany, such as rickets and osteomalacia in the early stages and acute pancreatitis, the serum phosphorus is usually low or low normal and rarely high. Confusion might arise with the tetany due to magnesium deficiency or in chronic renal failure, in which retention of phosphorus will produce a high serum phosphorus with low serum calcium, but the differentiation should be obvious on clinical grounds (eg, uremia).

In primary hyperaldosteronism with tetany (due to alkalosis) there is associated hypertension and hypokalemia with inability to concentrate the urine. Hypomagnesemia must be considered if tetany fails to respond to calcium, especially in critically ill patients.

The physical signs of pseudohypoparathyroidism without the abnormal blood chemical findings are seen in certain dysplasias ("pseudopseudohypoparathyroidism").

In order to differentiate true hypoparathyroidism, which responds to parathyroid extract, from pseudohypoparathyroidism, which does not respond, the Ellsworth-Howard test (phosphaturia after administration of parathyroid hormone intravenously) may be performed. The parathyroid hormone resistance has been demonstrated to be due to failure of activation of renal adenylate cyclase with defective excretion of cAMP after administration of parathyroid hormone. Medullary carcinoma of the thyroid is rarely associated with hypocalcemia in spite of excess calcitonin.

At times hypoparathyroidism is misdiagnosed as idiopathic epilepsy, choreoathetosis, or brain tumor (on the basis of brain calcifications, convulsions, choked disks) or, more rarely, as "asthma" (on the basis of stridor and dyspnea). Other causes of cataracts and basal ganglia calcification also enter into the differential diagnosis.

## Treatment

**A. Emergency Treatment for Acute Attack (Hypoparathyroid Tetany):** This usually occurs after surgery and requires immediate treatment.

1. Be sure an adequate airway is present.

2. Calcium gluconate, 10–20 mL of 10% solution intravenously, may be given slowly until tetany ceases. Ten to 50 mL of 10% calcium gluconate may be added to 1 L of 5% glucose in water or saline and administered by slow intravenous drip. The rate should be so adjusted that the serum calcium is raised above 7 mg/dL and maintained between 8 and 9 mg/dL. *Note:* Do not raise serum calcium above 10.5 mg/dL, or irreversible tissue calcification will occur.

3. Calcium salts should be given orally as soon as possible to supply 1–2 g of calcium daily. Calcium carbonate (40% calcium) is effective and is the calcium salt of choice at present. OsCal, a preparation of calcium carbonate containing 250 mg of calcium, is well tolerated; the dosage is 4–8 tablets per day. Other available calcium preparations include Tums (200-mg tablets), Calcimax (325-mg tablets), and Caltrate (600-mg tablets). Other calcium preparations, such as calcium lactate or gluconate, have low calcium content and are more expensive. Calcium citrate (Citracal) is better absorbed in patients with achlorhydria and is a safer preparation in patients who de-velop hypercalciuria, since it lessens the danger of renal stones. The dose is 6–10 tablets daily.

4. Dihydrotachysterol (Hytakerol) and calci-ferol–Give either compound as soon as oral calcium is begun. Pure crystalline preparations of dihydrota-chysterol in tablets of 0.125, 0.2, and 0.4 mg are available. The initial dose is 0.8–2.4 mg daily for several days. Calciferol, 80,000–160,000 units (2–4 mg) daily, is almost as effective (though slower to act) and probably should be used in most patients. 1,25-Dihydroxycholecalciferol (calcitriol, Rocaltrol) is highly effective in hypoparathyroid tetany in doses of 1–3 $\mu$g/d. It acts most rapidly in reversing hypocalcemia and should be used initially in severe tetany, such as after thyroid or parathyroid surgery. (See Table 18–12.)

5. Phenytoin and phenobarbital have been shown to control overt and latent tetany without alteration in calcium levels. These agents may be used as adjuncts in the management of refractory patients.

**B. Maintenance Treatment:**

1. High-calcium, low-phosphate diet (omit milk and cheese).

2. Calcium salts (as above) are continued.

3. Dihydrotachysterol, 0.2–1 mg daily, to maintain blood calcium at normal level.

4. Calciferol, 40,000–200,000 units (1–5 mg) daily, is the drug of choice at present (rather than dihydrotachysterol) for the majority of patients. In some cases, up to 7 or 8 mg of calciferol daily may be needed. Its action is probably similar to that of dihydrotachysterol, and it can certainly be substituted adequately clinically. The initial action of vitamin D appears to be slower. However, the cost to the patient is less than with dihydrotachysterol. It accumulates in the body over prolonged periods, and serum calcium levels should be checked periodically. *Note:* Corticosteroids are effective antidotes in vitamin D intoxication. The active metabolites of vitamin D (see Table 18–12) may be used if there is unusual resistance to calciferol and in pseudohypoparathyroidism.

5. Aluminum hydroxide gels may be employed to help lower the serum phosphate level in the initial stages of treatment. They are rarely required for chronic therapy.

6. Chlorthalidone, 50 mg/d, combined with a low-sodium diet, may control mild hypoparathyroidism without the use of vitamin D, which would cause more complications.

*Caution:* Phenothiazine drugs should be administered with caution in hypoparathyroid patients, since they may precipitate dystonic reactions. Furosemide should be avoided, since it may enhance hypocalcemia.

## Prognosis

The outlook is fair if prompt diagnosis is made and treatment instituted. Some changes (eg, in the electroencephalogram) are reversible by appropriate treatment, but the dental changes, cataracts, and brain calcifications are permanent. They may be in part genetically determined and not related to hypocalcemia per se. Although treatment of the immediate acute attack is simple and effective, long-term therapy is tedious and expensive, since a good preparation of parathyroid hormone is not available. Adequate control by a fairly intelligent patient is required to avoid undertreatment or overtreatment. Periodic blood chemical evaluation is required, since sudden changes in calcium levels may call for modification of the treatment schedule. Sudden appearance of hypercalcemia, especially in children, may be due to Addison's disease.

Unrecognized or late cases may find their way into mental institutions.

Ahn TG et al: Familial isolated hypoparathyroidism: A molecular genetic analysis of 8 families with 23 affected persons. *Medicine* 1986;**65**:73.

Along U, Chan JC: Hypocalcemia from deficiency of and resistance to parathyroid hormone. *Adv Pediatr* 1985;**32**:439.

Burckhardt P: Idiopathic hypoparathyroidism and autoimmunity. *Horm Res* 1982;**16**:304.

Burnstein MI et al: Metabolic bone disease in pseudohypoparathyroidism: Radiologic features. *Radiology* 1985;**155**:351.

Haussler MR, Cordy PE: Metabolites and analogues of vitamin D: Which for what? *JAMA* 1982;**247**:841.

Levine MA et al: Resistance to multiple hormone in patients with pseudohypoparathyroidism: Association with deficient activity of guanine nucleotide regulatory protein. *Am J Med* 1983;**74**:545.

Nusynowitz ML, Frame B, Kolb FO: The spectrum of the hypoparathyroid states: A classification based on physiologic principles. *Medicine* 1976;**55**:105.

Okano K et al: Comparative efficacy of various vitamin D metabolites in the treatment of various types of hypoparathyroidism. *J Clin Endocrinol Metab* 1982;**55**:238.

Okazaki T et al: Ossification of the paravertebral ligaments: A frequent complication of hypoparathyroidism. *Metabolism* 1984;**33**:710.

Recker RR: Calcium absorption and achlorhydria. *N Engl J Med* 1985;**313**:70.

Spiegel AM et al: Pseudohypoparathyroidism: The molecular basis for hormone resistance: A retrospective. (Editorial.) *N Engl J Med* 1982;**307**:679.

Zaloga GP, Chernow B: Hypocalcemia in critical illness. *JAMA* 1986;**256**:1924.

# HYPERPARATHYROIDISM

## Essentials of Diagnosis

- Renal stones, nephrocalcinosis, polyuria, polydipsia, hypertension, uremia, intractable peptic ulcer, constipation.
- Bone pain, cystic lesions, and, rarely, pathologic fractures.
- Serum and urine calcium elevated; urine phosphate high with low to normal serum phosphate; alkaline phosphatase normal to elevated.
- "Band keratopathy" on slit lamp examination of cornea.
- X-ray: subperiosteal resorption, loss of lamina dura of teeth, renal parenchymal calcification or stones, bone cysts, chondrocalcinosis.
- Elevated levels of parathyroid hormone.

## General Considerations

Primary hyperparathyroidism is a relatively rare disease, but its incidence appears to be increasing; it is potentially curable if detected early. Recent surveys suggest that hyperfunction of the parathyroids, often as asymptomatic hypercalcemia, may be present in 0.1% of patients examined. (*Note:* It should always be suspected in obscure bone and renal disease, especially if nephrocalcinosis or calculi are present.) At least 5% of renal stones are associated with this disease. A past history of neck radiotherapy may be of etiologic importance in some cases.

About 80% of cases of primary hyperparathyroidism are caused by a single adenoma (or, in rare cases, 2 adenomas); 15–20% are caused by primary hypertrophy and hyperplasia of all 4 glands; and 2% are caused by carcinoma of one gland. Recent findings suggest that chief cell hyperplasia may be more common than previously reported. Multiple neoplasms, often familial, of the pancreas, pituitary, thyroid, and adrenal glands may be associated with primary hyperparathyroidism due to tumor or, more commonly, due to hyperplasia of the parathyroids (multiple endocrine adenomatosis types I, IIa, and IIb; see Table 18–17).

Secondary hyperparathyroidism is almost always associated with hyperplasia of all 4 glands, but on rare occasions an autonomous tumor may arise in hyperplastic glands ("tertiary hyperparathyroidism"). It is most commonly seen in chronic renal disease but is also found in rickets, osteomalacia, and acromegaly.

Hyperparathyroidism causes excessive excretion of calcium and phosphate by the kidneys; this eventually produces either calculus formation within the urinary tract or, less commonly, diffuse parenchymal calcification (nephrocalcinosis). (The 2 types rarely coexist.) If the excessive demands for calcium are met by dietary intake, the bones may be spared. If calcium intake is not adequate, bone disease may occur. This may show either diffuse demineralization, pathologic fractures, or cystic bone lesions throughout the skeleton ("osteitis fibrosa cystica"). Factors other than the calcium intake, eg, the level of circulating 1,25-dihydroxyvitamin D, may determine whether bone or stone disease will be present in hyperparathyroidism.

## Clinical Findings

**A. Symptoms and Signs:** The manifestations of hyperparathyroidism may be divided into those referable to (1) skeletal involvement, (2) renal and urinary tract damage, and (3) hypercalcemia per se. Since the adenomas are small and deeply located, only about 5% are palpable. Hyperparathyroidism may be associated with a thyroid adenoma or carcinoma. Some patients have surprisingly few symptoms, and the disease is discovered fortuitously by blood chemical findings.

**1. Skeletal manifestations**–These may vary from simple back pain, joint pains, painful shins, and similar complaints, to actual pathologic fractures of the spine, ribs, or long bones, with loss of height and progressive kyphosis. At times an epulis of the jaw (actually a "brown tumor") may be the telltale sign of osteitis fibrosa. Clubbing of the fingers due to fracture and telescoping of the tips occurs more rarely.

**2. Urinary tract manifestations**–Polyuria and polydipsia occur early in the disease. Sand, gravel, or stones containing calcium oxalate or phosphate may be passed in the urine. Secondary infection and obstruction may cause nephrocalcinosis and renal damage, leading eventually to renal failure.

**3. Manifestations of hypercalcemia**–Thirst, anorexia, and nausea and vomiting are outstanding symptoms. Often one finds a past history of peptic ulcer, with obstruction or even hemorrhage. There may be stubborn constipation, asthenia, anemia, and weight loss. Hypertension is commonly found. Some patients present primarily with neuromuscular disorders such as muscle weakness, easy fatigability, or paresthesias. Depression and psychosis may occur. Of unusual interest is hypermotility of joints. The fingernails and toenails may be unusually strong and thick. Calcium may precipitate in the corneas ("band keratopathy"). In secondary (renal) hyperparathyroidism, calcium also precipitates in the soft tissues, especially around the joints. Recurrent pancreatitis occurs in some patients.

**B. Laboratory Findings:** Serum calcium (especially ionized calcium) is usually high (adjust for serum protein); the serum phosphate is low or normal; the urinary calcium is often high but at times is normal or low. There is an excessive loss of phosphate in the urine in the presence of low to low normal serum phosphate (low tubular reabsorption of phosphate [below 80–90%]); the alkaline phosphatase is elevated only if clinical bone disease is present (in about 25% of cases). The plasma chloride and uric acid levels may be elevated. (In secondary hyperparathyroidism, the serum phosphate is high as a result of renal retention, and the calcium is usually low or normal.) Radioimmunoassays for parathyroid hormone are available to confirm the diagnosis in most cases and to establish the diagnosis of "normocalcemic hyperparathyroidism." A "normal" parathyroid hormone level in the presence of mild hypercalcemia is still compatible with the diagnosis of primary hyperparathyroidism, since hypercalcemia should suppress parathyroid hormone. Since the circulating hormone is heterogeneous, there are still technical problems with any assay procedure.

A great number of special tests have been devised to demonstrate abnormal phosphate dynamics in primary hyperparathyroidism. None of these are as consistently reliable as several accurately performed serum calcium determinations combined with a good parathyroid hormone assay, which demonstrate hypercalcemia for which no other cause can be detected. Control of the dietary phosphate is important, since high phosphate intake may normalize borderline high serum calcium levels. Measurement of nephrogenous cyclic adenosine monophosphate can be used as a biologic test of parathyroid hormone function. Other highly sensitive and specific bioassay procedures are being developed.

**C. Imaging:** Radiography rarely demonstrates the tumor on barium swallow; at times, special angiography may demonstrate it. Signs of bone disease include diffuse demineralization, subperiosteal resorption of bone (especially in the radial aspects of the fingers), and often loss of the lamina dura of the teeth. There may be cysts throughout the skeleton, mottling of the skull ("salt and pepper appearance"), or pathologic fractures. Articular cartilage calcification (chondrocalcinosis) is sometimes found. One may find calculi in the urinary tract or diffuse stippled calcifications in the region of the kidneys (nephrocalcinosis). Soft tissue calcifications around the joints and in the blood vessels may be seen in renal osteitis.

Angiography may locate ectopic and intrathoracic tumors. High-resolution ultrasonography may help locate fair-sized adenomas; CT scan may locate aberrant tumors. Enlarged parathyroid glands have been located with the technetium-thallium subtraction scan (see Gooding reference, below). Bone densitometry may show loss of trabecular bone not seen on routine x-ray.

**D. Other Examinations:** Electrocardiography may show a shortened QT interval. Slit lamp examination of the eye may show corneal calcification ("band keratopathy").

The localization of parathyroid tumors by selective radioimmunoassay for parathyroid hormone via venous catheter is rarely done only after an unsuccessful prior neck exploration.

## Complications

Although the striking complications are those associated with skeletal damage (eg, pathologic fractures), the serious ones are those referable to renal damage. Urinary tract infection due to stone and obstruction may lead to renal failure and uremia. If the serum calcium level rises rapidly (eg, due to dehydration or salt restriction), "parathyroid poisoning" may occur, with acute cardiac and renal failure and rapid precipitation of calcium throughout the soft tissues. Peptic ulcer and pancreatitis may be intractable before surgery. Pancreatic islet cell adenoma with hypoglycemia may be associated, or ulcerogenic pancreatic tumor may coexist. Hypertension is frequently found. Reversible changes in glucose tolerance and insulin secretion have been reported. There may be associated hyperthyroidism, thyroiditis, or thyroid carcinoma. There is also an increased incidence of hyperuricemia and gouty arthritis. Pseudogout may complicate hyperparathyroidism both before and after surgical removal of tumors. Subcutaneous, soft tissue, and extensive vascular calcification—as well as dermal necrosis—may occur in secondary hyperparathyroidism due to renal insufficiency.

## Differential Diagnosis (Table 18–13)

The combination of high calcium and low phosphate in the serum, high urinary phosphate and calcium, and normal or high serum alkaline phosphatase is almost pathognomonic of hyperparathyroidism. Only rarely has this combination been seen in multiple myeloma, metastatic cancer (kidney, bladder, thyroid), and hyperthyroidism. The most common problem is the differentiation of idiopathic hypercalciuria with renal stones from primary hyperparathyroidism with borderline serum calcium levels. If renal damage is present, the typical picture may be obscured, ie, the serum phosphate may not be low. An increasing number of granulomatous disorders (eg, sarcoidosis, berylliosis, silicosis, candidiasis, tuberculosis) are being reported with hypercalcemia due to ectopic production of 1–25 dihydroxyvitamin $D_3$. A similar mechanism may cause the hypercalcemia of some lymphomas. They usually respond to the administration of corticosteroids, which usually does not affect the hypercalcemia of primary hyperparathyroidism. Chlorothiazides may raise the serum calcium level. Hypercalcemia due to hypervitaminosis A must be considered as a possibility. If bone disease is present, the typical subperiosteal resorption may differentiate osteitis fibrosa from nonmetabolic bone disease (eg, neoplasm) and from osteoporosis. Bone biopsy may at times settle the diagnosis.

Nonmetastasizing carcinomas (eg, of the lung, kidney, or ovary) have been described with blood chemical changes identical with those seen in hyperparathyroidism; these changes are often reversible upon removal or chemotherapy of these tumors, which appear to produce a parathyroidlike humoral agent or other bone resorptive factors, such as prostaglandins, or transforming or epidermal growth factors. If significant hypercalcemia is produced by a disorder other than hyperparathyroidism, the parathyroid hormone level should be low or undetectable, since the parathyroid glands are suppressed. In actual practice, this is not always the case, because of difficulties with the assay and the fact that disorders producing hypercalcemia may coexist with hyperparathyroidism (eg, sarcoidosis, hyperthyroidism, breast carcinoma). Familial hyperplasia of the parathyroids and of other endocrine glands requiring surgical treatment has been seen. Another syndrome, **familial hypocalciuric hypercalcemia** (benign familial hypercalcemia), runs a relatively benign course, is not reversed by subtotal resection of the parathyroid glands, and is best treated conservatively. However, this syndrome may be associated with severe juvenile familial parathyroid hyperplasia, which may require immediate subtotal parathyroidectomy to reverse severe hypercalcemia.

## Treatment

**A. Surgical Measures:** A parathyroid tumor should be removed surgically. Multiple tumors may be present; the tumor may be in the thyroid gland or in an ectopic site, eg, the mediastinum. Hyperplasia of all glands requires removal of 3 glands and subtotal resection of the fourth before cure is likely. Success is related to the expertness of the surgery and follow-up care. Total parathyroidectomy with transplantation of a normal amount of functioning parathyroid tissue into the forearm is a new experimental approach. It is useful when total thyroidectomy is required and in instances of severe primary or secondary parathyroid hyperplasia. It simplifies the management of recurrent hypercalcemia and permits avoidance of permanent hypocalcemia, which is common in such situations. After surgery, the patient may, in the course of several hours or days, develop tetany (usually transient) as a result of rapid fall of blood calcium even though the calcium level may fall only to the normal or low normal range. *Caution:* Be certain that an adequate airway is present. Therapy is as for hypoparathyroid tetany (see p 710). Prolonged hypocalcemia due to recalcification of the "hungry" skeleton may require large amounts of calcium and vitamin D. Additional magnesium salts may be required postoperatively.

**B. Fluids:** A large fluid intake is necessary so that a diluted urine will be excreted to minimize the formation of calcium phosphate renal stones.

**C. Treatment of Hypercalcemia:** Force fluids both orally and parenterally (sodium chloride given intravenously is most helpful); mobilize the patient; reduce calcium intake; and add extra phosphate orally. Cortisone therapy is usually not effective in this type of hypercalcemia. Furosemide is especially effective; ethacrynic acid may be helpful. Chlorothiazides should not be given. If renal function is impaired, hemodialysis may be lifesaving if only for a short time. Mithramycin effectively reduces the hypercalcemia due to hyperparathyroidism or cancer, but this drug is quite toxic. Calcitonin combined with glucocorticoids has been used in the treatment of hypercalcemia, but its value is uncertain. Intravenous etidronate (a diphosphonate) has been used successfully to reverse the hypercalcemia of cancer with minimal side effects (see Canfield reference, below). The patient with hypercalcemia is very sensitive to the toxic effects of digitalis. Propranolol may be useful in preventing the adverse cardiac effects of hypercalcemia.

**D. Medical Treatment of Mild Hyperparathyroidism:** Since this disorder is more frequently recognized by routine chemical screening procedures, a number of patients with relatively mild hypercalcemia and few symptoms are encountered. They are best managed by forcing fluids; avoiding immobilization and chlorothiazides; adding phosphate preparations if renal function is good; and giving estrogenic or progestational hormones if postmenopausal. If the patient cannot be followed periodically or becomes symptomatic—eg, passes a stone or shows progressive bone disease—neck exploration must be considered (see Bilezikian 1982 reference, below).

## Prognosis

The disease is usually a chronic progressive one unless treated successfully by surgical removal of the abnormal parathyroid glands. There are at times unexplained exacerbations and partial remissions. Completely asymptomatic patients with mild hypercalcemia may be followed by means of serial calcium determinations and treated medically as outlined above. (See Scholz reference, below.)

Spontaneous cure due to necrosis of the tumor has been reported but is exceedingly rare. The prognosis is directly related to the degree of renal impairment. The bones, in spite of severe cyst formation, deformity, and fracture, will heal completely if a tumor is successfully removed, but this may take several years. Significant renal damage, however, may progress even after removal of an adenoma, and life expectancy is materially reduced. Secondary hyperparathyroidism not infrequently results due to irreversible renal impairment. In carcinoma of the parathyroid (rare), the prognosis is not necessarily hopeless. The presence of pancreatitis increases the mortality rate. If hypercalcemia is severe, the patient may suddenly die in cardiac arrest or may develop irreversible acute renal failure. However, early diagnosis and cure of this disease in an increasing number of patients have led to dramatic recovery. In some patients, reversal of bizarre neuromuscular disorders (neuropathy, asthenia) occurs. Improvement in mentation is often but not always seen after successful surgery. Prolonged postoperative follow-up must be stressed to ensure that the state of hyperparathyroidism has been reversed.

The distressing bone disease of secondary hyperparathyroidism due to renal failure (renal osteodystrophy) can be partially prevented and treated by careful monitoring of the phosphate and parathyroid hormone levels. Resistance to vitamin D can now be overcome by the newer biologically active derivatives, eg, 1,25-dihydroxycholecalciferol and 1α-hydroxycholecalciferol. "Tertiary hyperparathyroidism," ie, hypercalcemia following correction of renal failure, is rarely seen in patients so managed, and parathyroidectomy is rarely required nowadays for this disorder.

Some patients with chronic renal failure have hypercalcemia due to aluminum intoxication rather than to autonomous hyperparathyroidism (pseudohyperparathyroidism).

Bilezikian JP: The medical management of primary hyperparathyroidism. *Ann Intern Med* 1982;**96**:198.

Bilezikian JP: Surgery or no surgery for primary hyperparathyroidism. (Editorial.) *Ann Intern Med* 1985;**102**:402.

Borer MS, Bhanot VK: Hyperparathyroidism: Neuropsychiatric manifestations. *Psychosomatics* 1985;**26**:597.

Broadus AE et al: A detailed evaluation of oral phosphate therapy in selected patients with primary hyperparathyroidism. *J Clin Endocrinol Metab* 1983;**56**:953.

Canfield RE (editor): Etidronate disodium: A new therapy for hypercalcemia of malignancy. (Proceedings of a Symposium.) *Am J Med* 1987;**82(2A)**:1.

Coe FJ, Favus MJ, Parks JH: Is estrogen preferable to surgery for postmenopausal women with primary hyperparathyroidism? (Editorial.) *N Engl J Med* 1986;**314**:1508.

Fitzpatrick LA, Bilezikian JP: Acute primary hyperparathyroidism. *Am J Med* 1987;**82**:275.

Gaz RD, Wang CA: Management of asymptomatic hyperparathyroidism. *Am J Surg* 1984;**147**:498.

Gooding GA et al: Parathyroid imaging: Comparison of double-tracer (Tl-101, Tc-99m) scintigraphy and high-resolution US. *Radiology* 1986;**161**:57.

Law WM, Heath H III: Familial benign hypercalcemia (hypocalciuric hypercalcemia): Clinical and pathogenic studies in 21 families. *Ann Intern Med* 1985;**102**:511.

Manolagas SC, Deftos LJ: The vitamin D endocrine system and the hematolymphopoietic tissue. (Editorial.) *Ann Intern Med* 1984;**100**:144.

Marcus R et al: Conjugated estrogens in the treatment of postmenopausal women with hyperparathyroidism. *Ann Intern Med* 1984;**100**:633.

Marx SJ, Fraser D, Rapoport A: Familial hypocalciuric hypercalcemia: Mild expression of the gene in heterozygotes and severe expression in homozygotes. *Am J Med* 1985;**78**:15.

McCall AR et al: Parathyroid autotransplantation in forty-four patients with primary hyperparathyroidism: The role of thallium scanning. *Surgery* 1986;**100**:614.

Netelenbos C, Lips P, van der Meer C. Hyperparathyroidism following irradiation of benign diseases of the head and neck. *Cancer* 1983;**52**:458.

Richardson ML et al: Bone mineral changes in primary hyperparathyroidism. *Skeletal Radiol* 1986;**15**:85.

Rizzoli R, Green J III, Marx SJ: Primary hyperparathyroidism in familial multiple endocrine neoplasia type 1: Long-term follow-up of serum calcium levels after parathyroidectomy. *Am J Med* 1985;**78**:467.

Saxe AW, Brennan MF: Reoperative parathyroid surgery for primary hyperparathyroidism caused by multiple-gland disease: Total parathyroidectomy and autotransplantation with cryopreserved tissue. *Surgery* 1982;**91**:616.

Scholz DA, Purnell DC: Asymptomatic primary hyperparathyroidism: 10-year prospective study. *Mayo Clin Proc* 1981;**56**:473.

Selby PL, Peacock M: Ethinyl estradiol and norethindrone in the treatment of primary hyperparathyroidism in postmenopausal women. *N Engl J Med* 1986;**314**:1481.

Shane E, Bilezikian JP: Parathyroid carcinoma: A review of 62 patients. *Endocr Rev* 1982;**3**:218.

Sharma OP: Hypercalcemia in sarcoidosis: The puzzle finally solved. (Editorial.) *Arch Intern Med* 1985;**145**:626.

Sherrard DJ, Ott SM, Andress DL: Pseudohyperparathyroidism: Syndrome associated with aluminum intoxication in patients with renal failure. *Am J Med* 1985;**79**:127.

Stark DD et al: Parathyroid imaging: Comparison of high-resolution CT and high-resolution sonography. *AJR* 1983;**141**:633.

# METABOLIC BONE DISEASE
## (Table 18–13)

## OSTEOMALACIA & RICKETS

### Essentials of Diagnosis

- Muscular weakness, listlessness.
- Aching and "bowing" of bones.
- Serum calcium low to normal; serum phosphate low; alkaline phosphatase elevated.
- "Pseudofractures" and "washed out" bone on x-ray.

### General Considerations

Osteomalacia is the adult form of rickets. It is a condition resulting from a calcium or phosphorus deficiency (or both) in the bone. It may be caused by insufficient absorption from the intestine, due either to a lack of calcium alone, or a lack of or resistance to the action of vitamin D.

Almost all forms of osteomalacia are associated with compensatory, secondary hyperparathyroidism initiated by the low calcium level. It is for this reason that most patients will show only slightly low serum calcium levels (compensated osteomalacia). In chronic uremic states, a mixed picture of osteomalacia and secondary hyperparathyroidism is seen ("renal osteodystrophy"). Aluminum intoxication incident to chronic dialysis therapy and therapy with phosphate binders may be an important factor. (See Nebeker reference, below.) Resistance to the action of vitamin D due to failure of its conversion to the biologically active forms, 25-hydroxycholecalciferol and 1,25-dihydroxycholecalciferol, by the liver and kidney, respectively, has been demonstrated in many clinical states as outlined in Table 18–11.

### Clinical Findings

**A. Symptoms and Signs:** Manifestations are variable, ranging from almost none in mild cases to marked muscular weakness and listlessness in advanced cases. There is usually mild aching of the bones, especially of long bones and ribs, and a tendency to bowing. In the very early and acute osteomalacias, a rapidly falling calcium level may be associated with clinical tetany, although this is rare. As compensation takes place, tetanic features are absent. Malabsorption syndromes may include osteomalacia. A low-potassium syndrome with muscular weakness and paralysis may be present with renal tubular disorders.

**B. Laboratory Findings:** Serum calcium is low or normal but never high. Serum phosphate is low (may be normal in early stages). The alkaline phosphatase is elevated except in the early phase and in a rare patient with hypophosphatasia. Urinary calcium and phosphate are usually low in absorptive disorders

**Table 18–11.** Causes of osteomalacia.*

**Vitamin D deficiency**
  Inadequate vitamin D in the diet.
  Inadequate sunlight exposure without dietary supplementation.
    House- or institution-bound people.
    Atmospheric smog.
    Chronic residence in far northern and far southern latitudes.
    Excessive covering of body with clothing.
  Gastrointestinal disease that interrupts the normal enterohepatic recycling of vitamin D and its metabolites, resulting in their fecal loss.
    Chronic steatorrhea (pancreatic).
    Malabsorption (gluten-sensitive enteropathy).
    Surgical resection of large parts of intestine.
    Biliary fistula formation.
  Impaired synthesis of $1,25(OH)_2D_3$ by the kidney.
    Nephron loss as in chronic kidney disease (see section on renal hyperparathyroidism).
    Functional impairment of $1,25(OH)_2D_3$ hydroxylase (eg, hypoparathyroidism).
    Congenital absence of $1,25(OH)_2D_3$ hydroxylase (vitamin D-dependency rickets type I).
    Suppression of $1,25(OH)_2D_3$ production by endogenously produced substances (cancer).
  Target cell resistance to $1,25(OH)_2D_3$-absent or diminished number of $1,25(OH)_2D_3$ receptors, vitamin D-dependency rickets type II.

**Phosphate deficiency**
  Dietary.
    Low intake of phosphate.
    Excessive aluminum hydroxide ingestion (phosphate binders).
  Impaired renal tubular reabsorption of phosphate.
    Other acquired and hereditary renal tubular disorders associated with renal phosphate loss (Fanconi's syndrome).
    Tumor-associated hypophosphatemia.
    X-linked hypophosphatemia.
    Adult-onset hypophosphatemia.

**Systemic acidosis**
  Chronic renal failure.
  Distal renal tubular acidosis.
  Ureterosigmoidoscopy.
  Chronic acetazolamide and ammonium chloride administration.

**Drug-induced osteomalacia**
  Excessive alcohol intake.
  Excessive diphosphonate administration.
  Excessive fluoride administration.
  Anticonvulsant administration (enhanced vitamin D metabolism).
  Aluminum, lead, cadmium excess.
  Outdated tetracyclines.

**Primary mineralization defects**
  Hypophosphatasia.
  Osteopetrosis.
  Fibrogenesis imperfecta ossium.

* Modified and reproduced, with permission, from Greenspan FS, Forsham PH (editors): *Basic & Clinical Endocrinology*, 2nd ed. Lange, 1986.

and high in renal lesions. The intravenous calcium infusion test demonstrates avidity of bone for calcium (80–90% retained) in osteomalacia due to malabsorption. The blood levels of 25-hydroxycholecalciferol and of 1,25-dihydroxycholecalciferol may be low.

Parathyroid hormone levels may be elevated. There is a decrease in bone mass as measured by more sophisticated techniques. Laboratory findings of the primary steatorrhea or renal disease may be present. Characteristics of renal tubular acidosis are described in Chapter 15. Hypomagnesemia is common in disorders of malabsorption.

**C. Imaging:** Involvement of the pelvis and long bones, with demineralization and bowing, is seen; less often, the spine and skull are involved as well. Fractures are rare except for "pseudofractures" (Milkman's syndrome). Nephrocalcinosis may be seen in patients with renal tubular acidosis. Bone scans may show increased uptake of tracer material and may locate lesions not visualized on conventional radiograms, eg, pseudofractures.

**D. Quantitative Bone Densitometry Measurements:** These are helpful in initial assessment of the degree of bone mineral loss and response to therapy. (See Wahner reference, below.)

**E. Bone Biopsy:** This may be the only way to make a diagnosis. Undecalcified sections must be used with special staining methods to show undecalcified osteoid and osteoblastic overactivity.

**Differential Diagnosis (Table 18–11)**

It is most important to recognize osteomalacia and consider it in the differential diagnosis of bone disease, since it is a potentially curable disease. The childhood forms may be mistaken for osteogenesis imperfecta or other nonmetabolic bone disorders.

The acute forms must be differentiated from other forms of tetany. The long-standing disease enters into the differential diagnosis of any metabolic or generalized nonmetabolic bone disease. The pseudofracture is often the only outstanding sign of latent osteomalacia. Osteoporosis may exist as well and may obscure the osteomalacia. At times the diagnosis is confirmed by a rise and subsequent fall of the serum alkaline phosphatase after treatment with vitamin D and calcium. Other causes of hypophosphatemia, eg, chronic alcoholism, enter into the differential diagnosis. Some

tumors induce phosphaturia and osteomalacia resistant to vitamin D (see Ryan reference, below). The joint aches and pains may be mistaken for some form of arthritis. The cachexia suggests malignant disease. Bone biopsy of the iliac crest with tetracycline labeling may establish the diagnosis of latent osteomalacia.

**Treatment**

**A. Specific Measures:**

**1. Rickets–**Vitamin D, even in small doses, is specific; 2000–5000 units daily is adequate unless resistance to vitamin D is present.

**2. Adult osteomalacia and renal rickets–**Vitamin D is specific, but very large doses are necessary to overcome the resistance to its calcium absorptive action and to prevent renal loss of phosphate. Give until an effect is noted on the blood calcium. The usual dose is 25,000–100,000 units daily. Doses up to 300,000 units or more daily may be necessary, but if the doses are over 100,000 daily, they must be used cautiously with periodic determination of serum and urine calcium; the serum phosphate may remain low. Crystalline dihydrotachysterol in doses of 0.4–1 mg daily may be an alternative medication in states associated with fat malabsorption.

**3. Pancreatic insufficiency–**See Chapter 11.

**4. Sprue syndrome–**See Chapter 11.

**5. Some rare forms of renal disease–**See Chapter 15.

**B. General Measures:** Provide a high-calcium diet and supplement with calcium carbonate, 3–6 g daily. Calcium citrate, 2–4 g daily, may be preferable in patients with gastric surgery or malabsorption. A high-phosphate diet or phosphate salts are of value in certain types of renal rickets. Magnesium salts may have to be added.

**C. Vitamin D Metabolites:** The increasing availability of the biologically active metabolites of calciferol, 25-hydroxycholecalciferol and 1,25-dihydroxycholecalciferol, will help in the treatment of osteomalacia resistant to vitamin D (eg, chronic liver disease and renal failure). (See Table 18–12.)

**Table 18–12.** Comparison of various vitamin D preparations.*

| | How Supplied | Physiologic Dose | Pharmacologic Dose† | Onset of Maximal Effect |
|---|---|---|---|---|
| Ergocalciferol (calciferol, vitamin $D_2$, Drisdol) | Capsules, 1200 $\mu$g | 10 $\mu$g/d | 1200 $\mu$g/d | 30 days |
| Dihydrotachysterol | Tablets, 125 $\mu$g, 200 $\mu$g, and 400 $\mu$g | 20 $\mu$g/d | 400 $\mu$g/d | 15 days |
| Calcifediol (25-hydroxycholecalciferol; Calderol) | Capsules, 20 $\mu$g and 50 $\mu$g | 5 $\mu$g/d | 50 $\mu$g/d | 15 days |
| Calcitriol (1,25-dihydroxycholecalciferol; Rocaltrol) | Capsules, 0.25 $\mu$g and 0.5 $\mu$g | 0.5 $\mu$g/d | 1 $\mu$g/d | 3 days |

* Modified and reproduced, with permission, from Kumar R, Riggs BL: Vitamin D in the therapy of disorders of calcium and phosphorus metabolism. *Mayo Clin Proc* 1981;**56:**327.
† Usual dose for treating hypoparathyroidism, osteomalacia due to malabsorption or vitamin D resistance, and renal osteodystrophy. One microgram of vitamin $D_2$ has an activity of 40 IU; 1200 $\mu$g is approximately 50,000 IU.

## Prognosis

The prognosis is usually excellent in the absorptive disorders if diagnosed early. This does not hold for certain of the vitamin D-resistant forms of osteomalacia or rickets or for Fanconi's syndrome, which respond slowly or not at all unless huge amounts of vitamin D are given. Calcitriol may heal the bone disease. Hypercalcemia may occur as a complication of therapy. It can be prevented by carefully monitoring the serum and urine calcium periodically; treat with corticosteroids once the disorder has become established. In the renal forms, the ultimate prognosis is that of the basic kidney disease. The greater availability of the metabolically active metabolites of vitamin D will greatly improve the ultimate outlook in this disorder.

Alfrey AC: Aluminum intoxication. (Editorial.) *N Engl J Med* 1984;**17:**1113.

Audran M, Kumar R: The physiology and pathophysiology of vitamin D. *Mayo Clin Proc* 1985;**60:**851.

Brenner RJ et al: Incidence of radiographically evident bone disease, nephrocalcinosis, and nephrolithiasis in various types of renal tubular acidosis. *N Engl J Med* 1982;**307:**217.

Chan YL et al: Dialysis osteodystrophy. *Medicine* 1985;**64:**296.

DeLuca HF: New developments in the vitamin D endocrine system. *J Am Diet Assoc* 1982;**80:**231.

Frame B, Potts JT Jr (editors): *Clinical Disorders of Bone and Mineral Metabolism.* Excerpta Medica, 1983.

Glorieux FH et al: Bone response to phosphate salts, ergocalciferol, and calcitriol in hypophosphatemic vitamin D-resistant rickets. *N Engl J Med* 1980;**303:**1023.

Meredith SC, Rosenberg IH: Gastrointestinal-hepatic disorders and osteomalacia. *Clin Endocrinol Metab* 1980;**9:**131.

Nebeker HG et al: Aluminum and renal osteodystrophy. *Ann Rev Med* 1986;**37:**79.

Norman AW, Roth J, Orci L: The vitamin D endocrine system: Steroid metabolism, hormone receptors, and biological response (calcium binding proteins). *Endocr Rev* 1982;**3:**331.

Parfitt AM, Oliver I, Villanueva AR: Bone histology in metabolic bone disease. The diagnostic value of bone biopsy. *Orthop Clin North Am* 1979;**10:**329.

Ryan EA, Reiss E: Oncogenous osteomalacia: Review of the world literature of 42 cases and report of two new cases. *Am J Med* 1984;**77:**501.

Spencer H, Kramer L: Antacid-induced calcium loss. (Editorial.) *Arch Intern Med* 1983;**143:**657.

Wahner HW: Assessment of metabolic bone disease: Review of new nuclear medicine procedures. *Mayo Clin Proc* 1985;**60:**827.

## OSTEOPOROSIS

### Essentials of Diagnosis

- Asymptomatic to severe backache.
- Spontaneous fractures and collapse of vertebrae without spinal cord compression, often discovered "accidentally" on radiography; loss of height.
- Serum calcium, phosphorus, and alkaline phosphatase normal.
- Demineralization, especially of spine and pelvis.

### General Considerations

Osteoporosis is the most common metabolic bone disease in the USA. Since the usual form of the disease is clinically evident in middle life and beyond and since women are more frequently affected than men, it is often termed "postmenopausal" or "senile" osteoporosis. It is characterized by an absolute decrease in the amount of bone present to a level below which it is capable of maintaining the structural integrity of the skeleton. The rate of bone formation is often normal, whereas the rate of bone resorption is increased. There is a greater loss of trabecular bone than compact bone, accounting for the primary features of the disease, ie, crush fractures of vertebrae, fractures of the neck of the femur, and fractures of the distal end of the radius. Whatever bone is present is normally mineralized. Osteoporosis may be produced secondarily by a number of disorders (see below), but more commonly it is primary and of unknown cause. The inheritance of low skeletal mass in young adult life (especially in white females), loss of sex hormones at the time of the menopause, the effects of aging, lack of activity, inadequate dietary calcium intake, impaired intestinal calcium absorption, a high phosphate intake, acid ash diet, inappropriate secretion of parathyroid hormone or calcitonin, or some combination of these factors have been considered as possible contributing causes.

### Etiology

**A. Principal Causes:**

1. Lack of activity, eg, immobilization as in paraplegia or rheumatoid arthritis. (Osteoblasts depend upon strains and stresses for proper function.) While a moderate amount of physical activity is of benefit both to prevent and treat osteoporosis, excess athletic activity, which leads to weight loss and amenorrhea, has been shown to cause rapid bone loss (see Heath 1985 and Marcus references, below).

2. Lack of estrogens (postmenopausal, physiologic, or postoophorectomy osteoporosis). (Females are deprived of estrogens relatively early in life. About 30% of women over 60 years of age have clinical osteoporosis. Some degree of osteoporosis is almost always present in senility.)

3. A chronic low intake of calcium has been suggested as of etiologic importance.

4. Malabsorption, at times with intestinal lactase deficiency or after gastrectomy, may be an important factor in elderly patients with osteoporosis.

5. Deficient production of 1,25-dihydroxyvitamin D may be a cause of some types.

**B. Less Common Causes:**

1. Developmental disturbances (eg, osteogenesis imperfecta).

2. Nutritional disturbances (eg, anorexia nervosa, protein starvation or excess, ascorbic acid deficiency, alcohol or caffeine excess).

3. Chronic calcium depletion is claimed by some investigators to cause osteoporosis. Long-standing renal hypercalciuria may lead to osteoporosis.

**Table 18–13.** Differential diagnosis of disorders of mineral metabolism.* (TRP = tubular reabsorption of phosphate.)

| Disease | Serum | | | | | Urine | | | Comment |
|---|---|---|---|---|---|---|---|---|---|
| | Calcium | Phosphorus | Alkaline Ptase | Urea or Creatinine | Parathyroid Hormone | Calcium | TRP | Hydroxy-proline | |
| Hyperparathyroidism Primary | ↑ | ↓ | ↑ or N | N or ↑ | ↑ | ↑ or N | ↓ | ↑ | Phalangeal subperiosteal resorption. |
| Secondary | ↓ or N | ↑ | ↑ | ↑ | ↑ | N or ↓ | ↓ | ↑ | |
| "Tertiary" | ↑ | N or ↓ | ↑ or N | ↑ or N | ↑ | ↑ or N | ↓ | ↑ | Tends to appear after renal transplantation. |
| Cancer | ↑ | ↑ or N or ↓ | ↑ or N | ↑ or N | ↑ or N or ↓ | ↑ | N or ↓ | ↑ | May be abnormal PTH in serum, or prostaglandin. |
| Sarcoid | ↑ or N | N or ↓ | ↑ or N | ↑ or N | ↓ | ↑ | N or ↓ | ↑ | Good response to corticosteroids. |
| Vitamin D intoxication | ↑ | ↑ or N | N | ↑ or N | ↓ | ↑ | N or ↓ | ↑ | Good response to corticosteroids. |
| Hyperthyroidism | ↑ or N | N or ↑ | N or ↑ | N | N or ↓ | ↑ | N | ↑ | Serum thyroxine increased. |
| Acute bone atrophy (immobilization) | ↑ or N | ↑ | N | N | N or ↓ | ↑ | N | N or ↑ | |
| Milk-alkali syndrome | ↑ | ↑ or N | N | ↑ | N or ↓ | N | N or ↓ | N or ↑ | Alkalosis despite renal insufficiency. |
| Idiopathic hypercalcemia of infancy | ↑ | ↑ or N | ↑ | ↑ | ? | ↑ | N or ↓ | ↑ | "Elfin" facies. |
| Rickets and osteomalacia Vitamin D deficiency | ↓ | ↓ | ↑↑ | N | ↑ | ↓ | ↓ | N | Irritability, muscular hypotonia. |
| Vitamin D "refractory" | N | ↓ | ↑↑ | ↑ or N | ↑ or N | ↓ | ↓ | N | Pseudofractures, short stature. |
| Hypophosphatasia | ↑ or N | N | ↓ | N | ? | ↑ or N | N | ↓ | Urinary phosphorylethanolamine increased; rickets. |
| Hypoparathyroidism | ↓ | ↑ | N | N | ↓ | ↓ | ↑ | N | |
| Pseudohypoparathyroidism | ↓ | ↑ | ↑ or N | N | ↑ or N | ↓ | ↑ | N or ↑ | Short ulnar metacarpals. |
| Pseudopseudohypoparathyroidism | N | N | N | N | N | N | N | N | Short ulnar metacarpals, short stature. |
| Osteoporosis, idiopathic or senile | N | N | N | N | N | N | N | N or ↑ | |
| Osteogenesis imperfecta | N | N | N or ↑ | N | N | N | N | ↑ or ↑ | Blue scleras; deafness. |
| Osteopetrosis | N or ↓ | N | N | N | N | N or ↓ | N | N or ↑ | Acid phosphatase increased. |
| Paget's disease | N | N | ↑↑ | N | N | N | N | ↑↑ | Cardiac output increased. |
| Fibrous dysplasia | N | N or ↓ | ↑ or N | N | N | N | N | ↑ or N | Brown spots. |

*Modified and reproduced, with permission, from Goldsmith RS: Laboratory aids in the diagnosis of metabolic bone disease. *Orthop Clin North Am* 1972;**3**:546.

4. Endocrine diseases–Lack of androgens (eunuchoidism, senility in men), hypopituitarism and hyperprolactinemia (secondary gonadal failure), acromegaly (cause unknown; possibly due to hypogonadism), thyrotoxicosis (not constant; causes excessive catabolism of skeletal tissue), excessive exogenous or endogenous ACTH or corticosteroids causing catabolism of bone (eg, Cushing's disease), and longstanding uncontrolled diabetes mellitus (rare).

5. Bone marrow disorders–The presence of abnormal cells in the bone marrow, such as in myeloma or leukemia, may stimulate osteoclastic activity and cause osteoporosis. This is in addition to the active replacement of the marrow with tumor cells. A bone marrow factor may also play an etiologic role in senile osteoporosis.

6. Prolonged use of heparin may lead to osteoporosis. Tobacco smoking may be an important factor (see Seeman reference, below).

7. Idiopathic osteoporosis occurs most commonly in young men and women and occasionally in older people. It does not respond well to therapy.

8. Idiopathic juvenile osteoporosis is rare and often shows spontaneous remission after puberty.

## Clinical Findings

**A. Symptoms and Signs:** Osteoporosis may first be discovered on x-ray examination. It may present as backache of varying degrees of severity or as a spontaneous fracture of collapse of a vertebra. Loss of height is common.

**B. Laboratory Findings:** Serum calcium, phosphate, and alkaline phosphatase are normal. The alkaline phosphatase may be slightly elevated in osteogenesis imperfecta and also in other forms of osteoporosis if there has been a recent fracture. Urinary calcium is high early, normal in chronic forms. Urinary hydroxyproline may be elevated in active osteoporosis and in adult osteogenesis imperfecta.

**C. Imaging:** The principal areas of demineralization are the spine and pelvis, especially in the femoral neck and head; demineralization is less marked in the skull and extremities. Compression of vertebrae is common. The lamina dura is preserved. Kidney stones may occasionally be seen in acute osteoporosis. The increasing availability of instruments for quantitating bone mineral mass with low radiation exposure (especially photon absorptiometry) makes screening for premature bone loss feasible and allows assessment of response to therapy. (See Wahner reference, below.)

## Differential Diagnosis

It is important not to confuse this condition with other metabolic bone diseases, especially osteomalacia and hyperparathyroidism; or with myeloma and metastatic bone disease, especially of the breast and uterus, which may be aggravated by estrogens. (See Table 18–13.) Bone scintiscans and biopsy may be required, since these conditions may coexist in the postmenopausal patient.

A rare case of hypophosphatasia may appear as "osteoporosis."

## Treatment

**A. Specific Measures:** Specific treatment varies with the cause; combined hormone therapy is usually used, although its effectiveness may be in preventing bone loss rather than increasing bone mass.

**1. Postclimacteric (mostly in females)–**Estrogens appear to decrease bone resorption. Before beginning estrogen therapy in a postmenopausal woman, perform a careful pelvic examination to rule out neoplasm or other abnormality and warn the patient or a relative that vaginal bleeding may occur. Administer estrogen daily except for the first 5–7 calendar days of each month, and then repeat the cycle. Any of the following may be used: (1) Estradiol (Estrace), 1–2 mg orally. (2) Ethinyl estradiol, 0.02–0.05 mg orally daily as tolerated. (3) Estrone sulfate and conjugated estrogenic substances (Amnestrogen, Premarin, etc) are well tolerated and widely used. The dosage is 0.625–1.25 mg orally daily. The long-acting injectable estrogen preparations may be useful. The addition of a progestin, eg, medroxyprogesterone acetate (Provera), 10 mg daily for the last week to 10 days of each estrogen cycle, may reduce some of the side effects. See discussion of menopause (Chapter 13) for dangers of estrogen therapy.

Anabolic steroids, commonly used in the past, are of questionable benefit except in the debilitated patient. For women, the dose must be kept low in order to avoid undesirable side effects (eg, hirsutism, hoarseness, clitoral enlargement, and liver impairment).

**2. Old age and idiopathic–**As for postclimacteric; both testosterone and estrogens may be used in both males and females. Use with caution in very old people. Calcium and vitamin D may be of similar help.

**3. Patients with malnutrition–**Adequate diet is of great importance. However, hormones may be used as above if response to diet alone is poor.

**4. Cushing's syndrome–**See p 727.

**5. Sodium fluoride** has been used in refractory osteoporotic patients, but it must be considered still an experimental procedure with significant side effects. Combined with calcium and vitamin D, it appears to enhance bone formation. Recurrent spinal fracture rates have been reduced. (See Bikle 1983 reference, below.)

**6. Phosphate supplements** may be of value in certain types of osteoporosis (eg, after fracture, myeloma), especially if combined with calcium.

**7. Calcitonin** (Calcimar) has been approved by the FDA for the treatment of osteoporosis in doses of 100 IU/d. It must be used parenterally and is expensive but may be an alternative to estrogen therapy when this drug is contraindicated or not tolerated (see Gruber reference, below).

**8. Miscellaneous agents–**The efficacy of growth hormone and diphosphonates is still under study. A novel experimental approach to restore bone mass is the combined use of human parathyroid hormone with 1,25-dihydroxyvitamin D (see Slovik 1986 reference, below).

**B. General Measures:** The diet should be adequate in protein, calcium (milk and milk products are desirable except in lactose intolerance), and vitamin D. Increased calcium intake by use of supplementary calcium salts (eg, calcium carbonate), up to 1–2 g calcium per day, is advisable. Additional vitamin D (2000–5000 units/d) may be needed if there is associated malabsorption or osteomalacia. A rare patient may require 1,25-dihydroxycholecalciferol. Thiazides may be useful if hypercalciuria is present. Patients should be kept active; bedridden patients should be given active or passive exercises. The spine must be adequately supported (eg, with a Taylor brace or corset), but rigid or excessive immobilization must be avoided. Elderly patients must be protected from falling.

## Prognosis

The prognosis is good for postclimacteric osteoporosis if estrogen therapy is started early and maintained for years. Spinal involvement is not reversible on x-ray, but progression of the disease is often halted. In general, osteoporosis is a crippling rather than a killing disease, and the prognosis is essentially that of the underlying disorder (eg, Cushing's syndrome). The idiopathic variety does not respond appreciably to any form of therapy except possibly fluoride. Careful periodic records of the patient's height will indicate if the disease has become stabilized. Periodic measurements of bone mass in a given individual, using modern techniques (eg, bone densitometry), may alert the physician to a progressive bone loss before clinical or x-ray evidence of osteoporosis occurs. Measures to prevent progressive loss of bone mass may be more effective than treatment of the clinical disease, which at present is costing several billions of dollars in medical care annually in the USA alone.

Aloia JF et al: Risk factors for postmenopausal osteoporosis. *Am J Med* 1985;**78**:95.

Avioli LV (editor): *The Osteoporotic Syndrome: Detection, Prevention, and Treatment.* Grune & Stratton, 1983.

Baylinck DJ: Glucocorticoid-induced osteoporosis. (Editorial.) *N Engl J Med* 1983;**309**:306.

Bikle DD: Fluoride treatment of osteoporosis: A new look at an old drug. (Editorial.) *Ann Intern Med* 1983;**98**:1013.

Bikle DD et al: Bone disease in alcohol abuse. *Ann Intern Med* 1985;**103**:42.

Cann CE et al: Quantitative computed tomography for prediction of vertebral fracture risk. *Bone* 1985;**6**:1.

Christiansen C, Riis BJ, Rodbro MD: Prediction of rapid bone loss in postmenopausal women. *Lancet* 1987;**1**:1105.

Cummings SR, Nevitt MC, Haber RJ: Prevention of osteoporosis and osteoporotic fractures. (Topics in Primary Care Medicine.) *West J Med* 1985;**143**:684.

Ettinger B, Genant HK, Cann CE: Postmenopausal bone loss is prevented by treatment with low-dosage estrogen with calcium. *Ann Intern Med* 1987;**106**:40.

Gambrell RD: The menopause: Benefits and risks of estrogen-progestogen replacement therapy. *Fertil Steril* 1982;**37**:457.

Gruber HE et al: Long-term calcitonin therapy in postmenopausal osteoporosis. *Metabolism* 1984;**33**:295.

Health and Public Policy Committee, American College of Physicians: Radiologic methods to evaluate bone mineral content. *Ann Intern Med* 1984;**100**:908.

Heath H III: Athletic women, amenorrhea, and skeletal integrity. (Editorial.) *Ann Intern Med* 1985;**102**:258.

Heath H III: Progress against osteoporosis. (Editorial.) *Ann Intern Med* 1983;**98**:1011.

Hillner BE, Hollenberg JP, Pauker SG: Postmenopausal estrogens in prevention of osteoporosis: Benefit virtually without risk if cardiovascular effects are considered. *Am J Med* 1986;**80**:115.

Marcus R et al: Menstrual function and bone mass in elite women distance runners: Endocrine and metabolic features. *Ann Intern Med* 1985;**102**:158.

Ott S: Should women get screening bone mass measurements? (Editorial.) *Ann Intern Med* 1986;**104**:874.

Perry HM III et al: Osteoporosis in young men: A syndrome of hypercalciuria and accelerated bone turnover. *Arch Intern Med* 1982;**142**:1295.

Richelson LS et al: Relative contributions of aging and estrogen deficiency to postmenopausal bone loss. *N Engl J Med* 1984;**311**:1273.

Riggs BL, Melton LJ III: Involutional osteoporosis. *N Engl J Med* 1986;**314**:1676.

Rigotti NA et al: Osteoporosis in women with anorexia nervosa. *N Engl J Med* 1984;**311**:1601.

Riis B, Thomsen K, Christiansen C: Does calcium supplementation prevent postmenopausal bone loss? A double-blind, controlled clinical study. *New Engl J Med* 1987;**316**:173.

Sakhaee K et al: Postmenopausal osteoporosis as a manifestation of renal hypercalciuria with secondary hyperparathyroidism. *J Clin Endocrinol Metab* 1985;**61**:368.

Seeman E et al: Risk factors for spinal osteoporosis in men. *Am J Med* 1983;**75**:977.

Slovik DM et al: Deficient production of 1,25-dihydroxyvitamin D in elderly osteoporotic patients. *N Engl J Med* 1981;**305**:372.

Slovik DM et al: Restoration of spinal bone in osteoporotic men by treatment with human parathyroid hormone (1–34) and 1,25-dihydroxyvitamin D. *J Bone Mineral Res* 1986;**1**:377.

Smith R: Idiopathic osteoporosis in the young. *J Bone Joint Surg [Br]* 1980;**62**:417.

Wahner HW, Dunn WL, Riggs BL: Assessment of bone mineral. Parts 1 and 2. *J Nucl Med* 1984;**25**:1134, 1241.

Wasnich RD et al: Thiazide effect on the mineral content of bone. *N Engl J Med* 1983;**309**:344.

# NONMETABOLIC BONE DISEASE

## POLYOSTOTIC FIBROUS DYSPLASIA (Osteitis Fibrosa Disseminata)

### Essentials of Diagnosis

- Painless swelling of involved bone or fracture with minimal trauma.
- Bone cysts or hyperostotic lesions; usually multi-

ple, but occasionally single, in segmental distribution.

## General Considerations

Polyostotic fibrous dysplasia is a rare disease that is frequently mistaken for osteitis fibrosa generalisata due to hyperparathyroidism, since both are manifested by bone cysts and fractures. Polyostotic fibrous dysplasia is not a metabolic disorder of bone but a congenital dysplasia in which bone and cartilage do not form but remain as fibrous tissue.

Polyostotic fibrous dysplasia with "brown spots" with ragged margins and true precocious puberty in the female is called **Albright's syndrome.** Hyperthyroidism and acromegaly may be present also.

## Clinical Findings

**A. Symptoms and Signs:** The manifestations are painless swelling of the involved bone (usually the skull, upper end of femur, tibia, metatarsals, metacarpals, phalanges, ribs, and pelvis), either singly or in multiple distribution, with cysts or hyperostotic lesions and at times with brown pigmentation of the overlying skin. Involvement is segmental and may be unilateral. True sexual precocity may occur in females, with early development of secondary sex characteristics and rapid skeletal growth but ultimately short stature.

**B. Laboratory Findings:** Calcium and phosphorus are normal; the alkaline phosphatase and urinary hydroxyproline may be elevated.

**C. Imaging:** Radiographs reveal rarefaction and expansion of the affected bones, at times with cystic changes, or hyperostosis (especially of base of the skull). Fractures and deformities may also be visible, eg, "shepherd's crook" deformity of the hip.

## Differential Diagnosis

The bone cysts and fractures should, by their distribution and skin pigmentation, be distinguished from those of hyperparathyroidism and neurofibromatosis. All other types of bone cyst and tumor must be considered also. The hyperostotic lesions of the skull must be distinguished from those of Paget's disease. Biopsy of bone may be required to settle the diagnosis.

## Complications

Shortening of the extremity or deformity (eg, shepherd's crook deformity of femur) may follow extensive involvement of bone. The involvement of the orbit may cause proptosis or even blindness. Thyrotoxicosis, hyperparathyroidism, Cushing's syndrome, acromegaly, and gynecomastia may be associated features. Osteomalacia may be present also, as a result of renal phosphaturia. It may be reversed by removal of dysplastic bone.

## Treatment

There is no treatment except for surgical correction of deformities, eg, fractures, expanding cyst in the orbit or femur. Calcitonin has been used in active disease, but the results are not conclusive.

## Prognosis

Most lesions heal, and the progression is slow. Since precocity is of the isosexual type, girls are susceptible to early pregnancy. They will ultimately be of short stature. On rare occasions, sarcomatous transformation of bone occurs.

Bell NH et al: Effect of calcitonin in Paget's disease and polyostotic fibrous dysplasia. *J Clin Endocrinol Metab* 1970;**31**:283.

Harris RI: Polyostotic fibrous dysplasia with acromegaly. *Am J Med* 1985;**78**:539.

# PAGET'S DISEASE
## (Osteitis Deformans)

## Essentials of Diagnosis

- Often asymptomatic. Bone pain may be the first symptom.
- Kyphosis, bowed tibias, large head, waddling gait, and frequent fractures that vary with location of process.
- Serum calcium and phosphate normal; alkaline phosphatase elevated; urinary hydroxyproline elevated.
- Dense, expanded bones on x-ray.

## General Considerations

Paget's disease is a nonmetabolic bone disease of unknown etiology, although it is believed that it may represent a benign neoplasm of bone-forming cells. A possible viral etiology has recently been suggested. It causes excessive bone destruction and repair—with associated deformities, since the repair takes place in an unorganized fashion. Up to 3% of persons over age 50 will show isolated lesions, but clinically important disease is much less common. There is a strong familial incidence of Paget's disease. A rare form occurs in young people ("juvenile Paget's disease").

## Clinical Findings

**A. Symptoms and Signs:** Often mild or asymptomatic. Deep "bone pain" is usually the first symptom. The bones become soft, leading to bowed tibias, kyphosis, and frequent fractures with slight trauma. The head becomes larger, and headaches are a prominent symptom. Increased vascularity over the involved bones causes increased warmth.

**B. Laboratory Findings:** The blood calcium and phosphorus are normal, but the alkaline phosphatase is usually markedly elevated. Urinary hydroxyproline and calcium are elevated in active disease.

**C. Imaging:** On radiographs the involved bones are expanded and denser than normal. Multiple fissure fractures may be seen in the long bones. The initial lesion may be destructive and radiolucent, especially in the skull ("osteoporosis circumscripta"). Technetium pyrophosphate bone scans are helpful in delineating activity of bone lesions.

## Differential Diagnosis

Differentiate from primary bone lesions such as osteogenic sarcoma, multiple myeloma, and fibrous dysplasia and from secondary bone lesions such as metastatic carcinoma and osteitis fibrosa cystica. If serum calcium is elevated, hyperparathyroidism may be present in some patients as well.

## Complications

Fractures are frequent and occur with minimal trauma. If immobilization takes place and there is an excessive calcium intake, hypercalcemia and kidney stones may develop. Associated hyperparathyroidism may also be present. Bony overgrowth may impinge on vital structures, especially nerves, causing deafness and blindness. Vertebral collapse may lead to spinal cord compression. A rare complication is a giant cell reparative granuloma of bone leading to bone destruction and soft tissue masses. Osteosarcoma may develop in long-standing lesions. Sarcomatous change is suggested by marked increase in bone pain, sudden rise in alkaline phosphatase, and appearance of a lytic lesion. The increased vascularity, acting like multiple arteriovenous fistulas, may give rise to high-output cardiac failure. Rheumatic manifestations and hyperuricemia with acute and chronic joint pain often complicate this disease, especially in joints near involved bone.

## Treatment

Mild cases require no treatment.

Supply a high-protein diet with adequate vitamin C intake. A high-calcium intake is desirable also unless the patient is immobilized, in which case calcium must be restricted. Vitamin D, 50,000 units 3 times a week, is helpful in some patients with marked osteoblastic overactivity (high serum alkaline phosphatase but low urinary calcium). Anabolic hormones, eg, estradiol valerate and testosterone enanthate (Deladumone), 1–3 mL/mo, may be given as for osteoporosis.

Three therapeutic agents have been introduced to reduce excessive bone resorption, with consequent fall of serum alkaline phosphatase and urinary hydroxyproline. They should be reserved for active and progressive disease. The calcitonins (porcine, human, and salmon) act by reducing osteoclastic activity. **Synthetic salmon calcitonin (Calcimar)** is given in doses of 50–100 IU subcutaneously daily or 3 times weekly for several months to years. Aside from local sensitivity reactions, systemic side effects—eg, flushing, nausea—are rare. It is expensive, and antibody formation is common. Escape from treatment (return of abnormal laboratory features or symptoms even though treatment is maintained) commonly occurs. **Synthetic human calcitonin (Cibacalcin)** has been recently released in the USA for the treatment of active Paget's disease. It is of use in patients who fail to respond to salmon calcitonin or have developed resistance due to antibodies. It is more expensive than other forms of therapy and causes side effects, including nausea and flushing, in as many as 20% of patients. The dose is 0.5 mg/d subcutaneously. The **diphosphonates** coat the bone crystal, making it less subject to excessive resorption. The diphosphonate EHDP (ethane-1-hydroxy-1-1-diphosphonic acid) is available as **etidronate disodium (Didronel)** in 200 and 400 mg tablets. The safest dose is 5 mg/kg daily for 90–180 days. In severe disease, 10 mg/kg/d may be used for 90 days, with rest periods before another course is given. Etidronate disodium is effective orally with minor side effects (eg, diarrhea), but it must only be used for short periods of time and in low dosage in order to avoid adverse effects on normal bone, eg, spontaneous fractures due to mineralizing defect. Newer diphosphonates (eg, 3-amino-1-hydroxypropylidene-1, 1-bisphosphonate [A.D.P.]) are equally effective and safer agents without adverse effects on bone but are not generally available in the USA. **Mithramycin,** an antitumor agent, works most rapidly in reducing activity of the bone disease, with rapid fall of the serum alkaline phosphatase level. It must be used as a slow intravenous infusion. Toxicity may be severe, and the drug should be used only in the most serious cases. Blood counts and liver function tests must be obtained throughout treatment. Response is at times so rapid that hypocalcemia occurs. Patients may respond to one agent after they have escaped from the beneficial effects of another. Combined or sequential therapy using several agents is under investigation. The choice of the best agent and the duration of treatment must be individualized.

## Prognosis

The prognosis of the mild form is good, but sarcomatous changes (in 1–3%) or renal complications secondary to hypercalciuria (in 10%) alter the prognosis unfavorably. In general, the prognosis is worse the earlier in life the disease starts. Fractures usually heal well. In the severe forms, marked deformity, intractable pain, and cardiac failure are found. The recently introduced therapeutic agents may improve the prognosis significantly, but osteogenic sarcoma is unresponsive to any form of therapy, including mithramycin.

Altman RD: Long-term follow-up of therapy with intermittent etidronate disodium in Paget's disease of bone. *Am J Med* 1985;**79**:583.

Altman RD, Singer F (editors): Proceedings of the Kroc Foundation Conference on Paget's Disease of Bone. *Arthritis Rheum* 1980;**10(Suppl):**23.

Cawley MI: Complications of Paget's disease of bone. *Gerontology* 1983;**29**:276.

Hoskins DJ: Paget's disease of bone: An update on management. *Drugs* 1985;**30:**156.

Jacobs TP: Diagnosis and management of Paget's disease. *Compr Ther* (March) 1986;**12:**30.

Krane SM: Etidronate disodium in the treatment of Paget's disease of bone. *Ann Intern Med* 1982;**96**:619.

Perry HM III, Droke DM, Avioli LV: Alternate calcitonin and etidronate disodium therapy for Paget's bone disease. *Arch Intern Med* 1984;**144**:929.

Schajowicz F, Santini AE, Berenstein M: Sarcoma complicating Paget's disease of bone: A clinicopathological study of 62 cases. *J Bone Joint Surg [Br]* 1983;**65**:299.

Singer FR, Mills BG: Evidence for a viral etiology of Paget's disease of bone. *Clin Orthop* 1983;**178**:245.

Strewler GJ: Paget's disease of bone. *West J Med* 1984;**140**:763.

Upchurch KS et al: Giant cell reparative granuloma of Paget's disease of bone: A unique clinical entity. *Ann Intern Med* 1983;**98**:35.

Wallach S: Treatment of Paget's disease. *Adv Intern Med* 1982;**27**:1.

Whyte MP, Daniels EH, Murphy WA: Osteolytic Paget's bone disease in a young man: Rapid healing with human calcitonin therapy. *Am J Med* 1985;**78**:326.

# DISEASES OF THE ADRENAL CORTEX

Total destruction of both adrenal cortices is not compatible with human life. The cortex regulates a variety of metabolic processes by means of secretion of some 30 steroid hormones, of which 2, cortisol and aldosterone, are of paramount importance.

The main stimulus for release of steroid hormones from the adrenal cortex appears to be adrenocorticotropic hormone (ACTH) from the anterior pituitary, which, in turn, is under the control of the hypothalamic corticotropin-releasing factor. The plasma free cortisol level, in turn, is one of the factors that regulates ACTH secretion. Aldosterone secretion, in contrast, is principally controlled by volume receptors, by angiotensin II, and also by the plasma potassium concentration. Clinical syndromes of adrenal insufficiency or excess may thus be due to primary lesions of the adrenal glands themselves or may be secondary to pituitary disorders. Although the differentiation is often important from the diagnostic standpoint, treatment is usually directed toward the cortical disorder itself, whether primary or secondary. Many of the steroids isolated from the adrenal cortex are not active, and some have more than one action. Transcortin, a plasma globulin, avidly binds cortisol and thus inactivates it. Estrogens increase transcortin levels. An active equilibrium exists between bound and free unbound cortisol. In general, the adrenocortical hormones have 3 types of activity:

**(1) Catabolic (glucocorticoids):** Cortisol and related steroids, the "stress hormones" of the adrenal cortex, are vital for survival. These steroids have a general "catabolic" action, increasing protein breakdown, inducing hyperaminoacidemia, and causing a negative nitrogen balance. They also increase gluconeogenesis and have an "anti-insulin" effect. They possess significant anti-inflammatory properties and alter the body's immune response.

**(2) Electrolyte-regulating (mineralocorticoids):** The principal hormone in this group is aldosterone. Its primary role is in retaining sodium and excreting potassium and thus "regulating" the extracellular fluid compartment and the blood pressure. It has minor effects on carbohydrate metabolism.

Most of the clinical features of both adrenal insufficiency and excess can be explained on the basis of the above types of activity. Since mixed pictures occur, however, and since excess of one type of activity may coexist with deficiency of another (eg, congenital adrenal virilism), exact physiologic correlation is difficult. Some phenomena, eg, the pigmentation of adrenal insufficiency, are not yet fully explained, and may be due to a pituitary intermedin or ACTH excess.

**(3) Anabolic (sex steroids):** Androstenedione and related $C_{19}$ steroids are protein builders and are also virilizing and androgenic, and represent the principal source of androgens in the female.

Improved chemical and radioimmunoassays of various hormones, stimulation and suppression tests, and refined radiologic procedures have facilitated accurate diagnosis of adrenal disorders. A problem seen with increased frequency is that of the patient who has no obvious symptoms of adrenal dysfunction but who is found to have an adrenal mass in a CT scan of the abdomen performed for an unrelated reason. Careful history taking, physical examination, and judicious use of the laboratory often allow the physician to determine the best course of therapy.

Copeland PM: The incidentally discovered adrenal mass. *Ann Intern Med* 1983;**98**:40.

James VHT, Few JD: Adrenocorticosteroids: Chemistry, synthesis, and disturbances in disease. *Clin Endocrinol Metab* 1985;**14**:867.

Streeten DHP et al: Normal and abnormal function of the hypothalmic-pituitary-adrenocortical system in man. *Endocr Rev* 1984;**5**:371.

## ADRENOCORTICAL HYPOFUNCTION
## (Adrenocortical Insufficiency)

### 1. ACUTE ADRENAL INSUFFICIENCY (Adrenal Crisis)

### Essentials of Diagnosis

- Onset of weakness, abdominal pain, high fever, confusion, nausea and vomiting, and diarrhea, with infection, or adrenal destruction, or cortisone withdrawal.
- Low blood pressure, dehydration, and increased skin pigmentation.
- Serum potassium high, sodium low, blood urea nitrogen high.
- Corticosteroids low in blood and urine.

## General Considerations

Acute adrenal insufficiency is a true medical emergency caused by sudden marked deprivation or insufficient supply of adrenocortical hormones. Crisis may occur in the course of chronic insufficiency in a known addisonian patient, or it may be the presenting manifestation of adrenal insufficiency. Acute crisis is more commonly seen in diseases of the cortex itself than in disorders of the pituitary gland causing secondary adrenocortical hypofunction.

Adrenal crisis may occur in the following situations: (1) Following stress, eg, trauma, surgery, infection, or prolonged fasting in a patient with latent insufficiency. (2) Following sudden withdrawal of adrenocortical hormone after replacement in a patient with chronic insufficiency or in a patient with temporary insufficiency due to suppression by exogenous glucocorticoids. (3) Following bilateral adrenalectomy or removal of a functioning adrenal tumor that had suppressed the other adrenal. (4) Following sudden destruction of the pituitary gland (pituitary necrosis), or when thyroid or insulin is given to a patient with panhypopituitarism. (5) Following injury to both adrenals by trauma, hemorrhage, anticoagulant therapy, thrombosis, infection, or, rarely, metastatic carcinoma. In overwhelming sepsis (principally meningococcemia), massive bilateral adrenal hemorrhage may occur (Waterhouse-Friderichsen syndrome).

## Clinical Findings

**A. Symptoms and Signs:** The patient complains of headache, lassitude, nausea and vomiting, abdominal pain, and often diarrhea. Confusion or coma may be present. Fever may be 40.6 °C (105 °F) or more. The blood pressure is low. Other signs may include cyanosis, petechiae (especially with meningococcemia), dehydration, abnormal skin pigmentation with sparse axillary hair, and lymphadenopathy.

**B. Laboratory Findings:** A high eosinophil count is often found in adrenal failure, but it is not specific. The blood glucose and serum sodium levels are low. Serum potassium and blood urea nitrogen are high. Hypercalcemia may be present. Blood culture may be positive (usually meningococci). Urinary and blood cortisol levels are very low. Plasma ACTH is markedly elevated if the patient has primary adrenal disease (generally higher than 200 pg/mL).

**C. Electrocardiographic Findings:** The ECG may show decreased voltage.

## Differential Diagnosis

This condition must be differentiated from other causes of coma and confusion, such as diabetic coma, cerebrovascular accident, and acute poisoning, and from other causes of high fever. The high serum potassium is not specific, but it should alert the physician to this possibility. The blood glucose is usually low, but the condition may coexist with diabetes mellitus, in which case the blood sugar is high, which may be misleading. Eosinophilia and lymphocytosis, which are usually absent in other emergencies, and low plasma cortisol help in the differentiation. (*Note:* If the diagnosis is suspected, draw blood sample for cortisol and treat with hydrocortisone, 100–300 mg intravenously, and saline *immediately,* without waiting for the results of laboratory tests.)

## Complications

Any of the progressive complications of the initiating disease may occur. The complications of treatment or those occurring during the course of treatment are discussed below.

When treatment is instituted, certain complications may be observed. Hyperpyrexia, loss of consciousness, generalized edema with hypertension, and flaccid paralysis due to low potassium have followed excessive use of intravenous fluids and corticosteroids. Psychotic reactions may occur with cortisone therapy.

## Treatment

The patient must be treated vigorously and observed constantly until well out of danger. (*Note:* It is better to overtreat than to undertreat.)

**A. Severe Crisis:**

**1. Emergency treatment**–Institute appropriate antishock measures (see Chapter 1), especially intravenous fluids and plasma, vasopressor drugs, and oxygen. Do not give narcotics or sedatives.

Give hydrocortisone phosphate or hydrocortisone sodium succinate, 100 mg intravenously immediately, and continue intravenous infusions of 50–100 mg every 6 hours for the first day. Give the same amount every 8 hours on the second day and then gradually reduce the dosage every 8 hours.

If hydrocortisone sodium succinate or hydrocortisone phosphate is not available, give cortisone acetate, 10–25 mg intramuscularly in 4 different sites (to a total of 40–100 mg), following with single injections of cortisone, 25–50 mg intramuscularly every 6 hours, and gradually lengthen the intervals of administration to 25 mg every 8 hours.

Give anti-infective agents as needed, eg, as for meningococcal meningitis. Monitor serum electrolytes and creatinine, blood urea nitrogen, and blood glucose.

**2. Convalescent treatment**–When the patient is able to take food by mouth, give oral hydrocortisone, 10–20 mg every 6 hours, and reduce dosage to maintenance levels as needed.

**B. Moderate Crisis:** If the patient's physical condition does not appear to be critical and is not associated with a significant degree of shock, the treatment outlined above may be modified by appropriate reduction in dosage. However, it is generally best to overtreat the patient in moderate crisis during the first 24 hours rather than risk undertreatment.

**C. Complications During Treatment:** Excessive use of intravenous fluids and corticosteroids may cause generalized edema with hypertension; flaccid paralysis due to potassium depletion and psychotic reactions may occur. Monitor blood pressure and ECGs throughout treatment.

1. Overhydration, usually due to sodium retention, may result in cerebral edema (with unconsciousness or convulsions) or pulmonary edema. Withhold sodium and fluids temporarily and treat for these conditions.

2. Hypokalemia—Flaccid paralysis, with low serum potassium, usually occurring on the second to fourth days of treatment, must be treated with potassium salts.

3. Hyperpyrexia is rare with present treatment methods.

4. For other complications of adrenal steroid therapy (eg, psychotic reactions), see p 747.

### Prognosis

Before replacement therapy and antibiotics became available, acute adrenal crisis was often rapidly fatal. Even today, if treatment is not early and vigorous, death occurs in several hours. Once the crisis has passed, the patient must be observed carefully to assess the degree of permanent adrenal insufficiency and to establish the cause if possible.

### 2. CHRONIC ADRENOCORTICAL INSUFFICIENCY (Addison's Disease)

### Essentials of Diagnosis

- Weakness, easy fatigability, anorexia; frequent episodes of nausea and vomiting, and diarrhea.
- Sparse axillary hair; increased skin pigmentation of creases, pressure areas, and nipples.
- Hypotension, small heart.
- Serum sodium and chloride are low. Serum potassium and blood urea nitrogen are elevated. Eosinophilia and lymphocytosis are present.
- Plasma cortisol levels are low to absent and fail to rise after administration of corticotropin. Urinary 17-ketosteroids and 17-hydroxycorticosteroids are low.
- Plasma ACTH level elevated.

### General Considerations

Addison's disease is a rare disorder due to progressive destruction of the adrenal cortices. It is characterized by chronic deficiency of hormones concerned with gluconeogenesis and with mineral metabolism, and causes often striking skin pigmentation. Electrolyte deficiencies may be the dominant manifestation. If chronic adrenal insufficiency is secondary to pituitary failure (atrophy, necrosis, tumor), lack of glycostasis is more commonly seen than electrolyte deficiencies, and skin pigmentary changes are not encountered. A syndrome of isolated aldosterone lack has been described, with persistent hyperkalemia, periodic paralysis, salt wasting, and acidosis. The majority of these patients have hypoaldosteronism on the basis of reduced renin production or release. This

syndrome is commonly seen in elderly diabetics with chronic renal failure.

The term Addison's disease should be reserved for adrenal insufficiency due to adrenocortical disease. Tuberculosis of the adrenals is no longer the most common cause, accounting today for less than one-third of cases. Idiopathic atrophy accounts for most of the other cases. There may be associated thyroiditis, hypoparathyroidism, hypogonadism, diabetes mellitus, pernicious anemia, and candidiasis. An autoimmune mechanism has been postulated for these and other causes of idiopathic atrophy.

Rare causes include metastatic carcinoma (especially of the breast or lung), coccidioidomycosis of the adrenal gland, syphilitic gummas, scleroderma, amyloid disease, and hemochromatosis. Bilateral adrenal hemorrhage may occur in patients taking anticoagulants, in patients in shock, or during open heart surgery, resulting in Addison's disease.

### Clinical Findings

**A. Symptoms and Signs:** The symptoms are weakness and fatigability, anorexia, nausea and vomiting, diarrhea, nervous and mental irritability, and faintness, especially after missing meals. Pigmentary changes consist of diffuse tanning over nonexposed as well as exposed parts or multiple freckles; or accentuation of pigment over pressure points and over the nipples, buttocks, perineum and recent scars. Black freckles may appear on the mucous membranes of the mouth. Seven to 15% of patients have associated vitiligo.

Other findings include hypotension with small heart, hyperplasia of lymphoid tissues, stiffness and calcification of the cartilages of the ear, scant to absent axillary and pubic hair (especially in women), absence of sweating, and at times costovertebral angle tenderness.

**B. Laboratory Findings:** The white count shows moderate neutropenia (about $5000/\mu L$), lymphocytosis (35–50%), and a total eosinophil count over $300/\mu L$. Hemoconcentration is present. Serum potassium and urea nitrogen are elevated; serum sodium is low. The serum sodium:potassium ratio is less than 30. Fasting blood glucose is low. Hypercalcemia may be present.

Low plasma cortisol (less than 5 $\mu g/dL$) at 8 AM is diagnostic, especially if accompanied by simultaneous elevation of the plasma ACTH level. Urinary 17-hydroxysteroids, 17-ketosteroids, and free cortisol are low.

Adrenal calcification on x-ray may be found in about 10% of cases, most frequently in granulomatous diseases such as tuberculosis and coccidioidomycosis.

**C. Special Tests:**

1. **The 8-hour intravenous corticotropin** test is the most specific and reliable diagnostic test. Each day, for 3–4 consecutive days, 25 units of corticotropin or 0.25 mg of the synthetic cosyntropin (Cortrosyn) is given in 1000 mL of physiologic saline by intravenous infusion. In primary Addison's disease,

the 24-hour urine 17-hydroxycorticosteroid values fail to rise; in adrenal insufficiency secondary to pituitary insufficiency or in patients who have had suppressive corticosteroid therapy, there is a slow, stepwise rise of 17-hydroxycorticosteroid levels after several days of stimulation. (*Note:* The patient suspected of having Addison's disease should be protected from untoward reactions during the test by the administration of 0.5 mg of dexamethasone without materially altering the urinary steroid levels.)

2. A more rapid test is the **plasma cortisol response to ACTH.** Plasma cortisol samples are obtained in the basal state and 45 minutes after intramuscular injection of 25 units of corticotropin or 0.25 mg of cosyntropin (Cortrosyn). If the plasma cortisol does not rise by at least 10 $\mu$g/dL, the diagnosis of primary or secondary adrenal insufficiency is likely.

3. Autoimmune antibodies to adrenal tissue may be found in idiopathic adrenal atrophy.

4. Plasma ACTH levels are high in primary adrenal insufficiency (> 200 pg/mL).

### Differential Diagnosis

Differentiate from anorexia nervosa, sprue syndrome, and malignant tumors. Weakness must be differentiated from that due to hyperparathyroidism, hyperthyroid myopathy, and myasthenia gravis; skin pigmentation from that of primary skin diseases, ethnic or racial pigmentation, and hemochromatosis.

### Complications

Any of the complications of the underlying disease (eg, tuberculosis) are more likely to occur, and the patient is susceptible to intercurrent infections that may precipitate crisis. Diabetes mellitus and, rarely, thyrotoxicosis may be associated. Thyroiditis, hypoparathyroidism, pernicious anemia, and ovarian failure, probably caused by an autoimmune disorder, may be associated with idiopathic adrenal failure. Hypercalcemia is most apt to occur in children, especially when the adrenocortical level is suddenly reduced.

The dangers of overzealous treatment as well as inadequate replacement must be guarded against. Psychoses, gastric irritation, and low-potassium syndrome may occur with corticosteroid treatment. Corticosteroid treatment may impair the patient's resistance to tuberculosis, which may spread. Excessive mineralocorticoid administration leads to hypertension, edema, and muscular weakness.

### Treatment

**A. Specific Therapy:** Replacement therapy should include a combination of glucocorticoids and mineralocorticoids. In mild cases, hydrocortisone alone may be adequate.

1. Hydrocortisone is the drug of choice. Most addisonian patients are well maintained on 15–25 mg of hydrocortisone orally daily in 2–3 divided doses. On this dosage, most of the metabolic abnor-

malities are corrected. Many patients, however, do not obtain sufficient salt-retaining effect and require desoxycorticosterone or fludrocortisone supplementation or extra dietary salt.

2. If hydrocortisone tablets are not available, cortisone acetate can be used. It is rapidly transformed in the liver to hydrocortisone. The dose is about 20% higher than that of hydrocortisone. Another effective and inexpensive glucocorticoid is prednisone, given in a dosage of 5–7.5 mg/d.

3. Fludrocortisone acetate has a potent sodium-retaining effect. The dosage is 0.05–0.1 mg orally daily or every other day, added to cortisone or hydrocortisone. If postural hypotension, hyperkalemia, or weight loss occurs, raise the dose. If weight gain, edema, hypokalemia, or hypertension ensues, lower the dose.

4. Desoxycorticosterone acetate controls electrolyte balance, and, since it has no other significant metabolic effect, it must be used in combination with cortisone or hydrocortisone. It is given intramuscularly initially. The usual dose is 1–4 mg intramuscularly daily. Desoxycorticosterone acetate is now rarely used for chronic therapy.

*Caution:* When using desoxycorticosterone acetate or fludrocortisone, avoid overdosage. Patients receiving these drugs should not be on low-potassium diets, because of the possibility that potassium deficiency may develop.

5. Sodium chloride in large doses (5–20 g daily) may be used to supplement hydrocortisone therapy instead of desoxycorticosterone acetate or if desoxycorticosterone acetate or fludrocortisone is not available.

**B. General Measures:** If replacement therapy is adequate, most patients need no special diets or precautions. Prevent exposure to infection. Treat all infections immediately and vigorously, and raise the dose of cortisone appropriately. The dose of glucocorticoid should also be raised in case of trauma, surgery, complicated diagnostic procedures, or other forms of stress. Patients are well advised to carry at all times a card or bracelet giving information about their disease and their need for hydrocortisone.

### Criteria of Adequate Therapy & Overdosage

**A. Adequate Therapy:**

1. Return of blood pressure to normal.
2. Maintenance of normal fasting blood glucose level.
3. Return of serum electrolytes to normal levels.
4. Weight gain (usually due to fluid).
5. Improvement of appetite and strength.
6. Increase in size of heart to normal.

**B. Overdosage:** Excessive administration of cortisone or desoxycorticosterone acetate must be avoided, especially in patients with cardiac or renal complications.

1. Signs and symptoms of cortisone overdosage are discussed on p 747.

2. Development of dependent edema, or excessive weight gain.

3. Development of hypertension.

4. Increase of diameter of heart above normal.

5. Development of signs of potassium deficiency (weakness followed by loss of muscle power and finally paralysis), especially if the patient is on a low-potassium diet.

## Prognosis

With adequate replacement therapy, the life expectancy of patients with Addison's disease is markedly prolonged. Active tuberculosis responds to specific chemotherapy. Withdrawal of treatment or increased demands due to infection, trauma, surgery, or other types of stress may precipitate crisis with a sudden fatal outcome unless large doses of parenteral corticosteroids are employed. Pregnancy may be followed by exacerbation of the disease. Psychotic reactions may interfere with management. Hyperkalemic paralysis is a rare but serious complication if potassium intake is not monitored.

The ultimate prognosis depends largely upon the intelligence of the patient and the availability of medical supervision. A fully active life is now possible for the majority of patients.

Burke CW: Adrenocortical insufficiency. *Clin Endocrinol Metab* 1985;**14:**947.

Melby JC: Diagnosis and treatment of primary aldosteronism and isolated hypoaldosteronism. *Clin Endocrinol Metab* 1985;**14:**977.

## ADRENOCORTICAL OVERACTIVITY

Overactivity of the adrenal secretions is caused either by bilateral hyperplasia or by adenoma or, more rarely, carcinoma of one adrenal. The clinical picture will vary with the type of secretion produced, but in general, 3 clinical disorders can be differentiated: (1) Cushing's syndrome, in which the glucocorticoids predominate; (2) the adrenogenital syndrome, in which the adrenal androgens predominate (feminizing tumors are rare); and (3) hyperaldosteronism, with mineralocorticoid excess. The clinical picture is most apt to be mixed in cases of malignant tumor and in bilateral hyperplasia. All syndromes of adrenal overactivity are far more common in females than in males.

## 1. CUSHING'S SYNDROME
### (Adrenocortical Hyperfunction)

## Essentials of Diagnosis

- Centripetal obesity, easy bruisability, psychosis, hirsutism, purple striae.
- Osteoporosis, hypertension.
- Hyperglycemia, glycosuria, low serum potassium and chloride, low total eosinophils, and lymphocytopenia.

- Elevated serum cortisol and urinary 17-hydroxysteroids. Abnormal suppression by exogenous dexamethasone.
- CT scan or MRI may reveal a small pituitary adenoma.

## General Considerations

The term Cushing's syndrome refers to hypercortisolism due to any cause. The primary lesion may be in the pituitary or the hypothalamus, with resultant hypersecretion of ACTH and anatomic or functional bilateral adrenal hyperplasia. It has been speculated that ACTH hypersecretion by the pituitary may be the result of autonomous ACTH-secreting adenoma or of increased release of corticotropin releasing factor by the hypothalamus. This is the most common form of the disorder (about 70%) and is usually referred to as Cushing's disease. Hypercortisolism may also be due to an autonomous adrenal tumor (adenoma or carcinoma) or to ectopic secretion of an ACTH-like material by a nonpituitary neoplasm.

Hypercortisolism due to a tumor of one adrenal is usually associated with atrophy of the contralateral gland. Carcinoma of the adrenal (5%) is always unilateral and often metastasizes late. A mixed picture with virilization is often present.

Adrenal rest tumors in the ovary rarely cause Cushing's syndrome; they are more commonly associated with virilizing syndromes. Carcinoma of the anterior pituitary is a rare cause of Cushing's disease.

Administration of corticotropin causes adrenal hyperplasia; administration of glucocorticoid causes adrenal atrophy associated with most features of Cushing's syndrome. These effects are partially reversible when medication is withdrawn.

Certain extra-adrenal malignant tumors (eg, bronchogenic oat cell carcinoma) may secrete ACTH or, more rarely, corticotropin-releasing factor and produce severe Cushing's syndrome with bilateral adrenal hyperplasia. Severe hypokalemia and hyperpigmentation are commonly found in this group.

## Clinical Findings

**A. Symptoms and Signs:** Cushing's syndrome causes "moon face" and "buffalo hump," obesity with protuberant abdomen, and thin extremities; a plethoric appearance; oligomenorrhea or amenorrhea (or impotence in the male); weakness, backache, headache; hypertension; mild acne and superficial skin infections; chloasmalike pigmentation (especially on the face), hirsutism (mostly of the lanugo hair over the face and upper trunk, arms, and legs), purple striae (especially around the thighs, breasts, and abdomen), and easy bruisability (eg, hematoma formation following venipuncture). Mental symptoms may range from increased lability of mood to frank psychosis.

**B. Laboratory Findings:** Glucose tolerance is low, often with glycosuria. The patient is resistant to the action of insulin. Urinary 17-hydroxycorticosteroids and plasma cortisol are high (the latter over

20 $\mu g/dL$). (*Note:* In patients receiving estrogens— eg, contraceptive pills—the plasma cortisol levels are elevated due to increase in cortisol-binding globulin. The usual diurnal variation in plasma cortisol levels is absent in Cushing's syndrome. Urinary free cortisol is always elevated. Urinary 17-ketosteroids are often low or normal in Cushing's syndrome due to adenoma; normal or high if the disorder is due to hyperplasia; and very high if due to carcinoma. Total eosinophils are low (under $50/\mu L$), lymphocytes are under 20%, and red and white blood cell counts are elevated. Serum $CO_2$ is high and serum $Cl^-$ and $K^+$ are low in some cases, especially those associated with malignant tumors.

**C. Imaging:** Osteoporosis of the skull, spine, and ribs is common. Nephrolithiasis may be present. CT scan or MRI easily demonstrates most adrenal tumors if any are present. Bilateral adrenal hyperplasia can also be visualized. Since the pituitary adenomas causing Cushing's disease are usually very small, they are always missed by conventional radiographic techniques, but many can be demonstrated by CT or MRI scans of the pituitary. Adrenal angiography or $^{131}I$-19-iodocholesterol scanning may demonstrate small adrenal tumors or hyperplastic glands.

**D. Electrocardiographic Findings:** The ECG may show signs of hypertension and hypokalemia and a short PR interval.

**E. Special Tests:** (*Note:* Exceptions to the following rules are occasionally seen.)

**1. Dexamethasone suppression tests**–These tests, originally described by Grant Liddle, are still very useful. Administering dexamethasone in low doses (0.5 mg every 6 hours for 2 days) separates patients with all forms of Cushing's syndrome from those who do not have the disorder. (A common problem is to decide whether an obese, hypertensive, slightly hirsute woman does or does not have hypercortisolism.) In patients with Cushing's syndrome, the 24-hour urinary 17-hydroxycorticosteroids are not reduced to less than 3.5 mg in the second day of dexamethasone administration as they are in normals.

Once it is clear that the patient has hypercortisolism, one proceeds to the high-dose dexamethasone suppression test (2 mg every 6 hours for 2 days). In patients with Cushing's *disease,* (pituitary hypersecretion of ACTH), the urinary 17-hydroxycorticosteroids are lowered to less than 50% of the baseline value. This does not occur in those with adrenal tumors or ectopic ACTH production.

A faster, less accurate screening test for Cushing's syndrome is administration of 1 mg of dexamethasone at midnight. In most normal subjects, plasma cortisol levels are suppressed the following morning to less than 5 $\mu g/dL$. Patients with Cushing's syndrome do not suppress to this value and should have additional work-up.

**2. ACTH stimulation test**–The administration of ACTH causes marked hypersecretion of plasma cortisol and urinary 17-hydroxycorticosteroids and 17-ketosteroids in Cushing's disease and often also in cases due to adrenal adenoma; but ACTH does not stimulate secretion in cases due to adrenal carcinoma or ectopic ACTH.

**3. Metyrapone (Metopirone) stimulation test**–Failure of 11-deoxycortisol (compound S) to rise after a 4-hour infusion or after an oral dose of 500 mg every hour for 6 doses indicates that the hypercortisolism is due to adrenal tumor or ectopic ACTH secretion.

**4. Direct assay of plasma ACTH**–ACTH is markedly decreased in cases of autonomous secretion of cortisol by an adrenal tumor (adenoma or carcinoma). It is high normal or elevated in patients with Cushing's disease and usually very high in those with ACTH-secreting ectopic tumors producing Cushing's syndrome and in Nelson's syndrome (see below).

**5. The urinary free cortisol test**–This test is very useful for the diagnosis of Cushing's syndrome, since, unlike the 17-hydroxycorticosteroids, free cortisol excretion is not affected by drugs, obesity, hyperthyroidism, etc.

**6. Corticotropin-releasing hormone test**–This new stimulation test is not yet generally available. It has proved useful in the differential diagnosis of hypercortisolism—and especially in the clarification of the mechanism of the hypercortisolism of depression, which is associated with decreased response of the pituitary to corticotropin-releasing hormone, whereas patients with Cushing's disease have plasma ACTH hyperresponsiveness to the same stimulus.

## Differential Diagnosis

A frequent problem is differentiating true Cushing's syndrome from obesity associated with diabetes mellitus, especially if there are hirsutism and amenorrhea. The distribution of fat, the presence or absence of muscle atrophy in the extremities, and the color and width of the striae often help but are not infallible signs. Dexamethasone suppression tests often clarify the diagnosis. Cushing's syndrome must be differentiated from the adrenogenital syndrome (see below), since the latter may be amenable to medical treatment unless it is caused by tumor. The 2 diseases may coexist. An elderly woman with osteoporosis, diabetes, and mild hirsutism may present a difficult problem in differentiation. Exogenous administration of corticosteroids must be kept in mind. Hypercortisolism secondary to alcoholism has been reported (pseudo-Cushing's syndrome).

In rare cases, the outstanding manifestation of Cushing's disease or syndrome may be only diabetes, osteoporosis, hypertension, or psychosis. Adrenal disease must be ruled out in patients with these disorders, especially in insulin-resistant diabetes mellitus, since early treatment may be curative. The dexamethasone suppression tests (see above) are most helpful in differentiation.

## Complications

The patient may suffer from any of the complications of hypertension, including congestive failure, cerebrovascular accidents, and coronary attacks, or of diabetes. Susceptibility to infections, especially of the skin and urinary tract, is increased. Compression fractures of the osteoporotic spine may cause marked disability. Renal colic may occur. Intractable peptic ulcer may be present. Most serious, perhaps, are the psychotic complications not infrequently observed in this disease. After adrenalectomy, hypercalcemia and pancreatitis may complicate the recovery. Pituitary enlargement (due to ACTH-secreting adenomas) and deepening skin pigmentation have been observed following adrenalectomy for hyperplasia (Nelson's syndrome), causing, at times, visual field abnormalities.

## Treatment

### A. Specific Measures:

1. Adrenal tumors are removed surgically. Total resection of both adrenals in patients with diffuse bilateral hyperplasia was the treatment of choice for rapidly advancing Cushing's disease. At present, the preferred initial therapy is transsphenoidal surgical removal of the ACTH-secreting pituitary adenoma. In selected cases, pituitary irradiation may be used, and there are a few patients who may respond well to pharmacologic inhibition of ACTH secretion. If these measures fail to produce a remission of the disease, total adrenalectomy is performed. Adequate preoperative medication and care are of utmost importance. The patient should receive all general measures listed below, plus adequate hormonal supplementation.

If bilateral adrenalectomy is contemplated, give high doses of cortisone, eg, cortisone acetate, 100–300 mg intramuscularly, or, preferably, 100–300 mg of hydrocortisone hemisuccinate (Solu-Cortef) in divided doses intramuscularly or intravenously, on the day of surgery; continue the intramuscular dosage for 1–2 days after surgery, then gradually decrease the dose and maintain on oral hydrocortisone as for Addison's disease. Because of the danger of precipitating heart failure, care must be taken to avoid excessive fluids and sodium.

In cases of unilateral tumor, the patient is prepared as for total adrenalectomy. After surgery, cortisol must be provided. Treatment with cortisol may have to be continued for weeks or months, since the contralateral gland has undergone atrophy because of ACTH suppression and may be slow to recover function.

2. X-ray therapy to the pituitary has been the treatment of choice in children with Cushing's disease. Transsphenoidal microadenomectomy is now preferred. Partial destruction of the pituitary by other means (proton beam, yttrium implant, cryotherapy) has been attempted. Hypophysectomy may be required for large adenomas.

Large numbers of patients with Cushing's disease have now been reported as "cured" following removal of ACTH-secreting pituitary microadenomas via a transsphenoidal approach. An experienced neurosurgeon is required. Long-term follow-up of these cases is lacking, but reports of recurrences are disturbing.

3. Removal of a malignant tumor producing Cushing's syndrome by ectopic secretion of ACTH should be attempted if feasible.

4. Chemical treatment by means of adrenocortical inhibitors has been largely unsuccessful. The least toxic of these, mitotane (Lysodren; *o,p'*-DDD), has limited use in inoperable carcinomas. Metyrapone and aminoglutethimide have been used to reduce adrenocortical overactivity, but the results are erratic. The antiserotonin drug cyproheptadine has been reported to induce remission of the disease, but this has not been universally confirmed.

5. A rare variant of Cushing's syndrome is bilateral nodular adrenal hyperplasia. These patients now have low or undetectable serum ACTH, do not suppress well with dexamethasone, and appear to have autonomous secretion of cortisol. Bilateral adrenalectomy is the treatment of choice.

**B. General Measures:** A high-protein diet should be given, although dietary attempts to correct the negative nitrogen balance are never successful. Potassium chloride administration may replace losses before and after surgery.

Insulin is usually unnecessary, as the diabetes is mild; however, if the hyperglycemia is severe, it should be given in spite of the insulin resistance usually present.

## Prognosis

This is a chronic disease that is subject to cyclic exacerbations (especially with pregnancy) and rare spontaneous remissions; it is a serious and often fatal disease unless discovered and treated early. A rather rapid course suggests a malignant tumor, but these may be dormant for years.

The best prognosis for total recovery is for patients in whom a benign adrenal adenoma has been removed and who have survived the postadrenalectomy state of adrenal insufficiency. Cushing's disease has a more guarded prognosis. Only 25–50% of patients with Cushing's *disease* respond to pituitary irradiation alone. Microsurgery of the pituitary, involving removal of small adenomas, may favorably alter the prognosis in the future. If extensive hypophysectomy is necessary to remove the ACTH-secreting tumor, panhypopituitarism supervenes. Diabetes insipidus, transient or permanent, may also ensue. The more extensive the surgical procedure, the more frequent will be the rate of postoperative complications. Bilateral adrenalectomy cures the hypercortisolism but is associated with high morbidity. Furthermore, it may be followed by severe hyperpigmentation and rapid growth of ACTH-secreting pituitary tumors (Nelson's syndrome) with visual complications and sometimes malignant transformation.

Complete adrenalectomy necessitates chronic replacement therapy with glucocorticoid and mineralocorticoid hormones. A small number of patients with

Cushing's disease treated with bilateral adrenalectomy have a subsequent recurrence of hypercortisolism. It is postulated that a small piece of adrenal tissue, either ectopic tissue or tissue left inadvertently by the surgeon, undergoes hyperplasia in response to the very high ACTH levels that are found after adrenalectomy.

Malignant extra-adrenal tumors are usually rapidly fatal, even after such drastic attempts at treatment as total adrenalectomy.

Carpenter PC: Cushing's syndrome: Update of diagnosis and management. *Mayo Clin Proc* 1986;**61**:49.

Chrousos GP et al: Clinical applications of corticotropin-releasing factor. *Ann Intern Med* 1985;**102**:344.

Daughaday WH: Cushing's disease and basophilic microadenomas. (Editorial.) *N Engl J Med* 1984;**310**:919.

Gold PW et al: Responses to corticotropin-releasing hormone in the hypercortisolism of depression and Cushing's disease: Pathophysiologic and diagnostic implications. *N Engl J Med* 1986;**21**:329.

Krieger DT: Physiopathology of Cushing's disease. *Endocr Rev* 1983;**4**:22.

Larsen JL et al: Primary adrenocortical nodular dysplasia, a distinct subtype of Cushing's syndrome: Case report and review of the literature. *Am J Med* 1986;**80**:976.

Orth DN: The old and the new in Cushing's syndrome. *N Engl J Med* 1984;**310**:649.

Streeten DH et al: Normal and abnormal function of the hypothalamic-pituitary-adrenocortical system in man. *Endocr Rev* 1984;**5**:371.

## 2. THE ADRENOGENITAL SYNDROME: PREPUBERTAL

Adrenal virilizing syndromes in infancy or childhood are of great interest to the pediatrician and may be due to excessive production of androgens by a tumor (benign or malignant) or, more commonly, to congenital adrenal hyperplasia.

### Congenital Adrenal Hyperplasia

The term congenital adrenal hyperplasia refers to a complex series of rare but well-studied enzymatic errors of metabolism, with deficient levels of different enzymes involved in the synthesis of cortisol. By far the most common forms are 21- and 11$\beta$-hydroxylase deficiencies, both characterized by excessive formation of adrenal androgens under the ACTH drive induced by hypocortisolism. This excess of androgens results in masculinization in the female (ranging from mild hirsutism and clitoral hypertrophy to frank pseudohermaphroditism) and in premature virilization in the male. In both entities, there is a variable degree of clinical hypocortisolism. In untreated 11$\beta$-hydroxylase deficiency, there is hypertension due to excessive formation of desoxycorticosterone, a metabolic precursor with potent mineralocorticoid activity. Hypertension never occurs in untreated 21-hydroxylase deficiency; on the contrary, a salt-losing form with clear-cut mineralocorticoid deficiency is present in approximately 50% of cases. In both enzymatic deficiencies, one finds high ACTH levels, plasma androgens, urinary pregnanetriol, and 17-ketosteroids. Specific diagnosis is made by demonstrating elevated plasma levels of the metabolic precursor immediately before the enzymatic block: 11-deoxycortisol in 11$\beta$-hydroxylase deficiency and 17-hydroxyprogesterone in 21-hydroxylase deficiency.

The fundamental step in the treatment of congenital adrenal hyperplasia is the administration of enough glucocorticoid to suppress ACTH and reverse the metabolic abnormalities. A mineralocorticoid is required in the salt-losing form. Plastic surgery may be necessary in females with ambiguous genitalia. It should be performed early in life.

New M, Levine LS: Congenital adrenal hyperplasia and related conditions. Chapter 47 in: *The Metabolic Basis of Inherited Disease,* 5th ed. Stanbury JB et al (editors). McGraw-Hill, 1983.

## 3. ADRENOGENITAL SYNDROME & VIRILIZING DISEASES OF WOMEN

### Essentials of Diagnosis

- Menstrual disorders and hirsutism.
- Regression or reversal of primary and secondary sex characteristics, with balding, hoarse voice, acne, and enlargement of the clitoris.
- Occasionally a palpable pelvic tumor.
- 17-Ketosteroids elevated in adrenal disorders, variable in others.
- Plasma testosterone often elevated.

### General Considerations

The diagnosis of virilizing disorders in women is more difficult than in young girls, since sources of abnormal androgens other than the adrenal exist, principally the ovaries. There is no interference with formation of the female genital tract or secondary sex characteristics, but rather a regression or sex reversal of varying degree. Although the diagnosis is readily apparent in a complete state of the virilizing syndrome (eg, the adult form of the congenital adrenogenital syndrome), the milder forms, presenting primarily with defeminization or merely hirsutism, may be caused by equally serious adrenal and ovarian disorders such as tumors. A sudden change in amount of hair (other than at puberty, pregnancy, or menopause) is of greater importance than hirsutism that has been present throughout life.

Besides adrenal hyperplasia and tumors, syndromes of androgen excess may be caused by the following disorders:

**(1) Ovarian disorders:** Stein-Leventhal syndrome (large, polycystic ovaries, most common), theca luteinization (thecosis ovarii), arrhenoblastoma, hilar cell tumor or hyperplasia, adrenal cell rests, dysgerminoma (rare).

**(2) Hypothalamic-pituitary disorders:** Acromegaly (eosinophilic adenoma), hyperostosis frontalis (Stewart-Morgagni-Morel syndrome).

**(3) Placental causes:** Pregnancy, choriocarcinoma.

**(4) Miscellaneous causes:** True hermaphroditism, thymic tumors, drugs (eg, testosterone).

## Clinical Findings

**A. Symptoms and Signs:** Symptoms include scant menstrual periods or amenorrhea, acne and roughening of the skin, odorous perspiration, and hoarseness or deepening of voice. Hirsutism is present over the face, body, and extremities, with thinning or balding of head hair. Musculature is increased and feminine contours are lost. The breasts and genitalia are atrophied, the clitoris and larynx enlarged. A tumor may rarely be palpable on pelvic examination (arrhenoblastoma, polycystic ovaries).

**B. Laboratory Findings:** Urinary 17-ketosteroid determination is the most important single test in the diagnosis of adrenogenital syndrome. It helps differentiate constitutional hirsutism from adrenal disorders, in which the 17-ketosteroids are significantly elevated. Very high levels favor a diagnosis of adrenal tumor. In arrhenoblastoma or Stein-Leventhal syndrome, 17-ketosteroids may be normal or moderately elevated. The dexamethasone suppression test may help distinguish between adrenal tumors, adrenal hyperplasia, and ovarian lesions. Elevated serum dehydroepiandrosterone sulfate levels suggest an adrenal lesion. LH levels are often elevated in the Stein-Leventhal syndrome. Plasma 11-deoxycortisol (compound S) and 17-hydroxyprogesterone assays, if available, are more accurate in determining enzymatic adrenal defects than the urinary 17-ketosteroid and pregnanetriol determinations.

The assay of the most potent androgen (testosterone) in the blood is the screening procedure of choice for virilized women.

**C. Imaging:** Ultrasonography is an accurate and noninvasive procedure to demonstrate ovarian enlargement. CT scan or MRI may reveal an adrenal tumor.

**D.** Laparoscopy is often helpful.

## Differential Diagnosis

Since hirsutism may be the only sign of adrenal tumor, all of the disorders characterized by excessive hair have to be considered in the differential diagnosis. From the practical standpoint, however, the diagnosis commonly depends upon whether one is dealing simply with racial, familial, or idiopathic hirsutism, where an unusual end organ sensitivity to endogenous androgen exists; or whether excessive amounts of male hormone are being produced. Recent evidence suggests that most cases of idiopathic hirsutism may be due to an ovarian abnormality in testosterone and androstenedione production and that the dexamethasone test is not reliable in differentiating between adrenal and ovarian sources of excess androgen. In general, if hirsutism is associated with enlargement

of the clitoris, deepening of the voice, frontal baldness, development of heavy musculature, or breast atrophy and amenorrhea and if the onset is rapid, one can assume that a tumor of the adrenal or ovary is present. In these circumstances, exploratory operation may be necessary in spite of equivocal laboratory findings. Although virilization is not the rule with Cushing's syndrome, a mixed picture is at times seen in malignant adrenal tumors and, more rarely, in hyperplasia.

## Complications

Aside from the known high incidence of malignancy in tumors causing virilization, the interference with femininity and consequent sterility may be irreversible. Diabetes and obesity may be complicating features. At times, mental disorders accompany states of defeminization.

## Treatment

Treatment varies with the cause of the androgen excess.

When ovarian or adrenal tumors are present, surgical removal is the treatment of choice. In cases of adrenal hyperplasia, especially starting in infancy, there may be associated manifestations of hypoadrenocorticism (eg, excessive salt and water loss and failure to maintain a fasting blood sugar). This condition is due to a congenital absence of hydroxylating enzymes of the adrenals. The "androgenic" compounds formed have no cortisol activity and are unable to suppress endogenous ACTH, hence the continued adrenal stimulation and large glands.

It has become clear that in addition to the classic presentations there are many cases of mild adrenal enzymatic deficiencies that may not be manifested clinically until adult life. "Late-onset" adrenal hyperplasia is now being recognized as a cause of hirsutism or menstrual abnormalities in some women. The most common variant is due to 21-hydroxylase deficiency. The serum concentration of 17-hydroxyprogesterone (the precursor just before the enzymatic block) is elevated.

Treatment with corticosteroids has proved valuable in reducing the activity of the glands (by suppressing endogenous ACTH) and in supplying exogenously needed corticosteroids. In adults, the drugs of choice appear to be prednisone or prednisolone, 5–15 mg daily orally, or dexamethasone, 0.5–1.5 mg daily orally, in divided doses; use the smallest dose that keeps the 17-ketosteroid, pregnanetriol, and 17-hydroxyprogesterone levels within the normal range.

The response of congenital adrenal hyperplasia to long-term corticosteroid therapy is gratifying, with lessening of virilization and hirsutism and eventually normal cyclic menstruation. Plastic repair (removal of the clitoris and repair of a urogenital sinus) is required. Corticosteroid therapy of milder forms of androgen excess (eg, simple hirsutism) is less successful. Estrogen therapy may be of some value but must be used in large dosage. A combination of estrogen-progestogen may be used for long-term suppression of ovarian androgens.

Measurement of the free, non-protein-bound fraction of serum testosterone is helpful in determining the optimal regimen in many cases of hirsutism of unclear origin.

New and still unproved forms of therapy include spironolactone and cimetidine. Androgen antagonists such as cyproterone acetate have been used successfully in experimental clinical trials but are not available in the USA for use in virilizing disorders.

## Prognosis

The outlook is favorable if a malignant tumor is removed early, since metastasis often occurs late. Glucocorticoid therapy may be of help in adrenal hyperplastic lesions. Fertility is often restored.

The ultimate fate of the virilized woman depends not only upon the underlying cause (ie, tumor or hyperplasia) but more particularly upon the age at onset of the virilizing influence and its duration. If virilization is of long standing, restoration of normal femininity or loss of hirsutism is unlikely even though the causative lesion is successfully removed.

*Note:* Many cases of simple hirsutism in females are not due to a readily demonstrable endocrine disease but to hereditary or racial factors and cannot be treated effectively with systemic medications or surgery. Epilation, preferably by electrolysis, is the treatment of choice.

Biffignandi P et al: Female hirsutism: Pathophysiological considerations and therapeutic implications. *Endocr Rev* 1984;**5**:498.

Chrousos GP et al: Late-onset 21-hydroxylase deficiency mimicking idiopathic hirsutism or polycystic ovarian disease. *Ann Intern Med* 1982;**96**:143.

Kuttenn F et al: Late onset adrenal hyperplasia in hirsutism. *N Engl J Med* 1985;**313**:224.

Kvedar JC et al: Hirsutism: Evaluation and treatment. *J Am Acad Dermatol* 1985;**12**:215.

Rittmaster RS, Loriaux DL: Hirsutism. *Ann Intern Med* 1987;**106**:95.

## PRIMARY HYPERALDOSTERONISM

### Essentials of Diagnosis

- Hypertension, polyuria, polydipsia, muscular weakness.
- Hypokalemia, hypernatremia, alkalosis.
- Elevated urinary aldosterone level and low plasma renin level.

### General Considerations

Primary hyperaldosteronism is a relatively rare disorder caused by aldosterone excess. It accounts for less than 2% of cases of hypertension. It is more common in females. The two main types of primary hyperaldosteronism are those due to adrenocortical adenoma (Conn's syndrome) and those due to macro- or micronodular cortical hyperplasia. Edema is rarely seen in primary hyperaldosteronism, but secondary hyperaldosteronism is often found in edematous states such as cardiac failure and hepatic cirrhosis.

### Clinical Findings

**A. Symptoms and Signs:** Hypertension, muscular weakness (at times with paralysis simulating periodic paralysis), paresthesias with frank tetanic manifestations, headache, polyuria (especially nocturnal), and polydipsia are the outstanding complaints. Edema is rarely present. On the other hand, some patients have only diastolic hypertension, without other signs or symptoms.

**B. Laboratory Findings:** Low serum potassium, hypernatremia, and alkalosis are characteristic, but at times the potassium level is normal. Various degrees of renal damage are manifested by proteinuria, alkaline urine, nephrocalcinosis, and low urine specific gravity unresponsive to vasopressin. Urinary and plasma aldosterone levels are markedly elevated, and plasma renin levels are low.

The best screening test in a patient with hypertension in whom primary aldosteronism is suspected is the determination of plasma renin after sodium depletion (diet or diuretic) and after several hours of being in the upright position. These stimuli normally increase renin production. In primary aldosteronism, the renin level characteristically remains *low*.

A high-sodium diet, saline infusion, or desoxycorticosterone acetate administration fails to suppress the elevated aldosterone levels.

**C. Electrocardiographic Findings:** Electrocardiographic changes are due to prolonged hypertension and hypokalemia.

**D. Imaging:** Cardiac hypertrophy due to hypertension is present. The tumors are usually small but can often be visualized by CT scan or MRI. Adrenal arteriography is rarely necessary today for visualization of adrenal adenomas. Adrenal vein catheterization for measurement of aldosterone and cortisol is sometimes necessary to confirm unilateral disease. $^{131}I$ iodocholesterol scanning can be used for the same purpose (dexamethasone is used to suppress ACTH-mediated steroid production).

**E. Other Findings:** The plasma volume is increased 30–50% above normal.

### Differential Diagnosis

This important reversible cause of hypertension must be considered in the differential diagnosis in any patient who shows muscular weakness and tetanic manifestations; and in the differential diagnosis of periodic paralysis, potassium- and sodium-losing nephritis, nephrogenic diabetes insipidus, and hypokalemia (be certain the patient has not been receiving diuretic agents). Excessive ingestion of licorice or laxatives may simulate hyperaldosteronism. The oral contraceptives may raise aldosterone secretion in some patients. Unilateral renal vascular disease producing secondary hyperaldosteronism with severe hypertension must be ruled out. Plasma renin activity is low in primary hyperaldosteronism and elevated in renal vascular disease. Excessive secretion of desoxycorticosterone and corticosterone may produce a similar clinical picture. Low renin levels are found in about 25% of cases of essential hypertension. Their response to diuretics and their prognosis are better than those of patients with hypertension associated with high renin levels. Excess of an as yet unidentified mineralocorticoid is thought by some to be responsible. Aldosteronism due to a malignant ovarian tumor has been reported.

It is important to differentiate primary aldosteronism due to an adenoma and that due to bilateral nodular hyperplasia, since the hypertension can be cured or greatly ameliorated by removal of the adenoma, whereas it usually does not respond after bilateral adrenalectomy in patients with hyperplasia. Subjects with adenoma tend to have lower serum potassiums, higher aldosterone levels, and lower renal vein renins. Postural studies are useful. Aldosterone and renin activity are determined with the patient in the recumbent position and again a few hours later after ambulation. In adenoma, the plasma aldosterone and renin levels do not change. In bilateral hyperplasia, both levels rise, reflecting the incomplete suppression of renin and its increase by assumption of the upright posture. In doubtful cases, adrenal vein catheterization may yield the diagnosis.

Recent studies raise the issue that a pituitary aldosterone stimulatory factor may exist and that its hyperproduction causes the aldosteronism of bilateral adrenal hyperplasia.

### Complications

All of the complications of chronic hypertension are encountered in primary hyperaldosteronism. Progressive renal damage is less reversible than hypertension.

### Treatment

Conn's syndrome (unilateral adrenal adenoma secreting aldosterone) is treated by surgical removal of the lesion. Bilateral adrenal hyperplasia is best treated with spironolactone. Bilateral adrenalectomy corrects the hypokalemia but not the hypertension and should *not* be performed. Antihypertensive agents may also be necessary. A rare type of hyperplasia responds well to dexamethasone suppression.

### Prognosis

The hypertension is reversible in about two-thirds of cases but persists or returns in spite of surgery in the remainder.

The prognosis is much improved by early diagnosis with chemical tests and scanning procedures.

Carey RM et al: Idiopathic hyperaldosteronism: A possible role for aldosterone stimulatory factor. *N Engl J Med* 1984;**311**:94.

Melby JC: Diagnosis and treatment of primary aldosteronism and isolated hypoaldosteronism. *Clin Endocrinol Metab* 1985;**14**:977.

Weinberger MH: Primary aldosteronism: Diagnosis and differentiation of subtypes. *Ann Intern Med* 1984;**100**:300.

# DISEASES OF THE ADRENAL MEDULLA

## PHEOCHROMOCYTOMA

### Essentials of Diagnosis

- "Spells" or "attacks" of headache, visual blurring, severe sweats, vasomotor changes in a young adult, weight loss.
- Hypertension, often paroxysmal ("spells") but frequently sustained.
- Postural tachycardia and hypotension; cardiac enlargement.
- Hypermetabolism with normal $T_4$.
- Elevation of plasma and urinary catecholamines or their metabolites.

### General Considerations

Pheochromocytoma is a rare disease characterized by paroxysmal or sustained hypertension due to a tumor of pheochrome tissue, located in either or both adrenals or anywhere along the sympathetic nervous chain, and rarely in such aberrant locations as the thorax, bladder, or brain. In about 10% of cases, the tumor involves both adrenal glands. Most tumors are sporadic; only 10–15% are familial. Bilateral adrenal tumors tend to occur more frequently in familial cases.

The following familial syndromes have been identified:

(1) Familial pheochromocytoma without other abnormalities.

(2) Pheochromocytoma associated with islet cell tumors of the pancreas.

(3) Pheochromocytoma associated with calcitonin-secreting medullary carcinoma of the thyroid and hyperparathyroidism (multiple endocrine neoplasia type II).

(4) Pheochromocytoma in association with medullary carcinoma of the thyroid and the syndrome of multiple mucosal neuromas, without hyperparathyroidism (multiple endocrine neoplasia type III).

(5) Pheochromocytoma with neurofibromatosis (Recklinghausen's disease).

(6) Pheochromocytoma with Hippel-Lindau disease (hemangioblastomas of retina, cerebellum, and other parts of the nervous system).

### Clinical Findings

**A. Symptoms and Signs:** Pheochromocytoma is manifested by attacks of severe headache, palpitation or tachycardia, profuse sweating, vasomotor changes (including pallor or flushing of the face or extremities), precordial or abdominal pain, nausea and vomiting, visual disturbances (including blurring or blindness), aphasia and loss of consciousness (rarely), increasing nervousness and irritability, increased appetite, dyspnea, angina, and loss of weight. Physical findings include hypertension, either in attacks or sustained, with cardiac enlargement; postural tachycardia (change of more than 20 beats/min) and postural hypotension; mild elevation of basal body temperature. Retinal hemorrhage or papilledema occurs occasionally.

**B. Laboratory Findings:** Hypermetabolism is present; $T_4$ and free $T_4$ are normal; and glycosuria or hyperglycemia (or both) may be present. Blood volume is usually contracted.

**C. Special Tests:** Pharmacologic provocative and suppressive tests that evaluate the rise or fall in blood pressure have become obsolete and are not recommended.

**1. Assay of urinary catecholamines on a 24-hour urine specimen**—and the simpler tests for 3-methoxy-4-hydroxymandelic acid (vanillylmandelic acid, VMA), or total metanephrines—are now generally available. Urinary catecholamines are usually elevated. One should remember that stress, catecholamine-containing topical nasal medications, many bronchodilators, and methyldopa will also produce abnormally high values. Since VMA determinations can also be affected by a number of drugs, avoidance of drug-taking during the urine collection is desirable. Antihypertensive agents such as thiazides, clonidine, and ganglionic blockers do *not* elevate VMA, metanephrines, or catecholamines.

Most patients with pheochromocytoma have clearcut elevations of urinary catecholamines (normal range up to 130 $\mu$g/24 h) and VMA (normal range, 2–7 mg/24 h). Occasionally there are patients with large tumors who have normal excretion of catecholamines but high VMA, presumably due to intratumoral metabolism of the catecholamines. Conversely, a very small, actively catecholamine-releasing tumor may be associated with normal VMA and very high urinary catecholamines. In any patient with pheochromocytoma, the secretion of catecholamines may be sporadic and intermittent.

**2. Direct assay of epinephrine and norepinephrine in blood and urine** during or following an attack is the most reliable test for pheochromocytoma associated with paroxysmal hypertension. High epinephrine levels favor tumor localization within the adrenal gland. Proper collection of specimens is essential. Determination of blood catecholamines via a venous catheter—a research procedure—will help localize ectopic lesions and paragangliomas.

**3. Clonidine suppression test**–This test of plasma catecholamines has recently been proposed to differentiate pheochromocytoma (no suppression) from essential hypertension. Experience is limited, and the test has not yet been proved useful.

**4. Imaging**– CT scan and MRI have been shown to be very accurate in the diagnosis of these tumors. Ultrasonography is useful in demonstrating adrenal or para-adrenal masses.

A radioactive scanning procedure has recently been described. Results seem encouraging, but experience is limited.

### Differential Diagnosis

Pheochromocytoma should always be suspected in any patient with labile hypertension, especially if some of the other features such as hypermetabolism or glycosuria are present in a young person. Because of such symptoms as tachycardia, tremor, palpitation, and hypermetabolism, pheochromocytoma may be confused with thyrotoxicosis. It should be considered in patients with unexplained acute anginal attacks. About 10% are mistakenly treated for diabetes mellitus because of the glycosuria. Pheochromocytoma may also be misdiagnosed as essential hypertension, myocarditis, glomerulonephritis or other renal lesions, toxemia of pregnancy, eclampsia, and psychoneurosis. It rarely masquerades as gastrointestinal hemorrhage and abdominal disorders of an emergency nature. Catecholamine determination has made the diagnosis much more accurate.

### Complications

All of the complications of severe hypertension may be encountered. Hypertensive crises with sudden blindness or cerebrovascular accidents are not uncommon. These may be precipitated by sudden movement, by manipulation during or after pregnancy, by emotional stress or trauma, or during surgical removal of the tumor. Cardiomyopathy may develop.

After removal of the tumor, a state of severe hypotension and shock (resistant to epinephrine and norepinephrine) may ensue with precipitation of renal failure or myocardial infarction. These complications can be avoided by judicious preoperative and operative use of catecholamine blocking agents such as phentolamine and phenoxybenzamine and by the use of blood or plasma to restore blood volume. Hypotension and shock may occur from spontaneous infarction or hemorrhage of the tumor; emergency surgical removal of the tumor is necessary in these cases.

On rare occasions, a patient dies as a result of the complications of diagnostic tests or during surgery. No patient with suspected pheochromocytoma should be subjected either to an invasive diagnostic procedure or to surgery unless there has been adequate blockade with phenoxybenzamine and, if necessary, with propranolol.

Cholelithiasis is often associated.

### Treatment

Surgical removal of the tumor or tumors is the treatment of choice. This may require exploration of the entire sympathetic chain as well as both adrenals. Administration of $\alpha$-adrenergic blocking drugs and blood or plasma before and during surgery has made this type of surgery a great deal safer in recent years. Give phenoxybenzamine, 10 mg orally ev y 12 hours, and increase the dose gradually until hypertension is controlled. The usual maintenance dose is 40–120 mg daily. Do not increase the dose further when postural hypotension and nasal stuffiness become manifest.

*After* appropriate α-adrenergic receptor blockade with phenoxybenzamine, the β-blocker propranolol can be employed to control tachycardia and other arrhythmias. Maintain adrenergic blockade for a minimum of 10 days or until optimal cardiac status is established. Monitor the ECG until it becomes stable. (It may take a week or even months to correct electrocardiographic changes in patients with catecholamine myocarditis, and it is prudent to defer surgery until then in such cases. An experienced anesthesiologist should always be present at surgery to prevent (and control if unavoidable) sudden changes in blood pressure, cardiac arrhythmias, etc.

Since there may be multiple tumors, it is essential to recheck urinary catecholamine levels postoperatively (1–2 weeks after surgery).

Long-term treatment with phentolamine is not successful. Oral phenoxybenzamine (Dibenzyline) has been successfully used as chronic treatment in inoperable carcinoma.

Alpha-methyl-L-tyrosine (metyrosine, Demser) is a competitive blocker in the synthesis of catecholamines. It is useful in the medical management of malignant or inoperable tumors. The initial dosage is 250 mg 4 times daily, increased daily by increments of 250–500 mg to a maximum of 4 g/d.

**Prognosis**

The prognosis depends upon how early the diagnosis is made. If the tumor is successfully removed before irreparable damage to the cardiovascular system has occurred, a complete cure is usually achieved. Complete cure (or improvement) may follow removal of a tumor that has been present for many years. Rarely, hypertension persists or returns in spite of successful surgery. Only a small percentage of tumors are malignant.

Before the advent of blocking agents, the surgical mortality rate was as high as 30%, but this has rapidly decreased. The importance of a team approach—endocrinologist, experienced anesthesiologist, and surgeon—cannot be overemphasized. In good hands, the surgical mortality rate is less than 3%.

If after removal of a tumor a satisfactory fall of blood pressure does not occur, always consider the presence of another tumor.

It has been estimated that in the USA alone about 800 deaths a year may be due to unrecognized pheochromocytoma.

Bravo EL, Gifford RW: Pheochromocytoma: Diagnosis, localization, and management. *N Engl J Med* 1984;**311**:1298.

Cryer PE: Physiology and pathophysiology of the human sym-

pathoadrenal neuroendocrine system. *N Engl J Med* 1980;**303**:436.

Pullerits J et al: Pheochromocytoma: A clinical review with emphasis on pharmacologic aspects. *Clin Invest Med* 1982;**5**:259.

Shapiro B et al: Iodine 131 metaiodobenzyl guanidine for the locating of suspected pheochromocytoma: Experience with 400 cases. *J Nucl Med* 1985;**26**:576.

# DISEASES OF THE PANCREATIC ISLET CELLS*

## ISLET CELL FUNCTIONING PANCREATIC TUMORS

The pancreatic islet is composed of several types of cells, each with distinct chemical and microscopic features: the A cell, B cell, and D cell.† The A cells (20%) secrete glucagon, the B cells (75%) secrete insulin, and the D cells (5%) secrete somatostatin. A fourth type, secreting "human pancreatic polypeptide," has been described recently. Each cell may give rise to benign or malignant neoplasms that are often multiple and usually present with a clinical syndrome related to hypersecretion of a native or ectopic hormonal product. Diagnosis of the tumor depends principally on specific assay of the hormone produced. In malignant insulinoma, an increase in plasma proinsulin—and, in the Zollinger-Ellison syndrome, the prohormone "big" gastrin—may be the most specific finding. The exact hormone responsible for the "pancreatic cholera" syndrome remains unknown, but a biologically active substance called vasoactive intestinal peptide (VIP) is often found both in the plasma and in the tumors of patients with this condition. Glucagon-secreting A cell tumors are rare; patients present with diabetes, anemia, weight loss, hypoaminoacidemia, and a chronic generalized skin rash (migratory necrolytic erythema). Somatostatinomas are very rare and are associated with weight loss, diabetes, malabsorption, and hypochlorhydria.

In addition to the native hormones, aberrant or ectopic hormones are often secreted by islet cell tumors, including ACTH, melanocyte-stimulating hormone, serotonin, and chorionic gonadotropin, with a variety of clinical syndromes. Islet cell tumors may be part of the syndrome of multiple endocrine adenomatosis type I (with pituitary and parathyroid adenomas).

Direct resection of the tumor (or tumors), which often spreads locally, is the primary form of therapy for all types of islet cell neoplasm except Zollinger-Ellison syndrome, where treatment choices include

---

* Diabetes mellitus and the hypoglycemic states are discussed in Chapter 19.

† Formerly called α, β, and δ cells.

blockade of acid secretion by the gastric mucosa with $H_2$ blocking agents or removal of the end organ (total gastrectomy). A new class of "acid pump" inhibitors (omeprazole) may become the therapy of choice for Zollinger-Ellison syndrome. Palliation of functioning malignant disease often requires both antihormonal and anticancer chemotherapy. The use of streptozocin, doxorubicin, and asparaginase, especially for malignant insulinoma, has produced some encouraging results, although these drugs are quite toxic.

Prognosis in these neoplasms is variable. Long-term survival in spite of widespread metastases has been reported. Earlier diagnosis by hormonal assay may lead to earlier detection and a higher cure rate.

Friesen SR: Tumors of the endocrine pancreas. *N Engl J Med* 1982;**306**:580.

Jensen RT et al: Zollinger-Ellison syndrome: Current concepts and management. *Ann Intern Med* 1983;**98**:59.

Kaplan EL et al: Endocrine tumors of the pancreas and their clinical syndromes. *Surg Annu* 1986;**18**:181.

Lamers BHW et al: Omeprazole in Zollinger-Ellison syndrome. *New England J Med* 1984;**310**:758.

Leichter SB: Clinical and metabolic aspects of glucagonoma. *Medicine* 1980;**59**:100.

Stacpoole PW et al: A familial glucagonoma syndrome: Genetic, clinical and biochemical features. *Am J Med* 1981;**70**:1017.

Zollinger RM: Gastrinoma: Factors influencing prognosis. *Surgery* 1985;**97**:49.

# DISEASES OF THE TESTES

## MALE HYPOGONADISM

Male hypogonadism may be classified according to time of onset, ie, prepubertal or postpubertal. It may also be classified as primary or secondary, depending on whether the lesion is in the testes (hypergonadotropic) or in the hypothalamic-pituitary area (hypogonadotropic).

The etiologic diagnosis of hypogonadism (eg, primary or secondary) is based on a careful history and physical examination and is confirmed by laboratory tests (Table 18–14).

## 1. PREPUBERTAL HYPOGONADISM

The diagnosis of hypogonadism cannot usually be made in boys under age 16 or 17, since it is difficult to differentiate from "physiologic" delay of puberty.

Prepubertal hypogonadism is most commonly due to a specific gonadotropic deficiency of the pituitary. It may be familial and associated with anosmia (Kallmann's syndrome) or hyposmia. It may also occur as a result of destructive lesions near the pituitary

**Table 18–14.** Causes of hypogonadism.

| Primary Hypogonadism (Hypergonadotropic) | Secondary Hypogonadism (Hypogonadotropic) |
|---|---|
| Klinefelter's syndrome | Kallmann's syndrome |
| Anorchia | Pituitary tumors |
| Surgical or accidental castration | Craniopharyngiomas |
| Viral infections (mumps) | Hypothalamic lesions |
| Tuberculosis | Hemochromatosis |
| Leprosy | Prader-Willi syndrome |
| Myotonic dystrophy | Laurence-Moon-Biedl syndrome |
| Ionizing radiation injury | |
| Chemotherapeutic agents | |

region (eg, suprasellar cyst) or, more rarely, as a result of destruction or malformation of the testes (prepubertal castration). Rare causes include Prader-Willi syndrome (obesity, hypogonadism, mental retardation, and hypotonia associated with deletions of chromosome 15), Laurence-Moon-Biedl syndrome (obesity, hypogonadism, polydactyly, retinitis pigmentosa), and Alström's syndrome (hypogonadism, nerve deafness, obesity, and retinitis pigmentosa).

In cases associated with a complete pituitary defect, the patient is of short stature or fails to grow and mature. Otherwise, the patient is strikingly tall due to overgrowth of the long bones due to delay in closure of epiphyseal plates. The external genitalia are underdeveloped, the voice is high-pitched, the beard does not grow, and the patient lacks libido and potency. In adult life he presents a youthful appearance, with obesity (often in girdle distribution), disproportionately long extremities (span exceeds height), lack of temporal recession of the hairline, and a small Adam's apple. Gynecomastia is occasionally seen (but apparent gynecomastia may be merely fat). The skin is fine-grained, wrinkled, and sallow, especially on the face. There is no acne or sebum production. The penis is small and the prostate undeveloped. Pubic and axillary hair are scant. The testes may be absent from the scrotum (cryptorchidism) or may be in the scrotum but very small. Rarely, and for unknown reasons, they may be entirely absent (anorchia).

Bone age is retarded. Anemia may be present. Urinary 17-ketosteroids are low or normal in testicular failure; very low or absent in primary pituitary failure. Serum FSH and LH are low in cases of hypothalamic or pituitary origin and elevated in patients with primary testicular failure. Serum testosterone is subnormal and is an excellent index of Leydig cell function.

The response to chorionic gonadotropin injections in cases due to pituitary failure will be maturation, elevation of plasma testosterone, and, occasionally, descent of cryptorchid testes. (In primary testicular failure, no such response occurs.) Testicular biopsy shows immature tubules and Leydig cells in hypopituitary patients.

Testosterone therapy can produce adequate secondary sexual characteristics in hypogonadal patients but will not induce spermatogenesis. To induce spermatogenesis in patients with *secondary* hypogonadism, a combination of an FSH preparation, eg, human menopausal gonadotropin (hMG [Pergonal]), with human chorionic gonadotropin (hCG) is usually required. This treatment is expensive. Spermatogenesis can occasionally be achieved with the use of hCG alone. Patients with prepubertal hypogonadism must be placed on testosterone and maintained for life on adequate doses. Long-acting testosterone preparations such as the enanthate or cypionate, 200–300 mg intramuscularly every 2–4 weeks, are employed. These doses are well tolerated, although gynecomastia may occur with prolonged therapy. It is due to conversion of testosterone to estradiol by peripheral aromatases. The use of oral synthetic androgenic preparations is less desirable, since they have a significant hepatotoxicity, especially when used for long periods of time. Recent reports demonstrating a dramatic response of FSH and LH to LH-releasing factor (GnRH, LHRH) seem to locate the defect in isolated hypogonadotropic hypogonadism to the hypothalamus and offer renewed hope for future treatment. Experimental use of pulsatile LHRH infusion to induce both puberty and spermatogenesis has been described.

Bray GA et al: The Prader-Willi syndrome: A study of 40 patients and review of the literature. *Medicine* 1983;**62**:59.
Lieblich JM et al: Syndrome of anosmia with hypogonadotropic hypogonadism (Kallmann's syndrome): Clinical and laboratory studies in 23 cases. *Am J Med* 1982;**73**:506.
Santoro N, Filicori M, Crowley WF: Hypogonadotropic disorders in men and women: Diagnosis and therapy with pulsatile gonadotropin releasing hormone. *Endocr Rev* 1986;**7**:11.
Wu FC: Male hypogonadism: Current concepts and trends. *Clin Obstet Gynecol* 1985;**12**:531.

## 2. KLINEFELTER'S SYNDROME

The most common primary developmental abnormality causing hypogonadism is Klinefelter's syndrome (seminiferous tubule dysgenesis). It afflicts one out of every 400–500 males. It is caused by the presence of one or more supernumerary X chromosomes and is usually recognized at or shortly after puberty. It is at times familial. Most commonly, there is only failure of the tubules with permanent sterility. The secretory function of the Leydig cells ranges from normal to definite failure. An abnormality in the LH feedback control as well as a disorder in steroidogenesis has been demonstrated in Klinefelter's syndrome.

The clinical findings are swelling of the breasts (gynecomastia), sterility, lack of libido and potency (rare), and at times lack of development of body hair, and female escutcheon. Excessive growth of long bones is present. There may be associated mental retardation. The testes are usually small (< 2 cm in longest diameter) and firm. The penis and prostate are usually normal. The ejaculate usually contains no spermatozoa, although an occasional case of sper-

matogenesis in a patient with a mosaic variant has been described. Urinary 17-ketosteroids are low normal or normal. Serum testosterone is usually low to normal. LH and FSH levels are invariably elevated. Serum estradiol is higher than normal. Testicular biopsy shows sclerosis of the tubules, nests of Leydig cells, and no spermatozoa. The cell karyotype is most commonly 47,XXY, with a chromatin-positive buccal smear. Mosaicism may have clinical features ranging from normal to the classic picture just described here. Chromosomal analysis is necessary to diagnose the condition. In mosaics with a normal 46,XY cell line, spermatogenesis may be present.

All causes of gynecomastia must be differentiated from Klinefelter's syndrome. Testicular size, plasma FSH, and, if necessary, chromosomal analysis will settle the diagnosis.

Testosterone replacement should be given if secondary sexual characteristics have failed to appear or if impotence and low blood testosterone develop later in life. There is no treatment for the infertility. If gynecomastia is disfiguring, plastic surgical removal is indicated.

Hsueh WA et al: Endocrine features of Klinefelter's syndrome. *Medicine* 1978;**57**:447.
Klinefelter HF: Klinefelter's syndrome: Historical background and development. *South Med J* 1986;**79**:1089.

## 3. POSTPUBERTAL HYPOGONADISM

Any pituitary lesion (eg, tumor, infection, necrosis) may lead to lack of gonadotropin; often, hypogonadism is an early sign. The testes may be damaged by trauma, x-ray irradiation, infection, or in other ways. Viral (mumps) and bacterial (gonorrhea, leprosy) orchitis usually affects only the seminiferous tubules and spermatogenesis, leaving Leydig cell function intact. Occasionally, low plasma testosterone and high LH are seen. Many drugs can affect testicular function—cyclophosphamide rapidly causes azoospermia, ketoconazole inhibits testosterone biosynthesis, and hepatic and renal failure are often associated with low testosterone levels. Myotonic dystrophy should be considered if myotonia, frontal baldness, and diabetes are present. States of malnutrition, anemia, and similar disorders may lead to functional gonadal underactivity. The male climacteric, although a disputed syndrome, probably does exist; it makes its appearance about 20 years later than the female menopause, although there is great individual variation.

The symptoms of acquired adult hypogonadism are varying degrees of loss of libido and potency; retardation of hair growth, especially of the face; vasomotor symptoms (flushing, dizziness, chills); lack of aggressiveness and interest; sterility; and muscular aches and back pain. Atrophy or hypoplasia of external genitalia and prostate is rare. The skin of the face is thin and finely wrinkled, and the beard is scant. Girdle type obesity and kyphosis of the spine are present.

Urinary and plasma testosterone levels are low. Urinary and serum FSH or LH are low in cases due to pituitary lesions and elevated in primary testicular failure. Serum prolactin is often elevated in hypothalamic or pituitary lesions, especially in pituitary tumors. In fact, the first manifestation of a prolactin-secreting pituitary tumor in a male may be impotence. The sperm count is low, or spermatozoa may be absent.

True adult hypogonadism must be differentiated from the far more commonly seen psychogenic lack of libido and potency. Measurement of plasma testosterone is useful in this regard. Confusion may also arise in men who are obese and have a sparse beard and small genitalia but normal sperm counts and urinary FSH ("fertile eunuchs"). These patients may represent examples of end-organ unresponsiveness or isolated lack of LH. The usual form of male infertility is "spermatogenic arrest." The disorder can only be diagnosed by testicular biopsy. Most of these patients have normal gonadotropin levels and are not benefited by therapy.

Acquired male hypogonadism is treated with androgens. Oral methyltestosterone or fluoxymesterone is effective, but these synthetic oral preparations are not recommended for chronic therapy because of their hepatotoxicity. They may cause peliosis hepatis and even hepatic tumors. It is preferable to use the long-acting injectable preparations of testosterone (cypionate, enanthate). The dose used is 200–400 mg every 3 weeks. Treatment of long-standing hypogonadism with androgens may precipitate anxiety and acute emotional problems that often require concomitant psychotherapy. Watch for acute urinary retention in older patients. In cases of hypogonadism due to hyperprolactinemia, excellent results may be achieved by administration of bromocriptine or, more permanently, with removal of a pituitary prolactin-secreting tumor.

In cases of *secondary* hypogonadism, it is possible to restore spermatogenesis in many patients with parenteral gonadotropin therapy (see previous section for details).

## Prognosis of Hypogonadism

If hypogonadism is due to a pituitary lesion, the prognosis is that of the primary disease (eg, tumor, necrosis). The prognosis for restoration of virility is good if testosterone is given. The sooner administration is started, the fewer stigmas of eunuchoidism remain (unless therapy is discontinued).

The prognosis for fertility is dismal for the overwhelming majority of patients with primary testicular failure (primary hypogonadism). In many subjects with gonadotropin deficiency, it is possible to induce spermatogenesis. It is only feasible in instances where the testicular elements are present but are unstimulated due to lack of pituitary tropic hormones.

Cryptorchidism should be corrected early, since the incidence of malignant testicular tumors is higher in ectopic testicles and the chance of ultimate fertility is lessened in long-standing cases, even after orchiopexy. The advantages of medical therapy with human chorionic gonadotropin or (recently) with gonadotropin-releasing hormone versus surgical orchiopexy are still controversial.

Bardin CW: Male hypogonadism. In: *Reproductive Endocrinology,* 2nd ed. Yen SSC, Jaffe RB (editors). Saunders, 1986.

Colodny AH: Undescended testes: Is surgery necessary? (Editorial.) *N Engl J Med* 1986;**314:**511.

Griffin JE: Diagnosis and management of male infertility. *Ann Intern Med* 1987;**32:**259.

Lipsett MB: Physiology and pathology of the Leydig cell. *N Engl J Med* 1980;**303:**682.

Morley JE: Impotence. *Am J Med* 1986;**80:**897.

Snyder PJ: Clinical use of androgens. *Annu Rev Med* 1984;**35:**207.

Wu FC: Male hypogonadism: Current concepts and trends. *Clin Obstet Gynecol* 1985;**12:**531.

## MALE HYPERGONADISM & TESTICULAR TUMORS*

In adults, almost all lesions causing male hypergonadism are functioning testicular tumors, which quite frequently are malignant. In children, male hypergonadism may take the form of true precocious puberty, due to pituitary or hypothalamic lesions; or pseudoprecocious puberty, due to lesions of the testes or adrenal glands.

## 1. PREPUBERTAL HYPERGONADISM (Table 18–15)

The symptoms and signs are premature growth of pubic and axillary hair, beard, and external genitalia and excessive muscular development. In true precocity due to pituitary or hypothalamic lesions, pituitary gonadotropins (FSH and LH) are secreted, the testicles enlarge, testosterone is secreted, and spermatogenesis occurs. In adrenal virilization or testicular tumor there is testicular atrophy, with or without palpable nodules; spermatogenesis does not take place. In childhood, interstitial cell tumors are the principal testicular tumors to be considered. Bilateral interstitial cell nodules are also rarely seen with adrenal hyperplasia. Deficiency of 11- or 21-hydroxylase causes isosexual precocity in the male only. Cases of hepatoma with true isosexual precocity due to gonadotropin secretion by the tumor have been reported. Rarely, severe hypothyroidism may be associated with precocious puberty.

In "idiopathic" precocious puberty, no cause is

---

* See also Tumors of the Testis in Chapter 15.

**Table 18–15.** Sexual precocity along isosexual pattern.

| Types and Causes | Characteristics |
|---|---|
| **Neurogenic**<br>Brain tumor<br>Encephalitis<br>Congenital defect<br>with hypothalamic<br>involvement<br>**Pituitary**<br>Idiopathic activation;<br>"constitutional"<br>type | Testes mature normally; spermatogenesis occurs; secondary characteristics normal; sex hormones excreted in normal adult amounts. |
| **Gonadal**<br>Interstitial cell tumor<br>of testis | Tumor in one gonad, the other gonad immature or atrophic; spermatogenesis does not occur; sex hormones excreted in excessive amounts. |
| **Adrenal**<br>Embryonic hyperplasia or tumor | Testes usually small and immature, occasionally containing aberrant adrenal tissue; no spermatogenesis; often results in adrenocortical insufficiency in males. |

ever found; it may be associated with a seizure disorder. The sexual activities of these children must be controlled to prevent socially undesirable conceptions. If precocity is due to hypothalamic or pituitary lesions, the prognosis is poor, since most of these tumors are not removable. Adrenal tumors and testicular tumors are often malignant.

Most patients with this syndrome who survive into adulthood will be short as a result of premature maturation and closure of their epiphyses.

## Treatment

In cases where the tumor is accessible, surgical removal is the treatment of choice. Bilateral adrenal hyperplasia that causes pseudoprecocious puberty can be successfully treated with glucocorticoid replacement, and normal development and spermatogenesis will occur following treatment. Thyroxine replacement therapy stops precocious development in the rare patient with hypothyroidism having this complication. Medroxyprogesterone (Provera) is the most frequently used drug in true isosexual precocity. It inhibits gonadotropin secretion and therefore prevents further stimulation of testicular function. The usual dose is 10–20 mg daily orally in divided doses. Check plasma testosterone levels to adjust dosage. The antiandrogen cyproterone acetate has also been used, with similar results. LHRH (GnRH) analogs have been synthesized and successfully used as antagonists to prevent release of gonadotropins, thus halting the process of precocious puberty. These agents may become the therapy of choice for true precocious puberty.

Boepple PA et al: Use of a potent, long-acting agonist of gonadotropin-releasing hormone in the treatment of precocious puberty. *Endocr Rev* 1985;**7**:24.

Ducharme JR, Collu R: Pubertal development: Normal, precocious and delayed. *Clin Endocrinol Metab* 1982;**11**:57.

Pescovitz OH et al: the NIH experience with precocious puberty: Diagnostic subgroups and response to short-term LHRH analogue therapy. *J Pediatr* 1986;**108**:47.

## 2. NEOPLASMS OF THE TESTES IN ADULTS (See also Chapter 15.)

Many or most testicular neoplasms are functioning (ie, productive of androgenic, estrogenic hormones, or of chorionic gonadotropin), and the majority are highly malignant. They are at times quite small and are clinically recognized because of their hormonal effects or because of the presence of metastases. The sudden appearance of gynecomastia in an otherwise healthy male should raise the possibility of testicular tumor. Ultrasonography is helpful in early diagnosis. In general, once hormonal manifestations have become pronounced, cure by surgical removal is unlikely. Some tumors are bilateral, eg, interstitial cell tumors. Often, a mixed picture is present. Gonadotropin-secreting bronchogenic carcinomas have been recently described.

The incidence of cancer in cryptorchidism is high.

## Treatment

If the diagnosis is made early, surgical removal may be curative; radiotherapy is feasible as a palliative measure in radiosensitive types. Chemotherapy may control the growth of choriocarcinomas.

The serum concentration of the beta subunit of human chorionic gonadotropin (hCG) is elevated in choriocarcinomas and, less commonly, in other testicular tumors. The response to therapy can be monitored in such cases by following the level of this glycoprotein.

Einhorn LH: Cancer of the testis: A new paradigm. *Hosp Pract* (April 15) 1986;**21**:165.

Hainsworth JD, Greco FA: Testicular germ cell neoplasms. *Am J Med* 1983;**75**:817.

## DISEASES OF THE OVARIES (See also Chapter 13.)

## FEMALE HYPOGONADISM

The outstanding symptom of female hypogonadism is amenorrhea (see below). Partial deficiencies, principally corpus luteum failure, may occur; these do not always cause amenorrhea but more often produce anovulatory periods or metrorrhagia.

Estrogenic failure has far-reaching effects, especially if it begins early in life (eg, Turner's syndrome).

Primary pituitary disorders are much less common causes of hypogonadism in the female than primary ovarian disorders and are often associated with other signs of pituitary failure.

Ovarian failure starting in early life will lead to delayed closure of the epiphyses and retarded bone age, often resulting in tall stature with long extremities. On the other hand, in ovarian agenesis due to chromosomal disorder, dwarfism is the rule (see below). In adult ovarian failure, changes are more subtle, with some regression of secondary sex characteristics, including breast atrophy, diminished vaginal secretions, changes in vaginal epithelium, etc. Vasomotor instability with ''hot flushes'' is a typical sign of estrogen secretory failure. In estrogenic deficiency of long standing in any age group, osteoporosis, especially of the spine, is almost always found, since estrogen protects bone against excessive resorption.

A relatively rare form of ovarian failure is seen in states of androgen excess originating in the adrenal cortex or ovary, when estrogens, though present in the body, are suppressed by the presence of large amounts of androgens (see p 743).

## 1. AMENORRHEA

Since regular menstruation depends upon normal function of the entire physiologic axis extending from the hypothalamus and pituitary to the ovary and the uterine lining, it is not surprising that menstrual disorders are among the most common presenting complaints of endocrine disease in women. Correct diagnosis depends upon proper evaluation of each component of the axis, and nonendocrine factors must also be considered.

If menstruation is defined as shedding of endometrium which has been stimulated by estrogen or by estrogen and progesterone which are subsequently withdrawn, it is obvious that amenorrhea can occur either when hormones are deficient or lacking (the hypohormonal or ahormonal type) or when these hormones, though present in adequate amounts, are never withdrawn (the continuous hormonal type).

Primary amenorrhea implies that menses have never been established. This diagnosis is not usually made before the age of about 16. Secondary amenorrhea means that menses once established have ceased (temporarily or permanently).

The most common type of hypohormonal amenorrhea is the menopause, or physiologic failure of ovarian function. The most common example of continuous hormonal amenorrhea is that due to pregnancy, when cyclic withdrawal is prevented by the placental secretions. These 2 conditions should always be considered before extensive diagnostic studies are undertaken.

The principal diagnostic aids that are used in the study of amenorrhea are as follows: (1) vaginal smear for estrogen effect; (2) endometrial biopsy; (3) ''medical D&C'' (see below); (4) basal body temperature determination; (5) urine determinations of 17-ketosteroids, FSH, pregnanediol, and pregnanetriol; (6) culdoscopy and gynecography; (7) chromosomal studies; (8) pelvic exploratory operation or laparoscopy and gonadal biopsy; (9) radioimmunoassays of FSH, LH, and prolactin, which are now available for specific diagnosis of certain types of amenorrhea; (10) plasma testosterone assay; (11) x-ray studies of the hypothalamic and pituitary areas; and (12) in young females, bone age.

Odell WD, Federman DD: Symposium on adolescent gynecology. 1. Physiology of sexual maturation and primary amenorrhea. *West J Med* 1979;**131**:401.

Rebar RW et al: Idiopathic premature ovarian failure: Clinical and endocrine characteristics. *Fertil Steril* 1982;**37**:35.

Tan SL et al: Recent advances in the management of patients with amenorrhea. *Clin Obstet Gynecol* 1985;**12**:725.

Yen SSC: Chronic anovulation. In: *Reproductive Endocrinology*, 2nd ed. Yen SSC, Jaffe RB (editors). Saunders, 1986.

### Primary Amenorrhea

Because of the frequency with which ''delayed puberty'' is found in otherwise normal females, the diagnosis of primary amenorrhea usually is not made until the patient is clearly beyond the age at which normal menarche occurs. In the USA, the mean age at menarche is 12½ years. If menses have not started by age 16, primary amenorrhea is definitely present, and the cause should be investigated.

Most cases of primary amenorrhea are of the hypohormonal or ahormonal type. Exact diagnosis is essential to rule out an organic lesion along the hypothalamic-pituitary-gonadal axis. The chromosomal sex pattern must be determined in many cases. Laparoscopy or pelvic exploration may be required to establish the diagnosis. In large series, the most common cause has always been Turner's syndrome.

The causes are as follows:

**(1) Hypothalamic causes:** Constitutional delay in onset, severe malnutrition, serious organic illness, lack of LHRH (GnRH).

**(2) Pituitary causes (with low or absent FSH):** Suprasellar cyst, pituitary tumors (eosinophilic adenomas, chromophobe adenomas, basophilic adenomas, craniopharyngiomas, etc), isolated lack of pituitary gonadotropins.

**(3) Ovarian causes (with high FSH):** Ovarian dysgenesis with XO karyotype (Turner's syndrome), mosaic variants, mixed gonadal dysgenesis (XO–XY karyotype), pure gonadal dysgenesis, etc. Rarely, ''resistant ovaries'' syndrome.

**(4) Uterine causes:** Malformations, congenital müllerian dysgenesis, imperforate hymen, hermaphroditism, unresponsive or atrophic endometrium.

**(5) Miscellaneous causes:** All forms of male pseudohermaphroditism (enzymatic defects in testosterone synthesis, androgen resistance syndromes), androgen excess syndromes (adrenal or ovarian tumors, adrenal enzymatic defects with excess androgen formation, such as 21- or 11-hydroxylase deficiencies, polycystic ovaries).

Since primary amenorrhea is only a manifestation of multiple and often complex underlying defects, treatment must be individualized according to the specific cause.

## Secondary Amenorrhea

Temporary cessation of menses is extremely common and usually does not require extensive endocrine investigation. In the childbearing age, pregnancy must be ruled out. In women beyond the childbearing age, menopause should be considered first. States of emotional stress, malnutrition, anemia, and similar disorders may be associated with temporary amenorrhea and correction of the primary disorder will usually also reestablish menses. Some women fail to menstruate regularly for prolonged intervals after stopping oral contraceptive pills. Lactation may be associated with amenorrhea, either physiologically or for abnormally prolonged periods after delivery. An increasing number of small prolactin-secreting pituitary tumors causing secondary amenorrhea and often lactation have been discovered by means of prolactin assays and pituitary imaging studies (see prolactin, p 688).

By the use of the "medical D&C," ie, the administration of progesterone with subsequent withdrawal, these amenorrheas can be arbitrarily divided into amenorrhea with negative D&C and amenorrhea with positive D&C. The former (with the exception of pregnancy) show an atrophic or hypoestrin type of endometrium; the latter show an endometrium of the proliferative type but lacking progesterone.

(1) Secondary amenorrhea with negative medical D&C may be due to the following causes: premature ovarian failure, pituitary tumor, pituitary infarction (Sheehan's syndrome). The measurement of serum FSH and LH is extremely helpful in separating ovarian causes (high gonadotropins) from hypothalamic-pituitary origin (low gonadotropins). Serum prolactin levels must be measured. Less common causes include virilizing syndromes such as arrhenoblastoma, Cushing's disease, Addison's disease, and miscellaneous causes such as anorexia nervosa, profound myxedema, and scarring of the uterine cavity with synechia formation (Asherman's syndrome).

(2) Secondary amenorrhea with positive medical D&C may be due to metropathia hemorrhagica, polycystic ovary syndrome, estrogen medication, estrogenic granulosa cell tumors (rare), and hyperthyroidism. A common cause is "psychogenic amenorrhea" related to emotional trauma (divorce, going to college, stressful new job, etc). Menses usually return in a few months without any specific therapy. Tonic elevation of serum LH with normal FSH is helpful in the diagnosis of polycystic ovary syndrome. Amenorrhea or oligomenorrhea is also often found in athletes (long-distance runners, dedicated ballet dancers, etc). De-

pletion of body fat due to strenuous exercise may play a role in the pathogenesis of this problem.

Some degree of overlap in these 2 groups is sometimes found.

The aim of therapy is not only to reestablish menses (although this is valuable for psychologic reasons) but also to attempt to establish the cause (eg, pituitary tumor) of the amenorrhea and to restore reproductive function.

Treatment depends upon the underlying disease. It is not necessary to treat all cases, especially temporary amenorrhea or irregular menses in unmarried girls or women. These cases usually are corrected spontaneously after marriage or the first pregnancy.

In patients whose response to progesterone is normal, the administration of this hormone during the last 5–10 days of each month, orally or parenterally, will correct the amenorrhea.

In patients who are unresponsive to progesterone and whose urinary gonadotropin levels are low, treatment of a pituitary lesion may restore menstruation; gonadotropins would appear to be of value, and human pituitary FSH has been used with some success experimentally. This, or gonadotropins from postmenopausal urine (menotropins, hMG), has given good results in secondary amenorrhea. Clomiphene citrate (Clomid) has been extensively and often successfully tried for the treatment of these patients. However, in current clinical practice, if attainment of pregnancy is not desirable, estrogen alone or in combination with progesterone is more commonly used. If gonadotropin levels are high, gonadotropins are of no value; treat with estrogens alone or with estrogens and progesterone. A commonly used schedule is the oral administration of 1.2 mg of conjugated estrogens from days 1 to 20 of each month and 10 mg of medroxyprogesterone daily during days 21 to 25. Corticosteroids may restore menstruation in virilizing disorders that are due to enzymatic abnormalities in cortisol biosynthesis. Wedge resection of the ovaries often restores regular menstruation in the polycystic ovary syndrome. The use of LHRH (GnRH) is under investigation at present and appears promising. In patients with the galactorrhea-amenorrhea syndromes associated with elevated prolactin levels, restoration of ovulatory menses has been achieved with the ergot derivative bromocriptine (bromoergocryptine). Transsphenoidal resection of small prolactin-producing pituitary adenomas likewise has resulted in restoration of fertility.

General measures include dietary management as required to correct overweight or underweight; psychotherapy in cases due to emotional disturbance; and correction of anemia and any other metabolic abnormality that may be present (eg, mild hypothyroidism).

## Hypothalamic Amenorrhea

Secondary hypothalamic amenorrhea, due to emotional or psychogenic causes, is far more common in young women than amenorrhea due to organic causes (except for pregnancy). It is probably mediated by a hypothalamic block of the release of pituitary gonadotropic hormones, especially LH. Pituitary FSH is still produced and is found in normal or low levels in the urine. Since some LH is necessary in the production of estrogen as well as FSH, a state of hypoestrinism with an atrophic endometrium will eventually result.

A history of psychic trauma just preceding the onset of amenorrhea can usually be obtained. The urinary FSH level is normal or low normal, and the 17-ketosteroid level is low normal. Plasma LH is low. Vaginal smear and endometrial biopsy show mild hypoestrin effects. The response to progesterone (medical D&C) is variable. The endometrium responds to cyclic administration of estrogens.

Menses often return spontaneously, after weight gain, or after several induced "cycles." Psychotherapy may be of value. Clomiphene citrate (Clomid) may be tried to reestablish menses. If amenorrhea persists for years, signs of estrogen deficiency will appear and must be treated.

It is most important to recognize this syndrome and not to mistake it for an organic type of amenorrhea with a very different prognosis.

Petrucco OM: Current investigation and therapy of secondary amenorrhea. *Drugs* 1986;**31**:550.

Tan SL: Recent advances in the management of patients with amenorrhea. *Clin Obstet Gynecol* 1985;**12**:725.

Yen SSC: Chronic anovulation. In: *Reproductive Endocrinology.* Yen SSC, Jaffe RB (editors). Saunders, 1986.

## 2. TURNER'S SYNDROME
### (Primary Ovarian Agenesis, Gonadal Dysgenesis)

Turner's syndrome is a chromosomal disorder associated with congenital absence of the ovaries and with short stature and other phenotypic anomalies. It represents the most common cause of primary amenorrhea. Patients with the classic syndrome lack one of the two X chromosomes.

The principal features include bilateral streak gonads, genital hypoplasia with infantile uterus, vagina, and breasts and primary amenorrhea; scant axillary and pubic hair; short stature, usually between 122 and 142 cm (48 and 56 inches); increased carrying angle of arms; webbing of neck (quite common); stocky "shield" chest with widely spaced nipples; cardiovascular disorders, especially coarctation of the aorta, congenital valve defects; osteoporosis and other skeletal anomalies (short fourth metacarpals, exostosis of tibia, etc) with increasing age; and prematurely senile appearance. Nevi are common. Lymphedema of hands and feet is seen in infants. There is an increased incidence of autoimmune thyroiditis and diabetes.

Serum FSH and LH are high. Bone age is retarded. The chromatin sex pattern most often shows a "nega-tive" buccal smear and 45,X chromosomal pattern. Mosaicism is common; most frequent is the 45,X, 46,XX chromosomal pattern.

Exploratory operation shows a "streak ovary" and, at times, islands of interstitial cells. The genital apparatus is entirely female but infantile in development.

The principal disorder to be differentiated is pituitary dwarfism. In this disorder, urinary and serum FSH is low or absent, and other signs of pituitary failure are present. Other forms of constitutional dwarfism, such as Laurence-Moon-Biedl syndrome, are ruled out by the FSH levels and lack of stigmas such as polydactyly, retinitis pigmentosa, and other signs of the disease. The short stature and occasional metacarpal deformities may resemble pseudohypoparathyroidism, but these patients menstruate normally. In Noonan's syndrome, a rare inherited disorder, the female patient has many similar phenotypic characteristics (short stature, shield chest, short neck), but cardiac lesions are in the right side of the heart (pulmonary stenosis is common), the ovaries are normal, the chromosomal pattern is 46,XX, and the serum FSH and LH are not elevated.

With administration of estrogens, some increase in height can be achieved, but this is almost never enough to increase stature significantly; androgens may also promote growth, especially fluoxymesterone in low doses. Some cases respond to administration of growth hormone.

Without treatment, growth will eventually cease, since the epiphyses will close spontaneously (though late). The administration of estrogen will develop the breasts and uterus and lead to anovulatory menses upon cyclic withdrawal. Administration of an oral progestogen such as medroxyprogesterone acetate (Provera) for the last 5–10 days of each cycle is recommended. Fertility can never be achieved.

The associated congenital cardiovascular anomalies may cause early death or may require surgical correction (eg, coarctation). Webbing of the neck can be corrected by plastic surgery.

Similar syndromes with different chromosomal patterns have been described. "Pure gonadal dysgenesis" has only "streak" gonads and sexual infantilism, with normal stature and normal 46,XX chromosomal pattern. "Mixed" or "atypical" gonadal dysgenesis has a "streak" gonad on one side and an abnormal gonad, prone to neoplasm, on the other side, making prophylactic removal a reasonable procedure. It is very often associated with XY mosaicism.

Brook CY: Turner syndrome. *Arch Dis Child* 1986;**61**:305.

Grumbach MM, Conte F: Disorders of sex differentiation. In: *Textbook of Endocrinology,* Wilson JD, Foster DW (editors). Saunders, 1985.

Jaffe RB: Disorders of sexual development. In: *Reproductive Endocrinology,* 2nd ed. Yen SSC, Jaffe RB (editors). Saunders, 1986.

## 3. MENOPAUSAL SYNDROME
### (See Chapter 13.)

## FEMALE HYPERGONADISM

Excesses of ovarian hormones are often encountered during the normal reproductive life of women, and most frequently give rise to irregular or excessive menstrual bleeding and, more rarely, to amenorrhea. Excesses before the age of puberty or after the menopause, however, should be thoroughly investigated, since the possibility of malignant lesions is great. Estrogen excess is more common than progesterone excess, which is seen in pregnancy and in chorioepithelioma. Other extra-ovarian sources of estrogens are malignant tumors of the adrenals, which secrete abnormal amounts of estrogens. Since these tumors usually produce excesses of androgens as well, their hyperestrogenic effects are rarely detectable clinically in the female. Another cause of hyperestrogenism is the ingestion or other use of hormones (eg, in face or vaginal creams).

## 1. PREPUBERTAL FEMALE HYPERGONADISM

It is important to differentiate lesions of the pituitary-hypothalamic region, which cause true precocious puberty (due to secretion of FSH and LH by the pituitary) from pseudoprecocity, in which endogenous or exogenous estrogens induce some pubertal changes, with concomitant *suppression* of pituitary gonadotropins. Constitutional true sexual precocity may be partial, consisting only of precocious breast development and early growth of public hair, or it may be associated with premature menarche as well. It is often familial. In McCune-Albright syndrome, true precocity is associated with polyostotic fibrous dysplasia and hyperpigmented skin patches (see Chapter 4).

Pseudoprecocious puberty may be caused by ovarian follicular cysts, granulosa cell tumors, other rare ovarian tumors, and exogenous estrogens. Pelvic sonograms are helpful in detection of ovarian masses. Granulosa cell tumors of the ovary cause uterine bleeding by virtue of their estrogenic secretions, but they do not cause ovulation, and these girls are not fertile. The same is usually true of choriocarcinoma. Both of these tumors are highly malignant.

Pseudoprecocious puberty may also be caused by ingestion of estrogens present in lotions, creams, etc, or even in foodstuffs.

An important point of the differentiation between true and pseudoprecocious puberty is that in true precocity ovulatory cycles may occur and the patient must be protected from pregnancy. The most useful guide to the differentiation is the serum FSH and LH determinations. FSH is not present in significant levels in girls before puberty and is absent in pseudoprecocious puberty, whereas girls with true precocious puberty secrete significant levels of FSH and LH and also have a pubertal response to the administration of LHRH.

The diagnosis of either true or pseudoprecocious puberty is important because many cases are due to tumors that must be found and removed if possible (Table 18–16). Unfortunately, most estrogen-secreting tumors are highly malignant, and tumors of the third ventricle and other lesions near the hypothalamus are quite difficult to remove.

Precocious development of breasts and early onset of menses may cause psychic disturbances. Short stature in adult life is the rule, since bone age is advanced and the epiphyses close prematurely. As adults these patients may suffer from excessive menstrual bleeding, which may cause anemia unless it is checked. Cystic mastitis is a chronic problem, and the incidence of uterine adenofibromas is high. It is not definitely known whether long-standing hyperestrinism causes a higher incidence of breast and genital tract cancer, but it may be an aggravating factor.

In case of tumor, the best treatment is surgical removal, but most are malignant and metastasize early. The prognosis for simple constitutional precocity is not so unfavorable, although these girls must be watched to prevent pregnancy. Recent reports on the use of progesterone (Depo-Provera) are encouraging but the response is variable and the possible adverse long-term effects of such treatment are uncertain. Long-acting analogs of LHRH (GnRH) have been used successfully to halt true precocious puberty in both girls and boys.

Boepple PA et al: Use of potent, long-acting agonist of gonadotropic-releasing hormone in the treatment of precocious puberty. *Endocr Rev* 1986;**7**:24.

Luder AS et al: Intranasal and subcutaneous treatment of central precocious puberty in both sexes with a long-acting analog of luteinising hormone-releasing hormone. *J Clin Endocrinol Metab* 1984;**58**:966.

**Table 18–16.** Hormones elaborated by actively secreting ovarian tumors.

| Type | Secretion |
|------|-----------|
| **Feminizing** | |
| Granulosa | Estrogen +++ |
| Theca cell | Estrogen ++ |
| Luteoma? | Estrogen + and/or progesterone |
| **Virilizing*** | |
| Arrhenoblastoma | Androgen +++ |
| Adrenal rest (lipoid cell) | Androgen ++ and corticosteroids |
| Hilar cell | Androgen +++ |
| **Miscellaneous** | |
| Choriocarcinoma | Gonadotropins ++++ and estrogens; TSH |
| Dysgerminoma* | Gonadotropins + and androgens? |
| Gynandroblastoma | Androgens ++ and estrogens +++ |
| Struma ovarii | Thyroxine + |

* Most women have complete amenorrhea with negative medical D&C, since the endometrium is atrophic.

Root AW et al: Isosexual precocity: Current concepts and recent advances. *Fertil Steril* 1986;**45**:749.

Styne DM, Grumbach M: Puberty in the male and female: Its physiology and disorders. In: *Reproductive Endocrinology*, 2nd ed. Yen SSC, Jaffe RB (editors). Saunders, 1986.

## 2. ADULT FEMALE HYPERGONADISM (Hyperestrogenism)

Estrogen excess in adult women may be isolated or combined with progesterone excess. Estrogen excess is characterized by menorrhagia or, rarely, amenorrhea. The vaginal smear shows estrogen excess. Lack of ovulation is demonstrated by the absence of mid-cycle temperature rise and LH rise. Sterility is the rule. The medical D&C is positive, ie, bleeding starts after a short course of progesterone. Endometrial biopsy shows a proliferative endometrium. The urinary and serum FSH levels are low.

Adult female hyperestrogenism may be caused by (1) states in which ovulation does not occur, leading to "metropathia hemorrhagica" or dysfunctional uterine bleeding; (2) liver disease, which interferes with the catabolism of estrogens; (3) drug administration (eg, estrogen creams or tablets); (4) granulosa cell and theca cell tumors (both types are usually present); and (5) polycystic ovary syndrome (see below).

Estrogen and progesterone excess often causes amenorrhea without other evidence of hypogonadism. Excess of both hormones may be due to the following: (1) Pregnancy. (2) Choriocarcinoma or teratoma. (3) Luteoma. (4) Malignant adrenal tumors (possibly). D&C is negative. Pregnanediol is found in the urine. Secretory endometrium is demonstrated on biopsy. The LH and FSH levels (actually chorionic gonadotropin) may be high and pregnancy tests positive. (5) Hyperhormonal effects with stromal luteinization may occur in postmenopausal women because of metastatic tumors in the ovaries (Krukenberg tumor) or as a result of ectopic production of chorionic gonadotropin by neoplasms.

Treatment depends upon the cause. Cyclic administration of progesterone, wedge resection of the ovary, or surgical removal of functioning tumors at times restores normal cyclic ovarian function. Recent reports of treatment of functional anovulation with human pituitary or urinary FSH, clomiphene, and LHRH (GnRH) are encouraging.

The prognosis is that of the underlying disease. Treatment with cyclic progesterone alone or with estrogen-progesterone is usually quite effective in temporary disorders of ovulation. Stubborn anovulation may persist, however, after cessation of therapy.

Aiman J et al: Androgen and estrogen secretion by normal and neoplastic ovaries in premenopausal women. *Obstet Gynecol* 1986;**68**:327.

## VIRILIZING DISORDERS OF THE OVARY (See also Adrenogenital Syndrome [above] and Chapter 13.)

### Polycystic Ovary Syndrome

This term is used to denote a heterogeneous group of disorders all characterized by bilateral polycystic ovaries but with variable incidence and degree of hirsutism, amenorrhea, and obesity. Patients may have only mild hirsutism or may present with signs and symptoms of virilization. Some women have normal menses; in others, anovulatory cycles and infertility are present. An occasional patient presents with primary amenorrhea. Conditions found to be associated with this syndrome include adrenal defects in the synthesis of cortisol, central nervous system lesions, thyroid diseases, and adrenal and ovarian tumors. In most cases, however, no associated disorder is found, and the exact mechanism of the syndrome remains unclear.

The eponym **Stein-Leventhal syndrome** is usually reserved for patients who have amenorrhea, hirsutism, and obesity associated with polycystic ovaries without other associated endocrine disease.

Patients with polycystic ovary syndrome usually have normal or elevated estrogen levels; frequently show a tonic elevation of serum LH; and often have elevated levels of plasma testosterone. Gonadal steroid-binding globulin levels in plasma are decreased, so that the free (active) fraction of testosterone is elevated even if the level of total testosterone is normal.

Urinary 17-ketosteroids are usually normal or modestly elevated. FSH is normal or low. Administration of progesterone results in withdrawal bleeding. The hirsutism has been shown to be related to abnormal production of testosterone and related compounds by the ovaries and possibly also by the adrenals. Glucose intolerance and elevated serum insulin levels (associated with peripheral insulin resistance) are often found, even in subjects who are not obese. Hereditary factors may be involved. Pelvic sonography is helpful in demonstrating bilateral enlargement of the ovaries. At operation, the enlarged ovaries are found to have many follicles on the surface and are surrounded by a thick capsule ("oyster ovaries").

Therapy must be individualized depending on the severity of the disorder, the presenting complaint, and any associated endocrine disease. Excess hair usually responds to oral contraceptive steroids. Glucocorticoid suppression (with small doses of dexamethasone at bedtime) is sometimes helpful. Combined adrenal and ovarian suppression has been reported to have additional beneficial effect. The dopamine agonist bromocriptine has been reported to improve the menstrual abnormalities and hirsutism of polycystic ovary syndrome. Experience is lacking for this use of the drug. If the patient wants to maintain fertility, several procedures are available. Wedge resection often restores ovulatory periods and fertility, but hirsutism is not helped by this procedure unless large doses of estrogens are also used. Recently, ovulation followed by pregnancy has been produced by human pituitary or urinary FSH and also by clomiphene. There is danger of rapid enlargement of the ovaries due to cyst formation and rupture if the dosage is not carefully controlled. Multiple pregnancies may occur.

### Diffuse Theca Luteinization

This disorder is similar to the Stein-Leventhal syndrome, but many follicles are not found in the ovaries. Hirsutism and often more marked virilization are associated with amenorrhea.

Excessive testosterone and androstenedione production has been demonstrated recently in ovarian slices removed surgically and also in blood and urine in these patients, which may explain the virilization.

There is a greater incidence of endometrial carcinoma in these patients, possibly related to continued estrogen stimulation.

### Ovarian Tumors

Several ovarian tumors can produce significant hirsutism and virilization: hilar cell tumors, teratomas, luteomas, and (most frequently) **arrhenoblastoma.** Arrhenoblastoma is associated with very high levels of serum testosterone. The 17-ketosteroids in urine are usually normal. Regional venous catheterization may be of great value in localization of the tumor before surgery.

Chang RJ et al: Associated nonovarian problems of polycystic ovarian disease: Insulin resistance. *Clin Obstet Gynaecol* 1985;**12**:675.

Rittmaster RS, Loriaux DL: Hirsutism. *Ann Intern Med* 1987;**106**:95.

Schriock E, Martin MC, Jaffe RB: Polycystic ovarian disease. *West J Med* 1985;**142**:519.

Spruce BA et al: Effect of bromocriptine in the polycystic ovary syndrome. *Clin Endocrinol* 1984;**20**:481.

# DISORDERS OF PLURIGLANDULAR INVOLVEMENT

Involvement of multiple endocrine glands in the same patient is becoming recognized with increasing frequency. Many of these disorders are familial, although sporadic cases are also seen. The syndromes may consist of excessive hormone formation, usually due to the presence of hormone-secreting tumors, or they may consist of failure of multiple endocrine glands.

# DISORDERS OF HORMONE EXCESS

Several familial syndromes with multiple gland involvement have been described. The most common one is multiple endocrine neoplasia (or adenomatosis) type I (MEN I or MEA I). In this condition, tumors of the pituitary gland, the parathyroid gland, and the pancreatic islets occur in the same patient, although not necessarily at the same time. The disorder is inherited as an autosomal dominant, but there is considerable phenotypic variability. Some individuals in the same family express the abnormality as children, whereas in others the clinical manifestations may not appear until late in adult life. The clinical manifestations of this syndrome are extremely variable, since the glandular tumors may secrete a variety of different hormones. The most common finding is hypercalcemia due to primary hyperparathyroidism. Either hyperplasia or adenoma of the parathyroid glands may be found. The clinical manifestations and laboratory findings are identical to those found in spontaneously occurring primary hyperparathyroidism. The pituitary gland tumors may secrete **prolactin** (galactorrhea-amenorrhea syndrome) or **growth hormone** (producing gigantism or acromegaly). The tumors of the pancreatic islets may produce **insulin,** giving all of the clinical manifestations found in a spontaneously occurring insulinoma, or **gastrin,** giving rise to gastric acid hypersecretion (Zollinger-Ellison syndrome). Elevation of serum gastrin (measured by radioimmunoassay) is characteristic of Zollinger-Ellison syndrome and is associated with increased hydrochloric acid secretion. Tumors of the pancreatic islets have also been described as secreting additional

**Table 18–17.** Multiple endocrine gland neoplasia or adenomatosis (MEA).*

| | Tissue Affected | Clinical Presentation |
|---|---|---|
| Type I (MEA I) | Parathyroid | Adenoma or hyperplasia |
| | Pancreas | Adenoma (often multiple) of islet cells, gastrinoma |
| | Pituitary | Adenoma (acromegaly, prolactinoma) |
| | Adrenal | Adenoma (cortical) |
| | Miscellaneous | Lipomas, thyroid tumors (other than medullary carcinoma) |
| Type II or IIa (MEA II) | Thyroid | Medullary carcinoma or C cell hyperplasia |
| | Adrenal | Pheochromocytomas |
| | Parathyroid | Hyperplasia or adenoma |
| Type III or IIb (MEA III) | Thyroid | Medullary carcinoma or C cell hyperplasia |
| | Adrenal | Pheochromocytomas (adenoma or hyperplasia) |
| | Neural tissue | Ganglioneuromas |
| | Somatic manifestations | Marfanoid habitus, thick lips, "blubbery tongue," megacolon |

* Modified after Deftos LJ: Calcitonin in clinical medicine. *Adv Intern Med* 1978;**23**:159.

peptide hormones such as substance P, secretin, vasoactive intestinal peptide (VIP), glucagon, and others. The glucagon-producing tumors are associated with a typical skin rash (migratory necrolytic erythema), with diabetes mellitus, and with very low levels of amino acids in plasma.

A separate disorder of familial hypersecretion of hormones is the so-called multiple endocrine neoplasia type II (MEN II or MEA II), or Sipple's syndrome. In this syndrome, one finds pheochromocytomas (often bilateral) associated with medullary carcinoma of the thyroid, a tumor that originates in the C cells of the thyroid. These cells are the remnants of the ultimobranchial body found in lower species, and they secrete calcitonin. The baseline levels of calcitonin in blood are often markedly elevated and are helpful in the diagnosis of these tumors as well as in monitoring the response to therapy. In members of affected families, one can demonstrate the presence of small calcitonin-producing tumors by stimulatory tests such as calcium infusion or pentagastrin administration that result in markedly elevated levels of calcitonin. In patients with MEA II, one may also find hypercalcemia, which is often due to parathyroid hyperplasia.

A few families have been described with the so-called MEA type III syndrome, which consists of pheochromocytomas and medullary carcinomas of the thyroid associated with multiple mucosal neuromas and a peculiar phenotypic appearance: bumpy lips, enlarged tongue, visible corneal nerves, marfanlike habitus, muscular hypotonia, etc.

Case reports of "overlap" between MEA I and MEA II have been published in the last few years, but the significance is not clear. A more meaningful association may be that of pheochromocytoma and islet cell tumors of the pancreas.

Although many theories have been proposed to explain the existence of these syndromes, none are consistent with the facts known at present (see references at end of next section).

## DISORDERS OF MULTIPLE ENDOCRINE DEFICIENCIES

It has long been known that primary adrenal insufficiency and primary thyroid failure could occur simultaneously in the same patient for unclear reasons (Schmidt's syndrome). It has been demonstrated that many of these patients have an autoimmune disorder, with formation of antibodies against cellular fractions of many endocrine glands. In addition to adrenal and thyroid failure, patients with these syndromes may have failure of the gonads, of the parathyroids, of the pituitary gland, of the insulin-secreting cells of the pancreatic islets, etc. There is often an association with pernicious anemia and with vitiligo and nontropical sprue as well as other autoimmune disorders. This syndrome has also been designated **polyglandular autoimmune syndrome type II** to differentiate it from **polyglandular autoimmune syndrome type I,** which is characterized by the appearance of mucocutaneous candidiasis (often in childhood), associated or followed by hypoparathyroidism and adrenal insufficiency. The type I condition occurs in siblings, without involvement of other generations in the family.

The basic mechanisms for the formation of autoantibodies are not clear at present. Although a familial tendency is often seen, many patients present with a sporadic disorder. An increased association of certain HLA antigens has been described in afflicted individuals with the type II disorder. No treatment other than hormone replacement is known at present.

A very rare syndrome involving endocrine systems is the POEMS syndrome, consisting of *P*olyneuropathy, *O*rganomegaly, *E*ndocrinopathy, *M*-protein, and *S*kin changes. The endocrine involvement includes diabetes mellitus, primary hypogonadism, and hyperpigmentation. The disorder is associated with sclerotic bone lesions, hepatosplenomegaly, and lymph node enlargement. The bone lesions contain plasma cells, and it is postulated that pathogenic immunoglobulins are produced there since radiation of the affected bone has resulted in resolution of the endocrine abnormalities.

Neufeld M, Maclaren NK, Blizzard RM: Two types of autoimmune Addison's disease associated with different polyglandular autoimmune (PGA) syndromes. *Medicine* 1981;**60:**355.

Pont A: Multiple endocrine neoplasia syndromes. *West J Med* 1980;**132:**301.

Rabinowe SL, Eisenbarth GS: Polyglandular autoimmunity. *Adv Intern Med* 1986;**31:**293.

Schimke RN: Genetic aspects of multiple endocrine neoplasia. *Annu Rev Med* 1984;**35:**25.

Trence DL, Morley JE, Handwerger BS: Polyglandular autoimmune syndromes. *Am J Med* 1984;**77:**107.

## CLINICAL USE OF CORTICOTROPIN (ACTH) & THE CORTICOSTEROIDS

Both pituitary adrenocorticotropin (ACTH), acting by adrenal stimulation, and the C-11-oxygenated adrenal steroids (corticosteroids) have been shown to have profound modifying effects on many pathologic processes, especially those associated with immunologic problems and inflammation. These effects cannot be entirely explained at present on the basis of the known metabolic and immunologic activities of these compounds.

These agents do not appear to "cure." Their action is primarily anti-inflammatory and appears to be related to multiple effects upon blood vessels, leukocytes, macrophages, fibroblasts, cell membrane permeability, etc, rather than to one discrete, all-encompassing effect. They suppress the inflammatory process but do not deal with the underlying cause of the disease process. When they are discontinued, the disease often recurs.

In general, these agents are interchangeable, and there is no support for the claim that a patient or a disease process may be responsive to one and not to another. Their duration of action varies. Both cause varying degrees of pituitary suppression, while the corticosteroids lead to adrenal atrophy after prolonged use as well. They should not be stopped suddenly, and during periods of stress (eg, surgery, trauma), additional amounts of rapidly acting steroids must be provided. Some patients become dependent on corticosteroids, and withdrawal is difficult.

## Toxicity & Side Reactions

These agents are potentially dangerous, but with proper precautions most of these dangers can be avoided (see below). Corticosteroids are generally contraindicated during early pregnancy, except in the adrenogenital syndromes.

**A. Hyperglycemia and glycosuria** (diabetogenic effect) is of major significance in the early or potential diabetic.

**B. Marked retention of sodium and water,** with subsequent edema, increased blood volume, and hypertension, is minimized by the use of the newer agents.

**C. Negative nitrogen and calcium balance** may occur, with loss of body protein and consequent osteoporosis.

**D. Potassium loss** may lead to hypokalemic alkalosis.

**E. Hirsutism and acne** are cosmetic problems that may be of greater concern to females. Amenorrhea may occur.

**F. Cushing's features or facies** may develop with prolonged administration.

**G. Peptic ulcer** may be produced or aggravated.

**H. Resistance to infectious agents** is lowered.

**I. Impotence and decreased libido** associated with decreased serum testosterone have been recently described.

## Techniques Employed to Correct or Minimize Dangers

(1) Always reduce the dosage as soon as consistent with the clinical response. Intermittent alternate-day use may be a preferable and safer method of treatment. This method works well with prednisone or prednisolone but not with longer-acting drugs such as dexamethasone.

(2) During the first 2 weeks of therapy, blood pressure and weight should be carefully observed. Take an initial complete blood count and sedimentation rate and repeat as indicated. Determine the urine glucose; if reducing substances are found in the urine, determine fasting blood glucose. Serum potassium, bicarbonate, and chloride should be checked occasionally if large doses of these hormones are to be given

over a period of more than several days. Measurement of plasma or urinary steroid levels is indicated if any question of lack of adrenal response to corticotropin arises.

(3) All patients should be on high-protein diets (100 g or more of protein daily) with adequate calcium intake.

(4) If edema develops, place the patient on a low-sodium diet (200–400 mg of sodium daily). Diuretics may be employed when strict sodium restriction is impossible.

(5) Potassium chloride, as 10% or 20% solution, effervescent tablets, or powder, 3–15 g daily in divided doses, should be administered if prolonged use or high dosage is employed.

(6) In cases of long-continued administration, anabolic preparations may be used to counteract the negative protein, calcium, and potassium balance. Unfortunately, the distressing osteoporosis cannot be prevented.

(7) Do not stop either ACTH or corticosteroids abruptly, since sudden withdrawal may cause a severe "rebound" of the disease process or a malignant necrotizing vasculitis. Also remember that glucocorticoids cause atrophy of the adrenal cortex through endogenous ACTH inhibition; sudden withdrawal may lead to symptoms of adrenal insufficiency.

(8) When treating mild disorders, giving corticosteroids during the daytime only or on alternate days causes less suppression of endogenous ACTH. When discontinuing therapy, withdraw evening dose first.

## Contraindications & Special Precautions

**A. Stress in Patients Receiving Maintenance Corticosteroids:** Patients receiving corticosteroids, especially the oral preparation (or even ACTH), must be carefully watched because suppression of endogenous ACTH interferes with the normal response to

**Table 18–18.** Systemic versus topical activity of corticosteroids.
(Hydrocortisone = 1 in potency.)

|  | Systemic Activity | Topical Activity |
|---|---|---|
| Prednisolone | 4–5 | 1–2 |
| Fluprednisolone | 8–10 | 10 |
| Triamcinolone | 5 | 1 |
| Triamcinolone acetonide | 5 | 40 |
| Dexamethasone | 30 | 10 |
| Betamethasone | 30 | 5–10 |
| Betamethasone valerate |  | 50–150 |
| Methylprednisolone | 5 | 5 |
| Fluocinolone acetonide |  | 40–100 |
| Flurandrenolone acetonide |  | 20–50 |
| Fluorometholone | 1–2 | 40 |

stressful situations (eg, surgery or infections). Patients should be warned of this danger and should carry identification cards showing what drug they are taking, the dosage, and the reason for taking it. Whenever such a situation occurs or is about to occur, the dosage of cortisone or hydrocortisone should be increased or parenteral corticosteroids given (or both). If oral cortisone or hydrocortisone can be administered, it must be administered in larger doses at least every 6 hours.

**B. Heart Disease:** These agents should be used with caution in patients with cardiac disease or hypertension. Blood pressure may be increased by sodium retention or by increases in plasma renin substrate. The increase in extracellular fluid may lead to cardiac decompensation. Always begin with small doses and place the patient on a low-sodium diet.

**C. Predisposition to Psychosis:** These drugs cause a sense of well-being and euphoria in most persons, but in predisposed patients, an acute psychotic reaction may occur. (Insomnia may be the presenting symptom.) In these cases the drug should be stopped or the dosage reduced, and the patient should be carefully observed and protected. Persons have committed suicide under the influence of these drugs.

**D. Effect on Peptic Ulcer:** Active peptic ulcer is a contraindication to the use of these drugs because of the danger of perforation or hemorrhage. These agents also tend to activate ulcers, and should be used only in emergency situations or with optimal antiulcer therapy in patients who have a history of peptic ulcer. Acute pancreatitis has been reported as well.

**E. Tuberculosis:** Active or recently healed tuberculosis is a contraindication to the use of these drugs unless intensive antituberculosis therapy is also carried out. A chest x-ray should be taken before and periodically during prolonged treatment with corticosteroids.

**F. Infectious Diseases:** Because these drugs tend to lower resistance and therefore to promote dissemination of infections, they must be used with caution, even when appropriate antibiotics are being given, in any acute or chronic infection.

**G. Myopathy:** A peculiar steroid myopathy has been reported, especially with the substituted steroids.

**H. Fatty Liver:** Fatty liver and fat embolism may occur.

**I. Diagnostic Errors:** Administration of these drugs may interfere with certain immune mechanisms that are of diagnostic value, eg, in skin tests and agglutination tests; they produce leukocytosis and lymphopenia, which may be confusing. The potent substituted corticosteroids (eg, dexamethasone) will suppress the urinary ketosteroids and hydroxycorticosteroid values. The signs and symptoms of infection may be masked by corticosteroid therapy. These drugs may also interfere with normal pain perception (eg, joint pain), which may lead to Charcot-like disintegration of the weight-bearing joints after local or systemic corticosteroid therapy.

**J. Withdrawal of Corticosteroids:** Prolonged use of these agents leads to combined pituitary-adrenal gland suppression that may last for as long as 1 year after stopping the drug. In the presence of infection, trauma, surgery, or other forms of stress, the patient may have signs of adrenal insufficiency unless given supplemental hydrocortisone.

Always withdraw corticosteroids *slowly* to minimize both flare-ups of the original disease and to prevent "steroid withdrawal reactions" (arthralgias, aches and pains, fatigue, nausea, fine desquamation of skin with a "chalky" appearance, etc).

---

# REFERENCES

DeGroot LJ et al: *Endocrinology.* 3 vols. Grune & Stratton, 1979.

Dillon RS: *Handbook of Endocrinology: Diagnosis and Management of Endocrine and Metabolic Disorders,* 2nd ed. Lea & Febiger, 1980.

Felig P et al (editors): *Endocrinology and Metabolism.* 2nd ed. McGraw-Hill, 1987.

Greenspan FS, Forsham PH (editors): *Basic & Clinical Endocrinology.* 2nd ed. Lange, 1986.

Hershman JM: *Endocrine Pathophysiology: A Patient Oriented Approach,* 2nd ed. Lea & Febiger, 1982.

Ingbar SH, Braverman LE (editors): *The Thyroid: A Fundamental and Clinical Text,* 5th ed. Lippincott, 1986.

McKusik VA: *Mendelian Inheritance in Man: Catalogue of Autosomal Dominant, Autosomal Recessive, and X-linked Phenotypes,* 6th ed. Johns Hopkins Univ Press, 1983.

Nordin BEC (editor): *Metabolic Bone and Stone Disease.* Churchill Livingstone, 1984.

Speroff L et al: *Clinical Gynecologic Endocrinology and Infertility,* 3rd ed. Williams & Wilkins, 1983.

Stanbury JB et al (editors): *The Metabolic Basis of Inherited Disease,* 5th ed. McGraw-Hill, 1983.

Troen P, Nankin HR (editors): *The Testis in Normal and Infertile Men.* Raven Press, 1977.

Wilson JD, Foster DW (editors): *Williams' Textbook of Endocrinology,* 7th ed. Saunders, 1985.

Yen SSC, Jaffe RB (editors): *Reproductive Endocrinology,* 2nd ed. Saunders, 1986.

# Diabetes Mellitus, Hypoglycemia, & Lipoprotein Disorders

# 19

*John H. Karam, MD*

## DIABETES MELLITUS

### Classification & Pathogenesis

Clinical diabetes mellitus represents a syndrome with disordered metabolism and inappropriate hyperglycemia due to either an absolute deficiency of insulin secretion or a reduction in its biologic effectiveness or both. It is classified into 2 major types in which age at onset is not a criterion (Table 19–1).

**A. Type I: Insulin-Dependent Diabetes Mellitus (IDDM):** This severe form is associated with ketosis in the untreated state. It occurs most commonly in juveniles but occasionally in adults, especially the nonobese and those who are elderly when hyperglycemia first appears. It is a catabolic disorder in which circulating insulin is virtually absent, plasma glucagon is elevated, and the pancreatic B cells fail to respond to all insulinogenic stimuli. Exogenous insulin is therefore required to reverse the catabolic state, prevent ketosis, reduce the hyperglucagonemia, and bring the elevated blood glucose level down.

Certain HLA antigens—B8, B15, DR3, and DR4—are strongly associated with the development of type I diabetes, particularly in northern Europeans. A DR2 antigen is associated with a reduced incidence of disease. Recently, a group of DQ antigens have been identified as being important in understanding susceptibility to IDDM. A particular variety of DQ apparently increases and others apparently decrease the susceptibility of patients with DR4 or even DR2 to develop IDDM. The genetic determinants of these antigens are located on the sixth human chromosome adjacent to immune response genes. A polymorphic region of DNA flanking the 5′ end of the insulin gene on chromosome 11 has also been shown to have an association with type I diabetes in a white population. In addition, circulating islet cell antibodies have been detected in as many as 85% of patients tested in the first few weeks of their diabetes, and when sensitive immunoassays are used, the majority of these patients also have detectable anti-insulin antibodies prior to receiving insulin therapy.

Because of these immune characteristics, type I diabetes is felt to result from an infectious or toxic environmental insult to pancreatic B cells of persons whose immune system is genetically predisposed to develop a vigorous autoimmune response against altered pancreatic B cell antigens. Extrinsic factors that affect B cell function include damage caused by viruses such as mumps or coxsackie B4 virus, by toxic chemical agents, or by destructive cytotoxins and antibodies released from sensitized immunocytes. An underlying genetic defect on chromosome 11 relating to B cell replication or function may predispose to development of B cell failure after viral infection; alternatively, specific HLA genes may increase susceptibility to a diabetogenic virus or be linked to certain immune response genes that predispose patients to a destructive autoimmune response against their own islet cells (autoaggression).

**B. Type II: Non-Insulin-Dependent Diabetes Mellitus (NIDDM):** This represents a heterogeneous group comprising milder forms of diabetes that occur predominantly in adults but occasionally in juveniles. Circulating endogenous insulin is sufficient to prevent

**Table 19–1.** Clinical classification of idiopathic diabetes mellitus syndromes.

| Type | Ketosis | Islet Cell Antibodies | HLA Association | Treatment |
|---|---|---|---|---|
| (I)  Insulin-dependent (IDDM) | Present | Present at onset | Positive | Insulin (mixtures of rapid- and intermediate-acting, at least twice daily) and diet |
| (II)  Non-insulin-dependent (NIDDM) (a) Nonobese | Absent | Absent | Negative | (1) Eucaloric diet alone (2) Diet plus insulin or sulfonylureas |
| (b) Obese | | | | (1) Weight reduction (2) Hypocaloric diet, plus sulfonylureas or insulin for symptomatic control only |

ketoacidosis but is often either subnormal or relatively inadequate in the face of increased needs owing to tissue insensitivity. Type II diabetes is defined in essentially negative terms: It is a *non*ketotic form of diabetes that is *not* linked to HLA markers on the sixth chromosome; it has *no* islet cell antibodies; and it is *not* dependent on exogenous insulin therapy to sustain life, thereby being termed "*non*-insulin-dependent diabetes mellitus" (*NIDDM*). In this "non-type I" group of diabetes is a wide assortment of heterogeneous disorders that include several rare instances wherein a defective insulin gene produces a biologically inadequate insulin as has been documented in only 9 families worldwide. However, in most cases of this type of diabetes, the cause is unknown.

An element of tissue insensitivity to insulin has been noted in most NIDDM patients irrespective of weight. In addition, there is an accompanying deficiency in the response of pancreatic B cells to glucose. Both the tissue resistance to insulin and the impaired B cell response to glucose appear to be further aggravated by increased hyperglycemia, and both defects are ameliorated by treatment that reduces the hyperglycemia toward normal. Attempts to establish genetic linkage of the insulin gene region of chromosome 11 with NIDDM have generally been unsuccessful.

Two subgroups of patients with type II diabetes are currently distinguished by the absence or presence of obesity:

**1. Nonobese NIDDM patients–**These patients generally show an absent or blunted early phase of insulin release in response to glucose; however, it may often be elicited in response to other insulinogenic stimuli such as acute intravenous administration of sulfonylureas, glucagon, or secretin. Among this heterogeneous subgroup may be certain unrecognized patients with a milder expression of type I diabetes who initially retain enough B cell function to avoid ketosis but later develop increasing dependency on insulin therapy. Also included within this subgroup are those with diabetes characterized as "maturity-onset diabetes of the young," whose strongly positive family history of a mild form of diabetes suggests an autosomal dominant transmission.

The hyperglycemia in this subgroup of patients often responds to oral hypoglycemic agents or, at times, to dietary therapy alone. Occasionally, insulin therapy is required to achieve satisfactory glycemic control even though it is not needed to prevent ketoacidosis.

Although residual insulin resistance may persist after therapeutic correction of the hyperglycemia in some cases, it does not seem to be clinically relevant to the treatment of nonobese NIDDM patients, who generally respond to appropriate therapeutic supplements of insulin in the absence of rare associated conditions such as lipoatrophy or acanthosis nigricans.

**2. Obese NIDDM patients–**This form of diabetes is secondary to extrapancreatic factors that produce insensitivity to endogenous insulin. It is characterized by nonketotic mild diabetes, mainly in adults but occasionally also in children. The primary problem is a "target organ" disorder resulting in ineffective insulin action (Table 19–2) that can secondarily influence pancreatic B cell function. Hyperplasia of pancreatic B cells is often present and probably accounts for the fasting hyperinsulinism and exaggerated insulin responses to glucose and other stimuli seen in the milder forms of this disorder. In more severe cases, secondary (but potentially reversible) failure of B cell secretion may result after exposure to prolonged fasting hyperglycemia. This phenomenon has been called "desensitization" of the pancreatic B cell. It is selective for glucose, and the B cell recovers sensitivity to glucose stimulation once the sustained hyperglycemia is corrected by any form of therapy, including diet, sulfonylureas, and insulin. Obesity is common in this type of diabetes as a result of excessive caloric intake, perhaps facilitated by hunger resulting from mild postprandial hypoglycemia after excess insulin release. In obese patients, insulin insensitivity is positively correlated with the presence of distended adipocytes, but liver and muscle cells also resist the deposition of additional glycogen and triglycerides in their storage depots.

Two major mechanisms have been proposed to account for the observed tissue insensitivity to insulin in obesity: Chronic overfeeding may lead to either (1) sustained B cell stimulation and hyperinsulinism, which in itself induces receptor insensitivity to insulin; or (2) a postreceptor defect associated with overdistended storage depots and a reduced ability to clear nutrients from the circulation. Consequent hyperinsulinism induces receptor insensitivity to insulin. When hyperglycemia develops, a specific glucose transporter protein within insulin target tissue becomes down-regulated after continuous activation. This contributes to further defects in postreceptor insulin action, thereby aggravating the hyperglycemia.

Regardless of the mechanism, a reduction in overfeeding can interrupt the cycle. In the first case, restricted diet would reduce islet stimulation of insulin release, thereby restoring insulin receptor sites and

**Table 19–2.** Factors reducing response to insulin.

---

**Prereceptor inhibitors:** Anti-insulin antibodies
**Receptor inhibitors:**
  Insulin receptor antibodies
  "Down regulation" of receptors by hyperinsulinism:
    Primary hyperinsulinism (B cell adenoma)
    Hyperinsulinism secondary to a postreceptor defect (obesity, Cushing's syndrome, acromegaly, pregnancy) or prolonged glycemia (diabetes mellitus, post-glucose tolerance test)
**Postreceptor influences:**
  Poor responsiveness of principal target organs; obesity; hepatic disease; muscle inactivity
  Hormonal excess: glucocorticoids, growth hormone, oral contraceptive agents, progesterone, human chorionic somatomammotropin, catecholamines, thyroxine

---

improving tissue sensitivity to insulin, whereas in the second situation, normal tissue sensitivity returns as storage depots become less saturated and as hyperglycemia is corrected.

**3. Patients with diabetes secondary to other causes**–In addition to obesity, chronic muscle inactivity or disease and liver disease have been associated with carbohydrate intolerance and hyperinsulinism in response to glucose.

Other secondary causes of carbohydrate intolerance include endocrine disorders—often specific endocrine tumors—associated with excess production of growth hormone, glucocorticoids, catecholamines, or glucagon. In all 4 situations, peripheral responsiveness to insulin is impaired. With excess of glucocorticoids, catecholamines, or glucagon, increased hepatic output of glucose is a contributory factor; in the case of catecholamines, decreased insulin release is an additional factor in producing carbohydrate intolerance.

A rare syndrome of extreme insulin resistance associated with acanthosis nigricans is divided into 2 groups on the basis of clinical and laboratory manifestations: Group A consists of younger women with androgenic features (hirsutism, amenorrhea, polycystic ovaries) in whom insulin receptors are deficient in number. Group B consists of older people, mostly women, in whom immunologic disease is suspected (high erythrocyte sedimentation rate, anti-DNA antibodies, and a circulating immunoglobulin that binds to insulin receptors, reducing their affinity to insulin).

Recently, the insulin receptor gene has been identified on chromosome 19. It has been sequenced and found to code for an integral membrane glycoprotein consisting of 2 alpha and 2 beta subunits. When insulin binds to the alpha subunit, it initiates phosphorylation reactions within its own beta subunit as well as on other cytosolic proteins. Characterization of the insulin receptor gene in patients with acanthosis nigricans and insulin resistance offers considerable promise for resolving the pathogenesis of these syndromes with severe insulin resistance.

## Epidemiologic Considerations

An estimated 5.5 million people in the USA are known to have diabetes, of which 440,000 have the insulin-dependent type. Use of the current "therapeutic" classification has been widely accepted throughout the world, but its deficiencies are apparent in many individual cases. For example, a 23-year-old nonobese woman whose mild diabetes is presently responding adequately to diet alone and who shows a low-normal C-peptide response to stimuli had presented with severe diabetes with ketosis and required insulin for several weeks following diagnosis. In addition, she has an associated autoimmune disorder, myasthenia gravis. From an etiologic standpoint, she has type I diabetes, but her present clinical status is "non-insulin dependent." The National Diabetes Data Group is reviewing the present classification

system so that such cases may be incorporated. Information about the epidemiology of mild adult-onset diabetes was a major contribution of the University Group Diabetes Program (UGDP). This study revealed that the vast majority of persons with mild adult-onset diabetes were obese and thus may well have represented a type of diabetes in which tissue insensitivity to insulin was a fundamental pathologic feature.

## Clinical Findings

The principal clinical features of the 2 major types of diabetes mellitus are listed for comparison in Table 19–3.

Patients with type I diabetes (IDDM) present with a characteristic symptom complex, as outlined below. An absolute deficiency of insulin results in excessive accumulation of circulating glucose and fatty acids, with consequent hyperosmolality and hyperketonemia. The severity of the insulin deficiency and the acuteness with which the catabolic state develops determine the intensity of the osmotic and ketotic excess.

Patients with type II diabetes (NIDDM) may or may not present with characteristic signs and symptoms. The presence of obesity or a strongly positive family history for mild diabetes suggests a high risk for the development of type II diabetes.

**A. Symptoms:**

**1. Type I diabetes (IDDM)**–Increased urination is a consequence of osmotic diuresis secondary to sustained hyperglycemia. This results in a loss of glucose as well as free water and electrolytes in the urine. Enuresis may signal the onset of diabetes in very young children. Thirst is a consequence of the hyperosmolar state, as is blurred vision, which often develops as the lenses and retinas are exposed to hyperosmolar fluids.

Weight loss despite normal or increased appetite is a common feature of IDDM when it develops subacutely over a period of weeks. The weight loss is initially due to depletion of water, glycogen, and triglyceride stores; thereafter, reduced muscle mass occurs as amino acids are diverted to form glucose and ketone bodies.

Lowered plasma volume produces dizziness and weakness due to postural hypotension when sitting or standing. Total body potassium loss and the gen-

**Table 19–3.** Clinical features of diabetes.

| | Diabetes Type I (IDDM) | Diabetes Type II (NIDDM) |
|---|---|---|
| Polyuria and thirst | ++ | + |
| Weakness or fatigue | ++ | + |
| Polyphagia with weight loss | ++ | − |
| Recurrent blurred vision | + | ++ |
| Vulvovaginitis or pruritus | + | ++ |
| Peripheral neuropathy | + | ++ |
| Nocturnal enuresis | ++ | − |
| Often asymptomatic | − | ++ |

eral catabolism of muscle protein contribute to the weakness.

Parethesias may be present at the time of diagnosis of type I diabetes, particularly when the onset is subacute. They reflect a temporary dysfunction of peripheral sensory nerves, which usually clears as insulin replacement restores glycemic levels closer to normal, suggesting neurotoxicity from sustained hyperglycemia.

When insulin deficiency is absolute and of acute onset, the above symptoms progress in an accelerated manner. Ketoacidosis exacerbates the dehydration and hyperosmolality by producing anorexia and nausea and vomiting, thus interfering with oral fluid replacement. As plasma osmolality exceeds 330 mosm/L (normal, 285–295 mosm/L), impaired consciousness ensues; increased osmolality has a better correlation with progression to coma and subsequent outcome than does lowered pH. With progression of acidosis, deep breathing with a rapid ventilatory rate (Kussmaul respiration) occurs in an attempt to eliminate carbonic acid. With worsening acidosis and increasing osmolality, the cardiovascular system may be unable to maintain compensatory vasoconstriction; severe circulatory collapse may result.

**2. Type II diabetes (NIDDM)–**Most patients with type II diabetes have an insidious onset of hyperglycemia and may be relatively asymptomatic initially. This is particularly true in obese patients, whose diabetes may be detected only after glycosuria or hyperglycemia is noted during routine laboratory studies. Chronic skin infections are common. Generalized pruritus and symptoms of vaginitis are frequently the initial complaints of women with NIDDM. Diabetes should be suspected in women with chronic candidal vulvovaginitis as well as in those who have delivered large babies (> 9 lb, or 4.1 kg) or have had polyhydramnios, preeclampsia, or unexplained fetal losses.

**B. Signs:**

**1. Type I diabetes (IDDM)–**The patient's level of consciousness can vary depending on the degree of hyperosmolality. When insulin deficiency develops relatively slowly and sufficient water intake is maintained to permit renal excretion of glucose and appropriate dilution of extracellular sodium chloride, patients remain relatively alert and physical findings may be minimal. When vomiting occurs in response to worsening ketoacidosis, dehydration progresses and compensatory mechanisms become inadequate to keep plasma osmolality below 320 mosm/L. Under these circumstances, stupor or even coma may occur. Evidence of dehydration in a stuporous patient with rapid deep breathing and the fruity breath odor of acetone suggests the diagnosis of diabetic ketoacidosis.

Postural hypotension indicates a depleted plasma volume; hypotension in the recumbent position is a serious prognostic sign. Loss of subcutaneous fat and muscle wasting are features of more slowly developing insulin deficiency. In occasional patients with slow, insidious onset of insulin deficiency, subcutaneous fat may be considerably depleted. An enlarged liver, eruptive xanthomas on the flexor surface of the limbs and on the buttocks, and lipemia retinalis indicate that chronic insulin deficiency has resulted in chylomicronemia, with circulating triglycerides elevated usually to over 2000 mg/dL.

**2. Type II diabetes (NIDDM)–**Nonobese patients with this mild form of diabetes often have no characteristic physical findings at the time of diagnosis. Obese diabetics may have any variety of fat distribution; however, diabetes seems to be more often associated in both men and women with localization of fat deposits on the upper segment of the body (particularly the abdomen, chest, neck, and face) and relatively less fat on the appendages, which may be quite muscular. Mild hypertension may be present in obese diabetics. In women, candidal vaginitis with a reddened, inflamed vulvar area and a profuse whitish discharge may herald the presence of diabetes.

**C. Laboratory Findings:**

**1. Urinalysis–**

**a. Glycosuria–**The Clinitest tablet placed in 5 drops of urine with 10 drops of water provides a rapid, semiquantitative estimate of the degree of glycosuria. A more specific and convenient method is the paper strip impregnated with glucose oxidase and a chromogen system (Clinistix, Diastix, TesTape), which is sensitive to as little as 0.1% glucose in urine. Diastix can be directly applied to the urinary stream, and differing color responses of the indicator strip reflect glucose concentration. This is sufficiently accurate in most patients to eliminate the need for the more cumbersome Clinitest tablets.

Certain common therapeutic agents interfere with both of these methods. When taken in large doses, ascorbic acid, salicylates, methyldopa (Aldomet), and levodopa can give false-positive Clinitest measurements, as can the presence of alkaptonuria; they give false-negative results when glucose oxidase paper strips are used, since these powerful reducing agents interfere with the color reaction and thus prevent accurate estimation of glucose in the urine of diabetics. Both of these methods are dependent upon a normal renal threshold for glucose as well as reliable bladder emptying for proper interpretation.

**b. Ketonuria–**Qualitative detection of ketone bodies can be accomplished by nitroprusside tests (Acetest or Ketostix). Although these tests do not detect β-hydroxybutyric acid, which lacks a ketone group, the semiquantitative estimation of ketonuria thus obtained is nonetheless usually adequate for clinical purposes.

**2. Blood Testing Procedures–**

**a. Glucose tolerance test–**

**(1) Methodology and normal fasting glucose–**Plasma or serum from venous blood samples may be used and has the advantage over whole blood of providing values for glucose that are independent of hematocrit and that reflect the glucose concentration to which body tissues are exposed. For these reasons, and because plasma and serum are more readily measured on automated equipment, plasma and serum glucose measurements are rapidly replacing the whole blood glucose determinations used heretofore in most laboratories. Fluoride anticoagulant in the collecting tube prevents enzymatic glycolysis by blood corpuscles and prevents pseudohypoglycemia, seen in states of extreme leukocytosis. If serum is used, samples should be refrigerated and separated within an hour after collection.

**(2) Criteria for laboratory confirmation of diabetes mellitus**–If the fasting plasma glucose level is over 140 mg/dL on more than one occasion, further evaluation of the patient with a glucose challenge is unnecessary. However, when fasting plasma glucose is less than 140 mg/dL in suspected cases, a standardized oral glucose tolerance test may be done. The National Diabetes Data Group recommends giving a 75-g glucose dose dissolved in 300 mL of water for adults (1.75 g/kg ideal body weight for children) after an overnight fast in subjects who have been receiving at least 150–200 g of carbohydrate daily for 3 days before the test.

Normal glucose tolerance is considered to be present when the fasting plasma glucose is below 115 mg/dL and the 2-hour value is below 140 mg/dL, with no value between zero time and 2 hours exceeding 200 mg/dL. However, a diagnosis of diabetes mellitus requires plasma glucose levels to be above 200 mg/dL at both 2 hours and at least one other time between zero time and 2 hours. Values above the normal standard that do not meet the criteria for diabetes are considered nondiagnostic, and the patient is described as having "impaired glucose tolerance." For proper evaluation of the test, the subjects should be normally active and free from acute illness. Medications that may impair glucose tolerance include diuretics, contraceptive drugs, glucocorticoids, nicotinic acid, and phenytoin.

Because of difficulties in interpreting oral glucose tolerance tests and the lack of standards related to aging, these tests are generally being replaced by documentation of fasting hyperglycemia as a means of diagnosing diabetes mellitus.

**b. Glycosylated hemoglobin (hemoglobin $A_1$) measurements**–Glycosylated hemoglobin is abnormally high in diabetics with chronic hyperglycemia and reflects their metabolic control. The major form of glycohemoglobin is termed hemoglobin $A_{1c}$, which normally comprises only 4–6% of the total hemoglobin. It is produced by a nonenzymatic reaction between glucose and the N-terminal amino acid of both $\beta$ chains of the hemoglobin molecule. The remaining glycohemoglobins (2–4% of the total) consist of phosphorylated glucose or fructose and are termed hemoglobin $A_{1a}$ and hemoglobin $A_{1b}$. Most laboratories measure the sum of these 3 glycohemoglobins and report it as hemoglobin $A_1$.

Since glycohemoglobins have a long half-life, they generally reflect the state of glycemia over the preceding 8 weeks, thereby providing an improved method of assessing diabetic control. When glycohemoglobins are measured in a reliable laboratory, they are extremely useful in monitoring the progress of patients. Measurements should be made in patients with either type of diabetes mellitus at 3- to 4-month intervals. In patients monitoring their own blood glucose levels, glycohemoglobin values provide a valuable check on the accuracy of monitoring. In patients who do not monitor their own blood glucose levels, glycohemoglobin values are essential for adjusting therapy.

Occasionally, fluctuations in hemoglobin $A_1$ are due to an acutely generated, reversible, intermediary (aldimine-linked) product that can falsely elevate glycohemoglobins when measured with "short-cut" chromatographic methods. This can be eliminated by using more intricate methods or by dialysis of the hemolysate before chromatography. When hemoglobin variants are present, such as negatively charged hemoglobin F, acetylated hemoglobin from high-dose aspirin therapy, or carbamylated hemoglobin produced by the complexing of urea with hemoglobin in uremia, falsely *high* "hemoglobin $A_1$" values are obtained with commonly used chromatographic methods. In the presence of positively charged hemoglobin variants such as hemoglobin S or C, or when the life span of red blood cells is reduced by increased hemolysis or hemorrhage, falsely *low* values for "hemoglobin $A_1$" result.

**Serum fructosamine** is formed by nonenzymatic glycosylation of serum proteins (predominantly albumin). Since serum albumin has a much shorter half-life than hemoglobin, serum fructosamine generally reflects the state of glycemic control for only the preceding 2 weeks. When abnormal hemoglobins or hemolytic states affect the interpretation of glycohemoglobin results or when a narrower time frame is required, such as for ascertaining glycemic control at the time of conception in a diabetic woman who has recently become pregnant, serum fructosamine assays offer some advantage. In most circumstances, however, glycohemoglobin assays remain the preferred method for assessing long-term glycemic control in diabetic patients.

**c. Self glucose monitoring**–Capillary blood glucose measurements performed by patients themselves, as outpatients, are extremely useful, particularly in IDDM patients in whom "tight" metabolic control is attempted. A portable battery-operated Glucometer II (Ames Co.) or Glucosan II (Lifescan, Inc.) provides a digital readout of the intensity of color developed when glucose oxidase paper strips are exposed to a drop of capillary blood for up to 60 seconds. Similar diagnostic strips made by Ames Co. (Visidex) or by Biodynamics Corp. (Chemstrip-bG) have 2 chromogen indicators that permit *visual* estimation of the glucose concentration when compared to a series of color standards. The Chemstrip-bG can be read by a reflectance meter (Accu-chek II). In self-monitoring of blood glucose, patients must prick their finger with a small lancet (Monolet, Ames Co.), which can be facilitated by a small plastic trigger device such as an Autolet (Ames Co.), Autoclix (Bio-Dynamics), or Penlet (Lifescan, Inc.).

**3. Capillary morphometry (biopsy of the quadriceps muscle)**–The basement membrane of capillaries from skeletal muscle tissue of the quadriceps area is abnormally thickened in cases of overt spontaneous diabetes in adults with fasting hyperglycemia of 140 mg/dL or more. Capillary morphometry appears to be less useful in diabetic children, being normal in as many as 60% of those below age 18.

The controversy about whether basement membrane thickening in diabetics can result from hyperglycemia alone with no genetic component appears to have been resolved by documented observation of thickened capillary basement membranes in the muscle of patients with acquired chronic hyperglycemia after ingestion of a diabetogenic toxin (Vacor rodenticide) during attempted suicide. While this finding establishes that glucose toxicity can produce abnormally thick membranes, it is still possible that the degree of abnormal thickening may depend on varying genetic susceptibility among diabetic patients. Moreover, it remains unclear whether a thickened capillary basement membrane of skeletal muscle has clinical significance, since it has not been possible to demonstrate a correlation between this marker and clinically evident renal dysfunction or renal mesangial changes associated with progressive diabetic nephropathy.

## Differential Diagnosis

Nondiabetic glycosuria (renal glycosuria) is a benign, asymptomatic condition wherein glucose appears in the urine despite a normal amount of glucose in the blood, either basally or during a glucose tolerance test. Its cause may vary from an autosomally transmitted genetic disorder to one associated with dysfunction of the proximal renal tubule (Fanconi's syndrome, chronic renal failure), or it may merely be a consequence of the increased load of glucose presented to the tubules by the elevated glomerular filtration rate during pregnancy. As many as 50% of pregnant women normally have demonstrable sugar in the urine, especially during the third and fourth months. This sugar is practically always glucose except during the late weeks of pregnancy, when lactose may be present.

Causes of hyperglycemia associated with end organ insensitivity to insulin include obesity, acromegaly, Cushing's syndrome, liver disease, muscle disorders (myotonic dystrophy), glucagonoma, lipoatrophy, hemochromatosis, and thyrotoxicosis. Pheochromocytoma can induce hyperglycemia by a variety of mechanisms, including end organ resistance, inhibition of insulin release, and hypersecretion of glucagon. Chronic pancreatitis reduces the number of functioning B cells and can result in a metabolic derangement very similar to that of genetic diabetes mellitus except that a concomitant reduction in pancreatic A cells may reduce glucagon secretion despite insulin deficiency, which often raises glucagon levels. Insulin-dependent diabetes is occasionally associated with Addison's disease and chronic thyroiditis (Schmidt's syndrome). This occurs particularly in women and probably represents an autoimmune disorder in which there are circulating antibodies to adrenocortical and thyroid tissue, thyroglobulin, and gastric parietal cells.

## Treatment

**A. Principles of Treatment of Diabetes:** Rational therapy of diabetes requires the application of principles derived from current knowledge concerning (1) the nature of the disease and (2) the mechanism of action and the efficacy and safety of available treatment regimens (diet, oral hypoglycemic drugs, and insulin). There is conflicting evidence about whether microangiopathy is related to the existence and duration of hyperglycemia or whether it reflects a separate, coexisting genetic disorder. Until this conflict is resolved, the therapeutic objective endorsed by the executive committee of the American Diabetes Association is to attempt to restore known metabolic derangements to normal in the hope that this approach will impede if not prevent the progression of microvascular disease.

The general principles of therapy emphasized in this chapter will be based on the classification of diabetes outlined in Table 19–1.

**Diet** will be prescribed individually to meet the needs of each type: caloric restriction for obese patients and regular spaced feedings with a bedtime snack for patients receiving hypoglycemic agents, especially insulin.

**Exercise** will also be encouraged as an adjunct to diet and insulin replacement in reducing hyperglycemia in the insulinopenic diabetic and to help achieve weight reduction in the insulin-insensitive obese diabetic.

Treatment of the insulinopenic diabetic will be directed toward normalization of the endocrine and metabolic abnormalities. In more severe cases, exogenous insulin replacement will be required, whereas in milder degrees of insulinopenia, an attempt to restore endogenous insulin release with sulfonylureas will have the advantage of causing insulin to be released intraportally and will not introduce immunogenic effects from administering exogenous insulin subcutaneously. Potential disadvantages of sulfonylurea therapy will be discussed in the section on safety of oral hypoglycemic agents.

Treatment of insulin-insensitive diabetes will be directed at the cause of tissue resistance, eg, weight reduction in cases of obesity and reduction of endocrine hypersecretion in cases of acromegaly or Cushing's syndrome.

**B. Treatment Regimens:**

**1. Diet**–A well-balanced, nutritious diet remains a fundamental element of therapy. However, in more than half of cases, diabetic patients fail to follow their diet. In prescribing a diet, it is important to relate dietary objectives to the type of diabetes. In obese patients with mild hyperglycemia, the major goal of diet therapy is weight reduction by caloric restriction. Thus, there is less need for exchange lists, emphasis on timing of meals, or periodic snacks, all of which are so essential in the treatment of insulin-requiring nonobese diabetics.

Because of the prevalence of obese patients with mild diabetes among the population of diabetics receiving therapy, this type of patient represents the most frequent and thus one of the most important challenges for the physician. Treatment requires an energetic, vigorous program directed by persons who are aware of the mechanisms by which weight reduction is known to effectively lower hyperglycemia and who are convinced of the profoundly beneficial effects of weight control on blood lipid levels as well as on hyperglycemia in obese diabetics. Weight reduction is an elusive goal that can only be achieved by close supervision of the obese patient.

**a. ADA diet**–Exchange lists for meal planning can be obtained from the American Diabetes Association and its affiliate associations or from the American Dietetic Association, 430 North Michigan Avenue, Chicago 60611. The ADA diet stresses the major goal of caloric restriction as a means of achieving or maintaining ideal weight. A prudent diet is recommended, which includes restriction of fat intake to 35% or less of the total calories and suggests that saturated fat be reduced to only one-third of this by substituting poultry, veal, and fish for red meats as a major protein source. At the same time, cholesterol is restricted to less than 300 mg daily. Carbohydrates may be consumed liberally (as much as 50–60% of total calories) as long as refined and simple sugars are avoided as snacks. Dietary sucrose need not aggravate postprandial hyperglycemia in diabetic patients if consumed as part of a mixed meal and in exchange for other carbohydrate components of the meal. Unrefined carbohydrates with a fiber content sufficient to provide 15–20 g of fiber daily are recommended for both type I and type II diabetic patients.

**b. Dietary fiber**–Plant components such as cellulose, gum, and pectin are indigestible by humans and are termed dietary "fiber." Insoluble fibers such as cellulose or hemicellulose, as found in bran, tend to increase intestinal transit time. In contrast, soluble fibers such as gums and pectins, as found in beans or apple skin, tend to decrease gastric and intestinal transit. However, regardless of the type of fiber, it has been clearly demonstrated that when fiber accompanies ingested carbohydrates, glucose absorption is slower and hyperglycemia is diminished. Although the ADA diet does not include fiber supplements such as added bran, it recommends food such as grain cereals and beans with relatively high fiber content as staple components of the diet in diabetics. High fiber content in the diet may also have a favorable effect on blood cholesterol levels.

**c. Glycemic index**–Jenkins and others have attempted to quantitate the relative glycemic contribution of various carbohydrate foods and have proposed a glycemic index. A patient is given a test food containing 50 g of carbohydrate and, on another occasion, a reference food such as glucose or white bread. (White bread is preferred because of its greater palatability and lesser tendency to slow gastric emptying by high tonicity.) The areas of blood glucose generated over a 3-hour period following ingestion of each food are compared to yield the glycemic index.

$$\text{Glycemic index} = \frac{\text{Blood glucose area of test food}}{\text{Blood glucose area of reference food}} \times 100$$

Differences in glycemic indices have been seen in both diabetic and nondiabetic patients. When white bread is assigned the value of 100, the mean glycemic index for a baked potato is 135; for table sugar (sucrose), 86; for spaghetti, 66; for kidney beans, 54; for ice cream, 52; and for lentils, 43. There is some controversy as to the value of this index, since the index of a food ingested alone may become considerably altered when it is ingested with fats and proteins during meals.

**d. Artificial sweeteners**–The nonnutritive sweetener saccharin continues to be available in certain foods and beverages despite recent warnings by the FDA about its potential long-term carcinogenicity to the bladder. A restriction on the use of saccharin in children and pregnant women is recommended; however, in patients with diabetes or obesity, physicians should determine on an individual basis its comparative benefit versus risk.

Nutritive sweeteners such as sorbitol and fructose have recently increased in popularity. Except for acute diarrhea induced by ingestion of large amounts of sorbitol-containing foods, their relative risk has yet to be established. Fructose represents a "natural" sugar substance that is a highly effective sweetener which induces only slight increases in plasma glucose levels.

Aspartame (NutraSweet) may prove to be the optimal sweetener for diabetic patients. It consists of 2 amino acids (aspartic acid and phenylalanine) that combine to produce a nutritive sweetener 180 times as sweet as sucrose.

**2. Oral hypoglycemic drugs**–These are of 2 major types: sulfonylureas and biguanides. Their modes of action are quite different, and considerable controversy exists over their mechanisms of action, therapeutic indications, and safety for long-term use. Only the sulfonylureas remain in use as oral hypoglycemic drugs in the USA.

**a. Sulfonylureas**–(Table 19–4) This group of drugs contains a sulfonic acid-urea nucleus which can be modified by chemical substitutions to produce agents that have similar qualitative actions but differ widely in potency. The mechanism of action of the sulfonylureas when they are acutely administered is due to their insulinotropic effect on pancreatic B cells. However, it remains unclear whether this well-documented *acute* action requires additional extrapancreatic effects such as an increase in insulin binding

**Table 19–4.** Sulfonylureas.

| | Tablet Size (mg) | Daily Dose | Duration of Action (hours) |
|---|---|---|---|
| Tolbutamide (Orinase)* | 250, 500 | 0.25–2 g in divided doses | 6–12 |
| Tolazamide (Tolinase)* | 100, 250, 500 | 0.1–1 g as single dose or in divided doses | 10–14 |
| Acetohexamide (Dymelor)* | 250, 500 | 0.25–1.5 g as single dose or in divided doses | 12–24 |
| Chlorpropamide (Diabinese)* | 100, 250 | 0.1–0.5 g as single dose | Up to 60 |
| Glyburide (Diaβeta, Micronase) | 1.25, 2.5, 5 | 1.25–20 mg | 10–24 |
| Glipizide (Glucotrol) | 5, 10 | 5–30 mg | 10–20 |

* Generic form available.

to receptors to explain more adequately the hypoglycemic effect of sulfonylureas during chronic administration.

Sulfonylureas are presently not indicated in the juvenile type ketosis-prone insulin-dependent diabetic, since these drugs seem to depend on functioning pancreatic B cells to produce their effect on blood glucose. There is apparently little, if any, potentiation of insulin effectiveness on long-term glycemic control when sulfonylureas are added.

The sulfonylureas seem most appropriate for use in the nonobese insulinopenic mild maturity-onset diabetic in whom acute administration restores the early phase of insulin release that is refractory to acute glucose stimulation. In obese mild diabetics and others with peripheral insensitivity to levels of circulating insulin, primary emphasis should be on weight reduction. When hyperglycemia in obese diabetics has been more severe, with consequent impairment of pancreatic B cell function, sulfonylureas may improve glycemic control until concurrent measures such as diet, exercise, and weight reduction can sustain the improvement without the need for oral drugs.

**(1) Tolbutamide** (Orinase) is supplied in tablets of 250 and 500 mg. It is rapidly oxidized in the liver to an inactive form, and its approximate duration of effect is relatively short (6–10 hours). Tolbutamide is probably best administered in divided doses (eg, 500 mg before each meal and at bedtime); however, some patients require only 1 or 2 tablets daily. Acute toxic reactions are rare, with skin rashes occurring infrequently. Because of its short duration of action, which is independent of renal function, tolbutamide is probably the safest agent to use in elderly patients, in whom hypoglycemia would be a particularly serious risk. Prolonged hypoglycemia has been reported rarely, mostly in patients receiving certain drugs (eg, dicumarol, phenylbutazone, or some of the sulfonam-

ides). The latter compounds apparently compete with sulfonylureas for oxidative enzyme systems in the liver, resulting in maintenance of high levels of unmetabolized, active sulfonylureas in the circulation.

**(2) Chlorpropamide** (Diabinese) is supplied in tablets of 100 and 250 mg. This drug, with a half-life of 32 hours, is slowly metabolized, with approximately 20–30% excreted unchanged in the urine. Since the metabolites retain hypoglycemic activity, elimination of the biologic effect is almost completely dependent on renal excretion, so that its use is contraindicated in patients with hepatic or renal insufficiency. The average maintenance dose is 250 mg daily, given as a single dose in the morning. Chlorpropamide is a potent agent that is occasionally effective in controlling hyperglycemia in NIDDM despite the failure of maximum therapeutic doses of other less potent sulfonylureas such as tolbutamide, tolazamide, and acetohexamide. Prolonged hypoglycemic reactions are more common than with tolbutamide, particularly in elderly patients, in whom chlorpropamide therapy should be monitored with special care. Doses in excess of 500 mg daily increase the risk of jaundice, which does not occur with the usual dose of 250 mg/d or less. A hyperemic flush may occur when alcohol is ingested by patients taking chlorpropamide. This alcohol flush appears within 8 minutes of ingesting the alcohol and lasts for 10–12 minutes and is believed to relate to the plasma level of chlorpropamide. Patients taking this drug chronically have a higher frequency of flushing after alcohol than persons given a single-dose challenge with chlorpropamide.

Hyponatremia is a complication of chlorpropamide therapy in some patients, apparently because chlorpropamide both stimulates vasopressin secretion and potentiates its action at the renal tubule. The antidiuretic effect of chlorpropamide is relatively unique, since 3 other sulfonylureas (acetohexamide, tolazamide, and glyburide) facilitate water excretion in humans. Hematologic toxicity (transient leukopenia, thrombocytopenia) occurs in less than 1% of patients.

**(3) Tolazamide** (Tolinase) is supplied in tablets of 100, 250, and 500 mg. It is comparable to chlorpropamide in potency but has a shorter duration of action and does not cause water retention. Tolazamide is more slowly absorbed than the other sulfonylureas, with effects on blood glucose not appearing for several hours. Its duration of action may last up to 20 hours, with maximal hypoglycemic effect occurring between the fourth and 14th hours. Tolazamide is metabolized to several compounds that retain hypoglycemic effects. If more than 500 mg/d is required, the dose should be divided and given twice daily. Doses larger than 1000 mg daily do not improve the degree of glycemic control.

**(4) Acetohexamide** (Dymelor) is supplied in tablets of 250 and 500 mg. Its duration of action is about 10–16 hours, being intermediate in action between tolbutamide and chlorpropamide. A dose of 0.25–1.5 g is given daily in one or 2 doses. Liver metabolism is rapid, but the metabolite produced remains active. Side effects are similar to those of the other sulfonylurea drugs.

**(5) Second-generation sulfonylureas (glyburide and glipizide)**—Glyburide and glipizide have similar chemical structures, with cyclic carbon rings at each end of the sulfonylurea nucleus; this causes them to be highly potent (100-fold more so than tolbutamide). These drugs should be used with caution in patients with cardiovascular disease or in elderly patients, in whom hypoglycemia would be especially dangerous.

Diabetic patients who have not responded to tolbutamide or even tolazamide often (not always) respond to the more potent first-generation sulfonylurea chlorpropamide or to either of the second-generation sulfonylureas. Unfortunately, substantial benefit has not always resulted when a maximum therapeutic dose of chlorpropamide has been replaced with that of a second-generation drug.

**(a) Glyburide (glibenclamide; Diaβeta, Micronase)**—Glyburide is available in 1.25-, 2.5-, and 5-mg tablets. The usual starting dose is 2.5 mg/d, and the average maintenance dose is 5—10 mg/d given as a single morning dose; maintenance doses higher than 20 mg/d are not recommended. Glyburide is metabolized in the liver into products with such low hypoglycemic activity that they are considered clinically unimportant. Although assays specific for the unmetabolized compound suggest a plasma half-life of only 1–2 hours, the biologic effects of glyburide are clearly persistent 24 hours after a single morning dose in diabetic patients.

Glyburide has few adverse effects other than its potential for causing hypoglycemia. Flushing has rarely been reported after ethanol ingestion. It does not cause water retention, as chlorpropamide does, but rather slightly enhances free water clearance. Glyburide is absolutely contraindicated in the presence of hepatic impairment and probably should not be used in patients with renal insufficiency.

**(b) Glipizide (Glucotrol)**—Glipizide is available in 5- and 10-mg tablets. For maximum effect in reducing postprandial hyperglycemia, this agent should be ingested 30 minutes before meals, since rapid absorption is delayed when the drug is taken with food. The recommended starting dose is 5 mg/d with up to 15 mg/d given as a single daily dose before breakfast. When higher daily doses are required, they should be divided and given before meals. The maximum recommended dose is 40 mg/d.

At least 90% of glipizide is metabolized in the liver to inactive products, and 10% is excreted unchanged in the urine. Glipizide therapy is therefore contraindicated in patients with hepatic or renal impairment, who would therefore be at high risk for hypoglycemia.

**b. Efficacy and safety of the oral hypoglycemic agents**—The University Group Diabetes Program (UGDP) reported that the number of deaths due to cardiovascular disease in diabetic patients treated with tolbutamide or the no longer used phenformin was excessive compared to either insulin-treated patients or those receiving placebos. Controversy persists about the validity of the conclusions reached by the UGDP because of the heterogeneity of the population studied, with its preponderance of obese subjects, and certain features of the experimental design such as the use of a fixed dose of oral drug.

**3. Insulin**—Insulin is indicated for type I (IDDM) diabetics as well as for nonobese type II diabetics with insulinopenia whose hyperglycemia does not respond to diet therapy either alone or combined with oral hypoglycemic drugs.

With the development of highly purified porcine insulin preparations, immunogenicity has been markedly reduced, and it might well be eliminated once adequate supplies of human insulin become available from recombinant DNA biosynthesis or from enzymatic conversion of pork insulin to that of human insulin structure. However, the problem of achieving optimal insulin delivery remains unsolved with the present state of technology. It has not been possible to reproduce the physiologic patterns of intraportal insulin secretion with subcutaneous injections of soluble or longer-acting insulin suspensions. Even so, with the help of appropriate modifications of diet and exercise and careful monitoring of capillary blood glucose levels at home, it has often been possible to achieve acceptable control of blood glucose by using portable insulin infusion pumps or variable mixtures of short- and longer-acting insulins injected at least twice daily.

**a. Characteristics of available insulin preparations**—Commercial insulin preparations differ with respect to the animal species from which they are obtained, their purity and solubility, and the time of onset and duration of their biologic action. In the fall of 1986, more than 40 different formulations of insulin were available in the USA.

**(1) Species of insulin**—Because the supply of pork insulin has been too limited to satisfy the insulin requirements of all diabetic patients, most commercial insulins contain the slightly more antigenic beef insulin, which differs by 3 amino acids from human insulin (in contrast to the single amino acid distinguishing pork and human insulins). Standard preparations of Iletin I (Eli Lilly) are mixtures containing 70% beef and 30% pork insulin. However, a limited supply of monospecies pork or beef insulin (Iletin II) has been available for use in certain patients with insulin allergy or immune insulin resistance. The production of highly purified insulins by Danish manufacturers has resulted in a substantial increase in the availability of porcine insulin. Human insulin can now be produced by recombinant DNA techniques (biosynthetic human insulin) or by enzymatic conversion of pork insulin to human insulin structure (semisynthetic human insulin), in which alanine, the terminal amino acid on the beta chain of pork insulin, is replaced by threonine. Human insulin prepared by the recombinant DNA method has been introduced for clinical use as Humulin (Eli Lilly) and dispensed as either Regular, NPH, or Lente Humulin. Human insulin prepared by enzymatic conversion of pork insulin is marketed by Squibb-Novo as well as by Nordisk. Novolin R (formerly Actrapid Human), a zinc suspension of human insulin, Novolin L (formerly Monotard Human), and an isophane suspension of human, Novolin N, are products of Squibb-Novo. The R, L, and N refer to the particular formulation (regular, lente, and NPH, respectively). Since human insulin tends to be slightly more hydrophilic than beef insulin, it was not until July 1987 that Eli Lilly was able to produce an ultralente formulation of human insulin with the required degree of insolubility characteristic of beef insulin products.

**(2) Purity of insulin**–Recent improvements in purification techniques with Sephadex gel columns have reduced or eliminated contaminating insulin precursors which had molecular weights greater than that of insulin and which were biologically inactive yet capable of inducing anti-insulin antibodies. The degree of purification in which proinsulin contamination is greater than 10 but less than 50 ppm characterizes the main form of insulin produced commercially in the USA by Eli Lilly as Iletin I. When proinsulin content is reduced to less than 10 ppm, manufacturers are entitled by FDA regulations to label the insulin as "purified." Such highly purified insulins are presently marketed in the USA by Eli Lilly, Squibb-Novo, and Nordisk. Because they are relatively free of impurities including even those whose molecular weight is comparable to that of insulin, they have been termed **single component** or **monocomponent insulin.** The Eli Lilly product is called Iletin II to identify this highly purified insulin, and it presently is available only as a monospecies pork or beef insulin. All human insulins are also highly purified.

The more purified insulins that have recently become available seem to preserve their potency quite well, so that refrigeration is recommended but not crucial. During travel, reserve supplies of insulin can thus be readily transported for weeks without losing potency if protected from extremes of heat or cold.

**(3) Concentration of insulin**–At present, most insulins are available in a concentration of 100 units/mL (U100), and all are dispensed in 10-mL vials. To accommodate children and occasional adults who may require small quantities, a U40 insulin continues to be available. However, with the popularity of "low-dose" (0.5-mL) disposable insulin syringes, there is less need for U40 insulin, since U100 can now be measured with acceptable accuracy in doses as low as 1–2 units. For use in rare cases of severe insulin resistance in which large quantities of insulin are required, a limited supply of U500 regular porcine insulin (Iletin II) is available from Eli Lilly.

**b. Insulin preparations**–Three principal types of insulins are available: (1) short-acting, with rapid onset of action; (2) intermediate-acting; and (3) long-acting, with slow onset of action (Fig 19–1). Short-acting insulin (unmodified insulin) is a crystalline zinc insulin provided in soluble form and thus is dispensed as a clear solution. All other commercial insulins have been specially modified to retain more prolonged action and are dispensed as turbid suspensions at neutral pH with either protamine in phosphate buffer (protamine zinc insulin and NPH) or varying concentrations of zinc in acetate buffer (ultralente and semilente). The use of protamine zinc insulin and semilente preparations is currently decreasing, and almost no indications for their use exist.

**(1) Regular insulin** (Regular Iletin I or II or Humulin [Eli Lilly], Insulin Injection, Actrapid, or Novolin-R [Squibb-Novo], Velosulin [Nordisk]) is a short-acting soluble crystalline zinc insulin whose effect appears within 15 minutes after subcutaneous injection and lasts 5–7 hours. It is the only type of insulin that can be administered intravenously or by infusion pumps. It is particularly useful in the treatment of diabetic ketoacidosis and when the insulin requirement is changing rapidly, such as after surgery or during acute infections.

**(2) Lente insulin** is a mixture of 30% semilente (an amorphous precipitate of insulin with zinc ions) with 70% ultralente insulin (an insoluble crystal of zinc and insulin)—Lente Iletin I or II and Humulin L (Eli Lilly), Lente Insulin, Monotard, Lentard, and Novolin-L (Squibb-Novo). Its onset of action is delayed for up to 2 hours (Fig 19–1), and because its duration of action often is less than 24 hours (with a range of 18–24 hours), most patients require at least 2 injections daily to maintain a sustained insulin effect. Lente insulin has its peak effect in most patients between 8 and 12 hours, but individual variations in peak response time must be considered when interpreting unusual or unexpected patterns of glycemic responses in individual patients. While lente insulin is the most widely used of the lente series, particularly in combination with regular insulin, there has recently been a resurgence of the use of ultralente in combination with multiple injections of regular insulin as a means of attempting optimal control in IDDM patients. Ultralente has a very slow onset of action with a prolonged duration (Fig 19–1), and its administration once or twice daily has been advocated to provide a basal level of insulin comparable to that achieved by basal endogenous secretion or the overnight infusion rate programmed into insulin pumps.

**(3) NPH (neutral protamine hagedorn or isophane) insulin** (NPH Iletin I and II or Humulin N [Eli Lilly], NPH Insulin, Protaphane and Novolin N [Squibb-Novo], Insulatard NPH Pork or Human [Nordisk]) is an intermediate-acting insulin whose onset of action is delayed by combining 2 parts soluble crystalline zinc with 1 part protamine zinc insulin. This produces equivalent amounts of insulin and protamine, so that neither is present in an uncomplexed form ("isophane").

The onset and duration of action of NPH insulin are comparable to those of lente insulin (Fig 19–1); it is usually mixed with regular insulin and given at

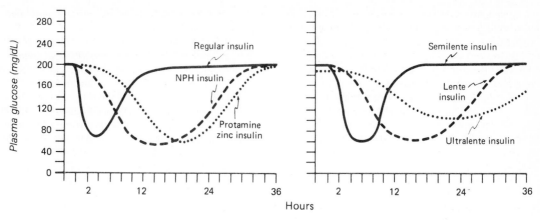

**Figure 19–1.** Extent and duration of action of various types of insulin (in a fasting diabetic). Duration of action is extended considerably when the dose of a given insulin formulation increases above the average therapeutic doses depicted here.

least twice daily for insulin replacement in IDDM patients.

**(4) Mixtures of insulin–**Since intermediate insulins require several hours to reach adequate therapeutic levels, their use in IDDM patients requires supplements of regular insulin preprandially. For convenience, these may be mixed together in the same syringe and injected subcutaneously in split dosage before breakfast and supper. When mixing insulin, it is necessary to inject into both bottles a quantity of air equivalent to the volume of insulin to be subsequently withdrawn. It is recommended that the regular insulin be withdrawn first, then the intermediate insulin. No attempt should be made to mix the insulins in the syringe, and the injection is preferably given immediately after loading the syringe. Mixtard (Nordisk) is a premixed pure pork insulin consisting of 30% regular insulin and 70% NPH insulin; Novolin 70/30 is an identical proportion of premixed NPH and regular human insulin.

Recent reports caution that insulin mixtures containing increased proportions of lente to regular insulins may retard the rapid action of admixed regular insulin, particularly if not injected immediately after mixing. The excess zinc in lente insulin may bind the soluble insulin and partially blunt its action, particularly when a relatively small proportion of regular insulin is mixed with lente (eg, 1 part regular to 1½ or more parts lente). NPH preparations that do not contain excess protamine do not delay absorption of admixed regular insulin. They are therefore preferable to lente when mixtures of intermediate and regular insulins are prescribed.

Occasional vials of NPH insulin have tended to show unusual clumping of their contents or "frosting" of the container, with considerable loss of bioactivity. The Eli Lilly Co. feels that this instability is a rare phenomenon which may not be restricted to biosynthetic NPH human insulin and might occur less frequently if NPH human insulin were refrigerated when not in use.

**c. Methods of insulin administration–**

**(1) Insulin syringes and needles–**Plastic disposable syringes with needles attached are available in 1-mL and 0.5-mL sizes. In cases where very low insulin doses are prescribed, as in young children, the specially calibrated 0.5-mL disposable syringe facilitates accurate measurement of U100 insulin in doses up to 50 units. The "low-dose" syringes have become increasingly popular, because diabetics generally should not take more than 50 units of insulin in a single injection, except in rare instances of extreme insulin resistance. Several recent reports have indicated that "disposable" syringes may be reused until blunting of the needle occurs (usually after 3–5 injections). Sterility adequate to avoid infection with reuse appears to be maintained by refrigerating syringes between uses. One concern, however, arises from a recent report that flecks of silicone may become suspended in insulin bottles in which disposable syringes have repeatedly been reused; the silicone flecks seem to reduce the activity of the insulin.

**(2) Site of injection–**Any part of the body covered by loose skin can be used, such as the abdomen, thighs, upper arms, flanks, and upper buttocks. Rotation of sites continues to be recommended to avoid delayed absorption when fibrosis or lipohypertrophy occurs from repeated use of a single site. However, as more highly purified insulins have become available, fibrosis is less of a problem. Moreover, considerable variability of absorption rates from different sites, particularly with exercise, may contribute to the instability of glycemic control in certain IDDM patients if injection sites are rotated too frequently in different areas of the body. Consequently, health professionals recommend limiting injection sites to a single region of the body and rotating sites within that region. The abdomen is recommended for subcutaneous injections, since regular insulin has been shown to absorb more rapidly from that site than from other subcutaneous sites.

**(3) Insulin delivery systems**–Efforts to administer soluble insulin by "closed-loop" systems (glucose-controlled insulin infusion system) have been successful for acute situations such as diabetic ketoacidosis or for administering insulin to diabetics during surgery. However, chronic use is precluded by the need for continually aspirating blood to reach an external glucose sensor and the large size of the computerized pump system.

Current research into smaller "open-loop" means of insulin delivery (insulin reservoir and pump programmed to deliver regular insulin at a calculated rate without a glucose sensor) has developed several relatively small pumps for subcutaneous, intravenous, or intraperitoneal infusion. With improving methods for patients' self-monitoring of blood glucose, these pump systems have become more useful for managing diabetics. However, at present, conventional methods of insulin administration with multiple subcutaneous injections of soluble, rapid-acting insulin and a single injection of long-acting insulin usually can provide as effective glycemic control in most cases as the more expensive open-loop systems if frequent self-monitoring of blood glucose is practiced.

To facilitate these multiple injection regimens, portable pen-sized injectors have been introduced which contain cartridges of U100 regular human insulin and retractable needles (NovoPen, Insuject). These injectors eliminate the need for patients to carry an insulin bottle and syringes during the day while adhering to a regimen of multiple injections of regular insulin supplementing a single injection of long-acting insulin.

**C. General Considerations in Treatment of Diabetes:** Patients with diabetes can have a full and satisfying life. However, "free" diets and unrestricted activity are still not advised for insulin-requiring diabetics. Until new methods of insulin replacement are developed that provide more normal patterns of insulin delivery in response to metabolic demands, multiple feedings will continue to be recommended, and certain occupations potentially hazardous to the patient or others will continue to be prohibited.

Exercise increases the effectiveness of insulin, and moderate exercise is an excellent means of improving utilization of fat and carbohydrate in diabetic patients. A judicious balance of the size and frequency of meals with moderate regular exercise can often stabilize the insulin dosage in diabetics who tend to slip out of control easily. Strenuous exercise could precipitate hypoglycemia in an unprepared patient, and diabetics must therefore be taught to reduce their insulin dosage in anticipation of strenuous activity or to take supplemental carbohydrate. Injection of insulin into a site farthest away from the muscles most involved in exercise may help ameliorate exercise-induced hypoglycemia, since insulin injected in the proximity of exercising muscle is much more rapidly mobilized.

All diabetic patients must receive adequate instruction on personal hygiene, especially with regard to care of the feet (see below), skin, and teeth. All infections—but especially pyogenic infections with fever and toxemia—provoke the release of high levels of insulin antagonists such as catecholamines or glucagon and thus bring about a marked increase in insulin requirements. Supplemental regular insulin is often required to correct hyperglycemia during infection.

Psychologic factors are of great importance in the control of diabetes, particularly when the disease is difficult to stabilize. One reason the diabetic may be particularly sensitive to emotional upset is that A cells of diabetics are hyperresponsive to physiologic levels of epinephrine, producing excessive levels of glucagon with consequent hyperglycemia.

Counseling should be directed at avoiding extremes of compulsive rigidity or self-destructive neglect.

## Steps in the Management of the Diabetic Patient

**A. Diagnostic Examination:** Any features of the clinical picture that suggest end organ insensitivity to insulin, such as obesity, must be identified. The family history should document not only the incidence of diabetes in other members of the family but also the age at onset, whether it was associated with obesity, and whether insulin was required. Other factors that increase cardiac risk, such as smoking history, presence of hypertension or hyperlipidemia, or oral contraceptive pill use, should be recorded.

Laboratory diagnosis should document fasting plasma glucose levels above 140 mg/dL or postprandial values consistently above 200 mg/dL and whether ketonuria accompanies the glycosuria. A glycohemoglobin measurement is useful for assessing the effectiveness of future therapy.

Baseline values of any observation that may help in the evaluation of future complications should be recorded. These include plasma triglycerides and cholesterol, electrocardiography, chest radiograph, renal function studies, peripheral pulses, and neurologic and ophthalmologic examinations.

**B. Patient Education:** Since diabetes is a lifelong disorder, education of the patient is probably the most important obligation of the physician who provides initial care. The best persons to manage a disease that is affected so markedly by daily fluctuations in environmental stress, exercise, diet, and infections are the patients themselves and their families. The "teaching curriculum" should include explanations by the physician of the nature of diabetes and its potential acute and chronic hazards and how they can be recognized early and prevented or treated. The importance of regular recording of tests for glucose on either capillary blood or double-voided urine specimens should be stressed and instructions on proper testing provided. Advice on personal hygiene, including detailed instructions on foot care, as well as individual instruction on diet and specific hypoglycemic therapy, should be provided. Patients should be told about community agencies, such as Diabetes Association chapters, that can serve as a continuing source of instruction. Finally, vigorous efforts should be made to persuade new diabetics who smoke to give up the habit, since occlusive peripheral vascular disease and debilitating retinopathy are less common in nonsmoking diabetic patients.

**C. Self-Monitoring of Blood Glucose:** Monitoring of blood glucose by patients has allowed greater flexibility in management while achieving improved glycemic control. It involves educating the patient to perform 3 essential steps.

1. The obtaining of a drop of capillary blood from the fingertip by means of a specially designed lancet. Automatic spring-loaded devices facilitate finger-pricking and ensure an adequate blood sample.

2. Application of the sample to the test strip and removal at the proper time.

3. Accurate quantitation of the color developed (either visually or with a colorimeter).

Self-monitoring of blood glucose is particularly indicated in brittle diabetics, those attempting "ideal" glycemic control such as during pregnancy, patients who have little or no early warning of hypoglycemic attacks, and those with dysfunctional bladders from diabetic neuropathy or altered renal thresholds for glucose. It is useful in educating patients on the glycemic effects of specific foods in their diet and reduces the likelihood of unexpected episodes of severe hypoglycemia in insulin-treated diabetics. It has proved to be an effective and safe clinical tool that in compliant patients can be a valuable component of their therapeutic options.

**D. Initial Therapy:** Treatment must be individualized on the basis of the type of diabetes and specific needs of each patient. However, certain general principles of management can be outlined for hyperglycemic states of different types.

**1. The obese NIDDM patient**–The most common type of diabetic patient is obese, is non-insulin-dependent, and has hyperglycemia because of insensitivity to normal or elevated circulating levels of insulin (insulinoplethoric diabetes).

**a. Weight reduction**–Treatment is directed toward achieving weight reduction, and prescribing a diet is only one means to this end. Cure can be achieved by reducing adipose stores, with consequent restoration of tissue sensitivity to insulin. The presence of diabetes with its added risk factors may motivate the obese diabetic to greater efforts to lose weight.

**b. Hypoglycemic agents**–All hypoglycemic agents, including insulin as well as oral hypoglycemic drugs, are not indicated for long-term use in the obese patient with mild diabetes. The weight reduction program can be upset by real or imagined hypoglycemic reactions when insulin therapy is used; it is also possible that administration of insulin to an obese patient who already has excessive circulating levels may have

the ill effects of maintaining insulin insensitivity of receptor sites as well as interfering with catabolic mechanisms during caloric deprivation. The obese diabetic who has been previously treated with conventional beef-pork insulin—often in interrupted fashion—and who requires high doses both to offset excess caloric intake and to overcome tissue insensitivity may develop immune insulin resistance. This not only increases the requirements for exogenous insulin but also impairs the effectiveness of endogenous insulin and may even precipitate ketosis.

Oral sulfonylureas have a role in the management of obese patients with hyperglycemia that does not respond to dietary measures and, particularly, of those with severe diabetes causing nocturia, blurred vision, or (in women) candidal vulvovaginitis. Insulin injections may be required if a trial of sulfonylurea therapy is ineffective. In such cases, short-term therapy (weeks or months) with either sulfonylureas or insulin may be indicated to ameliorate symptoms until simultaneous caloric restriction leading to weight reduction can occur.

Although combinations of sulfonylureas with insulin are no more effective than insulin alone in IDDM, the data for NIDDM are insufficient to resolve this important question.

**2. The nonobese patient**–In the nonobese diabetic, mild to severe hyperglycemia is usually due to refractoriness of B cells to glucose stimulation (insulinopenic diabetes). Treatment depends on whether insulinopenia is mild (NIDDM) or severe, with ketoacidosis (IDDM).

**a. Diet therapy**–If hyperglycemia is mild, normal metabolic control can occasionally be restored by means of multiple feedings of a diet limited in simple sugars and with a caloric content sufficient to maintain ideal weight. Restriction of saturated fats and cholesterol is also strongly advised.

**b. Oral hypoglycemic agents**–When diet therapy is not sufficient to correct hyperglycemia, a trial of sulfonylureas to improve insulin release is often successful in nonobese patients with mild nonketotic diabetes. Once the dosage of one of the more potent sulfonylureas reaches the upper recommended limit in a compliant patient without maintaining blood glucose below 200 mg/dL during the day, insulin therapy is indicated.

**c. Insulin treatment**–The patient requiring insulin therapy should be initially regulated under conditions of optimal diet and normal daily activities. In patients with IDDM, information and counseling should be provided about the advantages of taking multiple injections of insulin in conjunction with self blood glucose monitoring. If tight control is attempted, urine glucose measurements are not sufficient, and at least 3 measurements of capillary blood glucose are required daily to avoid frequent hypoglycemic reactions.

**(1) Conventional split-dose insulin mixtures**–A typical initial dose schedule in a 70-kg patient taking 2200 kcal divided into 6 or 7 feedings

# INSTRUCTIONS IN THE CARE OF THE FEET
## FOR PERSONS WITH DIABETES MELLITUS OR VASCULAR DISTURBANCES

### Hygiene of the Feet

(1) Wash feet daily with mild soap and luke-warm water. Dry thoroughly between the toes by pressure. Do not rub vigorously, as this is apt to break the delicate skin.

(2) When feet are thoroughly dry, rub well with vegetable oil to keep them soft, prevent excess friction, remove scales, and prevent dryness. Care must be taken to prevent foot tenderness.

(3) If the feet become too soft and tender, rub them with alcohol about once a week.

(4) When rubbing the feet, always rub upward from the tips of the toes. If varicose veins are present, massage the feet very gently; never massage the legs.

(5) If the toenails are brittle and dry, soften them by soaking for one-half hour each night in lukewarm water containing 1 tbsp of powdered sodium borate (borax) per quart. Follow this by rubbing around the nails with vegetable oil. Clean around the nails with an orangewood stick. If the nails become too long, file them with an emery board. File them straight across and no shorter than the underlying soft tissues to the toe. Never cut the corners of the nails. (The podiatrist should be informed if a patient has diabetes.)

(6) Wear low-heeled shoes of soft leather that fit the shape of the feet correctly. The shoes should have wide toes that will cause no pressure, fit close in the arch, and grip the heels snugly. Wear new shoes one-half hour only on the first day and increase by 1 hour each day following. Wear thick, warm, loose stockings.

### Treatment of Corns & Calluses

(1) Corns and calluses are due to friction and pressure, most often from improperly fitted shoes and stockings. Wear shoes that fit properly and cause no friction or pressure.

(2) To remove excess calluses or corns, soak the feet in lukewarm (not hot) water, using a mild soap, for about 10 minutes and then rub off the excess tissue with a towel or file. Do not tear it off. Under no circumstances must the skin become irritated.

(3) Do not cut corns or calluses. If they need attention it is safer to see a podiatrist.

(4) Prevent callus formation under the ball of the foot (a) by exercises, such as curling and stretching the toes several times a day; (b) by finishing each step on the toes and not on the ball of the foot; and (c) by wearing shoes that are not too short and that do not have high heels.

### Aids in Treatment of Impaired Circulation (Cold Feet)

(1) Never use tobacco in any form. Tobacco contracts blood vessels and so reduces circulation.

(2) Keep warm. Wear warm stockings and other clothing. Cold contracts blood vessels and reduces circulation.

(3) Do not wear circular garters, which compress blood vessels and reduce blood flow.

(4) Do not sit with the legs crossed. This may compress the leg arteries and shut off the blood supply to the feet.

(5) If the weight of the bedclothes is uncomfortable, place a pillow under the covers at the foot of the bed.

(6) Do not apply any medication to the feet without directions from a physician. Some medicines are too strong for feet with poor circulation.

(7) Do not apply heat in the form of hot water, hot water bottles, or heating pads without a physician's consent. Even moderate heat can injure the skin if circulation is poor.

(8) If the feet are moist or the patient has a tendency to develop athlete's foot, a prophylactic dusting powder should be used on the feet and in shoes and stockings daily. Change shoes and stockings at least daily or oftener.

### Treatment of Abrasions of the Skin

(1) Proper first-aid treatment is of the utmost importance even in apparently minor injuries. Consult a physician immediately for any redness, blistering, pain, or swelling. Any break in the skin may become ulcerous or gangrenous unless properly treated by a physician.

(2) Dermatophytosis (athlete's foot), which begins with peeling and itching between the toes or discoloration or thickening of the toenails, should be treated immediately by a physician or podiatrist.

(3) Avoid strong irritating antiseptics such as tincture of iodine.

(4) As soon as possible after any injury, cover the area with sterile gauze, which may be purchased at drugstores. Only fine paper tape or cellulose tape (Scotch Tape) should be used on the skin if adhesive retention of the gauze is required.

(5) Elevate and, as much as possible until recovery, avoid using the foot.

might be 10 units of regular and 20 units of NPH insulin in the morning and 5 units of regular and 5 units of NPH insulin in the evening. The morning urine or capillary blood glucose (or both) gives a measure of the effectiveness of NPH insulin administered the previous evening; the noon urine or blood glucose reflects the effects of the morning regular insulin; and the 5:00 PM and 9:00 PM sugars represent the effects of the morning NPH and evening regular insulins, respectively. A properly educated patient might be taught to adjust insulin dosage by observing the pattern of glycemia and glycosuria and correlating it with the approximate duration of action and the time of peak effect after injection of the various insulin preparations (Fig 19–1). Adjustments to correct hyperglycemia should be made gradually and preferably not more often than every 3 days.

**(2) Intensive insulin therapy–**In cases where conventional split doses of insulin mixtures cannot maintain near normalization of blood glucose without hypoglycemia, particularly at night, multiple injections of insulin may be required. An increasingly popular regimen consists of reducing or omitting the evening dose of intermediate insulin and adding a portion of it at bedtime. For example, 10 units of regular insulin mixed with 10 units of NPH insulin in the morning, 8–10 units of regular insulin before the evening meal, and 6 units of NPH insulin at bedtime might be more efficacious than the conventional split-dose regimen mentioned above.

In cases where hypoglycemia occurs unexpectedly and at inconsistent times day or night, variable or delayed insulin absorption from large subcutaneous depots containing regular and NPH insulin may be a contributing factor. Reducing the size and changing the character of the depots by administering small doses of regular insulin more frequently (eg, 4 times a day), with one injection of a long-acting insulin (eg, ultralente insulin) at bedtime has often been most helpful in reducing the frequency and severity of hypoglycemia in patients attempting near normalization of blood glucose. This regimen has become more

convenient with the advent of pen-injectors (see p 760) and gives greater flexibility regarding meal patterns and diet than conventional therapy with split-dose insulin mixtures. Certain patients do not accept multiple injections of regular insulin but often prefer continuous subcutaneous infusions with portable open-loop insulin pumps, which require subcutaneous needle insertion only every 48 hours.

**(3) Management of early morning hyperglycemia in IDDM–**One of the more difficult therapeutic problems in managing patients with IDDM is determining the proper adjustment of insulin dose when the prebreakfast blood glucose level is high.

**(a) Somogyi effect–**Patients with IDDM may develop nocturnal hypoglycemia, which may in turn stimulate a surge of counterregulatory hormones (Somogyi effect) to produce high blood glucose levels by 7:00 AM. A lowered dosage of intermediate insulin given the night before is indicated.

**(b) Waning of circulating insulin levels–**A possibly more common cause of prebreakfast hyperglycemia is the waning of circulating insulin levels. This would suggest that *more,* rather than less, intermediate insulin should be given the evening before. The Somogyi effect and the waning of insulin levels are not mutually exclusive; if they occur together, more severe hyperglycemia develops.

**(c) Dawn phenomenon–**The recently described dawn phenomenon is found in as many as 75% of IDDM patients and occurs in most NIDDM and normal subjects as well. It is characterized by reduced tissue sensitivity to insulin developing between 5:00 AM and 8:00 AM. Recent evidence suggests that this phenomenon is evoked by spikes of growth hormone released hours before, at the onset of sleep. When the dawn phenomenon occurs alone, it may produce only mild hyperglycemia in the early morning, but when it is associated with either the Somogyi effect or the waning phenomenon, or both, the hyperglycemia may be more severe. Table 19–5 shows that diagnosis of the cause of prebreakfast hyperglycemia can be facilitated by the self-monitoring of blood

**Table 19–5.** Typical patterns of overnight blood glucose levels and serum free immunoreactive insulin levels in prebreakfast hyperglycemia due to various causes in IDDM.

| | Blood Glucose (mg/dL) | | | Free Immunoreactive Insulin (μU/mL) | | |
|---|---|---|---|---|---|---|
| | 10:00 PM | 3:00 AM | 7:00 AM | 10:00 PM | 3:00 AM | 7:00 AM |
| Somogyi effect | 90 | 40 | 200 | High | Slightly high | Normal |
| Dawn phenomenon | 110 | 110 | 150 | Normal | Normal | Normal |
| Waning of insulin dose plus dawn phenomenon | 110 | 190 | 220 | Normal | Low | Low |
| Waning of insulin dose plus dawn phenomenon plus Somogyi effect | 110 | 40 | 380 | High | Normal | Low |

glucose at 3:00 AM in addition to the usual bedtime and 7:00 AM measurements.

**(d) Therapy of prebreakfast hyperglycemia–** When a particular pattern emerges from monitoring blood glucose levels overnight, appropriate therapeutic measures can be taken. The Somogyi effect can be treated by reducing the dose of intermediate insulin, giving a portion of it at bedtime, or supplying more food at bedtime. When the dawn phenomenon alone is present, the dosage of intermediate insulin can be divided between dinnertime and bedtime, or when insulin pumps are used, the basal infusion rate can be increased (eg, from 0.8 unit/h to 1 unit/h from 6:00 AM until breakfast). With waning insulin levels, either increasing the evening dose or shifting it from dinnertime to bedtime, or both, can be effective.

**d. Acceptable levels of glycemic control–** Limited data are available concerning the level of glucose control needed to avoid diabetic complications. Postprandial blood glucose levels below 200 mg/dL have been advocated by retrospective analysis of 2 populations of NIDDM-patients. A reasonable aim of therapy is to approach normal glycemic excursions without provoking severe or frequent hypoglycemia. What has been considered ''acceptable'' control includes blood glucose levels of 60–130 mg/dL before meals and after an overnight fast and levels no higher than 180 mg/dL 1 hour after meals and 140 mg/dL 2 hours after meals. In NIDDM patients with milder forms of insulinopenia who require insulin therapy, a single morning injection of a small dose of intermediate insulin may suffice to supplement their own endogenous insulin secretion.

## Indications for Purified Insulins

Human insulin or purified insulins are indicated when insulin of conventional purity has been associated with allergy, immune resistance, or lipoatrophy. Also, they would seem to be preferable in any patient undergoing insulin therapy for the first time, since the absence of anti-insulin antibodies would facilitate the measurement of therapeutic levels of circulating insulin as a guide for optimal management. In patients with NIDDM whose therapy with insulin is to be for a limited time (eg, in gestational diabetes or during acute infections or surgery), human insulin or purified insulin would reduce the risks of immunologic sensitization to future exposures to insulin.

## Complications of Insulin Therapy

**A. Hypoglycemia:** Hypoglycemic reactions, the most common complication of insulin therapy, may result from delay in taking a meal or unusual physical exertion. With more patients attempting ''tight'' control without frequent capillary glucose home monitoring, this complication is likely to become even more frequent. In older diabetics, in those taking only longer-acting insulins, and often in those maintaining euglycemia on infusion pumps, autonomic counter-regulatory responses are less readily elicited responses, and the manifestations are mainly from impaired function of the central nervous system, ie, mental confusion, bizarre behavior, and ultimately coma. Even focal neurologic deficits mimicking stroke may be observed. More rapid development of hypoglycemia from the effects of regular insulin causes signs of autonomic hyperactivity, both adrenergic (tachycardia, palpitations, sweating, tremulousness) and parasympathetic (nausea, hunger), that may progress to coma and convulsions. These symptoms are blunted in patients receiving beta-blocking agents for angina or hypertension. Though not absolutely contraindicated, these drugs must be used with great caution in insulin-requiring diabetics.

Because of the potential danger of insulin reactions, the diabetic patient should carry packets of table sugar or a candy roll at all times for use at the onset of hypoglycemic symptoms. Recently, tablets containing 3 g of glucose have become available (dextrosol). The educated patient soon learns to take the amount of glucose needed and avoids the excess that may occur with eating candy or drinking orange juice, causing very high hyperglycemia. An ampule of glucagon (1 mg) should be provided to every diabetic receiving insulin therapy, and family or friends should be instructed how to inject it in the event that the patient is unconscious or refuses food. An identification bracelet, necklace, or card in the wallet or purse should be carried by every diabetic receiving hypoglycemic drug therapy (see box).

All of the manifestations of hypoglycemia are rapidly relieved by glucose administration. In a case of mild hypoglycemia in a patient who is conscious and able to swallow, orange juice, glucose tablets, or any sugar-containing beverage or food may be given. If more severe hypoglycemia has produced uncon-

---

**I Am a Diabetic and Take Insulin**

If I am behaving peculiarly but am conscious and able to swallow, give me sugar or hard candy or orange juice slowly. If I an unconscious, call an ambulance immediately, take me to a physician or a hospital, and notify my physician. *I am not intoxicated.*

My name _____

Address _____

Telephone _____

Physician's name _____

Physician's address _____

Telephone _____

sciousness or stupor, the treatment of choice is to give 20–50 mL of 50% glucose solution by intravenous infusion over a period of 2–3 minutes. If intravenous therapy is not available, 1 mg of glucagon injected intramuscularly will usually restore the patient to consciousness within 15 minutes to permit ingestion of sugar. If the patient is stuporous and glucagon is not available, small amounts of honey or syrup can be inserted within the buccal pouch, but, in general, oral feeding is contraindicated in unconscious patients. Rectal administration of syrup or honey (30 mL per 500 mL of warm water) has been effective.

**B. Immunopathology of Insulin Therapy:** At least 5 molecular classes of insulin antibodies are produced during the course of insulin therapy in diabetes, including IgA, IgD, IgE, IgG, and IgM.

**1. Insulin allergy–**Insulin allergy, or immediate-type hypersensitivity, is a rare condition in which local or systemic urticaria is due to histamine release from tissue mast cells sensitized by adherence of anti-insulin IgE antibodies. In severe cases, anaphylaxis results. A subcutaneous nodule appearing several hours later at the site of insulin injection and lasting for up to 24 hours has been attributed to an IgG-mediated complement-binding Arthus reaction. Because sensitivity is often to noninsulin protein contaminants, the new highly purified insulins have reduced markedly the incidence of insulin allergy, especially of the local variety. Furthermore, when only human insulin has been used from the onset of insulin therapy, insulin allergy is exceedingly rare. When allergy to beef or, more rarely, pork insulin is present, a species change (eg, to pure pork or human insulin) may correct the problem although in many cases cross-reaction between human and animal insulins results in persistent allergic responses. Antihistamines, corticosteroids, and even desensitization may be required, especially for systemic hypersensitivity. A kit containing various dilutions of pure beef or pork insulin is distributed on request by the Eli Lilly Co. for allergy testing and insulin desensitization.

**2. Immune insulin resistance–**All insulin-treated patients develop a low titer of circulating IgG anti-insulin antibodies that neutralize to a small extent the action of insulin. In some diabetic patients, principally those with some degree of tissue insensitivity to insulin (such as in the obese) and with a history of interrupted exposure to therapy with beef insulin, a high titer of circulating IgG anti-insulin antibodies develops. This results in extremely high insulin requirements—often more than 200 units daily. This is often a self-limited condition and may clear spontaneously after several months. However, in cases where the circulating antibody is specifically more reactive with beef insulin—a more potent immunogen in humans than pork insulin—changing the patient to a less antigenic insulin (pork or human) may make possible a dramatic reduction in insulin dosage or at least may shorten the duration of immune resistance. Other forms of therapy include sulfated beef

insulin (a chemically modified form of beef insulin containing an average of 6 sulfate groups per molecule) and immunosuppression with corticosteroids. In some adults, the foreign insulin can be completely discontinued and the patient maintained on diet along with oral sulfonylureas. This is possible only when the circulating antibodies do not effectively neutralize endogenous (human) insulin.

**C. Lipodystrophy at Injection Sites:** Atrophy of subcutaneous fatty tissue leading to disfigurement and scarring may rarely occur at the site of injection. This complication results from an immune reaction, and it has become rarer with the development of highly concentrated, pure insulin preparations of neutral pH. Injection of these preparations directly into the atrophic area often results in restoration of normal contours. Lipohypertrophy, on the other hand, is not a consequence of immune responses but rather seems to be due to the pharmacologic effects of insulin being deposited in the same location repeatedly. It can occur with purified insulins and is best treated by avoiding the hypertrophic areas. Rotation of injection sites will prevent lipohypertrophy.

## Chronic Complications of Diabetes

**A. Ocular Complications:**

**1. Diabetic cataracts–**Premature cataracts occur in diabetic patients. These opacities resemble those found in elderly patients with "senile" cataracts but occur at a younger age and seem to correlate with both the duration of diabetes and the severity of chronic hyperglycemia. Nonenzymatic glycosylation of lens protein is twice as high in diabetic patients as in age-matched nondiabetic persons and may contribute to the premature occurrence of cataracts.

**2. Diabetic retinopathy–**Three main categories exist: background, or "simple," retinopathy, consisting of microaneurysms, hemorrhages, exudates, and retinal edema; proliferative retinopathy with arteriolar ischemia manifested as cotton-wool spots (small infarcted areas of retina); and proliferative, or "malignant," retinopathy, consisting of newly formed vessels. Proliferative retinopathy is a leading cause of blindness in the USA. Recent experience suggests that extensive "scatter" xenon or argon photocoagulation and focal treatment of new vessels reduce severe visual loss in those cases in which proliferative retinopathy is associated with *recent* vitreous hemorrhages or in which extensive new vessels are located on or near the optic disk. Macular edema has also responded to this therapy with improvement in visual acuity.

**B. Diabetic Nephropathy:** Capillary basement membrane thickening of renal glomeruli produces varying degrees of glomerulosclerosis and renal insufficiency. Diffuse glomerulosclerosis is more common than nodular intercapillary glomerulosclerosis (Kimmelstiel-Wilson syndrome); both produce heavy proteinuria.

**1. Microalbuminuria–**New methods of detecting small amounts of urinary albumin using a sensitive immunoassay have permitted detection of microgram concentrations—in contrast to the less sensitive dip-stick strips, whose minimal detection limit is 0.3–0.5%. Conventional 24-hour urine collections, in addition to being inconvenient for patients, also show wide variability of albumin excretion, since several factors such as sustained erect posture, dietary protein, and exercise tend to increase albumin excretion rates. For these reasons, most laboratories prefer to screen patients with a timed overnight urine collection beginning at bedtime, when the urine is discarded and the time noted. The collection is ended the next morning at the time the bladder is emptied, and this urine, as well as any urine voided overnight, is assayed for albumin. Normal subjects excrete less than 15 $\mu$g/min during overnight urine collections; values of 20 $\mu$g/min or higher are considered to represent abnormal microalbuminuria.

Three clinical trials in diabetic patients have demonstrated that subsequent renal failure can be predicted by urinary albumin excretion rates exceeding 30 $\mu$g/min. Increased microalbuminuria correlates with increased levels of blood pressure, and this may explain why increased proteinuria in diabetic patients is associated with an increase in cardiovascular deaths even in the absence of renal failure. Careful glycemic control as well as a low-protein diet (0.6 g/kg/d) have been reported to reduce both the hyperfiltration and the elevated microalbuminuria in patients in the early stages of diabetes and those with incipient diabetic nephropathy.

**2. Progressive diabetic nephropathy**–The clinical syndrome of progressive diabetic nephropathy consists of proteinuria of varying severity occasionally leading to the full-blown nephrotic syndrome with hypoalbuminemia, edema, and an increase in circulating betalipoproteins. In contrast to all other renal disorders, the proteinuria associated with diabetic nephropathy does not diminish with progressive renal failure (patients continue to excrete 10–11 g daily as creatinine clearance diminishes). As renal failure progresses, there is an elevation in the renal threshold at which glycosuria appears.

Hypertension develops with progressive renal involvement, and the processes of coronary and cerebral atherosclerosis, with all of the sequelae of those disorders, seem to be accelerated in diabetics.

Once diabetic nephropathy has progressed to the stage of hypertension, proteinuria, or early renal failure, glycemic control is not beneficial in influencing its course. In this circumstance, antihypertensive medications, dietary protein restriction, and drugs that inhibit angiotensin I converting enzyme inhibitor (eg, captopril, enalapril) are recommended.

Dialysis has been of limited value in the treatment of renal failure due to diabetic nephropathy. At present, experience in renal transplantation—especially from related donors—is more promising and is the treatment of choice in cases where there are no contraindications such as severe cardiovascular disease.

**C. Gangrene of the Feet:** The incidence of gangrene of the feet in diabetics is 20 times the incidence in matched controls. The factors responsible for its development are ischemia, peripheral neuropathy, and secondary infection. Occlusive vascular disease of the lower extremities involves both microangiopathy and atherosclerosis of large and medium-sized arteries. If both feet feel cool, a good blood supply might still be present, but if one foot is cooler than the other, occlusive arterial disease is usually present in the cooler one. Cigarette smoking should be avoided, and prevention of foot disease (see p 762) should be emphasized, since treatment is difficult once ulceration and gangrene have developed. Amputation of the lower extremities is sometimes required.

Beta blockers are relatively contraindicated in patients with ischemic foot ulcers, because these drugs reduce peripheral blood flow.

**D. Diabetic Neuropathy:** Peripheral and autonomic neuropathy, the 2 most common chronic complications of diabetes, are poorly understood. Peripheral neuropathy is generally bilateral, symmetric, and associated with dulled perception of vibration, pain, and temperature, particularly in the lower extremities. At times, discomfort of the lower extremities can be incapacitating. Both motor and sensory nerve conduction are delayed in peripheral nerves, and ankle jerks may be absent.

Contrasting with this axonal neuropathic process is ischemic neuropathy resulting from small vessel disease of the vasa nervorum. Femoral and cranial nerves are commonly involved, and motor abnormalities predominate. Skeletal muscle atrophy may be prominent, especially in the thighs. This condition is occasionally referred to as diabetic amyotrophy.

With autonomic neuropathy, there is evidence of postural hypotension, resting tachycardia, decreased cardiovascular response to Valsalva's maneuver, alternating bouts of diarrhea (particularly nocturnal) and constipation, inability to empty the bladder, and impotence. Impotence due to neuropathy differs from the psychogenic variety in that the latter may be intermittent (erections occur under special circumstances), whereas diabetic impotence is usually persistent; aortoiliac occlusive disease may contribute to this problem.

There is no consistently effective treatment other than optimal control of the diabetes. Ophthalmoplegias spontaneously resolve within 6–9 weeks. Diarrhea associated with autonomic neuropathy has occasionally responded to broad-spectrum antibiotic therapy, although it often undergoes spontaneous remission. Gastric atony may be so severe as to require gastrojejunal anastomosis. Metoclopramide may be used orally or intravenously to improve gastric motility when cholinergic activity is diminished but not when it is absent. The physician should be familiar with side effects of metoclopramide; somnolence is a common adverse effect. Bethanechol (Urecholine) has occasionally improved emptying of the atonic urinary bladder. Impotence is usually permanent. Mineralocorticoid therapy and pressure suits have reportedly been of some help in patients with orthostatic hypotension occurring as a result of loss of postural reflexes. Amitriptyline, 50–75 mg at bedtime, has been recommended for pain associated with diabetic neuropathy. Dramatic relief has often resulted within 48–72 hours. Mild to moderate drowsiness is a side effect that generally improves with time. This drug should not be continued if improvement has not occurred after 5 days of therapy.

**E. Skin and Mucous Membrane Complications:** Chronic pyogenic infections of the skin may occur, especially in poorly controlled diabetic patients. Eruptive xanthomas can develop in long-standing uncontrolled cases. An unusual lesion termed **necrobiosis lipoidica diabeticorum** is usually located over the anterior surfaces of the legs or the dorsal surfaces of the ankles.

"Shin spots" are not uncommon in adult diabetics. They are brownish, rounded, painless atrophic lesions of the skin in the pretibial area. Candidal infection can produce erythema and edema of intertriginous areas below the breasts, in the axillas, and between the fingers. It causes vulvovaginitis in most chronically uncontrolled diabetic females with persistent glucosuria and is a frequent cause of pruritus.

While antifungal creams containing nystatin offer immediate relief of vulvovaginitis, recurrence is frequent unless measures are taken to eliminate the persistent glucosuria.

**F. Special Situations:**

**1. Insulin replacement during surgery–**During major surgery and in the immediate recovery period in patients with insulin-requiring diabetes, 5% dextrose in physiologic saline should be infused intravenously at a rate of 100–200 mL/h with regular human insulin (25 units/250 mL normal saline) infused into the intravenous tubing at a rate of 2–3 units/h. The patient's blood glucose should be monitored every 2 hours initially and the rates of insulin or dextrose adjusted to maintain blood glucose values between 120 and 190 mg/dL. Insulin replacement should be regulated to avoid hypoglycemia while restricting hyperglycemia to levels unlikely to result in significant loss of glucose and electrolytes in the urine.

**2. Pregnancy and the diabetic patient–**Several features distinguish the management of diabetics during pregnancy from the general therapy of diabetes. These include the following: (1) Oral hypoglycemic agents are contraindicated. (2) Weight reduction is not advised, since fetal nutrition can be adversely affected. (3) Intensive insulin therapy with frequent self-monitoring of blood glucose is generally recommended to improve the likelihood of having healthy normal babies. Every effort should be made, utilizing multiple injections of insulin or a continuous infusion of insulin by pump, to maintain near-normalization of fasting and preprandial blood glucose values while avoiding hypoglycemia. Glycohemoglobin should be maintained in the normal range.

Since many diabetic pregnancies persist beyond the expected term—or because the infants are usually large and hydramnios may be present—it has been suggested that pregnancy be terminated early (at 37–38 weeks), especially if glycemic control during pregnancy has been inadequate (eg, glycohemoglobin >10%). There is a present trend away from elective cesarean section and toward induction of labor.

## Prognosis

The effect of diabetic control on the development of complications remains an unresolved controversy. The observation that supposedly well-controlled diabetics often have elevated levels of hemoglobin $A_{1c}$, a result of sustained hyperglycemia, indicates the ineffectiveness of present conventional therapeutic methods for controlling hyperglycemia. Until pancreatic islet transplants or improved insulin delivery systems are available, this important question of control affecting complications may not be resolved. Korean patients who developed chronic hyperglycemia after accidental ingestion of Vacor, a rodenticide with potent toxicity for pancreatic B cells, were examined 6–7 years after the onset of their acquired diabetes. More than half of them showed thickened muscle capillary basement membranes, while 44% showed retinopathy and 28% had proteinuria. These findings suggest that hyperglycemia associated with insulin deficiency can itself be responsible for microvascular changes in diabetic patients. Recent intervention trials in small groups of IDDM patients with background or proliferative retinopathy have shown that despite 1 year of "tight" glycemic control with insulin pumps, worsening of the retinopathy continued. A large-scale prevention trial involving 25 centers in the USA is under way to determine if "tight" glycemic control in IDDM can delay or prevent the *onset* of microvascular disease. Until these questions are resolved, the prognosis remains uncertain.

The period between 10 and 20 years after onset of diabetes seems to be a critical one. If the patient survives this period without fulminating complications, there is a strong likelihood that reasonably good health will continue. In addition to poorly understood factors relating to differences in individual susceptibility to development of long-term complications of hyperglycemia, it is clear that the diabetic patient's intelligence, motivation, and awareness of the potential complications of the disease contribute significantly to the ultimate outcome.

Ai E, Coonan P: The treatment of diabetic retinopathy. *Ann Rev Med* 1987;**38**:279.

Bennett PH: The diagnosis of diabetes: New international classification and diagnostic criteria. *Annu Rev Med* 1983;**34**:295.

Binder C et al: Insulin pharmacokinetics. *Diabetes Care* 1984;**7**:188.

Bolli GB, Gerich JE: The dawn phenomenon: A common occurrence in both non–insulin-dependent and insulin-dependent diabetes mellitus. *N Engl J Med* 1984;**310**:746.

Bolli GB et al: Glucose counterregulation and waning of insulin in the Somogyi phenomenon (posthypoglycemic hyperglycemia). *N Engl J Med* 1984;**311**:1214.

Brink SJ, Stewart C: Insulin pump treatment in insulin-dependent diabetes mellitus. *JAMA* 1986;**255**:617.

Coustan DR et al: A randomized clinical trial of the insulin pump vs intensive conventional therapy in diabetic pregnancies. *JAMA* 1986;**255**:631.

Cryer PE, White NH, Santiago JV: The relevance of glucose counterregulatory systems to patients with insulin-dependent diabetes mellitus. *Endocr Rev* 1986;**7**:131.

DCCT Research Group: The diabetes control and complications trial (DCCT): Results of feasibility study. *Diabetes Care* 1987;**10**:1.

Eisenbarth GS: Genes, generator of diversity, glycoconjugates, and autoimmune beta cell insufficiency in type I diabetes. *Diabetes* 1987;**36**:355.

Ellis EN et al: Relationship of muscle capillary basement membrane to renal structure and function in diabetes mellitus. *Diabetes* 1986;**35**:421.

Feingold KR, Siperstein MD: Diabetic vascular disease. *Adv Intern Med* 1986;**31**:309.

Feingold KR et al: Muscle capillary basement membrane width in patients with Vacor-induced diabetes mellitus. *J Clin Invest* 1986;**78**:102.

Firth RG, Bell PM, Rizza RA: Effects of tolazamide and exogenous insulin on insulin action in patients with non-insulin-dependent diabetes mellitus. *N Engl J Med* 1986;**314**:1280.

Garvey WT et al: The effect of insulin treatment on insulin secretion and insulin action in type II diabetes mellitus. *Diabetes* 1985;**34**:222.

Goetz FC et al: Renal transplantation in diabetes. *Clin Endocrinol Metab* 1986;**15**:807.

Heine RJ et al: Absorption kinetics and action profiles of mixtures of short- and intermediate-acting insulins. *Diabetologia* 1984;**27**:558.

Lean MEJ, James WPT: Prescription of diabetic diets in the 1980s. *Lancet* 1986;**1**:723.

Melander A: Clinical pharmacology of sulfonylureas. *Metab Clin Exper* 1987;**36(Suppl)**:12.

Nathan DM et al: The clinical information value of the glycosylated hemoglobin assay. *N Engl J Med* 1984;**77**:211.

Niakan E, Harati Y, Comstock JP: Diabetic autonomic neuropathy. *Metabolism* 1986;**35**:224.

Peden N, Newton RW, Feely J: Oral hypoglycemic agents. *Br Med J* 1983;**286**:1564.

Raskin P, Rosenstock J: Blood glucose control and diabetic complications. *Ann Intern Med* 1986;**105**:254.

Rizza RA: New modes of insulin administration: Do they have a role in clinical diabetes? (Editorial.) *Ann Intern Med* 1986;**105**:126.

Rosenstock J, Friberg T, Raskin P: Effect of glycemia control on microvascular complications in patients with type I diabetes mellitus. *Am J Med* 1986;**81**:1012.

Schade DS et al: The etiology of incapacitating, brittle diabetes. *Diabetes Care* 1985;**8**:12.

Simonson DC et al: Effect of glyburide on glycemic control, insulin requirement, and glucose metabolism in insulin-treated diabetic patients. *Diabetes* 1987;**36**:136.

Taylor R: Insulin receptors and the clinician. *Br Med J* 1986;**292**:919.

Viberti G, Keen H: The patterns of proteinuria in diabetes mellitus. *Diabetes* 1984;**33**:686.

Winegrad AI: Does a common mechanism induce the diverse complications of diabetes? *Diabetes* 1987;**36**:396.

The Working Group of Hypertension in Diabetes: Statement on hypertension in diabetes mellitus. (Two parts.) *Arch Intern Med* 1987;**147**:830, 1165.

Zatz R, Brenner BM: Pathogenesis of diabetic microangiopathy: The hemodynamic view. *Am J Med* 1986;**80**:443.

## DIABETIC COMA

Coma may be due to a variety of causes not directly related to diabetes, eg, cerebrovascular accidents, alcohol or other drug toxicity, and head trauma. However, certain major causes of coma directly related to diabetes require differentiation: (1) Hypoglycemic coma resulting from excessive doses of insulin or oral hypoglycemic agents. (2) Hyperglycemic coma associated with either severe insulin deficiency (diabetic ketoacidosis) or mild to moderate insulin deficiency (hyperglycemic nonketotic hyperosmolar coma). (3) Lactic acidosis associated with diabetes, particularly in diabetes stricken with severe infections or with cardiovascular collapse.

A physical examination is essential to resolve the differential diagnosis. Patients in coma due to hypoglycemia are generally flaccid and hypothermic and have quiet breathing—in contrast to patients with acidosis, who appear dehydrated and whose respirations are rapid and deep. The laboratory remains the final arbiter in confirming the diagnosis, but a rapid estimation can be made of blood glucose concentration with paper strips (Chemstrips bG, Visidex) and of plasma ketones with either crushed Acetest tablets or Ketostix paper strips.

## 1. DIABETIC KETOACIDOSIS

Diabetic ketoacidosis may be the initial manifestation of type I diabetes or may result from increased insulin requirements in type I diabetes patients during the course of infection, trauma, myocardial infarction, or surgery. Recently, diabetic ketoacidosis has been found to be one of the more common serious complications of insulin pump therapy, occurring in approximately one per 80 patient months of treatment. Many patients who monitor capillary blood glucose regularly ignore urine ketone measurements, which would signal the possibility of insulin leakage or pump failure before serious illness develops. Poor compliance, either for psychologic reasons or because of inadequate patient education, is one of the most common causes of diabetic ketoacidosis, particularly when episodes are recurrent.

### Clinical Findings

**A. Symptoms and Signs:** As opposed to the acute onset of hypoglycemic coma, the appearance of diabetic ketoacidotic coma is usually preceded by a day or more of polyuria and polydipsia associated with marked fatigue, nausea and vomiting, and, finally, mental stupor that can progress to frank neurologic coma. On physical examination, evidence of dehydration in a stuporous patient with rapid deep breathing and a "fruity" breath odor of acetone would strongly suggest the diagnosis. Hypotension with tachycardia indicates profound dehydration and salt depletion.

**B. Laboratory Findings:** (Table 19–6) Glycos-

**Table 19–6.** Laboratory diagnosis of coma in diabetic patients.

| | Urine | | Plasma | | |
|---|---|---|---|---|---|
| | Glucose | Acetone | Glucose | Bicarbonate | Acetone |
| **Related to diabetes** | | | | | |
| Hypoglycemia | 0* | 0 or + | Low | Normal | 0 |
| Diabetic ketoacidosis | + + + + | + + + + | High | Low | + + + + |
| Nonketotic hyperglycemic coma | + + + + | 0 | High | Normal or slightly low | 0 |
| Lactic acidosis | 0 or + | 0 or + | Normal or low or high | Low | 0 or + |
| **Unrelated to diabetes** | | | | | |
| Alcohol or other toxic drugs | 0 or + | 0 or + | May be low | Normal or low† | 0 or + |
| Cerebrovascular accident or head trauma | + or 0 | 0 | Often high | Normal | 0 |
| Uremia | 0 or + | 0 | High or normal | Low | 0 or + |

\* Leftover urine in bladder might still contain glucose from earlier hyperglycemia.
† Alcohol can elevate plasma lactate as well as keto acids to reduce pH.

uria of 4+ and strong ketonuria with hyperglycemia, ketonemia, low arterial blood pH, and low plasma bicarbonate are typical of diabetic ketoacidosis. Serum potassium is often elevated despite total body potassium depletion resulting from protracted polyuria or vomiting. Elevation of serum amylase is common but often represents salivary as well as pancreatic amylase, thereby correlating poorly as an indicator of acute pancreatitis. Multichannel chemical analysis of serum creatinine (SMA-6) is falsely elevated by nonspecific chromogenicity of keto acids and glucose. Most laboratories can correct for these interfering substances on request.

## Complications

The 2 major metabolic aberrations of diabetic ketoacidosis are hyperglycemia and ketoacidemia, both due to insulin lack associated with hyperglucagonemia.

**A. Hyperglycemia:** Hyperglycemia results from increased hepatic production of glucose as well as diminished glucose uptake by peripheral tissues. Hepatic glucose output is a consequence of increased gluconeogenesis resulting from insulinopenia as well as from an associated hyperglucagonemia. Hyperglycemia produces an osmotic overload in the kidney, causing diuresis, with a critical loss of electrolytes and a disproportionate loss of free water in the urine with intracellular dehydration.

**B. Ketoacidemia:** Ketoacidemia represents the effect of insulin lack at multiple enzyme loci. Insulin lack associated with elevated levels of growth hormone and glucagon contributes to an increase in lipolysis from adipose tissue and in hepatic ketogenesis. In addition, there is evidence that reduced ketolysis by insulin-deficient peripheral tissues contributes to the ketoacidemia. The only true "keto" acid present is acetoacetic acid, which, along with its by-product acetone, is measured by nitroprusside reagents (Acetest and Ketostix). The sensitivity for acetone, however, is poor, requiring over 10 mmol, which is sel-

dom reached in the plasma of ketoacidotic subjects—although this detectable concentration is readily achieved in urine. Thus, in the plasma of ketotic patients, only acetoacetate is measured by these reagents. The more prevalent β-hydroxybutyric acid has no ketone group and is therefore not detected by conventional nitroprusside tests. This takes on special importance with associated circulatory collapse, wherein an increase in lactic acid can shift the redox state to increase β-hydroxybutyric acid at the expense of the readily detectable acetoacetic acid. Bedside diagnostic reagents would then be unreliable, suggesting no ketonemia in cases where β-hydroxybutyric acid is a major factor in producing the acidosis.

## Treatment

**A. Prevention:** Education of diabetic patients to recognize the early symptoms and signs of ketoacidosis has done a great deal to prevent severe acidosis. Urine ketones should be measured in patients with signs of infection or in insulin pump-treated patients when capillary blood glucose is unexpectedly and persistently high. When heavy ketonuria and glycosuria persist on several successive examinations, supplemental regular insulin should be administered and liquid foods such as lightly salted tomato juice and broth should be ingested to replenish fluids and electrolytes. The patient should be instructed to contact the physician if ketonuria persists, and especially if vomiting develops or if appropriate adjustment of the infusion rate on an insulin pump does not correct the hyperglycemia and ketonuria. In juvenile-onset diabetics, particularly in the teen years, recurrent episodes of severe ketoacidosis often indicate poor compliance with the insulin regimen, and these patients will require intensive family counseling.

**B. Emergency Measures:** If ketosis is severe, the patient should be placed in the hospital for correction of the hyperosmolarity as well as the ketoacidemia. Severe hyperosmolarity correlates closely with central nervous system depression and coma, whereas prolonged acidosis can compromise cardiac output and reduce vascular tone; this contributes to circulatory collapse in the dehydrated patient.

**1. Therapeutic flow sheet**–One of the most important steps in initiating therapy is to start a flow sheet listing vital signs and the time sequence of diagnostic laboratory values in relation to therapeutic maneuvers. Indices of the metabolic defects include urine glucose and ketones as well as arterial pH, plasma glucose, acetone, bicarbonate, and electrolytes. One physician should be responsible for maintaining this therapeutic flow sheet and prescribing therapy. An indwelling catheter is required in all comatose patients but should be avoided if possible in a fully cooperative diabetic because of the risk of introducing bladder infection. Fluid intake and output should be recorded. Gastric intubation is recommended in the comatose patient to correct the commonly associated dilatation gastric that may lead to vomiting and aspiration. The patient should not receive sedatives or narcotics.

**2. Insulin replacement**–Only regular insulin should be used initially in all cases of severe ketoacidosis, and it should be given immediately after the diagnosis is established. Regular insulin can be given in a loading dose of 0.3 unit/kg as an intravenous bolus followed by 0.1 unit/kg/h, either continuously infused or injected intramuscularly; this is sufficient to replace the insulin deficit in most patients. Replacement of insulin deficiency helps correct the acidosis by reducing the flux of fatty acids to the liver, reducing ketone production by the liver, and also improving removal of ketones from the blood. Insulin treatment reduces the hyperosmolarity by reducing the hyperglycemia. It accomplishes this by increasing removal of glucose through peripheral utilization as well as by decreasing production of glucose by the liver. This latter effect is accomplished by direct inhibition of gluconeogenesis and glycogenolysis, as well as by lowered amino acid flux from muscle to liver and reduced hyperglucagonemia.

Doses of insulin as low as 0.1 unit/kg, given hourly either by slow intravenous drip or intramuscularly, are as effective in most cases as the much higher doses previously recommended and appear to be safer. When a continuous infusion of insulin is used, 25 units of regular human insulin should be placed in 250 mL of physiologic saline and the first 50 mL of solution flushed through to saturate the tubing before connecting it to the intravenous line. An I-Vac or Harvard pump provides a reliable infusion rate. The insulin dose should be "piggy-backed" into the fluid line so the rate of flow can be changed without altering the insulin delivery rate. For optimal effects, continuous low-dose insulin infusions should always be preceded by a rapid intravenous loading dose of regular insulin, 0.3 unit/kg, to prime the tissue insulin receptors. If the plasma glucose level fails to fall at least 10% in the first hour, a repeat loading dose is recommended. Insulin therapy is greatly facilitated when plasma glucose can be measured within a few minutes of sampling. The availability of instruments for rapid and accurate glucose analysis (Beckman or Yellow Springs glucose analyzer) has contributed much to achieving optimal insulin replacement. Rarely, a patient with insulin resistance is encountered, and this requires doubling the insulin dose every 2–4 hours if hyperglycemia does not improve after the first 2 doses of insulin. One must be alert to the danger of anaphylactic shock in resistant patients requiring very high doses of insulin if it is given intravenously.

**3. Fluid and electrolyte replacement**–In most patients, the fluid deficit is 4–5 L. Initially, normal saline solution is the solution of choice to help reexpand the contracted vascular volume in the dehydrated patient, thereby improving renal capability to excrete hydrogen ions. The use of sodium bicarbonate has been questioned by some because of the following potential consequences: (1) Hypokalemia from rapid potassium shifts into cells. (2) Tissue anoxia from reduced dissociation of oxygen from hemoglobin when acidosis is rapidly reversed. (3) Cerebral acidosis resulting from a reduction of cerebrospinal fluid pH. However, these considerations are relatively less important in certain clinical settings, and 1–2 ampules of sodium bicarbonate (44 meq per 50-mL ampule) added to a bottle of *hypotonic* saline solution should probably be administered whenever the blood pH is 7.0 or less or blood bicarbonate is below 9 meq/L. Once the pH reaches 7.2, no further bicarbonate should be given, since it aggravates rebound metabolic alkalosis as ketones are metabolized. Alkalosis causes potassium shifts that increase the risk of cardiac arrhythmias. In the first hour, at least 1 L of normal saline should be infused, and fluid should be given thereafter at a rate of 300–500 mL/h with careful monitoring of serum potassium. If the blood glucose is above 500 mg/dL, 0.45% saline solution may be used after the first hour, since the water deficit exceeds the sodium loss in uncontrolled diabetes with osmotic diuresis. When blood glucose falls to 250 mg/dL or less, 5% glucose solutions should be used to maintain blood glucose between 200 and 300 mg/dL. Glucose administration has the dual advantage of preventing hypoglycemia and also of reducing the likelihood of cerebral edema, which could result from too rapid a decline in hyperglycemia. Insulin therapy should be continued every 2–4 hours until ketonemia has cleared.

**4. Potassium and phosphate replacement**–Total body potassium loss from polyuria as well as from vomiting may be as high as 200 meq. However, because of shifts from cells due to the acidosis, serum potassium is usually normal or high until after the first few hours of treatment, when acidosis improves and serum potassium returns into cells. Potassium in doses of 20–30 meq/h should be infused within 3–4 hours after beginning therapy, or sooner if initial serum potassium is inappropriately low. An ECG can be of help in monitoring the patient and reflecting the state of potassium balance at the time, but it should not replace accurate laboratory measurements.

Foods high in potassium content can be prescribed when the patient has recovered sufficiently to take food orally. (Tomato juice and grapefruit juice contain 14 meq of potassium per 240 mL, and a medium-sized banana 10 meq.)

Because severe hypophosphatemia also develops during insulin therapy of diabetic ketoacidosis, some phosphate can be replaced as the potassium salt, but only a small amount. The potassium need is several times that of phosphate, and replacing phosphorus ions too rapidly (while meeting potassium requirements) can precipitate serum calcium and induce tetany. Potassium and phosphate should be replaced separately most of the time.

A significant therapeutic benefit of phosphate replacement has not been documented in at least 2 clinical trials. However, certain potential advantages have been suggested. Treatment of hypophosphatemia helps to restore the buffering capacity of the plasma, thereby facilitating renal excretion of hydrogen; and it corrects the impaired oxygen dissociation from hemoglobin by regenerating 2,3-diphosphoglycerate. To minimize the risk of inducing tetany from an overload of phosphate replacement, an average deficit of 40–50 mmol phosphate in adults with diabetic ketoacidosis should be replaced by intravenous infusion *at a rate not to exceed 3 mmol/h.*

A stock solution available from Abbott Laboratories provides a mixture of 1.12 g $KH_2PO_4$ and 1.18 g $K_2HPO_4$ in a 5-mL single-dose vial representing 22 meq potassium and 15 mmol phosphate (27 meq). Five milliliters of this stock solution in 2 L of either 0.45% saline or 5% dextrose in water, infused at 400 mL/h, will replace the phosphate at the optimal rate of 3 mmol/h and will provide 4.4 meq of potassium per hour. If serum phosphate remains below 2.5 mg/dL, a repeat 5-hour infusion of potassium phosphate at a rate of 3 mmol/h would be reasonable. Although it remains controversial whether phosphate replacement is beneficial, the total body deficit can be safely replaced in the above manner without risk of tetany.

**5. Treatment of associated infection**–Appropriate antibiotics should be given if acute bacterial infection, often a precipitating cause of diabetic ketoacidosis, is present. Acute cholecystitis and pyelonephritis may be particularly severe in these patients.

**Prognosis**

The frequency of deaths due to diabetic ketoacidosis has been dramatically reduced by improved therapy of young diabetics, but this complication remains a significant risk in the aged and in patients in profound coma in whom treatment has been delayed. Acute myocardial infarction or infarction of the bowel following prolonged hypotension has a high mortality rate. A serious prognostic sign is renal shutdown, and prior kidney dysfunction worsens the prognosis considerably because the kidney plays a key role in compensating for massive shifts of pH and electrolytes. pH lowering has less prognostic significance than hyperosmolaity. Cerebral edema has been reported to occur rarely as metabolic deficits return to normal. This is best prevented by avoiding sudden reversal of marked hyperglycemia to hypoglycemia, since massive fluid shifts into cerebral tissue can occur as a consequence of osmotically active particles accumulating within neurons during hyperglycemia. Maintaining glycemic levels of 200–300 mg/dL for the initial 24 hours after correction of severe hyperglycemia reduces the risk of cerebral edema.

## 2. NONKETOTIC HYPERGLYCEMIC COMA

This second most common form of hyperglycemic coma is characterized by severe hyperglycemia in the absence of significant ketosis, with hyperosmolarity and severe dehydration. It occurs in patients with mild or occult diabetes, and most patients are at least middle-aged to elderly. Underlying renal insufficiency or congestive heart failure is common, and the presence of either worsens the prognosis. A precipitating event such as pneumonia, burns, cerebrovascular accident, or recent operation is often present. Certain drugs such as phenytoin, diazoxide, glucocorticoids, and diuretics have been implicated in its pathogenesis, as have procedures associated with glucose loading such as peritoneal dialysis.

**Pathogenesis**

A partial or relative insulin deficiency may initiate the syndrome by reducing glucose utilization of muscle, fat, and liver while inducing hyperglucagonemia and increasing hepatic glucose output. With massive glycosuria, obligatory water loss ensues. If a patient is unable to maintain adequate fluid intake because of an associated acute or chronic illness or has suffered excessive fluid loss (eg, from burns or therapy with diuretics), marked dehydration results. As plasma volume contracts, renal insufficiency develops, and the resultant limitation of glucose loss leads to increasingly high blood glucose concentrations. A severe hyperosmolarity develops that causes mental confusion and finally coma. It is not clear why ketosis is virtually absent under these conditions of insulin insufficiency, although reduced levels of growth hormone may be associated along with portal vein insulin concentrations sufficient to restrain ketogenesis.

**Clinical Findings**

**A. Symptoms and Signs:** Onset may be insidious over a period of days or weeks, with weakness, polyuria, and polydipsia. The lack of toxic features of ketoacidosis may retard recognition of the syndrome and delay therapy until dehydration becomes more profound than in ketoacidosis. Reduced intake of fluid is not an uncommon historical feature, due to either inappropriate lack of thirst, gastrointestinal upset, or inaccessibility of fluids to elderly, bedridden patients. Lethargy and confusion develop, progressing to convulsions and deep coma. Physical examination confirms the presence of profound dehydration in a lethargic or comatose patient without Kussmaul respirations.

**B. Laboratory Findings:** Severe hyperglycemia is present, with blood glucose values ranging from 800 to 2400 mg/dL. In mild cases, where dehydration is less severe, dilutional hyponatremia as well as urinary sodium losses may reduce serum sodium to 120–125 meq/L, which protects to some extent against extreme hyperosmolarity. However, once dehydration progresses further, serum sodium can exceed 140 meq/L, producing serum osmolarity readings of 330–440 mosm/kg. Ketosis and acidosis are usually absent or mild. Prerenal azotemia is the rule, with blood urea nitrogen elevations to 90 mg/dL being typical.

A convenient method of estimating serum osmolality is as follows (normal values in humans are 280–300 mosm/L):

$$mosm/L = 2[Na^+] + \frac{Glucose\ (mg/dL)}{18} + \frac{BUN\ (mg/dL)}{2.8}$$

These calculated estimates are usually 10–20 meq/L lower than values recorded by standard cryoscopic techniques in patients with diabetic coma.

## Treatment

**A. Saline:** Fluid replacement is of paramount importance in treating nonketotic hyperglycemic coma. If circulatory collapse is present, fluid therapy should be initiated with isotonic saline. In all other cases, hypotonic (0.45%) saline appears to be preferable as the initial replacement solution because the body fluids of these patients are markedly hyperosmolar. As much as 4–6 L of fluid may be required in the first 8–10 hours. As long as blood pressure and urine output are maintained, hypotonic saline can be continued; however, as insulin therapy further lowers plasma glucose concentration, a reduced solute content of the vascular compartment may necessitate isotonic saline to avoid hypotension. Careful monitoring of the patient is required for proper sodium and water replacement. Once blood glucose reaches 250 mg/dL, fluid replacement should include 5% dextrose in either water, 0.45% saline solution, or 0.9% saline solution. The rate of dextrose infusion should be adjusted to maintain glycemic levels of 250–300 mg/dL in order to reduce the risk of cerebral edema. An important end point of fluid therapy is to restore urine output to 50 mL/h or more.

**B. Potassium:** With the absence of acidosis, there may be no initial hyperkalemia unless associated renal failure is present; thus, less potassium is lost in the urine during the initial stages of glycosuria. This results in less severe total potassium depletion than in diabetic ketoacidosis, and less potassium replacement is therefore needed. However, because initial serum potassium is usually not elevated and because it declines rapidly as a result of the sensitivity of the nonketotic patient to insulin, it has been recommended that potassium replacement be initiated earlier than in ketotic patients, assuming that no renal insufficiency or oliguria is present. Potassium chloride (10 meq/L) can be added to the initial bottle of fluids administered if the patient's serum potassium is not elevated.

**C. Phosphate:** When hypophosphatemia develops during insulin therapy, phosphate replacement can be given as described for ketoacidotic patients (at 3 mmol/h).

**D. Insulin:** Less insulin may be required to reduce the hyperglycemia in nonketotic patients as compared to those with diabetic ketoacidotic coma. In fact, fluid replacement alone can reduce hyperglycemia considerably. An initial dose of only 15 units intravenously and 15 units subcutaneously of regular insulin is usually quite effective, and in most cases subsequent doses need not be greater than 10–25 units subcutaneously every 4 hours.

## Prognosis

The overall mortality rate of hyperglycemic, hyperosmolar, nonketotic coma is more than 10 times that of diabetic ketoacidosis, chiefly because of its higher incidence in older patients, who may have compromised cardiovascular systems or associated major illnesses. (When patients are matched for age, the prognoses of these 2 hyperglycemic emergencies are reasonably comparable.) When prompt therapy is instituted, the mortality rate can be reduced from nearly 50% to that related to the severity of coexistent disorders.

## 3. LACTIC ACIDOSIS

Lactic acidosis is characterized by accumulation of excess lactic acid in the blood. Normally, the principal sources of this acid are the erythrocytes (which lack enzymes for aerobic oxidation), skeletal muscle, skin, and brain. Conversion to glucose and oxidation principally by the liver but also by the kidneys represent the chief pathways for its removal. Overproduction of lactic acid (tissue hypoxia), deficient removal (hepatic failure), or both (circulatory collapse) can cause accumulation of excess lactic acid. Lactic acidosis is not uncommon in any severely ill patient suffering from cardiac decompensation; respiratory or hepatic failure; acute septicemia; acute infarction of lung, bowel, or extremities; leukemia; or terminal metastatic cancer. Hyperlactanemia has been produced by toxic overdoses of phenformin or alcohol. With the discontinuation of phenformin therapy in the USA, lactic acidosis in patients with diabetes mellitus has become uncommon, but it still must be considered in the acidotic diabetic, especially if the patient is seriously ill.

## Clinical Findings

**A. Symptoms and Signs:** The main clinical features of lactic acidosis are marked hyperventilation and mental confusion leading to stupor and coma. When lactic acidosis is secondary to tissue hypoxia or vascular collapse, the clinical presentation is variable, being that of the prevailing catastrophic illness. However, in the idiopathic, or spontaneous, variety, the onset is rapid (usually over a few hours), blood pressure is normal, peripheral circulation is good, and there is no cyanosis.

**B. Laboratory Findings:** Plasma bicarbonate and blood pH are quite low, indicating the presence of severe metabolic acidosis. Ketones are usually absent from plasma and urine or at least not prominent. The first clue may be a high anion gap (serum sodium minus the sum of chloride and bicarbonate anions [in meq/L] should be no greater than 15). A higher value indicates the existence of an abnormal compartment of anions. If this cannot be clinically explained by an excess of keto acids (diabetes), inorganic acids (uremia), or anions from drug overdosage (salicylates, methyl alcohol, ethylene glycol), then lactic acidosis is probably the correct diagnosis. In the absence of azotemia, hyperphosphatemia may be a clue to the presence of lactic acidosis. The diagnosis is confirmed by demonstrating, in a sample of blood that is promptly chilled and separated, a plasma lactic acid concentration of 7 mmol/L or higher (values as high as 30 mmol/L have been reported). Normal plasma values average 1 mmol/L, with a normal lactate/pyruvate ratio of 10:1. This ratio is greatly exceeded in lactic acidosis.*

## Treatment

Aggressive treatment of the precipitating cause of lactic acidosis is the main component of therapy. An adequate airway and good oxygenation should be assured. If hypotension is present, fluids and, if appropriate, pressor agents must be given to restore tissue perfusion. Empiric antibiotic coverage should be given after culture samples are obtained in any patient in whom the cause of the lactic acidosis is not apparent.

Alkalinization with intravenous sodium bicarbonate to keep the pH above 7.2 is generally needed in the emergency treatment of severe lactic acidosis. Massive doses may be required (as much as 2000 meq in 24 hours has been used); however, there is no evidence that the mortality rate is favorably affected by their use, and the matter is at present controversial. Hemodialysis may be useful in cases where large sodium loads are poorly tolerated. Dichloroacetate, an anion that facilitates pyruvate removal by activating pyruvate dehydrogenase, reverses certain types of lactic acidosis in animals and may prove useful in treating some types of lactic acidosis in humans. If hypoxemia

---

* In collecting samples, it is essential to rapidly chill and separate the blood to remove red cells, whose continued glycolysis at room temperature is a common source of error in reports of high plasma lactate. Frozen plasma remains stable for subsequent assay.

is the precipitating factor, vigorous treatment is indicated.

## Prognosis

The mortality rate of spontaneous lactic acidosis approaches 80%. It is slightly lower when lactic acidosis is due to potentially reversible causes such as phenformin, when alkalinization need be maintained only until the drug effect is dissipated. The prognosis in most cases is that of the primary disorder that produced the lactic acidosis.

Foster DW, McGarry JD: The metabolic derangements and treatment of diabetic ketoacidosis. *N Engl J Med* 1983;**309**:159.

Fulop M: The treatment of severely uncontrolled diabetes mellitus. *Adv Intern Med* 1984;**29**:327.

Kreisberg RA: Pathogenesis and management of lactic acidosis. *Annu Rev Med* 1984;**35**:181.

Narins RG, Cohen JJ: Bicarbonate therapy for organic acidosis: The case for its continued use. *Ann Intern Med* 1987;**106**:615.

Morris LR, Murphy MB, Kitabchi AE: Bicarbonate therapy in severe ketoacidosis. *Ann Intern Med* 1986;**105**:836.

Stacpoole PW: Lactic acidosis: The case against bicarbonate therapy. *Ann Intern Med* 1986;**105**:276.

Wachtel TJ, Silliman RA, Lamberton P: Predisposing factors for the diabetic hyperosmolar state. *Arch Intern Med* 1987;**147**:499.

---

# THE HYPOGLYCEMIC STATES

---

Spontaneous hypoglycemia in adults is of 2 principal types: fasting and postprandial. Fasting hypoglycemia is often subacute or chronic and usually presents with neuroglycopenia as its principal manifestation; postprandial hypoglycemia is relatively acute and is often heralded by symptoms of adrenergic discharge (sweating, palpitations, anxiety, tremulousness).

## Differential Diagnosis
## (See Table 19–7.)

**Fasting hypoglycemia** may occur in certain endocrine disorders, such as hypopituitarism, Addison's disease, or myxedema; in disorders related to liver malfunction, such as acute alcoholism or liver failure; and in instances of renal failure, particularly in patients requiring dialysis. These conditions are usually obvious, with hypoglycemia being only a secondary feature. When hypoglycemia is a primary manifestation developing in adults without apparent endocrine disorders or inborn metabolic diseases from childhood, the principal diagnostic possibilities include (1) hyperinsulinism, due to either pancreatic B cell tumors or surreptitious administration of insulin (or sulfonylureas); and (2) hypoglycemia due to non-insulin-producing extrapancreatic tumors.

**Postprandial (reactive) hypoglycemia** may be

**Table 19–7.** Common causes of hypoglycemia in the absence of clinically obvious endocrine or hepatic disorders.

**Fasting hypoglycemia**
  Hyperinsulinism
    Pancreatic B cell tumor
    Surreptitious administration of insulin or sulfonylureas
  Extrapancreatic tumors
**Postprandial (reactive) hypoglycemia**
  Early hypoglycemia (alimentary)
    Postgastrectomy
    Functional (increased vagal tone)
  Late hypoglycemia (occult diabetes)
    Delayed insulin release due to B cell dysfunction
  Counterregulatory deficiency
  Idiopathic
**Alcohol hypoglycemia**
**Immunopathologic hypoglycemia**
  Idiopathic anti-insulin antibodies (which release their bound insulin)
  Antibodies to insulin receptors (which act as agonists)

classified as early (within 2–3 hours after a meal) or late (3–5 hours after eating). Early, or alimentary, hypoglycemia occurs when there is a rapid discharge of ingested carbohydrate into the small bowel followed by rapid glucose absorption and hyperinsulinism. It may be seen after gastrointestinal surgery and is particularly associated with the dumping syndrome after gastrectomy. In some cases, it is functional and may represent overactivity of the parasympathetic nervous system mediated via the vagus nerve. Rarely, it results from defective counterregulatory responses such as deficiencies of growth hormone, glucagon, cortisol, or autonomic responses.

**Alcohol hypoglycemia** may occur after a period of fasting or within several hours after drinking ethanol in combination with sugar-containing mixers. In either case, blood ethanol may be below levels usually associated with legal standards relating to being "under the influence."

**Immunopathologic hypoglycemia** is an extremely rare condition in which anti-insulin antibodies or antibodies to insulin receptors develop spontaneously. In the former case, the mechanism is unclear, but it may relate to increasing dissociation of insulin from circulating pools of bound insulin. When antibodies to insulin receptors are found, most patients do not have hypoglycemia but rather severe insulin-resistant diabetes and acanthosis nigricans. However, during the course of the disease in these patients, certain anti-insulin receptor antibodies with agonist activity mimicking insulin action predominate, producing severe hypoglycemia.

**Factitious hypoglycemia** is self-induced hypoglycemia due to surreptitious administration of insulin or sulfonylureas.

## 1. HYPOGLYCEMIA DUE TO PANCREATIC B CELL TUMORS

Fasting hypoglycemia in an otherwise healthy adult is most commonly due to an adenoma of the islets of Langerhans. Ninety percent of such tumors are single and benign, but multiple adenomas can occur as well as malignant tumors with functional metastases. B cell hyperplasia as a cause of fasting hypoglycemia is not well documented in adults. Adenomas may be familial and have been found in conjunction with tumors of the parathyroids and pituitary (Wermer's syndrome; multiple endocrine adenomatosis type I).

### Clinical Findings

**A. Symptoms and Signs:** The signs and symptoms are those of subacute or chronic hypoglycemia, which may progress to permanent and irreversible brain damage. Delayed diagnosis has often resulted in prolonged psychiatric care or treatment for psychomotor epilepsy before the true diagnosis was established. In long-standing cases, obesity can result as a consequence of overeating to relieve symptoms.

Whipple's triad is characteristic of hypoglycemia regardless of the cause. It consists of (1) a history of hypoglycemic symptoms, (2) an associated fasting blood glucose of 40 mg/dL or less, and (3) immediate recovery upon administration of glucose. The hypoglycemic symptoms in insulinoma often develop in the early morning or after missing a meal. Occasionally, they occur after exercise. They typically begin with evidence of central nervous system glucose lack and can include blurred vision or diplopia, headache, feelings of detachment, slurred speech, and weakness. Personality and mental changes vary from anxiety to psychotic behavior, and neurologic deterioration can result in convulsions or coma. Sweating and palpitations may not occur.

**B. Laboratory Findings:** B cell adenomas do not reduce secretion in the presence of hypoglycemia, and the critical diagnostic test is to demonstrate inappropriately elevated serum insulin levels at a time when hypoglycemia is present. A reliable serum insulin level of 11 μU/mL or more in the presence of blood glucose values below 40 mg/dL is diagnostic of inappropriate hyperinsulinism. Other causes of hyperinsulinemic hypoglycemia must be considered, including factitious administration of insulin or sulfonylureas. An elevated circulating proinsulin level is characteristic of most B cell adenomas and does not occur in factitious hyperinsulinism.

**C. Diagnostic Tests:**

1. Prolonged fasting under hospital supervision until hypoglycemia is documented is probably the most dependable means of establishing the diagnosis, especially in males. In patients with insulinoma, the blood glucose levels often drop below 40 mg/dL after an overnight fast. In normal male subjects, the blood glucose does not fall below 55–60 mg/dL during a 3-day fast. In contrast, in premenopausal women who have fasted for only 24 hours, the plasma glucose falls normally to such an extent that it must drop to values lower than 35 mg/dL (and < 30 mg/dL by 36 hours) to be significant. After 36 hours of fasting, premenopausal females normally achieve such low

levels of glucose that clinical evaluation of this test for insulinoma becomes quite difficult. In these cases, however, the women are not symptomatic, presumably owing to the development of sufficient ketonemia to supply energy needs to the brain. Insulinoma patients, on the other hand, become symptomatic when plasma glucose drops to subnormal levels, since inappropriate insulin secretion restricts ketone formation. Moreover, the demonstration of a nonsuppressed insulin level ($\geq 11$ units/mL) in the presence of hypoglycemia and of an *increasing* ratio of insulin to glucose (ie, glucose falls more rapidly than does insulin) suggests the diagnosis of insulinoma, since normal females show a falling insulin-to-glucose ratio during a fast. If hypoglycemia does not develop in a male patient after 72 hours of fasting terminated with moderate exercise, insulinoma must be considered an unlikely diagnosis.

2. Suppression of C peptide during insulin-induced hypoglycemia is the basis of a diagnostic test for insulinoma. This small peptide connecting A and B chains of insulin is released in equimolar quantities with endogenous insulin and thus reflects endogenous insulin secretion, which cannot be directly monitored during insulin infusion. Whereas normal persons suppress their C peptide levels to 50% or more during hypoglycemia induced by 0.1 unit of insulin per kilogram body weight per hour, absence of suppression suggests the presence of an autonomous insulin-secreting tumor.

3. In contrast to normal subjects, whose proinsulin concentration is less than 20% of the total immunoreactive insulin, patients with insulinoma have elevated levels of proinsulin representing 30–90% of total immunoreactive insulin. Sensitive new assays for human proinsulin, incorporating specific monoclonal antibodies, offer considerable potential for the evaluation of patients with suspected insulinoma, although experience with their diagnostic usefulness is limited at present.

4. Stimulation tests with pancreatic B cell secretagogues such as tolbutamide, glucagon, or leucine are generally not needed in most cases if basal insulin is found to be nonsuppressible and therefore inappropriately elevated during fasting hypoglycemia. However, in occasional patients with a relatively fixed level of circulating insulin that is only barely inappropriate, stimulation may be helpful, bearing in mind that false-negative results can occur if the tumor is poorly differentiated and agranular.

Intravenous glucagon (1 mg over 1 minute) can be useful in patients with "borderline" fasting inappropriate hyperinsulinoma. A rise above baseline of 200 μU/mL or more at 5 and 10 minutes strongly suggests insulinoma, although poorly differentiated tumors may not respond. Glucagon has the advantage over tolbutamide of correcting rather than provoking hypoglycemia during stimulation testing and is diagnostic in 60–70% of patients with insulinoma.

**D. Preoperative Localization of B Cell Tumors:** Pancreatic arteriography has been disappointing, with an accuracy rate of only 20% and a false-positive rate of about 5%. CT scan and MRI are not helpful in the preoperative localization of insulinoma because they do not distinguish small tumors within the pancreas. However, intraoperative ultrasound is proving to be a valuable means of localizing small tumors within the pancreas not palpable at laparotomy.

Percutaneous transhepatic pancreatic vein catheterization with insulin assay is useful for localizing small insulinomas. However, this is a painful invasive procedure and is useful only if performed by angiographers experienced with this technique. It offers promise in helping localize small B cell tumors, particularly in the head of the pancreas, where they may be difficult to see or palpate at the time of surgery. It may also detect multiple tumors or islet cell hyperplasia preoperatively. Further experience with this technique is needed to determine its reliability and accuracy.

### Treatment

**A. Surgical Measures:** Operation is the treatment of choice, preferably by a surgeon who is experienced at mobilizing the pancreas and exploring adequately the posterior surface of the head and body as well as the tail. Blood glucose should be monitored throughout surgery, and 10% dextrose in water should be infused at a rate of 100 mL/h or faster. In cases where the diagnosis has been established but no adenoma is located, subtotal pancreatectomy is usually indicated, including the entire body and tail of the pancreas. Total pancreatectomy is seldom required now in view of the efficacy of long-term therapy with diazoxide in most patients with insulinomas. Recent development of the "closed loop" artificial pancreas permits monitoring of plasma glucose and infusion of dextrose. This not only protects against hypoglycemia but also may aid in determining whether all insulin-secreting tumors have been removed, at which time the dextrose infusion stops and blood glucose rises.

**B. Diet and Chemotherapy:** In patients with inoperable functioning islet cell carcinoma or in patients in whom subtotal removal of the pancreas has failed to produce cure, reliance on frequent feedings is necessary. Since most tumors are not responsive to glucose, carbohydrate feedings every 2–3 hours are usually effective in preventing hypoglycemia, although obesity may become a problem. Glucagon should be available for emergency use as indicated in the discussion of treatment of diabetes. Diazoxide, 300–600 mg daily orally, has been useful with concomitant thiazide diuretic therapy to control sodium retention characteristic of diazoxide. When patients are unable to tolerate diazoxide because of side effects such as gastrointestinal upset, hirsutism, or edema, the calcium channel blocker verapamil may be beneficial in view of its inhibitory effect on insulin release from insulinoma cells. Streptozocin is useful in decreasing insulin secretion in islet cell carcinomas, and effective doses have been achieved without the undue renal toxicity that characterized early experience.

## Prognosis

When insulinoma is diagnosed early and cured surgically, complete recovery is likely, although brain damage following severe hypoglycemia is not reversible. A significant increase in survival rate has been shown in streptozocin-treated patients with islet cell carcinoma, with reduction in tumor mass as well as decreased hyperinsulinism.

## 2. HYPOGLYCEMIA DUE TO EXTRAPANCREATIC TUMORS

These rare causes of hypoglycemia include mesenchymal tumors such as retroperitoneal sarcomas, hepatomas, adrenocortical carcinomas, and miscellaneous epithelial type tumors. The tumors are frequently large and readily palpated or visualized on urograms.

Laboratory diagnosis depends upon fasting hypoglycemia associated with serum insulin levels that are generally below 10 μU/mL. The mechanism of these tumors' hypoglycemic effect remains obscure. Although they do not release immunoreactive insulin, it has been suggested that they may produce certain insulinlike substances similar to the somatomedins or growth factors.

The prognosis for these tumors is generally poor, and surgical removal should be attempted when feasible. Dietary management of the hypoglycemia is the mainstay of medical treatment, since diazoxide is usually ineffective.

## 3. POSTPRANDIAL HYPOGLYCEMIA (Reactive Hypoglycemia)

### Postgastrectomy Alimentary Hypoglycemia

Reactive hypoglycemia following gastrectomy is a consequence of hyperinsulinism resulting from rapid gastric emptying of ingested food that produces overstimulation of vagal reflexes and overproduction of beta-cytotropic gastrointestinal hormones. Symptoms result from adrenergic hyperactivity in response to the hypoglycemia. Treatment consists of more frequent feedings with smaller portions of less rapidly assimilated carbohydrate and more slowly absorbed fat and protein.

### Functional Alimentary Hypoglycemia

This syndrome is classified as functional when no postsurgical explanation exists for the presence of early alimentary type reactive hypoglycemia. It is most often associated with chronic fatigue, anxiety, irritability, weakness, poor concentration, decreased libido, headaches, hunger after meals, and tremulousness. However, most patients with these symptoms do not have hypoglycemia; furthermore, even in those who have documented early hypoglycemia, it is likely to be only a secondary manifestation of their nervous imbalance, with consequent vagal overactivity causing increased gastric emptying and early hyperinsulinism.

Indiscriminate use and overinterpretation of glucose tolerance tests have led to an unfortunate tendency to overdiagnose functional hypoglycemia. As many as a third or more of *normal* subjects have hypoglycemia with or without symptoms during a 4-hour glucose tolerance test. Thus, the nonspecificity of glucose tolerance testing makes it a highly unreliable tool for evaluating patients with suspected episodes of postprandial hypoglycemia. Accordingly, to increase diagnostic reliability, hypoglycemia should preferably be documented during a spontaneous symptomatic episode accompanying routine daily activity, with clinical improvement following feeding. Personality evaluation suggesting hyperkinetic compulsive behavior in thin, anxious patients, particularly females, supports this diagnosis in patients with a compatible history.

In patients with documented postprandial hypoglycemia on a functional basis, there is no harm and occasional benefit in reducing the proportion of carbohydrate in the diet while increasing the frequency and reducing the size of meals; however, it should not be expected that these maneuvers will cure the neurasthenia, since the reflex response to hypoglycemia may be only one component of a generalized primary nervous hyperactivity. Support and mild sedation should be the mainstays of therapy, with dietary manipulation only an adjunct.

### Late Hypoglycemia (Occult Diabetes)

This condition is characterized by a delay in early insulin release from pancreatic B cells, resulting in initial exaggeration of hyperglycemia during a glucose tolerance test. In response to this hyperglycemia, an exaggerated insulin release produces a late hypoglycemia 4–5 hours after ingestion of glucose. These patients are usually quite different from those with early hypoglycemia, being more phlegmatic, often obese, and frequently having a family history of diabetes mellitus.

In obese patients, treatment is directed at weight reduction to achieve ideal weight. Like all patients with postprandial hypoglycemia, regardless of cause, these patients often respond to reduced carbohydrate intake with multiple, spaced, small feedings high in protein. They should be considered early diabetics and advised to have periodic medical evaluations.

## 4. ALCOHOL HYPOGLYCEMIA

### Fasting Hypoglycemia After Ethanol

During the postabsorptive state, normal plasma glucose is maintained by hepatic glucose output derived from both glycogenolysis and gluconeogenesis. With prolonged starvation, glycogen reserves become depleted within 18–24 hours and hepatic glucose output becomes totally dependent on gluconeogenesis. Under these circumstances, a blood concentration of ethanol as low as 45 mg/dL (considerably below the California legal "under the influence" level of 100 mg/dL) can induce profound hypoglycemia by blocking gluconeogenesis. Neuroglycopenia in a patient whose breath smells of alcohol may be mistaken for alcoholic stupor. Prevention consists of adequate food intake during ethanol ingestion and avoidance of excess ethanol, which could lead to vomiting or anorexia. Therapy consists of glucose administration to replenish glycogen stores until gluconeogenesis resumes.

## Postethanol Reactive Hypoglycemia

When sugar-containing soft drinks are used as mixers to dilute alcohol in beverages (gin and tonic, rum and cola), there seems to be a greater insulin release than when the soft drink alone is ingested and a tendency for more of a late hypoglycemic overswing to occur 3–4 hours later. Prevention would consist of avoiding sugar mixers while ingesting alcohol or ensuring supplementary food intake to provide sustained absorption.

## 5. FACTITIOUS HYPOGLYCEMIA

Factitious hypoglycemia may be difficult to document. A suspicion of self-induced hypoglycemia is supported when the patient is associated with the health professions or has access to insulin or sulfonylurea drugs taken by a diabetic member of the family. The triad of hypoglycemia, high immunoreactive insulin, and suppressed plasma C peptide immunoreactivity is pathognomonic of exogenous insulin administration. Demonstration of circulating antibodies supports this diagnosis in suspected cases. When sulfonylureas are suspected as a cause of factitious hypoglycemia, a chemical test of the plasma to detect the presence of these drugs may be required to distinguish laboratory findings from those of insulinoma.

## 6. IMMUNOPATHOLOGIC HYPOGLYCEMIA

This rare cause of hypoglycemia, documented in isolated case reports, may occur as 2 distinct disorders: one associated with spontaneous development of circulating anti-insulin antibodies and another associated with antibodies to insulin receptors, in which the antibodies apparently have agonist capabilities.

Casparie AF, Elving LD: Severe hypoglycemia in diabetic patients: Frequency, causes, prevention. *Diabetes Care* 1985;**8**:141.

Dons RF et al: Anomalous glucose and insulin responses in patients with insulinoma: Caveats for diagnosis. *Arch Intern Med* 1985;**145**:1861.

Fischer KF, Lees JA, Newman JH: Hypoglycemia in hospitalized patients: Causes and outcomes. *N Engl J Med* 1986;**315**:1245.

Merimee TJ: Insulin-like growth factors in patients with nonislet cell tumors and hypoglycemia. *Metabolism* 1986;**35**:360.

Rifkin MD, Weiss SM: Intraoperative sonographic identification of nonpalpable pancreatic masses. *J Ultrasound Med* 1984;**3**:409.

Ulbrecht JS et al: Insulinoma in a 94-year-old woman: Long-term therapy with verapamil. *Diabetes Care* 1986;**9**:186.

Unger RH: Insulin-glucagon relationships in the defense against hypoglycemia. *Diabetes* 1983;**32**:575.

Williams HE: Alcoholic hypoglycemia and ketoacidosis. *Med Clin North Am* 1984;**68**:33.

# DISTURBANCES OF LIPID METABOLISM

The principal circulating lipids in humans are of 4 types: (1) triglycerides, (2) free cholesterol, (3) cholesteryl esters, and (4) phospholipids. These are transported as spherical macromolecular complexes termed **lipoproteins,** wherein an inner core of hydrophobic lipids (triglycerides and cholesteryl esters) is encased by a membrane of unimolecular thickness consisting of various proteins (apolipoproteins, or simply apoproteins) in association with hydrophilic lipids (free cholesterol and phospholipids).

## Classification of Lipoproteins

Specific differences among the various lipoprotein classes depend on the amount each class contains of each of the 4 lipids (this affects their size and density) and on the nature of the apoprotein in their membrane. These differences allow for classification of lipoproteins on the basis of ultracentrifugal density, with those containing mostly triglyceride being termed **very low density lipoproteins (VLDL)** and those containing mostly cholesterol called **low-density lipoproteins (LDL);** when the total lipid content is slightly less than the weight of protein in the membrane, the density is **high (HDL).**

When classified on the basis of their mobility on paper electrophoresis, LDL are termed betalipoproteins; VLDL, prebetalipoproteins; and HDL, alphalipoproteins. These 3 classes of lipoproteins are normally present in fasting sera. Chylomicrons constitute a fourth class, normally present only after ingestion of fat. These are of such low density that they float even without centrifugation, and because of their large size and proportionately low protein content, they fail to migrate on paper electrophoresis.

## Metabolism
## of Lipoproteins

Chylomicrons, which carry ingested fat, and VLDL, which contain triglyceride converted from endogenous fatty acids and ingested carbohydrate, are transported in plasma to fat depots, where they are cleared by an enzyme, lipoprotein lipase, attached to capillary endothelium. The normal end products of both chylomicrons and VLDL are "remnant" particles of very low density that contain different B apoproteins in their membranes. The B apoprotein of chylomicron remnants (B-48) is smaller than that of VLDL remnants (B-100), and studies of apoprotein metabolism indicate that chylomicron remnants are completely metabolized by the liver, while VLDL remnants are further hydrolyzed by hepatic lipase and either removed by the liver or converted to LDL and then returned to the circulation. Low-density lipoproteins are responsible for transporting cholesteryl esters to peripheral tissues where the transported cholesterol can be used for membrane synthesis, thus sparing these tissues in their endogenous production

of cholesterol. High-density lipoproteins contribute to lipid transport by transferring apoprotein C-II to VLDL particles and chylomicrons, which activates lipoprotein lipase; they also participate in the removal of cholesterol either from aging cell membranes or from tissue deposits by providing apoprotein A-I, which activates a circulating enzyme, lecithin-cholesterol acyltransferase (LCAT). This produces cholesteryl esters that are subsequently removed by the HDL and either recycled via remnant lipoproteins and LDL for resynthesis of cell membrane or taken to the liver for excretion as biliary cholesterol or bile salts.

## Lipoprotein Disorders

An excess or deficiency of certain lipoproteins can result from primary genetic disorders or may be secondary to acquired metabolic dysfunction. Until more information becomes available to permit classification on the basis of cause, the use of electrophoresis to define various phenotypes has been accepted by WHO (Table 19–8). These phenotypes, together with their acquired (secondary) counterparts, probably in-

Table 19–8. Major categories of primary hyperlipidemia.*

| Type | Lipoprotein Abnormalities and Defect | Appearance of Serum† | Cholesterol Elevation‡ | Triglyceride Elevation‡ | Clinical Presentation | Rule Out |
|------|------|------|------|------|------|------|
| I | Fasting chylomicronemia (due to lipoprotein lipse or apoprotein C-II deficiency). Rare. | Creamy layer over clear infranate | Elevated (to about 10% of triglyceride level) | Often 1000–10,000 or more | Creamy blood, lipemic retina, eruptive xanthomas, hepatosplenomegaly, recurrent abdominal pain; onset in childhood. | Pancreatitis, diabetes. |
| IIA | Hyperbetalipoproteinemia (lack of a cell surface receptor involved in degrading LDL). Common. | Clear | Usually 300–600 but may be higher | None | Xanthelasma, tendon xanthomas, accelerated atherosclerosis; detectable in childhood. | Hypothyroidism, nephrotic syndrome, hepatic obstruction. |
| IIB | Familial combined lipidemia (both LDL and VLDL elevation). Quite common. | Turbid | Usually 250–600 | Usually 200–600 | Relatively common. Severe forms are like IIA; milder forms associated with obesity or diabetes. | Same as IIA. |
| III | Dysbetalipoproteinemia (lipidemia due to excess of remnants; apoprotein E abnormality). Rare. | Turbid | Highly variable (from near normal to over 1000) | Highly variable (175–1500 in same patient) | Planar xanthomas, tuberous xanthomas appear in adult. Relatively uncommon. Hyperglycemia, hyperuricemia. | Hepatic disease, diabetes. |
| IV | Hyperprebetalipoproteinemia (delay in clearance or overproduction of VLDL). Common. | Turbid | 300–800 | 200–5000 | Most common, usually in adults. Eruptive xanthomas; accelerated vascular disease, mild glucose intolerance, hyperuricemia. | Nephrotic syndrome, hypothyroidism, glycogen storage disease; oral contraceptives. |
| V | Mixed lipemia (both chylomicronemia and VLDL); defects similar to I and IV. Rare. | Creamy layer over turbid infranate | 300–1000 | Usually 500–10,000 or more | Adulthood mainly; recurrent abdominal pain, eruptive xanthomas, hepatosplenomegaly. | Insulin-deficient diabetes, pancreatitis, alcoholism. |

* Modified from Levy RI, Morganroth J, Rifkind BM: Treatment of hyperlipidemia. *N Engl J Med* 1974;**290**:1295.
† Refrigerated serum overnight at 4°C.
‡ mg/dL. Normal cholesterol, 150–250 mg/dL; triglycerides, <150 mg/dL.

clude the main types of hyperlipidemia seen clinically. These "types" should not be considered disease entities but may be useful for determining the most rational therapy.

### A. Primary Genetic Hyperlipoproteinemias:

**1. Type I hyperlipoproteinemia (hyperchylomicronemia; Bürger-Grütz disease)**–This autosomal recessive condition is the rarest form of familial hyperlipoproteinemia and is characterized by massive chylomicronemia when a patient is on a normal diet and complete disappearance of the chylomicronemia a few days after fat is eliminated from the diet. Postheparin lipolytic activity is absent in the serum in most cases, indicating that the defect is a deficiency of lipoprotein lipase. Several families have been reported to have a deficiency of C-II apoprotein, which interferes with normal activation of lipoprotein lipase and in the case of homozygotes results in marked hyperchylomicronemia. Lipemia retinalis is seen when serum triglycerides exceed 2500 mg/dL. Serum cholesterol is often quite high, since it accounts for as much as 10% of the weight of chylomicron particles; however, LDL cholesterol is subnormal. Spurious hyponatremia may result from displacement of plasma water by high fat content during routine blood sampling. Pancreatitis is the major hazard, and patients with this disorder may not have accelerated atherosclerosis despite hypercholesterolemia. The diagnosis is suspected in children with recurrent abdominal pain, especially when hepatosplenomegaly is present. Eruptive xanthomas and creamy serum that separates into a creamy supernate and a clear infranate confirm the diagnosis.

Treatment consists of a fat-restricted diet (10–20 g daily), and the response is usually good.

**2. Type IIA (hyperbetalipoproteinemia)**–This disorder results from the presence of defective LDL receptors in homozygotes and a reduced number of normal LDL receptors in heterozygotes; this interferes with clearance of betalipoproteins. This receptor defect also prevents normal feedback inhibition of cholesterol synthesis by cholesterol released after internalization of betalipoproteins. It is one of the commonest of familial hyperlipoproteinemias and is transmitted as an autosomal dominant, at least in the severe variety. Milder forms may be caused by dietary indiscretion. The major clinical manifestations of this disorder include an accelerated atherosclerosis, early myocardial infarction, and the presence of tendon xanthomas and xanthelasma. The diagnosis is based on hypercholesterolemia in the presence of clear serum after overnight incubation at 4 °C. Total serum cholesterol is elevated, with a normal serum triglyceride and normal HDL cholesterol level—indicating that LDL-cholesterol accounts for the elevated serum cholesterol. Dietary restriction of saturated fat and cholesterol is seldom of help in severe cases; vigorous measures, including oral administration of combinations of bile acid-binding resins with either nicotinic acid or with inhibitors of hydroxymethyl glutaryl-coenzyme A reductase have recently been shown to restore serum cholesterol to normal in highly compliant patients. Jejunoileal bypass surgery has been reported to reduce serum cholesterol by 50% or more but in general, this procedure has produced discouraging results. Chronic plasma-exchange therapy is expensive and inconvenient but can lower cholesterol and reduce the size of xanthomas. In mild cases, dietary management alone may be satisfactory.

**3. Type IIB (mixed hyperbeta- and hyperprebetalipoproteinemia)**–This familial combined hyperlipidemia is quite common and often alternates with the IIA pattern in affected relatives. In some cases, hyperlipidemia is particularly sensitive to caloric intake and the composition of the diet and may represent several different disorders. When the combined pattern is present in affected members, both the triglyceride/cholesterol ratio and the electrophoretic pattern are indistinguishable from those of type III disease, as is the character of serum turbidity after overnight incubation at 4 °C. Ultracentrifugal analysis confirms the diagnosis by showing both an LDL and a VLDL elevation, whereas in type III, a "floating beta" particle is obtained. Patients with this disorder are at high risk for coronary artery disease.

**4. Type III (hyper-"remnant"-lipoproteinemia; dysbetalipoproteinemia)**–This rare disorder results from absence of the apoprotein E-3, which normally activates hepatic lipase to clear chylomicron remnants and transforms VLDL remnants to LDL. In its place is an abnormal isoform (E-2) that binds poorly to hepatic lipase. This results in accumulation of lipoprotein remnants of intermediate density (IDL), which have flotation characteristics on ultracentrifugation in the lower range of VLDL but have the electrophoretic mobility of betalipoproteins (B-VLDL, or floating betas). A reduction in LDL concentration is a consequence of the impairment of VLDL-remnant catabolism and is characteristic of this disorder.

The genetic mode of transmission of dysbetalipoproteinemia suggests a mendelian-recessive trait; however, its expression as hyperlipidemia seems to require precipitating factors such as obesity or hypothyroidism. It occurs predominantly in adults and is rare in premenopausal women, since estrogens seem to reduce accumulation of the "remnant" particles. Patients are often obese and may have tuberous xanthomas, xanthelasma, and accelerated atherosclerosis. Planar xanthomas on the palms have been considered diagnostic. Treatment is especially gratifying in type III disease. Reduction to ideal weight in the obese patient and maintenance on a low-cholesterol diet may produce dramatic improvement, and total correction of hyperlipoproteinemia may result, especially in response to the addition of clofibrate, 1 g twice daily, to the dietary regimen. Estrogen therapy can also produce a dramatic increase in removal of these remnant particles, even though it does not affect the abnormal apoprotein E distribution.

**5. Type IV (hyperprebetalipoproteinemia)**–This type of lipemia is endogenous as compared to type I hyperlipoproteinemia and represents a failure in removal of prebetalipoproteins produced by the liver, either in normal amounts or excessively.

Since carbohydrate intake induces production of this lipoprotein from esterification of endogenous fatty acids, it has been termed carbohydrate-induced hyperlipemia. It is a common disorder, usually in adults, and often associated with caloric excess, obesity, and hyperuricemia. Chylomicronemia can occasionally develop, especially if alcohol or fat intake is excessive, and eruptive xanthomas may occur. Treatment is directed at weight reduction in the obese, avoiding high carbohydrate or alcohol intake and caloric excess. Although clofibrate, 1 g twice daily, is occasionally beneficial, recent concern about its long-term toxicity precludes its use in this disorder, where slight benefits do not justify the overall risk.

**6. Type V (mixed lipemia)–**This is a rare disorder wherein excessive prebetalipoproteins and chylomicrons are present. Onset is usually in early adult life and is characterized by recurrent abdominal pain, pancreatitis, hepatosplenomegaly, eruptive xanthomas, and glucose intolerance. The disorder is markedly aggravated by alcohol excess.

Therapy is similar to that for type IV except that fat restriction is necessary as in type I.

**B. Secondary Hyperlipoproteinemias:** In all cases of hyperlipoproteinemia, secondary forms should be ruled out before a diagnosis of primary genetic hyperlipoproteinemia is made. In uncontrolled diabetes mellitus, circulating levels of lipoprotein are often elevated along with glucose. Since lipoprotein lipase is an insulin-dependent enzyme, elevated levels of both chylomicrons and VLDL result from diabetes in which insulin levels are low (insulinopenic diabetes) or ineffective (insulin-insensitive diabetes). Replacement of deficient insulin or restriction of caloric intake to restore effectiveness of endogenous insulin in obese diabetics facilitates clearance of these lipoproteins. In addition, when lipemia is resolving after insulin replacement in insulin-deficient diabetics, an increase of betalipoproteins inevitably follows clearance of the larger triglyceride-carrying particles because of the much longer half-life of the betalipoproteins. Hyperbetalipoproteinemia is commonly a consequence of hypothyroidism or mild forms of nephrotic syndrome.

Hyperprebetalipoproteinemia and mixed lipemia can result from hypopituitarism, lipodystrophy, renal failure with azotemia, severe hypothyroidism, hypergammaglobulin disorders, or advanced nephrotic syndrome (with serum albumin below 2 g/dL). These lipemic manifestations are seen in genetically predisposed persons with mild diabetes mellitus or hyperestrogenemia (as in pregnancy or with oral contraceptive therapy) or in those who use alcohol excessively.

Dysbetalipoproteinemia can become apparent during hypothyroidism and revert to a latent state with thyroid replacement.

*Antihypertensive therapy and serum lipods.* Antihypertensive agents such as thiazide diuretics and β-adrenergic blockers have an adverse effect on serum lipids, tending so slightly raise serum levels of LDL cholesterol and triglycerides while at the same time lowering HDL cholesterol. Prazosin and clonidine have been reported to have a beneficial effect on serum lipids by lowering serum LDL cholesterol and triglycerides while raising levels of HDL cholesterol. Angiotensin-converting enzyme inhibitors, calcium channel blockers, and captopril have no demonstrable effects on serum lipids.

## Relationship of Lipoproteins to Atheroma (Fig 19–2)

Studies suggest that the arterial wall intima is permeable to small molecular complexes in inverse proportion to their size. Elastin, a component of arterial wall, has a demonstrable affinity for apoprotein B, which is present on all lipoproteins except HDL. Accordingly, small lipoproteins such as HDL, LDL, and certain of the smaller VLDL and remnants may enter through defects and tears in the intimal walls of arteries, where all except HDL adhere to elastin, which retards their exit and allows their accumulation. This would explain why chylomicrons, owing to their large size, are not considered atherogenic in type I disorders despite severe hypercholesterolemia and why hypertension, aging, and hyperlipidemia, either individually or (especially) in combination, could exaggerate normal atherogenic processes.

A number of recent studies have documented a consistent negative correlation between plasma concentration of HDL cholesterol and clinically evident atherosclerosis. In its transit through the wall of the artery, HDL may incorporate cholesteryl esters into its central core for recycling onto cell membranes or for transport to excretory systems in the liver. The presumed role of HDL in clearing cholesterol from tissues may account for the observed increase in risk of atherosclerosis when HDL levels are rela-

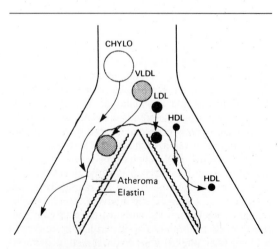

**Figure 19–2.** Lipoproteins and atheromas.

tively low, as in obesity, diabetes, and hyperlipidemic disorders and in males, especially when physically inactive. Conversely, in persons with a lower than normal risk of atherosclerosis, such as chronic alcoholics, women of childbearing age, and marathon runners, there is a high level of HDL. The "scavenger" role of HDL in clearing cholesterol from tissues could slow down atherogenesis and thereby contribute to the apparent protective effect of high plasma HDL in relation to atherosclerosis.

## Diagnostic Evaluation of Hypercholesterolemia:

In most adult patients, a fasting serum cholesterol measurement is indicated. In those at high risk, such as relatives of patients with a strongly positive family history of myocardial infarction, children as well as other adult members of the family should be screened. If the total serum cholesterol is above 200 mg/dL, a further assessment by measuring a repeat serum cholesterol along with an HDL cholesterol and a serum triglyceride measurement would permit indirect estimation of the LDL cholesterol concentration based on the following approach: After an overnight fast, total serum cholesterol is generally composed of the cholesterol contained within 3 major lipoprotein particles: LDL, HDL, and VLDL. HDL cholesterol can readily be measured in most clinical laboratories using a simple modification of the same assay used to quantitate the total serum cholesterol. The VLDL cholesterol must be indirectly estimated as follows: In the average-sized VLDL particle, there is a ratio of 5:1 (by weight) of triglyceride to cholesterol. Thus, it is possible to estimate the VLDL cholesterol content by taking one-fifth of the serum triglyceride value. This estimate is inapplicable in 2 situations: chylomicrons have higher ratios (8:10) of triglyceride to cholesterol, and in the rare type III disorder, remnant particles have a lower ratio of 1:1 or 2:1.

When fasting levels of triglycerides are moderately elevated in the serum in association with an elevated serum cholesterol to give a triglyceride:cholesterol ratio of 1:1 or 2:1, the most probable diagnosis statistically is the mixed hyperlipidemic disorder familial combined hyperlipidemia, characterized by elevation of both LDL and VLDL, rather than the rare type III disorder characterized by increased numbers of remnant particles. Although certain clinical features such as distinctive planar xanthomas may identify the patient with dysbetalipoproteinemia, for a definite laboratory diagnosis, analytic ultracentrifugation with fractionation of the various lipoproteins is helpful in distinguishing these 2 disorders. Similarly, genetic analysis of DNA for the presence of alleles for apoprotein $E_2$ is informative or diagnostic.

As long as fasting serum triglyceride levels are below 600–800 mg/dL (lower than would be expected from chylomicronemia) and there are no clinical suggestions of dysbetalipoproteinemia (type III), the following equation provides an indirect estimate of LDL cholesterol ($LDL_c$):

$$LDL_c = \text{Total cholesterol} - HDL_c + \frac{\text{Serum triglyceride}}{5}$$

Values of LDL cholesterol above 150 mg/dL in adults would generally increase risk factors to a degree that would justify a recommendation for a modified diet initially and, if this is not effective, consideration of a subsequent trial of drug therapy—assuming that secondary causes of LDL elevation are not identified.

## Treatment

Treatment of the secondary hyperlipoproteinemias consists, where possible, of treatment of the primary disorder, eg, hypothyroidism, nephrotic syndrome, obstructive jaundice, or estrogen excess due to use of oral contraceptives. In primary hyperlipoproteinemia, no one diet is effective in all the lipid transport disorders. Similarly, none of the pharmacologic agents are universally effective. An understanding of lipid transport mechanisms and drug actions has improved the therapeutic approach to the hyperlipidemic patient.

**A. Diet Therapy:** When chylomicrons are elevated, total fat intake should be reduced (including polyunsaturated fats). In all other hyperlipidemias, certain general principles apply: Calories are restricted to achieve or maintain ideal body weight; alcohol is avoided; and daily cholesterol intake is limited to 300 mg, which results in an increase in high-affinity LDL receptors on cell membranes. Reduction of saturated fatty acids in the diet to no more than 10% of the total caloric intake is recommended, with a shift of the ratio of polyunsaturated to saturated fatty acid from the usual 1:5 to 2:1. Unsaturated fats improve palatability when saturated fats have to be restricted and may have a beneficial role in reducing platelet factors that promote an increased coagulability of blood.

Recently, epidemiologic studies from the Netherlands indicate that over a 20-year follow-up period, mortality rates from coronary heart disease were more than 50% lower among those who consumed at least 30 g of fish per day than in those who did not eat fish. Moreover, a specific triglyceride-lowering effect has been produced by dietary fish oils containing highly unsaturated fatty acids of the omega-3 family (in which the first of 5 or 6 double bonds begins at the third carbon from the methyl terminal). Remarkable improvement of hypertriglyceridemia in type IIb patients as well as in type V hyperlipemic patients occurred after salmon fillets and fish oil supplements were included in their diet for 4 weeks. Vegetable oil (containing omega-6 linoleic acid) had much less effect in type IIb patients and actually increased the triglyceride levels in type V patients. Application of these principles of diet to the general population as a means of reducing the risk of atherosclerosis remains a controversial subject.

**B. Hypolipidemic Drugs:** Several major classes of drugs are currently in use:

**1. Nicotinic acid**—Nicotinic acid reduces lipolysis and diminishes production of VLDL and is equally effective at lowering LDL. The dosage is 100 mg 3 times daily initially, gradually building up to a level of 3–7 g daily taken with meals. Cutaneous flushing and pruritus, as well as gastrointestinal upsets, are major side effects, but the flushing is transient and readily tolerated if the patient is warned to anticipate it. Aspirin may help alleviate flushing. Nicotinic acid is particularly useful in primary hyperbetalipoproteinemia when combined with resins that bind bile acids, but it may be effective in all types of primary hyperlipoproteinemia except type I.

**2. Clofibrate (chlorphenoxyisobutyrate)**–Clofibrate has many known effects in the body and both decreases the synthesis of VLDL and increases its catabolism. It is most effective in type III remnant excess but is of occasional value also in disorders with increased VLDL (IIB, IV, V). In cases of hyperbetalipoproteinemia, its effects have been less impressive. The dosage is 1.5–2 g daily. Side effects are few, but myositis has been reported, especially if hypoalbuminemia is present, as in lipidemia associated with nephrotic syndrome. Pharmacokinetic interactions with anticoagulants may occur. A major risk is increased frequency of cholelithiasis and a possible association with gastrointestinal cancer. The National Collaborative Coronary Drug Project in the USA showed no beneficial effects of clofibrate on mortality rates in men recovering from myocardial infarction; in fact, more arrhythmias occurred in those receiving this drug. Although an international WHO study of 5000 men documented its slight efficacy in reducing the incidence of nonfatal myocardial infarctions, use of clofibrate was associated with a 36% greater mortality rate due to noncardiovascular causes. For these reasons, West Germany has banned the drug, and in the USA the FDA has recommended label revision to include a special warning on clofibrate's risk.

**3. Gemfibrozil**–Gemfibrozil is an analog of clofibrate. Its action is similar to that of clofibrate in reducing very high serum triglyceride concentrations that do not respond to usual dietary measures. In doses of 1200 mg/d (two 300-mg tablets before breakfast and dinner), gemfibrozil inhibits lipolysis in adipose tissue and decreases fat uptake by the liver. This has been found to reduce hepatic triglyceride synthesis and lower VLDL triglycerides. It also stimulates synthesis of HDL particles to raise plasma HDL levels, but it is of little use in lowering LDL cholesterol levels in cases of hypercholesterolemia. Its long-term safety has not yet been established.

**4. Resins to absorb bile acids (cholestyramine, colestipol)**–Cholestyramine is an insoluble resin that absorbs bile acids and is thus able to increase cholesterol catabolism and enhance LDL removal. It is not very palatable, and 16–32 g/d is required in 2–4 divided doses, preferably in orange juice or applesauce. Gastrointestinal side effects, especially constipation, are common. Similar doses of colestipol, a recently introduced resin, are as effective as cholestyramine while being more palatable. VLDL

excess is not helped and may be aggravated by these agents. They are the drugs of choice in treating types IIA and IIB, particularly when combined with nicotinic acid. In a recent prospective cross-over trial of patients with type IIA hypercholesterolemia, combined therapy with colestipol and nicotinic acid resulted in complete and sustained normalization of LDL levels.

**5. Probucol**–Probucol is reported to modestly lower serum cholesterol levels by as yet undefined mechanisms. Cardiotoxicity in animals and reduction of HDL cholesterol levels in addition to LDL cholesterol levels make further trials necessary before the benefit-to-risk ratio can be properly assessed.

**6. HMG-CoA reductase inhibitors**–Fugure therapy for patients with elevated LDL cholesterol will soon include drugs that competitively inhibit HMG-CoA reductase, the rate-limiting enzyme in cholesterol biosynthesis. Reduction in biosynthesis of cholesterol induces increased numbers of high-affinity LDL receptors on cell membranes which result in increased clearance of LDL from serum. In homozygous cases of familial hyperbetalipoproteinemia, these agents are ineffective owing to the absence of functioning LDL receptors. However, in heterozygotes, clinical trials have shown them to be quite effective in lowering LDL cholesterol as much as 40% in conjunction with diet and as much as 65% when combined with other drugs such as nicotinic acid or bile sequestrants. Side effects are surprisingly minimal, with only myositis reported in approximately 0.5% and subclinical serum transaminase elevations in 1.5%. FDA approval for lovastatin (mevinolin; Mevacor) was given in 1987 and is pending for several similar analogs.

Grundy SM, Vega GL, Bilheimer DW: Influence of combined therapy with mevinolin and interruption of bile-acid reabsorption on low density lipoproteins in heterozygous familial hypercholesterolemia. *Ann Intern Med* 1985;**103:**339.

Havel RJ: Functional activities of hepatic lipoprotein receptors. *Annu Rev Physiol* 1986;**48:**119.

Havel RJ, Yamada N, Shames DM: Role of apolipoprotein E in lipoprotein metabolism. *Am Heart J* 1987;**113:**470.

Hoeg JM, Gregg RE, Brewer HB Jr: An approach to the management of hyperlipoproteinemia. *JAMA* 1986;**255:**512.

Kane JP, Havel RJ: Treatment of hypercholesterolemia. *Annu Rev Med* 1986;**37:**427.

Kromhout D, Bosschieter EB, Coulander CD: The inverse relation between fish consumption and 20-year mortality from coronary heart disease. *N Engl J Med* 1985;**312:**1205.

The Lovastatin Study Group: Therapeutic response to lovastatin in non-familial hypercholesterolemia. *JAMA* 1986;**256:**2829.

Nikkila EA et al: Prevention of progression of coronary atherosclerosis by treatment of hyperlipidemia: A seven-year prospective angiographic study. *Br Med J* 1984;**289:**207.

Phillipson BE et al: Reduction of plasma lipids, lipoproteins, and apoproteins by dietary fish oils in patients with hypertriglyceridemia. *N Engl J Med* 1985;**312:**1210.

Rohlfing JJ, Brunzell JD: The effects of diuretics and adrenergic-blocking agents on plasma lipids. *West J Med* 1986;**145:**210.

Taylor WC et al: Cholesterol reduction and life expectancy: A model incorporating multiple risk factors. *Ann Intern Med* 1987;**106:**605.

Tran ZV, Weltman A: Differential effects of exercise on serum lipid and lipoprotein levels seen with changes in body weight: A meta-analysis. *JAMA* 1985;**254:**919.

Weinberger MH: Antihypertensive therapy and lipids: Evidence, mechanisms, and implications. *Arch Intern Med* 1985;**145:**1102.

Williams RR et al: Evidence that men with familial hypercholesterolemia can avoid early coronary death. *JAMA* 1986;**255:**219.

## REFERENCES

Alberti KGMM, Krall LP (editors): *The Diabetes Annual II.* Elsevier, 1987.

Bergman M (editor): *Principles of Diabetes Management.* Medical Examination, 1987.

Felig P et al (editors): *Endocrinology and Metabolism,* 2nd ed. McGraw-Hill, 1987.

Keen H, Jarrett J (editors): *Complications of Diabetes,* 2nd ed. Arnold, 1982.

Kohler PO (editor): *Clinical Endocrinology.* Wiley, 1986.

Marble A et al (editors): *Joslin's Diabetes Mellitus,* 12th ed. Lea & Febiger, 1985.

Pickup JC (editor): *Brittle Diabetes.* Blackwell Mosby, 1985.

Rifkin H (editor): *The Physician's Guide to Type II Diabetes (NIDDM): Diagnosis and Treatment.* American Diabetes Association, 1984.

Schilfgaarde RV, Persijn GG, Sutherland DER: *Organ Transplantation in Diabetics.* Grune & Stratton, 1984.

Wilson JD, Foster DW (editors): *Williams Textbook of Endocrinology,* 7th ed. Saunders, 1985.

# 20

# Nutrition

*Robert B. Baron, MD*

## NUTRITIONAL REQUIREMENTS

Approximately 40 nutrients are required by the human body. Nutrients are considered essential if they cannot be synthesized by the body and if a deficiency causes recognizable abnormalities that disappear when the deficit is corrected. Required nutrients include the essential amino acids, water-soluble vitamins, fat-soluble vitamins, minerals, and the essential fatty acids. The body also requires an adequate energy substrate, a small amount of metabolizable carbohydrate, indigestible carbohydrate (fiber), additional nitrogen, and water.

Most of the required nutrients are harmful when consumed in excessive amounts. Thus, a range of acceptable intake levels can be established for most of them.

Nutritional requirements are most commonly expressed as the average daily amounts of nutrients a population group should consume. Requirements for any given individual cannot be stated, because of the great range of biologic variability. In the USA, the most widely used estimates of nutritional requirements are the Recommended Dietary Allowances (RDAs)—"the levels of intake of essential nutrients considered, in the judgment of the Committee on Dietary Allowances of the Food and Nutrition Board [of the National Academy of Sciences] on the basis of available scientific knowledge, to be adequate to meet the known nutritional requirements of practically all healthy persons."

RDAs have been established for energy and protein; the water-soluble vitamins thiamine, riboflavin, niacin, folacin, and vitamin $B_{12}$; the fat-soluble vitamins A, D, and E; and the minerals calcium, phosphorus, magnesium, iron, zinc, and iodine (Table 20–1).

The RDA Committee has also established "estimated safe and adequate intakes" for 12 additional nutrients. These include vitamin K, pantothenic acid, and biotin; the trace elements copper, chromium, fluoride, manganese, molybdenum, and selenium; and the electrolytes sodium, potassium, and chloride (Table 20–2).

The RDAs exceed the actual requirements of most individuals in the population because they are stated as 2 standard deviations above the estimated mean requirement. Therefore, a dietary intake of less than the RDA of a specific nutrient is not necessarily inadequate for a given individual—it increases the *risk* of an inadequate intake. For most clinical situations, two-thirds of the RDA is considered an adequate nutritional intake.

The RDAs for energy are treated in a different manner. Because energy needs vary so greatly among individuals, the RDA Committee sets forth estimates of the average needs of the population rather than recommended intakes for individuals. About half of the population will require more energy than the RDA and half will require less.

Nutritional requirements vary not only from one individual to the next but from one day to the next in any given subject. They differ also with age, sex, and body size and during pregnancy and lactation. Different RDAs have been developed for different age and sex groups. Requirements vary also with such clinical circumstances as premature birth, aging, metabolic disorders, infections, chronic illness, medications, extremes of climate and physical activity, and the route of ingestion. The RDAs do not cover such situations—they are intended only for healthy populations.

The RDAs represent recommendations based on the best information available. They are updated approximately every 5 years.

Other Western nations have established similar recommendations which in some instances are considerably different from those developed for the USA.

## ENERGY

The human body requires energy to support normal functions and physical activity, growth, and repair of damaged tissues. Energy is provided by oxidation of dietary protein, fat, carbohydrate, and alcohol. Oxidation of 1 g of each provides 4 kcal of energy from protein and carbohydrate, 9 kcal from fat, and 7 kcal from alcohol.

Energy requirements vary greatly between individuals even under basal conditions. Age, size, sex, growth, physical activity, environmental factors, and disease all affect energy requirements.

In healthy individuals, energy expenditure is primarily determined by 3 factors: basal energy expendi-

**Table 20–1.** Recommended daily dietary allowances.[1] (Revised 1980.) Designed for the maintenance of good nutrition of practically all healthy people in the USA.

| | | Weight | | Height | | | Fat-Soluble Vitamins | | | Water-Soluble Vitamins | | | | | | | Minerals | | | | | |
|---|---|---|---|---|---|---|---|---|---|---|---|---|---|---|---|---|---|---|---|---|---|---|
| Age (years) | | (kg) | (lb) | (cm) | (in) | Protein (g) | Vita-min A (μg RE)[2] | Vita-min D (μg)[3] | Vita-min E (mg α-TE)[4] | Vita-min C (mg) | Thia-min (mg) | Ribo-flavin (mg) | Niacin (mg NE)[5] | Vita-min B6 (mg) | Fola-cin[6] (μg) | Vita-min B12 (μg) | Cal-cium (mg) | Phos-phorus (mg) | Magne-sium (mg) | Iron (mg) | Zinc (mg) | Iodine (μg) |
| Infants | 0.0–0.5 | 6 | 13 | 60 | 24 | kg × 2.2 | 420 | 10 | 3 | 35 | 0.3 | 0.4 | 6 | 0.3 | 30 | 0.5[7] | 360 | 240 | 50 | 10 | 3 | 40 |
| | 0.5–1.0 | 9 | 20 | 71 | 28 | kg × 2.0 | 400 | 10 | 4 | 35 | 0.5 | 0.6 | 8 | 0.6 | 45 | 1.5 | 540 | 360 | 70 | 15 | 5 | 50 |
| Children | 1–3 | 13 | 29 | 90 | 35 | 23 | 400 | 10 | 5 | 45 | 0.7 | 0.8 | 9 | 0.9 | 100 | 2.0 | 800 | 800 | 150 | 15 | 10 | 70 |
| | 4–6 | 20 | 44 | 112 | 44 | 30 | 500 | 10 | 6 | 45 | 0.9 | 1.0 | 11 | 1.3 | 200 | 2.5 | 800 | 800 | 200 | 10 | 10 | 90 |
| | 7–10 | 28 | 62 | 132 | 52 | 34 | 700 | 10 | 7 | 45 | 1.2 | 1.4 | 16 | 1.6 | 300 | 3.0 | 800 | 800 | 250 | 10 | 10 | 120 |
| Males | 11–14 | 45 | 99 | 157 | 62 | 45 | 1000 | 10 | 8 | 50 | 1.4 | 1.6 | 18 | 1.8 | 400 | 3.0 | 1200 | 1200 | 350 | 18 | 15 | 150 |
| | 15–18 | 66 | 145 | 176 | 69 | 56 | 1000 | 10 | 10 | 60 | 1.4 | 1.7 | 18 | 2.0 | 400 | 3.0 | 1200 | 1200 | 400 | 18 | 15 | 150 |
| | 19–22 | 70 | 154 | 177 | 70 | 56 | 1000 | 7.5 | 10 | 60 | 1.5 | 1.7 | 19 | 2.2 | 400 | 3.0 | 800 | 800 | 350 | 10 | 15 | 150 |
| | 23–50 | 70 | 154 | 178 | 70 | 56 | 1000 | 5 | 10 | 60 | 1.4 | 1.6 | 18 | 2.2 | 400 | 3.0 | 800 | 800 | 350 | 10 | 15 | 150 |
| | 51+ | 70 | 154 | 178 | 70 | 56 | 1000 | 5 | 10 | 60 | 1.2 | 1.4 | 16 | 2.2 | 400 | 3.0 | 800 | 800 | 350 | 10 | 15 | 150 |
| Females | 11–14 | 46 | 101 | 157 | 62 | 46 | 800 | 10 | 8 | 50 | 1.1 | 1.3 | 15 | 1.8 | 400 | 3.0 | 1200 | 1200 | 300 | 18 | 15 | 150 |
| | 15–18 | 55 | 120 | 163 | 64 | 46 | 800 | 10 | 8 | 60 | 1.1 | 1.3 | 14 | 2.0 | 400 | 3.0 | 1200 | 1200 | 300 | 18 | 15 | 150 |
| | 19–22 | 55 | 120 | 163 | 64 | 44 | 800 | 7.5 | 8 | 60 | 1.1 | 1.3 | 14 | 2.0 | 400 | 3.0 | 800 | 800 | 300 | 18 | 15 | 150 |
| | 23–50 | 55 | 120 | 163 | 64 | 44 | 800 | 5 | 8 | 60 | 1.0 | 1.2 | 13 | 2.0 | 400 | 3.0 | 800 | 800 | 300 | 18 | 15 | 150 |
| | 51+ | 55 | 120 | 163 | 64 | 44 | 800 | 5 | 8 | 60 | 1.0 | 1.2 | 13 | 2.0 | 400 | 3.0 | 800 | 800 | 300 | 10 | 15 | 150 |
| Pregnant | | | | | | +30 | +200 | +5 | +2 | +20 | +0.4 | +0.3 | +2 | +0.6 | +400 | +1.0 | +400 | +400 | +150 | 8 | +5 | +25 |
| Lactating | | | | | | +20 | +400 | +5 | +3 | +40 | +0.5 | +0.5 | +5 | +0.5 | +100 | +1.0 | +400 | +400 | +150 | 8 | +10 | +50 |

Reference: *Recommended Dietary Allowances*, 9th ed. Food and Nutrition Board, National Research Council—National Academy of Sciences, 1980.

[1] The allowances are intended to provide for individual variations among most normal persons as they live in the United States under usual environmental stresses. Diets should be based on a variety of common foods in order to provide other nutrients for which human requirements have been less well defined.

[2] Retinol equivalents. 1 retinol equivalent = 1 μg retinol or 6 μg β-carotene.

[3] As cholecalciferol. 10 μg cholecalciferol = 400 IU of vitamin D.

[4] α-Tocopherol equivalents. 1 mg α-tocopherol = 1 α-TE.

[5] 1 NE (niacin equivalent) is equal to 1 mg of niacin or 60 mg of dietary tryptophan.

[6] The folacin allowances refer to dietary sources as determined by *Lactobacillus casei* assay after treatment with enzymes (conjugases) to make polyglutamyl forms of the vitamin available to the test organism.

[7] The recommended dietary allowance for vitamin $B_{12}$ in infants is based on average concentration of the vitamin in human milk. The allowances after weaning are based on energy intake (as recommended by the American Academy of Pediatrics) and consideration of other factors, such as intestinal absorption.

[8] The increased requirement during pregnancy cannot be met by the iron content of habitual North American diets or by the existing iron stores of many women; therefore, the use of 30–60 mg of supplemental iron is recommended. Iron needs during lactation are not substantially different from those of nonpregnant women, but continued supplementation of the mother for 2–3 months after parturition is advisable in order to replenish stores depleted by pregnancy.

**Table 20–2.** Estimated safe and adequate daily dietary intakes of selected vitamins and minerals.*

| | Age (years) | Vitamins | | | Trace Elements | | | | | | Electrolytes | | |
|---|---|---|---|---|---|---|---|---|---|---|---|---|---|
| | | Vitamin K (μg) | Biotin (μg) | Pantothenic Acid (mg) | Copper (mg) | Manganese (mg) | Fluoride (mg) | Chromium (mg) | Selenium (mg) | Molybdenum (mg) | Sodium (mg) | Potassium (mg) | Chloride (mg) |
| Infants | 0–0.5 | 12 | 35 | 2 | 0.5–0.7 | 0.5–0.7 | 0.1–0.5 | 0.01–0.04 | 0.01–0.04 | 0.03–0.06 | 115–350 | 350–925 | 275–700 |
| | 0.5–1 | 10–20 | 50 | 3 | 0.7–1.0 | 0.7–1.0 | 0.2–1.0 | 0.02–0.06 | 0.02–0.06 | 0.04–0.08 | 250–750 | 425–1275 | 400–1200 |
| Children and adolescents | 1–3 | 15–30 | 65 | 3 | 1.0–1.5 | 1.0–1.5 | 0.5–1.5 | 0.02–0.08 | 0.02–0.08 | 0.05–0.1 | 325–975 | 550–1650 | 500–1500 |
| | 4–6 | 20–40 | 85 | 3–4 | 1.5–2.0 | 1.5–2.0 | 1.0–2.5 | 0.03–0.12 | 0.03–0.12 | 0.06–0.15 | 450–1350 | 775–2325 | 700–2100 |
| | 7–10 | 30–60 | 120 | 4–5 | 2.0–2.5 | 2.0–3.0 | 1.5–2.5 | 0.05–0.2 | 0.05–0.2 | 0.10–0.3 | 600–1800 | 1000–3000 | 925–2775 |
| | 11+ | 50–100 | 100–200 | 4–7 | 2.0–3.0 | 2.5–5.0 | 1.5–2.5 | 0.05–0.2 | 0.05–0.2 | 0.15–0.5 | 900–2700 | 1525–4575 | 1400–4200 |
| Adults | | 70–140 | 100–200 | 4–7 | 2.0–3.0 | 2.5–5.0 | 1.5–4.0 | 0.05–0.2 | 0.05–0.2 | 0.15–0.5 | 1100–3300 | 1875–5625 | 1700–5100 |

* From: *Recommended Dietary Allowances*, 9th ed. Food and Nutrition Board, National Research Council—National Academy of Sciences, 1980.

ture (BEE), diet-induced thermogenesis (DIT), and physical activity.

The BEE is the amount of energy required to maintain basic physiologic functions. It is measured under a defined set of cirumstances. The subject must be in a warm room, awake, and at rest and must not have eaten for 12 hours. In healthy persons, the BEE can be estimated by the Harris-Benedict equation:

For men,

$$BEE = 66 + (13.7 \times \text{weight in kg}) + (5 \times \text{height in cm}) - (6.8 \times \text{age in years})$$

For women,

$$BEE = 655 + (9.5 \times \text{weight in kg}) + (1.7 \times \text{height in cm}) - (4.7 \times \text{age in years})$$

The Harris-Benedict equation will correctly predict measured BEE in 90% ± 10% of healthy subjects. In clinical practice, patients rarely meet the strict criteria for basal status. Energy expenditure measured in individuals at rest without food for 2 hours is the resting metabolic expenditure (RME) and is about 10% greater than BEE.

Diet-induced thermogenesis (DIT) is the amount of energy expended during and following the ingestion of food. The precise cause of this increase in energy expenditure is still uncertain. DIT averages approximately 10% of the BEE.

Physical activity has a major impact on energy expenditure. The average energy expenditure per hour by adults engaged in typical activities is shown in Table 20–3.

Daily recommended energy intakes for healthy individuals are shown in Table 20–4.

## PROTEIN

Protein is required for growth and for maintenance of body structure and function. Although the nutritional requirement is commonly stated in grams of protein, the true requirement is for 9 **essential amino**

**acids** plus additional nitrogen for protein synthesis. The essential amino acids are leucine, isoleucine, lysine, methionine, phenylalanine, threonine, tryptophan, valine, and histidine.

Adequate protein must be consumed each day to replace essential amino acids lost through protein turnover. On a protein-free diet, the average male loses 3.8 g of nitrogen per day—equivalent to 24 g of protein. Allowing for differences in protein quality and utilization and for individual variability, the RDA for protein is 56 g/d for men and 45 g/d for women.

Amino acids are required by the body in a specific pattern very similar to that found in egg protein. Proteins that most closely resemble this pattern are commonly referred to as "high-quality" (milk, eggs, other animal proteins), while others with lower amounts of one or more amino acids are considered to be of "lower quality" (seeds, grains, other vegetable proteins). Actually, the amino acid composition of various food proteins represents a continuum of quality. Proteins of "lower quality" can be ingested with other "low-quality" proteins to provide amounts of deficient amino acids sufficient to make up a protein intake of high quality.

Protein and energy requirements are closely related. Diets that provide insufficient energy will require additional protein to maintain nitrogen equilibrium.

## CARBOHYDRATE

As long as adequate energy and protein are provided in the diet, there is no specific requirement for dietary carbohydrate. A small amount of carbohydrate—approximately 100 g/d—is necessary to prevent ketosis. In practice, however, most dietary energy should be provided by carbohydrate. In the USA, the average diet contains 45% of calories as carbohydrate. Current recommendations are to increase carbohydrate intakes to 55–60% of total calories in the diet.

Dietary carbohydrates include simple sugars, complex carbohydrates (starches), and undigestible car-

**Table 20–3.** Average energy calories expended per hour by adults at selected weights engaged in various activities.*

| Activity | 54 kg (120 lbs) | 64 kg (140 lbs) | 73 kg (160 lbs) | 82 kg (180 lbs) | 91 kg (200 lbs) | 100 kg (220 lbs) |
|---|---|---|---|---|---|---|
| Sleeping: Reclining | 50 | 58 | 69 | 78 | 86 | 99 |
| Very light: Sitting | 73 | 83 | 103 | 115 | 127 | 150 |
| Light: Walking on level, shopping, light housekeeping | 143 | 166 | 200 | 225 | 250 | 290 |
| Moderate: Cycling, dancing, skiing, tennis | 226 | 262 | 307 | 345 | 382 | 430 |
| Heavy: Walking uphill, shoveling, swimming, playing basketball or football | 440 | 512 | 598 | 670 | 746 | 840 |

*Note:* Range of rate of expenditure of calories per minute of activity (for a 70-kg man or a 58-kg woman): Sleeping, 0.9–1.2; very light, 1.5–2.5; light, 2–4.9; moderate, 5–7.4; heavy, 6–12.
* Data from: *Recommended Dietary Allowances*, 9th ed. National Academy of Sciences—National Research Council, 1980. Adapted from McArdle WD, Katch FI, Katch VL: *Exercise Physiology: Energy, Nutrition and Human Performance.* Lea & Febiger, 1981.

**Table 20–4.** Mean heights and weights and recommended energy intake.*

| Category | Age (years) | Weight (kg) | Weight (lb) | Height (cm) | Height (in) | Energy Needs (With Range) (kcal) | | Energy Needs (With Range) (MJ) |
|---|---|---|---|---|---|---|---|---|
| Infants | 0.0–0.5 | 6 | 13 | 60 | 24 | kg × 115 | (95–145) | kg × 0.48 |
|  | 0.5–1.0 | 9 | 20 | 71 | 28 | kg × 105 | (80–135) | kg × 0.44 |
| Children | 1–3 | 13 | 29 | 90 | 35 | 1300 | (900–1800) | 5.5 |
|  | 4–6 | 20 | 44 | 112 | 44 | 1700 | (1300–2300) | 7.1 |
|  | 7–10 | 28 | 62 | 132 | 52 | 2400 | (1650–3300) | 10.1 |
| Males | 11–14 | 45 | 99 | 157 | 62 | 2700 | (2000–3700) | 11.3 |
|  | 15–18 | 66 | 145 | 176 | 69 | 2800 | (2100–3900) | 11.8 |
|  | 19–22 | 70 | 154 | 177 | 70 | 2900 | (2500–3300) | 12.2 |
|  | 23–50 | 70 | 154 | 178 | 70 | 2700 | (2300–3100) | 11.3 |
|  | 51–75 | 70 | 154 | 178 | 70 | 2400 | (2000–2800) | 10.1 |
|  | 76+ | 70 | 154 | 178 | 70 | 2050 | (1650–2450) | 8.6 |
| Females | 11–14 | 46 | 101 | 157 | 62 | 2200 | (1500–3000) | 9.2 |
|  | 15–18 | 55 | 120 | 163 | 64 | 2100 | (1200–3000) | 8.8 |
|  | 19–22 | 55 | 120 | 163 | 64 | 2100 | (1700–2500) | 8.8 |
|  | 23–50 | 55 | 120 | 163 | 64 | 2000 | (1600–2400) | 8.4 |
|  | 51–75 | 55 | 120 | 163 | 64 | 1800 | (1400–2200) | 7.6 |
|  | 76+ | 55 | 120 | 163 | 64 | 1600 | (1200–2000) | 6.7 |
| Pregnancy |  |  |  |  |  | +300 |  |  |
| Lactation |  |  |  |  |  | +500 |  |  |

* From: *Recommended Dietary Allowances,* 9th ed. Food and Nutrition Board, National Research Council—National Academy of Sciences, 1980.

bohydrates (dietary fiber). Although simple sugars and complex carbohydrates provide equal amounts of calories, the bulk of dietary carbohydrates should be derived from starches. Sugars—particularly sucrose—are concentrated sources of calories without other sources of essential nutrients. Sucrose consumption is also thought to be an important factor in the development of tooth decay. Complex carbohydrates, when unrefined, provide carbohydrate calories and vitamins, minerals, and dietary fiber.

Dietary fiber is that portion of plant foods that cannot be digested by the human intestine. Fiber increases the bulk of the stool and facilitates excretion. Epidemiologic evidence suggests that diets high in dietary fiber are associated with a lower incidence of digestive diseases. The ingestion of dietary fiber also results in lower blood sugar levels in diabetics and in lower serum cholesterol levels.

## FAT

Dietary fat is the most concentrated source of food energy. Like energy from dietary carbohydrate, energy derived from fat can support protein synthesis. Dietary fat also provides the essential fatty acid linoleic acid. Other than the need for adequate quantities of linoleic acid, there is no specific requirement for dietary fat as long as the diet provides adequate nutrients oxidizable for energy. Although the average American diet contains 40% of calories as fat, current recommendations are to limit dietary fat to 30% or less of total calories. Diets containing as little as 5–10% of total calories as fat appear to be safe and well tolerated.

Dietary fats are composed chiefly of fatty acids and dietary cholesterol. Fatty acids contain either no double bonds (saturated), one double bond (monounsaturated), or more than one double bond (polyunsaturated). Typical American diets contain predominantly saturated fatty acids. Current recommendations are to equalize the intake of saturated, monounsaturated, and polyunsaturated fatty acids. Saturated fatty acids are associated with increased dietary cholesterol, while polyunsaturated fatty acids lower serum cholesterol. Monounsaturated fatty acids, which were previously thought to have no significant effect on serum cholesterol, have recently been shown to lower it. Saturated fats are solid at room temperature and in general are derived from animal foods; unsaturated fats are liquid at room temperature and in general are derived from plant foods.

The polyunsaturated fatty acid **linoleic acid** is an essential nutrient, required by the body for the synthesis of arachidonic acid, the major precursor of prostaglandins. Deficiencies of linoleic acid result in dermatitis, hair loss, and impaired wound healing. For individuals with average energy requirements, approximately 5 g of linoleic acid per day—1–2% of total calories—is required to prevent essential fatty acid deficiency. The polyunsaturated fatty acid **linolenic acid** is also an essential fatty acid in some mammalian species, but its role in human nutrition is unclear. Most foods that contain linoleic acid also contain linolenic acid. If there is a human requirement for linoleic acid, it would be met by diets that provide adequate linoleic acid.

**Cholesterol** is a major constituent of cell membranes. It is synthesized easily by the body and is not an essential nutrient. Diets that contain large amounts of cholesterol partially inhibit endogenous cholesterol synthesis and can increase serum cholesterol concentrations. Average American diets contain 600 mg/d of cholesterol. Current recommendations are to limit dietary cholesterol to 300 mg or less per day. Patients with hypercholesterolemia should limit cholesterol intake to 100–200 mg/d.

## VITAMINS

Vitamins are a heterogeneous group of organic molecules required by the body for a variety of essential metabolic functions. They are grouped as **water-soluble vitamins:** thiamine, riboflavin, niacin, pyridoxine, cobalamin (vitamin $B_{12}$), folacin, pantothenic acid, biotin, and ascorbic acid (vitamin C); and **fat-soluble vitamins:** A, D, E, and K. Major characteristics of vitamins are summarized in Tables 20–5 and 20–6. Disorders of vitamin metabolism are discussed on pp 803–807.

## MINERALS

The body also requires a number of inorganic minerals, commonly grouped as the **major minerals** calcium, magnesium, and phosphorus; the **electrolytes** sodium, potassium, and chloride; and the **trace elements** iron, zinc, copper, manganese, molybdenum, fluoride, iodine, cobalt, chromium, and selenium. Major characteristics of minerals are summarized in Table 20–7.

## DRUG-NUTRIENT INTERACTIONS

Many commonly used medications can have important effects on nutritional requirements. Chronic therapy with a variety of drugs can induce nutrient deficiencies by appetite suppression, intestinal malabsorption, and alterations in nutrient metabolism. The effects of selected drugs on nutrient absorption and metabolism are summarized in Table 20–8.

## DIETARY RECOMMENDATIONS

Prior to 1977, the emphasis in nutrition education and diet planning was to ensure that the RDAs were met by diets that contained a wide variety of foods. The most important dietary education tool used for this purpose was *The Four Food Groups,* published by the United States Department of Agriculture and the National Dairy Council. According to this model, 2 servings per day from both the milk group and the meat group and 4 servings per day from both the fruit and vegetable group and the cereal group would meet the minimal nutritional requirements for most individuals.

Although this model does ensure that the RDAs are met by a variety of foods, it does not guarantee that the individual foods selected are of high quality. The effects of food processing on the nutrient density of food, the balance of macronutrients (percentages of fat, carbohydrate, and protein), and the character of macronutrients (simple versus complex carbohydrate; saturated versus unsaturated fat) are omitted.

Since 1977, literally dozens of governmental, professional, and public health agencies and associations have published dietary recommendations that attempt to deal with these issues. Although attention has been directed to the differences between these reports, most agree on the basic principles of eating a wide variety of foods; increasing the consumption of foods containing complex carbohydrates; restricting the intake of sugar, fat (particularly saturated fat, ie, animal fat), cholesterol, salt, and alcohol; and maintaining an ideal body weight. Major features of some of these reports are summarized in Table 20–9.

The most important of these publications has been *Dietary Goals for the United States,* a United States Senate report that recommends specific changes in the percentages of total macronutrients, types of macronutrients, and quantities of dietary cholesterol and sodium (Table 20–10). To meet these goals, the report recommends specific changes in food selection and preparation, as follows: (1) increased consumption of fruits and vegetables and whole-grain cereals; (2) decreased consumption of beef and pork and increased consumption of poultry and fish; (3) decreased consumption of foods high in fat and partial substitution of polyunsaturated fat for saturated fat; (4) substitution of nonfat milk for whole milk; (5) decreased consumption of butterfat, eggs, and other foods with high cholesterol content; (6) decreased consumption of sugar and foods with high sugar content; and (7) decreased consumption of salt and foods with high salt content.

Similar percentages of macronutrients and changes in food selection and preparation have also been recommended for the prevention of coronary artery disease and cancer and for the treatment of diabetes, hypertension, obesity, and lipid disorders.

The controversy surrounding these recommendations relates not to the dietary recommendations as such but to their application. Most authorities urge that the recommendations be made to the public at large; others feel they should be limited to individual patients at risk for a particular disorder such as coronary artery disease or hypertension. At present, it seems reasonable to recommend that all persons be screened for risk factors for chronic illness and advised to change their diets if they are at risk. Patients at low risk may be well advised to change their dietary habits to maintain that low risk profile, but this is less important. Since all individuals do not have equal access to medical care, risk factor screening, and dietary counseling, it also seems reasonable to make these recommendations to the public at large.

**Table 20–5.** Essential water-soluble vitamins: Summary of major characteristics.[*]

| Vitamin | Coenzymes | Biochemical or Physiologic Function[1] | Deficiency Syndrome or Symptoms[2] (and Associated Diet) | Sources[3] | Stability[4] |
|---|---|---|---|---|---|
| Niacin (nicotinic acid, nicotin-amide) | Nicotinamide adenine dinucleotide (NAD); nicotinamide adenine dinucleotide phos-phate (NADP). | Electron (hydrogen) transfer reactions carried out by de-hydrogenase enzymes, eg, pyruvate dehydrogenase, glyceraldehyde-3-phosphate dehydrogenase. | Pellagra (milled corn). | Protein foods containing tryptophan, in addition to niacin sources in note[3]. | Stable. |
| Thiamin (vitamin $B_1$) | Thiamin pyrophosp-hate (TPP). | Oxidative decarboxylation of $\alpha$-ketoacids (pyruvate and $\alpha$-ketoglutarate dehydrogenases) and 2-ketosugars (transketolases). | Beriberi (milled rice); Wer-nicke-Korsakoff syndrome (alcohol). Antagonized by thiaminase in raw fish. | | Stable in acid solution. |
| Riboflavin (vitamin $B_2$) | Flavin adenine dinu-cleotide (FAD); flavin mononucleotide (FMN). | Electron (hydrogen) transfer reactions (eg, pyruvate de-hydrogenase, acyl-CoA de-hydrogenase). | Cheilosis. | | Stable in acid solution. Light-sensi-tive. |
| Pantothenic acid | CoA. | Acyl transfer reactions (citrate synthase, choline acetylase, etc). | | | Stable in neutral solu-tion. |
| Vitamin $B_6$, pyridoxine, pyridoxal, pyridoxamine | Pyridoxal phosphate (PLP). | Transamination and decar-boxylation via Schiff's base (many aminotransferase and decarboxylase enzymes). | Low serum levels are asso-ciated with pregnancy and oral contraceptive agents. Antagonized by isoniazid, penicillamine, and other drugs. | | Stable in acid solution. Light-sensi-tive. |
| Biotin | N-Carboxybiotinyl ly-sine. | $CO_2$ transfer reactions of car-boxylase coenzymes (pyru-vate carboxylase, acetyl-CoA carboxylase). | Induced by avidin, a pro-tein in raw egg whites, or by antibiotic therapy. | Synthesized by intestinal micro-organisms. | |
| Vitamin $B_{12}$ (cobalamin) | Methylcobalamin; 5'-deoxyadenosyl co-balamin. | Methylation of homocysteine to methionine; conversion of methylmalonyl-CoA to succi-nyl-CoA. | Megaloblastic anemia, methylmalonic aciduria, peripheral neuropathy (strict vegetarian diet). Per-nicious anemia induced by lack of intrinsic factor. | Animal foods (meat, dairy) only. | Stable in neutral solu-tions. |
| Folic acid (folacin) | Derivatives of tetrahy-drofolic acid. | One-carbon transfer reac-tions, eg, purine nucleotide and thymidylate synthesis. | Megaloblastic anemia. | | |
| Ascorbic acid (vitamin C) | Unknown. | Antioxidant; collagen biosyn-thesis; tyrosine catabolism (?). | Scurvy (lack of fresh fruits and vegetables). | Fresh fruits (especially citrus) and vegetables. | Especially unstable to heat. Easily oxidized in the presence of copper or iron. |

[*] Reproduced, with permission, from Martin DW Jr et al: *Harper's Review of Biochemistry,* 20th ed. Lange, 1985.

[1] The metabolism of most water-soluble vitamins is similar. They are absorbed in the intestine, stored bound to enzymes and transport proteins, and excreted in urine when plasma levels exceed kidney thresholds. The one notable exception is vitamin $B_{12}$, which requires intrinsic factor (synthesized by gastric parietal cells) for absorption in the distal ileum, is stored in milligram amounts in the liver, and is excreted in bile (and reabsorbed via the enterohepatic circulation) as well as in urine.

[2] Excess intake of water-soluble vitamins is not usually toxic. Exceptions: Excess nicotinic acid—but not nicotinamide—causes vascular dilatation of skin ("flushing"); megadose intake of ascorbic acid has been reported to produce diarrhea, oxalate kidney stones, and a variety of other toxic symptoms; high-dose pyridoxine (5 g/d) has caused sensory ataxia, sensory nerve dysfunction, and axonal degeneration in a few cases. Deficiency of these vitamins affects actively metabolizing tissues; symptoms usually include disorders of the digestive and nervous systems, skin, and blood cells.

[3] Unless otherwise stated, a varied intake of adequate amounts of foods from the following groups will meet nutritional requirements for water-soluble vitamins: whole-grain cereals, legumes, leafy green vegetables, meat, and dairy products.

[4] Stability refers to survival of vitamin activity during normal food preparation, cooking, and storage. Unless noted to the contrary, water-soluble vitamins are unstable to heat, strong acid or alkali solutions, and prolonged storage. These vitamins all dissolve in cooking water.

**Table 20–6.** Essential fat-soluble vitamins: Summary of major characteristics.*

| Vitamin/Provitamin[1] | Metabolism[2] | Active Metabolite: Physiologic Function | Deficiency Syndrome or Symptoms | Toxicity Syndrome or Symptoms | Sources[3] |
|---|---|---|---|---|---|
| Vitamin A<br>Provitamin:<br>$\beta$-carotene<br>Vitamin: retinol | Transported in lymph as retinyl esters in blood bound to retinol-binding protein and prealbumin. | 11-*Cis* retinal: constituent of rhodopsin and other light-receptor pigments. Unknown metabolites (retinoic acid?): required for growth and differentiation of epithelial, nervous, and bone tissues. | Children: poor dark adaptation, xerosis, keratomalacia, growth failure, death.<br>Adults: night blindness, xeroderma. | Hypervitaminosis A: headache, dizziness, nausea, skin sloughing, bone pain. | Highly pigmented vegetables (containing carotenes), fortified margarine. |
| Vitamin D<br>Provitamins: ergosterol (plants, yeast) and 7-dehydrocholesterol (skin)<br>Vitamins $D_2$ (ergocalciferol) and $D_3$ (cholecalciferol) | Provitamins converted to vitamins by ultraviolet irradiation. Vitamins hydroxylated in liver to 25-hydroxyvitamin D and in kidney to 1,25-dihydroxy-vitamin D and other metabolites. | 1,25-Dihydroxy-vitamin $D_3$ is major hormonal regulator of bone mineral (calcium and phosphorus) metabolism. | Children: rickets.<br>Adults: osteomalacia. | Hypervitaminosis D: hypercalcemia, hypercalciuria, nephrocalcinosis. | Fortified milk; sunlight on skin. |
| Vitamin E<br>tocopherols, tocotrienols | Generally unknown. | Active metabolite unknown. Functions as an antioxidant. | Children: anemia in premature infants.<br>Adults: no known syndrome. | Undefined. Megadose intake reported to induce blurred vision, headaches. | Vegetable seed oils are major source. |
| Vitamin K<br>$K_1$ (phylloquinone), $K_2$ (menaquinone), others | Generally undefined. | Active metabolite unknown but probably hydroquinone derivative. Activates blood clotting factors II, VII, IX, and X by $\gamma$-carboxylating glutamic acid residues; also carboxylates bone and kidney proteins. | Infants: hemorrhagic disease of newborn.<br>Adults: defective blood clotting. Deficiency symptoms can be produced by coumarin anticoagulants and by antibiotic therapy. | Can be induced by water-dispersible analogs: hemolytic anemia, liver damage. | Synthesized by intestinal bacteria. |

* Reproduced, with permission, from Martin DW Jr et al: *Harper's Review of Biochemistry,* 20th ed. Lange, 1985.

[1] The fat-soluble vitamins are insoluble in water but dissolve in fats and oils. They are relatively stable to normal cooking temperatures but are slowly inactivated by ultraviolet light and by oxidation.

[2] Absorption of fat-soluble vitamins requires dietary fat and bile; malabsorption or biliary obstruction leads to deficiency. Transport is via lipoproteins or specific transport proteins. Storage is mainly in liver, some in adipose tissue. These vitamins are excreted in bile and either reabsorbed via the enterohepatic circulation or excreted in feces. Some metabolites may be excreted in urine.

[3] Food sources of all fat-soluble vitamins include leafy green vegetables, vegetable seed oils, and fat-containing meat and dairy products, in addition to the specific sources listed here.

Birens BA et al: Linoleic acid versus linolenic acid: What is essential? *JPEN* 1983;**7**:473.

Cummings JH: Dietary fiber. *Am J Clin Nutr* 1987;**45 (Suppl)**:1040.

Daly JM et al: Human energy requirements: Overestimation by a widely used prediction equation. *Am J Clin Nutr* 1985;**42**:1170.

Grundy SM, Nestel PJ: Fat and cholesterol. *Am J Clin Nutr* 1985;**45(Suppl)**:1037.

Hautvast JGAJ: Proteins and selected vitamins. *Am J Clin Nutr* 1987;**45(Suppl)**:1044.

Isaksson B, Brubacher GB: Selected minerals. *Am J Clin Nutr* 1987;**45(Suppl)**:1043.

Jackson AA: Amino acids: Essential and non-essential? *Lancet* 1983;**1**:1034.

Macdonald I: Simple and complex carbohydrates. *Am J Clin Nutr* 1987;**45(Suppl)**:1039.

O'Dell BL: Bioavailability of trace elements. *Nutr Rev* 1984;**42**:301.

Owen OE et al: A reappraisal of caloric requirements in healthy women. *Am J Clin Nutr* 1986;**44**:1.

Roe DA: Nutrient and drug interactions. *Nutr Rev* 1984;**42**:141.

Schneider EL et al: Recommended Dietary Allowances and the health of the elderly. *New Engl J Med* 1986;**314**:157.

Select Committee on Nutrition and Human Needs, United States Senate: *Dietary Goals for the United States,* 2nd ed. US Government Printing Office, 1977.

Suter PM, Russell RM: Vitamin requirements of the elderly. *Am J Clin Nutr* 1987;**45**:501.

Willet WC, MacMahon B: Diet and cancer. (2 parts.) *N Engl J Med* 1984;**310**:633.

**Table 20–7.** Essential minerals and trace elements: Summary of major characteristics.*

| Elements | Functions | Metabolism[1] | Deficiency Disease or Symptoms | Toxicity Disease or Symptoms[2] | Sources[3] |
|---|---|---|---|---|---|
| **Minerals: required intake > 100 mg/d** | | | | | |
| Calcium | Constituent of bones, teeth; regulation of nerve, muscle function. | Absorption requires calcium-binding protein. Regulated by vitamin D, parathyroid hormone, calcitonin, etc. | Children: rickets. Adults: osteomalacia. May contribute to osteoporosis. | Occurs with excess absorption due to hypervitaminosis D or hypercalcemia due to hyperparathyroidism, or idiopathic hypercalcemia. | Dairy products, beans, leafy vegetables. |
| Phosphorus | Constituent of bones, teeth, ATP, phosphorylated metabolic intermediates. Nucleic acids. | Control of absorption unknown (vitamin D?). Serum levels regulated by kidney reabsorption. | Children: rickets. Adults: osteomalacia. | Low serum $CA^{2+}/P_i$ ratio stimulates secondary hyperthyroidism; may lead to bone loss. | Phosphate food additives. |
| Sodium | Principal cation in extracellular fluid. Regulates plasma volume, acid-base balance, nerve and muscle function, $Na^+, K^+$-ATPase. | Regulated by aldosterone. | Unknown on normal diet; secondary to injury or illness. | Hypertension (in susceptible individuals). | Table salt; salt added to prepared food. |
| Potassium | Principal cation in intracellular fluid; nerve and muscle function, $Na^+, K^+$-ATPase. | Also regulated by aldosterone. | Occurs secondary to illness, injury, or diuretic therapy; muscular weakness, paralysis, mental confusion. Low $Na^+/K^+$ ratio may predispose to hypertension. | Cardiac arrest, small bowel ulcers. | |
| Chloride | Fluid and electrolyte balance; gastric fluid. | | Infants fed salt-free formula. Secondary to vomiting, diuretic therapy, renal disease. | | Table salt. |
| Magnesium | Constituent of bones, teeth; enzyme cofactor (kinases, etc). | | Secondary to malabsorption or diarrhea, alcoholism. | Depressed deep tendon reflexes and respiration. | Leafy green vegetables (containing chlorophyll). |
| **Trace elements: required intake < 100 mg/d** | | | | | |
| Chromium | Trivalent chromium, a constituent of "glucose tolerance factor." | Undefined. | Impaired glucose intolerance; secondary to parenteral nutrition. | | |
| Cobalt | Constituent of vitamin $B_{12}$. | As for vitamin $B_{12}$. | Vitamin $B_{12}$ deficiency. | | Foods of animal origin. |
| Copper | Oxidase enzymes: cytochrome C oxidase, tyrosinase, ferroxidase, etc. | Transported by albumin; bound to ceruloplasmin. | Anemia (hypochromic, microcytic); secondary to malnutrition, Menke's syndrome. | Rare; secondary to Wilson's disease. | |
| Iodine | Thyroxine, triiodothyronine. | Stored in thyroid as thyroglobulin. | Children: cretinism. Adults: goiter and hypothyroidism, myxedema. | Thyrotoxicosis, goiter. | Iodized salt, seafood. |
| Iron | Heme enzymes (hemoglobin, cytochromes, etc). | Transported as transferrin; stored as ferritin or hemosiderin; excreted in sloughed cells and by bleeding. | Anemia (hypochromic, microcytic). | Siderosis; hereditary hemochromatosis. | Iron cookware. |
| Manganese | Hydrolase, decarboxylase, and transferase enzymes. Glycoprotein and proteoglycan synthesis. | | Unknown in humans. | Inhalation poisoning produces psychotic symptoms and parkinsonism. | |
| Molybdenum | Oxidase enzymes (xanthine oxidase). | | Secondary to parenteral nutrition. | | |
| Selenium | Glutathione peroxidase. | Synergistic antioxidant with vitamin E. | Marginal deficiency when soil content is low; secondary to parenteral nutrition, protein-energy malnutrition. | Megadose supplementation induces hair loss, dermatitis, and irritability. | |

**Table 20–7 (cont'd).** Essential minerals and trace elements: Summary of major characteristics.*

| Elements | Functions | Metabolism[1] | Deficiency Disease or Symptoms | Toxicity Disease or Symptoms[2] | Sources[3] |
|---|---|---|---|---|---|
| **Trace elements: required intake < 100 mg/d (cont'd)** | | | | | |
| Zinc | Cofactor of many enzymes: lactic dehydrogenase, alkaline phosphatase, carbonic anhydrase, etc. | | Hypogonadism, growth failure, impaired wound healing, decreased taste and smell acuity; secondary to acrodermatitis enteropathica, parenteral nutrition. | Gastrointestinal irritation, vomiting. | |
| Fluoride[4] | Increases hardness of bones and teeth. | | Dental caries; osteoporosis(?). | Dental fluorosis. | Drinking water. |

* Reproduced, with permission, from Martin DW Jr et al: *Harper's Review of Biochemistry,* 20th ed. Lange, 1985.
[1] In general, minerals require carrier proteins for absorption. Absorption is rarely complete; it is affected by other nutrients and compounds in the diet (eg, oxalates and phytates that chelate divalent cations). Transport and storage also require special proteins. Excretion occurs in feces (unabsorbed minerals) and in urine, sweat, and bile.
[2] Excess mineral intake produces toxic symptoms. Unless otherwise specified, symptoms include nonspecific nausea, diarrhea, and irritability.
[3] Mineral requirements are met by a varied intake of adequate amounts of whole-grain cereals, legumes, leafy green vegetables, meat, and dairy products.
[4] Fluoride is essential for rat growth. While not proved to be strictly essential for human nutrition, fluorides have a well-defined role in prevention and treatment of dental caries.

# ASSESSMENT OF NUTRITIONAL STATUS (Table 20–11)

The prevention and treatment of nutritional problems requires the identification of patients at risk for the development of malnutrition and the identification of patients who already show symptoms and signs of malnutrition. Unfortunately, no single biochemical test or clinical technique is sufficiently accurate to serve as a reliable test for malnutrition. Current techniques of nutritional assessment utilize a combination of methods, including evaluation of dietary intake, anthropometric measurements, clinical examination, and laboratory tests. Some patients require serial measurements and close observation to confirm the diagnosis of malnutrition. Current recommendations for nutritional assessment are summarized in Table 20–13.

## DIETARY HISTORY

Virtually all patients undergoing a complete history and physical examination should be asked screening dietary questions to help identify those high-risk patients who require further evaluation. Of particular importance are the regularity and availability of meals; who does the shopping and food preparation; recent changes in appetite level, intake, or body weight; use of special diets or dietary supplements; use of alcohol, drugs, or medications; food preferences and food allergies; and the presence of illnesses that affect nutritional intakes, losses, or requirements. Elderly and adolescent patients, pregnant or lactating women, and the poor and socially isolated are at particular risk for nutritional problems.

Further quantification of dietary intake can be performed using a variety of techniques. **Twenty-four-hour diet recalls** can be performed quickly and easily and provide rough estimates of nutrient intakes. Patients are asked to describe their dietary intake over the last 24 hours, including snacks, beverages, and alcohol. Questions should be asked also about food preparation. Intake can then be rapidly assessed by determining the numbers of servings ingested from each group and by evaluating the quality of food within each group. Problems with this technique include inaccurate reporting by patients, difficulties in estimating serving sizes, and the usual problems of generalizing from inadequate data: in this case, a single day's intake. These problems can be partially solved by showing the patient serving-size models and by repeating the procedure several times or different occasions.

More accurate quantitative information can be obtained by asking patients to complete a **3- to 5-day diet record.** Nutrient composition can then be analyzed with the aid of standard handbooks or computer software. Although this technique is prospective and less likely to be invalidated by memory lapses, omissions are still common as well as the usual difficulties in estimating serving sizes. Furthermore, 3–5 days may not be truly representative of long-term intakes because of random and seasonal variations and changes in eating behavior induced by the fact itself of record-keeping.

**Table 20–8.** Effect of drugs on nutrient absorption and metabolism.*

| Drug | Effect |
|---|---|
| **Antacids** | |
| Aluminum antacids | Decrease absorption of phosphate. |
| Others | Alkaline destruction of thiamine; some decrease absorption of vitamin A, iron; steatorrhea. |
| **Anticonvulsants** | |
| Phenobarbital | Decreases serum folate, vitamins $B_6$, $B_{12}$; increases catabolism of vitamin D and metabolites. |
| Phenytoin | Decreases serum folate, vitamins $B_6$, $B_{12}$, calcium; increases catabolism of vitamin D and metabolites. |
| Primidone | Decreases serum folate, vitamins $B_6$, $B_{12}$; decreases calcium absorption; increases catabolism of vitamin D and metabolites. |
| **Antimicrobials** | |
| Neomycin | Binds bile acids; decreases absorption of fat, carotene, vitamins A, D, K, $B_{12}$, potassium, sodium, calcium, nitrogen. |
| Salicylazosulfapyridine | Decreases absorption of folate. |
| Aminosalicylic acid | Decreases absorption of folate, vitamin $B_{12}$, iron, cholesterol, fat. |
| Chloramphenicol | Increases need for vitamins $B_2$, $B_6$, $B_{12}$. |
| Penicillin | Hypokalemia; renal potassium wasting. |
| Tetracycline | Decreases absorption of fat, amino acids, calcium, iron, magnesium, zinc. |
| Cycloserine | May decrease absorption of calcium, magnesium; may decrease serum folate, vitamins $B_6$, $B_{12}$; decreases protein synthesis. |
| Isoniazid | Vitamin $B_6$ deficiency. |
| Sulfonamides | Decrease absorption of folate; decrease serum folate, iron. |
| Nitrofurantoin | Decreases serum folate. |
| **Antimitotics** | |
| Methotrexate | Decreases absorption of folate, vitamin $B_{12}$. |
| Colchicine | Decreases absorption of vitamin $B_{12}$, carotene, fat, sodium, potassium, cholesterol, lactose, nitrogen. |
| **Cathartics** | |
| Phenolphthalein | Malabsorption, hypokalemia, deficiency of vitamin D, calcium. |
| Mineral oil | Malabsorption, decreased absorption of vitamins A, D, K. |
| **Diuretics** | Some cause hypokalemia, hypomagnesemia; may increase urinary excretion of vitamins $B_1$, $B_6$, calcium, magnesium, potassium. |
| **Hypocholesterolemics** | |
| Cholestyramine | Binds bile acids; decreases absorption of fat, carotene, vitamins A, D, K, $B_{12}$, folate, iron. |
| Clofibrate | Decreases absorption of carotene, vitamine $B_{12}$, iron, glucose. |
| **Hypotensives** | |
| Hydralazine | Vitamin $B_6$ deficiency. |
| **Oral contraceptives** | Vitamin $B_6$, folate deficiency; may increase the need for other nutrients. |

* Reproduced, with permission, from Thiele VF: *Clinical Nutrition,* 2nd ed. Mosby, 1980.

## ANTHROPOMETRICS

Anthropometric measurement is a method of assessing nutritional status by estimating body composition, particularly fat stores and skeletal muscle. The most commonly used measurements are those of height and weight, the triceps skin fold, and the mid arm muscle circumference.

Evaluation of body weight is the most useful anthropometric technique. Body weight in relationship to height should be checked against reference tables of "desirable weights" (Table 20–12) and expressed as **relative weight:**

$$\text{Relative weight} = \frac{\text{Current actual weight}}{\text{"Desirable weight"}} \times 100$$

Relative weights in excess of 120% are defined as obesity. Recent change in body weight is a better index of undernutrition than low relative weight. Changes in body weight are best expressed as the percentage of usually weight lost per unit of time:

$$\frac{\text{Percentage change}}{\text{in body weight}} = \frac{\text{Usual weight} - \text{Current weight}}{\text{Usual weight}} \times 100$$

A loss of 10% or more of usual weight within a period of 1–2 months is generally considered to be predictive of a poor clinical outcome.

Estimates of fat stores and skeletal protein can be performed by measurements of the triceps skin fold (TSF) and the mid arm muscle circumference (MAMC). The **triceps skin fold** is measured midway

**Table 20–9.** Dietary recommendations: Summary of recent reports from selected federal and health agencies. (Nearly all of these reports also advise alcohol restriction and maintenance of ideal body weight.)*

| | Recommendation | | | | | |
|---|---|---|---|---|---|---|
| | Eat a Variety of Foods | Increase Complex Carbohydrates (% kcal) | Restrict Sugar (% kcal) | Restrict Fat (% kcal) | Restrict Cholesterol (mg/d) | Restrict Salt (g/d) |
| US Senate: Dietary Goals, 1977 | Not discussed | R (48%) | R (10%) | R (30%) | R (300 mg) | R (5 g) |
| USDA, USDHHS: Dietary Guidelines, 1980 | R | R | R | R | R | R |
| Food, Nutrition Board (NAS): Toward Healthful Diets, 1980 | R | R (For persons with diabetes) | R (For weight control) | R (For weight control, otherwise 40%) | No specific recommendation | R (3–8 g) |
| American Diabetes Association: Special Report, 1979 | Not discussed | R (50–60%) | R | R (20–30%) | R | R |
| American Heart Association: Recommendations, 1982 | Not discussed | R | Not discussed | R (30–35%) | R (300 mg or less) | R |
| National Research Council: Diet, Nutrition, Cancer, 1982 | R | R | Not discussed | R (30% or less) | Not discussed | R (salt-cured foods) |
| American Cancer Society: Special Report, 1984 | Not discussed | R | Not discussed | R (30% or less) | Not discussed | R (salt-cured foods) |
| NIH Committee on high blood pressure: Report, 1984 | Not discussed | Not discussed | Not discussed | R (to lower CHD risk) | Not discussed | R (5 g) |
| American Heart Association, Committee on Hyperlipoproteinemia: Recommendations, 1984 | Not discussed | R | Not discussed | R (30% or less) | R (300 mg or less) | R |

R = recommended. CHD = congestive heart disease.
* Reproduced, with permission, from Nestle MN: *Nutrition in Clinical Practice.* Jones, 1985. Jones Medical Publications, 355 Los Cerros Drive, Greenbrae, CA 94904.

between the acromial process of the scapula and the olecranon process of the elbow. Unfortunately, great variations in TSF exist in normal persons, which means that any one measurement is unreliable as a means of diagnosing undernutrition or obesity.

The **mid arm muscle circumference** is measured at the same level as the TSF and then derived from the following equation:

$$\text{MAMC} = \text{Mid arm circumference} - (0.314 \times \text{TSF})$$

The MAMC can also be compared to standard values but has limitations similar to those mentioned with respect to the TSF.

## LABORATORY TESTS

**Serum albumin** is the most important test for the diagnosis of protein-calorie undernutrition. Most patients with severe protein depletion will have abnormally low serum albumin levels. Unfortunately, many nonnutritional conditions can also cause low levels of serum albumin—particularly liver disease and severe illness in general. Other serum proteins with shorter half-lives (transferrin, prealbumin, etc) may

more accurately reflect short-term changes in nutritional status but suffer from similar shortcomings.

Qualitative and quantitative tests of cellular immunity are also abnormal in many patients with protein-calorie undernutrition. Measurements of the **total lymphocyte count** and **delayed hypersensitivity reactions** to common skin test antigens are commonly used but are nonspecific; ie, abnormalities may be due to nonnutritional factors.

Excretion of urinary creatinine can be used as a rough measure of skeletal protein. The **creatinine-height index** measures 24-hour excretion of creatinine for a given body size and can be compared to sex-specific standards. Unfortunately, this test is also confounded by a number of nonnutritional factors, particularly renal disease, which affects creatinine excretion.

Thus, the use of laboratory tests to diagnose protein-calorie malnutrition is limited by confounding factors that make the tests unreliable for differentiating malnutrition from nonnutritional health disorders. The judicious interpretation of these tests, however—particularly the serum albumin—may help to confirm the diagnosis of protein-calorie undernutrition in selected patients. Despite their uncertain diagnostic utility, these tests are useful prognostic indicators. Pa-

**Table 20–10.** Dietary goals for the USA. Current and recommended intakes of carbohydrate, fat, and protein as percent of total energy consumption, and of cholesterol and salt.*

| | Percentage of Total Energy | |
|---|---|---|
| | Current Diet | Dietary Goals |
| **Carbohydrate, total** | 46 | 58 |
| Complex carbohydrate and naturally occurring sugars | 28 | 48 |
| Sugars, refined and processed | 18 | 10 |
| **Protein, total** | 12 | 12 |
| **Fat, total** | 42 | 30 |
| Saturated | 16 | 10 |
| Monounsaturated | 19 | 10 |
| Polyunsaturated | 7 | 10 |
| **Cholesterol, mg/d** | 600 | 300 |
| **Salt, g/d** | 6–18 | 5 |

* Data from Select Committee on Nutrition and Human Needs, US Senate: *Dietary Goals for the US,* 2nd ed. US Government Printing Office, 1977.

tients with abnormal nutritional assessment parameters have a markedly increased risk of poor clinical outcomes. Combining the tests into quantitative indices further improves their prognostic validity.

Laboratory tests can also be used to diagnose abnormalities in vitamin and mineral deficiencies. Nutrient levels can be measured directly in blood, saliva, and other body tissues or can be evaluated by measuring nutrient-specific biochemical reactions. Most of these tests are unavailable in hospital laboratories and require referral to specialized facilities.

## CLINICAL EXAMINATION

Clinical evaluation is the most important aspect of the assessment of nutritional status. A careful **nutritionally focused history and physical examination** should be performed on each patient at risk for nutri-

**Table 20–11.** Recommendations for nutritional assessment.

**Nutritionally focused history**
  Intake history
  Weight history
  Functional status
**Nutritionally focused physical examination**
  Muscle mass
  Fat stores
  Volume status
  Signs of micronutrient deficiency
**Interpretation of readily available laboratory data**
  Serum albumin
  Serum transferrin
  Total lymphocyte count
**Observation**
  Dietary intake as a function of estimated needs
  Changes in body weight
  Serial clinical assessment

tional problems. The history emphasizes recent reduction in dietary intake, weight loss, and evaluation of the patient's functional status. The physical examination focuses on muscle wasting, fat stores, volume status, and signs of micronutrient deficiencies (Table 20–13). This type of clinical assessment has recently been demonstrated to be more accurate than techniques relying primarily on laboratory tests or anthropometry.

Despite these techniques, it is difficult to diagnose malnutrition, especially in hospitalized patients. Continued close observation is often necessary. Monitoring dietary intakes during hospitalization can be quite helpful. **Calorie counts** by registered dietitians can be used to estimate energy and protein intakes for comparison with estimated requirements. Serial measurements of body weight and serial clinical assessments should also be performed.

Detsky AS et al: Evaluating the accuracy of nutritional assessment techniques applied to hospitalized patients: Methodology and comparisons. *JPEN* 1984;**8**:153.

Krantzler NJ et al: Methods of food intake assessment: An annotated bibliography. *J Nutr Educ* 1982;**14**:108.

McLaren DS, Meguid MM: Nutritional assessment at the crossroads. *JPEN* 1983;**7**:575.

Twomey P, Ziegler D, Rombeau J: Utility of skin testing in nutritional assessment: A critical review. *JPEN* 1982;**6**:50.

# NUTRITIONAL DISORDERS

## PROTEIN-CALORIE UNDERNUTRITION

Protein-calorie undernutrition occurs as a result of a relative or absolute deficiency of calories and protein. For most developing nations, protein-calorie undernutrition remains the most important nutritional problem and among the most significant of all health problems. Classically, protein-calorie undernutrition has been described as 2 distinct syndromes. **Kwashiorkor,** caused by a deficiency of protein in the presence of adequate calories, is typically seen in weaning infants at the birth of a sibling in areas where foods containing protein are insufficiently abundant. **Marasmus,** caused by combined protein and calorie deficiency, is most commonly seen where adequate quantities of food are not available.

In industrialized societies, protein-calorie undernutrition is most commonly seen among hospitalized medical and surgical patients. As many as 20% of all patients admitted to hospital have significant protein-calorie undernutrition. In these patients, protein-calorie undernutrition is caused either by decreased intake of calories and protein, increased nutrient losses, or increased nutrient requirements dictated by the underlying illness. Some of the disorders that

**Table 20–12.** Reference height and body weight ranges for adult males and females.*†

| Height, Men and Women | | Weight, lb (kg) | | | | | |
|---|---|---|---|---|---|---|---|
| | | Men | | | Women | | |
| in | cm | Small Frame | Medium Frame | Large Frame | Small Frame | Medium Frame | Large Frame |
| 58 | 147 | . . . | . . . | . . . | 102–111 (46–50) | 109–121 (49–55) | 118–131 (54–59) |
| 59 | 150 | . . . | . . . | . . . | 103–113 (47–51) | 111–123 (50–56) | 120–134 (54–61) |
| 60 | 152 | . . . | . . . | . . . | 104–115 (47–52) | 113–126 (51–57) | 122–137 (55–62) |
| 61 | 155 | . . . | . . . | . . . | 106–118 (48–54) | 115–129 (52–59) | 125–140 (57–64) |
| 62 | 158 | 128–134 (58–61) | 131–141 (59–64) | 138–150 (63–68) | 108–121 (49–55) | 118–132 (54–60) | 128–143 (58–65) |
| 63 | 160 | 130–136 (59–62) | 133–143 (60–65) | 140–153 (64–69) | 111–124 (50–56) | 121–135 (55–61) | 131–147 (59–67) |
| 64 | 163 | 132–138 (60–63) | 135–145 (61–66) | 142–156 (64–71) | 114–127 (52–58) | 124–138 (56–63) | 134–151 (61–68) |
| 65 | 165 | 134–140 (61–64) | 137–148 (62–67) | 144–160 (65–73) | 117–130 (53–59) | 127–141 (58–64) | 137–155 (62–70) |
| 66 | 168 | 136–142 (62–65) | 139–151 (63–68) | 146–164 (66–74) | 120–133 (54–60) | 130–144 (59–65) | 140–159 (64–72) |
| 67 | 170 | 138–145 (63–66) | 142–154 (64–69) | 149–168 (68–76) | 123–136 (56–62) | 133–147 (60–67) | 143–163 (65–74) |
| 68 | 173 | 140–148 (64–67) | 145–157 (66–71) | 152–172 (69–78) | 126–139 (57–63) | 136–150 (62–68) | 146–167 (66–76) |
| 69 | 175 | 142–151 (64–68) | 148–160 (67–73) | 155–176 (70–80) | 129–142 (59–64) | 139–153 (63–69) | 149–170 (68–77) |
| 70 | 178 | 144–154 (65–69) | 151–163 (68–74) | 158–180 (72–82) | 132–145 (60–66) | 142–156 (64–71) | 152–173 (69–78) |
| 71 | 181 | 146–157 (66–71) | 154–166 (70–75) | 161–184 (73–83) | 135–148 (61–67) | 145–159 (66–72) | 155–176 (70–80) |
| 72 | 183 | 149–160 (68–73) | 157–170 (71–77) | 164–188 (74–85) | 138–151 (63–68) | 148–162 (67–73) | 158–179 (71–81) |
| 73 | 185 | 152–164 (69–74) | 160–174 (73–79) | 168–192 (76–87) | . . . | . . . | . . . |
| 74 | 188 | 155–168 (70–76) | 164–178 (74–81) | 172–197 (78–89) | . . . | . . . | . . . |
| 75 | 190 | 158–172 (72–78) | 167–182 (76–83) | 176–202 (80–92) | . . . | . . . | . . . |
| 76 | 193 | 162–176 (73–80) | 171–187 (78–85) | 181–207 (82–94) | . . . | . . . | . . . |

* From: Metropolitan Life Foundation: 1983 Metropolitan height and weight tables. *Stat Bull Metropol Life Insur Co* 1983;**64**:2.
† Ages 25 through 59, for 5 lb of indoor clothing for men and 3 lb of indoor clothing for women, and 1-in heels for both.

**Table 20–13.** Clinical signs that may be due to nutrient deficiency.

| Clinical Sign | Nutrient | Clinical Sign | Nutrient |
|---|---|---|---|
| **Hair** | | **Mouth (cont'd)** | |
| Transverse depigmentation | Protein, copper | Atrophic lingual papillae | Niacin, iron, riboflavin, folate, vitamin $B_{12}$ |
| Easily pluckable | Protein | | |
| Sparse and thin | Protein, zinc, biotin | Hypogeusia | Zinc, vitamin A |
| **Skin** | | Tongue fissuring | Niacin |
| Dry, scaling | Zinc, vitamin A, essential fatty acids | **Neck** | |
| | | Goiter | Iodine |
| Flaky paint dermatitis | Protein, niacin, riboflavin | **Chest** | |
| Follicular hyperkeratosis | Vitamins A and C | Thoracic rosary | Vitamin D |
| Perifollicular petechiae | Vitamin C | **Yeart** | |
| Petechiae, purpura | Vitamins C and K | High-output failure | Thiamine |
| Pigmentation, desquamation | Niacin | Decreased output | Protein-calorie |
| Nasolabial seborrhea | Niacin, riboflavin, pyridoxine | **Abdomen** | |
| Pallor | Iron, folate, vitamin $B_{12}$, copper | Hepatosplenomegaly | Protein-calorie |
| | | Distention | Protein-calorie |
| Scrotal/vulvar dermatoses | Riboflavin | Diarrhea | Niacin, folate, vitamin $B_{12}$ |
| Subcutaneous fat loss | Calorie | **Extremities** | |
| **Nails** | | Muscle tenderness, pain | Thiamine, vitamin C |
| Spooning | Iron | Muscle wasting | Protein-calorie |
| Transverse lines, ridging | Protein-calorie | Edema | Protein, thiamine |
| **Head** | | Bone tenderness | Vitamin D, vitamin C, calcium, phosphorus |
| Temporal muscle wasting | Protein-calorie | | |
| Parotid enlargement | Protein | **Neurologic** | |
| **Eyes** | | Hyporeflexia | Thiamine |
| Night blindness | Vitamin A, zinc | Decreased position and vibratory sense | Vitamin $B_{12}$, thiamine |
| Corneal vascularization | Riboflavin | | |
| Xerosis, Bitot spots, keratomalacia | Vitamin A | Paresthesias | Vitamin $B_{12}$, thiamine, niacin |
| | | Confabulation, disorientation | Thiamine |
| Conjunctival inflammation | Riboflavin | Dementia | Niacin |
| **Mouth** | | Ophthalmoplegia | Thiamine, phosphorus |
| Glossitis (scarlet, raw) | Niacin, pyridoxine, riboflavin, vitamin $B_{12}$, folate | Tetany | Calcium, magnesium |
| | | **Other** | |
| Bleeding gums | Vitamin C, riboflavin | Delayed wound healing | Zinc, protein-calorie, vitamin C |
| Cheilosis | Riboflavin | | |
| Angular stomatitis | Riboflavin, iron | | |

may lead to protein-calorie undernutrition are shown in Table 20–14. Few patients are sick enough to require acute hospitalization without manifesting some of these risk factors.

## Pathophysiology

Protein-calorie undernutrition results in important pathophysiologic changes that can affect virtually every organ system. The most obvious results are loss of body weight, adipose stores, and skeletal muscle mass. Weight losses of 5–10% are usually tolerated without significant loss of physiologic function; losses of 35–40% of body weight usually result in death. Loss of protein from skeletal muscle and internal organs is usually proportionate to weight loss. Protein mass is lost from the liver, gastrointestinal tract, kidneys, and heart.

As protein-calorie undernutrition progresses, organ dysfunction may develop. Hepatic synthesis of serum proteins decreases, and depressed levels of circulating proteins may be observed. Cardiac output and contractility are decreased, and the ECG may show decreased voltage and a rightward axis shift. Autopsies of patients who die with severe undernutrition show myofibrillar atrophy and interstitial edema of the heart.

The lungs are affected primarily by weakness and atrophy of the muscles of respiration. Vital capacity and tidal volume are depressed, and mucociliary clearance is abnormal. The gastrointestinal tract is most importantly affected by mucosal atrophy and loss of villi of small intestine, resulting in a decrease in absorptive capacity. Intestinal disaccharidase deficiency

**Table 20–14.** Causes of protein-calorie malnutrition in hospitalized patients.

| |
|---|
| **Decreased oral intake** |
| Anorexia |
| Nausea |
| Dysphagia |
| Pain |
| Obstruction |
| Poor dentition |
| Poverty |
| Old age |
| Social isolation |
| Substance abuse |
| Depression |
| **Increased nutrient losses** |
| Malabsorption |
| Diarrhea |
| Bleeding |
| Glycosuria |
| Nephrosis |
| Fistula drainage |
| Protein-losing enteropathy |
| **Increased nutrient requirements** |
| Fever |
| Infection |
| Neoplasms |
| Surgery |
| Trauma |
| Burns |
| Medications |

and mild pancreatic insufficiency can also develop and result in malabsorption.

Changes in immunologic function are among the most important changes seen in protein-calorie undernutrition. The total lymphocyte count is commonly decreased, primarily because of a reduction in circulating T cells. T cell function is also depressed. Changes in B cell function are more variable. Other aspects of immunologic function are also affected, including total complement activity, granulocyte function, and anatomic barriers to infection. Virtually every phase of wound healing is also affected.

## Clinical Findings

Patients with severe protein-calorie malnutrition—particularly children in developing countries—commonly exhibit signs of the classic syndromes of kwashiorkor and marasmus. The child with severe kwashiorkor will have marked edema, ascites, and muscle wasting. Lethargy, irritability, anorexia, and growth failure are common. The blood pressure and pulse are depressed, and the temperature may be low. The skin shows a "flaky paint" dermatitis, with dry, hyperpigmented lesions. The hair is sparse, dry, and depigmented. Cheilosis, stomatitis, and conjunctivitis are usually present. The liver is commonly enlarged. Laboratory manifestations include hypoalbuminemia, anemia (usually normochromic normocytic unless other deficiencies are present), and a decreased total lymphocyte count. Liver enzymes are most commonly normal, and BUN and the serum creatinine, cholesterol, potassium, magnesium, and calcium are usually low.

Patients with marasmus also exhibit growth retardation and muscle wasting. In contrast to kwashiorkor, there is no edema or ascites or specific dermatitis. Subcutaneous fat is usually absent and the skin dry and loose, giving the child a "skin and bones" appearance. Weakness and irritability are common, but there is usually less lethargy than is the case with kwashiorkor, and the appetite may be normal or increased. Blood pressure, pulse, and temperature are depressed. Laboratory values are more likely to be normal than in kwashiorkor—particularly serum albumin and other serum protein levels.

Most patients with protein-calorie undernutrition do not manifest the classic syndromes of kwashiorkor and marasmus but have intermediate syndromes. Similarly, most hospitalized patients in industrialized nations have less characteristic signs of malnutrition. In these instances, the features of malnutrition are often obscured by the underlying disease. Detection of hospitalized patients with protein-calorie undernutrition requires identification of high-risk patients, application of current techniques of nutritional assessment, and close observation of every patient's nutritional status during the course of hospitalization.

The diagnosis of protein-calorie undernutrition is particularly difficult in 2 further circumstances. Patients with significant obesity often appear to be overnourished because of their excess adipose stores.

Rapid weight loss, however—particularly when due to illness—commonly results in depletion of skeletal and visceral protein and can lead to the pathophysiologic abnormalities described above. In such patients, significant weight loss and depletion of serum proteins may be the only clues to protein depletion. Acutely ill patients—particularly those who are "hypermetabolic" and unable to eat—may develop visceral protein depletion rapidly without manifesting significant weight loss or other signs of undernutrition. In these patients, signs of hypermetabolism and decreased levels of serum protein may be the only clues to the diagnosis of undernutrition.

## Treatment

The treatment of severe protein-calorie undernutrition is a slow process requiring great care. Initial efforts should be directed at correcting fluid and electrolyte abnormalities and any significant acute infections. Of particular concern is depletion of potassium, magnesium, and calcium and acid-base abnormalities. The second phase of treatment is directed at repletion of protein, energy, and micronutrients. Treatment should be started with modest quantities of protein and calories calculated according to the patient's actual body weight. Adult patients can initially be given 0.8 g of protein and 30 kcal per kilogram. Concomitant administration of vitamins and minerals is necessary. Either the enteral or parenteral route can be used, although the former is of course preferable. Enteral fat and lactose are usually withheld initially. Patients with less severe protein-calorie undernutrition can be given calories and protein simultaneously with the correction of fluid and electrolyte abnormalities. Similar quantities of protein and calories are recommended for initial treatment.

All patients initially treated for protein-calorie undernutrition require close follow-up. Both calories and protein can be advanced as tolerated. Adult patients can be advanced to 1.5 g/kg/d of protein and 40 kcal/kg/d.

Patients who are refed too rapidly can develop a number of untoward clinical sequelae. During refeeding, circulating potassium, magnesium, phosphorus, and glucose move intracellularly and can result in low serum levels of each. The administration of water and sodium in combination with carbohydrate refeeding can overload hearts with depressed cardiac function and result in congestive heart failure. Enteral refeeding can result in malabsorption and diarrhea due to abnormalities in the gastrointestinal tract.

Refeeding edema is a benign condition that must be differentiated from congestive heart failure. Changes in renal sodium reabsorption and poor skin and blood vessel integrity result in the development of edema in dependent areas without other signs of congestive heart failure. Treatment is with reassurance, elevation of the dependent area, and modest sodium restriction. Diuretics are usually ineffective and should not be utilized.

The prevention and early detection of protein-calorie malnutrition in hospitalized patients require constant awareness of that possibility by the physicians and others responsible for their care. Each patient admitted to the hospital should be screened for risk factors. Patients at risk require formal assessment of nutritional status and close observation of dietary intake, body weight, and nutritional requirements during the hospital stay.

The prevention of protein-calorie malnutrition in the developing world is, of course, a more complex problem. Most important is the redistribution of food and food-related resources from industrialized nations to the still developing ones. Poverty—not overpopulation or world food shortages—is the primary cause of most of the world's undernutrition.

The distribution of infant formula to the developing world to replace traditional breast feeding practices has had a deleterious effect in many nations and should be discouraged.

Baron RB: Malnutrition in hospitalized patients: Diagnosis and treatment. *West J Med* 1986;**144:**63.

Garre MA, Boles JM, Youinou PY: Current concepts in immune derangement due to undernutrition. *JPEN* 1987;**11:**309.

Golden MHN, Jackson AA: Chronic severe undernutrition. In: *Nutrition Review's Present Knowledge in Nutrition,* 5th ed. Nutrition Foundation, 1984.

Keys A et al: *The Biology of Human Starvation.* Univ Minnesota Press, 1950.

Rennie MJ, Harrison R: Effects of injury, disease, and malnutrition on protein metabolism in man: Unanswered questions. *Lancet* 1984;**1:**323.

## OBESITY

Obesity is one of the most common disorders in medical practice and among the most frustrating and difficult to manage. Little progress has been made in obesity treatment in the last 25 years, yet major changes have occurred in our understanding of its causes and its implications for health.

### Definition & Measurement

Adipose tissue is a normal component of the human body, and obesity is defined as an excess of adipose tissue. The exact criterion for how much is too much is controversial. Accurate quantification of body fat requires sophisticated techniques not usually available in clinical practice. In most situations, physical examination is sufficient to detect excess body fat. Two methods commonly used for more quantitative evaluation are relative weight (RW) and body mass index (BMI).

**Relative weight (RW)** is the measured body weight divided by the "desirable weight." Desirable weight is defined as the midpoint value recommended for a "medium-frame" person in the 1983 Metropolitan Life Insurance Tables (Table 20–12). This technique does not differentiate between patients with excess fat or "excess" muscle.

The **body mass index (BMI),** more accurately

reflects the presence of excess adipose tissue. BMI is calculated by dividing measured body weight in kilograms by the height in meters squared. The "normal" BMI is 20–25 kg/m$^{2.}$

Most authors currently consider relative weights over 120% (BMI > 27.5) to constitute mild obesity, relative weights of 140–200% (BMI 30–40) moderate obesity, and relative weights over 200% (BMI > 40) severe or "morbid" obesity. Other factors, however, are also probably important. Recent data suggest that excess fat around the waist and flank is a greater health hazard than fat in the thighs and buttocks. Obese patients with high waist-hip ratios (>1.0) have a significantly greater risk of diabetes mellitus, stroke, coronary artery disease, and early death than equally obese patients with waist-hip ratios less than 1.0. Age is also an important factor. As age increases, moderate increases in body weight are not associated with increased mortality rates.

About 25% of people in the USA have relative weights in excess of 120%. Blacks—particularly black women—are more apt to be obese than whites, and the poor are more obese than the rich regardless of race.

## Health Consequences of Obesity

Obesity is associated with significant increases in both morbidity and mortality. A great many disorders occur with greater frequency in obese people. The most important common of these are hypertension, type II diabetes mellitus, hyperlipidemia, coronary artery disease, degenerative joint disease, and psychosocial disability; but certain cancers (colon, rectum, and prostate in men; uterus, biliary tract, breast, and ovary in women), thromboembolic disorders, digestive tract diseases (gallstones, reflux esophagitis), and skin disorders are also more prevalent in the obese, and surgical and obstetric risks are greater as well. Obese patients also have a greater risk of pulmonary functional impairment, endocrine abnormalities, proteinuria, and increased hemoglobin concentration.

The death rate increases in proportion to the degree of obesity: Relative weights of 130% are associated with an excess mortality rate of 35% and relative weights of 150% a greater than 2-fold excess death rate. Patients with "morbid" obesity (relative weight > 200%) have as much as a 10-fold increase in death rate.

## Etiology

Until recently, obesity was considered to be the direct result of a sedentary lifestyle plus chronic ingestion of excess calories. Obese people were *blamed* for being obese—by their friends and families, their employers, their physicians, and even by themselves. Although these factors are undoubtedly the principal cause of obesity in many cases, there is now evidence that many other factors may also be involved. In laboratory animals, for example, a variety of hypothalamic abnormalities can lead to obesity. Genetic

factors are also important. A recent study of 540 adopted children demonstrated a close relationship between their body mass index and that of their biologic parents. No such relationship was found between the children and their adoptive parents. Many metabolic abnormalities have recently been described in obese patients that may also be the cause—rather than the effect—of obesity.

Further research will probably permit classification of obese patients into subgroups according to different etiologic features. It is also possible that specific methods of treatment will be developed. Given our imperfect understanding of the causes of obesity, it is essential not to hold the patients personally responsible for their condition.

## Medical Evaluation of the Obese Patient

The history and physical examination are the most important parts of the evaluation of obese patients. Historical information should be obtained about age at onset, recent weight changes, family history of obesity, occupational history, eating and exercise behavior, cigarette and alcohol use, previous weight loss experience, and psychosocial factors. Particular attention should be directed at use of laxatives, diuretics, hormones, nutritional supplements, and over-the-counter medications.

Physical examination should assess the degree and distribution of body fat, overall nutritional status, and signs of secondary causes of obesity.

Less than 1% of obese patients have an identifiable secondary cause of obesity. Hypothyroidism and Cushing's syndrome are important examples that can usually be diagnosed by physical examination in patients with unexplained recent weight gain. Some patients with ambiguous physical findings may require further endocrinologic evaluation, including serum TSH determination and dexamethasone suppression testing.

All obese patients should be evaluated for medical consequences of their obesity. Fasting levels of glucose, cholesterol, and triglycerides should be measured.

## Treatment

There is no single effective method of treatment for obesity. Using conventional techniques, only 20% of patients will lose 20 lb and maintain the loss for over 2 years; 5% will maintain a 40-lb loss. Continued close provider-patient contact appears to more important for success of treatment than the specific features of any given treatment regimen. Careful patient selection will improve success rates and lessen frustration of both patients and therapists. Only sufficiently motivated patients should enter treatment programs.

Most successful programs employ a multidisciplinary approach to weight loss, with hypocaloric diets, behavior modification or other strategies to change eating behavior, aerobic exercise, and social support. Emphasis must be on *maintenance* of weight loss.

Dietary instructions should incorporate the same principles that apply to healthy people who are not obese, ie, a low-fat, high-complex carbohydrate, high-fiber diet. This is achieved by emphasizing intake of a wide variety of predominantly "unprocessed" foods. Special attention is usually paid to limiting foods that provide large amounts of calories without other nutrients, ie, fat, sucrose, and alcohol. There is no advantage to diets that restrict carbohydrates, advocate large amounts of protein or fats, or recommend ingestion of foods one at a time.

Long-term changes in eating behavior are required to maintain weight loss. Although formal **behavior modification** programs are available to which patients can be referred, the clinician caring for obese patients can teach a number of useful behavioral techniques. The most important technique is to emphasize planning and record keeping. Patients can be taught to plan menus and exercise sessions and to record their actual behavior. Record keeping not only aids in behavioral change; the availability of records also helps the health care provider to make specific suggestions for problem solving. Patients can be taught to recognize "eating cues" (emotional, situational, etc) and how to avoid or control them. Reward systems and refundable financial contracts are also useful for many patients.

**Exercise** offers a number of advantages to patients trying to lose weight and keep it off. Aerobic exercise directly increases the daily energy expenditure and is particularly useful for long-term weight maintenance. Exercise will also preserve lean body mass and partially prevent the decrease in basal energy expenditure seen with semistarvation.

**Social support** is essential for a successful weight loss program. Continued close contact with the therapist, family and peer group involvement, etc, are useful techniques for reinforcing behavioral change and preventing social isolation.

Patients with severe obesity may require more aggressive treatment regimens. Diets very low in calories (400–500 kcal/d) result in rapid weight loss and marked improvement in obesity-related metabolic complications. Side effects such as fatigue, orthostatic hypotension, and fluid and electrolyte disorders are common and require regular supervision by a physician. Patients are commonly maintained on such programs for 4–6 months and lose an average of 2–4 pounds a week. Long-term weight maintenance is not so reliable and requires concurrent behavior modification and exercise.

Gastroplasty can also be used in selected patients with severe complications of obesity. Significant weight loss is almost always achieved, but the perioperative mortality rate averages 2%. Mechanical and nutritional complications are common.

A recent development in the treatment of obesity is the gastric bubble, a small polyurethane cylinder placed in the stomach and designed to produce early satiety. Although short-term weight loss can be achieved, complications such as ulcers, obstruction, and spontaneous deflation are common. No data are available about long-term weight maintenance.

Anderson T et al: Randomized trial of diet and gastroplasty compared with diet alone in morbid obesity. *N Engl J Med* 1984;**310:**352.

Atkinson RL et al: A comprehensive approach to outpatient obesity management. *J Am Diet Assoc* 1984;**84:**439.

Brownell KD: The physiology and physiology of obesity: Implications for screening and treatment. *J Am Diet Assoc* 1984;**84:**406.

Cole HM: Diagnostic and therapeutic technology assessment: Garren gastric bubble. *JAMA* 1986;**256:**3282.

Greenwood MRC (editor): *Obesity: Contemporary Issues in Clinical Nutrition.* Churchill Livingstone, 1983.

Henry RR et al: Metabolic consequences of very low calorie diet therapy in obese noninsulin dependent diabetic and nondiabetic subjects. *Diabetes* 1986;**35:**155.

Hocking MP et al: Jejunoileal bypass for morbid obesity: Late followup in 100 cases. *N Engl J Med* 1983;**308:**995.

Knapp TR: A methodical critique of the "ideal weight" concept. *JAMA* 1983;**250:**506.

NIH Consensus Development Panel on the Health Implications of Obesity: Health implications of obesity. *Ann Intern Med* 1984;**151:**103.

Russ CS, Wolfe BM: Obesity: Current concepts and therapy. *Pract Gastroenterol* 1987;**11:**20.

Simopoulous AP, Van Itallie TB: Body weight, health and longevity. *Ann Intern Med* 1984;**100:**285.

Stunkard AJ et al: An adoption study of human obesity. *New England J Med* 1986;**314:**193.

Stunkard AJ, Steller E (editors): *Eating and Its Disorders.* Raven Press, 1984.

Visocan OJ, Dworkin MF, Klein LW: Effect of long-term group support on weight-loss maintenance. *J Nutr Educ* 1985;**17:**3.

Wadden TA, Stunkard AJ, Brownell KD: Very low calorie diets: Their efficacy, safety and future. *Ann Intern Med* 1983;**99:**675.

# EATING DISORDERS

## ANOREXIA NERVOSA

Anorexia nervosa characteristically begins in the years between mid adolescence and young adulthood. Over 95% of patients are females, most commonly from the middle and upper socioeconomic strata. The diagnosis is based on the loss of 25% or more of body weight, a distorted body image, and fear of weight gain or of loss of control over food intake. Other medical or psychiatric illnesses that can account for anorexia and weight loss must be excluded.

The prevalence of anorexia nervosa is estimated to be about one per 100,000 in the population at large, but in Caucasian adolescent girls from middle and upper class families the rate may be as high as 1:200. Many other adolescent girls have features of the disorder without the severe weight loss.

The cause of anorexia nervosa is not known. Although multiple endocrinologic abnormalities exist in these patients, most authorities believe they are secondary to malnutrition and not primary disorders. Most authors favor a primary psychiatric origin, but no single psychiatric hypothesis satisfactorily explains all cases. The patient characteristically comes from a family whose members are highly goal- and achievement-oriented. Interpersonal relationships may be inadequate or destructive. The parents are usually overly directive and concerned with slimness and physical fitness, and most discussion centers around dietary matters. One theory holds that the patient's refusal to eat is an attempt to regain control of her body in defiance of parental control. The patient's unwillingness to inhabit an "adult body" may also represent a rejection of adult responsibilities and the implications of adult interpersonal relationships. Patients are commonly perfectionistic in behavior and exhibit obsessional personality characteristics. Marked depression or anxiety may be present.

### Clinical Findings

**A. Symptoms and Signs:** Clinically, patients with anorexia nervosa may exhibit severe emaciation and may complain of cold intolerance or constipation. Amenorrhea is almost always present. Bradycardia, hypotension, and hypothermia may be present in severe cases. Examination demonstrates loss of body fat, dry and scaly skin, and increased lanugo body hair. Parotid enlargement and edema may also be present.

**B. Laboratory Findings:** Laboratory findings are variable but may include anemia, leukopenia, electrolyte abnormalities, and elevations of BUN and serum creatinine. Serum cholesterol levels are often increased. Endocrine abnormalities included depressed levels of luteinizing and follicle-stimulating hormones and impaired response of LH to luteinizing hormone-releasing hormone.

### Treatment

The goal of treatment is restoration of normal body weight and resolution of psychologic difficulties. Hospitalization is usually necessary. Treatment programs conducted by experienced teams are successful in about two-thirds of cases, restoring normal weight and menstruation. One-half continue to experience difficulties with eating behavior and psychiatric problems. Occasional patients with anorexia develop obesity after treatment. Two to 6% of patients die from the complications of the disorder or commit suicide.

Various treatment methods have been used without clear evidence of superiority of one over another. Supportive care by physicians and nurses is probably the most important feature of therapy. Structured behavioral therapy, intensive psychotherapy, and family therapy may be tried. A variety of medications including tricyclic antidepressants and lithium carbonate are effective in some cases. Patients with severe malnutrition must be hemodynamically stabilized and may require enteral or parenteral feeding. Forced feed-

ings should be reserved for life-threatening situations, since the goal of treatment is to reestablish normal eating behavior.

Dempsey DT: Weight gain and nutritional efficacy in anorexia nervosa. *Am J Clin Nutr* 1984;**39**:236.

Heroz DB, Copeland PM: Eating disorders. *N Engl J Med* 1985;**313**:295.

Huse DM, Lucas AR: Dietary patterns in anorexia nervosa. *Am J Clin Nutr* 1984;**39**:236.

Laroca FEF (editor): Symposium on eating disorders. *Psychiatr Clin North Am* 1984;**7**:199.

Winston DH: Treatment of severe malnutrition in anorexia nervosa with enteral tube feedings. *Nutritional Support Services* 1987;**7**:24.

## BULIMIA & BULIMAREXIA

Bulimia is the episodic uncontrolled ingestion of large quantities of food. When combined with purging, either by self-induced vomiting or abuse of diuretics or cathartics, the disorder is called bulimarexia, or the binge-purge syndrome.

Like anorexia, bulimia and bulimarexia are predominantly disorders of young, white middle- and upper-class women. It is more difficult to detect than anorexia, and some studies have estimated the prevalence to be 40–50% in college-age women. As many as 10% of college-age men may also be bulimics.

Patients with bulimia typically consume large quantities of easily ingested high-calorie foods, usually in secrecy. Some patients may have several such episodes a day for a few days; others report regular and persistent patterns of binge eating. Binging is usually followed by vomiting, cathartics, or diuretics and is usually accompanied by feelings of guilt or depression. Periods of binging may be followed by intervals of self-imposed starvation. Body weights may fluctuate but generally are within 20% of desirable weights.

Some patients with bulimia also have a cryptic form of anorexia nervosa with significant weight losses and amenorrhea. Family and psychologic issues are generally similar to those encountered among patients with anorexia nervosa. Bulimics, however, have a higher incidence of premorbid obesity, greater use of cathartics and diuretics, and more impulsive or antisocial behaviors. Weights are closer to normal, and menstruation is usually preserved.

Depending on the type and severity of abnormal behavior, a variety of medical complications can occur. Gastric dilatation and pancreatitis have been reported after binges. Vomiting can result in poor dentition, pharyngitis, esophagitis, aspiration, and electrolyte abnormalities. Cathartic and diuretic abuse also commonly result in electrolyte abnormalities or dehydration. Constipation and hemorrhoids are common.

Treatment of bulimia and bulimarexia requires supportive care and psychotherapy. Individual, group, family, and behavioral therapy have all been utilized with modest success. Antidepressants may be helpful in some patients. Although death from bulimia is rare, the long-term psychiatric prognosis in severe bulimia is worse than the prognosis in anorexia nervosa, which suggests that the underlying psychiatric disorder may be more severe.

Harris RT: Bulimarexia and related serious eating disorders with medical complications. *Ann Intern Med* 1983;**99**:800.
Killen JD et al: Self-induced vomiting and laxative and diuretic use among teenagers: Precursors of the binge-purge syndrome? *JAMA* 1986;**255**:1447.
See also references under Anorexia Nervosa, above.

# DISORDERS OF VITAMIN METABOLISM

*Milton J. Chatton, MD*

The body's requirement for vitamins may vary considerably depending upon age, sex, physical activity, diet, metabolic rate, state of health, drug therapy, individual habits such as smoking or use of alcohol, use of contraceptives, and other factors affecting vitamin absorption, utilization, and excretion. Vitamin deficiencies are almost always multiple, although a particular symptom complex may predominate.

Early signs of vitamin deficiency are usually nonspecific, vague, and mild and are easily misinterpreted or missed entirely.

The treatment of multiple vitamin deficiencies consists of giving an adequate balanced diet and vitamin supplementation as indicated. Vitamins used therapeutically for specific deficiencies are usually given in 5–10 times the amounts required for daily maintenance.

Vitamin deficiencies of hereditary origin, should be distinguished from the acquired vitamin deficiencies. Almost a dozen rare vitamin-dependent genetic diseases, involving 5 different vitamins (thiamine, nicotinamide, pyridoxine, vitamin $B_{12}$, and vitamin D), have been described. The vitamin dependencies do not respond to physiologic replacement therapy but only to large (pharmacologic) doses of the needed vitamin.

Large doses of some vitamins (eg, vitamins A, C, D, K, niacin, and pyridoxine) are toxic and may cause illness, particularly when continued for long periods. The use of very large doses of vitamins for the treatment of a variety of disorders ("megavitamin therapy") is rarely warranted and potentially hazardous.

Alhadeff L, Gualtieri CT, Lipton M: Toxic effects of water-soluble vitamins. *Nutr Rev* 1984;**42**:33.
Rudman D, Williams PJ: Megadose vitamins: Use and misuse. *N Engl J Med* 1983;**309**:488.

# FAT-SOLUBLE VITAMINS

## 1. VITAMIN A

Vitamin A is an alcohol of high molecular weight that is stored in the liver. Most of it is derived from conversion of beta-carotene in foods to vitamin A, mainly by the mucosa of the small intestine but also by the liver. It is necessary for normal function and structure of all epithelial cells and for the synthesis of visual purple in the retinal rods (hence for vision in dim light). The recent epidemiologic observation that dietary carotene intake is inversely related to the incidence of lung cancer—perhaps owing to the vitamin's role in maintaining epithelial integrity—is of great potential significance and requires further evaluation. Carotene only is present in leafy green and yellow fruits and vegetables; vitamin A and, at times, carotene are present in whole milk, butter, eggs, fish, and liver oil. Actually, vitamin A itself is quite rare in foods; therefore, most is derived from carotene-bearing plant sources. The recommended daily allowances for adults are 5000 International Units (or USP units) for men and 4000 IU for women; during pregnancy and lactation, 5000–6000 IU.

### Hypovitaminosis A

**A. Clinical Findings:** Mild or early manifestations consist of dryness of the skin, tunnel vision, night blindness, and follicular hyperkeratotis. Severe or late manifestations are xerophthalmia, atrophy and keratinization of the skin, and keratomalacia.

**B. Tests for Deficiency:** Dark adaptation is impaired. A low serum value ($< 20~\mu g/dL$) of vitamin A may be found but is not diagnostic. A therapeutic test with 25,000–75,000 IU daily for 4 weeks may be helpful.

**C. Treatment:** Give oleovitamin A, 15,000–25,000 units once or twice daily. If an absorption defect is present, it may be necessary to administer bile salts with the vitamin A or to give the same dosage in oil intramuscularly (50,000 units/mL in sesame oil).

### Hypervitaminosis A

This disorder is rare in adults, but it may occur as a result of chronic excessive ingestion of vitamin A. Current enthusiasm for large doses of vitamins is expected to increase the incidence of vitamin A toxicity. The minimal toxic adult dose is about 75,000–100,000 units daily for 6 months; when ingested over a period of 8 years, a daily dose of 40,000 units may cause toxicity in adults.

**A. Clinical Findings:** Anorexia, loss of weight, dry and fissured skin, brittle nails, hair loss, gingivitis, cheilosis, hypercalcemia, hyperostosis, and periosteal elevation of bone, bony resorption, hepatomegaly, cirrhosis, splenomegaly, anemia, and central nervous system manifestations.

**B. Tests of Excess:** Serum levels of vitamin

A over 400 $\mu$g/dL are found (normal, 20–80 $\mu$g/dL).

**C. Treatment:** Withdraw the medicinal source.

Goodman DS: Vitamin A and retinoids in health and disease. *N Engl J Med* 1984;**310:**1023.

Olson JA: Recommended dietary intakes of vitamin A in humans. *Am J Clin Nutr* 1987;**45:**704.

Shepherd AN et al: Primary biliary cirrhosis, dark adaptometry, electro-oculography, and vitamin A state. *Br Med J* 1984;**289:**1484.

Vijayaraghavan K et al: Impact of massive doses of vitamin A on incidence of nutritional blindness. *Lancet* 1984;**2:**149.

Willett WC et al: Relation of serum vitamins A and E and carotenoids to the risk of cancer. *N Engl J Med* 1984;**310:**436.

## 2. VITAMIN D

Vitamin D is the generic name for a family of sterols that have varying degrees of antirachitic potency. The 2 most important of these sterols are ergocalciferol (vitamin $D_2$) and cholecalciferol (vitamin $D_3$). The human body can synthesize provitamin $D_3$ (7-dehydrocholesterol), which can be converted photochemically to vitamin $D_3$ by ultraviolet irradiation of the skin. Natural sources of vitamin D include liver and viscera of fish, livers of fish-eating animals, egg yolks, and butter.

Vitamin $D_3$ is transformed in the body to the biologically much more active metabolites 25-hydroxyvitamin $D_3$ and 1,25-dihydroxyvitamin $D_3$. These compounds, formed by the sequential hydroxylation of cholecalciferol by the liver and kidneys, are considerably more potent than the parent vitamin.

Vitamin D and its metabolites, together with parathyroid hormone and calcitonin, play an essential hormonal role in calcium homeostasis. The D vitamins maintain normal blood calcium transport in the intestine, mobilizing calcium from and to the bones, and control urinary phosphorus excretion.

Impaired metabolism of vitamin D or altered sensitivity of target tissues (intestine and bone) to the vitamin has been described in a wide variety of bone diseases and other disorders associated with abnormal calcium metabolism, eg, malabsorption, liver disease, renal failure, rickets, parathyroid disorders, and sarcoidosis.

There is, therefore, a wide spectrum of responsiveness to vitamin D. Some patients may require more than 50 times the therapeutic dose to correct manifestations of vitamin D deficiency (eg, vitamin D-resistant rickets), whereas others (eg, those with hyperparathyroidism) are hypersensitive even to doses below the recommended daily allowance.

### Hypovitaminosis D

Hypovitaminosis D is usually due to inadequate dietary intake, lack of sunlight, or an intestinal absorption defect (eg, pancreatitis, sprue), hepatic disease, or renal disease.

**A. Clinical Findings:** Deficiency of vitamin D leads to osteomalacia in children (rickets) or infantile tetany. Some cases of adult osteomalacia appear to be associated with gastrointestinal disorders and with increased requirements of vitamin D.

**B. Tests for Deficiency:** Serum calcium and phosphorus may be normal or decreased, and serum alkaline phosphatase is generally increased. The urinary calcium is usually low.

**C. Treatment:** See Osteomalacia (p 716). Simple dietary increase of vitamin D is relatively ineffective in treating the deficiencies encountered in the malabsorption syndromes and in biliary cirrhosis.

### Hypervitaminosis D

This disorder is usually caused by prolonged ingestion of 5000–150,000 units daily.

**A. Clinical Findings:** The manifestations of hypercalcemia are present and may progress to renal damage and metastatic calcification.

**B. Tests of Excess:** Serum calcium elevation ($>$11.5 mg/dL) occurs if large doses of vitamin D are taken. (Always consider other causes of hypercalcemia.)

**C. Treatment:** Withdraw the medicinal source. Complete recovery, although it may be slow, will occur if overtreatment is discontinued in time. Prednisone will dramatically reduce hypercalcemia that is due to vitamin D intoxication. Treatment of hypercalcemia may be required (see p 1063).

Avioli LV, Haddad JG: The vitamin D family revisited. *N Engl J Med* 1984;**311:**47.

Fraser DR: The physiological economy of vitamin D. *Lancet* 1983;**1:**969.

Manolagas SC, Deftos LJ: The vitamin D endocrine system and the hematolymphopoietic tissue. *Ann Intern Med* 1984;**100:**144.

Rinkleman RD, Butler WT: Vitamin D and skeletal tissues. *J Oral Pathol* 1985;**14:**181.

## 3. VITAMIN K

The K vitamins are fat-soluble chemical compounds necessary for the synthesis by the liver of blood coagulation factors II (prothrombin), VII, IX, and X. The similarity of the chemical structure of vitamin K to that of coenzyme Q suggests that the K vitamins may also be involved in the oxidative phosphorylation process in cellular mitochondria.

Vitamin K is widely distributed in foods. The naturally occurring form is called vitamin $K_1$. Vitamin K is also synthesized by microorganisms in the intestines and, since it differs from $K_1$ somewhat in chemical structure, is referred to as vitamin $K_2$. A third form of the vitamin, prepared synthetically, is known as vitamin $K_3$ (menadione).

The daily requirement of vitamin K is not known but is probably quite low. Vitamin K depletion due to dietary deficiency alone is extremely rare.

## Hypovitaminosis K

Hypovitaminosis K may result from biliary obstruction or medical or surgical disorders of the small bowel that interfere with the absorption of fat. Longterm therapy with antibiotics or nonabsorbable sulfonamides that interfere with microorganism synthesis of vitamin K may also cause vitamin K deficiency.

A bleeding tendency or uncontrollable hemorrhage may occur. The coagulation defect may be aggravated by ingestion of drugs that depress prothrombin synthesis (eg, coumarins, salicylates). Prolongation of the prothrombin time as well as abnormal tests for coagulation factors VII, IX, and X may be demonstrated.

Successful treatment of the defective coagulation is dependent upon a functioning hepatic parenchyma, and vitamin K therapy is of no avail if liver disease is severe.

## Hypervitaminosis K

Large doses of water-soluble vitamin K (derivative of $K_3$; menadione) to infants—particularly premature infants—may cause hemolytic anemia, hyperbilirubinemia, hepatomegaly, and even death. In adults with G6PD deficiency, ordinary doses of menadione or derivatives may cause hemolytic reactions.

Krasinski SD et al: The prevalence of vitamin K disorders in chronic gastrointestinal disorders. *Am J Clin Nutr* 1985;**41**:639.
Olson JA: Recommended dietary intakes of vitamin K in humans. *Am J Clin Nutr* 1987;**45**:687.

## 4. VITAMIN E
## (Tocopherol)

Vitamin E is a natural antioxidant that plays a role in the normal physiology of animals and probably also of humans, although its exact role in humans is unclear. Hemolytic anemia due to vitamin E deficiency occurs in small premature infants who are given artificial formulas containing iron and high concentrations of unsaturated fatty acids. Vitamin E deficiency has been reported in malabsorption and maldigestion disorders of different types including chronic exocrine pancreatic insufficiency, advanced hepatobiliary disease, and intestinal resection. Deficiency may also occur in retinitis pigmentosa, myopathies, neuropathies, cystic fibrosis, and hereditary abetalipoproteinemia. The antioxidant property of vitamin E has been utilized to counteract the harmful effects of excess of free radicals or pro-oxidants that occur in certain hereditary metabolic disorders or as a result of body stresses such as hyperoxia, ionizing radiation, and exposure to various drugs and toxins. The vitamin is widely held to be a panacea for a great variety of disorders; these claims cannot be scientifically substantiated. Recommended daily allowances for adults (based upon the usual range of intake of vitamin E) are 10 mg of $\alpha$-tocopherol for men and 8 mg of $\alpha$-tocopherol for women, with 10 mg of $\alpha$-tocopherol

during pregnancy and lactation. The requirement of the vitamin may be related to the polyunsaturated fatty acid content in body tissue.

Bieri JG, Corash L, Hubbard VS: Medical uses of vitamin E. *N Engl J Med* 1983;**308**:1063.
Sokol RJ et al: Vitamin E deficiency in adults with chronic liver disease. *Am J Clin Nutr* 1985;**41**:66.

## WATER-SOLUBLE VITAMINS: VITAMIN B COMPLEX*

The members of the vitamin B complex are intimately associated in occurrence in food as well as in function (eg, as coenzymes). As a result of this close interrelationship, nutritional deficiency of a single B vitamin rarely exists except under experimental conditions. Deficiency of a single member of the B complex can lead to impaired metabolism of the others. Hence, although certain clinical features may predominate in the absence of a single member of the complex, this does not mean that the deficiency can be entirely corrected by replacing that factor alone. All members of the B complex must be provided.

## 1. VITAMIN B₁
## (Thiamine Hydrochloride)

Vitamin $B_1$ is a constituent of the enzyme that decarboxylates pyruvic acid and alpha-ketoglutaric acid and is important for normal carbohydrate oxidation. Dietary sources are liver, lean pork, kidney, and whole grain cereals. Steaming or exposure to moist heat reduces the thiamine content of foods. The daily dietary allowances are about 1.2–1.4 mg/d.

## Hypovitaminosis B₁
## (Beriberi)

Hypovitaminosis $B_1$ results from an inadequate intake due usually to idiosyncrasies of diet or excessive cooking or processing of foods. The increased need for vitamin $B_1$ during fever, high carbohydrate intake, alcoholism, or thyrotoxicosis may lead to deficiency.

**A. Clinical Findings:** Mild or early manifestations consist of vague multiple complaints and include anorexia, formication, muscle cramps, calf tenderness, paresthesias, and hyperactivity followed later by hypoactivity of knee and ankle jerks.

Severe or late manifestations (beriberi) are anorexia, polyneuritis, subcutaneous edema, paralyses (particularly in the extremities), and cardiac insufficiency manifested by tachycardia, dyspnea, edema, and nonspecific electrocardiographic changes. A particularly virulent form of beriberi heart disease,

---

* Vitamin $B_{12}$ is discussed on p 300.

probably associated with metabolic acidosis, is referred to as Shoshin beriberi in the Orient.

**B. Treatment:** Give thiamine hydrochloride, 20–50 mg orally, intravenously, or intramuscularly daily in divided doses for 2 weeks and then 10 mg daily orally. The clinical response to thiamine injection within 24–48 hours is one of the best criteria for a diagnosis of thiamine deficiency. An alternative is to give dried yeast tablets (brewer's yeast), 30 g 3 times daily.

Campbell CH: The severe lactic acidosis of thiamine deficiency: Acute pernicious or fulminating beriberi. *Lancet* 1984;**2**:446.

Daney M et al: Blood thiamine and thiamine ester concentrations in alcoholic and nonalcoholic liver diseases. *Br Med J* 1984;**289**:79.

## 2. RIBOFLAVIN (Vitamin B₂)

Riboflavin serves principally as a coenzyme for hydrogen transfer in the electron transport system of the respiratory chain. It is abundant in milk and milk products, leafy green vegetables, liver, kidneys, and heart. The daily dietary allowances for adults are 1.5–1.8 mg; in pregnancy and lactation, 1.5–2 mg.

### Hypovitaminosis B₂ (Ariboflavinosis)

The etiologic factors in ariboflavinosis are similar to those in thiamine deficiency, but inadequate intake of milk is an important contributing factor. Riboflavin deficiency has been reported in women taking oral contraceptives. The manifestations of deficiency are highly variable and usually occur along with those of thiamine and niacin deficiency but may occur earlier.

**A. Clinical Findings:** Mild or early manifestations are oral pallor, superficial fissuring at the angles of the mouth, conjunctivitis and photophobia, lack of vigor, malaise, weakness, and weight loss. Severe or late manifestations consist of cheilosis (fissuring at the angles of the mouth), fissuring of the nares, magenta tongue, moderate edema, anemia, dysphagia, corneal vascularization and circumcorneal injection, and seborrheic dermatitis.

**B. Treatment:** Give riboflavin, 40–50 mg intravenously, intramuscularly, or orally daily until all symptoms have cleared. An alternative is to give dried yeast tablets (brewer's yeast), 30 g 3 times daily.

Belko A et al: Effects of aerobic exercise and weight loss on riboflavin requirements of moderately obese, marginally deficient young women. *Am J Clin Nutr* 1984;**40**:553.

Garry PJ et al: Nutritional status in a healthy elderly population: Riboflavin. *Am J Clin Nutr* 1982;**36**:902.

## 3. NICOTINIC ACID (Niacin) & NICOTINAMIDE (Niacinamide)

Niacin and niacinamide function in important enzyme systems concerned with reversible oxidation and reduction by hydrogen transfer. They are present in liver, yeast, meat, whole-grain cereals, and peanuts. Nicotinic acid may be synthesized in the body from tryptophan. Therefore, adequate protein intake virtually ensures adequate nicotinic acid. Sixty milligrams of tryptophan produce 1 mg of nicotinic acid.

The daily allowances for adults are 13–20 mg. Niacin may be used therapeutically as a vasodilating agent for headaches, myalgias, neurologic disorders, and edema of the labyrinth (100 mg or more daily in divided doses). Because niacin decreases the synthesis of low-density lipoprotein and lowers serum cholesterol, it can be used pharmacologically to treat hypercholesterolemia and hypertriglyceridemia. Doses as high as 3–7 g/d are usually necessary (see Chapter 17). There is no strong evidence that high doses of niacin or niacinamide help in the treatment of schizophrenia. Niacinamide does not possess the vasodilating or lipid-lowering effects of niacin.

### Pellagra

The etiologic factors in deficiency of these components of the B complex are similar to those of thiamine deficiency.

**A. Clinical Findings:** Mild or early manifestations consist of multiple vague complaints; a reddened, roughened skin, and redness and hypertrophy of the papillae of the tongue. Severe or late manifestations are marked roughening of the skin when exposed to light and friction, diarrhea, abdominal distention, scarlet red tongue with atrophy of papillae, stomatitis, depression, rigidity, and dementia.

**B. Treatment:** Give nicotinamide (niacinamide), 50–500 mg intravenously, intramuscularly, or orally daily until symptoms subside. Nicotinic acid (niacin) is less often used because of its vasodilating effect; the dosage is similar. Give therapeutic doses of thiamine, riboflavin, and pyridoxine also. An alternative is to give dried yeast tablets (brewer's yeast), 30 g 3 times daily.

### Nicotinic Acid Poisoning

Large oral doses of nicotinic acid may cause flushing and burning of the skin and dizziness but are usually not harmful. After intravenous administration, hypotension may be severe. Anaphylaxis occurs rarely.

Leads From MMWR: Niactin intoxication from pumpernickel bagels—New York. *JAMA* 1983;**250**:160.

Rabbani GH et al: Reduction of fluid loss in cholera by nicotinic acid: A randomized controlled trial. *Lancet* 1983;**2**:1439.

Shelley WB, Shelley ED: Nicotinic acid-responsive photosensitivity. *Lancet* 1984;**2**:576.

### Folic Acid

Folic acid is essential for the metabolism of cell

nuclear materials. Signs of folic acid deficincy appear rapidly, since minimal folic acid is stored in the body. Cells with rapid turnover such as bone marrow and the gastrointestinal mucosa demonstrate abnormalities first. A megaloblastic anemia is commonly seen. The recommended daily allowance for adults is 400 $\mu$g. This is increased to 800 $\mu$g in pregnancy and to 600 $\mu$g in lactation.

Folate deficiency has been described most commonly in persons with chronic alcoholism, in the elderly, and in patients taking oral contraceptives and anticonvulsant drugs.

Herbert V: Recommended dietary intakes of folate in humans. *Am J Clin Nutr* 1987;**45:**661.

## Pyridoxine Hydrochloride
## (Vitamin B<sub>6)</sub>

Pyridoxine is important in transamination and decarboxylation of amino acids. Deficiency of the vitamin may result in an anemia with intramedullary hemolysis (see p 302). The recommended daily allowance for adults is about 2 mg. It may relieve nervous symptoms and weakness in pellagrins when niacin fails and may relieve glossitis and cheilosis when riboflavin fails. The therapeutic dosage is 10–50 mg intravenously or intramuscularly daily with other factors of the B complex. Large doses of pyridoxine have been advocated for the prevention and treatment of premenstrual syndrome. An irreversible sensory neuropathy has been described, however, in patients taking large doses (>300 mg daily).

Berger A, Schaumburg HH: More on neuropathy from pyridoxine abuse. *New Engl J Med* 1984;**311:**986.

Natta CL, Reynolds RD: Apparent vitamin B<sub>6</sub> deficiency in sickle anemia. *Am J Clin Nutr* 1984;**40:**235.

Schaumburg H et al: Sensory neuropathy from pyridoxine abuse: A new megavitamin syndrome. *N Engl J Med* 1983;**309:**445.

## WATER-SOLUBLE VITAMINS:
## VITAMIN C (Ascorbic Acid)

Vitamin C is involved in the formation and maintenance of intercellular structures (dentine, cartilage, collagen, bone matrix). Its biochemical action is not clear. It may play a specific role in hydroxylation of proline in collagen, which may be related to connective tissue functioning and wound healing. Dietary sources include citrus fruits, tomatoes, paprika, bell peppers, and all leafy green vegetables. The ascorbic acid content of foods is markedly decreased by cooking, alkalies, and contact with copper utensils. The recommended allowance for adults in the USA is 45 mg daily; for pregnant or lactating women, 60 mg daily.

Ascorbic acid in doses of 0.5 g or more has been advocated for the prevention of neoplastic disease and in the treatment of certain poisonings, but proof of its value is lacking. Large doses have also been recommended for the prevention or palliation of the common cold, but recent studies suggest that massive vitamin C prophylaxis does not result in significantly fewer colds. Although large doses of vitamin C are relatively safe, diarrhea and flatulence are common side effects. An increased risk of kidney stones has also been reported.

## Hypovitaminosis C
## (Scurvy)

Scurvy is usually due to inadequate intake of vitamin C but may occur with increased metabolic needs. The disease is seen frequently in formula-fed infants, food faddists, and the elderly. Vitamin C concentration in tissues has been reported to be decreased in healthy women taking oral contraceptives.

**A. Clinical Findings:** Mild or early manifestations are edema and hemorrhage of the gingivae, and hyperkeratotic hair follicles. Severe or late manifestations consist of severe muscle changes, swelling of the joints, rarefaction of bone, a marked bleeding tendency, extravasation of blood into fascial layers, anemia, loosening or loss of the teeth, and poor wound healing.

**B. Treatment:** Give sodium ascorbate injection, 100–500 mg intramuscularly daily, or ascorbic acid, 100–500 mg orally daily, as long as deficiency persists.

Olson JA, Hodges RE: Recommended dietary intakes of vitamin C in humans. *Am J Clin Nutr* 1987;**45:**693.

Reuler JB, Broudy VC, Cooney TG: Adult scurvy. *JAMA* 1985;**253:**805.

Wittes RE: Vitamin C and cancer. *New Engl J Med* 1985; **312:**178.

## DIET THERAPY

Specifid therapeutic diets can be designed to facilitate the medical management of many common illnesses. In most cases, consultation with a registered dietitian is necessary in order to design and implement major dietary changes. Physicians should be familiar with the indications for special diets and their basic composition to facilitate patient referrals and to maximize patient compliance.

Diet therapy is a difficult process, and not all patients are able to cooperate fully. Before starting specific dietary changes, one should assess the patient's motivation for change in eating habits. Patients who are not adequately motivated or who for other reasons are unable to change their diets should not be started on diet therapy, since embarking on a course that can only fail will interfere with other aspects of the therapeutic relationship between doctor and patient. Requesting the patient to record dietary intake for 3–5 days may provide useful insight into the patient's motivation.

Prescribed diets should take into account personal food preferences, cultural habits, and eating behavior. Changes should be introduced gradually. Close follow-up and a close patient-therapist relationship are necessary for sustained dietary change.

Therapeutic diets can be divided into 3 groups: (1) diets that alter the consistency of food; (2) diets that restrict or otherwise modify dietary components; and (3) diets that supplement dietary components.

## DIETS THAT ALTER CONSISTENCY

### Clear Liquid Diet

This diet provides adequate water, up to 1000 kcal as simple sugar, and some electrolytes. It is fiber-free and requires minimal digestion or intestinal motility.

A clear liquid diet is useful for patients with resolving postoperative ileus, acute gastroenteritis, partial intestinal obstruction, and as preparation for diagnostic gastrointestinal procedures. It is commonly used as the first diet for patients who have been taking nothing by mouth for long periods. Because of the low calorie and minimal protein content of the clear liquid diet, it should be used only for short periods.

### Full Liquid Diet

The full liquid diet provides adequate water and can be designed to provide adequate calories and protein. Vitamins and minerals—especially folic acid, iron, and vitamin $B_6$—may be inadequate and should be provided in the form of supplements. Diary products, soups, eggs, and soft cereals are used to supplement clear liquids. Commercial oral supplements can also be incorporated into the diet or used alone.

This diet is low in residue and can be used in many instances instead of the clear liquid diet described above—especially in patients with difficulty in chewing or swallowing, with partial obstructions, or in preparation for some diagnostic procedures. Full liquid diets are commonly used following clear liquid diets to "advance" diets in patients who have been taking nothing by mouth for long periods.

### Mechanical Soft Diet

This diet includes foods permitted in the liquid diets as well as foods containing easily digested protein and carbohydrates. Eggs, cottage cheese, ground meat, crackers, refined cereals and grains, skinless potatoes and starches, cooked skinless fruits and vegetables, and cakes and cookies are included.

The diet is low in residue. It can be designed to meet all other nutritional requirements. It is most commonly used for patients who have difficulty with chewing and swallowing or with partial intestinal obstruction. Mechanical soft diets that restrict spices and seasonings—the **bland diet**—have traditionally been used for patients with peptic disease. There is no evidence that such diets are useful, and they should no longer be prescribed.

## DIETS THAT RESTRICT NUTRIENTS

Diets can be designed to restrict (or eliminate) virtually any nutrient or food component. The most commonly used restricted diets are those that limit sodium, fat, and protein. Other restrictive diets and their most common therapeutic indications are listed in Table 20–15.

### Sodium-Restricted Diets

Low-sodium diets are useful in the management of hypertension and in conditions in which sodium retention and edema are prominent features, particularly congestive heart failure, chronic liver disease, and chronic renal failure. Sodium restriction is beneficial with or without diuretic therapy. When used in conjunction with diuretics, sodium restriction allows lower dosage of the diuretic medication and may prevent side effects. Potassium excretion, in particular, is directly related to distal renal tubule sodium delivery, and sodium restriction will decrease diuretic-related potassium losses.

Typical American diets contain about 4–6 g (175–260 meq) of sodium per day. Typical sodium-restricted diets contain 2000 mg (88 meq), 1000 mg (44 meq), and 500 mg (22 meq) of sodium per day. Diets containing intermediate quantities of sodium can also be designed.

Dietary sodium includes sodium naturally occurring in foods, sodium added during food processing, and sodium added by the consumer during cooking and at the table. About a third of current dietary intake is derived from each. Diets that allow 2000 mg of sodium daily are easiest to design and imple-

**Table 20–15.** Diets that restrict nutrients.

| | Common Indication |
|---|---|
| Sodium-restricted | Hypertension, congestive heart failure, chronic liver disease, chronic renal failure |
| Fat-restricted | Malabsorption syndromes |
| Fat- and cholesterol-restricted | Hyperlipidemia, diabetes |
| Protein-restricted | Hepatic encephalopathy, chronic renal failure |
| Calorie-restricted | Obesity, diabetes (type II) |
| Lactose-restricted | Lactose intolerance |
| Potassium-restricted | Chronic renal failure |
| Gluten-restricted | Celiac sprue |
| Phosphate-restricted | Chronic renal failure |
| Copper-restricted | Wilson's disease |
| Oxalate-restricted | Hyperoxaluria |
| Elimination diets | Food allergies |
| Salicylate-restricted | Chronic urticaria |
| Tyramine-restricted | Monoamine oxidase inhibitor use |
| Amino acid-restricted | Amino acid disorders, eg, phenylketonuria |

ment. Such diets generally eliminate added salt, most processed foods, and selected foods with particularly high sodium content. Patients who follow such diets for 2–3 months lose their craving for salty foods and can often continue to restrict their sodium intake indefinitely. Many patients with mild hypertension will normalize their blood pressure with this 2000-mg sodium diet.

Diets allowing 1000 mg and 500 mg of salt require, in addition to the restrictions outlined above, restrict more commonly eaten foods. Special "low-sodium" products are now available to facilitate such diets. These diets are difficult for most people to follow and are generally reserved for hospitalized patients and highly motivated outpatients—most commonly those with severe liver disease and ascites.

### Fat-Restricted Diets

Traditional fat-restricted diets are useful in the treatment of fat malabsorption syndromes. Such diets will improve the symptoms of diarrhea with steatorrhea independently of the primary physiologic abnormality by limiting the quantity of fatty acids that reach the colon. The degree of fat restriction necessary to control symptoms must be individualized. Patients with severe malabsorption can be limited to 40–60 g of fat per day. Diets containing 60–80 g of fat per day can be designed for patients with less severe abnormalities.

In general, fat-restricted diets require broiling, baking, or boiling meat and fish; discarding the skin of poultry and fish and using those foods as the main protein source; using nonfat dairy products; and avoiding desserts, sauces, and gravies.

### Low-Cholesterol, Low-Saturated Fat Diets

Diets low in cholesterol and saturated fats are fat-restricted diets that also restrict saturated fats and dietary cholesterol. Such diets are the mainstay of dietary treatment of hyperlipidemia (see Chapter 19). Similar diets are recommended also for diabetes (Chapter 19) and for the prevention of coronary artery disease (Chapter 8). Current recommendations for the prevention of cancer by dietary modification also include fat restriction.

These diets limit total fat intake to 20–30% of total calories. Saturated fat intake is limited to 10% or less of total calories. In practice, the fat intake with these diets is similar to that achieved with traditional fat-restricted diets. In addition, dietary cholesterol intake is limited to 300 mg or less per day.

### Protein-Restricted Diets

Protein-restricted diets are most commonly used in patients with hepatic encephalopathy due to chronic liver disease and in chronic renal failure. Patients with selected inborn errors of amino acid metabolism and other abnormalities resulting in hyperammonemia also require protein restriction.

Protein restriction is intended to limit the produc-tion of nitrogenous waste products. Energy intake must be adequate to facilitate the efficient use of dietary protein. Proteins must be of high biologic value and be provided in sufficient quantity to meet minimal requirements. For most patients, the diet should contain at least 0.5 g/kg/d of protein. Patients with encephalopathy who fail to respond to this degree of restriction are unlikely to respond to more severe restriction.

## DIETS THAT SUPPLEMENT NUTRIENTS

Diets that supplement specific nutrients can also be designed. Such diets and their most common therapeutic indications are shown in Table 20–16.

### High-Fiber Diet

Dietary fiber is a diverse group of plant contituents that are resistant to digestion by the human digestive tract. Typical American diets contain about 5–10 g of dietary fiber per day. Epidemiologic evidence has suggested that populations consuming greater quantities of fiber have a lower incidence of certain gastrointestinal disorders, including diverticulitis and colon cancer. Most authorities currently recommend higher intakes of dietary fiber for health maintenance.

Diets high in dietary fiber (20–35 g/d) are also commonly used in management of a variety of gastrointestinal disorders, particularly the irritable bowel syndrome and recurrent diverticulitis. Diets high in fiber may also be useful to reduce blood sugar in patients with diabetes and to reduce cholesterol levels in patients with hypercholesterolemia. Such diets include greater intakes of fresh fruits and vegetables, whole grains, legumes and seeds, and bran products. For some patients, the addition of psyllium seed (2 tsp per day) or natural bran (½ cup per day) may be preferable.

### High-Potassium Diets

Potassium-supplemented diets are used most commonly to compensate for potassium losses caused by diuretics. Although potassium losses can be partially prevented by using lower doses of diuretics, concurrent sodium restriction, and potassium-sparing diuretics, some patients require additional potassium to prevent hypokalemia. Preliminary epidemiologic and experimental evidence suggests that high-potas-

**Table 20–16.** Diets that supplement nutrients.

|  | Common Indication |
|---|---|
| Protein- and calorie-supplemented | Protein-calorie undernutrition |
| High-fiber | Diverticulitis, irritable bowel |
| High-potassium | Diuretic use |
| High-calcium | Osteoporosis |

sium diets may also have a direct antihypertensive effect. Typical American diets contain about 3 g (80 meq) of potassium per day. High-potassium diets commonly contain 4.5–7 g (120–180 meq) of potassium per day.

Most fruits, vegetables, and their juices contain high concentrations of potassium. Supplemental potassium can also be provided with potassium-containing salt substitutes or as potassium chloride in solution or capsules, but this is rarely necessary if the above measures are followed to prevent potassium losses and supplement dietary potassium.

## High-Calcium Diets

Additional intakes of dietary calcium have recently been recommended for the prevention of postmenopausal osteoporosis, the prevention and treatment of hypertension, and the prevention of colon cancer. Although the evidence in each case is preliminary, most authorities currently recommend intakes of 1 g of calcium per day for most adults and 1.5 g/d for postmenopausal women. Current USA intakes are approximately 700 mg/d.

Low-fat and nonfat dairy products are the mainstay of supplemental calcium intakes. Patients with lactose intolerance who cannot tolerate liquid dairy products may be able to tolerate nonliquid products such as cheese and yogurt. Leafy green vegetables and canned fish with bones also contain high concentrations of calcium, although the latter is also very high in sodium.

Anderson JW et al: Hypocholesterolemic effects of oat-bran or bran intake for hypercholesterolemic men. *Am J Clin Nutr* 1984;**40:**1146.

Beauchamp GK, Bertino M, Engelman K: Modification of salt taste. *Ann Intern Med* 1983;**98:**763.

Eastwood MA, Passmore R: Dietary fiber. *Lancet* 1983;**2:**202.

Ettinger B, Genant HK, Cann CE: Postmenopausal bone loss is prevented by treatment with low-dosage estrogen with calcium. *Ann Intern Med* 1987;**106:**40.

Glomset JA: Fish, fatty acids and human health. *N Engl J Med* 1985;**312:**1253.

Grundy SM: Comparison of monounsaturated fatty acids and carbohydrate for lowering cholesterol. *New Engl J Med* 1986;**314:**745.

Herold PM, Kinsella JE: Fish oil consumption and decreased risk of cardiovascular disease. *AM J Clin Nutr* 1986;**43:**566.

Holliday MA: Nutritional aspects of renal disease in children and adults. *Hosp Pract* (March) 1983;**18:**179.

Kaplan N: Nondrug treatment of hypertension. *Ann Intern Med* 1985;**102:**359.

Lipkin M, Newmark H: Effect of added dietary calcium on colonic epithelial-cell proliferation in subjects at high risk for familial colon cancer. *N Engl J Med* 1985;**313:**1381.

Lugar SW, McCormick E: Breakfast of champions or of hypertensives? *New Engl J Med* 1986;**314:**1052.

McCarron DA: Is calcium more important than sodium in the pathogenesis of hypertension? *Hypertension* 1985;**7:**607.

Peters WL, Goroll AH: The evaluation and treatment of hypercholesterolemia in primary care practice. *J Gen Intern Med* 1986;**1:**183.

Sleisenger MH (editor): Malabsorption and nutritional support. *Clin Gastroenterol* 1983;**12:**323.

Van Horn LV et al: Serum lipid response to oat product intake with a fat-modified diet. *J Am Diet Assoc* 1986;**86:**759.

# NUTRITIONAL SUPPORT

Nutritional support is the provision of nutrients to patients who cannot meet their nutritional requirements by eating standard diets. Nutrients may be delivered enterally, using oral nutritional supplements, nasogastric and nasoduodenal feeding tubes, and tube enterostomies; or parenterally, using lines or catheters placed in peripheral or central veins, respectively. Current nutritional support techniques permit adequate nutrient delivery to virtually any patient. Nutrition support should only be utilized, however, if it is likely to improve the patient's clinical outcome. The financial costs and risks of side effects must be balanced against the potential advantages of improved nutritional status in each clinical situation.

The rational use of nutritional support requires a full understanding of its indications, a knowledge of how to select the best method for nutritional support in individual cases, a knowledge of how to select the best solution for the individual patient, and how to monitor patients to prevent untoward side effects.

## INDICATIONS FOR NUTRITIONAL SUPPORT

The precise indications for nutritional support remain controversial. Most authorities agree that nutritional support is indicated for at least 4 groups of adult patients: (1) those with inadequate bowel syndromes; (2) those with severe prolonged hypercatabolic states (eg, due to extensive burns, multiple trauma); (3) those requiring prolonged therapeutic bowel rest; and (4) those with severe protein-calorie undernutrition with a treatable disease who have sustained a loss of over 25% of body weight.

It has been difficult to prove the efficacy of nutritional support in the treatment of most other conditions. Over 70 randomized controlled clinical trials have been conducted in an attempt to address this question. In most cases it has not been possible to show a clear advantage of treatment by means of nutritional support over treatment without such support. Unfortunately, most of these studies have design flaws and do not disprove the effectiveness of nutritional support. Better-designed randomized controlled studies of larger scale are now in progress.

The American Society for Parenteral and Enteral Nutrition (ASPEN) has published recommendations for the rational use of nutritional support. These are shown in Table 20–17. The recommendations emphasize the need to individualize the decision to begin

**Table 20–17.** Indications and contraindications for nutritional support.*

1. Normally nourished patients who are eating sufficiently—no additional therapy.
2. Normally nourished patients who are not eating sufficiently for a period of less than 5–7 days—no further therapy. For a period of over 5–7 days, enteral and/or parenteral nutrition support to meet requirements should be considered.
3. Malnourished patients who are eating sufficiently—no further therapy.
4. Malnourished patients who are not eating sufficiently—enteral and/or parenteral nutrition support to meet requirements should be considered.
5. Selected patients who are hypermetabolic may require specialized nutrition therapy before 5–7 days.

* Reprinted from: *Standards for Nutrition Support: Hospitalized Patients.* American Society for Parenteral and Enteral Nutrition (ASPEN), 1984.

nutritional support, carefully weighing the risks and costs against the benefit to each patient. They also demonstrate the advantages of nutritional assessment in identifying high-risk malnourished patients.

## NUTRITIONAL SUPPORT METHODS

Selection of the most appropriate nutritional support method involves consideration of gastrointestinal function, the anticipated duration of nutritional support, and the ability of each method to meet the patient's nutritional requirements. The method chosen should meet the patient's nutritional needs with the lowest risk and lowest cost possible. For most patients, enteral feeding is safer and cheaper and offers significant physiologic advantages. An algorithm for selection of the most appropriate nutritional support method is presented in Fig 20–1.

The simplest **enteral nutritional support** method

is oral feeding. Careful attention to patient preferences, timing of meals, diagnostic procedures and use of medications, and the use of foods brought to the hospital by family and friends can often significantly increase oral intake. Patients unable to eat enough at regular mealtimes to meet their nutritional requirements can be given **oral supplements** as snacks or to replace low-calorie beverages. Supplements of differing nutritional composition are available for the purpose of individualizing the diet in accordance with specific clinical requirements. Fiber and lactose content, caloric density, protein level, and amino acid profiles can all be modified as necessary.

Patients unable to take oral nutrients who have functioning gastrointestinal tracts and who meet the criteria for nutritional support are candidates for **tube feedings.** Small-bore feeding tubes are placed via the nose into the stomach or duodenum. Patients able to sit up in bed who can protect their airways can be fed into the stomach. Because of the increased risk of aspiration, patients who cannot adequately protect their airways should be fed nasoduodenally. Feeding tubes can be passed into the duodenum by leaving an extra length of tubing and placing the patient in the right decubitus position. Metoclopramide, 10 mg intravenously, can be given 20 minutes prior to insertion and continued every 6 hours thereafter to facilitate passage through the pylorus. Occasional patients will require fluoroscopy or endoscopic guidance to insert the tube distal to the pylorus. Placement of nasogastric and, particularly, nasoduodenal tubes should be confirmed radiographically before delivery of feeding solutions.

Feeding tubes can also be placed directly into the gastrointestinal tract using **tube enterostomies.** Most tube enterostomies are placed in patients who require long-term enteral nutritional support. The most common application is the surgical placement of gastrostomies and jejunostomies. Gastrostomies have the ad-

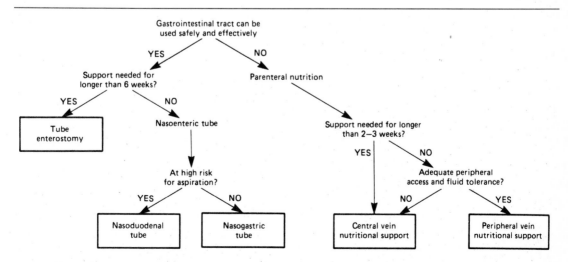

**Figure 20–1.** Nutritional support method decision tree.

vantage of allowing bolus feedings, while jejunostomies require continuous infusions. Gastrostomies—like nasogastric feeding—should only be used in patients at low risk for aspiration. Gastrostomies can also be placed percutaneously with the aid of endoscopy. These tubes can then be advanced to jejunostomies. Tube enterostomies can also be used in patients with unrelievable obstructions.

Patients who require nutritional support but whose gastrointestinal tracts are nonfunctional should receive **parenteral nutritional support.** Most patients receive parenteral feedings via a central vein—most commonly the subclavian vein. Peripheral veins can be used in some patients, but because of the high osmolality of parenteral solutions this is rarely tolerated for long periods.

**Peripheral vein nutritional support** is most commonly used in patients with nonfunctioning gastrointestinal tracts who require immediate support but whose clinical status is expected to improve within 1–2 weeks, allowing enteral feeding. Peripheral vein nutritional support is administered via standard intravenous lines. Solutions should always include lipid and dextrose in combination with amino acids to provide adequate nonprotein calories. Serious side effects are infrequent, but there is a high incidence of phlebitis and infiltration of intravenous lines.

**Central vein nutritional support** is most commonly delivered via intravenous catheters placed percutaneously using aseptic technique. Proper placement in the superior vena cava is documented radiographically before the solution is allowed to start running. Catheters must be carefully maintained by experienced nursing personnel and not used for anything other than nutritional support.

## NUTRITIONAL REQUIREMENTS

Each patient's nutritional requirements should be determined independently of the method chosen. In most situations, solutions of equal nutrient value can be designed for delivery via enteral and parenteral routes, but differences in absorption must be considered. A complete nutritional support solution must contain water, energy, amino acids, electrolytes, vitamins, and minerals (see Nutritional Requirements at the beginning of this chapter).

### Water

For most patients, water requirements can be calculated by allowing 1500 mL for the first 20 kg of body weight plus 20 mL for every kilogram over 20. Additional losses should be replaced as they occur. For average-sized adult patients, fluid needs are about 30–35 mL/kg, or approximately 1 mL/kg of energy required (see below).

### Energy

Energy requirements can be estimated by one of 3 methods: (1) by using standard equations to calculate basal energy expenditure (BEE) plus additional calories for activity and illness; (2) by applying a simple calculation based on calories per kilogram of body weight; or (3) by measuring energy expenditure with indirect calorimetry.

Measurement of the basal energy expenditure (BEE) by the Harris-Benedict equation is described earlier in this chapter. For undernourished patients, actual body weight should be used; whereas for obese patients, ideal body weight should be used. For most patients, an additional 20–50% of BEE is administered as nonprotein calories to accommodate energy expenditures during activity or relating to the illness. Occasional patients are noted to have energy expenditures greater than 150% of BEE.

Energy requirements can be estimated also by multiplying actual body weight in kilograms (for obese patients, ideal body weight) by 30–35 kcal.

Both of these methods provide imprecise estimates of actual energy expenditures. Studies using indirect calorimetry have demonstrated that as many as 30–40% of patients will have measured expenditures 10% above or below estimated values. For accurate determination of energy expenditure, indirect calorimetry should be used. Unfortunately, calorimeters are available in only a few medical centers. This means that patients must be closely monitored and regularly reassessed to determine whether estimates are close enough for clinical purposes.

### Protein

Protein and energy requirements are closely related. If adequate calories are provided, most patients can be given 0.8–1.2 g of protein per kilogram per day. Patients undergoing moderate to severe stress should receive up to 1.5 g/kg/d. As in the case of energy requirements, actual weights should be used for normal and underweight patients and ideal weights for patients with significant obesity.

Patients who are receiving protein without adequate calories will catabolize protein for energy rather than utilizing it for protein synthesis. Thus, when energy intake is low, excess protein is needed for nitrogen balance. If both energy and protein intakes are low, extra energy will have a more significant positive effect on nitrogen balance than extra protein.

### Electrolytes & Minerals

Requirements for sodium, potassium, and chloride vary widely. Most patients require 45–145 meq/d of each. The actual requirement in individual patients will depend on the patient's cardiovascular, renal, endocrine, and gastrointestinal status as well as measurements of serum concentration.

Patients receiving enteral nutritional support should receive adequate vitamins and minerals according to the recommended daily allowances (Tables 20–1 and 20–2). Most premixed enteral solutions provide adequate vitamins and minerals as long as adequate calories are administered.

Patients receiving parenteral nutritional support

require smaller amounts of minerals: calcium, 10–15 meq/d; phosphorus, 15–20 meq per 1000 nonprotein calories; and magnesium, 16–24 meq/d. Most patients receiving nutritional support do not require supplemental iron because body stores are adequate. Iron nutrition should be monitored closely by following the hemoglobin concentration, MCV, and iron studies. Parenteral administration of iron is associated with a number of adverse effects and should be reserved for iron-deficient patients unable to take oral iron.

Patients receiving parenteral nutritional support should be given the trace elements zinc (about 5 mg/d) and copper (about 2 mg/d). Patients with diarrhea will require additional zinc to replace fecal losses. Additional trace elements—especially chromium, manganese, and selenium—are provided to patients receiving long-term parenteral nutrition.

Parenteral vitamins are provided daily. Standardized multivitamin solutions are currently available to provide adequate quantities of vitamins A, $B_{12}$, C, C, E, thiamine, riboflavin, niacin, pantothenic acid, pyridoxine, folic acid, and biotin. Vitamin K is not given routinely but administered when the prothrombin time becomes abnormal.

### Essential Fatty Acids

Patients receiving nutritional support should be given 2–4% of their total nonprotein calories as linoleic acid to prevent essential fatty acid deficiency. Most prepared enteral solutions contain adequate linoleic acid. Patients receiving parenteral nutrition should be given 500 mL of intravenous fat (emulsified soybean or safflower oil) about 2–3 times a week. Intravenous fat can also be used as an energy source in place of dextrose.

## ENTERAL NUTRITIONAL SUPPORT SOLUTIONS

Most patients who require enteral nutritional support can be given commercially prepared enteral solutions (Table 20–18). Nutritionally complete solutions have been designed to provide adequate proportions of water, energy, protein, and micronutrients. Nutritionally incomplete solutions are also available to provide specific macronutrients (eg, protein, carbohydrate, and fat) to supplement complete solutions for patients with unusual requirements or to design solutions that are not available commercially.

Nutritionally complete solutions are characterized as follows: (1) by osmolality (isotonic or hypertonic), (2) by lactose content (present or absent), (3) by the molecular form of the protein component (intact proteins; peptides or amino acids), (4) by the quantity of protein and calories provided, and (5) by fiber content (present or absent). For most patients, isotonic solutions containing no lactose or fiber are preferable. Such solutions generally contain relatively higher quantities of fat and intact protein. Most commercial

**Table 20–18.** Enteral solutions.

**Complete**
Blenderized (eg, Compleat, Compleat-Modified, Vitaneed)
Whole protein, lactose-containing (eg, Meritene, Sustagen)
Whole protein, lactose-free, low-residue:
  1 kcal/mL (eg, Ensure, Entrition, Isocal, Osmolite)
  1.5 kcal/mL (eg, Ensure Plus, Sustacal HC)
  2 kcal/mL (eg, Isocal HCN, Magnacal, TwoCal HN)
  High-nitrogen: > 16% total calories from protein (eg, Ensure HN, Isotein HN, Sustacal)
Whole protein, lactose-free, high-residue:
  1 kcal/mL (eg, Enrich)
Defined (elemental) formulas (eg, Vital, Vivonex)
"Disease-specific" formulas:
  Renal failure: with essential amino acids (eg, Amin-Aid, Travasorb Renal)
  Malabsorption: with medium-chain triglycerides (eg, Portagen, Travasorb MCT)
  Respiratory failure: with > 50% calories from fat (eg, Pulmocare)
  Hepatic encephalopathy: with high amounts of branched-chain amino acids (eg, Hepatic-Aid II, Travasorb Hepatic)
**Incomplete** (modular)
Protein (eg, Nutrisource Protein, Promed, Propac)
Carbohydrate (eg, Nutrisource Carbohydrate, Polycose, Sumacal)
Fat (eg, MCT Oil, Microlipid, Nutrisource Lipid)
Vitamins (eg, Nutrisource Vitamins)
Minerals (eg, Nutrisource Minerals)

isotonic solutions contain 1000 kcal and about 37–45 g of protein per liter.

Solutions containing hydrolyzed proteins or crystalline amino acids and with no significant fat content are called elemental solutions, since macronutrients are provided in their most "elemental" form. These solutions have been designed for patients with malabsorption, particularly pancreatic insufficiency and limited fat absorption. Elemental diets are extremely hypertonic and often result in more severe diarrhea. Their use should be limited to patients who cannot tolerate isotonic solutions.

Although formulas have been designed for specific clinical situations—solutions containing primarily essential amino acids (for renal failure), medium-chain triglycerides (for fat malabsorption), more fat (for respiratory failure and $CO_2$ retention), and more branched-chain amino acids (for hepatic encephalopathy and severe trauma)—they have not been shown to be superior to standard formulas for most patients.

Enteral solutions should be administered via continuous infusion, preferably with an infusion pump. Feedings should be started at full strength at about 25–33% of the estimated final infusion rate. Feedings can be advanced by similar amounts every 12 hours as tolerated.

### Complications of Enteral Nutritional Support

Minor complications of tube feedings occur in 10–15% of patients. Gastrointestinal complications include diarrhea (most common), inadequate gastric emptying, emesis, esophagitis, and occasionally gastrointestinal bleeding. Diarrhea associated with tube feeding may be due to intolerance to the osmotic load or to one of the macronutrients (eg, fat, lactose) in the solution. Patients being fed in this way may also have diarrhea from other causes (as side effect of antibiotics or other drugs; associated with infection, etc), and these possibilities should always be investigated in appropriate circumstances.

Mechanical complications of tube feedings are potentially the most serious. Of particular importance are aspiration and aspiration pneumonia. All patients receiving nasogastric tube feedings are at risk for these life-threatening complications. Limiting nasogastric feedings to those patients who can adequately protect their airway and careful monitoring of patients being fed by tube should limit these serious complications to 1–2% of cases. Minor mechanical complications are common and include tube obstruction, and dislodgment.

Metabolic complications during enteral nutritional support are common but in most cases easily managed. The most important problem is hypernatremic dehydration, most commonly seen in elderly patients unable to respond to thirst. Abnormalities of potassium, glucose, and acid-base balance may also occur.

## PARENTERAL NUTRITIONAL SUPPORT SOLUTIONS

Parenteral nutritional support solutions can be designed to deliver adequate nutrients to virtually any patient. The basic parenteral solution is composed of dextrose, amino acids, and water. Electrolytes, minerals, trace elements, vitamins, and medications can also be added. Most commercial solutions contain the monohydrate form of dextrose that provides 3.4 kcal/g. Crystalline amino acids are available in a variety of concentrations, so that a broad range of solutions can be made up that will contain specific amounts of dextrose and amino acids as required.

Typical solutions for central vein nutritional support contain 25–35% dextrose and 2.75–4.25% amino acids depending upon the patient's estimated nutrient and water requirements. These solutions typically have osmolalities in excess of 1800 mosm/L and require infusion into a central vein.

Solutions with lower osmolalities can also be designed for infusion into peripheral veins. Typical solutions for peripheral infusion contain 5–10% dextrose and 2.75–4.25% amino acids. These solutions have osmolalities between 800 and 1200 mosm/L and result in a high incidence of thrombophlebitis and line infiltration. These solutions will provide adequate protein for most patients but inadequate energy. Additional energy must be provided in the form of emulsified soybean or safflower oil. Such intravenous fat solutions are currently available in 10% and 25% solutions providing 1.1 and 2.2 kcal/mL, respectively. Intravenous fat solutions are isosmotic and well tolerated by peripheral veins. Typical patients are given 500 mL of a 10% or 20% solution each day. As much as 60% of total nonprotein calories can be administered in this manner.

Intravenous fat can also be provided to patients receiving central vein nutritional support. In this instance, dextrose concentrations should be decreased to provide a fixed concentration of energy. Intravenous fat has been shown to be equivalent to intravenous dextrose in providing energy to "spare protein." Intravenous fat is associated with less glucose intolerance, less production of carbon dioxide, and less fatty infiltration of the liver and has been increasingly utilized in patients with hyperglycemia, respiratory failure, and liver disease. Intravenous fat has also been increasingly used in patients with large estimated energy requirements. Recent studies suggest that the maximum glucose utilization rate is approximately 5–7 mg/min/kg. Patients who require additional calories can be given them as fat to prevent excess administration of dextrose. Intravenous fat can also be used to prevent essential fatty acid deficiency. The optimal ratio of carbohydrate and fat in parenteral nutritional support has not been determined.

Infusion of parenteral solutions should be started slowly to prevent hyperglycemia and other metabolic complications. Typical solutions are given initially at a rate of 50 mL/h and advanced by about the same amount every 24 hours.

## COMPLICATIONS OF PARENTERAL NUTRITIONAL SUPPORT

Complications of central vein nutritional support occur in up to 50% of patients. Although most are minor and easily managed, about 5% of patients will develop significant complications. Complications of central vein nutritional support can be divided into catheter-related complications and metabolic complications.

Catheter-related complications can occur during insertion or while the catheter is in place. Pneumothorax, hemothorax, arterial laceration, air emboli, and brachial plexus injury can occur during catheter placement. The incidence of these complications is inversely related to the experience of the physician performing the procedure but will occur in 1–2% of cases even in major medical centers. Each catheter placement should be documented by chest radiograph prior to initiation of nutritional support.

Catheter thrombosis and catheter-related sepsis are the 2 most important complications of indwelling catheters. Patients with indwelling central vein catheters who develop signs of sepsis without an apparent source should have their lines removed immediately, the tip cultured, and antibiotics begun empirically. Patients with less significant fevers without an apparent source should have their lines removed and be observed without antibiotics. Catheter-related sepsis occurs in 2–3% of patients even if maximal efforts are made to prevent infection.

Metabolic complications of central vein nutritional support occur in over 50% of patients (Table 20–

19). Most are minor and easily managed, and termination of support is seldom necessary.

## PATIENT MONITORING DURING NUTRITIONAL SUPPORT

Every patient receiving enteral or parenteral nutritional support should be followed closely. Formal nutritional support teams composed of a physician, a nurse, a dietitian, and a pharmacist have been shown to decrease the rate of complications.

Patients should be monitored both for the adequacy of treatment and to prevent complications or detect them early when they occur. Because estimates of nutritional requirements are imprecise, frequent reassessment is necessary. Daily intakes should be recorded and compared with estimated requirements. Body weight, hydration status, and overall clinical status should be followed. Patients who do not appear to be responding as anticipated can be evaluated for nitrogen balance by means of the following equation:

$$\text{Nitrogen balance} = \frac{\text{24-hour protein intake (g)}}{6.25} - \text{24-hour urinary nitrogen (g)} + 4$$

Patients with positive nitrogen balances can be continued on their current regimens; patients with negative balances should receive moderate increases in calorie and protein intake and then be reassessed.

Feeding tubes and catheters should be examined often to avoid mechanical and infectious complications.

Monitoring for metabolic complications should include urine glucose determination every 6 hours and daily measurements of electrolytes; serum glucose, phosphorus, magnesium, calcium, and creatinine; and BUN until the patient is stabilized. Once the patient is stabilized, electrolytes, phosphorus, calcium, magnesium, and glucose should be checked at least twice weekly. Serum folate, zinc, and copper should be checked at least once a month.

**Table 20–19.** Metabolic complications of parenteral nutritional support.

| Complication | Common Causes | Possible Solutions |
|---|---|---|
| Hyperglycemia | Too rapid infusion of dextrose, "stress," glucocorticoids. | Decrease glucose infusion. Insulin. Replacement of dextrose with fat. |
| Hyperosmolar non-ketotic dehydration | Severe, undetected hyperglycemia. | Insulin, hydration, potassium. |
| Hyperchloremic metabolic acidosis | High chloride administration. | Decrease chloride. |
| Azotemia | Excessive protein administration. | Decrease amino acid concentration. |
| Hyperphosphatemia, hypokalemia, hypomagnesemia | Extracellular to intracellular shifting with refeeding. | Increase solution concentration. |
| Liver enzyme abnormalities | Lipid trapping in hepatocytes, fatty liver. | Decreased dextrose. |
| Acalculous cholecystitis | Biliary stasis. | Oral fat. |
| Zinc deficiency | Diarrhea, small bowel fistulas. | Increase concentration. |
| Copper deficiency | Biliary fistulas. | Increase concentration. |

Ashkenazi J et al: Perioperative nutritional support. *Nutr Internat* 1987;**3**:12.

Baron RB: Nutrition support of the critically ill obese patient. *Top Clin Nutr* (Apr) 1986;**1**:71.

Batuman V et al: Renal and electrolyte effects of total parenteral nutrition. *JPEN* 1985;**9**:546.

Cataldi-Betcher EL et al: Complications occurring during enteral nutrition support: A prospective study. *JPEN* 1983;**7**:546.

Cerra FB et al: Branched-chain metabolic support: A prospective, randomized, double-blind trial in surgical stress. *Ann Surg* 1984;**199**:286.

Cerra FB: Hypermetabolism, organ failure, and metabolic support. *Surgery* 1987;**101**:1.

Dalton MJ et al: Consultative total parenteral nutrition teams: The effect on the incidence of total parenteral nutrition-related complications. *JPEN* 1984;**8**:146.

Dempsey DT et al: Treatment effects of parenteral vitamins in total parenteral nutrition patients. *JPEN* 1987;**11**:229.

Dudrick SJ et al: 100 patient-years of ambulatory home total parenteral nutrition. *Ann Surg* 1984;**199**:770.

Hill GL, Church J: Energy and protein requirements of general surgical patients requiring intravenous nutrition. *Br J Surg* 1984;**71**:1.

Howard L, Michalek AV: Home parenteral nutrition (HPN). *Ann Rev Nutr* 1984;**4**:69.

Koretz RL: What supports nutritional support? *Dig Dis Sci* 1984;**29**:577.

Koretz RL, Meyer JH: Elemental diets: Facts and fantasies. *Gastroenterology* 1983;**78**:393.

Mamel JJ: Percutaneous endoscopic gastrostomy: A review. *Nutr Clin Pract* 1987;**2**:65.

Muggia-Sullam M et al: Postoperative enteral versus parenteral nutritional support in gastrointestinal surgery: A matched prospective study. *Am J Surg* 1985;**149**:106.

Muller JM et al: Indications and effects of preoperative parenteral nutrition. *World J Surg* 1986;**10**:63.

Murphy LM, Lipman TO: Central venous catheter care in parenteral nutrition: A review. *JPEN* 1987;**11**:190.

Robin AP et al: Influence of parenteral carbohydrate on fat oxidation in surgical patients. *Surgery* 1984;**95**:608.

Rombeau JL, Caldwell MD: *Enteral Nutrition.* Saunders, 1984.

Rombeau JL, Caldwell MD: *Parenteral Nutrition.* Saunders, 1986.

Ryan JA Jr, Page CP: Intrajejunal feeding: Development and current status. *JPEN* 1984;**8**:187.

Select Committee on Standards of Professional Practice: *Standards for Nutrition Support: Hospitalized Patients.* American Society for Parenteral and Enteral Nutrition (ASPEN), 1984.

Stabile BE et al: Intravenous mixed amino acids and fats do not stimulate exocrine pancreatic secretion. *Am J Physiol* 1984;**246**:G274.

## REFERENCES

Alpers DH, Clouse RE, Stenson WF: *Manual of Nutritional Therapeutics*. Little, Brown, 1983.

Food & Nutrition Board, National Academy of Sciences-National Research Council: *Recommended Dietary Allowances*, 9th ed. Publication 1694, Washington DC, 1980.

Martin DW Jr et al: *Harper's Review of Biochemistry*, 20th ed. Lange, 1985.

Nestle M: *Nutrition in Clinical Practice*. Jones Medical Publications, 1985

Oson RE et al: *Nutrition Review's Present Knowledge in Nutrition*, 5th ed. The Nutrition Foundation, 1984.

Ordy JM, Harman D, Alfin-Slater RB (editors): *Aging: Nutrition in Gerontology*. Vol 26 of *Aging*. Raven Press, 1984.

Pennington JAT, Church HN: *Bowes and Church's Food Values of Portions Commonly Used,* 14th ed. Lippincott, 1985.

Rombeau JL, Caldwell MD: *Enteral Nutrition*. Saunders, 1985.

Rombeau JL, Caldwell MD: *Parenteral Nutrition*. Saunders, 1986.

Silberman H, Eisenberg D: *Parenteral and Enteral Nutrition for the Hospitalized Patient*. Appleton-Century-Crofts, 1982.

Stunkard AJ, Stellar LE: *Eating and Its Disorders*. Raven Press, 1984.

Taylor KB, Anthony LE: *Clinical Nutrition*. McGraw-Hill, 1983.

Yetiv JZ: *Popular Nutritional Practices: A Scientific Appraisal*. Popular Medicine Press, 1986.

# Introduction to Infectious Diseases

# 21

*Ernest Jawetz, MD, PhD, & Moses Grossman, MD*

Infections can and do involve all human organ systems. In a book organized, as this one is, principally by organ system, many important infectious disease entities are discussed in the chapters devoted to specific anatomic areas. Thus, pneumonias are discussed in Chapter 7, infective endocarditis in Chapter 8, and urinary tract infections in Chapter 15. Other important infections are described under the headings of their etiologic agents in Chapters 22–27.

In this introductory chapter, we wish to focus on a few broad problems of infectious disease that touch upon many facets of diagnosis and treatment. To minimize duplication, we will refer to other areas of this book for more detailed or supplementary information.

## FEVER OF UNDETERMINED ORIGIN (FUO)

Fever of undetermined origin is defined as an illness of at least 3 weeks' duration with fever over 38 °C (100.4 °F) as the principal symptom. This "diagnosis" should not be entertained until diagnostic procedures, including repeated cultures of blood, tissues, and urine, skin and serologic tests, search for neoplasm or evidence of collagen vascular disease, etc, have failed to establish a specific etiologic diagnosis. Most cases of FUO are eventually found to represent atypical manifestations of common diseases rather than exotic illnesses.

## Etiologic Considerations

It is important to proceed systematically in approaching this difficult diagnostic problem. Concerted efforts must be made to identify disorders in the following 4 categories:

**A. Infectious Processes:** It is well to consider systemic infections and localized infections separately. The former include tuberculosis, disseminated mycoses, infective endocarditis, infectious mononucleosis, cytomegalovirus infection, toxoplasmosis, brucellosis, salmonellosis, and many other less common diseases.

The most common form of localized infection is an obscure abscess. Liver, spleen, kidney, brain, and bone are organs where an abscess may be difficult to find. A collection of pus may form in the peritoneal cavity or in the subdiaphragmatic, subhepatic, paracolonic, or other areas. Cholangitis, urinary tract infec-

tion, dental abscess, or a collection of pus in a paranasal sinus may cause prolonged fever.

**B. Neoplasms:** Many cancers may present with obscure fever as a major symptom. The most common of these are lymphoma and leukemia.

**C. Autoimmune Disorders:** Juvenile rheumatoid arthritis is an example of a disease in which fever continues for a long time as almost the only symptom. This may also occur in system lupus erythematosus, polyarteritis nodosa, and other autoimmune disorders.

**D. Miscellaneous Causes:** Many other diseases can cause prolonged fever, eg, sarcoidosis, other noncaseating granulomas, pulmonary embolization, chronic liver disease, and familial Mediterranean fever. At times the fever may be factitious or self-induced.

## Approach to Diagnosis

The key to diagnosis often lies in careful daily physical examination of the patient, repeated review of the medical history, and dogged pursuit of any abnormal finding (eg, an enlarged lymph node, a questionable chest x-ray). Systematic examination by ultrasound, computed tomography (CT scan), and radio-nuclide scan (including tagged white cell scan) may reveal abdominal or retroperitoneal lymphadenopathy or tumor or abscess in pelvis or abdomen. If these and other studies remain noncontributory, biopsy of a lymph node or of the liver may reveal abnormalities. Rarely, exploratory laparotomy may be considered.

If any tissue is obtained, optimal use of it must be made for touch preparations, microbiologic cultures, and histologic examination.

It is most important to diagnose those diseases for which effective treatment is available and early institution of therapy may be curative.

With the passage of time, the true cause of fever often becomes apparent; thus, it may be helpful to repeat tests that previously were noncontributory. About 10% of cases of FUO remain undiagnosed. Therapeutic trials without diagnosis are seldom indicated. There is little benefit (or harm) in suppressing the fever as such, but doing so may make the patient more comfortable.

Dinarello CA, Wolff SM: Molecular basis of fever in humans. *Am J Med* 1982;**72**:799.

Larson EB et al: Fever of undetermined origin: Diagnosis and follow-up of 105 cases, 1970–1980. *Medicine* 1982;**61**:269.

Pizzo PA et al: Prolonged fever in children: Review of 100 cases. *Pediatrics* 1975;**55**:468.

Quinn MJ et al: Computed tomography of the abdomen in evaluation of patients with fever of unknown origin. *Radiology* 1980;**136**:407.

## INFECTIONS IN THE IMMUNOCOMPROMISED PATIENT

A description of the cellular basis of immune responses, the role of various host responses in maintaining health, and the methods used for detection of deficiencies in the immune system can be found in Chapter 33. Immunodeficiency may be congenital but more often is due to suppression of the immune system by diseases or drugs. Deficiencies of polymorphonuclear cells, T lymphocytes, or B lymphocytes tend to predispose the host to infection with different agents. Thus, polymorphonuclear cell deficiency predisposes particularly to infection with gram-negative enteric bacteria, staphylococci, and fungi; B lymphocyte deficiency and hypogammaglobulinemia to infection with extracellular encapsulated organisms, eg, pneumococci or *Haemophilus* sp; and T lymphocyte deficiency to infection with intracellular bacteria (eg, mycobacteria, *Listeria, Legionella*), fungi (*Candida, Cryptococcus, Aspergillus,* etc), protozoa (*Pneumocystis carinii,* etc), and viruses (cytomegalovirus, herpes simplex, etc).

Many opportunistic organisms (ie, organisms that rarely produce invasive infections in an uncompromised host) do not produce disease except in the immunodeficient host. Such hosts are often infected with several opportunists simultaneously.

Infections caused by common organisms may present uncommon clinical manifestations. Determination of the specific infecting agents is essential for effective treatment.

### Immunodeficient Hosts

Patients deficient in normal immune defenses fall into several groups:

(1) Congenital defects of cellular or humoral immunity or a combination of both, eg, Wiskott-Aldrich syndrome. These are usually children.

(2) Patients with cancer, particularly lymphoreticular cancer.

(3) Patients receiving immunosuppressive therapy. These include patients with neoplastic disease and transplant recipients who are receiving corticosteroids, other immunosuppressive drugs, or radiation treatment.

(4) Patients who have very few polymorphonuclear cells ($< 500/\mu L$) or those whose polymorphonuclear cells do not function normally with respect to phagocytosis or the intracellular killing of microorganisms (eg, chronic granulomatous disease).

(5) A larger group of patients who are not classically immunodeficient but whose host defenses are seriously compromised by prior splenectomy, debilitating illness, diabetes mellitus, surgical or other invasive procedures (eg, intravenous drug abuse or intravenous hyperalimentation), burns, or massive antimicrobial therapy.

(6) Patients with variants of the acquired immunodeficiency syndrome (AIDS). This profound disturbance in T lymphocyte subpopulations produces extreme susceptibility to opportunistic infections and to rapidly disseminating Kaposi's sarcoma and other neoplasms, with an exceedingly high death rate. See AIDS discussion, p. 834.

### Infectious Agents

**A. Bacteria:** Any bacterium pathogenic for humans can infect an immunosuppressed host. Furthermore, noninvasive and nonpathogenic organisms (opportunists) may also cause disease in such cases. Examples include gram-negative bacteria—particularly *Pseudomonas, Serratia, Proteus, Providencia*—and *Nocardia*. Many come from the hospital environment and are resistant to antimicrobial drugs. Mycobacteria—both *Mycobacterium tuberculosis* and atypical organisms—must be considered.

**B. Fungi:** *Candida, Aspergillus, Cryptococcus, Mucor,* and others can all cause disease in immunosuppressed hosts. Candidiasis is the most common and is often found in patients receiving intensive antimicrobial therapy.

**C. Viruses:** Cytomegalovirus is the most common, but varicella-zoster and herpes simplex viruses are also important. Vaccinia virus may cause serious problems, and its use is contraindicated.

**D. Protozoa:** *Pneumocystis carinii* is an important cause of pneumonia in many immunodeficient patients. This diagnosis must be made early, because reasonably effective therapy is available. *Toxoplasma gondii* is also important and is susceptible to therapy.

*Cryptosporidium* may cause chronic, severe diarrhea.

### Approach to Diagnosis

A systematic approach is necessary, including the following steps:

(1) Review carefully the patient's current immune status, previous antimicrobial therapy, and *all* previous culture reports.

(2) Obtain pertinent cultures for bacteria, fungi, yeasts, and viruses.

(3) Consider which of the serologic tests for fungal, viral, and protozoal diseases are pertinent.

(4) Consider special diagnostic procedures, eg, lung biopsy, bronchopulmonary lavage, transbronchial biopsy to demonstrate *Pneumocystis*. Quantitation of T lymphocyte subpopulations by monoclonal antibodies in immunofluorescence tests may help.

(5) Consider whether the infection (eg, candidiasis) is superficial or systemic. Therapeutic considerations are quite different in each case.

## Approach to Treatment

*Caution:* It is essential to avoid aggravating the patient's other problems and to avoid gross alterations of the host's normal microbial flora.

Take measures to improve host defenses, correct electrolyte imbalance, offer adequate caloric intake, etc. Improve the patient's immune status whenever possible. This includes temporary decrease in immunosuppressive drug dosage in transplant patients and modification of chemotherapy in cancer patients.

Injection of immune globulin USP (human gamma globulin) at regular intervals can compensate for certain B cell deficiencies. Granulocyte transfusions are only rarely able to tide the patient over a prolonged period of neutropenia.

Antimicrobial drug therapy should be specific and lethal for the infecting agent. Combinations of antimicrobial drugs may be necessary, since multiple infectious agents may be involved.

Thus, empiric combined therapy may have to be started promptly in the immunosuppressed patient with a pulmonary infiltrate or fever. This often includes a cephalosporin (eg, cefoperazone or cefotaxime, 2 g every 4 hours in intravenous infusion) plus an aminoglycoside (eg, amikacin, 15 mg/kg/d) and even trimethoprim with sulfamethoxazole (16 tablets daily orally or appropriate doses intravenously) for possible *Pneumocystis* organisms. Amphotericin B may at times be started empirically on suspicion rather than on definitive proof of systemic mycosis.

Peterson PK et al: Infectious diseases in hospitalized renal transplant recipients. *Medicine* 1982;**61**:360.

Press DW et al: Hickman catheter infections in patients with malignancies. *Medicine* 1984;**63**:189.

Prober CG et al: Open lung biopsy in immunocompromised children with pulmonary infiltrates. *Am J Dis Child* 1984;**138**:60.

Schimpf SC, Klastersky J, Goya H (editors): Therapy for immunocompromised patients. *Am J Med* 1986;**80(Suppl 5C)**:1. [Entire issue.]

van der Meer JWM, van den Broek JP: Present status of the management of patients with defective phagocyte function. *Rev Infect Dis* 1984;**6**:107.

Wheeler RR et al: Esophagitis in the immunocompromised host. *Rev Infect Dis* 1987;**9**:88.

Young LS: Empirical antimicrobial therapy in the neutropenic host. *N Engl J Med* 1986;**315**:580.

## NOSOCOMIAL INFECTIONS

Nosocomial infections are by definition those acquired in the course of hospitalization. Historical examples are "childbed fever" after delivery and wound gangrene after surgical operations. These were largely controlled by the development of aseptic techniques, the introduction of sterile materials and sterile surgical methods, and the rise of bacteriologic diagnosis.

At present in the USA, 3–7% of patients who enter the hospital free from infection acquire a nosocomial infection. Very rarely, a virulent, highly communicable organism such as Lassa fever virus is transmitted from an undiagnosed patient to others in the hospital. Generally, patients acquire hospital infections with common organisms because of their own great susceptibility to infection or because of procedures carried out in the hospital.

Nosocomial infections can be attributed principally to the following aspects of contemporary medical care:

(1) Many hospitalized patients (especially in tertiary care hospitals, which have the highest nosocomial infection rate) are compromised because of deficiencies in their immunologic responses. These may be congenital but commonly are acquired as a result of the administration of drugs for the treatment of cancer, for maintenance of transplants, or for suppression of autoimmune processes. The very young and the elderly are particularly susceptible to infection.

(2) Many aspects of medical care now require the use of invasive techniques for diagnosis, monitoring, and therapy. Examples are the indwelling urinary catheter; intravascular lines used for measurements, infusions of fluids or drugs, or parenteral alimentation; drainage tubes; and shunts.

(3) Materials administered in intensive care may themselves be vectors of infection: Intravenous solutions or their containers may be contaminated; respirators and humidifiers may introduce microorganisms into particularly susceptible lungs; plastic tubing may carry infectious agents into the body, etc.

(4) The massive use of antimicrobial drugs contributes to the selection of drug-resistant microorganisms both in the individual patient and in the hospital environment. Thus, nosocomial infections are often attributable to members of the endogenous human microflora or free-living microorganisms that happen to be particularly resistant to antimicrobial drugs, presenting difficult management problems. Such organisms often are not established human "pathogens" but can be classed as "opportunists."

The principal anatomic sites of hospital-acquired infection are the urinary tract, surgical wounds, the respiratory tract, and skin sites where indwelling needles or tubes penetrate. Most notorious among nosocomial infections are those due to gram-negative enteric bacteria, staphylococci, or mycotic organisms that develop in patients with granulocyte counts below 500/$\mu$L as a result of cancer chemotherapy or organ transplant. In such patients, bloodstream invasion often occurs without a well-defined portal of entry. Patients with markedly depressed cell-mediated immunity may also develop viral infections in the hospital, eg, varicellazoster, cytomegalovirus, hepatitis, and others. They are likewise open to opportunists like *Legionella, Nocardia,* and other bacteria and protozoa, eg, *Pneumocystis carinii.*

The management of the immunodeficient patient is outlined on p 817. In nosocomial infections, it is particularly important to be alert to the possibility of infection, maintain continuous surveillance of patients at high risk (eg, by nurse epidemiologists), and have a well-defined, regularly updated program for diagnosis and treatment (through the hospital infection control committee). Continuing education of all hospital personnel and information about possible sources of infection among personnel are essential to maintain awareness of the many problems. The high-risk areas of hospitals include the nursery (especially the intensive care nursery), operating and recovery rooms, intensive care and coronary care units, cancer chemotherapy areas, hemodialysis and transplantation units, and all areas where postoperative patients are cared for.

Garibaldi RA et al: Infections among patients in nursing homes. *N Engl J Med* 1981;**305**:731.

Haley RW et al: The efficacy of infection surveillance and control programs in preventing nosocomial infections. *Am J Epidemiol* 1985;**121**:183.

Maki DG: Nosocomial bacteremia: An epidemiologic overview. *Am J Med* 1981;**70**:719.

McGowan JE Jr: Antimicrobial resistance in hospital organisms and its relation to antibiotic use. *Rev Infect Dis* 1983;**5**:1033.

Prince A et al: Management of fever in patients with central vein catheters. *Pediatr Infect Dis* 1986;**5**:20.

## INFECTIONS OF THE CENTRAL NERVOUS SYSTEM

Infections of the central nervous system can be caused by almost any infectious agent but most commonly are due to bacteria, mycobacteria, fungi, spirochetes, and viruses. Certain symptoms and signs are more or less common to all types of central nervous system infection: headache, fever, sensorial disturbances, neck and back stiffness, positive Kernig and Brudzinski signs, and cerebrospinal fluid abnormalities. In patients presenting with these manifestations, the possibility of central nervous system infection must be considered.

Such an infection constitutes a *medical emergency*. Immediate diagnostic steps must be instituted to establish the specific cause. Normally, these include the history, physical examination, blood count, blood culture, lumbar puncture with careful study and culture of the cerebrospinal fluid, and a chest film when the patient's condition permits. A nasopharyngeal culture is also helpful. The cerebrospinal fluid must be examined for cell count, glucose, and protein, and a smear must be stained for bacteria (and acid-fast organisms when appropriate) and cultured for pyogenic organisms and for mycobacteria and fungi when indicated. Counterimmunoelectrophoresis and latex agglutination can detect antigens of encapsulated organisms. In bacterial meningitis, prompt therapy is essential to prevent death and minimize serious sequelae.

If a space-occupying lesion (brain abscess, subdural empyema) is suspected, its presence may be confirmed by CT scan, which ideally should precede lumbar puncture.

## Etiologic Classification

Central nervous system infections can be divided into several categories that usually can be readily distinguished from each other by cerebrospinal fluid examination as the first step toward etiologic diagnosis (Table 21–1).

**A. Purulent Meningitis:** Due to infection with meningococci (40% of cases), pneumococci, streptococci, *Haemophilus influenzae,* staphylococci, and other pyogenic organisms. Postoperative meningitis is often caused by staphylococci, gram-negative enteric bacteria, or fungi.

**B. Granulomatous Meningitis:** Due to *Mycobacterium tuberculosis; Coccidioides, Cryptococcus, Histoplasma,* and other fungi; or *Treponema pallidum* (meningovascular syphilis).

**C. Aseptic Meningitis:** Aseptic meningitis is much more benign, caused principally by viruses—especially mumps virus, the enterovirus group (including coxsackieviruses and echoviruses), and herpesviruses. Poliomyelitis virus was a common cause of aseptic meningitis before the introduction of vaccination. Infectious mononucleosis may be accompanied by aseptic meningitis. Leptospiral infection is usually placed in the aseptic group because of the lymphocytic cellular response and its relatively benign course. This type of meningitis also occurs during secondary syphilis.

**D. Encephalitis:** Due to herpesviruses, arboviruses, and many other viruses. Produces disturbances of the sensorium, seizures, and many other manifestations. Cerebrospinal fluid may be entirely normal or may show some lymphocytes.

**E. Partially Treated Bacterial Meningitis:** Bacterial meningitis may present with the same course and some of the same cerebrospinal fluid findings as aseptic meningitis following partly effective antimicrobial therapy.

**F. "Neighborhood" Reaction:** As noted in Table 21–1, this term denotes a purulent infectious process in close proximity to the central nervous system that spills some of the products of the inflammatory process—pus or protein—into the cerebrospinal fluid. Such an infection might be a brain abscess, osteomyelitis of the vertebrae, epidural abscess, subdural empyema, etc.

**G. Meningitis in the Neonate:** In newborn infants, meningitis often accompanies sepsis and is most often caused by group B beta-hemolytic streptococci, gram-negative rods (most commonly *Escherichia coli*), *Listeria monocytogenes,* and *Haemophilus influenzae;* it fails to show the typical signs of meningitis present in children or adults. Fever and neck signs are often absent. Instead, the infant is irritable, lethargic, and anorexic. Antimicrobial therapy is directed to enteric bacteria and streptococci.

**H. Noninfectious Meningeal Irritation:** Meningismus, presenting with the classic signs of meningeal irritation with totally normal cerebrospinal fluid findings, may occur in the presence of other infections such as pneumonia, shigellosis, etc. Meningeal inva-

**Table 21–1.** Typical cerebrospinal fluid findings in various central nervous system diseases.

| Diagnosis | Cells/μL | Glucose (mg/dL) | Protein (mg/dL) | Opening Pressure |
|---|---|---|---|---|
| Normal[1] | 0–5 lymphocytes | 45–85 | 15–45 | 70–180 mm H$_2$O |
| Purulent meningitis (bacterial)[2] | 200–20,000 polymorphonuclear neutrophils | Low (< 45) | High (> 50) | ++++ |
| Granulomatous meningitis (mycobacterial, fungal)[2,3] | 100–1000, mostly lymphocytes | Low (< 45) | High (> 50) | +++ |
| Aseptic meningitis, viral or meningoencephalitis[3,4] | 100–1000, mostly lymphocytes | Normal | Moderately high (> 50) | Normal to + |
| Spirochetal meningitis[3] | 25–2000, mostly lymphocytes | Normal or low | High (> 50) | + |
| "Neighborhood" reaction[5] | Variably increased | Normal | Normal or high | Variable |

[1] Cerebrospinal fluid glucose must be considered in relation to blood glucose level. Normally, cerebrospinal fluid glucose is 20–30 mg/dL lower than blood glucose, or 50–70% of the normal value of blood glucose.
[2] Organisms in smear of culture of cerebrospinal fluid; counterimmunoelectrophoresis or latex agglutination may be diagnostic.
[3] Polymorphonuclear neutrophils may predominate early.
[4] Viral isolation from cerebrospinal fluid early; antibody titer rise in paired specimens of serum.
[5] May occur in mastoiditis, brain abscess, epidural abscess, sinusitis, septic thrombus, brain tumor. Cerebrospinal fluid culture results usually negative.

sion by neoplastic cells may present both with physical findings of meningeal irritation and with increased cells and lowered cerebrospinal fluid glucose.

**I. Brain Abscess:** Brain abscess presents as a space-occupying lesion; symptoms may include vomiting, fever, and neurologic manifestations. If brain abscess is suspected, a CT scan should precede lumbar puncture.

### Treatment

Treatment consists of supporting circulation, ventilation, the airway, and other life-support functions that may be compromised by infection and resulting disturbance of the central nervous system. Increased intracranial pressure due to brain edema often requires therapeutic attention. In the case of purulent meningitis proper, antimicrobial treatment is imperative. Since the identity of the causative microorganism may remain unknown or doubtful for a few days, initial antibiotic treatment as listed in Table 21–2 should be directed against the microorganisms most common for each age group.

Peltola H: Meningococcal disease: Still with us. *Rev Infect Dis* 1983;**5:**71.
Tarber MG, Sande MA: Principles in the treatment of bacterial meningitis. *Am J Med* 1984;**76(Suppl 5A):**224.

### GRAM-NEGATIVE BACTEREMIA & SEPSIS

Overwhelming gram-negative bacteremia with high mortality was typical of the great pestilences of the past such as plague and typhoid. Although environmental control has greatly reduced this threat, the rare case of plague today (originating from infected rodents and their fleas) can be as devastating as in the past. More commonly, sporadic meningococcemia (originating in the respiratory tract of asymptomatic persons) requires emergency diagnosis and treatment and may nevertheless end in death within a few hours.

Recently, bacteremia and sepsis caused by gram-negative bacteria and fungi—especially in hospitals—have increased greatly in incidence. Factors responsible for this shift are larger numbers of debilitated or immunodeficient patients; more extensive surgical procedures; greater use of invasive diagnostic and therapeutic procedures; and the relentless selection pressure of antimicrobial drugs within individual patients and within hospital populations, which favors the survival and proliferation of drug-resistant gram-negative bacteria, yeasts, and fungi in a hospital setting.

The following are among the most frequent events leading up to gram-negative bacteremia and sepsis:

(1) Urinary tract infection, cystoscopy, catheterization (especially with an indwelling catheter), and urologic surgery.

**Table 21–2** Initial antimicrobial therapy for purulent meningitis of unknown cause.

| Age Group | Optimal Therapy (Intravenous Dose/24 Hours) | |
|---|---|---|
| Adult* | Penicillin | 24 million units |
| Child older than 7 years | Penicillin or ampicillin | 360,000 units/kg 300 mg/kg |
| Infant and child up to 7 years‡ | Ampicillin† and chloramphenicol | 300 mg/kg 100 mg/kg |
| Neonate (up to 3 months)‡ | Ampicillin and gentamicin | 200 mg/kg 5–6 mg/kg |

\* In penicillin allergy, chloramphenicol is the best alternative therapy.
† Combination designed to include coverage of ampicillin-resistant *Haemophilus influenzae* meningitis.
‡ Cefotaxime, ceftriaxone, and cefuroxime are suitable alternative drugs for initial therapy but must be combined with ampicillin.

(2) Tracheostomy, use of respirators with aerosol, use of endotracheal tubes.

(3) Intravenous infusion (plastic catheter needle) without changing site frequently; thrombophlebitis; contaminated solutions; intravenous drug abuse by addicts.

(4) Postsurgical infection, especially during antimicrobial therapy.

(5) Infected burns, wounds; delivery or abortion; perforation of an abdominal viscus.

(6) Severe neutropenia, eg, due to cancer with or without chemotherapy.

(7) Organ transplantation with its attendant immunosuppression.

### Clinical Findings

**A. Symptoms and Signs:** The onset might be with a shaking chill followed by an abrupt rise of fever. Alternatively, the patient may only appear flushed and anxious, with moderate temperature elevation. Soon there may be a fall in blood pressure or even frank shock with greatly impaired organ perfusion (kidney, brain, heart), anuria, nitrogen retention, acidosis, circulatory collapse, and death.

Unless the sequence of clinical signs can be reversed early, the mortality rate may be 50% or higher.

**B. Laboratory Findings:** Initial leukopenia may be present and is often followed by moderate leukocytosis. Proteinuria may precede a drastic reduction in urine volume. There may be evidence of metabolic acidosis or respiratory alkalosis and of disseminated intravascular coagulation (see p 335).

### Treatment

The consequences of irreversible gram-negative shock are so grave that the clinician must constantly be on guard (see list of predisposing factors, above). Whenever a suspicion of gram-negative bacteremia arises, samples for blood cultures must be taken immediately and a survey of potential sources of infection (catheters, infusions, thrombophlebitis, abscesses) must be carried out. Prompt elimination of these sources is often the most important step in the management of bacteremic shock. Gram-positive bacteremia may occasionally also precipitate shock.

**A. Antibiotics:** Suspected or proved gram-negative bacteremia must be promptly and intensively treated with antimicrobial drugs. Selection of the best initial drug depends on the most likely source and type of organism and on the pattern of drug susceptibility that prevails in a given locality in a given year. In 1986–87, drugs used initially often include a new cephalosporin (eg, cefotaxime, cefoperazone, or ceftriaxone, 12 g/d) and an aminoglycoside (eg, amikacin, 15 mg/kg/d). If *Bacteroides fragilis* or another anaerobe is suspected of originating from bowel or the female genital tract, metronidazole, 500 mg 4 times daily, or cefoxitin, 12 g/d, might be a drug of choice. If *Pseudomonas* sp are likely, ticarcillin, 18 g/d, plus amikacin, 15 mg/kg/d, or ceftazidime, 6 g/d, may be started.

**B. Management of Shock:** (See also discussion in Chapter 1.) Management of bacteremic shock is directed at maintenance of organ perfusion, ventilation, correction of acidosis, and improvement of cardiac function. Central venous pressure or pulmonary artery wedge pressure is monitored to prevent fluid overload (see p 11). Plasma volume expanders (blood plasma, dextran, electrolyte solutions) are given to maintain organ perfusion and correct the prominent lactic acidosis but avoid pulmonary edema. Cardiac output may be increased by dopamine. This sympathomimetic amine dilates mesenteric and renal vessels (and thus increases renal blood flow and urine output) in addition to increasing cardiac output if infused in doses of 2–10 μg/kg/min. Vasoconstrictors such as norepinephrine may further restrict organ perfusion and are therefore used sparingly in the early treatment of bacteremic shock. Very large doses of corticosteroids (eg, hydrocortisone, 2–5 g intravenously) have been administered with claimed benefit. In one controlled human study, methylprednisolone, 30 mg/kg injected in 20 minutes intravenously and repeated only once 4 hours later, markedly reduced the death rate from septic shock. Thus, a dose-related effect is possible. Heparinization may be considered in disseminated intravascular coagulation.

The opiate antagonist naloxone has been given experimentally to counteract the observed rise in endorphin blood levels during shock. The role of naloxone in human shock is uncertain. There is evidence that antibody to the core glycolipid of gram-negative enteric bacteria can protect against shock and death in gram-negative sepsis. Antibody to *Pseudomonas aeruginosa* types may be beneficial in burn patients.

### Prognosis

Persistent gram-negative bacteremia has a high mortality rate—often over 50%. Bad prognostic signs include hypothermia during bacteremia, severe underlying disease, azotemia, and shock. Failure to drain collections of pus adequately usually interferes with the response to antimicrobial therapy.

Guerrant RL et al: Campylobacteriosis in man: Pathogenic mechanisms and review of 91 blood stream infections. *Am J Med* 1978;**65**:584.

Sande M, Root RR: Septic shock: *Newer Concepts in Pathophysiology and Treatment.* Churchill Livingstone, 1985.

Sheagren JN: Septic shock and corticosteroids. *N Engl J Med* 1981;**305**:456.

Yu VL: *Serratia marcescens:* Historical perspective and clinical review. *N Engl J Med* 1979;**300**:887.

Ziegler EJ et al: Treatment of gram-negative bacteremia and shock with human antiserum to a mutant *E coli. N Engl J Med* 1982;**307**:1225.

## NONTUBERCULOUS ATYPICAL MYCOBACTERIAL DISEASES

About 10% of mycobacterial infections seen in clinical practice are not caused by *Mycobacterium tuberculosis* but by "atypical" mycobacteria. These organisms have distinctive laboratory characteristics, occur in the environment, are not communicable from person to person, and are often strikingly resistant to antituberculosis drugs. Some representative species and clinical presentations are listed here. (See also p 154.)

*Mycobacterium kansasii* can produce pulmonary disease resembling tuberculosis, but the illness is less severe. Treatment is with ethambutol plus rifampin plus isoniazid, at least initially. *Mycobacterium marinum* produces skin granulomas but rarely systemic dissemination; initial treatment is with a tetracycline. *Mycobacterium scrofulaceum* and, less commonly, *Mycobacterium intracellulare* are prominent causes of cervical adenitis in children; excision is the management of choice. The *Mycobacterium avium-intracellulare* complex produces widespread asymptomatic infection and occasional pulmonary disease in the USA, Australia, and elsewhere. Most infected persons are well, but those who do become ill (especially immunodeficient persons, eg, AIDS patients) present a formidable treatment problem. Multiple drugs (rifampin, ethambutol, amikacin, cycloserine, etc) may be effective, and other drugs, eg, Ansamycin, clofazimine can be selected by sensitivity tests. Excisional surgery is sometimes successful. *Mycobacterium fortuitum* and similar organisms may produce skin ulcers after accidental inoculation and, rarely, lung disease. They are usually resistant to antimycobacterial drugs, but amikacin and tetracycline may be effective.

## Diagnosis

Nontuberculous atypical mycobacterial disease is suspected when acid-fast bacilli are found on smears, but the patient is not as ill as one might expect with tuberculosis and has no history of contact with tuberculosis, and nobody else in the family has the disease. Chest films may be negative, and the PPD-S test often produces less than 10 mm of induration. Specific diagnosis depends on cultural identification of the organism. This may take 1–4 weeks.

## Treatment

The management of pulmonary disease is described on p 155. Cervical adenitis presumptively due to atypical mycobacteria is best managed by surgical excision, thus facilitating culture and histologic examination. The effective use of antimicrobial agents requires specific bacteriologic diagnosis and tests for drug sensitivity.

Iseman MD et al: Diseases due to *Mycobacterium avium-intracellulare. Chest* 1985;**87**:1395.

Margileth AM: Management of nontuberculous (atypical) mycobacterial infections in children and adolescents. *Pediatr Infect Dis* 1985;**4**:119.

Woods GL, Washington JA: Mycobacteria other than *M tuberculosis:* Review of microbiologic and clinical aspects. *Rev Infect Dis* 1987;**9**:275.

## ANAEROBIC INFECTIONS

A large majority of the bacteria that make up the normal human flora are anaerobes. Prominent members of the normal microbial flora of the mouth (anaerobic spirochetes, *Bacteroides,* fusobacteria), the skin (anaerobic diphtheroids), the large bowel (*Bacteroides,* anaerobic streptococci, clostridia), and the female tract (*Bacteroides,* anaerobic streptococci, fusobacteria) may produce disease when displaced from their normal sites into tissues or closed body spaces.

Certain characteristics are suggestive of anaerobic infections: (1) They tend to involve mixtures of organisms, frequently several anaerobes. (2) They tend to form closed-space infections, either in discrete abscesses (lung, brain, pleura, peritoneum) or by burrowing through tissue layers. (3) Pus from anaerobic infections often has a foul odor. (4) Septic thrombophlebitis and metastatic suppurative lesions are frequent and often require surgical drainage in addition to antimicrobial therapy. (Most of the important anaerobes except *Bacteroides fragilis* are highly sensitive to penicillin G, but the diminished blood supply that favors proliferation of anaerobes because of reduced tissue oxygenation also interferes with the delivery of antimicrobials to the site of anaerobic infection.) (5) Bacteriologic examination may yield negative results or only inconsequential aerobes unless rigorous anaerobic culture conditions are used, employing collection methods and media suitable for fastidious organisms.

The following is a brief listing of important types of infections that are most commonly caused by anaerobic organisms. Treatment of all of these infections consists of surgical exploration and judicious excision in conjunction with administration of antimicrobial drugs.

### Upper Respiratory Tract

*Bacteroides melaninogenicus* together with anaerobic spirochetes is commonly involved in periodontal infections. These organisms, fusobacteria, and peptostreptococci are responsible for a substantial percentage of cases of chronic sinusitis and probably of peritonsillar abscess, chronic otitis media, and mastoiditis. Hygiene and drainage are usually more important in treatment than antimicrobials, but penicillin G is the drug of choice.

### Chest Infections

Aspiration of saliva (which contains $10^8$ anaerobic organisms per milliliter in addition to aerobes) may lead to pneumonitis, necrotizing pneumonia, lung abscess, and empyema. While polymicrobial infection is the rule, anaerobes—particularly *B melaninogenicus,* fusobacteria, and peptostreptococci—are common etiologic agents. All of these organisms are susceptible to penicillin G and tend to respond to drug treatment combined with surgical drainage when indicated.

The relatively penicillin-resistant *Bacteroides fragilis* is found in about 20% of anaerobic chest infections, but these still usually respond to penicillin G, 10 million units daily intravenously. Occasionally, clindamycin or chloramphenicol is required.

## Central Nervous System

While anaerobes only rarely produce meningitis, they are a common cause of brain abscess, subdural empyema, or septic central nervous system thrombophlebitis. The organisms reach the central nervous system by direct extension from sinusitis, otitis, or mastoiditis or by hematogenous spread from chronic lung infections. Antimicrobial therapy (eg, penicillin, 20 million units intravenously, and chloramphenicol, 0.5 g orally every 6 hours) or metronidazole, 7.5 mg intravenously every 8 hours, is an important adjunct to surgical drainage. It appears that some small, multiple brain abscesses can be treated with metronidazole alone and may heal without surgical drainage.

## Intra-abdominal Infections

In the colon there are up to $10^{11}$ anaerobes per gram of content—predominantly *B fragilis*, clostridia, and peptostreptococci. These organisms play a central etiologic role in most intra-abdominal abscesses following trauma to the colon, diverticulitis, appendicitis, or perirectal abscess and may also participate in hepatic abscess and cholecystitis, often in association with aerobic coliform bacteria. The gallbladder wall may be infected with clostridia as well. In infections associated with perforation of the lower bowel, penicillin G may be ineffective because of the resistance of *B fragilis;* chloramphenicol, clindamycin, or metronidazole may be the drug of choice to aid in localization and supplement drainage.

Although the normal flora of the upper intestinal tract is more sparse than that of the colon, anaerobes comprise a large portion of it.

## Female Genital Tract & Pelvic Infections

The normal flora of the vagina and cervix includes several species of *Bacteroides*, peptostreptococci, group B streptococci, lactobacilli, coliform bacteria, and, occasionally, spirochetes and clostridia. These organisms commonly cause genital tract infections and may disseminate from there.

While salpingitis is commonly caused by gonococci and chlamydiae, tubo-ovarian and pelvic abscesses are associated with anaerobes in a majority of cases. Postpartum infections may be caused by aerobic streptococci or staphylococci, but in most instances anaerobes are found, and the most severe cases of postpartum or postabortion sepsis are associated with clostridia and *Bacteroides*. These have a high mortality rate, and treatment requires both antimicrobials (penicillin, metronidazole, cefoxitin, doxycycline) and abscess drainage or early hysterectomy.

## Bacteremia & Endocarditis

Anaerobes are probably responsible for 5–10% of cases of bacteremia seen in general hospitals. Most of these originate in the gastrointestinal tract and the female genital tract and—until now—have been associated with a high mortality rate. Endocarditis due to anaerobic and microaerophilic streptococci and *Bacteroides* originates in the same sites. Rigorous anaerobic cultures to identify the causative organism and institute specific and adequate treatment are essential in patients whose "routine" blood cultures in clinical endocarditis have remained negative. Most cases of streptococcal endocarditis can be effectively treated with 20–60 million units of penicillin G daily, but optimal therapy of other types of anaerobic bacterial endocarditis must rely on laboratory guidance. Anaerobic corynebacteria (*Propionibacterium*), clostridia, and *Bacteroides* occasionally cause endocarditis. *Bacteroides* bacteremia may cause disseminated intravascular coagulation.

## Skin & Soft Tissue Infections

Anaerobic infections in the skin and soft tissue usually follow trauma, inadequate blood supply, or surgery and are commonest in areas that are contaminated by oral or fecal flora. There is often rapidly progressive tissue necrosis and a putrid odor.

**Bacterial synergistic gangrene** is a painful ulcerating lesion that commonly follows laparotomy performed as part of the management of intra-abdominal infections but produces little fever or systemic toxicity. It is usually caused by a mixture of anaerobic streptococci and *Staphylococcus aureus*. It requires wide excision of the discolored skin and (later) skin grafts, but recovery is the rule.

**Synergistic necrotizing cellulitis** progresses more rapidly, with high fever and often positive blood cultures for peptostreptococci, *Bacteroides*, and aerobic gram-negative bacteria. It occurs with greatest frequency on the perineum and the lower extremities and has a high mortality rate. Excision of necrotic tissue must be combined with antimicrobial drugs (eg, gentamicin plus clindamycin) to attempt early control.

**Necrotizing fasciitis** is a mixed anaerobic or aerobic infection that rapidly dissects deep fascial planes and produces severe toxicity with a mortality rate of up to 30%. Anaerobic streptococci and *S aureus* are the commonest etiologic organisms. Extensive surgical incisions through fascial planes are needed.

**Nonclostridial crepitant cellulitis** is an infection of subcutaneous or deeper tissues with peptostreptococci and coliform bacteria that leads to gas formation in tissue, with minimal toxicity, lack of muscle involvement, and a good prognosis. Improved perfusion, incision and drainage, and antimicrobial drugs (eg, ampicillin) are often successful.

Bartlett JG: Recent developments in the management of anaerobic infections. *Rev Infect Dis* 1983;**5**:235.

Dunn DL, Simmons RL: The role of anaerobic bacteria in intraabdominal infections. *Rev Infect Dis* 1984;**6**:S139.

Mathisen GE et al: Brain abscess and cerebritis. *Rev Infect Dis* 1984;**6**:S101.

Swenson RM: Rationale for identification and susceptibility testing of anaerobic bacteria. *Rev Infect Dis* 1986;**8**:809.

Zaleznik DF, Kasper DL: The role of anaerobic bacteria in abscess formation. *Annu Rev Med* 1982;**33**:217.

## ANIMAL & HUMAN BITE WOUNDS

About 1% of emergency room visits in urban areas are for animal and human bites. Cats produce the highest percentage of bacterial infections (30–50%), many of which are caused by *Pasteurella multocida*. About 5% of dog bites result in bacterial infections, often with the gram-negative DF-2 organisms that present in 10% of dog mouth flora. They may lead to sepsis and peripheral gangrene. Both *Pasteurella multocida* and DF-2 are susceptible to penicillin and may occur in mixed infections. Human bites are associated with bacterial infection in 15–20% of cases. Tetanus prophylaxis must be considered in all bite wounds (see p 873) and rabies prophylaxis in animal bites (see p 847).

All bites, especially human bites, introduce a mixed complex anaerobic and aerobic flora into the wound. These wounds must be irrigated intensively and debrided. There is little evidence that "prophylactic" antimicrobial drugs are valuable. When bacterial infection is already evident, administration of penicillin G, warm soaks, and elevation and immobilization of the wounded area are advisable. Initial Gram stains and cultures from the wound may direct the choice of antibiotic. Clindamycin or cefoxitin may be desirable when lack of response suggests anaerobes, and nafcillin is indicated if lactamase-producing staphylococci are present. Hospitalization must be considered for major human bites to permit close observation, surgical intervention, or parenteral therapy.

Aghabanian RV, Conte JE: Mammalian bite wounds. *Ann Emerg Med* 1980;**9**:79.

Brown CG: Dog bites: The controversy continues. *Am J Emerg Med* 1985;**3**:83.

Kalb R et al: Cutaneous infection in dog bite wounds associated with fulminant DF-2 septicemia. *Am J Med* 1985;**78**:687.

## SEXUALLY TRANSMITTED DISEASES

Some infectious diseases are transmitted most commonly—or most efficiently—by sexual contact. The frequency of some of these infections (eg, gonorrhea) has increased markedly in recent years as a result of changing patterns of sexual behavior. Others (eg, herpetic and chlamydial genital infections) are only now beginning to be appreciated as important systemic infections with a primarily sexual mode of transmission. Rectal and pharyngeal infections caused by these microorganisms are common as a result of varied sexual practices.

Most of the infectious agents that cause sexually transmitted diseases are fairly easily inactivated when exposed to a harsh environment. They are thus particularly suited to transmission by contact with mucous membranes. They may be bacteria (eg, gonococci), spirochetes (syphilis), chlamydiae (nongonococcal urethritis, cervicitis), viruses (eg, herpes simplex, hepatitis B virus, cytomegalovirus, AIDS virus), or protozoa (eg, *Trichomonas*). In most infections caused by these agents, early lesions occur on genitalia or other sexually exposed mucous membranes; however, wide dissemination may occur, and involvement of nongenital tissues and organs may mimic many noninfectious disorders. All sexually transmitted diseases have subclinical or latent phases that may play an important role in long-term persistence of the infection or in its transmission from infected (but largely asymptomatic) persons to other contacts. Laboratory examinations are of particular importance in the diagnosis of such asymptomatic patients. Simultaneous infection by several different agents is common.

For each patient, there are one or more sexual contacts who require diagnosis and treatment. As a rule, sexual partners should be treated simultaneously to avoid prompt reinfection. Finding a sexually transmitted disease in a child strongly suggests sexual abuse, and the case should be reported to the authorities. The commonest sexually transmitted diseases are gonorrhea,* syphilis,* condyloma acuminatum, chlamydial genital infections, cytomegalovirus and herpesvirus genital infections, *Trichomonas* vaginitis,* chancroid,* granuloma inguinale,* scabies, and lice. However, shigellosis, hepatitis, amebiasis, giardiasis, cryptosporidiasis, salmonellosis, and campylobacteriosis may also be transmitted by sexual (oral-anal) contact, especially in homosexual males. The same population is a high-risk group for acquisition of AIDS (see p 834) by sexual contact and with appallingly high mortality rate.

Clinical and epidemiologic details and methods of diagnosis and treatment are discussed for each infection separately elsewhere in this book (see Index).

Centers for Disease Control: Sexually transmitted diseases: Treatment guidelines. *MMWR* 1985;**34**:75S.

Holmes KK et al: *Sexually Transmitted Diseases.* McGraw-Hill, 1984.

Quinn TC et al: The etiology of anorectal infections in homosexual men. *Am J Med* 1981;**71**:395.

## INFECTIONS IN DRUG ADDICTS

The abuse of parenterally administered narcotic drugs has increased enormously. There are an esti-

---

* Reportable to public health authorites.

mated 300,000 or more narcotic addicts in the USA, mostly in or near large urban centers. Consequently, many physicians and hospitals serving such urban and suburban populations are faced with the diagnosis and treatment of problems that are closely related to drug abuse. Infections are a large part of these problems.

## Common Infections That Occur With Greater Frequency in Drug Users

(1) Skin infections are associated with poor hygiene and multiple needle punctures, commonly due to *S aureus*.

(2) Hepatitis is nearly universal among habitual drug users and is transmissible both by the parenteral and by the fecal-oral route. Many addicts experience hepatitis twice.

(3) Aspiration pneumonia and its complications (lung abscess, empyema, brain abscess) are due to anaerobes, *Nocardia,* and other organisms.

(4) Pulmonary septic emboli may originate in venous thrombi or right-sided endocarditis.

(5) Sexually transmitted diseases are not directly related to drug abuse but, for social reasons, occur with greater frequency in population groups that are also involved in drug abuse.

(6) AIDS has a high incidence among intravenous drug abusers.

(7) Infective endocarditis (see below).

## Infections Rare in USA Except in Drug Users

(1) Tetanus: Drug users now form a majority of cases of tetanus in the USA. Tetanus develops most commonly in the unimmunized female addict who injects drugs subcutaneously ("skin-popping").

(2) Malaria: Needle transmission occurs from addicts who acquired the infection in malaria-endemic areas outside the USA.

(3) Melioidosis: This chronic pulmonary infection caused by *Pseudomonas pseudomallei* is occasionally seen in debilitated drug users.

## Infective Endocarditis

The organisms that cause infective endocarditis in those who use drugs intravenously are most commonly *S aureus, Candida* (especially *Candida parapsilosis*), *Streptococcus faecalis,* and gram-negative bacteria (especially *Pseudomonas* and *Serratia marcescens*).

Involvement of the left side of the heart is somewhat more frequent than involvement of the right side, and infection of more than one valve is not infrequent. Right-sided involvement, especially in the absence of murmurs, is often suggested by manifest pulmonary emboli. The diagnosis must be established by blood culture. Until the etiologic organism is known, treatment must be directed against the most probable organism—especially *S aureus.* Many strains of *S aureus* in those who use drugs intrave-

nously are nafcillin-resistant. Vancomycin is the drug of choice.

## Osteomyelitis

Osteomyelitis involving vertebral bodies, sternoclavicular joints, and other sites usually results from hematogenous distribution of injected organisms or septic venous thrombi. Pain and fever precede roentgenologic changes by several weeks. While staphylococci, often methicillin-resistant, are common organisms, *Serratia, Pseudomonas,* and other organisms rarely encountered in "spontaneous" bone or joint disease are found in addicts who use drugs intravenously.

Chandrasekar PH, Narula AP: Bone and joint infections in intravenous drug abusers. *Rev Infect Dis* 1986;**8**:904.

Levine DP et al: Bacteremia in narcotic addicts: Infective endocarditis. *Rev Infect Dis* 1986;**8**:374.

Sapico FL, Montgomerie JZ: Vertebral osteomyelitis in intravenous drug abusers: Report of three cases and review of the literature. *Rev Infect Dis* 1980;**2**:196.

Scalcini MC, Sanders CV: Endocarditis from human to human transmission of *Staphylococcus aureus. Arch Intern Med* 1980;**140**:111.

## DIAGNOSIS OF VIRAL INFECTIONS

In the diagnosis of viral infections, the current state of clinical knowledge and laboratory technology allows specific identification in the vast majority of cases. Diagnoses such as "viral syndrome," "viral diarrhea," or "flu syndrome" are not helpful.

Some viral illnesses present a clear-cut clinical syndrome (chickenpox, measles, mumps) that identifies the virus involved. Laboratory assistance is required only for confirmation in atypical cases or for the differential diagnosis of similar syndromes.

In some instances, the clinical picture has a number of features that are suggestive of viral infection in general but could be caused by any one of a number of viruses. Such a "viral" picture is seen in aseptic meningitis. The viruses involved in aseptic meningitis include mumps and several enteroviruses; the specific viral diagnosis can only be made with laboratory assistance. In the case of the respiratory tract, viral infections also have certain features in common—widespread involvement of the respiratory epithelium with redness and clear nasal secretion, absence of a purulent response—and, if pneumonia is present, it is more apt to be interstitial pneumonia.

Sometimes the statistical predilection of one of the respiratory viruses for an anatomic site allows one to make an "educated guess." For example, respiratory syncytial virus is the most common cause of bronchiolitis, and parainfluenza virus is the most common cause of croup. However, specific identification of the virus involved can only be made in the laboratory.

At times, accurate diagnosis is of such import to

the patient (rubella during pregnancy) or the community (hepatitis) that rapid laboratory confirmation of the suspected diagnosis is essential.

Diagnosis of viral illnesses requires the close collaboration of the clinician and the laboratory virologist. Knowing which specimens are most likely to be productive, when they should be obtained, and what to do with them in the laboratory depends on the virologist's understanding of the suspected diagnosis, the timetable of the illness, and the clinician's awareness of laboratory capabilities and limitations.

## Laboratory Considerations

There are 3 basic laboratory techniques for making a viral diagnosis:

**A. Isolation and Identification of the Virus:** This requires prompt transport (best on wet ice) to the laboratory and inoculation of the appropriate specimen into a suitable cell culture or into a live animal. A variety of techniques are then utilized to determine the presence and nature of the particular virus. At times this can be done very simply (eg, in the case of herpes simplex); at times it may be laborious, time-consuming, and expensive (eg, in the case of coxsackievirus). The isolation of virus from a specimen that is normally free of virus (eg, cerebrospinal fluid, lung biopsy) or from a pathologic lesion (herpes or varicella vesicle) has great diagnostic significance. However, finding a virus in the nasopharynx or in the stool may denote carriage rather than disease; in this case, additional evidence of a rise in antibody titer will be necessary before a specific diagnosis can be made.

**B. Microscopic Methods:** This entails the microscopic examination of cells, body fluids, or aspirates to demonstrate either the presence of the virus or specific cytologic changes peculiar to one virus or a group of viruses (eg, multinucleate giant cells at the base of herpesvirus lesions; rotavirus structures seen in electron micrographs or diarrheal stools). Immunofluorescence methods are particularly useful in many viral illnesses (rabies, varicella, herpes simplex, respiratory syncytial virus, etc) to identify antigen in cells from the patient. Viruses lead an obligate intracellular existence; therefore, it is important to examine scraped cells rather than exudates or transudates.

**C. Serologic Methods:** During viral illnesses, specific antibodies develop. The timing of rise in titer and persistence of antibodies varies. A 4-fold rise in antibody titer during the course of the illness is usually considered significant evidence of disease. Since a single serum titer is not particularly helpful, many laboratories will not do the test until paired sera (taken 2–3 weeks apart) are available. It is not practical to do serologic tests for a large number of viruses in any patient. Thus, the use of this method requires a specific suspicion of which virus might be involved.

Jawetz E, Melnick JL, Adelberg EA: *Review of Medical Microbiology,* 17th ed. Appleton-Lange, 1987.

McIntosh K et al: Summary of a workshop on new and useful methods in viral diagnosis. *J Infect Dis* 1980;**142**:793.

## HERPESVIRUSES OF HUMANS

This large group of DNA viruses shares common features that are important in the general clinical patterns manifested in humans. The better-defined clinical pictures are described under the specific disease entities. The most important herpesviruses in human disease states are herpes simplex type 1, herpes simplex type 2, varicella-zoster, cytomegalovirus, and EB-infectious mononucleosis virus.

Each virus tends to produce subclinical primary infection more often than clinically manifest illness. Each tends to persist in a latent state (evidenced only by persistent immunologic reactivity) for the rest of the person's life. Reactivation producing a clinical recurrence of disease may follow a known or unrecognized triggering mechanism. In herpes simplex and varicella-zoster, the virus is latent in sensory ganglia, and reactivation is followed by the appearance of lesions in the distal sensory nerve distribution. As a result of the suppression of cell-mediated immunity by disease, drugs, or radiation, reactivation of virus may lead to widespread disseminated lesions on and within affected organs and the central nervous system. Severe or even fatal illness may also occur in the newborn or the immunodeficient child.

Herpesviruses can infect the fetus and induce serious congenital malformations. They have also been linked to neoplasia (eg, cervical carcinoma, Burkitt's lymphoma), but the relationship remains uncertain. Primary or recurrent herpesvirus infections that involve epithelial surfaces may lead to prolonged shedding of virus and its spread to contacts of the infected person.

Several drugs can inhibit replication of herpesviruses. Of these, idoxuridine and trifluorothymidine are effective in humans when applied topically to herpetic keratitis, but they are too toxic for systemic use. Vidarabine (adenine arabinoside) and acyclovir (acycloguanosine) can be given topically or systemically. Acyclovir, 15 mg/kg/d, has been used intravenously in disseminated herpes simplex or herpetic encephalitis. The latter should be diagnosed by brain biopsy with immunofluorescent stain and culture of virus. If the diagnosis is made very early before onset of coma, the mortality rate can be significantly reduced. However, many of the survivors are not neurologically normal. Because of the need for rapid treatment and the difficulty of brain biopsy, many suspected cases of herpetic encephalitis receive drug therapy prior to the establishment of the diagnosis.

Acyclovir, 15 mg/kg/d intravenously, is more effective than vidarabine and has low toxicity. It is clearly beneficial in symptomatic primary genital infections (particularly in females) and in disseminating herpetic mucocutaneous lesions of immunosuppressed patients or newborns. It can limit varicella lesions in immunocompromised patients if used early. Oral acyclovir (200 mg 5 times daily) can be effective systemically in such patients and can also be used to reduce the frequency and severity of recurrent herpetic lesions.

Topical acyclovir (5%) applied to primary genital herpetic lesions can reduce viral shedding and local pain and shorten healing time, but it has little effect on recurrent lesions. It helps in treating mucocutaneous lesions in immunocompromised patients (see Chapter 28). No drug available in 1987 affects the recurrence rate of herpetic lesions following a course of treatment.

Balfour HH: Acyclovir and other chemotherapy for herpes group viral infections. *Annu Rev Med* 1984;**35**:279.
Corey L, Spear PG: Infections with herpes simplex viruses. (2 parts.) *N Engl J Med* 1986;**314**:686, 749.
Whitley RH et al: Vidarabine versus acyclovir therapy in herpes simplex encephalitis. *N Engl J Med* 1986;**314**:144.

## SLOW VIRUSES

Several animal diseases (scrapie, visna) are caused by viruses that are definitely communicable but replicate in the host very slowly—for months without producing symptoms. Eventually, they produce progressive disease and death. At least 4 human degenerative diseases are believed to be caused by similar "slow" viruses.

**Kuru** and **Creutzfeldt-Jakob disease** are spongiform encephalopathies. The virus can be transmitted by brain or eye tissue, and perhaps by other forms of contact, to humans, chimpanzees, and monkeys. After many weeks or months, the diseases pursue an inexorable downhill course and end in death. Kuru is characterized by cerebellar ataxia, tremors, dysarthria, and emotional lability; Creutzfeldt-Jakob disease by progressive dementia, myoclonic fasciculations, ataxia, and somnolence. Little is known about the characteristics of the causative viruses. There is no specific treatment, and prevention is limited to avoidance of specific risks (contamination by affected brain tissue, transplant of cornea from patient).

**Subacute sclerosing panencephalitis (SSPE)** is a slowly progressive demyelinating disorder of the central nervous system, ending in death. Altered measles viruses have been grown from brain tissue, and the cerebrospinal fluid antibody to measles is high.

**Progressive multifocal leukoencephalopathy (PML)** is an extremely rare progressive demyelinating neurologic disease that occurs particularly in persons immunosuppressed by drugs or disease. Certain papovaviruses (eg, JC virus) have been grown from brain tissue of patients with PML. However, a large percentage (60%) of a normal population has serum antibodies to the same virus, suggesting that disease production must have another determinant.

It is possible that other degenerative central nervous system diseases in humans (eg, multiple sclerosis) may be caused by "slow" viruses.

Bockman JM et al: Creutzfeld-Jakob disease prion proteins in human brains. *New Engl J Med* 1985;**312**:73.
Brown P et al: Diagnosis of Creutzfeld-Jakob disease by Western blot identification of marker protein in human brain tissue. *New Engl J Med* 1986;**314**:547.

## MISCELLANEOUS RESPIRATORY INFECTIONS

Infections of the respiratory tract are perhaps the most common human ailments. While they are a source of discomfort, disability, and loss of time for most average adults, they are a substantial cause of morbidity and serious illness in young children and in the elderly. Specific associations of certain groups of viruses with certain disease syndromes have been established. Many of these viral infections run their natural course in older children and in adults, without specific treatment and without great risk of bacterial complications. In young infants and in the elderly, or in persons with impaired respiratory tract reserves, bacterial superinfection increases morbidity and mortality rates.

### Common Cold

This familiar syndrome is characterized mainly by nasal obstruction and discharge, sore throat, sneezing, hoarseness, and varying degrees of malaise, cough, sinusitis, and otitis. Fever is usually absent in adults but may be present in small children. Rhinoviruses, coronaviruses, parainfluenza viruses, and others may be the etiologic agents. All of these exist in multiple antigenic types, and recurrence of infection is common. Secondary bacterial infection is more common in children (15%) than in adults and may produce purulent sinusitis, otitis media, or tracheobronchitis.

Treatment is largely palliative, and its true merits are poorly established. Aspirin (two 325-mg tablets every 4–8 hours in adults) tends to act as an analgesic. Phenylephrine, 0.25% solution as nose drops 4 times daily, or methylhexamine or propylhexedrine inhalers may temporarily relieve nasal congestion. Sedative cough mixtures may suppress the annoying and incapacitating cough at some stages. There is no solid support for the claim that ascorbic acid (1–4 g daily) can prevent the common cold or markedly alter its severity. Antimicrobial drugs have no place in the management of the common cold unless secondary bacterial infection is unequivocally present. Antihistamines are of value only in allergic or vasomotor rhinitis.

### Croup
### (Laryngotracheobronchitis)

This is most commonly a parainfluenza virus infection of small children, with anatomic localization in the subglottal area. It produces hoarseness, a "seal bark" cough, and signs of upper airway obstruction with inspiratory stridor, xiphoid and suprasternal retraction, but no pain on swallowing. It must be differentiated from epiglottitis due to *Haemophilus influenzae*. Treatment includes hydration, steam inhalation (hot or cold), and alertness to the possibility of complete airway obstruction. Should that emergency occur, intubation or tracheostomy is lifesaving.

### Epiglottitis

This is a medical emergency requiring urgent attention to the airway. It occurs most commonly in children 1–6 years old, who develop a swollen, "cherry-red" epiglottis and airway obstruction with fever, pain on swallowing, and a "croupy" cough. Lateral neck x-ray can help to establish swelling of the epiglottis. Direct laryngoscopy may precipitate obstruction and must therefore be performed only in a setting where immediate intubation can be done expertly. Epigottitis sometimes occurs in adults with pale erythematous swelling of the supraglottic region. In adults, laryngoscopy is less likely to precipitate an airway crisis, and for that reason immediate intubation is not critical.

Treatment consists of airway maintenance, antimicrobials (either ampicillin plus chloramphenicol, or cefuroxime) and close observation.

### Bronchiolitis

This viral infection is caused most often by respiratory syncytial virus in children under 2 years of age. It results in a "ball valve" obstruction to expiration at the level of the bronchiole, resembling bronchial asthma in pathophysiology. Clinical signs include low-grade fever, severe tachypnea (up to 100 respirations per minute), an expiratory wheeze, overinflation of lungs, depressed diaphragm, decreased air exchange, and greatly increased work of breathing. Foreign body aspiration and bronchial asthma may have to be considered in differential diagnosis.

Treatment consists of hydration, humidification of inspired air, and—with rising blood $P_{CO2}$—the possible need for ventilatory support. In infants, the clinical course of respiratory syncytial viral infections can be favorably modified by use of aerosolized ribavirin.

### Pneumonia

Upon first contact with a patient suspected of having acute pneumonitis, the physician must promptly undertake steps toward a specific etiologic diagnosis and arrive at a decision whether to administer antimicrobial drugs. Specific types of pneumonia are described in Chapter 7; the general approach to the patient with pneumonitis of unknown cause acquired in the community is outlined here.

The principal initial differentiation must be between bacterial and nonbacterial pneumonias. Characteristically, bacterial pneumonia is associated with sudden onset, chills, high fever, pleuritic chest pain, tachypnea, blood-tinged or purulent sputum, and polymorphonuclear leukocytosis. None of these symptoms are common in viral or mycoplasmal pneumonia.

Diagnosis rests on history (aspiration or prior upper respiratory infection, rate of progression, pain); physical and x-ray findings of consolidation or pleural effusion; white blood cell count and differential; blood culture; and examination of sputum. The latter must include an immediate Gram stain (the possibility of many polymorphonuclear cells, many squamous epithelial cells [suggesting salivary admixture], prevalent microorganisms) and culture (normal flora versus one predominant type of pathogen). Unless a likely pathogen is found promptly in severe pneumonia, transtracheal aspiration, fiberoptic bronchoscopy, or even lung biopsy must be considered to obtain an optimal specimen. This is especially important in immunocompromised hosts whose pneumonia is likely to be due to multiple, often opportunistic organisms.

Initial therapy is directed at the most probable pathogen. Since pneumococci account for 60–80% of cases of typical bacterial pneumonia acquired outside the hospital, procaine penicillin G, 600,000 units intramuscularly twice daily, is often appropriate. Other prevailing causes of bacterial pneumonia are staphylococci in 5–15% of cases and gram-negative bacteria in 15–20%. Mycoplasmal pneumonia is common in teenagers and young adults. Therapeutic choices are given on p 149. If the evidence favors nonbacterial etiology, antimicrobial drug treatment is generally not advisable.

For high-risk individuals, pneumococcal polysaccharide vaccines can be given as prophylaxis. Its efficacy is not great in children under 3 years and in old people.

Denny FW et al: Croup: An 11 year study in a pediatric practice. *Pediatrics* 1983;**71**:871.

Dick EC et al: Interruption of rhinovirus colds among human volunteers using virucidal paper handkerchiefs. *J Infect Dis* 1986;**153**:325.

Hall CB et al: Ribavirin treatment of respiratory syncytial viral infections in infants with underlying cardiopulmonary disease. *JAMA* 1985;**254**:3047.

Mayosmith MF et al: Acute epiglottitis in adults. *N Engl J Med* 1986;**314**:1134.

### ACUTE GASTROINTESTINAL SYNDROMES: NAUSEA, VOMITING, & DIARRHEA

Acute disturbances of gastrointestinal function have a wide variety of causes. Often, however, they are associated with the acquisition of infectious agents or toxins produced by them. Many common causes of acute bacterial gastroenteritis, "food poisoning," and "traveler's diarrhea" are described—together with their etiologic agents in Chapter 23 and listed in Table 23–1, and the epidemiologic setting and management of these disorders are briefly outlined.

Three categories of "infectious diarrheas" deserve

mention, although there is much overlap between them.

(1) The first is induced by enterotoxins produced by microorganisms (*Staphylococcus aureus*, *Clostridium perfringens*, *Vibrio cholerae*, *Bacillus cereus*, *Escherichia coli*, etc). There is an absence of inflammation, and no leukocytes are found in feces. The principal site of involvement is the proximal small bowel; the incubation period between exposure and symptoms is brief; and there is generally no fever. Rotavirus diarrheas of small children and parvovirus (Norwalk viruses) or *Giardia lamblia* diarrheas of adults probably belong in the same category.

(2) A second category is caused by infectious agents that invade superficial tissues, penetrate epithelium of lower small bowel and colon, and induce an inflammatory response. Leukocytes and red blood cells are found in the feces. Fever is commonly present, but blood cultures tend to be negative. Etiologic agents include some *Shigella* spp and invasive *E coli* associated with dysentery, *Salmonella* spp and *Vibrio parahaemolyticus* associated with enterocolitis, and *Campylobacter jejuni* and *Entamoeba histolytica* producing colitis.

(3) In a third category are invasive enteric fevers involving the distal small bowel, such as those caused by *Salmonella typhi* or *Yersinia enterocolitica*. Frequently, there is a long incubation period, prolonged systemic illness, and positive blood cultures. Invasive *Entamoeba histolytica* with spread to visceral organs may fit here at times.

Other disorders, eg, antibiotic-associated colitis caused by a necrotizing toxin of *Clostridium difficile*, are distinct entities. Enterovirus infections (eg, with poliovirus, coxsackieviruses, and echoviruses) often have diarrhea as a presenting symptom, and virus circulates in the blood, but the gastrointestinal localization is only part of a systemic viral dissemination. These are discussed in the next chapter.

A broad ("gay bowel") syndrome of enterocolitis encountered especially in homosexual males has received much attention. It is transmitted as a result of oral-anal-genital sexual practices and includes a wide variety of infectious agents ranging from viruses (hepatitis, herpes simplex), chlamydiae (*Chlamydia trachomatis*), and bacteria (*Shigella*, *Salmonella*, *Campylobacter*, *Neisseria gonorrhoeae*) to protozoa (*G lamblia*, *E histolytica*, *Cryptosporidium* sp), among others. Thus, it is necessary to consider the sexual practices of an individual who presents with an acute gastrointestinal tract syndrome to undertake proper diagnostic steps. In AIDS patients, diarrhea without a demonstrable cause appears to be common.

In all forms of acute gastrointestinal syndromes, restoration of fluid and electrolyte balance is an essential early therapeutic goal. When an etiologic diagnosis can be formulated, the decision to use antimicrobial or antiparasitic drugs depends on the clinical status of the patient and on the epidemiologic setting. In some disorders in categories (1) and (2), avoidance of anti-infective drugs is desirable (as discussed under individual headings in subsequent chapters).

## KAWASAKI SYNDROME

Kawasaki syndrome, also called mucocutaneous lymph node syndrome, is a febrile illness of unknown cause. It occurs mainly in children under 5 years of age. Prominent features are prolonged fever, cracked lips, conjunctivitis, pharyngitis, strawberry tongue, a maculopapular red rash and edema of extremities with desquamation on hands and feet, lymphadenopathy, and angiitis of coronary arteries in up to 30% of cases. There may be thrombocytosis or electrocardiographic changes preceding a coronary occlusion or aneurysm formation.

First reported in Japan, outbreaks have also occurred in Hawaii, Massachusetts, and elsewhere. In these outbreaks, the majority of patients experienced antecedent respiratory illness.

Treatment is with aspirin, 100 mg/kg/d until afebrile. Immune globulin USP, 400 mg/kg/d intravenously for 4 days, may reduce the frequency of coronary artery abnormalities. One to 3 percent of patients have died.

Hicks RV, Melish ME: Kawasaki syndrome. *Pediatr Clin North Am* 1986;**33**:1151.

Newburger JW et al: The treatment of Kawasaki syndrome with intravenous gamma globulin. *N Engl J Med* 1986;**315**:341.

## ACTIVE IMMUNIZATION AGAINST INFECTIOUS DISEASES

Every individual—child or adult—should be adequately immunized against infectious diseases. The schedule of administration, dose, and recommended method of choice vary with each product and change often. Always consult the manufacturer's package insert and follow its recommendations.

The schedule for active immunizations in childhood (Table 21–3) is adapted from *Report,* 20th ed., by the Committee on Control of Infectious Diseases, American Academy of Pediatrics, 1986.

### Recommended Immunization of Adults for Travel

Every adult, whether traveling or not, must be immunized with tetanus toxoid. Purified toxoid "for adult use" must be used to avoid reactions. Every adult should also receive primary or booster vaccination for poliomyelitis (oral live trivalent vaccine). Every traveler must fulfill the immunization require-

**Table 21–3.** Recommended schedule for active immunization of children.*

| Normal Infants and Children[1] | | Those Not Immunized in Infancy (7–18 Years) | |
|---|---|---|---|
| **Age** | **Product Administered or Test Recommended** | **Schedule** | **Product Administered** |
| 2 months | DTP,[2] TOPV[3] | Initial | Td,[7] TOPV |
| 4 months | DTP, TOPV | 1 month later | Measles vaccine, mumps, vaccine, rubella vaccine |
| 6 months | DTP, TOPV[4] | 2 months later | Td, TOPV |
| 15–19 months | DTP, TOPV, *H influenzae* type b;[5] measles vaccine, mumps vaccine, rubella vaccine;[6] tuberculin test[7] | 6–12 months later | Td, TOPV |
| 4–6 years (School entry) | DTP, TOPV; tuberculin test | 14–16 years of age | Td |
| Every 10 years thereafter | Td[8] | Every 10 years thereafter | Td |

* Follow manufacturer's directions for dose and precautions. A physician may choose to obtain informed consent for immunizations.
[1] A child who experiences any type of seizure after immunization should receive only diphtheria-tetanus (DT) vaccine subsequently.
[2] **DTP:** Toxoids of diphtheria and tetanus, aluminum-precipitated or aluminum hydroxide-absorbed, combined with pertussis bacterial antigen. Three doses intramuscularly at 4- to 8-week intervals. Fourth dose intramuscularly about 1 year later. Not suitable for children over 7 years old.
[3] **TOPV:** Trivalent (types I, II, and III) oral live poliomyelitis virus vaccine. Inactivated trivalent vaccine (Salk type) preferred for immunodeficient children, children with immunodeficient members of the household, and for those initially immunized after age 18, but not recommended for others.
[4] Optional dose, if exposure to wild poliomyelitis virus is anticipated.
[5] **Haemophilus influenzae** type b vaccine is recommended for all children aged 2–5 years and for children aged 18–23 months who are at high risk (eg, those with asplenia or immunosuppression and those in day-care programs).
[6] These are live vaccines of attenuated viruses grown in cell culture. They may be administered as a mixture or singly at 1-month intervals. Persons who received measles vaccine (inactivated) before 1968 or before age 15 months should be reimmunized with measles vaccine. Some physicians prefer to give rubella vaccine to prepubertal females (age 10–14 years). These live vaccines are not recommended for severely immunodeficient children.
[7] It is desirable to give a tuberculin test prior to measles vaccination and at intervals thereafter, depending on probable risk of exposure.
[8] **Td:** Tetanus toxoid and diphtheria toxoid, purified, suitable for adults. It should be given ever 7–10 years.
**References:**
Committee on Control of Infectious Diseases: *Report,* 20th ed. American Academy of Pediatrics, 1986.
General recommendations on immunization. *MMWR* (Jan 14) 1983;**32:**1.
Polysaccharide vaccine for prevention of *Haemophilus influenzae* type b disease. *MMWR* 1985;**34:**201.

ments of the health authorities of different countries. These are listed in Centers for Disease Control: *Health Information for International Travel 1982*. US Government Printing Office, 1982.

The following are suggestions for travel in different parts of the world.

## Tetanus

Booster injection of 0.5 mL tetanus toxoid, for adult use, every 7–10 years, assuming completion of primary immunization. (All countries.)

## Diphtheria

Because diphtheria is still prevalent in many parts of the world, a booster injection of diphtheria toxoid for adult use is indicated. This is usually given in combination with tetanus toxoid (Td), for adults.

## Smallpox

As of 1980, smallpox has been eradicated from the world. Since then, a valid vaccination certificate has not been required of travelers. Military personnel, however, continue to be vaccinated in the USA.

## Traveler's Diarrhea

See Chapter 23.

## Typhoid

Suspension of killed *Salmonella typhi* can provide effective immunity. Two doses are given 4 weeks or more apart. A single booster dose is given every 3 years for probable exposure. (Many countries.)

Paratyphoid vaccines are probably ineffective and are not recommended at present.

## Yellow Fever

Live attenuated yellow fever virus, 0.5 mL subcutaneously. WHO certificate requires registration of manufacturer and batch number of vaccine. Vaccination available in USA only at approved centers. Vaccination must be repeated at intervals of 10 years or less. (Africa, South America.)

## Cholera

Suspension of killed vibrios, including prevalent antigenic types. Two injections are given intramuscularly 2–6 weeks apart. This must be followed by booster injections every 6 months during periods of possible exposure. Protection depends largely on booster doses. WHO certificate is valid for 6 months only. (Middle Eastern countries, Asia, occasionally others.) Benefit doubtful.

## Plague

Suspension of killed plague bacilli given intramuscularly, 3 injections 4 or more weeks apart. A single booster injection 6 months later is desirable. (Some areas in South America, Southeast Asia, occasionally others.)

## Typhus

Suspension of inactivated typhus rickettsiae can give some protection. However, no approved vaccine was available in the USA or Canada in 1987.

## Measles

Persons born since 1957 who have not had live measles vaccine (after age 15 months) and who do not have a convincing history of clinical measles should receive measles vaccine (see above).

## Hepatitis A

No active immunization available. Temporary passive immunity may be induced by the intramuscular injection of human gamma globulin, 0.02 mL/kg every 2–3 months, or 0.1 mL/kg every 6 months. Recommended for all parts of the world where environmental sanitation is poor and the risk of exposure to hepatitis A is high through contaminated food and water and contact with infected persons.

## Hepatitis B

While not directly travel-related, postexposure prophylaxis against hepatitis is mentioned here. An inactivated hepatitis B vaccine is available for use in persons at high risk who have no anti-HBs antibody. It might be considered for travelers to hyperendemic areas. (China, Southeast Asia.)

## Pneumococcal Pneumonia

Elderly travelers, especially those with chronic obstructive respiratory disease or other chronic illnesses, may be given the 23-type pneumococcal vaccine, 0.5 mL intramuscularly once, several weeks before departure.

## Meningococcal Meningitis

If travel is contemplated to an area where meningococcal meningitis is highly endemic or epidemic, polysaccharide vaccines from types A, C, W-135, and Y may be indicated. Follow manufacturer's dosage recommendations. (Africa, South America.)

## Malaria

Take chloroquine phosphate, 500 mg once weekly, beginning 1 week prior to arrival in malaria-endemic area and continuing for 6 weeks after leaving it. Immunization not available. (In Southeast Asia, Africa, and South America, chloroquine-resistant *Plasmodium falciparum* may be present; pyrimethamine-sulfadoxine mixture may be required.)

## Rabies

For travelers to areas where rabies is common in domestic animals (eg, India, parts of South America), preexposure prophylaxis with human diploid cell vaccine should be considered. It usually consists of 3 injections given 1 week apart, with a booster 3 weeks later. Such primary immunization can, very rarely, sensitize recipients to the vaccine.

Advisory Committee on Immunization Practices, Centers for Disease Control: Diphtheria, tetanus and pertussis: Guidelines for vaccine prophylaxis and other preventive measures. *MMWR* 1985;**34:**602.

Centers for Disease Control: *Health Information for International Travel 1982.* US Government Printing Office, 1982.

Centers for Disease Control: Prevention of malaria in travelers, 1982. *MMWR* 1982;**31(Suppl).** [Entire issue.]

Centers for Disease Control: Revised recommendations for preventing malaria in travelers to areas with chloroquine-resistant *Plasmodium falciparum. MMWR* 1985;**34:**185.

DuPont HL et al: Treatment of travelers' diarrhea with trimethoprim/sulfamethoxazole and with trimethoprim alone. *N Engl J Med* 1982;**307:**841.

Fulginiti VA (editor): *Immunization in Clinical Practice.* Lippincott, 1982.

Goodman RA, Orenstein WA, Hinman AR: Vaccination and disease prevention for adults. *JAMA* 1982;**248:**1607.

# HYPERSENSITIVITY TESTS & DESENSITIZATION

## Tests for Hypersensitivity

Before injecting antitoxin, materials derived from animal sources, or drugs (eg, penicillin) to which a patient has reacted in the past, test for hypersensitivity. If both tests described below are negative, desensitization is not necessary, and a full dose of the material may be given. If any test is positive, desensitization is necessary or alternative drugs should be used.

**A. Intradermal Test:** Inject 0.1 mL of a 1:10 dilution of the antitoxin (or other material) intradermally on the flexor surface of the forearm. A large wheal and surrounding areola appearing within 5–20 minutes constitute a positive test.

**B. Conjunctival Test:** Instill 1 drop of a 1:10 dilution of the antitoxin into the conjunctival sac of one eye as a test dose and 1 drop of physiologic saline into the other eye as a control. Conjunctival redness, itching, and lacrimation appearing within 5–20 minutes in the test eye constitute a positive test if the control is negative.

## Desensitization

### A. Precautionary Measures:

1. If extreme hypersensitivity is suspected, it is advisable to perform desensitization or use an alternative drug.

2. An antihistaminic drug should be administered before desensitization is begun, in order to lessen any reaction that might occur. An airway device must be available.

3. Epinephrine, 1 mL of 1:1000 solution, must be ready for immediate administration.

### B. Desensitization Method: The following plan may be used in desensitization. Give doses of antitoxin intramuscularly at 30-minute intervals and observe closely for reactions.

**First dose:** 0.1 mL (1:10 dilution)
**Second dose:** 0.2 mL (1:10 dilution)
**Third dose:** 0.5 mL (1:10 dilution)
**Fourth dose:** 0.1 mL (undiluted)
**Fifth dose:** 0.2 mL (undiluted)
**Sixth dose:** 0.5 mL (undiluted)
**Seventh dose:** 1 mL (undiluted)
**Eighth and subsequent doses:** 1 mL (undiluted) every 30 minutes until the total amount of antitoxin is given.

## Treatment of Reactions

### A. Mild: If a mild reaction occurs, drop back to the next lower dose and continue with desensitization. If a severe reaction occurs, administer epinephrine (see below) and discontinue the antitoxin unless treatment is urgently needed. If desensitization is imperative, continue slowly, increasing the dosage of the antitoxin more gradually.

### B. Severe: If manifestations of a severe reaction appear, give 0.5–1 mL of 1:1000 epinephrine into an intravenous drip of 5% dextrose in water at once. The symptoms include urticaria, angioneurotic edema, dyspnea, coughing, choking, and shock. Observe the patient closely and repeat epinephrine as necessary.

Corticosteroids may be used (eg, hydrocortisone, 100 mg intravenously), but their effect begins only after 18 hours.

Norman PS: Specific therapy in allergy. *Med Clin North Am* 1974;**58**:111.

Sherman WB: *Hypersensitivity: Mechanism and Management.* Saunders, 1968.

# REFERENCES

Centers for Disease Control: Sexually transmitted diseases: Treatment guidelines 1985. *MMWR* 1985;**34**:75S.

Dupont ML, Pickering LK: *Infections of the Gastrointestinal Tract.* Plenum Medical Book Co, 1980.

Feigin RD, Cherry JD: *Textbook of Pediatric Infectious Diseases.* Saunders, 1981.

Jawetz E, Melnick JL, Adelberg EA: *Review of Medical Microbiology,* 17th ed. Appleton-Lange, 1986.

Mandell GL, Douglas RG Jr, Bennett JE: *Principles and Practice of Infectious Disease,* 2nd ed. Wiley, 1985.

# 22

# Infectious Diseases: Viral & Rickettsial

*Moses Grossman, MD, & Ernest Jawetz, MD, PhD*

---

## VIRAL DISEASES*

---

### ACQUIRED IMMUNODEFICIENCY SYNDROME (AIDS, ARC)

#### Essentials of Diagnosis

- Lymphadenopathy, weight loss, diarrhea, hematologic abnormalities (thrombocytopenia, anemia, neutropenia), neurologic abnormalities.
- Opportunistic infections or neoplasms (Kaposi's sarcoma, lymphoma).
- Defective cell-mediated immunity (without a previously recognized cause) manifested by an abnormal CD4/CD8 T cell ratio.
- Evidence of infection with a human immunodeficiency retrovirus (HIV).

#### General Considerations

AIDS has been recognized only since 1980 but has now reached worldwide distribution. It has afflicted mainly the following high-risk groups: homosexual or bisexual men with multiple partners, abusers of intravenous drugs, central African natives, and the sexual partners of any of these groups; recipients of factor VII concentrate (hemophiliacs) and of blood transfusions donated by persons infected with HIV; and infants of HIV-seropositive mothers who abuse intravenous drugs.

The disease is caused by a group of retroviruses called human immunodeficiency viruses (HIV) that attack CD4 (helper) T lympocytes and severely damage the immune system. The best-studied of these viruses (HTLV III/LAV/ARV; HIV-1) causes most cases of AIDS in the Western world, whereas HIV-2 is prevalent in western Africa. Other types exist also. All of these retroviruses have multiple antigenic variants. Cofactors may influence HIV infection and the development of AIDS, but their nature and role are uncertain.

#### Clinical Findings

**A. Symptoms and Signs:** The onset of AIDS is insidious, with fatigue, weight loss, diarrhea, fever, and lymphadenopathy for months before there is any manifestation of opportunistic infection or cancer. Oral candidiasis and spreading lesions casued by herpesviruses are common. An abrupt onset of severe illness tends to be precipitated by an opportunistic infection (see Complications). The presence of such an opportunistic infection or neoplasm is an essential feature of the diagnosis. About half of AIDS patients have serious central nervous system involvement, including dementia and encephalopathy produced by HIV itself, a central nervous system neoplasm (eg, lymphoma), or a central nervous system infection (eg, toxoplasmosis).

There are 3 groups of patients: (1) patients with evident AIDS, as defined by CDC for epidemiologic purposes and requiring the presence of an opportunistic infection or Kaposi's sarcoma; (2) patients with the AIDS-related complex (ARC) (see below); and (3) asymptomatic persons who have been infected with an HIV retrovirus as evidenced by the presence of antibodies in serum or virus in blood or genital secretions. It is not known how many such individuals will develop the full-blown syndrome—or when—but epidemiologic evidence supports the assumption that half may do so.

AIDS-related complex (ARC) may include lymphadenopathy, unexplained fever, weight loss, and hematologic and neurologic abnormalities in a person without the full picture of AIDS or in a member of a high-risk group.

AIDS in young children is usually acquired by vertical transmission from an infected mother. Kaposi's sarcoma is rare, whereas opportunistic infections are similar to those in adults. There may be additional manifestations, eg, lymphocytic infiltrative pneumonia.

**B. Laboratory Findings:** The lymphocyte count is often low (<500 $\mu$/L), with markedly depressed number of CD4 (helper) T cells. T cell counting is done with the aid of monoclonal antibodies directed at T cell surface receptors. The ratio of helper/inducer (CD4) T cells to suppressor/killer (CD8) T cells (see p 1084) is 1.5 or greater in normal persons; in AIDS patients, the ratio is 1.0 or less (often <0.5). This severe deficiency in cell-mediated immunity results

---

\* Herpesviruses are discussed in Chapter 21.

in extreme susceptibility to opportunistic infections and neoplasms; it also severely hampers attempts to provide treatment.

The presence of antibodies to an AIDS retrovirus is an indicator of infection and is useful for screening blood donors and for epidemiologic studies. However, it is *not* diagnostic of AIDS. Antibodies are determined by an ELISA method, but confirmation by a second technique (eg, Western blot) is essential to avoid false-positives. Antibody determination in individuals has many medicolegal implications (eg, insurability) and must always be accompanied by informed consent, appropriate counseling, and follow-up.

Isolation of HIV viruses remains a research procedure. Tests for the presence of antigen are being developed.

## Complications

Complications attributable to severe deficiency in cell-mediated immunity are an essential feature of the diagnosis of AIDS. Among the commonest opportunistic pathogens are *Pneumocystis carinii* (causing pneumonia), *Toxoplasma gondii* (cerebral mass), *Cryptosporidium* sp (diarrhea), *Candida* sp (esophagitis), *Cryptococcus neoformans* (meningitis), herpes and varicella viruses (skin and mucous membrane lesions), and many others, including the agents of histoplasmosis, tuberculosis, etc.

Among the commonest cancers are Kaposi's sarcoma (localized or disseminated) and lymphoreticular neoplasms. Women with AIDS who become pregnant have an aggravation of their own disease and a 50% chance of giving birth to an infected infant with a major illness and a high risk of death in infancy.

Patients die from complications in spite of appropriate therapy; thus, *Pneumocystis* pneumonia has a mortality rate of about 80% within 2 years. While temporary remissions of infections or neoplasms have been achieved, nothing has been shown to have a major impact on the overall prognosis of the disease.

## Treatment

Treatment includes supportive care, especially nutrition, moral support, the management of opportunistic infections, and the possible use of drugs that inhibit HIV replication. The first such drug directed at HIV is azidothymidine (AZT, zidovudine, Retrovir; see Chapter 28), which can slow virus production, reduce symptoms, and extend life but which also has major side effects. Other drugs aimed at retroviruses are being tested. However, since the virus is incorporated into host cell genomes, eradication of the viral infection cannot be expected, and it is likely to persist for life. Antiviral treatment can only be expected to prevent clinical expression of HIV infection and perhaps to reduce HIV excretion and infectivity.

The major specific treatment efforts are directed at opportunistic infections and neoplasms. (For prevention and treatment of *Pneumocystis* pneumonia, see p 921.) Cytomegalovirus infections may sometimes respond to DHPG (a guanine derivative) or to ganciclovir (see Chapter 28), both investigational drugs. Multidrug treatment of *Mycobacterium avium* complex infections may achieve remissions. Neoplasms also require aggressive management by radiotherapy and chemotherapy.

## Prevention & Control

The mainstay of prevention must be education about the mode of HIV spread, the major risk factors, and methods of risk reduction. Measures have been taken in the Western world to reduce the risk of HIV transmission by transfusions and blood products. In the USA, the risk of infection from blood transfusion has been reduced to one infection per 0.5–1 million transfusions. Blood factors used in management of hemophilia can be rendered noninfectious by heat treatment.

To reduce HIV transmission by sexual contact, the use of condoms and the avoidance of sexual practices associated with high risk are of greatest importance. HIV viruses are transmitted *only* by intimate sexual contact and through blood (but not insect bites) or blood products and not by ordinary contact in household, family, school, or health care settings. Precautions applicable to hepatitis B virus should be used in managing AIDS patients and avoiding contact with their blood, removed tissues, and genital secretions. Because most HIV-infected individuals are asymptomatic and thus unrecognized, such precautions may have to apply to blood and body fluids from all patients in the future, especially in areas or populations of high HIV prevalence.

Patients with a diagnosis of AIDS are reportable to local health departments or to the National AIDS Activity Center, CDC, Atlanta. Updated information on AIDS can be obtained by telephoning (800) 342-2437 or (404) 329-3472.

Immunization against HIV retroviruses is not available now and is not likely to become available in the near future.

## Prognosis

It has been estimated that over 1.5 million persons in the USA show serologic evidence of infection with HIV retroviruses. Most of these people are presently healthy. Over 40,000 persons have developed AIDS, and about half of those have died. The eventual mortality rate of the full-blown AIDS syndrome is probably near 100%. A smaller number have developed ARC. There is a long latency period until infection with HIV retroviruses is expressed as disease. The precise relationship of ARC to AIDS remains unsettled, particularly the neurologic manifestations of ARC.

It is likely that factors other than retrovirus infection determine whether disease will develop. It is not known what proportion of currently HIV-infected persons will develop ARC or AIDS. While in the Western world HIV transmission was initially most evident among homosexual males with multiple partners, heterosexual transmission is becoming increasingly evident and in some areas (eg, central and western Africa) appears to be the principal mode of spread of the epidemic.

Blaser MJ, Cohn DL: Opportunistic infection in patients with AIDS: Clues to the epidemiology of AIDS and the relative virulence of pathogens. *Rev Infect Dis* 1986;**8:**21.

Clavel F et al: Human immunodeficiency virus type 2 infection associated with AIDS in West Africa. *New Engl J Med* 1987;**316:**1180.

Clumeck N et al: AIDS in African patients. *N Engl J Med* 1984;**310:**492.

Conte JE et al: Infection control guidelines for patients with AIDS. *N Engl J Med* 1983;**309:**740.

Curran JW et al: AIDS associated eith transfusions. *N Engl J Med* 1984;**310:**69.

Fauci AS et al: NIH Conference: The acquired immunodeficiency syndrome: An update. *Ann Intern Med* 1985;**102:**800.

Friedland GM et al: Lack of transmission of HTLV III/LAV infection to household contact of patients with AIDS or ARC with oral candidiasis. *N Engl J Med* 1986;**314:**344.

Gallo RC et al: Frequent detection and isolation of cytopathic retroviruses (HTLV-III) from patients with AIDS and at risk for AIDS. *Science* 1984;**224:**500.

Harris C et al: Immunodeficiency in female sexual partners of men with AIDS. *N Engl J Med* 1983;**308:**1181.

Landesman SH, Ginzburg HM, Weiss SH: The AIDS epidemic. *N Engl J Med* 1985;**312:**521

Laurence J et al: Lymphadenopathy-associated viral antibody in AIDS. *N Engl J Med* 1984;**311:**1269.

Levy JA et al: Isolation of AIDS-associated retrovirus from cerebrospinal fluid and brain of patients with neurological symptoms. *Lancet* 1985;**2:**586.

MMWR (Centers for Disease Control, Atlanta): [Periodic reports on latest developments in epidemiology and management of patients with AIDS.]

Noble GR et al: International Conference on Acquired Immunodeficiency Syndrome, April, 1985, Atlanta, Georgia. *Ann Intern Med* 1985;**103:**653. [Entire issue.]

Piot P et al: Acquired immunodeficiency syndrome in a heterosexual population in Zaire. *Lancet* 1984;**2:**65.

Weiss SH et al: HTLV III infection among health care workers. *JAMA* 1985;**254:**2089.

Weiss SH et al: Screening test for HTLV-III antibodies: Specificity, sensitivity, and applications. *JAMA* 1985;**253:**221.

## MEASLES (Rubeola)

### Essentials of Diagnosis

- Prodrome of fever, coryza, cough, conjunctivitis, photophobia, Koplik's spots.
- Rash: brick-red, irregular, maculopapular; onset 3 days after onset of prodrome; face to trunk to extremities.
- Leukopenia.
- Exposure 10–14 days previously.

### General Considerations

Measles is an acute systemic viral (paramyxovirus) infection transmitted by inhalation of infective droplets. Its highest incidence is in young children. One attack confers permanent immunity. Communicability is greatest during the preeruptive stage but continues as long as the rash remains.

### Clinical Findings

**A. Symptoms and Signs:** Fever is often as high as 40 – 40.6 °C (104 –105 °F). It persists through the prodrome and rash (about 7 days), but may remit briefly at the onset of rash. Malaise may be marked. Coryza resembles that seen with upper respiratory infections (nasal obstruction, sneezing, and sore throat). Cough is persistent and nonproductive. There is conjunctivitis, with redness, swelling, photophobia, and discharge.

Koplik's spots are pathognomonic of measles. They appear about 2 days before the rash and last 1–4 days as tiny "table salt crystals" on the dull red mucous membranes of the cheeks and often on inner conjunctival folds and vaginal mucous membranes. The pharynx is red, and a yellowish exudate may appear on the tonsils. The tongue is coated in the center; the tip and margins are red. Moderate generalized lymphadenopathy is common. Splenomegaly occurs occasionally.

The rash usually appears first on the face and behind the ears 4 days after the onset of symptoms. The initial lesions are pinhead-sized papules which coalesce to form the brick-red, irregular, blotchy maculopapular rash and which may further coalesce in severe cases to form an almost uniform erythema on some areas of the body. By the second day, the rash begins to coalesce on the face as it appears on the trunk. On the third day, the rash is confluent on the trunk, begins to appear on the extremities, and begins to fade on the face. Thereafter, it fades in the order of its appearance. Hyperpigmentation remains in fair-skinned individuals and severe cases. Slight desquamation may follow.

Atypical measles is a syndrome occurring in children, adolescents, or adults who have received inactivated measles vaccine or who received live measles vaccine before age 12 months and as a result have developed hypersensitivity rather than protective immunity. When they are infected with wild measles virus, such individuals develop high fever, unusual rashes (papular, hemorrhagic), headache, arthralgias and pneumonitis, often with severe illness and a substantial mortality rate.

**B. Laboratory Findings:** Leukopenia is usually present unless secondary bacterial complications exist. Febrile proteinuria is present. Virus can be recovered from nasopharyngeal washings and from blood. A 4-fold rise in serum antibody supports the diagnosis.

### Complications

**A. Central Nervous System Complications:** Encephalitis occurs in approximately 1:1000 to 1:2000 cases. Its onset is usually 3–7 days after the rash. Vomiting, convulsions, coma, and a variety of severe neurologic signs and symptoms develop. Treatment is symptomatic and supportive. There is an appreciable mortality rate, and many patients are left with

**Table 22–1.** Diagnostic features of some acute exanthems.

| Disease | Prodromal Signs and Symptoms | Nature of Eruption | Other Diagnostic Features | Laboratory Tests |
|---|---|---|---|---|
| Measles (rubeola) | 3–4 days of fever, coryza, conjunctivitis, and cough. | Maculopapular, brick-red; begins on head and neck; spreads downward. In 5–6 days rash brownish, desquamating. See atypical measles. | Koplik's spots on buccal mucosa. | White blood count low. Virus isolation in cell culture. Antibody tests by hemagglutination inhibition or neutralization. |
| Atypical measles | Same as measles. | Maculopapular centripetal rash, becoming confluent. | History of measles vaccination. | Measles antibody present in past, with titer rise during illness. |
| Rubella (German measles) | Little or no prodrome. | Maculopapular, pink; begins on head and neck, spreads downward, fades in 3 days. No desquamation. | Lymphadenopathy, postauricular or occipital. | White blood count normal or low. Serologic tests for immunity and definitive diagnosis (hemagglutination inhibition). |
| Chickenpox (varicella) | 0–1 day of fever, anorexia, headache. | Rapid evolution of macules to papules, vesicles, crusts; all stages simultaneously present; lesions superficial, distribution centripetal. | Lesions on scalp and mucous membranes. | Specialized complement fixation and virus neutralization in cell culture. Fluorescent antibody test of smear of lesions. |
| Scarlet fever | ½–2 days of malaise, sore throat, fever, vomiting. | Generalized, punctate, red; prominent on neck, in axilla, groin, skinfolds; circumoral pallor; fine desquamation involves hands and feet. | Strawberry tongue, exudative tonsillitis. | Group A hemolytic streptococci cultures from throat; antistreptolysin O titer rise. |
| Exanthem subitum | 3–4 days of high fever. | As fever falls by crisis, pink maculopapules appear on chest and trunk; fade in 1–3 days. | | White blood count low. |
| Erythema infectiosum | None. Usually in epidemics. | Red, flushed cheeks; circumoral pallor; maculopapules on extremities. | "Slapped face" appearance. | White blood count normal. |
| Meningococcemia | Hours of fever, vomiting. | Maculopapules, petechiae, purpura. | Meningeal signs, toxicity, shock. | Cultures of blood. Cerebrospinal fluid. High white blood count. |
| Rocky Mt. spotted fever | 3–4 days of fever, chills, severe headaches. | Maculopapules, petechiae, initial distribution centripetal (extremities to trunk). | History of tick bite. | Agglutination (OX19, OX2), complement fixation. |
| Typhus fevers | 3–4 days of fever, chills, severe headaches. | Maculopapules, petechiae, initial distribution centrifugal (trunk to extremities). | Endemic area, lice. | Agglutination (OX19), complement fixation. |
| Infectious mononucleosis | Fever, adenopathy, sore throat. | Maculopapular rash resembling rubella, rarely papulovesicular. | Splenomegaly, tonsillar exudate. | Atypical lymphocytes in blood smears; heterophil agglutination. Monospot test. |
| Enterovirus infections | 1–2 days of fever, malaise. | Maculopapular rash resembling rubella, rarely papulovesicular or petechial. | Aseptic meningitis. | Virus isolation from stool or cerebrospinal fluid; complement fixation titer rise. |
| Drug eruptions | Occasionally fever. | Maculopapular rash resembling rubella, rarely papulovesicular. | | Eosinophilia. |
| Eczema herpeticum | None. | Vesiculopustular lesions in area of eczema. | | Herpes simplex virus isolated in cell culture. Multinucleate giant cells in smear of lesion. |
| Kawasaki disease | Fever, adenopathy, conjunctivitis. | Cracked lips, strawberry tongue, maculopapular polymorphous rash, peeling skin on fingers and toes. | Edema of extremities. Angiitis of coronary arteries. | Thrombocytosis, electrocardiographic changes. |

permanent sequelae. Subacute sclerosing panencephalitis is a very late form of central nervous system complication, the measles virus acting as a "slow virus" to produce this degenerative central nervous system disease years after the initial infection.

**B. Respiratory Tract Disease:** Early in the course of the disease, bronchopneumonia or bronchiolitis due to the measles virus may occur and result in serious difficulties with ventilation.

**C. Secondary Bacterial Infections:** Immediately following measles, secondary bacterial infection—particularly cervical adenitis, otitis media, and pneumonia—occurs in about 15% of patients.

**D. Tuberculosis:** Measles produces temporary anergy to the tuberculin skin test; there may be exacerbations in patients with tuberculosis.

## Prevention

Attenuated live virus vaccine can greatly reduce the incidence of measles. Its use has virtually eliminated endemic measles in the USA. It is important to immunize all children, including children in those areas of the world where the incidence and mortality rate of measles remain high. Combined virus vaccines (measles-mumps-rubella) are available and effective. Measles immunity is lasting if the vaccine is given at age 15 months or older. Complications of vaccination are negligible.

When susceptible individuals are exposed to measles, the live virus vaccine can prevent disease if given within 24 hours of exposure. This is rarely feasible in a household. Later, gamma globulin (0.25 mL/kg [0.1 mL/lb] body weight) can be injected for prevention of clinical illness. This must be followed by active immunization 3 months later.

## Treatment

**A. General Measures:** Isolate the patient for the week following onset of rash and keep at bed rest until afebrile. Give aspirin, saline eye sponges, vasoconstrictor nose drops, and a sedative cough mixture as necessary.

**B. Treatment of Complications:** Secondary bacterial infections are treated with appropriate antimicrobial drugs. Postmeasles encephalitis can only be treated symptomatically.

## Prognosis

The mortality rate of measles in the USA is 0.2%, but it may be as high as 10% in underdeveloped areas. Death are due principally to encephalitis (15% mortality rate) and bacterial pneumonia.

Bloch AB et al: Health impact of measles vaccination in the United States. *Pediatrics* 1985;**76**:524.

Dave KH: Measles in India. *Rev Infect Dis* 1983;**5**:406.

Martin DB et al: Atypical measles in adolescents and young adults. *Ann Intern Med* 1979;**90**:877.

Ofosu-Amaah S: The control of measles in tropical Africa. *Rev Infect Dis* 1983;**5**:546.

## EXANTHEM SUBITUM (Roseola Infantum)

Although this illness is commonly diagnosed in clinical practice, laboratory confirmation is not available. Rotaviruses have been implicated as etiologic agents. The disease has been transmitted by blood filtrates.

The typical clinical picture is sudden development of very high fever (up to 41°C [106°F]) and irritability in a young child (age 6 months to 3 years). Febrile convulsions occur commonly. The physical findings are limited to postoccipital and postauricular lymphadenopathy. It is essential to rule out other causes of high fever. The febrile state continues for 3 days. As the temperature drops, an evanescent, very transient maculopapular rash appears. The white blood count may be slightly elevated initially, but as the disease progresses, leukopenia is invariably present.

Treatment is purely symptomatic. Aspirin or acetaminophen and tepid sponges will serve to keep the temperature down. Convulsions are usually very brief but may require anticonvulsant medication.

The prognosis is excellent. There are no reported deaths, and no sequelae occur.

## ERYTHEMA INFECTIOSUM (Fifth Disease)

This acute, communicable viral illness is common and occurs in focal and community-wide outbreaks. It is caused by a human parvovirus (HPV—a 20-nm DNA virus). The initial manifestation of illness is a distinctive fiery red appearance of the cheeks ("slapped cheeks"), with circumoral pallor. A few days later, there is a red, lacy, maculopapular rash on the trunk which may wax and wane for several days. Malaise, headache, and pruritus occur, but fever is rare. At the time of the rash, there may be arthralgia, synovitis, and arthritis, particularly in females. The arthritis is symmetric and involves mainly the hands, wrists, and knees. It usually resolves in 4 weeks but may last for months. HPV is also implicated in aplastic crisis, especially in sickle cell disease, and may cause disturbances in pregnancy.

The diagnosis is clinical but may be confirmed by an elevated titer of IgM anti-HPV antibodies in serum. Scarlet fever is the main differential diagnosis. The prognosis is excellent. Besides arthritis, which is common in some outbreaks, encephalitis has been described as a rare complication. Treatment is symptomatic.

Chorba T et al: The role of parvovirus B19 in aplastic crisis and erythema infectiosum. *J Infect Dis* 1986;**154**:383.

Whitley RJ: Parvovirus infection. *N Engl J Med* 1985;**313**:112.

## RUBELLA (German Measles)

### Essentials of Diagnosis

- No prodrome; mild symptoms (fever, malaise, coryza) coinciding with eruption.
- Posterior cervical and postauricular lymphadenopathy.
- Fine maculopapular rash of 3 days' duration; face to trunk to extremities.
- Leukopenia.
- Exposure 14–21 days previously.
- Arthralgia, particularly in young women.

### General Considerations

Rubella is a systemic viral disease transmitted by inhalation of infective droplets. It is only moderately communicable. One attack usually confers permanent immunity. The incubation period is 14–21 days (average, 16 days). The disease is transmissible for 1 week before the rash appears.

The clinical picture of rubella is difficult to distinguish from other viral illnesses such as infectious mononucleosis, echovirus infections, and coxsackievirus infections. Definitive diagnosis can only be made by isolating the virus or by serologic means.

The principal importance of rubella lies in the devastating effect this virus has on the fetus in utero, producing teratogenic effects and a continuing congenital infection.

## Clinical Findings

**A. Symptoms and Signs:** Fever and malaise, usually mild, accompanied by tender suboccipital adenitis, may precede the eruption by 1 week. Mild coryza may be present. Joint pain (polyarthritis) occurs in about 25% of adult cases. These symptoms usually subside in less than 7 days.

Posterior cervical and postauricular lymphadenopathy is very common. Erythema of the palate and throat, sometimes blotchy, may be noted. A fine, pink maculopapular rash appears on the face, trunk, and extremities in rapid progression (2–3 days) and fades quickly, usually lasting 1 day in each area. Rubella without rash may be at least as common as the exanthematous disease. Diagnosis can be suspected when there is epidemiologic evidence of the disease in the community but requires laboratory confirmation.

**B. Laboratory Findings:** Leukopenia may be present early and may be followed by an increase in plasma cells. Virus isolation and serologic tests of immunity (rubella virus hemagglutination inhibition and fluorescent antibody tests) are available. Definitive diagnosis is based on a 4-fold rise in the antibody titer.

## Complications

**A. Complications in Pregnancy:** It is important to know whether rubella antibodies are present at the beginning of pregnancy.

If a pregnant woman is exposed to a possible case of rubella, an immediate hemagglutination-inhibiting rubella antibody level should be obtained. If antibodies are found, there is no reason for concern. If no antibodies are found, careful clinical and serologic follow-up is essential. If the occurrence of rubella in the expectant mother can be confirmed, therapeutic abortion may be considered. Judgment in this regard is tempered by personal, religious, legal, and other considerations. The risk to the fetus is highest in the first trimester but continues into the second.

**B. Congenital Rubella:** An infant acquiring the infection in utero may be normal at birth but more likely will have a wide variety of manifestations, including growth retardation, maculopapular rash, thrombocytopenia, cataracts, deafness, congenital heart defects, organomegaly, and many other manifestations. Viral excretion in the throat and urine persists for many months despite high antibody levels. The diagnosis is confirmed by isolation of the virus. A specific test for IgM rubella antibody is useful for making this diagnosis in the newborn. Treatment is directed to the many anomalies.

## Prevention

Live attenuated rubella virus vaccine (eg, RA 27/3) should be given to all girls before the menarche. When adult women are immunized, they must not be pregnant, and the absence of antibodies should be established. (In the USA, about 80% of 20-year-old women are immune to rubella.) Birth control must be practiced for at least 3 months after the use of the vaccine. Arthritis may follow administration of rubella vaccine.

## Treatment

Give aspirin or acetaminophen as required for symptomatic relief. Encephalitis and thrombocytopenic purpura can only be treated symptomatically.

## Prognosis

Rubella (other than the congenital form) is a mild illness and rarely lasts more than 3–4 days. Congenital rubella, on the other hand, has a high mortality rate, and the congenital defects associated with it require many years of medical and surgical management.

Chantler JK et al: Persistent rubella virus infection associated with chronic arthritis in children. *N Engl J Med* 1985;**313**:1117.

Herrman KL: Available rubella serologic tests. *Rev Infect Dis* 1985;**7**:S108.

Hinman AR et al: Rational strategy for rubella vaccination. *Lancet* 1983;**1**:39.

International symposium on the prevention of congenital rubella infection. *Rev Infect Dis* 1985;**7**(**Suppl 1**):1.

Preblud SR: some current issues relating to rubella vaccine. *JAMA* 1985;**254**:253.

# CYTOMEGALOVIRUS DISEASE

The vast majority of cytomegalovirus infections are clinically inapparent. The virus (human herpesvirus 5) can be cultured from the salivary glands of 10–25% of healthy individuals, from the cervix of 10% of healthy women, and from the urine of 1% of all newborns. Cytomegalovirus infection occurs in 85–95% of homosexual men and is sexually transmitted. In such individuals, cytomegalovirus infection may result in immunosuppression. In immunocompetent individuals, cytomegalovirus infection results in clinical disease in only a minority of cases.

## Clinical Findings

**A. Classification:** Three important clinical entities are recognized.

**1. Perinatal disease**—Intrauterine infection results in serious disease, with jaundice, hepatosplenomegaly, thrombocytopenia, and purpura. Of congenitally infected children, more than 15% develop a hearing deficit and up to 30% have mental retardation. Infection acquired soon after birth is asymptomatic but may induce neurologic deficits later.

**2. Acute acquired cytomegalovirus disease**—The clinical picture is that of infectious mononucleosis with fever, malaise, muscle and joint pains, generalized lymphadenopathy, and an enlarged liver. Pharyngitis and respiratory symptoms are not pronounced. Laboratory findings include atypical lymphocytes and abnormal liver function tests. In contrast to Epstein-Barr herpesvirus infection, the heterophil antibody test is negative. This disease is common after massive blood transfusions, including those given to infants. In intensive care nurseries, up to 30% of infants acquire cytomegalovirus infection.

**3. Disease in the immunosuppressed host–** In immunocompromised persons, cytomegalovirus can cause an opportunistic severe pneumonia. Cytomegalovirus infection itself can result in immunosuppression and may provide a favorable environment for spread of other opportunistic pathogens (eg, *Pneumocystis carinii* pneumonia, disseminated herpes simplex lesions). Most male homosexuals with multiple sexual contacts have cytomegalovirus infection, including those who develop AIDS. Some such persons have repeated infections with different strains.

**B. Laboratory Findings:** (In addition to those listed above.) In neonatal infections, urine often shows typical "owl eye" cells, which are renal epithelial cells with intranuclear inclusions. From urine, cervical secretions, semen, saliva, blood, and various tissues, cytomegalovirus can be grown in cell culture. Serologic tests are used to determine the incidence of infection in various groups. A significant titer rise is the only indication of recent infection.

## Treatment

Control fever, pain, and convulsions with appropriate drugs. Although specific antiviral drug therapy is not established, 2 experimental drugs—DHPG and ganciclovir—have yielded some benefits, albeit with significant toxicity (see Chapter 28). Hyperimmune cytomegalovirus globulin given intravenously to bone marrow transplant recipients may have some prophylactic value.

Meyers JD et al: Risk factors for CMV infection after human marrow transplantation. *J Infect Dis* 1986;**153**:479.

Onorato IM et al: Epidemiology of cytomegaloviral infection: Recommendations for prevention and control. *Rev Infect Dis* 1985;**7**:479.

Stagno S, Whitley RJ: Herpesvirus infections of pregnancy: Cytomegalovirus infections. *N Engl J Med* 1985;**313**:1270.

Winston DJ et al: Intravenous immune globulin for prevention of CMV infection and interstitial pneumonia after bone marrow transplantation. *Ann Intern Med* 1987;**106**:12.

# VARICELLA (Chickenpox) & HERPES ZOSTER (Shingles)

## Essentials of Diagnosis

- Fever and malaise just before or with eruption.
- Rash: pruritic, centripetal, papular, changing to vesicular, pustular, and finally crusting.
- Leukopenia.
- Exposure 14–20 days previously.

## General Considerations

Varicella is a viral (human herpesvirus 3) disease spread by inhalations of infective droplets or contact with lesions. Most cases occur in children. One attack confers permanent immunity. The incubation period of varicella is 10–20 days (average, 14 days).

Herpes zoster is caused by the same virus and occurs in individuals who were infected with chickenpox earlier.

## Clinical Findings

### A. Varicella:

**1. Symptoms and signs–**Fever and malaise are usually mild in children and more severe in adults. Itching is characteristic of the eruption. Vesicular lesions, quickly rupturing to form small ulcers, may appear first in the oropharynx. The rash is most prominent on the face, scalp, and trunk but to a lesser extent commonly involves the extremities (centripetal). Maculopapules change in a few hours to vesicles that quickly become pustular and eventually form crusts. New lesions may erupt for 1–5 days, so that all stages of the eruption are generally present simultaneously. The crusts usually slough in 7–14 days. The vesicles and pustules are superficial, elliptic, and have slightly serrated borders.

The distribution and evolution of varicella distinguish it from herpes zoster.

**2. Laboratory findings–**Leukopenia is common. Multinucleated giant cells may be found in scrapings of the base of the vesicles. Virus isolation is possible.

**B. Herpes Zoster:** This syndrome is caused by the same virus as varicella. Usually a single, unilateral dermatome is involved. Pain, sometimes very severe, may precede the appearance of the skin lesions. The lesions follow the distribution of a nerve root. Thoracic and lumbar roots are most common, but cervical roots and the trigeminal nerve may be involved. The skin lesions are similar to those of chickenpox and develop in the same way from maculopapules to vesicles to pustules. Antibody levels are higher and more persistent in zoster than they are in varicella.

## Complications

Secondary bacterial infection of the lesions is common and may produce a pitted scar. Cellulitis, erysipelas, and surgical scarlet fever may occur.

Pneumonia of the interstitial type occurs more often in adults and may lead to alveolar capillary block, hypoxia, and sometimes death.

Encephalitis occurs infrequently. It tends to exhibit cerebellar signs—ataxia and nystagmus. Most patients recover without sequelae.

Varicella in immunosuppressed patients (eg, children with leukemia receiving antileukemic drugs or children with kidney transplants) is often very severe and may be fatal. Chickenpox contracted during the first or second trimester of pregnancy carries a small risk of a distinctive pattern of congenital malformations in the fetus. If a mother develops varicella within 5 days of delivery, the newborn is at great risk of severe disease and should receive varicella-zoster immune globulin (VZIG).

In immunosuppressed patients, herpes zoster may disseminate, producing skin lesions beyond the dermatome, visceral lesions, and encephalitis. This is a serious, sometimes fatal complication.

### Prevention
VZIG is effective in preventing chickenpox in exposed susceptible immunosuppressed individuals. A live attenuated vaccine for immunocompromised susceptible children appears to be safe and effective.

VZIG may be obtained by calling the nearest regional Red Cross Blood Center or the Centers for Disease Control, Atlanta.

### Treatment
**A. General Measures:** Isolate the patient until primary crusts have disappeared, and keep at bed rest until afebrile. Hospital patients with varicella-zoster should be placed in isolation rooms, and personnel entering the room should wear gowns, gloves, and masks. Keep the skin clean by means of frequent tub baths or showers when afebrile. Calamine lotion locally and antihistaminics may relieve pruritus. If antipyretics are necessary, acetaminophen rather than aspirin should be given.

**B. Treatment of Complications:** Secondary bacterial infection of local lesions may be treated with bacitracin-neomycin ointment; if lesions are extensive, appropriate antimicrobial therapy may be indicated. Varicella encephalitis and varicella pneumonia are treated symptomatically. Corticosteroids may have a beneficial effect in the latter. Bacterial pneumonia is treated with appropriate antibiotics.

In the management of varicella and zoster in the immunosuppressed host, vidarabine (adenine arabinoside) or acyclovir can be beneficial (see Chapter 28) when administered during the first 5 days of disease. VZIG is not helpful for clinical therapy but only for prevention.

### Prognosis
The total duration from onset of symptoms to disappearance of crusts rarely exceeds 2 weeks. Fatalities are rare except in immunosuppressed patients.

Orenstein WO et al: Prophylaxis of varicella in high risk children: Dose response of zoster immune globulin. *J Pediatr* 1981;**98**:368.

Plotkin S: Varicella vaccine: A point of decision. *Pedriatrics* 1986;**78**:705.

Shepp DH: Treatment of varicella-zoster virus infection in severely immunocompromised patients. *New Engl J Med* 1986;**314**:208.

Weller T: Varicella and herpes zoster. (2 parts.) *N Engl J Med* 1983;**309**:1362, 1434.

## VARIOLA
### (Smallpox, Variola Major)

Smallpox was a highly contagious viral (poxvirus) disease characterized by severe headache, fever, and prostration and accompanied by a centrifugal rash developing from macules to papules to vesicles to pustules.

Immunization with vaccinia virus culminating in a worldwide effort by WHO has apparently succeeded in eradicating smallpox from the world as of 1979. While no more cases are expected, an isolated case may occur as a result of infection from laboratory-stored variola virus. If a case is suspected, the nearest public health facility must be contacted as an emergency measure, so that the diagnosis can be promptly established and suitable containment initiated.

## VACCINIA

The efficacy of vaccination was the essential factor in the eradication of smallpox. Since the world has been declared free of smallpox, civilian vaccination is now indicated only for laboratory workers working with smallpox virus or closely related viruses. Vaccination is still practiced among military forces. Smallpox vaccination is no longer required for international travel.

Any form of immunosuppression is an absolute contraindication to smallpox vaccination. Eczema in the patient or family member (including a past history of eczema), other forms of dermatitis, and burns also contraindicate vaccination. Smallpox vaccine should *never* be used ''therapeutically.''

Complications range from minor rashes to life-threatening complications such as postvaccinal encephalitis, vaccinia necrosum, and eczema vaccinatum. Vaccinia can be transmitted from military personnel and their families to contacts. Assistance with the management of such complications may be obtained through the Centers for Disease Control.

US Public Health Service Advisory Committee on Immunization Practices: Smallpox vaccine. *MMWR* 1985;**34**:341.

## MUMPS (Epidemic Parotitis)

### Essentials of Diagnosis
- Painful, swollen salivary glands, usually parotid.
- Orchitis, meningoencephalitis, pancreatitis.
- Cerebrospinal fluid lymphocytic pleocytosis in meningoencephalitis.
- Exposure 14–21 days previously.

### General Considerations
Mumps is a viral (paramyxovirus) disease spread by respiratory droplets that usually produces inflammation of the salivary glands and, less commonly, orchitis, meningoencephalitis, pancreatitis, and oophoritis. Most patients are children. The incubation period is 14–21 days (average, 18 days). Infectivity precedes the symptoms by about 1 day, is maximal for 3 days, and then declines until the swelling is gone.

## Clinical Findings

**A. Symptoms and Signs:** Fever and malaise are variable but are often minimal in young children. High fever usually accompanies orchitis or meningoencephalitis. Pain and swelling of one or both (75%) of the parotid or other salivary glands occurs, usually in succession 1–3 days apart. Occasionally, one gland subsides completely (usually in 7 days or less) before others become involved. Orchitis occurs in 25% of men. Headache and lethargy suggest meningoencephalitis. Upper abdominal pain and nausea and vomiting suggest pancreatitis. Lower abdominal pain in females suggests oophoritis.

Tender parotid swelling is the commonest physical finding. Edema is occasionally marked. Swelling and tenderness of the submaxillary and sublingual glands are variable. The orifice of Stensen's duct may be reddened and swollen. Neck stiffness and other signs of meningeal irritation suggest meningoencephalitis. Testicular swelling and tenderness (unilateral in 75%) denote orchitis. Epigastric tenderness suggests pancreatitis. Lower abdominal tenderness and ovarian enlargement may be noted in mumps oophoritis, but the diagnosis is often difficult. Salivary gland involvement must be differentiated from lymph node involvement in the anterior cervical space.

**B. Laboratory Findings:** Relative lymphocytosis may be present, but the blood picture is not typical. Serum amylase is commonly elevated with or without pancreatitis. Lymphocytic pleocytosis of the cerebrospinal fluid is present in meningoencephalitis, which may be asymptomatic. The diagnosis is confirmed by isolating mumps virus from saliva or demonstrating a 4-fold rise in complement-fixing antibodies in paired sera.

## Differential Diagnosis

Swelling of the parotid gland may be due to causes other than mumps; calculi in the parotid ducts and a reaction to iodides may produce such swelling. Parotitis may also be produced by pyogenic organisms, particularly in debilitated individuals. Swelling of the parotid gland has to be differentiated from inflammation of the lymph nodes that are located more posteriorly and inferiorly than the parotid gland.

## Complications

The "complications" of mumps are simply other manifestations of the disease less common than inflammation of the salivary glands. These usually follow the parotitis but may precede it or occur without salivary gland involvement: meningoencephalitis (30%), orchitis (25% of adult males), pancreatitis, oophoritis, thyroiditis, neuritis, myocarditis, and nephritis.

Aseptic meningitis is common during the course of mumps, often occurs without salivary gland involvement, and is the most common viral meningitis. This is a very benign self-limited illness. Occasionally, however, encephalitis develops. This is associated with cerebral edema, serious neurologic manifestations, and sometimes death. Deafness may develop (rarely) as a result of eighth nerve neuritis.

## Prevention

Mumps live virus vaccine is safe and highly effective. It is recommended for routine immunization for children over age 1 year, either alone or in combination with other virus vaccines. Its use has markedly decreased the incidence of mumps in the USA. The mumps skin test is less reliable in determining immunity than are serum neutralization titers. Mumps hyperimmune globulin may be considered for passive protection of certain exposed susceptibles. However, its effectiveness is uncertain.

## Treatment

**A. General Measures:** Isolate the patient until swelling subsides and keep at bed rest during the febrile period. Give aspirin or codeine for analgesia as required and alkaline aromatic mouthwashes.

**B. Treatment of Complications:**

**1. Meningoencephalitis–**The treatment of aseptic meningitis is purely symptomatic. The management of encephalitis requires attention to cerebral edema, the airway, and maintenance of vital functions.

**2. Orchitis–**Suspend the scrotum in a suspensory or toweling "bridge" and apply ice bags. Incision of the tunica may be necessary in severe cases. Give codeine or morphine as necessary for pain. Pain can also be relieved by injection of the spermatic cord at the external inguinal ring with 10–20 mL of 1% procaine solution. Reduce inflammatory reaction with hydrocortisone sodium succinate, 100 mg intravenously, followed by 20 mg orally every 6 hours for 2–3 days.

**3. Pancreatitis–**Symptomatic relief only and parenteral fluids if necessary.

**4. Oophoritis–**Symptomatic treatment only.

## Prognosis

The entire course of the infection rarely exceeds 2 weeks. Fatalities (due to encephalitis) are very rare.

Orchitis often makes the patient very uncomfortable but very rarely results in sterility.

Koplan JP, Preblud SR: A benefit-cost analysis of mumps vaccine. *Am J Dis Child* 1982;**136**:362.

Sullivan KM et al: Effectiveness of mumps vaccine in a school outbreak. *Am J Dis Child* 1985;**139**:909.

## POLIOMYELITIS

### Essentials of Diagnosis

- Muscle weakness, headache, stiff neck, fever, nausea and vomiting, sore throat.
- Lower motor neuron lesion (flaccid paralysis) with

decreased deep tendon reflexes and muscle wasting.

● Cerebrospinal fluid shows excess cells. Lymphocytes predominate; rarely more than 500/$\mu$L.

## General Considerations

Poliomyelitis virus (enterovirus) is present in throat washings and stools, and infection probably can be acquired by the respiratory droplet route or by ingestion. Since the introduction of effective vaccine, poliomyelitis has become a rare disease in developed areas of the world.

Three antigenically distinct types of poliomyelitis virus (I, II, and III) are recognized, with no cross-immunity between them.

The incubation period is 5–35 days (usually 7–14 days). Infectivity is maximal during the first week, but virus is excreted in stools for several weeks.

## Clinical Findings

### A. Symptoms and Signs:

**1. Abortive poliomyelitis**–The symptoms are fever, headache, vomiting, diarrhea, constipation, and sore throat.

**2. Nonparalytic poliomyelitis**–Headache, neck, back, and extremity pain; fever, vomiting, abdominal pain, lethargy, and irritability are present. Muscle spasm is always present in the extensors of the neck and back and often in hamstring and other muscles. The muscles may be tender to palpation.

**3. Paralytic poliomyelitis**–Paralysis may occur at any time during the febrile period. Tremors, muscle weakness, constipation, and ileus may appear. Paralytic poliomyelitis may be divided into 2 forms, which may coexist: (1) spinal poliomyelitis, with weakness of the muscles supplied by the spinal nerves; and (2) bulbar poliomyelitis, with weakness of the muscles supplied by the cranial nerves and variable "encephalitis" symptoms. Bulbar symptoms include diplopia (uncommon), facial weakness, dysphagia, dysphonia, nasal voice, weakness of the sternocleidomastoid and trapezius muscles, difficulty in chewing, inability to swallow or expel saliva, and regurgitation of fluids through the nose. The most life-threatening aspect of bulbar poliomyelitis is respiratory paralysis.

Paralysis of the shoulder girdle often precedes intercostal and diaphragmatic paralysis, which leads to diminished chest expansion and decreased vital capacity. Cyanosis and stridor may appear later as a result of hypoxia. Paralysis may quickly become maximal or may progress over a period of several days until the temperature becomes normal.

Deep tendon reflexes are diminished or lost, often asymmetrically, in areas of involvement.

In bulbar poliomyelitis there may be loss of gag reflex, loss of movement of palate and pharyngeal muscles, pooling of secretions in the oropharynx, deviation of tongue, and loss of movement of the vocal cords.

Lethargy or coma may be due to encephalitis or hypoxia, most often caused by hypoventilation.

Hypertension, hypotension, and tachycardia may occur. Convulsions are rare.

**B. Laboratory Findings:** The white blood cell count may be normal or mildly elevated. Cerebrospinal fluid pressure and protein are normal or slightly increased; glucose not decreased; cells usually number fewer than 500/$\mu$L (predominantly lymphocytes; polymorphonuclear cells may be elevated at first). Cerebrospinal fluid is normal in 5% of patients. The virus may be recovered from throat washings (early) and stools (early and late). Neutralizing and complement-fixing antibodies appear during the first or second week of illness.

## Differential Diagnosis

Nonparalytic poliomyelitis is very difficult to distinguish from other forms of aseptic meningitis due to other enteroviruses. The distinction is made by laboratory means. Acute infectious polyneuritis (Guillain-Barré) and paralysis from a tick bite may initially resemble poliomyelitis but are easily distinguishable on the basis of clinical and laboratory findings.

## Complications

Urinary tract infection, atelectasis, pneumonia, myocarditis, and pulmonary edema may occur.

## Prevention

Oral live trivalent virus vaccine (Sabin) is easily administered, safe, and very effective in providing local gastrointestinal immunity as well as a good level of circulating antibody. It is essential for primary immunization of all infants. Routine immunization of adults in the USA is not recommended because of the low incidence of the disease. However, adults who are exposed to poliomyelitis or plan to travel to endemic areas should receive oral poliovaccine. Inactivated ("killed") poliomyelitis virus vaccine (Salk) should be given to immunodeficient or immunosuppressed individuals and members of their households.

## Treatment

Cranial nerve involvement must be detected promptly. Maintain comfortable but changing positions in a "polio bed": firm mattress, foot board, sponge rubber pads or rolls, sandbags, and light splints. Change of position, hot packs for the extremities, and analgesic drugs usually control muscle spasm and pain. Fecal impaction and urinary retention (especially with paraplegia) must be managed. In cases of respiratory paralysis or weakness, intensive care is needed. Maintain a clear airway, remove secretions, and maintain ventilation—if necessary by intubation and mechanical assistance.

To prevent future deformity, active exercise is avoided during fever but passive range-of-motion exercises are carried out, as well as frequent changes in position. As soon as the fever has subsided, early mobilization and active exercise under skilled direction is begun. Early bracing and splinting may be helpful.

## Prognosis

During the febrile period, paralysis may develop or progress. Mild weakness of small muscles is more likely to regress than severe weakness of large muscles. Bulbar poliomyelitis carries the highest mortality rate (up to 50%). New muscle weakness may develop years after recovery from acute paralytic poliomyelitis, with signs of chronic and new denervation. This is due to dysfunction of surviving motor neurons—not new infectious activity.

Dalakas MC et al: A long-term follow-up of patients with post-poliomyelitis neuromuscular symptoms. *N Engl J Med* 1986;**314:**959.
Hovi T et al: Outbreak of paralytic poliomyelitis in Finland: Widespread circulation of antigenically altered poliovirus type 3 in a vaccinated population. *Lancet* 1986;**1:**1427.
Nikowane BM et al: Vaccine-associated paralytic poliomyelitis. *JAMA* 1987;**257:**1335.

## ENCEPHALITIS

### Essentials of Diagnosis

- Fever, malaise, stiff neck, sore throat, and nausea and vomiting, progressing to stupor, coma, and convulsions.
- Signs of an upper motor neuron lesion (exaggerated deep tendon reflexes, absent superficial reflexes, pathologic reflexes, spastic paralysis).
- Cerebrospinal fluid protein and pressure often increased, with lymphocytic pleocytosis.

### General Considerations

**A. Viral Encephalitis:** While arboviruses (Table 22–2) are the principal causes, many other viruses may produce encephalitis. Herpes simplex produces "masslike" lesions in the temporal lobes. Rabies virus invariably produces encephalitis; mumps virus, poliovirus, and other enteroviruses can cause aseptic meningitis or meningoencephalitis.

**B. Encephalitis Accompanying Exanthematous Diseases of Childhood:** This may occur in the course of measles, varicella, infectious mononucleosis, and rubella.

**C. Encephalitis Following Vaccination:** Encephalitis of the demyelinating type may follow use of certain immunizing agents. These include vaccines against smallpox, rabies, and pertussis.

**D. Toxic Encephalitis:** Toxic encephalitis due to drugs, poisons, or bacterial toxins (*Shigella dysenteriae* type 1) may be clinically indistinguishable from infectious encephalitis.

**E. Reye's Syndrome:** See p 849.

### Clinical Findings

**A. Symptoms and Signs:** The symptoms are fever, malaise, sore throat, nausea and vomiting, lethargy, stupor, coma, and convulsions. Signs include stiff neck, signs of meningeal irritation, tremors, convulsions, cranial nerve palsies, paralysis of extremities, exaggerated deep reflexes, absent superficial reflexes, and pathologic reflexes.

**B. Laboratory Findings:** The white blood cell count is variable. Cerebrospinal fluid pressure and protein content are often increased; glucose is normal; lymphocytic pleocytosis may be present (polymorphonuclears may predominate early in some forms). The virus may sometimes be isolated from blood or, rarely, from cerebrospinal fluid. Serologic tests of blood may be diagnostic in a few specific types of encephalitis. A CT scan of the brain may reveal the temporal lobe lesions indicative of herpesvirus.

### Differential Diagnosis

Mild forms of encephalitis must be differentiated from aseptic meningitis, lymphocytic choriomeningitis, and nonparalytic poliomyelitis; severe forms from cerebrovascular accidents, brain tumors, brain abscess, and poisoning.

### Complications

Bronchial pneumonia, urinary retention and infection, and decubitus ulcers may occur. Late sequelae are mental deterioration, parkinsonism, and epilepsy.

### Prevention

Effective measures include vigorous mosquito control and active immunization against childhood infectious diseases. Special inactivated virus vaccines have been prepared for high-risk persons.

**Table 22–2.** Arbovirus (arthropod-borne) encephalitis.

| Disease | Geographic Distribution | Vector; Reservoir | Comment |
|---|---|---|---|
| California encephalitis | Throughout USA | Mosquitoes; small mammals | Mainly in children |
| Eastern (equine) encephalitis | Eastern part of North, Central, and South America | Mosquitoes; birds, small rodents | Often occurs in horses in the area |
| St. Louis encephalitis | Western and central USA, Florida | Mosquitoes; birds (including domestic fowl) | |
| Venezuelan encephalitis | South America | Mosquitoes | Rare in USA |
| Western (equine) encephalitis | Throughout western hemisphere | Mosquitoes; birds | Often occurs in horses in the area; particularly affects young children |

## Treatment

Although specific therapy for the majority of causative entities is not available, vigorous supportive measures can be helpful. Such measures include reduction of intracranial pressure (by the use of mannitol and glucocorticoids), the control of convulsions, maintenance of the airway, administration of oxygen, and attention to adequate nutrition during periods of prolonged coma. After 72 hours of conventional intravenous nutrition, a nasogastric tube must be inserted and intestinal feedings begun.

Prevention or early treatment of decubiti, pneumonia, and urinary tract infections is important. Give anticonvulsants as needed.

Acyclovir is an effective drug for biopsy-proved herpes simplex encephalitis if administered early in the disease before onset of coma. It has no effect on other viral encephalitides (see Chapter 28).

## Prognosis

The prognosis should always be guarded, especially in younger children. Sequelae may become apparent late in the course of what appears to be a successful recovery.

Arvin AM et al: Management of the patient with herpes simplex encephalitis. *Pediatr Infect Dis* 1987;**6**:2.

Johnson RT: The pathogenesis of acute viral encephalitis and postinfectious encephalomyelitis. *J Infect Dis* 1987;**155**:359.

## LYMPHOCYTIC CHORIOMENINGITIS

### Essentials of Diagnosis

- "Influenzalike" prodrome of fever, chills, malaise, and cough, followed by meningitis with associated stiff neck.
- Kernig's sign, headache, nausea, vomiting, and lethargy.
- Cerebrospinal fluid: slight increase of protein, lymphocytic pleocytosis (500–1000/$\mu$L).
- Complement-fixing antibodies within 2 weeks.

### General Considerations

Lymphocytic choriomeningitis is a viral (arenavirus) infection of the central nervous system. The reservoir of infection is the infected house mouse, although naturally infected guinea pigs, monkeys, dogs, and swine have been observed. Pet hamsters may be a source of infection. The virus is shed by the infected animal via oronasal secretions, urine, and feces, with transmission to humans probably through contaminated food and dust. The incubation period is probably 8–13 days to the appearance of systemic manifestations and 15–21 days to the appearance of meningeal symptoms. The disease is not communicable from person to person. Complications are rare.

This disease is principally confined to the eastern seaboard and northeastern states of the USA.

### Clinical Findings

**A. Symptoms and Signs:** The prodromal illness is characterized by fever, chills, headache, myalgia, cough, and vomiting; the meningeal phase by headache, nausea and vomiting, and lethargy. Signs of pneumonia are occasionally present during the prodromal phase. During the meningeal phase there may be neck and back stiffness and a positive Kernig sign (meningeal irritation). Severe meningoencephalitis may disturb deep tendon reflexes and may cause paralysis and anesthesia of the skin.

The prodrome may terminate in complete recovery, or meningeal symptoms may appear after a few days of remission.

**B. Laboratory Findings:** Leukocytosis may be present. Cerebrospinal fluid lymphocytic pleocytosis (total count is often 500–3000/$\mu$L) may occur, with slight increase in protein and normal glucose. Complement-fixing antibodies appear during or after the second week. The virus may be recovered from the blood and cerebrospinal fluid by mouse inoculation.

### Differential Diagnosis

The influenzalike prodrome and latent period help distinguish this from other aseptic meningitides, meningismus, and bacterial and granulomatous meningitis. A history of exposure to mice is an important diagnostic clue.

### Treatment

Treat as for encephalitis.

### Prognosis

Fatality is rare. The illness usually lasts 1–2 weeks, although convalescence may be prolonged.

Biggar RJ et al: Lymphocytic choriomeningitis outbreak associated with pet hamsters. *JAMA* 1975;**232**:494.

## DENGUE
## (Breakbone Fever, Dandy Fever)

### Essentials of Diagnosis

- Sudden onset of high fever, chills, severe aching, headache, sore throat, prostration, and depression.
- Biphasic fever curve: initial phase, 3–4 days; remission, few hours to 2 days; second phase, 1–2 days.
- Rash: maculopapular, scarlatiniform, morbilliform, or petechial; on extremities to torso, occurring during remission or second phase.
- Leukopenia.

### General Considerations

Dengue is a viral (group B arbovirus, togavirus) disease transmitted by the bite of the *Aedes* mosquito. It may be caused by one of several serotypes widely distributed between latitudes 25° north and 25° south. It occurs only in the active mosquito season (warm weather). The incubation period is 3–15 days (usually 5–8 days).

## Clinical Findings

**A. Symptoms and Signs:** Dengue begins with a sudden onset of high fever (often of the saddleback type), chilliness, and severe aching ("breakbone") of the head, back, and extremities, accompanied by sore throat, prostration, and depression. There may be conjunctival redness and flushing or blotching of the skin. The initial febrile phase lasts 3–4 days, typically but not inevitably followed by a remission of a few hours to 2 days. The skin eruption appears in 80% of cases during the remission or during the second febrile phase, which lasts 1–2 days and is accompanied by similar but usually milder symptoms than in the first phase. The rash may be scarlatiniform, morbilliform, maculopapular, or petechial. It appears first on the dorsum of the hands and feet and spreads to the arms, legs, trunk, and neck but rarely to the face. The rash lasts 2 hours to several days and may be followed by desquamation. Petechial rashes and gastrointestinal hemorrhages occur in a high proportion of cases (mosquito-borne hemorrhagic fever) in Southeast Asia. These probably involve an immunologic reaction (immune complex disease).

Before the rash appears, it is difficult to distinguish dengue from malaria, yellow fever, or influenza. With the appearance of the eruption, which resembles rubella, the diagnosis is usually clear.

**B. Laboratory Findings:** Leukopenia is characteristic. Thrombocytopenia occurs in the hemorrhagic form of the disease. Virus may be recovered from the blood during the acute phase. Serologic diagnosis must consider the several viruses that can produce this clinical syndrome.

## Complications

Depression, pneumonia, iritis, orchitis, and oophoritis are rare complications. Shock occurs in hemorrhagic dengue.

## Prevention

Available prophylactic measures include control of mosquitoes by screening and insect repellents. An effective vaccine has been developed but has not been produced commercially.

## Treatment

Treat shock by expanding circulating blood volume. Give salicylates as required for discomfort. Permit gradual restoration of activity during prolonged convalescence.

## Prognosis

Fatalities are rare. Convalescence is slow.

Halstead SB: The pathogenesis of dengue: Molecular epidemiology in infectious disease. *Am J Epidemiol* 1981;**114**:632.

Malinson MD, Waterman SH: Dengue fever in the United States. *JAMA* 1983;**249**:496.

# RIFT VALLEY FEVER

Rift Valley fever is a viral disease of sheep and cattle, chiefly in Africa, transmitted to humans probably by mosquito bites. It is not contagious. The clinical manifestations are closely similar to those of dengue: acute prostration, fever (often saddleback in type), myalgia and arthralgia, gastrointestinal distress, and sometimes hepatitis. The course is usually brief and self-limited.

There is no effective treatment. Complete recovery is the rule.

Meegan JM, Shope RE: Emerging concepts in Rift Valley fever. *Perspect Virol* 1981;**11**:267.

# COLORADO TICK FEVER

## Essentials of Diagnosis

- Fever, chills, myalgia, headache, prostration.
- Leukopenia.
- Second attack of fever after remission lasting 2–3 days.
- Onset 3–6 days following tick bite.

## General Considerations

Colorado tick fever is an acute viral (orbivirus) infection transmitted by *Dermacentor andersoni* bites. The disease is limited to the western USA and is most prevalent during the tick season (March to August). The incubation period is 3–6 days.

## Clinical Findings

**A. Symptoms and Signs:** The onset of fever (to 38.9–40.6 °C [102–105 °F]) is abrupt, sometimes with chills. Severe myalgia, headache, photophobia, anorexia, nausea and vomiting, and generalized weakness are prominent symptoms. Abnormal physical findings are limited to an occasional faint rash. Fever continues for 3 days, followed by a remission of 2–3 days and then by a full recrudescence lasting 3–4 days. In an occasional case there may be 2 or 3 bouts of fever.

Influenza, Rocky Mountain spotted fever, and other acute leukopenic fevers must be differentiated.

**B. Laboratory Findings:** Leukopenia (2000–3000/$\mu$L) with a shift to the left occurs. Viremia may be demonstrated by inoculation of blood into mice or by fluorescent antibody staining of the patient's red cells (with adsorbed virus). Complement-fixing antibodies appear during the third week after onset of the disease.

## Complications

Aseptic meningitis or encephalitis occurs rarely. Asthenia may follow, but fatalities are very rare.

## Treatment

No specific treatment is available. Aspirin or codeine may be given for pain.

## Prognosis

The disease is self-limited and benign.

Goodpasture HC et al: Colorado tick fever: Clinical, epidemiologic and laboratory aspects of 228 cases in Colorado in 1973–74. *Ann Intern Med* 1978;**88**:303.

## HEMORRHAGIC FEVERS

This is a diverse group of illnesses resulting from virus infections and perhaps immunologic responses to them. The common clinical features include high fever; hemorrhagic diathesis with petechiae or purpura; and bleeding from the nose, gastrointestinal tract, and genitourinary tract, with thrombocytopenia, leukopenia, and marked toxicity, often leading to shock and death. The viruses may be tick-borne (eg, Omsk hemorrhagic fever, Russia; Kyasanur Forest hemorrhagic fever, India), mosquito-borne (eg, Chikungunya hemorrhagic fever, yellow fever, dengue), or zoonotic (often derived from rodents, eg, Junin hemorrhagic fever, Argentina; Machupo hemorrhagic fever, Bolivia; Lassa hemorrhagic fever, West Africa). This last (zoonotic) group includes Marburg hemorrhagic fever (from contact with African vervet monkeys) and Ebola hemorrhagic fever in central Africa.

Persons who present with symptoms compatible with those of hemorrhagic fever and who have traveled from a possible endemic area should be strictly isolated for diagnosis and symptomatic treatment. Conclusive diagnosis may be made by growing the virus from blood obtained early in the disease or by showing a significant specific antibody titer rise. Isolation is particularly important, because some of these infections are highly transmissible to close contacts, including medical personnel, and carry a mortality rate of 50–70%.

For most of these entities, no specific treatment is available. Lassa fever can be effectively treated with intravenous ribavirin if started early (see Chapter 28). It is more important to differentiate hemorrhagic fever from such easily treated entities as meningococcemia and Rocky Mountain spotted fever.

Monath TP: Lassa fever: New issues raised by field studies in West Africa. *J Infect Dis* 1987;**155**:433.
Simpson DIH: Viral haemorrhagic fevers of man. *Bull WHO* 1978;**56**:819.
Viral hemorrhagic fever: Initial management of suspected and confirmed cases. *MMWR* 1983;**32**:275.
Zhi-Yi X et al: Epidemiological studies of hemorrhagic fevers with renal syndrome. *J Infect Dis* 1985;**152**:137.

## RABIES

### Essentials of Diagnosis

- Paresthesia, hydrophobia, rage alternating with calm.
- Convulsions, paralysis, thick tenacious saliva.
- History of animal bite.

### General Considerations

Rabies is a viral (rhabdovirus) encephalitis transmitted by infected saliva that gains entry into the body by a bite or an open wound. Bats, skunks, and foxes are extensively infected. Dogs and cats may be infected. Rodents are unlikely to have rabies. The virus gains entry into the salivary glands of dogs 5–7 days before their death from rabies, thus limiting their period of infectivity. The incubation period may range from 10 days to 2 years but is usually 3–7 weeks. The virus travels in the nerves to the brain, multiplies there, and then migrates along the efferent nerves to the salivary glands.

Rabies is almost uniformly fatal. The most common clinical problem confronting the physician is the management of a patient bitten by an animal. (See Prevention.)

### Clinical Findings

**A. Symptoms and Signs:** There is usually a history of animal bite. Pain appears at the site of the bite, followed by tingling. The skin is quite sensitive to changes of temperature, especially air currents. Attempts at drinking cause extremely painful laryngeal spasm, so that the patient refuses to drink (hydrophobia). The patient is restless and behaves in a peculiar manner. Muscle spasm, laryngospasm, and extreme excitability are present. Convulsions occur, and blowing on the back of the patient's neck will often precipitate a convulsion. Large amounts of thick tenacious saliva are present.

**B. Laboratory Findings:** Biting animals who are apparently well should be kept under observation. Sick or dead animals should be examined for rabies. The diagnosis of rabies in the brain of a rabid animal may be made rapidly by the fluorescent antibody technique.

### Prevention

Since the disease is almost always fatal, prevention is the only available approach. Immunization of household dogs and cats and active immunization of persons with an unusual degree of exposure (eg, veterinarians) are important. However, the most important common decisions concern handling animal bites.

**A. Local Treatment of Animal Bites and Scratches:** Thorough and repeated flushing and cleansing of wounds with soap and water are important. If rabies immune globulin or antiserum is to be used, a portion should be infiltrated locally around the wound (see below). Wounds caused by animal bites should not be sutured.

**B. The Biting Animal:** A dog or cat should be captured, confined, and observed by a veterinarian for 7–10 days. A wild animal, if captured, should be sacrificed and the head shipped on ice to the nearest laboratory qualified to examine the brain for rabies. When the animal cannot be examined, skunks, bats, coyotes, foxes, and raccoons should be presumed to be rabid. The rabies potential of bites by other animals must be evaluated individually.

**C. Postexposure Immunization:** The physician must reach a decision based on the recommendations of the USPHS Advisory Committee but should also be influenced by the circumstances of the bite, the extent and location of the wound, the presence of rabies in the region, the type of animal responsible for the bite, etc. (Consultation is provided by the Rabies Investigation Unit, Centers for Disease Control, Atlanta.) Treatment includes both passive antibody and vaccine. The optimal form of passive immunization is human rabies immune globulin (20 IU/kg). Up to 50% of the globulin should be used to infiltrate the wound; the rest is administered intramuscularly. If the human gamma globulin is not available, equine rabies antiserum (40 IU/kg) can be used after appropriate tests for horse serum sensitivity. Two inactivated preparations of rabies vaccine are currently licensed. The human diploid cell rabies vaccine is preferred. It is given as 5 injections intramuscularly on days 0, 3, 7, 14, and 28 after exposure. The vaccine effectively produces a regular antibody response. Allergic reactions are rare. The vaccine can be obtained through state health departments.

Only if diploid cell vaccine is not available should duck embryo vaccine be used. It must be given as a series of 23 injections during the 2 weeks after exposure, as indicated in the package insert. Its efficacy is probably low. When duck embryo vaccine is used, rabies immune globulin must be given concurrently.

Preexposure prophylaxis with 3 injections of diploid cell vaccine is recommended for persons at high risk of exposure (veterinarians, animal handlers, etc). Simultaneous chloroquine prophylaxis for malaria may diminish the antibody response.

**Treatment**

This very severe illness with an almost universally fatal outcome requires skillful intensive care with attention to the airway, maintenance of oxygenation, and control of seizures.

**Prognosis**

Once the symptoms have appeared, death almost inevitably occurs after 2–3 days as a result of cardiac or respiratory failure or generalized paralysis.

Anderson LJ et al: Human rabies in the United States 1960–1979. *Ann Intern Med* 1984;**100**:728.

Compendium of animal rabies vaccines, 1984: Recommendations for immunization procedures. *MMWR* 1983;**32**:665.

Pappaioanou M et al: Antibody response to preexposure human diploid cells rabies vaccine given concurrently with chloroquine. *N Engl J Med* 1986;**314**:280.

Recommendation of the Immunization Practices Advisory Committee: Rabies prevention—United States, 1984. *MMWR* 1984;**33**:393.

Warrell DA et al: Pathophysiologic studies in human rabies. *Am J Med* 1976;**60**:180.

## YELLOW FEVER

### Essentials of Diagnosis

- Sudden onset of severe headache, aching in legs, and tachycardia. Later, bradycardia, hypotension, jaundice, hemorrhagic tendency ("coffee-ground" vomitus).
- Proteinuria, leukopenia, bilirubinemia, bilirubinuria.
- Endemic area.

### General Considerations

Yellow fever is a viral (group B arbovirus, togavirus) infection transmitted by the *Aedes* and jungle mosquitoes. It is endemic to Africa and South America (tropical or subtropical), but epidemics have extended far into the temperate zone during warm seasons. The mosquito transmits the infection by first biting an individual having the disease and then biting a susceptible individual after the virus has multiplied within the mosquito's body. The incubation period in humans is 3–6 days.

### Clinical Findings

**A. Symptoms and Signs:**

**1. Mild form**–Symptoms are malaise, headache, fever, retro-orbital pain, nausea, vomiting, and photophobia. Bradycardia may be present.

**2. Severe form**–Symptoms are the same as in the mild form, with sudden onset and then severe pains throughout the body, extreme prostration, bleeding into the skin and from the mucous membranes ("coffee-ground" vomitus), oliguria, and jaundice. Signs include tachycardia, erythematous face, and conjunctival redness during the congestive phase, followed by a period of calm (on about the third day) with a normal temperature and then a return of fever, bradycardia, hypotension, jaundice, hemorrhages (gastrointestinal tract, bladder, nose, mouth, subcutaneous), and later delirium. The short course and mildness of the icterus distinguish yellow fever from leptospirosis. The mild form is difficult to distinguish from infectious hepatitis.

**B. Laboratory Findings:** Leukopenia occurs, although it may not be present at the onset. Proteinuria is present, sometimes as high as 5–6 g/L, and disappears completely with recovery. With jaundice there are bilirubinuria and bilirubinemia. The virus may be isolated from the blood by intracerebral mouse inoculation (first 3 days). Antibodies appear during and after the second week.

### Differential Diagnosis

It may be difficult to distinguish yellow fever from leptospirosis and other forms of jaundice on clinical evidence alone.

## Prevention

Transmission is prevented through mosquito control. Live virus vaccine is highly effective and should be provided for persons living in or traveling to endemic areas. (See Chapter 21.)

## Treatment

Treatment consists of giving a liquid diet, limiting food to high-carbohydrate, high-protein liquids as tolerated; intravenous glucose and saline as required; analgesics and sedatives as required; and saline enemas for obstipation.

## Prognosis

The mortality rate is high in the severe form, with death occurring most commonly between the sixth and the ninth days. In survivors, the temperature returns to normal by the seventh or eighth day. The prognosis in any individual case should be guarded at the onset, since sudden changes for the worse are common. Hiccup, copious black vomitus, melena, and anuria are unfavorable signs.

Monath TP: Yellow fever: A medically neglected disease. *Rev Infect Dis* 1987;**9**:165.

## INFLUENZA

### Essentials of Diagnosis

- Abrupt onset with fever, chills, malaise, cough, coryza, and muscle aches.
- Aching, fever, and prostration out of proportion to catarrhal symptoms.
- Leukopenia.

### General Considerations

Influenza (orthomyxovirus) is transmitted by the respiratory route. Although sporadic cases occur, epidemics and pandemics appear at varying intervals, usually in the fall or winter. Antigenic types A and B produce clinically indistinguishable infections, whereas type C is usually a minor illness. The incubation period is 1–4 days.

It is difficult to diagnose influenza in the absence of a classic epidemic. The disease resembles many other mild febrile illnesses but is always accompanied by a cough.

### Clinical Findings

**A. Symptoms and Signs:** The onset is usually abrupt, with fever, chills, malaise, muscular aching, substernal soreness, headache, nasal stuffiness, and occasionally nausea. Fever lasts 1–7 days (usually 3–5). Coryza, nonproductive cough, and sore throat are present. Signs include mild pharyngeal injection, flushed face, and conjunctival redness.

**B. Laboratory Findings:** Leukopenia is common. Proteinuria may be present. The virus may be isolated from the throat washings by inoculation of embryonated eggs or cell cultures. Complement-fixing and hemagglutination-inhibiting antibodies appear during the second week.

### Complications

Influenza causes necrosis of the respiratory epithelium, which predisposes to secondary bacterial infections. Frequent complications are acute sinusitis, otitis media, purulent bronchitis, and pneumonia.

Pneumonia is commonly due to bacterial infection with pneumococci or staphylococci and rarely to the influenza virus itself. The circulatory system is not usually involved, but pericarditis, myocarditis, and thrombophlebitis sometimes occur.

**Reye's syndrome** is a rare and severe complication of influenza and other viral diseases (eg, varicella, coxsackievirus, echovirus), particularly in young children. It consists of rapid development of hepatic failure and encephalopathy, and there is a 30% fatality rate. The pathogenesis is unknown; aspirin may be a risk factor. Hypoglycemia, elevation of serum transaminases and blood ammonia, prolonged prothrombin time, and change in mental status all occur within 2–3 weeks after onset of the virus infection. Histologically, the periphery of liver lobules shows striking fatty infiltration and glycogen depletion. Treatment is supportive and directed to the management of cerebral edema.

### Prevention

Polyvalent influenza virus vaccine given twice (1–2 weeks apart) exerts moderate temporary protection. Partial immunity lasts a few months to 1 year. Current vaccine (as of June 1987) is composed of A/Taiwan/1/86 (HINI), B/Ann Arbor/1/86, and A/Leningrad/360/86 (H3N2) (*MMWR* 1987;**36**:193). It is possible that changes may be announced after this book goes to the printer. Vaccination is recommended every year for persons with chronic respiratory insufficiency, cardiac disease, or other debilitating illness. Effective chemoprophylaxis for epidemiologically or virologically confirmed influenza A consists of amantadine hydrochloride, 200 mg orally daily. This markedly reduces the incidence of infection in individuals exposed to influenza A if begun immediately and continued for 10 days. The drug does not prevent other types of influenza or other viral diseases.

### Treatment

Bed rest to reduce complications is important. Analgesics and a sedative cough mixture may be used. Antibiotics should be reserved for treatment of bacterial complications. If antipyretics are needed, acetaminophen rather than aspirin should be used, especially in children. Ribavirin by aerosol has helped severely ill patients with influenza A or B.

### Prognosis

The duration of the uncomplicated illness is 1–7 days, and the prognosis is excellent. Purulent bronchitis and bronchiectasis may result in chronic pulmonary disease and fibrosis that persist throughout life. Most fatalities are due to bacterial pneumonia. Pneumococcal pneumonia is most common, but staphylococcal pneumonia is most serious. In recent epidemics, the mortality rate has been low except in debilitated persons—especially those with severe heart disease.

If the fever persists for more than 4 days, if the cough becomes productive, or if the white blood cell count rises to about 12,000/$\mu$L, secondary bacterial infection should be ruled out or verified and treated.

Baine WB et al: Severe illness with influenza B. *Am J Med* 1980;**68**:181.

Gregg MB et al: Influenza-related mortality. *JAMA* 1978;**239**:115.

Hirsch MS, Swartz MN: Drug therapy: Antiviral agents. *N Engl J Med* 1980;**302**:903.

# INFECTIOUS MONONUCLEOSIS
## (EB Virus Infection)

### Essentials of Diagnosis

- Fever, sore throat, malaise, lymphadenopathy.
- Frequently splenomegaly, occasionally maculopapular rash.
- Positive heterophil agglutination test (Monospot).
- "Atypical" large lymphocytes in blood smear; lymphocytosis.
- Hepatitis frequent, and occasionally myocarditis, neuritis, encephalitis.

### General Considerations

Infectious mononucleosis is an acute infectious disease due to the Epstein-Barr (EB) herpesvirus (human herpesvirus 4). It is universal in distribution and may occur at any age but usually occurs between the ages of 10 and 35, either in an epidemic form or as sporadic cases. Its mode of transmission is probably by saliva. The incubation period is probably 5–15 days.

### Clinical Findings

**A. Symptoms and Signs:** Symptoms are varied but typically include fever; discrete, nonsuppurative, slightly painful, enlarged lymph nodes, especially those of the posterior cervical chain; and, in approximately half of cases, splenomegaly. Sore throat is often present, and toxic symptoms (malaise, anorexia, and myalgia) occur frequently in the early phase of the illness. A maculopapular or occasionally petechial rash occurs in less than 50% of cases. Exudative pharyngitis, tonsillitis, or gingivitis may occur.

Common manifestations of infectious mononucleosis are hepatitis with hepatomegaly, nausea, anorexia, and jaundice; central nervous system involvement with headache, neck stiffness, photophobia, pains of neuritis, and occasionally even Guillain-Barré syndrome; pulmonary involvement with chest pain, dyspnea, and cough; and myocardial involvement with tachycardia and arrhythmias.

The varying symptoms of infectious mononucleosis—especially sore throat, hepatitis, rash, and lymphadenopathy—raise difficult problems in differential diagnosis.

**B. Laboratory Findings:** Initially, there is a granulocytopenia followed within 1 week by a lymphocytic leukocytosis. Many lymphocytes are atypical, ie, are larger than normal adult lymphocytes, stain more darkly, and frequently show vacuolated, foamy cytoplasm and dark chromatin in the nucleus.

The mononucleosis spot test and the heterophil (sheep cell agglutination) test usually become positive in infectious mononucleosis before the fourth week after onset of the illness. Titer rises in antibodies directed at several EB virus antigens can be detected by immunofluorescence. During acute illness, there is always a rise in antibody to EB virus capsid antigen (VCA). A false-positive VDRL or RPR test occurs in 10% of cases.

In central nervous system involvement, the cerebrospinal fluid may show increase of pressure, abnormal lymphocytes, and protein.

With myocardial involvement, the electrocardiographic studies may show abnormal T waves and prolonged PR intervals.

Liver function tests are commonly abnormal.

### Differential Diagnosis

Causes of pharyngitis with exudate include diphtheria and adenovirus, herpes simplex, gonococcal, and streptococcal infections. Cytomegalovirus infection may be indistinguishable from infectious mononucleosis due to EB virus, but the heterophil antibody and Monospot tests are negative. The same applies to toxoplasmosis and rubella.

### Complications

These usually consist of secondary throat infections, often streptococcal, and (rarely) rupture of the spleen or hypersplenism. Very rarely, there may be a variety of neurologic involvements, eg, myelitis.

EB virus infections rarely may result in the production of B cell lymphomas. A special case, Burkitt's lymphoma of the jaw in African children, regularly shows the presence of EB viral antigens. The etiologic role of EB virus in this neoplasm is not established. While Burkitt's lymphoma in Africa responds to radiation therapy or anticancer chemotherapy, the effect of antiviral drugs is unknown. The rare cases of Burkitt's lymphoma in the USA are much more invasive, respond poorly to therapy, and are not regularly associated with EB virus. EB virus has also been associated with nasopharyngeal carcinoma in some populations, but again, the role of the virus is unclear.

### Chronic Epstein-Barr Virus Infection

A syndrome characterized by severe malaise, fatigue, mild elevation of body temperature, and other nonspecific symptoms in previously healthy young adults has been linked with persistent elevation of anti-EBV antibodies. Other laboratory data, including the erythrocyte sedimentation rate, are normal.

To date, evidence for the existence of chronic EBV infection is only inferential. Reproducibility of the serologic tests within and between laboratories has been inconsistent, and asymptomatic patients have been noted to have antibody levels within the range of those thought to have the disorder. At present, the diagnosis of chronic EBV infection is made only after exclusion of similar better-characterized illnesses. Current serologic testing is unreliable, and precise identification of the disease must await more accurate testing techniques.

Antiviral drugs have little in vitro activity against Epstein-Barr virus. Therapy for suspected chronic EBV infection is supportive and symptomatic.

## Treatment

**A. General Measures:** No specific treatment is available. The patient requires support and reassurance because of the frequent feeling of lassitude and the duration of symptoms. Symptomatic relief can be afforded by the administration of aspirin, and hot saline or 30% glucose throat irrigations or gargles 3 or 4 times daily. In severely ill patients, symptomatic relief can be obtained through a short course of corticosteroids. Diagnosis must be well established.

**B. Treatment of Complications:** Hepatitis, myocarditis, and encephalitis are treated symptomatically. Rupture of the spleen requires emergency splenectomy. Frequent vigorous palpation of the spleen is unwise.

## Prognosis

In uncomplicated cases, fever disappears in 10 days and lymphadenopathy and splenomegaly in 4 weeks. The illness sometimes lingers for 2–3 months.

Death is uncommon; when it does occur it is usually due to splenic rupture or hypersplenic phenomena (severe hemolytic anemia, thrombocytopenic purpura) or to encephalitis.

Andiman WA: Epstein-Barr virus associated syndromes. *Pediatr Infect Dis* 1984;**3**:198.

Chronic fatigue possibly related to Epstein-Barr virus: Nevada. *MMWR* 1986;**35**:350.

Jones JF et al: Evidence for active Epstein-Barr virus infection in patients with persistent unexplained illnesses: Elevated anti-early antigen antibodies. *Ann Intern Med* 1985;**102**:1.

Lymphoma in organ transplant recipients. (Editorial.) *Lancet* 1984;**1**:601.

Straus SE et al: Persistent illness and fatigue in adults with evidence of Epstein-Barr virus infection. *Ann Intern Med* 1985;**102**:7.

Sugden B: Epstein-Barr virus: A human pathogen inducing lymphoproliferation in vivo and in vitro. *Rev Infect Dis* 1982;**4**:1048.

Sumaya CV et al: Epstein-Barr virus infectious mononucleosis in children. *Pediatrics* 1985;**75**:1003.

## COXSACKIEVIRUS INFECTIONS

Coxsackievirus infections cause several clinical syndromes. As with other enteroviruses, infections are most common during the summer. Two groups, A and B, are defined by their differing behavior after injection into suckling mice. There are more than 50 serotypes.

### Clinical Findings

**A. Symptoms and Signs:** The clinical syndromes associated with coxsackievirus infection may be described briefly as follows:

**1. Summer grippe (coxsackie A and B)**–A febrile illness, principally of children, which lasts 1–4 days; minor symptoms and respiratory tract infection are often present.

**2. Herpangina (coxsackie A2, 4, 5, 6, 7, 10)**– Sudden onset of fever, which may be as high as 40.6 °C (105 °F), sometimes with febrile convulsions; headache, myalgia, vomiting; and sore throat, characterized early by petechiae or papules on the soft palate that become shallow ulcers in about 3 days and then heal.

**3. Epidemic pleurodynia (coxsackie B1, 2, 3, 4, 5)**–Sudden onset of recurrent pain in the area of diaphragmatic attachment (lower chest or upper abdomen); fever is often present during attacks of pain; headache, sore throat, malaise, nausea; tenderness, hyperesthesia, and muscle swelling of the involved area; orchitis, pleurisy, and aseptic meningitis may occur. Relapse may occur after recovery.

**4. Aseptic meningitis (coxsackie A2, 4, 7, 9, 10, 16; B viruses)**–Fever, headache, nausea, vomiting, stiff neck, drowsiness, cerebrospinal fluid lymphocytosis without chemical abnormalities; rarely, muscle paralysis. See also Viral Meningitis.

**5. Acute nonspecific pericarditis (coxsackie B types)**–Sudden onset of anterior chest pain, often worse with inspiration and in the supine position; fever, myalgia, headache; pericardial friction rub appears early; pericardial effusion with paradoxic pulse, increased venous pressure, and increase in heart size may appear; electrocardiographic and x-ray evidence of pericarditis is often present. One or more relapses may occur.

**6. Myocarditis (coxsackie B3, 4, and others)**–Heart failure in the neonatal period may be the result of myocarditis associated with infection acquired in utero. Adult heart disease may be caused by coxsackievirus group B.

**7. Hand, foot, and mouth disease**–Coxsackievirus type A16 and several other types produce an illness characterized by stomatitis and a vesicular rash on the hands and feet. This may take an epidemic form.

**B. Laboratory Findings:** Routine laboratory studies show no characteristic abnormalities. Neutralizing antibodies appear during convalescence. The virus may be isolated from throat washings or stools inoculated into suckling mice.

## Treatment & Prognosis

Treatment is symptomatic. With the exception of myocarditis, all of the syndromes caused by coxsackieviruses are benign and self-limited.

Centers for Disease Control: Enteroviral disease in the United States, 1970–79. *J Infect Dis* 1982;**146**:103.

Schiff GM: Coxsackievirus B epidemic at a boys' camp. *Am J Dis Child* 1979;**133**:782.

## ECHOVIRUS INFECTIONS

Echoviruses are enteroviruses that produce several clinical syndromes, particularly in children. Infection is most common during the summer.

Over 20 serotypes have been demonstrated. Types 4, 6, and 9 cause aseptic meningitis, which may be associated with rubelliform rash. Types 9 and 16 cause an exanthematous illness (Boston exanthem) characterized by a sudden onset of fever, nausea, and sore throat, and a rubelliform rash over the face and trunk that persists 1–10 days. Orchitis may occur. Type 18 causes epidemic diarrhea, characterized by a sudden onset of fever and diarrhea in infants. Types 18 and 20 cause common respiratory disease (see Chapter 6). Myocarditis has also been reported.

As is true of the other enterovirus infections also, the diagnosis is best established by correlation of the clinical, epidemiologic, and laboratory evidence. The virus produces cytopathic effects in tissue culture and can be recovered from the feces, throat washings, blood, and cerebrospinal fluid. A 4-fold rise in antibody titer signifies systemic infection.

Treatment is purely symptomatic. The prognosis is excellent, although occasional mild paralysis has been reported following central nervous system infection.

Jarvis WR et al: Echovirus type 7 meningitis in young children. *Am J Dis Child* 1981;**135**:1009.

## ADENOVIRUS INFECTIONS

Adenoviruses (there are more than 30 antigenic types) produce a variety of clinical syndromes. These infections are self-limited and most common among military recruits, although sporadic cases occur in civilian populations. The incubation period is 4–9 days.

There are 5 clinical types of adenovirus infection:

**(1) The common cold:** Many infections produce rhinitis, pharyngitis, and mild malaise without fever and are indistinguishable from other infections that produce the common cold syndrome.

**(2) Acute undifferentiated respiratory disease, nonstreptococcal exudative pharyngitis:** Fever lasts 2–12 days and is accompanied by malaise and myalgia. Sore throat is often manifested by diffuse injection, a patchy exudate, and cervical lymphade-nopathy. Cough is sometimes accompanied by rales and x-ray evidence of pneumonitis (primary atypical pneumonia) (especially with types 4 and 7 in military recruits). Conjunctivitis is often present.

**(3) Pharyngoconjunctival fever:** Fever and malaise, conjunctivitis (often unilateral), and mild pharyngitis.

**(4) Epidemic keratoconjunctivitis:** Unilateral conjunctival redness, mild pain, and tearing, with a large preauricular lymph node. Keratitis leads to subepithelial opacities (especially with types 8, 19, or 37).

**(5) Acute hemorrhagic cystitis in children:** (Often associated with type 11.)

Vaccines are not available for general use. Live oral vaccines containing attenuated type 4 and type 7 have been used in military personnel.

Treatment is symptomatic.

Fox JP et al: Observations of adenovirus infections. *Am J Epidemiol* 1977;**105**:362.

## RICKETTSIAL DISEASES (RICKETTSIOSES)

The rickettsioses are a group of febrile diseases caused by infection with rickettsiae. Rickettsiae, once thought to be viruses, are small obligate intracellular bacteria that are parasites of arthropods. In arthropods, rickettsiae grow in the cells lining the gut, often without harming the host. Human infection results either from the bite of the specific arthropod or from contamination with its feces. In humans, rickettsiae grow principally in endothelial cells of small blood vessels, producing vasculitis, necrosis of cells, thrombosis of vessels, skin rashes, and organ dysfunctions.

Different rickettsiae and their vectors are endemic in different parts of the world, but 2 or more types may coexist in the same geographic area. A summary of epidemiologic features is given in Table 22–3. The clinical picture is variable but usually includes a prodromal stage followed by fever, rash, and prostration. Isolation of rickettsiae from the patient is cumbersome and difficult and can be undertaken only by specialized laboratories. Laboratory diagnosis relies on the development of nonspecific antibodies to certain *Proteus* strains (Weil-Felix reaction) and of specific antibodies detected by complement fixation or immunofluorescence tests.

### Prevention & Treatment

Preventive measures are directed at control of the vector, specific immunization when available, and (occasionally) drug chemoprophylaxis. All rickettsiae can be inhibited by tetracyclines or chloramphenicol. All early clinical infections respond in some degree

**Table 22–3.** Rickettsial diseases.*

| Disease | *Rickettsia* | Geographic Area of Prevalence | Insect Vector | Mammalian Reservoir | Weil-Felix Agglutination | | |
|---|---|---|---|---|---|---|---|
| | | | | | OX19 | OX2 | OXK |
| **Typhus group** Epidemic typhus | *Rickettsia prowazekil* | South America, Africa, Asia, North America(?)† | Louse | Humans | + + | ± | − |
| Murine typhus | *Rickettsia typhi* | Worldwide; small foci | Flea | Rodents | + + | − | − |
| Scrub typhus | *Rickettsia tsutsugamushi* | Southeast Asia, Japan | Mite‡ | Rodents | − | − | + + |
| **Spotted fever group** Rocky Mountain spotted fever (RMSF) | *Rickettsia rickettsii* | Western Hemisphere | Tick‡ | Rodents, dogs | + | + | − |
| Fièvre boutonneuse Kenya tick typhus South African tick fever Indian tick typhus | *Rickettsia conorii* | Africa, India, Mediterranean countries | Tick‡ | Rodents, dogs | + | + | − |
| Queensland tick typhus | *Rickettsia australis* | Australia | Tick‡ | Rodents, marsupials | + | + | − |
| North Asian tick typhus | *Rickettsia sibirica* | Siberia, Mongolia | Tick‡ | Rodents | + | + | − |
| Rickettsialpox | *Rickettsia akari* | USA, Korea, USSR | Mite‡ | Mice | − | − | − |
| RMSF-like | *Rickettsia canada* | North America | Tick‡ | Rodents | ? | ? | − |
| **Other** Q fever | *Coxiella burnetii* | Worldwide | None§ | Cattle, sheep, goats | − | − | − |
| Trench fever | *Rochalimaea quintana* | Rare | Louse | Humans | ? | ? | ? |

* Reproduced, with permission, from Jawetz E, Melnick JL, Adelberg EA: *Review of Medical Microbiology,* 17th ed. Appleton-Lange, 1987.
† Contact with flying squirrels or their ectoparasites.
‡ Also serve as arthropod reservoir by maintaining rickettsiae through transovarian transmission.
§ Human infection results from inhalation of dust.

to treatment with these drugs. Treatment usually consists of giving either tetracycline hydrochloride or chloramphenicol, 0.5 g orally every 4–6 hours for 4–10 days (50 mg/kg daily). In seriously ill patients, initial treatment may consist of 1 g of tetracycline or chloramphenicol intravenously. Supportive measures may include parenteral fluids, sedation, oxygen, and skin care. The vector (louse, tick, mite) must be removed from patients by appropriate measures.

## EPIDEMIC LOUSE-BORNE TYPHUS

### Essentials of Diagnosis

- Prodrome of malaise and headache followed by abrupt chills and fever.
- Severe, intractable headaches, prostration, persisting high fever.
- Maculopapular rash appears on the fourth to seventh days on the trunk and in the axillas, spreading to the rest of the body but sparing the face, palms, and soles.
- Laboratory confirmation by *Proteus* OX19 agglutination and specific serologic tests.

### General Considerations

Epidemic louse-borne typhus is due to infection with *Rickettsia prowazekii,* a parasite of the body louse that ultimately kills the louse. Transmission is greatly favored by crowded living conditions, famine, war, or any circumstances that predispose to heavy infestation with lice. When the louse sucks the blood of a person infected with *R prowazekii,* the organism becomes established in the gut of the louse and grows there. When the louse is transmitted to another person (through contact or clothing) and has a blood meal, it defecates simultaneously, and the infected feces are rubbed into the itching bite wound. Dry, infectious louse feces may also enter the respiratory tract and result in human infection. A deloused and bathed typhus patient is no longer infectious for other humans.

In a person who recovers from clinical or subclinical typhus infection, *R prowazekii* may survive in lymphoid tissues for many years. Years later, such a person may have recrudescence of disease without exogenous exposure to lice or to the infectious agent. Such a recrudescence (Brill's disease) can serve as a source of infection for lice. Recently, cases of *R prowazekii* infection have occurred in the USA after contact with flying squirrels or their ectoparasites.

### Clinical Findings

**A. Symptoms and Signs:** Prodromal malaise, cough, headache, and chest pain begin after an incubation period of 10–14 days. There is then an abrupt onset of chills, high fever, and prostration, with "influenzal symptoms" progressing to delirium and stupor. The headache is intractably severe, and the fever is unremitting for many days.

Other findings consist of conjunctivitis, flushed face, rales at the lung bases, and often splenomegaly. A macular rash (that soon becomes papular) appears first in the axillas and then over the trunk, spreading to the extremities but rarely involving the face, palms, or soles. In severely ill patients, the rash becomes hemorrhagic, and hypotension becomes marked. There may be renal insufficiency, stupor, and delirium. In spontaneous recovery, improvement begins 13–16 days after onset with rapid drop of fever.

**B. Laboratory Findings:** The white blood cell count is variable. Proteinuria and hematuria commonly occur. Serum obtained 5–12 days after onset of symptoms usually shows agglutinating antibodies for *Proteus* OX19 (rarely also OX2)—*R prowazekii* shares antigens with these *Proteus* strains—and specific antibodies for *R prowazekii* antigens demonstrated by complement fixation, microagglutination, or immunofluorescence. A titer rise is most significant. In primary rickettsial infection, early antibodies are IgM; in recrudescence (Brill's disease), early antibodies are predominantly IgG, and the Weil-Felix test is negative.

**C. Imaging:** Radiographs of the chest may show patchy consolidation.

### Differential Diagnosis

The prodromal symptoms and the early febrile stage are not specific enough to permit diagnosis in nonepidemic situations. The rash is usually sufficiently distinctive for diagnosis, but it may be missing in 5–10% of cases and may be difficult to observe in dark-skinned persons. A variety of other acute febrile diseases may have to be considered.

Brill's disease (recrudescent epidemic typhus) has a more gradual onset than primary *R prowazekii* infection, fever and rash are of shorter duration, and the disease is milder and rarely fatal.

### Complications

Pneumonia, vasculitis with major vessel obstruction and gangrene, circulatory collapse, myocarditis, and uremia may occur.

### Prevention

Prevention consists of louse control with insecticides, particularly by applying chemicals to clothing or treating it with heat, and frequent bathing. Immunization with vaccines consisting of inactivated egg-grown *R prowazekii* gives some protection against severe disease, although the efficacy is limited. This vaccine is not available in the USA or Canada in 1985. An improved cell culture vaccine is being developed. Live attenuated (strain E) vaccine is under investigation.

### Treatment

See p 852.

### Prognosis

The prognosis depends greatly upon age and immunization status. In children under age 10, the disease is usually mild. The mortality rate is 10% in the second and third decades but may reach 60% in the sixth decade. Effective vaccination can convert a potentially serious disease into a relatively mild one.

Duma RJ et al: Epidemic typhus in the United States associated with flying squirrels. *JAMA* 1981;**245**:2318.

Ormsbee R et al: Serologic diagnosis of epidemic typhus fever. *Am J Epidemiol* 1977;**105**:261.

Philip RN et al: Immunofluorescence test for the serologic study of Rocky Mountain spotted fever and typhus. *J Clin Microbiol* 1976;**3**:51.

### ENDEMIC FLEA-BORNE TYPHUS (Murine Typhus)

*Rickettsia typhi* (*R mooseri*) is transmitted from rat to rat through the rat flea (rarely, the rat louse). Humans acquire the infection when bitten by an infected flea, which releases infected feces while sucking blood.

Flea typhus resembles Brill's disease (recrudescent epidemic typhus) in that it has a gradual onset and the fever and rash are of shorter duration (6–13 days) and the symptoms less severe than in louse-borne typhus. The rash is maculopapular, concentrated on the trunk, and fades fairly rapidly. Even without antibiotic treatment, flea typhus is a mild disease. Pneumonia or gangrene is rare. Fatalities are rare and limited to the elderly.

Complement-fixing or immunofluorescent antibodies can be detected in the patient's serum with specific *R typhi* antigens. There is a rising titer of agglutinating antibodies to *Proteus* OX19.

Preventive measures are directed at control of rats and their ectoparasites. Insecticides are first applied to rat runs, nests, and colonies, and the rats are then poisoned or trapped. Finally, buildings must be made ratproof. Antibiotic treatment need not be intensive because of the mildness of the natural disease. An experimental vaccine was fairly effective, but it is not commercially available now.

### SPOTTED FEVERS (Tick Typhus)

Tick-borne rickettsial infections occur in many different regions of the world and have been given regional or local names, eg, Rocky Mountain spotted fever in North America, Queensland tick typhus in Australia, boutonneuse fever in North Africa, Kenya tick typhus, etc. The causative agents are all antigenically related to *Rickettsia rickettsii,* and all are transmitted by hard (ixodid) ticks and have cycles in nature that involve dogs, rodents, or other animals. Rickettsiae are often transmitted from one generation of ticks to the next (transovarian transmission) without passage through a vertebrate host. Patients infected with spotted fevers usually develop antibodies to *Proteus* OX19 and OX2 in low titer, in addition to specific rickettsial antibodies, detected best by immunofluorescence, microagglutination, or complement fixation.

Control of spotted fevers involves prevention of tick bites, specific immunization when available, and antibiotic treatment of patients.

## 1. ROCKY MOUNTAIN SPOTTED FEVER

### Essentials of Diagnosis

- Exposure to tick bite in endemic area.
- "Influenzal" prodrome followed by chills, fever, severe headache, widespread aches and pains, restlessness, and prostration; occasionally, delirium and coma.
- Red macular rash appears between the second and sixth days of fever, first on the wrists and ankles and then spreading centrally; it may become petechial.
- Laboratory confirmation by agglutination of *Proteus* OX19 and OX2 and by specific antibodies with complement fixation and immunofluorescence.

### General Considerations

The causative agent, *Rickettsia rickettsii,* is transmitted to humans by the bite of the wood tick, *Dermacentor andersoni,* in the western USA and by the bite of the dog tick, *Dermacentor variabilis,* in the eastern USA. Other hard ticks transmit the rickettsia in the southern USA and in Central and South America and are responsible for transmitting it among rodents, dogs, porcupines, and other animals. Most human cases occur in late spring and summer. In the USA, most cases occur in the eastern third of the country.

### Clinical Findings

**A. Symptoms and Signs:** Three to 10 days after the bite of an infectious tick, anorexia, malaise, nausea, headache, and sore throat occur. These progress, with chills, fever, myalgia, aches in bones, joints, and muscles, abdominal pain, nausea and vomiting, restlessness, insomnia, and irritability. Cough and pneumonitis may develop. Delirium, lethargy, stupor, and coma may appear. The face is flushed and the conjunctivas infected. Between days 2 and 6 of fever, a rash appears first on the wrists and ankles, spreading centrally to the arms, legs, and trunk. The rash is initially small, red, and macular but becomes larger and petechial. It spreads for 2–3 days. In some cases there is splenomegaly, hepatomegaly, jaundice, gangrene, myocarditis, or uremia.

**B. Laboratory Findings:** Leukocytosis, proteinuria, and hematuria are common. Rickettsiae can sometimes be isolated in special laboratories from blood obtained in the first few days of illness. A rise in antibody titer during the second week of illness can be detected by specific complement fixation, immunofluorescence, and microagglutination tests or by the Weil-Felix reaction with *Proteus* OX19 and OX2. Antibody response may be suppressed if antimicrobial drugs are given very early.

### Differential Diagnosis

The early signs and symptoms of Rocky Mountain spotted fever are shared with many other infections. The rash may be confused with that of measles, typhoid, or meningococcemia. The suspicion of the latter requires blood cultures and cerebrospinal fluid examination.

### Prevention

Protective clothing, tick-repellent chemicals, and the removal of ticks at frequent intervals are helpful. Vaccines of inactivated *R rickettsii* grown in eggs or in cell culture have given moderate protection but are not commercially available in the USA or Canada in 1985.

### Treatment & Prognosis

In mild, untreated cases, fever subsides at the end of the second week. The response to chloramphenicol or tetracycline (see Chapter 28) is prompt if the drugs are started early.

The mortality rate for Rocky Mountain spotted fever varies strikingly with age. In untreated elderly persons it may be 70%; in children, less than 20%.

Donohue JF: Lower respiratory involvement in Rocky Mountain spotted fever. *Arch Intern Med* 1980;**140**:223.

Melnick CG et al: Rocky Mountain spotted fever: Clinical, laboratory and epidemiologic features in 262 cases. *J Infect Dis* 1984;**150**:480.

Walker DH et al: Rocky Mountain spotted fever mimicking acute cholecystitis. *Arch Intern Med* 1985;**145**:2195.

Woodward TE: Rocky Mountain Spotted Fever: Epidemiological and early clinical signs are keys to treatment and reduced mortality. *J Infect Dis* 1984;**150**:465

## 2. OTHER SPOTTED FEVERS

Tick-borne rickettsial infections in Africa, Asia, and Australia may resemble Rocky Mountain spotted fever but cover a wide spectrum from very mild to very severe. In many cases, a local lesion develops at the site of the tick bite (eschar), often with painful enlargement of the regional lymph nodes.

### RICKETTSIALPOX

*Rickettsia akari* is a parasite of mice, transmitted by mites (*Allodermanyssus sanguineus*). Upon close contact of mice with humans, infected mites may transmit the disease to humans. Rickettsialpox has an incubation period of 7–12 days. The onset is sudden, with chills, fever, headache, photophobia, and disseminated aches and pains. The primary lesion is a red papule that vesicates and forms a black eschar. Two to 4 days after onset of symptoms, a widespread papular eruption appears that becomes vesicular and forms crusts that are shed in about 10 days. Early lesions may resemble those of chickenpox.

Leukopenia and a rise in antibody titer with rickettsial antigen in complement fixation tests are often present. However, the Weil-Felix test is negative.

Treatment with tetracycline produces rapid improvement, but even without treatment the disease is fairly mild and self-limited. Control requires the elimination of mice from human habitations after insecticide has been applied to suppress the mite vectors.

Brettman LR et al: Rickettsialpox: Report of an outbreak and contemporary review. *South Afr Med J* 1981;**60:**363.

Wong B et al: Rickettsialpox: Case report and epidemiologic review. *JAMA* 1979;**242:**1998.

## SCRUB TYPHUS
## (Tsutsugamushi Disease)

### Essentials of Diagnosis

- Exposure to mites in endemic area of Southeast Asia, the western Pacific, and Australia.
- Black eschar at site of bite, with regional and generalized lymphadenopathy.
- Conjunctivitis and a short-lived macular rash.
- Frequent pneumonitis, encephalitis, and cardiac failure.
- Laboratory confirmation with agglutinins to *Proteus* OXK and specific antibodies by immunofluorescence.

### General Considerations

Scrub typhus is caused by *Rickettsia tsutsugamushi* (*R orientalis*), which is principally a parasite of rodents transmitted by mites. The infectious agent can be transmitted from one generation of mites to the next (transovarian transmission) without a vertebrate host. The mites may spend much of their life cycle on vegetation but require a blood meal to complete maturation. At that point, humans coming in contact with infested vegetation are bitten by mite larvae and are infected.

### Clinical Findings

**A. Symptoms and Signs:** After an incubation period of 1–3 weeks, there is a nonspecific prodrome, with malaise, chills, severe headache, and backache. At the site of the mite bite a papule develops that vesicates and forms a flat black eschar. The regional lymph nodes are enlarged and tender, and there may be generalized adenopathy. Fever rises gradually, and a generalized macular rash appears at the end of the

first week of fever. The rash is most marked on the trunk and may be fleeting or may last for a week. The patient appears obtunded, confused, and out of contact with the environment. During the second or third week, pneumonitis, myocarditis, and cardiac failure may develop.

**B. Laboratory Findings:** Blood obtained during the first few days of illness may permit isolation of the rickettsia by mouse inoculation in specialized laboratories. The Weil-Felix test usually shows a rising titer to *Proteus* OXK during the second week of illness. The complement fixation test is often unsatisfactory, but immunofluorescence with specific antigens is diagnostic.

### Differential Diagnosis

Leptospirosis, typhoid, dengue, malaria, and other rickettsial infections may have to be considered. When the rash is fleeting and the eschar not evident, laboratory results are the best guide to diagnosis.

### Prevention

Efforts must be made in endemic areas to minimize contact between humans and infected mites. Repeated application of long-acting miticides can make endemic areas safe. When this is not possible, insect repellents on clothing and skin provide some protection. For short exposure, chemoprophylaxis with chloramphenicol can prevent the disease but permits infection. No effective vaccines are available at present.

### Treatment & Prognosis

Without treatment, fever may subside spontaneously after 2 weeks, but the mortality rate may be 10–30%. Early treatment with chloramphenicol or tetracyclines can virtually eliminate deaths.

### TRENCH FEVER

Trench fever is a self-limited, louse-borne relapsing febrile disease caused by *Rochalimaea* (*Rickettsia*) *quintana*. This organism grows extracellularly in the louse intestine and is excreted in feces. Humans are infected when infected louse feces enter defects in skin. No animal reservoir except humans has been demonstrated.

This disease has occurred in epidemic forms in louse-infested troops and civilians during wars, and in endemic form in Central America. Onset is abrupt, with fever lasting 3–5 days, often followed by relapses. The patient becomes weak and complains of severe pain behind the eyes and in the back and legs. Lymphadenopathy and splenomegaly may appear, as well as a transient maculopapular rash. Subclinical infection is frequent, and a carrier state may occur. The differential diagnosis includes dengue, leptospirosis, malaria, relapsing fever, and typhus fever.

*R quintana* is the only rickettsia that has been grown on artificial media without living cells. The organism can be cultivated on agar containing 10%

fresh blood and has been recovered from blood cultures of patients. In volunteers, such agar-grown rickettsiae caused typical disease. The Weil-Felix test is negative, but a specific complement fixation test and a specific enzyme immunoassay are available.

The illness is self-limited, and recovery regularly occurs without treatment.

Hollingdale MR et al: Enzyme immunoassay of antibody to *Rochalimaea quintana. J Infect Dis* 1978;**137**:578.

## Q FEVER

### Essentials of Diagnosis

- An acute or chronic febrile illness with severe headache, cough, prostration, and abdominal pain.
- Extensive pneumonitis, hepatitis, or encephalopathy; rarely endocarditis.

### General Considerations

*Coxiella burnetii* is unique among rickettsiae in that it is usually transmitted to humans not by arthropods but by inhalation of infectious aerosols or ingestion of infected milk. It is a parasite of cattle, sheep, and goats, in which it produces mild or subclinical infection. It is excreted by cows and goats principally through the milk and placenta and by sheep through feces, placenta, and milk. Dry feces and milk, dust contaminated with them, and the tissues of these animals contain large numbers of infectious organisms that are spread by the airborne route. Inhalation of contaminated dust and of droplets from infected animal tissues is the main source of human infection. There is an occupational risk for animal handlers, slaughterhouse workers, veterinarians, etc. *Coxiella* is resistant to heat and drying, perhaps because the organism forms endosporelike structures. Thus, it survives in dust, on the fleece of infected animals, or in inadequately pasteurized milk. Spread from one human to another does not seem to occur even in the presence of florid pneumonitis, but fetal infection can occur.

### Clinical Findings

**A. Symptoms and Signs:** After an incubation period of 1–3 weeks, a febrile illness develops with headache, prostration, and muscle pains, occasionally with a nonproductive cough, abdominal pains, or jaundice. Physical signs of pneumonitis are slight. Hepatitis may be severe. Endocarditis occurs

rarely, but must always be considered in cases of culture-negative endocarditis with a suggestive epidemiologic background. At times, signs of encephalopathy are present. The clinical course may be acute or chronic and relapsing.

**B. Laboratory Findings:** Laboratory examination often shows leukopenia and a diagnostic rise in specific complement-fixing antibodies to *Coxiella* phase 2. The Weil-Felix test is negative. Liver function tests are often abnormal. In Q fever endocarditis, there is a titer of 1:200 or more by complement fixation or immunofluorescence with phase I antigen of *C burnetii*. Isolation of the organism from blood or sputum is rarely attempted.

**C. Imaging:** Radiographs of the chest show variable pulmonary infiltration.

### Differential Diagnosis

Viral, mycoplasmal, and bacterial pneumonias; viral hepatitis; brucellosis; tuberculosis; psittacosis; and other animal-borne diseases must be considered. The history of exposure to animals or animal dusts or animal tissues (eg, in slaughterhouses) should lead to appropriate specific serologic tests.

### Prevention

Prevention must be based on detection of the infection in livestock, reduction of contact with infected animals or dusts contaminated by them, special care during contact with animal tissues, and effective pasteurization of milk. A vaccine of formalin-inactivated phase 1 *Coxiella* is being developed for persons at high risk of infection and appears to be protective.

### Treatment & Prognosis

Treatment with tetracyclines can suppress symptoms and shorten the clinical course but does not always eradicate the infection. Even in untreated patients, the mortality rate is usually low, except with endocarditis.

Haldane EV et al: Endocarditis due to Q fever in Nova Scotia. *J Infect Dis* 1983;**148**:978.

Janigan DT et al: An inflammatory pseudotumor of the lung in Q fever pneumonia. *N Engl J Med* 1983;**308**:86.

Marmion BP et al: Vaccine prophylaxis of abattoir-associated Q fever. *Lancet* 1984;**2**:1411.

Meiklejohn G et al: Cryptic epidemic of Q fever in a medical school. *J Infect Dis* 1981;**144**:107.

Raoult D et al: Q fever endocarditis in the South of France. *J Infect Dis* 1987;**155**:570.

Tobin MJ et al: Q fever endocarditis. *Am J Med* 1982;**72**:396.

# 23

# Infectious Diseases: Bacterial

*Moses Grossman, MD, & Ernest Jawetz, MD, PhD*

## STREPTOCOCCAL SORE THROAT; STREPTOCOCCAL SKIN INFECTIONS

### Essentials of Diagnosis

- Abrupt onset of sore throat, fever, malaise, nausea, and headache.
- Throat red and edematous, with or without exudate; cervical nodes tender.
- Presence of scarlatiniform rash or pyoderma or erysipelas.
- Diagnosis confirmed by leukocytosis, throat or skin culture, and rise in antibody titer.

### General Considerations

Beta-hemolytic group A streptococci are the most common bacterial cause of exudative pharyngitis, and they also cause skin infections. Respiratory infections are transmitted by droplets; skin infections are transmitted by contact. Either may be followed by suppurative and nonsuppurative (rheumatic fever, glomerulonephritis) complications. If group A streptococci produce erythrogenic toxin, they may cause scarlet fever rashes in susceptible persons.

Beta-hemolytic group B streptococci are often carried in the female genital tract and thus may infect the newborn. Group B streptococci are a common cause of neonatal sepsis, meningitis, and pneumonia.

### Clinical Findings

**A. Symptoms and Signs:**

**1. Streptococcal sore throat**–"Strep throat" is characterized by a sudden onset of fever, sore throat, severe pain on swallowing, enlarged and tender cervical lymph nodes, malaise, and nausea. Children may vomit or convulse. The pharynx, soft palate, and tonsils are red and edematous, and there may be a purulent exudate. If scarlet fever rash occurs, the skin is diffusely erythematous, with superimposed fine red papules. The rash is most intense in the groin and axillas, blanches on pressure, and may become petechial. It fades in 2–5 days, leaving a fine desquamation. In scarlet fever, the face is flushed, with circumoral pallor; and the tongue is coated, with enlarged red papillae (strawberry tongue).

**2. Streptococcal skin lesions**–Impetigo begins as a papule that rapidly becomes a vesicle and a pustule with a thick, amber-colored crust. There is little redness, and the crusts appear "stuck on" the skin. Pyoderma is often chronic but produces little discomfort. It may become progressive in hot, humid climates.

Streptococci may enter the skin and subcutaneous tissues through abrasions or wounds and may produce progressive erysipelas (fever, chills, rapidly progressive edema and erythema, with a sharp advancing margin) or "surgical scarlet fever"—ie, wound infection with streptococci that produce erythrogenic toxin in a patient without antitoxin, who then develops signs of scarlet fever.

**3. Neonatal group B streptococcal infections**–Group B streptococci are often part of the normal vaginal flora and thus may infect the newborn, particularly if the mother lacks specific antibody. Group B streptococcal infection during the first month of life may present as fulminant sepsis, meningitis, or respiratory distress syndrome. Group B streptococci may be inhibited but not killed by penicillin, and such "tolerance" may prevent their eradication from the mother or infant.

**B. Laboratory Findings:** Leukocytosis with an increase in polymorphonuclear neutrophils is a regular early finding. The presence of large numbers of group A streptococci in throat, wound, or skin lesions can be detected by culture (and bacitracin disk inhibition) or by the more rapid antigen detection tests. The urine often contains protein and red cells. In 1–3 weeks after onset of infection, there is a rise in antibodies, particularly to streptolysin O, hyaluronidase, streptokinase, deoxyribonuclease, and other streptococcal antigenic products. Elevated antibody levels may continue for months after the infection. In pyoderma, antihyaluronidase is the most commonly elevated antibody; in streptococcal pharyngitis, it is antistreptolysin O (ASO). Group B streptococcal infections in newborns are identified by culture of blood, cerebrospinal fluid, or respiratory tract specimens; latex agglutination can identify the antigen.

### Complications

The suppurative complications of streptococcal sore throat include sinusitis, otitis media, mastoiditis, peritonsillar abscess, and suppuration of cervical lymph nodes, among others. Streptococcal skin infections (erysipelas; see Chapter 4) may lead to bacteremia and sepsis.

The outstanding nonsuppurative complications are rheumatic fever (0.05–3%) and glomerulonephritis (0.2–20%). Rheumatic fever may follow recurrent infections with any type of group A streptococci and begins 1–4 weeks after the onset of streptococcal sore throat. Glomerulonephritis follows a single infection with a nephritogenic strain of *Streptococcus* group

A (eg, types 4, 12, 2, 49, and 60), more commonly on the skin than in the throat, and begins 1–3 weeks after the onset of the infection.

## Differential Diagnosis

Streptococcal sore throat resembles (and cannot be reliably distinguished clinically from) the pharyngitis caused by adenoviruses; herpesviruses; and other agents, including gonococci. It may be confused with infectious mononucleosis, with generalized adenopathy, splenomegaly, atypical lymphocytes, and a positive serologic (Monospot) test; diphtheria, characterized by a more confluent pseudomembrane; candidiasis, which shows white patches of exudate and less erythema; and necrotizing ulcerative gingivostomatitis (Vincent's fusospirochetal disease), with shallow ulcers in the mouth. The petechial rash of scarlet fever must be distinguished from that of meningococcemia; the typical scarlet fever rash resembles the rash of sunburn, drug reactions, rubella, echovirus infections, and toxic shock syndrome.

## Prevention

Benzathine penicillin G, 1.2 million units as a single intramuscular injection every 4 weeks, is the method of choice to prevent reinfection with group A streptococci in persons who have suffered an initial attack of rheumatic fever. Prophylaxis with sulfadiazine, 1 g orally daily, or penicillin G, 200,000–400,000 units orally daily, is also acceptable but offers less reliable prophylaxis against rheumatic fever recurrences than benzathine penicillin G given intramuscularly. These regimens are administered continuously for 5 or more years.

There is no definite prophylaxis against glomerulonephritis except the very early eradication of nephritogenic streptococci, especially in contacts.

Neonatal group B streptococcal disease can be prevented by intrapartum intravenous ampicillin administration to mothers with positive prenatal vaginal cultures.

## Treatment

**A. Specific Measures:** Antimicrobial treatment is often given without proof of streptococcal origin if fever and leukocytosis accompany a sore throat with tender cervical adenopathy.

1. Benzathine penicillin G, 1.2 million units intramuscularly as a single dose, is optimal therapy and usually eradicates the streptococci.

2. Penicillin V, 400,000 units orally 3 times daily, must be taken for 10 days, and this regimen is not easily enforced, since the patient becomes asymptomatic in 2–4 days. Penicillin lozenges are worthless. Topical treatment of skin infections is undesirable.

3. Patients hypersensitive to penicillin may be treated with erythromycin, 0.5 g 4 times daily (40 mg/kg/d) for 10 days.

**B. General Measures:** Aspirin and gargling with warm saline solution relieves sore throat. Bed rest is desirable until the patient is afebrile. Diet may be modified to reduce discomfort, and fluids may be forced during fever.

**C. Treatment of Complications:** The suppurative complications usually respond promptly to antistreptococcal treatment, and incision and drainage of abscesses is rarely needed. Rheumatic fever is best prevented by prompt treatment of severe streptococcal infections. Its treatment is discussed in Chapter 8.

The treatment of glomerulonephritis is discussed in Chapter 15.

## Prognosis

Most streptococcal infections are self-limited. Severe illness or death is rare today except in untreated streptococcal pneumonia or sepsis. Treatment with antimicrobials shortens the course of sore throat, fever, and systemic symptoms to some extent. If adequate penicillin or erythromycin levels are maintained for 10 days, group A streptococci will be eliminated. This can prevent rheumatic fever if treatment is started during the first week after infection. In the USA, rheumatic fever now follows only 0.05% of group A streptococcal infections even without antistreptococcal treatment, perhaps because "rheumatologic streptococci" that share antigens with heart tissues are now rare. Glomerulonephritis can sometimes be prevented if antistreptococcal drugs are given on epidemiologic grounds, ie, before onset of renal signs or symptoms in contacts of patients infected with nephritogenic strains. The mortality rate is high in newborns with group B streptococcal infection, and relapses occur after penicillin treatment.

Boyer KM, Gotoff SP: Prevention of neonatal group B streptococcal disease with selective intrapartum chemoprophylaxis. *N Engl J Med* 1986;**314:**1665.

Pass MA, Gray BM, Dillon HC: Puerperal and perinatal infections with group B streptococci. *Am J Obstet Gynecol* 1982;**143:**147.

Randolph MF et al: Effect of antibiotic therapy on the clinical course of streptococcal pharyngitis. *J Pediatr* 1985;**106:**870.

Wannamaker LW: Changes and changing concepts in the biology of group A streptococci and in the epidemiology of streptococcal infections. *Rev Infect Dis* 1979;**1:**967.

## STAPHYLOCOCCAL TOXIC SHOCK SYNDROME

Staphylococci cause many soft tissue and organ system infections. Some strains of staphylococci elaborate toxins that can cause 3 important entities: "scalded skin syndrome" in children, toxic shock syndrome in adults, and enterotoxin food poisoning (see p 867). Toxic shock syndrome is characterized by abrupt onset of high fever, vomiting, and watery diarrhea. Sore throat, myalgias, and headache are often complaints. Hypotensive shock with renal and cardiac failure are ominous manifestations in severe cases. A diffuse macular erythematous rash and nonpurulent conjunctivitis are common, and desquamation, especially of palms and soles, is typical as the victim recovers. Reported fatality rates vary and may be as high as 15%. Although toxic shock syndrome has occurred in children 8–17 years old and in males, the great majority of cases (90% or more) have been reported in women of childbearing age. Of these, 95% have begun within 5 days of the onset of a menstrual period in women who have used tampons. If a woman recovers from the syndrome, she should stop using tampons. Outbreaks have also developed in surgical patients.

*Staphylococcus aureus* has been isolated from various sites, including the nasopharynx, vagina, or rectum or from wounds, but blood cultures are negative. It is probable that toxic shock syndrome is caused by a toxin produced by some strains of staphylococci, now called toxic shock syndrome toxin (TSST 1) and apparently identical with enterotoxin F and exotoxin C.

Important aspects of treatment include rapid rehydration, antistaphylococcal drugs, and management of renal or cardiac insufficiency.

Bartlett P et al: Toxic shock syndrome associated with surgical wound infections. *JAMA* 1982;**247**:1448.
Hirsch ML, Kass EH: An annotated bibliography of toxic shock syndrome. *Rev Infect Dis* 1986;**8(Suppl 1)**:1.
Schlech WF et al: Risk factors for development of toxic shock syndrome. *JAMA* 1982;**248**:835.

# DIPHTHERIA

## Essentials of Diagnosis

- Tenacious gray membrane at portal of entry.
- Sore throat, nasal discharge, hoarseness, malaise, fever.
- Myocarditis, neuritis.
- Smear and culture confirm the diagnosis.

## General Considerations

Diphtheria is an acute infection, caused by *Corynebacterium diphtheriae*, that usually attacks the respiratory tract but may involve any mucous membrane or skin wound. The organism usually gains entry through the respiratory tract and is spread chiefly by respiratory secretions from patients with active disease or healthy carriers. The incubation period is 2–7 days. Myocarditis and late neuritis caused by an exotoxin are also characteristic.

## Clinical Findings

### A. Symptoms and Signs:

**1. Pharyngeal diphtheria**–Characteristically, a tenacious gray membrane forms on the tonsil and pharyngeal walls, surrounded by a narrow zone of erythema and a wider zone of edema. Early manifestations are mild sore throat, fever, and malaise, followed rapidly by severe signs of toxemia and prostration. Edema of the pharynx may add to the difficulty of breathing and swallowing.

If myocarditis develops, there is a rapid thready pulse along with indistinct heart sounds, cardiac arrhythmia, and, finally, cardiac decompensation with falling blood pressure, hepatic congestion, and associated nausea and vomiting.

In toxic neuritis the cranial nerves are involved first, causing nasal speech, regurgitation of food through the nose, diplopia, strabismus, and inability to swallow, resulting in pooling of saliva and respiratory secretions. The neuritis may progress to involve the intercostal muscles and those of the extremities. Sensory manifestations are much less prominent than motor weakness.

**2. Nasal diphtheria**–An occasional case will be limited to nasal infection only, producing a serosanguineous discharge but few constitutional symptoms.

**3. Laryngeal diphtheria**–This may occur as an extension of pharyngeal disease or separately. The signs and symptoms are those of upper airway obstruction in a progressively more toxic patient.

**4. Cutaneous diphtheria**–More common in tropical countries; lesions resemble impetigo.

### B. Laboratory Findings:
Polymorphonuclear leukocytosis may be present. Bacterial culture will confirm the diagnosis. Throat smears are often unreliable. Albuminocytologic dissociation of the cerebrospinal fluid is noted in postdiphtheritic neuritis. Proteinuria as a result of toxic nephritis is not uncommon.

### C. Electrocardiographic Findings:
In myocarditis, the ECG may show an arrhythmia, PR prolongation, heart block, and inversion of T waves.

## Differential Diagnosis

Diphtheria must be differentiated from streptococcal pharyngitis, infectious mononucleosis, adenovirus or herpes simplex infection, Vincent's infection, and candidiasis. A presumptive diagnosis of diphtheria must be made on clinical grounds without waiting for laboratory verification, since emergency treatment is needed.

## Complications

The most common and most serious complications are myocarditis and toxic neuritis, the latter often producing paralysis of the soft palate and external muscles of the eyes as well as limb muscles.

## Prevention

Active immunization with diphtheria toxoid is part of routine childhood immunization (usually as DTP) with appropriate booster injections.

Adults should continue to receive booster injections every 10 years following childhood immunization. In order to avoid major reactions, only the "adult type" toxoid (Td) should be used.

Susceptibility to diphtheria can be determined by intradermal injection of 0.1 mL of a solution containing a standard amount of diphtheria toxin (Schick test).

Exposed susceptibles should receive a booster dose of toxoid (start active immunization if not previously immune), full doses of erythromycin or penicillin, and daily throat inspections.

## Treatment

### A. Specific Measures:

**1. Diphtheria antitoxin**–Antitoxin must be given in all cases when diphtheria cannot be ruled out. The intravenous route is preferable in all but patients who are sensitive to horse serum. Conjunctival and skin tests for serum sensitivity should be done in all cases and desensitization carried out if necessary.

The dose of antitoxin is purely empiric: for mild early pharyngeal or laryngeal disease, 20–40 thousand units; for moderate nasopharyngeal disease, 40–60 thousand units; for severe, extensive, or late (3 days or more) disease, 80–100 thousand units. Diphtheria equine antitoxin can be obtained from the Centers for Disease Control.

**2. Antimicrobial therapy**–Antibiotics are a useful adjunct to antitoxin, suppressing *C diphtheriae* and eliminating hemolytic streptococci, which are frequent secondary invaders. Penicillin and erythromycin are equally effective if given for 7–10 days.

**3. Corticosteroids**–Corticosteroids may be appropriate in 2 situations: (a) to diminish edema or obstruction in laryngeal diphtheria; and (b) to reduce the severity or incidence of acute myocarditis.

**B. General Measures:** The patient should remain at absolute bed rest for at least 3 weeks until the danger of developing myocarditis has passed.

Give a liquid to soft diet as tolerated, hot saline or 30% glucose throat irrigations 3–4 times daily, and aspirin or codeine as required for relief of pain.

### C. Treatment of Complications:

**1. Myocarditis**–No definitive treatment is known. Oxygen by tent or mask may be needed. Hypertonic glucose solution, 100 mL of 20% solution daily, may be of value. Digitalis and quinidine should be reserved for arrhythmias with rapid ventricular rate. It may be necessary to treat for shock (see Chapter 1).

**2. Neuritis**–Nasal feeding should be attempted if paralysis of deglutition is present. Tracheostomy and the use of a mechanical respirator may be necessary. Corrective splinting and physical therapy may be of value.

**3. Respiratory tract obstruction**–Croupy cough, stridor, and dyspnea suggest laryngeal obstruction. Suction of membrane and secretions under direct laryngoscopy may help. Intubation or tracheostomy should be performed before cyanosis appears.

**4. Skin infection**–A chronic skin ulceration due to *C diphtheriae* is particularly apt to occur in warm, humid climates and can be followed by myocarditis and neuritis. Treatment is as for pharyngeal disease.

**D. Treatment of Carriers:** Eradication of organisms from a carrier is difficult. Erythromycin followed by a course of penicillin may be successful. Tonsillectomy is a last resort.

## Prognosis

The mortality rate varies between 10 and 30%; it is higher in older people and when treatment has been delayed. Myocarditis that appears early is often fatal. A conduction disturbance or the appearance of an arrhythmia implies a poor prognosis. Neuritis is rarely fatal unless respiratory muscle paralysis occurs. Myocarditis and neuritis will subside slowly but completely if the patient survives.

Dobie RA, Tobey DN: Clinical features of diphtheria in the respiratory tract. *JAMA* 1979;**242**:2197.

Hodes HL: Diphtheria. *Pediatr Clin North Am* 1979;**26**:445.

# PERTUSSIS
# (Whooping Cough)

## Essentials of Diagnosis

- Paroxysmal cough ending in a high-pitched inspiratory "whoop."
- Two-week prodromal catarrhal stage of malaise, cough, coryza, and anorexia.
- Predominantly in infants under age 2 years.
- Absolute lymphocytosis.
- Culture confirms diagnosis.

## General Considerations

Pertussis is an acute infection of the respiratory tract caused by *Bordetella* (*Haemophilus*) *pertussis*. It is transmitted by respiratory droplets from infected individuals, now often adults with mild illness. The incubation period is 7–17 days. Infectivity is greatest early in the disease and decreases until the organisms disappear from the nasopharynx (after about 1 month). Infants are most commonly infected; half of all cases occur before age 2 years.

## Clinical Findings

**A. Symptoms and Signs:** Physical findings are minimal or absent. Fever, if present, is low-grade. The symptoms of classic pertussis last about 6 weeks and are divided into 3 consecutive stages.

**1. Catarrhal stage**–The onset is insidious, with lacrimation, sneezing, and coryza, anorexia and malaise, and a hacking night cough that tends to become diurnal.

**2. Paroxysmal stage**–This follows the beginning of the catarrhal stage by 10–14 days and is characterized by rapid consecutive coughs usually followed by a deep, hurried, high-pitched inspiration (whoop). Paroxysms may involve 5–15 coughs before a breath is taken and may occur up to 50 times in 24 hours. Stimuli such as fright or anger, crying, sneezing, inhalation of irritants, and overdistention of the stomach may produce the paroxysms. The cough is productive of copious amounts of thick mucus. Vomiting is common during the paroxysms.

**3. Convalescent stage**–This stage usually begins 4 weeks after the onset of the illness with a decrease in the frequency and severity of paroxysms of cough.

**B. Laboratory Findings:** The white count is usually 15–20 thousand/$\mu$L (rarely, to 50,000), 60–80% lymphocytes. The clinical diagnosis can be confirmed by taking the culture with a nasopharyngeal wire swab and planting it on fresh special media. A specific immunofluorescent stain of the nasopharyngeal swab dried onto a slide may aid in the diagnosis. The organism is recovered in only about half of clinically diagnosed patients.

### Differential Diagnosis

Several types of adenovirus and *Haemophilus* can produce a clinical picture essentially indistinguishable from that caused by *B pertussis*. Respiratory chlamydial infections may produce a syndrome resembling pertussis in infants under age 4 months. *B pertussis* infection may resemble viral pneumonia, influenza, or acute bronchitis in older persons. The lymphocytosis may suggest acute leukemia.

### Complications

Asphyxia, the most common complication, occurs most frequently in infants and may lead to convulsions and brain damage. The increased intracranial pressure during a paroxysm may also lead to brain damage by causing cerebral hemorrhage. Pneumonia, atelectasis, interstitial and subcutaneous emphysema, and pneumothorax may occur as a result of damaged respiratory mucosa, inspissated mucus, or increased intrathoracic pressure.

### Prevention

Active immunization with pertussis vaccine is recommended for all infants, usually combined with diphtheria and tetanus toxoids (DTP). The newborn derives little or no immunity from the mother. Because of the mildness of the disease in older individuals, neither primary nor booster immunization is recommended after age 6 years. Occasionally, neurologic disturbances may occur after DTP injection. Such rare individuals should subsequently receive DT immunization without the pertussis component (see Chapter 21).

Infants and susceptible adults with significant exposure to pertussis should receive prophylaxis with erythromycin (40 mg/kg/d). Those previously immunized should receive a booster dose of vaccine.

### Treatment

**A. Specific Measures:**

**1. Antibiotics**—Give erythromycin, 50 mg/kg daily orally for 10 days. Erythromycin may shorten the course of carriage. Antibiotics are of doubtful value at the paroxysmal coughing stage.

**2. Corticosteroids**—In severe pertussis, corticosteroids given for 4–6 days may diminish the intensity of paroxysms.

**B. General Measures:**

**1. Nutrition**—Frequent small feedings may be

necessary. Feeding can be repeated if vomiting occurs shortly after a meal. Parenteral fluids may be used to ensure adequate fluid intake in severe cases.

**2. Cough**—Sedative and expectorant cough mixtures are of only slight benefit.

**3. Nursing care**—In very young infants, a paroxysm will often terminate with an apneic spell instead of a whoop. Careful observation, skilled nursing care, cardiorespiratory monitoring for apnea, and avoidance of stimuli that trigger paroxysms are most important in the young infant.

**C. Treatment of Complications:** Pneumonia, usually due to secondary invaders, should be treated with erythromycin, ampicillin, or other appropriate antibiotic, depending upon specific bacteriologic diagnosis. Oxygen is often required.

Convulsions may require 100% oxygen inhalation, lumbar puncture, and anticonvulsive medication.

### Prognosis

In children under age 1 year, the mortality rate until recently was over 20%; this rate has been reduced to 1–2% with antibacterial therapy. Bronchiectasis is a fairly common sequela, and brain damage may result.

Bass JW: Pertussis: Current status of prevention and treatment. *Pediatr Infect Dis* 1985;**4**:614.

Hinman AR, Kaplan JP: Pertussis and pertussis vaccine. *JAMA* 1984;**251**:3109.

Immunization Practices Advisory Committee, Centers for Disease Control: Diphtheria, tetanus, and pertussis: Guidelines for vaccine prophylaxis and other preventive measures. *MMWR* 1985;**34**:405.

## MENINGITIS

### 1. MENINGOCOCCAL MENINGITIS

#### Essentials of Diagnosis

- Fever, headache, vomiting, confusion, delirium, convulsions.
- Petechial rash of skin and mucous membranes.
- Neck and back stiffness with positive Kernig and Brudzinski signs.
- Purulent spinal fluid with gram-negative intracellular and extracellular organisms.
- Culture of cerebrospinal fluid, blood, or petechial aspiration confirms the diagnosis.
- Shock and disseminated intravascular clotting may occur.

#### General Considerations

Meningococcal meningitis is caused by *Neisseria meningitidis* of groups A, B, C, Y, W-135, and others. A varying (15–40%) segment of the population are nasopharyngeal carriers of meningococci, but relatively few develop disease. Infection is transmitted by droplets, and many factors probably play a role in determining clinical illness—including prior immunity, physical stress, and immediately antecedent viral infections. The clinical illness may take the form of meningococcemia (a fulminant form of septicemia without meningitis), both meningococcemia and meningitis, or predominantly meningitis. Chronic recurrent meningococcemia with fever, rash, and arthritis can occur. The development of meningococcal disease is favored by complement deficiencies (especially C7–C9).

## Clinical Findings

**A. Symptoms and Signs:** High fever, chills, and headache; back, abdominal, and extremity pains; and nausea and vomiting are present. In severe cases, rapidly developing confusion, delirium, and coma occur. Twitchings or frank convulsions may also be present.

Nuchal and back rigidity are present, with positive Kernig and Brudzinski signs. A petechial rash is found in most cases. Petechiae may vary from pinhead-sized to large ecchymoses or even areas of skin gangrene that may later slough if the patient survives. These petechiae are found in any part of the skin, mucous membranes, or the conjunctiva but never in the nail beds, and they usually fade in 3–4 days. The increased intracranial pressure will cause the anterior fontanelle to bulge (if not closed) and may produce Cheyne-Stokes or Biot's respiration.

Shock due to the effects of endotoxin may be present and is a bad prognostic sign.

**B. Laboratory Findings:** Leukocytosis is usually marked and occurs very early in the course of the disease. The urine may contain protein, casts, and red cells. Lumbar puncture reveals a cloudy to frankly purulent cerebrospinal fluid, with elevated pressure, increased protein, and decreased glucose content. The fluid usually contains more than 100 cells/$\mu$L, with polymorphonuclear cells predominating and containing gram-negative intracellular diplococci. The absence of organisms in a gram-stained smear of the cerebrospinal fluid sediment does not rule out the diagnosis. The capsular polysaccharide can often be demonstrated in cerebrospinal fluid or urine by latex agglutination. The organism is usually demonstrated by smear or culture of the cerebrospinal fluid, oropharynx, blood, or aspirated petechiae.

Disseminated intravascular coagulation is an important complication of meningococcal infection. Assay of factor V and factor VIII activity (low), fibrin split products (elevated), and platelet count (low) help in establishing this diagnosis.

## Differential Diagnosis

Meningococcal meningitis must be differentiated from other meningitides. In small infants, the clinical manifestations of meningeal infection may be erroneously diagnosed as upper respiratory infection or other acute infections.

Other bacterial infections (*Haemophilus,* pneumococcal, staphylococcal) or rickettsial or echovirus infection may also produce a petechial rash.

## Complications

Arthritis, cranial nerve damage (especially the eighth nerve, with resulting deafness), and hydrocephalus may occur as complications. Myocarditis, nephritis, and intravascular coagulation may occur in severe cases.

## Prevention

Effective polysaccharide vaccines for groups A, C, Y, and W-135 are available. A and C vaccine has reduced the incidence of infections with these meningococcus groups in military recruits. The vaccines are effective for control of epidemics in civilian populations.

Outbreaks in closed populations are best controlled by administering antimicrobials that reduce meningococcal carriage. Sulfonamides are not useful, because many strains of meningococci are sulfonamide-resistant. Penicillin and ampicillin do not eliminate carriage. Rifampin (600 mg twice a day for 2 days for adults; 10 mg/kg twice a day for 2 days for children 1 month to 12 years; 5 mg/kg twice a day for 2 days for infants) is the drug of choice.

**Exposed contacts.** Household members are at increased risk and may be given rifampin prophylaxis for 2 days. Day-care center contacts are treated in the same manner. School and work contacts should not be treated. Hospital contacts should be treated only if intensive and intimate exposure has occurred, eg, giving mouth-to-mouth resuscitation.

Accidentally discovered carriers, without known close contact with a case of meningococcal disease, are generally not given prophylactic antimicrobials.

## Treatment

**A. Specific Measures:** Antimicrobial therapy by the intravenous route must be started immediately. If meningococcus is established or strongly suspected as the infectious agent, aqueous penicillin G is the agent of choice (24 million units/24 h for adults; 400,000 units/kg/24 h for children). One-fourth of the dose is given rapidly intravenously and the rest by continuous drip or in divided doses every 4 hours. If the possibility of *Haemophilus influenzae* meningitis has not been ruled out, treat as discussed on p 864. If the patient is allergic to penicillin, chloramphenicol, 100 mg/kg daily, is the preferred alternative drug. The older cephalosporins are unsuitable in meningitis, but newer ones (eg, cefuroxime, cefotaxime) are effective. Treatment should be continued for 7–10 days by the intravenous route or until the patient is afebrile for 5 days.

**B. General Measures:** Hypovolemic shock is the most serious complication of meningococcal infections. Volume expansion with isotonic electrolyte solution is the initial approach while monitoring central venous pressure. Isoproterenol or dopamine is added to the infusion if the patient fails to respond.

Vital signs must be monitored. Ventilatory assistance may be required. If cerebral edema is present—and particularly if herniation of the brain through the foramen magnum is imminent—intravenous mannitol (2 g/kg) or urea (0.5 g/kg) may temporarily decrease the intracranial pressure.

Corticosteroids have no established role in the management of meningitis. In the presence of shock, high-dose (30 mg/kg) prednisone may be beneficial.

Heparinization should be considered if there is evidence of intravascular coagulation. An initial dose of 50 units/kg intravenously is given; thereafter, an attempt is made to keep the clotting time at 20–30 minutes.

## Prognosis

If the patient survives the first day, the prognosis is excellent. Sequelae are less common than in other forms of purulent meningitis.

Band JD et al: Trends in meningococcal disease in the United States, 1975–1980. *J Infect Dis* 1983;**148:**754.

Centers for Disease Control: Meningogoccal vaccines. *MMWR* 1985;**34:**256.

Ellison RT et al: Prevalence of congenital or acquired complement deficiency in patients with sporadic meningococcal disease. *N Engl J Med* 1983;**308:**913.

Shapiro ED: Prophylaxis of meningitis. *Med Clin North Am* 1985;**69:**269.

## 2. PNEUMOCOCCAL, STREPTOCOCCAL, & STAPHYLOCOCCAL MENINGITIS

The symptoms are similar to those of meningococcal meningitis, but a preceding infection is usually present, and a focus is often demonstrable in the lungs (pneumococcal), the middle ear, or sinuses. The cerebrospinal fluid must be cultured and examined to determine the causative agent.

Specific treatment of pneumococcal and streptococcal meningitis consists of aqueous penicillin, 1 million units added every 2 hours to a continuous intravenous infusion.

Staphylococcal meningitis is treated with intravenous nafcillin (12 g/24 h or 300 mg/kg/24 h) in divided doses. When the organism is definitely penicillin-sensitive, penicillin G is preferred. The duration of therapy must be between 2 and 4 weeks. Complications, including ventriculitis, arachnoiditis, cerebrospinal fluid block, and hydrocephalus, are more common in these forms of meningitis than in meningococcal meningitis.

McCabe WR: Empiric therapy for bacterial meningitis. *Rev Infect Dis* 1983;**5(Suppl 1):**574.

## 3. *HAEMOPHILUS INFLUENZAE* MENINGITIS

*Haemophilus influenzae* meningitis occurs most frequently in children under age 6 years. It may present for several days as an apparent respiratory infection; however, headache, irritability, fever, malaise, vomiting, unexplained leukocytosis, and nuchal and back rigidity should suggest meningitis. Lumbar puncture may reveal gram-negative pleomorphic rods in the purulent spinal fluid smear or culture. The latex agglutination test on cerebrospinal fluid may confirm the presence of specific *Haemophilus influenzae* type b capsular polysaccharide. If culture is positive, assay for beta-lactamase production is necessary. It is not possible to distinguish *Haemophilus influenzae* meningitis from other purulent meningitides on the basis of the symptoms and signs. Identification of the organism is necessary for optimal treatment.

## Prevention

An *H influenzae* type b polysaccharide vaccine is recommended for children 2–5 years old and for those 18–23 months old at high risk (eg, asplenia, immunosuppression).

Close contacts in the household or day-care center under 4 years of age should receive antimicrobial prophylaxis with rifampin (20 mg/kg/d for 4 days).

## Treatment

**A. Specific Measures:** The rising prevalence of ampicillin-resistant strains (5 to > 20%) requires that 2 antimicrobial drugs be used initially—sodium ampicillin, 300 mg/kg/d intravenously (one-fourth of the dose given immediately and the remainder in divided doses every 4 hours), and chloramphenicol, 100 mg/kg/d intravenously. The antibiotics should be given separately and not in a mixed injection. As soon as the antibiotic susceptibility of the *H influenzae* isolate has been established (the test for β-lactamase production is best and fastest), one of the 2 antibiotics should be stopped and the remaining agent continued for 10–14 days until the patient is clinically well. Cefuroxime (150 mg/kg/d), cefotaxime, and ceftriaxone are equally effective and are drugs of choice when the *H influenzae* is resistant to both ampicillin and chloramphenicol.

**B. General Measures:** Management is similar to that described above for meningococcal meningitis. Shock is less likely to occur, but subdural effusion and other complications are more common.

## Prognosis

The case fatality rate is about 5%. One must aim not only at survival but at prevention of sequelae, including the more subtle forms of central nervous system damage.

American Academy of Pediatrics: Diagnosis and treatment of meningitis. *Pediatrics* 1986;**78:**959.

Immunization Practices Advisory Committee, Centers for Disease Control: Prevention of *Haemophilus influenzae* type b disease. *MMWR* 1986;**35:**170.

Jacobs RF et al: A prospective randomized comparison of cefotaxime vs. ampicillin and chloramphenicol for bacterial meningitis in children. *J Pediatr* 1985;**107:**129.

## 4. TUBERCULOUS MENINGITIS

### Essentials of Diagnosis

- Gradual onset of listlessness, irritability, and anorexia.
- Headache, vomiting, coma, convulsions; neck and back rigidity.
- Tuberculous focus may be evident elsewhere.
- Cerebrospinal fluid shows several hundred lymphocytes, low glucose, and high protein.

### General Considerations

Tuberculous meningitis is caused by hematogenous spread of tubercle bacilli from a focus usually in the lungs or the peritracheal, peribronchial, or mesenteric lymph nodes, or it may be a consequence of miliary spread. Its greatest incidence is in children age 1–5 years.

### Clinical Findings

**A. Symptoms and Signs:** The onset is usually gradual, with listlessness, irritability, anorexia, and fever, followed by headache, vomiting, convulsions, and coma. In older patients, headache and behavioral changes are prominent early symptoms.

Nuchal rigidity, opisthotonos, and paralysis occur as the meningitis progresses. Paralysis of the extraocular muscles is common. Ophthalmoscopic examination may show choroid tubercles. General physical examination may reveal evidence of tuberculosis elsewhere. The tuberculin skin test may be negative in miliary tuberculosis.

**B. Laboratory Findings:** The spinal fluid is frequently yellowish, with increased pressure; 100–500 cells/$\mu$L (early, polymorphonuclear neutrophils; later, lymphocytes); increased protein; and decreased glucose. On standing, the cerebrospinal fluid may form a web and pellicle from which organisms may be demonstrated by smear and culture. Moderate leukocytosis is common. Chest x-ray often reveals a tuberculous focus.

### Differential Diagnosis

Tuberculous meningitis may be confused with any other type of meningitis, but the gradual onset and evidence of tuberculosis elsewhere often point to the diagnosis.

Fungal and other granulomatous meningitides or rare neoplasms must be considered also.

### Complications

Residual brain damage may result in motor paralysis, convulsive states, mental impairment, and abnormal behavior. The incidence of these complications increases the later therapy is started.

### Prevention

Early identification of tuberculin converters and children with primary tuberculosis, and treatment with isoniazid at that stage, is the key to preventing tuberculous meningitis.

### Treatment

Early institution of antituberculosis therapy is essential for survival and to minimize sequelae. Thus, presumptive diagnosis and treatment are often necessary while awaiting confirmation by culture.

**A. Specific Measures:** Give isoniazid, 10 mg/kg/d (up to a total of 300 mg/d); rifampin, 600 mg/d; and ethambutol, 15 mg/kg/d. All are given orally, and each can be given as a single daily dose. Treatment should be continued for 18–24 months. In addition, give streptomycin, 1 g intramuscularly daily for 2 weeks, and then continue twice weekly for 60–90 days. Corticosteroid treatment (60 mg of prednisone or equivalent daily) is used initially until improvement is established and then gradually discontinued.

*Caution:* Ethambutol rarely causes retinal neuropathy. Visual acuity should be tested monthly with a Snellen chart. Peripheral neuropathy due to isoniazid can be prevented by giving pyridoxine, 50 mg orally daily. The incidence of isoniazid hepatitis increases with age.

**B. General Measures:** Treat symptoms as they arise and maintain good nutrition and adequate fluid intake. Treat hyponatremia due to inappropriate antidiuretic hormone secretion that may be present.

### Prognosis

The natural course of the untreated disease is death within 6–8 weeks. With early diagnosis and treatment, the recovery rate may reach 90%; if treatment is not instituted until the disease has reached the late stage, the survival rate is 25–30%. Serious neurologic sequelae are frequent.

Alvarez S, McCabe WR: Extrapulmonary tuberculosis revisited: A review of experience at Boston City and other hospitals. *Medicine* 1984;**63**:25.

Daniel TM: New approaches to the rapid diagnosis of tuberculous meningitis. *J Infect Dis* 1987;**155**:599.

Klein NC et al: Mycobacterial meningitis: Retrospective analysis 1970–1983. *Am J Med* 1985;**79**:29.

## SALMONELLOSIS

Salmonellosis includes infection by any of approximately 1600 serotypes of salmonellae. Three general clinical patterns are recognized: (1) enteric fever, the best example of which is typhoid fever, due to *Salmonella typhi*; (2) acute enterocolitis, caused by *Salmonella typhimurium* and many other types; and (3) the "septicemic" type, characterized by bacteremia and focal lesions, exemplified by infection with *Salmonella choleraesuis*. Any serotype may cause any of these clinical patterns. All are transmitted by ingestion of the organism in contaminated food or drink.

# 1. TYPHOID FEVER

## Essentials of Diagnosis

- Gradual onset of malaise, headache, sore throat, cough, and finally "pea soup" diarrhea or constipation.
- Slow (stepladder) rise of fever to maximum and then slow return to normal.
- Rose spots, relative bradycardia, splenomegaly, and abdominal distension and tenderness.
- Leukopenia; blood, stool, and urine culture positive for *Salmonella typhi* (group D).
- Elevated or rising specific agglutination titers.

## General Considerations

Typhoid fever is caused by *Salmonella typhi,* which enters the patient via the gastrointestinal tract, where it penetrates the intestinal wall and produces inflammation of the mesenteric lymph nodes and the spleen. Bacteremia occurs, and the infection then localizes principally in the lymphoid tissue of the small intestine (particularly within 60 cm of the ileocecal valve). Peyer's patches become inflamed and may ulcerate, with involvement greatest during the third week of disease. The organism may localize in the lungs, gallbladder, kidneys, or central nervous system. Infection is transmitted by consumption of contaminated food or drink. The sources of most infections are chronic carriers with persistent gallbladder or urinary tract infections. The incubation period is 5–14 days.

## Clinical Findings

**A. Symptoms and Signs:** The onset is usually insidious but may be abrupt, especially in children, with chills and high fever. The course of classic untreated typhoid fever can be divided into 3 stages.

**1. Prodromal stage**–The patient develops increasing malaise, headache, cough, general body aching, sore throat, and epistaxis. Frequently there is abdominal pain, constipation or diarrhea, and vomiting. The fever ascends in a stepladder fashion and is generally higher in the evening than in the morning.

**2. Fastigium**–After about 7–10 days, the fever stabilizes, varying less than 1.1 °C (2 °F) during the day, and the patient becomes quite sick. "Pea soup" diarrhea or severe constipation or marked abdominal distension is common. In severe cases, the patient lies motionless and unresponsive, with eyes half-shut, appearing wasted and exhausted (the "typhoid state"), but can usually be aroused.

**3. Stage of defervescence**–If the patient develops no complications, improvement occurs gradually. Fever declines in a stepladder fashion to normal in 7–10 days. The patient becomes more alert, and abdominal symptoms disappear. However, relapse may occur up to 2 weeks after defervescence.

During the early prodrome, physical findings are slight. Later, splenomegaly, abdominal distension and tenderness, relative bradycardia, dicrotic pulse, and occasionally meningismus, systolic murmur, and gallop rhythm appear. The rash (rose spots) commonly appears during the second week of disease. The individual spot, found principally on the trunk, is a pink papule 2–3 mm in diameter that fades on pressure. It disappears over a period of 3–4 days.

**B. Laboratory Findings:** Blood cultures may be positive in the first week and remain positive for a variable period thereafter. Stools are positive for the organism after the first week; the urine may be positive at any time.

During the second week, antibodies appear in the blood and continue to rise in titer until the end of the third week. If an anamnestic response to other infectious diseases or recent vaccination is ruled out, an O (somatic) antibody titer of 1:160 is presumptively diagnostic; a rising titer (as demonstrated by 2 specimens taken approximately a week apart) is diagnostic.

Moderate anemia and leukopenia are the rule.

## Differential Diagnosis

Enteric fever can be produced by other *Salmonella* species (eg, *Salmonella paratyphi*).

Typhoid fever must be distinguished from other prolonged fevers associated with normal or depressed white count. Examples include tuberculosis, viral pneumonia, psittacosis, infective endocarditis, brucellosis, Q fever, and campylobacteriosis. *Yersinia enterocolitica* infection can produce enteritis with fever, diarrhea, vomiting, abdominal pain, and mesenteric adenitis, which may mimic appendicitis.

## Complications

Complications occur in about 30% of untreated cases and account for 75% of all deaths. Intestinal hemorrhage is most likely to occur during the third week and is manifested by a sudden drop in temperature, rise in pulse, and signs of shock followed by dark or fresh blood in the stool. Intestinal perforation is most likely to occur during the third week. Sudden rigor, drop in temperature, and increase in pulse rate, accompanied by abdominal pain and tenderness, may be noted. Less frequent complications are urinary retention, pneumonia, thrombophlebitis, myocarditis, psychosis, cholecystitis, nephritis, spondylitis (typhoid spine), and meningitis.

## Prevention

Active immunization should be provided for household contacts of a typhoid carrier, for travelers to endemic areas, and during epidemic outbreaks.

Typhoid vaccine is administered in 2 injections subcutaneously, not less than 4 weeks apart. The usual procedure is to revaccinate twice only at 4-year intervals. (See Chapter 21.) An experimental live attenuated vaccine of strain Ty21 has given promising results.

Environmental hygiene control requires protection of food and water and adequate waste disposal.

Carriers must not be permitted to work as food handlers.

## Treatment

**A. Specific Measures:** Ampicillin, chloramphenicol, and trimethoprim-sulfamethoxazole may be effective. All can be given orally or intravenously depending on the patient's condition. The choice depends on the prevailing susceptibility of *S typhi* in the region and on specific laboratory susceptibility tests. (See Chapter 28.)

**B. General Measures:** Give a high-calorie, low-residue diet. Hydrocortisone, 100 mg intravenously every 8 hours, may tide over severely toxic patients. Maintain skin care.

Parenteral fluids may be necessary to supplement oral intake and maintain urine output. Abdominal distention may be relieved by abdominal stupes. Vasopressin and neostigmine must be used with great caution because of the danger of perforation. Strict linen, stool, and urine isolation must be observed.

**C. Treatment of Complications:** Secondary pneumonia may be treated with antibiotics, depending on the etiologic agent.

Transfusions should be given as required for hemorrhage. If perforation occurs, immediate surgery is required; anticipate and treat shock (see Chapter 1) before it becomes manifest.

**D. Treatment of Carriers:** Chemotherapy is usually ineffective in abolishing the carrier state. However, a trial of ampicillin first and then chloramphenicol is worthwhile. Cholecystectomy may be effective.

## Prognosis

The mortality rate of typhoid fever is about 2% in treated cases. Elderly or debilitated persons are likely to do poorly. The course is milder in children.

With complications, the prognosis is poor. Relapses occur in up to 15% of cases. A residual carrier state frequently persists in spite of chemotherapy.

## 2. *SALMONELLA* ENTEROCOLITIS

By far the most common form of salmonellosis is acute enterocolitis. The commonest causative serotypes are *Salmonella typhimurium, Salmonella derby, Salmonella heidelberg, Salmonella infantis, Salmonella newport, Salmonella agona,* and *Salmonella enteritidis*. The incubation period is 8–48 hours after ingestion of contaminated food or liquid.

Symptoms and signs consist of fever (often with chills), nausea and vomiting, cramping abdominal pain, and diarrhea, which may be bloody. The disease persists over a course of 3–5 days. Differentiation must be made from viral gastroenteritis, food poisoning, shigellosis, amebic dysentery, acute ulcerative colitis, and acute surgical abdominal conditions. Leukocytosis is usually not present. The organisms can be cultured from the stools, but not from blood.

The disease is usually self-limited, but bacteremia with localization in joints or bones may occur, especially in young infants and in patients with sickle cell disease.

Treatment in the uncomplicated case of enterocolitis is symptomatic only. Antimicrobial therapy does not ameliorate clinical symptoms and does not shorten—may even prolong—the shedding time of organisms. Young, malnourished, or immunocompromised infants, severely ill patients, those with sickle cell disease, and those in whom bacteremia is suspected should be treated with ampicillin (100 mg/kg intravenously or orally) or chloramphenicol (50–100 mg/kg orally).

## 3. SEPTICEMIC SALMONELLOSIS

Rarely, *Salmonella* infection may be manifested by prolonged or recurrent fever accompanied by bacteremia and by localization and abscess formation in one or more sites—such as the bones, joints, pleura, pericardium, endocardium, meninges, and lungs. Treatment is as for typhoid fever and should include drainage of accessible lesions.

Blaser MJ, Newman LS: A review of human salmonellosis. 1. Infective dose. *Rev Infect Dis* 1982;**4**:1096.

Edelman R, Levine MM: Summary of an International Workshop on Typhoid Fever. *Rev Infect Dis* 1986;**8**:329.

Hoffman SL et al: Reduction of mortality in chloramphenicol-treated severe typhoid fever by high-dose dexamethasone. *N Engl J Med* 1984;**310**:82.

Klotz SA et al: Typhoid fever. *Arch Intern Med* 1984;**144**:533.

Nelson JD et al: Treatment of salmonella gastroenteritis with ampicillin, amoxicillin or placebo. *Pediatrics* 1980;**65**:1125.

## "FOOD POISONING" & ACUTE ENTEROCOLITIS

Food poisoning is a nonspecific term often applied to the syndrome of acute anorexia, nausea, vomiting, or diarrhea that is attributed to food intake, particularly if it afflicts groups of people and is not accompanied by fever. (See Acute Gastrointestinal Syndromes in Chapter 21.) The actual cause of such acute gastrointestinal upsets might be emotional stress, viral or bacterial infections, food intolerance, inorganic (eg, sodium nitrite) or organic (eg, mushroom, shellfish) poisons, or drugs (eg, antimicrobials). More specifically, food poisoning may refer to toxins produced by bacteria growing in food (staphylococci, clostridia, *Bacillus cereus*) or to acute food infections with short incubation periods and a mild course (*Salmonella* enterocolitis [see above]) or to infection with enterotoxigenic *Escherichia coli*, shigellae, or vibrios (*Vibrio cholerae,* El Tor vibrios, marine vibrios including *Vibrio parahaemolyticus, Vibrio vulnificus*). *Campylobacter jejuni* and *Yersinia enterocolitica* may produce similar clinical enterocolitis and can be identified only by special stool culture methods. Adenoviruses rotaviruses, and Norwalk-type viruses may produce a similar syndrome. *E coli* O157:H7 is an infrequent cause of hemorrhagic colitis. Some prominent features of some of these "food poisonings" are listed in Table 23–1. In general, the diagnosis must be suspected when groups of people who have shared a meal develop acute vomiting or diarrhea. Food and stools must be secured for bacteriologic and toxicologic examination. In febrile patients, blood cultures are indicated.

Treatment usually consists of replacement of fluids and electrolytes and, very rarely, management of hypovolemic shock and respiratory embarrassment. If botulism is suspected, polyvalent antitoxin must be administered.

Antimicrobial drugs are not indicated unless a specific microbial agent producing progressive systemic involvement can be identified. Antimicrobial drugs may in fact aggravate anorexia and diarrhea and may prolong microbial carriage and excretion.

*Note:* Iodochlorhydroxyquin (Entero-Vioform, Vioform) is not useful for prophylaxis or treatment of any of these disorders and may be harmful.

Blacklow NR, Cukor G: Viral gastroenteritis. *N Engl J Med* 1981;**304**:397.

Blaser MJ, Reller LB: *Campylobacter* enteritis. *N Engl J Med* 1981;**305**:1444.

DeWitt TG et al: Clinical predictors of acute bacterial diarrhea in young children. *Pediatrics* 1985;**76**:551.

Fekety R: Recent advances in management of bacterial diarrheas. *Rev Infect Dis* 1983;**5**:246.

Marks MI et al: *Yersinia enterocolitica* gastroenteritis: A prospective study of clinical, bacteriologic and epidemiologic features. *J Pediatr* 1980;**96**:26.

Spika JS et al: Chloramphenicol-resistant *Salmonella newport* traced through hamburger to dairy farms. *N Engl J Med* 1987;**316**:565.

Terranova W, Blake PA: *Bacillus cereus* food poisoning. *N Engl J Med* 1978;**298**:143.

## CHOLERA

### Essentials of Diagnosis

- Sudden onset of severe, frequent diarrhea, up to 1 L per hour.
- The liquid stool (and occasionally vomitus) is gray, turbid, and without fecal odor, blood, or pus ("rice water stool").
- Rapid development of marked dehydration, acidosis, hypokalemia, and hypotension.
- History of sojourn in endemic area or contact with infected person.
- Positive stool cultures and agglutination of vibrios with specific sera.

### General Considerations

Cholera is an acute diarrheal disease caused by *Vibrio cholerae* or related vibrios. A pandemic of cholera is in progress. The infection is acquired by the ingestion of food or drink contaminated by feces from cases or carriers containing large numbers of vibrios. The infective dose is near $10^7$–$10^9$ vibrios.

The vibrios grow in the small intestine (particularly the ileum) and produce a powerful exotoxin. The toxin activates adenylate cyclase, resulting in increased concentration of cyclic adenosine monophosphate in the gut wall. This produces massive hypersecretion of water and chloride into the gut lumen and reduces reabsorption of sodium. This results in massive diarrhea of up to 15 L/24 h, which is fatal in 50% of patients if untreated. The incubation period is 1–5 days. Only a small minority of exposed persons become ill.

### Clinical Findings

**A. Symptoms and Signs:** The spectrum of severity of illness is wide. Typical cases have an explosive onset of frequent, watery stools that soon lose all fecal appearance and odor. They are grayish, turbid, and liquid, containing degenerated epithelium and mucus but few leukocytes or red blood cells. A typical stool may be 7 L/24 h, containing $Na^+$, 125 meq/L; $K^+$, 20 meq/L; and $HCO_3^-$, 45 meq/L. Vomiting may also occur early. As a result, the patient rapidly becomes dehydrated and acidotic, with sunken eyes, hypotension, subnormal temperature, rapid and shallow breathing, muscle cramps, oliguria, shock, and coma.

**B. Laboratory Findings:** Blood studies reveal marked hemoconcentration, with rising specific gravity of plasma, metabolic acidosis, and often elevation of nonprotein nitrogen. The serum potassium may be normal in spite of severe potassium loss.

The vibrios can be easily grown from the stool—never from blood—and can be identified by agglutination with known specific serum.

### Differential Diagnosis

Cholera must be distinguished from other causes of severe diarrhea and dehydration, particularly diarrheas due to shigellae, enterotoxigenic *E coli*, viruses, and protozoa in endemic areas.

### Prevention

Cholera vaccine gives only limited protection and is of no value in controlling outbreaks. The vaccine is given in 2 injections 1–4 weeks apart (see package insert). A booster dose is given every 6 months when cholera is a hazard. Better vaccines, including toxoids, are being investigated. At present, cholera vaccination is not required of travelers entering the USA.

In endemic areas, all water, other drinks, food, and utensils must be boiled or avoided. Effective decontamination of excreta is essential, but strict isolation of patients is unnecessary and quarantine is undesirable. In countries with high standards of sanitation and public health, the importation of cholera rarely leads to outbreaks of significant size.

### Treatment

Water and electrolyte losses must be restored promptly and continuously, and acidosis must be corrected. Diarrheal loss and hemoconcentration must

**Table 23–1.** Acute bacterial diarrheas and "food poisoning."

| Organism | Incubation Period (Hours) | Vomiting | Diarrhea | Fever | Epidemiology | Pathogenesis | Clinical Features |
|---|---|---|---|---|---|---|---|
| Staphylococcus | 1–8, rarely up to 18 | +++ | + | – | Staphylococci grow in meats, dairy, bakery products and produce enterotoxin. | Enterotoxin acts on receptors in gut that transmit impulse to medullary centers. | Abrupt onset, intense vomiting for up to 24 hours, regular recovery in 24–48 hours. Occurs in persons eating the same food. No treatment usually necessary except to restore fluids and electrolytes. |
| Bacillus cereus | 1–8, rarely up to 18 | +++ | ++ | – | Reheated fried rice causes vomiting or diarrhea. | Enterotoxins formed in food or in gut from growth of B cereus. | After 1–6 hours, mainly vomiting. After 8–16 hours, mainly diarrhea. Both self-limited to less than 1 day. |
| Clostridium perfringens | 8–16 | ± | +++ | – | Clostridia grow in rewarmed meat dishes and produce enterotoxin. | Enterotoxin produced in food and in gut causes hypersecretion in small intestine. | Abrupt onset of profuse diarrhea; vomiting occasionally. Recovery usual without treatment in 1–4 days. Many clostridia in cultures of food and feces of patients. |
| Clostridium botulinum | 24–96 | ± | Rare | – | Clostridia grow in anaerobic foods and produce toxin. | Toxin absorbed from gut blocks acetylcholine at neuromuscular junction. | Diplopia, dysphagia, dysphonia, respiratory embarrassment. Treatment requires clear airway, ventilation, and intravenous polyvalent antitoxin (see p 874). Toxin present in food and serum. Mortality rate high. |
| Escherichia coli (some strains) | 24–72 | ± | ++ | – | Organisms grow in gut and produce toxin. May also invade superficial epithelium. | Toxin* causes hypersecretion in small intestine ("traveler's diarrhea").† | Usually abrupt onset of diarrhea; vomiting rare. A serious infection in neonates. In adults, "traveler's diarrhea" is usually self-limited in 1–3 days. Use diphenoxylate (Lomotil) but no antimicrobials. |
| Vibrio para-haemolyticus | 6–96 | + | ++ | ±† | Organisms grow in seafood and in gut and produce toxin, or invade. | Hypersecretion in small intestine; stools may be bloody. | Abrupt onset of diarrhea in groups consuming the same food, especially crabs and other seafood. Recovery is usually complete in 1–3 days. Food and stool cultures are positive. |
| Vibrio cholerae (mild cases) | 24–72 | + | +++ | – | Organisms grow in gut and produce toxin. | Toxin* causes hypersecretion in small intestine. Infective dose: $10^7$–$10^9$ organisms. | Abrupt onset of liquid diarrhea in endemic area. Needs prompt replacement of luids and electrolytes (see p 868) IV or orally. Tetracyclines shorten excretion of vibrios. Stool cultures positive. |
| Shigella spp (mild cases) | 24–72 | ± | ++ | + | Organisms grow in superficial gut epithelium and gut lumen and produce toxin. | Organisms invade epithelial cells, blood, mucus, and PMNs in stools. Infective dose: $10^2$–$10^3$ organisms. | Abrupt onset of diarrhea, often with blood and pus in stools, cramps, tenesmus, and lethargy. Stool cultures are positive. In severe cases, give trimethoprim-sulfamethoxazole, ampicillin, or chloramphenicol. Do not give opiates. Restore fluids. Often mild and self-limited. |
| Salmonella spp | 8–48 | ± | ++ | + | Organisms grow in gut. Do not produce toxin. | Superficial infection of gut, little invasion. Infective dose: $10^5$ organisms. | Gradual or abrupt onset of diarrhea and low-grade fever. No antimicrobials unless systemic dissemination is suspected. Stool cultures are positive. Prolonged carriage is frequent. |
| Clostridium difficile | ? | – | +++ | + | Associated with antimicrobial drugs, eg, clindamycin. | Toxin causes epithelial necrosis in colon; pseudomembranous colitis (see p 386). | Especially after abdominal surgery, abrupt bloody diarrhea, and fever. Toxin in stool. Oral vancomycin useful in therapy. |
| Campylobacter jejuni | 2–10 days | – | +++ | + | Organism grows in jejunum and ileum. | Invasion and toxin production uncertain. | Fever, diarrhea; PMNs and fresh blood in stool, especially in children. Usually self-limited. Special media needed for culture at 43°C. Erythromycin in severe cases with invasion. Usual recovery in 5–8 days. |
| Yersinia entero-colitica | ? | ± | ++ | ÷ | Fecal-oral transmission (occasionally). Food-borne. ?In pets. | Gastroenteritis or mesenteric adenitis. Occasional bacteremia. Toxin† produced. | Severe abdominal pain, diarrhea, fever; PMNs and blood in stool; polyarthritis, erythema nodosum in children. If severe, give tetracycline or gentamicin. Keep stool at 4°C before culture. |

* Toxin stimulates adenylate cyclase activity and increases cAMP concentration in gut; this increases secretion of chloride and water and reduces reabsorption of sodium.
† Heat-stable toxin activates guanylate cyclase and results in hypersecretion.

be measured continuously. In moderately ill patients, it may be possible to provide replacement by oral fluids given in the same volume as that lost. A suitable oral solution contains NaCl, 4 g/L; NaHCO₃, 4 g/L; KCl, 1–2 g/L; and glucose, 21 g/L. In more severely ill patients or those unable to take fluids by mouth, replacement must be by intravenous fluids. A suitable intravenous solution contains Na$^+$, 133 meq/L; Cl$^-$, 98 meq/L; K$^+$, 13 meq/L; and HCO₃$^-$, 48 meq/L. Initially, this solution is infused at a rate of 50–100 mL/min until circulating blood volume and blood pressure are restored. It may then be given more slowly to replace lost stool volume. In children, more potassium and less sodium are lost, and potassium must be replaced. An older method relied on the degree of hemoconcentration to direct fluid replacement: For every 0.001 increase in plasma specific gravity above 1.025, 4 mL/kg of mixed isotonic sodium lactate and saline (1:2 ratio) were infused.

Tetracycline, 0.5 g orally every 6 hours for 3–5 days, and perhaps doxycycline, 200 mg orally as a single dose, suppresses vibrio growth in the gut and shortens the time of vibrio excretion.

Whenever cholera is suspected, the Health Department must be notified by telephone.

### Prognosis

The untreated disease lasts 3–5 days, with a mortality rate ranging from 20% to 80%. With prompt and competent treatment, the mortality rate is 1% or less.

Miller CJ, Feachem RG, Drassar BS: Cholera epidemiology in developed and developing countries. *Lancet* 1985;**1**:261.
Morris JG Jr, Black RE: Cholera and other vibrioses in the United States. *N Engl J Med* 1985;**312**:343.
Wang F: The acidosis of cholera. *N Engl J Med* 1986;**315**:1591.

## BACILLARY DYSENTERY (Shigellosis)

### Essentials of Diagnosis

- Diarrhea, often with blood and mucus.
- Cramps.
- Fever, malaise, prostration, clouded sensorium.
- Pus in stools; organism isolated on stool culture.

### General Considerations

*Shigella* dysentery is a common disease, often self-limited and mild but occasionally serious, particularly in the first 3 years of life. Poor sanitary conditions promote the spread of *Shigella*. *Shigella sonnei* is the leading cause of this illness in the USA, followed by *Shigella flexneri*. *Shigella dysenteriae* causes the most serious form of the illness. Shigellae are invasive organisms: The infective dose is $10^2$–$10^3$ organisms. Recently, there has been a rise in strains resistant to multiple antibiotics.

### Clinical Findings

**A. Symptoms and Signs:** The illness usually starts abruptly, with diarrhea, lower abdominal cramps, and tenesmus. The diarrheal stool often is mixed with blood and mucus. Systemic symptoms are fever (in young children, up to 40 °C [104 °F]), chills, anorexia and malaise, headache, lethargy, and, in the most severe cases, meningismus, coma, and convulsions. As the illness progresses, the patient becomes progressively weaker and more dehydrated. The abdomen is tender. Sigmoidscopic examination reveals an inflamed, engorged mucosa with punctate, sometimes large areas of ulceration.

**B. Laboratory Findings:** The white blood count shows an increase in polymorphonuclear cells with a pronounced shift to the left. The stool shows many leukocytes (even gross pus and mucus) and many red blood cells (or gross blood). Stool culture is positive for shigellae in most cases, blood culture in 2–3%.

### Differential Diagnosis

Bacillary dysentery must be distinguished from *Salmonella* enterocolitis, enterotoxigenic *E coli*, *Campylobacter* enteritis, *Y enterocolitica* and vibrio infections, and viral diarrhea (caused by rotaviruses in young children and Norwalk viruses in adults). Amebic dysentery may be similar clinically and is diagnosed by finding amebas in the fresh stool specimen. Ulcerative colitis in the adolescent and adult is an important cause of bloody diarrhea.

### Complications

Dehydration, acidosis, and electrolyte imbalance occur in infancy. Temporary disaccharidase deficiency may follow the diarrhea. Arthritis is an uncommon complication.

### Treatment

**A. Specific Measures:** Treatment of shock, restoration of circulating blood volume, and renal perfusion are lifesaving in severe cases. The current antimicrobial agent of choice is trimethoprim-sulfamethoxazole, ampicillin (100 mg/kg/d) (but not amoxicillin), or chloramphenicol. Shigellae resistant to ampicillin and chloramphenicol are increasing in frequency. Drugs should not be continued beyond the beginning of marked improvement even if stool cultures remain positive. At times, single doses of tetracycline (2 g orally) or ampicillin (100 mg/kg) have given satisfactory results. Since the majority of cases are mild and self-limited, the use of even mildly toxic antibiotics cannot be justified.

**B. General Measures:** Parenteral hydration and correction of acidosis and electrolyte disturbances are essential in all moderately or severely ill patients. After the bowel has been at rest for a short time, clear fluids are given for 2–3 days. The diet should then be soft, easily digestible, and given in small frequent feedings, avoiding whole milk and high-residue and fatty foods.

Antispasmodics (eg, tincture of belladonna) are helpful when cramps are severe. Drugs that inhibit intestinal peristalsis (paregoric, diphenoxylate with atropine [Lomotil]) may ameliorate symptoms but prolong fever, diarrhea, and excretion of *Shigella* in feces. The patient should be placed on effective stool isolation precautions both in the hospital and in the home to limit spread of infection.

### Prognosis

The prognosis is excellent in all but very young or debilitated patients if intravenous rehydration is available. The recent importation into the USA of the more virulent *S dysenteriae* from Central America—which may be ampicillin- and chloramphenicol-resistant—may make this illness a greater threat.

Centers for Disease Control: Shigellosis: United States, 1983. *MMWR* 1984;**33**:616.
Levine MM: Bacillary dysentery: Mechanisms and treatment. *Med Clin North Am* 1982;**66**:623.

## TRAVELER'S DIARRHEA

Whenever a person travels from one country to another, particularly if the change involves a marked difference in climate, social conditions, or sanitation standards and facilities, diarrhea is likely to develop within 2–10 days. There may be up to 10 or even more loose stools per day, often accompanied by abdominal cramps, nausea, occasionally vomiting, and, rarely, fever. The stools do not usually contain mucus or blood, and aside from weakness, dehydration, and occasionally acidosis, there are no systemic manifestations of infection. The illness usually subsides spontaneously within 1–5 days; rarely, it lasts 2–3 weeks.

Bacteriologic cultures of stools rarely reveal salmonellae or shigellae. Contributory causes may at times include unusual food and drink, change in living habits, occasional viral infections (enteroviruses or rotaviruses), and change in bowel flora. A significant number of cases of traveler's diarrhea are caused by acquisition of strains of *Escherichia coli* that produce a potent enterotoxin. This enterotoxin is released by the organisms growing in the small intestine, attaches to ganglioside receptors on intestinal villi, stimulates adenylate cyclase, and increases cyclic adenosine monophosphate concentration in the gut wall. As a result, there is hypersecretion of water and electrolytes into the gut, distention, and massive diarrhea. Strains of *E coli* that elaborate a heat-labile enterotoxin and are prevalent in a given environment appear to be particularly responsible, but heat-stable toxins (which activate guanylate cyclase) can also be involved. Some individuals are not susceptible because the multiplication of these organisms is limited in them; others are perhaps resistant to the enterotoxin because of prior exposure.

For most individuals the affliction is short-lived, and its effects may be further reduced by opiates or diphenoxylate with atropine (Lomotil). Antimicrobial drugs generally are not indicated and, indeed, may aggravate the diarrhea. For prophylaxis, bismuth subsalicylate suspension (Pepto-Bismol), 60 mL 4 times daily, has been suggested; or doxycycline, 200 mg on the first day of travel followed by 100 mg daily for 5–10 days. However, the risk of favoring colonization by drug-resistant *Shigella* or *Salmonella* is recognized. Many travelers might prefer to use caution with food and drink and take 160 mg trimethoprim plus 800 mg sulfamethoxazole daily for 3–5 days if traveler's diarrhea should develop. In all cases, water and electrolyte balance must be restored.

DuPont HL, Ericsson CD, Johnson PC: Chemotherapy and chemoprophylaxis of travelers' diarrhea. *Ann Intern Med* 1985;**102**:260.
DuPont HL et al: Prevention of travelers' diarrhea by the tablet formulation of bismuth subsalicylate. *JAMA* 1987;**257**:1347.
Gorbach SL, Edelman R: Travelers' diarrhea (NIH Consensus Development Conference). *Rev Infect Dis* 1986;**255**:S227.
Mathewson JJ et al: A newly recognized cause of travelers' diarrhea: Enteroadherent *Escherichia coli. J Infect Dis* 1985;**151**:471.

## BRUCELLOSIS

### Essentials of Diagnosis

- Insidious onset: easy fatigability, headache, arthralgia, anorexia, sweating, irritability.
- Intermittent fever, especially at night, which may become chronic and undulant.
- Cervical and axillary lymphadenopathy; hepatosplenomegaly.
- Lymphocytosis, positive blood culture, elevated agglutination titer.

### General Considerations

The infection is transmitted from animals to humans. *Brucella abortus* (cattle), *Brucella suis* (hogs), and *Brucella melitensis* (goats) are the main agents. Transmission to humans occurs by contact with infected meat (slaughterhouse workers), placentae of infected animals (farmers, veterinarians), or ingestion of infected unpasteurized milk or cheese. Organisms may enter through abraded skin or mucous membranes or via the respiratory tract. The incubation period varies from a few days to several weeks. The disorder may become chronic and persist for years. In the USA, brucellosis is very rare except in the midwestern states (from *B suis*) and in occasional outbreaks associated with consumption of goat cheese from Mexico.

### Clinical Findings

**A. Symptoms and Signs:** The onset may be acute, with fever, chills, and sweats, but often the disease begins so insidiously that it may be weeks before the patient seeks medical care for weakness and exhaustion upon minimal activity. Symptoms also include headache, abdominal pains with anorexia and constipation, and arthralgia, sometimes associated with periarticular swelling but not local heat. The fever may be septic, sustained, low-grade, or even absent but is more often of the intermittent type preceded by chilliness, rising during the evening hours and falling with a sweat (night sweat) in the early morning hours. The chronic form may assume an undulant nature, with periods of normal temperature between acute attacks, and the above symptoms plus emotional instability and weight loss may persist for years, either continuously or intermittently.

Physical findings are minimal. Half of cases have peripheral lymph node enlargement and splenomegaly; hepatomegaly is less common.

**B. Laboratory Findings:** The white count is usually normal to low, with a relative or absolute lymphocytosis. Early in the course of infection, the organism can be recovered from the blood, cerebrospinal fluid, urine, and bone marrow; later, this may be difficult. An agglutination titer greater than 1:100 (and especially a rising titer) supports the diagnosis. A prozone phenomenon (serum agglutinates in high but not in low dilution) is common. IgG antibody indicates active disease, whereas IgM antibody may persist after recovery. The intradermal skin test is of no value. Liver enzyme levels are often elevated.

### Differential Diagnosis

Brucellosis must be differentiated from any other acute febrile disease, especially influenza, tularemia, Q fever, and enteric fever. In its chronic form it resembles Hodgkin's disease, tuberculosis, and malaria. The chronic form may also simulate psychoneurosis, so that the latter is sometimes incorrectly given a diagnosis of chronic brucellosis.

### Complications

The most frequent complications are bone and joint lesions such as spondylitis and suppurative arthritis (usually of a single joint), subacute infective endocarditis, encephalitis, and meningitis. Less common complications are pneumonitis with pleural effusion, hepatitis, and cholecystitis. Abortion in humans is no more common with this disease than with any other acute bacterial disease during pregnancy. Pancytopenia is rare.

### Prevention

Prevention is by destruction of infected dairy animals, immunization of susceptible animals, and pasteurization of milk and milk products.

### Treatment

**A. Specific Measures:** Tetracycline, 2 g orally daily for 21 days, is the treatment of choice. Streptomycin, 0.5 g intramuscularly every 12 hours, is occasionally given at the same time as tetracycline. Relapse may require re-treatment. Ampicillin or trimethoprim-sulfamethoxazole may be effective.

**B. General Measures:** Place patient at bed rest during the acute febrile stage; maintain adequate nutrition.

### Prognosis

In a few cases, brucellosis may remain active for many years as an intermittent illness, but about 75% of patients recover completely within 3–6 months, and fewer than 20% have residual disease after 1 year. Treatment has considerably shortened the natural course of the disease. Brucellosis is rarely fatal in either the acute or the chronic form.

Young EJ: Human brucellosis. *Rev Infect Dis* 1983;**5**:821.

## GAS GANGRENE

### Essentials of Diagnosis

● Sudden onset of pain and edema in an area of wound contamination.
● Brown to blood-tinged watery exudate, with skin discoloration of surrounding area.
● Gas in the tissue by palpation or x-ray.
● Organisms in culture or smear of exudate.
● Prostration and systemic toxicity.

### General Considerations

Gas gangrene or clostridial myositis is produced by entry of one of several clostridia (*Clostridium perfringens, Clostridium ramosum, Clostridium bifermentans, Clostridium histolyticum, Clostridium novyi,* etc) into devitalized tissues. It grows and produces toxins under anaerobic conditions, resulting in shock, hemolysis, and myonecrosis. Alpha toxin (lecithinase) of *C perfringens* is the most potent. *Clostridium difficile,* an infrequent member of the normal gut flora, produces a toxin that can lead to pseudomembranous colitis, especially after antibiotic administration (see Chapter 21).

### Clinical Findings

**A. Symptoms and Signs:** The onset of gas gangrene is usually sudden, with rapidly increasing pain in the affected area accompanied by a fall in blood pressure, and tachycardia. The temperature may be elevated, but not proportionate to the severity of the inflammation. In the last stages of the disease, severe prostration, stupor, delirium, and coma occur.

The wound becomes swollen, and the surrounding skin is pale as a result of fluid accumulation beneath it. This is followed by a discharge of a brown to blood-tinged, serous, foul-smelling fluid from the wound. As the disease advances, the surrounding tissue changes from pale to dusky and finally becomes deeply discolored, with coalescent, red, fluid-filled vesicles. Gas may be palpable in the tissues. In clostridial sepsis, hemolysis and jaundice are common, often complicated by acute renal failure.

**B. Laboratory Findings:** Gas gangrene is a clinical rather than a bacteriologic diagnosis. Culture of the exudate confirms the diagnosis, and stained smears of the exudate showing the typical gram-positive rods (usually as part of a mixed flora) are valuable. Neither demonstration of clostridia in the smear from the wound nor the presence of gas is sufficient to make this diagnosis. The clinical picture must be present.

**C. Imaging:** Radiography may show gas in the soft tissues spreading along fascial planes.

## Differential Diagnosis

Other types of infection can cause gas formation in the tissue, eg, *Enterobacter, Escherichia,* and mixed anaerobic infections including *Bacteroides* and peptostreptococci. Clostridia may produce serious puerperal infection with hemolysis.

## Treatment

**A. Specific Measures:** Give penicillin, 2 million units every 3 hours as a bolus into an intravenous infusion. Polyvalent gas gangrene antitoxin is available but of dubious benefit.

**B. Surgical Measures:** Adequate surgical debridement and exposure of infected areas is essential. Radical surgical excision may be necessary. Hyperbaric oxygen therapy, if available, may be beneficial when used in conjunction with other measures. A tetanus toxoid booster injection should be given.

## Prognosis

Without treatment, the mortality rate is very high.

Darke SG et al: Gas gangrene and related infection: Classification, clinical features and aetiology, management and mortality: A report of 88 cases. *Br J Surg* 1977;**64:**104.

## TETANUS

### Essentials of Diagnosis

- Jaw stiffness followed by spasms of jaw muscles (trismus).
- Stiffness of the neck and other muscles, dysphagia, irritability, hyperreflexia.
- Finally, painful convulsions precipitated by minimal stimuli.
- History of wound and possible contamination.

### General Considerations

Tetanus is an acute intoxication by the neurotoxin elaborated by *Clostridium tetani.* Spores of this organism are ubiquitous in soil. When introduced into a wound in the presence of necrotic tissue and impaired circulation, the spores germinate. Spores may enter clean wounds. In the newborn, infection enters through the umbilical stump. The vegetative bacteria elaborate a toxin, tetanospasmin, that blocks the action of inhibitory mediators at spinal synapses and also interferes with neuromuscular transmission. As a result, minor stimuli result in uncontrolled spasms, and reflexes are enormously exaggerated. The incubation period is 5 days to 15 weeks, with the average being 8–12 days.

In the USA today, female heroin users ("skin poppers") are particularly at risk.

## Clinical Findings

**A. Symptoms and Signs:** Occasionally, the first symptom is pain and tingling at the site of inoculation, followed by spasticity of the group of muscles nearby, and this may be all that happens. More frequently, however, the presenting symptoms are stiffness of the jaw, neck stiffness, dysphagia, and irritability. Hyperreflexia develops later, with spasms of the jaw muscles (trismus) or facial muscles and rigidity and spasm of the muscles of the abdomen, neck, and back. Painful tonic convulsions precipitated by minor stimuli are common. The patient is awake and alert during the entire course of the illness. During convulsions the glottis and respiratory muscles go into spasm, so that the patient is unable to breathe and cyanosis and asphyxia may ensue. The temperature is only slightly elevated.

**B. Laboratory Findings:** The diagnosis of tetanus is made clinically. There is usually a polymorphonuclear leukocytosis.

## Differential Diagnosis

Tetanus must be differentiated from various acute central nervous system infections. Trismus may occasionally develop with the use of phenothiazines. Strychnine poisoning should also be considered.

## Complications

Airway obstruction and anoxia are common. Urinary retention and constipation may result from spasm of the sphincters. Respiratory arrest and cardiac failure are late, life-threatening events.

## Prevention

Active immunization with tetanus toxoid should be universal. It is an essential part of childhood immunization, usually given as DTP (see p 831). For adults, give Td toxoid as recommended by manufacturers. Booster doses of toxoid should be given about every 10 years or at the time of a major injury.

Passive immunization should be used in nonimmunized individuals and those whose immunization status is uncertain whenever the wound is contaminated, major, or likely to have devitalized tissue. Tetanus immune globulin, 250 units intramuscularly, is the preferred agent. Tetanus antitoxin (equine or bovine) in a dose of 3000–5000 units should be used (after testing for serum hypersensitivity) only if tetanus immune globulin is not available. Active immunization with tetanus toxoid should be started concurrently. Table 23–2 provides a guide to prophylactic management.

Adequate debridement of wounds is an essential preventive measure. In suspect cases, benzathine penicillin G, 1.2 million units intramuscularly, may be a reasonable adjunctive measure.

## Treatment

**A. Specific Measures:** Give tetanus immune globulin, 5000 units intramuscularly; this antitoxin does not cause sensitivity reactions. If tetanus immune

**Table 23–2.** Guide to tetanus prophylaxis in wound management (United States, 1985). (Modified from *MMWR* 1985;**34:** 405.)

| History of Absorbed Tetanus Toxoid (Doses) | Clean, Minor Wounds | | All Other Wounds* | |
|---|---|---|---|---|
| | Td | TIG | Td | TIG |
| Unknown or <3 | Yes | No | Yes | Yes |
| ≥3 | Not† | No | Not‡ | No |

Td = tetanus toxoid and diphtheria toxoid, adult form. Use only this preparation (Td-adult) in children older than 6 years.
TIG = tetanus immune globulin.
* Such as, but not limited to, wounds contaminated with dirt, feces, soil, saliva, etc; puncture wounds; avulsions; and wounds resulting from missiles, crushing, burns, and frostbite.
† Yes, if more than 10 years since last dose.
‡ Yes, if more than 5 years since last dose. (More frequent boosters are not needed and can accentuate side effects.)

globulin is not available, give tetanus antitoxin, 100,000 units intravenously, after testing for horse serum sensitivity. The value of antitoxin treatment has been questioned.

**B. General Measures:** Place the patient at bed rest and minimize stimulation. Sedation and anticonvulsant therapy are essential. Experience from areas of high incidence suggests that most convulsions can be eliminated by treatment with chlorpromazine (50–100 mg 4 times daily) or diazepam combined with a sedative (amobarbital, phenobarbital, or meprobamate). Mild cases of tetanus can be controlled with one or the other rather than both. Only rarely is general curarization required. Other recommended anticonvulsant regimens are tribromoethanol, 15–25 mg/kg rectally every 1–4 hours as needed; and amobarbital sodium, 5 mg/kg intramuscularly as needed. Paraldehyde, 4–8 mL intravenously (2–5% solution), may be combined with barbiturates. Penicillin is of value but should not be substituted for antitoxin.

Give intravenous fluids as necessary. Tracheostomy may be required for laryngeal spasm. Assisted respiration is required in conjunction with curarization. Hyperbaric oxygen therapy is of no established value.

**Prognosis**

The mortality rate is higher in very small children and very old people; with shorter incubation periods; with shorter intervals between onset of symptoms and the first convulsion; and with delay in treatment. If trismus develops early, the prognosis is grave. The overall mortality rate is about 40%. Contaminated lesions about the head and face are more dangerous than wounds on other parts of the body.

If the patient survives, recovery is complete.

Edmondson RS, Flowers MW: Intensive care in tetanus: Management, complications and mortality in 100 cases. *Br Med J* 1979;**1:**1401.

Immunization Practices Advisory Committee, Centers for Disease Control: Diphtheria, tetanus and pertussis: Guidelines for vaccine prophylaxis and other preventive measures. *MMWR* 1985;**34:**405.

# BOTULISM

## Essentials of Diagnosis

- Sudden onset of cranial nerve paralysis, diplopia, dry mouth, dysphagia, dysphonia, and muscle weakness progressing to respiratory paralysis.
- History of recent ingestion of home-canned, smoked, or unusual foods.
- Demonstration of toxin in serum or food.

## General Considerations

Botulism is food poisoning caused by ingestion of the toxin (usually type A, B, or E) of *Clostridium botulinum*, a strict anaerobic spore-forming bacillus found widespread in soil. Canned, smoked, or vacuum-packed anaerobic foods are involved—particularly home-canned vegetables, smoked meats, and vacuum-packed fish. The toxins block the release of acetylcholine from nerve endings. Clinically, there is early nervous system involvement leading to respiratory paralysis. The mortality rate in untreated cases is high. Botulism may follow wound infection.

## Clinical Findings

**A. Symptoms and Signs:** Twelve to 36 hours after ingestion of the toxin, visual disturbances appear, particularly diplopia and loss of power of accommodation. Other symptoms are dry throat and mouth, dysphagia, and dysphonia. There may be nausea and vomiting, particularly with type E toxin. Muscle weakness is prominent. The edrophonium (Tensilon) test gives typical results, and respiration is impaired, but the sensorium remains clear and the temperature normal. Progressive respiratory paralysis may lead to death unless mechanical assistance is provided.

**Infant botulism.** Infants in the first few months of life may present with weakness, generalized hypotonicity, and electromyographic findings compatible with botulism. Both botulinus organisms and toxin are found in the stool but not in serum. The cause of this syndrome is not known, but honey fed to infants has been incriminated.

**B. Laboratory Findings:** Most routine determinations are within normal limits. Toxin in the patient's serum and in suspected foods may be shown by mouse inoculation and identified with specific antiserum.

## Differential Diagnosis

Cranial nerve involvement suggests bulbar poliomyelitis, myasthenia gravis, stroke, infectious neuronitis, or tick paralysis. Nausea and vomiting may suggest intestinal obstruction or other types of food poisoning.

## Complications

The dysphagia may cause aspiration pneumonia; such infection and respiratory paralysis are the usual causes of death.

## Prevention

Home-canned vegetables must be sterilized to destroy spores. Sterilization standards for commercial canned or vacuum-packed foods must be strictly enforced. Boiling food for 20 minutes can inactivate the toxin, but punctured or swollen cans or jars with defective seals should be discarded. Early and adequate treatment of wounds prevents wound botulism.

## Treatment

As soon as the clinical diagnosis of botulism is suspected, the Centers for Disease Control should be consulted (central number: [404] 329–3311). That agency can ship pentavalent (A, B, C, D, E) botulinus antitoxin by air or can request release of trivalent (A, B, E) antitoxin from one of several regional quarantine centers in the USA. The Centers for Disease Control can also assay for toxin in the patient's serum or stool, as well as the suspect food item. Two vials of antitoxin are administered to the patient if tests for hypersensitivity are negative.

Adequate ventilation and oxygenation must be maintained by good respiratory drainage (elevate foot of bed), removal of respiratory obstruction by aspiration or tracheostomy, and mechanical respirator if necessary.

Parenteral fluids or alimentation are given as necessary. Give nothing by mouth while swallowing difficulty persists. If pneumonitis develops, appropriate antimicrobials are used.

Guanidine hydrochloride, 15–35 mg/kg/d orally, has been used experimentally with occasional benefit.

The removal of unabsorbed toxin from the gut may be attempted if it can be done very soon after ingestion of the suspected toxin. Any remnants of suspected foods must be saved for analysis. Persons who might have eaten the suspected food must be located and observed.

## Prognosis

If good ventilation can be maintained and the toxin promptly neutralized, the mortality rate may be substantially lower than the 30–70% that is to be expected in untreated patients. If the patient survives the attack of botulism, there are no neurologic residua.

Arnon SS: Infant botulism: Anticipating the second decade. *J Infect Dis* 1986;**154**:201.

Bartlett JC: Infant botulism in adults. *N Engl J Med* 1986;**315**:254.

Dowell VR: Botulism and tetanus: Selected epidemiologic and microbiologic aspects. *Rev Infect Dis* 1984;**6**:5202.

Simpson LL: The action of botulinal toxin. *Rev Infect Dis* 1979;**1**:656.

## ANTHRAX

Anthrax is a disease of sheep, cattle, horses, goats, and swine caused by *Bacillus anthracis,* a gram-positive spore-forming aerobe transmitted to humans by entry through broken skin or mucous membranes or, less commonly, by inhalation. Human infection is rare. It is most apt to occur in farmers, veterinarians, and tannery and wool workers. Several clinical forms have been observed. Rarely, other gram-positive spore-forming bacilli (eg, *Bacillus cereus*) are found in sepsis, meningitis, or endocarditis. *B cereus* produces an enterotoxin.

## Clinical Findings

**A. Symptoms and Signs:**

**1. Cutaneous anthrax ("malignant pustule")**–An erythematous papule appears on an exposed area of skin and becomes vesicular, with a purple to black center. The area around the lesion is swollen or edematous and surrounded by vesicles. The center of the lesion finally forms a necrotic eschar and sloughs. Regional adenopathy, variable fever, malaise, headache, and nausea and vomiting may be present. After the eschar sloughs, hematogenous spread and sepsis may occur, at times manifested by shock, cyanosis, sweating, and collapse. Hemorrhagic meningitis may also occur.

Anthrax sepsis sometimes develops without a skin lesion.

**2. Pulmonary anthrax ("woolsorter's disease")**–This follows the inhalation of spores from hides, bristles, or wool. It is characterized by fever, malaise, headache, dyspnea, and cough; congestion of the nose, throat, and larynx; and evidence of pneumonia or mediastinitis. Very rarely, gram-positive spore-forming aerobic bacilli other than *B anthracis* (eg, *B cereus*) can produce a similar disease.

**B. Laboratory Findings:** The white count may be elevated or low. Sputum or blood culture may be positive for *B anthracis*. Smears of skin lesions show gram-positive encapsulated rods, and cultures should be attempted. Antibodies may be detected by an indirect hemagglutination test.

## Treatment

Give penicillin G, 10 million units intravenously daily; or, in mild, localized cases, tetracycline, 0.5 g orally every 6 hours.

## Prognosis

The prognosis is excellent in the cutaneous form of the disease if treatment is given early. Sepsis and pulmonary anthrax have a grave prognosis. Bacteremia is a very unfavorable sign.

LaForce FM: Woolsorters' disease in England. *Bull NY Acad Med* 1978;**54**:956.

## TULAREMIA

### Essentials of Diagnosis

- Fever, headache, nausea, and prostration.
- Papule progressing to ulcer at site of inoculation.
- Enlarged regional lymph nodes.
- History of contact with rabbits, other rodents, and biting arthropods (eg, ticks in summer) in endemic area.

- Confirmed by culture of ulcer, lymph node aspirate, or blood.

## General Considerations

Tularemia is an infection of wild rodents—particularly rabbits and muskrats—with *Francisella* (*Pasteurella*) *tularensis*. It is transmitted from animals to humans by contact with animal tissues (eg, trapping muskrats, skinning rabbits); by the bite of certain ticks and biting flies; by consumption of infected, undercooked meat; or by drinking contaminated water. Infection in humans often produces a local lesion and widespread organ involvement but may be entirely asymptomatic. The incubation period is 2–10 days.

## Clinical Findings

**A. Symptoms and Signs:** Fever, headache, and nausea begin suddenly, and a local lesion—a papule at the site of inoculation—develops and soon ulcerates. Regional lymph nodes become enlarged and tender and may suppurate. The local lesion may be on the skin of an extremity (ulceroglandular) or in the eye. Pneumonia may develop from hematogenous spread of the organism or may be primary after inhalation of infected aerosols. Following ingestion of infected meat or water, an enteric form (typhoidal) may be manifested by enteritis, stupor, and delirium. In any type of involvement, the spleen may be enlarged and tender and there may be rashes, generalized aches, and prostration. Asymptomatic infection is not rare.

**B. Laboratory Findings:** The white blood count is slightly elevated or normal. Culture of blood, an ulcerated lesion, or lymph node aspirate yields the organisms in special culture media early in the illness. A positive agglutination test (more than 1:80) develops in the second week after infection and may persist for several years. A delayed type skin test (read in 48 hours) becomes positive within a few days after infection; about 50% of patients have a positive skin test when first seen. The skin test (positive is more than 5 mm induration) is highly specific; it remains positive longer after infection than does the agglutination test, but skin test material is rarely available.

## Differential Diagnosis

Tularemia must be differentiated from rickettsial and meningococcal infections, cat-scratch disease, infectious mononucleosis, and various pneumonias and fungal diseases. Epidemiologic considerations, positive skin tests, and rising agglutination titers are the chief differential points.

## Complications

Hematogenous spread to any organ may produce severe problems, particularly meningitis, perisplenitis, pericarditis, and pneumonia.

## Treatment

Streptomycin, 0.5 g intramuscularly every 6–8 hours, together with tetracycline, 0.5 g orally every 6 hours, is administered until 4–5 days after the patient becomes afebrile. Chloramphenicol may be substituted for tetracycline in the same dosage. Adequate fluid intake is essential, and oxygen may be required. Suppurating lymph nodes may be aspirated but should not be incised during the first week if the process is still localized. Later in the disease, drainage of fluctuant nodes may be needed and is safe after proper chemotherapy for several days.

## Prognosis

The mortality rate of untreated ulceroglandular tularemia is 5%; that of tularemic pneumonia, 30%. Early chemotherapy is promptly effective and prevents fatalities. Skin tests and agglutination tests suggest that subclinical infection is common in outbreaks of tularemia.

## Prevention

Awareness of the risk of infection through contact with potentially infected rodents, biting insects, or water supply is helpful.

Evans ME et al: Tularemia: A 30-year experience with 88 cases. *Medicine* 1985;**64**:251.

Markowitz LE et al: Tick-borne tularemia. *JAMA* 1985;**254**:2922.

## PLAGUE

### Essentials of Diagnosis

- Sudden onset of high fever, malaise, muscular pains, and prostration.
- Axillary or inguinal lymphadenitis (bubo).
- Bacteremia, sepsis, and pneumonitis may occur.
- History of exposure to rodents in endemic area.
- Positive smear and culture from bubo and positive blood culture.

### General Considerations

Plague is an infection of wild rodents with *Yersinia* (*Pasteurella*) *pestis,* a small gram-negative rod. It is transmitted from one rodent to another and from rodents to humans by the bites of fleas. Plague bacilli grow in the gut of the flea and obstruct it. When the hungry flea sucks blood, it regurgitates organisms into the bite wound. Feces of fleas may also transmit the infection. If a plague victim develops pneumonia, the infection can be transmitted by droplets to other persons and an epidemic may be started in this way. The incubation period is 2–10 days.

Following the flea bite, the organisms spread through the lymphatics to the lymph nodes, which become greatly enlarged (bubo). They may then reach the bloodstream to involve all organs. When pneumonia or meningitis develops, the outcome is often fatal.

### Clinical Findings

**A. Symptoms and Signs:** The onset is usually sudden, with high fever, malaise, tachycardia, intense headache, and generalized muscular aches. The patient appears profoundly ill and very anxious. Delirium may ensue. If pneumonia develops, tachypnea, productive cough, blood-tinged sputum, and cyanosis also occur. Meningeal signs may develop. A pustule or ulcer at the site of inoculation and signs of lymphangitis may occur. Axillary, inguinal, or cervical lymph nodes become enlarged and tender and may eventually suppurate and drain. With hematogenous spread, the patient may rapidly become toxic and comatose, with purpuric spots (black plague) appearing on the skin.

Primary plague pneumonia results from the inhalation of bacilli in droplets coughed up by another patient with plague pneumonia. This is a fulminant pneumonitis with bloody, frothy sputum and sepsis and is usually fatal in unimmunized persons unless treatment is started within a few hours of onset.

**B. Laboratory Findings:** Peripheral white counts range from 12 to 20 thousand/μL. The plague bacillus may be found in smears from aspirates of buboes examined with Gram's or immunofluorescent stain. Cultures from bubo aspirate or pus and blood are positive but may grow slowly. In convalescing patients, an antibody titer rise may be demonstrated by agglutination tests.

**C. Imaging:** Pulmonary infiltration in a person suspected of having plague implies a grave prognosis and should lead to strict isolation.

### Differential Diagnosis

The lymphadenitis of plague is most commonly mistaken for the lymphadenitis accompanying staphylococcal or streptococcal infections of an extremity, sexually transmitted diseases such as lymphogranuloma venereum or syphilis, and tularemia. The systemic manifestations resemble those of enteric or rickettsial fevers, malaria, or influenza. The pneumonia resembles other severe gram-negative or staphylococcal pneumonias.

### Prevention

Periodic surveys of rodents and their ectoparasites in endemic areas provide guidelines for the need for extensive rodent and flea control measures. Total eradication of plague from wild rodents in an endemic area ("sylvatic plague") is rarely possible.

Drug prophylaxis may provide temporary protection for persons exposed to the risk of plague infection, particularly by the respiratory route. Tetracycline hydrochloride, 500 mg orally 1–2 times daily for 5 days, can accomplish this.

Plague vaccines—both live and killed—have been used for many years, but their efficacy is not clearly established. The USP formol-killed suspension gives some protection. It is given as directed by the manufacturer, usually in 2 doses 4 weeks apart, followed by a booster dose. For continued exposure, subsequent boosters are given every 6–12 months.

### Treatment

Therapy must be started promptly when plague is suspected. Give streptomycin, 1 g intramuscularly, immediately, and then 0.5 g intramuscularly every 6–8 hours. Tetracycline, 2 g daily orally (parenterally if necessary), is given at the same time. Intravenous fluids, pressor drugs, oxygen, and tracheostomy are used as required.

### Prognosis

If the diagnosis can be made and treatment started relatively early, most patients with bubonic plague will recover. In untreated cases, the mortality rate may range from 20 to 60%. When gross sepsis, pneumonia, and shock supervene, the outlook is poor. Primary pneumonic plague is almost invariably fatal unless treated intensively within hours of onset.

Mann JM et al: Peripatetic plague. *JAMA* 1982;**247**:47.
Werner SB et al: Primary plague pneumonia contracted from a domestic cat at South Lake Tahoe, Calif. *JAMA* 1984;**251**:929.

## LEPROSY

### Essentials of Diagnosis

- Pale, anesthetic macular—or nodular and erythematous—skin lesions.
- Superficial nerve thickening with associated sensory changes.
- History of residence in endemic area in childhood.
- Acid-fast bacilli in skin lesions or nasal scrapings, or characteristic histologic nerve changes.

### General Considerations

Leprosy is a chronic infectious disease caused by the acid-fast rod *Mycobacterium leprae*. The mode of transmission is unknown but probably involves prolonged exposure in childhood. Only rarely have adults become infected (eg, by tattooing). The disease is endemic in tropical and subtropical Asia, Africa, Central and South America and the Pacific regions, and the southern USA.

### Clinical Findings

**A. Symptoms and Signs:** The onset is insidious. The lesions involve the cooler body tissues: skin, superficial nerves, nose, pharynx, larynx, eyes, and testicles. Skin lesions may occur as pale, anesthetic macular lesions 1–10 cm in diameter; discrete erythematous, infiltrated nodules 1–5 cm in diameter; or a diffuse skin infiltration. Neurologic disturbances are manifested by nerve infiltration and thickening, with resultant anesthesia, neuritis, paresthesia, trophic ulcers, and bone resorption and shortening of digits. In untreated cases, disfigurement due to the skin infiltration and nerve involvement may be extreme.

The disease is divided clinically and by laboratory tests into 2 distinct types: lepromatous and tuberculoid. In the lepromatous type, the course is progressive and malignant, with nodular skin lesions; slow, symmetric nerve involvement; abundant acid-fast bacilli in the skin lesions; and a negative lepromin skin test. The patient has impaired cellular immunity. In the tuberculoid type, the course is benign and nonprogressive, with macular skin lesions, severe asymmetric nerve involvement of sudden onset with few bacilli present in the lesions, and a positive lepromin skin test. Intermediate (''borderline'') cases are frequent. Eye involvement (keratitis and iridocyclitis), nasal ulcers, epistaxis, anemia, and lymphadenopathy may occur.

**B. Laboratory Findings:** Laboratory confirmation of leprosy requires the demonstration of acid-fast bacilli in scrapings from slit skin smears or the nasal septum. Biopsy of skin or of a thickened involved nerve also gives a typical histologic picture.

*M leprae* has not been grown in culture media, but it multiplies in experimentally injected mouse foot pads and in armadillos.

### Differential Diagnosis

The skin lesions of leprosy often resemble those of lupus erythematosus, sarcoidosis, syphilis, erythema nodosum, erythema multiforme, and vitiligo. Nerve involvement, sensory dissociation, and resulting deformity may require differentiation from syringomyelia and scleroderma.

### Complications

Intercurrent pulmonary tuberculosis is common in the lepromatous type, probably because of deficient cellular immunity. Amyloidosis may occur with long-standing disease.

### Prevention

Experimental vaccines made from animal-grown *M leprae* are promising for the immunization of children. Drugs and vaccines are being tested for prophylaxis in family contacts of patients with lepromatous leprosy.

### Treatment

Drugs should be given cautiously, with slowly increasing doses, and must be withheld when they induce an exacerbation called ''lepra reaction'': fever, progressive anemia with or without leukopenia; severe gastrointestinal symptoms, allergic dermatitis, hepatitis, or mental disturbances; or erythema nodosum. It is important, therefore, to observe temperature, blood counts, and biopsy changes in lesions at regular intervals. Corticosteroids are valuable in lepra reactions. The duration of treatment must be guided by progress, preferably as judged by biopsy. Treatment must be continued for several years or indefinitely, because recrudescence may occur after cessation of therapy. No isolation procedures are warranted for patients under treatment.

Dapsone (DDS) is given orally, 50–100 mg/d. It is widely used because of efficacy, low cost, and low toxicity. DDS-resistant *M leprae* is found in 10–30% of patients on long-term treatment and occasionally in untreated persons. The likelihood of DDS resistance is reduced if rifampin is given simultaneously. If fever, granulocytopenia, or jaundice develops, DDS is discontinued and clofazimine is given. Rifampin, 10 mg/kg/d up to 600 mg/d orally, is given together with a second drug (eg, DDS). Rifampin is effective but costly. Clofazimine, 1–4 mg/kg/d orally, is given mainly in DDS-resistant lepromatous leprosy. Thalidomide, 100–400 mg/d orally, is valuable for management of erythema nodosum of leprosy (ENL) in nonpregnant patients. Corticosteroids are also useful. Surgical care of extremities can prevent deformity.

### Prognosis

Untreated lepromatous leprosy is progressive and fatal in 10–20 years. In the tuberculoid type, spontaneous arrest usually occurs in 1–3 years; it may, however, produce crippling deformities.

With treatment, the lepromatous type regresses slowly (over a period of 3–8 years). Recovery from the tuberculoid type is more rapid. Recrudescences are always possible, and it may be safe to assume that the bacilli are never eradicated. Deformities persist after complete recovery and may markedly interfere with function and appearance.

Levy L, Noordene SK, Sansarri CQ: Increase in prevalence of leprosy caused by dapsone-resistant *Mycobacterium leprae. MMWR* (Jan 8) 1982;**30**:637.

Shepard CC: Leprosy today. *N Engl J Med* 1982;**307**:1640.

## CHANCROID

Chancroid is an acute, localized, sexually transmitted disease caused by the short gram-negative bacillus *Haemophilus ducreyi*. Infection occurs by sexual contact, although nonvenereal inoculation has occurred in medical personnel through contact with chancroid patients. The incubation period is 3–5 days.

The initial lesion at the site of inoculation is a vesicopustule that breaks down to form a painful, soft ulcer with a necrotic base, surrounding erythema, and undermined edges. Multiple lesions—started by autoinoculation—and inguinal adenitis often develop. The adenitis is usually unilateral and consists of tender, matted nodes of moderate size with overlying erythema. The nodal mass softens, becomes fluctuant, and may rupture spontaneously. With lymph node involvement, fever, chills, and malaise may develop. These signs occur more commonly in men, whereas no external signs may be evident in women, although they can serve as sources of infection for contacts.

Swabs from lesions are best cultured on chocolate agar with 1% Isovitalex and vancomycin, 3 μg/mL, to yield *Haemophilus ducreyi*. The chancroid skin test may become positive and remain positive for life. Mixed sexually transmitted disease is very common (including syphilis and herpes), as is infection of the ulcer with fusiforms, spirochetes, and other organisms.

Balanitis and phimosis are frequent complications. Chancroid must be differentiated from other genital ulcers. The chancre of syphilis is clean and painless, with a hard base.

Treat with erythromycin, 0.5 g orally 4 times daily for 10 days, or with trimethoprim-sulfamethoxazole for 7 days. Cleaning the ulcers with soap and water promotes healing. Fluctuant buboes may be aspirated by needle. Chancroid tends to respond to treatment and to be self-limited.

Plummer FA et al: Single dose therapy of chancroid with trimethoprim-sulfametrole. *N Engl J Med* 1983;**309**:67.

## GONORRHEA

### Essentials of Diagnosis

- Purulent urethral discharge, especially in men, with dysuria, yielding positive smear.
- Cervicitis with purulent discharge, or asymptomatic, yielding positive culture.
- Epididymitis, prostatitis, periurethral inflammation, proctitis in men.
- Vaginitis, salpingitis, proctitis in women.
- Fever, arthritis, skin lesions, conjunctivitis, pharyngitis.
- Gram-negative intracellular diplococci seen in a smear from the male urethra or cultured from any site, particularly the urethra, cervix, and rectum.

### General Considerations

Gonorrhea is the most prevalent reportable communicable disease in the USA, with an estimated 2.5 million or more infectious cases annually. It is caused by *Neisseria gonorrhoeae,* a gram-negative diplococcus typically found inside polymorphonuclear cells. It is most commonly transmitted during sexual activity and has its greatest incidence in the 15- to 29-year-old age group. The incubation period is usually 2–8 days.

### Clinical Findings

**A. Symptoms and Signs:**

**1. Men**–Initially, there is burning on urination and a serous or milky discharge. One to 3 days later, the urethral pain is more pronounced and the discharge becomes yellow, creamy, and profuse, sometimes blood-tinged. Without treatment, the disorder may regress and become chronic or progress to involve the prostate, epididymis, and periurethral glands with acute, painful inflammation. This in turn becomes chronic, with prostatitis and urethral strictures. Rectal infection is common in homosexual men. Unusual sites of primary infection (eg, the pharynx) must always be considered. Systemic involvement is listed below. Asymptomatic infection is common.

**2. Women**–Dysuria, frequency, and urgency may occur, with a purulent urethral discharge. Vaginitis and cervicitis with inflammation of Bartholin's glands are common. Most often, however, the infection is asymptomatic, with only slightly increased vaginal discharge and moderate cervicitis on examination. Infection may remain as a chronic cervicitis—a main reservoir of gonococci in any community. It may progress to involve the uterus and tubes with acute and chronic salpingitis and with ultimate scarring of tubes and sterility. In pelvic inflammatory disease, anaerobes and chlamydiae often accompany gonococci. Rectal infection is common both as spread of the organism from the genital tract and as a result of infection by anal coitus. Systemic involvement is listed below.

**B. Laboratory Findings:** Smears of urethral discharge in men, especially during the first week after onset, usually show typical gram-negative diplococci in polymorphonuclear leukocytes. Smears are less often positive in women. Cultures are essential in all cases where gonorrhea should be suspected and gonococci cannot be shown in gram-stained smears. This applies particularly to cervical, rectal, pharyngeal, and joint specimens. Specimens of pus or secretions are streaked on a selective medium such as Thayer-Martin or Transgrow. The latter is suitable for transport if a laboratory is not immediately available. The medium must be 20 °C when inoculated and must be incubated at 37 °C in a 10% $CO_2$ atmosphere (closed Transgrow bottle; Thayer-Martin in candle jar). Colonies are identified by oxidase test, Gram's stain, or immunofluorescence. No good serologic test is available.

### Differential Diagnosis

The chief alternatives to acute gonococcal urethritis or cervicitis are nongonococcal urethritis; cervicitis or vaginitis due to *Chlamydia trachomatis, Gardnerella (Haemophilus) vaginalis, Trichomonas, Candida,* and many other agents associated with sexually transmitted diseases; pelvic inflammatory disease, arthritis, proctitis, and skin lesions. Often, several such agents coexist in a patient. Reiter's disease (urethritis, conjunctivitis, arthritis) may mimic gonorrhea or coexist with it.

### Complications

The forms of local extension of the initial infection have been described. Systemic complications follow the dissemination of gonococci from the primary site (eg, genital tract) via the bloodstream. Gonococci that produce bacteremia and dissemination are resistant to serum but usually sensitive to penicillin. They belong to certain nutritionally deficient auxotypes. In contrast, strains producing local gonorrhea are susceptible to the bactericidal action of serum but often drug-resistant. Gonococcal bacteremia is associated with intermittent fever, arthralgia, and skin lesions ranging from maculopapular to pustular or hemorrhagic. Rarely, gonococcal endocarditis or meningitis develops. Arthritis and tenosynovitis are common complications, particularly involving the knees, ankles, and wrists. Several joints are commonly involved. Gonococci can be isolated from less than half of patients with gonococcal arthritis. In the others, some immunologic reaction may be responsible. Gonococcal arthritis may be accompanied by iritis or conjunctivitis, with negative cultures. The most common form of eye involvement is direct inoculation of gonococci into the conjunctival sac. This may occur during passage through an infected birth canal, leading to ophthalmia neonatorum, or by autoinoculation of a person with genital infection. The purulent conjunctivitis may rapidly progress to panophthalmitis and loss of the eye unless treated promptly.

## Prevention

Prevention is based on education, mechanical or chemical prophylaxis, and early diagnosis and treatment. The condom, if properly used, can reduce the risk of infection. Effective drugs taken in therapeutic doses within 24 hours of exposure can abort an infection, but prophylaxis with penicillin is no longer effective; in fact, penicillin prophylaxis contributes to the selection of penicillinase-producing gonococci. Intensive search for sex contacts by public health agencies must rely on physician reporting. Contacts are sometimes given full treatment for gonorrhea on epidemiologic grounds, without individual diagnosis, to reduce the reservoir of infection.

Ophthalmic infection of the newborn is prevented by the instillation of 0.5% erythromycin ointment, 1% tetracycline ointment, or 1% silver nitrate solution into each conjunctival sac immediately after birth. Ceftriaxone, 125 mg intramuscularly once, is effective against both eye and systemic infections.

## Treatment

The choice of drug reflects the emergence of tetracycline resistance and the increase in penicillin resistance among gonococci.

**A. Uncomplicated Gonorrhea:** All sexual partners should be treated.

For urethritis or cervicitis, give amoxicillin, 3 g orally, plus probenecid, 1 g orally, once; or ceftriaxone, 125–250 mg intramuscularly once. Anal gonorrhea in women responds to the same drugs, but in males only ceftriaxone is effective. Pharyngeal gonorrhea responds to ceftriaxone in the same dosage or to trimethoprim-sulfamethoxazole, 9 regular tablets orally for 5 days.

If coexistent chlamydial infection is suspected, the above courses should be followed by erythromycin or tetracycline, 500 mg 4 times daily orally, for 7 days. The latter is sometimes given concurrently.

Several alternative regimens are available, eg, procaine penicillin G, 4.8 million units intramuscularly once with probenecid, 1 g orally once.

**B. Penicillin-Resistant Gonorrhea:** β-Lactamase-producing gonococci are increasing in frequency. For such infections, give ceftriaxone, 125–250 mg intramuscularly once, or spectinomycin or cefoxitin, 2 g intramuscularly once, with probenecid, 1 g orally once.

**C. Follow-Up:** Single-dose intramuscular treatment presents no problem of patient compliance, which may be doubtful in the case of multidose oral treatment. Urethral, rectal, or pharyngeal specimens should be obtained from men 1 week after treatment. Cervical, rectal, or pharyngeal specimens should be obtained from women 7–14 days after completion of treatment. Serologic tests for syphilis are desirable 1 and 3 months later. All sexual partners should be followed after treatment.

**D. Treatment of Complications:** Salpingitis, prostatitis, bacteremia, arthritis, ophthalmia, and other complications in adults should be treated with penicillin G, 10 million units intravenously daily, for 5–10 days. Alternative drugs are ceftriaxone, or cefotaxime, or cefoxitin, 2–4 g intravenously daily for 10 days.

Postgonococcal urethritis or cervicitis is treated with tetracycline or erythromycin, 0.5 g orally 4 times daily, for 7–10 days. Gonococcal ophthalmia requires both topical and systemic drugs. Pelvic inflammatory disease requires cefoxitin, 2 g parenterally, once or twice daily until improvement is noted, each dose being accompanied by probenecid, 1 g orally. Concurrent treatment for chlamydial infection may be indicated. Alternative drug choices exist.

Additional supportive treatment is needed for most complications. Prostatitis may be relieved by hot sitz baths or diathermy; acute epididymitis requires bed rest, cold and support to the scrotum, and analgesics. Acute salpingitis requires bed rest during the acute stage, and surgical evaluation if chronic pain and signs of inflammation continue. Aspiration of joints may be necessary to relieve high pressure; physical therapy must be started when inflammation subsides.

## Prognosis

The regimens given above cure 95% of acute gonococcal infections, although the steady rise in resistance to drugs is responsible for an increasing number of relapses that require re-treatment. The complications of gonorrhea may cause irreversible damage (urethral stricture, persistent tubo-ovarian abscess, valve destruction in endocarditis, peritoneal adhesions with intestinal obstruction, sterility, etc) requiring surgical treatment.

Follow-up examinations cannot distinguish failures of chemotherapy from reinfection. Furthermore, the patient with acute gonorrhea may have undetected syphilis, genital herpes, or chlamydial infection from the same exposure or from more than one infected source. All of these must be detected by laboratory procedures in repeated follow-up. The recommended parenteral penicillin schedules are probably curative for most cases of coexisting syphilis. Patients treated with other antimicrobials will require additional penicillin treatment if serologic tests for syphilis become positive during 4 months following treatment for gonorrhea.

Centers for Disease Control: Sexually transmitted diseases: Treatment guidelines 1985. *MMWR* 1985;**34**:81S.

Jaffe HW et al: Infections due to penicillinase-producing *Neisseria gonorrheae* in the United States. *J Infect Dis* 1981;**144**:191.

O'Brien JP, Goldenberg DL, Rice PA: Disseminated gonococcal infection: A prospective analysis of 49 patients and a review of pathophysiology and immune mechanisms. *Medicine* 1983;**62**:395.

Rice RJ, Thompson SE: Treatment of uncomplicated infections due to *N gonorrhoeae. JAMA* 1986;**255**:1739.

Treatment of sexually transmitted diseases. *Med Lett Drugs Ther* 1986;**28**:21.

## GRANULOMA INGUINALE

Granuloma inguinale is a chronic, relapsing granulomatous anogenital infection due to *Calymmatobacterium (Donovania) granulomatis,* which is related to *Klebsiella* and occurs intracellularly. The pathognomonic cell, found in tissue scrapings or secretions, is large (25–90 $\mu$m) and contains intracytoplasmic cysts filled with bodies (Donovan bodies) that stain deeply with Wright's stain.

The incubation period is 8 days to 12 weeks.

The onset is insidious. The lesions occur on the skin or mucous membranes of the genitalia or perineal area. They are relatively painless infiltrated nodules that soon slough. A shallow, sharply demarcated ulcer forms, with a beefy-red friable base of granulation tissue. The lesion spreads by contiguity. The advancing border has a characteristic rolled edge of granulation tissue. Large ulcerations may advance onto the lower abdomen and thighs. Scar formation and healing may occur along one border while the opposite border advances. The process may become indolent.

The characteristic Donovan bodies are found in scrapings from the ulcer base or on histologic sections. The microorganism may also be cultured on special media. A specific complement fixation test is not widely available.

Superinfection with spirochete-fusiform organisms is common. The ulcer then becomes purulent, painful, foul-smelling, and extremely difficult to treat. Other sexually transmitted diseases may coexist. Rare complications include superimposed malignancy and secondary elephantoid swelling of the genitalia.

Initial treatment consists of tetracycline or ampicillin, 2 g orally daily for 2 weeks.

With antimicrobial therapy, most cases can be cured. In resistant or untreated cases, massive extension of the lesion may occur, with resulting anemia, cachexia, and death.

Washing the genitalia with soap and water immediately after intercourse may reduce the likelihood of infection. A serologic test for syphilis must be performed to rule out the existence of this disease.

Kuberski T: Granuloma inguinale. *Sex Transm Dis* 1980;**7**:29.

## CAT-SCRATCH DISEASE

### Essentials of Diagnosis

- A primary infected ulcer or papule-pustule at site of inoculation (30% of cases).
- Regional lymphadenopathy that often suppurates.
- History of scratch by cat at involved area.
- Positive intradermal test.

### General Considerations

This is an acute infection that occurs worldwide and is more common in children and young adults in contact with cats or dogs. It may be transmitted by a scratch or other injury, but some proved cases lack such a history. The cause (based on morphologic and immunologic evidence) appears to be a small gram-negative bacterium seen in lesions, especially on the walls of capillaries and inside macrophages.

### Clinical Findings

**A. Symptoms and Signs:** A few days after the scratch, about one-third of patients develop a primary lesion at the site of inoculation. This primary lesion appears as an infected, scabbed ulcer or a papule with a central vesicle or pustule. One to 3 weeks later, symptoms of generalized infection appear (fever, malaise, headache), and the regional lymph nodes become enlarged without evidence of lymphangitis. The nodes may be tender and fixed, with overlying inflammation; or nontender, discrete, and without evidence of surrounding inflammation. Suppuration may occur, with the discharge of sterile pus. While the course is usually benign, some adults have fever and severe systemic symptoms for weeks.

Lymph node enlargement must be differentiated from that of lymphoma, tuberculosis, lymphogranuloma venereum, and acute bacterial infection.

**B. Laboratory Findings:** The sedimentation rate is elevated, the white blood cell count is usually normal, and the pus from the nodes is sterile. Intradermal skin testing with antigen prepared from the pus is positive (tuberculinlike reaction) in most cases. Lymph node morphology is fairly characteristic; excisional biopsy confirms the diagnosis.

### Complications

Encephalitis occurs rarely. Macular or papular rashes and erythema nodosum are occasionally seen.

### Treatment

There is no specific treatment. Available antimicrobial drugs are ineffective. Surgical removal of a large node or aspiration of liquid contents usually produces an amelioration of symptoms and fever.

### Prognosis

The disease is benign and self-limiting. Symptoms may continue for 5 days to 2 weeks.

Margileth AM: Cat scratch disease update. *Am J Dis Child* 1984;**138**:711.

Margileth AM et al: Systemic cat scratch disease. *J Infect Dis* 1987;**155**:390.

## BARTONELLOSIS
### (Oroya Fever, Carrión's Disease)

Bartonellosis, an acute or chronic infection that occurs in the high Andean valleys of Colombia, Ecuador, and Peru, is caused by a gram-negative, very pleomorphic bacterium (*Bartonella bacilliformis*), which is transmitted to humans by the bite of *Phlebotomus*. The organism is parasitic in humans in red cells and cells of the reticuloendothelial system. The initial stage (Oroya fever) exhibits intermittent or remittent fever, malaise, headache, and bone and joint pains. The disease becomes more apparent with the rapid progression of severe macrocytic anemia, hemorrhagic lymph nodes, and hepatosplenomegaly. Masses of organisms fill the cytoplasm of vascular endothelial cells, resulting in occlusion and thrombosis. In favorable cases, Oroya fever lasts 2–6 weeks and subsides. In those who survive, the eruptive stage of the disease (verruga peruana) commonly begins 2–8 weeks later. Verruga may also appear in the absence of Oroya fever, possibly because of a mild, subclinical first stage. Multiple miliary and nodular hemangiomas appear in crops, particularly on the face and limbs. The lesions bleed easily, sometimes ulcerate, usually persist for 1–12 months, finally heal without scar formation, and produce little systemic reaction. In early Oroya fever, the organisms are best demonstrated by blood culture. Later, *Bartonella* organisms appear in red cells in large numbers. The severe macrocytic, hypochromic anemia (hemoglobin as low as 3–5 g/dL) of Oroya fever is accompanied by jaundice, marked reticulocytosis, and numerous megaloblasts and normoblasts. In verrugous lesions, the organisms may be demonstrated in endothelial cells.

Chloramphenicol or a tetracycline, 2 g daily orally, has been effective and has reduced the mortality rate in these patients. Transfusion may be necessary if the anemia is severe. The *Phlebotomus* vector should be controlled.

Dooley JR: Haemotropic bacteria in man. *Lancet* 1980;**2**:1237.

Schultz MG: A history of bartonellosis (Carrión's disease). *Am J Trop Med Hyg* 1968;**17**:503.

## CHLAMYDIAL INFECTIONS

Chlamydiae are a large group of obligate intracellular parasites closely related to gram-negative bacteria. They are assigned to 2 species—*Chlamydia psittaci* and *Chlamydia trachomatis*—on the basis of intracellular inclusions, sulfonamide susceptibility, antigenic composition, and disease production. *C psittaci* causes psittacosis in humans and many animal diseases. *C trachomatis* causes many different human infections involving the eye (trachoma, inclusion conjunctivitis), the genital tract (lymphogranuloma venereum, nongonococcal urethritis, cervicitis, salpingitis), or the respiratory tract (pneumonitis). A few specific diseases are described.

## LYMPHOGRANULOMA VENEREUM

### Essentials of Diagnosis
- Evanescent primary genital lesion.
- Lymph node enlargement, softening, and suppuration, with draining sinuses.
- Proctitis and rectal stricture in women or homosexual men.
- Systemic, joint, eye, and central nervous system involvement may occur.
- Positive complement fixation test and sometimes positive skin test.
- Elevated serum globulin.

### General Considerations

Lymphogranuloma venereum is an acute and chronic sexually transmitted disease caused by *Chlamydia trachomatis* types $L_1$-$L_3$. After the genital lesion disappears, the infection spreads to lymph channels and lymph nodes of the genital and rectal areas. The disease is acquired during intercourse or through contact with contaminated exudate from active lesions. The incubation period is 5–21 days. Inapparent infections and latent disease are not uncommon in promiscuous individuals.

### Clinical Findings
**A. Symptoms and Signs:** In men, the initial vesicular or ulcerative lesion (on the external genitalia) is evanescent and often goes unnoticed. Inguinal buboes appear 1–4 weeks after exposure, are often bilateral, and have a tendency to fuse, soften, and break down to form multiple draining sinuses, with extensive scarring. Proctoscopic examination is important for diagnosis and in evaluating therapy. In women, the genital lymph drainage is to the perirectal glands. Early anorectal manifestations are proctitis with tenesmus and bloody purulent discharge; late manifestations are chronic cicatrizing inflammation of the rectal and perirectal tissue. These changes lead to obstipation and rectal stricture and, occasionally, rectovaginal and perianal fistulas. They are also seen in homosexual men.

Systemic invasion may occur, causing fever, arthralgia, arthritis, skin rashes, conjunctivitis, and iritis. Nervous system invasion causes headache and meningeal irritation. Pneumonia can develop in laboratory workers who inhale aerosols of the organisms.

**B. Laboratory Findings:** The intradermal skin

test (Frei test) and the complement fixation test may be positive, but cross-reaction with other chlamydiae occurs. A positive reaction may reflect an old (healed) infection; however, high complement fixation titers usually imply active infection. Specific immunofluorescence tests for antibody can be performed. Skin tests with commercial antigens are unreliable. The serum globulin levels are greatly elevated in chronic lymphogranuloma venereum. A nontreponemal test for syphilis (VDRL) may be falsely positive.

### Differential Diagnosis

The early lesion of lymphogranuloma venereum must be differentiated from the lesions of syphilis, genital herpes, and chancroid; lymph node involvement must be distinguished from that due to tularemia, tuberculosis, plague, neoplasm, or pyogenic infection; rectal stricture must be differentiated from that due to neoplasm and ulcerative colitis.

### Complications

Lymphatic involvement and blocking may cause marked disfiguration of the external genitalia (elephantiasis) as well as extensive scarring. Rectal stricture resists treatment and may require colostomy.

### Treatment

**A. Specific Measures:** The antibiotics of choice are the tetracyclines, 0.25–0.5 g orally 4 times daily, or minocycline, 0.1 g twice daily for 10–20 days. Sulfadiazine, 1 g 3 times daily for 2–3 weeks or longer, has little effect on the chlamydial infection but reduces bacterial complications.

**B. Local and General Measures:** Place the patient at bed rest, apply warm compresses to buboes, and give analgesics. Aspirate fluctuant nodes with aseptic care. Plastic operations may be necessary in the chronic anorectal form of the disease. Rectal strictures should be treated by repeated gentle dilation, although in some cases this may be impossible, and colon shunting procedures may be necessary.

### Prognosis

Prompt early treatment will cure the disorder and prevent late complications; the longer treatment is delayed, the more difficult it is to eradicate the infection and to reverse the pathologic changes. There may be a higher incidence of rectal carcinoma in persons with anorectal lymphogranuloma venereum.

Quinn TC et al: *Chlamydia trachomatis* proctitis. *N Engl J Med* 1981;**305**:195.

Sowmini CN et al: Minocycline in the treatment of lymphogranuloma venereum. *J Am Vener Dis Assoc* 1976;**2**:19.

Walzer PD, Armstrong D: Lymphogranuloma venereum presenting as supraclavicular and inguinal lymphadenopathy. *Sex Transm Dis* 1977;**4**:12.

## CHLAMYDIAL GENITAL & NEONATAL INFECTIONS

Some males develop symptomatic or asymptomatic anterior urethritis from which gonococci cannot be isolated by available laboratory tests. This is referred to as nongonococcal urethritis. *Chlamydia trachomatis* immunotypes D-K can be isolated in about 50% of such cases by appropriate techniques. In other cases, a mycoplasma, *Ureaplasma urealyticum*, can be grown as a possible etiologic agent. In still others, gonococcal urethritis is diagnosed and treated; afterwards, gonococci can no longer be found, but postgonococcal urethritis persists. Some of the latter cases can be attributed to chlamydiae or mycoplasmas that were present originally in a mixed infection. Occasionally, epididymitis, prostatitis, or proctitis is caused by chlamydial infection.

The female sexual partners of men with chlamydial nongonococcal urethritis often are infected with the same organisms symptomatically or asymptomatically. Chlamydiae are often recovered from the cervix, and there may be overt cervicitis, salpingitis, or pelvic inflammatory disease. Males or females with genital chlamydial infection may infect the eye through finger contact and develop a follicular conjunctivitis (''inclusion conjunctivitis'') that may become chronic and lead to pannus formation.

If a pregnant woman has chlamydial genital tract infection, the baby often acquires chlamydiae during passage through the birth canal. This may remain asymptomatic or may lead to the appearance of neonatal inclusion conjunctivitis (see p 100) during the first 2 weeks after birth. This conjunctivitis in the newborn may regress spontaneously, after topical treatment of the eye, or may remain chronic and lead to permanent changes in the conjunctiva or cornea.

The newborn infected with chlamydiae may also develop involvement of the respiratory tract with chlamydial pneumonitis appearing during the first 2–6 months of life. This chlamydial pneumonitis (see Chapter 7) is often afebrile and associated with eosinophilia, hyperinflation of the lungs, and marked hypoxia. Chlamydial pneumonitis has also been seen in immunosuppressed adults.

The diagnosis of chlamydial infection relies on the isolation of chlamydiae in specially treated cell cultures or on the demonstration of chlamydial particles by immunofluorescence (with monoclonal antibodies) in secretions or surface scrapings. Occasionally, there is a significant rise in specific antibodies in serum or secretions. Neonatal pneumonitis produces high titers of antichlamydial IgM antibody.

Proof or strong suspicion of chlamydial genital infection should lead to antimicrobial treatment of both sex partners. Drugs of choice are tetracycline hydrochloride or erythromycin, 0.5 mg 4 times daily orally for 10–14 days, or doxycycline, 100 mg orally daily for 10–14 days. Erythromycin is used in pregnant females. Neonatal inclusion conjunctivitis can be managed by topical tetracycline into the conjunctival sac, but systemic erythromycin, 40 mg/kg/d, is preferred and is also the treatment of choice for chlamydial pneumonitis. Both conjunctivitis and pneumonitis can be prevented in the newborn by diagnosis and treatment of maternal infection during pregnancy.

Nongonococcal urethritis not caused by chlamydiae but associated with *Ureaplasma* has been linked to infertility. It may be treated with trimethoprim-sulfamethoxazole, 2 tablets twice daily, or doxycycline, 0.1 g twice daily, for 2 weeks.

Alexander ER, Harrison MR: Role of *Chlamydia trachomatis* in perinatal infection. *Rev Infect Dis* 1983;**5**:713.

Brunham RC et al: Mucopurulent cervicitis: The ignored counterpart in women of urethritis in men. *N Engl J Med* 1984;**311**:1.

Puolakkainen M et al: Chlamydial pneumonitis and its serodiagnosis in infants. *J Infect Dis* 1984;**149**:598.

Schachter J: Chlamydial infections. (3 parts.) *N Engl J Med* 1978;**298**:428, 490, 540.

Schachter J et al: Experience with routine use of erythromycin for chlamydial infections in pregnancy. *N Engl J Med* 1986;**314**:227.

Schachter J et al: Prospective study of perinatal transmission of *Chlamydia trachomatis*. *JAMA* 1986;**255**:3374.

Tam MR et al: Culture-independent diagnosis of *Chlamydia trachomatis* using monoclonal antibodies. *N Engl J Med* 1984;**310**:1146.

Taylor-Robinson D, McCormack WM: The genital mycoplasmas. (2 parts.) *N Engl J Med* 1980;**302**:1003, 1063.

Tipple MA et al: Clinical characteristics of the afebrile pneumonia associated with *C trachomatis* infection in infants less than 6 months of age. *Pediatrics* 1979;**63**:192.

# PSITTACOSIS
# (Ornithosis)

## Essentials of Diagnosis

- Fever, chills, malaise, prostration; cough, epistaxis; occasionally, rose spots and splenomegaly.
- Slightly delayed appearance of signs of pneumonitis.
- Isolation of chlamydiae or rising titer of complement-fixing antibodies.
- Contact with infected bird (psittacine, pigeons, many others) 7–15 days previously.

## General Considerations

Psittacosis is acquired from contact with birds (parrots, parakeets, pigeons, chickens, ducks, and many others). Human-to-human spread is rare, except with special strains of *C psittaci* (eg, TWAR), which can produce acute upper or lower tract respiratory infections.

## Clinical Findings

**A. Symptoms and Signs:** The onset is usually rapid, with fever, chills, headache, backache, malaise, myalgia, epistaxis, dry cough, and prostration. Signs include those of pneumonitis, alteration of percussion note and breath sounds, and rales. Pulmonary findings may be absent early. Rose spots, splenomegaly, and meningismus are occasionally seen. Delirium, constipation or diarrhea, and abdominal distress may occur. Dyspnea and cyanosis may occur later.

**B. Laboratory Findings:** The white count is normal or decreased, often with a shift to the left. Proteinuria is frequently present. The organism may be isolated from the blood and sputum by inoculation of mice or cell cultures. Antibodies appear during the second week and can be demonstrated by complement fixation or immunofluorescence. Antibody response may be suppressed by early chemotherapy.

**C. Imaging:** The radiographic findings in typical psittacosis are those of central pneumonia that later becomes widespread or migratory. Psittacosis is indistinguishable from viral pneumonias by radiography.

## Differential Diagnosis

This disease can be differentiated from acute viral, mycoplasmal, or rickettsial pneumonias only by the history of contact with potentially infected birds and by laboratory tests. Rose spots and leukopenia suggest typhoid fever.

## Complications

Myocarditis, secondary bacterial pneumonia.

## Treatment

Treatment consists of giving tetracycline, 0.5 g orally every 6 hours or 0.5 g intravenously every 12 hours for 14–21 days. Give oxygen and sedation as required.

## Prognosis

Psittacosis may vary from a mild respiratory infection (especially in children) to a severe, protracted illness. The mortality rate with early treatment is very low.

Grayston, JT et al A new *C. psittaci* strain (TWAR) isolated in acute respiratory tract infections. *N Engl J Med* 1986;**315**:161.

McPhee SJ et al: Psittacosis. West J Med 1987;**146**:91.

# Infectious Diseases: Spirochetal

# 24

*Moses Grossman, MD, & Ernest Jawetz, MD, PhD*

## SYPHILIS

### NATURAL HISTORY & PRINCIPLES OF DIAGNOSIS & TREATMENT

Syphilis is a complex infectious disease caused by *Treponema pallidum,* a spirochete capable of infecting any organ or tissue in the body and causing protean clinical manifestations. Transmission occurs most frequently during sexual contact, through minor skin or mucosal lesions; sites of inoculation are usually genital but may be extragenital. The organism is extremely sensitive to heat and drying but can survive for days in fluids; therefore, it can be transmitted in blood from infected persons. Syphilis can be transferred via the placenta from mother to fetus after the tenth week of pregnancy (congenital syphilis).

The immunologic response to infection is complex, but it provides the basis for most clinical diagnoses. The infection induces the synthesis of a number of antibodies, some of which react specifically with pathogenic treponemes and some with components of normal tissues (see below). If the disease is untreated, sufficient defenses develop to produce a relative resistance to reinfection; however, in most cases these immune reactions fail to eradicate existing infection and may contribute to tissue destruction in the late stages. Patients treated early in the disease are fully susceptible to reinfection.

The natural history of acquired syphilis is generally divided into 2 major clinical stages: (1) early, or infectious, syphilis and (2) late syphilis. The 2 stages are separated by a symptom-free latent phase during the first part of which (early latency) the infectious stage is liable to recur. Infectious syphilis includes the primary lesions (chancre and regional lymphadenopathy); the secondary lesions (commonly involving skin and mucous membranes, occasionally bone, central nervous system, or liver); relapsing lesions during early latency; and congenital lesions. The hallmark of these lesions is an abundance of spirochetes; tissue reaction is usually minimal. Late syphilis consists of so-called benign (gummatous) lesions involving skin, bones, and viscera; cardiovascular disease (principally aortitis); and a variety of central nervous sys-

tem and ocular syndromes. These forms of syphilis are not contagious. The lesions contain few demonstrable spirochetes, but tissue reactivity (vasculitis, necrosis) is severe and suggestive of hypersensitivity phenomena.

As a result of intensive public health efforts during and after World War II, there was a reduction in the incidence of infectious syphilis. With the marked increase in all sexually transmitted diseases since the 1970s, there has been a rise in the number of reported cases of syphilis. In the 1980s, the incidence of infectious syphilis is particularly high among homosexual males. Reinfection in treated persons is common. No appreciable rise in the incidence of congenital syphilis has been reported yet.

### Laboratory Diagnosis

The infectious agent of syphilis cannot be cultured in vitro. Diagnostic measures must rely mainly on serologic testing, microscopic detection of *T pallidum* in lesions, and other examinations (biopsies, lumbar puncture, x-rays) for evidence of tissue damage.

**A. Serologic Tests for Syphilis:** There are 2 general categories of serologic tests for syphilis: (1) nontreponemal tests, which use a component of normal tissue (eg, beef heart cardiolipin) as an antigen to measure nonspecific antibodies (reagin) formed in the blood of patients with syphilis; and (2) treponemal tests, which employ live or killed *T pallidum* as antigen to detect antibodies specific for pathogenic treponemes.

**1. Nontreponemal antigen tests**—Commonly employed nontreponemal antigen tests are of 2 types: (1) flocculation (VDRL, RPR) and (2) complement fixation (Kolmer, Wassermann). The flocculation tests are easy, rapid, and inexpensive to perform and are therefore used primarily for routine (often automated) screening for syphilis. Quantitative expression of the reactivity of the serum, based upon titration of dilutions of serum, may be valuable in establishing the diagnosis and in evaluating the efficacy of treatment.

The VDRL test (the nontreponemal test in widest use) generally becomes positive 4–6 weeks after infection, or 1–3 weeks after the appearance of a primary lesion; it is almost invariably positive in the secondary stage. The VDRL titer is usually high ($> 1:32$) in secondary syphilis and tends to be lower ($< 1:4$) or even negative in late forms of syphilis. A falling titer in treated early or latent syphilis suggests satisfactory response to treatment. These serologic tests are not highly specific and must be closely correlated with other clinical and laboratory findings. The tests are positive in patients with nonsexually transmitted treponematoses (see below). More importantly, "false-positive" serologic reactions are frequently encountered in a wide variety of nontreponemal states, including collagen diseases, infectious mononucleosis, malaria, febrile diseases, leprosy, drug addiction, old age, and possibly pregnancy. False-positive reactions are usually of low titer and transient and may be distinguished from true positives by specific treponemal antibody tests. The rapid plasma reagin (RPR) test is a simple, rapid, and reliable substitute for the traditional VDRL test and gives comparable results. It is suitable for automated screening tests.

**2. Treponemal antibody tests**–The fluorescent treponemal antibody absorption (FTA-ABS) test is the most widely employed treponemal test. It measures antibodies capable of reacting with killed *T pallidum* after absorption of the patient's serum with extracts of nonpathogenic treponemes. The FTA-ABS test is of value principally in determining whether a positive nontreponemal antigen test is "false-positive" or is indicative of syphilis. Because of its great sensitivity, particularly in the late stages of the disease, the FTA-ABS test is also of value when there is clinical evidence of syphilis but the routine serologic test for syphilis is negative. The test is positive in most patients with primary syphilis and in virtually all with secondary syphilis, and it usually remains positive permanently in spite of successful treatment. False-positive FTA-ABS tests occur rarely in systemic lupus erythematosus and in other disorders associated with abnormal globulins. A treponemal passive hemagglutination (TPHA) test is comparable in specificity and sensitivity to the FTA-ABS test but may become positive somewhat later in infection.

Final decision about the significance of the results of serologic tests for syphilis must be based upon a total clinical appraisal.

**B. Microscopic Examination:** In infectious syphilis, *T pallidum* may be shown by darkfield microscopic examination of fresh exudate from lesions or material aspirated from regional lymph nodes. The darkfield examination requires considerable experience and care in the proper collection of specimens and in the identification of pathogenic spirochetes by characteristic morphology and motility. Repeated examinations may be necessary. Spirochetes usually are not found in late syphilitic lesions by this technique.

An immunofluorescent staining technique for demonstrating *T pallidum* in dried smears of fluid taken from early syphilitic lesions is available. Slides are fixed and treated with fluorescein-labeled antitreponemal antibody that has been preabsorbed with nonpathogenic treponemes. The slides are then examined for fluorescing spirochetes in an ultraviolet microscope. Because of its simplicity and convenience to physicians (slides can be mailed), this technique has replaced darkfield microscopy in most health departments and medical center laboratories.

**C. Spinal Fluid Examination:** The cerebrospinal fluid findings in neurosyphilis usually consist of elevation of total protein and gamma globulins, increase in the cell count, and a positive reagin test (VDRL). False-positive reagin tests rarely occur in the cerebrospinal fluid. Improvement of the cerebrospinal fluid findings is of great prognostic value.

Cerebrospinal fluid examination is mandatory in all cases of secondary syphilis or latent syphilis not previously adequately treated. Asymptomatic neurosyphilis (ie, positive cerebrospinal fluid findings without symptoms) requires prolonged penicillin treatment as given for symptomatic neurosyphilis. Adequate treatment is indicated by gradual decrease in cerebrospinal fluid cell count, protein concentration, and VDRL titer. Rarely, serologic tests of cerebrospinal fluid may remain positive for years after adequate treatment of neurosyphilis even though all other parameters have returned to normal. In the presence of high-titer serum FTA-ABS, there may be a positive FTA test on cerebrospinal fluid in the absence of neurosyphilis.

## Treatment

### A. Specific Measures:

**1. Penicillin,** as benzathine penicillin G or aqueous procaine penicillin G, is the drug of choice for all forms of syphilis and other spirochetal infections. Effective tissue levels must be maintained for several days or weeks because of the spirochete's long generation time. Penicillin is highly effective in early infections and variably effective in the late stages. The principal contraindication is hypersensitivity to the penicillins. The recommended treatment schedules are included below in the discussion of the various forms of syphilis.

**2. Other antibiotic therapy**–Oral tetracyclines and erythromycins are effective in the treatment of syphilis for patients who are sensitive to penicillin. Tetracycline, 30–40 g, or erythromycin, 30–40 g, is given over a period of 10–15 days in early syphilis; twice as much is recommended for syphilis of more than 1 year's duration. Experience with these drugs in the treatment of syphilis is limited, and some failures have been reported. Careful follow-up is therefore mandatory.

**B. Local Measures (Mucocutaneous Lesions):** Local treatment is usually not necessary. No local antiseptics or other chemicals should be applied to a suspected syphilitic lesion until specimens for microscopy have been obtained.

**C. Public Health Measures:** Patients with infectious syphilis must abstain from sexual activity until rendered noninfectious by antibiotic therapy. All cases of syphilis must be reported to the appropriate public health agency for assistance in identifying, investigating, and treating all contacts.

**D. Epidemiologic Treatment:** Patients who have been exposed to infectious syphilis within the preceding 3 months, as well as others who on epidemiologic grounds present a high risk for syphilis, should be treated as for early syphilis. Every effort should be made to establish a diagnosis in these persons.

## Complications of Specific Therapy

The Jarisch-Herxheimer reaction is ascribed to the sudden massive destruction of spirochetes by drugs and release of toxic products and is manifested by fever and aggravation of the existing clinical picture. It is most likely to occur in early syphilis. Treatment should not be discontinued unless the symptoms become severe or threaten to be fatal or unless syphilitic laryngitis, auditory neuritis, or labyrinthitis is present, where the reaction may cause irreversible damage.

The reaction may be prevented or modified by simultaneous administration of corticosteroids. It usually begins within the first 24 hours and subsides spontaneously within the next 24 hours of penicillin treatment.

## Follow-Up Care

Patients who receive treatment for early syphilis should be followed clinically and with periodic quantitative VDRL tests for at least 1 year. Patients with all other types of syphilis should be under similar observation for 2 or more years.

## Prevention

Avoidance of sexual contact is the only reliable method of prophylaxis but is an impractical public health measure for obvious reasons.

**A. Mechanical:** The standard rubber condom is effective but protects covered parts only. The exposed parts should be washed with soap and water as soon after contact as possible. This applies to both sexes.

**B. Antibiotic:** If there is known exposure to infectious syphilis, abortive penicillin therapy may be used. Give 2.4 million units of procaine penicillin G intramuscularly in each buttock once. Treatment of gonococcal infection with penicillins is probably effective against incubating syphilis in most cases. However, other antimicrobial agents (eg, spectinomycin) may be ineffective in aborting preclinical syphilis. In view of the increasing use of antibiotics other than penicillin for gonococcal disease, patients treated for gonorrhea should have a serologic test for syphilis 3–6 months after treatment.

**C. Vaccine:** No vaccine against syphilis exists now or is likely to become available soon.

## Course & Prognosis

The lesions associated with primary and secondary syphilis are self-limiting and resolve with few or no residua. Late syphilis may be highly destructive and permanently disabling and may lead to death. With treatment, the nontreponemal serologic tests usually return to negative in early syphilis. In late latent and late syphilis, serofastness is not uncommon even after adequate treatment. In broad terms, if no treatment is given, about one-third of people infected with syphilis will undergo spontaneous cure, about one-third will remain in the latent phase throughout life, and about one-third will develop serious late lesions.

Brown ST et al: Serological response to syphilis treatment. *JAMA* 1985;**253:**1296.

Centers for Disease Control: Sexually transmitted diseases: Treatment guidelines 1985. *MMWR* 1985;**34:**94S.

Jaffe HW et al: Tests for treponemal antibody in CSF. *Arch Intern Med* 1978;**138:**252.

Johnson RC: The spirochetes. *Annu Rev Microbiol* 1977;**31:**89.

Lee TJ, Sparling PF: Syphilis: An algorithm. *JAMA* 1979; **242:**1187.

# CLINICAL STAGES OF SYPHILIS

## 1. PRIMARY SYPHILIS

### Essentials of Diagnosis

- History of sexual contact (often unreliable).
- Painless ulcer on genitalia, perianal area, rectum, pharynx, tongue, lip, or elsewhere 2–6 weeks after exposure.
- Nontender enlargement of regional lymph nodes.
- Fluid expressed from lesion contains *T pallidum* by immunofluorescence or darkfield microscopy.
- Serologic test for syphilis often positive.

### General Considerations

This is the stage of invasion and may pass unrecognized. The typical lesion is the chancre at the site or sites of inoculation, most frequently located on the penis, labia, cervix, or anorectal region. Anorectal lesions are especially common among male homosexuals. The primary lesion occurs occasionally in the oropharynx (lip, tongue, or tonsil) and rarely on the breast or finger. The chancre starts as a small erosion 10–90 days (average, 3–4 weeks) after inoculation that rapidly develops into a painless superficial ulcer with a clean base and firm, indurated margins, associated with enlargement of regional lymph nodes, which are rubbery, discrete, and nontender. Bacterial infection of the chancre may occur and may lead to pain. Healing occurs without treatment, but a scar may form, especially with secondary bacterial infection.

### Laboratory Findings

The serologic test for syphilis is usually positive 1–2 weeks after the primary lesion is noted; rising titers are especially significant when there is a history of previous infection. Immunofluorescence or darkfield microscopy shows treponemes in at least 95% of chancres. The spinal fluid is normal at this stage.

The syphilitic chancre may be confused with chancroid, lymphogranuloma venereum, genital herpes, or neoplasm. Any lesion on the genitalia should be considered a possible primary syphilitic lesion.

## Treatment

Give benzathine penicillin G, 1.2 million units in each buttock for a total dose of 2.4 million units once. Sometimes a dose of the same size is given twice more at weekly intervals, especially when a typical lesion was not observed by the physician. Other regimens of penicillin, or other drugs, are less desirable.

Fiumara NJ: Treatment of seropositive primary syphilis: An evaluation of 196 patients. *Sex Transm Dis* 1977;**4:**92.

## 2. SECONDARY SYPHILIS

### Essentials of Diagnosis

- Generalized maculopapular skin rash.
- Mucous membrane lesions, including patches and ulcers.
- Weeping papules (condylomas) in moist skin areas.
- Generalized nontender lymphadenopathy.
- Fever.
- Meningitis, hepatitis, osteitis, arthritis, iritis.
- Many treponemes in scrapings of mucous membrane or skin lesions by immunofluorescence or darkfield microscopy.
- Serologic tests for syphilis always positive.

### General Considerations & Treatment

The secondary stage of syphilis usually appears a few weeks (or up to 6 months) after development of the chancre, when sufficient dissemination of *T pallidum* has occurred to produce systemic signs (fever, lymphadenopathy) or infectious lesions at sites distant from the site of inoculation. The most common manifestations are skin and mucosal lesions. The skin lesions are nonpruritic, macular, papular, pustular, or follicular (or combinations of any of these types), although the maculopapular rash is the most common. The skin lesions usually are generalized; involvement of the palms and soles is especially suspicious. Annular lesions simulating ringworm are observed in blacks. Mucous membrane lesions range from ulcers and papules of the lips, mouth, throat, genitalia, and anus ("mucous patches") to a diffuse redness of the pharynx. Both skin and mucous membrane lesions are highly infectious at this stage. Specific lesions—**condylomata lata**—are fused, weeping papules on the moist areas of the skin and mucous membranes.

Meningeal (aseptic meningitis or acute basilar meningitis), hepatic, renal, bone, and joint invasion, with resulting cranial nerve palsies, jaundice, nephrotic syndrome, and periostitis may occur. Alopecia (moth-eaten appearance), iritis, and iridocyclitis may also occur. A transient myocarditis may be manifested by temporary electrocardiographic changes.

All serologic tests for syphilis are positive in almost all cases. The cutaneous and mucous membrane lesions often show *T pallidum* on microscopic examina-tion. There is usually a transient cerebrospinal fluid involvement, with pleocytosis and elevated protein, although only 5% of cases have positive serologic cerebrospinal fluid reactions. There may be evidence of hepatitis or nephritis (immune complex type). Circulating immune complexes exist in the blood and are deposited in blood vessel walls.

Skin lesions may be confused with the infectious exanthems, pityriasis rosea, and drug eruptions. Visceral lesions may suggest nephritis or hepatitis due to other causes. The diffusely red throat may mimic other forms of pharyngitis.

Treatment is as for primary syphilis unless central nervous system disease is present, in which case treatment is as for neurosyphilis (see below). Isolation of the patient is important.

Fiumara NJ: Treatment of secondary syphilis: An evaluation of 204 patients. *Sex Transm Dis* 1977;**4:**96.
Gamble CN, Readan JB: Immunopathology of syphilitic glomerulonephritis. *N Engl J Med* 1975;**292:**449.
Jorizzo JL et al: Role of circulating immune complexes in human secondary syphilis. *J Infect Dis* 1986;**153:**1014.

## 3. RELAPSING SYPHILIS

The essentials of diagnosis are the same as in secondary syphilis.

The lesions of secondary syphilis heal spontaneously, but secondary syphilis may relapse if undiagnosed or inadequately treated. These relapses may include any of the findings noted under secondary syphilis: skin and mucous membrane, neurologic, ocular, bone, or visceral. Unlike the usual asymptomatic neurologic involvement of secondary syphilis, neurologic relapses may be fulminating, leading to death. Relapse is almost always accompanied by a rising titer in quantitative serologic tests; indeed, a rising titer may be the first or only evidence of relapse. About 70% of relapses occur during the first year after infection.

Treatment is as for primary syphilis unless central nervous system disease is present.

## 4. LATENT ("HIDDEN") SYPHILIS

### Essentials of Diagnosis

- No physical signs.
- History of syphilis with inadequate treatment.
- Positive treponemal serologic tests for syphilis.

### General Considerations & Treatment

Latent syphilis is the clinically quiescent phase during the interval after disappearance of secondary lesions and before the appearance of tertiary symptoms. Early latency is defined as the first 4 years after infection, during which time infectious lesions may recur ("relapsing syphilis"); after 4 years, the patient is said to be in the late latent phase. Transmission to the fetus, however, can probably occur in any phase. There are (by definition) no clinical manifestations during the latent phase, and the only significant laboratory findings are positive serologic tests. A diagnosis of latent syphilis is justified only when the cerebrospinal fluid is entirely negative, x-ray and physical examination shows no evidence of cardiovascular involvement, and false-positive tests for syphilis have been ruled out. The latent phase may last from months to a lifetime.

It is important to differentiate latent syphilis from a false-positive serologic test for syphilis, which can be due to the many causes listed above.

Treatment is with benzathine penicillin G, 2.4 million units 3 times at 7-day intervals. If there is evidence of cerebrospinal fluid involvement, treat as for neurosyphilis. Only a small percentage of serologic tests will be appreciably altered by treatment with penicillin. The treatment of this stage of the disease is intended to prevent the late sequelae.

Ducas J, Robson HG: Cerebrospinal fluid penicillin levels during therapy for latent syphilis. *JAMA* 1981;**246**:2583.

## 5. LATE (TERTIARY) SYPHILIS

### Essentials of Diagnosis

- Infiltrative tumors of skin, bones, liver (gummas).
- Aortitis, aneurysms, aortic insufficiency.
- Central nervous system disorders, including meningovascular and degenerative changes, paresthesias, shooting pains, abnormal reflexes, dementia, or psychosis.

### General Considerations

This stage may occur at any time after secondary syphilis, even after years of latency. Late lesions probably represent, at least in part, a delayed hypersensitivity reaction of the tissue to the organism and are usually divided into 2 types: (1) a localized gummatous reaction, with a relatively rapid onset and generally prompt response to therapy ("benign late syphilis"); and (2) diffuse inflammation of a more insidious onset that characteristically involves the central nervous system and large arteries, is often fatal if untreated, and is at best arrested by treatment. Gummas may involve any area or organ of the body but most often the skin or long bones. Cardiovascular disease is usually manifested by aortic aneurysm, aortic insufficiency, or aortitis. Various forms of diffuse or localized central nervous system involvement may occur.

Late syphilis must be differentiated from neoplasms of the skin, liver, lung, stomach, or brain; other forms of meningitis; and primary neurologic lesions.

Treatment is as for latent syphilis. Reversal of positive serologic tests does not usually occur. A second course of penicillin therapy may be given if necessary. There is no known method for reliable eradication of the treponeme from humans in the late stages of syphilis. Viable spirochetes are occasionally found in the eyes, in cerebrospinal fluid, and elsewhere in patients with "adequately" treated syphilis, but claims for their capacity to cause progressive disease are speculative.

Although almost any tissue and organ may be involved in late syphilis, the following are the most common types of involvement.

### Skin

Cutaneous lesions of late syphilis are of 2 varieties: (1) multiple nodular lesions that eventually ulcerate or resolve by forming atrophic, pigmented scars; and (2) solitary gummas that start as painless subcutaneous nodules, then enlarge, attach to the overlying skin, and eventually ulcerate.

### Mucous Membranes

Late lesions of the mucous membranes are nodular gummas or leukoplakia, highly destructive to the involved tissue.

### Skeletal

Bone lesions are destructive, causing periostitis, osteitis, and arthritis with little or no associated redness or swelling but often marked myalgia and myositis of the neighboring muscles. The pain is especially severe at night.

### Eyes

Late ocular lesions are gummatous iritis, chorioretinitis, optic atrophy, and cranial nerve palsies, in addition to the lesions of central nervous system syphilis.

### Respiratory System

Respiratory involvement by late syphilis is caused by gummatous infiltrates into the larynx, trachea, and pulmonary parenchyma, producing discrete pulmonary densities. There may be hoarseness, respiratory distress, and wheezing secondary to the gummatous lesion itself or to subsequent stenosis occurring with healing.

### Gastrointestinal System

Gummas involving the liver produce the usually benign, asymptomatic **hepar lobatum.** Occasionally a picture resembling Laennec's cirrhosis is produced by liver involvement. Infiltration into the stomach wall causes "leather bottle" stomach with epigastric distress, inability to eat large meals, regurgitation, belching, and weight loss.

### Cardiovascular System

Cardiovascular lesions (10–15% of late syphilitic lesions) are often progressive, disabling, and life-threatening. Central nervous system lesions are often present also. Involvement usually starts as an arteritis in the supracardiac portion of the aorta and progresses to cause one or more of the following: (1) Narrowing of the coronary ostia with resulting decreased coronary circulation, angina, cardiac insufficiency, and acute myocardial infarction. (2) Scarring of the aortic valves, producing aortic insufficiency with its water-hammer pulse, aortic diastolic murmur, frequently aortic systolic murmur, cardiac hypertrophy, and eventually congestive heart failure. (3) Weakness of the wall of the aorta, with saccular aneurysm formation and associated pressure symptoms of dysphagia, hoarseness, brassy cough, back pain (vertebral erosion), and occasionally rupture of the aneurysm. Recurrent respiratory infections are common as a result of pressure on the trachea and bronchi.

Treatment of cardiac problems requires first consideration, after which penicillin G is given as for latent syphilis.

## Neurosyphilis

Neurosyphilis (15–20% of late syphilitic lesions; often present with cardiovascular syphilis) is also a progressive, disabling, and life-threatening complication. It develops more commonly in men than in women and in whites than in blacks. There are 4 clinical types.

**(1) Asymptomatic neurosyphilis:** This form is characterized by spinal fluid abnormalities (positive spinal fluid serology, increased cell count, occasionally increased protein) without symptoms or signs of neurologic involvement.

**(2) Meningovascular syphilis:** This form is characterized by meningeal involvement or changes in the vascular structures of the brain (or both), producing symptoms of low-grade meningitis (headache, irritability); cranial nerve palsies (basilar meningitis); unequal reflexes; irregular pupils with poor light and accommodation reflexes; and, when large vessels are involved, cerebrovascular accidents. The cerebrospinal fluid shows increased cells ($100–1000/\mu L$), elevated protein, and usually a positive serologic test for syphilis. The symptoms of acute meningitis are rare in late syphilis.

**(3) Tabes dorsalis:** This form is a chronic progressive degeneration of the parenchyma of the posterior columns of the spinal cord and of the posterior sensory ganglia and nerve roots. The symptoms and signs are impairment of proprioception and vibration sense, Argyll Robertson pupils (which react poorly to light but well to accommodation), and muscular hypotonia and hyporeflexia. Impairment of proprioception results in a wide-based gait and inability to walk in the dark. Paresthesias, analgesia, or sharp recurrent pains in the muscles of the leg ("shooting" or "lightning" pains) may occur. Crises are also common in tabes: gastric crises, consisting of sharp abdominal pains with nausea and vomiting (simulating an acute abdomen); laryngeal crises, with paroxysmal cough and dyspnea; urethral crises, with painful bladder spasms; and rectal and anal crises. Crises may begin suddenly, last for hours to days, and cease abruptly. Neurogenic bladder with

overflow incontinence is also seen. Painless trophic ulcers may develop over pressure points on the feet. Joint damage may occur as a result of lack of sensory innervation (Charcot joint). The cerebrospinal fluid may have a normal or increased cell count ($3–200/\mu L$), elevated protein, and variable results of serologic tests.

**(4) General paresis:** This is a generalized involvement of the cerebral cortex with insidious onset of symptoms. There is usually a decrease in concentrating power, memory loss, dysarthria, tremor of the fingers and lips, irritability, and mild headaches. Most striking is the change of personality; the patient becomes slovenly, irresponsible, confused, and psychotic. Combinations of the various forms of neurosyphilis (especially tabes and paresis) are not uncommon. The cerebrospinal fluid findings resemble those of tabes dorsalis.

**Special considerations in treatment of neurosyphilis.** It is most important to prevent neurosyphilis by prompt diagnosis, adequate treatment, and follow-up of early syphilis. Lumbar puncture should be performed on all patients with syphilis in the secondary or later stages. In the presence of definite cerebrospinal fluid or neurologic abnormalities, treat for neurosyphilis. The pretreatment clinical and laboratory evaluation should include neurologic, ocular, psychiatric, and cerebrospinal fluid examinations.

There is no simple established treatment schedule for neurosyphilis. The minimum therapy is as given for latent syphilis, but acute or treatment-resistant neurosyphilis is often treated with larger doses of short-acting penicillin (eg, aqueous penicillin G, 20 million units intravenously daily for 10–14 days).

All patients must have spinal fluid examinations at 3-month intervals for the first year and every 6 months for the second year following completion of antisyphilis therapy. Response may be gauged by clinical improvement and effective and persistent reversal of cerebrospinal fluid changes. A second course of penicillin therapy may be given if necessary. Not infrequently, there is progression of neurologic symptoms and signs despite high and prolonged doses of penicillin. It has been postulated that these treatment failures are related to the unexplained persistence of viable *T pallidum* in central nervous system or ocular lesions in at least some cases.

Luxon L, Lees AJ, Greenwood RJ: Neurosyphilis today. *Lancet* 1979;**1**:90.

Rein MF: Treatment of neurosyphilis. *JAMA* 1981;**246**:2613.

Tramont EC: Persistence of *T pallidum* following penicillin G therapy. *JAMA* 1976;**236**:2206.

## 6. SYPHILIS IN PREGNANCY

All pregnant women should have a nontreponemal serologic test for syphilis at the time of the first prenatal visit. Seroreactive patients should be evaluated promptly. Such evaluation includes the history (including prior therapy), a physical examination, a quantitative nontreponemal test, and a confirmatory treponemal test. If the FTA-ABS test is nonreactive and there is no clinical evidence of syphilis, treatment may be withheld. Both the quantitative nontreponemal test and the FTA-ABS test should be repeated in 4 weeks. If the diagnosis of syphilis cannot be excluded with reasonable certainty, the patient should be treated as outlined below.

Patients for whom there is documentation of adequate treatment for syphilis in the past need not be re-treated unless there is clinical or serologic evidence of reinfection (eg, 4-fold rise in titer of a quantitative nontreponemal test).

In women suspected of being at increased risk for syphilis, a second nontreponemal test should be performed during the third trimester.

The preferred treatment is with penicillin in dosage schedules appropriate for the stage of syphilis (see above). Penicillin prevents congenital syphilis in 90% of cases, even when treatment is given late in pregnancy.

For patients definitely known to be allergic to penicillin, the drug of second choice is erythromycin (base, stearate, or ethylsuccinate) in dosage schedules appropriate for the stage of syphilis. Such treatment is safe for the mother and the child, but the efficacy is not clearly established. Therefore, the documentation of penicillin allergy is particularly important before a decision is made not to use the first-choice drug. Erythromycin estolate and tetracycline are not recommended because of potential adverse effects on the mother and the fetus.

The infant should be evaluated immediately, as noted below, and at 6–8 weeks of age.

Centers for Disease Control: Sexually transmitted diseases: Treatment guidelines 1985. *MMWR* 1985;**34:**94S.

Jones JE Jr, Harris RE: Diagnostic evaluation of syphilis during pregnancy. *Obstet Gynecol* 1979;**124:**705.

Mescola L et al: Inadequate treatment of syphilis in pregnancy. *Am J Obstet Gynecol* 1984;**150:**945.

## 7. CONGENITAL SYPHILIS

Congenital syphilis is a transplacentally transmitted infection that occurs in infants of untreated or inadequately treated mothers. The physical findings at birth are quite variable: The infant may have many or only minimal signs or even no signs until 6–8 weeks of life (delayed form). The most common findings are on the skin and mucous membranes—serous nasal discharge (snuffles), mucous membrane patches, maculopapular rash, condylomas. These lesions are infectious; *T pallidum* can easily be found microscopically, and the infant must be isolated. Other common findings are hepatosplenomegaly, anemia, or osteochondritis. These early active lesions subsequently heal, and if the disease is left untreated it produces the characteristic stigmas of syphilis—interstitial ker-

atitis, Hutchinson's teeth, saddle nose, saber shins, deafness, and central nervous system involvement.

The serologic evaluation for syphilis in newborn infants is complicated by the transplacental acquisition of maternal antibody (IgG). Evaluation of a newborn suspected of having congenital syphilis includes the history of maternal therapy, a careful physical examination, hematocrit (for possible anemia), and x-rays of long bones. It is particularly important to follow the infant every 2–3 weeks over a period of 4 months to watch for developing physical signs; a sustained rise or fall in VDRL titer during this time will reveal the need for treatment.

Infants should be treated at birth if maternal treatment was inadequate, unknown, or done with drugs other than penicillin or if adequate follow-up of the infant cannot be assured.

Infants with congenital syphilis should always have a cerebrospinal fluid examination before therapy. If the diagnosis of congenital neurosyphilis cannot be excluded, the infant should be treated with aqueous penicillin G, 50,000 units/kg intramuscularly or intravenously daily in 2 divided doses for 10 days, or with aqueous procaine penicillin G, 50,000 units/kg intramuscularly daily for a minimum of 10 days. If the cerebrospinal fluid is perfectly normal and the spinal fluid VRDL is negative, the infant may be treated with benzathine penicillin G, 50,000 units/kg intramuscularly in a single dose. Antibiotics other than penicillin are not recommended for congenital syphilis.

The quantitative nontreponemal test (VDRL) should be repeated 3, 6, and 12 months after therapy to establish falling titers.

Bryan EM, Nicholson E: Congenital syphilis. *Clin Pediatr* 1981;**20:**81.

Mescola L et al: Congenital syphilis revisited. *Am J Dis Child* 1985;**139:**575.

# NONSEXUALLY TRANSMITTED TREPONEMATOSES

A variety of treponemal diseases other than syphilis occur endemically in many tropical areas of the world. They are distinguished from disease caused by *T pallidum* by their nonsexual transmission, their relatively high incidence in certain geographic areas and among children, and their tendency to produce less severe visceral manifestations. As in syphilis, organisms can be demonstrated in infectious lesions with darkfield microscopy or immunofluorescence but cannot be cultured in artificial media; the serologic tests for syphilis are positive; the diseases have primary, secondary, and sometimes tertiary stages; and penicillin is the drug of choice. There is evidence that infection with these agents may provide partial resistance to syphilis and vice versa. Treatment with penicillin in doses appropriate to primary syphilis (eg, 2.4 million units of benzathine penicillin G intramuscularly) is generally curative in any stage of the nonsexually transmitted treponematoses. In cases of penicillin hypersensitivity, tetracycline is usually the recommended alternative.

## YAWS
## (Frambesia)

Yaws is a contagious disease largely limited to tropical regions that is caused by *Treponema pertenue*. It is characterized by granulomatous lesions of the skin, mucous membranes, and bone. Yaws is rarely fatal, although if untreated it may lead to chronic disability and disfigurement. Yaws is acquired by direct nonsexual contact, usually in childhood, although it may occur at any age. The "mother yaw," a painless papule that later ulcerates, appears 3–4 weeks after exposure. There is usually associated regional lymph-adenopathy. Six to 12 weeks later, similar secondary lesions appear and last for several months or years. Painful ulcerated lesions on the soles are frequent and are called "crab yaws." Late gummatous lesions may occur, with associated tissue destruction involving large areas of skin and subcutaneous tissues. The late effects of yaws, with bone change, shortening of digits, and contractions, may be confused with similar changes occurring in leprosy. Central nervous system, cardiac, or other visceral involvement is rare.

Burke JP et al (editors): International Symposium on Yaws and Other Endemic Treponematoses. *Rev Infect Dis* 1985;**7**:217.
Hopkins DR: Yaws in the Americas, 1950–1975. *J Infect Dis* 1977;**136**:548.

## PINTA

Pinta is a nonsexually transmitted spirochetal infection caused by *Treponema carateum*. It occurs endemically in rural areas of Latin America, especially in Mexico, Colombia, and Cuba, and in some areas of the Pacific. A nonulcerative, erythematous primary papule spreads slowly into a papulosquamous plaque showing a variety of color changes (slate, lilac, black). Secondary lesions resemble the primary one and appear within a year after it. These appear successively, new lesions together with older ones; are commonest on the extremities; and later show atrophy and depigmentation. Some cases show pigment changes and atrophic patches on the soles and palms, with or without hyperkeratosis, that are indistinguishable from "crab yaws." Very rarely, central nervous system or cardiovascular disease is observed late in the course of infection.

## ENDEMIC SYPHILIS
## (Bejel, Skerljevo, Etc)

Endemic syphilis is an acute and chronic infection caused by an organism indistinguishable from *T pallidum*. It has been reported in a number of countries, particularly in the eastern Mediterranean area, often with local names: bejel in Syria, Saudi Arabia, and Iraq; skerljevo in Bosnia; and dichuchwa, njovera, and siti in Africa. It also occurs in Southeast Asia. The local forms have distinctive features. Moist ulcerated lesions of the skin or oral or nasopharyngeal mucosa are the most common manifestations. Generalized lymphadenopathy and secondary and tertiary bone and skin lesions are also common. Deep leg pain points to osteoperiostitis. Cardiovascular and central nervous system involvement is rare.

Pace JL, Csonka GW: Endemic non-venereal syphilis (bejel) in Saudi Arabia. *Br J Vener Dis* 1984;**60**:293.

---

# MISCELLANEOUS SPIROCHETAL DISEASES

---

## RELAPSING FEVER

Relapsing fever is endemic in many parts of the world. The main reservoir is rodents, which serve as the source of infection for ticks (eg, *Ornithodoros*). The distribution and seasonal incidence of the disease are determined by the ecology of the ticks in different areas. In the USA, infected ticks are found throughout the West, especially in mountainous areas, but clinical cases are uncommon in humans.

The infectious organism is a spirochete, *Borrelia recurrentis*. It may be transmitted transovarially from one generation of ticks to the next. The spirochetes occur in all tissues of the tick, and humans can be infected by tick bites or by rubbing crushed tick tissues or feces into the bite wound. Tick-borne relapsing fever is endemic but is not transmitted from person to person. Different species (or strain) names have been given to *Borrelia* in different parts of the world where the organisms are transmitted by different ticks.

When an infected person harbors lice, the lice become infected with *Borrelia* by sucking blood. A few days later, the lice serve as a source of infection for other persons. Large epidemics may occur in louse-infested populations, and transmission is favored by crowding, malnutrition, and cold climate.

### Clinical Findings
**A. Symptoms and Signs:** There is an abrupt onset of fever, chills, tachycardia, nausea and vomiting, arthralgia, and severe headache. Hepatomegaly and splenomegaly may develop, as well as various

types of rashes. Delirium occurs with high fever, and there may be various neurologic and psychic abnormalities. The attack terminates, usually abruptly, after 3–10 days. After an interval of 1–2 weeks, a relapse occurs, but often it is somewhat milder. Three to 10 relapses may occur before recovery.

**B. Laboratory Findings:** During episodes of fever, large spirochetes are seen in blood smears stained with Wright's or Giemsa's stain. The organisms can be cultured in special media but rapidly lose pathogenicity. The spirochetes can multiply in injected rats or mice and can be seen in their blood.

A variety of anti-*Borrelia* antibodies develop during the illness; sometimes the Weil-Felix test and nontreponemal serologic test for syphilis may also be positive. Cerebrospinal fluid abnormalities occur in patients with meningeal involvement. Mild anemia and thrombocytopenia are common, but the white blood cell count tends to be normal.

## Differential Diagnosis

The manifestations of relapsing fever may be confused with malaria, leptospirosis, meningococcemia, yellow fever, typhus, or rat-bite fever.

## Prevention

Prevention of tick bites (as described for rickettsial diseases) and delousing procedures applicable to large groups can prevent illness. Arthropod vectors should be controlled if possible.

An effective means of chemoprophylaxis has not been developed.

## Treatment

A single dose of tetracycline or erythromycin, 0.5 g orally, or a single dose of procaine penicillin G, 600,000 units intramuscularly, probably constitutes adequate treatment. Jarisch-Herxheimer reactions may occur and must be managed.

## Prognosis

The overall mortality rate is usually about 5%. Fatalities are most common in old, debilitated, or very young patients. With treatment, the initial attack is shortened and relapses are largely prevented.

Butler T et al: *Borrelia recurrentis* infection. *J Infect Dis* 1978;**137**:573.
Edell TA et al: Tick-borne relapsing fever in Colorado. *JAMA* 1979;**241**:2279.
Malison MD: Relapsing fever. *JAMA* 1979;**241**:2819.

## RAT-BITE FEVER
## (Spirillary Rat-Bite Fever, Sodoku)

Rat-bite fever is an uncommon acute infectious disease caused by *Spirillum minor*. It is transmitted to humans by the bite of a rat. Inhabitants of rat-infested slum dwellings and laboratory workers are at greatest risk.

## Clinical Findings

**A. Symptoms and Signs:** The original rat bite, unless secondarily infected, heals promptly, but 1 to several weeks later the site becomes swollen, indurated, and painful; assumes a dusky purplish hue; and may ulcerate. Regional lymphangitis and lymphadenitis, fever, chills, malaise, myalgia, arthralgia, and headache are present. Splenomegaly may occur. A sparse, dusky-red maculopapular rash appears on the trunk and extremities in many cases, and there may be frank arthritis.

After a few days, both the local and systemic symptoms subside, only to reappear again in a few more days. This relapsing pattern of fever of 24–48 hours alternating with an equal afebrile period may persist for weeks. The other features, however, usually recur only during the first few relapses.

**B. Laboratory Findings:** Leukocytosis is often present, and the nontreponemal test for syphilis is often falsely positive. The organism may be identified in darkfield examination of the ulcer exudate or aspirated lymph node material; more commonly, it is observed after inoculation of a laboratory animal with the patient's exudate or blood. It has not been cultured in artificial media.

## Differential Diagnosis

Rat-bite fever must be distinguished from the rat bite-induced lymphadenitis and rash of streptobacillary fever. Reliable differentiation requires an increasing titer of agglutinins against *Streptobacillus moniliformis* or identification of the causative organism. Rat-bite fever may also be distinguished from tularemia rickettsial disease, *Pasteurella multocida* infections, and relapsing fever by identification of the causative organism.

## Treatment

Treat with procaine penicillin G, 300,000 units intramuscularly every 12 hours; or tetracycline hydrochloride, 0.5 g every 6 hours for 2–3 days. Give supportive and symptomatic measures as indicated.

## Prognosis

The reported mortality rate is about 10%, but this should be markedly reduced by prompt diagnosis and antimicrobial treatment.

Cole JS et al: Rat-bite fever. *Ann Intern Med* 1969;**71**:979.

## LEPTOSPIROSIS

Leptospirosis is an acute and often severe infection that frequently affects the liver or other organs and is caused by reservoirs of *Leptospira interrogans*. The 3 most common reservoirs of infection are *Leptospira icterohaemorrhagiae* of rats, *Leptospira canicola* of dogs, and *Leptospira pomona* of cattle and swine. Several other varieties can also cause the disease, but *L icterohaemorrhagiae* causes the most severe illness. The disease is worldwide in distribution, and the incidence is higher than usually supposed. The leptospirae are often transmitted to humans by the ingestion of food and drink contaminated by the urine of the reservoir animal. The organism may also enter through minor skin lesions and probably via the conjunctiva. Many infections have followed bathing in contaminated water. The disease is an occupational hazard among sewer workers, rice planters, and farmers. The incubation period is 2–20 days.

## Clinical Findings

**A. Symptoms and Signs:** There is a sudden onset of fever to 39–40 °C (102.2–104 °F), chills, abdominal pains, vomiting, and myalgia, especially of the calf muscles. Extremely severe headache is usually present. The conjunctiva is markedly reddened. The liver may be palpable, and in about 50% of cases (most commonly in *L icterohaemorrhagiae* infections [''Weil's disease'']), jaundice is present on about the fifth day and may be associated with nephritis. Capillary hemorrhages and purpuric skin lesions may also appear. The illness is often biphasic. After initial improvement, the second phase develops at the time that IgM antibodies appear. It manifests itself often as ''aseptic meningitis'' with intense headache, stiff neck, and pleocytosis. Nephritis and hepatitis may also recur until the illness resolves.

Pretibial fever occurred during World War II at Fort Bragg, USA. In pretibial fever, there is patchy erythema on the skin of the lower legs or generalized rash occurring with fever.

Leptospirosis with jaundice must be distinguished from hepatitis, yellow fever, and relapsing fever.

**B. Laboratory Findings:** The leukocyte count may be normal or as high as 50,000/μL, with neutrophils predominating. The urine may contain bile, protein, casts, and red cells. Oliguria is not uncommon, and in severe cases uremia may occur. In cases with meningeal involvement, organisms may be found in the cerebrospinal fluid. The organism may be identified by darkfield examination of the patient's blood (during the first 10 days) or by culture on a semisolid medium (eg, Fletcher's EMJH) for 1–6 weeks. The organism may also be grown from the urine from the tenth day to the sixth week. Specific agglutination titers develop after 7 days and may persist at high levels for many years; specific serologic tests are of particular value in diagnosis of the milder, anicteric forms and of aseptic meningitis. A rapid diagnosis can be made by the determination of specific IgM with the DOT-ELISA method. Serum CPK is usually elevated in leptospirosis patients and normal in hepatitis patients.

## Complications

Myocarditis, aseptic meningitis, renal failure, and massive hemorrhage are not common but are the usual causes of death. Iridocyclitis may occur.

## Treatment

Various antimicrobial drugs, including penicillin and tetracyclines, show antileptospiral activity. Penicillin has been given, but its therapeutic effect is in doubt, despite observed Jarisch-Herxheimer reactions. Observe for evidence of renal failure, and treat as necessary. Effective prophylaxis consists of doxycycline, 200 mg orally, given once weekly during the risk of exposure.

## Prognosis

Without jaundice, the disease is almost never fatal. With jaundice, the mortality rate is 5% for those under age 30 and 30% for those over age 60.

McLain JB et al: Doxycycline therapy for leptospirosis. *Ann Intern Med* 1984;**100**:696.

Pappas MG et al: Rapid serodiagnosis of leptospirosis using IgM-specific DOT-ELISA. *Am J Trop Med Hyg* 1985; **34**:346.

Takafuji ET et al: An efficacy trial of doxycycline chemoprophylaxis against leptospirosis. *N Engl J Med* 1984;**310**:497.

## LYME DISEASE

This illness, named after the town of Lyme, Connecticut, occurs typically in summer. It presents with the unique skin lesion erythema chronicum migrans, often accompanied by headache, stiff neck, fever, myalgias, arthralgias, or lymphadenopathy. Weeks or months later, some patients have neurologic symptoms and frank arthritis, which may recur for several years. The disease has been reported from 3 areas in the USA (the Northeast, the northern Midwest, and the Pacific Coast) and in Europe and Australia.

The disease is transmitted by a small ixodid tick, often *Ixodes dammini* (*I pacificus* on the west coast of the United States; *I ricinus* in Europe), that carries spirochetes (*Borrelia burgdorferi*). The nymphal stage seems to be responsible for transmitting the disease. The wild animal reservoir includes deer and a variety of rodents. The same spirochetes *(B burgdorferi)* have been recovered from the blood and cerebrospinal fluid of patients, who also develop specific IgM antibodies to the spirochetes 3–6 weeks after onset of illness. In patients with arthritis and other complications, high titers of IgG antibody are found, and it is probable that the late complications are a manifestation of antigen-antibody complex deposition.

Penicillin or tetracycline given early in the acute illness terminates it abruptly and prevents late arthritis and other complications. About half of patients with established arthritis will have a permanent resolution if treated with benzathine penicillin, 2.4 million units per week for 3 weeks.

Benach JL et al: Spirochetes isolated from the blood of two patients with Lyme disease. *N Engl J Med* 1983;**308**:740.

Campagna J et al: Lyme disease in northern California. *West J Med* 1983;**139**:319.

Hardin JA et al: Immune complexes and the evolution of Lyme arthritis. *N Engl J Med* 1979;**301:**1358.

Malawista SE, Steere AC: Lyme disease: Infectious in origin, rheumatic in expression. *Adv Intern Med* 1986;**31:**147.

Meyerhoff J: Lyme disease. *Am J Med* 1983;**75:**663.

Steere AC et al: Neurologic abnormalities of Lyme disease. *Ann Intern Med* 1983:**99:**767.

Steere AC et al: Successful parenteral penicillin therapy of established Lyme arthritis. *N Engl J Med* 1985;**312:** 869.

Steere AC et al: Treatment of the early manifestations of Lyme disease. *Ann Intern Med* 1983;**99:**22.

# Infectious Diseases: Protozoal

*Robert S. Goldsmith, MD, MPH, DTM&H*

## AMEBIASIS

### Essentials of Diagnosis

- Mild to moderate amebic colitis: recurrent diarrhea and abdominal cramps, sometimes alternating with constipation. Mucus may be present but no blood.
- Severe amebic colitis: semiformed to liquid stools streaked with blood and mucus; fever; colic; prostration. In fulminant cases, ileus, perforation, peritonitis, hemorrhage.
- Hepatic amebiasis: hepatic enlargement, pain, and tenderness; fever.
- Laboratory findings: amebas in stools or in abscess aspirate. Serologic tests positive with severe colitis or hepatic abscess. Radiologic methods show size and location of abscess.

### General Considerations

Amebiasis is caused by the protozoan parasite *Entamoeba histolytica*. The organisms either live as commensals in the lumen of the large intestine without causing disease (the asymptomatic chronic carrier) or invade the colon wall causing acute dysentery or chronic diarrhea of variable severity. The organisms may also be carried by the blood to the liver, where they produce hepatic abscesses. Rarely, they are carried to the lungs, brain, or other organs or invade the perianal skin.

*E histolytica* exists as 2 forms in feces: cysts (10–14 μm) and motile trophozoites (12–50 μm). In the absence of diarrhea, trophozoites encyst in the large bowel. Trophozoites passed into the environment die rapidly, but cysts remain viable in soil and water for several weeks to months at appropriate temperature and humidity.

The infection is present worldwide but is most prevalent and severe in tropical areas, where rates may exceed 40% under conditions of crowding, poor sanitation, and poor nutrition. It is estimated that invasive amebiasis causes between 40,000 and 100,000 deaths annually worldwide. In temperate areas, amebiasis tends to be a mild, chronic disease that often remains undiagnosed. In the USA, seropositive rates up to 2–5% have been reported in some populations.

Humans are the only known host and are universally susceptible. Only cysts are infectious, the source of infection being persons who eliminate cysts in their feces—asymptomatic carriers and those with chronic diarrhea. On ingestion, cysts survive gastric acidity, but trophozoites are destroyed.

Transmission generally occurs through ingestion of cysts from fecally contaminated food or water. Flies and other arthropods also serve as mechanical vectors; to an undetermined degree, transmission results from contamination of food by the hands of food handlers. Where human excrement is used as fertilizer, it is often a source of food contamination. Person-to-person contact is important in transmission; therefore, all household members as well as an infected person's sexual partner should have their stools examined. Amebiasis is rarely epidemic, but urban outbreaks have occurred because of common-source water contamination. Sexual transmission of *E histolytica* and other intestinal protozoa has reached epidemic proportions among male homosexuals in some urban areas. In closed institutions such as mental institutions, prevalence rates as high as 50% have been reported.

It is undetermined whether strains differ with regard to invasiveness or whether all strains under the right conditions can become invasive. The circumstances under which commensals become invasive is little understood. Malnutrition probably predisposes to enhanced virulence. Corticosteroids and other immunosuppressive drugs often convert a commensal infection to an invasive one. Women in late pregnancy and the puerperium are especially susceptible. Isoenzyme analysis of isolates has shown 22 zymodemes from different parts of the world, of which 9 have been associated with tissue invasiveness. In culture, these traits have been stable. Tissue invasion elicits both humoral (IgM and IgG) antibodies and a cellular immune response, but humoral antibody titers do not correlate with protective immunity.

The characteristic intestinal lesion is the amebic ulcer, which can occur anywhere in the large bowel (including the appendix) and sometimes in the terminal ileum but predominates in the cecum, descending colon, and the rectosigmoid colon—areas of greatest fecal stasis. Trophozoites invade the colonic mucosa by means of their ameboid movement and proteolytic secretions and induce necrosis to form the characteristic flask-shaped ulcers. Usually the ulcers are limited to the outer muscular layer, but when this has been penetrated to the serous layer, bowel perforation may result and lead to local abscess or generalized peritonitis. In fulminating cases, the ulceration may be extensive, and the bowel becomes thin and friable. Hepatic abscesses range in size from a few millimeters to 15 cm or larger, usually are single but may be multiple, occur more often in the right lobe and in the upper portion of that lobe, and are more common in men.

## Clinical Findings

**A. Symptoms and Signs:** Amebiasis has protean clinical manifestations that can be classified into intestinal and extraintestinal lesions and further subdivided into the clinical syndromes described below. Some patients have an acute onset of intense diarrhea as early as 8 days (commonly 2–4 weeks) after infection. Others may have an asymptomatic intestinal infection for months to several years before either intestinal symptoms or a liver abscess appear. Transition may occur from one type of intestinal infection to another, and each may give rise to hepatic abscess, or the intestinal infection may clear spontaneously.

**1. Intestinal amebiasis–**

**a. Asymptomatic infection–**In most infected persons, the organism lives as a commensal, and the patient is without symptoms.

**b. Mild to moderate colitis (nondysenteric colitis)–**This may follow acute disease or be the initial manifestation. The patient passes only a few stools a day, which are semiformed and have a strong fetid odor; mucus may be present, but the stools are free of blood. There may be abdominal cramps, flatulence, chronic fatigue, and weight loss. Characteristically, there are periods of remission and recurrence that may last days to weeks or longer, and during remission the patient may have constipation. Abdominal examination may show hyperperistalsis and tenderness and fullness due to gaseous distention of the colon. In some patients with chronic infection, the colon is thick and palpable, particularly over the cecum and descending colon.

**c. Severe colitis (dysenteric colitis)–**As the severity of intestinal infection increases, the number of stools increases, they change from semiformed to liquid with an unpleasant odor, and streaks of blood and mucus begin to appear. With larger numbers of stools, 10–20 or more, little fecal material is present, but blood (fresh or dark), mucus, and bits of necrotic tissue become increasingly evident. With increasing severity, the patient may become prostrate and show signs of toxicity, with fever up to 40.5 °C (105 °F), and have colic, tenesmus, vomiting, generalized abdominal tenderness, and nonspecific hepatic enlargement and tenderness. Rare complications include appendicitis, bowel perforation (followed by peritonitis, pericolonic abscess, retroperitoneal fecal cellulitis, fistula to the abdominal surface), and fulminating colitis (with paralytic ileus, hypotension, massive mucosal sloughing, and hemorrhage). Death may follow.

**d. Localized ulcerative lesions of the colon–**Sometimes the bowel ulcerations are limited to the rectal area, which may result in the passage of formed stools with bloody exudate. Bowel ulcerations limited to the cecum may cause pain with little diarrhea and simulate acute appendicitis. Amebic appendicitis itself, in which the appendix is extensively involved but not the remainder of the large bowel, is rare.

**e. Localized granulomatous lesions of the colon (ameboma)–**This occurs as a result of excessive production of granulation tissue in response to amebic infection, either in the course of dysentery or slowly in chronic intestinal infection. These masses may present as an irregular tumor (single or multiple) that projects into the bowel or as an annular constricting mass up to several centimeters in length. Clinical findings (pain, obstructive symptoms, and hemorrhage) and x-ray findings may simulate bowel carcinoma or lymphogranuloma venereum. At endoscopy, the mass is deep red and bleeds easily, and biopsy specimens show granulation tissue and *E histolytica*. Surgical removal of the lesion without antiamebic treatment is likely to result in the death of the patient.

**f. Postdysenteric colitis–**This is an uncommon sequela of severe amebic colitis. Following adequate treatment, diarrhea continues and the mucosa may be reddened and edematous, but no ulcers or organisms are found. Most such cases are self-limited, with permanent remission in weeks to months. Uncommonly, the diarrhea may be profound and unremitting and in some instances probably represents ulcerative colitis triggered by the amebic infection.

**2. Extraintestinal amebiasis–**

**a. Hepatic amebiasis–**Amebic liver abscess, although a relatively infrequent consequence of intestinal amebiasis, is not uncommon given the large number of intestinal infections. A large percentage of patients with liver abscess do not have concurrent intestinal symptoms nor can they recall having had chronic intestinal symptoms. The onset of symptoms can be sudden or gradual, ranging from a few days to many months. Cardinal manifestations are fever (often high), pain (continuous, stabbing, or pleuritic, and sometimes severe), and an enlarged and tender liver. Patients may also experience malaise or prostration, sweating, chills, anorexia, and weight loss. The liver enlargement may present subcostally, in the epigastrium, as a localized bulging of the rib cage, or, as a result of enlargement against the dome of the diaphragm, it may produce coughing and findings at the right lung base (dullness to percussion, rales, and diminished breath sounds). Intercostal tenderness is common. Localizing signs may be an area of edema or a point of maximum tenderness. Without prompt treatment, the hepatic abscess may rupture into the pleural, peritoneal, or pericardial space or other contiguous organs, and death may follow.

**b. Nonspecific hepatic enlargement–**A low-grade, nonspecific enlargement of the liver—in which amebic liver infection is not present—may accompany invasive amebic bowel disease. It disappears with eradication of the amebic bowel infection but without use of specific drugs required to eradicate an amebic liver infection.

**3. Other extraintestinal infections–**Metastatic

infection may rarely occur throughout the body, particularly the lungs, brain, perianal skin, and genitalia.

**B. Laboratory Findings:** *E histolytica* trophozoites and cysts in stool specimens are difficult to detect. Three specimens obtained under optimum conditions and tested by skilled personnel will probably detect only 80% of amebic infections. Three additional tests will raise the diagnosis rate to about 90%. Trophozoites predominate in liquid stools, and cysts predominate in formed stools.

A standard procedure is to collect 3 specimens at 2-day intervals or longer, with one of the 3 obtained after a laxative. They should be collected in a clean container without having come in contact with urine or toilet water. Because trophozoites rapidly autolyze, specimens should be examined within about 30 minutes or should immediately be mixed with a preservative. Polyvinyl alcohol is commonly used but is a poison; therefore, a child-proof bottle should be provided and labeled as such.

If the patient has received specific therapy, antibiotics, antimalarials, antidiarrheal preparations containing bismuth or kaolin, magnesium hydroxide, barium, or mineral oil, specimen collection should be delayed 10–14 days.

In mild intestinal amebiasis, there are usually no findings by sigmoidoscopy. In severe disease, sigmoidoscopy commonly aids diagnosis by permitting detection of ulcerative lesions (from 1 mm to 2 cm) with intact intervening mucosa and collection of exudate for examination. Exudate should be collected with a glass pipette (not cotton) or obtained by scraping with a metal instrument. The colon should not be cleansed before sigmoidoscopy, since this washes exudate from ulcers and destroys trophozoites. In some centers, rectal biopsy has enhanced diagnosis; the specimens are best examined by immunofluorescence methods. Where possible, in vitro culture of amebas can be attempted.

Finding trophozoites that contain ingested red blood cells is diagnostic for invasive *E histolytica,* but they may be confused with the occasional macrophage also containing red blood cells. *E histolytica* cysts and trophozoites must be differentiated from the other pathogenic intestinal protozoa: *Giardia lamblia, Dientamoeba fragilis, Balantidium coli, Sarcocystis* species, and *Isospora belli;* and from the nonpathogens: *Endolimax nana, Entamoeba coli, Entamoeba polecki, Entamoeba hartmanni, Iodamoeba bütschlii, Trichomonas hominis, Chilomastix mesnili,* and other flagellates. Leukocytes and macrophages are relatively scarce (in contrast to bacillary dysentery) unless there is concomitant bacillary infection. Charcot-Leyden crystals may be present.

In dysentery, the white blood cell count can reach 20,000 or higher, but it is not elevated in mild colitis. A low-grade eosinophilia is occasionally present. Serologic testing for amebiasis is specific and usually positive if there has been substantial tissue invasion (as occurs in liver amebic abscess or severe intestinal infection); with relatively little tissue invasion (as

in mild or asymptomatic intestinal infection), only a few patients are positive. The indirect hemagglutination test is sensitive and apparently produces no false-positive reactions. Positive titers persist for several years after successful treatment. Test results from central laboratories may not be available for 1–3 weeks, but immunodiffusion tests can provide results in hours to 2 days. The antibody detected by immunodiffusion tests disappears within several months after successful treatment.

In amebic liver abscess, serologic tests will be positive, but the stools may or may not contain the parasite. The white count ranges from 15,000 to 25,000/µL (25% < 10,000; 10% > 25,000). Eosinophilia is not present. Liver function test abnormalities, when present, are usually low-grade. In many patients, aspiration is indicated for diagnosis and, if the abscess is large, for therapy as well to prevent rupture. The risks are hemorrhage and bacterial infection; therefore, aspiration should be done under strict aseptic conditions. Divide the aspirate into serial 30- to 50-mL aliquots, but examine only the last sample. Add 10 units of streptodornase per milliliter, mix, incubate for 30 minutes at 37 °C, centrifuge for 5 minutes at 1000 rpm, and then examine for trophozoites.

**C. Imaging:** Procedures used to locate and define liver lesions include chest radiograph and fluoroscopy, radioisotope scanning, ultrasonography, CT scanning, and in some cases arteriography.

### Differential Diagnosis

Amebiasis should be considered in persons residing in or in travelers returning from endemic areas and in individuals intimately associated with known cases. Amebiasis should be included in the differential diagnosis of most cases of acute and chronic diarrhea (including persons with only mild changes in bowel habits who have an exposure history), liver abscess, annular lesions of the colon, and skin lesions in the perianal area. All patients with inflammatory bowel disease should be tested by stool examination and serology, because of the risk of overwhelming amebic disease if corticosteroid therapy were to be given.

### Prevention & Control

Prevention is effected through education about personal hygiene, sanitary disposal of human feces, protection of rural and urban water supplies against fecal contamination, and control of flies and protection of foods against contamination by flies.

### Treatment

Amebiasis may present in many different clinical forms (see above). The choice of drug depends on the clinical presentation and the site of drug action. Treatment may require the concurrent or sequential use of several drugs. Table 25–1 outlines a preferred and an alternative method of treatment for each clinical type of amebiasis. No drugs are recommended as safe or effective for chemoprophylaxis.

**Table 25–1.** Treatment of amebiasis.

| | Drug(s) of Choice | Alternative Drug(s) |
|---|---|---|
| Asymptomatic intestinal infection | Diloxanide furoate[1,2] | Iodoquinol (diiodohydroxyquin)[3] |
| Mild to moderate intestinal infection (non-dysenteric colitis) | (1) Metronidazole[4]<br>**plus**<br>(2) Diloxanide furoate[1,2] or iodoquinol[3] | (1) Diloxanide furoate[1,2] or iodoquinol[3]<br>**plus**<br>(2) A tetracycline[5]<br>**followed by**<br>(3) Chloroquine[6]<br>**or**<br>(1) Paromomycin[7]<br>**followed by**<br>(2) Chloroquine[6] |
| Severe intestinal infection (dysentery) | (1) Metronidazole[8]<br>**plus**<br>(2) Diloxanide furoate[1,2] or iodoquinol[3]<br>**If parenteral therapy is needed initially**<br>(1) Intravenous metronidazole[9] until oral therapy can be started<br>(2) Then give oral metronidazole[8] plus diloxanide furoate[1,2] or iodoquinol[3] | (1) A tetracycline[5]<br>**plus**<br>(2) Diloxanide furoate[1,2] or iodoquinol[3]<br>**followed by**<br>(3) Chloroquine[10]<br>**or**<br>(1) Dehydroemetine[1,11] or emetine[11]<br>**followed by**<br>(2) A tetracycline[5] plus diloxanide furoate[1,2] or iodoquinol[3]<br>**followed by**<br>(3) Chloroquine[10] |
| Hepatic abscess | (1) Metroidazole[8,9]<br>**plus**<br>(2) Diloxanide furoate[1,2] or iodoquinol[3]<br>**followed by**<br>(3) Chloroquine[10] | (1) Dehydroemetine[1,12] or emetine[12]<br>**plus**<br>(2) Chloroquine[13]<br>**plus**<br>(3) Diloxanide furoate[1,2] or iodoquinol[3] |
| Ameboma or extraintestinal infection | As for hepatic abscess, but not including chloroquine | As for hepatic abscess, but not including chloroquine |

[1] Available in the USA only from the Parasitic Disease Drug Service, Centers for Disease Control, Atlanta 30333. Telephone requests may be made by calling the central number (404) 329–3311 days; (404) 329–2888 nights, weekends, and holidays (emergencies only).

[2] Diloxanide furoate, 500 mg 3 times daily with meals for 10 days (for children, 20 mg/kg in 3 divided doses daily for 10 days).

[3] Iodoquinol (diiodohydroxyquin), 650 mg 3 times daily for 21 days (for children, 30–40 mg/kg (maximum 2 g) in 3 divided doses daily for 21 days).

[4] Metronidazole, 750 mg 3 times daily for 10 days (for children, 35 mg/kg in 3 divided doses daily for 10 days).

[5] A tetracycline, 250 mg 4 times daily for 10 days; in severe dysentery, give 500 mg 4 times daily for the first 5 days, then 250 mg 4 times daily for 5 days. Tetracycline should not be used during pregnancy or in children under 8 years of age; in older children, give 20 mg/kg in 4 divided doses daily for 10 days).

[6] Chloroquine, 500 mg (salt) daily for 7 days (for children, 16 mg/kg [salt] daily for 7 days).

[7] Paromomycin, 25–30 mg/kg (base) (maximum 3 g) in 3 divided doses after meals daily for 5–10 days (for children, the same dosage). Use only for mild disease.

[8] Metronidazole, 750 mg 3 times daily for 5–10 days (for children, 35–50 mg/kg in 3 divided doses daily for 10 days).

[9] An intravenous metronidazole is available; change to oral medication as soon as possible. See manufacturer's recommendation for dosage.

[10] Chloroquine, 500 mg (salt) daily for 14 days (for children, 16 mg/kg [salt] daily for 14 days).

[11] Dehydroemetine or emetine, 1 mg/kg subcut (preferred) or IM daily for the least number of days necessary to control severe symptoms (usually 3–5 days) (maximum daily dose of dehydroemetine is 90 mg; of emetine, 65 mg).

[12] Dehydroemetine or emetine, 1 mg/kg subcut (preferred) or IM daily for 8–10 days (maximum daily dose of dehydroemetine is 90 mg; of emetine, 65 mg).

[13] Chloroquine, 500 mg (salt) twice daily for 2 days IM and then 500 mg daily for 21 days (for children, 16 mg/kg [salt] daily for 21 days).

The **tissue amebicides** dehydroemetine and emetine act on organisms in the bowel wall and in other tissues but not on amebas in the bowel lumen. Chloroquine is active principally against amebas in the liver. The **luminal amebicides** diloxanide furoate, iodoquinol, and paromomycin act on organisms in the bowel lumen but are ineffective against amebas in the bowel wall or other tissues. Oral tetracycline inhibits the bacterial associates of *E histolytica* and thus has an indirect effect on amebas in the bowel lumen and bowel wall but not in other tissues. Given parenterally, antibiotics have little antiamebic activity at any site.

Metronidazole is unique in that it is effective both in the bowel lumen and in the bowel wall and other tissues. However, metronidazole when used alone for bowel infections is not sufficient as a luminal amebicide, for it fails to cure up to 50% of infections.

**A. Asymptomatic Intestinal Infection:** Cure rates with a single course of diloxanide furoate or iodoquinol are 80–85%. Usually in asymptomatic infection, a tissue amebicidal drug is not given to prevent liver infection. Other alternatives for treatment or re-treatment are paromomycin or metronidazole plus iodoquinol or diloxanide furoate.

## B. Mild to Moderate Intestinal Infection:

When iodoquinol is used, concomitant use of a tetracycline probably increases intestinal cure rates. It is less well established that adding a tetracycline to diloxanide furoate therapy increases effectiveness. Chloroquine is used to destroy trophozoites carried to the liver or to eradicate an undetected early-stage amebic liver abscess; the minimum dose needed to accomplish this is not known. In endemic areas where intestinal infection and reinfection are common yet hepatic abscess is rare (eg, in urban communities where intestinal amebiasis is sexually transmitted among male homosexuals but hepatic amebiasis is uncommon), it is probably unnecessary to use chloroquine in the treatment of mild intestinal disease.

## C. Severe Intestinal Infection:
Fluid and electrolyte therapy and opiates to control bowel motility are necessary adjuncts in severe amebic dysentery.

## D. Hepatic Abscess:
When metronidazole is given for 10 days, early or late treatment failure occurs rarely. If a satisfactory clinical response has not occurred within 2–3 days, especially if the abscess has been adequately drained, therapy should be changed to the alternative mode of treatment: dehydroemetine (or emetine) plus chloroquine. When the clinical response to metronidazole is adequate, it is suggested that a 2-week course of chloroquine follow to prevent late failures. The need for adding this course of chloroquine remains to be evaluated. Either mode of treatment also requires a luminal amebicide (diloxanide furoate or iodoquinol), whether or not the organism is found in the stool.

Since a comparative trial of metronidazole with and without aspiration has not been reported, the indications for therapeutic aspiration are still controversial. Aspiration is clearly indicated when the diagnosis is in doubt, if rupture of a large abscess is impending, or if there is a lack of response to therapy.

## E. Adverse Drug Reactions:
Dehydroemetine and emetine are general protoplasmic poisons having adverse effects on many tissues and a narrow range between therapeutic and toxic effects; dehydroemetine may be the safer of the 2 drugs. Metronidazole has been found to induce neoplasms in rodents and to be mutagenic in the *Salmonella* test system and thus may be carcinogenic. However, based on current evidence, some authorities consider the drug to be essentially free of cancer risk. The other nitroimidazoles have similar mutagenic action in the *Salmonella* test system. The halogenated hydroxyquinolines have been increasingly implicated in the production of neurotoxicity. The tetracyclines should not be used for children under age 8 years; use erythromycin stearate instead, even though it is somewhat less effective.

## Follow-Up Care

Follow-up examination consists of study of at least 3 stools at 2- to 3-day intervals, starting 2–4 weeks after the end of treatment. For some patients, sigmoidoscopy and reexamination of stools within 3 months may be indicated.

## Prognosis

The mortality rate from untreated amebic dysentery or hepatic abscess may be high. With modern chemotherapy instituted early in the course of the disease, the prognosis is good.

Allason-Jones E et al: *Entamoeba histolytica* as a commensal parasite in homosexual men. *N Engl J Med* 1986;**315**:353.

Davis A, Pawlowski ZS: Amoebiasis and its control. *Bull WHO* 1985;**63**:417.

Goldmeier D et al: Is *Entamoeba histolytica* in homosexual men a pathogen? *Lancet* 1986;**1**:641.

Guerrant RL: Introduction, current status, and research questions in: *The Global Problems of Amebiasis: Current Status, Research Needs, and Opportunities for Progress. Rev Infect Dis* 1986;**8**:218.

Ravdin JI: Pathogenesis of disease caused by *Entamoeba histolytica*: Studies of adherence, secreted toxins, and contact-dependent cytolysis. *Rev Infect Dis* 1986;**8**:247.

Ravdin JI, Guerrant RL: Current problems in diagnosis and treatment of amebic infections. In: *Current Clinical Topics in Infectious Diseases*. Remington JS, Swartz MN (editors). McGraw-Hill, 1986.

Thompson JE, Forlenza S, Verma R: Amebic liver abscess: A therapeutic approach. *Rev Infect Dis* 1985;**7**:171.

## PATHOGENIC FREE-LIVING AMEBAS

### Primary Amebic Meningoencephalitis

Primary amebic meningoencephalitis is a fulminating, purulent meningoencephalitis that resembles bacterial meningitis and is rapidly fatal. The disease is rare but probably has worldwide distribution. More than 130 cases have been recognized in the past 15 years, mostly in children and young adults. The responsible organisms are free-living ameboflagellates of the genus *Naegleria;* most cases have been due to *Naegleria fowleri.*

*N fowleri* is a thermophilic organism found in fresh and polluted warm lake water, domestic water supplies, swimming pools, thermal water, and sewers. Most patients give a history of exposure to fresh water, eg, swimming in surface water or in swimming pools, especially heated water. Dust is also a possible source of infection. Nasal and throat swabs have shown a human carrier state, and serologic surveys suggest that inapparent infections occur.

The organism apparently invades the central nervous system through the cribriform plate. The incubation period is not established but appears to vary from 1 to 14 days. Early symptoms include headache, fever, and lethargy, often associated with rhinitis and pharyngitis. Vomiting, disorientation, and other signs of meningoencephalitis develop within 1 or 2 days, followed by coma and then death on the fifth or sixth day. A few victims have been shown at autopsy to have a nonspecific myocarditis.

Lumbar or ventricular fluid contains several hundred to 25,000 leukocytes/$\mu$L, 50–100% of which are neutrophils. Erythrocytes are present in most cases, up to several thousand per microliter. Protein is usually moderately elevated and glucose moderately reduced. If conventional examinations for bacteria and fungi are negative, the fluid must then be examined for free-living amebas to make the specific diagnosis. A simple wet mount examined by an ordinary optical microscope with the aperture restricted or condensor down will enhance contrast and refractility; a warm stage is not needed. The fluid should not be centrifuged or refrigerated, as this tends to immobilize the amebas. Their brisk motility distinguishes them from leukoctyes of various types, which they otherwise closely resemble. In fixed stained smears, the amebas may also be recognized by their distinctive "targetlike" large nucleolus in the center of the nucleus. Culture and mouse inoculation studies should be performed. Serologic testing for antibody and circulating antigen is experimental.

Precise species identification is based on morphology, demonstration of flagellate transformation (*Naegleria* only), immunofluorescent antibody studies, immunoelectrophoretic antigen patterns, and isoenzyme studies.

Only 2 well-documented survivors are reported in the literature. One patient was treated with intravenous and intrathecal amphotericin B in large doses and the other with a combination of amphotericin B, miconazole, and rifampin. Experimental studies have shown a marked synergistic effect in vitro and in vivo between amphotericin B and either tetracycline or rifampin.

### *Acanthamoeba* Infections

Free-living amebas of the genus *Acanthamoeba* are found in soil and in fresh, brackish, and thermal water as trophozoites (15–45 μm) or cysts (10–25 μm). They have been recognized only recently as human pathogens, causing a number of poorly defined syndromes: (1) a subacute and chronic focal granulomatous necrotizing meningoencephalitis that invariably has led to death in weeks to months, (2) skin lesions that resemble deep fungal infections, (3) granulomatous dissemination to many tissues, and (4) uveitis and corneal ulceration leading to blindness. Portals of entry may include the skin, eyes, or respiratory tract. A commensal nasal carrier state is established, and immunocompromised patients may have increased susceptibility.

In the encephalitis syndrome, cerebrospinal fluid lymphocytes have been described. Antemortem diagnosis has been made via biopsy specimens. The presence of cysts or mitotic division in tissue section may be pathognomonic of *Acanthamoeba* infection.

The clinical features suggestive of *Acanthamoeba* keratitis are (1) severe ocular pain, (2) partial or 360-degree paracentral stromal ring infiltrate; (3) recurrent corneal epithelial breakdown, and (4) a corneal lesion refractory to the usual medications. The diagnosis can be confirmed by vigorously scraping the cornea with a swab or platinum-tipped scapula; the material is microscopically examined after staining with Giemsa's or trichrome stain and is also placed in culture on nonnutrient agar seeded with *Escherichia coli*.

There is no effective treatment at present. In vitro studies show that some strains are sensitive to ketoconazole, miconazole, sulfonamides, clotrimazole, pentamidine, paromomycin, flucytosine, and other drugs but not to amphotericin B. Ophthalmic keratitis has been treated with success in some instances by use of ketoconazole, miconazole, propamidine, isethionate, and neomycin.

Ferrante A: Amphotericin B doses for primary amoebic meningoencephalitis. *Lancet* 1986;**2**:35.

Jones DB: *Acanthoamoeba*—the ultimate opportunist? *Am J Ophthalmol* 1986;**102**:527.

Martinez AJ: *Free-Living Amebas: Natural History, Prevention, Diagnosis, Pathology, and Treatment of Disease*. CRC Press, 1985.

Martinez AJ, Janitschke K: *Acanthamoeba*, an opportunistic microorganism: A review *Infection* 1985;**13**:251.

## BABESIOSIS
### (Piroplasmosis)

*Babesia* are tick-borne protozoal parasites that affect wild and domestic animals worldwide. Babesiosis in humans is a rare intraerythrocytic infection caused by 2 *Babesia* species and characterized by fever, chills, myalgia, and hemolytic anemia. The infection has been recognized only in Europe (*Babesia divergens*) and North America (*Babesia microti*), with most infections reported from the northeastern coastal region of the USA. Serosurveys show frequent subclinical *B microti* infections. Humans are infected as a result of *Ixodes* tick bites, but transmission from blood transfusion has also been reported. The parasite apparently enters the red blood cells without passing through an exoerythrocytic stage. Multiplication, cell rupture, and infection of other cells can result in hemolytic anemia, hemoglobinuria, and acute renal necrosis. Splenectomized persons are apparently more susceptible to infection and have more severe illness.

The incubation period is 1–4 weeks, but patients usually do not recall the tick bite. *B microti* infection lasts a few weeks to a month; the illness is characterized by irregular fever, chills, diaphoresis, myalgia, and fatigue but is without malarialike periodicity of symptoms. Most patients have a moderate hemolytic anemia, and some have hepatosplenomegaly. Although parasitemia may continue for months, with or without symptoms, the disease is self-limited and most patients recover without sequelae.

The few reported infections with *B divergens* have been in patients who have undergone splenectomy. These infections progress rapidly with high fever, severe hemolytic anemia, jaundice, hemoglobinuria, and renal failure; death usually follows.

Diagnosis is by identification of the intraerythrocytic parasite on Giemsa-stained thick or thin blood smears; no gametocytes and no intracellular pigment are seen. Repeated smears may be necessary. The organism must be differentiated from malarial parasites, particularly *Plasmodium falciparum*. Isolation of the parasite can be attempted by inoculating patient blood into hamsters or gerbils. Serologic tests are available; serologic cross-reactions occur between *Babesia* and malaria parasites, but antibody titers are generally highest to the infecting organism.

No drug treatment is satisfactory. The only patients who have recovered from *B divergens* infections have been managed with blood transfusions and renal dialysis. As *B microti* infections in patients with intact spleen are usually self-limiting, most infections can be treated symptomatically. In splenectomized patients, however, limited experience suggests that quinine plus clindamycin may be useful; exchange transfusion has also been successful in several patients.

Gombert ME et al: Human babesiosis: Clinical and therapeutic considerations. *JAMA* 1982;**248:**3005.

Rosner F et al: Babesiosis in splenectomized adults: Review of 22 reported cases. *Am J Med* 1984;**76:**696.

Smith RP et al: Transfusion-acquired babesiosis and failure of antibiotic treatment. *JAMA* 1986;**256:**2276.

Steketee RW et al: Babesiosis in Wisconsin: A new focus of disease transmission. *JAMA* 1985;**253:**2675.

## MALARIA

### Essentials of Diagnosis

- History of exposure to malaria.
- Paroxysms (often periodic) of sequential chills, fever, and sweating.
- Headache, myalgia, splenomegaly; anemia, leukopenia.
- Characteristic parasites in erythrocytes, identified in thick or thin blood films.
- *Complications of falciparum malaria:* Cerebral findings (mental disturbances, neurologic findings, convulsions), hemolytic anemia, dysenteric or choleralike stools, dark urine, anuria.

### General Considerations

Four species of the genus *Plasmodium* are responsible for human malaria. Although the infection is generally limited to the tropics and subtropics, many imported cases occur in the USA and other countries free of malaria transmission. Malaria is known to exist in parts of Mexico, Haiti, Central and South America, Africa, the Middle East, Turkey, the Indian subcontinent, Southeast Asia, China, the Malay archipelago, and Oceania. The most common parasites, *Plasmodium vivax* and *Plasmodium falciparum*, are found through the malaria belt. *Plasmodium malariae* is widely distributed but is less common. *Plasmodium ovale* is rare, but in West Africa it seems to replace *P vivax*.

Malaria is transmitted from human to human by the bite of infected female *Anopheles* mosquitoes. Congenital transmission and transmission by blood transfusion or the use of contaminated needles by drug abusers also occur.

The mosquito becomes infected by taking blood containing the sexual forms of the parasite (micro- and macrogametocytes). After a developmental phase in the mosquito, sporozoites develop that are inoculated into humans when the mosquito next feeds. The first stage of development in humans, the exoerythrocytic stage, takes place in the liver. Subsequently, parasites escape from the liver into the bloodstream, invade red blood cells, multiply, and 48 hours later (or 72 with *P malariae*) cause the red cells to rupture, releasing a new crop of parasites. This cycle of invasion, multiplication, and red cell rupture may be repeated many times. Symptoms do not appear until several of these erythrocytic cycles have been completed. The incubation period varies considerably, depending upon the species and strain of parasite, the intensity of the infection, and the immune status of the host. The usual incubation period is 8–20 days for *P falciparum*, and almost all cases will develop within 2 months of infection; 12–18 days for *P vivax* and *P ovale*, but initial attacks may occur up to 8 months after infection; and 24–30 days for *P malariae*. If untreated, *P falciparum* infections usually terminate spontaneously in 6–8 months but can persist for up to 3 years; *P vivax* and *P ovale* infections can persist without treatment for as long as 5 years; and *P malariae* infections have lasted for as long as 40 years.

*P falciparum* and *P malariae* have only one cycle of liver cell invasion and multiplication. Liver infection ceases spontaneously in less than 4 weeks; thereafter, multiplication is confined to the red cells. Thus, treatment that eliminates these species from the red cells will cure the infection. *P vivax* (and presumably *P ovale*) have, however, a dormant hepatic stage (the hypnozoite) that is responsible for subsequent relapses. Cure of *P vivax* and *P ovale* infections, therefore, requires treatment to eradicate parasites both from the red cells and from the liver.

### Clinical Findings

**A. Symptoms and Signs:** The paroxysms of malaria are closely related to events in the bloodstream. The chill, lasting from 15 minutes to an hour, begins as a generation of parasites rupture their host red cells and escape into the blood. Nausea, vomiting, and headache are common at this time. The succeeding hot stage, lasting several hours, is accompanied by a spiking fever, sometimes reaching 40 °C (104 °F) or higher. During this stage, the parasites presumably invade new red cells. The third, or sweating stage, concludes the episode. The fever subsides and the patient frequently falls asleep, to awake feeling relatively well. In *P vivax* (benign tertian malaria), *P ovale*, and *P falciparum* (malignant tertian malaria) infections, red cells are ruptured and paroxysms occur every 48 hours. In *P malariae* infections (quartan malaria), the cycle takes 72 hours. Early, the cycles are frequently asynchronous and the fever patterns irregular. As the disease progresses, splenomegaly and, to a lesser extent, hepatomegaly appear.

*P falciparum* infection is more serious than the others because of the high frequency of severe or fatal complications. *P falciparum* malaria may also be more difficult to recognize clinically. It often presents as a flulike illness with nonspecific symptoms of fever, headache, myalgia, nausea, diarrhea, and abdominal pain or discomfort. The fever may be low-grade, continuous, or with daily spikes and may occur without chills or rigors. Parasites are sometimes difficult to find on blood smears.

**B. Laboratory Findings:** The thick and thin blood film, stained with Giemsa's stain, is the mainstay of malaria diagnosis. The thin film is used primarily for species differentiation after the presence of an infection is detected on a thick film. Because the level of parasitemia varies from hour to hour, especially for *P falciparum* infections, blood should be examined several times a day for 2–3 days. In all but *P falciparum* infections, the number of red cells infected seldom exceeds 2% of the total cells. Very high red cell infection rates may occur with *P falciparum* infection (20–30% or more). For this reason, anemia is frequently much more severe in *P falciparum* malaria. The anemia is normocytic, with poikilocytosis and anisocytosis. During paroxysms, there may be transient leukocytosis; leukopenia develops subsequently, with a relative increase in large mononuclear cells. During attacks, hepatic function tests often become abnormal, but the tests revert to normal with treatment or spontaneous recovery. Hemolytic jaundice and thrombocytopenia may develop in severe infections.

There are no specific blood chemical findings. In *P malariae* infections, a form of nephrosis, with protein and casts in the urine, sometimes occurs in children. Severe *P falciparum* infections may cause renal damage.

Serologic tests are not used in the diagnosis of acute malaria but may be of value occasionally in the diagnosis of low-level infections that are long-standing and relapsing. A titer of 1:64 in the indirect immunofluorescence test indicates that the patient has acquired malaria at some time in the past.

**Differential Diagnosis**

Uncomplicated malaria, particularly when modified by partial immunity, must be distinguished from a variety of other causes of fever, splenomegaly, anemia, or hepatomegaly. Some diseases often considered in the diagnosis of malaria in the tropics include urinary tract infections, typhoid fever, infectious hepatitis, dengue, kala-azar, influenza, amebic liver abscess, leptospirosis, and relapsing fever. Examination of multiple blood films is essential to differentiate atypical malaria from some of the above.

**Complications**

Serious complications of malaria occur primarily in *P falciparum* infections, particularly in persons who have experienced repeated attacks with inadequate treatment. These complications include cerebral

malaria with headache, convulsions, delirium, and coma; hyperpyrexia, closely resembling heat hyperpyrexia; gastrointestinal disorders resembling cholera or acute bacillary dysentery; and algid malaria, which resembles acute adrenal insufficiency. Blackwater fever must be considered apart from other complications of *P falciparum* infections. This acute intravascular hemolytic condition develops in patients with long-standing *P falciparum* infections and a history of irregular quinine dosage. The principal findings are profound anemia, jaundice, fever, and hemoglobinuria. The mortality rate may be as high as 30%, primarily as a result of anuria and uremia.

**Treatment &
Chemoprophylaxis
(Table 25–2)**

Consultation with a center working on malaria is important for obtaining up-to-date information on malaria prophylaxis and treatment. Sources of information and advice in the USA include state health departments and the Centers for Disease Control in Atlanta, Georgia: telephone (404) 452-4046 (for emergencies only, on nights and weekends, call [404] 329-2888).

**A. Drug Classification:** The antimalarial drugs can be classified according to their selective action on different phases of the parasite's life cycle. Except for the action of the antifolates (pyrimethamine and proguanil* [chloroguanide*]) that prevent maturation of the pre-erythrocytic hepatic schizonts of *P falciparum,* none of the drugs prevent infection (ie, are true causal prophylactic drugs), but they do prevent attacks or effect cure. The blood schizonticidal drugs, which destroy circulating plasmodia and thus prevent attacks, include quinine; chloroquine and amodiaquine,* which are 4-aminoquinolines; and pyrimethamine and proguanil. Primaquine destroys the persisting liver stage (the hypnozoite) of *P vivax* and *P ovale,* preventing relapses from these parasites; it is also used to destroy the gametocytes of *P falciparum.* Chloroquine destroys the gametocytes of *P vivax, P malariae,* and *P ovale* but not those of *P falciparum.* Drug combinations that have come into use to treat *P falciparum* malaria resistant to chloroquine include Fansidar (pyrimethamine plus sulfadoxine) and Maloprim* (pyrimethamine plus dapsone).

**B. Indications, Limitations, and Adverse Reactions of Selected Drugs:**

**1. Chloroquine phosphate**—Chloroquine (Aralen) is used in chemoprophylaxis to prevent attacks (to suppress symptoms) of all forms of malaria but does not prevent infection. *P falciparum* and *P malariae* infections are terminated (suppressive cure) if chloroquine is taken weekly for 6 weeks, because these infections have no persistent exoreythrocytic phase. However, in *P vivax* and *P ovale* infections, which have a persistent liver phase, delayed initial attacks or relapses may occur after chloroquine is stopped; use of primaquine eradicates the liver phase.

---

* Not available in the USA but available in some other countries.

Chloroquine is also the drug of choice for treating acute attacks of malaria, but cure occurs only with *P falciparum* and *P malariae*. Cure for *P vivax* and *P ovale* requires primaquine to eradicate the liver phase of the infections. Chloroquine hydrochloride is used for parenteral treatment, but only until oral treatment can be started. This drug must not be used in young children, in whom it may cause hypotension or sudden death.

Although capable of causing ocular damage when used in large doses for prolonged periods for collagen disease, chloroquine is usually well tolerated when used for malaria prophylaxis or treatment. Gastrointestinal symptoms, mild headache, pruritus (especially in blacks), anorexia, malaise, and urticaria may occur; taking the drug after meals may reduce side effects. Rare reactions include impaired hearing, psychosis, convulsions, blood dyscrasias, skin reactions, and hypotension. A total cumulative dosage of 100 g (base) theoretically may be critical in the development of ocular, ototoxic, and myopathic effects. A recent WHO paper, however, presented the view that weekly administration of 0.5 g (of salt) of chloroquine could be continued for up to 7 years. Pregnancy is not a contraindication to use of chloroquine.

Certain antacids and antidiarrheal agents (kaolin, calcium carbonate, and magnesium trisilicate) have been shown to interfere with absorption of chloroquine and should not be taken within about 4 hours of taking the drug.

**2. Primaquine phosphate**–Primaquine is used (1) to prevent relapse of disease by eliminating persistent liver forms of *P vivax* or *P ovale* (''radical cure'') in patients who have had an acute attack and (2) for prophylactic use for individuals returning from an endemic area who have probably been exposed to malaria (see below).

Primaquine is generally well tolerated. Occasional side effects of the drug are gastrointestinal disturbances, dizziness, or neutropenia. Primaquine should not be used in pregnancy.

All patients should be tested for glucose-6-phosphate dehydrogenase (G6PD) deficiency before therapy is begun and followed carefully during treatment; this is because primaquine may cause mild, self-limited hemolysis or marked hemolysis or methemoglobinemia in persons with certain variants of G6PD deficiency or other hereditary erythrocytic pentose phosphate pathway defects that render red blood cells unusually vulnerable to drug-induced lysis. G6PD deficiency is most common among blacks or persons of Mediterranean or Asian extraction. Stop the drug if reddening or darkening of the urine occurs. For individuals deficient in G6PD, it is usually safe to give primaquine phosphate, 78.9 mg (45 mg base), and chloroquine phosphate, 0.5 g (0.3 g base) weekly, for 8 weeks. However, for persons suspected of having the Mediterranean or Canton forms of G6PD deficiency, it may be preferable not to give primaquine but to treat attacks of malaria with chloroquine as they occur.

Primaquine is also used occasionally to eliminate gametocytes of *P falciparum* from patients and thus prevent their transmission to mosquitoes; the dosage is either 45 mg (base) once or 15 mg/d for 5 days.

**3. Quinine**–Oral quinine is used to treat malaria due to chloroquine-resistant strains of *P falciparum*. Although quinine alone will control an acute attack, in many infections—particularly with strains from southeast Asia—it fails to prevent recurrence. Addition of pyrimethamine-sulfadoxine or other drugs (see Table 25–2) lowers the rate of occurrence.

Parenteral quinine (dihydrochloride) is used in the treatment of severe attacks of malaria due to *P falciparum* strains sensitive or resistant to chloroquine. It should be used with extreme caution and only for patients who cannot take the medication orally; appropriate oral therapy should be started as soon as possible.

Oral quinine (sulfate) is occasionally used in prophylaxis where *P falciparum* has become resistant to both chloroquine and pyrimethamine-sulfadoxine.

Quinine toxicity (cinchonism) includes nausea, vomiting, diarrhea, abdominal pain, tinnitus, decreased auditory acuity, blurred vision, and, less often, hypotension or hives or other allergic reactions. Severe toxicity, including agranulocytosis, thrombocytopenia, hypoprothrombinemia, or massive acute hemolysis and renal failure (blackwater fever), is very rare. Desired plasma quinine levels are about 5–10 $\mu$g/mL. Plasma quinine determinations and reduction in dosage to avoid serious toxicity are crucial in patients with renal insufficiency.

**4. Mefloquine**–Mefloquine is a new quinoline methanol derivative. It has minimal side effects and is effective against the blood schizonts of all forms of malaria, including most but not all chloroquine-resistant or multidrug-resistant strains of *P falciparum*. The drug has no effect on the liver forms of parasites or on gametocytes. Side effects, which include dizziness and gastrointestinal symptoms, are usually mild but last a few days. Although resistance can also develop to mefloquine, no resistance has been reported to the combination of quinine and mefloquine. Mefloquine in combination with Fansidar has been undergoing clinical tests.

**C. Parasite Resistance to Drugs:** Strains of *P falciparum* resistant to chloroquine have been reported in rural areas of the following: (1) **Central and South America**—Bolivia, Brazil, Colombia, Ecuador, French Guiana, Guyana, Panama (east of the Canal Zone), Peru (north), Surinam, Venezuela; (2) **Africa**—Angola, Benin, Burundi, Central African Republic, Comoros, Gabon, Kenya, Madagascar, Malawi, Mozambique, Namibia, Rwanda, Sudan (north), Tanzania, Uganda, Zaire (northeast), Zambia (northeast); (3) **Asia**—Burma, China (Hainan Island and southern provinces), Indonesia, Kampuchea, Laos, Malaysia, Philippines, Thailand, Vietnam; (4) **Indian subcontinent**—Bangladesh (north and east), India, Pakistan (Rawalpini), Sri Lanka; and (5) **Ocea-**

**Table 25–2.** Chemoprophylaxis and treatment of malaria in nonimmune populations.

## CHEMOPROPHYLAXIS

| Chemoprophylaxis of all species (except chloroquine-resistant *P falciparum*) | Chemoprophylaxis of *P falciparum* strains resistant to chloroquine but sensitive to pyrimethamine-sulfadoxine (Fansidar)[1] |
|---|---|
| **Prevention of attacks while in endemic area**<br>Chloroquine phosphate, 500 mg (salt)[3,4] once weekly. | **Prevention of attacks while in endemic area[2]**<br>For **long-term exposure** (>3–4 weeks)—pyrimethamine, 25 mg, *plus* sulfadoxine, 500 mg (Fansidar),[1,3] weekly, *plus* chloroquine phosphate, 500 mg (salt)[4] weekly to prevent attacks due to *P vivax* and *P malariae*.<br>For **short-term exposure** (<3–4 weeks)—see text. |
| **Prevention of attacks after leaving endemic area**<br>Chloroquine phosphate, 500 mg (salt) once weekly for 6 weeks *plus* primaquine phosphate, 26.3 mg (salt)[2,4,5,6] daily for 14 days.<br>**or**<br>Chloroquine phosphate 500 mg (salt), *plus* primaquine phosphate, 78.9 mg (salt)[2,4,5,6] once weekly for 8 weeks. | **Prevention of attacks after leaving endemic area[2]**<br>Pyramethamine, 25 mg, *plus* sulfadoxine, 500 mg (Fansidar),[1] once weekly for 6 weeks.<br><br>**plus**<br>Chloroquine and primaquine by one of the 2 methods in the left-hand column to eradicate *P vivax, P ovale,* and *P malariae* infection. |

## TREATMENT

| Treatment of all species (except chloroquine-resistant *P falciparum*) | Treatment of *P falciparum* strains resistant to chloroquine but sensitive to antifolate-sulfonamide combinations |
|---|---|
| **Oral treatment**<br>Chloroquine phosphate, 1 g (salt)[4] as initial dose, then 0.5 g in 6 hours, then 0.5 at 24 and 48 hours,<br><br>**followed by**<br>Primaquine phosphate, 26.3 mg (salt)[5] daily for 14 days if the infection is due to *P vivax* or *P ovale*. | **Oral treatment**<br>Quinine sulfate, 650 mg 3 times daily for 3–7 days;[7] on the first day, give pyrimethamine, 75 mg, and sulfadoxine, 1500 mg (Fansidar),[1]<br>**or**<br>Quinine sulfate, 650 mg 3 times daily for 3–7 days,[7] *plus* pyrimethamine, 25 mg twice daily for 3 days, and sulfadiazine, 500 mg 4 times daily for 5 days.<br>**or**<br>Quinine sulfate, 650 mg 3 times daily for 3–7 days,[7] *plus either tetracycline,*[9] 250–500 mg 4 times daily for 7 days, or doxycycline,[9] 100 mg twice daily for 7 days. |
| **Parenteral treatment of severe attacks**<br>Quinine dihydrochloride.[5] Start oral chloroquine therapy as soon as possible; follow with primaquine if the infection is due to *P vivax* of *P ovale*.<br>**or**<br>Chloroquine hydrochloride, 250 mg (salt)[10] intramuscularly; repeat every 6 hours, but start oral chloroquine therapy as soon as possible; follow with primaquine if the infection is due to *P vivax* of *P ovale*. | **Parenteral treatment of severe attacks**<br>Quinine dihydrochloride.[8] Start oral therapy with quinine plus a second drug (see above) as soon as possible. |

---

[1] One tablet of Fansidar contains 25 mg of pyrimethamine plus 500 mg of sulfadoxine. Fansidar is available in the USA and generally can be obtained in the endemic area. See text for contraindications. Advise travelers to discontinue use of Fansidar immediately in the event of side effects.

[2] Chemoprophylaxis with Fansidar or primaquine should only be used if there is likelihood of exposure (see text).

[3] Before leaving home, patients should take a test dose to detect possible idiosyncratic reactions. The first dose of the drug should be started 1–2 weeks before entering the endemic area. It is essential that the drug be continued weekly for 6 weeks after leaving the endemic area.

[4] 500 mg of chloroquine phosphate salt = 300 mg of chloroquine base.

[5] 26.3 mg of primaquine phosphate salt = 15 mg of primaquine base.

[6] Chloroquine alone, when taken for 6 weeks after leaving the endemic area, is curative for *P falciparum* and *P malariae,* but primaquine is needed to eradicate the persistent exoerythrocytic (liver) stages of *P vivax* and *P ovale*. Start primaquine only after returning home; continue chloroquine weekly until that time and during primaquine therapy. Only travelers likely to be exposed to infection require primaquine (see text). Patients should be screened for G6PD deficiency before use of primaquine.

[7] Although quinine sulfate is usually given for 3 days, it may be continued for 7 days in areas of Southeast Asia where diminished sensitivity to quinine has been noted.

[8] Quinine dihydrochloride is available in the USA from the Parasitic Disease Drug Service, Centers for Disease Control, Atlanta 30333. Telephone requests may be made by calling (404) 452–4046 days; (404) 329-2888 nights, weekends, and holidays. Give 10 mg/kg (salt) in 500 mL of normal saline or 5% glucose intravenously slowly over 4 hours; repeat every 8 hours until oral therapy is possible. Blood pressure and ECG should be monitored frequently. If it is known with certainty that the patient has not already taken the medication, a higher initial loading dose of quinine is given (20 mg/kg). In an emergency, when parenteral quinine or chloroquine is unavailable, quinidine gluconate has been used; 800 mg is diluted in 250 mL of 5% dextrose and administered very slowly intravenously under electrocardiographic monitoring; repeat every 8 hours. Widening of the QRS interval requires discontinuation.

[9] Contraindicated in children under 8 years of age and in pregnancy.

[10] 250 mg of chloroquine hydrochloride salt = 200 mg of chloroquine base; parenteral use of the drug is contraindicated in young children.

nia—Papua New Guinea, Solomon Islands, and Vanuatu.

Resistance in urban areas has been reported in all countries listed under Africa, the Indian subcontinent, and Oceania; in southeast Asia in Kampuchea, Laos (except Vientiane), the Philippines, Thailand, and Vietnam; in the interior of the Amazon River region; and in some parts of Ecuador.

Drug-resistant strains of *P falciparum* may be only partially resistant to 4-aminoquinolines, manifested by a temporary subsidence of symptoms and decrease in parasitemia, followed by recrudescences of symptoms and patent parasitemia after several days to weeks.

*P falciparum* resistance to pyrimethamine and proguanil is common in most endemic areas, but the degree and distribution of resistance are not accurately known. Strains of *P falciparum* resistant to pyrimethamine-sulfadoxine have been established or suspected in Thailand, Papua New Guinea, Irian Jaya, Indonesia, Kenya, Colombia, Kampuchea, Tanzania, and parts of Brazil.

Some strains of *P falciparum* in southeast Asia have shown decreased sensitivity to quinine and mefloquine.

Strains of *P vivax* resistant to pyrimethamine, including the pyrimethamine-containing drugs Fansidar and Maloprim, have been reported in many areas of the world, particularly southeast Asia. However, resistance of *P vivax*, *P malariae,* and *P ovale* to chloroquine and other 4-aminoquinolines has not been observed. Radical cure of *P vivax* with primaquine often requires a larger dosage (22.5 mg [base] for 14 days) in areas of the southwest Pacific and for some strains in Thailand.

## 1. CHEMOPROPHYLAXIS
### (See Table 25–2.)

Adults and children at whatever age, including breastfed infants, require prophylaxis, but no method is 100% effective. Travelers to malarious areas must be warned that malaria symptoms can develop as early as 8 days after first exposure in an endemic area and that malaria is a possible diagnosis if they develop fever and other symptoms even when taking prophylactics regularly. Travelers should also be reminded of the need to use other protective measures when mosquitoes are biting (chiefly between dusk and dawn)—eg, wear clothing that covers most of the body, apply insect repellents (N,N-diethyl-*m*-toluamide [deet]) and reapply it at frequent intervals (1–2 hours); use mosquito nets and screens; and spray the living and sleeping quarters with pyrethrum-containing agents to kill mosquitoes.

## Chemoprophylaxis in Regions Where *P falciparum* Is Sensitive to 4-Aminoquinolines

**A. Chloroquine (Aralen):** Chemoprophylaxis

for nonimmune visitors or temporary residents for all forms of malaria (except in regions where *P falciparum* is resistant to 4-aminoquinolines) is 500 mg chloroquine salt weekly beginning 1–2 weeks before departure for the malarious area and continuing for 6 weeks after last exposure. If a person has been infected with *P vivax* or *P ovale*, relapse may occur for up to several years after stopping chloroquine prophylaxis. Elimination (radical cure) of the persistent liver phase of these parasites is only possible with primaquine. Some experts prefer to avoid the risk of primaquine toxicity and to rely instead on surveillance to detect cases when they occur, particularly when exposure was limited or doubtful. However, when there is a high probability of exposure, primaquine can be given at some point in the 6-week postexposure period at a dosage of 26.3 mg (salt) daily for 14 days. An alternative regimen, in which primaquine is better tolerated, is 500 mg chloroquine salt and 78.9 mg primaquine salt weekly for 8 weeks. Pregnant women should receive chloroquine but not primaquine. For persons intolerant of chloroquine, hydroxychloroquine (Plaquenil) is sometimes better tolerated at a dosage of 400 mg of the salt weekly and for 6 weeks after leaving the endemic area.

**B. Proguanil\* (Chloroguanide,\* Paludrine\* ) and Pyrimethamine (Daraprim):** The status of proguanil in chemoprophylasis is uncertain, as drug-resistant strains of *P vivax* and *P falciparum* usually appear wherever the drug is extensively used; nevertheless, some evidence suggests that proguanil remains effective against pre-erythrocytic stages when effectiveness is lost against blood forms. The prophylactic dose of proguanil is 100 mg (200 mg for a limited period in highly endemic areas) daily and for 6 weeks after departure from the endemic area; when necessary primaquine is used to eradicate *P vivax* and *P ovale*. Some physicians are prescribing proguanil and chloroquine combined for prophylaxis.

**C. Pyrimethamine (Daraprim):** Prophylaxis using pyrimethamine alone is no longer considered to be adequate because of widespread resistance.

**D. Amodiaquine\* (Basoquin,\* Camoquin,\* Flavoquine):** Amodiaquine, a 4-aminoquinoline similar in structure to chloroquine, has been shown to cause agranulocytosis and toxic hepatitis and is no longer recommended in prophylaxis.

**E. Chemoprophylaxis for Indigenes in Endemic Areas:** Chemoprophylaxis is recommended for semi-immune pregnant women, but *mass* prophylaxis of children under 5 years is not recommended.

## Chemoprophylaxis in Regions Where *P falciparum* Is Resistant to 4-Aminoquinolines But Sensitive to Antifolate-Sulfonamide Combinations

For prevention of falciparum malaria in most areas of the world where *P falciparum* is resistant to chloro-

---

\* Not available in the USA but available in some other countries.

quine, the drug of choice is a synergistic combination of a long-acting sulfonamide or sulfone with a folic acid antagonist (eg, pyrimethamine or trimethoprim). Current experience has led to the combination of pyrimethamine, 25 mg, and sulfadoxine, 500 mg, as one agent in use for this purpose. This fixed-dose combination is available in the USA under the trade name Fansidar and in other countries as Fansidar or Falcidar.

Because the antifolate-sulfonamide or sulfone combinations are only weakly blood schizonticidal for *P vivax* or *P ovale,* it is recommended that—in addition to a combination drug—500 mg of chloroquine (salt) be taken weekly while in an endemic area and for 6 weeks after leaving. Primaquine is also given to achieve radical cure of *P vivax* or *P ovale,* but under the indications and precautions described above.

**A. Pyrimethamine-Sulfadoxine (Fansidar):** The Centers for Disease Control reported that since Fansidar became available in the USA in 1982, 24 cases of severe reactions (erythema multiforme, Stevens-Johnson syndrome, and toxic epidermal necrolysis) have occurred, including 7 deaths. The risk of death is estimated to be about one in 11,000–25,000 users. All of the reactions occurred after a series of weekly doses of Fansidar (1–7 doses); all but one of the patients were concurrently taking chloroquine. Other adverse reactions include serum sickness-like reactions, urticaria, exfoliative dermatitis, and hepatitis. Additional side effects are those associated with the individual components of the drug. Pyrimethamine in high doses for prolonged periods has caused megaloblastic anemia due to folate deficiency, but this has not happened when the drug has been used for weekly prophylaxis for malaria. The antifolate effect may be exacerbated by poor nutrition, concurrent use of antimicrobials (including sulfonamides), and pregnancy. Adverse effects of sulfonamides include hypersensitivity reactions, blood dyscrasias, hepatitis, toxic nephrosis, and central nervous system symptoms.

Fansidar is contraindicated for individuals with known sulfonamide sensitivity or folate deficiency; in infants under 2 months of age; and in pregnancy, when it may interfere with folic acid metabolism. It should be used with caution in the presence of impaired renal or hepatic function, in patients with G6PD deficiency (hemolysis occurs in some), and in those with severe allergic disorders or bronchial asthma. Adequate fluid intake should be maintained to prevent crystalluria and stone formation. Periodic blood counts (for leukopenia) and urinalysis (for crystalluria) are desirable during prolonged prophylaxis (over 6 months). Children should be given supplementary calcium folinate.

Because of risks of serious side effects, the Centers for Disease Control (see *MMWR* 1985;**34:**185) recommends that Fansidar only be used in chemoprophylaxis when exposure to infection is likely. Chemoprophylaxis is not warranted, for example, for individuals traveling through or living in urban areas that are free of transmission. Additionally, persons traveling through rural endemic areas during the daytime only (when mosquitoes are not biting) have a low probability of exposure. Under these circumstances, individuals should instead carry Fansidar with them and use it in the event of symptoms as described under short-term travel.

**1. Use in long-term travel or residence (> 3–4 weeks)**–For individuals who will be significantly exposed to infection, Fansidar is given weekly and for 6 weeks after leaving the endemic area. Chloroquine is given concurrently to provide chemoprophylaxis against the other *Plasmodium* species, since in many areas of the world, *P vivax* is resistant to the pyrimethamine in Fansidar.

The Centers for Disease Control warns that "physicians who advise such travelers and expatriate residents must take into consideration individual living conditions while in [the country], the availability of local medical care, and when possible, local malaria transmission patterns. . . . The potential benefit of [routine prophylaxis] must be weighed against the risk of a possible serious or fatal adverse reaction. If weekly use of Fansidar is prescribed, the traveler should be advised to discontinue it immediately in the event of a possible ill effect, especially if any mucocutaneous signs or symptoms, such as pruritus, erythema, rash, orogenital lesions, or pharyngitis, develop."

**2. Use in short-term travel (< 3–4 weeks)**– The Centers for Disease Control advises that individuals traveling through an endemic area for only a short time should keep in their possession a single treatment dose of Fansidar (3 tablets = 75 mg of pyrimethamine and 1500 mg of sulfadoxine) to be taken "promptly in the event of an illness with fever during or after their travel *when professional medical care is not readily available.* It must be emphasized to travelers that such presumptive self-treatment . . . is only a temporary measure and that professional medical follow-up care as soon as possible is imperative. They should also be advised to continue weekly chloroquine prophylaxis after presumptive treatment with Fansidar." After the patient has left the endemic area, primaquine can be given according to the guidelines presented above to provide radical cure of *P vivax* and *P ovale* infection.

**B. Alternative Drugs, Particularly for Regions Where *P falciparum* Is Resistant to Both 4-Aminoquinolines and the Antifolate-Sulfonamide Combinations:** For each of the following regimens, primaquine treatment can be considered after the patient has left the endemic area, according to the guidelines presented above to provide radical cure for *P vivax* and *P ovale* infection.

**1. Doxycycline**–Limited studies in Thailand suggest that the tetracyclines when used alone, such as doxycycline (100 mg daily while in the endemic area and for 6 weeks after leaving), are effective against *P falciparum.* Chloroquine must be given concurrently for protection against the other species of plasmodia. Doxycycline is particularly appropriate for short-term use; its efficacy and safety for prolonged use have not been evaluated. Photosensitivity is a potential side effect of doxycycline; the drug is contraindicated in pregnancy and for children under 8 years of age.

**2. Pyrimethamine-dapsone (Maloprim*)**– Because of its potential toxicity, this drug is not recommended for routine prophylaxis. Each tablet contains pyrimethamine, 12.5 mg, plus dapsone, 100 mg. The dosage is 2 tablets per week before entering the endemic area, 1 tablet weekly while exposed, and 1 tablet weekly for 6 weeks after leaving. Hemolytic anemia, methemoglobinemia, agranulocytosis, and bone marrow red cell aplasia have rarely been associated with dapsone used as an antimalarial agent; periodic hemograms are recommended when Maloprim is used for longer than 6 months. Some persons sensitive to sulfonamides may also be sensitive to dapsone. *P falciparum* resistant to Maloprim has been reported from Kenya and Tanzania. Chloroquine should be given with Maloprim, because the latter is not effective against *P vivax*.

**3. Pyrimethamine-Sulfalone (Matakelfin*)**– This is another combination available in some countries.

**4. Quinine**–For selected areas and patients, quinine sulfate, 325 mg twice daily and for 6 weeks after leaving the endemic area, may be indicated for prophylaxis. Chloroquine is not taken concurrently.

**5. Mefloquine**–A major concern at present is that excessive use of mefloquine will result in the development of new strains of *P falciparum* resistant to it. Therefore, mefloquine is best reserved for treatment of *P falciparum* infections resistant to chloroquine and to the antifolate-sulfonamide combinations. For selected patients, however, mefloquine can be used prophylactically against resistant strains of *P falciparum* (it also provides suppressive chemoprophylaxis against *P vivax* but not radical cure) at a dosage of 250 mg (base) weekly for adults, and 4–6 mg (base)/kg weekly for children. Combination therapy has been recommended by some with sulfadoxine-pyrimethamine, but this involves the hazard of potentially serious adverse reactions of sulfadoxine.

## 2. CHEMOTHERAPY
(Table 25–2)

### Treatment of All Forms of Malaria Except *P falciparum* Strains Resistant to 4-Aminoquinolines & Other Drugs

**A. Elimination of Asexual Erythrocytic Parasites:** Infection by all 4 species of malaria is treated with oral chloroquine. An alternative drug for oral

treatment is amodiaquine, though chloroquine is preferred.

Early diagnosis and prompt treatment are essential in *P falciparum* infection, as death can occur within 1–2 days after initial presentation. In monitoring the therapeutic response, it is essential also to determine the density of parasites on the blood smear (as a measure of the severity of infection) and to recheck the patient at regular intervals. If symptoms caused by *P falciparum* do not begin to respond to chloroquine within about 48 hours or if there is increasing asexual parasitemia after 1–2 days (in the presence of adequate drug ingestion and retention), parasite resistance to the drug must be assumed and treatment changed to quinine and another drug (Table 25–2).

Severe disease is usually due to *P falciparum* infection. If patients cannot effectively absorb the drug because of vomiting or severe diarrhea—or if they are comatose or have a high parasite count (100,000/ µL, or parasites in 1–2% of red cells)—give quinine intravenously (Table 25–2) and start oral treatment with chloroquine as soon as possible. Chloroquine hydrochloride intramuscularly (contraindicated in young children) is a more toxic alternative parenteral drug. If neither parenteral quinine nor chloroquine is available, quinidine gluconate can be used (see footnotes to Table 25–2).

**B. Eradication of *P vivax* or *P ovale* Infections:** This is accomplished with a standard course of primaquine. In some parts of the world (see above), partial resistance of *P vivax* requires a higher dose of primaquine or a second course of treatment.

**C. Elimination of Persistent Gametocytemia:** Gametocytes of *P vivax*, *P ovale*, and *P malariae* are eliminated by chloroquine. Gametocytes of *P falciparum* are eliminated by a single dose of 26.3 mg of primaquine salt.

**D. Treatment of Semi-Immunes:** Treatment of attacks in semi-immune patients generally requires shorter courses.

### Treatment of Falciparum Malaria Acquired in Areas Where *P falciparum* Is Resistant to 4-Aminoquinolines But Sensitive to Antifolate-Sulfonamide Combinations

**A. Quinine Plus an Antifolate-Sulfonamide or Tetracycline:** For patients whose falciparum infection originated in an endemic area where *P falciparum* is known to be resistant to chloroquine or when chloroquine resistance is emerging, start treatment with oral quinine and a second drug (Table 25–2). Quinine is a rapidly acting blood schizonticide, whereas the other drugs are slower-acting. If the patient is severely ill, begin with parenteral quinine and start oral quinine as soon as possible.

**B. Quinine Plus Mefloquine:** An alternative treatment is oral quinine given as in Table 25–2 plus oral mefloquine; 18–20 mg/kg (total, 750–1250 mg). Up to 750 mg can be given as a single dose; the

---

* Not available in the USA but available in some other countries.

remainder is given in 250- to 500-mg increments at 8-hour intervals.

## Treatment of Falciparum Malaria Acquired in Areas Where *P falciparum* Is Resistant to Both 4-Aminoquinolines & Antifolate-Sulfonamide Combinations

Treatment is with quinine plus a tetracycline or with quinine plus mefloquine.

## 3. FOLLOW-UP FOR *P FALCIPARUM* MALARIA

Blood films should be checked daily until parasitemia clears; check weekly thereafter for 4 weeks to observe for recrudescence of infection.

## 4. SPECIAL MEASURES FOR TREATMENT OF SEVERE *P FALCIPARUM* MALARIA

For details on the management of severe and complicated falciparum malaria, see the WHO review article (1986) cited below. In initial management, it is crucial to achieve an effective concentration of quinine as soon as possible by giving the drug slowly intravenously, preferably with an initial loading dose (Table 25–2). Quinine treatment must be continued for at least 3 days after disappearance of asexual parasitemia. For patients who remain severely ill from the third day of treatment onward, the dose of quinine should be reduced by one-third until there is clinical improvement.

Corticosteroids were recently shown to be deleterious in cerebral malaria and should no longer be used. Heparin therapy is also no longer recommended, since its use may be hazardous and since its indication—ie, disseminated intravascular coagulation—is rare in severe malaria. If there is proof of disseminated intravascular coagulation, however, heparin therapy may be considered. Rehydration of the patient should be carried out with caution, particularly in the first 24 hours, since overhydration may precipitate pulmonary edema. In general, 2–3 L of fluid is required the first day, followed by 10–20 mL/kg/d; intake and output should be carefully recorded. Dialysis may be necessary for renal failure. Blood glucose levels should be monitored during the acute and early convalescent period, since hypoglycemia (unrelated to starvation) may be severe and life-threatening, especially during quinine therapy. Anticonvulsants (diazepasm) may be needed; hyperpyrexia should be controlled symptomatically. Severe anemia is an indication for transfusion of packed red blood cells.. Recent reports suggest that the survival of patients with parasitemias greater than $10^6/\mu L$ may be increased by exchange transfusion.

## Prognosis

The uncomplicated and untreated primary attack of *P vivax, P ovale,* or *P falciparum* malaria usually lasts 2–4 weeks; that of *P malariae* about twice as long. Each type of infection may subsequently relapse (once or many times) before the infection terminates spontaneously. With modern antimalarial drugs, the prognosis is good for most malaria infections, but in *P falciparum* infections, when complications such as cerebral malaria and blackwater fever develop, the prognosis is poor even with treatment.

Bruce-Chwatt LJ: *Essential Malariology,* 2nd ed. Wiley, 1985.

Centers for Disease Control: Malaria prevention recommendations. *Health Information for International Travel.* HHS Publication No. (CDC) 85–8280, 1985.

Centers for Disease Control: Revised recommendations for preventing malaria in travelers to areas with chloroquine-resistant *Plasmodium falciparum. MMWR* 1985;**34**:185.

Cook GC: *Plasmodium falciparum* infection: Problems in prophylaxis and treatment in 1986. *Quart J Med* 1986;**61**:1091.

Hall A, Yardumian A, Marsh A: Exchange transfusion and quinine concentrations in falciparum malaria. *Br Med J* 1985;**291**:1169.

Malaria prophylaxis: Two problem regions. (Editorial.) *Br Med J* 1984;**288**:1216.

Peters W, Richards WHG (editors): *Antimalarial Drugs: Handbook of Experimental Pharmacology,* Vol 68. Part I: Biological background, experimental methods, and drug resistance. Part II: Current antimalarials and new drug developments. Springer, 1984.

Peto TEA, Gilks CF: Strategies for the prevention of malaria in travellers: Comparison of drug regimens by means of risk-benefit analysis. *Lancet* 1986;**1**:1256.

Phillips RE: Warrell DA: The pathophysiology of severe falciparum malaria. *Parasitol Today* 1986;**2**:271.

Phillips RE et al: Intravenous quinidine for the treatment of severe falciparum malaria: Clinical and pharmacokinetic studies. *N Engl J Med* 1985;**312**:1273.

Strickland GT (Editor): Malaria. In: *Clinics in Tropical Medicine and Communicable Diseases.* Saunders, 1986.

Warrell DA et al: Dexamethasone proves deleterious in cerebral malaria: A double-blind trial in 100 comatose patients. *N Engl J Med* 1982;**306**:313.

WHO Malaria Action Programme: Severe and complicated malaria. *Trans Roy Soc Trop Med Hyg* 1986;**80(Suppl)**:1.

WHO Scientific Group: *Advances in Malaria Chemotherapy.* Technical Report Series No. 711. World Health Organization, 1984.

World Health Organization: *WHO Expert Committee on Malaria.* Eighteenth Report. Technical Report Series 735. WHO, Geneva, 1984.

Wyler DJ: Malaria: Resurgence, resistance, and research. (2 parts.) *N Engl J Med* 1983;**308**:875, 934.

## AFRICAN TRYPANOSOMIASIS (Sleeping Sickness)

### Essentials of Diagnosis

● History of exposure to tsetse flies. Chancre in *T b rhodesiense* infections.

*Hemolymphatic stage:* (Usually absent or unnoticed in *T b gambiense* infections.)

- Irregular fevers, headache, joint pains, malaise, pruritus, papular skin rash, edema.
- Posterior cervical or generalized lymphadenopathy.
- Trypanosomes in blood or lymph node aspirate.

*Meningoencephalitic stage:*

- Insomnia, motor and sensory disorders, abnormal reflexes, somnolence to coma.
- Trypanosomes and increased white count and protein in cerebrospinal fluid.

## General Considerations

Rhodesian and Gambian trypanosomiasis are caused by *Trypanosoma brucei rhodesiense* and *Trypanosoma brucei gambiense,* respectively, both hemoflagellates morphologically indistinguishable from the third member of the group, *Trypanosoma brucei brucei,* a pathogen of animals but not of humans. All are transmitted by bites of tsetse flies (*Glossina* species), which inhabit shaded areas along streams and rivers. Sleeping sickness in humans occurs locally throughout tropical Africa from south of the Sahara to about 20° south latitude. *T b gambiense* infections occur in the moist sub-Saharan savannah and riverine forests of west and central Africa up to the eastern Rift Valley. *T b rhodesiense* occurs to the east of the Rift Valley in the savannah of east and southeast Africa and along the shores of Lake Victoria. The annual incidence of cases is estimated to be 10,000–20,000. Without treatment, the disease is almost always fatal. Rhodesian sleeping sickness is primarily a zoonosis of game animals. Cattle and sheep may also serve as incidental reservoirs. Within the sylvatic cycle, humans are infected only sporadically; but epidemics have occurred in which the transmission cycle is probably human-to-fly-to-human. Gambian sleeping sickness is a human disease with human-to-fly-to-human transmission in which humans serve as reservoir hosts. The recent demonstration that domestic pigs and wild animals are naturally infected with a *T b gambiense*-like strain suggests a domestic or wild animal cycle for the organism.

## Clinical Findings

**A. Symptoms and Signs:** The first stage of infection, the trypanosomal chancre, is a local, pruritic, painful inflammatory reaction (3–10 cm) with regional lymphadenopathy that appears about 48 hours after the tsetse fly bite and lasts 2–4 weeks. Chancres have been reported only in some patients with *T b rhodesiense* infections.

The second stage, the hemolymphatic stage, usually begins 3–10 days later with invasion of the blood stream and reticuloendothelial system. High fever, severe headache, joint pains, and malaise recur at irregular intervals corresponding to waves of parasitemia. Between febrile episodes there are symptom-free periods that last up to 2 weeks. Transient rashes, often pruritic and papular or circinate, and scattered areas of firm edema may appear. There may be tachycardia, myalgias and arthralgias, mild enlargement

of the liver and spleen, and edemas (peripheral, pleural, ascites, etc). Findings may not be present early in Gambian infection. Enlarged, rubbery, and painless lymph nodes occur in 75% of patients, particularly those of the posterior cervical group (Winterbottom's sign) in Gambian infection. With progression of the disease, there is increasing weight loss and debilitation. Signs of myocardial involvement appear early in Rhodesian infection, and the patient may succumb to myocarditis before signs of central nervous system invasion appear.

The meningoencephalitic stage appears within a few weeks or months of onset of Rhodesian infection but in Gambian sleeping sickness develops more insidiously, starting 6 months to several years after onset. Insomnia, anorexia, personality changes, apathy, and headaches are among the early findings. Tremors, disturbances of speech, gait, and reflexes, and somnolence appear late. The patient becomes severely emaciated and, finally, comatose. Death often results from secondary infection.

**B. Laboratory Findings:** Definitive diagnosis is made by finding the organism in the bite lesion, blood, lymph node, bone marrow aspirate, or cerebrospinal fluid. Although trypanosomes are often difficult to find in peripheral blood, specimens should be examined daily for 15 days (1) for motile organisms in wet films, (2) after staining thick and thin films, and (3) after concentration by centrifugation of heparinized blood (the buffy coat is examined.) Other diagnostic techniques employing blood samples include Millipore filtration, DEAE cellulose separation of trypanosomes, and inoculation of culture medium and mice or rats. Aspirate lymph nodes that are still soft (not yet fibrosed) by the "massage" technique; organisms on wet films or stained smears are seen more often with *T b gambiense* than *T b rhodesiense* infections. The cerebrospinal fluid contains increased cells (lymphocytes) and an elevated protein level. Wet films and stained smears of centrifuged cerebrospinal fluid may show trypanosomes in advanced cases; also inoculate the fluid into an experimental animal and culture medium. Serologic tests may be useful, but false-negative results may occur, particularly for brief periods after high parasitemia.

Other findings include anemia, increased sedimentation rate, thrombocytopenia, reduced total serum protein, increased serum globulin, and an elevated IgM level. The latter begins to rise shortly after infection and may reach 10–20 times normal. However, normal or low levels of IgM in acute disease do not rule out the infection. An elevated IgM in the cerebrospinal fluid is nearly pathognomonic and differentiates trypanosomiasis from other diseases causing elevated serum IgM levels; however, false-negative results have been reported in cases of central nervous system involvement.

## Differential Diagnosis

Trypanosomiasis may be mistaken for a variety

of other diseases, including malaria, kala-azar, tuberculosis, cerebral tumors, encephalitis, and cerebral syphilis. Serologic tests for syphilis may be falsely positive in trypanosomiasis. Malaria, suggested by fever and splenomegaly, may be ruled out by blood examinations; kala-azar can usually be ruled out clinically without resorting to spleen or marrow puncture. Other central nervous system conditions are differentiated by neurologic examination and lumbar puncture findings.

## Prevention

Prevention in endemic areas should include wearing long sleeves and trousers, avoiding dark-colored clothing, and using mosquito nets while sleeping. Repellents have no effect. Pentamidine is the drug of choice for chemoprophylaxis of sleeping sickness, but it is effective with certainty only against the Gambian type. In Rhodesian infection, pentamidine may lead to suppression of early symptoms, resulting in recognition of the disease too late in its course for effective treatment. Excretion of pentamidine isethionate from the body is slow; one intramuscular injection (4 mg/kg, maximum 300 mg) will protect against Gambian infection for 3–6 months. The drug is potentially toxic and should only be used for persons at high risk (ie, those with constant, heavy exposure to tsetse flies in areas with known transmission of Gambian disease). Performing serologic tests every 6 months during exposure and for 3 years afterward is the safest method for detecting the disease at an early stage.

## Treatment

**A. Specific Measures:** Suramin and pentamidine do not cross the blood-brain barrier and therefore can only be used in the early stage of the disease. Melarsoprol is used for central nervous system involvement, but drug resistance does occur. Many investigators believe that only patients in whom trypanosomes are found should be treated with these potentially toxic drugs. However, see Apted reference below for arguments for considering treatment with melarsoprol in the absence of parasitologic proof when serologic tests are positive and the cerebrospinal fluid cell count and protein are elevated. In the USA, suramin and melarsoprol are available only from the Parasitic Disease Drug Service, Centers for Disease Control, Atlanta 30333. Call (404) 329–3670. α-Difluoromethylornithine, an inhibitor of ornithine decarboxylase, is being tested clinically for the clearing of both peripheral and central nervous system parasites.

**1. Early disease: hemolymphatic stage–**

**a. Suramin sodium** is a drug of choice in the early stages of trypanosomiasis before the central nervous system is invaded. It is administered intravenously as a freshly prepared 10% solution in distilled water. Start treatment with a test dose of 100 mg; then give 20 mg/kg body weight (maximum, 1 g) every 5–7 days. The usual course is 5 injections,

and it should not exceed 7. Because of occasional renal toxicity, frequent urinalyses are essential during therapy. Discontinue if red blood cells, casts, or significant amounts of protein occur in urine. About one person in 20,000 has an idiosyncratic reaction with vomiting, seizures, and shock; rare fatalities have been reported. The drug is contraindicated in renal disease.

**b. Pentamidine isethionate–** This drug, a diamidine, is a somewhat less effective alternative to suramin in treating early trypanosomiasis. It is administered as a 2% solution intramuscularly. Pain, induration, or sterile abscess may occur at the injection site. Vomiting, hypotension, hypoglycemia, syncope, and peripheral neuritis are rare. Use with caution in renal disease. Administer in doses of 3–4 mg (base)/kg (maximum, 300 mg); the powder, which must be freshly dissolved in 2–3 mL of water, is given intramuscularly daily or every other day for 7–10 injections.

**2. Late disease: central nervous system involvement–**

**a. Melarsoprol (Mel B)** is the trivalent arsenical melarsen oxide coupled with dimercaprol (BAL) to reduce toxicity. The drug has only a narrow margin of safety; in approximately 10% of cases, reactive and hemorrhagic encephalopathy develops and may be fatal. The drug is prepared as a 3.6% solution in propylene glycol and must be given intravenously. A recommended schedule is 3 series of 3 daily injections, each series separated by an interval of 7–10 days. Each injection is 3.6 mg/kg (maximum 200 mg). If the patient is a poor risk, start with 1.8 mg/kg and increase over the first 3 days. Pretreatment is given with pentamidine for 1 day for *T b gambiense* infections or with suramin for 2 days for *T b rhodesiense* infections.

Melarsonyl potassium (Mel W) is a water-soluble alternative compound effective against *T b gambiense,* but the results against *T b rhodesiense* have been inconclusive.

**b. Alternative drugs–** Nitrofurazone may be tried when melarsoprol has not been successful. It is given in a dosage of 0.5 g 3–4 times daily for 5–7 days. Side effects include polyneuropathy.

**B. General Measures:** Good nursing care, treatment of anemia and concurrent infections, and correction of malnutrition are essential in the management of advanced trypanosomiasis. Following treatment, patients should be monitored for signs of central nervous system involvement at 3- and then 6-month intervals for 3 years.

## Prognosis

Relapses may occur for 2 years after treatment. If untreated, most cases of African trypanosomiasis are fatal. With treatment, the prognosis is excellent, even in Rhodesian infection, if therapy is started before onset of central nervous system symptoms; if started late, irreversible brain damage or death is common.

Apted FIC: Present status of chemotherapy and chemoprophylaxis of human trypanosomiasis in the eastern hemisphere. *Pharmacol Ther* 1980;**11**:391.

Gutteridge WE: Existing chemotherapy and its limitations. *Br Med Bull* 1985;**41**:162.

Meshnick SR: Chemotherapy of African trypanosomiasis. Pages 165–200 in: *Parasitic Diseases*. Vol 2:*Chemotherapy*. Mansfield JM (editor). Marcel Dekker, 1984.

Molyneux DH, de Raadt P, Seed JR: African human trypanosomiasis. Pages 39–62 in: *Recent Advances in Tropical Medicine*. Gilles HM (editor). Churchill Livingstone, 1984.

Trypanosomiasis: I. *Salivaria*. A review of recent abstracts. (Special Article.) *Trop Dis Bull* (Feb) 1986;**83**:R1.

WHO Expert Committee: *The African Trypanosomiases*. Technical Report Series No. 635. World Health Organization, 1979.

## AMERICAN TRYPANOSOMIASIS (Chagas' Disease)

### Essentials of Diagnosis

*Acute stage*

- Principally in children. Inflammatory lesion at site of inoculation.
- Prolonged fever, signs of myocarditis, hepatosplenomegaly, lymphadenopathy.
- Parasites in blood, positive serologic tests, abnormal ECG.

*Chronic stage*

- Cardiac abnormalities: arrhythmias, heart failure, abnormal ECG.
- Gastrointestinal abnormalities in some regions: dysphagia, severe constipation, megaesophagus or megacolon by radiography.
- Parasites recovered by xenodiagnosis or hemoculture, positive serologic tests.

### General Considerations

Chagas' disease is caused by *Trypanosoma cruzi,* a protozoan parasite of humans and wild and domestic animals, *T cruzi* occurs only in the Americas; it is found in wild animals from southern South America to northern Mexico, Texas, and the southwestern USA. Though human infection is less widespread, an estimated 12 million people are infected, mostly in rural areas. In many countries of Latin America, particularly South America, Chagas' disease is the most important cause of heart disease.

The infection is transmitted by many species of triatomine bugs that become infected by ingesting blood with circulating trypanosomes from infected animals or humans. Multiplication occurs in the digestive tract of the bug; infective forms are eliminated in feces. Infection in humans is through "contamination" with bug feces; the parasite penetrates the skin (generally through the bite wound) or the conjunctiva. Transmission can also occur by blood transfusion or in utero.

The trypanosomes first multiply close to the point of entry, assuming a leishmanial form. They then enter the bloodstream as trypanosomes and later invade the heart and other tissues, where they assume a leishmanial form. Multiplication causes cellular destruction, inflammation, and fibrosis. Infection continues for many years, probably for life.

### Clinical Findings

**A. Symptoms and Signs:** The acute state, seen principally in children, lasts 2–4 months and leads to death in up to 10% of cases. The earliest findings are at the site of inoculation either in the eye—Romaña's sign (unilateral bipalpebral edema, conjunctivitis, local lymphadenopathy)—or in the skin—a chagoma (furunclelike lesion with local lymphadenopathy). Subsequent findings include fever, malaise, headache, hepatomegaly, mild splenomegaly, and generalized lymphadenopathy. Acute myocarditis may lead to biventricular failure, but arrhythmias are rare. Meningoencephalitis is limited to young children and often is fatal.

A latent period may last from 10 to 30 years in which the patient is asymptomatic but in which serologic tests and sometimes parasitologic examination confirm the presence of the infection.

The chronic stage is usually manifested by cardiac disease in the third and fourth decades of life, characterized by arrhythmias, congestive heart failure (mainly right-sided), and thromboembolic phenomena arising from a ventricle. Sudden cardiac arrest in young persons may occur and is attributed to ventricular fibrillation. Megacolon and megaesophagus, caused by damage to nerve plexuses in the bowel or esophageal wall, occur in some areas of Chile, Argentina, and Brazil. Symptoms include dysphagia, regurgitation, and constipation.

**B. Laboratory Findings:** Appropriate selection of tests allows a definitive parasitologic diagnosis in most acute cases and in up to 40% of chronic ones. In the acute stage, trypanosomes should be looked for in the blood by examination of anticoagulated fresh blood for motile organisms and by examination of the following stained preparations: thick, blood films, buffy coat after centrifugation of 5–10 mL of heparinized blood, and sediment from centrifuged supernatant clotted blood. In the chronic stage, the parasite can only be detected by culture or xenodiagnosis. The latter consists of permitting uninfected laboratory-reared bugs of the local major vector to feed on the patients and then examining their intestinal contents for trypanosomes. In both acute and chronic infection, blood should also be cultured using Nicolle-Novy-MacNeal medium and inoculated into laboratory mice or rats 3–10 days old. *Trypanosoma rangeli,* a nonpathogenic blood trypansome also found in humans in Central America and northern South America, must not be mistaken for *T cruzi.* Serologic tests are of presumptive value when positive; more than one test should be used. Antibodies of the IgM class are usually elevated in the acute stage but normal in the chronic stage. The most important electrocardiographic abnormalities are complete right bundle branch block, conduction defects, and arrhythmias.

Radiologic examination may show cardiac enlargement and megaesophagus or megacolon.

## Treatment

Treatment of Chagas' diseases is unsatisfactory. Cures are usually possible in the acute phase. In the chronic phase, although parasitemia and xenodiagnosis become negative, treatment does not alter the serologic reaction, cardiac function, or progression of the disease. Benznidazole is preferred over nifurtimox in treatment.

Benznidazole is administered as an oral dose of 5–7 mg/kg/d for 60 days. Side effects include nausea, headache, anorexia, abdominal pain, and weight loss; exfoliative dermatitis, thrombocytopenia, and allergic purpura are rare. The drug is not available in the USA.

Nifurtimox is given orally in a dosage of 8–16 mg/kg/d in 3 divided does for 50–120 days. It generally produces anorexia, weight loss, tremors, and peripheral neuritis. Hallucinations and convulsions are rare. Children tolerate the drug better than adults. In the USA, nifurtimox is available only from the Parasitic Disease Drug Service, Centers for Disease Control, Atlanta 30333 (call [404] 329-3670).

In advanced cardiac failure, diuretics are usually very effective, but digitalis is not well tolerated and may need to be discontinued. Arrhythmias require selected use of quinidine, procainamide, intravenous lidocaine, or amiodarone.

## Prognosis

Acute infections in infants and young children are often fatal, particularly when the central nervous system is involved. Adults with chronic cardiac infections also may ultimately succumb to the disease. Mortality rates are not known, because infections are often unrecognized.

Apt W: Treatment of Chagas' disease. *Rev Med Chil* 1985;**113**:162.

Gutteridge WE: Chemotherapy of Chagas' disease. Pages 47–57 in: *Perspectives in Trypanosomiasis Research. Proceedings of the Twenty-First Trypanosomiasis Seminar, London 1981.* Baker JR (editor). Chinchester Research Studies Press, 1982.

Marsden PD: Chagas's disease: Clinical aspects. In: *Recent Advances in Tropical Medicine.* Gilles HM (editor). Churchill Livingstone, 1984.

Trypanosomiasis: II *Stercoraria.* A review of recent abstracts. (Special Article.) *Trop Dis Bull* (March) 1986;**83**:R29.

## LEISHMANIASIS

The leishmaniae are intracellular protozoal parasites. The leishmanial diseases are caused by different species of *Leishmania* in different parts of the world and often result in significant morbidity and mortality. The clinical manifestations of leishmaniasis may be classified as (1) visceral, (2) cutaneous, and (3) mucocutaneous. The disease is a zoonosis transmitted by bites of sandflies (*Phlebotomus* species) from wild or domestic animal reservoirs to humans, except in the case of Indian kala-azar, which is transmitted directly from human to human. The leishmaniae have 2 distinct forms in their life cycle: (1) In infected mammalian hosts, the parasite is found in its amastigote form (2–3 μm in length) within mononuclear phagocytes; (2) in the sandfly vector, the parasite converts to and is then transmitted as a flagellated extracellular promastigote.

Bryceson ADM: Therapy in man. In: *The Leishmanias in Biology and Medicine.* Peters W, Killick-Kendrick R (editors). Academic Press, 1987.

Chang, KP, Bray RS (editors): *Leishmaniasis, Vol 1 of series: Human Parasitic Diseases.* Ruitenberg EJ, MacInnis AJ (series editors). Elsevier, 1985.

Marr JJ: The chemotherapy of leishmaniasis. Pages 201–228 in: *Parasitic Diseases.* Vol 2: *Chemotherapy.* Mansfield JM (editor). Marcel Dekker, 1984.

Pearson RD et al: The immunobiology of leishmaniasis. *Rev Infect Dis* 1983;**5**:907.

World Health Organization: *Report of a WHO Expert Committee: The Leishmaniases.* WHO Tech Rep Ser No. 701, 1985.

## 1. VISCERAL LEISHMANIASIS (Kala-Azar)

### Essentials of Diagnosis

- Insidious or acute onset with fever.
- Marked splenomegaly, hepatomegaly.
- Anemia, leukopenia, and wasting.
- Pigmentation of skin on forehead and hands.
- Leishman-Donovan bodies in splenic or sternal puncture smears.
- Elevated serum globulins (IgG) and total proteins.

### General Considerations

Visceral leishmaniasis is geographically widespread. It is caused mainly by 2 species: *Leishmania donovani* in the Indian region and *Leishmania infantum* in the USSR, China, Middle East, Mediterranean basin, and Africa. It also occurs in South America, where the agent has been tentatively designated *Leishmania chagasi.* In each locale, the disease has its own peculiar clinical and epidemiologic features, and in some places it may also occur in epidemics. Although humans are the major reservoir, animal reservoirs such as the dog are important. The incubation period varies from weeks to months.

### Clinical Findings

**A. Symptoms and Signs:** A local lesion at the site of the bite may precede systemic manifestations but usually is inapparent. The onset may be acute or insidious. Fever often peaks twice daily with chills and sweats, weakness, weight loss, cough, or diarrhea. Usually, there is marked enlargement of the spleen, with discomfort in the left hypochondrium, and the liver is somewhat enlarged.

Eventually, the spleen becomes huge, hard, and

nontender. Generalized lymphadenopathy is common. Hyperpigmentation of skin, especially on hands, feet, abdomen, and forehead, is marked in light-skinned patients (kala-azar = black sickness). In blacks, there may be warty eruptions or skin ulcers. There may be bleeding from nose and gums, jaundice, ascites, and wasting; death is often due to intercurrent infections.

Post-kala-azar dermal leishmaniasis may appear 1–2 years after apparent cure (up to 10 years in India and China). This may simulate leprosy as multiple hypopigmented macules or nodules develop on preexisting lesions. Erythematous patches may appear on the face. Leishmaniae are present in the skin. The condition responds well to additional courses of antimony.

**B. Laboratory Findings:** There is usually progressive leukopenia (seldom over 3000/μL after the first 1–2 months), with lymphocytosis and monocytosis. Occasional leukocytosis, due to concurrent sepsis, may be confusing. Associated with the hypersplenism are a normochromic anemia and a low platelet count. Diagnosis must always be confirmed by demonstrating Leishman-Donovan bodies in blood or in aspirates of sternal marrow, liver, or spleen by stained smears; by culture in Nicolle-Novy-MacNeal medium; or by inoculation into hamsters. Buffy coat preparations of centrifuged blood may also show the organism. Serologic tests are useful, for they seldom give false-negative results. Some cross-reactions do occur. Diagnosis is supported by an increase in total serum proteins up to and greater than 10 g/dL, mainly hypergammaglobulinemia due to increased IgG. The *Leishmania* skin test is negative in active visceral leishmaniasis but becomes positive after recovery.

### Differential Diagnosis

Acute or subacute kala-azar may resemble enteric fever (but there is no toxemia) or malaria (response to antimalarial therapy may aid the diagnosis, since concomitant malaria parasites may be present in the blood in kala-azar) and other causes of splenomegaly, eg, brucellosis and lymphoma.

Chronic cases may also be confused with infectious mononucleosis, leukemia, anemias due to other causes, and tuberculosis. Post-kala-azar dermatitis may resemble leprosy.

### Treatment

Visceral leishmaniasis in India usually responds well to pentavalent antimonials or pentamidine, but the former are usually necessary in areas where *L infantum* or *L chagasi* is the causative agent. The Sudanese, East African, and South American forms are generally less susceptible to drug therapy, and childhood kala-azar is occasionally completely resistant to treatment. Amphotericin B may be used as the last resort for such patients.

When giving antimonials, fresh solutions only should be used, and the ampules must be stored away from heat. Intravenous injection must be given slowly over 5 minutes through a 22- to 23-gauge needle.

(1) Sodium antimony gluconate (sodium stibogluconate) treatment begins with a 0.2-g test dose, followed by 10 mg/kg/d (maximum 600 mg/d) as 5% solution intramuscularly or intravenously for 10 days. In China, India, and Sudan, one 6- to 10-day course is usually sufficient; in other regions (such as Kenya), several courses may be needed. Formerly, rest intervals of 2–4 weeks were advocated between courses. Recent work suggests (1) that rest periods are not only unnecessary but may increase the likelihood of relapse and of induced drug resistance and (2) that higher doses are well tolerated. The drug is available in the USA only from the Parasitic Disease Drug Service, Centers for Disease Control, Atlanta 30333 (call [404] 329–3670).

(2) Pentamidine isethionate, 2–4 mg/kg intravenously or (preferably) intramuscularly, is given daily or on alternate days (up to 15 injections). Pentamidine is not available in the USA for this indication.

(3) Stilbamidine isethionate is used only in antimony-resistant cases and must be given with great care because it is unstable and may produce immediate reactions or delayed trigeminal hyperesthesia. The initial adult dose is 25 mg intravenously daily, increasing by 10–20 mg daily to 2 mg/kg daily. The most that should be given is about 10 injections or a total of about 15 mg/kg.

(4) Amphotericin B is dissolved in 500 mL of 5% dextrose and injected slowly intravenously over 6 hours on alternate days. The initial dose is 0.5 mg/kg/d, which is gradually increased to 1 mg/kg/d until a total of about 30 mg/kg is given. Patients must be closely monitored in hospital, because side effects may be severe.

(5) Allopurinol is undergoing clinical trials for the treatment of kala-azar resistant to sodium antimony gluconate.

### Prognosis

Without treatment, kala-azar is usually fatal. Therapy is usually effective, but relapses may occur after 2 or more years and require additional courses of therapy. Keep the patient under observation for at least 12 months; the spleen, blood studies, and body weight should return to normal.

See also references above.

Rees PG et al: The treatment of kala-azar: A review with comments drawn from experience in Kenya. *Trop Geogr Med* 1985;**37**:37.

Smith DH: Visceral leishmaniasis—human aspects. Pages 79–87 in: *Recent Advances in Tropical Medicine.* Gilles HM (editor). Churchill Livingstone, 1984.

Thakur CP et al: Comparison of regimens of treatment with sodium stibogluconate in kala-azar. *Br Med J* 1984;**288**:895.

### 2. CUTANEOUS LEISHMANIASIS

Cutaneous leishmaniasis may present as self-healing ulcers (Oriental sore), as chronic mutilating ulcers, or, rarely, as disseminated cutaneous leishmaniasis that is nonulcerating and resembles lepromatous leprosy.

Cutaneous leishmaniasis is caused by *Leishmania tropica* in the USSR, India, Middle East, Mediterranean basin, and Africa; by *Leishmania aethiopica* in Ethiopia and Kenya; by *Leishmania mexicana* subspecies in Mexico and Guatemala ("chiclero's ulcer") and in South America; by *Leishmania peruviana* (uta) in the Peruvian and Argentinian highlands; and by *Leishmania braziliensis* subspecies in South and Central America. *Leishmania tropica major* infection is a rural acute disease characterized by a wet, rapidly ulcerating sore; *Leishmania tropica minor* infection is an urban chronic disease that produces a dry sore which ulcerates only slowly or not at all.

Disseminated cutaneous leishmaniasis is a rare syndrome caused by *L mexicana* subspecies in the Amazon region of Brazil and in Venezuela. It appears to be incurable. Long-standing nodular, nonulcerative skin lesions are widely disseminated. As in the case of leprosy, there is a state of impaired cell-mediated immunity, and parasites are usually abundant in smears and sections. The Montenegro skin test is negative. A form of diffuse cutaneous leishmaniasis also occurs in Ethiopia and the Sudan.

In cutaneous leishmaniasis, cutaneous swellings appear about 2–8 weeks after bites of sandflies. The swellings may ulcerate and discharge pus, or they may remain dry. Dry and moist forms are caused by locally distinct leishmania species, with the dry forms having longer incubation periods.

Lesions tend to heal spontaneously over a period of months to 2 years, but secondary infection may lead to gross extension and disfigurement, especially if the lesion is on the face.

Leishmania species cannot be detected in purulent discharge but may be seen in stained scrapings from the cleaned edge of the ulcer or in material aspirated after the injection of saline under the margin of the ulcer. Under sterile conditions, aspirate may be inoculated into NNN medium or into hamsters. The skin test is positive early. Serologic tests may be helpful.

Single lesions of Old World leishmaniasis (Oriental sore) may be cleaned, covered, and left to heal spontaneously. Local heat often helps the healing process. Carbon dioxide snow, infrared therapy, the intralesional instillation of a pentavalent antimony compound or quinacrine, or radiotherapy is often effective. Antibiotics may be required for secondary infections. Sodium antimony gluconate as for visceral leishmaniasis may be effective with indolent ulcers. Metronidazole and cycloguanil pamoate have given variable results. Rifampin, ketoconazole, and topical use of imidazoles and paromomycin are being tested.

Lesions caused by *L aethiopica* have been treated only with pentamidine in the past, because of poor response to conventional doses of pentavalent antimonials; however, high-dose antimonial therapy has recently been reported as effective.

The milder forms of solitary nodules and ulcers due to *L mexicana* from Mexico and Central America seldom require treatment. Metronidazole at dosage levels used to treat amebiasis, or cycloguanil pamoate, 5 mg/kg as a single repository injection, may be tried to speed healing. If necessary, use sodium antimony gluconate, 10 mg/kg/d (maximum 600 mg/d) intramuscularly or intravenously for 6–10 days. If there is any suspicion that a lesion is caused by *L braziliensis,* it should be treated with sodium antimony gluconate.

See also references above.

Chulay JD et al: High-dose sodium stibogluconate treatment of cutaneous leishmaniasis in Kenya. *Trans R Soc Trop Med Hyg* 1983;**77:**717.

Currie M: Treatment of cutaneous leishmaniasis by curettage. *Br Med J* 1983;**287:**1099.

El-On J et al: Topical treatment of cutaneous leishmaniasis. *J Invest Dermatol* 1986;**87:**284.

Manson-Bahr PEC: Cutaneous leishmaniasis. Pages 88–101 in: *Recent Advances in Tropical Medicine.* Gilles HM (editor): Churchill Livingstone, 1984.

Oster CN et al: American cutaneous leishmaniasis: A comparison of three sodium stibogluconate treatment schedules. *Am J Trop Med Hyg* 1985;**34:**856.

Viallet J et al: Response to ketoconazole in two cases of long-standing cutaneous leishmaniasis. *Am J Trop Med Hyg* 1986;**35:**491.

## 3. MUCOCUTANEOUS (NASO-ORAL) LEISHMANIASIS

*Leishmania braziliensis* causes severe naso-oral lesions (espundia) in lowland forest areas of South America and Central America. The initial lesion, single or multiple, is on exposed skin; it is initially papular (can be pruriginous or painful), then nodular, and later may ulcerate. Nonulcerating tumors may become wartlike or papillomatous. Healing follows with scarring within several months to a year. Naso-oral involvement is either by direct extension or, more often, metastatically to the mucosa; it may appear concurrently with the initial lesion, shortly after healing, or after many years. The mucosa of the anterior part of the nasal septum is generally the first area to be involved. Extensive destruction of the soft tissues and cartilage of the nose, oral cavity, and lips may follow and may extend to the larynx and pharynx. Gross and hideous destruction and marked suffering can result. Severe bacterial infection is common. Regional lymphangitis, lymphadenitis, fever, weight loss, keratitis, and anemia may be present. In blacks, large polypoid masses may affect the lips and cheeks. Death may result from inanition or bacterial infection.

Diagnosis is by finding Leishman-Donovan bodies in scrapings, biopsy specimen, or aspirated tissue juice; the organism also grows with difficulty in Novy-MacNeal-Nicolle medium or after hamster inoculation. The Montenegro skin test is useful. If an injection of a suspension of killed leptomonads produces a fully developed papule in 2–3 days that disappears after a week, the diagnosis is fairly certain. Antibodies are detectable in most cases and disappear with radical cure.

Specific treatment should be combined, if necessary, with local or systemic antibiotics or sulfonamides. Give sodium antimony gluconate, 10 mg/kg/d (maximum 600 mg/d) intramuscularly or intravenously for 6–10 days. Established naso-oral lesions are often difficult to cure. Two additional courses can be given. If initial treatment fails, use amphotericin B, 0.25–1 mg/kg, by slow intravenous infusion daily or every 2 days for up to 8 weeks. In some areas, pyrimethamine, 50 mg/d for 15 days, plus folinic acid, 6 mg/d, has appeared promising; the course is repeated up to 4 times, with 15-day intervals between courses. Nifurtimox (Lampit) is undergoing clinical trials.

See also references above.

Marsden PD: Mucosal leishmaniasis (''espundia'' Escomel, 1911) *Trans R Soc Trop Med Hyg* 1986;**80:**859.

Sampaio RNR, Sampaio JHD, Marsden PD: Pentavalent antimonial treatment in mucosal leishmaniasis. *Lancet* 1985;**1:**1097.

## GIARDIASIS

### Essentials of Diagnosis

- Most infections are asymptomatic.
- In some cases, acute or chronic diarrhea, mild to severe, with bulky, greasy, frothy, malodorous stools, free of blood and pus. Lassitude.
- Upper abdominal discomfort, cramps, distension, and excessive flatus.
- Cysts and occasionally trophozoites in stools.
- Trophozoites in duodenal fluid.

### General Considerations

Giardiasis is a protozoal infection of the upper small intestine caused by the flagellate *Giardia lamblia.* Often the infection is asymptomatic, but it may present as acute or chronic diarrhea or rarely as a malabsorption syndrome. The parasite occurs worldwide, and the infection is considered the most common intestinal protozoal pathogen in the USA and Europe. Persons of all ages are affected, but occurrence is particularly high among children. Prevalence rates of up to 20% have been reported in lower economic groups, and giardiasis is a well-recognized problem in special groups including travelers, campers, male homosexuals, and persons with impaired immune states.

The organism occurs in feces as a symmetric, heart-shaped flagellated trophozoite measuring 10–25 μm × 6–12 μm and as a cyst measuring 8–13 μm × 6–11 μm. Only the cyst form is infectious by the oral route; trophozoites are destroyed by gastric acidity. Most infections are sporadic, resulting from cysts transmitted by person-to-person contact, by anal-oral sexual contact, or as a result of fecal contamination of water or food. Multiple infections are common in households, and outbreaks occur in nursery schools and mental institutions and as a result of contamination of water supplies. Humans are the reservoir for *Giardia,* but dogs and beavers have been implicated as a source of infection.

After the cysts are ingested, trophozoites emerge in the duodenum and jejunum. They can cause epithelial damage, atrophy of villi, hypertrophic crypts, and extensive cellular infiltration of the lamina propria by lymphocytes, plasma cells, and neutrophils. It is likely that hypogammaglobulinemia, low secretory IgA levels in the gut, achlorhydria, and malnutrition favor the development of illness. Serum antibodies have been demonstrated, usually in association with symptomatic disease.

### Clinical Findings

**A. Symptoms and Signs:** The clinical forms of giardiasis are (1) asymptomatic infection, (2) acute diarrhea, (3) chronic diarrhea, and (4) malabsorption syndrome. A large proportion of patients remain asymptomatic cyst carriers, and their infection clears spontaneously. The incubation period is usually 1–3 weeks but may be longer. The illness may begin gradually or be sudden and severe. The acute phase may last days or weeks, but it is usually self-limited, although cyst excretion may continue. In a few patients, the disorder may become chronic and last for years, but it does not appear to last indefinitely.

In both the acute and chronic forms of the disease, diarrhea ranges from mild to severe; most often it is mild. There may be no complaints other than of one bulky, loose bowel movement a day, often after breakfast. With larger numbers of movements, the stools become increasingly watery and may contain mucus but are usually free of blood and pus; they are copious, frothy, malodorous, and greasy, tending to float in the toilet bowl. The diarrhea may be continuous or recurrent; if it is recurrent, stools may be normal to mushy during intervening days, or the patient may be constipated. Other less common gastrointestinal symptoms are anorexia, nausea and vomiting, midepigastric discomfort and cramps (often after meals), belching, flatulence, borborygmus, and abdominal distention. Weight loss and weakness are common, but low-grade fever is less common. Headache, urticaria, and myalgia are rare.

A malabsorption syndrome develops in a few patients, either in the acute phase, when diarrhea persists for more than a few weeks, or in the chronic phase. There may be rapid and marked weight loss and debility, particularly in the acute stage. Malabsorption that is reversible with treatment has been confirmed for fat- and protein-losing enteropathy and vitamin $B_{12}$, D-xylose, and lactase deficiency. Other reversible disturbances occur less frequently.

With treatment and successful eradication of the infection, there are no sequelae. Without treatment, severe malabsorption may rarely contribute to death from other causes.

**B. Laboratory Tests:** Diagnosis is achieved through identifying cysts or trophozoites in feces or duodenal fluid. Detecting the organism can be difficult, because the number of cysts passed in the feces varies considerably from day to day, and at the onset of infection, patients may have symptoms for about a week before organisms can be detected.

If clinically warranted, diagnostic accuracy can be increased by proceeding as follows: (1) routine stool examinations → (2) examination of upper intestinal fluid by the duodenal string test (Entero-Test) or by duodenal aspiration → (3) duodenal biopsy. Three stool specimens should be examined at intervals of 2 days or longer. Unless they can be submitted within an hour, specimens should be preserved immediately in a fixative. Stool specimens obtained with a purge do not increase the sensitivity of parasite detection. Use of barium, antibiotics, antacids, kaolin products, or oily laxatives may temporarily reduce the number of parasites or interfere with detection, requiring a delay in further examination for about 10 days. Duodenal aspirate should be concentrated by centrifugation at 500 rpm for 5 minutes and be examined by wet mount after permanent staining. Biopsy specimens should first be pressed onto a slide to obtain a mucosal imprint for staining and then be sectioned for histologic examination. Procedures are being developed to detect *Giardia* antigen in feces.

Serologic tests are not available for diagnosis. The hemogram is usually normal. Eosinophilia is rare. Radiologic examination of the small bowel is usually normal in asymptomatic and mildly ill persons but may show nonspecific findings of altered motility, thickened mucosal folds, and barium column segmentation in patients with marked symptoms.

## Treatment

**A. Specific Measures:** Symptomatic patients should be treated; asymptomatic patients should usually be treated, since they can transmit the infection to others and may occasionally become symptomatic themselves. In selected instances of asymptomatic infection, it is often best to wait a few weeks before starting treatment to see if the infection will clear spontaneously.

Treatment can be carried out effectively with tinidazole or metronidazole (both are nitroimidazole compounds) or with quinacrine or furazolidone. Occasional treatment failures require re-treatment with an alternative drug. Tinidazole, where available, is the drug of choice, based on reports that it is effective as a single dose. Furazolidone is the least effective but in the USA the most convenient pediatric preparation.

All of these drugs occasionally have unpleasant side effects. In addition, furazolidone induces mammary tumors in rats, metronidazole increases the rate of naturally occurring tumors in rodents, and both metronidazole and tinidazole are mutagens in the *Salmonella* test system. These findings suggest that these drugs may carry risk factors for carcinogenicity.

**1. Tinidazole (Fasigyn)** (not available in the USA), 2 g given once, has had reported cure rates of 90–100%. The drug was formerly given in a dosage of 150 mg twice daily for 7 days. Adverse reactions consist of mild gastrointestinal side effects in about 10% of patients; headache and vertigo are less common.

**2. Metronidazole (Flagyl)**–Adults receive 250 mg 3 times daily for 5–10 days; children receive 5 mg/kg 3 times daily for 5 days. Cure rates are generally between 85 and 95%. Metronidazole may cause gastrointestinal symptoms, headache, and a metallic taste. Patients must be warned that alcohol may cause a disulfiramlike reaction. Liquid suspensions for pediatric use are available only outside the USA.

**3. Quinacrine (Mepacrine, atabrine)**–For adults and children over 8 years of age, give 100 mg 3 times daily after meals for 5–7 days; for younger children, give 2 mg/kg 3 times daily (maximum 300 mg/d) for 5–7 days. (The drug has a bitter taste, and young children tend to tolerate it poorly.) Cure rates are 80–95%. Gastrointestinal symptoms, headache, and dizziness are common; harmless yellowing of the skin is infrequent. Toxic psychosis and exfoliative dermatitis are rare. Quinacrine is contraindicated in psoriasis or in persons with a history of psychosis.

**4. Furazolidone (Furoxone)**–Adults receive 100 mg 4 times daily for 10 days; children receive 1.25 mg/kg 4 times daily for 10 days. Cure rates range from 72 to 90%. The drug is prepared as a pediatric suspension. Gastrointestinal symptoms, fever, headache, rash, and a disulfiramlike reaction with alcohol occur. Furazolidone can cause mild hemolysis in glucose-6-phosphate dehydrogenase-deficient persons. Hypersensitivity reactions have occurred rarely, including hypotension, urticaria, and serum sickness.

In follow-up, it is best to wait about 2 weeks before rechecking 2 or more stools at weekly intervals.

**B. Prevention and Control:** There is no effective chemoprophylaxis for giardiasis. Individual treatment of small quantities of water with iodine tablets or drops probably makes drinking water safe, except in the case of very cold water.

Dupont HL, Sullivan PS: Giardiasis: The clinical spectrum, diagnosis and therapy. *Ped Infect Dis* 1986;**5**:131.

Erlandsen SL, Meyer EA (editors): *Giardia and Giardiasis.* Plenum Press, 1984.

Gillon J: Giardiasis: Review of epidemiology: Pathogenetic mechanisms and host responses. *Q J Med* 1984;**209**:29.

Rosoff JD, Stibbs HH: Isolation and identification of a *Giardia lamblia*-specific stool antigen (GSA 65) useful in coprodiagnosis of giardiasis. *J Clin Microbiol* 1986;**23**:905.

Smith PD: Pathophysiology and immunology of giardiasis. *Annu Rev Med* 1985;**36**:295.

Speelman P: Single-dose tinidazole for the treatment of giardiasis. *Antimicrob Agents Chemother* 1985;**27**:227.

## BALANTIDIASIS

*Balantidium coli* is a large ciliated intestinal protozoon found throughout the world, particularly in the tropics. Infection results from ingestion of viable cysts passed in stools of humans or swine, the reservoir hosts. In the new host, the cyst wall dissolves, and the trophozoite may invade the mucosa and submucosa of the large bowel and terminal ileum, causing abscesses and irregularly rounded ulcerations. Many cases are asymptomatic and probably need not be treated. Chronic recurrent diarrhea, alternating with constipation, is the most common clinical manifestation, but attacks of severe dysentery with bloody mucoid stools, tenesmus, and colic may occur intermittently. Diagnosis is made by finding trophozoites in liquid stools and cysts in formed stools. The treatment of choice is tetracycline hydrochloride, 500 mg 4 times daily for 10 days. The alternative drug is iodoquinol (diiodohydroxyquin), 650 mg 3 times daily for 21 days. Occasional success has also been reported with metronidazole, 750 mg 3 times daily for 10 days; paromomycin, ampicillin, and carbarsone.

In properly treated mild to moderate symptomatic cases, the prognosis is good, but in spite of treatment, fatalities have occurred in severe infections as a result of intestinal perforation or hemorrhage.

Dorfman S, Rangel O, Bravo LG: Balantidiasis: Report of a fatal case with appendicular and pulmonary involvement. *Trans R Soc Trop Med Hyg* 1984;**78**:833.

Knight R: Giardiasis, isosporiasis and balantidiasis. *Clin Gastroenterol* 1978;**7**:31.

## TOXOPLASMOSIS

### Essentials of Diagnosis

*Acute primary infection:*
- Fever, malaise, headache, lymphadenopathy, myalgia, arthralgia, stiff neck, sore throat; occasionally, rash, hepatosplenomegaly, retinochoroiditis, confusion; in various combinations.
- Positive serologic tests with high and rising IgG and IgM.
- Isolation of *T gondi* from blood or body fluids; tachyozoites in histologic sections of tissue or cytologic preparations of body fluids.

*Acute primary or recrudescent infection in immunocompromised patients:*
- Retinochoroiditis, encephalitis, pneumonitis, myocarditis; sometimes other findings (above).
- Positive IgG titers moderately high; IgM antibody usually absent.
- Laboratory findings (above).

### General Considerations

*Toxoplasma gondii,* an obligate intracellular protozoan, is found worldwide in humans and in many species of animals and birds. The parasite is a coccidian of cats, the definitive host, and exists in 3 forms: The trophozoite (tachyzoite) is the rapidly proliferating form seen in the tissues and body fluids in the acute stage. The trophozoites can enter and multiply in most mammalian nucleated cells. The cyst (bradyzoite), containing viable trophozoites, is the latent form that can persist indefinitely in the host in the chronic stage and is found particularly in muscle and nerve tissue. The oocyst is the form passed only in the feces of the cat family. In the intestinal epithelium of cats, a sexual cycle occurs, with subsequent release of oocysts. Human infection occurs by ingestion of oocysts in soil (by soil-eating children), by ingestion of cysts in raw or undercooked meat (adults), by transplacental transmission, or, rarely, by direct inoculation of trophozoites, as in blood transfusion.

### Clinical Findings

**A. Symptoms and Signs:** The incubation period after ingestion of *Toxoplasma* cysts or oocysts is 1–2 weeks, though a large proportion of primary infections are asymptomatic. Generally, both asymptomatic and symptomatic infections persist on recovery as chronic infections.

The clinical manifestations of toxoplasmosis may be grouped into 4 syndromes: primary infection in the normal host, congenital infection, retinochoroiditis, and primary infection or reactivated disease in the immunologically compromised host.

Most symptomatic primary infections in the normal host are mild, acute, febrile multisystem illnesses that resemble infectious mononucleosis. The illness includes the following features in various combinations: fever, malaise, myalgia, arthralgia, headache, sore throat, generalized lymphadenopathy (especially cervical), and maculopapular rash. Hepatosplenomegaly may occur. Rarely, severe cases include pneumonitis, meningoencephalitis, hepatitis, myocarditis, and retinochoroiditis. Symptoms may fluctuate, but most patients recover spontaneously over 1–2 months.

Congenital transmission occurs only as a result of acute infection in a nonimmune woman during pregnancy. Infection has been detected in up to 1% of women during pregnancy; approximately 15–60% of such infections, varying by trimester, are transmitted to the fetus, but only a small percentage result in abortions or stillbirths or in active disease in liveborn infants. Though fetal infection may occur in any trimester, it is more severe early in pregnancy. Signs of congenital toxoplasmosis may be present at birth or may develop during the first months of life: microcephaly, internal hydrocephalus, seizures, mental retardation, hepatosplenomegaly, pneumonitis, rash, fever, retinochoroiditis, and cerebral calcification. Psychomotor and learning disorders, hearing loss, and retinochoroiditis may not be apparent for years.

Retinochoroiditis develops gradually weeks to years after congenital infection (the preponderant form and generally bilateral) or rarely after an acquired infection in a young child (generally unilateral). Primary infections in older children and adults rarely progress to late retinochoroiditis. The inflammatory process persists for weeks to months as focally necrotic retinal lesions with blurred margins. With healing, white or dark-pigmented scars may result.

Infection in the immunologically compromised host may present as a disseminated disease, particularly in patients given immunosuppressive drugs or patients with lymphoreticular, hematologic, or other cancers or with acquired immunodeficiency syndrome (AIDS). Encephalitis is the most common manifestation; pneumonitis, myocarditis, and other forms of systemic disease may also occur.

**B. Laboratory Findings:** Diagnosis depends principally on serologic test results. However, toxoplasmosis can be diagnosed occasionally by histologic examination of tissue or isolation of the parasite in mice or tissue culture. The organism may be directly identified by staining bone marrow aspirates, cerebrospinal fluid sediment, sputum, blood (buffy coat from centrifuged blood), and other tissue or body fluids, or placental tissue. The demonstration of cysts does not establish a causal relationship to clinical illness, since cysts may be found in both acute and chronic illness. Only finding tachyzoites in blood or body fluids confirms active infection. However, the presence of cysts in the placenta, fetus, or newborn indicates congenital infection; finding numerous cysts in sections from active cases suggests active infection. Leukocyte counts are normal or reduced, often with lymphocytosis or monocytosis with rare atypical cells, but there is no heterophil antibody. Chest radiographs may show interstitial pneumonia.

Serologic tests—the Feldman-Sabin dye test, the complement fixation test, ELISA, and indirect immunofluorescence and other tests—can be conducted on blood, cerebrospinal fluid, and other body fluids. In acute acquired toxoplasmosis, the diagnosis is established serologically by a 4-fold rise in serologic titers by any test or by a single high titer (1:160) of IgM antibodies. A presumptive diagnosis is supported by a single very high titer ($\geq$ 1:1000) of IgG antibodies; however, these antibodies may persist for years. In immunocompetent persons, a negative Feldman-Sabin dye test virtually excludes the diagnosis of acute toxoplasmosis, but high titers can persist for years after recovery. For the IgM indirect fluorescent antibody test, however, negative results can occur in up to 25% of acute cases. In patients with AIDS or cancer, serologic methods for diagnosis of reactivated toxoplasmosis may give false-negative results. The diagnosis of congenital infection is supported by a high titer of IgM antibodies in cord blood; the presence of specific IgM antibody is diagnostic. The presence of IgG antibodies may indicate only transplacental passage from the mother.

Where available, the following new methods may be useful in diagnosis: Testing for antigenemia has been used to demonstrate acute infection, and lymphocyte transformation to *Toxoplasma* antigens has provided a specific and sensitive indicator of prior infection.

## Treatment

Asymptomatic infections in normal hosts are not treated except in children under 5 years of age.

Symptomatic patients should be treated until manifestations of the illness have subsided and there is serologic evidence that immunity has been acquired.

Although most episodes of retinochoroiditis are self-limited, treatment is generally given because the clinical course cannot be predicted with certainty.

Immunocompromised patients with active infection (primary or recrudescent) must be treated. Therapy should continue for 4–6 weeks after cessation of symptoms—which may require up to a 6-month course, to be followed by drug prophylaxis as long as immunosupression persists. Chronic asymptomatic infection in these patients usually need not be treated, but prophylaxis may be started after a significant increase in antibody titer is noted.

Treatment is also indicated in congenitally infected infants with or without symptoms.

Treatment of women who become infected during pregnancy is controversial because of possible toxic effects on the fetus. Because early treatment reduces (but does not eliminate) the incidence of fetal infection, most workers feel that treatment is justified.

For details on management of congenital infections and those occurring during pregnancy, see specialized texts.

The treatment of choice is pyrimethamine, 75 mg/d for 3 days, then 25 mg daily, plus either trisulfapyrimidine (2–6 g/d in divided doses) or sulfadiazine (100 mg/kg/d [maximum 6 g/d] in 4 divided doses). In the treatment of severe disease in immunodeficient patients, the dose of pyrimethamine may be increased to 50 mg/d. The usual sulfonamide precautions must be observed, and folinic acid, 3–10 mg/d in divided doses, is given to avoid the hematologic effects of folate deficiency. Platelet and white blood cell counts should be performed at least twice weekly. Spiramycin is in use in Europe at a dosage of 2–4 g in 4 divided doses and is safe in pregnancy. Trimethoprim-sulfamethoxazole is being used but with unreliable results.

Clindamycin (300 mg 4 times daily) is being tested; because it is concentrated in the ocular choroid, it has had particular use in the treatment of ocular disease. Corticosteroids may also be required in the management of ocular disease.

## Prevention

Pregnant women should have their serum examined for *Toxoplasma* antibody. If the IgM test is negative and the conventional tests less than 1:1000, no further evaluation is necessary. Those with negative titers by conventional tests should take measures to prevent infection—preferably by having no further contact with cats and not eating raw meats. Vegetables and fruits should be thoroughly washed or cooked and the hands washed after handling raw meat.

Freezing of meat to −20 °C for 2 days or heating to 60 °C kills cysts in tissues. Under appropriate environmental conditions, oocysts passed in cat feces can remain infective for a year or more. Thus, children's play areas, including sand boxes, should be protected from cat and dog feces; hand washing is indicated after contact with soil potentially contaminated by animal feces.

Farkash AE et al: CNS toxoplasmosis in acquired immune deficiency syndrome: A clinical-pathological-radiological review of 12 cases. *J Neurology Neurosurg Psychiat* 1986;**49**:744.

Frenkel JK: Toxoplasmosis. *Pediatr Clin North Am* 1985; **32**:917.

Hall SM: The diagnosis of toxoplasmosis. *Br Med J* 1984; **289**:570.

Henderson JB et al: The evaluation of new services: Possibilities for preventing congenital toxoplasmosis. *Int J Epidemiol* 1984;**13**:65.

Hughes HPA: Toxoplasmosis: The need for improved diagnostic techniques and accurate risk assessment. *Cur Top Microbiol Immunol* 1985;**120**:105.

McCabe RE, Remington JS: The diagnosis and treatment of toxoplasmosis. *Eur J Clin Microbiol* 1983;**2**:95.

## COCCIDIOSIS: ISOSPORIASIS, CRYPTOSPORIDIOSIS, SARCOCYSTOSIS

Coccidiosis is an intestinal infection usually accompanied by diarrhea and abdominal discomfort and caused by coccidia of 3 genera: *Isospora*, *Cryptosporidium*, and *Sarcocystis*. Rarely, sarcocystiasis also presents as transient painful muscular and subcutaneous swellings. Although these infections occur worldwide, they are recognized only sporadically.

### General Considerations

**A. Isosporiasis:** Isosporiasis, caused by *Isospora belli*, is considered host-specific for humans, with transmission directly from person to person. Infection is by the fecal-oral route following ingestion of oocysts. Sporozoites excyst and invade jejunal and duodenal epithelial cells, in which they undergo both a sexual and an asexual cycle, resulting in the liberation of unsporulated oocysts, $20-30 \times 10-20$ µm, into the feces.

The incubation period is 7–11 days. Some patients remain asymptomatic. Most symptomatic infections follow a benign, self-limited course lasting a few weeks or months. The principal findings are diarrhea, abdominal pain, flatulence, low-grade fever, vomiting, malaise, and anorexia. Infrequently, the disease is protracted or recurrent; when severe, there may be intense diarrhea, steatorrhea, malabsorption, and weight loss. Several deaths have been reported. Isosporiasis has been seen in patients with acquired immunodeficiency syndrome (AIDS).

The diagnosis is made by finding the parasite in feces or duodenal aspirates or by duodenal biopsy. Diagnosis by stool examination is often difficult, for the organisms may be scanty even in the presence of significant symptoms. The laboratory should be notified of the need to search for the organisms, so that special concentration techniques will be used. Because of their buoyancy, oocysts must be looked for just beneath the coverslip of the preparation. Although the peroral duodenal string test or duodenal aspiration may also assist in diagnosis, frequently diagnosis can be made only after duodenal biopsy and search of multiple serial sections. Some patients have marked steatorrhea, and up to 50% of patients with isosporiasis have eosinophilia.

**B. Cryptosporidiosis:** Cryptosporidiosis is a well-known cause of diarrhea in many animal species and only recently has been recognized as a cause of diarrhea in humans, with about half of the cases in immunologically competent persons and half in immunosuppressed persons. However, information is accumulating to show that the infection may be an unrecognized cause of mild gastroenteritis worldwide, including cases of traveler's diarrhea, and that it is one of the causes of acute childhood diarrhea in developing countries. Fecal-oral transmission from animals to humans may be an important mode of infection. Human-to-human transmission is presumed to occur. Outbreaks in day-care centers and clustering in families have been reported. Infective oocysts (4 µm in diameter) shed in feces by a host proliferate sexually and asexually in the new host. The organisms attach to the microvillous borders of enterocytes of the small and large bowel and are also found free within mucosal crypts. Other epithelial surfaces are sometimes infected, including the gallbladder and respiratory tract, but the parasite is not invasive. Clinically, in immunocompetent persons, the disease is characterized by watery diarrhea (without gross or microscopic blood), low-grade fever, abdominal cramps, and, sometimes, anorexia and weight loss. The infection is self-limited and lasts a few days to about 2 weeks. Occasionally, a malabsorption syndrome has been described. In immunologically deficient patients, however, especially those with AIDS, the illness is characterized by chronic, profuse, choleralike watery diarrhea and by fever, marked weight loss, and lymphadenopathy. The diarrhea may persist for months and contribute to death.

Diagnosis is by detection of oocysts in stool by a variety of flotation, concentration, and staining methods or by mucosal biopsy. In AIDS patients, the organism should also be looked for in sputum and specimens obtained from lung tissue. An immunofluorescence serologic test is in use at some centers.

**C. Sarcocystosis:** *Sarcocystis* is a 2-host coccidian. Human disease occurs as 2 syndromes, both rare: (1) an enteric infection in which humans are the definitive host and (2) a muscle infection in which humans are an intermediate host. In the enteric form of the disease, sporocysts passed in human feces are not infective for humans but must be ingested by cattle or pigs. Humans become infected by eating poorly cooked beef or pork containing oocysts of *Sarcocystis bovihominis* or *Sarcocystis suihominis*, respectively. (Formerly, the causative agent was known as *Isospora hominis*.) Organisms enter intestinal epithelial cells and are transformed into oocysts that release sporocysts into the feces. The fecal stage of the parasite is more mature than that of *I belli*—the oocyst has lost its wall and appears as single or paired sporocysts. Clinically, the intestinal infection is often asymptomatic or causes mild, protracted diarrhea. Diagnosis is by stool examination using a fecal flotation method.

The muscle form of sarcocystosis results when humans ingest sporocysts in feces from an infected carnivore that has eaten prey which harbored sarcocysts. The sporocysts liberate sporozoites that invade the intestinal wall and are disseminated to skeletal muscle. This results in subcutaneous and muscular inflammation lasting several days to 2 weeks and the finding of swellings at these sites, sometimes associated with eosinophilia. Sarcocysts are often asymptomatic, however, such as those found incidentally at autopsy in cardiac muscle.

### Treatment

Instances of effective treatment for isosporiasis have been described using (1) sulfadiazine, 4 g, and pyrimethamine, 35–75 mg, in 4 divided doses daily for 3 weeks; or (2) trimethoprim-sulfamethoxazole, 2–8 tablets daily for 3 weeks (tablets contain trimethoprim, 80 mg, and sulfamethoxazole, 400 mg). No treatment has been effective in cryptosporidiosis or sarcocystosis.

Beaver PC, Gadgil K, Morera P: *Sarcocystis* in man: A review and report of five cases. *Am J Trop Med Hyg* 1979;**28**:819.

Fayer R, Ungar BL: *Cryptosporidium* spp. and cryptosporidiosis. *Microbiol Rev* 1986;**50**:458.

Kobayashi LM et al: *Isospora* infection in a homosexual man. *Diagn Microbiol Infect Dis* 1985;**3**:363.

Ma P: Cryptosporidium—biology and diagnosis. *Adv Exp Med Biol* 1986;**202**:135.

Mata L: *Cryptosporidium* and other protozoa in diarrheal disease in less developed countries. *Pediatr Infect Dis* 1986;**5**:117.

Navin TR, Juranek DD: Cryptosporidiosis: Clinical, epidemiologic, and parasitologic review. *Rev Infect Dis* 1984;**6**:313.

Stehr-Green JK et al: Shedding of oocysts in immunocompetent individuals infected with *Cryptosporidium*. *Am J Trop Med Hyg* 1987;**36**:338.

## PNEUMOCYSTOSIS
### (*Pneumocystis carinii* Pneumonia)

*Pneumocystis carinii* infection occurs as an asymptomatic process in most of the population by a young age. Overt infection, pneumocytosis, is an acute interstitial plasma cell pneumonia. The disease occurs worldwide; although rare in the general population, it occurs in larger numbers among 2 groups: (1) as epidemics of primary infections among prematures or among debilitated or marasmic infants on wards or in nursing homes, and (2) as sporadic cases among older children and adults who have an abnormal or altered immune status. Most childhood-adult cases

are assumed to be due to reactivation of latent infection in the presence of immunosuppression; they occur in the presence of immunosuppression; they occur generally in patients with cancer or severe malnutrition and debility, in patients treated with immunosuppressive or cytotoxic drugs or irradiation for the management of organ transplants and cancer, patients receiving adrenocorticosteroid therapy, and patients with acquired immunodeficiency syndrome (AIDS) (see Chapter 21). In the USA, *Pneumocystis* pneumonia occurs in about 60% of AIDS patients and is a major cause of death in patients with the syndrome.

The organism, which appears to be a protozoan with intra- and extracellular stages, has 3 forms: cysts, sporozoites, and trophozoites. The thick-walled cyst is 4–6 μm in diameter and contains 8 sporozoites; when released from the cyst, these sporozoites become pleomorphic trophozoites, which are 2–5 μm in diameter. Although the mode of transmission in primary infection is unknown, some evidence suggests airborne transmission. Following asymptomatic primary infection, latent and presumably inactive organisms are sparsely distributed in the alveoli. The organism has been found in lung tissue of many wild and domestic animals.

In the sporadic form of the disease associated with deficient cell-mediated immunity, the onset is abrupt, with high fever, tachypnea, mild nonproductive cough, intercostal retractions, and cyanosis. Without treatment, the course usually is one of rapid deterioration and death. In the infantile form of the disease, the patient is generally free of fever and may show eosinophilia.

With rare exceptions, pathologic findings are limited to the pulmonary parenchyma. Pulmonary physical findings may be slight (including no rales) and disproportionate to the degree of illness and to the radiologic findings. Radiographic findings include bilateral or asymmetric alveolar infiltrates, pulmonary consolidation, nodular infiltrates in the periphery, and other atypical findings. The blood gases usually show impaired diffusion and severe hypoxemia with minimal (or no) $CO_2$ retention, resulting in uncompensated respiratory alkalosis.

Specific diagnosis depends on morphologic demonstration of the organism in clinical specimens using specific stains. Sputum, transtracheal aspirates, bronchial washings, and bronchial brushing and sometimes gastric aspirates provide relatively low yields of the organisms, in contrast with the approximately 80% yields using procedures that sample the parenchymal compartments—bronchoalveolar lavage, transbronchial biopsy, transthoracic aspiration, endobronchial brushing, and open lung biopsy. Diffuse gallium citrate (Ga 67) accumulation on chest radiograph may provide early recognition of *P carinii* infection. Serologic tests, including tests to detect antigenemia, are not helpful in diagnosis at present.

The treatment of choice for *Pneumocystis* pneumonia is trimethoprim-sulfamethoxazole. Trimethoprim, 20 mg/kg, plus sulfamethoxazole, 100 mg/kg, is given daily orally in 4 equal doses for 14 days. A prolonged course may be required for some patients with AIDS. When possible, blood levels should be monitored; optimum peak therapeutic blood levels are 3–5 μg/mL of trimethoprim and 100–150 μg/mL of sulfamethoxazole. If necessary, an intravenous preparation can be used (follow the manufacturer's directions). Sulfonamide precautions must be observed. Patients with AIDS have a high frequency of hypersensitivity reactions to trimethoprim-sulfamethoxazole—fever, rashes (sometimes severe), malaise, and leukopenia. Because of the hypoxia usually associated with this disease, oxygen therapy may be indicated to maintain the $P_{O_2}$ at 70 mm Hg or higher. The fraction of inspired oxygen ($F_{i02}$) should be kept below 50 vol% if possible to avoid oxygen toxicity.

Pentamidine, which is more toxic than trimethoprim-sulfamethoxazole, is used to treat patients who have had adverse reactions or who fail to respond to the latter drug. Pentamidine causes side effects in nearly 50% of patients, including severe renal reactions, hypoglycemia, hypotension, liver function abnormalities, thrombocytopenia, and reactions at the injection site. Pentamidine isethionate is administered intramuscularly or intravenously as a single daily dose of 4 mg (salt)/kg/d for 12–14 days. To avoid hypotension and sterile injection site abscesses, some groups administer the drug only intravenously by diluting it in 100 mL of fluid and giving it slowly over 1 hour. α-Difluoromethylornithine is undergoing early clinical trials as an alternate mode of treatment.

Chemoprophylaxis for high-risk immunocompromised patients consists of oral trimethoprim-sulfamethoxazole in one-fourth of the therapeutic dose given in 2 divided doses. Persons with G6PD deficiency should not receive such prophylaxis.

In the absence of early and adequate treatment, the fatality rate for the endemic infantile form of pneumocystosis is 20–50%; for the sporadic form in immunodeficient persons, the fatality rate is nearly 100%. Early treatment reduces the mortality rate to about 3% in the former and 25% in the latter forms of infection. Recurrences may be seen after trimethoprim-sulfamethoxazole treatment or pentamidine treatment. Resistance to trimethoprim-sulfamethoxazole occurs sometimes during recurrence.

Hughes WT: *Pneumocystis carinii* pneumonitis. *Chest* 1984; **85:**810.

Kaufman DL: *Pneumocystics carinii* pneumonia. *Adv Exp Med Biol* 1986;**202:**153.

Pearson RD, Hewlett EL: Pentamidine for the treatment of *Pneumocystis carinii* pneumonia and other protozoal diseases. *Ann Intern Med* 1985;**103:**782.

Peters SG, Prakash UB: *Pneumocystis carinii* pneumonia. Review of 53 cases. *Am J Med* 1987:**82:**73.

Ruskin J: Newer developments in diagnosis and treatment of *Pneumocystis* infections. Pages 194–215 in: *Current Clinical Topics in Infectious Diseases.* Remington JS, Swartz MN (editors). McGraw-Hill, 1986.

Young LS (editor): Pneumocystis carinii: *Pathogenesis, Diagnosis, Treatment.* Marcel Dekker, 1984.

# REFERENCES

Adams ARD, Maegraith BG: *Clinical Tropical Diseases,* 8th ed. Blackwell, 1984.

Banks BJ: Antiparasitic agents. *Annu Rep Med Chem* 1984;**19:**147.

Beaver PC, Jung RC, Cupp EW: *Clinical Parasitology,* 9th ed. Lea & Febiger, 1984.

Benenson AS (editor): *Control of Communicable Diseases in Man,* 14th ed. Lucas, Springfield, Virginia, 1985.

Binford CH, Connor DH (editors): *Pathology of Tropical and Extraordinary Diseases.* Vols 1 and 2. Armed Forces Institute of Pathology, 1976.

Brown HW, Neva FA: *Basic Clinical Parasitology,* 5th ed. Appleton-Century-Crofts, 1983.

Bruckner DA: Serologic and intradermal tests for parasitic infections. *Pediatr Clin North Am* 1985;**32:**1063.

Campbell WC, Rew RS (editors): *Chemotherapy of Parasitic Disease.* Plenum, 1986.

Draper CC, Lillywhite JE: Immunodiagnosis of tropical parasitic infections. Pages 267–289 in: *Recent Advances in Tropical Medicine.* Gilles HM (editor). Churchill Livingstone, 1984.

Drugs for parasitic infections. *Med Lett Drugs Ther* (January 31) 1986;**28:**9.

Goldsmith RS: Infectious diseases: Helminthic. Chap 55 in: *Basic & Clinical Pharmacology,* 3rd ed. Katzung BG (editor). Appleton-Lange, 1986.

Hoskins DW: Drugs for intestinal parasitism. In: *Drugs of Choice.* Modell W (editor). Mosby, 1984.

James DM, Gilles HM: *Human Antiparasitic Drugs: Pharmacology and Usage.* Wiley, 1985.

Jelliffe DB, Stanfield JP (editors) *Diseases of Children in the Subtropics and Tropics,* 3rd ed. Arnold, 1978.

Manson-Bahr PEC, Apted FIC: *Manson's Tropical Diseases,* 18th ed. Baillière Tindall, 1982.

Marchalonis JJ (editor): Immunobiology of parasites and parasitic infections. *Contemp Top Immunobiol* 1984;**12.** [Entire issue.]

Marcial-Rojas RA (editor): *Pathology of Protozoal and Helminthic Diseases With Clinical Correlation.* Williams & Wilkins, 1971.

Markell EK, Voge M, John DT (editors): *Medical Parasitology,* 6th ed. Saunders, 1986.

Most H: Treatment of parasitic infections of travelers and immigrants. *N Engl J Med* 1984;**310:**298.

Pearson RD, Hewlett EL, Guerrant RL: *Tropical Diseases in North America.* Year Book, 1984.

Seidel JS: Treatment of parasitic infections. *Pediatr Clin North Am* 1985;**32:**1077.

Steele JH (editor-in-chief): *CRC Handbook Series in Zoonoses. Section C: Parasitic Zoonoses.* Vol 3. Hillyer GV, Hopla CE (volume editors). CRC Press, 1982.

Strickland GT: *Hunter's Tropical Medicine,* 6th ed. Saunders, 1984.

Vanden Bossche H, Thienpont D, Jassens PG (editors): *Chemotherapy of Gastrointestinal Helminths.* Springer, 1985.

Walls KW, Wilson M: Immunoserology in parasitic infections. *Lab Res Methods Biol Med* 1983;**8**:191.

Warren KS, Mahmoud AAF: *Tropical and Geographic Medicine* McGraw-Hill, 1984.

WHO Scientific Group: *Intestinal Protozoan and Helminthic Infections*. Technical Report Series No. 666. World Health Organization, 1981.

## TREMATODE (FLUKE) INFECTIONS

### SCHISTOSOMIASIS
### (Bilharziasis)

**Essentials of Diagnosis**
- Acute phase: Abrupt onset (2–6 weeks postexposure) of abdominal pain, weight loss, headache, malaise, chills, fever, myalgia, diarrhea (sometimes bloody), dry cough, hepatomegaly, and eosinophilia.
- Chronic phase: Either (1) diarrhea, abdominal pain, blood in stool, hepatomegaly or hepatosplenomegaly, and bleeding from esophageal varices (*Schistosoma mansoni* or *Schistosoma japonicum* infection); or (2) terminal hematuria, urinary frequency, and urethral and bladder pain (*Schistosoma haematobium* infection).
- Depending on species, characteristic eggs in feces, urine, or scrapings or biopsy of rectal or bladder mucosa.

**General Considerations**

Schistosomiasis is found in many tropical and subtropical areas of the world and is of great public health importance, particularly in rural areas. Three blood flukes (trematodes) are responsible for the disease. *Schistosoma mansoni*, which causes intestinal schistosomiasis, is widespread in Africa and occurs in the Arabian peninsula, northeastern South America, and the Caribbean (including Puerto Rico but not Cuba). Vesical (urinary) schistosomiasis, caused by *Schistosoma haematobium*, is found throughout the Middle East and Africa. Asiatic intestinal schistosomiasis, due to *Schistosoma japonicum*, is important in China and the Philippines, and a small focus is present in Sulawesi, Indonesia. Transmission of *S japonicum* in Japan has been interrupted.

Various species of snails, the intermediate hosts, are infected by larvae hatched from eggs that reach fresh water in feces or urine. After development, infective larvae (cercariae) leave the snails, enter water, and penetrate human skin or mucous membranes that come in contact with the water. In humans, the schistosomula in the larval stage reach the portal circulation in the liver, where they rapidly mature. After

a few weeks, adult worms pair, mate, and migrate mainly to terminal venules of specific veins, where females deposit their eggs. By means of their lytic secretions, some eggs reach the lumen of the bowel or bladder and are passed with feces or urine. Others are retained in the bowel or bladder wall, while still others are carried in the circulation to the liver, lung, and (less often) other tissues. Except for the allergic response in the acute syndrome (see below), disease is due to granuloma formation around eggs retained in the tissues and subsequent fibrous tissue replacement. Live worms produce no lesions and rarely produce symptoms. The type or degree of tissue damage and symptoms vary with the intensity of infection (worm burden), degree of host reactivity, site of egg deposition, and duration of infection. Egg accumulation in the liver can result in periportal fibrosis followed by portal hypertension. Eggs in the lung may lead to lung scarring, bronchiectasis, emphysema, and cor pulmonale.

*S mansoni* worms migrate to the inferior mesenteric veins. The adult males are 9–12 mm × 1–1.2 mm; the females are longer but have a smaller diameter. Many eggs lodge in the bowel wall, where they induce granulomas, fibrosis, ulcers, and polyps. Eggs are frequently carried to the liver and sometimes to the lungs, spinal cord, and other tissues where they may cause local symptoms. For *S mansoni*, the prepatent period—cercarial penetration until the appearance of eggs in feces—is about 50 days. The life span of the worms is 5–20 years or more.

*S japonicum* adults lie in terminal branches of the superior and inferior mesenteric veins in the small and large bowel walls. Eggs are passed in the stool or lodge in the bowel wall, provoking changes similar to those noted above. Because greater numbers of eggs are produced by *S japonicum*, the resulting disease is more extensive and severe. Eggs are frequently carried to the liver and lung (and occasionally to the central nervous system and other organs), and cirrhosis and portal hypertension are common.

The adult *S haematobium* matures in the venous plexuses of the bladder, rectum, prostate, and uterus. Eggs are passed in the urine or retained in the tissues, particularly the bladder wall and the female genital organs. Some eggs may reach the liver, lungs, and other tissues.

A number of animal schistosomes sometimes infect humans. *Schistosoma intercalatum* causes human disease in central Africa, and *Schistosoma mekongi* has recently been recognized in humans in a limited area along the Mekong River in Thailand, Cambodia, and Laos.

Many mammals serve as reservoirs for *S japonicum*. However, the few mammals found infected with *S mansoni* or *S haematobium* are of little epidemiolgic significance.

## Clinical Findings

### A. Symptoms and Signs:

**1. Cercarial dermatitis**–Although the significance is not often recognized, the first sign of infection is an itchy erythematous or petechial rash at sites of penetration of the cercariae. The findings last 2–5 days.

**2. Acute schistosomiasis (Katayama fever)**–This syndrome, primarily an allergic phenomenon, may occur as a result of infection with all 3 schistosomes, though it is rare in the case of *S haematobium*. In addition to fever, malaise, urticaria, diarrhea, cough, and eosinophilia, the liver and spleen may be temporarily enlarged. The patient again becomes asymptomatic in 2–8 weeks.

**3. Chronic schistosomiasis**–This stage begins 6 months to several years after infection as lesions develop around eggs embedded in the tissues. Early in the course of *S mansoni* and *S japonicum* infections, frequent findings include diarrhea, dysentery, and abdominal pain. With subsequent slow progression over 5–15 years or longer, the following may appear: anorexia, weight loss, polypoid intestinal tumors, and features of portal hypertension (contracted liver, splenomegaly, pancytopenia, esophageal varices) and hepatic insufficiency. Chronic salmonellosis or the nephrotic syndrome may also occur. Complications that may lead to death include hematemesis, hepatic coma, intercurrent infection, and possibly adenocarcinoma of the bowel.

Early symptoms of urinary tract disease are frequency and dysuria, followed by terminal hematuria and proteinuria. Frank hematuria may be recurrent; obstruction of the ureteral orifices may lead to hydronephrosis. Sequelae may include bladder polyp formation, cystitis, pyelitis, pyelonephritis, urolithiasis, nephrotic syndrome, renal failure, and death. Severe liver, lung, genital, or neurologic disease is rare. Many cases of bladder cancer have been associated with vesicular schistosomiasis.

### B. Laboratory Findings:

Definitive diagnosis is made by finding characteristic eggs in excreta or by mucosal or liver biopsy. In *S haematobium* infection, eggs may be found in the urine, in tissues obtained from the vesical mucosa, or less frequently in stools. Eggs are sought in urine specimens collected between 9:00 AM and 2:00 PM or in 24-hour collections. They are processed either by examination of the sediment or preferably by membrane filtration. In *S mansoni* and *S japonicum* infections, eggs may be found in stool specimens by direct examination, but some form of concentration is usually necessary; repeated examinations are often needed to find eggs in light infections. If results are negative—in selected cases only (because of the risks of biopsy)—proceed to rectal mucosal biopsy of suspicious lesions or take biopsy specimens at 2–3 sites of normal mucosa. Biopsy specimens should be examined as crush preparations between 2 glass slides. The Kato thick smear or membrane filtration method is useful to quantitate fecal egg output in order to estimate severity of infection and to follow response to therapy. When eggs are found, their viability should be determined, since dead eggs are retained in the tissues for months. Rarely, liver biopsy may be necessary for diagnosis.

Screening for infection is possible by skin or serologic testing, but neither is sufficiently sensitive or specific to be used as the sole criterion for diagnosis.

Serologic tests become positive a few weeks after infection, but both false-positive and false-negative reactions may occur. Microscopic hematuria may be present in *S haematobium* infection, and in advanced disease, lower abdominal x-rays may show calcification of the bladder wall or ureters. Eosinophilia is common during the migration of the immature flukes, but the count usually returns to normal later.

## Differential Diagnosis

Schistosomiasis mansoni or japonicum should be considered in all unresponsive gastrointestinal disorders in persons who have been in endemic areas. Early intestinal schistosomiasis may be mistaken for amebiasis, bacillary dysentery, or other causes of diarrhea and dysentery. Later, the various causes of portal hypertension or of bowel papillomas and polyps must be considered. Vesical schistosomiasis must be differentiated from other causes of hematuria, prostatic disease, genitourinary tract cancer, and bacterial infections of the urinary tract.

## Complications

Among the many complications of these diseases are transverse myelitis (*S mansoni* eggs in the spinal cord); seizures, optic neuritis, paralysis, and mental disorders (*S japonicum* eggs in the brain); liver failure, variceal bleeding, and colon neoplasms (*S mansoni*, *S japonicum*); liver failure, uremia, and bladder neoplasms (*S haematobium*); chronic pulmonary disease (periarteritis and endarteritis, primarily due to *S mansoni* eggs); and persistent *Salmonella* infection of the bowel (*S masoni*) or bladder (*S haematobium*).

## Treatment

### A. Medical Treatment:

The development of the new drugs metrifonate, oxamniquine, and praziquantel now makes it possible to treat infections caused by all schistosome species without the concern for serious side effects that was experienced with the older drugs.

Treatment should be given only if live ova are identified. The drugs of choice for the treatment of *S haematobium* infections are metrifonate or praziquantel; for *S mansoni,* oxamniquine or praziquantel;

**Table 26–1.** Drugs for the treatment of helminthic infections.

| Infecting Organism | Drug of Choice | Alternative Drugs |
|---|---|---|
| **Roundworms (nematodes)** | | |
| *Ascaris lumbricoides* (roundworm) | Pyrantel pamoate | Piperazine, mebendazole, levamisole,[1] bephenium,[1] or albendazole[1,2] |
| *Trichuris trichiura* (whipworm) | Mebendazole | Oxantel-pyrantel pamoate[1,2] or albendazole[1,2,4] |
| *Necator americanus* (hookworm) *Ancylostoma duodenale* (hookworm) | Pyrantel pamoate[3] or mebendazole | Bephenium,[1] tetrachloroethylene,[1] levamisole,[1] or albendazole[1,2,4] |
| Combined infection with *Ascaris, Trichuris,* and hookworm | Mebendazole or oxantel-pyrantel pamoate[1,2] | Albendazole[1,2,4] |
| Combined infection with *Ascaris* and hookworm | Mebendazole or pyrantel pamoate | Bephenium[1] or albendazole[1,2,4] |
| *Strongyloides stercoralis* (threadworm) | Thiabendazole | Albendazole,[1,2,4] mebendazole,[3,4] or cambendazole[1,2,4] |
| *Enterobius vermicularis* (pinworm) | Mebendazole or pyrantel pamoate | Pyrvinium pamoate or albendazole[1,2] |
| *Trichinella spiralis* (trichinosis) | ACTH, corticosteroids, and thiabendazole[4] or mebendazole[3,4] | None |
| *Trichostrongylus* species | Pyrantel pamoate[3] or mebendazole[3] | Bephenium[1] or levamisole[1] |
| Cutaneous larva migrans (creeping eruption) | Thiabendazole | Diethylcarbamazine[4,5] or albendazole[1,2,4] |
| Visceral larva migrans | Thiabendazole[3,4] or mebendazole[3,4] | Diethylcarbamazine[4,5] |
| *Angiostrongylus cantonensis* | Levamisole[1,4] | None |
| *Wuchereria bancrofti* (filariasis), *Brugia malayi* (filariasis), tropical eosinophilia, and *Loa loa* (loiasis) | Diethylcarbamazine[5] | None |
| *Onchocerca volvulus* (onchocerciasis) | Diethylcarbamazine[5] plus suramin[6] | Ivermectin[1,2,4] |
| *Dracunculus medinensis* (guinea worm) | Metronidazole[3] | Thiabendazole[3] or mebendazole[3,4] |
| Intestinal capillariasis | Mebendazole[3] | Thiabendazole[3] |
| **Flukes (trematodes)** | | |
| *Schistosoma haematobium* (bilharziasis) | Praziquantel | Metrifonate[1] |
| *Schistosoma mansoni* | Praziquantel | Oxamniquine |
| *Schistosoma japonicum* | Praziquantel | Niridazole[1] |
| *Clonorchis sinensis* (liver fluke) *Opisthorchis* species | Praziquantel[3] | Mebendazole[3,4] or albendazole[1,2,4] |
| *Paragonimus westermani* (lung fluke) | Praziquantel[3] | Bithionol[6] |
| *Fasciola hepatica* (sheep liver fluke) | Bithionol[6] | Emetine, dehydroemetine,[6] or praziquantel[3,4] |
| *Fasciolopsis buski* (large intestinal fluke) | Praziquantel[3] or niclosamide[3] | Dichlorophen,[1,4] tetrachloroethylene,[1] or bephenium[1] |
| *Heterophyes heterophyes* and *Metagonimus yokogawai* (small intestinal flukes) | Praziquantel[3] or niclosamide[3] | Bephenium[1] or tetrachloroethylene[1] |
| **Tapeworms (cestodes)** | | |
| *Taenia saginata* (beef tapeworm) | Niclosamide | Praziquantel,[3] dichlorophen,[1] paromomycin,[3] or mebendazole[3,4] |
| *Diphyllobothrium latum* (fish tapeworm) | Niclosamide | Praziquantel,[3] dichlorophen,[1] or paromomycin[3] |
| *Taenia solium* (pork tapeworm) | Niclosamide[3] | Praziquantel[3] or mebendazole[3,4] |
| Cysticercosis (pork tapeworm larval stage) | Praziquantel[2,3] | Albendazole[1,2,4] |
| *Hymenolepis nana* (dwarf tapeworm) | Praziquantel[3] | Niclosamide or paromomycin[3] |
| *Hymenolepis diminuta* (rat tapeworm) *Dipylidium caninum* | Niclosamide[3] | Praziquantel[3,4] |
| *Echinococcus granulosus* (hydatid disease) *Echinococcus multilocularis* | Albendazole[1,2,4] | Mebendazole[2,3,4] |

[1] Not available in the USA.
[2] Undergoing clinical investigation.
[3] Available in the USA but not approved for this indication.
[4] Effectiveness not established or not at a high level.
[5] Available in the USA from Lederle Laboratories, telephone (914) 753–5000.
[6] Available in the USA only from the Parasitic Disease Drug Service, Parasitic Diseases Branch, Centers for Disease Control, Atlanta 30333. Telephone (404) 329–3311 during the day, (404) 329-2888 nights, weekends, and holidays (emergencies only).

and for *S japonicum, S mekongi,* and *S intercalatum,* praziquantel.

After treatment, periodic laboratory follow-up is essential, starting at 3 months and continuing at intervals for 1 year. The decision to repeat treatment depends on the intensity of live ova output and on whether reinfection is likely. In light of the safety and efficacy of modern drugs, patients in nonendemic areas should have their infections eradicated.

**1. Praziquantel,** a pyrazino isoquinoline compound, is given orally and has the unique characteristic of being effective against all human schistosome species. The drug is effective in adults and children and is well tolerated by patients in the hepatosplenic stage of advanced schistosomiasis; its safety in children under 4 years of age, however, has not been established. More than 10,000 patients were treated in 31 study groups at various dosage schedules; cure rates at 6 months for *S haematobium, S mansoni,* and *S japonicum* infections were 87%, 80%, and 84%, respectively, with marked reduction in ovum counts in those not cured.

The manufacturer's recommended dosage to treat all forms of schistosomiasis is 20 mg/kg 3 times daily for 1 day. Lower dosages have been reported to be highly effective in some parts of the world and for some species. Tablets are taken after a meal with water and should not be chewed. The interval between doses should be no less than 4 and no more than 6 hours.

The drug is free of embryologic toxicity and mutagenic or carcinogenic potential. There are no laboratory test abnormalities. Mild and transient side effects persisting for hours to 1 day are common and include malaise, headache, dizziness, and anorexia. Less frequent are fatigue, drowsiness, nausea, vomiting, generalized abdominal pain, loose stools, pruritus, urticaria, arthralgia and myalgia, and low-grade fever. The drug should not be used in pregnancy, and because of drug-induced dizziness, patients should not drive and should be cautioned if their work requires physical coordination or alertness. In areas where cysticercosis may coexist with an infection being treated with praziquantel, treatment is best carried out in a hospital.

**2. Metrifonate** is a highly effective oral drug and a drug of choice for the treatment of *S haematobium* infections, but it is not effective against *S mansoni* or *S japonicum.* The drug is a cholinesterase inhibitor and at therapeutic dosages in humans produces prolonged depression of blood cholinesterase activity, which is not known to be associated with any significant disturbance of organ structure or function. In the treatment of *S haematobium* infections, the dosage is 7.5–10 mg/kg (maximum 600 mg) once and then repeated twice at 2-week intervals. Cure rates at this schedule in various clinical trials ranged from 44 to 93%. Those not cured showed marked reduction in ovum counts. Some studies reported no side effects; others noted mild and transient findings (up to 12 hours), including gastrointestinal symptoms,

headache, bronchospasm, weakness, and vertigo. One case of organophosphate poisoning following a standard dose has been reported. Metrifonate is not available in the USA.

**3. Oxamniquine** is a highly effective oral drug and a drug of choice for the treatment of *S mansoni* infections and is both safe and effective in the advanced (hepatosplenic) form of the disease. The drug is not effective against *S haematobium* or *S japonicum.* It is a tetrahydroquinoline derivative. The dosage for strains of *S mansoni* in the western hemisphere is 12–15 mg/kg given once; for children under 30 kg, 20 mg/kg is given in 2 divided doses in 1 day, with an interval of 2–8 hours between doses. Cure rates are 70–95% with a marked reduction in egg excretion in those not cured. For most African strains, the total dosage for adults and children varies by region from 40 to 60 mg/kg in divided doses over 2–3 days. Dizziness persisting for about 6 hours is common. Less frequent side effects are drowsiness, nausea and vomiting, diarrhea, abdominal pain, and headache. An orange or red discoloration of the urine may occur. Rarely reported side effects are central nervous system stimulation with behavioral changes, hallucinations, or seizures; patients should be observed for 2 hours after ingestion of the drug for appearance of these findings. Since the drug makes some patients dizzy or drowsy, it should be used with caution in patients whose work or activity requires mental alertness. The drug has shown mutagenic and embryocidal effects and is contraindicated in pregnancy.

**4. Niridazole,** a nitrothiazole derivative, is an effective oral drug for treating *S mansoni* and *S haematobium* infections and may be tried against *S japonicum.* However, because of its toxicity, its use is being discontinued.

**5. Antimonial drugs** (eg, sodium antimony dimercaptosuccinate [stibocaptate], stibophen, tartar emetic) should no longer be used in the treatment of schistosomiasis if praziquantel, oxamniquine, or metrifonate is available, since the antimonials are significantly more toxic and require a longer course of therapy. Nevertheless, tartar emetic, in spite of its potential for serious toxicity, may occasionally be needed as a third alternative drug in the treatment of *S japonicum* infection.

**B. Surgical Measures:** In selected instances, corrective surgery may be indicated for removal of papillomas, polyps, and early carcinoma. As a last resort in patients who have repeated episodes of variceal bleeding, splenorenal anastomosis is done rather than portacaval shunts, which are associated with a high level of chronic portal systemic encephalopathy. Recent trials suggest that distal splenorenal shunt and eosphagogastric devascularization with splenectomy is a more successful procedure. Severe pancytopenia is an indication for splenectomy. Filtering of *S mansoni* adults from the portal system should be considered whenever splenectomy is contemplated. Thousands of worms have been removed in this way from a single patient.

## Prognosis

With treatment, as long as reinfection does not occur, the prognosis is excellent in early and light infections. There is evidence of reversibility of some pathologic features: shrinkage or elimination of bladder and bowel ulcerations and granulomas. In advanced disease with extensive involvement of the intestines, liver, bladder, or other organs, the outlook is poor even with treatment.

Archer S: The chemotherapy and schistosomiasis. Ann Rev Pharmacol Toxicol 1985;**25**:485.

Bennett JL, Depenbusch JW: The chemotherapy of schistosomiasis. Pages 73–117 in: Parasitic Diseases. Vol 2: Chemotherapy. Mansfield JM (editor). Marcel Dekker, 1984.

Damian RT: Immunity in schistosomiasis: A holistic view. Contemp Top Immunobiol 1984;**12**:359.

Davis A: Recent advances in schistosomiasis. Quart J Med 1986;**58**:95.

De Cock KM: Progress Report. Hepatosplenic schistosomiasis: A clinical review. Gut 1986;**27**:734.

McMahon JE: A comparative trial of praziquantel, metrifonate and niridazole against Schistosoma haematobium. Ann Trop Med Parasitol 1983;**77**:139.

Raia S, Mies S, Luiz Macedo AL: Portal hypertension in schistosomiasis. Clin Gastroenterol 1985;**14**:57.

Raia S, Mies S, Luiz Macedo AL: Surgical treatment of portal hypertension in schistosomiasis. World J Surg 1984;**8**:738.

Schistosomiasis: A review of recent abstracts. Tropical Disease Bulletin 1985;**82**:R1-R3.

## FASCIOLOPSIASIS

The large intestinal fluke, *Fasciolopsis buski,* is a common parasite of humans and pigs in central and south China, Taiwan, Southeast Asia, Indonesia, eastern India, and Bangladesh. When eggs shed in stools reach water, they hatch to produce free-swimming larvae that penetrate and develop in the flesh of snails. Cercariae escape from the snails and encyst on various water plants. Humans are infected by eating these plants uncooked (usually water chestnuts, bamboo shoots, or caltrops). Adult flukes (length 2–7.5 cm) mature in about 3 months and live in the small intestine attached to the mucosa or buried in mucous secretions.

After an incubation period of several months, manifestations of gastrointestinal irritation appear in all but light infections. Symptoms in severe infections include nausea, anorexia, upper abdominal pain, and diarrhea, sometimes alternating with constipation. Ascites and edema of the face and body may occur later. Intestinal stasis, ileus, and partial obstruction have been described.

Leukocytosis with moderate eosinophilia is common. The diagnosis depends on finding characteristic eggs or, occasionally, flukes in the stools. No serologic test is available. Because the adult worms live for only 6 months, absence from the endemic area for 6 months or more makes the diagnosis unlikely.

The drug of first choice is praziquantel. A recommended dosage is 20 mg/kg given once. Alternative drugs are tetrachloroethylene, administered as for hookworm disease, and niclosamide, administered as for taeniasis but given every other day for 3 doses. Where available, dichlorophen or bephenium can also serve as an alternative drug.

In rare cases—particularly in children—heavy infections with severe toxemia have resulted in death from cachexia or intercurrent infection. With these exceptions, the prognosis is good with proper treatment.

Bunnag D, Radomoyos P, Harinasuta T: Field trial on the treatment of fasciolopsiasis with praziquantel. Southeast Asian J Trop Med Public Health 1983;**14**:216.

Idris M et al: The treatment of fasciolopsiasis with niclosamide and dichlorophen. J Trop Med Hyg 1980;**83**:71.

## FASCIOLIASIS

Infection by *Fasciola hepatica,* the sheep liver fluke, results from ingestion of encysted metacercariae on watercress or other aquatic vegetables or ingestion of encysted metacercariae with water. A wide range of herbivorous mammals are reservoir hosts. The illness in humans is prevalent in sheep-raising countries, particularly where raw salads are eaten. Eggs of the worm, passed in host feces, release a miracidium that infects snails; the snails subsequently release cercariae that in turn encyst to complete the life cycle.

In infection in humans, metacercariae excyst from eggs, penetrate and migrate through the liver, and mature in the bile ducts, where they cause inflammatory and obstructive changes. The leaf-shaped adult flukes measure 3 cm $\times$ 1.5 cm. Although the infection is usually mild, 3 clinical syndromes can develop: acute, chronic latent, and chronic obstructive. The acute illness is associated with migration of immature larvae through the liver. Cardinal features are an enlarged and tender liver, high fever, leukocytosis, and high eosinophilia. Pain may be present in the epigastrium or right upper quadrant, and the patient may experience headache, anorexia, and vomiting. In severe illnesses, the patient may be prostrated, wasted, and jaundiced. A variety of allergic symptoms, including myalgia and urticaria, may be present. Anemia may occur, plus leukocytosis up to 35,000, with eosinophilia to 90%. Hypergammaglobulinemia is common; other liver function tests may be abnormal. Early diagnosis is difficult in the acute phase, because ova are not found in the feces for 3–4 months.

In the chronic latent phase, many infected persons are relatively free of symptoms. Others have variable degrees of pain in the epigastrium or right upper quadrant, vomiting or diarrhea, and hepatomegaly. Leukocytosis, eosinophilia, and altered liver function are sometimes seen. The chronic obstructive phase takes place if the extrahepatic bile ducts are occluded, producing a clinical picture similar to that of choledocholithiasis. Occasionally, adult flukes migrate and produce symptoms in ectopic sites. Diagnosis is by detecting characteristic eggs in the feces; repeated examinations may be necessary. Sometimes the diagnosis can only be made by finding eggs in biliary drainage and, in rare instances, only after liver biopsy or at surgical exploration. In some regions of the world, spurious infections are common (but transient) as a result of ingestion of egg-containing cow or sheep liver. Serologic tests are often useful in diagnosis, particularly in the acute phase. Cross-reactions occur with other helminths.

Bithionol, given as for paragonimiasis, is the drug of choice. Side effects occur in up to 40% of patients but are generally mild and transient; gastrointestinal symptoms and headache are the most common symptoms. If bithionol is not available, use emetine hydrochloride, 1 mg/kg body weight intramuscularly up to a maximum of 65 mg daily for 10 days. Dehydroemetine may be less toxic than emetine; the dosage is 1 mg/kg intramuscularly or subcutaneously for 10 days (maximum daily dose, 90 mg). For any of the drugs, the destruction of parasites followed by release of antigen in sensitized patients may evoke clinical symptoms.

Reports on the effectiveness of praziquantel have been variable. Although the drug has been generally ineffective when used for 1–2 days, it has been suggested that it should be tried on an investigational basis at a dosage of 25 mg/kg 3 times daily for 7 days.

Bithionol and dehydroemetine are available in the USA only from the Parasitic Disease Drug Service, Centers for Disease Control, Atlanta 30333.

In endemic areas, aquatic plants should not be eaten raw; washing does not destroy the metacercariae, but cooking will. Drinking water must be boiled or purified.

Boray JC: Fascioliasis. Pages 71–88 in: *CRC Handbook Series in Zoonoses.* Steele JH (editor). Section C: *Parasitic Zoonoses.* Vol III. Hillyer GV (editor). CRC Press, 1982.

Knobloch J et al: Human fascioliasis in Cajamarca/Peru. I. Diagnostic methods and treatment with praziquantel. *Trop Med Parasitol* 1985;**36**:88.

Rivera JV, Bermúdez RH: Radionuclide imaging of the liver in human fascioliasis. *Clin Nucl Med* 1984;**9**:450.

## CLONORCHIASIS & OPISTHORCHIASIS

Infection by *Clonorchis sinensis,* the liver fluke, is endemic in areas of Japan, Korea, China, Taiwan, and southeast Asia. Opisthorchiasis is caused by worms of the genus *Opisthorchis,* generally either *O felineus* (central, eastern, and southern Europe, east Asia, southeast Asia, India) or *O viverrini* (Thailand, Laos, Vietnam). Clinically and epidemiologically, opisthorchiasis and clonorchiasis are identical.

Certain snails are infected as they ingest eggs shed into water in human or animal feces. Larval forms escape from the snails, penetrate the flesh of various freshwater fish, and encyst. Fish-eating mammals, including dogs and cats, are of great importance in maintaining the natural cycle. Human infection results from eating such fish, either raw or undercooked. Pickling, smoking, or drying may not suffice to kill the metacercariae. In humans, the ingested parasites excyst in the duodenum and ascend the bile ducts into the bile capillaries, where they mature and remain throughout their lives, shedding eggs in the bile. In the chronic stage of infection, there is progressive bile duct thickening, periductal fibrosis, dilatation, biliary stasis, and secondary infection. Little fibrosis occurs in the portal tracts. Occasionally, adults inhabit the pancreatic duct.

Most patients harbor few parasites and are asymptomatic. Among symptomatic patients, an acute and chronic syndrome occurs. Acute symptoms follow entry of immature worms into the biliary ducts and may persist for several months. Symptoms include malaise, low-grade fever, high leukocytosis and eosinophilia, an enlarged, tender liver, and pain in the hepatic area or epigastrium. The acute syndrome is difficult to diagnose, since ova may not appear in the feces until 3–4 weeks after onset of symptoms.

In chronic infections, findings include weakness, anorexia, epigastric pain, diarrhea, prolonged low-grade fever, progressive hepatomegaly, and intermittent episodes of right upper quadrant pain and localized hepatic area tenderness. Cholangiocarcinoma has been linked with late *Clonorchis* infection.

Complications of clonorchiasis are usually localized. Intrahepatic bile duct calculi may develop, leading to recurrent pyogenic cholangitis, biliary abscess, or endophlebitis of the portal-venous branches. Although focal initially, recurrent pyogenic cholangitis gradually results in destruction of the liver parenchyma, fibrosis, and, in a few patients, cirrhosis with ascites, anasarca, and jaundice. Rarely, a severe form of pancholangitis has been described. Flukes may also enter the pancreatic duct, causing acute pancreatitis.

The diagnosis is established by finding characteristic eggs in stools or duodenal aspirate. During the chronic stage of infection, leukocytosis varies according to intensity of infection; eosinophilia may be present. In advanced disease, liver function tests will indicate parenchymal damage. Transhepatic cholangiograms may show alternating stricture and dilatation of the biliary tree. Serologic tests are sometimes available.

The drug of choice is praziquantel. For *Clonorchis* infections, "apparent" cure rates (disappearance of ova) at 2 months posttreatment ranged from 87 to 100% of patients given a 1-day course consisting of 25 mg/kg 3 times at 4- to 6-hour intervals. However, some patients failed to be cured when reexamined at 1 year. No failures were reported at 1 year among an equivalent group treated for 2 days. Praziquantel may be more effective against *Opisthorchis* infections; at 2 months, the 1-day course of treatment resulted in 98–100% cure rates. (See under Schistosomiasis for side effects.) Albendazole, undergoing early clinical trials in the treatment of opisthorchiasis, may prove to be a useful alternative drug. Chloroquine is no longer recommended because of its potential toxicity and lack of efficacy.

The disease is rarely fatal, but patients with advanced infections and impaired liver function may succumb more readily to other diseases. The prognosis is good for light to moderate infections.

Chen M-G et al: Praziquantel in 237 cases of clonorchiasis sinensis. *Chin Med J* 1983;**96:**935.

Pungpark S et al: Clinical features in severe opisthorchiasis viverrini. *Southeast Asia J Trop Med Pub Health* 1985;**16:**405.

Pungpark S, Bunnag D, Harinasuta T: Albendazole in the treatment of opisthorchiasis and concomitant intestinal helminthic infections. *Southeast Asian J Trop Med Public Health* 1984;**15:**44.

Sun T: Pathology and immunology of *Clonorchis sinensis* infection of the liver. *Ann Clin Lab Sci* 1984;**14:**208.

## PARAGONIMIASIS

*Paragonimus westermani*, the lung fluke, commonly infects humans throughout the Far East, and foci are present in West Africa, Southeast Asia, South Asia, the Pacific Islands, Indonesia, and New Guinea. Many carnivores and omnivores in addition to humans serve as reservoir host for the adult fluke (8–16 × 4–8 × 3–5 mm). A number of other *Paragonimus* species can also infect humans in China, Japan, and Central and South America. Eggs reaching water, either in sputum or feces, hatch in 3–6 weeks. The miracidia penetrate snails and develop, and the emergent cercariae encyst in the tissues of crabs and crayfish. When these crustaceans are eaten raw or pickled—or when crabs are crushed and food vessels or fingers are contaminated by metacercariae that are later ingested—immature flukes excyst in the small intestine and penetrate the peritoneal cavity. Most migrate through the diaphragm and enter the peripheral lung parenchyma; some may lodge in the peritoneum, the intestinal wall, the liver, or other tissues but the brain is the most commonly invaded site. In the lungs, the parasite becomes encapsulated by granulomatous fibrous tissue. The lesion, which usually opens into a bronchiole, may subsequently rupture, resulting in expectoration of eggs, blood, and inflammatory cells. Eggs from lung cysts may also enter the general circulation and be carried throughout the body, where they produce granulomas in the tissues.

The majority of light and moderate infections are asymptomatic. The onset of symptoms is usually insidious, marked by low-grade fever, cough, or hemoptysis. The cough is dry at first; later a rusty or blood-flecked viscous sputum is produced. Pleuritic chest pain is common. The condition is chronic and slowly progressive. Dyspnea, signs of bronchitis and bronchiectasis, weakness, malaise, and weight loss may be seen in heavy infections. Parasites in the peritoneal cavity or intestinal wall may cause abdominal pain, diarrhea, or dysentery. Those in the central nervous system, depending on their location, may provoke seizures, palsies, or meningoencephalitis.

Diagnosis is by finding characteristic eggs in sputum, feces, or pleural fluid. Various serologic tests are available. Eosinophilia and low-grade leukocytosis are common. Chest x-rays may show a patchy infiltrate, nodular shadows, calcified spots, or pleural thickening or effusion. Cerebral paragonimiasis can result in intracranial calcifications.

Praziquantel is a drug of choice for the treatment of pulmonary infections at a dosage of 25 mg/kg after meals 3 times daily for 2 days. Cure rates of about 90% can be anticipated. (See under Schistosomiasis for side effects, p 927.) Bithionol remains a second drug of choice; 30–50 mg/kg body weight, should be given on alternate days for 10–15 doses (20–30 days). The daily dose should be divided into a morning and evening dose. Cure rates of over 95% have been reported. Side effects are frequent but generally mild and transient. Gastrointestinal symptoms, particularly diarrhea, occur in most patients. Liver function should be tested serially. Antibiotics may be necessary to control secondary pulmonary infection. Bithionol is available in the USA only from the Parasitic Disease Drug Service, Centers for Disease Control, Atlanta 30333.

In the acute stages of cerebral paragonimiasis, particularly meningitis, bithionol may be effective. In the chronic stage, when the drug by itself is unlikely to be effective, surgical removal of parasites is indicated when possible, as well as chemotherapy.

Johnson RJ et al: Paragonimiasis: Diagnosis and the use of praziquantel in treatment. *Rev Infect Dis* 1985;**7:**200.

Singh TS, Mutum SS, Razaque MA: Pulmonary paragonimiasis: Clinical features, diagnosis and treatment of 39 cases in Manipur. *Trans Roy Soc Trop Med Hyg* 1986;**80:**967.

Vanijanonta S, Bunnag D, Harinasuta T: Radiological findings in pulmonary paragonimiasis heterotremus. *Southeast Asian J Trop Med Public Health* 1984;**15:**122.

## CESTODE INFECTIONS

### TAPEWORM INFECTIONS
### (See also Cysticercosis and Echinococcosis.)

#### Classification

A number of species of adult tapeworms have been recorded as parasites of the human intestinal tract, but only 6 infect humans frequently. The large tapeworms are *Taenia saginata* (the beef tapeworm, up to 25 m in length), *Taenia solium* (the pork tapeworm, 7 m), and *Diphyllobothrium latum* (the fish tapeworm, 10 m). The small tapeworms are *Hymenolepis nana* (the dwarf tapeworm, 25–40 mm), *Hymenolepsis diminuta* (the rodent tapeworm, 20–60 cm), and *Dipylidium caninum* (the dog tapeworm, 10–70 cm). Four of the 6 tapeworms occur worldwide; the pork and fish tapeworms have more limited distribution. Humans are the only definitive host of 3 of the parasites: *T saginata, T solium,* and *H nana.*

An adult tapeworm consists of a head (scolex), a neck, and a chain of individual segments (proglottids). The scolex is the attachment organ and generally, in humans, lodges in the upper part of the small intestine.

**A. Beef Tapeworm:** Gravid segments of *T saginata* detach themselves from the chain and are passed in the feces to soil. When the proglottids or eggs are ingested by grazing cattle, the eggs hatch to release embryos that encyst in muscle as cysticerci. Humans are infected by eating undercooked beef containing viable cysticerci. In the human intestines, the cysticercus develops into an adult worm.

**B. Pork Tapeworm:** This tapeworm is particularly prevalent in Mexico, Latin America, the Iberian Peninsula, the Slavic countries, Africa, southeast Asia, India, and China. The worm is no longer found in northwestern Europe; in the USA and Canada, the infection is rare, usually found in imported cases. The life cycle of *T solium* is similar to that of *T saginata* except that the pig is the normal host of the larval stage. Humans become infected with the adult parasite when they eat undercooked pork. Humans are also the intermediate host when they become infected with the larval stage (see Cysticercosis, below) by accidentally ingesting eggs in human feces. Transmission of eggs may occur as a result of autoinfection (hand to mouth), direct person-to-person transfer, or ingestion of food or drink contaminated by eggs.

**C. Fish Tapeworm:** *D latum* is found in temperate and subarctic lake regions in many areas of the world, including Europe, the USA, Alaska and Canada, Japan, the Middle East, central and southern Africa, and southern South America. The intermediate hosts of the fish tapeworm are various species of freshwater crustaceans and fish. Eggs passed in human feces that reach water are taken up first by crustaceans that in turn are eaten by fish. Human infection results from eating raw or inadequately cooked brackish or freshwater fish, including salmon.

**D. Dwarf Tapeworm:** The *H nana* life cycle is unusual in that both larval and adult stages of the worms are found in the human intestine and there is no intermediate host. Adult worms (2.5–5 cm) expel infective eggs in the intestinal lumen, which when passed in the feces are immediately infective. Transmission is in most cases directly from person to person and only infrequently by fomites, water, or food. Internal autoinfection occurs when larvae hatch within the intestine, invade the mucosa, develop for a time, and then return to the lumen to mature.

**E. Rodent Tapeworm:** *H diminuta* is a common parasite of rodents. Many arthropods (eg, rat fleas, beetles, and cockroaches) serve as intermediate hosts. Humans are infected by accidentally swallowing the infected arthropods, usually in cereals or stored products.

**F. Dog Tapeworm:** *D caninum* infection generally occurs in young children in close association with infected dogs or cats. Transmission results from swallowing the infected intermediate hosts, fleas, or lice.

Multiple infections are the rule for small tapeworms and may occur for *D latum* infections; however, it is rare for a person to harbor more than one or 2 of the taeniae.

### Clinical Findings

**A. Signs and Symptoms:**

**1. Large tapeworms–**Large tapeworm infections are generally asymptomatic. Occasionally, vague gastrointestinal symptoms (eg, nausea, diarrhea, abdominal pain) and systemic symptoms (eg, fatigue, hunger, dizziness) have been attributed to the infections. Rarely, vomiting of segments or obstruction of the bile duct, pancreatic duct, or appendix has been described.

Among persons harboring the fish tapeworm, 1–2% develop a hyperchromic macrocytic megaloblastic anemia accompanied by thrombocytopenia and mild leukopenia. Gastric acidity is normal. The anemia is a result of the worm's competing with the host for vitamin $B_{12}$. Clinical findings include glossitis, dyspnea, tachycardia, and neurologic findings (weakness, numbness, paresthesias, disturbances of motility and coordination, and impairment of deep sensibilities). For unknown reasons, the anemia occurs mostly in the Scandinavian countries.

**2. Small tapeworms–**Light infections by *H nana, H diminuta,* and *D caninum* are also generally asymptomtic. Heavy infections, particularly with *H nana,* may, however, cause diarrhea, abdominal pain, anorexia, vomiting, weight loss, and irritability, particularly in young children.

**B. Laboratory Findings:** Infection by a beef or pork tapeworm is often discovered by the patient finding one or more segments in stool, clothing, or bedding. To determine the species of worm, segments must be flattened between glass slides and examined microscopically for anatomic detail. Enzyme electrophoresis of glucose phosphate isomerase is also able to distinguish between *T saginata* and *T solium.* The presence of eggs in the stools is infrequent, but the perianal swab test with cellophane tape, as used to diagnose pinworm, is sometimes useful in detecting the eggs of *T saginata.* The eggs look alike and do not differentiate between the species.

The diagnosis of fish tapeworm is by finding characteristic operculated eggs in stool; repeat examinations may be necessary. Proglottids are passed occasionally, and their internal morphology is also diagnostic. In fish tapeworm–induced macrocytic anemia, the marrow may be megaloblastic, the presence of hydrochloric acid in the stomach differentiates the anemia from pernicious anemia.

The diagnosis of *H nana* and *H diminuta* is by finding characteristic eggs in feces; proglottids are usually not seen, because they disintegrate in the bowel. *D caninum* is usually diagnosed following detection of proglottids (the size of melon seeds) in feces or after their active migration through the anus.

Serologic tests are not available for diagnosis of intestinal tapeworm infections.

## Differential Diagnosis

Fish tapeworm anemia may mimic pernicious anemia, but the presence of gastric hydrochloric acid and positive stool examinations will establish the diagnosis. Cysticercosis should be considered in all cases of epilepsy in patients who have lived in an endemic area for the pork tapeworm.

## Complications

Pork tapeworm infection may be complicated by cysticercosis if the patient's hands are contaminated and eggs are unknowingly transferred to the mouth. For such a patient, vomiting is also a hazard in that eggs may be propelled up the small intestine into the stomach, where they may hatch.

## Treatment

Niclosamide is the drug of choice for the treatment of all of the adult tapeworm infections except *H nana* infection, for which it is an alternative drug. Other alternative drugs are praziquantel, paromomycin, dichlorophen, and mebendazole. Quinacrine and aspidium oleoresin are no longer recommended, because of their potential toxicity.

The drug of choice for the treatment of *H nana* infection is praziquantel.

The anemia and neurologic manifestations of *D latum* infection respond to vitamin $B_{12}$ treatment.

**A. Specific Measures for the Treatment of Adult Tapeworm Infections:** Pre- and posttreatment purges are no longer used for any of the following drugs, except for the treatment of *T solium*.

**1. Niclosamide–**For *T saginata*, *T solium*, and *D latum* infections, only a single treatment is required and results in over 95% cure rates. The drug should be administered in the morning before the patient has eaten. The adult dosage is 4 tablets (2 g). Children weighing more than 34 kg are given 3 tablets; children 11–34 kg, 2 tablets. The tablets *must be chewed thoroughly* and swallowed with water. Eating may be resumed in 2 hours. For *T solium* infection, although niclosamide appears to cause little degeneration of mature segments, it may be useful to give a moderate purgative 2–3 hours after treatment to eliminate segments from the bowel. The patient must be instructed about the need for careful washing of the hands and perianal area and for safe disposal of feces for 4 days following therapy.

For *H nana* and *H diminuta* infections, one mode of therapy is to treat with niclosamide daily for 5–7 days; some workers repeat the course in 5 days. Cure rates are about 75%.

Niclosamide rarely causes side effects.

**2. Praziquantel–***H nana* infections are treated only once with 15–25 mg/kg; 86% of 473 persons were cured when treated with 15 mg/kg; 94% of 521 persons were cured when treated with 25 mg/kg.

*T saginata* and *T solium* infections treated with a single 10 mg/kg dose of praziquantel resulted in cure rates over 97%. Although 10 mg/kg will probably be satisfactory in the treatment of *D latum* infection, in reports to date, a single dose of 25 mg/kg resulted in 95% cure rates. Praziquantel appears to cause rapid degeneration of gravid proglottids.

**3. Paromomycin,** an antibiotic not appreciably absorbed from the gastrointestinal tract, is effective for the treatment of *T saginata* in an adult dosage of 1 g every 15 minutes for 4 doses. For children give 11 mg/kg every 15 minutes for 4 doses. In the USA, paromomycin is considered an investigational drug for the treatment of tapeworm infections. The treatment course for *H nana* is 45 mg/kg daily (to a maximum of 4 g) for 5–7 days. Gastrointestinal side effects are common but not severe. Because vomiting may occur, do not use the drug to treat *T solium* infections.

**4. Dichlorophen** given for 2 days is also an effective drug for *T saginata*, *T solium*, and *D latum*. The dosage is 75 mg/kg (to a maximum of 6 g) taken on an empty stomach in the morning without prior dietary restrictions (except for avoiding alcohol) or purgatives. Breakfast may follow in 2 hours. Because of the risk of drug-induced vomiting, dichlorophen should not be used in the treatment of *T solium* infection. Dichlorophen is not available in the USA.

**5. Mebendazole,** at a dosage of 300 mg twice daily for 3 days, appears to be effective therapy for *T solium;* the drug has a theoretic advantage over niclosamide in that proglottids are expelled intact after therapy. Reports have varied on the effectiveness of the drug for *T saginata*.

**B. Follow-Up Care:** Except following mebendazole administration, a disintegrating worm is usually passed within 24–48 hours of treatment. Since efforts are not generally made to recover and identify the scolex, cure can be presumed only if regenerated segments have not reappeared 3–5 months later. If it is preferred that parasitic cure be established immediately, the head (scolex) must be found in posttreatment stools. A laxative is given 2 hours after treatment, and stools are collected in a preservative for 24 hours. To facilitate examination, toilet paper must be disposed of separately.

## Prognosis

Because the prognosis is often poor in cerebral cysticercosis, the eradication of a *T solium* infection is a matter of much greater urgency than that of the other tapeworm infections, which are usually benign.

# CYSTICERCOSIS

Human cysticercosis is infection by the larval (cysticercus) stage of the tapeworm *Taenia solium* (see above), which forms cysts in the tissues. Locations of the cysts in order of frequency are the central nervous system, the subcutaneous tissues and striated muscle, the globe of the eye, and, rarely, other tissues. Cysts reach 5–10 mm in soft tissues but may be larger in the central nervous system. Cysticerci complete their development within 3–4 months after larval entry and can live for many years. The parasite causes little or no inflammatory reaction until it dies, at which time the cyst capsule becomes distended with fluid and increases in size; subsequently, it is replaced by fibrous tissue or undergoes calcification. Both living and calcified cysts may be present in the same organ.

## Clinical Findings

**A. Signs and Symptoms:** Up to 50% of central nervous system cysticerci are asymptomatic; cysticerci in other locations are usually asymptomatic as well, even in the presence of heavy infection.

**1. Neurocysticercosis–**One or more of the following syndromes (in order of frequency) may be present: (a) Epilepsy. (b) Intracranial hypertension (intense headache, nausea, vomiting, papilledema, diplopia, progressive loss of visual acuity leading to blindness). (c) Mental disturbances. (d) Meningeal syndrome: The basilar membranes, principally the arachnoid, are affected. Extensive adhesive arachnoiditis may be manifested by intracranial hypertension, obstructive hydrocephalus, arterial thrombosis, and cranial nerve involvement, most often the optic nerve. (e) Ventricular cysts: Cysts may float freely within the ventricles or cerebral aqueduct or may be attached to the ventricular wall. They are usually asymptomatic but cause increased intracranial pressure as a result of intermittent or total blockage. (f) Racemose cysts: These are rare aberrant forms that are multiple-branched, nonencysted, lack a scolex, and may reach over 10 cm in diameter. They generally are found in the ventricular and subarachnoid spaces, where they cause marked adhesive arachnoiditis and often obstructive hydrocephalus. (g) Spinal cord cysts: There can be extraspinal or intraspinal and cause arachnoiditis or pressure symptoms.

**2. Ophthalmocysticercosis–**Usually there is a single cyst. Presenting symptoms include periorbital pain, scotomas, and progressive deterioration of visual acuity. Findings include disk hemorrhage and edema, retinal detachment, iridocyclitis, and chorioretinitis.

**3. Subcutaneous and muscular cysticercosis–**These cysts present as fixed nodules that tend to appear at different times. Some nodules will collapse and disappear or reappear after a period of time.

**B. Laboratory Tests:** Definitive diagnosis is by finding the parasite on histologic section of specimens removed by excisional biopsy of skin or subcutaneous tissues. Patients should be thoroughly examined by palpation for pea-sized nodules.

**1. Imaging–**Plain radiographs of soft tissues may detect oval or linear calcified lesions (4–10 × 2–5 mm). The lesions are usually multiple, sometimes in the hundreds, and the long axes of the cysts are nearly always in the plane of the surrounding muscle fibers.

Plain skull films may demonstrate intracranial hypertension as well as one or more cerebral calcifications (generally 5–10 mm; sometimes 1–2 mm when only the scolex is calcified). Computed tomography is the the most useful procedure, as it detects both uncalcified and calcified cysts, edema, intracranial hypertension, and enhancement signs when contrast medium is used. Often a combination of different CT images is found, owing to different stages of development among cysticerci. MRI is useful. Spinal cysticercosis is evaluated by myelography or MRI.

**2. Immunologic tests–**Immunologic tests are useful adjuncts in diagnosis. Differentiation of cysticercosis from echinococcosis is possible by the immunoelectrophoresis and agar gel double diffusion tests but not by the indirect hemagglutination test. Sometimes a patient may have a positive serologic test but a negative test on cerebrospinal fluid; even a negative test with both fluids does not rule out cysticercosis. Patients presenting with only calcified lesions are generally serologically negative.

**3. Other tests–**The cerebrospinal fluid in neurocysticercosis typically shows increased protein, decreased glucose, and a cellular reaction consisting mainly of lymphocytes and eosinophils; eosinophilia over 20% is diagnostically important. Though the patient usually no longer harbors a tapeworm at the time cysticercosis is diagnosed, stools should be examined over several days by the patient for the passage of proglottids and by the laboratory for proglottids and eggs.

## Treatment

When living parasites are present in the central nervous system, medical treatment with praziquantel (which crosses the blood-brain barrier) is usually preferred to surgical removal of the lesion. However, praziquantel has no effect on calcified parasites, whether or not the patient is symptomatic. Albendazole has recently been described as having some effectiveness in treatment.

**A. Specific Measures:**

**1. Praziquantel–**The dosage for praziquantel is 50 mg/kg/d in 3 divided doses for 14 days, or 75 mg/kg/d for 10 days. To avoid or diminish the inflammatory reaction that follows death of the parasites in brain tissue, a steroid such as prednisone, 30 mg/d in 2–3 divided doses, starting 1–2 days before praziquantel and continuing for 3–4 days afterward, should be given. Others advocate use of steroids only for selected patients, based on the initial response to praziquantel. Use of anticonvulsant drugs must be continued during praziquantel treatment and probably for a considerable time afterward.

Side effects, which occur in about one-third of patients treated with combined praziquantel and steroids—and in about 90% given praziquantel without steroids—include increased intracranial pressure, headache, vomiting, mental changes, and convulsions. The side effects are usually mild and generally subside within 48–72 hours. In some cases, however, severity may require the following additional measures: (1) steroids in higher doses, (2) mannitol, (3) anticonvulsants if not used concomitantly, and (4) diuretics.

Fifty percent of praziquantel-treated patients are clinically cured (clearing of symptoms and disappearance of lesions by cerebral tomograms). Of the remainder, many have amelioration of symptoms, including intracranial hypertension and seizures. In ventricular and spinal cysticercosis, however, little or no response is achieved. When hydrocephalus is present, surgical shunt is required, even where the parasites have been destroyed.

At 3 months, the patient should be assessed clinically and by cerebral tomograms to determine whether a second treatment is necessary.

**2. Surgery**–Surgery has successfully removed orbital, cisternal, and ventricular cysts and, if accessible, cerebral, meningeal, or spinal cord cysts. Ocular cysticercosis is treated by surgical removal of cysts. Praziquantel is contraindicated for a cyst attached to the retina, as destruction of the larva may damage the retina inrreversibly.

**B. General Measures:** Symptomatic treatment of neurocysticercosis is based on the use of steroids for cerebral edema and anticonvulsants for seizures.

## Prognosis

The fatality rate for untreated neurocysticercosis is about 50%; survival time from onset of symptoms ranges from days to many years. Drug treatment has reduced the mortality rate to 6–16%. Surgical procedures to relieve intracranial hypertension along with use of steroids to reduce edema improve the prognosis for those not effectively treated by praziquantel.

Escobedo F et al: Albendazole therapy for neurocysticercosis. *Arch Intern Med* 1987;**147**:738.

Hamrick HJ et al: Two cases of dipylidiasis (dog tapeworm infection) in children: Update on an old problem. *Pediatrics* 1983;**72**:114.

Martinez-Lopez M, Quiroz y Ferrari F: Cysticercosis. *J Clin Neuro Ophthalmol* 1985;**5**:127.

Nash TE, Neva FA: Recent advances in the diagnosis and treatment of cerebral cysticercosis. *N Engl J Med* 1984;**311**:1492.

Richards F, Schantz PM: Treatment of *Taenia solium* infections. *Lancet* 1985;**1**:1264.

Ruttenber AJ et al: Diphyllobothriasis associated with salmon consumption in Pacific coast states. *Am J Trop Med Hyg* 1984;**33**:455.

Sotelo J et al: Therapy of parenchymal brain cysticercosis with praziquantel. *N Engl J Med* 1984;**310**:1001.

Von Bonsdorff B: *Diphyllobothriasis in Man.* Academic Press, 1977.

# ECHINOCOCCOSIS/HYDATIDOSIS (Hydatid Disease)

Human echinococcosis results from parasitism by the larval stage of 2 *Echinococcus* species: *Echinococcus granulosus* (cystic hydatid disease) and *Echinococcus multilocularis* (alveolar hydatid disease). Very rarely, *Echinococcus vogeli* (polycystic hydatid disease) has been reported from northern South America and Panama. Echinococcosis is a zoonosis in which humans are an intermediate host of the larval stage of the parasite. The definitive host is a carnivore that harbors the adult tapeworm in the small intestine; the carnivore becomes infected by ingesting the larval form in tissue of the intermediate host. The intermediate hosts, including humans but chiefly herbivorous mammals, become infected by ingesting tapeworm eggs passed in carnivore feces. The larval stages are referred to as hydatid cysts.

## 1. CYSTIC HYDATID DISEASE (Unilocular Hydatid Disease)

### Essentials of Diagnosis

- Avascular cystic tumor of liver, lung, or, infrequently, bone, brain, or other organs as detected by radiologic and nuclear medicine procedures.
- Positive serologic tests.
- History of exposure to dogs associated with livestock in a hydatid-endemic region.

### General Considerations

Human infection with *E granulosus* occurs principally where dogs are used to herd grazing animals, particularly sheep. The disease is common throughout southern South America, the Mediterranean littoral, the Middle East, central Asia, and East Africa. Foci of endemicity are in eastern Europe, Iceland, Russia, Australasia, India, and the United Kingdom. In North America, endemic foci have been reported from the western USA, the lower Mississippi Valley, Alaska, and northwestern Canada.

There are at least 2 geographic strains of the parasite. The pastoral strain—which is more pathogenic to humans—has a transmission cycle in which dogs are the definitive host and sheep (usually), but also cattle, hogs, and other domestic livestock are intermediate hosts. The sylvatic, or northern, strain is maintained in wolves and wild ungulates (moose and reindeer) in northern Alaska, Canada, Scandinavia, and Eurasia.

Human infection occurs when eggs passed in dog feces are accidentally swallowed. Embryos liberated from the eggs penetrate the intestinal mucosa, enter the portal bloodstream, and are carried to the liver where they are trapped and become hydatid cysts

(65% of all cysts). Some larvae reach the lung (25%) and develop into pulmonary hydatids. Infrequently, cysts form in the brain, bones, skeletal muscles, kidneys, spleen, or other tissues. Cysts of the sylvatic strain tend to localize in the lungs.

The wall of the cyst has 3 layers. The inner germinal layer gives rise within the cyst to scoleces, brood capsules, and daughter cysts. The supporting intermediate layer is an acellular laminated membrane. These 2 layers are derived from the parasite. The outer, granulomatous adventitial layer is produced by the host. The disease becomes evident because of cyst pressure or release of cyst contents. In the liver, cysts may increase in size 1–5 cm in diameter per year and become enormous, but symptoms generally do not develop until they reach about 10 cm. Some cysts die spontaneously. Part or all of the adventitial layer may calcify, which does not necessarily mean cyst death. Calcification may also occur in some splenic cysts but probably does not occur in lung cysts.

## Clinical Findings

**A. Symptoms and Signs:** A liver cyst may remain silent for 10–20 or more years until it becomes large enough to be palpable, to be visible as an abdominal swelling, to produce pressure effects, or to produce symptoms due to leakage or rupture. There may be right upper quadrant pain, nausea, and vomiting. The effects of pressure may result in cholangitis and secondary infection, which may lead to obstructive jaundice, cirrhosis, and portal hypertension. If a cyst ruptures suddenly, anaphylaxis and death may occur. If fluid and hydatid particles escape slowly, allergic manifestations may result, including a rise in the eosinophil count. Rupture can occur into the pleural, pericardial, or peritoneal space or into the duodenum, colon, or renal pelvis. Dissemination of scoleces may be followed by the development of multiple secondary cysts. A characteristic clinical syndrome may follow intrabiliary extrusion of cyst contents—jaundice, biliary colic, and urticaria.

Pulmonary cysts cause no symptoms until they leak; become large enough to obstruct a bronchus, causing segmental collapse; or erode a bronchus and rupture. Brain cysts produce symptoms earlier and may cause seizures or symptoms of increased intracranial pressure. Cysts in the bone marrow or spongiosa do not have an adventitial layer, are irregular in shape, erode osseous tissue, and may present as pain or as spontaneous fracture. The bones most often affected are the vertebrae; many of these cases develop epidural extension with compression of the spinal cord and paraplegia. Because 20% of patients have multiple cysts, each patient should be screened for cysts in the liver, spleen, kidneys, lungs, brain, bones, skin, tongue, vitreous, and other tissues.

**B. Imaging:** Scintillation scan, CT scan, and ultrasound examination are used to detect a cystic mass in the liver. The mass can be further defined by angiography, which may show the "halo" sign. Radiographs of the abdomen may show spotty calcified densities

or a calcified cyst wall in the liver or spleen. Chest films may show a pulmonary lesion. An intravenous urogram or full body or bone scan may detect other cysts at other sites.

**C. Laboratory Findings:** Two or 3 serologic tests should be done. The finding of an arc-5 in the counterimmunoelectrophoresis test and a high titer in the indirect hemagglutination test is particularly useful to confirm the diagnosis. But 5–10% of intact liver cysts and up to 50% of intact lung cysts may give a negative serologic result. The disappearance within about a year of arc-5 or seroconversion from positive to negative in the complement fixation or immunofluorescent tests frequently occurs and is indicative of complete surgical removal of a cyst. Because of its poor specificity, the Casoni intracutaneous skin test should probably be abandoned.

Eosinophilia is uncommon except after cyst rupture. Liver function tests are usually normal. Diagnostic aspiration of suspected hydatid cysts should never be undertaken because of the danger of leakage or rupture. Confirmation of the diagnosis is possible only by examination of cyst contents after surgical removal.

## Differential Diagnosis

Hydatid cysts of the liver need to be differentiated from bacterial and amebic abscesses. Hydatid cysts in any site may be mistaken for a variety of malignant and nonmalignant tumors and cysts. In the lung, a cyst may be confused with an advanced tubercular lesion. Allergic symptoms arising from cyst leakage may resemble those associated with many other diseases.

## Treatment

**A. Surgical Treatment:** The current definitive treatment is surgical removal of cysts where their location permits it. All lung cysts should be removed but not all liver cysts. Operative treatment of liver cysts involves 2 major problems: (1) selection of a method to sterilize and remove cyst contents without spillage, and (2) management of the remaining cavity. Germicidal solutions include cetrimide (5%), hypertonic saline (20%), silver nitrate, and sodium hypochlorite. Curettage, lavage, and instillation of chemical sterilization substances are indicated treatment of bone cysts but may not be effective.

**B. Drug Treatment:** In some cases because of the extent or location of cysts or the patient's general condition, surgery may not be indicated. Under such conditions, mebendazole may be tried. When used at high doses for several months, marked regression and apparent death of cysts have occurred in some patients. In other patients, however, cysts were either stable or continued to grow and if removed were viable. A suggested dosage of mebendazole is 50 mg/kg/d in 3 divided doses for 3 months, with many patients requiring repeated courses. When possible, mebendazole levels should be monitored; serum levels in excess of 100 mg/L 1–2 hours after an oral dose may be necessary for parasite killing. In unresponsive cases, it is possible that plasma levels of mebendazole are insufficient; some researchers, therefore, give up to 200 mg/kg/d. Occasional side effects with treatment include pruritus, rash, alopecia, reversible leukopenia, gastric irritation, musculoskeletal pain, fever, and acute pain in the cyst area; 6 cases of glomerulonephritis and 3 of agranulocytosis (with one death) have been reported.

Treatment with albendazole, a benzimidazole derivative, is experimental. Following oral administration, the drug is readily absorbed and can be measured in the blood and in the fluid of cysts. Of 40 patients treated with 7–10 mg/kg for 1–2 months and followed for 30 months, some showed improvement, with shrinkage or disappearance of cysts; in 2 patients, failures were evident from viable protoscoleces found postoperatively. Side effects included fever (5 patients), reversible leukopenia (one patient), reversible transaminase elevations (several), and cyst leakage with an anaphylactic reaction (in one patient 2 weeks after stopping of treatment).

In endemic areas, prophylactic treatment of pet dogs is with 5 mg/kg of praziquantel at monthly intervals.

### Prognosis

Patients may live for years with relatively large hydatid cysts before the condition is diagnosed. Liver and lung cysts often can be removed surgically without great difficulty, but in patients with cysts in less accessible sites the prognosis is less favorable. Surgical mortality rates vary from 2 to 10%, and postoperative recurrence of cysts may be seen in some patients. The prognosis is always grave in secondary echinococcosis. About 15% of patients eventually die because of the disease or its complications.

### 2. ALVEOLAR HYDATID DISEASE (Multilocular Hydatid Disease)

Alveolar hydatid disease results from infection by the larval form of *Echinococcus multilocularis*. The life cycle involves foxes as definitive host and microtine rodents as intermediate host. Domestic dogs and cats can also become infected with the adult tapeworm when they eat infected wild rodents. Human infection is by accidental ingestion of tapeworm eggs passed in fox or dog feces. The disease in humans has been reported in parts of central Europe, much of Siberia, northwestern Canada, and western Alaska. A single case has been reported in Minnesota. The primary localization of alveolar cysts is in the liver, where they may extend locally or metastasize to other tissues. The larval mass has poorly defined borders and behaves like a neoplasm; it infiltrates and proliferates indefinitely by exogenous budding of the germinative membrane, producing an alveoluslike pattern of microvesicles, ie, irregular, thin, peripheral layers of dense fibrous tissue, necrotic cavities containing an amorphous material, and focal calcification. X-rays

show hepatomegaly and characteristic scattered areas of radiolucency often outlined by 2- to 4-mm calcific rings. Serologic tests are the same as for cystic hydatid disease and cannot distinguish between the species. Treatment is by surgical removal of the entire larval mass, when possible. Ninety percent of patients with nonresectable masses die within 10 years. Long-term mebendazole therapy (40 mg/kg/d) inhibits growth of the parasite and has extended patient survival, but larval tissue is not completely destroyed.

Davis A, Pawloski ZS, Dixon H: Multicentre clinical trials of benzimidazolecarbamates in human echinococcosis. *Bull WHO* 1986;**64**:383.

Kammerer WS, Schantz PM: Long-term follow-up of human hydatid disease (*Echinococcus granulosus*) treated with a high-dose mebendazole regimen. *Am J Trop Med Hyg* 1984;**33**:132.

Man, dogs, and hydatid disease. (Editorial.) *Lancet* 1987;**1**:21.

Morris DL, Chinnery JB, Hardcastle JD: Can albendazole reduce the risk of implantation of spilled scoleces? An animal study. *Trans Roy Soc Trop Med Hyg* 1986;**80**:481.

Morris DL et al: Albendazole: Objective evidence of response in human hydatid disease. *JAMA* 1985;**253**:2053.

Schantz PM: Effective medical treatment for hydatid disease? *JAMA* 1985;**253**:2095.

# NEMATODE (ROUNDWORM) INFECTIONS

## ANGIOSTRONGYLIASIS

### 1. ANGIOSTRONGYLIASIS CANTONENSIS (Eosinophilic Meningoencephalitis)

A nematode of rats, *Angiostrongylus cantonensis*, is the causative agent of a form of eosinophilic meningoencephalitis reported from Hawaii and other Pacific islands, south and southeast Asia, Australia, and Madagascar. It has also been reported from Japan, Egypt, Cuba, and Puerto Rico. Human infection results from the ingestion of infected larvae contained in faw food—either infected mollusks (the intermediate host) or transport hosts (crabs, shrimp, fish) that have ingested mollusks. Drinking water and fresh vegetables can also become contaminated with infective larvae, as can fingers during the collection and preparation of snails for cooking.

The incubation period is about 2 weeks. The larvae (0.5 × 0.025 mm) usually invade the central nervous system, producing signs and symptoms of meningoencephalitis, including headache, fever, neck stiffness, nausea and vomiting, and multiple neurologic findings, particularly asymmetric transient paresthesias and cranial and other nerve palsies. A characteristic feature is spinal fluid pleocytosis, consisting largely of eosinophils. Occasionally, the parasite can be recovered from spinal fluid. Peripheral eosinophilia and a low-grade leukocytosis are common. Serologic and skin tests have been developed but are not specific. Ocular infection has been reported from Thailand.

No specific treatment is available; levamisole or thiabendazole can be tried. Corticosteroids have not influenced the course of the disease. The illness usually persists for weeks to months, the parasite dies, and the patient then recovers spontaneously, usually without sequelae. However, fatalities have been recorded.

## 2. ANGIOSTRONGYLIASIS COSTARICENSIS

*Angiostrongylus costaricensis* has been identified in humans in Mexico, Central America, Venezuela, Brazil, and USA (Texas). The known geographic range of the parasite in rats extends from northern South America to Texas. The normal definitive hosts are rat species, and the intermediate host is a slug that contaminates the food of humans with the infective third-stage larvae. Adult worms mature in the mesenteric vessels, where they cause arteritis, thrombosis, and ischemic necrosis; their eggs lodged in capillaries give rise to eosinophilic granulomas. The granulomas are most commonly localized in the appendix but may also be found in the terminal ileum, the cecum, the first part of the ascending colon, and the regional lymph nodes. Patients have fever, right lower quadrant abdominal pain and a mass, leukocytosis, and eosinophilia. Incomplete or complete obstruction, infarction, and an inflammatory reaction are the most common complications. A serologic test has been described but is not very useful. The disease usually simulates acute appendicitis, which can, in fact, be caused by the parasite. Intra-abdominal mass can mimic tumor. There is no specific treatment. Operative treatment is frequently necessary.

Ko RC et al: First report of human angiostrongyliasis in Hong Kong diagnosed by computerized axial topography (CAT) and enzyme-linked immunosorbent assay. *Trans R Soc Trop Med Hyg* 1984;**78**:354.

Kuberski T, Wallace GD: Clinical manifestations of eosinophilic meningitis due to *Angiostrongylus cantonensis*. *Neurology* 1979;**29**:1566.

Morera P et al: Visceral larva migrans-like syndrome caused by *Angiostrongylus costaricensis*. *Am J Trop Med Hyg* 1982;**31**:67.

## ASCARIASIS

### Essentials of Diagnosis

- Pulmonary phase: Transient cough, dyspnea, wheezing; allergic findings (eosinophilia, urticaria, asthma); transient pulmonary infiltrates.
- Intestinal phase: Vague upper abdominal discomfort, occasional vomiting, abdominal distention.
- Eggs in stools; worms passed per rectum, nose, or mouth.

### General Considerations

*Ascaris lumbricoides,* the largest of the intestinal roundworms, is also the most common of the intestinal helminths. It is cosmopolitan in distribution and is found in high prevalence wherever there are low standards of hygiene and sanitation or where human feces are used as fertilizer. The infection is specific for humans and occurs in all age groups, but young children have the highest worm burdens. The adult worms live in the upper small intestine. After fertilization, the female produces enormous numbers of eggs that are carried out to the soil in feces. In the soil, the eggs become infective in 2–3 weeks and thereafter can survive for up to 7 years. Infection occurs through ingestion of mature eggs in fecally contaminated food and drink. The eggs hatch in the small intestine, releasing motile larvae that penetrate the wall of the small intestine and reach the right heart via the mesenteric venules and lymphatics. From the heart they move to the lung, burrow through the alveolar walls, and migrate up the bronchial tree into the pharynx, down the esophagus, and back to the small intestine. The larvae mature and female egg production begins about 60–75 days after ingestion of the infective eggs. The large adult worms (20–40 cm × 3–6 mm), may live for 1 year or more.

### Clinical Findings

**A. Symptoms and Signs:** Migrating larvae in the lung cause capillary and alveolar damage, which may result in low-grade fever, cough, blood-tinged sputum, wheezing, rales, dyspnea, substernal pain, areas of local pulmonary consolidation, and allergic findings (eosinophilia, urticaria, asthma, angioneurotic edema). Rarely, larvae lodge ectopically in the brain, kidney, eye, spinal cord, etc, and may cause unusual symptoms.

Small numbers of adult worms in the intestine usually produce no symptoms. With heavy infection, vague abdominal discomfort (preprandial or postprandial) and colic may occur, particularly in children. The worms may also migrate with heavy infections; adult worms may be coughed up, vomited, or passed out through the nose. They may also force themselves into the common bile duct, the pancreatic duct, the appendix, diverticula, and other sites, which may lead to cholangitis, cholecystitis, pyogenic liver abscess, or pancreatitis. With very heavy infestations, masses of worms may cause intestinal obstruction, volvulus, or intussusception. During typhoid fever, bowel perforation may occur.

It is important that *Ascaris* infections be cured prior to bowel surgery because the worms have been known to break open suture lines postoperatively. Because anesthesia stimulates the worms to become hypermotile, they should be removed in advance for patients undergoing elective surgery.

**B. Imaging:** Chest radiographs may show scattered, patchy, ill-defined asymmetric infiltrations (Löffler's pneumonia).

**C. Laboratory Findings:** The diagnosis usually

depends upon finding the characteristic eggs in stool specimens. Occasionally, an adult worm spontaneously passed per rectum or orally reveals a previously unsuspected infection. There are no characteristic alterations of the blood picture during the intestinal phase. The diagnosis is sometimes established by chance, when radiologic examination of the abdomen (with or without barium) shows characteristic findings. Serologic tests are not useful, because of low specificity.

During the pulmonary phase, the number of eosinophils may reach 30–50% and remain high for about a month; larvae may occasionally be found in sputum.

### Differential Diagnosis

Pulmonary ascariasis with eosinophilia must be differentiated from nonparasitic causes (asthma, Löffler's syndrome, eosinophilic pneumonia, systemic lupus erythematosus, Hodgkin's disease) and parasitic causes (tropical pulmonary eosinophilia, toxocariasis, strongyloidiasis, hookworm disease, paragonimiasis). *Ascaris*-induced pancreatitis, appendicitis, diverticulitis, etc, must be differentiated from other causes of inflammation of these tissues; postprandial dyspepsia may simulate duodenal ulcer, hiatal hernia, gallbladder disease, or pancreatic disease.

### Treatment

Pyrantel pamoate is the drug of choice in treatment of ascariasis. None of the drugs listed below require pre- or posttreatment purges. Stools should be rechecked at 2 weeks and patients re-treated until all ascarids are removed. Ascariasis, hookworm, and trichuriasis infections, which often occur together, may be treated simultaneously by mebendazole or oxantel-pyrantel pamoate in countries where this drug combination is available. Ascariasis and hookworm combined may be treated with mebendazole, pyrantel pamoate, or bephenium.

**A. Pyrantel Pamoate:** Pyrantel pamoate is highly effective when administered as a single oral dose of 10 mg of base per kg body weight (maximum, 1 g). In various studies, cure rates of 85–100% have been reported. It may be given before or after meals. Infrequent side effects include vomiting, diarrhea, headache, dizziness, drowsiness, and rash. Experience with this drug is limited in children under age 2 years.

**B. Piperazine:** Many brands of syrups and tablets of piperazine salts are available; in solution, all form piperazine hexahydrate. Usually, each milliliter of syrup contains the equivalent of 100 mg of piperazine hexahydrate; tablets usually contain 250 or 500 mg. The dosage for piperazine (as the hexahydrate) is 75 mg/kg body weight (maximum, 3.5 g) for 2 days in succession, giving the drug orally before or after breakfast. For heavy infestations, treatment should be continued for 4 days in succession or the 2-day course should be repeated after 1 week.

Gastrointestinal symptoms and headache occur occasionally with piperazine; central nervous system symptoms, including temporary ataxia and exacerbation of seizures, are rarely reported. Allergic symptoms have been attributed to piperazine. The drug should not be used for patients with hepatic or renal insufficiency or with a history of seizures or chronic neurologic disease. Piperazine may be used in the last trimester of pregnancy.

**C. Mebendazole:** Mebendazole is effective when given in a dosage of 100 mg twice daily before or after meals for 3 days. Gastrointestinal side effects are infrequent, but worms may appear occasionally at the nose or mouth of children under age 5. The drug is contraindicated in pregnancy, and experience is limited in children under age 2 years.

**D. Levamisole:** This drug is highly effective (with cure rates of 86–100%) as a single oral dose of 150 mg; children should receive a single dose of 3 mg/kg. Levamisole is the levorotatory isomer of tetramisole. Side effects from levamisole—nausea, vomiting, abdominal cramps, headache, and dizziness—are mild and transient and occur in some patients. The drug has immunomodulating and immunostimulating properties that are currently under investigation. Levamisole is not available in the USA.

**E. Bephenium Hydroxynaphthoate:** Bephenium is less effective than the other drugs and has more side effects. Reported cure rates after one dose (5 g for older children and adults; 2.5 g for children under 22 kg) vary from 30 to 82%. However, a 3-day course, as for hookworm infection, may be effective for mixed infections with both parasites. Bephenium is no longer marketed in the USA.

**F. Albendazole:** At a dosage of 400 mg taken once, 96–100% of persons with light infections were cured, but only 85–89% of those with heavy infections were cured. To increase cure rates, an appropriate dosage remains to be determined. Albendazole is not available in the USA.

### Prognosis

The complications caused by wandering adult worms, plus the possibility of intestinal obstruction, require that all *Ascaris* infections be treated and completely eradicated.

Crompton DWT, Nesheim MC, Pawloski ZS (editors): *Ascariasis and Its Public Health Significance.* Taylor & Francis, 1985.

Jessen, K, Al Mofleh I, Al Mofarreh M: Endoscopic treatment of ascariasis causing acute obstructive cholangitis. *Hepatogastroenterology* 1986;**33:**275.

Pawlowski ZS: Ascariasis: Host-pathogen biology. *Rev Infect Dis* 1982;**4:**806.

### CUTANEOUS LARVA MIGRANS (Creeping Eruption)

Creeping eruption, prevalent throughout the tropics and subtropics, is caused by larvae of the dog and cat hookworms, *Ancylostoma braziliense* and *Ancylostoma caninum;* a number of other animal hookworms have rarely been implicated. It is a common infection of humans in the southeastern USA, particularly where people come in contact with moist sandy soil (beaches, children's sand piles) contaminated by dog or cat feces.

The larvae may invade any skin surface, but the hands or feet are usually affected. Soon after invasion, minute itchy erythematous papules appear at the sites of entry. Two or 3 days later, characteristic serpiginous eruptions begin to form as larval migration starts. Hundreds of lesions may occur on a single patient. These intensely pruritic lesions may persist for several months as slow migration continues. The parasite usually lies slightly ahead of the advancing border of the eruption. Vesiculation and crusting commonly occur in the later stages. Eosinophilia is common. Eventually, if not killed by treatment, the larvae die and are absorbed.

Simple transient cases may not require treatment. The larvae must be killed to provide relief in severe or persistent cases. Thiabendazole, given as for strongyloidiasis, is very effective and the drug of choice. Progression of the lesions and itching are usually stopped within 48 hours, but if active lesions are still present at that time, repeat treatment. Thiabendazole cream (15% in a hygroscopic base) applied topically daily for 5 days may also be effective. As alternative drugs for patients who cannot tolerate thiabendazole, diethylcarbamazine or albendazole can be tried, but their effectiveness has not been established. Antihistamines are helpful in controlling pruritus, and antibiotic ointments may be necessary to treat secondary infections.

Cypress RH: Cutaneous larva migrans. Pages 213–219 in: Steele JH (editor): CRC Handbook Series in Zoonoses. Section C: *Parasitic Zoonoses*, Vol III, Schultz MG (editor). CRC Press, 1982.

## DRACUNCULIASIS
## (Guinea Worm Infection, Dracunculosis, Dracontiasis)

*Dracunculus medinensis* is a nematode parasite found only in humans. It occurs predominantly in rural farming communities in tropical countries in the northern hemisphere, notably the Indian subcontinent; west and central Africa (Cameroon to Mauritania, Uganda, southern Sudan); and Saudi Arabia, Iran, and Yemen. All ages are affected, and the prevalence may reach 60% in some areas. Infection occurs by swallowing water containing the infected intermediate host, the crustacean *Cyclops* (water fleas), which is common in wells and ponds in the tropics. Larvae escape from the crustacean in the human host and mature in subcutaneous connective tissue. After mating, the male worm dies and the gravid female, now 1 m or more in length, moves to the surface of the body. The head of the worm reaches and penetrates the dermis, where it provokes a blister that ruptures on contact with water. Intermittently over 2–3 weeks, the uterus discharges great numbers of larvae, whenever the ulcer comes in contact with water. Larvae that reach water are eaten by the water fleas. Most adult worms are gradually extruded; some worms retract and reemerge; and others die in the tissues, disintegrate, and may provoke a severe inflammatory reaction. Infection does not induce protective immunity.

### Clinical Findings

**A. Symptoms and Signs:** The incubation period is silent and lasts 9–14 months. The usual infection is with a single worm, but multiple infections occur. Several hours before the head appears at the skin surface, local erythema, burning, pruritus, and tenderness often develop in the area where emergence is to take place. In some patients there may also be a 24-hour systemic allergic reaction, including generalized urticaria and pruritus, fever, nausea, vomiting, and dyspnea. As the blister forms and ruptures, these symptoms subside. After rupture, the tissues surrounding the ulceration frequently become indurated, reddened, and tender. Since 90% of the lesions appear on the leg or foot, the patient often must give up walking and work. Uninfected ulcers heal in 4–6 weeks.

In some patients, a worm may first be recognized as a visible or palpable cordlike structure under the skin. Some patients present with a deep "cold" abscess at the site of a dying worm.

**B. Laboratory Findings:** When an emerging adult worm is not visible in the ulcer, the diagnosis may be made by detection of larvae in smears from discharging sinuses. Immersion of an ulcer in cold water stimulates larval expulsion. Eosinophilia is usually present. Skin and serologic tests are not useful. Calcified worms can be recognized on radiographs.

### Complications

Secondary infections, including tetanus, are common. Deep abscess may result; ankle and knee joint infection with resultant deformity are common complications. If the worm is broken during removal, sepsis almost always results, leading to cellulitis, abscess formation, or septicemia. The worm rarely reaches ectopic sites. Epidural localization has resulted in abscesses leading to paraplegia.

### Treatment

Prevention of tetanus is essential; all persons in an endemic area should be actively immunized.

**A. General Measures:** The patient should be at bed rest with the affected part elevated. Cleanse the lesion and control secondary infection with antibiotics.

**B. Manual Extraction:** Traditional extraction of emerging worms by gradually rolling them out a few centimeters each day on a small stick is still useful, especially when done along with chemotherapy. The ulcer should be dressed daily.

**C. Chemotherapy:** Three drugs—niridazole, metronidazole, and thiabendazole—are effective (failure rate, 25%) both in alleviating symptoms (due to their anti-inflammatory action) and in reducing the duration of infection (by expediting spontaneous extrusion of worms or facilitating their manual extraction). The drugs do not kill the adult or larvae.

**1. Niridazole,** 25–35 mg/kg/d for 7–10 days, provokes fever, gastrointestinal symptoms, and headache; neuropsychiatric and cardiologic reactions are very rare. Simultaneous administration of antihistamines relieves some side effects.

**2. Metronidazole,** 35–40 mg/kg/d for 3–5 days or 25 mg/kg daily for 10–20 days, is devoid of serious side effects but may cause mild gastrointestinal symptoms, headache, fatigue, and a bitter taste. The drug produces disulfiramlike reactions when alcohol is ingested.

**3. Thiabendazole,** 50–100 mg/kg/d for 2–3 days after meals, frequently causes transient gastrointestinal disturbances and dizziness.

**D. Surgical Removal:** Preemergent female worms can be surgically removed intact under local anesthesia if they are not firmly embedded in deep fascia or around tendons. Abscesses should be incised.

Hopkins DR: The campaign against dracunculiasis. *Lancet* 1985;**1**:96.

Kake OO, Elemile T, Enahoro F: Controlled comparative trial of thiabendazole and metronidazole in the treatment of dracontiasis. *Ann Trop Med Parasitol* 1983;**77**:151.

## ENTEROBIASIS (Pinworm Infection)

### Essentials of Diagnosis

- Nocturnal perianal and vulval pruritus, insomnia, irritability, restlessness.
- Vague gastrointestinal symptoms.
- Eggs demonstrable by cellulose tape test; worms visible on perianal skin or in stool.

### General Considerations

*Enterobius vermicularis,* a short (8–13 mm in length) spindle-shaped roundworm, is worldwide in distribution and is one of the most common causes of helminthic infection. Humans are the only host for the parasite. Young children are affected more often than adults, and multiple infections are common in households with young children. The adult worms inhabit the cecum and adjacent bowel areas and lie loosely attached to the mucosa. When the fertilized female worms become gravid, they migrate through the anus to the perianal skin, where eggs are deposited in large numbers. The females die after oviposition. The eggs become infective in a few hours and may then infect others or be autoinfective, if transferred to the mouth by contaminated food, drink, fomites, or hands. After being swallowed, the eggs hatch in the duodenum, and the larvae migrate down to the cecum. Retroinfection occasionally occurs when the eggs hatch on the perianal skin and the larvae migrate through the anus into the large intestine. The development of a mature ovipositing female from an ingested egg requires about 3–4 weeks. Eggs can remain viable for up to 2–3 weeks outside the host. In the absence of reinfection, the natural history of enterobiasis without treatment is one of spontaneous cure, since the life span of the worms is 30–45 days.

### Clinical Findings

**A. Symptoms and Signs:** Many patients are asymptomatic. The most common and most important symptom is perianal pruritus (particularly at night), due to the presence of the female worms or deposited eggs. This must be distinguished from similar pruritus due to mycotic infections, allergies, hemorrhoids, proctitis, fissures, strongyloidiasis, and other conditions. Insomnia, restlessness, enuresis, and irritability are common symptoms, particularly in children. Many mild gastrointestinal symptoms—abdominal pain, nausea, vomiting, diarrhea, anorexia—have also been attributed to enterobiasis, although the association is difficult to prove. At night, worms may occasionally be seen near the anus. Perianal scratching may result in excoriation and impetigo. Adults sometimes report a "crawling" sensation in the anal area. Rarely, worm migration results in ectopic inflammation or granulomatous reaction (including appendicitis) or, in young girls, vulvovaginitis, urethritis, endometritis, salpingitis, and pelvic granuloma. Recurrent urinary tract infections have also been associated with the infection.

**B. Laboratory Findings:** Diagnosis is by finding eggs on the perianal skin (eggs are seldom found on stool examination). The most reliable method is by applying a short strip of sealing cellulose pressure-sensitive tape (eg, Scotch Tape) to the perianal skin and then spreading the tape on a slide for low-power microscopic study. Three such preparations made on consecutive mornings before bathing or defecation will establish the diagnosis in about 90% of cases. Before the diagnosis can be ruled out, 5–7 such examinations are necessary. Nocturnal examination of the perianal area or gross examination of stools may reveal adult worms, which should be placed in preservative or saline for laboratory examination. The worms can sometimes be seen on anoscopy. Eosinophilia is rare.

### Treatment

**A. General Measures:** Symptomatic patients should be treated, and in some situations all members of the patient's household should be treated concurrently, since for each overt case there are usually several inapparent cases. However, treatment of all nonsymptomatic cases is not necessary. Careful washing of hands with soap and water after defecation and again before meals is important. Fingernails should be kept trimmed close and clean, scratching of the perianal area avoided, and the hands kept away from the mouth. Ordinary washing of bedding will usually kill pinworm eggs. Recurrence is frequent in children because of continued exposure outside the home.

**B. Specific Measures:** Since eggs deposited in a moist environment remain infective for 2–3 weeks, the following drugs are recommended every 2 weeks for 3 doses (only 2 doses has been the standard approach to therapy).

**1. Pyrantel pamoate** is a highly effective drug (with cure rates of over 95%) and a drug of choice. It is administered in a single oral dose of 10 mg of the base per kilogram body weight (maximum, 1 g); repeat after 2 and 4 weeks. It may be given before or after meals. Infrequent side effects include vomiting, diarrhea, headache, dizziness, drowsiness, and rash. Experience with this drug is still limited in children under age 2.

**2. Mebendazole** is highly effective and also a drug of choice. It is administered as a single 100-mg oral dose, irrespective of body weight. It may be given with or without food and should be chewed for best effect. Repeat treatment after 2 and 4 weeks. Gastrointestinal side effects are infrequent. The drug has not yet been adequately studied in children under age 2 and should not be used in pregnancy.

**3. Pyrvinium pamoate** in syrup is given as a single dose of 5 mg/kg body weight (maximum, 0.25 g) and is repeated after 2 and 4 weeks. Pyrvinium is well tolerated, but it may cause gastrointestinal symptoms and dizziness in some persons, particularly older children and adults. Posttreatment stools are often stained red for several days, and the tablets must be swallowed intact to avoid temporary staining of the teeth. For these reasons it is viewed as an alternate drug in enterobiasis treatment.

**4. Other drugs**–Treatment with **albendazole** (not available in the USA) resulted in cure rates of 100% in multiple studies in which it was given once only at a single dose of 400 mg. If albendazole is used, treatment should be repeated at least once at 2 weeks. **Piperazine citrate** is no longer recommended in this text for the treatment of pinworms because the course of treatment requires 1 week. **Thiabendazole** is not recommended because of its frequent side effects, which in rare cases may be severe.

## Prognosis

Although annoying, the infection is benign. Cure is readily attainable with one of several effective drugs, but reinfection is common.

Mogensen K, Pahle E, Kowalski K: *Enterobius vermicularis* and acute appendicitis. *Acta Chir Scand* 1985;**151**:705.

Wagner ED, Eby WC: Pinworm prevalence in California elementary school children, and diagnostic methods. *Am J Trop Med Hyg* 1983;**32**:998.

## FILARIASIS

### Essentials of Diagnosis

- Recurrent attacks of lymphangitis, lymphadenitis, fever, orchitis.
- Hydrocele, chyluria, acute or chronic lymphedema; elephantiasis of legs, arms, genitalia, or breasts.
- Characteristic microfilariae in the blood, chylous urine, or hydrocele fluid.
- Eosiniphilia; positive serologic tests.

### General Considerations

Filariasis is caused by infection with one of 3 filiarial nematodes: *Wuchereria bancrofti, Brugia malayi,* and *Brugia timori.* *W bancrofti* is widely distributed in the tropics and subtropics of both hemispheres and on Pacific islands and is transmitted by species of *Culex, Aedes,* and *Anopheles* mosquitoes. *Brugia malayi* is transmitted by the bite of certain *Mansonia* and *Anopheles* mosquitoes of south India, Sri Lanka, southeast Asia, south China, the northern coastal areas of China, and South Korea. *B timori* is found on the southeast islands of Indonesia.

No animal reservoir hosts are known for *W bancrofti* or *B timori;* cats, monkeys, and other animals may harbor the swamp species of *B malayi.* Mosquitoes become infected by ingesting microfilariae with a blood meal; at subsequent feedings, they can infect new susceptible hosts. Over months, adult worms (females, 8–9 cm × 0.2–0.3 mm) mature and live in or near superficial and deep lymphatics and lymph nodes and produce large numbers of viviparous circulating microfilariae, which may be seen in the blood starting 6–12 months after infection. Adult females live and reproduce for 5–10 years. The pathologic changes in the lymph vessels are due to the host's immunologic reaction to developing and mature adult worms. Living microfilariae generally cause no lesions, with the possible exception of tropical pulmonary eosinophilia. Rapid death of microfilariae, however, does produce findings (see below), and an abscess may form at the site of a dying adult worm.

Several other species of filarial worms infect humans, usually without causing important findings. *Mansonella perstans* and *M streptocerca* are found in west and central Africa and produce nonperiodic circulating microfilariae. Those of *M streptocerca* also appear in the skin. Mild allergic symptoms (pruritus, hives, fever, and Calabar swellings [for *M perstans*]) have been described. Eosinophilia is generally present, but serologic tests are negative. *M ozzardi* is found in tropical Central and South America and the West Indies and produces nonperiodic circulating microfilariae. Though generally asymptomatic, fever, pruritic-maculopapular skin lesions, and eosinophilia have been reported. Infection with *Dirofilaria immitis,* the dog heartworm, has been reported in the USA, Japan, and Australia. Nodules have been found in the skin or as solitary 1–2 cm "coin" lesions in the periphery of the lungs. The serologic test for filariasis is positive.

Tropical pulmonary eosinophilia is probably due to sequestered microfilariae of *W bancrofti* or *B malayi* in the lungs. The condition is characterized by miliary lesions on chest films, episodic asthmatic coughing or wheezing, eosinophilia, high IgE levels, positive serologic tests, and a response to diethylcarbamazine treatment.

## Clinical Findings

**A. Symptoms and Signs:** Many infections remain asymptomatic. Early manifestations are inflammatory; those of later stages are obstructive. In typical early cases, episodes of fever, with or without inflammation of lymphatics and nodes, occur at irregular intervals and last for several days. Persistent lymph node enlargement is most common in *B malayi* but occurs in some *W bancrofti* infections. Funiculitis, epididymitis, and orchitis as well as involvement of pelvic, abdominal, or retroperitoneal lymphatics may also occur intermittently. The number and severity of these attacks, and the extent of later changes, depend primarily upon the intensity of the infection, which is related to the length of residence in an endemic area.

Obstructive phenomena, arising from interference with normal lymphatic flow, include hydrocele, scrotal lymphedema, lymphatic varices, and elephantiasis. Chyluria may result from rupture of distended lymphatics into the urinary tract. In the early stages of elephantiasis, the tissues of the affected part are edematous and soft; later, with skin hypertrophy and subcutaneous connective tissue proliferation, the part becomes hard. As the swelling enlarges, sometimes to enormous size, the skin surface becomes thickened and nodular and fissures. Bancroftian elephantiasis frequently involves the legs and genitalia, less often the arms and breasts; in *B malayi* infections, elephantiasis of the legs below the knees is most common and the genitals and breasts are rarely affected.

Hydrocele and elephantoid tissue changes in persons residing in endemic areas are usually filarial in origin. Elephantiasis in those who have visited endemic areas only briefly is rarely due to filariasis.

**B. Laboratory Findings:** Diagnosis is by finding microfiliriae in the blood. They are rare in the first 2–3 years after infection, abundant as the disease progresses, and again rare in the advanced obstructive stage. Microfiliariae of *W bancrofti* are found in the blood chiefly at night (nocturnal periodicity), except for a nonperiodic variety in the South Pacific. *B malayi* microfilariae are usually nocturnally periodic but in southeast Asia may be semiperiodic (present at all times, with a slight nocturnal rise). Anticoagulated blood specimens are collected at times related to the periodicity of the local strain (10:00 PM to 2:00 AM for nocturnal strains). Specimens may be stored at ambient temperatures. They should be examined initially by wet film for motile larvae and by Giemsa-stained thin smears for specific morphology. If these are negative, the blood specimens should be concentrated by the Knott concentration or membrane filtration technique. If all of these are negative, the oral administration of 12 mg/kg of diethylcarbamazine often produces positive blood specimens when examined in 1 hour. This test must be done with extreme caution in areas where onchocerciasis or loiasis may be present, because of potential severe reactions due to massive destruction of microfilariae of these species. Microfilariae may also be found in hydrocele, lymphatic, ascitic, and pleural fluids.

Serologic tests may be helpful in diagnostic screening, but false-positive and false-negative reactions occur. An indirect hemagglutination titer of 1:128 and a bentonite flocculation titer of 1:5 in combination are considered significant titers. Most active clinical cases have higher titers. Lymphangiography is helpful in differential diagnosis. Removal of lymph nodes for diagnosis may further impair drainage from the affected area and is contraindicated.

## Differential Diagnosis

Diagnosis of the early febrile and inflammatory episodes may be difficult, particularly when the patient has moved away from an endemic area, because attacks of lymphangitis, adenitis, and fever are transitory and microfilariae may be rare in the blood. The retrograde progression of filarial lymphangitis contrasts with the proximal spread of acute bacterial lymphangitis. Superficial phlebitis may resemble filarial lymphangitis. Filarial funiculitis, orchitis, and epididymitis may suggest gonococcal infection, but there is no urethral discharge in the uncomplicated case. Among the late manifestations, elephantiasis may be confused with hernia, Milroy's disease, multiple lipomatosis, severe congestive heart failure, venous thrombosis, and chronic obstructive lesions of the lymphatics, which may produce nonfilarial elephantiasis of the extremities. Milroy's congenital elephantiasis usually involves both legs below the knees, the skin is smooth, and there is no eosinophilia.

## Treatment

**A. General Measures:** Patients with attacks of lymphangitis should be treated during a quiescent period between attacks; bed rest is indicated during the inflammatory episodes. Antibiotics should be given for secondary infections, particularly abscesses over inflamed nodes. Suspensory bandaging is a valuable palliative measure for orchitis, epididymitis, and scrotal lymphedema. Treat mild edema of a limb with rest, elevation, and use of an elastic stocking or pressure bandage from below upward. Chyluria usually requires only rest. Hydroceles may be aspirated.

**B. Surgical Measures:** Hydroceles are treated by excision or eversion of the hydrocele sac; small hydroceles may benefit from a locally injected sclerosing agent (eg, tetracycline). Surgical removal of the elephantoid scrotum, vulva, or breast is relatively easy, and results are usually satisfactory. Surgery for limb elephantiasis is difficult; results are often disappointing.

**C. Specific Measures:** Diethylcarbamazine rapidly kills microfilariae in the blood but only slowly kills adult worms or injures them, reducing their ability to reproduce. *W bancrofti* infections are treated with diethylcarbamazine (salt), 2 mg/kg orally 3 times a day after meals for 2–4 weeks. To reduce the incidence of allergic reactions from dying microfilariae, a single dose (2 mg/kg) is administered on the first day, 2 doses on the second day, and 3 doses on the third day and thereafter. For *B malayi*, the same schedule should be used, but individual doses should start at 1 mg/kg once on the first day and gradually increase to 2 mg/kg 3 times daily by the fourth to fifth day.

Antihistamines may be given for the first 4–5 days of diethylcarbamazine therapy to reduce the incidence of "allergic" reactions. If severe reactions occur, start corticosteroids and temporarily lower or interrupt doses of diethylcarbamazine.

Blood should be checked for microfilariae several weeks after treatment is completed; if any are still present, a course may be repeated at intervals of 3–4 weeks. However, since the initial treatment does not kill all adult worms, microfilariae may reappear in 3–12 months. Cure may require subsequent courses of treatment over 1–2 years.

Only a few mild side effects can be attributed directly to the drug: headache, malaise, anorexia, and weakness are most frequent. Reactions to dying microfilariae are usually mild or absent for *W bancrofti* and more intense for *B malayi*. Nevertheless, even in *W bancrofti* infection, about 25% of patients experience generalized reactions including headache, gastrointestinal symptoms, cough, chest pains, muscle or joint pain, malaise, fever, and papular rash. Local reactions may occur around dying adult or immature worms, including lymphangitis, lymphadenitis, and lymph abscess. These reactions are most common from the third day of treatment onward and may last as long as 10 days.

In prophylaxis of filariasis caused by *W bancrofti* and *B malayi*, 50 mg of diethylcarbamazine monthly has been recommended.

### Prognosis

In early and mild cases, the prognosis is good with treatment and if the patient avoids reinfection. Drug treatment will not significantly influence the course of advanced filariasis.

Kochar AS: Human pulmonary dirofilariasis: Report of three cases and brief review of the literature. *Am J Clin Pathol* 1985;**84**:19.

Ottesen EA: Efficacy of diethylcarbamazine in eradicating infection with lymphatic-dwelling filariae in humans. *Rev Infect Dis* 1985;**7**:341.

Recent advances in research on filariasis. *Trans R Soc Trop Med Hyg* 1984;**78(Suppl)**:1.

Taylor AER, Denham DA: Immunology and diagnosis of filariasis. *Trop Dis Bull* 1986;**83**:R2.

WHO Expert Committee on Filariasis: *Lymphatic Filariasis,* fourth report. Technical Report Series No. 702. World Health Organization, 1984.

## GNATHOSTOMIASIS

Gnathostomiasis is an infection with the larval stage of the nematode parasite *Gnathostoma spinigerum*. It is most common in Thailand and Japan but is also reported from southeast Asian countries, Indonesia, China, India, and Israel. Humans are infected by ingestion of larvae in raw, marinated, or inadequately cooked freshwater fish, chicken or other fowl, frogs, or rarely pork. Within 24–48 hours, larval migration through the intestinal wall can cause acute epigastric pain, vomiting, urticaria, and eosinophilia. The worm then migrates to subcutaneous and other tissues but is unable to mature.

The most common manifestation is a pruritic subcutaneous swelling up to 25 cm across, occasionally accompanied by stabbing pain. The swelling may appear on any body surface, remain in that area for days or weeks, or move continuously. Occasionally the worm becomes visible under the skin.

Internal organs, the eye, and the cervix may also be invaded. Spontaneous pneumothorax, leukorrhea, hematemesis, hematuria, hemoptysis, paroxysmal coughing, and edema of the pharynx with dyspnea have been reported as complications. Invasion of the brain can result in encephalitis, paralysis, subarachnoid hemorrhage, cerebrospinal fluid eosinophilia, and other findings. Spinal cord invasion can result in myelitis and severe nerve root pain.

A high eosinophilia accompanies the infection. Skin-testing antigens and serologic tests are available but unsatisfactory, since cross-reactions with other nematodes are common. Final diagnosis usually rests upon identification of the worm.

Surgical removal of the worm when it appears close to the skin surface or in the eye is the only effective treatment. Although chemotherapy has not proved successful, diethylcarbamazine (as for filariasis), thiabendazole, or mebendazole should be tried. Courses of prednisolone have provided temporary relief of symptoms.

Ollague W et al: Human gnathostomiasis in Ecuador (nodular migratory eosinophilic panniculitis). *Internat J Dermatol* 1984;**23**:647.

## HOOKWORM DISEASE

### Essentials of Diagnosis

*Early findings:* (Not commonly recognized.)
- Dermatitis: pruritic, erythematous, papulovesicular eruption at site of larval invasion.
- Pulmonary migration of larvae: transient episodes of coughing, asthma, fever, blood-tinged sputum, high eosinophilia.

*Later findings:*
- Intestinal symptoms: anorexia, diarrhea, abdominal discomfort.
- Anemia (hypochromic microcytic): fatigue, apathy, pallor, deformed nails, dyspnea on exertion,

palpitations, syncope, peripheral edema, heart failure.

● Characteristic eggs and occult blood in the stool.

## General Considerations

Hookworm disease, widespread in the moist tropics and subtropics, is caused by *Ancylostoma duodenale* and *Necator americanus*. Probably a quarter of the world's population is infected, and in many areas hookworms are a major cause of general debility, retardation of growth of children, and increased susceptibility to infections. Deaths of many children occur from infections that could normally be tolerated, such as malaria, measles, and those that cause diarrhea. The infection is rare in regions with less than 1000 mm of rainfall annually. In the Western Hemisphere and tropical Africa, *Necator* was the prevailing species, and in the Far East, India, China, and the Mediterranean area, *Ancylostoma* was prevalent, but both species have now become widely distributed. Humans are the only host for both species.

The adult worms are approximately 1 cm long. Eggs produced by the female worms are passed in the stool and must fall on warm, moist soil if hatching followed by larval development is to take place. Larvae remain infective for hours to about a week, depending on environmental conditions. Following skin penetration, the larvae migrate in the bloodstream to the pulmonary capillaries, break into the alveoli, and then are carried by ciliary action upward to the bronchi, trachea, and mouth. After being swallowed, they reach and attach to the mucosa of the upper small bowel, where they develop into adult worms. *Ancylostoma* infections can probably also be acquired by ingestion of the larvae in food or water. Adult *Ancylostoma* survive about a year; *Necator* about 3–5 years.

## Clinical Findings

**A. Symptoms and Signs:** Ground itch, the first manifestation of infection, is a pruritic erythematous dermatitis, either maculopapular or vesicular, associated with the invasion of infective larvae. Severity of the dermatitis is a function of the number of invading larvae and the sensitivity of the host. Scratching may result in secondary infection. *Strongyloides* infection and creeping eruption caused by nonhuman hookworm species must be considered in the differential diagnosis at this stage. The pulmonary phase, in which there is larval migration through the lungs, is sometimes characterized by dry cough, asthmatic wheezing, blood-tinged sputum, and low-grade fever.

Two or more weeks after skin invasion, maturing and adult worms attach to the mucosal villi of the duodenum and upper jejunum. In heavy infections, worms may reach the ileum. A large proportion of patients who have light infections and adequate iron intake remain asymptomatic. In heavy infections, however, there may be anorexia, diarrhea, vague abdominal pain, and ulcerlike epigastric symptoms. Severe illness results from blood loss caused by worms

sucking blood at their attachment sites. Depending on the host's dietary intake of iron, severe anemia may result if 30 or more *Ancylostoma* or 100 or more *Necator* worms are present. Marked protein loss may also occur, resulting in hypoalbuminemia and edema. There are conflicting reports of malabsorption in some severe cases. Severe anemia (hemoglobin levels as low as 2 g/dL) may result in pallor, thinning of the hair, deformed nails, pica, cardiac decompensation, edema, ascites, and other clinical manifestations. Young children are especially likely to be seriously affected; a protuberant abdomen is common, and kwashiorkor may be precipitated. Stunted growth and possibly some degree of mental retardation may occur.

Reduction in worm loads after the first decade of life suggests that a moderate degree of immunity develops.

**B. Laboratory Findings:** The diagnosis depends upon demonstration of characteristic eggs in the feces. The stool usually contains occult blood; the severity of the hypochromic microcytic anemia with a low serum iron and a high iron-binding capacity will depend upon the worm burden. This can be estimated by quantitative egg counts: light infections, up to 2000 ova per gram of feces; moderate, 2000–5000; heavy, over 5000. Eosinophilia (as high as 30–60% of a total white blood count reaching $17,000/\mu L$) is usually present in the early months of the infection but is not marked in the chronic stage.

## Treatment

**A. General Measures:** The need for anthelmintic treatment for light infections was in the past controversial, since light infections do not injure the well-nourished patient and iron loss is replaced if the patient is receiving adequate dietary iron. However, the recent development of safe anthelmintics makes it reasonable to treat all patients initially, irrespective of the intensity of infection. Re-treatment is often necessary at 2-week intervals, until the worm burden is reduced to a low level, as estimated by semiquantitative egg counts.

If anemia is present, provide iron medication and a diet high in protein and vitamins: continue for at least 3 months after the anemia has been corrected in order to replace iron stores. Blood transfusion may be necessary.

**B. Specific Measures:** If ascariasis and hookworm infections are both present, either give mebendazole for the combined infection or piperazine first to eradicate *Ascaris,* followed by a drug to eradicate hookworms.

**1. Pyrantel pamoate** is one of the drugs of first choice. In *Ancylostoma duodenale* infections, pyrantel given as a single dose, 10 mg of the base per kilogram body weight (maximum 1 g), produces cures in 76–98% of cases and a marked reduction in the worm burden in the remainder. However, for *Necator americanus* infections a single dose may give a satisfactory cure rate in light infection, but for moderate or heavy infection a 3-day course is necessary. If the species is unknown, treat as for necatoriasis. Side effects are infrequent, mild, and transient, including gastrointestinal symptoms, drowsiness, and headache. The drug is given before or after meals, without purges.

**2. Mebendazole** is also a drug of choice for treatment of *Necator* and *Ancylostoma* infections. When it is given at a dosage of 100 mg twice daily for 3 days, reported cure rates for both species range from 35 to 95%. The drug is given before or after meals, without purges. Therapy is remarkably free of side effects; gastrointestinal symptoms occur infrequently. The drug should not be used in pregnancy, and experience with the drug in children under 2 years is limited.

**3. Bephenium hydroxynaphthoate** is used only as an alternative drug for hookworm infection because it may cause nausea and vomiting and has a bitter taste. The drug is given on an empty stomach, and food is then withheld for 2 hours. For young children, however, the taste may be disguised when mixed with a flavored vehicle such as chocolate milk or orange juice. For *Ancylostoma* infections, give 5 g of the granules (2.5 g base) twice daily for 1 day, repeating in 2 weeks if necessary. For children weighing less than 22 kg, give half this dose. Do not use in pregnancy. *Necator* is generally more resistant to bephenium, but the same dose for 3 days may reduce the worm load to acceptable levels. *Do not follow with a purge.* Bephenium is no longer marketed in the USA.

**4. Tetrachloroethylene** is an effective alternative drug for *Necator* and may be used for *Ancylostoma*. **Caution:** Be sure to correct severe anemia before giving this drug. Tetrachloroethylene is contraindicated in patients with alcoholism, chronic gastrointestinal disorders, severe constipation, or hepatic disease and in patients undergoing heavy metal therapy. It is generally recommended that ascarids be removed from the intestinal tract before tetrachloroethylene is used. Eliminate fatty food for 24 hours before and 3 days after medication. Give tetrachloroethylene, 0.12 mL/kg body weight (not more than 5 mL) in soluble gelatin capsules containing 1 mL, in the morning on an empty stomach. The patient should be kept at bed rest for 4 hours after treatment, and then may resume eating. Side effects may be reduced by giving the drug at bedtime, also on an empty stomach. Two or more treatments at 4-day intervals may be required. Saline purgation following treatment is no longer recommended. Note that the drug may deteriorate if not adequately refrigerated at ambient tropical temperatures.

**5. Albendazole,** given orally once only at a dosage of 400 mg, resulted in the cure of 86–95% of patients with *Ancylostoma* infection and markedly reduced the worm burden in those not cured. Cure rates for patients with *Necator* infection were 33–90%; a satisfactory dosage schedule remains to be determined.

### Prognosis

If the disease is recognized before serious secondary complications appear, the prognosis is favorable. With iron therapy, improved nutrition, and administration of an anthelmintic, complete recovery is the rule.

Gilles HM: Selective primary health care: Strategies for control of disease in the developing world. XVII. Hookworm infection and anemia. *Rev Infect Dis* 1985;**7**:111.

Gilman RH: Hookworm disease: Host-pathogen biology. *Rev Infect Dis* 1982;**4**:824.

Rossignol JF, Maisonneuve H: Albendazole: Placebo-controlled study in 870 patients with intestinal helminthiasis. *Trans R Soc Med Hyg* 1983;**77**:707.

Sharma S, Charles ES: Chemotherapy of hookworm infections. *Prog Drug Res* 1982;**26**:9.

## LOIASIS

Loiasis is caused by the filarial nematode *Loa loa*. The infection occurs in humans and monkeys in rain and swamp forest areas of West Africa from Nigeria to Angola and throughout the Congo river watershed of central Africa eastward to southwest Sudan and western Uganda. The vector and intermediate hosts are *Chrysops* spp, day-biting flies that become infected when they ingest a blood meal that contains microfilariae. When the fly feeds again, it can infect a new host.

Many infected individuals remain symptom-free. In others, symptoms may appear within a year, though microfilariae may not be found for several years. Some previously unexposed persons may develop extreme hyperresponsiveness and be amicrofilaremic. Symptoms are due to the adult worm (female, 4–7 cm × 0.5 mm), which lives for years and migrates in subcutaneous tissues. The first definite signs of the disease are Calabar swellings or the migration of a worm beneath the conjunctiva. Calabar swellings are temporary subcutaneous edematous reactions, often several inches in diameter, and may be painful, erythematous, and pruritic. The swelling may migrate a few inches before disappearing; more often, it remains in one place for several days and then subsides. The reaction occurs most frequently on the hands and forearms and around the eyes, but it may appear anywhere. Some patients experience Calabar swellings at infrequent intervals, others as often as twice a week. Systemic symptoms sometimes occur, including generalized urticaria, erythema, and pruritus; low-grade fever; and edema of a whole leg. Migrating worms are sometimes visible in the subcutaneous tissues. Migration across the eye may produce pain, intense conjunctivitis, and eyelid swelling. Dying adult worms may elict local sterile abscesses. Loiasis has been etiologically associated with endomyocardial fibrosis.

Microfilariae in the blood do not induce symptoms. Rarely, however, they enter the central nervous system and may cause encephalitis or myelitis; the larvae can also induce lesions in the retina, heart, and other tissues.

The microfilariae, which have a diurnal periodicity, are found in daytime blood films (20–30% of patients). Serologic tests may be useful but show cross-reactions with other filarial diseases. The eosinophil count is elevated, varying between 10% and 40% or more.

Although surgical removal of adult worms from the eye or skin is sometimes possible, this is not recommended. The most satisfactory treatment is with diethylcarbamazine, which kills microfilariae rapidly and adults slowly. Give 1 mg/kg once on the first day and gradually increase to 2 mg/kg 3 times daily by the fourth or fifth day; continue treatment up to a total of 72 mg/kg. The drug should be given after meals. This gradual increase in dosage reduces the risk of allergic reactions (fever, urticaria, rashes, pruritus, arthralgia, hematuria, proteinuria, encephalitis), which are common because of the rapid killing of microfilariae. Antihistamines given for the first 4–5 days may reduce the incidence of such reactions, but corticosteroids should be started and the doses of diethylcarbamazine lowered temporarily if severe reactions occur. Allergic reactions are more likely to be severe in patients with pretreatment microfilaria counts greater than 25 per microliter of blood; such patients should be given a concurrent course of a corticosteroid. Adult worms tend to appear under the skin, where they die, form small nodules, and are gradually absorbed. Several courses of treatment may be necessary.

The prognosis is good with treatment. A second course may be required. Without treatment, loiasis is annoying and uncomfortable but rarely life-endangering. Fatal encephalitis is rare.

*Loa loa*—a pathogenic parasite. (Editorial.) *Lancet* 1986;**2**:554.

Nutman TB et al: *Loa loa* infection in temporary residents of endemic regions: Recognition of a hyperresponsive syndrome with characteristic clinical manifestations. *J Infect Dis* 1986;**154**:10.

Paleologo FP, Neafie RC, Connor DH: Lymphadenitis caused by *Loa loa. Am J Trop Med Hyg* 1984;**33**:395.

## ONCHOCERCIASIS

Humans and *Simulium* black flies are the natural hosts of *Onchocerca volvulus*, a filarial nematode found in many parts of tropical Africa and in localized areas of the southwestern Arabian peninsula, southern Mexico, Guatemala, Venezuela, Colombia, and northwestern Brazil. An estimated 20–50 million persons (95% of them in Africa) are afflicted. Eye lesions, with visual impairment and even blindness (an estimated half million cases of the latter), are the principal effects. The biting fly introduces infective larvae that develop slowly into adults (2.3–5 cm × 0.25–0.5 mm) in the subcutaneous tissues of humans. Flies are infected in turn by picking up microfilariae while biting. Adult worms may live for 10–15 years, commonly within fibrous subcutaneous nodules. Microfilariae—motile, migratory, and nonperiodic—may be found in the skin, subcutaneous tissues, and lymphatics; in the eye (cornea, anterior chamber, and other structures); and occasionally in the blood, urine, and cerebrospinal fluid. Most tissue damage is in the skin or eyes and is caused by dead or dying microfilariae. Their life span is about 6–30 months.

### Clinical Findings

**A. Symptoms and Signs:** Intensity of infection determines the extent and severity of the clinical picture. The prepatent period to appearance of microfilariae in the skin is 10–20 months (range, 7–34 months). Many persons remain asymptomatic; in others, the incubation period for appearance of symptoms can extend up to several years. Skin manifestations appear in up to 40% of patients. Localized or generalized pruritus is common and may be severe, causing scratching, skin excoriation, and lichenification. Depending on the part of the world where it occurs and on the stage of the disease, a variety of pigmentary changes, papules, focal edema, dryness with scaling, atrophy, and acute inflammation resembling erysipelas may appear. Subcutaneous nodules appear at a later stage of infection. Few patients have more than 3–6 palpable nodules. These are painless, freely movable, and between 0.5 and 1 cm in diameter. An unknown proportion are deeply situated and are not palpable. Common sites are over bony prominences on the trunk, thighs, shoulders, arms, and head. In Africa, nodules are commonly distributed around the pelvis, but in Central America about 50% are on the head. Generalized lymphadenopathy may be present.

The severity of eye lesions and the development of blindness are related to the intensity of infection, especially the density of microfilariae found in the head region and near the eye. The types of eye lesions seen are "fluffy" corneal opacities (punctate keratitis), sclerosing keratitis, anterior uveitis (with secondary glaucoma; secondary cataract may also result), chorioretinitis, optic neuritis, and postneuritic optic atrophy. Common findings are itching, photophobia, and visual impairment, including contraction of visual fields and night blindness.

In some regions, weight loss, elephantiasis, pendulous skin and lymph nodes in the inguinal areas, and hernia may be late sequelae of the infection.

**B. Laboratory Findings:** The diagnosis is made by demonstrating microfilariae in skin snips or shavings. The snips are performed by tenting the skin with a needle and cutting off a bit of skin above the needle tip with a razor. Blood-free shavings may also be cut with a razor blade from the top of a ridge of skin firmly pressed between thumb and forefinger. Corneoscleral punches facilitate the procedure. The snip or shaving is examined in a drop of saline under a coverslip on a slide; many microfilariae emerge from the snip with 30–60 minutes. Sensitivity is increased if the specimen is incubated for 24 hours in a moist-chamber Petri dish. Shavings or snips should be taken from several sites over bony prominences. In Africa, the best sites are the iliac crest and calves; in Central and South America, the deltoid and scapular areas. Care should be taken to prevent bleeding, since in some geographic regions the specimen may be contaminated by the simultaneous presence of blood microfilariae. (The 2 types of microfilariae can be distinguished by staining.) However, specimens must be of sufficient thickness to include the outer parts of the dermal papillae—the level where microfilariae are most likely to be found. In west Africa, *Onchocerca* microfilariae must be distinguished from *Mansonella perstans* microfilariae, which are also found in the skin.

The Mazzotti challenge test, using a small dose of diethylcarbamazine (50 mg), may be useful in diagnosis in patients in whom microfilariae are not found. A skin reaction begins in 15 minutes to 24 hours. In addition, in 2–4 hours microfilariae may appear and should be looked for in the blood and urine. The test should be used only in selected patients and with appropriate safeguards because severe reactions may occur. In patients who show a negative reaction but in whom suspicion of infection is high, a second test dose of 150–200 mg should be given.

Aspiration of nodules will often reveal microfilariae. Adult worms may be demonstrated in excised nodules by histopathologic methods or after collagenase digestion. In patients with eye lesions, microfilariae can sometimes be seen in the cornea and anterior chamber by slit lamp examination. Eosinophilia of 15–50% is common. Skin and serologic tests are usually positive, but cross-reactions occur with other forms of filariasis.

## Treatment

The preferred treatment of onchocerciasis consists of surgical removal of nodules on or near the head, the use of suramin in selected patients to kill adult worms, and the use of diethylcarbamazine before and after suramin to destroy microfilariae slowly. Two drugs that reduce embryogenesis are under investigation for treatment of onchocerciasis: ivermectin and injectable flubendazole. Neither drug is available in the USA.

**A. Nodulectomy:** As many nodules as possible should be excised surgically, particularly when nodules are located close to the eyes. Some are deep in the subcutaneous tissues and cannot be detected by palpation.

**B. Diethylcarbamazine:** This drug kills the microfilariae of onchocerciasis but not the adult worms. Only a few mild, occasional side effects can be attributed directly to the drug: headache, malaise, weakness; less often, vomiting. However, mild to severe allergic symptoms are frequent owing to release of foreign protein from dying microfilariae and may start within 30 minutes. Severe reactions are more likely if microfilariae are producing symptoms in the skin, if microfilariae or nodules are close to the eyes, and

if skin concentrations of microfilariae are high (over 100/mg). Treatment should begin with low doses and increase progressively. The following is one type of dosage schedule for heavy infections, with the drug to be given after meals: Initially, give 25 mg once and wait several days for the reaction to subside; then give 25 mg daily for 2 days; then 50 mg twice daily for 2 days; then 100 mg twice daily for 2 days; then 200 mg twice daily for 7 days.

When reactions to diethylcarbamazine have nearly ceased, suramin treatment is started and is continued weekly until completed. About 3–4 weeks after completing the course of suramin, remaining microfilariae in the skin are killed by giving a course of diethylcarbamazine, 200 mg twice daily for 3–5 days, and repeating the course at 3- to 4-week intervals until pruritic skin reactions no longer occur.

In mild infections, symptomatic relief may be provided by antihistamines and analgesics. However, all patients with heavy infections, skin reactions, or ocular complications should receive corticosteroids starting 1 day before treatment and continuing for 3–7 days, at which time the dosage is to be reduced gradually.

Use of diethylcarbamazine in the form of ocular inserts and as 1% lotion applied locally to the skin is under clinical study.

**C. Suramin sodium** is effective in eradicating infection by killing the adult worms, but it has potential renal toxicity (proteinuria, casts, red cells) and can produce a variety of other serious side effects. Fatal reactions have occurred. Its usage requires hospitalization, expert consultation, and close attention to cautions and contraindications. Before starting suramin, all patients should have a course of diethylcarbamazine to eliminate most microfilariae. Then an initial dose of 0.1 g of suramin is given intravenously slowly over 3 minutes. If tolerated, subsequent dosages are 1 g given intravenously weekly for 4–7 weeks depending upon the severity of the disease. Suramin is available in the USA only from the Parasitic Disease Drug Service, Centers for Disease Control, Atlanta 30333.

**D. Ivermectin:** Ivermectin appears to be at least as effective as diethylcarbamazine in reducing the number of microfilariae in the skin and anterior chamber, but it does so more slowly and with significant reduction in systemic and ocular reactions. The reduction in microfilariae also persists longer. After a single 200–$\mu$g/kg dose of ivermectin, skin microfilariae density decreased to near zero after a month and then gradually increased to 2–10% of the pretreatment level by 12 months; counts in the anterior chamber fell to near zero at 3 months.

## Prognosis

With chemotherapy, progression of the disease usually can be checked. The prognosis is unfavorable only for those patients who are seen for the first time with already far advanced ocular onchocerciasis.

Buck AA (editor): *Onchocerciasis: Symptomatology, Pathology, Diagnosis.* World Health Organization, 1974.

Dadzie KY et al: Ocular findings in a double-blind study of ivermectin versus diethylcarbamazine versus placebo in the treatment of onchocerciasis. *Br J Opththalmol* 1987;**71**:78.

Francis H, Awadzi K, Ottesen EA: The Mazzotti reaction following treatment of onchocerciasis with diethylcarbamazine: Clinical severity as a function of infection intensity. *Am J Trop Med Hyg* 1985;**34**:529.

Greene BM et al: Comparison of ivermectin and diethylcarbamazine in the treatment of onchocerciasis. *N Engl J Med* 1985;**313**:133.

O'Day J, Mackenzie CD: Ocular onchocerciasis: Diagnosis and current clinical approaches. *Trop Doct* 1985;**15**:87.

Pearson CA: Awareness of onchocerciasis. *Lancet* 1986;**2**:805.

## STRONGYLOIDIASIS

### Essentials of Diagnosis

- Pruritic dermatitis at sites of larval penetration.
- Diarrhea, epigastric pain, nausea, malaise, weight loss.
- Cough, rales, transient pulmonary infiltrates.
- Eosinophilia; characteristic larvae in stool specimens, duodenal aspirate, or sputum.

### General Considerations

Strongyloidiasis is an infection caused by the small nematode *Strongyloides stercoralis* (2–2.5 nm × 30–50 $\mu$m). The major symptoms result from adult parasitism, principally in the duodenum and jejunum, or from larval migration through the pulmonary and cutaneous tissues. *Strongyloides,* unlike most other helminths infecting humans, multiplies within the host; this can result in persistence of infection at a low level as well as in overwhelming infection (hyperinfection syndrome) with severe intestinal ulceration, malabsorption, and other complications that can lead to death.

The parasite is an infection of humans, but dogs, cats, and primates have been found naturally infected with strains indistinguishable from those of humans. The disease is endemic in tropical and subtropical areas; although the prevalence is generally low, in some areas rates of disease exceed 25%. In temperate areas, including the USA, the disease occurs sporadically. Multiple infections in households are common, and prevalence in institutions, particularly mental institutions, may be high. Hospital staff should be protected from contact with feces and sputum from infected patients.

The parasite is uniquely capable of maintaining its life cycle both within the human host and in soil. Infection occurs when filariform larvae penetrate the skin, enter the bloodstream, and are carried to the lungs, where they escape from capillaries into alveoli and ascend the bronchial tree to the glottis. The larvae are then swallowed and carried to the duodenum and upper jejunum, where maturation to the adult stage takes place. The parasitic female, generally held to be parthenogenetic, matures and lives embedded in the mucosa, where its eggs are laid and hatch. Rhabditiform larvae, which are noninfective, emerge, and most migrate into the intestinal lumen to leave the host via the feces. The life span of the adult worm may be as long as 5 years.

In the soil, the rhabditiform larvae metamorphose into the infective (filariform) larvae. However, the parasite also has a free-living cycle in soil, in which some rhabditiform larvae develop into adults that produce eggs from which rhabditiform larvae emerge to continue the life cycle.

Autoinfection, which probably occurs at a low rate in most infections, is an important factor in determining worm burden and is responsible for persistence of asymptomatic or symptomatic strongyloidiasis in individuals for many years after they leave an endemic area. Internal autoinfection takes place in the lower bowel when some rhabditiform larvae, instead of passing with the feces, develop into filariform larvae that penetrate the intestinal mucosa, enter the intestinal lymphatic and portal circulation, are carried to the lungs, and return to the small bowel to complete the cycle. This process is accelerated by constipation and other conditions that reduce bowel motility. In addition, an external autoinfection cycle can occur as a result of fecal contamination of the perianal area.

In the hyperinfection syndrome, autoinfection is greatly increased, resulting in a marked increase in the intestinal worm burden and in massive dissemination of filariform larvae to the lungs and most other tissues, where they can cause local inflammatory reactions and granuloma formation. Occasionally, in the lungs and elsewhere, larvae metamorphose into adults. Hyperinfection is generally initiated under conditions of depressed host cellular immunity, especially in debilitated, malnourished persons and in patients receiving immunosuppressive therapy, particularly corticosteroids. However, the syndrome can occur in individuals who show no obvious predisposing cause. Penetration of the bowel wall by filariform larvae can result in gram-negative septicemia.

### Clinical Findings

**A. Signs and Symptoms:** The time from penetration of the skin by filariform larvae until rhabditiform larvae appear in the feces is 3–4 weeks. The severity of infection ranges from asymptomatic to fatal. Although an acute syndrome can sometimes be recognized in which cutaneous symptoms are followed by pulmonary and then intestinal symptoms, most patients have chronic symptoms that continue for years or sometimes for life. Symptoms may be continuous, or exacerbations may recur at irregular intervals.

**1. Cutaneous manifestations–**In acute infection, filariform larvae usually invade the skin of the feet. The reaction in unsensitized patients may be minimal, with only a macule or papule, but in sensitized patients there may be focal edema, inflammation, petechiae, serpiginous or urticarial tracts, and intense itching. In chronic infections, stationary urticaria or larva currens, characterized by transient eruptions that migrate in serpiginous tracts, may occur.

**2. Intestinal manifestations**–Symptoms range from mild to severe, the most common being diarrhea, abdominal pain, and flatulence. Anorexia, nausea, vomiting, and epigastric tenderness may be present. The diarrhea may alternate with constipation, and in severe cases the feces contain mucus and blood. The pain is often epigastric in location and may mimic the burning, dull cramp, or ache of duodenal ulcer. Malabsorption or a protein-losing enteropathy can result from a large intestinal worm burden.

**3. Pulmonary manifestations**–With migration of larvae through the lungs, bronchi, and trachea there may be a dry cough and throat irritation without further difficulty, or a low-grade fever, bronchitis, dyspnea, wheezing, asthma, and hemoptysis. As the disease becomes more marked, bronchopneumonia and pleural effusion can occur, accompanied by progressive dyspnea; the cough may become productive of an odorless, mucopurulent sputum; miliary abscesses can develop.

**4. Other findings**–Severe infection may present with fever, malaise, and weakness leading to prostration and emaciation.

**5. Hyperinfection syndrome**–Massive increase in the intestinal worm burden with intense dissemination of larvae to the lungs and other tissues can result in the following complications: severe diarrhea with generalized abdominal pain and distention, bronchopneumonia, pleural effusion, pericarditis and myocarditis, hepatic granulomas, cholecystitis, ulcerating lesions at all levels of the gastrointestinal tract, paralytic ileus, perforation and peritonitis, gram-negative septicemia, meningitis, cachexia, shock, and death.

**B. Laboratory Findings:** Eggs are seldom found in feces. Diagnosis is by finding the larval stages in feces or duodenal fluid. Rhabditiform larvae may be found in recently passed stool specimens; filariform larvae will be present in specimens held in the laboratory for some hours or if the specimen is processed by stool culture. Three specimens, preserved or unpreserved, should be collected at 2-day intervals or longer, since the number of larvae in feces may vary considerably from day to day. Each specimen should be examined by direct microscopy, and in addition, to increase sensitivity of testing, one or more should be processed by the Baermann concentration method. Stool specimens used in the Baermann procedure must be unpreserved; they can be received in the laboratory up to 48 hours after passage if held at refrigerated but nonfreezing temperatures. Stool specimens can also be put into culture for 7–10 days to increase the number of larvae.

Although larvae cannot be found in the stools of 25% or more of infected patients, the diagnosis can often be made by examination of duodenal mucus for rhabditiform larvae or ova. Mucus is obtained by means of the duodenal string test or by duodenal intubation and aspiration. Duodenal biopsy is seldom

indicated but will confirm the diagnosis in most patients. Occasionally, filariform or rhabditiform larvae can be detected in sputum during the pulmonary phase of the disease.

In chronic low-grade intestinal strongyloidiasis, the white blood cell count is often normal, with a slightly elevated percentage of eosinophils. However, with increasing larval migration, eosinophilia may reach 50% and leukocytosis 20,000/$\mu$L. Mild anemia may be present. Serum IgE immunoglobulins may be elevated. New ELISA and immunofluorescent serologic tests are promising; earlier tests by other methods were not. In the hyperinfection syndrome, there may be findings of hypoproteinemia, malabsorption, and abnormal liver function. Ova and rhabditiform and filariform larvae may be present in sputum, and filariform larvae in the urine; eosinopenia, when present, is thought to be a poor prognostic sign.

Small bowel x-rays early in the disease may show inflammation and irritability, with prominent mucosal folds; there may be a dilatation, delay, and ulcerative duodenitis. Later in the disease, the findings can resemble those in nontropical and tropical sprue, or there may be narrowing, rigidity, and diminished peristalsis. During pulmonary migration of larvae, fine nodulation or irregular patches of pneumonitis may be seen.

## Differential Diagnosis

Because of varied signs and symptoms, the diagnosis of strongyloidiasis is often difficult, especially in nonendemic areas. The disease should always be considered in patients with unexplained eosinophilia. Eosinophilia plus one or more of the following factors should further enhance consideration of the diagnosis: endemic area exposure, duodenal ulcer-like pain, persistent or recurrent diarrhea, recurrent coughing or wheezing, and transient pulmonary infiltrates. The duodenitis and jejunitis of strongyloidiasis can mimic giardiasis, cholecystitis, and pancreatitis. Transient pulmonary infiltrates must be differentiated from tropical pulmonary eosinophilia and Löffler's syndrome. The diagnosis should be considered among the many causes of malabsorption in the tropics.

## Treatment

Since *Strongyloides* can multiply in humans, treatment should continue until the parasite is eradicated. Patients receiving immunosuppressive therapy should be examined for the presence of the infection before and probably at intervals during treatment. In concurrent infection with *Strongyloides* and *Ascaris* or hookworm (which is common), eradicate *Ascaris* and hookworms first and *Strongyloides* subsequently.

**A. Thiabendazole:** Thiabendazole is the drug of choice. An oral dose of 25 mg/kg (maximum, 1.5 g) is given after meals twice daily for 2–3 days. A 5- to 7-day course of treatment is needed for disseminated infections. Tablet and liquid formulations are available; tablets should be chewed. Side effects, including headache, weakness, vomiting, vertigo, and decreased mental alertness, occur in as many as 30% of patients and may be severe. These symptoms are lessened if the drug is taken after meals. Other potentially serious side effects occur rarely. Erythema multiforme and the Stevens-Johnson syndrome have been associated with thiabendazole therapy; in severe cases, fatalities have occurred.

**B. Alternative Drugs:** Albendazole is undergoing clinical trials. At a dosage of 400 mg/d for 3 days, cure rates in several studies were 48–81%. At this dosage, the drug is nearly free of side effects. If thiabendazole cannot be tolerated, mebendazole (500 mg 3 times daily for 14 days), cambendazole, or levamisole can be tried, but their efficacy is based on limited trials. In 6 studies (459 patients) in which cambendazole was given orally (with a meal) one time only at a dose of 5 mg/kg, cure rates ranged from 90 to 100%. Side effects (nausea, vomiting, headache, dizziness) were mild and transient in up to 20% of cases.

## Prognosis

The prognosis is favorable except in the hyperinfection syndrome. Infections associated with emaciation, advanced liver disease, cancer, immunologic disorders, or the use of immunosuppressive drugs may be difficult to treat. In selected instances, a 2-day course of treatment with thiabendazole once monthly can be tried to control infections that cannot be eradicated.

Bicalho SA, Leao OJ, Pena Q Jr: Cambendazole in the treatment of human strongyloidiasis. *Am J Trop Med Hyg* 1983; **32:**1181.

Davidson RA, Fletcher RH, Chapman LE: Risk factors for strongyloidiasis: A case-control study. *Arch Intern Med* 1984;**144:**321.

Neva FA: Biology and immunology of human strongyloidiasis. *J Infect Dis* 1986;**153:**397.

Wilson KH, Kauffman CA: Persistent *Strongyloides stercoralis* in a blind loop of the bowel: Successful treatment with mebendazole. *Arch Intern Med* 1983;**143:**357.

## TRICHINOSIS
## (Trichinelliosis, Trichinellosis)

### Essentials of Diagnosis

- History of ingestion of raw or inadequately cooked meat, especially pig or bear.
- First week: diarrhea, cramps, malaise.
- Second week to 1–2 months: muscle pain and tenderness, fever, periorbital and facial edema, conjunctivitis.
- Eosinophilia and elevated serum enzymes.
- Positive skin and serologic tests.
- History of ingestion of raw or inadequately cooked pork (including boar) or bear meat.
- Larvae present in muscle biopsy.

### General Considerations

Trichinosis is caused by the nematode *Trichinella spiralis*. Adult worms (2–3.6 mm × 75–90 μm) live in the intestines of humans, pigs, bears, rats, and most carnivores, including marine animals; fowl are resistant to infection. Viviparous larvae liberated by the females enter striated muscle, are encysted, and live for years. In the natural life cycle, these larvae develop into a new generation of adults when parasitized muscle is ingested by a new host. Pigs generally become infected by feeding on uncooked food scraps or, less often, by eating infected rats.

Humans usually acquire the infection by eating encysted larvae in raw or undercooked pork or pork products. Cases occur sporadically or in outbreaks. Sometimes the source of infection is the flesh of wild animals, particularly bear or walrus in far northern areas or bush pigs in Africa. Ground beef has also been contaminated by adulteration with pork or inadvertently in common meat grinders. Gastric juices liberate the encysted larvae, which rapidly mature and mate. The adult female burrows into the mucosa of the small intestine. Within 4–5 days, she begins to discharge larvae that are disseminated via the lymphatics and bloodstream to most body tissues. Larvae that reach striated muscle encyst and remain viable for months to years, those that reach other tissues are rapidly destroyed.

Although trichinosis is present wherever pork is eaten, the disease is a greater problem in many temperate areas than in the tropics. In the USA, there has been a marked reduction in the prevalence of trichinosis both in humans and in pigs. Nevertheless, the annual incidence of infection is estimated to be over 150,000 cases, although most are asymptomatic or so mild as to elude diagnosis.

### Clinical Findings

**A. Symptoms and Signs:** The incubation period is generally from 2 to 12 days (range, 12 hours to 28 days). Depending upon the intensity of infection, the tissues invaded, the immune status of the host, the age of the host (children have less severe infections), and, perhaps, the strain of the parasite. Infection ranges from (1) asymptomatic, in which eosinophilia may be recognized only by chance; to (2) a mild febrile illness in which there may be one or more mild, short-lasting symptoms; to (3) a severe disease with multiple system involvement that rarely progresses to a fulminating fatal illness.

In the pathogenesis of the disease, 3 clinical stages can be differentiated: intestinal, muscle invasion, and convalescence. The intestinal stage can be asymptomatic or symptomatic and lasts from 1 to 7 days. Diarrhea, abdominal cramps, and malaise are the major findings; nausea and vomiting occur less frequently; and constipation is occasionally present. Fever and leukocytosis are rarely found during the first week.

The stage of muscular invasion, which is the result of larval migration and muscle penetration, begins at the end of the first week. It lasts about 6 weeks, corresponding with the death of the worms. Parasitized muscles show an intense inflammatory reaction. Clinical findings include fever (low-grade to marked); muscle pain (especially upon movement) and muscle tenderness, edema, and spasm; periorbital and facial edema; sweating; photophobia and conjunctivitis; weakness or prostration; pain on swallowing; dyspnea, coughing, and hoarseness; subconjunctival, retinal, and nail splinter hemorrhages; and rashes and formication. The most frequently parasitized muscles and sites of findings are the masseters, the tongue, the diaphragm, the intercostal muscles, and the extraocular, laryngeal, paravertebral, nuchal, deltoid, pectoral, gluteus, biceps, and gastrocnemius muscles. Inflammatory reactions around larvae that reach tissues other than muscle may result in a broad range of findings, including the development of meningitis, encephalitis, myocarditis, bronchopneumonia, nephritis, and peripheral and cranial nerve disorders.

The stage of convalescence generally begins in the second month but in severe infections may not begin before 3 months or longer. Vague muscle pains and malaise may persist for several more months. Permanent muscular atrophy has been reported.

**B. Laboratory Findings:** The diagnosis is supported or confirmed by findings of eosinophilia, positive serologic tests, and detection of larvae in muscle biopsy specimens.

Leukocytosis and eosinophilia appear during the second week after ingestion of infected meat. The proportion of eosinophils rises to a maximum of 20–90% in the third or fourth week and then slowly declines to normal over the next few months.

Serologic tests can detect most clinically manifest cases but are not sufficiently sensitive to detect low-level infections involving only a few larvae per gram of muscle. More than one test should be used and then repeated, since it is important to observe seroconversion from a negative to a positive titer or to a rising titer. The bentonite flocculation (BF) test (positive titer, ≥ 1:5) is highly sensitive and is considered nearly 100% specific. It becomes positive in the third or fourth week and reaches a maximum titer at about 2 months. The immunofluorescence test (positive titer ≥ 16), is also highly sensitive, though less specific than the BF test; it may become positive in the second week. Other tests are available at some laboratories.

In most persons with moderate infections, the BF test is negative within 2–3 years after infection. The intradermal test, which becomes positive within 3 weeks, is no longer recommended, as it may remain positive for years and batches of antigen vary in potency.

Adult worms may be looked for in feces, although they are seldom found. In the second week, there are occasional larvae in blood, duodenal washings, and, rarely, in centrifuged spinal fluid. In the third to fourth weeks, definitive diagnosis becomes possible through biopsy of skeletal muscle (particularly gastrocnemius and pectoralis), preferably at a site of swelling or tenderness. Portions of the specimen should be examined microscopically by compression between glass slides, by digestion, and by preparation of many histologic sections. If biopsy is done too early, there are 2 possible risks: larvae may not be detectable because they have not yet coiled, and young larvae may be digested in the course of the digestion test. Myositis even in the absence of larvae is a significant finding.

Nonspecific laboratory findings include elevation of serum enzymes (creatinine phosphokinase, lactate dehydrogenase, and serum transaminases). Serum aldolase may be very high. The low sedimentation rate is a useful diagnostic clue. There may be a marked hypergammaglobulinemia with reversal of the albumin/globulin ratio.

**C. Imaging:** Chest films during the acute phase may show disseminated or localized infiltrates. Calcified muscle cysts are not detectable radiologically.

**D. Electrocardiographic Findings:** ECGs should be examined for signs of myocarditis.

## Complications

The more important complications are allergic granulomatous reactions in the lungs, encephalitis, and cardiac failure.

## Differential Diagnosis

Mild infections and those with atypical symptoms are often difficult to diagnose; because of its protean manifestations, trichinosis may resemble many other diseases. Eosinophilia, muscle pain and tenderness, and fever should lead the physician to consider collagen vascular disorders.

## Prevention

Public health measures to prevent feeding of uncooked garbage to hogs and animal inspection (not in the USA) by various techniques have significantly reduced the frequency and intensity of infection in the USA and other countries. The chief safeguard against trichinosis is adequate cooking of pork at the newly recommended temperature of 77 °C. Alternatively, larvae can be made nonviable by freezing meat at −15 °C (5 °F) for 20 days. Recent reports indicate that *T spiralis* in arctic sylvatic animals is resistant to freezing.

## Treatment

The treatment of trichinosis is principally supportive, since most cases recover spontaneously without sequelae. If the patient is still in the intestinal phase of the disease, thiabendazole is indicated at an oral dosage of 25 mg/kg (maximum 1.5 g) twice daily after meals for 3–5 days. Side effects may occur (see under Strongyloidiasis, above). Unless the patient is severely ill, corticosteroids are contraindicated in the intestinal phase.

In the stage of larval invasion of muscle, severe infections require hospitalization and high doses of corticosteroids for 24–48 hours, followed by lower doses for several days or weeks to control symptoms. Thiabendazole has been tried in the muscle stage with equivocal relief of muscle pain or tenderness or lysis of fever. However, further trials are recommended.

Initial reports suggest some success for mebendazole efficacy against adult worms in the intestinal tract, migrating larvae, and larvae in muscle using the following schedule: 200–400 mg 3 times daily for 3 days, followed by 400–500 mg 3 times daily for 10 days. Albendazole is undergoing clinical tests.

## Prognosis

Death may rarely occur in 2–3 weeks in overwhelming infections; more often, it occurs in 4–8 weeks from a major complication such as cardiac failure or pneumonia.

Campbell WC (editor): *Trichinella and Trichinosis.* Plenum Press, 1983.

Levin ML: Treatment of trichinosis with mebendazole. *Am J Trop Med Hyg* 1983;**32:**980.

Viallet J et al: Arctic trichinosis presenting as prolonged diarrhea. *Gastroenterology* 1986;**91:**938.

## TRICHURIASIS
## (Trichocephaliasis, Whipworm)

### Essentials of Diagnosis

- Most infections are silent; heavy infections may cause chronic diarrhea, lower abdominal cramps, flatulence, hematochezia, tenesmus, and rectal prolapse.
- Characteristic barrel-shaped eggs and (less commonly) adult worms are found in the stool.

### General Considerations

*Trichuris trichiura* is a common intestinal parasite of humans throughout the world, particularly in the subtropics and tropics. Persons of all ages are affected, but infection is heaviest and most frequent in children. The small slender worms, 30–50 mm in length, attach themselves by means of their anterior whiplike end to the mucosa of the large intestine, particularly the cecum. Eggs passed in the feces require 2–4 weeks for larval development after reaching the soil before becoming infective; thus, person-to-person transmission is not possible. Infections are acquired by ingestion of the infective egg. The larvae hatch in the small intestine and mature in the large bowel but do not migrate through the tissues.

### Clinical Findings

**A. Symptoms and Signs:** Light (fewer than 10,000 eggs per gram of feces) to moderate infections rarely cause symptoms. Heavy infections (usually 30,000 or more eggs per gram of feces) may be accompanied by a variety of symptoms arising from irritation of the mucosa. Most common are lower abdominal cramps, tenesmus, diarrhea, distention, flatulence, nausea, vomiting, and weight loss. In heavy infections, most often found in malnourished young chil-

dren, rectal prolapse and hematochezia or chronic occult blood loss may occur. Sometimes, adult worms are seen in stools. Invasion of the appendix, with resulting appendicitis, is rare.

**B. Laboratory Findings:** Diagnosis is by identification of characteristic eggs and, sometimes, adult worms in stools. Eosinophilia (5–20%) is common with all but light infections, and severe hypochromic anemia may be present with heavy infections.

### Treatment

**A. Mebandazole:** Patients with asymptomatic light infections do not require treatment. For those with heavier or symptomatic infections, give mebendazole, 100 mg twice daily before or after meals for 3 days. It may be therapeutically advantageous for the tablets to be chewed before swallowing. Cure rates of 60–80% and higher are reported after one course of treatment, with marked reduction in ova counts in the remaining patients. For severe trichuriasis, a longer course of treatment (up to 6 days) or a repeat course will often be necessary. Gastrointestinal side effects from the drug are rare. The drug is contraindicated in pregnancy, and experience with it is limited in children under age 2.

**B. Oxantel Pamoate:** Oxantel pamoate is an analog of pyrantel pamoate and acts only on *T trichiura.* Cure rates of 57–100% have been reported in various trials. One treatment schedule is 15 mg/kg (base) daily for 2 days for patients with mild to moderate intensity of infection. For patients with severe infection, give 10 mg/kg (base) daily for 5 days. Oxantel pamoate is also marketed in combination with pyrantel pamoate as oxantel-pyrantel, which combines the efficacy of both drugs to provide broad-spectrum anthelmintic action against trichuriasis, hookworm, ascariasis, pinworm, and trichostrongyliasis infections. Neither oxantel nor oxantel-pyrantel is available in the USA.

**C. Albendazole,** given orally at a single dose of 400 mg, resulted in cure rates of 33–90%, with marked reduction in egg counts in those not cured; an appropriate dosage to achieve higher cure rates in moderate to heavy infections remains to be determined.

**D. Thiabendazole** should *not* be used, because it is not effective and is potentially toxic.

Gilman RH et al: The adverse consequences of heavy *Trichuris* infection. *Trans R Soc Trop Med Hyg* 1983;**77:**432.

Rossignol JF, Maisonneuve H: Benzimidazoles in the treatment of trichuriasis: A review. *Ann Trop Med Parasitol* 1984; **78:**135.

### VISCERAL LARVA MIGRANS
### (Toxocariasis)

Most cases of visceral larva migrans are due to *Toxocara canis,* an ascarid of dogs and other canids, but in a few cases *Toxocara cati* in domestic cats has been implicated and rarely *Belascaris procyonis* of raccoons. The adult worms live in the intestinal tracts of their respective hosts and release large numbers of eggs in the stool. Puppies (2 weeks to 6 months) and lactating bitches (up to 6 months after parturition) are responsible for most *T canis* eggs passed to the environment. The chief mode of transmission among dogs and the reservoir mechanism of the disease is transplacental and in milk following reactivation of dormant tissue larvae during pregnancy of an infected bitch. The life cycle of *T cati* is similar, but transplacental transmission does not occur.

Human infections are sporadic and probably occur worldwide. Infection is generally in dirt-eating young children who ingest *T canis* eggs from soil or sand contaminated with dog feces, most often from puppies. Direct contact with infected animals does not produce infection, as the eggs require a 3- to 4-week extrinsic incubation period to become infective; thereafter, eggs in soil remain infective for months to years. In humans, hatched larvae are unable to mature and continue to migrate through the tissues for up to 6 months. Eventually they lodge in various organs, particularly the lungs and liver, less often the brain, eyes, and other tissues, where they produce eosinophilic granulomas (up to 1 cm in diameter).

## Clinical Findings

**A. Acute Infection:** Fever, cough, wheezing, hepatomegaly, and sometimes splenomegaly and lymphadenopathy are present. A variety of other findings may occur when such organs as the heart, eyes, and kidneys are invaded. The acute phase may last 2–3 weeks, but resolution of all physical and laboratory findings may take 18 months.

Eosinophil counts of 30–80% and marked leukocytosis are common. The white count may exceed 100,000/$\mu$L. Hyperglobulinemia occurs when the liver is extensively invaded and is a useful clue in diagnosis. An ELISA test is the most specific (92%) and sensitive (78%) serologic test and permits a presumptive diagnosis. Nonspecific isohemagglutinin titers (anti-A and anti-B) are usually greater than 1:1024. Chest radiographs may show infiltration. With central nervous system involvement, the cerebrospinal fluid may show eosinophils. No parasitic forms can be found by stool examination.

Specific diagnosis can only be made by liver biopsy to search for *Toxocara* larvae, but the procedure is seldom justified. When indicated, laparoscopy may permit direct biopsy of a granuloma.

**B. Ocular Toxocariasis:** Most cases occur in children, most commonly aged 5–10 years, who present with visual loss. The principal pathologic entity is eosinophilic granuloma of the retina that resembles retinoblastoma; until the recent development of the ELISA test, this resulted in the enucleation of many eyes. The most common clinical findings are a diffuse, painless endophthalmitis; posterior pole granuloma; and a peripheral inflammatory mass. Uncommonly seen are an iris nodule, optic nerve granuloma, uniocular pars planitis, and a migrating retinal nematode. Ocular toxocariasis is generally not associated with peripheral eosinophilia, hypergammaglobulinemia, or isohemagglutinin elevation. Serum ELISA tests may be positive, but a negative test does not rule out the diagnosis. If doubt exists about whether a patient with a positive serum ELISA test has retinoblastoma, examination of the vitreous humor for ELISA antibody and eosinophils can be helpful. High-resolution CT scanning of the orbit should be done.

## Treatment & Prognosis

Disease in humans is best prevented by periodic treatment of puppies, kittens, and nursing dog and cat mothers, starting at 2 weeks postpartum, repeating at weekly intervals for 3 weeks and then every 6 months. Children should be supervised to prevent dirt-eating; their hands should be washed after playing in soil and sand; and play areas should be protected from animal feces.

**A. Acute Infection:** There is no specific treatment, but thiabendazole, levamisole, diethylcarbamazine, or mebendazole should be tried. The cortisones, antibiotics, antihistamines, and analgesics may be needed to provide symptomatic relief. Symptoms may persist for months but generally clear within 1–2 years, and the ultimate prognosis is usually good.

**B. Ocular Toxocariasis:** Treatment includes corticosteroids (subconjunctival applications may be preferable to oral usage), vitrectomy for vitreous traction, laser photocoagulation, and an anthelmintic drug. Partial or total permanent visual impairment is rare.

Bekhti A: Mebendazole in toxocariasis. *Ann Intern Med* 1984;**100**:463.

Cypess RH: Visceral larva migrans. Pages 205–212 in: CRC Handbook Series in Zoonoses, Steele JH (Editor); Section C: *Parastic Zoonoses,* Vol II, Schultz MG (Editor). CRC Press, 1982.

Glickman LT, Shofer FD: Zoonotic visceral and ocular larva migrans. *Vet Clin North Am Small Animal Practice* 1987;**17**:39.

Molk R: Ocular toxocariasis: A review of the literature. *Ann Ophthalmol* 1983;**15**:216.

Schantz PM, Glickman LT: Toxocaral visceral larva migrans. *N Engl J Med* 1978;**298**:436.

Shields JA: Ocular toxocariasis: A review. *Surv Ophthalmol* 1984;**28**:361.

## REFERENCES
### (See also Chapter 25 references.)

Reeder MM, Palmer PE (editors): *The Radiology of Tropical Disease With Epidemiological, Pathological, and Clinical Correlation.* Williams & Wilkins, 1980.

Steele JH (editor): *CRC Handbook Series in Zoonoses.* Section C: *Parasitic Zoonoses.* Vol 3. Hillyer GV, Hopla CE (editors). CRC Press, 1982.

WHO Expert Committee: *Parasitic Zoonoses.* Technical Report Series, No. 637. World Health Organization, 1979.

# Infectious Diseases: Mycotic*

**27**

*Carlyn Halde, PhD*

## COCCIDIOIDOMYCOSIS

### Essentials of Diagnosis

- Influenzalike illness with malaise, fever, backache, headache, and cough.
- Pleural pain.
- Arthralgia and periarticular swelling of knees and ankles.
- Erythema nodosum or erythema multiforme.
- Dissemination (rare) may result in meningitis or granulomatous lesions in any or all organs.
- X-ray findings vary widely from pneumonitis to cavitation.
- Positive skin test, serologic tests useful; sporangia containing endospores demonstrable in sputum or tissues.

### General Considerations

Coccidioidomycosis should be considered in the diagnosis of any obscure illness in a patient who has lived in or visited an endemic area.

Infection results from the inhalation of arthroconidia of *Coccidioides immitis,* a mold that grows in soil in certain arid regions of the southwestern USA, in Mexico, and in Central and South America.

About 60% of infections are subclinical and unrecognized other than by the subsequent development of a positive coccidioidin skin test. In the remaining cases, symptoms may be of severity warranting medical attention. Fewer than 1% show dissemination, but among these patients the mortality rate is high.

### Clinical Findings

**A. Symptoms and Signs:** Symptoms of primary coccidioidomycosis occur in about 40% of infections. These vary from mild to severe and prostrating and resemble those due to viral, bacterial, or other mycotic infections. The onset (after an incubation period of 10–30 days) is usually that of a respiratory tract illness with fever and occasionally chills. Pleural pain is common and usually severe. Nasopharyngitis may be followed by bronchitis accompanied by a dry or slightly productive cough. Weakness and anorexia may become marked, leading to prostration. A morbilliform rash may appear 1–2 days after the onset of symptoms.

Arthralgia accompanied by periarticular swellings, often of the knees and ankles, is common. Erythema

nodosum may appear 2–20 days after onset of symptoms. Erythema multiforme may appear on the upper extremities, head, or thorax. Breath sounds may become bronchial in nature, especially in the severely ill patient. Persistent pulmonary lesions, varying from cavities and abscesses to parenchymal nodular densities or bronchiectasis, occur in about 5% of diagnosed cases.

About 0.1% of white and 1% of nonwhite patients are unable to localize or control infection caused by *C immitis.* Symptoms in progressive coccidioidomycosis depend upon the site of dissemination. Any or all organs may be involved. Pulmonary findings usually become more pronounced, with mediastinal and hilar lymph node enlargement, cough, and increased sputum production. Pulmonary abscesses may rupture into the pleural space, producing an empyema. Extension to bones and skin may take place, and pericardial and myocardial extension is not unusual.

Lesions in the bones are often in the bony prominences and the ends of long bones. The ankle, wrist, and elbow joints are commonly involved. Meningitis occurs in 30–50% of disseminated cases. Subcutaneous abscesses and verrucous skin lesions are especially common in fulminating cases. Lymphadenitis may occur and may progress to suppuration. Mediastinal and retroperitoneal abscesses are not uncommon.

**B. Laboratory Findings:** In primary coccidioidomycosis, there may be moderate leukocytosis and eosinophilia and an elevated sedimentation rate. A persisting elevated or increasing sedimentation rate is a sign of progressive disease. The coccidioidin skin test becomes positive early after infection. Serologic testing is useful for both diagnosis and prognosis. The combination of latex agglutinate test (IgM) and immunodiffusion test (IgG) is useful for screening, but the complement fixation test is needed for confirmation and quantitation. An initial eosinophilia of 15% or higher together with a persistent rising complement fixation titer is a bad prognostic sign. A rising complement fixation titer may herald dissemination weeks before it is otherwise evident. Demonstrable antibodies in spinal fluid are pathognomonic for coccidioidal meningitis. Spinal fluid findings include increased cell count with lymphocytosis and reduced sugar. Sporangia filled with endospores may be found in clinical specimens. These should be cultured only by trained technicians using safety precautions because of the danger of laboratory infection.

**C. Imaging:** Radiographic findings vary, but

---

* Superficial mycoses are discussed in Chapter 4.

patchy and nodular infiltrations are the most common. Hilar lymphadenopathy may be visible. There may be primary pleural effusion and thin-walled cavities.

## Complications

Pulmonary infiltrations persisting for 6 or more weeks should be suspected of possible progression, especially with increase in area, enlargement of mediastinal and hilar nodes, cavity enlargement, and hemoptysis. Progressive disease is more likely to appear in blacks, Filipinos, and Mexicans. Immunodeficient patients or pregnant women of any race are also more vulnerable to dissemination.

## Treatment

Bed rest is the most important therapeutic measure for the primary infection. This should be continued until there is a complete regression of fever, a normal sedimentation rate, clearing or stabilization of pulmonary radiologic findings, and a lowering of the complement fixation titer. These precautions are especially important for patients in whom the rate of dissemination is high. General symptomatic therapy is given as needed.

There is no specific therapy for patients with disseminated disease. Amphotericin B has proved effective in some patients and should be tried. The drug is suspended in 500 mL of 5% dextrose in distilled water (not saline) and administered intravenously over a 4-hour period. Toxic properties (including renal toxicity) suggest that the adult dose should not exceed 0.5–1 mg/kg. Therapy should begin with 1 mg/d, increasing by 5-mg increments to 25–35 mg/d or to 40–60 mg/d in the acutely ill. As the illness stabilizes, continue at 25–35 mg/d, decreasing with poor tolerance or increasing with poor clinical response. Therapy should continue to a total dose of 2.5–3 g. (See p 986 for precautions in the use of this drug.) Coccidioidal meningitis has been controlled with oral ketoconazole, 800–1200 mg/d, with or without intrathecal amphotericin B. Ketoconazole, at a lower dose, is continued indefinitely.

The best monitor of renal function is a creatinine clearance test done before treatment and once a week during treatment. Determine the blood urea nitrogen periodically.

Thoracic surgery is indicated for giant, infected, or ruptured cavities. Surgical drainage is also useful for subcutaneous abscesses. Excisional surgery may be used to remove any focus of proliferating sporangia. Amphotericin B is advisable following extensive surgical manipulation of infected tissue.

## Prognosis

The prognosis is good, but persistent pulmonary cavities may present complications. Nodules, cavities, and fibrotic residuals may rarely progress after long periods of stability or regression. Oral ketoconazole, 200–800 mg daily 1–2 hours before breakfast, is used in amphotericin B failure; however, therapy must be continued for 6 months or longer after recovery in order to prevent relapse.

Bayer AS: Fungal pneumonias; pulmonary coccidioidal syndromes. 1. Primary and progressive primary coccidioidal pneumonias; diagnostic, therapeutic, and prognostic considerations. 2. Miliary, nodular, and cavitary pulmonary coccidioidomycosis; chemotherapeutic and surgical considerations. *Chest* 1981;**79:**575, 686.

Bronneman DA et al: Coccidioidomycosis in the acquired immunodeficiency syndrome. *Ann Intern Med* 1987;**106:**372.

Goodpasture HC: Treatment of central nervous system fungal infection with ketoconazole. *Arch Int Med* 1985;**145:**879.

Hermans PE, Keys TF: Antifungal agents used for deep-seated mycotic infections. *Mayo Clin Proc* 1983;**58:**223.

Labadie EL, Hamilton RH: Survival improvement in coccidioidal meningitis by high dose intrathecal amphotericin B. *Arch Intern Med* 1986;**146:**2013.

# HISTOPLASMOSIS

## Essentials of Diagnosis

- Asymptomatic to severe respiratory symptoms with malaise, fever, cough, and chest pain.
- Ulceration of naso- and oropharynx.
- Hepatomegaly, splenomegaly, and lymphadenopathy.
- Anemia and leukopenia.
- Diarrhea in children.
- Positive skin test; positive serologic findings; small budding fungus cells found within reticuloendothelial cells; culture confirms diagnosis.

## General Considerations

Histoplasmosis is caused by *Histoplasma capsulatum,* a mold that has been isolated from soil in endemic areas (central and eastern USA, eastern Canada, Mexico, Central America, South America, Africa, and Southeast Asia). Infection takes place presumably by inhalation of spores. These convert into small budding cells that are engulfed by phagocytic cells in the lungs. The organism proliferates and may be carried by the blood to other areas of the body.

## Clinical Findings

**A. Symptoms and Signs:** Most cases of histoplasmosis are asymptomatic or mild and so are unrecognized. Past infection is recognized by the development of a positive histoplasmin skin test and occasionally by pulmonary and splenic calcification. Symptomatic infections may present mild influenza, like characteristics, often lasting 1–4 days. Signs and symptoms of pulmonary involvement are usually absent even in patients who subsequently show areas of calcification on chest x-ray. Moderately severe infections are frequently diagnosed as atypical pneumonia. These patients have fever, cough, and mild chest pain lasting 5–15 days. Physical examination is usually negative. Radiographic findings are variable and nonspecific.

Severe infections have been divided into 3 groups:

(1) Acute histoplasmosis frequently occurs in epidemics. It is a severe disease with marked prostration, fever, and occasional chest pain but no particular symptoms relative to the lungs even when x-rays show severe disseminated pneumonitis. The illness may last from 1 week to 6 months but is almost never fatal. (2) Acute progressive histoplasmosis is usually fatal within 6 weeks or less. Symptoms usually consist of fever, dyspnea, cough, loss of weight, and prostration. Diarrhea is usually present in children. Ulcers of the mucous membranes of the oropharynx may be present. The liver and spleen are nearly always enlarged, and all the organs of the body are involved. (3) Chronic progressive histoplasmosis may continue for years. It is usually seen in older patients with chronic obstructive lung disease. The lungs show chronic progressive changes, often with cavities. The disease closely resembles chronic tuberculosis, and occasionally the patient has both diseases. Chronic histoplasmosis appears to be primarily confined to the lungs, but all organs of the body are involved in the terminal stage.

**B. Laboratory Findings:** In the moderately to severely ill patient, the sedimentation rate is elevated. Leukopenia is present, with a normal differential count or neutropenia. Most patients with progressive disease show a progressive hypochromic anemia. Precipitating and complement-fixing antibodies can be demonstrated, and a change in titer is of use in prognosis.

## Treatment

There is no specific therapy. Bed rest and supportive care are indicated for the primary form. Normal activities should not be resumed until fever has subsided. Resection of lung tissue containing cavities has been useful. Amphotericin B (as for coccidioidomycosis) in a low total dose (150–500 mg) has given excellent results in severe acute pulmonary disease. Chronic histoplasmosis rarely relapses after a total dose of 2500 mg. In clinical trials, oral ketoconazole, 200 mg 30 minutes before breakfast, appeared useful for treatment of disseminated or progressive cavitary histoplasmosis in hosts who are not compromised but was not effective in compromised hosts.

## Prognosis

The prognosis is excellent for primary pulmonary histoplasmosis and poor in untreated generalized infection. Most cavities resolve with time and therapy.

Lowell JR, McLarty JW: Factors relating to recurrence of chronic pulmonary histoplasmosis following treatment with amphotericin B. *Am J Med Sci* 1983;**285**:13.

Mandell W, Goldberg DM, Neu HC: Histoplasmosis in patients with acquired immunodeficiency syndrome. *Am J Med* 1986;**81**:974.

Slama TG: Treatment of disseminated and progressive cavitary histoplasmosis with ketoconazole. (In: Symposium on ketoconazole therapy.) *Am J Med* 1983;**74(Suppl 1B)**:70.

# BLASTOMYCOSIS

*Blastomyces dermatitidis* causes this chronic systemic fungus infection. The disease occurs more often in men and in a geographically delimited area of the central and eastern USA and Canada. A few cases have been found in Mexico and Africa.

Mild or asymptomatic cases are rarely found. When dissemination takes place, lesions are most frequently seen on the skin, in bones, and in the urogenital system, although any or all organs or tissues of the body may be attacked.

Little is known concerning the mildest pulmonary phase of this disease. Cough, moderate fever, dyspnea, and chest pain are evident in symptomatic patients. These may disappear or may progress to a marked degree, with bloody and purulent sputum production, pleurisy, fever, chills, loss of weight, and prostration. Even serious pulmonary disease may be self-limiting. Radiologic studies usually reveal massive densities projecting irregularly from the mediastinal nodes, which are markedly enlarged. Raised, verrucous cutaneous lesions that have an abrupt downward sloping border are usually present in disseminated blastomycosis. The surface is covered with miliary pustules. The border extends slowly, leaving a central atrophic scar. In some patients, only cutaneous lesions are found. These may persist untreated for long periods, with a gradual decline in the patient's health. Bones—often the ribs and vertebrae—are frequently involved. These lesions appear both destructive and proliferative on radiography. Epididymitis, prostatitis, and other involvement of the male urogenital system may occur. Central nervous system involvement is not a common complication. The viscera may be invaded, but rarely the gastrointestinal tract.

Laboratory findings usually include leukocytosis, hypochromic anemia, and elevated sedimentation rate. The organism is found in clinical specimens as a 5- to 20-$\mu$m, thick-walled cell that may have a single bud. It grows readily on culture. Complement-fixing antibody titer is variable but useful for prognosis.

There is no specific therapy for blastomycosis. Amphotericin B (as for coccidioidomycosis) in a total dose of 1.5–2 g appears to be the best drug available for treatment. Ketoconazole is an effective alternative in immunocompetent patients with nonmeningeal disease. Large abscesses or bronchopleural fistulas require drainage or correction, but resection of residual lung cavities is not indicated.

Careful follow-up for early evidence of relapse should be made for several years so that therapy may be resumed or another drug instituted. Patients whose disease is limited to localized cutaneous lesions have the best prognosis in that they show a better immunologic response to their infection.

Ismail MA, Lerner SA: Disseminated blastomycosis in a pregnant woman: Review of amphotericin B usage during pregnancy. *Am Rev Respir Dis* 1982;**126**:350.

Kinasewitz GT, Penn RL, George RB: The spectrum and significance of pleural disease in blastomycosis. *Chest* 1984; **86:**580.

McManus EJ, James JM: The use of ketoconazole in the treatment of blastomycosis. *Am Rev Respir Dis* 1985;**133:**141.

National Institute of Allergy and Infectious Diseases Mycoses Study Group: Treatment of blastomycosis and histoplasmosis with ketoconazole: Results of a prospective randomized clinical trial. *Ann Int Med* 1985;**103:**861.

## PARACOCCIDIOIDOMYCOSIS
### (South American Blastomycosis)

*Paracoccidioides brasiliensis* infections have been found only in patients who have resided in South or Central America or Mexico. Long asymptomatic periods enable patients to travel far from the endemic areas. Ulceration of the nasoand oropharynx is usually the first symptom. Papules ulcerate and enlarge both peripherally and deeper into the subcutaneous tissue. Extensive coalescent ulcerations may eventually result in destruction of the epiglottis, vocal cords, and uvula. Extension to the lips and face may occur. Eating and drinking are extremely painful. Skin lesions, usually on the face, may occur. Variable in appearance, they may have a necrotic central crater with a hard hyperkeratotic border. Lymph node enlargement may follow mucocutaneous lesions, eventually ulcerating and forming draining sinuses. Lymph node enlargement may be the presenting symptom, with subsequent suppuration and rupture through the skin. In some patients, gastrointestinal disturbances are first noted. Although the liver and spleen become enlarged, there is a lack of specific gastrointestinal symptoms. Cough, sometimes with sputum, indicates pulmonary involvement, but the signs and symptoms are often mild, even though radiographic findings indicate severe parenchymatous changes in the lungs.

The extensive ulceration of the upper gastrointestinal tract prevents sufficient intake and absorption of food. Most patients become cachectic early. Death may result from respiratory failure or malnutrition.

Laboratory findings include elevated sedimentation rate, leukocytosis with a neutrophilia showing a shift to the left, and sometimes eosinophilia and monocytosis. Serologic results are variable. A high titer usually indicates progressive disease; a descending titer is a favorable sign. The fungus is found in clinical specimens as a spherical cell that may have many buds arising from it. Colonial and cellular morphology are typical on culture.

The prognosis for paracoccidioidomycosis treated with amphotericin B and sulfonamides has been poor, with 32% mortality after 1–2 years. Trials with oral ketoconazole, 200–400 mg daily 1–2 hours before breakfast, show a clinical response within 1 month and effective control after 6 months. The rare relapse responded to resumed ketoconazole therapy. No deaths and 91.6% sustained remissions were observed in 24 patients in the following 1–2 years.

Restrepo A et al: Treatment of paracoccidioidomycosis with ketoconazole: A three-year experience. (In: Symposium on ketoconazole therapy.) *Am J Med* 1983;**74(Suppl 1B):**48.

Restrepo A et al: Itraconazole in the treatment of paracoccidioidomycosis: A preliminary report. In: First International Symposium on Itraconazole. *Rev Infect Dis* 1987;**9(Suppl 1):**S51.

## SPOROTRICHOSIS

Sporotrichosis is a chronic fungal infection caused by *Sporothrix schenckii*. It is worldwide in distribution; most patients are people whose occupation brings them in contact with soil, plants, or decaying wood. Infection takes place when the organism is introduced by trauma into the skin—usually on the hand, arm, or foot.

The most common form of sporotrichosis begins with a hard, nontender subcutaneous nodule. This later becomes adherent to the overlying skin, ulcerates (chancriform), and may persist for a long time. Within a few days to weeks, similar nodules usually develop along the lymphatics draining this area, and these may ulcerate. The lymphatic vessels become indurated and are easily palpable. The infection usually ceases to spread before the regional lymph nodes are invaded, and blood-borne dissemination is rare. The general health of the patient is not affected. Some patients complain of considerable pain. Skin infection may not spread through the lymphatics but may appear only as warty or papular, scaly lesions that may become pustular.

Pulmonary sporotrichosis presents no characteristic findings. Patients may be asymptomatic, although pleural effusion, hilar adenopathy, fibrosis, caseous nodularity, and cavitation have been reported.

Disseminated sporotrichosis presents a picture of multiple, hard subcutaneous nodules scattered over the body. These become soft but rarely rupture spontaneously. Lesions may also develop in the bones, joints, muscles, and viscera.

Cultures are needed to establish diagnosis. A skin test with heat-killed vaccine or sporotrichin is positive.

Potassium iodide taken orally in increasing dosage promotes rapid healing, although the drug is not fungicidal. Give as the saturated solution, 5 drops 3 times a day, after meals, increasing by 1 drop per dose until 40 drops 3 times a day are being given. Continue until signs of the active disease have disappeared. The dosage is then decreased by 1 drop per dose until 5 drops are being given, and then is discontinued. Care must be taken to reduce the dosage if signs of iodism appear. Concurrent topical heat therapy has been useful. Oral ketoconazole has been effective in isolated cases of lymphocutaneous infection. Amphotericin B intravenously (as for coccidioidomycosis) has been effective in systemic infection. Surgery is usually contraindicated except for simple aspiration of secondary nodules.

The prognosis is good for all forms of sporotrichosis except the disseminated type.

England DM, Hochholzer L: *Sporothrix* infection of the lung without cutaneous disease: Primary pulmonary sporotrichosis. *Arch Pathol Lab Med* 1987;**111**:298.

Restrepo A et al: Itraconazole therapy in lymphangitic and cutaneous sporotrichosis. *Arch Dermatol* 1986;**122**:413.

Spiers EM et al: Sporotrichosis masquerading as pyoderma gangrenosum. *Arch Dermatol* 1987;**122**:691.

## CHROMOBLASTOMYCOSIS

Chromoblastomycosis is a chronic, principally tropical cutaneous infection caused by several species of closely related black molds (*Fonsecaea* spp and *Phialophora* sp). In nature, these fungi grow as filamentous saprophytes in soil and on decaying vegetation.

The disease progresses slowly before the development of clinically characteristic lesions.

Lesions occur most frequently on a lower extremity but may occur on the hands, arms, and elsewhere. The lesion begins as a papule or ulcer. Over a period of months to years the lesions enlarge to become vegetating, papillomatous, verrucous, elevated nodules with a cauliflowerlike appearance or widespread dry verrucous plaques. The latter lesions spread peripherally with a raised, verrucous border, leaving central atrophic scarring. The surface of the active border contains minute abscesses. Satellite lesions may appear along the lymphatics. There may be extensive secondary bacterial infection, with a resulting foul odor. Some patients complain of itching. Elephantiasis may result if there are marked fibrosis and lymph stasis in the limb.

The fungus is seen as brown, thick-walled, spherical, sometimes septate cells in pus. The type of reproduction found in culture determines the species.

Oral flucytosine, 150 mg/kg/d, thiabendazole, 25 mg/kg/d, itraconazole, 200 mg/d, and ketoconazole have proved effective. Surgical excision and skin grafting may be useful.

Prolonged topical heat therapy or intralesional amphotericin B have been successful.

Borelli D: A clinical trial of itraconazole in the treatment of deep mycoses and leishmaniasis. In: First International Symposium on Itraconazole. *Rev Infect Dis* 1987;**9(Suppl 1)**:S57.

McGinnis MR: Chromoblastomycosis and phaeohyphomycosis: New concepts, diagnosis, and mycology. *J Am Acad Dermatol* 1983;**8**:1.

## MYCETOMA
## (Maduromycosis & Actinomycotic Mycetoma)

Maduromycosis is the term used to describe mycetoma caused by the true fungi. Actinomycotic mycetoma is caused by *Nocardia* and *Actinomadura* spp. The many species of causative agents are found in soil. Organisms are introduced by trauma in barefoot people. Mycetoma may occur on the hands and other parts of the body also. With time, the subcutaneous lesions develop sinuses that drain to the surface as well as deep into muscle and bone. Granules (dense colonies of the agent in tissue) drain out in the pus.

The disease begins as a papule, nodule, or abscess that over months to years progresses slowly to form multiple abscesses and sinus tracts ramifying deep into the tissue. The entire area becomes indurated, and the skin becomes discolored. Open sinuses or atrophic scars are scattered over its surface. Secondary bacterial infection may result in large open ulcers. Radiographs show destructive changes in the underlying bone. Extensive fibrosis in the tissue causes elephantiasis. Pain is not a serious complaint until the disease is far advanced.

The agents occur as white, yellow, red, or black granules in the tissue or pus. Microscopic examination assists in the diagnosis. The granules of *Nocardia* and *Actinomadura* consist of delicate, gram-positive branching filaments 1 μm in diameter. Maduromycosis caused by the true fungi has granules consisting of filaments 5 μm in diameter sometimes cemented to large thick-walled cells.

The prognosis is good for patients with actinomycotic mycetoma, since they usually respond well to sulfonamides and sulfones, especially if treated early. Give trimethoprim-sulfamethoxazole, 2 tablets twice a day. Dapsone (Avlosulfon), 100 mg twice daily after meals, and other sulfones have been reported to be effective. All of these medications must be taken for long periods of time and continued for several months after clinical cure to prevent a relapse. Surgical procedures such as drainage assist greatly in healing.

There is no specific therapy for maduromycosis, and at present the prognosis is poor. Early trials indicate that itraconazole may have use. Sulfones have been reported to be effective in isolated cases. Surgical excision of early lesions may prevent spread. Amputation is necessary in far-advanced cases.

Borelli D: A clinical trial of itraconazole in the treatment of deep mycoses and leishmaniasis. In: First International Symposium on Itraconazole. *Rev Infect Dis* 1987;**9(Suppl 1)**:S57.

Tight RR, Bartlett MS: Actinomycetoma in the United States. *Rev Infect Dis* 1981;**3**:1139.

## ACTINOMYCOSIS*

*Actinomyces israelii* and other species of *Actinomyces* occur in the normal flora of the mouth and tonsillar crypts. *A israelii* and related species play a role in the production of normal dental plaque and also grow in tonsillar crypts. They are anaerobic, gram-positive, branching filamentous bacteria (1 μm in diameter) that may fragment into bacillary forms. In diseased tissue, these filaments are seen as a compact mass called a ''sulfur granule.'' When introduced

---

* Included in this chapter by convention, since these organisms were thought for many years to be fungi.

into traumatized tissue and associated with other anaerobic bacteria, these actinomycetes become pathogens. Hard, indurated, granulomatous suppurative lesions develop that give rise to sinus tracts.

The most common site of infection is the cervicofacial area (about 60% of cases), and infection typically follows extraction of a tooth or other trauma. Lesions may develop in the gastrointestinal tract or lungs following ingestion or aspiration of the fungus from its endogenous source in the mouth.

Cervicofacial actinomycosis develops slowly. The area becomes markedly indurated, and the overlying skin becomes reddish or cyanotic. The surface is irregular. Abscesses developing within and eventually draining to the surface persist for long periods. Sulfur granules may be found in the pus. There is usually little pain unless there is marked secondary infection. Trismus indicates that the muscles of mastication are involved. Radiography reveals eventual involvement of the bone, with rarefaction as well as some proliferation of the underlying bone.

Abdominal actinomycosis usually causes pain in the ileocecal region, spiking fever and chills, intestinal colic, vomiting, and weight loss. Irregular masses in the ileocecal area or elsewhere in the abdomen may be palpated. Pelvic inflammatory disease caused by actinomycetes is associated with prolonged use of an intrauterine contraceptive device. Sinuses draining to the exterior may develop. Radiography may reveal the mass or enlarged viscera. Vertebrae and pelvic bones may be invaded.

Thoracic actinomycosis begins with fever, cough, and sputum production. The patient becomes weak, loses weight, and may have night sweats and dyspnea. Pleural pain may be present. Multiple sinuses may extend through the chest wall, to the heart, or into the abdominal cavity. Ribs may be involved. Radiography shows massive areas of consolidation, frequently at the bases of the lungs.

The sedimentation rate may be elevated in patients with progressive disease. Anemia and leukocytosis are usually present. The anaerobic, gram-positive organism may be demonstrated as a granule or as scattered branching gram-positive filaments in the pus. Anaerobic culture is necessary to distinguish *Actinomyces* species from *Nocardia* species. Specific identification by culture is necessary to avoid confusion with nocardiosis, because specific therapy differs radically.

Penicillin G is the drug of choice. Ten to 20 million units are given via a parenteral route for 4–6 weeks. Continue treatment with penicillin V orally. Prolonged massive therapy is necessary in order to push effective levels of the drug into the abscesses where the organism is found. Sulfonamides may be added to the regimen, as well as streptomycin, which will control associated gram-negative organisms. Broad-spectrum antibiotics should be considered only if sensitivity tests show that the organism is resistant to penicillin. Immediate amelioration of symptoms or prompt improvement cannot be expected because of the chronic nature of this disease. Therapy should be continued for weeks to months after clinical manifestations have disappeared in order to ensure cure. Surgical procedures such as drainage and resection are of great benefit.

With penicillin and surgery, the prognosis is good. The difficulties of diagnosis, however, may permit extensive destruction of tissue before therapy is started.

Mongiardo N et al: Primary hepatic actinomycosis. *J Infect* 1986;**12**:65.

## OPPORTUNISTIC FUNGUS INFECTIONS

Debilitating diseases and often the drugs used in their treatment (corticosteroids, antibiotics, antimetabolites), as well as pregnancy and other altered physiologic states, may render a patient susceptible to invasion by many species of fungi that ordinarily are unable to cause disease. These factors may also cause infections due to the pathogenic fungi to be more serious. Early diagnosis and treatment are essential.

### 1. CANDIDIASIS

*Candida albicans* may be cultured in small numbers from the mouth, vagina, and feces of most people. It is more frequent in debilitated individuals. Thrush, vaginitis, cutaneous lesions (frequently in intertriginous areas), onychia, and paronychia are common. These are discussed elsewhere in this book. Yeasts are frequent secondary invaders in other infections. Patients most susceptible to the development of systemic candidiasis are (1) those with hematologic cancer, (2) those immunosuppressed by disease or therapy, (3) postoperative patients, and (4) those who have undergone prolonged antibiotic therapy.

Systemic infection is of 2 types. Endocarditis, which almost always affects previously damaged heart valves, usually follows heart surgery or inoculation by contaminated needles or catheters. Splenomegaly and petechiae are usual, and emboli are common. In the other type of systemic infection, upper gastrointestinal tract candidiasis is usually the source. Dissemination follows antibiotic or cytotoxic chemotherapy for serious debilitating disease; the eyes, kidneys, spleen, lungs, liver, and heart are most commonly involved. Fungiuria is usual in renal disease; however, especially in older persons, *Candida* can be found in the bladder or as a urethral saprophyte.

Bronchial or pulmonary infection is nearly always superimposed on other serious underlying disease.

If fungemia is suspected, an eye examination should be performed; if ocular lesions are noted, vigorous antifungal therapy should be instituted. The typical lesion of *Candida* chorioretinitis appears as a fluffy white area on the chorioretina and is commonly accompanied by an overlying vitreous haze.

*Candida albicans* is seen as gram-positive budding cells (2.5–6 μm) and as a pseudomycelium. It grows readily in culture. It is the most common cause of systemic disease, but *Candida tropicalis, Candida parapsilosis,* and *Torulopsis glabrata* are not uncommon. Many species may cause endocarditis. Serologic tests aid in diagnosis and prognosis.

Intravenous administration of amphotericin B (as for coccidioidomycosis) is necessary in serious systemic infections. When combined with flucytosine (Ancobon), 150 mg/kg/d orally, lower doses of this toxic drug may be used and still prevent emergence of resistant organisms. Associated oral, gastrointestinal, and cutaneous lesions should be treated with clotrimazole, nystatin, or miconazole mouthwash, tablets, and lotions. Gentian violet, 1%, in 10–20% alcohol, is also effective for oral, cutaneous, and vaginal lesions. Antibiotic therapy should be discontinued if possible. The correction of underlying factors may be sufficient to control candidiasis without specific therapy. Management of the severely immunocompromised patient includes prophylaxis with ketoconazole, clotrimazole, or nystatin.

Response to chemotherapy is poor in endocarditis. Valve replacement is usually necessary. In other systemic infections, the prognosis is good only if the underlying predisposing factors are corrected.

Smego RA, Perfect JR, Durack DT: Combined therapy with amphotericin B and 5-fluorocytosine for *Candida* meningitis. *Rev Infect Dis* 1984;**6**:791.

Walch TJ, Gray WC: *Candida* epiglottitis in immunocompromised patients. *Chest* 1987;**91**:482.

## 2. CRYPTOCOCCOSIS

*Cryptococcus neoformans,* an encapsulated budding yeast that has been found worldwide in soil and on dried pigeon dung, causes cryptococcosis. Disseminated infection usually involves the central nervous system.

Infections are acquired by inhalation. In the lung the infection may remain localized, heal, or disseminate. Upon dissemination, lesions may form in any part of the body, but involvement of the central nervous system is most common and is the usual cause of death. Generalized meningoencephalitis occurs more frequently than localized granuloma in the brain or spinal cord. Solitary localized lesions may develop in the skin and, rarely, in the bones and other organs.

Spontaneous resolution of some pulmonary cases of cryptococcosis has been reported. The incidence of fatal cases, on the other hand, is increasing as a result of increased numbers of infections in susceptible debilitated individuals (especially in leukemia and lymphoma).

In pulmonary cryptococcosis there are no specific signs or symptoms, and many patients are nearly asymptomatic. The patient may present with a subacute respiratory infection with low-grade fever, pleural pain, and cough. There may be sputum production. Physical examination usually reveals signs of bronchitis or pulmonary consolidation. Radiographs commonly show a solitary, moderately dense infiltration in the lower half of the lung field, with little or no hilar enlargement. More diffuse pneumonic infiltration, also in the lower lung fields, or extensive peribronchial infiltration or miliary lesions, may also occur.

Central nervous system involvement usually presents a history of recent upper respiratory or pulmonary infection. Increasingly painful headache is usually the first and most prominent symptom. Vertigo, nausea, anorexia, ocular disorders, and mental deterioration develop. Nuchal rigidity is present, and Kernig's and Brudzinski's signs are positive. Patellar and Achilles reflexes are often diminished or absent.

Acneiform lesions enlarge slowly and ulcerate, often coalescing with other lesions to cover a large area. Bone lesions are painful, and the area is often swollen. Eye involvement may result from direct extension along the subarachnoid space into the optic nerve.

A mild anemia, leukocytosis, and increased sedimentation rate are found. Spinal fluid findings include increased pressure, many white cells (usually lymphocytes), budding encapsulated fungus cells, increased protein and globulin, and decreased sugar and chlorides. Cryptococcal antigen in cerebrospinal fluid may be the only evidence for establishing a diagnosis in a living patient. Marked depletion of serum opsonins and complement occurs during fungemia.

A combination of amphotericin B (0.3 mg/kg/d administered as for coccidioidomycosis) and flucytosine (Ancobon), 150 mg/kg/d divided into 4 equal doses and given every 6 hours, may be curative in a 6-week regimen with a more rapid sterilization of cerebrospinal fluid. Experimental studies in mice show the combination of oral flucytosine and ketoconazole to be superior in cryptococcal meningitis. Oral ketoconazole is effective for nonmeningeal cryptococcosis. Surgical resection of pulmonary granulomas has been successful.

Craven PC, Graybill JR: Combination of oral flucytosine and ketoconazole as therapy for experimental cryptococcal meningitis. *J Infect Dis* 1984;**149**:584.

Polsky D et al: Intraventricular therapy of cryptococcal meningitis via a subcutaneous reservoir. *Am J Med* 1986;**81**:24.

Zugar A et al: Cryptococcal disease in patients with the acquired immunodeficiency syndrome: Diagnostic features and outcome of treatment. *Ann Intern Med* 1986;**104**:234.

## 3. NOCARDIOSIS*

*Nocardia asteroides* and *Nocardia brasiliensis,* aerobic filamentous soil bacteria, cause pulmonary and systemic nocardiosis. Bronchopulmonary abnor-

---

* Included in this chapter by convention, since these organisms were thought for many years to be fungi.

malities predispose to colonization, but infection is unusual without underlying immunosuppressive disease.

Pulmonary involvement usually begins with malaise, loss of weight, fever, and night sweats. Cough and production of purulent sputum are the chief complaints. Radiography shows massive areas of consolidation, usually at the base of both lungs. Small areas of rarefaction caused by abscess formation within these consolidated masses may lead to multiple cavities. The lesions may penetrate to the exterior through the chest wall, invading the ribs. Pleural adhesions are common.

Dissemination may involve any organ. Lesions in the brain or meninges are most frequent, and such dissemination may occur following any minor pulmonary symptoms. Dissemination is common in immunocompromised patients.

An increased sedimentation rate and leukocytosis with increase in neutrophils are found in systemic nocardiosis. *N asteroides* is usually found as delicate, branching, gram-positive filaments that may be partially acid-fast. Identification is made by culture.

Give trimethoprim-sulfamethoxazole, 2–8 tablets twice a day orally, depending on the patient's weight and renal function and the severity of disease. Sensitivity tests should be used to determine the appropriate antibiotic, which should be administered concurrently if needed. Response is slow, and therapy should be continued for months after all clinical manifestations have disappeared. In experimental cerebral nocardiosis of the rat, imipenem-cilastatin and amikacin appear more effective than trimethoprim-sulfamethoxazole or minocycline for treatment. Surgical procedures such as drainage and resection may be urgently required.

The prognosis in systemic nocardiosis is poor when diagnosis and therapy are delayed.

Meier, B et al: Successful treatment of a pancreatic *Nocardia asteroides* abscess with amikacin and surgical drainage. *Antimicrob Agents Chemother* 1986;**29**:150.

Gombert ME et al: Therapy of experimental cerebral nocardiosis with imipenem, amikacin, trimethoprim-sulfamethoxazole, and minocycline. *Antimicrob Agents Chemother* 1986; **30**:270.

Moeller CA, Burton CS: Primary lymphocutaneous *Nocardia brasiliensis* infection. *Arch Dermatol* 1986;**122**:1180.

## 4. ASPERGILLOSIS

*Aspergillus fumigatus* is the usual cause of aspergillosis, although many species may cause a wide spectrum of disease. Burn eschar and detritus in the external ear canal are often colonized by these fungi. Mere colonization of an ectatic bronchus to form a compact mass of mycelium ("fungus ball") is usually associated with some immunity, and the fungus rarely adheres to or penetrates the wall of the bronchus. A pulmonary toilet regimen appears the most effective management for patients with *Aspergillus*-colonized cavities.

Allergic bronchopulmonary aspergillosis results from colonization but leads to bronchiectasis and pulmonary fibrosis. Early diagnosis and effective steroid therapy are extremely important. Steroids may work by inhibiting toxic antigen-antibody reactions, which reduces the volume of bronchial sputum, making a less suitable culture medium for the growth of the fungus in the bronchi.

Invasive aspergillosis is a serious form of the disease in patients with cancer and marked granulocytopenia. First growing in necrotic tissue or pulmonary cavities produced by other causes, the hyphae most commonly invade pulmonary parenchyma, with subsequent hematologic dissemination to kidney and other organs. Early diagnosis by biopsy or serologic study is crucial. Amphotericin B instituted within 96 hours of onset of clinical infection has achieved the most favorable outcome. Daily doses as high as 0.8–1 mg/kg for the first 2 weeks have been used for fulminant infections. Concurrent flucytosine therapy is sometimes helpful. Experimental studies with itraconazole show promise. Management requires reduction of corticosteroid and cytotoxic chemotherapy, if possible. Thoracotomy with wedge resection is done for relapsing or medically recalcitrant lesions.

*Aspergillus* is recognized in tissue and sputum as dichotomously branched, septate hyphae. Serologic tests may be helpful in diagnosis.

Kravitz SP, Berry PL: Successful treatment of *Aspergillus* peritonitis in a child undergoing continuous cycling peritoneal dialysis. *Arch Intern Med* 1986;**14**:2061.

Slavin RG, Gottlieb CC, Avioli LV: Grand Rounds: Allergic bronchopulmonary aspergillosis. *Arch Intern Med* 1986, **146**:1799.

Van Cutsem J et al: Itraconazole, a new triazole that is orally active in aspergillosis. *Antimicrob Agents Chemother* 1984;**26**:527.

## 5. MUCORMYCOSIS

The term "mucormycosis" (zygomycosis, phycomycosis) is applied to opportunistic infections caused by members of the genera *Rhizopus, Mucor, Absidia,* and *Cunninghamella*. These appear in tissues as broad, branching nonseptate hyphae that may show a special affinity for blood vessels. Biopsy is almost always required for diagnosis. Sinus, orbit, and brain infections are most often associated with acidosis (usually diabetic). Pulmonary disease occurs in patients with leukemia or lymphoma or those who are seriously compromised in other ways (transplant patients). Cutaneous lesions occur as complications of burn wounds and as nosocomial infections from contaminated surgical tape. High-dosage amphotericin B therapy initiated early, control of diabetes or other underlying condition, and extensive surgical removal of necrotic, nonperfused tissue are essential features of good management. The prognosis is poor.

Rangel-Guerra R, Martinez HR, Saenz G: Mucormycosis: Report of 11 cases. *Arch Neurol* 1985;**42**:578.

## 6. MYCOTIC KERATITIS

*Candida albicans, Fusarium,* or *Aspergillus* is most often responsible for mycotic keratitis. Trauma to the cornea followed by corticosteroid and antibiotic therapy is often a predisposing factor. Prompt withdrawal of corticosteroids, removal of the infected necrotic tissue, other surgical procedures, and application of natamycin or ketoconazole are useful in management. Amphotericin B and flucytosine are used for fungal endophthalmitis. Natamycin does not penetrate corneal epithelium adequately for treatment of deep fungal keratitis or intraocular infections.

## REFERENCES

Dismukes WE et al: Treatment of systemic mycoses with ketoconazole: Emphasis on toxicity and clinical response in 52 patients. *Ann Intern Med* 1983;**98**:13.

Drugs for treatment of systemic fungal infections. *Med Lett Drugs Ther* 1986;**28**:4.

Holleran WM, Wilbur JR, DeGregorio MW: Empiric amphotericin B in patients with acute leukemia. *Rev Infect Dis* 1985;**7**:619.

Jones BR et al: Recognition and chemotherapy of oculomycosis. In: Symposium on antifungal therapy. Cartwright RY (editor). *Postgrad Med J* 1979;**55**:625.

Rippon JW: *Medical Mycology,* 2nd ed. Saunders, 1982.

Salaki JS, Louria DB, Chmel H: Fungal and yeast infections of the central nervous system. *Medicine* 1984;**63**:108.

Sanitato JJ, Kelley CG, Kaufman HE: Surgical management of peripheral fungal keratitis (keratomycosis). *Arch Ophthalmol* 1984;**102**:1506.

Travis LB, Roberts GD, Wilson WR: Clinical significance of *Pseudallescheria boydii:* A review of 10 years experience. *Mayo Clin Proc* 1985;**60**:531.

Weitzman I: Saprophytic molds as agents of cutaneous and subcutaneous infection of the immunocompromised host. *Arch Dermatol* 1986;**122**:1161.

# 28

# Anti-infective Chemotherapeutic & Antibiotic Agents

*Ernest Jawetz, MD, PhD, & Richard A. Jacobs, MD, PhD*

## Some Rules for Antimicrobial Therapy

Antimicrobial drugs are used on a very large scale, and their proper use gives striking therapeutic results. On the other hand, they can create serious untoward reactions and should therefore be administered only upon proper indication.

Drugs of choice and alternative drugs are presented in Table 28–1.

The following steps are required in each patient.

**A. Etiologic Diagnosis:** Formulate an etiologic diagnosis based on clinical observations. It is evident that microbial infections are best treated early. Therefore, the physician must attempt to decide on clinical grounds (1) whether the patient has a microbial infection that can be favorably influenced by antimicrobial drugs and (2) the most probable kind of microorganisms causing such infection (''best guess'').

**B. "Best Guess":** (Table 28–2) Select a specific antimicrobial drug on the basis of past experience for empiric therapy. Based on a ''best guess,'' the physician should choose a drug or combination of drugs that is likely to be effective against the suspected microorganisms.

**C. Laboratory Control:** Before beginning antimicrobial drug treatment, obtain meaningful specimens for laboratory examination to determine the causative infectious organism and, if desirable, its susceptibility to antimicrobial drugs.

**D. Clinical Response:** Based on the clinical response of the patient, evaluate the laboratory reports and consider the desirability of changing the antimicrobial drug regimen. Laboratory results should not automatically overrule clinical judgment. The isolation of an organism that confirms the initial clinical impression is useful. Conversely, laboratory results may contradict the initial clinical impression and may force its reconsideration. If the specimen was obtained from a site that is normally devoid of bacterial flora and not exposed to the external environment (eg, blood, cerebrospinal fluid, pleural fluid, joint fluid), the recovery of a microorganism is a significant finding even if the organism recovered is different from the clinically suspected etiologic agent, and this may force a change in antimicrobial treatment. On the other hand, the isolation of unexpected microorgan-

isms from the respiratory tract, gut, or surface lesions (sites that have a complex flora) must be critically evaluated before drugs are abandoned that were judiciously selected on the basis of an initial ''best guess'' for empiric treatment.

**E. Drug Susceptibility Tests:** Some microorganisms are fairly uniformly susceptible to certain drugs; if such organisms are isolated from the patient, they need not be tested for drug susceptibility. For example, group A hemolytic streptococci and most pneumococci and clostridia respond predictably to penicillin. On the other hand, some organisms (eg, enteric gram-negative rods) are so variable as to warrant drug susceptibility testing when they are isolated from a significant specimen.

Antimicrobial drug susceptibility tests may be done on solid media as ''disk tests,'' in broth in tubes, or in wells of microdilution plates. The latter method yields results expressed as MIC (minimal inhibitory concentration), and the technique can be modified to give MBC (minimal bactericidal concentration) results. In some infections, the MIC or MBC permits a better estimate of the amount of drug required for therapeutic effect in vivo.

Disk tests usually indicate whether an isolate is susceptible or resistant to serum concentrations of drug achieved in vivo with conventional dosage regimens, thus providing valuable guidance in selecting therapy. When there appear to be marked discrepancies between test results and clinical response of the patient, the following possibilities must be considered:

1. Choice of inappropriate drug, dosage, or route of administration.

2. Failure to drain a collection of pus or to remove a foreign body.

3. Failure of a poorly diffusing drug to reach the site of infection (eg, central nervous system) or to reach intracellular phagocytosed bacteria.

4. Superinfection in the course of prolonged chemotherapy. After suppression of the original infection or of normal flora, a second type of microorganism may establish itself against which the originally selected drug is ineffective.

5. Emergence of drug-resistant or tolerant organisms.

6. Participation of 2 or more microorganisms in

**Table 28–1.** Drug selection, 1986–1987. ($\pm$ = alone or combined with)

| Suspected or Proved Etiologic Agent | Drug(s) of First Choice | Alternative Drug(s) |
|---|---|---|
| **Gram-negative cocci** | | |
| Gonococcus | Amoxicillin + probenecid, ceftriaxone | Spectinomycin, cefoxitin |
| Meningococcus | Penicillin,[1] ceftriaxone | Sulfonamide,[2] chloramphenicol |
| **Gram-positive cocci** | | |
| Pneumococcus (*Streptococcus pneumoniae*) | Penicillin[1] | Erythromycin,[3] cephalosporin[4] |
| Streptococcus, hemolytic, groups A, C, G | Penicillin[1] | Erythromycin,[3] cephalosporin[4] |
| *Streptococcus viridans* | Penicillin,[1] $\pm$ aminoglycosides[5] | Cephalosporin,[4] vancomycin |
| *Staphylococcus*, non-penicillinase-producing | Penicillin[1] | Cephalosporin,[4] vancomycin |
| *Staphylococcus*, penicillinase-producing | Penicillinase-resistant penicillin[6] | Vancomycin, cephalosporin[4] |
| *Streptococcus faecalis;* streptococcus, hemolytic, group B | Ampicillin + aminoglycoside[5] | Vancomycin |
| **Gram-negative rods** | | |
| *Acinetobacter* (*Mima-Herellea*) | Aminoglycoside[5] $\pm$ imipenem | Minocycline, TMP-SMX[7] |
| *Bacteroides,* oropharyngeal strains | Penicillin,[1] clindamycin | Metronidazole, cephalosporin[4,8] |
| *Bacteroides,* gastrointestinal strains | Metronidazole, clindamycin | Cefoxitin, chloramphenicol |
| *Brucella* | Tetracycline[9] + streptomycin | TMP-SMX[7] |
| *Campylobacter* | Erythromycin[3] | Tetracycline[9] |
| *Enterobacter* | Newer cephalosporins[8] | Aminoglycoside,[5] TMP-SMX[7] |
| *Escherichia coli* (sepsis) | Aminoglycoside[5] $\pm$ ampicillin | Newer cephalosporins,[8] TMP-SMX[7] |
| *Escherichia coli* (first urinary tract infection) | Sulfonamide,[10] TMP-SMX[7] | Ampicillin, cephalosporin[4] |
| *Haemophilus* (meningitis, respiratory infections) | Ampicillin + chloramphenicol | Newer cephalosporins[8] |
| *Klebsiella* | Newer cephalosporins,[8] aminoglycoside[5] | Chloramphenicol, TMP-SMX[7] |
| *Legionella* sp (pneumonia) | Erythromycin[3] $\pm$ rifampin | TMP-SMX[7] |
| *Pasteurella* (*Yersinia*) (plague, tularemia) | Streptomycin, tetracycline[9] | Chloramphenicol |
| *Proteus mirabilis* | Ampicillin | Newer cephalosporins,[8] aminoglycoside[5] |
| *Proteus vulgaris* and other species | Newer cephalosporins[8] | Aminoglycosides[5] |
| *Pseudomonas aeruginosa* | Aminoglycoside[5] + ticarcillin | Newer cephalosporins[8] $\pm$ aminoglycoside |
| *Pseudomonas pseudomallei* (melioidosis) | Tetracycline,[9] TMP-SMX[7] | Chloramphenicol |
| *Pseudomonas mallei* (glanders) | Streptomycin + tetracycline[9] | Chloramphenicol |
| *Salmonella* | Chloramphenicol, ampicillin | TMP-SMX[7] |
| *Serratia, Providencia* | Newer cephalosporins,[8] aminoglycoside[5] | TMP-SMX[7] |
| *Shigella* | TMP-SMX,[7] chloramphenicol | Ampicillin, tetracycline[9] |
| *Vibrio* (cholera, sepsis) | Tetracycline[9] | TMP-SMX[7] |
| **Gram-positive rods** | | |
| *Actinomyces* | Penicillin[1] | Tetracycline[9] |
| *Bacillus* (eg, anthrax) | Penicillin[1] | Erythromycin[3] |
| *Clostridium* (eg, gas gangrene, tetanus) | Penicillin[1] | Metronidazole, cephalosporin[4] |
| *Corynebacterium* | Erythromycin[3] | Penicillin,[1] cephalosporin[4] |
| *Listeria* | Ampicillin + aminoglycoside[5] | Tetracycline,[9] TMP-SMX[7] |
| **Acid-fast rods** | | |
| *Mycobacterium tuberculosis* | INH + rifampin, INH + ethambutol[11] | Other antituberculosis drugs |
| *Mycobacterium leprae* | Dapsone + rifampin, clofazimine | Ethionamide |
| *Mycobacteria,* atypical | Rifampin + ethambutol + INH | Combinations |
| *Nocardia* | Sulfonamide[2] | Minocycline |
| **Spirochetes** | | |
| *Borrelia* (Lyme disease, relapsing fever) | Tetracycline[9] | Penicillin[1] |
| *Leptospira* | Penicillin[1] | Tetracycline[9] |
| *Treponema* (syphilis, yaws, etc) | Penicillin[1] | Erythromycin,[3] tetracycline[9] |
| **Mycoplasmas** | Erythromycin[3] | Tetracycline[9] |
| **Chlamydiae** (*C trachomatis, C psittaci*) | Tetracycline[9] | Erythromycin[3] |
| **Rickettsiae** | Tetracycline[9] | Chloramphenicol |

[1] Penicillin G is preferred for parenteral injection; penicillin V for oral administration—to be used only in treating infections due to highly sensitive organisms.

[2] Oral sulfisoxazole and trisulfapyrimidines are highly soluble in urine; parenteral sodium sulfadiazine can be injected intravenously in treating severely ill patients.

[3] Erythromycin estolate is best absorbed orally but carries the highest risk of hepatitis; erythromycin stearate and erythromycin ethylsuccinate are also available.

[4] Older cephalosporins are cephalothin, cefazolin, cephapirin, and cefoxitin for parenteral injection; cephalexin and cephradine can be given orally.

[5] Aminoglycosides—gentamicin, tobramycin, amikacin, netilmicin—should be chosen on the basis of local patterns of susceptibility.

[6] Parenteral nafcillin or oxacillin; oral dicloxacillin, cloxacillin, or oxacillin.

[7] TMP-SMX is a mixture of 1 part trimethoprim and 5 parts sulfamethoxazole.

[8] Newer cephalosporins (1987) include cefotaxime, cefoperazone, cefuroxime, ceftriaxone, ceftazidime, ceftizoxime, and still others.

[9] All tetracyclines have similar activity against microorganisms. Dosage is determined by rates of absorption and excretion of various preparations.

[10] First choice for previously untreated urinary tract infection is a highly soluble sulfonamide (see Note 2). TMP-SMX[7] is acceptable.

[11] Either or both.

**Table 28–2.** Examples of empiric choice of antimicrobials in acutely ill adults pending identification of causative organism.

| Suspected Clinical Diagnosis | Likely Etiologic Agents | Drugs of Choice | Alternative Drugs |
|---|---|---|---|
| (a) Meningitis, bacterial | Pneumococcus, meningococcus | Penicillin G, 2 million units IV every 2 hours | Chloramphenicol, 0.5 g IV every 6 hours, or cefuroxime, 1.5 g IV every 6 hours |
| (b) Meningitis, postoperative or posttraumatic | *Staphylococcus aureus,* pneumococcus, gram-negative bacteria | Penicillin G as in (a) + nafcillin, 1.5 g IV every 4 hours, + gentamicin, 1.7 mg/kg IV every 8 hours, + gentamicin,* 8 mg intrathecally once daily | Vancomycin, 0.5 g IV every 6 hours, + cefotaxime,† 3 g IV every 6 hours. |
| (c) Brain abscess | Mixed anaerobes, pneumococci, streptococci | Penicillin G as in (a) + chloramphenicol as in (a) | Metronidazole, 750 mg IV 3 times daily, + penicillin G as in (a) |
| (d) Pneumonia, acute, community-acquired, severe | Pneumococci, *Mycoplasma pneumoniae* | Penicillin G, 1 million units IV every 8 hours | Erythromycin, 0.5 g orally or IV 4 times daily |
| (e) Pneumonia, postoperative | *S aureus, Klebsiella,* mixed anaerobes | Nafcillin as in (b) + gentamicin* as in (b) + penicillin G as in (d) | Cefotaxime,† 2 g IV every 8 hours |
| (f) Pneumonia in chronic lung disease, aspiration | Pneumococci, *Haemophilus influenzae, S aureus,* mixed anaerobes | Ampicillin, 1 g IV every 6 hours, + nafcillin as in (b) | Cefuroxime† as in (a) + clindamycin, 600 mg IV every 8 hours |
| (g) Endocarditis, acute (including prosthetic or IV drug user) | *S aureus, Streptococcus faecalis,* gram-negative aerobic bacteria | Penicillin G as in (a) + nafcillin as in (b) + gentamicin* as in (b) | Gentamicin* as in (b) + vancomycin as in (b) |
| (h) Septic thrombophlebitis (eg, IV tubing, IV shunts) | *S aureus,* gram-negative aerobic bacteria | Nafcillin as in (b) + gentamicin* as in (b) | Vancomycin as in (b) + gentamicin* as in (b) |
| (i) Osteomyelitis | *S aureus* | Nafcillin as in (b) | Vancomycin as in (b) |
| (j) Septic arthritis | *S aureus, Neisseria gonorrhoeae* | Nafcillin as in (b) + penicillin G as in (a) | Vancomycin as in (b) + ceftriaxone,† 2 g IV every 12 hours |
| (k) Urinary tract infection, first episode, community-acquired | *Escherichia coli* | Sulfisoxazole, 1 g orally 4 times daily for 1–3 days | Ampicillin, 0.5 g orally 4 times daily for 1–3 days |
| (l) Pyelonephritis with flank pain and fever (recurrent UTI) | *E coli, Klebsiella, Enterobacter, Pseudomonas* | Gentamicin* as in (b) | Cefotaxime,† 2 g IV every 8 hours |
| (m) Suspected sepsis in neutropenic patient receiving cancer chemotherapy | *S aureus, Pseudomonas, Klebsiella, E coli* | Ticarcillin, 18 g IV daily + gentamicin* as in (b) + nafcillin as in (b) | Cefotaxime* as in (e) + vancomycin as in (b) + gentamicin as in (b) |
| (n) Intra-abdominal sepsis (eg, postoperative, peritonitis, cholecystitis) | Gram-negative aerobic bacteria, *Bacteroides,* anaerobic bacteria, streptococci, clostridia | Ampicillin as in (f) + gentamicin* as in (b) + metronidazole as in (c) | Clindamycin as in (f) + gentamicin* as in (b) |

* Depending on local drug susceptibility pattern, use tobramycin, 5–7 mg/kg/d, or amikacin, 15 mg/kg/d, in place of gentamicin.
† Cefotaxime, cefuroxime, ceftriaxone, ceftazidime, ceftizoxime, cefoperazone, or others, depending on local susceptibility patterns (see text).

the infectious process, of which only one was originally detected and used for drug selection.

**F. Adequate Dosage:** Adequacy of therapy is usually assessed by a favorable clinical response. In most infections, either a bacteriostatic or a bactericidal agent can be used. In some infections (eg, infective endocarditis), it is mandatory to kill the infecting organism to achieve a cure, and proper choice of drug and dose can be judged by "serum assay." Two days after initiation of a drug regimen, serum is obtained from the patient 1–2 hours after a drug dose. Dilutions of this serum are inoculated with the organism originally isolated from the patient, and antibacterial activity is estimated. If an adequate dose of a proper drug is being given, the serum will be bactericidal in a dilution of 1:5 or more. When potentially toxic drugs (eg, aminoglycosides, vancomycin) are used, the serum levels of the drug should be measured to avoid toxicity and ensure appropriate dosage. In patients with altered clearance of drugs, the dose or frequency of administration must be adjusted. This can sometimes be done by reference to dosage nomograms or formulas, but it is best to measure levels directly and adjust therapy accordingly (Table 28–3).

In renal failure, dosage must be adjusted as shown in Table 28–4.

**G. Duration of Antimicrobial Therapy:** Gener-

**Table 28–3.** Blood levels of some commonly used antibiotics at therapeutic dosages in adults.*

| | Route | Daily Dose | Expected Mean Concentration per mL Blood or per gram Tissue |
|---|---|---|---|
| Penicillin | IM | 0.6–1 million units | 1 unit (0.6 $\mu$g) |
| | Oral | 0.6 million units | 0.2 unit |
| Nafcillin | IV | 6–12 g | 5–30 $\mu$g |
| Dicloxacillin | Oral | 2–4 g | 3–12 $\mu$g |
| Ampicillin | Oral | 2–3 g | 3–4 $\mu$g |
| | IV | 4–6 g | 10–40 $\mu$g |
| Amoxicillin | Oral | 2 g | 8–10 $\mu$g |
| Carbenicillin | IV | 30 g | 100–200 $\mu$g |
| Ticarcillin | IV | 18 g | 100–200 $\mu$g |
| Tetracyclines | Oral | 2 g | 6–8 $\mu$g |
| Chloramphenicol | Oral | 2 g | 8–10 $\mu$g |
| Erythromycin | Oral | 2 g | 0.5–2 $\mu$g |
| Amikacin | IM | 1 g | 20–30 $\mu$g |
| Gentamicin, tobramycin | IM | 0.3 g | 3–6 $\mu$g |
| Vancomycin | IV | 2 g | 10–20 $\mu$g |
| Clindamycin | IV | 2.4 g | 3–6 $\mu$g |

* For cephalosporins, see text and Table 28–5.

ally, effective antimicrobial treatment results in reversal of the clinical and laboratory parameters of active infection and marked clinical improvement. However, varying periods of treatment may be required for cure. This is influenced by such factors as (1) the type of infecting organism (bacterial infections can be cured more rapidly than fungal or mycobacterial ones), (2) the location of the process (eg, endocarditis and osteomyelitis require prolonged therapy), and (3) the immunocompetence of the patient.

The following examples are illustrative: Streptococcal pharyngitis requires 10 days of effective penicillin levels to eradicate the organism. Acute uncomplicated gonorrhea can be cured in males in 24 hours. Endocarditis due to viridans streptococci is curable in 2–4 weeks; that caused by staphylococci requires 5–6 weeks of treatment. Acute uncomplicated cystitis in women often responds to a single dose of drug. Pneumococcal pneumonia and meningococcal meningitis require penicillin for only 3 days after complete defervescence.

To minimize untoward reactions from drugs and the risk of superinfection, treatment should be continued only as long as needed to eradicate the infection.

**H. Adverse Reactions:** All antimicrobials can cause adverse effects. Most commonly these are (1) hypersensitivity reactions (eg, fever, rashes, anaphylaxis), (2) direct toxicity (eg, diarrhea, vomiting, im-

pairment of renal or hepatic function, neurotoxicity), or (3) superinfection by drug-resistant microorganisms. Physicians prescribing antimicrobials must be familiar with the adverse effects associated with specific drugs.

When an adverse reaction develops, the physician must assess its severity and prognosis in the context of the infection being treated. If the infection is life-threatening and treatment cannot be stopped, the reactions must be managed symptomatically (especially if mild) or another drug must be chosen that does not cross-react with the offending one. (Table 28–1). If the infection is less severe, it may be possible to stop all antimicrobials and follow the patient carefully.

**I. Oral Antibiotics:** The absorption of oral penicillins, cephalosporins, macrolides, tetracyclines, lincomycins, etc, is impaired by food. Therefore, these oral drugs must be given between meals.

**J. Intravenous Antibiotics:** When an antibiotic must be administered intravenously (eg, for life-threatening infection or to sustain very high blood levels), the following cautions should be observed:

(1) Give in neutral solution (pH 7.0–7.2) of sodium chloride (0.9%) or dextrose (5%) in water.

(2) Give alone without admixture of any other substance in order to avoid chemical and physical incompatibilities (which are frequent). Help from the clinical pharmacist will avoid physiologic incompatibilities, a few of which are mentioned in the discussions of individual drugs.

(3) Administer by intermittent (every 2–6 hours) addition to the intravenous infusion ("bolus injection") to avoid inactivation (by temperature, changing pH, etc) and prolonged vein irritation from high drug concentration, which favors thrombophlebitis.

(4) The infusion site must be changed every 48 hours to reduce the chance of superinfection.

Bennett WM et al: Drug prescribing in renal failure: Dosing guidelines for adults. *Am J Kidney Dis* 1983;**3**:155.

Calderwood SB, Moellering RC: Common adverse effects of antibacterial agents on major organ systems. *Surg Clin North Am* 1980;**60**:65.

Mills J, Barriere SL, Jawetz E: Clinical use of antimicrobials. Chapter 52 in: *Basic & Clinical Pharmacology*, 3rd ed. Katzung BG (editor). Appleton-Lange, 1987.

Neu HC (guest editor): Impact of the patient at risk on current and future antimicrobial therapy. *Am J Med* 1984;**76**(No. 5A). [Entire issue.]

# PENICILLINS

The penicillins are a large group of antimicrobial substances, all of which share a common chemical nucleus (6-aminopenicillanic acid) that contains a $\beta$-lactam ring essential to their biologic activity. All $\beta$-lactam antibiotics inhibit formation of microbial cell walls. In particular, they block the final transpepti-

**Table 28–4.** Use of antibiotics in patients with renal failure.*

| | | Approximate Half-Life in Serum | | Proposed Dosage Regimen in Renal Failure | | Significant Removal of Drug by Dialysis (H = Hemodialysis; P = Peritoneal Dialysis) |
|---|---|---|---|---|---|---|
| | Principal Mode of Excretion or Detoxification | Normal | Renal Failure† | Initial Dose‡ | Give Half of Initial Dose at Interval of | |
| Penicillin G | Tubular secretion | 0.5 h | 6 h | 4 g IV | 8–12 h | H, P no |
| Ampicillin | Tubular secretion | 1 h | 8 h | 6 g IV | 8–12 h | H yes, P no |
| Carbenicillin, ticarcillin | Tubular secretion | 1.5 h | 16 h | 3–4 g IV | 12–18 h | H, P yes |
| Nafcillin | Liver 80%, kidney 20% | 0.5 h | 2 h | 2 g IV | 4–6 h | H, P no |
| Amikacin | Glomerular filtration | 2.5 h | 2–3 d | 15 mg/kg IM | 3 d | H, P yes |
| Tobramycin, gentamicin | Glomerular filtration | 2.5 h | 2–4 d | 3 mg/kg IM | 2–3 d | H, P yes§ |
| Vancomycin | Glomerular filtration | 6 h | 6–9 d | 1 g IV | 5–8 d | H, P no |
| Tetracycline | Glomerular filtration | 8 h | 3 d | 1 g orally or 0.5 g IV | 3 d | H yes, P no |
| Chloramphenicol | Mainly liver | 3 h | 4 h | 1 g orally or IV | 8 h | H, P no |
| Erythromycin | Mainly liver | 1.5 h | 5 h | 1 g orally or IV | 8 h | H, P no |
| Clindamycin | Glomerular filtration and liver | 2.5 h | 4 h | 600 mg IV or IM | 8 h | H, P no |

* For cephalosporins, see text and Table 28–5.
† Considered here to be marked by creatinine clearance of 10 mL/min or less.
‡ For a 60-kg adult with a serious systemic infection. The "initial dose" listed is administered as an intravenous infusion over a period of 1–8 hours, or as 2 intramuscular injections during an 8-hour period, or as 2–3 oral doses during the same period.
§ Aminoglycosides are removed irregularly in peritoneal dialysis. Gentamicin is removed 60% in hemodialysis.

dation reaction in the synthesis of cell wall mucopeptide (peptidoglycan), and they activate autolytic enzymes in the cell wall. These reactions result in cell death.

## Antimicrobial Activity

The initial step in penicillin action is the binding of the drug to receptors, penicillin-binding proteins, some of which are transpeptidation enzymes. The penicillin-binding proteins of different organisms differ in number and in affinity for a given drug. After penicillins have attached to receptors, peptidoglycan synthesis is inhibited because the activity of transpeptidation enzymes is blocked. The final bactericidal action is the removal of an inhibitor of the autolytic enzymes in the cell wall, which activates the enzymes and results in cell lysis. Organisms that are defective in autolysin function are inhibited but not killed by β-lactam antibiotics ("tolerance"). Organisms that produce β-lactamases (penicillinases) are resistant to some penicillins because the β-lactam ring is broken and the drug inactivated. Only organisms that are actively synthesizing peptidoglycan (in the process of multiplication) are susceptible to β-lactam antibiotics. Nonmultiplying organisms or those lacking cell walls (L forms) are not susceptible but may act as "persisters."

One million units of penicillin G equals 0.6 g. Other penicillins are prescribed in grams. A blood level of 0.01–1 μg/mL of penicillin G or ampicillin is lethal for a majority of susceptible microorganisms.

Most β-lactamase-resistant penicillins are 5–50 times less active.

Penicillins can be arranged into groups:

1. Highest activity against gram-positive bacteria; little activity against most gram-negative rods. Susceptible to hydrolysis by β-lactamases, eg, penicillin G, benzathine penicillin.

2. Relatively resistant to β-lactamases but less active against gram-positive organisms and inactive against gram-negative ones, eg, nafcillin.

3. Relatively high activity against both gram-positive and gram-negative organisms but destroyed by β-lactamases (penicillinases), eg, ampicillin, amoxicillin, carbenicillin, ticarcillin, piperacillin.

4. Stable to gastric acid and suitable for oral administration, eg, penicillin V, cloxacillin, ampicillin.

## Resistance

Resistance to penicillins falls into several categories:

1. Production of β-lactamases, eg, by staphylococci, gonococci, *Haemophilus*, coliform organisms.

2. Lack of penicillin receptors (eg, resistant pneumococci) or impermeability of cell envelope so that penicillins cannot reach receptors (eg, metabolically inactive bacteria).

3. Failure of activation of autolytic enzymes in the cell wall; "tolerance," eg, in staphylococci, group B streptococci.

4. Cell wall-deficient (L) forms or mycoplasmas, which do not synthesize peptidoglycans.

## Absorption, Distribution, & Excretion

After parenteral administration, absorption of most penicillins is complete and rapid. Because of the irritation and consequent local pain produced by the intramuscular injection of large doses, administration by the intravenous route (intermittent bolus addition to a continuous infusion) is often preferred. After oral administration, only a portion of the dose is absorbed—from 5 to 35%, depending upon acid stability, binding to foods, and the presence of buffers. In order to minimize binding to foods, oral penicillins should not be preceded or followed by food for at least 1 hour.

After absorption, penicillins are widely distributed in body fluids and tissues. This varies to some extent with the degree of protein binding exhibited by different penicillins. Penicillin G and ampicillin are moderately protein-bound (40–60%), whereas cloxacillin and nafcillin are highly protein-bound (95–98%). With parenteral doses of 5–10 million units (3–6 g) of penicillin G per 24 hours, injected in divided doses intramuscularly or added to intravenous infusions, average serum levels of the drug reach 1–10 units (0.6–6 µg)/mL. A rough relationship of 6 g given parenterally per day yielding serum levels of 1–6 µg/mL also applies to other penicillins. The highly serum-bound penicillins yield, on the average, lower levels of free drug than less strongly bound penicillins.

Special dosage forms of penicillin permit delayed absorption to yield low blood and tissue levels for long periods. The best example is benzathine penicillin G. After a single intramuscular injection of 1.2 million units (0.75 g), serum levels in excess of 0.03 unit/mL are maintained for 10 days and levels in excess of 0.005 unit/mL for 3 weeks. The latter is sufficient to protect against beta-hemolytic streptococcal infection; the former, to treat an established infection with these organisms. Procaine penicillin also has delayed absorption, yielding levels for 24 hours.

In many tissues, penicillin concentrations are equal to those in serum. Lower levels are found in the eye, prostate, and central nervous system. However, with active inflammation of the meninges, as in bacterial meningitis, penicillin levels in the cerebrospinal fluid exceed 0.2 µg/mL with a daily parenteral dose of 12 g. Thus, pneumococcal and meningococcal meningitis may be treated with systemic penicillin, and intrathecal injection is contraindicated. Penetration into inflamed joints is likewise sufficient for treatment of infective arthritis caused by susceptible organisms.

Most of the absorbed penicillin is rapidly excreted by the kidneys into the urine; small amounts are excreted by other channels. About 10% of renal excretion is by glomerular filtration and 90% by tubular secretion, to a maximum of about 2 g/h in an adult.

Tubular secretion can be partially blocked by probenecid (Benemid), 0.5 g (10 mg/kg) every 6 hours orally, to achieve higher systemic levels. Renal clearance is less efficient in the newborn, so that proportionately smaller doses result in higher systemic levels and are maintained longer than in the adult. Individuals with impaired renal function likewise tend to maintain higher penicillin levels longer.

Renal excretion of penicillin results in very high levels in the urine. Thus, systemic daily doses of 6 g of penicillin may yield urine levels of 500–3000 µg/mL; this is enough to suppress not only gram-positive but also many gram-negative bacteria in the urine (provided they produce little β-lactamase).

Penicillin is also excreted into sputum and milk to levels of 3–15% of those present in the serum. This is the case in both humans and cattle. The presence of penicillin in the milk of cows treated for mastitis presents a problem in allergy.

## Indications, Dosages, & Routes of Administration

**A. Penicillin G:** This is the drug of choice for infections caused by pneumococci, streptococci, meningococci, non-β-lactamase-producing staphylococci and gonococci, *Treponema pallidum* and many other spirochetes, *Bacillus anthracis* and other gram-positive rods, clostridia, *Actinomyces,* and *Bacteroides* (except *Bacteroides fragilis*).

**1. Intramuscular or intravenous–**Most of the above-mentioned infections respond to aqueous penicillin G in daily doses of 0.6–5 million units (0.36–3 g) administered by intermittent intramuscular injection every 4–6 hours. Much larger amounts (6–24 million units) can be given by intermittent intravenous infusion every 2–4 hours in serious or complicated infections due to these organisms. Sites for such intravenous administration are subject to thrombophlebitis and superinfection and must be rotated every 2 days and kept scrupulously aseptic. In enterococcal endocarditis, an aminoglycoside is given simultaneously with large doses of a penicillin.

**2. Oral–**Penicillin V is indicated only in minor infections (eg, of the respiratory tract or its associated structures) in daily doses of 1.6–6.4 million units (1–4 g). About one-fifth of the oral dose is absorbed, but oral administration is so unreliable that it should not be relied upon in seriously ill patients.

**3. Intrathecal–**With high serum levels of penicillin, adequate concentrations reach the central nervous system and cerebrospinal fluid for the treatment of central nervous system infection. Therefore, and because injection of more than 10,000 units of penicillin G into the subdural space may cause convulsions, intrathecal injection has been virtually abandoned.

**4. Topical–**Penicillins are highly sensitizing and should not be applied to the skin. Rarely, solutions of penicillin (eg, 100,000 units/mL) are instilled into a joint or wound or into the pleural space.

**B. Benzathine Penicillin G:** This penicillin is

a salt of very low water solubility. It is injected intramuscularly to establish a depot that yields low but prolonged drug levels. A single injection of 1.2 million units intramuscularly is satisfactory for treatment of beta-hemolytic streptococcal pharyngitis. An injection of 1.2–2.4 million units every 3–4 weeks provides satisfactory prophylaxis for rheumatics against reinfection with group A streptococci. Syphilis can be treated with benzathine penicillin, 2.4 million units intramuscularly weekly for 1–3 weeks, depending on the stage of the disease. There is no indication for using this drug by mouth. Procaine penicillin G is another repository form for maintaining drug levels for up to 24 hours. For highly susceptible infections, 600,000 units intramuscularly is given once daily. For uncomplicated gonorrhea, 4.8 million units of procaine penicillin is given once intramuscularly with probenecid, 1 g orally.

**C. Ampicillin, Amoxicillin, Carbenicillin, Ticarcillin, Piperacillin, Mezlocillin, Azlocillin:** These drugs have greater activity against gram-negative aerobes than penicillin G but are destroyed by penicillinases (β-lactamases).

Ampicillin, 500 mg orally every 6 hours, is used to treat common urinary tract infections with susceptible gram-negative bacteria or mixed secondary bacterial infections of the respiratory tract (eg, sinusitis, bronchitis, otitis). Ampicillin, 300 mg/kg/d intravenously, is a current choice for bacterial meningitis in children, especially if the disease is caused by *Listeria* or *H influenzae*. However, β-lactamase-producing *Haemophilus* organisms are now occurring more frequently; therefore, either chloramphenicol is given concurrently or ceftriaxone or cefuroxime is used.

Ampicillin is ineffective against *Enterobacter, Pseudomonas,* and indole-positive *Proteus* infections. In systemic *Salmonella* infections (including typhoid and paratyphoid fevers), ampicillin, 6–12 g/d intravenously, is effective therapy if the organism is susceptible. Prolonged oral administration of ampicillin can eradicate the organism from the stool in some chronic carriers. For *Salmonella* gastroenteritis, antimicrobial therapy is usually not needed. In severely malnourished children with salmonellosis, ampicillin, 100 mg/kg/d intramuscularly, was effective.

Amoxicillin (500 mg orally every 8 hours) is better absorbed than ampicillin. The spectrum, activity, and side effects are comparable. A single dose of amoxicillin, 3 g orally, plus probenecid, 1 g orally, is effective in uncomplicated gonorrhea. Bacampicillin and pivampicillin have therapeutic effects comparable to those of ampicillin but can be administered orally every 12 hours (400–800 mg) to achieve adequate tissue concentrations.

Carbenicillin resembles ampicillin but has more marked activity against *Pseudomonas* and *Proteus,* although *Klebsiella* organisms are usually resistant. Ticarcillin resembles carbenicillin but gives higher tissue levels. In susceptible populations of *Pseudomonas* organisms, resistance to these drugs may emerge

rapidly. Therefore, in *Pseudomonas* sepsis (eg, burns, leukemia), carbenicillin, 30 g/d (300–500 mg/kg/d), or ticarcillin, 18 g/d (200–300 mg/kg/d), intravenously is usually combined with tobramycin, 5–7 mg/kg/d, to delay emergence of resistance and perhaps to obtain synergistic effects. Carbenicillin indanyl sodium is acid-stable and can be given orally for urinary tract infections.

Piperacillin, mezlocillin, and azlocillin all resemble ticarcillin but are somewhat more active against some gram-negative aerobes, especially *Pseudomonas*. Hetacillin is converted to ampicillin in vivo and has no advantage.

**D. β-Lactamase-Resistant Penicillins:** Methicillin, oxacillin, cloxacillin, dicloxacillin, nafcillin, and others are relatively resistant to destruction by β-lactamase. These drugs are limited to the treatment of infections due to β-lactamase-producing staphylococci. The combination of amoxicillin or ticarcillin with clavulanate can also be effective in infections due to β-lactamase-producing *Haemophilus* sp or *Branhamella catarrholis,* particularly sinusitis and otitis media.

**1. Oral**–Oxacillin, cloxacillin, dicloxacillin, or nafcillin may be given in doses of 0.25–0.5 g every 4–6 hours in mild or localized staphylococcal infections (50–100 mg/kg/d for children). Food must not be given within an hour of these doses, because it interferes with absorption.

**2. Intravenous**–For serious systemic staphylococcal infections, nafcillin, 6–12 g, is administered intravenously in 4–6 divided doses daily. The dose for children is nafcillin, 50–100 mg/kg/d. Eighty percent of nafcillin is excreted into the biliary tract, and only 20% is cleared by tubular secretion. Thus, the action of nafcillin is little affected by renal failure.

## Adverse Effects

The penicillins undoubtedly possess less direct toxicity than any other antibiotics. Most of the serious side effects are due to hypersensitivity.

**A. Allergy:** All penicillins are cross-sensitizing and cross-reacting. Any preparation containing penicillin may induce sensitization, including foods or cosmetics. In general, sensitization occurs in proportion to the duration and total dose of penicillin received in the past. The responsible antigenic determinants appear to be degradation products of penicillins, particularly penicilloic acid and products of alkaline hydrolysis (minor antigenic determinants) bound to host protein. Skin tests with penicilloyl-polylysine, with minor antigenic determinants, and with undegraded penicillin can identify many hypersensitive individuals. Among positive reactors to skin tests, the incidence of subsequent immediate severe penicillin reactions is high. Although many persons develop IgG antibodies to antigenic determinants of penicillin, the presence of such antibodies is not correlated with allergic reactivity (except rare hemolytic anemia), and serologic tests have little predictive value. A history of a penicillin reaction in the past is not reliable;

however, it there is a history of a severe reaction (anaphylaxis), the drug should be administered with caution (airway, 0.1% epinephrine in syringe, competent personnel available, intravenous fluids running), or a substitute drug should be given.

Allergic reactions may occur as typical anaphylactic shock, typical serum sickness type reactions (urticaria, fever, joint swelling, angioneurotic edema, intense pruritus, and respiratory embarrassment occurring 7–12 days after exposure), and a variety of skin rashes, oral lesions, fever, interstitial nephritis, eosinophilia, hemolytic anemia, other hematologic disturbances, and vasculitis. The incidence of hypersensitivity to penicillin is estimated to be 1–5% among adults in the USA but is negligible in small children. Acute anaphylactic life-threatening reactions are fortunately very rare (0.05%). Ampicillin produces maculopapular skin rashes more frequently than other penicillins, but some ampicillin rashes are not allergic in origin. Methicillin and other penicillins can induce nephritis with primary tubular lesions associated with anti-basement membrane antibodies. Nafcillin is less nephrotoxic than methicillin.

Individuals known to be hypersensitive to penicillin can at times tolerate the drug during corticosteroid administration. "Desensitization" is only infrequently warranted.

**B. Toxicity:** Since the action of penicillin is directed against a unique bacterial structure, the cell wall, it is virtually without effect on animal cells. The toxic effects of penicillin G are due to the direct irritation caused by intramuscular or intravenous injection of exceedingly high concentrations (eg, 1 g/mL). Such concentrations may cause local pain, induration, thrombophlebitis, or degeneration of an accidentally injected nerve. All penicillins are irritating to the central nervous system. There is no indication for intrathecal administration at present. In rare cases, a patient with renal insufficiency receiving large doses may exhibit signs of cerebrocortical irritation as a result of passage of unusually large amounts of penicillin into the central nervous system. With doses of this magnitude, direct cation toxicity ($Na^+$, $K^+$) can also occur. Potassium penicillin G contains 1.7 mEq of $K^+$ per million units (2.8 mEq/g), and potassium may accumulate in renal failure. Carbenicillin contains 4.7 mEq of $Na^+$ per gram—a risk in heart failure.

Large doses of penicillins given orally may lead to gastrointestinal upset, particularly nausea and diarrhea. This is most pronounced with the broad-spectrum penicillins—ampicillin or amoxicillin—and may be due to overgrowth of staphylococci, *Pseudomonas,* clostridia, or yeasts or to toxin production by *C difficile.* Superinfections in other organ systems may occur with penicillins as with any other antibiotic. Methicillin, nafcillin, and carbenicillin can cause granulocytopenia. Carbenicillin and ticarcillin can produce hypokalemic alkalosis and elevation of serum transaminases and can damage platelets or induce hemostatic defects leading to bleeding tendency.

Finegold SM et al: Comparative trial of bacampicillin and amoxicillin in bacterial infections of the lower respiratory tract. *Rev Infect Dis* 1981;**3:**150.

Nolan CM, Abernathy RS: Nephropathy associated with methicillin therapy. *Arch Intern Med* 1977;**137:**997.

Parker CW: Drug allergy. (3 parts.) *N Engl J Med* 1975; **292:**511, 732, 957.

Roselle GA et al: Clinical trial of the efficacy and safety of ticarcillin and clavulanic acid. *Antimicrob Agents Chemother* 1985;**27:**291.

Wendel GD et al: Penicillin allergy and desensitization in serious infections during pregnancy. *N Engl J Med* 1985;**312:**1229.

## CEPHALOSPORINS

The cephalosporins are structurally related to the penicillins. They consist of a β-lactam ring attached to a dihydrothiazoline ring. Substitutions of chemical groups at various positions on the basic structure have resulted in a proliferation of drugs with varying pharmacologic properties and antimicrobial activities.

The mechanism of action of cephalosporins is analogous to that of the penicillins: (1) binding to specific penicillin-binding proteins that serve as drug receptors on bacteria, (2) inhibition of cell wall synthesis, and (3) activation of autolytic enzymes in the cell wall that result in bacterial death. Resistance to cephalosporins may be due to poor permeability of the drug into bacteria, lack of penicillin-binding proteins, or degradation by β-lactamases.

Cephalosporins have been divided into 3 major groups or "generations" (Table 28–5) based mainly on their antibacterial activity: First-generation cephalosporins have good activity against aerobic gram-positive organisms and many community-acquired gram-negative organisms; second-generation drugs have a slightly extended spectrum against gram-negative bacteria, and some are active against anaerobes; and third-generation cephalosporins have less activity against gram-positives but are extremely active against most gram-negative bacteria. Not all cephalosporins fit neatly into this grouping, and there are exceptions to the general characterization of the drugs in the individual classes; however, the generational classification of cephalosporins is useful for discussion purposes.

**Table 28–5.** Major groups of cephalosporins.

| First Generation | Second Generation | Third Generation |
|---|---|---|
| Cephalothin | Cefamandole | Cefotaxime |
| Cephapirin | Cefuroxime | Ceftizoxime |
| Cefazolin | Cefonicid | Ceftriaxone |
| Cefalexin* | Ceforanide | Ceftazidime |
| Cephradine* | Cefaclor* | Cefoperazone |
| Cefadroxil* | Cefoxitin | Moxalactam |
| | Cefotetan | |

* Oral agents.

## 1. FIRST-GENERATION CEPHALOSPORINS

### Antimicrobial Activity

These drugs are very active against gram-positive cocci, including pneumococci, viridans streptococci, group A hemolytic streptococci, and *S aureus.* Like all cephalosporins, they are inactive against entero-cocci and methicillin-resistant staphylococci. Among gram-negative bacteria, *E coli, K pneumoniae,* and *P mirabilis* are usually sensitive except for some hospital-acquired strains. There is very little activity against such gram-negatives as *P aeruginosa,* indole-positive *Proteus* sp, *Enterobacter* spp, *Serratia marcescens, Citrobacter* spp, and *Acinetobacter* spp. Anaerobic cocci are usually sensitive, but *Bacteroides fragilis* is not.

### Pharmacokinetics & Administration

**A. Oral:** Cephalexin, cephradine, and cefadroxil are absorbed from the gut to a variable extent. After a 500-mg oral dose, serum levels range from 15 to 20 $\mu$g/mL. Urine concentrations are usually very high, but in other tissues the levels are variable and usually lower than in the serum. Cephalexin and cephradine are given orally in doses of 0.25–0.5 g 4 times daily (15–30 mg/kg/d). Cefadroxil has a longer half-life and can be given in doses of 0.5–1 g twice daily. Dosage should be reduced in renal insufficiency: for $Cl_{cr}$ 20–50 mL/min, give half the normal dose; for $Cl_{cr}$ < 20 mL/min, give one-fourth the normal dose.

**B. Intravenous:** Cefazolin has a longer half-life than cephalothin or cephapirin. After an intravenous infusion of 1 g, the peak serum level of cefazolin is 90–120 $\mu$g/mL, whereas cephalothin and cephapirin reach levels of 40–60 $\mu$g/mL. The usual doses of cefazolin for adults are 1–2 g intravenously every 8 hours (50–100 mg/kg/d) and for cephalothin and cephapirin 1–2 g every 4–6 hours (50–200 mg/kg/d). In patients with impaired renal function, dosage adjustment somewhat as for oral dosage is needed.

**C. Intramuscular:** Both cephapirin and cefazolin can be given intramuscularly, but pain on injection is less with cefazolin.

### Clinical Uses

Although the first-generation cephalosporins have a broad spectrum of activity and are relatively non-toxic, they are rarely the drugs of choice. Oral drugs are indicated for treatment of urogenital infections in patients who are allergic to sulfonamides or penicillins, and they can be used for minor staphylococcal infections in penicillin-allergic patients. Oral cephalosporins may also be preferred for minor polymicrobial infections (eg, cellulitis, soft tissue abscess). Oral cephalosporins should not be relied on in serious systemic infections.

Intravenous first-generation cephalosporins penetrate most tissues well and are the drugs of choice for surgical prophylaxis, particularly surgery undertaken for placement of a prosthesis. More expensive second- and third-generation cephalosporins offer no advantage over the first-generation drugs for surgical prophylaxis and should not be used for that purpose.

Other major uses of intravenous first-generation cephalosporins include infections for which they are the least toxic drugs (eg, *Klebsiella* infections) and infections in persons with a history of *mild* penicillin allergy (not anaphylaxis).

First-generation cephalosporins do not penetrate into the cerebrospinal fluid and cannot be used to treat meningitis.

## 2. SECOND-GENERATION CEPHALOSPORINS

Second-generation cephalosporins are a heterogeneous group with marked individual differences in activity, pharmacokinetics, and toxicity. In general, all of them are active against organisms also covered by first-generation drugs, but they have an extended gram-negative coverage. *Enterobacter* spp, indole-positive *Proteus,* and *Klebsiella* spp (including cephalothin-resistant strains) are usually sensitive. Cefamandole, cefuroxime, cefonicid, ceforanide, and cefaclor are active against *H influenzae,* including β-lactamase-producing strains, but have little activity against *Serratia* and *B fragilis.* In contrast, cefoxitin and cefotetan are active against *B fragilis* and some strains of *Serratia* but have poor activity against *Enterobacter* and *H influenzae.* Against gram-positive organisms, these drugs are less active than the first-generation cephalosporins. Like the latter, second-generation drugs have no activity against *P aeruginosa* or enterococci.

### Pharmacokinetics & Administration

**A. Oral:** Only cefaclor can be given orally; it is available as capsules (0.25 or 0.5 g) and in suspension (0.125 or 0.25 g/5 mL). The usual dose is 10–15 mg/kg/d in 3 or 4 divided doses for adults and 20–40 mg/kg/d up to a maximum of 1 g/d for children.

**B. Intravenously and Intramuscularly:** These agents can be injected. After an intravenous infusion of 1 g, serum levels range from 75 to 125 $\mu$g/mL. (Cefonicid reaches 200–250 $\mu$g/mL.) Because of differences in drug half-life and protein binding, intervals between doses vary greatly (see Table 28–6). For cefoxitin or cefamandole (short half-lives), the interval is 4–6 hours: cefoxitin, 50–200 mg/kg/d; cefamandole, 75–200 mg/kg/d.

Drugs with longer half-lives can be injected less frequently: cefuroxime, 0.75–1.5 g every 8–12 hours; cefotetan, 1–2 mg every 8–12 hours; cefonicid or ceforanide, 1–2 g (15–30 mg/kg/d) once or twice daily. In renal failure, dosage adjustments are required.

### Clinical Uses

Because of its activity against β-lactamase-produc-

**Table 28–6.** Pharmacology of the cephalosporins.

| Drug | Peak Serum Level (\mu\g/mL) After 1 g IV | Serum Half-Life (min) | Total Daily Dose (g) | Dosage Interval (Hours) | Dosage Adjustments in Renal Failure | | |
|---|---|---|---|---|---|---|---|
| | | | | | Moderate (Cl$_{cr}$ 10–50 mL/min) | Severe (Cl$_{cr}$ < 10 mL/min) | Post-Hemodialysis Dose |
| Cephalothin, cephapirin | 40–60 | 40 | 4–12 | 4–6 | 1–2 g every 6–12 hours | 1 g every 12 hours | 1 g |
| Cefazolin | 90–120 | 90 | 2–6 | 8 | 0.5–1 g every 12 hours | 0.5 g daily | 0.5 g |
| Cephalexin, cephradine* | 15–20 | 50–60 | 1–4 | 6 | 0.25–0.5 g every 8–12 hours | 0.25–0.5 g daily | 0.5 g |
| Cefadroxil* | 15 | 75 | 1–2 | 12–24 | 1 g daily | 0.5 g daily | 0.5 g |
| Cefamandole, cefoxitin | 60–80 | 45 | 4–12 | 6–8 | 1 g every 12 hours | 1–2 g daily | 0.5 g |
| Cefuroxime | 80–100 | 80 | 1.5–6 | 6–12 | 1 g every 12 hours | 1–2 g daily | 0.5 g |
| Cefonicid | 200–250 | 240 | 1–2 | 24 | 0.5 g daily | 1 g every 72 hours | 0.25 g |
| Ceforanide | 125 | 180 | 2–4 | 12 | 1 g daily | 1 g every 48 hours | 0.25 g |
| Cefaclor* | 15–20 | 50 | 1–3 | 6–8 | 0.5 g every 8–12 hours | 0.25–0.5 g every 12–24 hours | 0.25–0.5 g |
| Cefotetan | 60–80 | 150 | 3–6 | 8–12 | 1 g every 8–12 hours | 0.5–1 g daily | 0.5 g |
| Cefotaxime | 40–60 | 60 | 4–12 | 6–8 | 1–2 g every 6–8 hours | 1–2 g every 12 hours | 1–2 g |
| Ceftizoxime | 80–100 | 100 | 3–12 | 8–12 | 0.5–1 g every 8–12 hours | 0.25–0.5 g every 12–24 hours | 0.5 g |
| Ceftriaxone | 150 | 480 | 1–4 | 12–24 | 1–2 g daily | 1–2 g daily | None |
| Ceftazidime | 100–120 | 120 | 2–9 | 8–12 | 1 g every 8–12 hours | 0.5–1 g daily | 0.5 g |
| Cefoperazone | 150 | 120 | 2–6 | 8–12 | 1–2 g every 12 hours | 1–2 g every 12 hours | None |
| Moxalactam | 60–100 | 120 | 2–8 | 6–12 | 0.5–1 g every 12 hours | 0.25–0.5 g every 12 hours | 0.5 g |

* Oral agents. Serum levels based on 0.5 g oral dose.

ing *H influenzae* and *B catarrhalis,* cefaclor is used to treat sinusitis and otitis media in patients who are allergic to ampicillin or amoxicillin or have not responded to treatment with those drugs. Cefuroxime is the only second-generation cephalosporin that crosses the blood-brain barrier in sufficient amounts to be useful for treatment of meningitis. It is often used to treat serious *H influenzae* infections, including meningitis. For meningitis in children, it should be combined with penicillin to cover possible *Listeria monocytogenes* infections and should be given every 6 hours.

Because of their activity against *B fragilis,* cefoxitin and cefotetan can be used to treat mixed anaerobic infections, eg, peritonitis and diverticulitis. Cefonicid and ceforanide have been promoted for use in surgical prophylaxis, but there is no evidence that they are more effective than first-generation cephalosporins, and they tend to be more expensive. Cefamandole, like cefuroxime, may be useful for the treatment of community-acquired pneumonia, but it has few other uses.

## 3. THIRD-GENERATION CEPHALOSPORINS

### Antimicrobial Activity

These drugs are active against staphylococci (not methicillin-resistant strains) but less so than first-generation cephalosporins. They have no activity against enterococci but may inhibit nonenterococcal streptococci. A major advantage of the new cephalosporins is their expanded gram-negative coverage. In addition to organisms inhibited by other cephalosporins, they are consistently active against *Enterobacter* spp, *Citrobacter freundii, Serratia marcescens, Providencia* spp, *Haemophilus* spp, and *Neisseria* spp, including β-lactamase-producing strains. Two drugs—ceftazidime and cefoperazone—have good activity against *P aeruginosa,* whereas the others inhibit only 40–60% of strains. *Listeria* spp, *Acinetobacter* spp, and non-*aeruginosa* strains of *Pseudomonas* are variably sensitive to third-generation cephalosporins. Only ceftizoxime and moxalactam have good activity against *B fragilis.*

### Pharmacokinetics & Administration

After an intravenous infusion of 1 g, serum levels

of these drugs range from 60 to 140 μg/mL. They penetrate well into body fluids and tissues and—with the exception of cefoperazone—reach levels in the cerebrospinal fluid that exceed those needed to inhibit most pathogens, including gram-negative rods. The half-life of these drugs is variable: ceftriaxone, 7–8 hours; cefoperazone, 2 hours; and the others, 1–1.7 hours. Consequently, ceftriaxone can be injected every 12–24 hours in a dose of 15–30 mg/kg/d (or 30–50 mg/kg every 12 hours in adult meningitis and 50 mg/kg every 12 hours in infants). Cefoperazone can be given every 8–12 hours in a dose of 25–100 mg/kg/d and the other drugs of the group every 6–8 hours in doses ranging from 2 to 12 g/d depending on the severity of the infection. Cefoperazone and ceftriaxone are eliminated primarily by biliary excretion, and no dosage adjustment is required in renal insufficiency. The other drugs are eliminated by the kidney and thus require dosage adjustments in renal insufficiency.

## Clinical Uses

Because of their penetration into the cerebrospinal fluid, third-generation cephalosporins—except cefoperazone—can be used to treat meningitis. Meningitis due to pneumococci, meningococci, *H influenzae*, and susceptible enteric gram-negative rods have been successfully treated. In childhood meningitis, third-generation cephalosporins should be combined with ampicillin until *Listeria monocytogenes* has been excluded as the etiologic agent. Because of the high inhibitory dose of third-generation cephalosporins against *Pseudomonas*, these drugs are not recommended in meningitis caused by this organism. The dosage for meningitis should be near the top of the recommended range, because cerebrospinal fluid levels of these drugs are only 10% of serum levels.

Apart from meningitis, other potential indications include (1) infections in which cephalosporins are the least toxic agent available; (2) sepsis of unknown cause in the immunocompetent patient; and (3) fever in the immunocompromised neutropenic patient, in which case the drug should be given in combination with an aminoglycoside.

Barriere SL, Flaherty JF: Third-generation cephalosporins: A critical evaluation. *Clin Pharmacol* 1984;**3**:351.

Mandell GL, Douglas G, Bennett JE: Cephalosporins. Chap 18, pp 180–187, in: *Principles and Practice of Infectious Diseases,* 3rd ed. Wiley, 1985.

Neu HC (editor): Advances in cephalosporin therapy—beyond the third generation. *Am J Med* 1985;**79**(Suppl 2A):1. [Entire issue.]

Neu HC: New antibiotics: Areas of appropriate use. *J Infect Dis* 1987;**155**:403.

## ADVERSE EFFECTS OF CEPHALOSPORINS

### Allergy

Cephalosporins are sensitizing, and a variety of hypersensitivity reactions occur, including anaphylaxis, fever, skin rashes, nephritis, granulocytopenia, and hemolytic anemia. The frequency of cross-allergy between cephalosporins and penicillins is not certainly known but is estimated to be about 6–10%. Persons with a history of anaphylaxis to penicillins should not receive cephalosporins.

### Toxicity

Local pain can occur after intramuscular injection, or thrombophlebitis after intravenous injection. Hypoprothrombinemia is a frequent adverse effect (40–68%) of cephalosporins that have a methylthiotetrazole group (eg, cefamandole, moxalactam, cefoperazone). Administration of vitamin K, 10 mg twice weekly, can pervent this complication. Moxalactam interferes with platelet function and has been associated with severe bleeding. Drugs containing the methylthiotetrazole ring can also cause severe disulfiramlike reactions, and use of alcohol or medications containing alcohol (eg, theophylline) must be avoided.

### Superinfection

Many newer cephalosporins have little activity against gram-positive organisms, particularly staphylococci and enterococci. Superinfection with these organisms—as well as with fungi—may occur.

## NEW BETA-LACTAM DRUGS

### Monobactams

These are drugs with a monocyclic β-lactam ring which are resistant to β-lactamases and active against gram-negative organisms (including *Pseudomonas*) but have no activity against gram-positive organisms or anaerobes. Aztreonam resembles aminoglycosides in activity. The usual dose is 1–2 g intravenously every 6–8 hours, providing peak serum levels of 100 μg/mL. Clinical uses of aztreonam are limited because of the availability of third-generation cephalosporins with a broader spectrum of activity and minimal toxicity.

### Carbapenems

This new class of drugs is structurally related to β-lactam antibiotics. Imipenem, the first drug of this type, has a wide spectrum with good activity against many gram-negative rods and gram-positive organisms and anaerobes. It is resistant to β-lactamases but is inactivated by dipeptidases in renal tubules. Consequently, it must be combined with cilastatin, a dipeptidase inhibitor, for clinical use.

The half-life of imipenem is 1 hour. Penetration into body tissues and fluids, including the cerebrospinal fluid, is good. The usual dose is 0.5–1 g intravenously every 6 hours. Dosage adjustment is required in renal insufficiency. For patients with $Cl_{cr}$ 10–30 mL/min, one-half the usual dose is given; for those with $Cl_{cr}$ 10 mL/min, 0.5 g is given every 12 hours. An additional dose is given after hemodialysis.

The role of imipenem in therapy has not been defined. It may be indicated in infections due to multi-drug-resistant organisms that are susceptible only to imipenem. Since *Pseudomonas* may rapidly develop resistance to imipenem used alone, simultaneous use of an aminoglycoside is required. The use of imipenem alone or in combination with an aminoglycoside in febrile neutropenic patients is under investigation.

The most common adverse effects of imipenem are nausea, vomiting, diarrhea, reactions at the infusion site, and skin rashes. Seizures can occur in patients with renal failure. Patients allergic to penicillins may be allergic to imipenem as well.

Barriere SL, Flaherty JF: Third-generation cephalosporins: A critical evaluation. *Clin Pharm* 1984;**3**:351.

Mandell GL, Douglas G, Bennett JE: Chap 18, p 180, in: *Principles and Practice of Infectious Diseases,* 3rd ed. Wiley, 1985.

Neu HC: New antibiotics: Areas of appropriate use. *J Infect Dis* 1987;**155**:403.

Neu HC (editor): Advances in cephalosporin therapy: Beyond the third generation. Am J Med 1985;**79(Suppl 2A)**:1. [Entire issue.]

Remington JS (editor): Carbapenems: A new class of antibiotics. *Am J Med* 1985;**78(Suppl 6A)**:1. [Entire issue.]

## ERYTHROMYCIN GROUP (Macrolides)

The erythromycins are a group of closely related compounds characterized by a macrocyclic lactone ring to which sugars are attached. There are several different members of the group.

Erythromycins inhibit protein synthesis and are bacteriostatic or bactericidal for gram-positive organisms—especially pneumococci, streptococci, and corynebacteria—in concentrations of 0.02–2 $\mu$g/mL. Chlamydiae, mycoplasmas, *Legionella*, and *Campylobacter* are also susceptible. Activity is enhanced at alkaline pH. There is complete cross-resistance among all members of the erythromycin group. Absorption of these drugs varies greatly. Basic erythromycins are more acid-labile than erythromycin stearates. Erythromycin estolate is among the best-absorbed oral preparations. Oral doses of 2 g/d result in blood levels of up to 2 $\mu$g/mL, and there is wide distribution of the drug in all tissues except the central nervous system. Erythromycins are excreted largely in bile; only 5% of the dose is excreted into the urine.

Erythromycins are drugs of choice in corynebacterial infections (diphtheria, sepsis caused by susceptible corynebacteria, erythrasma); in respiratory, genital, or ocular chlamydial infections; and in pneumonias caused by *Mycoplasma* and *Legionella* (see Chapter 7). The erythromycins are useful as substitutes for penicillin in persons with streptococcal and pneumococcal infections who are allergic to penicillin. In rheumatic persons taking penicillin, erythromycin can be given prior to dental procedures as prophy-

laxis. Spiramycin can be of benefit in *Cryptosporidium* diarrhea.

### Dosages

**A. Oral:** Erythromycin base, stearate, or estolate, 0.25–0.5 g every 6 hours (for children, 40 mg/kg/d), or erythromycin ethylsuccinate, 0.4–0.6 g every 6 hours is the usual dose. A combination of erythromycin and sulfisoxazole is available for acute otitis media in children. Sometimes erythromycin is given orally together with neomycin for preoperative preparation of the colon as prophylaxis.

**B. Intravenous:** Erythromycin lactobionate or gluceptate, 0.5 g every 12 hours.

### Adverse Effects

Nausea, vomiting, and diarrhea may occur after oral intake. Erythromycins, particularly the estolate, can produce acute cholestatic hepatitis (fever, jaundice, impaired liver function), probably as a hypersensitivity reaction. Most patients recover from this, but hepatitis recurs if the drug is re-administered. Erythromycins can increase the effects of oral anticoagulants and of digoxin.

Ginsburg CM, Eichenwald HF: Erythromycin: Review of its uses in pediatrics. *J Pediatr* 1976;**89**:872.

Schachter J et al: The routine use of erythromycin for chlamydial infections in pregnancy. *N Eng J Med* 1986;**314**:276.

## TETRACYCLINE GROUP

The tetracyclines are a large group of drugs with common basic chemical structures, antimicrobial activity, and pharmacologic properties. Microorganisms resistant to this group show extensive cross-resistance to all tetracyclines.

### Antimicrobial Activity

Tetracyclines are inhibitors of protein synthesis and are bacteriostatic for many gram-positive and gram-negative bacteria. They are strongly inhibitory for the growth of mycoplasmas, rickettsiae, chlamydiae, and some protozoa (eg, amebas). Equal concentrations of all tetracyclines in blood or tissue have approximately equal antimicrobial activity. However, there are great differences in the susceptibility of different strains of a given species of microorganism, and laboratory tests are therefore important. Because of the emergence of resistant strains, tetracyclines have lost some of their former usefulness. *Proteus* and *Pseudomonas* are regularly resistant; among coliform bacteria, *Bacteroides,* pneumococci, staphylococci, streptococci, shigellae, and vibrios, strains resistant to tetracyclines are increasingly common.

### Absorption, Distribution, & Excretion

Tetracyclines are absorbed somewhat irregularly from the gut. Absorption is limited by the low solubility of the drugs and by chelation with divalent cations, eg, $Ca^{2+}$ or $Fe^{2+}$. A large proportion of orally administered tetracycline remains in the gut lumen, modifies intestinal flora, and is excreted in feces. With full systemic doses, levels of active drug in serum reach $5-8$ $\mu$g/mL. The drugs are widely distributed in tissues and body fluids, but the levels in central nervous system, cerebrospinal fluid, and joint fluids are only $3-10\%$ of serum levels. Tetracyclines are specifically deposited in growing bones and teeth, bound to calcium.

Absorbed tetracyclines are excreted mainly in bile and urine. Up to 20% of oral doses may appear in the urine after glomerular filtration. Urine levels may be $5-50$ $\mu$g/mL or more. With renal failure, doses of tetracyclines must be reduced or intervals between doses increased. Up to 80% of an oral dose appears in the feces.

Demeclocycline, methacycline, minocycline, and doxycycline are well absorbed from the gut but are excreted more slowly than other drugs in the tetracycline group. This may lead to accumulation and prolonged blood levels. Renal clearance ranges from 9 mL/min for minocycline to 90 mL/min for oxytetracycline. Doxycycline does not accumulate greatly in renal failure and can be used in uremia. Minocycline appears in respiratory secretions.

### Indications, Dosages, & Routes of Administration

At present, tetracyclines are drugs of choice in chlamydial, rickettsial, and *Vibrio* infections. They are effective in mycoplasmal pneumonia, plague, brucellosis, Lyme disease, leptospirosis, and some other bacterial infections and in amebiasis. For prophylaxis of meningococcal disease, minocycline, 200 mg daily for 5 days, is effective, but rifampin is preferred.

**A. Oral:** Tetracycline hydrochloride and oxytetracycline are dispensed in 250-mg capsules. Give $0.25-0.5$ g orally every 6 hours (for children, $20-40$ mg/kg/d). In acne vulgaris, 0.25 g once or twice daily for many months is prescribed by dermatologists. Tetracycline hydrochloride, 2 g/d, or doxycycline, 100 mg twice daily, given orally for 7 days, can eradicate acute gonorrhea and also be effective against chlamydial infections. Doxycycline, 100 mg twice daily, can accomplish the same effect. Usually, however, chlamydial infections are treated for longer periods (eg, 14 days). A single 200-mg dose of doxycycline may stop the shedding of vibrios in cholera, and a single 2.5-g dose of tetracycline hydrochloride may control enteric infection due to *Shigella*. Doxycycline, 200 mg once weekly, is effective prophylaxis against leptospirosis.

Demeclocycline and methacycline are long-acting tetracyclines available in capsules containing 50 or 150 mg. Give $0.15-0.3$ g orally every 6 hours (for children, $12-20$ mg/kg/d). Doxycycline and minocycline are available in capsules containing 50 or 100 mg or as powder for oral suspension. Give doxycycline, 100 mg every 12 hours on the first day and 100 mg/d for maintenance. Give minocycline, 200 mg for the first dose and then 100 mg every 12 hours.

**B. Intravenous:** Several tetracyclines are formulated for parenteral administration in individuals unable to take oral medication. The dose is generally similar to the oral dose (see package insert).

**C. Topical:** Topical tetracycline, 1%, in ointment, can be applied to conjunctival infections.

### Adverse Effects

**A. Allergy:** Hypersensitivity reactions with fever or skin rashes are uncommon.

**B. Gastrointestinal Side Effects:** Gastrointestinal side effects, especially diarrhea, nausea, and anorexia, are common. These can be diminished by reducing the dose or by administering tetracyclines with food or carboxymethylcellulose, but sometimes they force discontinuance of the drug. After a few days of oral use, the gut flora is modified so that drug-resistant bacteria and yeasts become prominent. This may cause functional gut disturbances, anal pruritus, and even enterocolitis with shock and death.

**C. Bones and Teeth:** Tetracyclines are bound to calcium deposited in growing bones and teeth, causing fluorescence, discoloration, enamel dysplasia, deformity, or growth inhibition. Therefore, tetracyclines should not be given to pregnant women or children under age 6 years.

**D. Liver Damage:** Tetracyclines can impair hepatic function or even cause liver necrosis, particularly during pregnancy, in the presence of preexisting liver damage, or with doses of more than 3 g intravenously.

**E. Kidney Damage:** Outdated tetracycline preparations have been implicated in renal tubular acidosis and other forms of renal damage. Tetracyclines may increase blood urea nitrogen when diuretics are administered.

**F. Other:** Tetracyclines, principally demeclocycline, may induce photosensitization, especially in blonds. Intravenous injection may cause thrombophlebitis, and intramuscular injection may induce local inflammation with pain. Minocycline induces vestibular reactions (dizziness, vertigo, nausea, vomiting), with a frequency of $35-70\%$ after doses of 200 mg daily. Demeclocycline inhibits antidiuretic hormone.

Barza M, Schiefe RT: Antimicrobial spectrum, pharmacology and therapeutic use of antibiotics. 1. Tetracyclines. *Am J Hosp Pharm* 1977;**34**:49.

Pickering LK et al: Single-dose tetracycline therapy for shigellosis in adults. *JAMA* 1978;**239**:853.

## CHLORAMPHENICOL

Chloramphenicol is a potent inhibitor of protein synthesis in bacteria and rickettsiae, arresting their growth. Resistant strains of organisms produce an enzyme that inactivates the drug. This enzyme is under control of a transmissible plasmid. There is no cross-resistance with other drugs.

After oral administration, chloramphenicol is rapidly and completely absorbed. Administration of 2 g/d orally to adults results in blood levels of 5–10 μg/mL. In children, chloramphenicol palmitate, 50 mg/kg/d orally, is hydrolyzed in the gut to yield free chloramphenicol and gives a blood level of 10 μg/mL. Chloramphenicol succinate, 25–50 mg/kg/d intravenously, yields free chloramphenicol by hydrolysis and gives blood levels comparable to those achieved by oral administration. After absorption, chloramphenicol is widely distributed to all tissues, including the eye and the central nervous system, where drug levels are similar to serum levels. It penetrates cells readily. Chloramphenicol is metabolized either by conjugation with glucuronic acid in the liver or by reduction to inactive aryl amines. In hepatic insufficiency, the drug may accumulate to toxic levels. Only 10% of active drug is excreted into the urine.

Because of its potential toxicity and the availability of effective new agents (eg, cephalosporins, quinolones), chloramphenicol is a drug of possible choice only in the following clinical circumstances: (1) Symptomatic *Salmonella* infections, eg, typhoid fever. Because many strains of *Salmonella* are resistant to chloramphenicol, trimethoprim-sulfamethoxazole is often used. The quinolones may become the drugs of choice. (2) Serious infections with *H influenzae* (meningitis, epiglottitis, pneumonia). However, several newer cephalosporins are active in such diseases, including those caused by *H influenzae* strains that produce β-lactamase; they are increasingly used for initial therapy unless the patient is known to be allergic to cephalosporins. (3) Meningococcal infections in patients hypersensitive to cephalosporins. (4) Anaerobic or mixed infections in the central nervous system, eg, brain abscess.

Topical chloramphenicol is occasionally used in ophthalmic infections. Chloramphenicol is rarely used as an alternative to tetracycline in rickettsial infections.

In serious systemic infection, give 0.5 g orally every 4–6 hours (for children, 30–50 mg/kg/d) for 7–21 days. Similar amounts are given intravenously.

## Adverse Effects

Nausea, vomiting, and diarrhea occur infrequently. The most serious adverse effects pertain to the hematopoietic system. Adults taking chloramphenicol in excess of 50 mg/kg/d regularly exhibit disturbances in red cell maturation within 1–2 weeks. There is anemia, rise in serum iron concentration, reticulocytopenia, and the appearance of vacuolated nucleated red cells in the bone marrow. These changes regress when the drug is stopped and are not related to the rare aplastic anemia.

Serious aplastic anemia is a rare consequence of chloramphenicol administration and represents a specific, probably genetically determined individual defect. It is seen more frequently with prolonged or repeated use. It tends to be irreversible. It has been estimated that fatal aplastic anemia occurs in one of 25–40 thousand courses of chloramphenicol treatment. Hypoplastic anemia may be followed by the development of leukemia.

Chloramphenicol inhibits the metabolism of certain drugs. Thus, it may prolong the action and raise blood concentration of tolbutamide, phenytoin, chlorpropamide, and warfarin sodium (Coumadin).

Chloramphenicol is specifically toxic for newborns, particularly premature infants. Because they lack the mechanism for detoxification of the drug in the liver, the drug may accumulate, producing the highly fatal "gray syndrome," with vomiting, flaccidity, hypothermia, and collapse. In full-term infants, the dose should be limited to less than 50 mg/kg/d; in prematures, the dose should be less than 30 mg/kg/d if the drug is employed at all.

Gump DW: Chloramphenicol: A 1981 view. *Arch Intern Med* 1981;**141:**573.

## AMINOGLYCOSIDES

Aminoglycosides are a group of bactericidal drugs sharing chemical, antimicrobial, pharmacologic, and toxic characteristics. At present, the group includes streptomycin, neomycin, kanamycin, amikacin, gentamicin, tobramycin, sisomicin, netilmicin, and others. All these agents inhibit protein synthesis in bacteria by attaching to and inhibiting the function of the 30S subunit of the bacterial ribosome. Resistance is based on (1) a deficiency of the ribosomal receptor (chromosomal mutant); (2) the enzymatic destruction of the drug (plasmid-mediated transmissible resistance of clinical importance) by acetylation, phosphorylation, or adenylylation; or (3) a lack of permeability to the drug molecule or failure of active transport across cell membranes. (This can be chromosomal, eg, streptococci are relatively impermeable to aminoglycosides; or it can be plasmid-mediated, eg, in gram-negative enteric bacteria.) Anaerobic bacteria are often resistant to aminoglycosides because transport across the cell membrane is an oxygen-dependent energy-requiring process.

All aminoglycosides are more active at alkaline than at acid pH. All are potentially ototoxic and nephrotoxic, though to different degrees. All can accumulate in renal failure; therefore, dosage adjustments must be made in uremia.

Aminoglycosides are used most widely against gram-negative enteric bacteria or when there is a suspicion of sepsis. In the treatment of bacteremia or endocarditis caused by fecal streptococci or by some gram-negative bacteria, the aminoglycoside is given together with a β-lactam drug to enhance permeability and facilitate the entry of the aminoglycoside. Aminoglycosides are selected according to recent susceptibility patterns in a given area or hospital until susceptibility tests become available on a specific isolate.

## General Properties of Aminoglycosides

Because of the similarities of the aminoglycosides, a summary of properties is presented briefly.

**A. Physical Properties:** Aminoglycosides are water-soluble and stable in solution. If they are mixed in solution with β-lactam antibiotics, they may form complexes and lose some activity.

**B. Absorption, Distribution, Metabolism, and Excretion:** Aminoglycosides are well absorbed after intramuscular or intravenous injection, but they are not absorbed from the gut. They are distributed widely in tissues and penetrate into pleural, peritoneal, or joint fluid in the presence of inflammation. They diffuse poorly into the eye, prostate, bile, central nervous system, or spinal fluid after parenteral injection.

There is no significant metabolic breakdown of aminoglycosides. The serum half-life is 2–3 hours. Excretion is almost entirely by glomerular filtration. Some representative mean blood or tissue concentrations following commonly used doses are shown in Table 28–1. Urine levels usually are 10–50 times higher. Aminoglycosides are removed fairly effectively by hemodialysis but irregularly by peritoneal dialysis.

**C. Dose and Effect of Impaired Renal Function:** In persons with normal renal function, the dose of kanamycin or amikacin is 15 mg/kg/d; that for gentamicin or tobramycin is 3–7 mg/kg/d, usually injected in 3 equal amounts every 8 hours.

In persons with impaired renal function, excretion is diminished and there is the danger of drug accumulation with increased side effects. Therefore, if the interval is kept constant, the dose has to be reduced, or the interval must be increased if the dose is kept constant (see Table 28–3). Nomograms have been constructed relating serum creatinine levels to adjustments of treatment regimens. One widely used formula uses a multiplication factor (kanamycin or amikacin = 9, gentamicin = 8, tobramycin = 6) times the serum creatinine value (mg/dL) to give the interval between doses in hours. However, there is considerable variation in aminoglycoside levels in different patients with similar creatinine values. Therefore, it is highly desirable to monitor drug levels in blood whenever possible to avoid severe toxicity when renal functional capacity is rapidly changing.

**D. Adverse Effects:** All aminoglycosides can cause varying degrees of ototoxicity and nephrotoxicity. Ototoxicity can present either as hearing loss (cochlear damage) that is noted first with high-frequency tones, or as vestibular damage, evident by vertigo, ataxia, and loss of balance. Nephrotoxicity is evident with rising serum creatinine levels or reduced creatinine clearance.

In very high doses, aminoglycosides can be neurotoxic, producing a curarelike effect with neuromuscular blockade that results in respiratory paralysis. Calcium gluconate or neostigmine can serve as an antidote to this reaction. Rarely, aminoglycosides cause hypersensitivity and local reactions.

Moellering RC, Siegenthaler WE (editors): Aminoglycoside therapy. The new decade: A worldwide perspective. *Am J Med* 1986;**80 (Suppl 6B):**1. [Entire issue.]

## 1. STREPTOMYCIN

Streptomycin is bactericidal for both gram-positive and gram-negative bacteria. However, resistance emerges so rapidly and has become so widespread that only a few specific indications for this drug remain. These are (1) plague and tularemia; (2) endocarditis caused by *S faecalis* or *Streptococcus viridans* (use in conjunction with a penicillin); (3) serious active tuberculosis (use with other antituberculosis drugs); (4) acute brucellosis (use with tetracycline). The usual dose is 0.5 g intramuscularly every 6–8 hours (20–40 mg/kg/d).

Streptomycin exhibits all the adverse effects typically associated with the aminoglycosides. It should not be given concurrently with other aminoglycosides, because excessive ototoxicity may occur. Dihydrostreptomycin is no longer used, because of severe ototoxicity.

## 2. NEOMYCIN & KANAMYCIN

These aminoglycosides are closely related, with similar activity and complete cross-resistance. The related paromomycin is used in amebiasis. Their systemic use has been abandoned because of oto- and nephrotoxicity.

Ointments containing 1–5 mg/g neomycin, often combined with bacitracin and polymyxin, can be applied to infected superficial skin lesions. The drug mixture covers most staphylococci and gram-negative bacteria likely to be present, but the efficacy of such topical treatment is in doubt. Solutions of neomycin 1–5 mg/mL, have been used for irrigation of infected joints or wounds. The total amount of drug must be kept below 15 mg/kg/d, because absorption can lead to systemic toxicity.

In preparation for elective bowel surgery, 1 g of neomycin is given orally every 4–6 hours for 1–2 days (often combined with erythromycin, 1 g) to reduce aerobic bowel flora. Action on gram-negative anaerobes is negligible. In hepatic coma, the coliform bacteria can be suppressed for prolonged periods by oral neomycin or kanamycin, 1 g every 6–8 hours, during reduced protein intake. This results in diminished ammonia production and intoxication.

Kanamycin is somewhat less toxic than neomycin. It is used for the same indications and in the same doses as neomycin for topical application and oral intake.

In addition to oto- and nephrotoxicity, which can result from systemic absorption, neomycin or kanamycin can give rise to allergic reactions when applied topically to skin or eye. Respiratory arrest has followed the instillation of 3–5 g of kanamycin into the peritoneal cavity after colonic surgery; this can be overcome by neostigmine.

## 3. AMIKACIN

Amikacin is a semisynthetic derivative of kanamycin. It is relatively resistant to several of the enzymes that inactivate gentamicin and tobramycin, and bacterial resistance is increasing only slowly. Many gram-negative enteric bacteria—including many strains of *Proteus, Pseudomonas, Enterobacter,* and *Serratia*—are inhibited by 1–20 μg/mL of amikacin in vitro. After injection of 500 mg of amikacin intramuscularly every 12 hours (15 mg/kg/d), peak levels in serum are 10–30 μg/mL. Some infections caused by gram-negative bacteria resistant to gentamicin respond to amikacin. Central nervous system infections require intrathecal or intraventricular injection of 1–10 mg daily.

Like all aminoglycosides, amikacin is nephrotoxic and ototoxic (particularly for the auditory portion of the eighth nerve). Its levels should be monitored in patients with renal failure.

Meyer RD: Drugs five years later: Amikacin. *Ann Intern Med* 1981;**95:**328.
Sarubbi FA, Hull JH: Amikacin serum concentrations: Prediction of levels and dosage guidelines. *Ann Intern Med* 1978;**89:**612.

## 4. GENTAMICIN

With doses of 3–7 mg/kg/d of this aminoglycoside, serum levels reach 3–8 μg/mL—sufficient for bactericidal effect against many strains of staphylococci, coliform organisms, and other gram-negative organisms. Enterococci are resistant unless a penicillin is also given. Gentamicin may be synergistic with penicillins active against *Pseudomonas, Proteus, Enterobacter, Klebsiella,* and other gram-negatives. Sisomicin resembles the C1a component of gentamicin.

### Indications, Dosages, & Routes of Administration

Gentamicin is used in severe infections caused by gram-negative bacteria. Included are sepsis, infected burns, pneumonia, and other serious infections. The dosage is 3–7 mg/kg/d intramuscularly (or intravenously) in 3 equal doses. In endocarditis or sepsis due to *S faecalis,* similar amounts of gentamicin are given in combination with penicillin. In renal failure, the suggested dose is 1 mg/kg intramuscularly every (8 × serum creatinine value [mg/dL]) hours. However, serum levels should be monitored by laboratory assay. About 2–3% of patients develop vestibular dysfunction and loss of hearing when peak serum levels exceed 10 μg/mL. For infected burns or skin lesions, creams containing 0.1% gentamicin are used. Such topical use should be restricted to avoid favoring

the development of resistant bacteria in hospitals. In meningitis due to gram-negative bacteria, 1–10 mg of gentamicin has been injected daily intrathecally or intraventricularly in adults. However, in neonatal gram-negative bacillary meningitis the benefit of either of these routes is in doubt, and intraventricular gentamicin is toxic.

McCracken GH et al: Intraventricular gentamicin therapy in gram-negative bacillary meningitis of infants. *Lancet* 1980;**1:**787.
Tablan CC et al: Renal and auditory toxicity of high-dose prolonged therapy with gentamicin and tobramycin in pseudomonas endocarditis. *J Infect Dis* 1984;**149:**257.

## 5. TOBRAMYCIN

Tobramycin closely resembles gentamicin in antibacterial activity and pharmacologic properties and exhibits partial cross-resistance. Tobramycin may be effective against some gentamicin-resistant gram-negative bacteria. A daily dose of 3–5 mg/kg is given in 3 equal amounts intramuscularly at intervals of 8 hours. In uremia, the suggested dose is 1 mg/kg intramuscularly every (6 × serum creatinine value [mg/dL]) hours. However, blood levels should be monitored. Tobramycin is somewhat less nephrotoxic than gentamicin, but their ototoxicity is similar.

Netilmicin shares many characteristics with gentamicin and tobramycin and can be given in a dose of 5–7 mg/kg/d. It may be less ototoxic and less nephrotoxic than the other aminoglycosides.

Smith CR et al: Double blind comparison of the nephrotoxicity and auditory toxicity of gentamicin and tobramycin. *N Engl J Med* 1980;**302:**1106.

## 6. SPECTINOMYCIN

Spectinomycin is an aminocyclitol antibiotic (related to aminoglycosides) for intramuscular administration. Its sole application is in the treatment of gonococci producing β-lactamase or of persons with gonorrhea who are hypersensitive to penicillin. One injection of 2 g (40 mg/kg) is given. About 5–10% of gonococci are probably resistant. There is usually pain at the injection site, and there may be nausea and fever.

Rettig PJ et al: Spectinomycin therapy for gonorrhea in prepubertal children. *Am J Dis Child* 1980;**134:**359.

## POLYMYXINS

The polymyxins are basic polypeptides that are bactericidal for most gram-negative aerobic rods, including *Pseudomonas.* Because of their poor distribution to tissues and substantial toxicity—and in view of the availability of better drugs—they are now rarely considered for systemic administration but are used topically only.

Solutions of polymyxin B sulfate, 1 mg/mL, can be applied to infected surfaces; injected into joint spaces, the pleural cavity, or subconjunctivally; or inhaled as aerosols. Ointments containing 0.5 mg/g of polymyxin B sulfate in a mixture with neomycin or bacitracin (or both) are often applied to superficial infected skin lesions. Polymyxins are inactivated by purulent exudates. They rarely cause local sensitization.

Davis SD: Polymyxins, colistin, vancomycin and bacitracin. In: Kagan BM (editor): *Antimicrobial Therapy,* 3rd ed. Saunders, 1980.

## ANTITUBERCULOSIS DRUGS

Singular problems exist in the treatment of tuberculosis and other mycobacterial infections. They tend to be exceedingly chronic but may give rise to hyperacute lethal complications. The organisms are frequently intracellular, have long periods of metabolic inactivity, and tend to develop resistance to any one drug. Combined drug therapy is usually employed to delay the emergence of this resistance. "First-line" drugs, often employed together in tuberculous meningitis, miliary dissemination, or severe pulmonary disease, are isoniazid, ethambutol, rifampin, and streptomycin. A series of "second-line" drugs will be mentioned only briefly. Most patients become noninfectious within 2–4 weeks after effective drug therapy is instituted. In active pulmonary tuberculosis without complications, treatment schedules including isoniazid and rifampin for 6–9 months are satisfactory.

American Thoracic Society: Treatment of tuberculosis and tuberculous infections in adults and children. *Am Rev Respir Dis* 1986;**134:**355.

## 1. ISONIAZID (INH)

Isoniazid is the hydrazide of isonicotinic acid (INH), the most active antituberculosis drug. Isoniazid in a concentration of 0.2 μg/mL or less inhibits and kills most tubercle bacilli. However, some "atypical" mycobacteria are resistant. In susceptible large populations of *Mycobacterium tuberculosis,* isoniazid-resistant mutants occur. Their emergence is delayed in the presence of a second drug. There is no cross-resistance between isoniazid, streptomycin, ethambutol, and rifampin.

Isoniazid is well absorbed from the gut and diffuses readily into all tissues, including the central nervous system, and into living cells. The inactivation of isoniazid—particularly its acetylation—is under genetic control. However, the speed of isoniazid acetylation has little influence over the selection of drug regimens. Isoniazid and its conjugates are excreted mainly in the urine.

## Indications, Dosages, & Routes of Administration

Isoniazid is the most widely used drug in tuberculosis. It should not be given as the sole drug in active tuberculosis. This favors emergence of resistance (up to 30% in some countries). In active, clinically manifest disease, it is given in conjunction with rifampin or ethambutol. The initial dose is 8–10 mg/kg/d orally (up to 20 mg/kg/d in smaller children); later, the dosage is reduced to 5–7 mg/kg/d or 15 mg/kg twice weekly. Dosage needs to be reduced only for very severe renal failure.

Children (or young adults) who convert from a negative to a positive tuberculin test but who have no evidence of an active lesion may be given 10 mg/kg/d (maximum: 300 mg/d) for 1 year as prophylaxis against the 5–15% risk of meningitis or miliary dissemination. For this "prophylaxis," isoniazid is given as the sole drug. Such isoniazid prophylaxis is also indicated in adults with positive tuberculin test results who must be immunosuppressed by cancer chemotherapy or for organ transplant.

Toxic reactions to isoniazid include insomnia, restlessness, fever, myalgia, hyperreflexia, and even convulsions and psychotic episodes. Some of these are attributable to a relative pyridoxine deficiency and peripheral neuritis and can be prevented by the administration of pyridoxine, 100 mg/d. Isoniazid can induce hepatitis. Progressive liver damage occurs rarely in patients under age 20; in 1.5% of persons between 30 and 50 years of age; and in 2.5% of older individuals. The risk of hepatitis is greater in alcoholics and in rapid rather than in slow acetylators of isoniazid and is an important determinant in the prophylactic use of isoniazid. Isoniazid can reduce the metabolism of phenytoin, increasing its blood level and toxicity.

Wolinsky E: Nontuberculous mycobacteria and associated diseases. *Am Rev Respir Dis* 1979;**119:**107.

## 2. ETHAMBUTOL

This is a synthetic, water-soluble, heat-stable compound, dispensed as the hydrochloride.

Many strains of *M tuberculosis* and of "atypical" mycobacteria are inhibited in vitro by ethambutol, 1–5 μg/mL. The mechanism of action is not known.

Ethambutol is well absorbed from the gut. About 20% of the drug is excreted in feces and 50% in the urine, in unchanged form. Excretion is delayed in renal failure. In meningitis, ethambutol appears in the cerebrospinal fluid.

Resistance to ethambutol emerges fairly rapidly among mycobacteria when the drug is used alone. Therefore, ethambutol, 15 mg/kg, is usually given as a single daily dose in combination with isoniazid.

Hypersensitivity to ethambutol occurs infrequently. It may cause a rise in the serum uric acid. The commonest side effects are visual disturbances: reduction in visual acuity, optic neuritis, and perhaps retinal damage occur in some patients receiving ethambutol, 25 mg/kg/d for several months. Most changes are reversible, but periodic visual acuity testing is mandatory. With doses of 15 mg/kg/d, side effects are rare.

Doster B et al: Ethambutol in the initial treatment of pulmonary tuberculosis. *Am Rev Respir Dis* 1973;**107:**177.

## 3. RIFAMPIN

Rifampin is a semisynthetic derivative of rifamycin. Rifampin, 1 μg/mL or less, inhibits many gram-positive cocci, meningococci, and mycobacteria in vitro. Gram-negative organisms are often more resistant. Highly resistant mutants occur frequently in susceptible microbial populations (1 in $10^6$–$10^8$ bacteria).

Rifampin binds strongly to DNA-dependent bacterial RNA polymerase and thus inhibits RNA synthesis in bacteria. Rifampin penetrates well into phagocytic cells and can kill intracellular organisms. Rifampin sometimes enhances the activity of amphotericin B against various fungi in vitro.

Rifampin given orally is well absorbed and widely distributed in tissues. It is excreted mainly through the liver and to a lesser extent in the urine. With oral doses of 600 mg, serum levels exceed 5 μg/mL for 4–6 hours, and urine levels may be 3–20 times higher.

In the treatment of tuberculosis, a single oral dose of 600 mg (10–20 mg/kg) is given daily or, later, twice weekly. In order to delay the rapid emergence of resistant microorganisms, combined treatment with isoniazid or ethambutol is required. Rifampin is effective for treatment of leprosy (see below). Rifampin, 600 mg twice daily for 2 days, can terminate the meningococcal carrier state, but rifampin-resistant strains emerge in 10% of subjects. Close contacts of children with manifest *H influenzae* infection (eg, in family or day-care center) can receive rifampin, 20 mg/kg/d for 4 days, as prophylaxis. Rifampin combined with trimethoprim-sulfamethoxazole can eradicate staphylococcal carriage in the nasopharynx. Synergistic action of rifampin with nafcillin against staphylococci in vitro is of uncertain clinical significance. With the exception of prophylaxis, rifampin should never be used alone.

Rifampin imparts an orange color to urine, sweat, and contact lenses. Occasional adverse effects include rashes, thrombocytopenia, impaired liver function, light chain proteinuria, and some impairment of immune response. In intermittent administration, rifampin must be given at least twice weekly to avoid a "flu syndrome," anemia, and other adverse affects. Rifampin increases the dose requirement for warfarin in anticoagulation and lowers serum levels of methadone, ketoconazole, and chloramphenicol.

Cox F et al: Rifampin prophylaxis for contacts of *Haemophilus influenzae* type B disease. *JAMA* 1981;**245:**1043.

Donta ST et al: Therapy of *Mycobacterium marinum* infections. *Arch Intern Med* 1986;**146:**902.

Farr B, Mandell GL: Rifampin. *Med Clin North Am* 1982;**66:**157.

## 4. STREPTOMYCIN

The general pharmacologic features and toxicity of streptomycin are described above. Streptomycin, 1–10 μg/mL, is inhibitory and bactericidal for most tubercle bacilli, whereas most "atypical" mycobacteria are resistant. All large populations of tubercle bacilli contain some streptomycin-resistant mutants. Therefore, streptomycin is employed only in combination with another antituberculosis drug.

Streptomycin penetrates poorly into cells and exerts its action mainly on extracellular tubercle bacilli. Since at any moment 90% of tubercle bacilli are intracellular and thus unaffected by streptomycin, treatment for many months is required.

For combination therapy in tuberculous meningitis, miliary dissemination, and severe organ tuberculosis, streptomycin is given intramuscularly, 1 g daily (30 mg/kg/d for children) for weeks or months. This is followed by streptomycin, 1 g intramuscularly 2–3 times a week for months. In tuberculous meningitis, intrathecal injections (1–2 mg/kg/d) are sometimes given in addition.

Prolonged streptomycin treatment may impair vestibular function and result in inability to maintain equilibrium. Later, some compensation usually occurs, so that patients can function fairly well.

## 5. SHORT-COURSE THERAPY

For uncomplicated pulmonary tuberculosis (and perhaps extrapulmonary disease), treatment for only 6–9 months can be satisfactory *provided that* both isoniazid and rifampin are administered. In adults, isoniazid, 300 mg, and rifampin, 600 mg, are given daily for 2–8 weeks, depending on the speed of sputum conversion and on the clinical and x-ray evidence of response. Subsequently, isoniazid, 15 mg/kg, and rifampin, 600 mg, can be given twice weekly. Ethambutol, 15 mg/kg/d, is given in addition if the patient resides in or has come from an area with a high level of initial drug resistance. Other regimens have been proposed. The addition of pyrazinamide, 30 mg/kg/d, for the first 2 months of treatment has been strikingly beneficial in some trials.

## 6. ALTERNATIVE DRUGS IN TUBERCULOSIS TREATMENT

The drugs listed alphabetically below are usually considered only in cases of drug resistance (clinical or laboratory) to "first-line" drugs and when expert guidance is available to deal with toxic side effects.

**Aminosalicylic acid (PAS),** closely related to *p*-aminobenzoic acid, inhibits most tubercle bacilli in concentrations of 1–5 μg/mL but has no effect on other bacteria. Resistant *M tuberculosis* will emerge rapidly unless another antituberculosis drug is present.

Aminosalicylic acid is readily absorbed from the gut. Doses of 8–12 g/d orally give blood levels of 10 μg/mL. The drug is widely distributed in tissues (except the central nervous system) and rapidly excreted into the urine. To avoid crystalluria, the urine should be kept alkaline.

Common side effects include anorexia, nausea, diarrhea, and epigastric pain. These may be diminished by taking the drug with meals and with antacids, but peptic ulceration may occur. Sodium aminosalicylate may be given parenterally. Hypersensitivity reactions include fever, skin rashes, granulocytopenia, lymphadenopathy, and arthralgias.

**Ansamycin,** 0.15–0.3 g/d, and **clofazimine,** 0.1 mg/kg/d, orally, are being used for experimental therapy in mycobacterial infections.

**Capreomycin,** 0.5–1.5 g/d intramuscularly, can perhaps substitute for streptomycin in combined therapy. It is nephrotoxic and ototoxic.

**Cycloserine,** 0.5–1 g/d orally, has been used alone or with isoniazid. It can induce a variety of central nervous system dysfunctions and psychotic reactions. These may be controlled by phenytoin, 100 mg/d orally. In smaller doses (15–20 mg/kg/d) it has been used in urinary tract infections.

**Ethionamide,** 0.5–1 g/d orally, has been used in combination therapy but produces marked gastric irritation.

**Pyrazinamide,** 0.75 g twice daily orally, has been used in combination therapy but may produce serious liver damage.

**Viomycin,** 2 g intramuscularly every 3 days, can occasionally substitute for streptomycin in combination therapy. It is nephrotoxic and ototoxic.

American Thoracic Society: Treatment of tuberculosis and other mycobacterial diseases. *Am Rev Respir Dis* 1983;**127**:790.

Dutt AK et al: Short-course chemotherapy for tuberculosis with mainly twice-weekly isoniazid and rifampin. *Am J Med* 1984;**104**:7.

## SULFONAMIDES & ANTIFOLATE DRUGS

Since the demonstration, in 1935, of the striking antibacterial activity of sulfanilamide, the molecule has been drastically altered in many ways. More than 150 different sulfonamides have been marketed at one time or another, the modifications being designed principally to achieve greater antibacterial activity, a wider antibacterial spectrum, greater solubility, or more prolonged action. Because of their low cost and their relative efficacy in some common bacterial infections, sulfonamides are still used widely. However, the increasing emergence of sulfonamide resistance (eg, among streptococci, gonococci, meningo-

cocci, and shigellae) and the higher efficacy of other antimantimicrobial drugs have curtailed the number of specific indications for sulfonamides as drugs of choice. The present indications for the use of these drugs can be summarized as follows:

**(1) First (previously untreated) infection of the urinary tract:** Many coliform organisms, which are the most common causes of urinary infections, are still susceptible to sulfonamides or to trimethoprimsulfamethoxazole.

**(2) *Chlamydia trachomatis* infections of eye and genital tract:** Sulfonamides may effectively suppress clinical activity, particularly in acute infections. They are ineffective in psittacosis.

**(3) Parasitic diseases:** The combination of a sulfonamide with trimethoprim is often effective for prophylaxis and treatment of *Pneumocystis carinii* pneumonia in immunodeficient individuals. The combination of a sulfonamide with pyrimethamine is employed in the treatment of toxoplasmosis and of chloroquine-resistant falciparum malaria.

**(4) Bacterial infections:** Sulfonamides are the drugs of choice in nocardiosis. In underdeveloped parts of the world, sulfonamides, because of their availability and low cost, may still be useful for the treatment of pneumococcal or staphylococcal infections; bacterial sinusitis, bronchitis, or otitis media; bacillary (*Shigella*) dysentery; and meningococcal infections. In many developed countries, however, sulfonamide resistance of the respective etiologic organisms is widespread.

Trimethoprim-sulfamethoxazole is a choice in *Pneumocystis* pneumonia, *Shigella* enteritis, systemic *Salmonella* infections, *Serratia* sepsis, recurrent urinary tract infections, and many other infections.

**(5) Leprosy:** Certain sulfones are the drugs of choice in leprosy.

### Antimicrobial Activity

The action of sulfonamides is bacteriostatic and is reversible upon removal of the drug or in the presence of an excess of *p*-aminobenzoic acid (PABA). Susceptible microorganisms require extracellular PABA in order to synthesize folic acid, an essential step in the formation of purines. Sulfonamides are structural analogs of PABA and can enter into the reaction in place of PABA, competing for the enzyme involved, so that nonfunctional analogs of folic acid are formed. As a result, further growth of the microorganism is inhibited. Animal cells and some sulfonamide-resistant microorganisms are unable to synthesize folic acid from PABA but depend on exogenous sources of preformed folic acid.

Trimethoprim, a substitued pyrimidine, is a folate antagonist. It inhibits dihydrofolate reductase of bacteria 50,000 times more efficiently than it inhibits the same enzyme of mammalian cells. In concentrations of 0.1–5 μg/mL it inhibits many gram-negative enteric bacteria found in urinary tract infections. A mixture of one part trimethoprim plus 5 parts sulfamethoxazole can result in sequential blocking of steps in the synthesis of purines. Some organisms carry plasmids that make them resistant to trimethoprim.

## Pharmacologic Properties

The soluble sulfonamides are readily absorbed from the gut, distributed widely in tissues and body fluids, and excreted primarily by glomerular filtration into the urine. Varying amounts of sulfonamides are acetylated by the liver or bound to plasma protein. A portion of the drug in the urine is acetylated, but enough active drug remains in the urine to permit effective treatment of urinary tract infections (usually 10–20 times the concentration present in the blood). In order to be therapeutically effective for systemic therapy, a sulfonamide must achieve a concentration of 8–12 mg/dL of blood. This is accomplished by full systemic doses listed below.

"Long-acting" sulfonamides (eg, sulfamethoxypyridazine) are readily absorbed after oral intake, but excretion is very slow, resulting in prolonged blood levels. These compounds cause more toxic reactions than short-acting sulfonamides and are not available in the USA.

"Insoluble" sulfonamides (eg, phthalylsulfathiazole) are absorbed to only a slight extent after oral administration and are largely excreted in the feces. Their action is limited to temporary suppression of intestinal flora.

For parenteral (usually intravenous) administration, sodium salts of several sulfonamides are used because of their greater solubility. Their distribution and excretion are similar to those of the orally administered, absorbed sulfonamides. Trimethoprim concentrates by nonionic diffusion in prostatic and vaginal fluids, which are more acidic than serum.

## Dosages & Routes of Administration

**A. Topical:** The application of sulfonamides to skin, wounds, or mucous membranes is undesirable because of the high risk of allergic sensitization or reaction and the low antimicrobial activity. Exceptions are the application of sodium sulfacetamide solution (30%) or ointment (10%) to the conjunctiva, and mafenide acetate cream (Sulfamylon) or silver sulfadiazine to control the flora of burn wounds.

**B. Oral:** For systemic disease, the soluble, rapidly excreted sulfonamides (eg, sulfadiazine, sulfisoxazole) are given in an initial dose of 2–4 g (40 mg/kg) followed by a maintenance dose of 0.5–1 g (20 mg/kg) every 4–6 hours. Trisulfapyrimidines USP may be given in the same total doses. Urine must be kept alkaline.

For uncomplicated symptomatic, previously untreated urinary tract infections in nonpregnant women, a single dose of sulfisoxazole, 1 g—or of trimethoprim, 320 mg, plus sulfamethoxazole, 1600 mg (2 tablets twice in 1 day)—is effective in 80–90% of cases. Trimethoprim by itself, 100 mg orally every 12 hours, may give sufficient urine levels to inhibit many organisms causing urinary tract infections.

However, the combination with sulfamethoxazole is more widely used in the USA. Half a tablet of this combination 3 times weekly serves as prophylaxis for recurrent urinary tract infections in some women.

For "intestinal surgery prophylaxis," insoluble sulfonamides (eg, phthalylsulfathiazole), 8–15 g/d, are given for 5–7 days before operations on the bowel. Salicylazosulfapyridine (sulfasalazine), 6 g/d, has been given in ulcerative colitis. The drug is split in the gut to yield sulfapyridine and salicylate. The latter may have anti-inflammatory action.

**C. Intravenous:** Sodium sulfadiazine can be injected intravenously in 0.5% concentration in 5% dextrose in water or physiologic saline solution in a total dose of 6–8 g/d (120 mg/kg/d). This is reserved for comatose individuals or those unable to take oral medication. The intravenous form of trimethoprim-sulfamethoxazole contains 80 mg of trimethoprim and 400 mg of sulfamethoxazole per 5-mL ampule in 40% propylene glycol, to be diluted with 125 mL of 5% dextrose in water. Up to 12–16 such ampules are given in *P carinii* pneumonia or gram-negative bacterial sepsis caused by susceptible organisms.

## Adverse Effects

Sulfonamides produce a wide variety of side effects—due partly to hypersensitivity, partly to direct toxicity—that must be considered whenever unexplained symptoms or signs occur in a patient who may have received these drugs. Except in the mildest reactions, fluids should be forced, and—if symptoms and signs progressively increase—the drugs should be discontinued. Precautions to prevent complications (below) are important.

**A. Systemic Side Effects:** Fever, skin rashes, urticaria; nausea, vomiting, or diarrhea; stomatitis, conjunctivitis, arthritis, exfoliative dermatitis; bone marrow depression, thrombocytopenia, hemolytic (in G6PD deficiency) or aplastic anemia, granulocytopenia, leukemoid reactions; hepatitis, polyarteritis nodosa, vasculitis, Stevens-Johnson syndrome; psychosis; and many others.

Trimethoprim can evoke similar side effects. It may precipitate folate deficiency.

Application of mafenide to burns may cause severe pain.

**B. Urinary Tract Disturbances:** Sulfonamides may precipitate in urine, especially at neutral or acid pH, producing hematuria, crystalluria, or even obstruction. They have also been implicated in various types of nephritis and nephrosis. Sulfonamides and methenamine salts should not be given together.

## Precautions in the Use of Sulfonamides

(1) There is cross-allergenicity among all sulfonamides. Obtain a history of past administration or reaction. Observe for possible allergic responses.

(2) Keep the urine volume above 1500 mL/d by forcing fluids. Check urine pH—it should be 7.5 or higher. Give alkali by mouth (sodium bicarbonate

or equivalent, 5–15 g/d). Examine fresh urine for crystals and red cells every 5–7 days.

(3) Check hemoglobin, white blood cell count, and differential count once weekly to detect possible disturbances early in high-risk patients.

Rubin RH, Swartz MN: Trimethoprim-sulfamethoxazole. *N Engl J Med* 1980;**303**:426.

Towner KJ et al: Increasing importance of plasmid-mediated trimethoprim resistance in enterobacteria. *Br Med J* 1980;**280**:517.

## SULFONES USED IN THE TREATMENT OF LEPROSY

A number of drugs closely related to the sulfonamides (eg, dapsone; diaminodiphenylsulfone, DDS) have been used effectively in the long-term treatment of leprosy. Dapsone may also be effective for *P carinii* pneumonia in AIDS. The clinical manifestations of both lepromatous and tuberculoid leprosy can often be suppressed by treatment extending over several years. It appears that 5–30% of *Mycobacterium leprae* organisms are resistant to dapsone in 1985. Consequently, initial combined treatment with rifampin is advocated.

### Absorption, Metabolism, & Excretion

All sulfones are well absorbed from the intestinal tract, are distributed widely in all tissues, and tend to be retained in skin, muscle, liver, and kidney. Skin involved by leprosy contains 10 times more drug than normal skin. Sulfones are excreted into the bile and reabsorbed by the intestine. Consequently, blood levels are prolonged. Excretion into the urine is variable, and the drug occurs in urine mostly as a glucuronic acid conjugate. Some persons acetylate sulfones slowly and others rapidly; this requires dosage adjustment.

### Dosages & Routes of Administration

See p 878 for recommendations.

### Adverse Effects

The sulfones may cause any of the side effects listed above for sulfonamides. Anorexia, nausea, and vomiting are common. Hemolysis, methemoglobinemia, or agranulocytosis may occur. If sulfones are not tolerated, clofazimine or amithiozone can be substituted.

Yawalkar SJ et al: Once-monthly rifampin plus daily dapsone in initial treatment of lepromatous leprosy. *Lancet* 1982;**1**:1199.

## SPECIALIZED DRUGS AGAINST BACTERIA

### 1. BACITRACIN

This polypeptide is selectively active against gram-positive bacteria. Because of severe nephrotoxicity upon systemic administration, its use has been limited to topical application on surface lesions, usually in combination with polymyxin or neomycin. Occasionally it is given orally for pseudomembranous colitis caused by toxin-producing *Clostridium difficile* (see below).

### 2. LINCOMYCIN & CLINDAMYCIN

These drugs resemble erythromycin (although different in structure) and are active against gram-positive organisms (except enterococci). Lincomycin, 0.5 g orally every 6 hours (30–60 mg/kg/d for children), or clindamycin, 0.15–0.3 g orally every 6 hours (10–40 mg/kg/d for children) yields serum concentrations of 2–5 μg/mL. The drugs are widely distributed in tissues. Excretion is through the bile and urine. The drugs are alternatives to erythromycin as substitutes for penicillin. Clindamycin is effective against most strains of *Bacteroides* and is a drug of choice in anaerobic infections, sometimes in combination with an aminoglycoside. Seriously ill patients are given clindamycin, 600 mg (20–30 mg/kg/d) intravenously during a 1-hour period every 8 hours. Success has also been reported in staphylococcal osteomyelitis. These drugs are ineffective in meningitis.

Common side effects are diarrhea, nausea, and skin rashes. Impaired liver function and neutropenia have been noted. If 3–4 g is given rapidly intravenously, cardiorespiratory arrest may occur. Bloody diarrhea with pseudomembranous colitis has been associated with the administration of clindamycin and other antibiotics. This antibiotic-associated colitis is due to a necrotizing toxin produced by *C difficile*. The organism is resistant to the antimicrobial, is selected out by its presence, and is favored in its growth and toxin production. *C difficile* is usually susceptible to—and can be treated with—vancomycin, (see below), bacitracin, or metronidazole given orally.

Bartlett JG: Anti-anaerobic antibacterial agents. *Lancet* 1982;**2**:478.

Larson HE et al: *Clostridium difficile* and the etiology of pseudomembranous colitis. *Lancet* 1978;**1**:1063.

### 3. METRONIDAZOLE

This is an antiprotozoal drug (see p 899) used for trichomonal and amebic infections. It also has striking antibacterial effects in anaerobic infections, in which the dose is 500–750 mg orally 3 or 4 times daily. In trichomoniasis and in *Gardnerella* (*Haemo-*

*philus*) vaginitis, 500 mg orally twice daily for 7 days is given. Metronidazole may also be effective for preparation of the colon before bowel surgery, though it has not yet been approved for this purpose because of possible carcinogenic effects. Oral metronidazole, 500 mg 3 times daily, is an effective alternative to vancomycin for treatment of antibiotic-associated colitis due to *C difficile*. Metronidazole can be given intravenously (7.5 mg/kg in 1 hour) 3 times daily or by rectal suppository. It is well absorbed by the latter route and gives drug levels comparable to those reached after intravenous administration. Simultaneous administration of barbiturates reduces the half-life of metronidazole. Metronidazole reaches high levels in brain tissue. It can sometimes cure small, multiple brain abscesses without surgical drainage.

Adverse effects including stomatitis, nausea, diarrhea, and disulfiram reactions may occur. With prolonged high doses, reversible peripheral neuropathy can develop.

Goldman P: Metronidazole. *N Engl J Med* 1980;**303**:1212.
Warner JF et al: Metronidazole therapy of anaerobic bacteremia, meningitis, and brain abscess. *Arch Intern Med* 1979;**139**:167.

## 4. VANCOMYCIN

This drug is bactericidal for most gram-positive organisms, particularly staphylococci and enterococci, in concentrations of 0.5–10 μg/mL. Resistant mutants are very rare, and there is no cross-resistance with other antimicrobial drugs. Vancomycin is not absorbed from the gut. It is given orally only for the treatment of antibiotic-associated enterocolitis. For systemic effect the drug must be administered intravenously, and for meningitis intrathecally. After intravenous injection of 0.5 g over a period of 20 minutes, blood levels of 10 μg/mL are maintained for 1–2 hours. Vancomycin is excreted mainly via the kidneys but may accumulate also in liver failure. In renal insufficiency, the half-life may be up to 8 days. Thus, only one dose of 0.5–1 g may be given every 4–8 days to a uremic individual undergoing hemodialysis.

Indications for parenteral vancomycin include staphylococcal or enterococcal endocarditis and serious methicillin-resistant infections due to *S aureus* or *S epidermidis*. Vancomycin, 0.5 g, is injected intravenously over a 20-minute period every 6–8 hours (for children, 20–40 mg/kg/d). Against streptococci, synergism with an aminoglycoside can occur. Vancomycin, 0.125–0.5 g orally 2–4 times daily, is effective in antibiotic-associated enterocolitis (see above).

Vancomycin is irritating to tissues; chills, fever, and thrombophlebitis sometimes follow intravenous injection. The drug is somewhat ototoxic and perhaps nephrotoxic. Rapid infusion may induce diffuse hyperemia ("red man syndrome") and can be avoided by extending infusions over 1 hour.

Tedesco F et al: Oral vancomycin for antibiotic-associated pseudomembranous colitis. *Lancet* 1978;**2**:226.
Wise RI: The Vancomycin Symposium: Summary and comments. *Rev Infect Dis* 1981;**3(Suppl):**S293.

## 5. QUINOLONES

Norfloxacin, ciprofloxacin, and other quinolones are analogs of nalidixic acid that inhibit DNA synthesis through inhibition of DNA gyrase. These drugs are active against gram-positive cocci (including enterococci and methicillin-resistant *S aureus*), gram-negative rods (including *P aeruginosa, Salmonella, Shigella, Campylobacter jejuni, Yersinia enterocolitica*), and intracellular organisms such as *Legionella, Brucella,* atypical mycobacteria, and others. Activity against anaerobes is variable.

Oral and intravenous preparations are available. After oral administration, quinolones are well absorbed and penetrate into tissues and fluids. Their half-life is 3–4 hours, permitting dosage 2–3 times daily. Initial results indicate that these drugs are useful for therapy of urinary tract infections and traveler's diarrhea and for prophylaxis against infection in neutropenic patients. Clinical uses are under investigation, and dosages are tentative.

Hooper DC, Wolfson JS: The fluoroquinolones: Pharmacology, clinical uses and toxicities in humans. *Antimicrob Agents Chemother* 1985;**28**:716.
Neu HC: New antibiotics: Areas of appropriate use. *J Infect Dis* 1987;**155**:403.

## URINARY ANTISEPTICS

These drugs exert antimicrobial activity in the urine but have little or no systemic antibacterial effect. Their usefulness is limited to urinary tract infections.

## 1. NITROFURANTOIN

Nitrofurantoin is bacteriostatic and bactericidal for both gram-positive and gram-negative bacteria in concentrations of 10–500 μg/mL. Microbial resistance does not emerge rapidly. The activity of nitrofurantoin is greatly enhanced at pH 6.5 or less.

Nitrofurantoin is rapidly absorbed from the gut, but levels in serum and tissues are negligible. Thus, there is no systemic antibacterial effect. The drug is rapidly excreted in urine, where concentrations may be 200–400 μg/mL. In renal failure, there is virtually no excretion into the urine and no therapeutic effect.

The average daily dose in urinary tract infections is 100 mg orally 4 times daily (for children, 5–10 mg/kg/d), taken with food. A single daily dose of

50–100 mg can prevent recurrent urinary tract infections in women.

Oral nitrofurantoin often causes nausea and vomiting. Hemolytic anemia occurs in G6PD deficiency. Hypersensitivity may produce skin rashes and pulmonary infiltration.

## 2. NALIDIXIC ACID & OXOLINIC ACID

Nalidixic acid is a synthetic urinary antiseptic that inhibits many gram-negative bacteria in concentrations of 1–50 μg/mL but has no effect on *Pseudomonas*. In susceptible bacterial populations, resistant mutants emerge fairly rapidly.

Nalidixic acid is readily absorbed from the gut. In the blood, virtually all drug is firmly bound to protein. Thus, there is no systemic antibacterial action. About 20% of the absorbed drug is excreted in the urine in active form to give urine levels of 20–200 μg/mL, which may produce false-positive tests for glucose.

The dose in urinary tract infections is 1 g orally 4 times daily (for children, 30–60 mg/kg/d). Adverse reactions include nausea, vomiting, rash, drowsiness, visual hallucinations, excitement, and, rarely, increased intracranial pressure with convulsions.

Oxolinic acid is similar to nalidixic acid. Cinoxacin, a drug related to nalidixic acid, can be effective in urinary tract infections in oral doses of 250 mg 4 times daily or 500 mg twice daily.

Brumfitt W, Hamilton-Miller JMT: Sulfonamides, nalidixic acid, oxolinic acid, methenamine and nitrofurans. In: *Antimicrobial Therapy,* 3rd ed. Kagan BM (editor): Saunders, 1980.

## 3. METHENAMINE MANDELATE & METHENAMINE HIPPURATE

These are salts of methenamine and mandelic acid or hippuric acid. The action of the drug depends on the liberation of formaldehyde and of acid in the urine and is enhanced by acetohydroxamic acid. The urinary pH must be below 5.5, and sulfonamides must not be given at the same time. The drug inhibits a variety of different microorganisms except those (eg, *Proteus*) that liberate ammonia from urea and produce strongly alkaline urine. The dosage is 2–6 g orally daily.

## 4. ACIDIFYING AGENTS

Urine with a pH below 5.5 tends to be antibacterial. Many substances can acidify urine and thus produce antibacterial activity. Ammonium chloride, ascorbic acid, methionine, and mandelic acid are sometimes used. The dose must be established for each patient by testing the urine for acid pH with test paper at frequent intervals.

## SYSTEMICALLY ACTIVE DRUGS IN URINARY TRACT INFECTIONS

Many antimicrobial drugs are excreted in the urine in very high concentration. For this reason, low and relatively nontoxic amounts of aminoglycosides, polymyxins, and cycloserine (see above) can produce effective urine levels. Many penicillins, cephalosporins, aminoglycosides, and trimethoprim-sulfamethoxazole can reach very high urine levels and can thus be effective in urinary tract infections.

Jawetz E: Urinary antiseptics. Chapter 51 in: *Basic & Clinical Pharmacology,* 3rd ed. Katzung BG (editor). Appleton-Lange, 1987.
Lohr JA et al: Prevention of recurrent urinary tract infections in girls. *Pediatrics* 1977;**59:**562.
Souney P, Polk BF: Single-dose therapy for urinary tract infections in women. *Rev Infect Dis* 1982;**4:**29.

## ANTIFUNGAL DRUGS

Most antibacterial substances have no effect on pathogenic fungi. Only a few drugs are known to be therapeutically useful in mycotic infections. Penicillins are used to treat actinomycosis; sulfonamides have been employed in nocardiosis.

## 1. AMPHOTERICIN B

Amphotericin B, 0.1–0.8 μg/mL, inhibits in vitro several organisms producing systemic mycotic disease in humans, including *Histoplasma, Cryptococcus, Coccidioides, Candida, Blastomyces, Sporothrix,* and others. This drug can be used for treatment of these systemic fungal infections. Intrathecal administration is necessary for the treatment of meningitis.

Amphotericin B solutions in 500 mL of 5% dextrose in water are given intravenously over a 4- to 8-hour period. The initial dose is 1–5 mg/d, increasing daily by 5-mg increments until a final dosage of 0.4–0.7 mg/kg/d is reached. This is usually continued daily or (in doubled doses) on alternate days for many weeks. In fungal meningitis, amphotericin B, 0.5 mg, is injected intrathecally 3 times weekly; continuous treatment (many weeks) with an Ommaya reservoir is sometimes employed. Relapses of fungal meningitis occur commonly. Combined treatment with flucytosine is beneficial in systemic candidiasis and cryptococcal meningitis. Amphotericin B can also be effective in *Naegleria* meningoencephalitis.

Amphotericin B is little removed by hemodialysis.

In impaired renal function, the amphotericin dose need not be reduced initially. However, if the drug further depresses renal function, the amphotericin dose is temporarily lowered (or even stopped for a few days) until renal function returns to its pretreatment level.

The intravenous administration of amphotericin

B usually produces chills, fever, vomiting, and headache. Tolerance may be enhanced by temporary lowering of the dose or administration of aspirin, diphenhydramine, phenothiazines, and corticosteroids. Therapeutically active amounts of amphotericin B commonly impair kidney and liver function and produce anemia (impaired iron utilization by bone marrow). Electrolyte disturbances (hypokalemia, distal tubular acidosis), shock, and a variety of neurologic symptoms also occur.

Drutz DJ, Catanzaro A: Coccidioidomycosis. *Am Rev Respir Dis* 1978;**117**:727.
Medoff G, Kobayashi GS: Strategies in the treatment of systemic fungal infections. *N Engl J Med* 1980;**302**:145.

## 2. GRISEOFULVIN

Griseofulvin is an antibiotic that can inhibit the growth of some dermatophytes but has no effect on bacteria or on the fungi that cause deep mycoses. Absorption of griseofulvin microsize, 1 g/d, gives blood levels of 0.5–1.5 $\mu$g/mL. The absorbed drug has an affinity for skin and is deposited there, bound to keratin. Thus, it makes keratin resistant to fungal growth, and the new growth of hair or nails is first free of infection. As keratinized structures are shed, they are replaced by uninfected ones. The bulk of ingested griseofulvin is excreted in the feces. Topical application of griseofulvin has little effect.

Give oral doses of 0.5–1 g/d (for children, 15 mg/kg/d) for 3–5 weeks if only the skin is involved and for 3–6 months or longer if the hair and nails are involved. Griseofulvin is most successful in severe dermatophytosis, particularly if caused by *Trichophyton rubrum*. Some strains of fungi are resistant.

An ultramicrosize particle formulation is better absorbed (Gris-PEG). The dose is 0.33–0.66 g orally daily for adults or 7.25 mg/kg/d for children.

Side effects include headache, nausea, diarrhea, photosensitivity, fever, skin rashes, and disturbances of hepatic, nervous, and hematopoietic systems. Griseofulvin increases the metabolism of coumarin anticoagulants, so that higher doses are needed. It is teratogenic and carcinogenic in rodents.

## 3. NYSTATIN

Nystatin inhibits *Candida* species upon direct contact. The drug is not absorbed from mucous membranes or gut. Nystatin in ointments, suspensions, etc, can be applied to buccal or vaginal mucous membranes to suppress a local *Candida* infection. After oral intake of nystatin, *Candida* in the gut is suppressed and the drug is excreted in feces. The only indication for the use of nystatin orally is for control of oral candidiasis, especially in immunosuppressed patients.

## 4. FLUCYTOSINE

5-Flucytosine inhibits some strains of *Candida, Cryptococcus, Aspergillus, Torulopsis,* and other fungi. Dosages of 3–8 g daily (150 mg/kg/d) orally produce good levels in serum and cerebrospinal fluid. Clinical remissions of meningitis or sepsis due to yeasts have occurred. However, resistant organisms are selected out rapidly, and flucytosine is therefore not employed as a single drug except in urinary tract infections.

In renal insufficiency, flucytosine may accumulate to toxic levels. It is effectively removed by hemodialysis. Toxic effects include bone marrow depression, abnormal liver function, loss of hair, and others. The side effects may be caused by conversion of flucytosine to 5-fluorouracil in the body. Combined use of flucytosine and amphotericin B in systemic candidiasis and cryptococcal meningitis has been shown to be of value.

Bennett JE et al: A comparison of amphotericin alone and combined with flucytosine in the treatment of cryptococcal meningitis. *N Engl J Med* 1979;**301**:126.

## 5. NATAMYCIN

Natamycin is a polyene antifungal drug effective against many different fungi in vitro. When combined with appropriate surgical measures, topical application of 5% ophthalmic suspension may be beneficial in the treatment of keratitis caused by *Fusarium, Cephalosporium,* or other fungi. The drug may also be effective in the treatment of oral or vaginal candidiasis. The toxicity after topical application appears to be low.

## 6. ANTIFUNGAL IMIDAZOLES

These antifungal drugs increase membrane permeability and inhibit lipid and enzyme synthesis. **Clotrimazole,** taken orally in 10-mg troches 5 times daily, can suppress oral candidiasis. It is too toxic for systemic use. **Miconazole** is used as a 2% cream in dermatophytosis and vaginal candidiasis. When used intravenously (30 mg/kg/d) it produced many serious side effects and was only moderately effective in controlling systemic mycoses.

**Ketoconazole** inhibits synthesis of sterols in fungal cell membranes, among other effects. It can be given orally in a single dose, 200–600 mg daily, preferably with food. It is well absorbed and reaches serum levels of 2–4 $\mu$g/mL, and it is metabolized in vivo. The dose remains the same in renal or hepatic failure. Absorption is impaired by antacid, cimetidine, or rifampin administration.

Ketoconazole dramatically improves chronic mucocutaneous candidiasis, vaginal candidiasis, paracoccidioidomycosis, and blastomycosis. It also has therapeutic benefits in noncavitary pulmonary coccidioidomycosis and histoplasmosis but not in meningitis due to these fungi. In disease of moderate severity, this oral antifungal drug has given encouraging results.

Adverse effects include nausea, vomiting, skin rashes, and occasional elevations in transaminase levels. Ketoconazole blocks the synthesis of adrenal steroids and testosterone and can cause gynecomastia and impotence.

Craven PC et al: High-dose ketoconazole for treatment of fungal infections of the central nervous system. *Ann Intern Med* 1983;**98**:160.

Dismukes WE et al: Treatment of systemic mycoses with ketoconazole. *Ann Intern Med* 1983;**98**:13.

NIH Mycoses Study Group: Treatment of blastomycosis and histoplasmosis with ketoconazole. *Ann Intern Med* 1985; **103**:861.

Pont A et al: Ketoconazole blocks adrenal steroid synthesis. *Ann Intern Med* 1982;**97**:370.

Restrepo A, Stevens DA, Utz JP (editors): Symposium on ketoconazole. *Rev Infect Dis* 1980;**2**:519.

Ross JB et al: Ketoconazole for treatment of chronic pulmonary coccidioidomycosis. *Ann Intern Med* 1982;**96**:440.

## ANTIMICROBIAL DRUGS USED IN COMBINATION

### Indications

Possible reasons for employing 2 or more antimicrobials simultaneously instead of a single drug are as follows:

(1) Prompt treatment in desperately ill patients suspected of having a serious microbial infection. A good guess about the most probable 2 or 3 pathogens is made, and drugs are aimed at those organisms. Before such treatment is started, adequate specimens must be obtained for identifying the etiologic agent in the laboratory. Suspected gram-negative or staphylococcal sepsis and bacterial meningitis in children are the foremost indications in this category at present.

(2) To delay the emergence of microbial mutants resistant to one drug in chronic infections by the use of a second or third non-cross-reacting drug. The most prominent examples are active tuberculosis of one or more organs, with large microbial populations.

(3) Mixed infections, particularly those following massive trauma or those involving vascular structures. Each drug is aimed at an important pathogenic microorganism.

(4) To achieve bactericidal synergism (see below). In a few infections, eg, enterococcal sepsis, a combination of drugs is more likely to eradicate the infection than either drug used alone. Unfortunately, such synergism is unpredictable. A given drug pair may be synergistic for only one microbial strain. Occasionally, simultaneous use of 2 drugs permits significant reduction in dose and thus avoids toxicity but still provides satisfactory antimicrobial action.

### Disadvantages

The following disadvantages of using antimicrobial drugs in combinations must always be considered:

(1) The doctor may feel that since several drugs are already being given, everything possible has been done for the patient. This attitude leads to relaxation of the effort to establish a specific diagnosis. It may also give a false sense of security.

(2) The more drugs are administered, the greater the chance for drug reactions to occur or for the patient to become sensitized to drugs.

(3) The cost is unnecessarily high.

(4) Antimicrobial combinations usually accomplish no more than an effective single drug.

(5) On very rare occasions, one drug may antagonize a second drug given simultaneously. Antagonism resulting in higher morbidity and mortality rates has been observed mainly in bacterial meningitis when a bacteriostatic drug (eg, tetracycline or chloramphenicol) was given prior to or with a bactericidal drug (eg, a penicillin or aminoglycoside). However, antagonism is usually limited by time-dose relationships and is overcome by an excess dose of one of the drugs in the pair and is therefore a very infrequent problem in clinical therapy.

### Synergism

Antimicrobial synergism can occur in several types of situations. Synergistic drug combinations must be selected by complex laboratory procedures.

(1) Sequential block of a microbial metabolic pathway by 2 drugs. Sulfonamides inhibit the use of extracellular $p$-aminobenzoic acid by some microbes for the synthesis of folic acid. Trimethoprim or pyrimethamine inhibits the next metabolic step, the reduction of dihydro- to tetrahydrofolic acid. The simultaneous use of a sulfonamide plus trimethoprim is effective in some bacterial infections (eg, urinary tract, enteric) and in some parasitic infections (*Pneumocystis* infection). Pyrimethamine plus a sulfonamide is used in toxoplasmosis and malaria.

(2) One drug may greatly enhance the uptake of a second drug and thereby greatly increase the overall bactericidal effect. Penicillins enhance the uptake of aminoglycosides by enterococci. Thus, a penicillin plus an aminoglycoside may be essential for the eradication of *S faecalis* or *Streptococcus* group B infections, particularly in sepsis or endocarditis. Similarly, ticarcillin plus gentamicin may be synergistic against some strains of *Pseudomonas*. Cell wall inhibitors (penicillins and cephalosporins) may also enhance the entry of aminoglycosides into other gram-negative bacteria and thus produce synergistic effects.

(3) One drug may affect the cell membrane and facilitate the entry of the second drug. The combined effect may then be greater than the sum of its parts. Polymyxins have been synergistic with trimethoprim-sulfamethoxazole or rifampin against *Serratia,* and amphotericin has been synergistic with flucytosine against *Candida* and *Cryptococcus*.

(4) One drug prevents the inactivation of a second

drug by microbial enzymes. Thus, inhibitors of β-lactamase (eg, clavulanic acid) can protect amoxicillin or ticarcillin from inactivation by β-lactamase-producing *H influenzae* and other organisms.

Jawetz E: The doctor's dilemma. In: *Current Clinical Topics in Infectious Diseases.* Remington JS, Swartz MN (editors). McGraw-Hill, 1981.

Rahal JJ: Antibiotic combinations: The clinical relevance of synergy and antagonism. *Medicine* 1978;**57**:179.

## ANTIMICROBIAL CHEMOPROPHYLAXIS

Anti-infective chemoprophylaxis implies the administration of antimicrobial drugs to prevent infection. In a broader sense, it also includes the use of antimicrobial drugs soon after the acquisition of pathogenic microorganisms (eg, after compound fracture) but before the development of signs of infection.

Useful chemoprophylaxis is limited to the action of a specific drug on a specific organism. An effort to prevent all types of microorganisms in the environment from establishing themselves only selects the most drug-resistant organisms as the cause of a resulting infection. In all proposed uses of prophylactic antimicrobials, the risk of the patient's acquiring an infection must be weighed against the toxicity, cost, inconvenience, and enhanced risk of superinfection resulting from the "prophylactic" drug.

### Prophylaxis in Persons of Normal Susceptibility Exposed to a Specific Pathogen

In this category, a specific drug is administered to prevent one specific infection. Outstanding examples are the injection of benzathine penicillin G, 1.2 million units intramuscularly once every 3–4 weeks, to prevent reinfection with group A hemolytic streptococci in patients who have had rheumatic fever; prevention of meningitis by eradicating the meningococcal carrier state with rifampin, 600 mg orally twice daily for 2 days, or minocycline, 100 mg every 12 hours for 5 days; prevention of *H influenzae* disease in contacts of patients with rifampin, 20 mg/kg/d for 4 days; prevention of syphilis by the injection of benzathine penicillin G, 2.4 million units intramuscularly, within 24 hours of exposure; prevention of plague pneumonia in contacts of patients with tetracycline, 0.5 g twice daily for 5 days; and prevention of clinical rickettsial disease (but not of infection) by the daily ingestion of 1 g tetracycline during exposure.

Early treatment of an asymptomatic infection is sometimes called "prophylaxis." Thus, administration of isoniazid, 6–10 mg/kg/d (maximum, 300 mg daily) orally for 6–12 months, to an asymptomatic person who converts from a negative to a positive tuberculin skin test may prevent later clinical active tuberculosis.

### Prophylaxis in Persons of Increased Susceptibility

Certain anatomic or functional abnormalities predispose to serious infections. It may be feasible to prevent or abort such infections by giving a specific drug for short periods. Some important examples are listed below:

**A. Heart Disease:** Persons with abnormalities of heart valves or with prosthetic valves are unusually susceptible to implantation of microorganisms circulating in the bloodstream. This bacterial endocarditis can sometimes be prevented if the proper drug can be used during periods of bacteremia. Large numbers of viridans streptococci are pushed into the circulation during dental procedures and operations on the mouth or throat. At such times, the increased risk warrants the use of a prophylactic antimicrobial drug aimed at viridans streptococci, eg, a penicillin administered 1 hour before and 6 hours after the procedure. (See Shulman reference, below.) It may be that an aminoglycoside should be given together with penicillin for optimal bactericidal effect. In persons hypersensitive to penicillin or those receiving daily doses of penicillin for prolonged periods (for rheumatic fever prophylaxis), erythromycin, 2 g daily orally, can be substituted to cover penicillin-resistant viridans streptococci in the throat.

Enterococci cause 5–15% of cases of bacterial endocarditis. They reach the bloodstream from the urinary or gastrointestinal tract or from the female genital tract. During surgical procedures in these areas, persons with heart valve abnormalities can be given prophylaxis directed against enterococci, eg, penicillin G, 5 million units, plus gentamicin, 3 mg/kg intramuscularly daily, beginning on the day of surgery and continuing for 2 days.

During and after cardiac catheterization, blood cultures may be positive in 10–20% of patients. Many of these persons also have fever, but very few acquire endocarditis. Prophylactic antimicrobials do not appear to influence these events.

**B. Respiratory Tract Disease:** Persons with functional and anatomic abnormalities of the respiratory tract—eg, emphysema or bronchiectasis—are subject to attacks of "recurrent chronic bronchitis." This is a recurrent bacterial infection, often precipitated by acute viral infections and resulting in respiratory decompensation. The most common organisms are pneumococci and *H influenzae*. Chemoprophylaxis consists of giving tetracycline or ampicillin, 1 g daily orally, during the "respiratory disease season." This is successful only in patients who are not hospitalized; otherwise, superinfection with *Pseudomonas, Proteus,* or yeasts is common. Similar prophylaxis of bacterial infection has been applied to children with mucoviscidosis who are not hospitalized. In spite of this, such children contract complicating infections caused by *Pseudomonas* and staphylococci. Trimethoprim-sulfamethoxazole is effective as a prophylactic against *Pneumocystis* pneumonia in immunocompromised persons.

**C. Recurrent Urinary Tract Infection:** In certain women who are subject to frequently recurring urinary tract infections, oral intake of nitrofurantoin, 100 mg, or trimethoprim (40 mg)-sulfamethoxazole (200 mg), daily or 3 times weekly, can markedly reduce the frequency of symptomatic recurrences over periods of many months—perhaps years—until resistant microorganisms appear.

Certain women frequently develop symptoms of cystitis after sexual intercourse. The ingestion of a single dose of antimicrobial drug (100 mg nitrofurantoin, 250 mg cephalexin, etc) can prevent this postcoital cystitis by early inhibition of growth of bacteria moved into the proximal urethra or bladder from the introitus during intercourse.

**D. Opportunistic Infections in Severe Granulocytopenia:** Patients with leukemia or neoplasm develop profound leukopenia while being given antineoplastic chemotherapy. When the neutrophil count falls below 500/$\mu$L, they become unusually susceptible to opportunistic infections, most often gram-negative sepsis. In some cancer centers, such individuals are given a drug combination (eg, vancomycin, gentamicin, cephalosporin) directed at the most prevalent opportunists at the earliest sign—or even without clinical evidence—of infection. This is continued for several days until the granulocyte count rises again. Retrospective studies suggest that there is some benefit to this procedure.

In other centers, such patients are given oral insoluble antimicrobials (neomycin + polymyxin + nystatin) during the period of granulopenia to reduce the incidence of gram-negative sepsis. Some benefit has been reported from this approach.

## Prophylaxis in Surgery

A major portion of all antimicrobial drugs used in hospitals is employed on surgical services with the stated intent of "prophylaxis." The administration of antimicrobials before and after surgical procedures is sometimes viewed as "banning the microbial world" both from the site of the operation and from other organ systems that suffer postoperative complications. Regrettably, the provable benefit of antimicrobial prophylaxis in surgery is much more limited.

Several general features of "surgical prophylaxis" merit consideration.

(1) In clean elective surgical procedures (ie, procedures during which no tissue bearing normal flora is traversed, other than the prepared skin), the disadvantages of "routine" antibiotic prophylaxis (allergy, toxicity, superinfection) generally outweigh the possible benefits.

(2) Prophylactic administration of antibiotics should generally be considered only if the expected rate of infectious complications approaches or exceeds 5%. An exception to this rule is the elective insertion of prostheses (cardiovascular, orthopedic), where a possible infection would have a catastrophic effect.

(3) If prophylactic antimicrobials are to be effective, a sufficient concentration of drug must be present at the operative site to inhibit or kill bacteria that might settle there. Thus, it is essential that drug administration begin 1–3 hours before operation.

(4) Prolonged administration of antimicrobial drugs tends to alter the normal flora of organ systems, suppressing the susceptible microorganisms and favoring the implantation of drug-resistant ones. Thus, antimicrobial prophylaxis should last only 1–3 days after the procedure to prevent superinfection.

(5) Systemic antimicrobial levels usually do not prevent wound infection, pneumonia, or urinary tract infection if physiologic abnormalities or foreign bodies are present.

In major surgical procedures, the administration of a "broad-spectrum" bactericidal drug from just before until 1 day after the procedure has been found effective. Thus, cefazolin, 1 g intramuscularly or intravenously given 2 hours before gastrointestinal, pelvic, or orthopedic procedures and again at 2, 10, and 18 hours after the end of the operation, reduces the risk of deep infections at the operative site. Similarly, in cardiovascular surgery, antimicrobials directed at the commonest organisms producing infection are begun just prior to the procedure and continued for 2 or 3 days thereafter. While this prevents drug-susceptible organisms from producing endocarditis, pericarditis, or similar complications, it may favor the implantation of drug-resistant bacteria or fungi.

Other forms of surgical prophylaxis attempt to reduce normal flora or existing bacterial contamination at the site. Thus, the colon is routinely prepared not only by mechanical cleansing through cathartics and enemas but also by the oral administration of insoluble drugs (eg, neomycin, 1 g, plus erythromycin base, 1 g every 6 hours) for one day before operation. In the case of a perforated viscus resulting in peritoneal contamination, there is little doubt that immediate treatment with an aminoglycoside, a penicillin, or clindamycin reduces the impact of seeded infection. Similarly, grossly infected compound fractures or war wounds benefit from a penicillin or cephalosporin plus an aminoglycoside. In all these instances, the antimicrobials tend to reduce the likelihood of rapid and early invasion of the bloodstream and tend to help localize the infectious process—although they generally are incapable of preventing it altogether. The surgeon must be watchful for the selection of the most resistant members of the flora, which tend to manifest themselves 2 or 3 days after the beginning of such "prophylaxis"—which is really an attempt at very early treatment.

In all situations where antimicrobials are administered with the hope that they may have a "prophylactic" effect, the risk from these same drugs (allergy, toxicity, selection of superinfecting microorganisms) must be evaluated daily, and the course of prophylaxis must be kept as brief as possible.

Topical antimicrobials (intravenous tube site catheter, closed urinary drainage, within a surgical wound, acrylic bone cement, etc) may have limited usefulness but must always be viewed with suspicion.

Hughes WT et al: Successful chemoprophylaxis for *Pneumocystis carinii* pneumonitis. *N Engl J Med* 1977;**297**:1419.

Jackson GG: Considerations of antibiotic prophylaxis in nonsurgical high risk patients. *Am J Med* 1981;**70**:467.

Joshi JH et al: Can antibacterial therapy be discontinued in persistently febrile granulocytopenic cancer patients? *Am J Med* 1984;**76**:450.

Kaiser AB: Antimicrobial prophylaxis in surgery. *N Engl J Med* 1986;**315**:1129.

Kaplan EL et al: AHA Committee Report: Prevention of rheumatic fever. *Circulation* 1977b;**55**:S1.

Shulman ST et al: Prevention of bacterial endocarditis. (Committee on Rheumatic Fever and Infective Endocarditis of the Council on Cardiovascular Disease.) *Circulation* 1984;**70**:1123A.

Storring RA et al: Oral non-absorbed antibiotics prevent infection in acute non-lymphoblastic leukemia. *Lancet* 1977;**2**:837.

## ANTIVIRAL CHEMOTHERAPY

Several compounds can influence viral replication and the development of viral disease.

**Amantadine hydrochloride,** 200 mg orally daily for 2–3 days before and 6–7 days after influenza A infection, reduces the incidence and severity of symptoms. It deserves wider use as a prophylactic in persons at high risk. The most marked untoward effects are insomnia, nightmares, and ataxia, especially in the elderly. Amantadine may accumulate and be more toxic in renal insufficiency. Rimantadine is equally effective and perhaps less toxic.

**Idoxuridine,** 0.1% solution or 0.5% ointment, can be applied topically every 2 hours to acute dendritic herpetic keratitis to enhance healing. It is also used, with corticosteroids, for stromal disciform lesions of the cornea to reduce the chance of acute epithelial herpes. Because of its toxicity for the cornea, it must not be used for more than 2–3 weeks. **Trifluridine** ointment (1%) is more effective than idoxuridine in herpetic keratitis but also more expensive.

**Vidarabine (adenine arabinoside),** 3% administered topically, is very effective in herpetic keratitis. Vidarabine, 15 mg/kg/d intravenously, provides systemic treatment for some herpesvirus infections. In immunocompromised patients it can reduce the dissemination of herpes zoster if begun before the fifth day of the skin eruption. In herpes simplex encephalitis it can reduce the mortality rate significantly if begun before the patient becomes comatose and continued for 10 days. About 40% of the survivors of herpes simplex encephalitis may resume a normal life, while the remainder suffer major neurologic sequelae. In neonatal herpes it can limit the spread of lesions. However, the incidence of cytomegalovirus pneumonia in recipients of bone marrow transplants or kidney transplants has not been reduced by prophylactic vidarabine. Topical vidarabine likewise has no effect on herpetic lesions of skin or mucous membranes.

The untoward effects of vidarabine include rashes, gastrointestinal disturbances, and neurologic abnormalities including tremors, ataxia, abnormal electroencephalogram, paresthesias, and encephalopathy. All of these are enhanced in renal failure.

**Methisazone,** 2–4 g orally given within 2 days after exposure to smallpox, protected against clinical disease. The drug is also effective against complications of vaccinia, which continue to occur in military personnel in the USA. The most serious adverse effect is profuse vomiting.

**Photodynamic inactivation** had been widely used as topical therapy for skin and mucous membrane lesions caused by herpes simplex. Controlled clinical studies failed to show a significant benefit from this treatment. There is no justification for its use.

**Acyclovir** is the least toxic antiviral drug, with therapeutic effects in infections due to herpes simplex and in herpes zoster-varicella infections. In herpes-infected cells, it is selectively active against viral DNA polymerase and thus inhibits virus proliferation. Given intravenously (15 mg/kg/d or 250 mg/m² every 8 hours), it can prevent or limit mucocutaneous herpes simplex in immunocompromised patients and can reduce pain and accelerate healing of herpes zoster and primary genital herpes simplex (in females), but it affects neither the establishment of latent infection nor the frequency of recurrence. In herpetic encephalitis and in neonatal herpetic dissemination, acyclovir is more effective than vidarabine. There is no significant effect on cytomegalovirus or EB virus infections, but acyclovir can arrest the progression of varicella and herpes zoster in immunocompromised patients.

Oral acyclovir, 200 mg 5 times daily, has therapeutic effects similar to those achieved with intravenous acyclovir, particularly in primary genital herpes simplex infections. When taken prophylactically for 4–6 months, oral acyclovir can reduce the frequency and severity of recurrent lesions during this period.

Topical 5% acyclovir ointment can be applied to mucocutaneous lesions caused by herpes simplex virus. It can shorten the period of pain and viral shedding in mucocutaneous oral lesions in immunosuppressed persons but not in patients with normal immunity. It can also be of benefit in primary but not in recurrent genital herpetic lesions by decreasing healing time of lesions and reducing pain.

**Ribavirin** aerosols sprayed into the respiratory tract early in influenza A and B infection of young adults or respiratory syncytial virus infections of small children resulted in a reduction of symptoms and more rapid recovery. Intravenous ribavirin can significantly lower the fatality rate of Lassa fever.

**Azidothymidine (AZT, Zidovudine; Retrovir)** is a synthetic thymidine analog that can be incorporated into DNA by the DNA polymerase (reverse transcriptase) of HIV/HTLV III/LAV. This terminates chain synthesis of viral DNA. HIV reverse transcriptase is about 100 times more susceptible to inhibition by AZT than the DNA polymerase of mammalian cells.

AZT is well absorbed from the gut; peak serum concentrations after 5 mg/kg by mouth are similar to those reached after 2.5 mg/kg intravenously in 1 hour. The drug is metabolized by the liver and excreted in the urine with a half-life of 1 hour. AZT appears to penetrate fairly well into the cerebrospinal fluid.

AZT appears to inhibit retrovirus synthesis and temporarily decrease the morbidity and mortality rates in patients with AIDS or ARC. Patients with AIDS have a temporary increase in T4 lymphocytes and a reduction in opportunistic infections. In patients with ARC, the increase in T4 lymphocytes persists longer.

The main adverse effects are anemia, granulocytopenia, thrombocytopenia due to bone marrow suppression, and the need for frequent transfusions. There may also be headaches, restlessness, agitation, and insomnia. It is likely that drugs which interfere with glucuronide conjugation in the liver (eg, acetaminophen, trimethoprim-sulfamethoxazole) will increase AZT toxicity.

In the treatment of AIDS, the dose suggested for AZT is 200 mg orally every 4 hours, perhaps to be reduced when adverse effects develop. Information is available through a "Retrovir Information Line" ([800] 843-9388, working hours, Eastern Standard Time).

**Investigational drugs for cytomegalovirus (CMV) infections.** While CMV has long been known as a cause of intrauterine infection and resulting defects, the increasing number of immunocompromised patients—especially those who receive organ transplants or antineoplastic drugs or suffer from AIDS—has drawn attention to the importance of CMV diseases, including retinitis and pneumonia with a high mortality rate. Two drugs are being investigated; both exhibit significant toxicity and neither is explicitly curative, but some remissions have been reported after their use.

**DHPG (9-[dihydroxy-2-propoxymethyl]guanine)** has been given to patients with confirmed CMV disease in doses of 5 mg/kg intravenously every 8–12 hours for 14 days. If started early—ie, before respiratory assistance was required—some improvement was noted in pneumonias, and virus shedding was reduced. Discontinuation of the drug, mainly because of marked neutropenia, was often followed by relapse. Some re-treatment with lower doses again produced improvement.

**Ganciclovir** is similar to acyclovir but markedly more effective against CMV in vitro. Patients with disseminated CMV disease were given 1–2.5 mg/kg every 8 hours as 1-hour infusions for 5–24 days.

Marked improvement occurred in retinitis and moderate improvement in pneumonia and gastrointestinal tract involvement. The major adverse effect was neutropenia, especially with higher doses, limiting treatment.

**Human interferons** have been prepared from stimulated lymphocytes or other cells and, more recently, by recombinant DNA technology. If given intravenously, $10^6$–$10^9$ units daily prevented dissemination of early herpes zoster in immunocompromised patients, prevented or delayed reactivation of herpes simplex after trigeminal root section, and suppressed viremia with hepatitis B virus. Interferons may have an adjunctive role in managing certain neoplasms or virus infections. Such preparations exhibit moderate antineoplastic and antiviral effects and, in high doses, significant toxicity. Possible practical use of this material is not yet evident.

Balfour HH et al: Acyclovir halts progression of herpes zoster in immunocompromised patients. *N Engl J Med* 1983;**308**:1448.

Bryson YB et al: Treatment of first episodes of genital herpes simplex virus infection with oral acyclovir. *N Engl J Med* 1983;**308**:916.

Collaborative DHPG Treatment Study Group: Treatment of serious cytomegalovirus with DHPG in patients with AIDS and other immunodeficiencies. *N Engl J Med* 1986;**314**:801.

Dolin R et al: A controlled trial of amantadine and rimantadine in the prophylaxis of influenza A infection. *N Engl J Med* 1982;**307**:580.

Laskin OL et al: Use of ganciclovir to treat serious cytomegalovirus infections in patients with AIDS. *J Infect Dis* 1987;**155**:323.

McClung HW et al: Ribavirin aerosol treatment of influenza B infection. *JAMA* 1983;**249**:2671.

McCormick JB et al: Lassa fever: Effective therapy with ribavirin. *N Engl J Med* 1986;**314**:20.

Redfield RR et al: Disseminated vaccinia in a military recruit with human immunodeficiency virus (HIV) disease. *N Engl J Med* 1987;**316**:673.

Reichman RC et al: Topically administered acyclovir in the treatment of recurrent herpes simplex genitalis. *J Infect Dis* 1983;**147**:336.

Reichman RC et al: Treatment of recurrent genital herpes simplex infections with oral acyclovir. *JAMA* 1984;**251**:2103.

Saral R et al: Acyclovir prophylaxis against herpes simplex infection in patients with leukemia. *Ann Intern Med* 1983;**99**:773.

Straus SE et al: Suppression of frequently recurring genital herpes with oral acyclovir. *N Engl J Med* 1984;**310**:1545.

Wade JC et al: Intravenous acyclovir to treat mucocutaneous herpes simplex virus infections after marrow transplantation. *Ann Intern Med* 1982;**96**:265.

Whitley RJ et al: Vidarabine versus acyclovir therapy in herpes simplex encephalitis. *N Engl J Med* 1986;**314**:144.

Wilson SZ et al: Treatment of influenza A (H1N1) virus infection with ribavirin aerosol. *Antimicrob Agents Chemother* 1984;**26**:200.

# REFERENCES

Barrett SP, Watt PJ: Antibiotics and the liver. *J Antimicrob Chemother* 1979;**5**:337.

Brown AE, Armstrong D (editors): Symposium on infectious complications of neoplastic disease. (2 parts.) *Am J Med* 1984;**76**:413, 631.

Committee on Infectious Diseases: *Report,* 20th ed. American Academy of Pediatrics, 1986.

Jawetz E, Melnick JL, Adelberg EA: *Review of Medical Microbiology,* 17th ed. Appleton-Lange, 1987.

Kagan BM: *Antimicrobial Therapy,* 3rd ed. Saunders, 1980.

Katzung BG (editor): *Basic & Clinical Pharmacology,* 3rd ed. Appleton-Lange, 1987.

Man and Drugs in the Third World: The doctor's viewpoint. (Workshop.) *Dan Med Bull* 1984;**31(Suppl 1).** [Entire issue.]

Neu HC: Changing patterns of hospital infections—implications for therapy: Changing mechanisms of bacterial resistance. *Am J Med* 1984;**77(1B)**:11.

Snavely SR, Hodges GR: The neurotoxicity of antibacterial agents. *Ann Intern Med* 1984;**101**:92.

# Disorders Due to Physical Agents

*Joseph LaDou, MD, Richard Cohen, MD, MPH, & Milton J. Chatton, MD*

## DISORDERS DUE TO COLD

Cold tolerance varies considerably among individuals. Factors that increase the likelihood of injury from exposure to cold include poor general physical conditioning, nonacclimatization, advanced age, systemic illness, poor tissue oxygenation, and the use of alcohol or other sedative drugs. High wind velocity ("windchill factor") increases the severity of cold injury at low temperatures.

### Cold Urticaria
Some persons have a familial or acquired hypersensitivity to cold and may develop urticaria upon even limited exposure to a cold wind. The urticaria usually occurs only on exposed areas, but in markedly sensitive individuals the response can be generalized. Immersion in cold water may result in severe systemic symptoms, including shock. Familial cold urticaria, manifested as a burning sensation of the skin occurring about 30 minutes after exposure to cold, does not seem to be a true urticarial disorder. In some patients with acquired cold urticaria, the disorder may be due to an underlying disease (eg, collagen disease, lymphoma, multiple myeloma) associated with cryoglobulinemia, which may result in purpura, Raynaud's phenomenon, and leg ulceration. Cold urticaria may be associated with cold hemoglobinuria as a complication of syphilis. In most cases of acquired cold urticaria, the cause is not known. The diagnosis is usually made by applying an ice cube to the skin: within a few minutes, an urticarial wheal appears at the site, accompanied by itching. Histamine and other mediators released in the cold urticaria response are similar to those found in allergic reactions. Antihistamines, however, are of limited value in preventing or treating attacks of cold urticaria.

### Raynaud's Phenomenon
See Chapter 9.

## SYSTEMIC HYPOTHERMIA

Systemic hypothermia may result from exposure (atmospheric or immersion) to prolonged or extreme cold. The condition may arise in otherwise healthy individuals in the course of occupational or recreational exposure or in victims of accidents.

Systemic hypothermia may follow exposure even to comparatively ordinary temperatures when there is altered homeostasis due to debility or disease. In colder climates, elderly and inactive individuals living in inadequately heated housing are particularly susceptible. Acute alcoholism is commonly a predisposing cause. Patients with cardiovascular or cerebrovascular disease, mental retardation, malnutrition, myxedema, and hypopituitarism are more vulnerable to accidental hypothermia. The use of sedative and tranquilizing drugs may be a contributing factor. Prolonged postoperative hypothermia with increased mortality rates after surgery has been reported, especially in elderly patients. Administration of large amounts of refrigerated stored blood (without rewarming) can cause systemic hypothermia.

### Pathogenesis
Systemic hypothermia is a reduction of core (rectal) body temperature below 35 °C. It causes reduced physiologic function—with decreased oxygen consumption and slowed myocardial repolarization, peripheral nerve conduction, gastrointestinal motility, and respirations—as well as hemoconcentration. The body defends itself against cold exposure by superficial blood vessel constriction and increased metabolic heat production.

### Clinical Findings
Early manifestations of hypothermia are not characteristic. There may be weakness, drowsiness, lethargy, irritability, confusion, and impaired coordination. A lowered body temperature may be the sole finding.

The internal (core) body temperature in accidental hypothermia may range from 25 to 35 °C (77–95 °F). Oral temperatures are useless, so a special rectal thermometer that reads as low as 25 °C is required. At rectal temperatures below 35 °C, the patient may become delirious, drowsy, or comatose and may stop breathing. Metabolic acidosis, pneumonia, ventricular fibrillation, hypoglycemia or hyperglycemia, and renal failure may occur. Abnormalities in cardiac rhythm are directly related to the lowering of core temperature. Progression of electrocardiographic abnormalities can also occur, including the pathognomonic "J" waves of Osborn. Death in systemic hypothermia usually results from cardiac arrest or ventricular fibrillation.

## Treatment

Patients with mild hypothermia (rectal temperature > 33 °C) who have been otherwise physically healthy usually respond well to a warm bed or to rapid rewarming with a warm bath or warm packs and blankets. A conservative approach is also usually employed in treating elderly or debilitated patients, using an electric blanket kept at 37 °C (98.6 °F).

Patients with moderate or severe hypothermia (core temperatures of < 32 °C [89.6 °F]) do not have the thermoregulatory shivering mechanism and so require active rewarming with individualized supportive care. Hypothermic victims should be transferred rapidly to a properly equipped emergency facility. They should be handled gently, because of the high incidence of occult associated trauma. The methods and rate of active rewarming are controversial. Aggressive rewarming should be attempted only by those experienced in the methods. Cardiopulmonary resuscitation may be necessary. The need for oxygen therapy, endotracheal intubation, controlled ventilation, warmed intravenous fluids, and treatment of metabolic acidosis should be dictated by careful clinical and laboratory monitoring during the rapid rewarming process. Cardiac rhythm should be monitored, and cardiac, central vascular, or chest trauma or stimulation (catheter, cannulas, etc) should be used judiciously because of the risk of inducing ventricular fibrillation during rewarming. Rectal core temperature should be recorded frequently and arterial blood gases measured as needed. It should be kept in mind that active rewarming is hazardous.

**Active External Rewarming Methods.** These are sometimes preferred when hypothermia is acute (eg, sudden, brief immersion in cold water). Although relatively simple and generally available, active external warming methods may cause marked peripheral dilation that predisposes to ventricular fibrillation and hypovolemic shock. Either heated blankets or warm baths may be used for active external rewarming. Rewarming by a warm bath is best carried out in a tub of stirred water at 40–42 °C (104–107.6 °F), with a rate of rewarming of about 1–2 °C/h. It is easier, however, to monitor the patient and to carry out diagnostic and therapeutic procedures when heated blankets are used for active rewarming.

**Active Internal (Core) Rewarming Methods.** Internal rewarming is suggested for patients with profound hypothermia of long duration, but the most effective methods are not clearly established. Repeated peritoneal dialysis may be employed with 2 L of warm (43 °C) potassium-free dialysate solution exchanged at intervals of 10–12 minutes until the rectal temperature is raised to about 35 °C. The administration of heated, humidified air through a face mask or endotracheal tube may be useful, either alone or as an adjunct to other rewarming techniques. Warm gastrointestinal irrigations and warm intravenous fluids are of limited value. Extracorporeal blood rewarming methods (eg, femorofemoral bypass) have been effectively employed in some medical centers to provide rapid cardiac rewarming with less likelihood of arrhythmias.

## Prognosis

With proper early care, more than 75% of otherwise healthy patients may survive moderate or severe systemic hypothermia. The risk of aspiration pneumonia is great in comatose patients. After obtaining at least one blood culture, consider use of antimicrobial drugs (see Chapter 7). The prognosis is grave if there are underlying predisposing causes or treatment is delayed.

## HYPOTHERMIA OF THE EXTREMITIES

Exposure of the extremities to cold produces immediate localized vasoconstriction followed by generalized vasoconstriction. When the skin temperature falls to 25 °C (77 °F), tissue metabolism is slowed, but the demand for oxygen is greater than the slowed circulation can supply, and the area becomes cyanotic. At 15 °C (59 °F), tissue metabolism is markedly decreased and the dissociation of oxyhemoglobin is reduced; this gives a deceptive pink, well-oxygenated appearance to the skin. Tissue damage occurs at this temperature. Tissue death may be caused by ischemia and thromboses in the smaller vessels or by actual freezing. Freezing (frostbite) does not occur until the skin temperature drops to –10 to –4 °C (14–24.8 °F) or even lower, depending on such factors as wind, mobility, venous stasis, malnutrition, and occlusive arterial disease.

## Prevention

"Keep warm, keep moving, and keep dry." Individuals should wear warm, dry clothing, preferably several layers, with a windproof outer garment. Wet clothing, socks, and shoes should be removed as soon as possible and replaced with dry ones. Extra socks, mittens, and insoles should always be carried in a pack when a person is in cold or icy areas. Cramped positions, constricting clothing, and prolonged dependency of the feet are to be avoided. Arms, legs, fingers, and toes should be exercised to maintain circulation. Wet and muddy ground and exposure to wind should be avoided. Good nutrition and skin cleanliness are necessary. Tobacco and alcohol should be avoided when the danger of frostbite is present.

## CHILBLAIN (Pernio)

Chilblains are red, itching skin lesions, usually on the extremities, caused by exposure to cold without actual freezing of the tissues. They may be associated with edema or blistering and are aggravated by warmth. With continued exposure, ulcerative or hemorrhagic lesions may appear and progress to scarring, fibrosis, and atrophy.

Treatment consists of elevating the affected part slightly and allowing it to warm gradually at room temperature. Do not rub or massage injured tissues or apply ice or heat. Protect the area from trauma and secondary infection.

## FROSTBITE

Frostbite is injury of the tissues due to freezing. In mild cases, only the skin and subcutaneous tissues are involved; the symptoms are numbness, prickling, and itching. With increasing severity, deep frostbite involves deeper structures, and there may be paresthesia and stiffness. Thawing causes tenderness and burning pain. The skin is white or yellow, loses its elasticity, and becomes immobile. Edema, blisters, necrosis, and gangrene may appear. Scintigraphy has been used to assess the degree of involvement in severe frostbite and to distinguish viable from nonviable tissue.

### Treatment
**A. Immediate Treatment:** Treat the patient for associated systemic hypothermia.

**1. Rewarming**–Superficial frostbite (frostnip) of extremities in the field can be treated by firm steady pressure with the warm hand (without rubbing), by placing fingers in the armpits, and, in the case of the toes or heels, by removing footwear, drying feet, rewarming, and covering with adequate dry socks or other protective footwear.

Rapid thawing at temperatures slightly above body heat may significantly decrease tissue necrosis. If there is any possibility of refreezing, the frostbitten part should not be thawed, even if this might mean prolonged walking on frozen feet. Refreezing results in increased tissue necrosis. It has been suggested that rewarming is best accomplished by immersing the frozen portion of the body for several minutes in water heated to 40–42 °C (104–107.6 °F) (*not warmer*). Water in this temperature range feels warm but not hot to the normal hand. Dry heat (eg, stove or open fire) is more difficult to regulate and is not recommended. After thawing has occurred and the part has returned to normal temperature (usually in about 30 minutes), discontinue external heat. Victims and rescue workers should be cautioned not to attempt rewarming by exercise or thawing of frozen tissues by rubbing with snow or ice water.

**2. Protection of the part**–Avoid trauma, eg, pressure or friction. Physical therapy is contraindicated in the early stage. Keep the patient at bed rest with the affected parts elevated and uncovered at room temperature. Do not apply casts, dressings, or bandages.

**3. Anti-infective measures**–It is very important to prevent infection after the rewarming process. Pro-

tect skin blebs from physical contact. Local infections may be treated with mild soaks of soapy water or povidone-iodine. Whirlpool therapy at temperatures slightly below body temperature twice daily for 15–20 minutes for a period of 3 or more weeks helps cleanse the skin and debrides superficial sloughing tissue. Antibiotics may be required for deep infections.

**4. Anticoagulants**–Early administration of heparin to prevent secondary thromboses is of questionable value.

**B. Follow-Up Care:** Gentle, progressive physical therapy to promote circulation is important as healing progresses. Buerger's exercises should be instituted as soon as tolerated. Vasodilating agents are of questionable value.

**C. Surgery:** Early regional sympathectomy (within 36–72 hours) has been reported to protect against the sequelae of frostbite, but the value of this measure is controversial. In general, other surgical intervention is to be avoided. *Amputation should not be considered until it is definitely established that the tissues are dead.* Tissue necrosis (even with black eschar formation) may be quite superficial, and *the underlying skin may sometimes heal spontaneously even after a period of months.*

### Prognosis
Recovery from frostbite is most often complete, but there may be increased susceptibility to discomfort in the involved extremity upon reexposure to cold.

## IMMERSION SYNDROME
## (Immersion Foot or Trench Foot)

Immersion foot (or hand) is caused by prolonged immersion in cool or cold water or mud. The affected parts are first cold and anesthetic. They become hot with intense burning and shooting pains during the hyperemic period and pale or cyanotic with diminished pulsations during the vasospastic period; blistering, swelling, redness, heat, ecchymoses, hemorrhage, or gangrene and secondary complications such as lymphangitis, cellulitis, and thrombophlebitis follow later.

Treatment is best instituted during the stage of reactive hyperemia. Immediate treatment consists of protecting the extremities from trauma and secondary infection and gradual rewarming by exposure to cool air (not ice or heat). Do not massage or moisten the skin or immerse the part in water. Bed rest is required until all ulcers have healed. Keep the affected parts elevated to aid in removal of edema fluid and protect pressure sites (eg, heels) with pillows. Antibiotics should be used if infection develops. Later treatment is as for Buerger's disease (see Chapter 9).

Ferguson J et al: Accidental hypothermia. *Emerg Med Clin North Am* 1983;**1**:619.

McCauley RL et al: Frostbite injuries: A rational approach based on the pathophysiology. *J Trauma* 1983;**23**:143.

Reuler JB: Hypothermia: Pathophysiology, clinical settings and management. *Ann Intern Med* 1978;**89**:519.

Wong KC: Physiology and pharmacology of hypothermia. *West J Med* 1983;**138**:227.

Zell SE, Kurtz KJ: Severe exposure hypothermia: A resuscitation protocol. *Ann Emerg Med* 1985;**14**:339.

# DISORDERS DUE TO HEAT

Four medical disorders can result from excessive exposure to hot environments (in order of increasing severity): heat syncope, heat cramps, heat exhaustion, and heat stroke. A stable internal temperature requires a balance between heat production and heat loss, which the hypothalamus regulates by calling for changes in muscle tone, vascular tone, and sweat gland function.

## Etiology

Sweat production and evaporation is a major mechanism of heat removal. Conduction (convection)—the direct transfer of heat from the skin to the surrounding air—also occurs, but with diminished efficiency as the ambient temperature rises. The passive transfer of heat from a warmer to a cooler object by radiation accounts for 65% of body heat loss under normal conditions. Radiant heat loss decreases as the temperature of the surrounding environment increases up to 37.2 °C (99 °F), the point at which heat transfer reverses direction. At normal temperatures, evaporation accounts for approximately 20% of the body's heat loss, but at high temperatures it becomes the major mechanism for dissipation of heat. This mechanism is also limited as humidity increases and is ineffective when relative humidity reaches 100%.

Health conditions that inhibit sweat production or evaporation and increase susceptibility to heat disorders include obesity, generalized skin diseases (miliaria), diminished cutaneous blood flow, dehydration, malnutrition, hypotension, and reduced cardiac output from heart disease. Medical disorders associated with debilitation and poor physical conditioning—with impaired sweating mechanism and inadequate circulatory vasodilatory response to heat—include severe infectious diseases, cancer, and malnutrition. Medications that impair the sweating mechanism are the anticholinergics, antihistamines, phenothiazines, tricyclic antidepressants, monoamine oxidase inhibitors, and diuretics; reduced cutaneous blood flow results from use of vasoconstrictors and β-adrenergic blocking agents; and dehydration results from use of alcohol. Illicit drugs—eg, phencyclidine, LSD, amphetamines, and cocaine—can cause increased muscle activity and thus generate increased body heat. Drug withdrawal syndrome may have the same effect.

## Prevention

Medical evaluation and monitoring should be used to identify individuals at increased risk of heat disorders. The general public should be made aware of the early signs and symptoms of heat disorders and should receive appropriate instruction in what constitutes proper attire in hot environments, alternating work and rest, and proper nutrition. It is not good practice to make salt tablets available for use without medical supervision, but close monitoring of fluid and electrolyte intake may be necessary in situations necessitating activity in hot environments. Workers should not begin work in hot areas without proper acclimatization and should be encouraged to take water frequently. Until acclimatization is complete, balanced electrolyte solutions at 1% saline solution should be used as drinking water.

Acclimatization is by scheduled regulated exposure to hot environments and by gradually increasing the duration of exposure and the work load, until the body adjusts by starting to produce sweat of lower salt content in greater amounts at lower ambient temperatures. Acclimatization is accompanied by increased plasma volume, cardiac output, and cardiac stroke volume and a slower heart rate.

## SPECIFIC SYNDROMES DUE TO HEAT EXPOSURE

### 1. HEAT SYNCOPE

Sudden unconsciousness can result from cutaneous vasodilatation with consequent systemic and cerebral hypotension. Systolic blood pressure is usually less than 100 mm Hg, and there is typically a history of vigorous physical activity for 2 hours or more just preceding the episode. The skin is typically cool and moist, and the pulse is weak.

Treatment consists of rest and recumbency in a cool place, with fluids by mouth (or intravenously if necessary). Predisposing causes should be identified and managed.

### 2. HEAT CRAMPS

Fluid and electrolyte depletion can result in slow, painful skeletal muscle contractions ("cramps") and even severe muscle spasms lasting 1–3 minutes, usually of the muscles being most heavily used. Cramping results from salt depletion as sweat losses are replaced with water alone. The skin is moist and cool, and the muscles are tender. There may be muscle twitching. The victim is alert, with stable vital signs, but may be agitated and complaining of pain. The body temperature may be normal or slightly increased. Involved muscle groups are hard and lumpy. There is almost always a history of vigorous activity just preceding the onset of symptoms. Laboratory evaluation may show low serum sodium and hemoconcentration.

The patient should be moved to a cool environment and given oral saline solution (4 tsp of salt per gallon of water) to replace both salt and water. *Because of their slower absorption, salt tablets are not recommended.* The victim may have to rest for 1–3 days with continued dietary salt supplementation before returning to work or resuming heavy activity in the heat.

## 3. HEAT EXHAUSTION

Heat exhaustion results from prolonged heavy activity with inadequate salt intake in a hot environment and is characterized by dehydration, sodium depletion, or isotonic fluid loss with accompanying cardiovascular changes.

The diagnosis is based on prolonged symptoms and a rectal temperature over 37.8 °C (100 °F), increased pulse rate—usually more than half again the patient's normal rate—and moist skin. Symptoms associated with heat syncope and heat cramps may also be present. The patient may be quite thirsty and weak, with central nervous system symptoms such as headache, fatigue, and, in cases due chiefly to water depletion, anxiety paresthesias, impaired judgment, hysteria, and in some cases psychosis. Hyperventilation secondary to heat exhaustion can lead to respiratory alkalosis. Heat exhaustion may progress to heat stroke if sweating ceases.

Treatment consists of placing the patient in a shaded, cool environment and providing adequate hydration and salt replenishment—orally, if possible. Physiologic saline or isotonic glucose solution can be administered intravenously in severe cases or when oral administration is not appropriate. Intravenous hypertonic saline may be necessary if sodium depletion is severe.

## 4. HEAT STROKE

Heat stroke is a life-threatening medical emergency resulting from failure of the thermoregulatory mechanism and is manifested by sudden loss of consciousness, high fever, and absence of sweating. Heat stroke is imminent when the core (rectal) temperature approaches 41 °C (106 °F). It is most likely to occur following excessive exposure to heat. Persons at greatest risk are the elderly or chronically infirm or those receiving medications that interfere with heat-dissipating mechanisms. Morbidity or even death can result from cerebral, cardiovascular, hepatic, or renal damage.

## Clinical Findings

**A. Symptoms and Signs:** Failure of the heat dissipation mechanism for any reason results in dizziness, weakness, emotional lability, nausea and vomiting, confusion, delirium, blurred vision, convulsions, collapse, and unconsciousness. The skin is hot and usually dry, and the pulse is strong initially. Blood pressure may be slightly elevated at first, but hypotension develops later. The core temperature is usually over 41°C. As with heat exhaustion, hyperventilation can occur, leading to respiratory alkalosis and compensatory metabolic acidosis.

**B. Laboratory Findings:** Laboratory evaluation reveals dehydration, leukocytosis, elevated BUN, hemoconcentration, and decreased serum potassium, calcium, and phosphorus; urine is concentrated, with elevated protein, tubular casts, and myoglobinuria. Thrombocytopenia, increased bleeding and clotting times, fibrinolysis, and consumption coagulopathy may also be present. Myocardial, hepatic, or renal damage may be identified by appropriate tests.

## Treatment

Treatment is aimed at rapidly reducing the core temperature and controlling the secondary effects. The preferred method of treatment is to place the patient in an ice water bath. Alternatively, the patient's clothing should be removed and the entire body sprinkled with cold water or 70% rubbing alcohol followed by fanning. The patient should be in the lateral recumbent position or supported in a hands-and-knees position to expose as much skin surface as possible to the air. Water should be applied in a finely atomized spray at 15 °C if a suitable device is available. Other alternatives include use of cold wet sheets or ice packs.

Treatment should be continued until the rectal temperature drops to 39 °C. The temperature remains stable in most cases, but it should continue to be monitored for 24 hours. Chlorpromazine (25–50 mg intravenously) can be used to control shivering and other muscular activity associated with increased heat load. Aspirin should not be given because of its anticoagulant effect.

Care must be taken to observe for and treat shock, maintain a patent airway, give oxygen as needed, identify and correct fluid and electrolyte imbalances, and support vital processes. Hypovolemic and cardiogenic shock must be carefully distinguished, and either or both may occur. Central venous or pulmonary artery wedge pressure should be monitored and intravenous fluids administered if indicated. Five percent dextrose in saline (500–1000 mL) may be given without overloading the circulation if hypovolemic shock is suspected.

The patient should also be observed for renal failure, rhabdomyolysis, cardiac arrhythmias, disseminated intravascular coagulation, and hepatic failure. Other medications appropriate for cardiac support should be considered. Corticosteroids have not been shown to be of value.

Fluid output should be monitored through the use of an indwelling urinary catheter.

Complications such as hepatic or cardiac failure or coagulopathy should be treated appropriately. Because sensitivity to high environmental temperature continues in some patients for prolonged periods following an episode of heat stroke, immediate reexposure should be avoided.

American Academy of Pediatrics Committee on Sports Medicine: Clinical heat stress and the exercising child. *Pediatrics* 1982;**69**:808.

Dinman BD, Horvath SM: Heat disorders in industry. *J Occup Med* 1984;**26**:489.

Johnson LW: Preventing heat stroke. *Am Fam Physician* (July) 1982;**26**:137.

Kilbourne EM et al: Risk factors for heatstroke: A case control study. *JAMA* 1982;**247**:3332.

Knochel JP: Environmental heat illness: An eclectic review. *Arch Intern Med* 1974;**133**:841.

Management of heat stroke. *Lancet* 1982;**2**:910.

Olson KR et al: Environmental and drug-induced hyperthermia. *Emerg Med Clin North Am* 1984;**2**:459.

Tucker LE et al: Classical heatstroke: Clinical and laboratory assessment. *South Med J* 1985;**78**:20.

# BURNS

*R. Laurence Berkowitz, MD*

The severe physical trauma caused by burns may result in intense pain, infection, metabolic disturbances, physical disfigurement and disability, and death.

Over 2 million injuries, 70,000 hospitalizations, and 9000 deaths occur from burns each year in the USA. Burns are the leading cause of accidental death in children. The tragedy is that burns are largely preventable.

Scalds are a common form of thermal injury to children and the elderly that can be partially prevented by regulating water temperatures (Table 29–1). Enforcement of the Flammable Fabric Act in the USA has reduced the incidence of flame injury to children. However, loose-fitting clothing of the elderly is a hazard near an open flame. Carelessness with burning cigarettes is a common cause of dwelling fires. Smoke alarms and other fire safety measures have helped

to save lives and prevent injury, but further safety legislation and public education are needed.

## CLASSIFICATION

Burns are classified by extent, depth, patient age, and associated illness or injury.

### Extent

The "rule of nines" (Fig 29–1) is useful for rapidly assessing the extent of a burn. More detailed charts based on age are available when the patient reaches the burn unit. Therefore, it is important to view the entire patient after cleaning soot to make an accurate assessment, both initially and on subsequent examinations. Only second- and third-degree burns are included in calculating the total burn surface area (TBSA), since first-degree burns usually do not represent significant injury in terms of prognosis or fluid and electrolyte management.

### Depth

Judgment of depth of injury is difficult. The **first-degree burn** may be red or gray but will demonstrate excellent capillary refill. First-degree burns are not blistered initially. If the wound is blistered, this represents a partial-thickness injury to the dermis, or a **second-degree burn.** However, a deep second-degree burn may have lost its blister and may actually appear hyperemic from fixed hemoglobin in the tissue. This redness will not have good refill and will not be as

**Table 29–1.** Temperatures at which tap water scalds may occur at various exposure times.

| Skin Temperature (°C) | (°F) | Time For Second-Degree Scald (seconds) |
|---|---|---|
| 65.6 | 150 | Any |
| 60.0 | 140* | 1.5* |
| 54.4 | 130 | 12 |
| 51.7 | 125 | 42 |
| 48.9 | 120 | 300 |

\* Note the risk at this common household temperature.

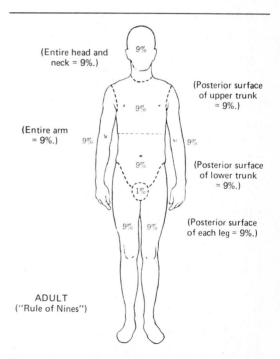

**Figure 29–1.** Estimation of body surface area in burns.

exquisitely sensitive as the hyperemia of the first-degree burn. The line between the partial- and full-thickness injury, or **third-degree burn,** may be rather indefinite. The initial vasoconstriction of a second-degree burn may make it appear more severe at first. Concerning healing properties of any second- or third-degree burn, the critical factors are blood supply and appendage population. In areas rich in vascularity, hair follicles, and sweat glands, the prospects for reepithelialization are good. Otherwise, even when the dermis is healthy, epithelialization may be slow and more scarring will result.

## Age of the Patient

As much as extent and depth of the burn, age of the victim plays a critical part. Even a relatively small burn in an elderly patient or infant may be fatal, as demonstrated in Fig 29–2.

## Associated Injuries & Illnesses

An injury commonly associated with burns is smoke inhalation. The products of combustion, not heat, are responsible for lower airway injury. Certain toxic substances from plastic products produce both hydrochloric acid and hydrocyanic acid. Electrical injury that causes burns may also produce cardiac arrhythmias that require immediate attention. Premorbid physical and psychosocial disorders that complicate recovery from burn injury include cardiac or pulmonary disease, diabetes, alcoholism, drug abuse, and psychiatric illness.

## Special Burn Care Units & Facilities

The American Burn Association and the American College of Surgeons have recommended that major burns be treated in specialized burn care facilities. They also advocate that even moderately severe burns be treated in a specialized facility or hospital where personnel have expertise in burn care. The American Burn Association has classified burn injuries as follows:

### A. Major Burn Injuries:

1. Partial-thickness burns over more than 25% of body surface area in adults or 20% in children.

2. Full-thickness burns over more than 10% of surface area in any age group.

3. Deep burns involving the hands, face, eyes, ears, feet, or perineum.

4. Burns complicated by inhalation injury.

5. Electrical and chemical burns.

6. Burns complicated by fractures and other major trauma.

7. Burns in poor-risk patients (extremes of age or intercurrent disease).

### B. Moderate Uncomplicated Burn Injuries:

1. Partial-thickness burns over 15–25% of body surface area in adults or 10–20% of body surface area in children.

2. Full-thickness burns over 2–10% of body surface area.

3. Burns not involving the specific conditions listed above.

### C. Minor Burn Injuries:

1. Partial-thickness burns over less than 15% of body surface area in adults or 10% in children.

2. Full-thickness burns over less than 2% of body surface area.

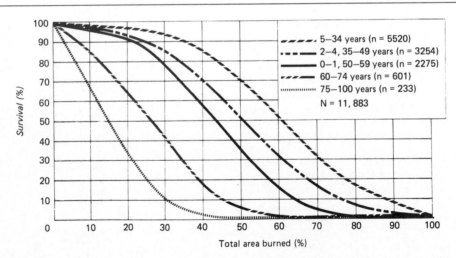

**Figure 29–2.** Sigmoid curves showing survival of humans as a function of total percentage of body surface burned and age. Survival curves estimated by probit analysis for 5 different age categories. (Reproduced, with permission, from Feller I, Flora JD Jr, Bawol R: Baseline results of therapy for burned patients. *JAMA* 1976;**236:**1943. Copyright 1976, American Medical Association.)

## INITIAL MANAGEMENT

### Airway

The physician or emergency medical technician should proceed as with any other trauma. The first priority is to establish an airway, then to evaluate the cervical spine and head injuries, and then to stabilize fractures. *The burn wound itself has a lower priority.* At some point during the initial management, endotracheal intubation should be considered for most major burn cases, regardless of the area of the body involved, for as fluid resuscitation proceeds, generalized edema develops, including the soft tissues of the upper airway and perhaps the lungs as well. *Tracheostomy is rarely indicated for the burn victim,* unless dictated by other circumstances. Inhalation injuries should be followed by serial blood gas determination and bronchoscopy. The use of corticosteroids is not recommended because of the potential for immunosuppression.

### Cooling the Wound

Cooling the victim for up to 20 minutes following the burn has been shown to reduce the depth of injury. Avoid prolonged application of cold water or ice packs to large surfaces, however, since they can cause systemic hypothermia and arrhythmias. Saline soaks at room temperature or cooler should be used. At the scene of an injury, a hose can be used for this purpose. Fire extinguishers and ice are not recommended, as further tissue injury may result.

### History

As soon as possible, obtain a detailed history of the circumstances of the injury, including locale, substances involved, and duration of exposure. The initial history may be extremely valuable, since medications, mental disturbances, confusion resulting from the injury, or the presence of an endotracheal tube may later prevent the recording of an accurate history.

### Vascular Access

Simultaneously with the above procedures, venous access must be sought, since the victim of a major burn is in hypovolemic shock. *A well-secured peripheral cutdown or femoral vein puncture is the preferred route of fluid administration,* though other sites may be used. A burn eschar, since it has been flame-sterilized, is an acceptable location for the initial cutdown. Femoral lines also provide rapid, safe access and can be replaced as soon as the patient is stable. An arterial line may also be useful for monitoring mean arterial pressure. The line may be placed initially in the femoral artery and later changed (as peripheral resistance decreases) to a safer site such as the dorsalis pedis, temporal, or radial arteries. Swan-Ganz catheters should be used in patients with preexisting cardiopulmonary disease and in severe burn cases to determine cardiac output and peripheral resistance. Once these parameters have been established, the catheter is usually removed.

## FLUID RESUSCITATION

### Crystalloids

Generalized capillary leak results from burn injury over more than 25% of the total body surface area. This often necessitates replacement of a large volume of fluid. An intravenous line is recommended in the management of deep partial-thickness and full-thickness burns that cover more than 20% of total body surface area in the adult and 10% in the child.

There are many guidelines for fluid resuscitation, eg, those of Evans, Brooke, Monafo (hypertonic saline), and Parkland (Baxter). In the first 24 hours, all of these fluids deliver approximately 0.5–0.6 meq of sodium per kilogram of body weight per percent of body surface area burned. The total amount of fluid in all but the hypertonic saline formula is roughly the same but differs in distribution. The Parkland formula is currently the most widely used in the USA. It relies upon the use of lactated Ringer's injection, which is available in every emergency room. For adults and children, the fluid requirement in the first 24 hours is estimated as 3–5 mL/kg body weight per percent of body surface area burned (Fig 29–3). The smaller amounts would be used in the elderly or those with less severe burns; the larger amounts would be used in children (who have a larger relative surface-to-volume ratio) and for treatment of deep electrical burns. Begin with 4 mL/kg body weight per percent of body surface area burned, and vary this amount according to the patient's response. *Remember that a formula is only a guideline and that blind adherence to any set of numbers can result in disaster.*

Half of the calculated fluid is given in the first 8-hour period. The remaining fluid, divided into 2 equal parts, is delivered over the next 16 hours. An extremely large volume of fluid may be required. For example, an injury over 40% of the total body surface area in a 70-kg victim may require 13 L *in the first 24 hours.* Calculate the first 8-hour period

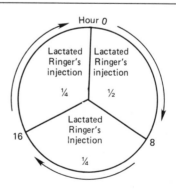

**Figure 29–3.** Half of the calculated crystalloid formula (lactated Ringer's injection [4mL/kg wt/% TBSA]) is given in the first 8 hours, beginning at the time of the injury. The remainder is given evenly over the ensuing 16 hours.

from the hour of injury, and catch up to that point if necessary.

## Colloids

After 24 hours, capillary leaks have sealed in the majority of cases, and plasma volume may be restored with colloids (plasma or albumin). The Parkland formula calls for 0.3–0.5 mL/kg body weight per percent of body surface area burned to be given over the first 8-hour period of the second 24 hours. Fluids given in the following 16 hours consist of dextrose in water in quantities sufficient to maintain adequate urine output (Fig 29–4). It is hoped that during the second 24-hour period the vascular system will hold colloids and draw off edema fluid, resulting in diuresis.

### Adequacy of Resuscitation

Mental alertness, urinary output, and the vital signs reflect the adequacy of fluid resuscitation. Mental alertness is important because it is the best indicator of adequate cerebral perfusion. Overmedication may cloud the sensorium during the resuscitation phase. Analgesics in the form of small doses of intravenous morphine should be used judiciously so as not to interfere with diagnosis. Renal perfusion is judged by urinary output. Adequate urinary output is 30–50 mL/h in adults and 1 mL/kg body weight/h in children. A smaller output represents inadequate renal perfusion. However, a larger output is unnecessary, and overloading results in edema in every organ. Keep edema at a minimum by maintaining a careful balance between input and output.

### Monitoring Fluid Resuscitation

A Foley catheter is essential for monitoring urinary output. *Diuretics have no part in this phase of patient management.* The use of mannitol may be indicated

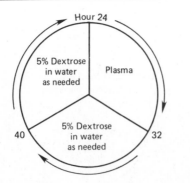

**Figure 29–4.** The colloid formula (aged plasma or 5% normal serum albumin [0.3–0.5 mL/kg wt/% TBSA]) is given as calculated between hours 24 and 32. In the remaining 16-hour period, 5% dextrose in water is given as needed to maintain a urine output of no less than 30 mL/h.

in the resuscitation of an electrical burn victim in whom myoglobin in the urine may precipitate in the kidneys. It should be used only until the urine is clear, and then discontinued.

### Escharotomy

As edema fluid accumulates, ischemia may develop under any constricting eschar of an extremity. Similarly, an eschar of the thorax or abdomen may limit respiratory excursion. Escharotomy incisions through the anesthetic eschar can save life and limb. *The penalty for failing to perform escharotomy can be great.*

## THE BURN WOUND

Treatment of the burn wound is based on several basic principles: (1) Prevent or delay infection. (2) Protect from desiccation and further injury those burned areas that will spontaneously reepithelialize in 7–10 days. (3) Excise and graft those burned areas that cannot spontaneously reepithelialize during this period.

### Systemic Prophylactic Antibiotics

Regardless of the severity of the burn, prophylactic systemic antibiotics are usually not recommended. Their effectiveness is unproved, and they have the disadvantage of favoring the growth of resistant organisms.

### Topical Antibiotics

Topical antibiotics delay or prevent infection. An ideal agent would readily penetrate the burn wound eschar, be effective against both gram-negative and gram-positive microorganisms as well as *Candida*, be painless and inexpensive, and have no deleterious side effects. Such an ideal agent does not currently exist. Silver sulfadiazine (Silvadene) is currently the most popular topical agent. It is painless, easy to apply, effective against most *Pseudomonas*, and a fairly good penetrator of eschar, but some microorganisms are resistant to it, and it may cause leukopenia or fever and delay epithelialization.

Mafenide (Sulfamylon) penetrates eschars better than silver sulfadiazine and is more effective against *Pseudomonas*. Mafenide inhibits carbonic anhydrase when used as a 10% solution and results in metabolic acidosis. It also delays epithelialization and may be painful. When diluted to a 5% solution, pain and metabolic side effects are lessened. It is useful primarily for deep burns, eg, electrical burns and burns of the ear or nose where cartilage is close to the surface, and when silver sulfadiazine is ineffective. It is best to limit the use of mafenide to no more than 10% of the total body surface area at any given time because of its metabolic effect.

Povidone-iodine is especially useful against *Candida* and both gram-positive and gram-negative microorganisms. However, it penetrates eschar poorly, is very desiccating to the wound surface, and is painful. Also, significantly high blood iodine levels have been demonstrated in patients receiving this agent.

Gentamicin and silver nitrate are no longer recommended as topical agents.

## Wound Closure

The goal of therapy after fluid resuscitation is closure of the wound. Nature's own blister is the best cover to protect wounds that spontaneously epithelialize in 7–10 days (ie, superficial second-degree burns). The serum in the blister nurses the surface of the **zone of stasis** until epithelialization takes place (Fig 29–5). Where the blister has been disrupted, human amnion, porcine heterografts (preferably fresh, or frozen and meshed), or collagen composite dressings (Biobrane) can substitute. Cadaver homografts can also serve this purpose if available.

Wounds that will not heal spontaneously in 7–10 days (ie, deep second-degree or third-degree burns) are best treated by excision and autograft; otherwise, granulation and infection may develop. Granulation is nature's signal that attempts to close the wound have failed. A "skin equivalent"—a patient's own skin cells grown in culture into multilayered sheets of epithelium—is currently being tested in some burn centers.

## PATIENT SUPPORT

During the wound closure phase, the patient must be supported in many ways. Most important is ade-

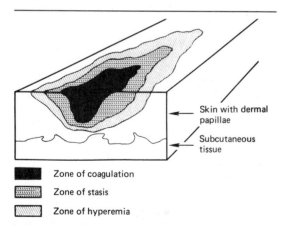

Skin with dermal papillae

Subcutaneous tissue

■ Zone of coagulation

▦ Zone of stasis

▨ Zone of hyperemia

**Figure 29–5.** The burn wound has 3 general zones of tissue death. The zone of necrosis or coagulation involves irreversible skin death. The intermediate zone of capillary stasis is vulnerable to desiccation and infection that can convert potentially salvageable tissue to full-thickness destruction and irreversible skin death. There is minimal cell involvement in the outermost hyperemic zone. (Modified from Zawacki BE: Reversal of capillary stasis and prevention of necrosis in burns. *Ann Surg* 1974;**180**:98. Redrawn, with permission from Artz CP, Moncrief JA, Pruitt BA: *A Team Approach.* Saunders, 1979.)

quate nutrition. Enteral feedings may begin once the ileus of the resuscitation period is relieved, which usually coincides with the subsidence of edema. The large nasogastric sump tube used to decompress stomach contents during resuscitation may now be replaced with a smaller, preferably soft Silastic tube. This will aid in delivering large quantities (4000–6000 kcal/d) that may be required during the wound closure period. The metabolic demands are immense. A useful guide is to provide 25 kcal/kg body weight plus 40 kcal per percent of burn surface area. Fat emulsions (Intralipid) given intravenously are useful during the resuscitation period to span the period of ileus.

Many enteral formulas are available. Eggs are a readily available source of protein and calories and are well tolerated by the patient. In many cases, more than 30 eggs per day are desirable. Early enteral feedings reduce the need for antacids and lessen the likelihood of development of Curling's ulcer, a life-threatening complication of burn injury. Gastric juice pH and hourly antacid delivery should be carefully monitored during the resuscitation phase. Cimetidine may be used to reduce acid production; however, undesirable side effects such as leukopenia and confusion in the elderly may result.

Pain plays a major role during the wound closure phase. The patient is more aware of pain during dressing changes and postsurgical periods. Hydrotherapy aids in dressing removal and joint range of motion, but it can be a source of wound contamination. Analgesics are essential, but overuse or underuse may be harmful. If intravenous morphine or other analgesics are required during dressing changes, the patient should be closely monitored. Methadone given on a regular basis in some cases has reduced the need for other intravenous narcotics.

### The Burn Team

The burn team consists of a group of highly skilled professionals—nurses, dietitians, physical therapists, occupational therapists, and counselors—who work closely with the physician in providing comprehensive services for the victim from the period of intensive care through recovery and rehabilitation. Careful attention is given to the complex problems encountered during the intensive care and recovery periods, including fluid and electrolyte abnormalities, infection, physical discomfort, malnutrition, immobility, and psychologic suffering.

Many of the residual physical and emotional problems in burn patients, eg, body disfigurement, impaired mobility, persistent itching, decreased ability to perspire, decreased skin sensitivity, and impairment of sexual enjoyment, require special individualized attention.

Demling RH: Fluid resuscitation after major burns. *JAMA* 1983;**250**:1438.

Fein A, Leff A, Hopewell PC: Pathophysiology and management of the complications resulting from fire and the inhaled products of combustion. *Crit Care Med* 1980;**8**:2.

First W et al: Long-term functional results of selective treatment of hand burns. *Am J Surg* 1985;**149**:516.

Fisher SV, Helm PA: *Rehabilitation of the Burn Patient.* Williams & Wilkins, 1984.

Gallico GG III et al: Permanent coverage of large burn wounds with autologous cultured human epithelium. *N Engl J Med* 1984;**311**:448.

Gillespie RW: The burn at first sight. *Emerg Med* (Feb 29) 1984;**16**:141.

Goodwin CW: Major burns. Chap 9, pp 163–175, in: *Principles of Trauma Care*, 3rd ed. Shires GT (editor). McGraw-Hill, 1985.

Kagan RJ et al: Serious wound infections in burned patients. *Surgery* 1985;**98**:640.

Luterman A, Curreri PW: Emergency protocol for the severely burned patient. *Hosp Med* (Oct) 1984;**20**:131.

Monafo WW, Crabtree JH, Galster AD: Hemodynamics and metabolic support of the severely burned patient. In: Shoemaker WC, Thompson WL, Holbrook PR (editors): *The Society of Critical Care Medicine: Textbook of Critical Care.* Saunders, 1984.

Shires GT, Black EA (editors): Frontiers in understanding burn injury: Proceedings of the NIH Conference. *J Trauma* (Sept) 1984;**24(Suppl)**:S1–204.

Supportive therapy in burn care. *J Trauma* 1981;**21(Suppl 8)**:665. [Entire issue.]

# ELECTRIC SHOCK

The possibility of life-threatening electrical injury exists in all electrified areas—home, school, industry, agriculture, recreation, and even in hospitals. Electric shock may result from carelessness, ignorance, faulty appliances and equipment, or from an act of nature—lightning. Dry skin provides a high-resistance barrier to ordinary levels of external electric current. Skin moistened with water, sweat, saline solution, or urine, however, has greatly reduced resistance to electric current. The effect of electric current may be a local unpleasant tingling or a painful sensation. The amount and type of current, the duration and area of exposure, and the pathway of the current through the body determine the degree of damage. If the current passes through the heart or brain stem, death may occur immediately owing to ventricular fibrillation or apnea. Current passing through skeletal muscle can cause contractions severe enough to result in bone fracture. Delayed electrical injuries include damage to the spinal cord and cataracts.

Direct current is much less dangerous than alternating current. Alternating current of high voltage with a very high number of cycles per second (hertz, Hz) may be less dangerous than a low voltage with fewer cycles per second. With alternating currents of 25–300 Hz, low voltages (< 220) tend to produce ventricular fibrillation; high voltages (> 1000), respiratory failure; intermediate voltages (220–1000), both. Domestic house current (AC) of 100 volts with low cycles (about 60 Hz) is, accordingly, dangerous to the heart, since it may cause ventricular fibrillation.

Electrical burns are of 3 distinct types: flash (arcing) burns, flame (clothing) burns, and the direct heating effect of tissues by the electric current. The latter lesions are usually sharply demarcated, round or oval, painless gray areas with inflammatory reaction. The superficial appearance of many discrete burns is deceptive; operation frequently discloses more extensive destruction than anticipated. Little happens for several weeks; sloughing then occurs slowly over a fairly wide area.

Electric shock may produce momentary or prolonged loss of consciousness. With recovery there may be muscular pain, fatigue, headache, and nervous irritability. The physical signs vary according to the action of the current. With ventricular fibrillation, no heart sounds or pulse can be found and the patient is unconscious. The respirations continue for a few minutes, becoming exaggerated as asphyxia occurs and then ceasing as death intervenes. With respiratory failure, respirations are absent and the patient is unconscious; the pulse can be felt, but there is a marked fall in blood pressure and the skin is cold and cyanotic.

Electric shock may be a hazard in routine hospital equipment that is usually considered to be harmless (eg, electrocardiographs, suction machines, electrically operated beds, x-ray units). Proper installation, utilization, and maintenance of equipment by qualified personnel should minimize this hazard. Battery-operated devices provide the maximum protection from accidental electric shock. Electrochemical cutaneous burns have been reported with direct current voltages as low as 3 volts.

**Treatment**

**A. Emergency Measures:** Free the victim from the current at once. This may be done in many ways, but the rescuer must be protected. Turn off the power, sever the wire with a dry wooden-handled axe, make a proper ground to divert the current, or drag the victim carefully away by means of dry clothing or a leather belt.

If breathing and pulses are absent, institute cardiopulmonary resuscitation immediately (see p 1108) and continue until spontaneous breathing and cardiac function return or rigor mortis is noted.

**Lightning Injury.** Victims of lightning injury, in whom coma may last for a few minutes to several days, should receive prompt and sustained artificial resuscitation. This should be continued as long as there is no clinical evidence of brain death.

**B. Hospital Measures:** Hospitalize the patient when revived and observe for shock, arrhythmia, sudden cardiac dilatation, secondary hemorrhage, acidosis, or myoglobinuria.

The unpredictable damage to deep tissues in electrical burns makes it difficult to assess the fluid requirements for patients who are in shock.

## Prognosis

Complications may occur in almost every part of the body. The most common cause of death in those who survive the original electric shock is systematic infection.

Amy BW et al: Lightning injury with survival in five patients. *JAMA* 1985;**253**:243.

Cooper MA: Electrical and lightning injuries. *Emerg Med Clin North Am* 1984;**2**:489.

Dixon GF: The evaluation and management of electrical injuries. *Crit Care Med* 1983;**11**:384.

Saffle JR, Crandall A, Warden GD: Cataracts: A long-term complication of electrical injury. *J Trauma* 1985;**25**:17.

# IONIZING RADIATION REACTIONS

The effects of ionizing radiation on the body have been observed in clinical use of x-rays and radioactive agents, after occupational or accidental exposure, and following the use of atomic weaponry. The harmful effects of radiation are determined by the extent of exposure, which in turn depends not only on the quantity of radiation delivered to the body but also the type of radiation (x-rays, neutrons, gamma rays, alpha or beta particles) to which tissues are exposed and the duration of exposure.

Tolerance to radiation is difficult to define, and there is no firm basis for evaluating radiation effects for all types and levels of radiation. The National Committee on Radiation Protection has set the maximum permissible radiation exposure for occupationally exposed workers over age 18 at 0.1 rem* per week for the whole body (but not to exceed 5 rem per year) and 1.5 rem per week for the hands. (For purposes of comparison, routine chest x-rays deliver from 0.1–0.2 rem.) If recommended limits for radiation safety in occupational workers or in clinical practice are exceeded, serious radiation injury may occur (see below).

Death after acute lethal radiation exposure is usually due to hematopoietic failure, gastrointestinal mucosal damage, central nervous system damage, or widespread vascular injury. Four hundred to 600 cgy of x-ray or gamma radiation applied to the entire body at one time may be fatal within 60 days; death is usually due to hemorrhage, anemia, and infection secondary to hematopoietic injury. Levels of 1000–3000 cgy to the entire body destroy gastrointestinal mucosa; this leads to toxemia and death within 2 weeks. Total body doses above 3000 cgy cause widespread vascular damage, cerebral anoxia, hypotensive shock, and death within 48 hours.

## ACUTE (IMMEDIATE) IONIZING RADIATION EFFECTS ON NORMAL TISSUES

### Clinical Findings

**A. Injury to Skin and Mucous Membranes:** Irradiation may cause erythema, epilation, destruction of fingernails, or epidermolysis.

**B. Injury to Deep Structures:**

**1. Hematopoietic tissues**–Injury to the bone marrow may cause diminished production of blood elements. Lymphocytes are most sensitive, polymorphonuclear leukocytes next most sensitive, and erythrocytes least sensitive. Damage to the blood-forming organs may vary from transient depression of one or more blood elements to complete destruction.

**2. Cardiovascular**–Pericarditis with effusion or constrictive carditis may occur after a period of months or even years. Myocarditis is less common. Smaller vessels (the capillaries and arterioles) are more readily damaged than larger blood vessels.

**3. Gonads**–In males, small single doses of radiation (200–300 R) cause temporary aspermatogenesis, and larger doses (600–800 R) may cause permanent sterility. In females, single doses of 200 R may cause temporary cessation of menses, and 500–800 R may cause permanent castration. Moderate to heavy irradiation of the embryo in utero results in injury to the fetus or in embryonic death and abortion.

**4. Respiratory tract**–High or repeated moderate doses of radiation may cause pneumonitis, often delayed for weeks or months.

**5. Salivary glands**–The salivary glands may be depressed by radiation, but relatively large doses may be required.

**6. Mouth, pharynx, esophagus, and stomach**–Mucositis with edema and painful swallowing of food may occur within hours or days after onset of irradiation. Gastric secretion may be temporarily (occasionally permanently) inhibited by moderately high doses of radiation.

**7. Intestines**–Inflammation and ulceration may follow moderately large doses of radiation.

**8. Endocrine glands and viscera**–Hepatitis and nephritis may be delayed effects of therapeutic radiation. The normal thyroid, pituitary, pancreas, adrenals, and bladder are relatively resistant to low or moderate doses of radiation.

**9. Brain and spinal cord**–The brain and spinal

---

* In radiation terminology, a rad is the unit of absorbed dose and a rem is the unit of any radiation dose to body tissue in terms of its estimated biologic effect. Roentgen (R) refers to the amount of radiation dose delivered to the body. For x-ray or gamma ray radiation, rems, rads, and roentgens are virtually the same. For particulate radiation from radioactive materials, these terms may differ greatly (eg, for neutrons, 1 rad = 10 rems). In the Système Internationale (SI) nomenclature, the rad has been replaced by the gray (Gy), and 1 rad = 0.01 Gy. The SI replacement for the rem is the Sievert (Sv), and 1 rem = 0.01 Sv.

cord may be damaged by high doses of radiation because of impaired blood supply.

**10. Peripheral and autonomic nerves–**These nerves are highly resistant to radiation.

**C. Systemic Reaction (Radiation Sickness):** The basic mechanisms of radiation sickness are not known. Anorexia, nausea, vomiting, weakness, exhaustion, lassitude, and in some cases prostration may occur, singly or in combination. Radiation sickness associated with x-ray therapy is most likely to occur when the therapy is given in large dosage to large areas over the abdomen, less often when given over the thorax, and rarely when therapy is given over the extremities. With protracted therapy, this complication is rarely significant. The patient's psychologic reaction to the illness or its treatment plays an important role in aggravating or minimizing such effect.

### Prevention

Persons handling radiation sources can minimize exposure to radiation by recognizing the importance of time, distance, and shielding. Areas housing x-ray and nuclear materials must be properly shielded. Inadequately trained personnel should not be permitted to work with x-ray and nuclear radiation. Any unnecessary exposures, diagnostic or therapeutic, should be avoided. X-ray equipment should be periodically checked for reliability of output, and proper filters should be employed. When feasible, it is advisable to shield the gonads, especially of young persons. Fluoroscopic examination should be performed as rapidly as possible, using an optimal combination of beam characteristics and filtration; the tube-to-table distance should be at least 45 cm, and the beam size should be kept to a minimum required by the examination. Special protective clothing may be necessary to protect against contamination with radioisotopes. In the event of accidental contamination, all clothing should be removed and the body vigorously bathed with soap and water. This should be followed by careful instrument (Geiger counter) check to localize the ionizing radiation.

No safe and effective radioprotectant drugs are as yet available.

### Emergency Treatment for Radiation Accident Victims

The need for emergency radiation accident care has grown because of the proliferation of radiation equipment and nuclear reactor plants (as emphasized by the recent Chernobyl disaster) and the increased transportation of radioactive materials. Hospitals have been asked to develop plans for managing patients who are accidentally exposed to ionizing radiation or to spillage or contamination with radioactive materials. The plans should provide for effective emergency care and disposition of victims and materials with the least possible risk of spreading radioactive contamination to personnel and facilities. Clinicians should be at least aware of the complexity of the problems involved. (See Leonard and USERDA references, below.)

### Treatment

The success of treatment of local radiation effects depends upon the extent, degree, and location of tissue injury. Treatment of systemic reactions is symptomatic and supportive. No truly effective antinauseant drug is available for the distressing nausea that frequently occurs. Chlorpromazine, 25–50 mg given deeply intramuscularly every 4–6 hours as necessary or 10–50 mg orally every 4–6 hours as necessary, may be of value. Dimenhydrinate, 100 mg, or perphenazine, 4–8 mg, 1 hour before and 1 and 4 hours after radiation therapy has been recommended. Simple, palatable foods and emotional support may help.

When radiation dosage levels are sufficient to cause damage to gastrointestinal mucosa, bone marrow, and other important tissues, good medical and nursing care may be lifesaving. Blood transfusions, bone marrow transplants, antibiotics, fluid and electrolyte maintenance, and other medical measures may support patients not too severely injured by radiation. Recovery obviously depends upon the severity of the injury. Patients with fulminant high-dose radiation syndrome—with cerebral anoxia and shock—fail to respond to treatment, and death occurs in 1–2 days.

## CHRONIC (DELAYED) EFFECTS OF EXCESSIVE DOSES OF IONIZING RADIATION

The risk of radiation exposure is a subject of much interest and controversy. There are concerns about possible delayed effects of exposure to medical radiation as well as those due to accidental environmental contamination. The chronic effects of radiation may be difficult to evaluate, because they take many years to become apparent. Furthermore, it is difficult to differentiate effects presumed to be due to radiation from abnormal conditions known to occur spontaneously in the population at large.

Skin scarring, atrophy and telangiectasis, obliterative endarteritis, pericarditis, pulmonary fibrosis, hepatitis, intestinal stenosis, nephritis, and other late effects of irradiation are known to occur.

The incidence of neoplastic disease, including leukemia, is increased in persons exposed to excessive radiation. The latency period between radiation therapy and the development of cancer may be 30 years or longer. Much of our knowledge of radiation-induced cancer in humans has been derived from follow-up studies of the survivors of the 1945 bombings in Japan during World War II. There is an increased incidence of thyroid cancer in patients who have received radiation therapy to the thymus. Prenatal irradiation may increase the risk of childhood cancer.

Microcephaly and other congenital abnormalities may occur in children exposed in utero, especially if the fetus was exposed during early pregnancy.

Abrams HL, Von Kaenel WE: Medical problems of survivors of nuclear war: Infection and the spread of communicable disease. *N Engl J Med* 1981;**305:**1226.

American Medical Association: *A Guide to the Hospital Management of Injuries Arising From Exposure to or Involving Ionizing Radiation.* American Medical Association, 1985.

Goldman M: Ionizing radiation and its risks. *West J Med* 1982;**137:**540.

Johnson CT: Cancer incidence in an area of radioactive fallout downwind from the Nevada test site. *JAMA* 1984;**251:**230.

Leonard RB: Emergency department radiation accident protocol. *Ann Emerg Med* 1980;**9:**462.

McKenna G, Glatstein E: When radiation therapy causes heart disease. *J Respir Dis* (June) 1984;**5:**96.

Milroy WC: Management of irradiated and contaminated casualty victims. *Emerg Med Clin North Am* 1984;**2:**667.

Schneider AB et al: Radiation-induced tumors of the head and neck following childhood irradiation: Prospective studies. *Medicine* 1985;**64:**1.

United States Energy Research and Development Administration: Emergency handling of radiation accident cases. Publication No. ERDA-17, 1975.

# DROWNING

Drowning is the fourth leading cause of accidental death in the USA. The number of deaths due to drowning could undoubtedly be significantly reduced if adequate preventive and first aid instruction programs were instituted.

The asphyxia of drowning is usually due to aspiration of fluid, but it may result from airway obstruction caused by laryngeal spasm while the victim is gasping under water. About 10% of victims develop laryngospasms after the first gulp and never aspirate water ("dry drowning"). The rapid sequence of events after submersion—hypoxemia, laryngospasm, fluid aspiration, ineffective circulation, brain injury, and brain death—may take place within 5–10 minutes. This sequence may be delayed for longer periods if the victim, especially a child, has been submerged in very cold water or if the victim has ingested significant amounts of barbiturates. Immersion in cold water can also cause a rapid fall in the victim's core temperature, so that systemic hypothermia and death may occur before actual drowning.

Past emphasis on differences in the pathophysiology of drowning in fresh water (hypotonic) and seawater (hypertonic), based upon observations in animal models, is of limited clinical significance in humans, since the amount of fluid aspirated is usually small. The primary effect in both cases is perfusion of poorly ventilated alveoli. The clinical presentation in both types of drowning is similar, and *cardiopulmonary resuscitation is the immediate requirement of rescue.*

A number of circumstances or primary events may precede near drowning and must be taken into consideration in management: (1) use of alcohol or other drugs (a contributing factor in an estimated 25% of adult drownings), (2) extreme fatigue, (3) intentional hyperventilation, (4) sudden acute illness (eg, epilepsy, myocardial infarction), (5) head or spinal cord injury sustained in diving, (6) venomous stings by aquatic animals, and (7) decompression sickness in deep water diving.

When first seen, the near-drowning victim may present with a wide range of clinical manifestations. Spontaneous return of consciousness often occurs in otherwise healthy individuals when submersion is very brief. Many other patients respond promptly to immediate ventilation. Other patients, with more severe degrees of near drowning, may have frank pulmonary failure, pulmonary edema, shock, anoxic encephalopathy, cerebral edema, and cardiac arrest. A few patients may be deceptively asymptomatic during the recovery period, only to deteriorate or die as a result of acute respiratory failure within the following 12–24 hours.

## Clinical Findings

**A. Symptoms and Signs:** The patient may be unconscious, semiconscious, or awake but apprehensive, restless, and complaining of headaches or chest pain. Vomiting is common. Examination may reveal cyanosis, trismus, apnea, tachypnea, and wheezing. A pink froth from the mouth and nose indicates pulmonary edema. Cardiovascular manifestations may include tachycardia, arrhythmias, hypotension, cardiac arrest, and circulatory shock.

**B. Laboratory Findings:** Urinalysis shows proteinuria, hemoglobinuria, and acetonuria. There is usually a leukocytosis. The $P_{a_{O_2}}$ is usually decreased and the $P_{a_{CO_2}}$ increased or decreased. The blood pH is decreased as a result of metabolic acidosis. Chest x-rays may show pneumonitis or pulmonary edema.

## Treatment

**A. First Aid:** Immediate measures to combat hypoxemia at the scene of the incident—with sustained effective ventilation, oxygenation, and circulatory support—are critical to survival with complete recovery.

1. If the victim is not breathing, clear the mouth and pharynx with the fingers, extend the victim's head, and institute immediate mouth-to-mouth or mouth-to-nose breathing.

2. Check carotid and femoral pulses. If pulses cannot be detected, institute cardiopulmonary resuscitation without delay (see p 1108).

3. Do not waste time attempting to drain water from the victim's lungs, since this measure is most often of no value. The Heimlich maneuver (subdiaphragmatic pressure) may clear the airway in a few persons, especially those who have gagged or vomited while aspirating water.

4. All near-drowning patients, with or without aspiration, should be hospitalized at least overnight for observation, chest x-rays, and serial arterial blood gas determinations. It may take 24 hours for pneu-

monitis or pulmonary edema to become evident. Call for assistance in moving the victim to the nearest hospital.

5. Do not discontinue basic life support for seemingly "hopeless" patients. Complete recovery has been reported after prolonged resuscitation efforts even when victims have had wide, fixed pupils.

**B. Hospital Care:** Careful observation of the patient; continuous monitoring of cardiorespiratory function; serial determination of arterial blood gases, pH, and electrolytes; and measurement of urinary output are required.

**1. Ensure optimal ventilation and oxygenation–**The danger of hypoxemia exists even in the alert, conscious patient who appears to be breathing normally. The proper assessment of oxygen requirements must be based upon initial and serial determination of arterial blood gases and pH. If the initial arterial blood gases and pH are within normal limits, there has probably been little or no alveolar damage due to aspiration, and full recovery usually occurs promptly. Chest radiographs are normal.

Endotracheal intubation is necessary for patients unable to maintain an open airway or normal blood gases and pH. If the victim does not have spontaneous respirations, intubation is required.

Initiate intermittent mandatory oxygen therapy with a volume ventilator. Positive end-expiratory pressure (PEEP) should be considered when the patient is unable to achieve a $P_{a_{O_2}}$ greater than 55 mm Hg when receiving less than 50% oxygen. Ventilatory support should be continued until normal arterial blood gases and pH have been established and can be maintained while the patient is breathing room air. Serial physical examinations and chest x-rays should be carried out to detect possible pneumonitis, atelectasis, and pulmonary edema. Bronchospasm due to aspirated material may require use of bronchodilators. Antibiotics should be given when there is x-ray or laboratory evidence of pneumonitis and other infections.

**2. Cardiovascular support–**Hypoxemia, acidosis, and hypothermia may cause myocardial depression, ventricular fibrillation, and cardiac arrest. Central venous pressure (or, preferably, pulmonary artery wedge pressure) may be monitored as a guide to determining whether vascular fluid replacement and cardiac drug therapy are needed. If low cardiac output persists after adequate intravascular volume is achieved, inotropic substances (eg, dopamine) should be considered. An increasing left ventricular pressure may indicate pulmonary edema and the need for fluid restriction, ventilatory modification, diuretics, and vasodilator drugs.

**3. Correction of blood pH and electrolyte abnormalities–**Metabolic acidosis is almost invariably present in near-drowning victims. Many authorities feel that patients who have been pulseless should routinely be given intravenous sodium bicarbonate (1 MEQ/kg) upon admission. This is advisable, but all subsequent bicarbonate administration should be based upon arterial blood gas and pH findings. Alkalosis is dangerous and should be avoided.

**4. Cerebral injury–**Some near-drowning patients may progress to irreversible central nervous system damage despite apparently adequate treatment of hypoxia and shock. Several types of measures to prevent cerebral injury have been employed with varying degrees of success—hypothermia, barbiturates, corticosteroids, osmolar agents (eg, mannitol), and readjustment of ventilatory assistance.

## Course & Prognosis

Victims of near drowning who have had prolonged hypoxemia should remain under close hospital observation for 2–3 days after all supportive measures have been withdrawn and clinical and laboratory findings have been stable. Residual complications of near drowning may include intellectual impairment, convulsive disorders, and pulmonary or cardiac disease.

Davis S, Ledman J, Kilgore J: Drownings of youth in a desert state. *West J Med* 1985;**143**:196.

Martin TG: Neardrowning and cold water immersion. *Ann Emerg Med* 1984;**13**:263.

Oakes DD et al: Prognosis and management of victims of near-drowning. *J Trauma* 1982;**22**:544.

Redding JS: Drowning and near drowning: Can the victim be saved? *Postgrad Med* (July) 1983;**74**:85.

Smith DS: Notes on drowning: The misunderstood, preventable tragedy. *Physicians Sportsmed* (July) 1984;**12**:66.

Yagil Y et al: Near drowning in the Dead Sea: Electrolyte imbalances and therapeutic implications. *Arch Intern Med* 1985;**145**:50.

# OTHER DISORDERS DUE TO PHYSICAL AGENTS

## DECOMPRESSION SICKNESS
## (Caisson Disease, Bends)

Decompression sickness has long been known as an occupational hazard for professional divers who are involved in deep-water exploration, rescue, salvage, or construction; and professional divers and their surface supporting teams are familiar with the prevention, recognition, and treatment of this disease. In recent years, the sport of scuba diving has become very popular, and a large number of untrained individuals are exposed to the hazards of decompression sickness.

At low depths the greatly increased pressure (eg, at 30 meters [100 ft] the pressure is 4 times greater than at the surface) compresses the respiratory gases into the blood and other tissues. During ascent from depths greater than 9 meters, gases dissolved in the blood and other tissues escape as the external pressure decreases. The appearance of symptoms depends on the depth and duration of submersion; the degree of physical exertion; the age, weight, and physical condition of the diver; and the rate of ascent. The size and number of gas bubbles (notably nitrogen) escaping from the tissues depends on the difference between the atmospheric pressure and the partial pressure of the gas dissolved in the tissues. The release of gas bubbles and (particularly) the location of their release determine the symptoms.

Decompression sickness may also occur in rapid ascents from sea level to high altitudes when there is no adequate pressurizing protection. Deep-sea and scuba divers may be vulnerable to air embolism if airplane travel is attempted too soon (within a few hours) after diving.

The onset of symptoms occurs within 30 minutes in half of cases and almost invariably within 6 hours. Symptoms, which are highly variable, include pain (largely in the joints), pruritic rash, visual disturbances, weakness or paralysis, dizziness or vertigo, headache, dyspnea, paresthesias, aphasia, and coma.

Early recognition and prompt treatment are extremely important. Continuous administration of oxygen is indicated as a first aid measure, whether or not cyanosis is present. Aspirin may be given for pain, but narcotics should be used very cautiously, since they may obscure the patient's response to recompression. Rapid transportation to a treatment facility for recompression, hyperbaric oxygen, hydration treatment of plasma deficits, and supportive measures are necessary not only to relieve symptoms but also to prevent permanent impairment. It has been recommended, however, that decompression symptoms be treated whenever they are seen—even up to 2 weeks postinjury—since it is still possible to completely alleviate symptoms. The physician should be familiar with the nearest compression center. The local public health department or nearest naval facility should be able to provide such information.

Davis JC et al: Altitude decompression sickness: Hyperbaric therapy results in 145 cases. *Aviat Space Environ Med* 1977;**48:**722.
Kizer KW: Diving medicine. *Emerg Med Clin North Am* 1984;**2:**513.
Myers RAM, Bray P: Delayed treatment of serious decompression sickness. *Ann Emerg Med* 1985;**14:**254.
Parell GJ et al: Management of inner ear barotrauma caused by scuba diving. *Otolaryngol Head Neck Surg* 1985;**93:**393.

## MOUNTAIN SICKNESS

Modern, rapid means of transportation have increased the number of unacclimatized individuals who are exposed to the effects of high altitude. Lack of sufficient time for acclimatization, increased physical activity, and varying degrees of health may be responsible for the acute and chronic disturbances that result from hypoxia at altitudes greater than 2000 meters. Marked individual differences in tolerance to hypoxia exist. Patients with sickle cell disease are at high risk of painful crises from altitude-induced hypoxemia; if they have had no previous mountain exposure, they should be advised to avoid mountains.

### Acute Mountain Sickness

Initial manifestations include dizziness, headache, lassitude, drowsiness, chilliness, nausea and vomiting, facial pallor, dyspnea, and cyanosis. Later, there is facial flushing, irritability, difficulty in concentrating, vertigo, tinnitus, visual (retinal hemorrhages may occur) and auditory disturbances, anorexia, insomnia, increased dyspnea and weakness on exertion, increased headaches (due to cerebral edema), palpitations, tachycardia, Cheyne-Stokes breathing, and weight loss. Voluntary, periodic hyperventilation may relieve symptoms. In most individuals, symptoms clear within 24–48 hours, but in some instances, if the symptoms are sufficiently persistent or severe, the patient must be returned to lower altitudes. Administration of oxygen will often relieve acute symptoms. Judicious use of sedatives may be of value for some adults with irritability and insomnia. Preventive measures include adequate rest and sleep the day before travel, reduced food intake, and avoidance of alcohol, tobacco, and unnecessary physical activity during travel. Acetazolamide (Diamox), 250 mg every 8 hours one day before, during, and several days after ascent, may prevent symptoms of acute mountain sickness or alleviate its severity.

### Acute High-Altitude Pulmonary Edema

This serious complication usually occurs at levels above 3000 meters. Early symptoms of pulmonary edema may appear within 6–36 hours after arrival at a high-altitude area—dry, incessant cough, dyspnea at rest, and substernal oppression. Later, wheezing, orthopnea, and hemoptysis may occur. Recognition of the early symptoms may enable the patient to climb down (or be assisted) to lower altitudes before incapacitating pulmonary edema develops. An early descent of even 500 or 1000 meters may result in improvement of symptoms. Physical findings include tachycardia, mild fever, tachypnea, cyanosis, and rales and rhonchi. The patient may become confused or even comatose, and the entire clinical picture may resemble severe pneumonia. Microthrombi are often found in the pulmonary capillaries. The white count is often slightly elevated, but the blood sedimentation rate is usually normal. Chest x-ray findings vary from irregular patchy exudate in one lung to nodular densities bilaterally or with transient prominence of the central pulmonary arteries. Transient, nonspecific electrocardiographic changes, occasionally showing right ventricular strain, may occur. Pulmonary arterial blood pressure is elevated, whereas pulmonary wedge pressure is normal. Treatment, which must often be given under field conditions, consists of rest in the semi-Fowler position and administration of 100% oxygen by mask at a rate of 6–8 L/min for 15–20 min. To conserve oxygen, lower flow rates may be used for the next 24–48 h until the victim recovers or can be evacuated to a lower altitude. Prompt descent (eg, by helicopter) may be lifesaving. Treatment for adult respiratory distress syndrome (see Chapter 7) may be required for some patients who have a prolonged course of pulmonary edema. Rapid digitalization and use of diuretics, corticosteroids, and other drugs have been recommended but are of no proved value. If bacterial pneumonia exists, appropriate antibiotic therapy should be given.

Preventive measures include education of prospective mountaineers regarding the possibility of serious pulmonary edema, optimal physical conditioning before travel, gradual ascent to permit acclimatization, and a period of rest and inactivity for 1–2 days after arrival at high altitudes. Acetazolamide (Diamox), 250 mg orally every 8 hours beginning the day before ascent and continuing for 3–4 days after arrival at high altitudes, may reduce the incidence and severity of pulmonary edema. Prompt medical attention with rest and high-flow oxygen if respiratory symptoms develop may prevent progression to frank pulmonary edema. Persons with a history of high-altitude pulmonary edema should be hospitalized for further observation if possible. Mountaineering parties at levels of 3000 meters or higher should carry a supply of oxygen and equipment sufficient for several days. Persons with symptomatic cardiac or pulmonary disease should avoid high altitudes.

## Acute High-Altitude Encephalopathy

High-altitude encephalopathy appears to be an extension of the central nervous symptoms of acute mountain sickness (see above). It usually occurs at elevations above 2500 meters (8250 ft) and is more common in unacclimated individuals. Clinical findings are due largely to hypoxemia and cerebral edema. Severe headaches, confusion, truncal ataxia, staggering gait, focal deficits, nausea and vomiting, and seizures may progress to obtundation and coma. Papilledema and retinal hemorrhages may be observed in about 50% of patients.

Early recognition of the encephalopathic symptoms is essential. Oxygen should be administered by mask. If descent is accomplished as quickly as possible, recovery is usually rapid and complete.

## Subacute Mountain Sickness

This occurs most frequently in unacclimatized individuals and at altitudes above 4500 meters. Symptoms, which are probably due to central nervous system anoxia without associated alveolar hyperventilation, are similar to but more persistent and severe than those of acute mountain sickness. There are additional problems of dehydration, skin dryness, and pruritus. The hematocrit may be elevated, and there may be electrocardiographic and chest x-ray evidence of right ventricular hypertrophy. Treatment consists

of rest, oxygen administration, and return to lower altitudes.

## Chronic Mountain Sickness (Monge's Disease)

This uncommon condition of chronic alveolar hypoventilation, which is encountered in residents of high-altitude communities who have lost their acclimatization to such an environment, is difficult to differentiate clinically from chronic pulmonary disease. The disorder is characterized by somnolence, mental depression, hypoxemia, cyanosis, clubbing of fingers, polycythemia (hematocrit often > 75%), signs of right ventricular failure, electrocardiographic evidence of right axis deviation and right atrial and ventricular hypertrophy, and x-ray evidence of right heart enlargement and central pulmonary vessel prominence. There is no x-ray evidence of structural pulmonary disease. Pulmonary function tests usually disclose alveolar hypoventilation and elevated $CO_2$ tension but fail to reveal defective oxygen transport. There is a diminished respiratory response to $CO_2$. Almost complete disappearance of all abnormalities eventually occurs when the patient returns to sea level.

Blume FD et al: Impaired osmoregulation at high altitude: Studies on Mt. Everest. *JAMA* 1984;**252**:524.

Comp RA, Levine BE: Acute high altitude illness. *Cont Educ* (Feb) 1985;**22**:107.

Dickinson JG: High altitude cerebral edema: Cerebral acute mountain sickness. *Semin Respir Med* 1983;**5**:151.

Houston CS: Altitude illness. *Emerg Med Clin North Am* 1984;**2**:503.

Houston CS: Altitude illness: The dangers of heights and how to avoid them. *Postgrad Med* (July) 1983;**74**:231.

Larson EB et al: Acute mountain sickness and acetazolamide: Clinical efficacy and effect on ventilation. *JAMA* 1982;**248**:328.

Meehan RT, Zavala DC: The pathophysiology of acute high-altitude illness. *Am J Med* 1982;**73**:395.

## MEDICAL EFFECTS OF AIR TRAVEL & SELECTION OF PATIENTS FOR AIR TRAVEL

The decision about whether or not it is advisable for a patient to travel by air depends not only upon the nature and severity of the illness but also upon such factors as the duration of flight, the altitude to be flown, pressurization, the availability of supplementary oxygen and other medical supplies, the presence of attending physicians and trained nursing attendants, and other special considerations. Air carriers in the USA cannot legally allow the use of personal (passenger-supplied) oxygen containers, but most major airlines will supply oxygen upon advance written request from the passenger's physician. Airline policies, charges, and other details must be checked with each carrier. Medical hazards or complications of modern air travel are remarkably uncommon; unless there is some specific contraindication (Table 29–2), air transportation may actually be the best means of

**Table 29–2.** Contraindications to commercial air travel.*

**Cardiovascular**
Within 4 weeks after myocardial infarction†
Within 2 weeks after cerebrovascular accident
Severe hypertension
Decompensated cardiovascular disease or restricted cardiac reserve‡
**Bronchopulmonary**
Pneumothorax
Congenital pulmonary cysts
Vital capacity less than 50%
**Eye, ear, nose, and throat**
Recent eye surgery
Acute sinusitis or otitis media
Surgical mandibular fixation (permanent wiring of jaw)
**Gastrointestinal tract**
Less than 10–14 days after abdominal surgery
Acute diverticulitis or ulcerative colitis
Acute esophageal varices
Acute gastroenteritis
**Neuropsychiatric**
Epilepsy (unless well controlled medically and cabin altitude does not exceed 2500 m [8000 ft])
Previous violent or unpredictable behavior
Recent skull fracture
Brain tumor
**Hematologic**
Anemia (hemoglobin < 8.5 g/dL or red blood cell count of 3 million/μL in an adult)
Sickle cell disease (except below 6800-m [22,500-foot] altitude)
Blood dyscrasias with active bleeding (hemophilia, leukemia)
**Pregnancy**
Beyond 240 days or with threatened miscarriage
**Miscellaneous**
Need for intravenous fluids or special medical apparatus†

* Slightly modified and reproduced, with permission, from *Mod Med* (June) 1982;**50**:196. Based on recommendations of the American Medical Association in *JAMA* 1982;**247**:1009.
† Consultation with an airline flight surgeon is suggested.
‡ In some cases, low-altitude flights can be made without supplemental oxygen in accordance with recommendations of the American College of Chest Physicians.

moving patients. The Air Transport Association of America defines an incapacitated passenger as "one who is suffering from a physical or mental disability and who, because of such disability or the effect of the flight on the disability, is incapable of self-care; would endanger the health or safety of such person or other passengers or airline employees; or would cause discomfort or annoyance of other passengers."

## Cardiovascular Disease

**A. Cardiac Decompensation:** Patients in congestive failure should not fly until they are compensated by appropriate treatment, or unless they are in a pressurized plane with 100% oxygen therapy available during the entire flight.

**B. Compensated Valvular or Other Heart Disease:** Patients should not fly above 2400–2800 m unless the aircraft is pressurized and oxygen is administered at altitudes of 2400 m or higher.

**C. Acute Myocardial Infarction, Convalescent and Asymptomatic:** At least 4 weeks of convalescence are recommended even for asymptomatic

patients if flying is contemplated. Ambulatory, stabilized, and compensated patients tolerate air travel well. Oxygen should be available.

**D. Angina Pectoris:** Air travel is inadvisable for patients with severe angina. In mild to moderate cases of angina, air travel may be permitted, especially in pressurized planes. Oxygen should be available.

## Respiratory Disease

**A. Nasopharyngeal Disorders:** Nasal allergies and infections predispose to development of aerotitis. Chewing gum, nasal decongestants, appropriate anti-infective treatment, and avoiding sleep on descent may prevent barotitis.

**B. Asthma:** Patients with mild asthma can travel without difficulty. Patients with status asthmaticus should not be permitted to fly.

**C. Congenital Pulmonary Cysts:** Patients should not travel unless cleared by physician.

**D. Tuberculosis:** Patients with active, communicable tuberculosis or pneumothorax should not be permitted to travel by air.

**E. Other Pulmonary Disorders:** Patients may be flown safely unless there is marked impairment of pulmonary function.

## Anemia

If hemoglobin is less than 8–9 g/dL, oxygen should be available. Patients with severe anemia should not travel by air until hemoglobin has been raised to a reasonable level. Patients with sickle cell anemia appear to be particularly vulnerable.

## Diabetes Mellitus

Diabetics who do not need insulin or who can administer their own insulin during flight may fly safely. "Brittle" diabetics who are subject to frequent episodes of hypoglycemia should be in optimal control before flying and should carry sugar or candy in case hypoglycemic reactions occur.

## Contagious Diseases

Patients with contagious diseases are not permitted to travel by scheduled passenger airlines at any time.

## Patients With Surgical Problems

Patients convalescing from thoracic or abdominal surgery should not fly until 10 days after surgery, and then only if the wound is healed and there is no drainage.

Colostomy patients may be permitted to travel by air providing they are nonodorous and colostomy bags are emptied before flight.

Patients with large hernias unsupported by a truss or binder should not be permitted to fly in nonpressurized aircraft because of an increased danger of strangulation.

Postsurgical or posttraumatic eye cases require pressurized cabins and oxygen therapy to avoid retinal damage due to hypoxia.

## Psychiatric Disorders

Severely psychotic, agitated, or disturbed patients should not be permitted to fly on scheduled airlines even when accompanied by a medical attendant.

Extremely nervous or apprehensive patients may travel by air if they receive adequate sedatives or tranquilizers before and during flight.

## Motion Sickness

Patients subject to motion sickness should receive sedatives or antihistamines (eg, dimenhydrinate or meclizine), 50 mg 4 times daily, before and during the flight. Small meals of easily digested food before and during flight may reduce the tendency to nausea and vomiting.

## Pregnancy

Pregnant women may be permitted to fly during the first 8 months of pregnancy unless there is a history of habitual abortion or premature birth. During the ninth month of pregnancy, a statement must be furnished that delivery is not due within 72 hours of destination time. Infants less than 1 week old should not be flown at high altitudes or for long distances.

AMA Commission on Emergency Medical Services: Medical aspects of transportation aboard commercial aircraft. *JAMA* 1982;**247:**1007.

Kusumi RK: Medical aspects of air travel. *Am Fam Physician* (June) 1981;**23:**125.

Mills FJ, Harding RM: Fitness to travel by air. 2. Specific medical considerations. *Br Med J* 1983;**286:**1340.

Schley WS: Barotrauma during air travel. *Hosp Med* (July) 1983;**19:**119.

Schwartz JS, Bencowitz HZ, Moser KM: Air travel hypoxemia with chronic obstructive pulmonary disease. *Ann Intern Med* 1984;**100:**473.

Voss MW: Air travel for the chronically ill and the elderly. *Am Fam Physician* (March) 1983;**27:**235.

# Poisoning

**30**

*Kent R. Olson, MD, & Robert H. Dreisbach, MD, PhD*

## DIAGNOSIS OF POISONING

Cases of poisoning generally fall into 3 specific categories: (1) exposure to a known poison, (2) exposure to an unknown substance that may be a poison, and (3) disease of undetermined cause in which poisoning must be considered as part of the differential diagnosis. The diagnosis, when not obvious, depends in great measure upon considering the possibility that poisoning has occurred. Once poisoning is included in the differential diagnosis, the physician will be more likely to take the necessary steps to confirm or reject this possibility.

In general, the steps leading to a diagnosis of poisoning are as follows:

(1) Question the patient, relatives and roommates, coworkers, etc, carefully concerning the presence of poisons in the environment or possible bites by venomous animals or insects. Be aware that the history from the patient is likely to be unreliable, especially in cases of attempted suicide.

(2) A physical examination and simple clinical laboratory tests are important, as outlined below.

(3) Take samples for laboratory evaluation of damage to specific organs and to confirm or rule out exposure to specific poisons. Gastric contents often have the highest concentration of poison and can be used to indicate the possibility but not the seriousness of poisoning.

### Poison Information Centers

Obtain the telephone number of the nearest poison information center, and record it for ready reference. Poison information centers are in most cases able to identify the ingredients of trade-named mixtures, give some estimate of their toxicity, suggest the necessary treatment, and make referrals to experienced toxicologists.

### DETERMINING DEGREE OF EXPOSURE TO KNOWN POISONS

In many cases of poisoning, the agent responsible is known and the physician's only problem is to deter-mine whether the degree of exposure is sufficient to require more than emergency or first aid treatment. The exact quantity of poison absorbed by the patient will probably not be known, but the physician may be able to estimate the greatest amount the patient could have absorbed by examining the container from which the poison was obtained and comparing the missing quantity with the known fatal dose. Reported minimum lethal doses (MLD) are useful indications of the relative hazards of poisonous substances, but the fatal dose may vary greatly. If the poison is known to cause serious or fatal poisoning, treatment for exposure to any quantity must be vigorous.

### SOURCES OF INFORMATION ABOUT POISONS

If a patient has been exposed to a substance whose ingredients are not known, the physician must identify the contents without delay. In addition to the regional poison information center, the following sources are suggested for identifying the contents of trade-named mixtures.

#### Books

Since available proprietary mixtures number in the hundreds of thousands, it is impractical to include all of these names in a single reference work. However, a number of books are useful in determining the contents of mixtures:

(1) Gosselin RE et al: *Clinical Toxicology of Commercial Products*, 5th ed. Williams & Wilkins, 1985. (Lists ingredients of 17,500 products.)

(2) *The Merck Index*, 10th ed. Merck, 1983.

(3) *American Drug Index* (annual publication). Lippincott.

(4) *Physicians' Desk Reference* (annual publication). Medical Economics, Inc. (Tablet and capsule identification guide.)

(5) Dreisbach RH: *Handbook of Poisoning: Prevention, Diagnosis, & Treatment*, 12th ed. Appleton-Lange, 1986. (Lists 6000 poisons and trade-named mixtures.)

(6) Goldfrank L et al: *Goldfrank's Toxicologic Emergencies*. Appleton & Lange, 1986.

(7) Haddad LM, Winchester JF (editors): *Clinical Management of Poisoning and Drug Overdose*. Saunders, 1983.

(8) Berg GL (editor): *Farm Chemical Handbook* (annual publication). Meister Publishing Co.

## Microfiche Poison Information Systems

(1) Rumack BH (editor): Poisindex. National Center for Poison Information, Denver, CO 80204. A microfiche information system. Revised quarterly.

(2) Likes KE (editor): Toxifile. Chicago Micro Corporation, Chicago, IL 60625. A microfiche information system.

## Other Sources of Information

(1) The manufacturer or the local representative. Another way to identify the contents of a substance is to telephone the manufacturer or the local distributor, who will be able to provide information concerning the type of toxic hazard to be expected from the material in question and what treatment should be given.

(2) Poisoning hotlines to manufacturers. Call the poison control center for the telephone number.

## SYSTEM EXAMINATION

A history and physical examination are essential for therapeutic purposes and may also provide valuable information for determining the cause and extent of a poisoning. Below are commonly seen symptoms and signs and poisons that may be causative.

### Vital Signs

**Tachycardia:** Amphetamines, cocaine, antihistamines, atropine, iron, theophylline, antidepressants.

**Bradycardia:** Digitalis, oleander, organophosphates, clonidine, beta blockers, calcium channel blockers (especially verapamil).

**Hyperthermia:** Amphetamines, cocaine, phencyclidine (PCP), atropine, salicylates, pentachlorophenol, monoamine oxidase inhibitors.

**Hypothermia:** Barbiturates, ethanol, narcotics, sedatives, insulin-induced hypoglycemia.

**Hyperventilation:** Salicylates, methanol, ethylene glycol, caffeine, theophylline.

**Respiratory depression:** Barbiturates, narcotics, sedatives, ethanol, antidepressants, organophosphates.

**Hypertension:** Amphetamines, cocaine, phenylpropanolamine, nicotine, phencyclidine (PCP), monoamine oxidase inhibitors.

**Hypotension:** Iron, nitrites, narcotics, antihypertensives, antidepressants, barbiturates, theophylline.

### Skin

**Cyanosis:** Methemoglobinemia (nitrites, chlorates, aniline), cyanide, carbon monoxide, apnea.

**Table 30–1.** Common causes of anion gap metabolic acidosis.*

| |
|---|
| **Salicylates** |
| **Alcohols** |
|   Ethanol (ketoacidosis) |
|   Methanol (formic acid) |
|   Ethylene glycol (oxalic acid) |
| **Lactic acidosis** |
|   Hypoperfusion (eg, iron) |
|   Hypoxia (eg, low $P_{O_2}$, carbon monoxide) |
| **Renal failure** |
| **Diabetic ketoacidosis** |

* Anion gap = $(NA^+ + K^+) - (HCO_3^- + Cl^-)$ = 12 – 16 meq/L.

**Flushing or redness:** Ethanol, carbon monoxide, cyanide, atropine.

**Jaundice:** *Amanita phalloides* mushrooms, acetaminophen, carbon tetrachloride and other halogenated hydrocarbons.

**Dry skin and mucous membranes:** Atropine, antihistamines, antidepressants.

**Sweaty skin:** Organophosphates, nicotine, amphetamines, cocaine, phencyclidine (PCP).

**Table 30–2.** Calculation of the osmolar gap in toxicology.*

The osmolar gap (Δosm) is determined by subtracting the calculated serum osmolality from the measured serum osmolality.

Calculated osmolality (osm) = $2(Na\,[meq/L]) + \dfrac{Glucose\,(mg/dL)}{18} + \dfrac{BUN\,(mg/dL)}{2.8}$

Δosm = Measured osmolality − Calculated osmolality

Serum osmolality may be increased by contributions of circulating alcohols and other low-molecular-weight substances. Since these substances are not included in the calculated osmolality, there will be a gap proportionate to their serum concentration and inversely proportional to their molecular weight:

Serum concentration (mg/dL) ≈ Δosm × $\dfrac{Molecular\,weight}{10}$

For ethanol (the commonest cause of Δosm), a gap of 30 mosm/L indicates an ethanol level of

$$30 \times 45/10 = 138 \approx 140\ mg/dL$$

| | Molecular Weight | Lethal Concentration (mg/dL) | Corresponding Δosm (mosm/L) |
|---|---|---|---|
| Ethanol | 46 | 350 | 75 |
| Methanol | 32 | 80 | 25 |
| Ethylene glycol | 62 | 200 | 35 |
| Isopropanol | 60 | 350 | 60 |

* Modified from Olson KR, Becker CE: Chapter 29 in: *Current Emergency Diagnosis & Treatment*, 2nd ed. Mills J et al (editors). Lange, 1985.
*Note:* Most laboratories use the freezing point method for calculating osmolality. If the vaporization point method is used, alcohols are driven off and their contribution to osmolality is lost.

## Mouth

**Dry mouth:** Atropine, antihistamines, antidepressants.

**Salivation:** Organophosphates, mercury, lead, caustics.

**Characteristic breath odors:** Ethanol, ammonia, camphor, paraldehyde, garlic (arsenic, organophosphates, arsine), bitter almond (cyanide), rotten eggs (hydrogen sulfide).

**Burns:** Acids, alkalies, paraquat.

## Eyes

**Ptosis:** Botulism, cholinergic excess, elapid type snakebite.

**Dilated pupils:** Atropine, amphetamines, cocaine, LSD, antidepressants.

**Constricted pupils:** Narcotics, clonidine, phenothiazines, organophosphates, pilocarpine.

**Oculogyric crises:** Antipsychotics.

## Abdomen

**Abdominal pain:** Black widow spider bite, lead, arsenic, organophosphates, *Amanita phalloides* mushrooms.

**Diarrhea:** Arsenic, *Amanita phalloides* mushrooms, organophosphates, colchicine.

**Hematemesis:** Corrosives, anticoagulants, iron, fluoride, theophylline.

## Neuromuscular System

**Delirium, hallucinations:** Ethanol (including withdrawal), cocaine, amphetamines, phencyclidine (PCP), atropine, LSD, salicylates, antihistamines.

**Coma:** Ethanol, barbiturates, sedative-hypnotic agents, antidepressants, antipsychotics, narcotics.

**Convulsions:** Antidepressants, theophylline, isoniazid, phenothiazines, antihistamines, camphor, amphetamines, cocaine, lindane, organophosphates, ethanol and other sedative withdrawal.

**Rigidity and cramps:** Strychnine, heat stroke, tetanus, black widow spider bite, phencyclidine (PCP).

## Laboratory, ECG, & Radiographic Studies

**Urine occult blood (eg, Hematest) positive:** (1) Naphthalene, arsine, chlorates, favism: hemoglobinuria. (2) Phencyclidine (PCP), amphetamines, convulsants, heat stroke: myoglobinuria. (3) Anticoagulants: hematuria.

**Urine Phenistix positive:** Salicylates, phenothiazines.

**Urine oxalate crystals:** Ethylene glycol, soluble oxalates.

**ECG:** (1) Ventricular arrhythmias—amphetamines, cocaine, antidepressants, theophylline, digitalis, procainamide; (2) AV block—antidepressants, digitalis, beta blockers, calcium channel blockers, quinidine, procainamide; (3) QRS prolongation—antidepressants, quinidine, procainamide, phenothiazines.

**Radiographs of abdomen (radiopaque pills or toxins):** Disk batteries, chloral hydrate, heavy metals, iodide, phenothiazines, antidepressants, sodium chloride, enteric-coated tablets. Visibility quite variable; normal radiograph does not rule out ingestion.

## SPECIAL LABORATORY TESTS

Toxicology screens (Table 30–3) are *not* comprehensive; they usually attempt to screen coarsely for a variety of common drugs but typically do not include some important drugs and toxins (eg, isoniazid, calcium channel blockers, beta blockers, newer antidepressants, etc). Laboratory methods vary widely and may have poor sensitivity *and* poor specificity. It is best to order specific drug determinations based on clinical suspicion. Remember that the most useful test is one whose result is likely to have an impact on therapy (see Table 30–4).

## PRINCIPLES OF TREATMENT OF POISONING

In emergency treatment of any suspected poisoning, the following general procedures should be carried out: (1) Remember that in suicide attempts, multiple drugs may have been ingested. Maintain airway and respiration, and support the circulation. (2) Place a large-bore intravenous catheter, and draw blood for complete blood count; glucose, electrolyte, and renal function tests; liver function tests; and tests for specific suspected toxins or toxicologic screening. In any case of drug overdose, even if the agent is known, an acetaminophen blood level should also

**Table 30–3.** Common drugs screened for in blood and urine in the toxicology laboratory.*

**Blood**
Acetaminophen, alcohols, barbiturates, benzodiazepines, cariosprodol, ethchlorvynol, glutethimide, meprobamate, methaqualone, phenytoin, salicylates.
**Urine**
Acetaminophen, alcohols, barbiturates, chlorpheniramine, cocaine, codeine, dextromethorphan, diphenhydramine, ethchlorvynol, lidocaine, meperidine, meprobamate, methadone, methyprylon, morphine, pentazocine, phencyclidine, phenothiazines, propoxyphene, salicylates, tricyclic antidepressants.

* **Note:** The urine screen is generally more comprehensive, detecting drugs of abuse (opiates, stimulants), antihistamines, and, in many cases, drugs also found in serum.

**Table 30–4.** Drugs for which immediate laboratory testing is recommended.*

| Drug or Toxin | Treatment |
|---|---|
| Acetaminophen | Use of specific antidote (acetylcysteine) based on serum level. |
| Carbon monoxide | High carboxyhemoglobin level indicates need for 100% oxygen. |
| Digitalis | On basis of serum digitalis and potassium levels, treatment with Fab antibody fragments may be indicated. |
| Ethanol | Low serum level may suggest nonalcoholic cause for coma (eg, trauma, other drugs, other alcohols). May also be used in monitoring ethanol therapy for methanol or ethylene glycol poisoning. |
| Ethylene glycol | High level and acidosis indicate need for hemodialysis and ethanol therapy. |
| Iron | Level may indicate need for chelation with deferoxamine. |
| Lithium | Serum levels and calculated half-life can guide decision to hemodialyze. |
| Methanol | Acidosis, high methanol level indicate need for hemodialysis, ethanol therapy. |
| Methemoglobin | Methemoglobinemia can be treated with methylene blue intravenously. |
| Salicylates | High level may indicate need for hemodialysis, alkaline diuresis. |
| Theophylline | Immediate hemoperfusion may be indicated based on serum level. |

* Some drugs or toxins may have profound and irreversible toxicity unless rapid and specific management is provided outside of routine supportive care. For these agents, laboratory testing may provide the serum level or other evidence required for administering a specific antidote or arranging for hemodialysis.

be obtained, since treatment is ineffective unless administered in the presymptomatic period. (3) Give specific antidote if one exists. (4) Remove poison by emesis or lavage, catharsis, and administration of activated charcoal as soon as possible.

## Supportive & Symptomatic Measures

The victim of acute poisoning must be kept under close observation in order to anticipate the immediate and delayed complications of the poisoning. Suicidal patients need special surveillance and should be seen by a psychiatrist.

**A. Respiratory Abnormalities:** Obtain arterial blood gases to measure adequacy of ventilation and oxygenation as soon as is feasible. Administer supplemental oxygen.

**1. Upper airway obstruction or depressed gag reflex**—Correct by positioning, suctioning, oropharyngeal airway, or endotracheal intubation.

**2. Respiratory depression**—Assist ventilation with mouth-to-mouth technique or bag/valve/mask. Perform intubation of the trachea with a cuffed endo-

tracheal tube. Stimulants (analeptic drugs) are of no value in poisoning.

**3. Methemoglobinemia**—If cyanosis persists despite ventilation and oxygen administration, consider methemoglobinemia. The presence of methemoglobinemia can be confirmed by determining the methemoglobin level or by noting that the blood is dark brown in color. Give 100% oxygen by mask, and methylene blue, 0.1 mL/kg of 1% solution slowly intravenously, in the presence of symptoms or if the methemoglobin level is over 30%.

**B. Circulatory Failure:**

**1. Shock**—The principal measures to be taken include recumbent position, warmth, and parenteral fluids. Saline solution is given in 200-mL boluses up to 1–2 L.

When hypotension does not respond to rehydration or is due to the cardiac depressant effects of toxins, administration of dopamine or dobutamine is recommended. A pulmonary artery catheter is useful in guiding the use of fluids and pressors in critically ill patients.

**2. Pulmonary edema**—Cardiac and noncardiac pulmonary edema may result from overhydration, although the latter is initiated by pulmonary capillary damage caused by hypotension, infection, or toxins. Ventilatory assistance, including positive end expiratory pressure (PEEP), may be needed to maintain adequate arterial oxygen saturation ($P_{O_2} > 55$ mm Hg) in noncardiac pulmonary edema. Furosemide may be helpful in both types.

**C. Coma:**

**1.** Glucose, 50%, 1 mL/kg intravenously after blood sample for serum glucose has been drawn, is administered empirically. In alcoholic or malnourished patients, give 100 mg of thiamine intramuscularly also to prevent Wernicke's syndrome.

**2.** Naloxone (Narcan), 0.4–1 mg intravenously, should be given. Up to 10–15 mg is occasionally required for massive narcotic overdose.

**D. Convulsions:** (See Table 30–5.)

**1.** Diazepam, 0.1–0.2 mg/kg intravenously, is given over 1–2 minutes.

**Table 30–5.** Important considerations in treating seizures.

**Hyperthermia**
Due to excessive muscle activity and exacerbated by anticholinergic effects of many drugs (eg, cyclic antidepressants). Temperature may rapidly rise to over 41°C (106°F), resulting in serious brain and other organ damage and further intractable seizure activity.

**Metabolic acidosis**
Due to anaerobic metabolism and generation of lactic acid as well as to respiratory acidosis due to impaired ventilation. Acidosis may exacerbate the cardiovascular effects of drugs such as cyclic antidepressants and may increase brain penetration by weak acids like salicylate.

**Rhabdomyolysis**
Due to muscle activity and hyperthermia. May result in myoglobinuria with deposition in the kidney and acute tubular necrosis.

2. Phenytoin may be given in doses of 100 mg intravenously in 15–30 minutes, up to a total of 1000 mg.

3. If these are unsuccessful, phenobarbital, pentobarbital, or other anticonvulsants may be useful, and neurologic consultation is essential. With prolonged or repeated seizures, hyperthermia and lactic acidosis may occur. Neuromuscular paralysis may be required to control seizure activity.

**E. Start Electrocardiographic Monitoring:** Obtain a 12-lead ECG, noting rate, rhythm, presence of arrhythmias, and PR, QRS, and QT intervals. Attach a continuous monitor for at least 6 hours if irregularities are present or overdose of tricyclic antidepressants or other cardiotoxic drug is suspected.

## Removal of Ingested Poison
## (See Table 30–6.)

*Caution:* Generally, gastric emptying is not used in poisonings due to corrosive agents or petroleum distillates; further injury may result. However, in certain cases, removal of the toxin may be more important than concern over possible complications of emesis or lavage. It is best to contact a toxicologist or regional poison center for advice.

**A. Emesis:** This is a convenient and a fairly effective way to evacuate gastric contents.

**1. Indications–**For removal of poison in conscious, cooperative patients and for promptness, since ipecac can be given in the home in the first few minutes after poisoning.

**2. Contraindications–**(1) Drowsy, unconscious, or convulsing patients. (2) Ingestion of kero-

sene or other hydrocarbons (danger of aspiration of stomach contents). (3) Ingestion of corrosive poisons. (4) Ingestion of rapidly acting convulsants, eg, cyclic antidepressants, strychnine, nicotine, camphor.

**3. Technique–**Give syrup of ipecac, 30 mL (15 mL in children), followed by ½ glass of water (120 mL). Repeat in 20 minutes if necessary. Dose should be 10 mL of syrup of ipecac in patients under 1 year of age. Ipecac may not be effective after charcoal has been given.

**B. Gastric Aspiration and Lavage:**

**1. Indications–**(1) For removal of ingested poisons when emesis is refused, contraindicated, or unsuccessful. (2) For collection and examination of gastric contents for identification of poison. (3) For convenient administration of antidotes. Danger of aspiration pneumonia is reduced by first protecting the airway with endotracheal intubation.

**2. Contraindications–**(1) Do not use lavage in stuporous or comatose patients with absent gag reflexes unless they are endotracheally intubated prior to lavage. (2) Some authorities advise against lavage when caustic material has been ingested; others regard it as essential to remove such material from the stomach.

**3. Technique–**Gently insert a lubricated, soft but noncollapsible stomach tube (at least 37–40F) through the mouth or nose into the stomach. Aspirate and save contents; then lavage repeatedly with 50–100 mL of fluid until return is clear. Always remove excess lavage fluid. Use lukewarm tap water or saline. For iron ingestion, use 1–2% bicarbonate solution.

**C. Adsorption:** Activated charcoal is effective for adsorbing almost all poisons. It is often sold in a suspension with water or 70% sorbitol. This preparation keeps well, it resuspends easily, the sorbitol does not interfere with adsorption, and the sorbitol acts as a cathartic. Give 60–100 g (about 2 coffee-cups full) orally after emesis, or use as lavage fluid. Activated charcoal is not effective for small, highly charged molecules such as sodium, lithium, potassium, or iron and is poorly effective for alcohols. Repeated doses may be useful for insuring complete gut decontamination and also may enhance elimination of theophylline, phenobarbital, digitalis, and carbamazepine overdoses.

**D. Catharsis:**

**1. Indications–**For removal of unabsorbed poisons, especially those that have passed into the intestine.

**2. Contraindications–**Do not use mineral oil or other oil-based cathartics. Avoid sodium-based cathartics in hypertension, renal failure, and congestive heart failure. Avoid magnesium-based cathartics in renal failure.

**3. Materials–**Sodium sulfate 10%, 1–2 mL/kg; magnesium sulfate 10%, 2–3 mL/kg; or sorbitol 70%, 1–2 mL/kg. Combine with activated charcoal, 60–90 g. Alternatives are magnesium citrate or magnesium sulfate.

**4. Technique–**A single dose is usually given.

**Table 30–6.** Outline for gastrointestinal decontamination (see text for details).

---

**Emesis**
Method: Give syrup of ipecac followed after 5–10 minutes with 1–2 glasses of warm water. If no emesis in 20 minutes, repeat dose.
Contraindications:
    (1) Comatose or convulsing patient.
    (2) Lethargic patient with absent gag reflex.
    (3) Ingestion of caustic agent.
    (4) Ingestion of hydrocarbon or petroleum distillate.
    (5) Ingestion of rapid-acting convulsant.
**Gastric lavage**
Method: Using a large (32F to 40F) orogastric or nasogastric tube, lavage repeatedly until return is clear.
Contraindications:
    (1) Comatose, convulsing, or lethargic patient with absent gag reflex, unless airway is protected with cuffed endotracheal tube.
    (2) Ingestion of highly caustic agent.*
**Activated charcoal**
Method: Use as a slurry given orally or via gastric tube. If given before ipecac, it may adsorb the ipecac.
**Cathartic**
Enhances gut motility and passage of charcoal.

---

* This is controversial. Some gastroenterologists recommend immediate gastric lavage after ingestion of liquid caustic substances.

**Table 30–7.** Some toxic agents for which there are "specific" antidotes.

| Toxic Agent | Specific Antidote |
|---|---|
| Acetaminophen | Acetylcysteine |
| Anticholinergics (eg, atropine) | Physostigmine |
| Anticholinesterases (eg, organophosphate pesticides, physostigmine) | Atropine and pralidoxime (2-PAM) |
| Carbon monoxide | Oxygen |
| Cyanide | Sodium nitrite, sodium thiosulfate |
| Heavy metals (eg, lead, arsenic, mercury, iron) | Specific chelating agents |
| Hydrogen sulfide | Sodium nitrite |
| Isoniazid | Pyridoxine (vitamin $B_6$) |
| Methanol (methyl alcohol) | Ethanol (ethyl alcohol) |
| Narcotics | Naloxone (Narcan) |
| Snake venom | Specific venom antisera |

Repeated doses of activated charcoal, 20–30 g in water, or 15–20 mL of sorbitol may hasten elimination of some drugs (eg, digitoxin, theophylline, phenobarbital). With repeated dosing, large stool volumes may result in dehydration or hypernatremia.

## Antidotes

Give "specific" antidotes when there is reasonable certainty of a specific diagnosis (Table 30–7). To effectively negate the physiologic effects of the toxic agent, the antidote must be given promptly. Keep in mind, however, that antidotes frequently have serious side effects of their own. The indications and dosages for specific antidotes are discussed in the respective sections for specific toxins. See also Table 30–8.

**Table 30–8.** Examples of ineffective or dangerous "antidotes."*

| "Antidote" | Application | Problems |
|---|---|---|
| Amphetamines, caffeine, or doxapram | Nonspecific arousal, eg, sedative overdose | Cardiac arrhythmias, seizures |
| Mineral oil | Petroleum distillate ingestion | Lipoid pneumonia |
| Physostigmine | Nonspecific arousal, eg, diazepam overdose, tricyclic antidepressants | Bradycardia, asystole, seizures |
| "Universal antidote" (burnt toast, tea) | Adsorbent in gut | Ineffective; aspiration; wastes time |
| Vinegar, other weak acids | Neutralization of alkali burns | Ineffective; may worsen injury |

* Reproduced, with permission, from Olson KR, Becker CE: Chapter 29 in: *Current Emergency Diagnosis & Treatment*, 2nd ed. Mills J et al (editors). Lange, 1985.

## Increased Drug Removal

**A. Diuretics:** Forced diuresis requires an adequate osmotic load and appropriate parenteral fluids and is hazardous. The risk of complications usually outweighs benefits. Basic drugs (eg, amphetamines, strychnine) are best excreted by maintaining an acid urine. Acidic drugs (eg, salicylates, phenobarbital) are best excreted with an alkaline urine. Other contraindications to osmotic diuresis include renal insufficiency, pulmonary edema, cardiac insufficiency, and persistent severe hypotension despite adequate fluid replacement. Acidification is contraindicated in the presence of rhabdomyolysis or myoglobinuria.

**B. Dialysis (Hemodialysis or Hemoperfusion):** The indications for dialysis are as follows: (1) Known or suspected potentially lethal amounts of a dialyzable drug (Table 30–9). (2) Poisoning with deep coma, apnea, severe hypotension, fluid and electrolyte or acid-base disturbance, or extreme body temperature changes which cannot be corrected by conventional measures. (3) Poisoning in patients with severe renal, cardiac, pulmonary, or hepatic disease who will not be able to eliminate the toxin by usual mechanisms.

Many of the substances that cannot be removed effectively by aqueous dialysis can be removed by hemoperfusion through specially designed coated resin or charcoal columns. Indications are the same as for dialysis. Peritoneal dialysis may occasionally be employed for acute poisonings when hemodialysis is not available, but it is very inefficient. Dialysis should usually augment rather than replace well-established emergency and supportive measures.

**Table 30–9.** Hemodialysis (HD) and hemoperfusion (HP).

| Toxin | Procedure | Indications* |
|---|---|---|
| Digitoxin | HP | Severe toxicity, Fab not available. |
| Ethylene glycol | HD | Acidosis, serum level > 100 mg/dL. |
| Lithium | HD | Severe symptoms, serum level > 2 meq/L (chronic) or > 4 meq/L (acute). |
| Methanol | HD | Acidosis, serum level > 50 mg/dL. |
| Paraquat | HP | Ingestion of known lethal dose. |
| Phenobarbital | HP | Intractable hypotension, acidosis despite maximal supportive care. |
| Salicylate | HD | Severe acidosis, CNS symptoms, level > 100 mg/dL (acute) or > 60 mg/dL (chronic). |
| Theophylline | HP | Seizures, serum level > 90–100 mg/L (acute) or > 40–60 mg/L (chronic). |

* Contact a regional poison center or a clinical toxicologist before undertaking these procedures. See text for further discussion of indications.

Goldfrank LR: *Toxicologic Emergencies,* 3rd Appleton-Century-Crofts, 1986.

Haddad LM, Winchester JF (editors): *Clinical Management of Poisoning and Drug Overdosage.* Saunders, 1983.

# TREATMENT OF COMMON SPECIFIC POISONINGS (Alphabetical Order)

## ACETAMINOPHEN

Acetaminophen is available in many over-the-counter and prescription items. Ingestion of 150 mg/kg or more in a single dose by an adult may cause liver damage within the first 12 hours, but symptoms and signs of liver damage may not appear for 24–48 hours. Peak plasma levels do not occur until 4 or more hours after ingestion. Patients with 4-hour plasma acetaminophen levels above 150 μg/mL are at risk of developing hepatic necrosis. Chronic ingestion of alcohol may result in toxicity with lower doses of acetaminophen (eg, 5 g/d) (Fig. 30–1). Blood acetaminophen levels should be determined in all patients with suspected drug overdose, since treatment is ineffective once signs of hepatotoxicity appear.

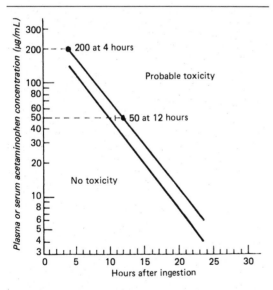

**Figure 30–1.** Nomogram for prediction of acetaminophen hepatotoxicity following acute overdosage. The upper line defines serum acetaminophen concentrations known to be associated with hepatotoxicity; the lower line defines serum levels 25% below those expected to cause hepatotoxicity. To give a margin for error, the lower line should be used as a guide to treatment. (Modified and reproduced, with permission, from Rumack BH, Matthew H: Acetaminophen poisoning and toxicity. *Pediatrics* 1975;**55**:871.)

## Treatment

Treatment should be started immediately in any patient with a 4-hour level > 150 μg/mL and is of doubtful value after 12 hours. Removal of the drug is by emesis or gastric lavage. Activated charcoal may adsorb the antidote; consult a poison center before using activated charcoal.

Give the specific antidote acetylcysteine (Mucomyst), 140 mg/kg orally of a 20% solution diluted to 5% in fruit juice or soda as a loading dose. Follow with 70 mg/kg orally every 4 hours for 3 days or until the plasma acetaminophen level is zero. If a dose is vomited within 1 hour, it should be repeated. If the patient has persistent vomiting, it may be necessary to give the drug by nasogastric or duodenal tube and to use antiemetics.

Rumack BH et al: Acetaminophen overdose: 662 cases with evaluation of acetylcysteine treatment. *Arch Intern Med* 1981;**141**:380.

Seeff LB et al: Acetaminophen hepatotoxicity in alcoholics. *Ann Intern Med* 1986;**104**:399.

## ACIDS, CORROSIVE

The strong mineral acids exert primarily a local corrosive effect on the skin and mucous membranes. In severe burns, circulatory collapse may result. Symptoms include severe pain in the throat and upper gastrointestinal tract, marked thirst, bloody vomitus; difficulty in swallowing, breathing, and speaking; discoloration and destruction of skin and mucous membranes in and around the mouth; and shock. Severe systemic metabolic acidosis may occur (see Table 30–10).

Inhalation of volatile acids, fumes, or gases such as chlorine, fluorine, bromine, or iodine causes severe irritation of the throat and larynx and may cause upper airway obstruction and noncardiogenic pulmonary edema.

**Table 30–10.** Common caustic agents.*

| Type | Examples | Injury |
|---|---|---|
| Concentrated alkalies | Clinitest tablets<br>Drain cleaners<br>Industrial-strength ammonia<br>Lye<br>Oven cleaners | Penetrating liquefaction necrosis |
| Concentrated acids | Etchers (hydrofluoric acid)<br>Pool disinfectants<br>Toilet bowl cleaners | Coagulation necrosis |
| Weaker cleaning agents | Cationic detergents (dishwasher detergents)<br>Household ammonia<br>Household bleach | Superficial burns and irritation; deep burns (rare) |

*Reproduced, with permission, from Olson KR, Becker CE: Chapter 29 in: *Current Emergency Diagnosis & Treatment,* 2nd ed. Mills J et al (editors). Lange, 1985.

## Treatment

**A. Ingested:** Dilute immediately by giving 200 mL of milk or water to drink. Do not give bicarbonate or carbonates.

Perform flexible endoscopic esophagoscopy promptly to determine the presence and extent of injury but do not attempt to pass beyond the injury. Perforation, peritonitis, and major bleeding are indications for surgery.

**B. Skin Contact:** Flood with water for 15 minutes. Use no chemical antidotes; the heat of the reaction may cause additional injury. For hydrofluoric acid burns, soak the affected area in magnesium sulfate solution or apply calcium gluconate; then arrange consultation with a plastic surgeon or other specialist. Binding of the fluoride ion may be achieved by injecting 0.5 mL of 10% calcium gluconate per square centimeter under the burned area.

**C. Eye Contact:** Anesthetize the conjunctiva and corneal surfaces with topical local anesthetic drops. Flood with water for 15 minutes, holding the eyelids open. Check pH with pH 6.0–8.0 test paper, and repeat irrigation, using normal saline, until pH is 7.0. Check for corneal damage with 1% fluorescein solution; consult an ophthalmologist about further treatment.

**D. Inhalation:** Remove from further exposure to fumes or gas. Check skin and clothing. Treat pulmonary edema.

Crain EF et al: Caustic ingestions: Symptoms as predictors of esophageal injury. *Am J Dis Child* 1984;**138**:863.

Trevino MA et al: Treatment of severe hydrofluoric acid exposures. *J Oral Med* 1983;**25**:861.

## ALCOHOL, ETHYL
## (See also p 661.)

The principal manifestations of ethyl alcohol (ethanol) poisoning are initial disinhibition, aggressiveness, nystagmus, and ataxia, followed by central nervous system depression. Alcohol poisoning must be differentiated from sedative or depressant poisoning and head injury and may even be associated with these clinical problems.

The MLD is 300 mL or 1 mL/kg in small children. The potentially lethal blood level is 300 mg/dL, although chronic alcohol abusers may tolerate much higher levels.

## Treatment of Severe
## Alcoholic Intoxication

**A. Emergency Measures:** Remove unabsorbed alcohol by gastric lavage. Activated charcoal is only minimally effective. Naloxone, 0.01 mg/kg intravenously, has been anecdotally reported to have an arousal effect in acute alcohol coma.

**B. General Measures:** (Similar to those for barbiturate poisoning.) Maintain the airway and adequate oxygenation and ventilation (determine arterial $P_{O2}$

and $P_{CO2}$). Keep the patient warm. If the patient is comatose and areflexic, treat as for barbiturate poisoning. Intubate the trachea, and maintain assisted mechanical ventilation.

Determine blood alcohol and glucose levels. Give glucose orally or intravenously if hypoglycemia is present and thiamine, 100 mg intramuscularly, concurrently with glucose administration.

Dialysis is rarely necessary.

Sellers EM et al: Alcohol intoxication and withdrawal. *N Engl J Med* 1976;**294**:757.

## ALCOHOL, METHYL

Methyl alcohol (methanol) is a central nervous system depressant that is metabolized to formic acid, which produces specific damage to the retinal cells and central nervous system as well as metabolic acidosis. The MLD is 30–60 mL. Symptoms include headache, dyspnea, nausea, vomiting, and visual disturbances ranging from white hazy vision to total blindness. Examination reveals hyperpnea, delirium, coma, and convulsions. Funduscopic examination may reveal papilledema or retinitis but is frequently normal. The serum osmolality and osmolar gap (Table 30–2) are often increased. Methanol can be detected in the serum and urine.

## Treatment

Empty the stomach by gastric lavage. Determine serum osmolality and calculate the osmolar gap (see Table 30–2). Measure $P_{O2}$, $P_{CO2}$, and pH. Give intravenous fluids and sodium bicarbonate to combat metabolic acidosis. Give ethanol, orally or intravenously, 7.5 mL/kg of a 10% solution as a loading dose, followed by 2.5 mL/kg of the 10% solution every hour for 3–4 days, to block the metabolism of methanol until it is excreted. Maintain blood ethanol level at 1 mg/mL. Dialysis is useful and is recommended when the serum methanol level exceeds 40 mg/dL (0.4 mg/mL).

Becker CE: Methanol poisoning. *J Emerg Med* 1983;**1**:51.

## ALKALIES

The strong alkalies are common ingredients of household cleaning compounds and may be suspected by their "soapy" texture. Those with solutions above pH 12.0 are particularly corrosive. Clinitest tablets and disk batteries are also a source. Alkalies cause liquefactive necrosis, which is deeply penetrating. Symptoms include burning pain in the upper gastrointestinal tract, nausea, vomiting, and difficulty in swallowing and breathing. Examination reveals destruction and edema of the affected skin and mucous membranes and bloody vomitus and stools. X-ray will reveal the presence of disk batteries in the esophagus or lower gastrointestinal tract.

The MLD is 1 g.

## Treatment

**A. Ingested:** Dilute immediately with 200 mL of water. Some gastroenterologists recommend immediate gastric lavage after ingestion of liquid caustic substances to remove residual material.

Immediate endoscopy is recommended to evaluate the extent of damage.

The use of corticosteroids to prevent stricture formation is controversial and is definitely contraindicated if there is evidence of esophageal perforation.

If x-ray reveals the location of ingested disk batteries in the esophagus, immediate endoscopic removal is mandatory.

**B. Skin Contact:** Wash with running water until the skin no longer feels soapy. Relieve pain and treat shock.

**C. Eye Contact:** Anesthetize the conjunctival and corneal surfaces with topical anesthetic. Wash with water continuously for 30 minutes, holding the lids open. Check pH with pH 6.0–8.0 test paper, and repeat irrigation, using normal saline, for additional 30-minute periods until the pH is 7.0. Check for corneal damage with 1% fluorescein solution; consult an ophthalmologist for further treatment.

Gaudreault P et al: Predictability of esophageal injury from signs and symptoms: A study of caustic ingestion in 378 children. *Pediatrics* 1983;**71**:767.

Mofenson HC et al: Ingestion of small flat disc batteries. *Ann Emerg Med* 1983;**12**:88.

## AMPHETAMINES & STIMULANTS (Amphetamine, Cocaine, Ephedrine, Phenylpropanolamine)

Manifestations are tachycardia, hypertension, dilated pupils, diaphoresis, psychosis, convulsions, cardiac arrhythmias, and hyperthermia. Phenylpropanolamine and other primarily alpha agonists can cause intense hypertension with reflex bradycardia. Intracranial hemorrhage may occur if blood pressure is not rapidly controlled. Myocardial infarction has occurred in patients with normal coronary arteries.

## Treatment

Remove ingested drug by emesis or gastric lavage followed by activated charcoal and catharsis. Give diazepam, 0.1–0.2 mg/kg intravenously over 2 minutes, and repeat as needed to control agitation or psychosis. Antihypertensive drugs may be useful to control severe hypertension. Rapid control of muscular hyperactivity and convulsions is necessary to lower the temperature in hyperthermic patients. Neuromuscular paralysis may be required.

Howard RE et al: Acute myocardial infarction following cocaine abuse in a young woman with normal coronary arteries. *JAMA* 1985;**254**:95.

## ANTICOAGULANTS

Warfarin and related compounds (including ingredients of many rodenticides) inhibit the clotting mechanism by blocking hepatic synthesis of vitamin K-dependent clotting factors. Abnormal bleeding occurs in many circumstances in patients receiving these drugs.

### Clinical Findings

Anticoagulants may cause hemoptysis, gross hematuria, bloody stools, hemorrhages into organs, widespread bruising, and bleeding into joint spaces. The prothrombin time is increased after administration of anticoagulants. After ingestion of brodifacoum and indanedione rodenticides, inhibition of clotting factor synthesis may persist for several weeks.

### Treatment

Discontinue the drug at the first sign of gross bleeding, and determine the prothrombin time. If the patient has ingested an acute overdose, remove by gastric lavage, by instillation of activated charcoal, and by catharsis, and give phytonadione (vitamin K), 5–10 mg subcutaneously. For more rapid effect, give 0.1 mg/kg slowly/intravenously as the diluted emulsion. If the patient is chronically anticoagulated and has strong medical indications for being maintained in that status (eg, prosthetic heart valve), give much smaller doses of vitamin K (1 mg intravenously) and fresh frozen plasma (or both) to titrate to the desired prothrombin time.

Lipton RA et al: Human ingestion of a "super superwarfarin" rodenticide resulting in a prolonged anticoagulant effect. *JAMA* 1984;**252**:3004.

O'Reilly RA: Drugs used in disorders of coagulation. Chapter 32 in: *Basic & Clinical Pharmacology*, 3rd ed. Katzung BG (editor). Appleton-Lange, 1986.

## ARSENIC

Arsenic is found in pesticides and industrial chemicals. Symptoms of poisoning usually appear within 1 hour after ingestion but may be delayed as long as 12 hours. They include abdominal pain, vomiting, watery diarrhea, and skeletal muscle cramps. Profound dehydration and shock may occur. In chronic poisoning, symptoms can be vague but often include those of peripheral sensory neuropathy. Urinary arsenic levels may be misleading and are falsely elevated after certain meals (eg, seafood).

The MLD of inorganic arsenic is 1 mg/kg. The MLD of alkyl methanearsonates is 0.1–0.5 g/kg.

### Treatment

**A. Emergency Measures:** Induce vomiting. Lavage with 2–4 L of warm tap water, and administer 60–100 g of activated charcoal.

**B. Antidote:** For symptomatic patients or those

with massive overdose, give dimercaprol injection (BAL), 10% solution in oil. Give immediately 2.5 mg/kg dimercaprol intramuscularly, then 2 mg/kg intramuscularly every 4 hours for 2 days. The side effects include nausea, vomiting, headache, generalized aches, and burning sensations around the head and face. These usually subside in 30 minutes. An antihistamine such as diphenhydramine, 25–50 mg orally, will reduce the side effects if given 30 minutes before dimercaprol.

Follow BAL with oral penicillamine, 100 mg/kg/d in 4 divided doses (maximum 1 g/d) for 1 week. If urinary arsenic excretion is above 50 μg in 24 hours, give penicillamine for an additional week. Hemodialysis will speed the removal of arsenic combined with dimercaprol if renal failure is present.

Hutton JT: Source, symptoms and signs of arsenic poisoning. *J Fam Pract* 1983;**17**:423.

## ATROPINE & ANTICHOLINERGICS

Atropine, scopolamine, belladonna, Lomotil, *Datura stramonium, Hyoscyamus niger,* some mushrooms, tricyclic antidepressants, and antihistamines are antimuscarinic agents with variable central nervous system effects. The patient complains of dryness of the mouth, thirst, difficulty in swallowing, and blurring of vision. The physical signs include dilated pupils, flushed skin, tachycardia, fever (although hypothermia has been reported), delirium, myoclonus, ileus, and flushed appearance. Antidepressants and antihistamines may induce convulsions.

### Treatment
**A. Emergency Measures:** Induce vomiting, or lavage with 2–4 L of water, preferably containing activated charcoal. *Do not* induce emesis in patients who have ingested antidepressants, because seizures may occur abruptly. Follow lavage with activated charcoal and cathartics.

**B. General Measures:** Treat respiratory failure as for barbiturate poisoning. Cool-water sponge baths and sedation are indicated to control high temperatures. If symptoms are severe (eg, hyperthermia or excessively rapid tachycardia), give physostigmine salicylate, 1 mg slowly intravenously over 5 minutes, with electrocardiographic monitoring, until symptoms are controlled. Arrhythmias and convulsions are a hazard with physostigmine administration, and it should not be used with antidepressant overdose. Physostigmine should be reserved specifically for atropine poisoning.

Pentel PR, Denowitz NL: Tricyclic antidepressant poisoning: Management of arrhythmias. *J Med Toxicol* 1986;**1**:101.

## BARBITURATES & OTHER DEPRESSANTS (Sedative-Hypnotics & Tranquilizers)

The barbiturates and other sedative-hypnotics are among the most common offenders in accidental as well as suicidal poisoning. Multiple drugs, including alcohol, may be involved.

Features of mild poisoning include drowsiness, ataxia, and nystagmus. There may be euphoria or irritability. Moderate poisoning causes stupor and shallow respirations. More severe poisoning may result in circulatory collapse, respiratory arrest, pulmonary edema, dilated and nonreacting pupils, hyporeflexia, coma, and death.

### Treatment
**A. Mild Poisoning:** Empty the stomach by inducing vomiting (if the patient is wide awake) or lavage. Follow with activated charcoal, 60–100 g.

**B. Moderate or Serious Poisoning:** Most patients will survive even days of unconsciousness if the airway is protected (usually with cuffed endotracheal tube). Patients should be placed in intensive care units, where monitoring of vital signs, tissue perfusion, state of consciousness, and reflexes is maintained on an ongoing basis.

Vasopressors (dopamine or dobutamine) may be useful if fluid replacement is ineffective in maintaining blood pressure. Hypothermia commonly occurs and when severe may cause bradycardia and dilated, fixed pupils. Central nervous system stimulants (analeptics or convulsant drugs) are contraindicated. They cause hyperthermia, cardiac arrhythmias, and convulsions.

Hemodialysis or hemoperfusion is usually reserved for patients with severe intoxication and unstable vital signs who cannot be stabilized with supportive measures. Dialysis or hemoperfusion is of no value for poisoning with drugs with very large volumes of distribution (eg, glutethimide).

Repeated doses of activated charcoal (20–30 g every 3–4 hours) may hasten elimination of phenobarbital.

Pond SM et al: Randomized study of the treatment of phenobarbital overdose with repeated doses of activated charcoal. *JAMA* 1984;**251**:3104.

## BETA-ADRENERGIC BLOCKING AGENTS

Overdose with β-adrenergic blocking agents such as propranolol results in hypotension, bradycardia, and variable heart block. Central nervous system toxicity includes coma, convulsions, and respiratory depression. Hypoglycemia and hyperkalemia may occur. In overdosage, beta selectivity is usually lost, and generalized beta blockade occurs. Drugs with membrane-depressant properties and high lipid solubility, such as propranolol, are more toxic.

## Treatment

Treatment includes gastric emptying and administration of activated charcoal. Symptomatic bradycardia or heart block may respond to atropine, isoproterenol, or intracardiac pacing. Hypotension may respond to intravenous fluids, dopamine, or norepinephrine. However, because of intense β-adrenergic receptor blockade, catecholamines may be ineffective. Glucagon activates adenylate cyclase and increases heart rate and myhocardial contractility independently of β-adrenergic receptors. It has successfully reversed beta-blocker overdose in doses of 50–70 μg/kg intravenously.

Weistein RS: Recognition and management of poisoning with beta-adrenergic blocking agents. *Ann Emerg Med* 1984;**13**:1123.

## CALCIUM CHANNEL-BLOCKING AGENTS

Overdosage with calcium channel-blocking agents may result in hypotension, bradycardia, and atrioventricular heart block. The various agents (verapamil, diltiazem, nifedipine) have differing effects on cardiac conduction and peripheral vascular resistance that may account for variable clinical manifestations of overdose.

## Treatment

Treatment includes gastric emptying followed by administration of activated charcoal. Atrioventricular block and bradycardia may be managed with atropine, isoproterenol, or intracardiac pacing. Hypotension may respond to supine positioning, intravenous fluids, and pressor agents. Intravenous calcium has been used successfully to reverse the negative inotropic effects of verapamil toxicity and may be given in doses of 10–20 mg/kg of calcium chloride.

Morris DL, Goldschlager N: Calcium infusion for reversal of adverse effects of intravenous verapamil. *JAMA* 1983;**249**:3212.

## CARBON MONOXIDE

Carbon monoxide poisoning results from unvented or inadequately vented combustion devices. Voluntary inhalation of carbon monoxide in exhaust fumes is often used for suicidal purposes. The gas exerts its toxic effect by combining with hemoglobin to form a relatively stable compound (carboxyhemoglobin) that prevents oxygen transport and utilization. Manifestations are headache, vomiting, syncope, seizures, and coma. Skin color varies from normal (in more than half) to flushed, cyanotic, or, uncommonly, cherry-pink. Blisters and bullous lesions may also occur. After apparent recovery persistent neurologic complications are common.

## Treatment

Give artificial respiration with 100% oxygen by tight-fitting mask or endotracheal tube for at least 1 hour or until carboxyhemoglobin levels are less than 10–15%. Hyperbaric oxygen may further hasten elimination of carbon monoxide but is often not readily available.

Olson KR: Carbon monoxide poisoning: Mechanisms, presentation, and controversies in management. *J Emerg Med* 1984;**1**:233.

## CHLORINATED INSECTICIDES (Chlorophenothane [DDT], Lindane, Toxaphene, Chlordane, Aldrin, Endrin)

DDT and other chlorinated insecticides are central nervous system stimulants that can cause poisoning by ingestion, inhalation, or direct contact. The MLD is about 20 g for DDT, 3 g for lindane, 2 g for toxaphene, 1 g for chlordane, and less than 1 g for endrin and aldrin. The manifestations of poisoning are nervous irritability, muscle twitching, convulsions, and coma. Arrhythmias may occur.

## Treatment

**A. Emergency Measures:** Do not induce emesis, since seizures may occur abruptly. Give activated charcoal at once, lavage with large quantities of warm tap water, and give a cathartic.

**B. General Measures:** For convulsions, give diazepam, 0.1 mg/kg slowly intravenously, or other anticonvulsants.

Telch J, Jarvis DA: Acute intoxication with lindane (gamma benzene hexachloride). *Can Med Assoc J* 1982;**126**:662.

## CLONIDINE & OTHER SYMPATHOLYTIC ANTIHYPERTENSIVES (Clonidine, Methyldopa, Prazosin)

Overdosage with these agents causes bradycardia, hypotension, miosis, respiratory depression, and coma. (Hypertension occasionally occurs after clonidine overdosage, a result of peripheral alpha effects of this drug in high doses.) Symptoms are usually resolved in less than 24 hours, and deaths are rare.

## Treatment

Empty the stomach by emesis or lavage. Give activated charcoal and a cathartic. Maintain the airway and support respiration if necessary. Symptomatic treatment is usually sufficient even in massive overdose. Maintain blood pressure with intravenous fluids. Dopamine can also be used. Atropine is usually effective for bradycardia.

## CYANIDES & HYDROCYANIC ACID

Hydrocyanic acid and the cyanides cause death by inactivation of cytochrome oxidase, preventing utilization of oxygen by the tissues. Cyanide is used in numerous industries and chemical laboratories and is produced in most fires as a component of toxic smoke. The clinical combination of cyanosis, asphyxia, and the odor of bitter almonds on the breath or in lavage fluid or vomitus is diagnostic. Respiration is first stimulated and later depressed. A marked drop in blood pressure may occur. The measured oxygen-hemoglobin saturation in the venous blood may be elevated, reflecting decreased oxygen utilization by cells.

The MLD is 0.05 g.

### Treatment

**A. Emergency Measures:** Use nitrites to form methemoglobin, which combines with cyanide to form less toxic cyanmethemoglobin. Give thiosulfates to convert cyanide to thiocyanate (see Table 30–11 and below).

1. Poisoning by inhalation—Place the patient in the open air in the recumbent position. Remove contaminated clothing.

2. Poisoning by ingestion—Induce vomiting immediately with a finger down the patient's throat. Do not wait until the lavage tube has arrived; death may occur within a few minutes.

3. Give amyl nitrate inhalations for 15–30 seconds every 2 minutes until intravenous antidotes are given.

**B. Antidote:** (Table 30–11.) Administration of nitrites must be based on hemoglobin levels. At 14 g/dL hemoglobin, give 0.4 mL/kg of 3% sodium nitrite intravenously and 1–2 mL/kg of 25% sodium thiosulfate intravenously. At lower hemoglobin levels, reduce the dosage of nitrite in exact proportion. Further administration of nitrite should not produce methemoglobin levels exceeding 40%. Sodium thiosulfate is relatively nontoxic and may be used as a single agent when the diagnosis is uncertain.

**C. General Measures:** Administration of 100% oxygen may be useful. Hyperbaric oxygen is of questionable value.

**Table 30–11.** Prepackaged cyanide antidote kit.*†

| Antidote | How Supplied | Dose |
|---|---|---|
| Amyl nitrite | 0.3 mL (aspirol inhalant) | Break 1–2 aspirols under patient's nose. |
| Sodium nitrite | 3 g/dL (300 mg in 10 mL [vials]) | 6 mg/kg intravenously (0.2 mL/kg) |
| Sodium thiosulfate | 25 g/dL (12.5 g in 50 mL [vials]) | 250 mg/kg intravenously (1 mL/kg) |

\* Reproduced, with permission, from Olson KR, Becker CE: Chapter 29 in: *Current Emergency Diagnosis & Treatment*, 2nd ed. Mills J et al (editors). Lange, 1985.
† In USA, manufactured by Eli Lilly & Co.

## DIGITALIS

Because digitalis, digitoxin, and related drugs have a prolonged action, poisoning is most likely to occur when large doses are given to patients who have previously received digitalis drugs. Chronic intoxication may also result from slow accumulation of the drug in patients receiving a maintenance dose if metabolic elimination is impaired (eg, digoxin toxicity in renal failure). Acute overdosage, as in a suicide attempt, may also result in toxicity.

### Clinical Findings

The manifestations of digitalis poisoning include anorexia, nausea, vomiting, delirium, bradycardia, and ventricular ectopy. The ECG may show a lengthened PR interval, heart block, ventricular extrasystoles, ventricular tachycardia, and a depressed ST segment. With acute ingestion of an overdose, toxicity is accompanied by hyperkalemia. With chronic intoxication, in contrast, the potassium level is usually depressed because of concomitant diuretic use.

The toxic serum level of digoxin is 2 ng/mL, though clinical toxicity generally correlates poorly with serum levels.

### Treatment

**A. Emergency Measures:** Discontinue digitalis and diuretics. In cases of acute ingestion, remove ingested digitalis by emesis or lavage followed by activated charcoal. Repeated administration of activated charcoal or cholestyramine resin can be used to bind digitoxin in the intestine. Do not give epinephrine or other stimulants. These may induce ventricular fibrillation.

**B. General Measures:** In the presence of hypokalemia, give potassium chloride slowly intravenously during electrocardiographic monitoring until the ECG shows improvement or evidence of potassium intoxication. Serum potassium must be determined before and during potassium administration. Severe hyperkalemia can be corrected by intravenous sodium bicarbonate, glucose with insulin, oral Kayexalate, or hemodialysis. Hyperkalemia (> 5 meq/L) may be an indication for digitalis-specific antibodies (see below). Phenytoin or lidocaine can be used to control arrhythmias. Ventricular pacing may be required for advanced atrioventricular block or bradycardia.

The use of digoxin-specific Fab antibody fragments is now possible. Call the nearest regional poison control center (or Burroughs-Wellcome, Inc) for information on availability.

Wenger TL et al: Treatment of 63 severely digitalis-toxic patients with digoxin-specific antibody fragments. *J Am Coll Cardiol* 1985;5(**Suppl A**):118A.

## ETHYLENE GLYCOL
## (Antifreeze)

The initial symptoms in massive dosage (over 100 mL in a single dose) are those of alcoholic intoxication. These symptoms then progress to stupor, anuria, and unconsciousness with convulsions. Smaller amounts (10–30 mL) result in anuria beginning 24–72 hours after ingestion. There is anion-gap metabolic acidosis and an elevation of the measured serum osmolality, as well as an increased osmolar gap (Table 30–2). The urine may show calcium oxalate crystals, protein, red cells, and casts. Hypocalcemia occasionally occurs.

### Treatment

Remove ingested glycol by gastric lavage or emesis, and follow with activated charcoal and catharsis. Give calcium gluconate, 10 mL of 10% solution intravenously, for symptomatic hypocalcemia. In the absence of renal impairment, force fluids to 4 L or more daily to increase excretion of glycol. Correct acidosis with sodium bicarbonate intravenously. Give ethanol as in methanol poisoning to prevent metabolism of ethylene glycol to glycolic acid and oxalic acid. Administer pyridoxine, 500 mg intravenously. Dialysis is mandatory for significant intoxication.

Brown CG et al: Ethylene glycol poisoning. *Ann Emerg Med* 1983;**12**:501.

## IRON

Iron salts are used extensively as antianemic agents in a large number of prescription and over-the-counter "blood tonic" drugs.

Acute poisoning is manifested by vomiting, tarry stools, diarrhea, tachycardia, hypotension, dehydration, acidosis, hyperglycemia, and coma. After serious ingestions, symptoms occur within 30–60 minutes. Following initial treatment, the patient may appear to improve for 6–12 hours. Symptoms then return, with cyanosis, pulmonary edema, shock, convulsions, anuria, hypoglycemia, and death in coma within 24–48 hours. Late sequelae include hepatic failure and pyloric stenosis. Doses exceeding 40–60 mg/kg of elemental iron may cause serious illness or death.

Chronic poisoning may occur after prolonged excess dosage of parenteral iron, causing exogenous hemosiderosis with damage to the liver and pancreas.

### Treatment

Draw blood for hemoglobin, white count, serum iron, total iron-binding capacity, electrolyte concentrations, blood typing, glucose, and serum iron test. Start an infusion of isotonic saline or dextrose solution to correct dehydration and maintain urinary output.

If the patient is clearly intoxicated (severe symptoms, serum iron elevated), give deferoxamine, 15 mg/kg/h intravenously (maximum 80 mg/kg per 12 hours), and maintain adequate blood volume. An orange-pink color to the urine indicates the presence of chelated free iron.

In patients not in shock or coma, induce emesis with syrup of ipecac. In all patients with severe toxicity or a history of massive ingestion (> 60 mg/kg), perform gastric lavage using sodium bicarbonate, 1–5%. Beware of inducing hypernatremia with large-volume lavage in small children. If a radiograph of the abdomen reveals a significant number of iron pills not removed by repeated emesis or lavage, consider gastrotomy.

Repeat deferoxamine after 12 hours if symptoms and iron determination warrant. Monitor blood pressure during administration of deferoxamine and reduce the rate of administration if blood pressure falls. In the presence of renal failure, dialysis must accompany deferoxamine use.

Lacouture PG et al: Emergency assessment of severity in iron overdose by clinical and laboratory methods. *J Pediatr* 1981;**99**:89.

## ISONIAZID

The characteristic findings in isoniazid (INH) overdosage are seizures and metabolic acidosis. Acidosis is often severe and out of proportion to the number of duration of seizures. The toxic dose is between 80 and 100 mg/kg. Symptoms occur within 1–2 hours after ingestion.

### Treatment

Empty the stomach by gastric lavage, and administer activated charcoal and a cathartic. Do not use ipecac because of the risk of abrupt onset of seizures.

Treat seizures with diazepam, 0.2 mg/kg intravenously. If this is not effective, give pyridoxine (vitamin $B_6$), 5–10 mg intravenously.

Wason S et al: Single high-dose pyridoxine treatment for isoniazid overdose. *JAMA* 1981;**246**:1102.

## LEAD

Lead poisoning may occur by ingestion (eg, paint chips) or by inhalation of lead dust or fumes. Toxicity rarely occurs after a single ingestion; more commonly, it results from chronic intake of lead-containing materials. Poisoning is manifested by anorexia, irritability, apathy, abdominal colic, vomiting, diarrhea, constipation, headache, leg cramps, black stools (lead sulfide), oliguria, stupor, convulsions, peripheral neuropathy, and coma. Chronic lead poisoning causes variable involvement of the central nervous system, the blood-forming organs, and the gastrointestinal tract.

Diagnostic laboratory tests include blood lead (>

50 μg/dL), blood erythrocyte protoporphyrin (EPP) > 100 μg/dL, urine coproporphyrin (> 500 μg/L), urine δ-aminolevulinic acid (> 13 mg/L), x-ray of abdomen (radiopaque paint), and x-ray of long bones in children (lead line). A blood lead level over 10 μg/dL indicates excessive exposure to lead. Levels above 50 μg/dL are consistent with serious intoxication.

The MLD is 0.5 g of absorbed lead.

### Treatment

Establish adequate urine flow (1 mL/kg/h). If renal failure has occurred, hemodialysis should accompany the use of antidotes.

Control convulsions with diazepam, 0.1 mg/kg intravenously.

Patients with blood lead levels above 70 μg/dL, including those with lead encephalopathy, give dimercaprol (BAL) and calcium disodium edetate (EDTA) as follows: Begin first with dimercaprol, 4 mg/kg intramuscularly, and repeat every 4 hours for 5 days (30 doses). Four hours after the first dimercaprol injection, give EDTA, 12.5 mg/kg (20% solution, with 0.5% procaine added) intramuscularly, in a different site from dimercaprol. Repeat every 4 hours for 5 days (30 doses). If symptoms have not improved by the fourth day, extend treatment to 7 days (42 doses each of both dimercaprol and EDTA). If blood lead is still above 70 μg/dL 14 days later, repeat the 5-day course of both drugs.

If blood lead is 50–70 μg/dL, give EDTA intramuscularly alone every 6 hours for a 5-day course (20 injections) if EDTA lead mobilization test is positive (24-hour urinary excretion exceeds 1 μg of lead per milligram of EDTA after giving EDTA, 25 mg/kg intramuscularly [maximum 1 g]).

Follow-up therapy (all cases)—Give penicillamine (Cuprimine) orally daily in 3 doses one-half hour before meals. The daily dosage is 100 mg/kg up to a maximum total of 1 g. Therapy should be continued for 1–2 months for adults and for 3–6 months for children. Blood lead should be below 50 μg/dL at the end of treatment.

Remove permanently from exposure, and provide an adequate diet with vitamin supplements.

Mielke HW et al: Lead concentrations in inner-city soils as a factor in the child lead problem. *Am J Public Health* 1983;**73**:1366.

## MERCURY

Acute mercury poisoning may occur by ingestion of inorganic mercuric salts or inhalation of metallic mercury vapor. Ingestion of the mercuric salts causes a metallic taste, salivation, thirst, a burning sensation in the throat, discoloration and edema of oral mucous membranes, abdominal pain, vomiting, bloody diarrhea, and shock. Direct nephrotoxicity causes acute renal failure. Inhalation of high concentrations of metallic mercury vapor causes acute fulminant chemical pneumonia. Chronic mercury poisoning causes weakness, ataxia, intention tremors, irritability, and depression. Chronic intoxication in children may be a cause of acrodynia. Exposure to alkyl (organic) mercury derivatives from contaminated fish or fungicides used on seeds has caused ataxia, tremors, and convulsions and catastrophic birth defects.

### Treatment

**A. Acute Poisoning:** There is no effective specific treatment for mercury vapor pneumonitis. For acute ingestion of mercuric salts, given dimercaprol (BAL) at once, as for arsenic poisoning. Ingested inorganic salts may be precipitated with egg whites or milk. Remove by emesis, lavage, and cathartic. Penicillamine, 100 mg/kg orally in divided doses (maximum 1 g/d), is also effective. Maintain urine output. Treat oliguria and anuria if they occur. Hemodialysis may be necessary to remove the mercury-Bal chelate if renal failure has already occurred.

**B. Chronic Poisoning:** Remove from exposure. Neurologic toxicity is not considered reversible with chelation, although some authors recommend a trial of penicillamine.

Jaffe KM et al: Survival after acute mercury vapor poisoning. *Am J Dis Child* 1983;**137**:749.

## MONOAMINE OXIDASE INHIBITORS (Isocarboxazid, Phenelzine)

Overdoses cause ataxia, excitement, hypertension, and tachycardia; later, fall of blood pressure and convulsions. Hyperthermia may also occur. Ingestion of tyramine-containing foods may cause a severe hypertensive reaction. These include aged cheese and red wines. Hypertensive reactions may also occur with any sympathomimetic drug. Fatal hyperthermia may occur if patients receiving monoamine oxidase inhibitors are given meperidine.

### Treatment

Remove ingested drug by gastric lavage, activated charcoal, and catharsis. Treat severe hypertension with nitroprusside, phentolamine, or other rapid-acting vasodilator. Treat hypotension with fluids and positioning, but avoid use of pressor agents. Treat hyperthermia with aggressive cooling. Neuromuscular paralysis may be required.

## MUSHROOMS

There are thousands of mushroom species that cause a variety of toxic effects. The most dangerous species of mushrooms are *Amanita phalloides, Amanita verna, Amanita virosa, Gyromitra esculenta,* and the *Galerina* species, all of which contain amanitin, a potent cytotoxin. Ingestion of part of one mushroom of a dangerous species may be sufficient to cause death.

The pathologic finding in fatalities from amanitin-containing mushroom poisoning is acute necrosis of the liver, kidneys, heart, and skeletal muscles.

## Clinical Findings
## (Table 30–12)
### A. Symptoms and Signs:
**1. Amanitin type cyclopeptides (Amanita phalloides, Amanita verna, Amanita virosa, and Galerina species)**–After a latent interval of 12–24 hours, severe abdominal cramps and vomiting begin and progress to profuse diarrhea, bloody vomitus and stools, painful tenderness and enlargement of the liver, jaundice, hepatic encephalopathy, and frequently renal failure. The fatality rate is about 20%. Cooking the mushrooms does *not* prevent poisoning.

**2. Gyromitrin type (Gyromitra and Helvella species)**–Toxicity is more common following ingestion of uncooked mushrooms. Vomiting, diarrhea, hepatic necrosis, convulsions, coma, and hemolysis may occur after a latent period of 8–12 hours. The fatality rate is probably less than 10%.

**3. Muscarinic type (Inocybe and Clitocybe species)**–Vomiting, diarrhea, bradycardia, hypotension, salivation, miosis, bronchospasm, and lacrimation occur shortly after ingestion. Cardiac arrhythmias may occur. The fatality rate is less than 5%.

**4. Anticholinergic type (eg, Amanita muscaria, Amanita pantherina)**–This type causes a variety of symptoms that may be atropinelike, including excitement, delirium, flushed skin, dilated pupils, and muscular jerking tremors, beginning 1–2 hours after ingestion. Fatalities are rare.

**5. Gastrointestinal irritant type (eg, Boletus, Cantharellus)**–Nausea, vomiting, and diarrhea occur shortly after ingestion. Fatalities are rare.

**6. Disulfiram type (Coprinus species)**–Disulfiramlike sensitivity to alcohol may persist for several days. Toxicity is characterized by flushing, hypotension, and vomiting after coingestion of alcohol.

**7. Hallucinogenic type (Psilocybe and Panaeolus species)**–Mydriasis, nausea and vomiting, and intense visual hallucinations occur 1–2 hours after ingestion. Fatalities are rare.

**B. Laboratory Findings:** (Type 1 or 2 mushrooms.) Creatinine and blood urea nitrogen may be elevated. Effects on the liver are revealed by increased transaminase and bilirubin levels and prothrombin time. The blood glucose should be monitored frequently when hepatotoxicity is present.

## Treatment
**A. Emergency Measures:** After the onset of symptoms, efforts to remove the toxic agent are probably useless, especially in cases of type 1 or type 2 poisoning, where there is a delay of 12 hours or more before symptoms occur. However, induction of vomiting is recommended for any recent ingestion of an unidentified or potentially toxic mushroom. Activated charcoal and a cathartic should also be given.

**B. General Measures:**
**1. Amanitin type cyclopeptides**–A variety of unproved antidotes have been suggested for amanitin type mushroom poisoning. The administration of thioctic acid has been recommended, but experimental results are equivocal. Administration of penicillin G and dexamethasone are also of unproved value.

Aggressive fluid replacement for diarrhea and intensive supportive care for hepatic failure are the mainstays of treatment. In severely poisoned patients,

**Table 30–12.** Poisonous mushrooms.*

| Toxin | Genus | Symptoms and Signs | Onset | Treatment |
|---|---|---|---|---|
| Amatoxin | *Amanita* (*A phalloides, A verna, A virosa*) | Severe gastroenteritis, followed by delayed hepatic and renal failure after 48–72 hours. | 6–24 hours. | Supportive. Correct dehydration. Thioctic acid is of unproved benefit. |
| Muscarine | *Inocybe, Clitocybe* | Muscarinic (salivation, miosis, bradycardia, diarrhea). | 30 minutes to 1 hour | Supportive. Give atropine, 0.5–2 mg intravenously, for severe cholinergic symptoms and signs. |
| Ibotenic acid, muscimol | *Amanita muscaria* ("fly agaric") | Anticholinergic (mydriasis, tachycardia, hyperpyrexia, delirium). | 30 minutes to 2 hours | Supportive. Give physostigmine, 0.5–2 mg intravenously, for severe anticholinergic symptoms and signs. |
| Coprine | *Coprinus* | Disulfiramlike effect occurs with ingestion of ethanol. | 30 minutes to 2 days | Supportive. Abstain from ethanol for 3–4 days. |
| Monomethylhydrazine | *Gyromitra* | Gastroenteritis; occasionally hemolysis, hepatic and renal failure. | 6–12 hours | Supportive. Correct dehydration. Pyridoxine, 2.5 mg/kg intravenously, may be helpful. |
| Psilocybin | *Psilocybe* | Hallucinations. | 15–30 minutes | Supportive. |
| Gastrointestinal irritants | Many species | Nausea and vomiting, diarrhea. | 30 minutes to 2 hours. | Supportive. Correct dehydration. |

* Modified and reproduced, with permission, from Becker CE et al: *West J Med* 1976;**125**:100.

liver function has been known to begin to return 6–8 days after exposure, followed by eventual complete recovery. Liver transplantation has been successful in one near-fatal case.

Interruption of enterohepatic circulation of the amanitin toxin by the administration of activated charcoal and laxatives may be of value. However, by the time this method is employed, most of the amanitin has already caused cellular damage and has already been excreted. Liver transplant may be the only hope for survival in gravely ill patients.

**2. Gyromitrin type**–For gyromitrin poisoning, give pyridoxine, 25 mg/kg intravenously.

**3. Muscarinic type**–For mushrooms producing predominantly muscarinic-cholinergic symptoms, give atropine, 0.005–0.01 mg/kg intravenously, and repeat as needed.

**4. Anticholinergic type**–For anticholinergic type, physostigmine, 0.5–1 mg intravenously, may calm extremely agitated patients and reverse peripheral anticholinergic manifestations, but it may also cause bradycardia, asystole, and seizures.

**5. Gastrointestinal irritant type**–Treat with antiemetics and intravenous or oral fluids.

**6. Disulfiram type**–For *Coprinus* ingestion, avoid alcohol. Treat alcohol reaction with fluids and supine position.

**7. Hallucinogenic type**–Provide a quiet, supportive atmosphere. Diazepam or haloperidol may be used for sedation.

Olson KR et al: *Amanita phalloides*–type mushroom poisoning. *West J Med* 1982;**137:**282.

Woodle ES et al: Orthotopic liver transplantation in a patient with *Amanita* poisoning. *JAMA* 1985;**253:**69.

## OPIOID NARCOTICS: see p 663 (Morphine, Heroin, Etc)

## PARAQUAT

Paraquat is used as a herbicide. Concentrated solutions of paraquat are highly corrosive to the oropharynx, esophagus, and stomach. The fatal dose after absorption may be as small as 4 mg/kg. If not rapidly fatal because of its corrosive effects, paraquat causes pulmonary edema and fibrosis with respiratory insufficiency, and renal damage with anuria. A urinary excretion rate over 1 mg/h indicates severe poisoning. Patients with plasma paraquat levels above 2 mg/L at 6 hours or 0.2 mg/L at 24 hours are likely to die.

### Treatment

Remove by emesis, gastric lavage, and catharsis. Clay (bentonite or fuller's earth) and activated charcoal are effective adsorbents. Whole gut lavage with a balanced salt/isosmolar solution (CoLyte, Go-LYTELY) has been recommended. Administer repeated doses of 60 g of activated charcoal by gastric tube every 2 hours. Charcoal hemoperfusion, 8 hours per day for 2–3 weeks, has been reported to be lifesaving. Supplemental oxygen should be withheld unless the $P_{O2}$ is less than 70 mm Hg. For further information and for rapid determination of paraquat levels, call the Chevron Poison Information Service, (415) 233–3737.

Landrigan PJ et al: Paraquat and marihuana: Epidemiologic risk assessment. *Am J Public Health* 1983;**73:**784.

## PESTICIDES: CHOLINESTERASE INHIBITOR (Organophosphates: Parathion, TEPP, Malathion, Thimet, Phosdrin, Systox, HETP, EPN, OMPA, Etc; Carbamates: Carbaryl, Aldicarb, Benomyl)

Inhalation, skin absorption, or ingestion of organophosphorus or carbamate pesticides causes marked inhibition of cholinesterase, resulting in continuous and excessive stimulation of the parasympathetic nervous system. Manifestations of acute poisoning appear within hours after exposure and include miosis, bronchorrhea and wheezing, sweating, salivation, lacrimation, vomiting, diarrhea, muscular twitchings, and convulsions. Pulse and blood pressure can be extremely variable.

The potency of available products is highly variable; for example, parathion is 100 times more toxic than malathion.

### Treatment

**A. Emergency Measures:** Maintain airway and give artificial respiration. If the material has been ingested, remove poison by induced vomiting or gastric lavage. Remove toxin from the skin (especially the hair and under the fingernails) by copious washing with soap and water. Remove and isolate contaminated clothing. Emergency personnel must avoid contamination. Counteract parasympathetic stimulation by giving atropine sulfate, 0.01–0.05 mg/kg intramuscularly or intravenously every 3–8 minutes until symptoms (especially bronchorrhea or bronchospasm) are relieved or signs of atropinization (dilated pupils, dry mouth) appear. Repeat as necessary to maintain complete atropinization. As much as 12 mg of atropine has been required in the first 2 hours. Give pralidoxime (Protopam), 25 mg/kg (maximum dose 1 g) slowly intravenously in aqueous solution. Protopam is a specific antidote that acts to remove the organophosphate from cholinesterase. It should be given every 8 hours until the intoxication has resolved. For some long-acting agents (eg, fenthion), this may require several days of treatment.

**B. General Measures:** Take a blood sample for determination of plasma and red cell cholinesterase levels. (This is of no practical value in immediate diagnosis or treatment of the acute episode but aids in confirmation of the diagnosis.)

Lotti M et al: Occupational exposure to the cotton defoliants DEF and merphos. *J Occup Med* 1983;**25**:517.

## PETROLEUM DISTILLATES (Petroleum Ether, Charcoal Lighter Fluid, Kerosene, Paint Thinner, Benzine, Gasoline, Etc)

Petroleum distillate toxicity occurs almost entirely as a result of pulmonary aspiration during or after ingestion. The intratracheal toxicity is 100 times the gastric toxicity. Some hydrocarbons—ie, those with aromatic or halogenated subunits—can cause severe systemic poisoning after oral ingestion. Most hydrocarbons can also cause systemic intoxication by inhalation, but only with very high concentrations of the vapors in an enclosed space. Chlorinated and fluorinated hydrocarbons (trichloroethylene, freons, etc) can cause ventricular arrhythmias by a mechanism of myocardial sensitization after inhalation.

Acute manifestations of aspiration pneumonitis are vomiting, coughing, and bronchopneumonia. Vertigo, muscular incoordination, irregular pulse, myoclonus, and convulsions occur with serious poisoning and may be due to hypoxemia or the systemic effects of some agents (eg, camphor).

## Treatment
### (See Table 30–13.)

Remove the patient to fresh air. Since aspiration is the primary danger with many common products, use of lavage or emesis is controversial. Removal of ingested hydrocarbon is usually suggested only if the preparation contains toxic solutes (eg, an insecticide) or is an aromatic or halogenated product. If lavage is done, prophylactic insertion of a cuffed endotracheal tube may be necessary to prevent aspiration. Watch the victim closely for 6–8 hours for signs of aspiration pneumonitis (cough, localized rales or rhonchi, tachypnea, and infiltrates on chest radiograph). The use of corticosteroids to treat pneumonitis is controversial. If fever occurs, give a specific antibiotic after identification of pathogens by laboratory studies.

Wasserman GS: Hydrocarbon poisoning. *Crit Care Q* 1982; **4**:33.

## PHENCYCLIDINE

Phencyclidine (PCP) was until recently one of the most commonly abused street drugs—second only to alcohol as a cause of emergency room visits for drug intoxication in many cities. It occurs under a variety of names or is misrepresented as other psychotomimetic agents. The drug has a wide range of toxic manifestations. Doses under 5 mg (adults) cause hyperactivity, horizontal and vertical nystagmus, incoordination, diaphoresis, flushing, rigidity, dissociative anesthesia, rhabdomyolysis with myoglobinuria, and wild movements. Doses over 10 mg cause, in addition, seizures, coma, hyperthermia, rhabdomyolysis, and myoglobinuria. Symptoms may persist for several days.

## Treatment

Maintain a quiet, calm atmosphere. Sedate the agitated patient with diazepam, 0.1 mg/kg intravenously, or haloperidol, 0.05–0.1 mg/kg intramuscularly. Endotracheal intubation and mechanical ventilation may be necessary. After gastric lavage and administration of a cathartic, restrict sensory input, prevent injuries, monitor vital signs, and maintain gastric suction. Repeated administration of activated charcoal,

**Table 30–13.** Clinical features of hydrocarbon poisoning.*

| Type | Examples | Risk of Pneumonia | Risk of Systemic Toxicity | Treatment |
|---|---|---|---|---|
| High-viscosity | Vaseline<br>Motor oil | Low | Low | None. |
| Low-viscosity, nontoxic | Furniture polish<br>Mineral seal oil<br>Kerosene<br>Lighter fluid | High | Low | Observe for pneumonia.<br>*Do not* induce emesis. |
| Low-viscosity, unknown systemic toxicity | Turpentine<br>Pine oil | High | Variable | Observe for pneumonia.<br>*Do not* induce emesis if less than 1–2 mL/kg was ingested. |
| Low-viscosity, known systemic toxicity | Camphor<br>Phenol<br>Chlorinated insecticides<br>Aromatic hydrocarbons<br>(benzene, toluene,<br>etc) | High | High | Induce emesis, or perform lavage.<br>Give activated charcoal. |

*Reproduced, with permission, from Olson KR, Becker CE: Chapter 29 in: *Current Emergency Diagnosis & Treatment*, 2nd ed. Mills J et al (editors). Lange, 1985.

30 g in sorbitol, may remove additional PCP secreted into the acidic stomach. Bear in mind, however, that repeated use of charcoal and cathartics may lead to dehydration and hypernatremia from massive fluid loss in stools. Control convulsions by giving diazepam, 0.1 mg/kg intravenously. Hyperthermia should be treated aggressively, with control of muscular rigidity or hyperactivity by paralysis with neuromuscular blockers and endotracheal intubation. Control hypertension by giving nitroprusside, 0.5–5 μg/kg/min intravenously.

Lowering blood pH removes PCP from the central nervous system by ion trapping but is hazardous and may promote myoglobinuric renal failure.

Krenzelok EP: Phencyclidine: A contemporary drug of abuse. *Crit Care Q* 1982;**4**:55.

## PHENOLS & DERIVATIVES

The phenols are present in carbolic acid, Lysol, cresol, and creosote. Hexachlorophene—2,2'-methylenebis(3,4,6-trichlorophenol)—is a widely used antiseptic (pHisoHex, etc). Pentachlorophenol is used as a wood preservative, and dinitrophenols are used as pesticides. They are local corrosives and also have marked systemic effects (after oral or dermal absorption) on the nervous and circulatory systems. Manifestations include corrosive injury to the upper gastrointestinal tract, nausea and vomiting, oliguria, and circulatory collapse. Convulsions and respiratory arrest may also occur. Pentachlorophenol and dinitrophenols, in addition, cause hyperthermia by interfering with oxidative phosphorylation.

### Treatment
**A. Ingestion:** Remove by gastric lavage, and then give activated charcoal and a cathartic. Do not give mineral oil, and do not use alcohol for lavage. Give supportive measures as outlined on pp 1015–1018. Lower the temperature with aggressive external cooling (tepid sponging and fanning) and ice water lavage.

**B. External Burns:** Wash with olive oil or soap and water (or both). Remove contaminated clothing.

Wood S et al: Pentachlorophenol poisoning. *J Oral Med* 1983;**25**:527.

## PHENOTHIAZINE TRANQUILIZERS
(Chlorpromazine, Promazine, Prochlorperazine, Etc)

Chlorpromazine and related drugs are synthetic chemicals derived in most instances from phenothiazine. They are used as antiemetics and psychic inhibitors and as potentiators of analgesic and hypnotic drugs.

### Clinical Findings
Minimum doses induce drowsiness and mild orthostatic hypotension in as many as 50% of patients. Larger doses cause obtundation, miosis, severe hypotension, tachycardia, stiffness of muscles, convulsions, and coma. Abnormal cardiac conduction may occur, resulting in prolongation of QRS or QT intervals (or both) and ventricular arrhythmias.

With therapeutic doses, some patients develop an acute extrapyramidal reaction similar to Parkinson's disease, with spasmodic contractions of the face and neck muscles, extensor rigidity of the back muscles, carpopedal spasm, and motor restlessness.

### Treatment
Remove overdoses by emesis or gastric lavage. Follow with activated charcoal and cathartic. For severe hypotension, treatment with fluids and pressor agents may be necessary. Control convulsions cautiously with diazepam, 0.1 mg/kg intravenously. Maintain cardiac monitoring. Hypotension and cardiac arrhythmias associated with widened QRS intervals on the ECG may respond to intravenous sodium bicarbonate as used for tricyclic antidepressants.

For extrapyramidal signs, give diphenhydramine, 0.5–4 mg/kg intravenously, or benztropine mesylate, 1–2 mg intramuscularly. Treatment with oral doses of these agents should be continued for 24–48 hours.

## QUINIDINE & QUININE

Manifestations of toxicity are tinnitus, diarrhea, arrhythmias, syncope, respiratory failure, and hypotension. The ECG may show widening of the QRS complex, a lengthened QT and PR interval, and premature ventricular beats. The MLD is 1 g. Associated toxicity due to digitalis may result from increased blood levels owing to concomitant quinidine administration. Repeated or massive ingestion of quinine causes visual loss associated with pallor of optic disks, narrowing of retinal vessels, and papilledema.

### Treatment
Remove ingested drug by gastric lavage followed by activated charcoal and catharsis. Raise blood pressure by administration of intravenous saline or dopamine. Intravenous administration of sodium lactate or sodium bicarbonate solution is said to reduce the cardiotoxic effects of quinidine. Ventricular tachycardia of the "torsade de pointes" variety may be treated with intravenous isoproterenol or overdrive pacing. There is no proved treatment for quinine-induced blindness; it often resolves spontaneously.

Swiryn S, Kim SS: Quinidine-induced syncope. *Arch Intern Med* 1983;**143**:314.

## SALICYLATE POISONING

Salicylate poisoning is most commonly caused by aspirin ingestion. Effects include acid-base disturbances, hypoprothrombinemia, hyperthermia, pulmonary and cerebral edema. Respiratory alkalosis appears first, later accompanied by metabolic acidosis. Severe poisoning after acute single overdose is associated with initial serum salicylate levels above 100 mg/dL (Fig 30–2). With chronic repeated overmedication, toxicity may occur with much lower levels.

Salicylates stimulate the respiratory center, producing hyperpnea, $CO_2$ loss, and respiratory alkalosis. In an effort to compensate, the kidneys excrete increased amounts of bicarbonate, potassium, and sodium. This contributes to development of metabolic acidosis and dehydration. Salicylates also interfere with carbohydrate metabolism, which results in the accumulation of fixed acids and ketones. When first seen, the patient may be alkalotic or acidotic. Diagnosis and treatment depend upon determination of serum $CO_2$, potassium, sodium, and chloride content and arterial pH. Urine pH is an unreliable indicator of acidosis or alkalosis.

The clinical picture may include a history of salicylate ingestion, hyperpnea, hyperthermia, tinnitus, vomiting, dehydration, spontaneous bleeding, convulsions, pulmonary edema, uremia, and coma. Salicylates may cause false-positive tests for ketonuria and glycosuria, or true ketonuria and glycosuria may be present. The Phenistix or ferric chloride test aids in diagnosis of salicylate ingestion. Prothrombin time may be prolonged owing to vitamin K antagonism.

The MLD for acute overdose is 150 mg/kg. However, repeated overmedication with only slightly supratherapeutic doses of salicylate may lead to severe intoxication. This so-called chronic or therapeutic intoxication often goes unrecognized initially and carries high morbidity and mortality rates.

Aspirin administration during certain viral infections (eg, varicella, influenza) is suspected of being a risk factor in the occurrence of Reye's syndrome.

### Treatment

**A. Emergency Measures:** After acute ingestion, empty the stomach by emesis or gastric lavage. Follow with activated charcoal and a cathartic. Salicylate may still be present in the stomach several hours after ingestion, especially if an enteric-coated formulation has been ingested.

**B. General Measures:** Salicylate poisoning can only be treated adequately with knowledge of the blood pH and the serum salicylate, sodium, potassium, and chloride levels. Hydration in the first hour should begin with 10 mL/kg of intravenous fluid prepared as follows: To each liter of 5% dextrose in 0.5-N saline solution, add 50 meq of sodium bicarbonate. After the first hour, modify this solution according to serum sodium and urine pH. Potassium replacement and supplementation will be necessary to achieve alkalinization of the urine in patients who are significantly dehydrated. A urine flow rate of 2–3 mL/kg/h is desirable. *The goal of rehydration is to establish a normal urine output; forced diuresis is not necessary, and overhydration may contribute to cerebral or pulmonary edema.* Maintenance of alkaline urine greatly speeds the excretion of salicylates but is difficult and dangerous to perform in seriously ill patients, especially those with chronic intoxication.

Phytonadione (vitamin K), 0.1 mg/kg intramuscularly, should be given once for hypoprothrombinemia. Reduce fever with tepid water sponge baths and fanning.

Hemodialysis may be lifesaving for critically ill patients with high serum salicylate concentrations, intractable acidosis or electrolyte abnormalities, persistent convulsions, or renal insufficiency.

Prescott LF et al: Diuresis or urinary alkalinisation for salicylate poisoning? *Br Med J* 1982;**285**:1383.

Proudfoot AT: Toxicity of salicylates. *Am J Med* (Nov 14) 1983;(**Suppl**):99.

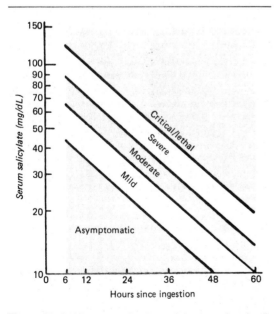

**Figure 30–2.** Nomogram for determining severity of salicylate intoxication. Absorption kinetics assume acute (one-time) ingestion of non–enteric-coated preparation. (Redrawn and reproduced, with permission, from Done AK: Salicylate intoxication: Significance of measurement of salicylate in blood in cases of acute ingestion. *Pediatrics* 1960;**26**:800.)

## SNAKE BITES

The venom of poisonous snakes and lizards may be predominantly neurotoxic (coral snake) or predominantly cytolytic (pit viper). Neurotoxins cause respiratory paralysis; cytolytic venoms cause tissue destruction by digestion and hemorrhage due to hemolysis and destruction of the endothelial lining of the blood vessels. The manifestations of cytolytic envenomation (eg, rattlesnake venom) are local pain, redness, swelling, and extravasation of blood. Perioral tingling, metallic taste, nausea and vomiting, hypotension, and coagulopathy may also occur. Neurotoxic envenomation may cause ptosis, dysphagia, diplopia, and respiratory arrest.

## Treatment

**A. Emergency Measures:** Immobilize the patient and the bitten part in a horizontal position immediately. Avoid manipulation of the bitten area. Transport the patient to a medical facility for definitive treatment. Do *not* give alcoholic beverages or stimulants; do *not* apply ice. The trauma to underlying structures resulting from incision and suction performed by unskilled people is probably not justified in view of the small amount of venom that can be recovered in this way (10% at most). Cryotherapy increases tissue loss.

**B. Specific Antidote and General Measures:**

**1. Pit viper (eg, rattlesnake) envenomation–** With local signs such as swelling, pain, and ecchymosis but no systemic symptoms, give 4–5 vials of polyvalent crotalid antivenin by intravenous drip. (This should be preceded by skin testing for horse serum sensitivity with the kit supplied.) For more serious envenomation with marked local effects and systemic toxicity (eg, hypotension, coagulopathy), 10–20 vials may be required. Epinephrine should be available for immediate use in the event of an allergic reaction. Specific antiserum therapy is more effective if given soon after the bite. Monitor vital signs and the blood coagulation profile. Type and cross-match blood. The adequacy of venom neutralization is indicated by improvement in signs and symptoms, and the rate of swelling slows. Serum sickness reactions are common after antivenin use, usually occur 5–10 days after antivenin administration, and may be treated with prednisone, 45–60 mg daily with tapering doses.

**2. Elapid (coral snake) envenomation–**Give 1–2 vials of specific antivenom as soon as possible.

To locate antisera for exotic snakes, call Poison Information Center, Tucson ([602] 626-6016).

Sivaprasad R, Cantini EM: Western diamondback rattlesnake (*Crotalus atrox*) poisoning. *Postgrad Med* (June) 1982;**71**:223.

## SPIDER BITES & SCORPION STINGS

The toxin of the less venomous species of spiders causes only local pain, redness, and swelling. That of the more venomous black widow spiders (*Latrodectus mactans*), causes generalized muscular pains, muscle spasms and rigidity. The brown recluse spider (*Loxosceles reclusa*) causes progressive local necrosis as well as hemolytic reactions (rare). Stings by most scorpions cause only local pain. Stings by the more toxic *Centruroides* species (found in the Southwestern USA) may cause muscle cramps, twitching and jerking, and occasionally convulsions.

## Treatment

**A. Black Widow Spider Bites:** Pain may be relieved with parenteral narcotics or muscle relaxants (eg, methocarbamol, 15 mg/kg). Calcium gluconate 10%, 0.1–0.2 mL/kg intravenously, may relieve muscle rigidity. Antivenin is rarely indicated, usually only for very young or elderly patients who do not respond to the above measures. Horse serum sensitivity testing is required.

**B. Brown Recluse Spider Bites:** Because bites occasionally progress to extensive local necrosis, some authorities recommend early excision of the bite site, whereas others use oral corticosteroids. Recently, interest has focused on the use of dapsone and colchicine and an antivenin is being developed. All of these treatments remain of unproved value.

**C. Scorpion Stings:** No specific treatment is available. For *Centruroides* stings, some toxicologists use a specific antivenom, but this is neither FDA-approved nor widely available.

## STRYCHNINE

Strychnine poisoning may result from ingestion or injection. The manifestations are tetanic muscle rigidity, opisthotonos, and respiratory muscle rigidity resulting in asphyxia. Although victims appear to be convulsing, they are usually awake.

## Treatment

**A. Emergency Measures:** Control tetanic rigidity or convulsions with neuromuscular paralysis using succinylcholine or pancuronium (the patient must be endotracheally intubated and will require mechanical ventilation). In less severe cases, give diazepam, 0.05–0.2 mg/kg (maximum 10 mg) slowly intravenously, and repeat as needed at 30-minute to 4-hour intervals. Perform gastric lavage, and then administer activated charcoal and a cathartic. Do not induce emesis, and do not lavage after twitching or convulsions have appeared unless succinylcholine or another neuromuscular blocker is being given. Severe metabolic acidosis, rhabdomyolysis, and myoglobinuria may occur. The urine should be alkalinized to prevent renal myoglobin deposition.

**B. General Measures:** Keep the patient quiet in a darkened room; avoid sudden stimuli.

Bloyd RE et al: Strychnine poisoning: Recovery from profound lactic acidosis, hyperthermia, and rhabdomyolysis. *Am J Med* 1983;**74**:507.

## THEOPHYLLINE, CAFFEINE

Overdoses occur most commonly from the therapeutic use of caffeine as a stimulant in newborns or theophylline (aminophylline, oxytriphylline) to improve respiration in older patients. Toxic levels may occur in patients receiving therapeutic theophylline levels if metabolic degradation of the drug is inhibited (ie, due to heart failure, liver disease, or concomitant use of erythromycin or cimetidine). Manifestations of intoxication include tachypnea, tremor, arrhythmias, and convulsions. Serious toxicity may occur with serum levels only moderately above the therapeutic range.

Acute single overdosage presents with similar toxicity and typically causes hypotension and hypokalemia as well. Seizures, arrhythmias, and death are likely only when plasma theophylline levels exceed 100 mg/L after acute single overdosage. Convulsions are often difficult to control with diazepam and phenytoin, and their persistence is an indication for hemoperfusion.

### Treatment

Remove ingested drug by emesis or lavage, and give activated charcoal and a cathartic. Repeated doses of charcoal may contribute to whole body elimination and can shorten the half-life. Control convulsions with diazepam, 0.1–0.2 mg/kg slowly intravenously, or phenytoin, 0.5 mg/kg/min intravenously to a total of 15 mg/kg. Tachycardia and hypotension may respond to propranolol, 0.03–0.06 mg/kg intravenously; however, propranolol is contraindicated in patients with asthma and COPD, who represent the majority of individuals receiving theophylline. Hemoperfusion is extremely effective and should be used if severe toxicity is present (level > 90–100 mg/L after acute ingestion, > 40–60 mg/L with chronic intoxication).

Olson KR et al: Theophylline overdose: Acute single ingestion vs. chronic repeated overmedication. *Am J Emerg Med* 1985;**3**:386.

Woo OF et al: Benefit of hemoperfusion in acute theophylline intoxication. *J Toxicol Clin Toxicol* 1984;**22**:411.

## TRICYCLIC ANTIDEPRESSANTS

Overdosage with the tricyclic antidepressants and newer tetracyclic analogues has profound effects on the heart and brain. Typical anticholinergic signs are common and consist of delirium, dilated pupils, and tachycardia. In addition, quinidinelike cardiotoxic effects result in hypotension and widening of the QRS and QT intervals on the ECG (exception: amoxapine) (Fig 30–3). Central effects of the antidepressants also include coma and seizures. The onset of seizures may be rapid and unexpected but is usually heralded by evidence of QRS widening.

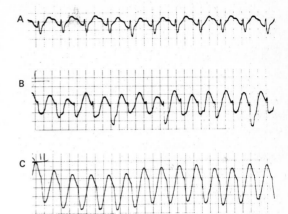

**Figure 30–3.** Cardiac arrhythmias resulting from tricyclic antidepressant overdose. *A:* Delayed intraventricular conduction results in prolonged QRS interval (0.18s). *B* and *C:* Supraventricular tachycardia with progressive widening of QRS complexes mimics ventricular tachycardia. (Reproduced, with permission, from Benowitz NL, Goldschlager N: Cardiac disturbances in the toxicologic patient. Page 71 in: *Clinical Management of Poisoning and Drug Overdose.* Haddad LM, Winchester JF [editors]. Saunders, 1983.)

### Treatment

Do not induce emesis, because of the danger of sudden deterioration. Perform gastric lavage and administer activated charcoal and a cathartic. Monitor the ECG continuously for at least 6–8 hours, and admit any patient with a QRS interval wider than 0.12 s or other evidence of toxicity. *Note:* Patients with amoxapine intoxication may have a normal ECG.

Seizures should be treated with standard anticonvulsants such as diazepam (0.1 mg/kg intravenously), phenytoin (15 mg/kg intravenously, no faster than 0.5 mg/kg/min), or phenobarbital (15 mg/kg intravenously). Neuromuscular paralysis may be needed to control muscular hyperactivity associated with hyperthermia or intractable acidosis.

Sodium bicarbonate (50-meq boluses) may reverse QRS widening, arrhythmias, and hypotension. Intubation and assisted ventilation should be used if there is airway compromise or respiratory acidosis.

Hypotension not responding to bicarbonate and ventilation may be treated with intravenous fluids (normal saline, up to 1–2 L) and, if needed, dopamine.

There is no role for physostigmine in antidepressant overdose. It may cause asystole and can aggravate seizures.

Boehnert MT, Lovejoy FH: Value of the QRS duration versus the serum drug level in predicting seizures and ventricular arrhythmias after an acute overdose of tricyclic antidepressants. *N Engl J Med* 1985;**313**:474.

Pentel PR, Benowitz NL: Tricyclic antidepressant poisoning: Management of arrhythmias. *J Med Toxicol* 1986;**1**:101.

• • •

## AIR POLLUTION & SMOKING

There is considerable evidence that the present levels of atmospheric contaminants that exist in many larger urban areas are sufficient to cause discomfort or significantly impair health. Toxicologic and epidemiologic studies suggest that the noxious nature of the atmosphere is usually due to a complex mixture of pollutants and to meteorologic factors.

Air pollutants are usually divided into 2 broad classes: (1) particulates (smoke, dust, ash, mists, and fumes that exist in the atmosphere in either a solid or liquid state) and (2) gases (eg, carbon monoxide, sulfur oxides, hydrogen sulfide, nitrogen oxides, and carbon compounds—particularly those reacting in the atmosphere to form photochemical smog).

The irritating effects of air pollution on the eye and upper respiratory tract are well known. Inhalation of irritant materials may interfere with lung function, aggravating chronic bronchitis, chronic constrictive ventilatory disease, pulmonary emphysema, and bronchial asthma. The particulate fraction contains a number of carcinogenic substances, and these could play a part in the rapidly changing incidence of different cancers.

The ill effects of atmospheric pollution are most obvious during acute episodes of unusually high pollution. Marked increases in the incidence of illnesses and deaths due to cardiorespiratory damage were reported in the Meuse Valley in Belgium in 1930; in Donora, Pennsylvania, in 1948; and in London in 1952 and 1962.

## ENVIRONMENTAL HAZARDS

A number of substances used in industry or as pesticides are under investigation for long-term low-concentration toxicity or carcinogenicity. Some of these agents are stable and persist as contaminants for months to years after use. A list of some of these substances and their suspected effects follows.

Asbestos—Pulmonary effects and mesotheliomas.

Chloroform—Liver cancer.

Chloromethyl methyl ether—Lung cancer.

4,4'-Diaminodiphenyl methane—Toxic hepatitis.

Formaldehyde—Respiratory damage, cancer.

n-Hexane—Neuropathy.

Kepone—Neurologic effects.

Methyl butyl ketone (MBK)—Neuropathy.

Mirex—Liver cancer.

Polybrominated biphenyl (PBB)—Birth defects, liver cancer.

Polychlorinated biphenyl (PCB)—Birth defects, liver cancer, melanoma.

Tetrachlorodibenzodioxin (TCDD, dioxin)—Birth defects, chloracne.

Vinyl chloride—Angiosarcoma of the liver.

Calesnick B: Dioxin and agent orange. *Am Fam Physician* (Feb) 1984;**29**:303.

Couri D, Milk M: Toxicity and metabolism of the neurotoxic hexacarbons, n-hexane 2-hexanone, 2,5-hexane dione. *Annu Rev Pharmacol Toxicol* 1982;**22**:145.

Jacobson JL et al: The transfer of polychlorinated biphenyls (PCBs) and polybrominated biphenyls (PBBs) across the human placenta and into maternal milk. *Am J Public Health* 1984;**74**:378.

Langauer-Lewowicka H et al: Vinyl chloride disease: Neurological disturbances. *Int Arch Occup Environ Health* 1983;**52**:151.

McCallum RI et al: Lung cancer associated with chloromethyl methyl ether manufacture: An investigation at two factories in the United Kingdom. *Br J Ind Med* 1983;**40**:384.

Schwartz EM, Rae WA: Effect of polybrominated biphenyls (PBB) on developmental abilities in young children. *Am J Public Health* 1983;**73**:277.

## REFERENCES

Adverse Reactions. A monthly report of adverse reactions to drugs and therapeutic devices by the Adverse Reactions Branch, Food and Drug Administration, US Department of Health and Human Services, Washington DC.

Adverse Reactions Titles. Excerpta Medica (monthly bibliography).

Baselt RC: *Disposition of Toxic Drugs and Chemicals in Man.* Biomedical Publications, 1982.

Clin-Alert. A weekly to fortnightly serial publication of all adverse drug reactions reported in the international medical literature. Science Editors, Inc., Louisville, Kentucky.

*Dangerous Properties of Industrial Materials Report.* Van Nostrand Reinhold. Bimonthly serial.

Dreisbach RH, Robertson WO: *Handbook of Poisoning: Prevention, Diagnosis & Treatment,* 12th ed. Appleton-Lange, 1987.

Dukes MNG (editor): *Meyler's Side Effects of Drugs,* 9th ed. Excerpta Medica, 1980.

FDA Drug Bulletin. Food and Drug Administration (monthly). US Department of Health and Human Services, Washington, DC.

Gilman AG et al (editors): *Goodman and Gilman's The Pharmacological Basis of Therapeutics,* 7th ed. Macmillan, 1985.

Goldfrank LR: *Toxicologic Emergencies,* 3rd ed. Appleton-Century-Crofts, 1986.

Gosselin RE et al (editors): *Clinical Toxicology of Commercial Products,* 5th ed. Williams & Wilkins, 1985.

Katzung BG (editor): *Basic & Clinical Pharmacology,* 3rd ed. Lange, 1987.

National Institute of Occupational Safety and Health: *Registry of Toxic Effects of Chemical Substances.* US Government Printing Office. (Annual publication.)

Rom WN: *Environmental and Occupational Medicine.* Little, Brown, 1983.

Sittig M: *Handbook of Toxic and Hazardous Chemicals.* Noyes, 1981.

# Medical Genetics

31

*Margaret S. Kosek, MD*

The rapid advance of the science of genetics in recent years has so many applications to clinical medicine that a knowledge of basic genetic principles is now a necessity for diagnostic purposes. Many cases of mental retardation, infertility, dwarfism, habitual abortion, and multiple congenital anomalies are associated with specific chromosomal defects. Cells of certain tumors have an abnormal chromosomal composition, in some instances a specific one. Many of the metabolic disorders are hereditary; and even in the case of some drug reactions, the problem lies not only with the drug but also with the patient, who has inherited an enzymatic defect that prevents normal detoxification. Future genetic investigation promises to increase our understanding of the causes and the mechanisms of individual responses to disease.

## INTRODUCTION TO MEDICAL GENETICS

Inherited characteristics are carried from generation to generation by the **chromosome,** a complex nucleic acid structure in the nucleus of the cell. Humans normally have 46 chromosomes, which are arranged in 23 pairs. One of these pairs determines the sex of the individual; these are the **sex chromosomes,** X and Y. Females have the pair XX and males the pair XY. The remaining 22 pairs are called **autosomes** (not sex determiners). Pairs of autosomes are **homologous,** ie, each member of a pair has the same configuration and constituent genetic loci as the other. The sex chromosomes, on the other hand, are **heterologous,** ie, the X chromosome differs in both size and total function from the Y chromosome.

Both the X and Y chromosomes have a genetic as well as sex-determining aspect, but the genetic information is more extensive on the X chromosome. The very small amount of genetic information on the Y chromosome has only recently been discovered.

### GENES

Chromosomes are composed of thousands of **genes,** which are the basic units of heredity. The gene is the information area for the transmission of an inherited trait. The genes are arranged in a linear fashion on the chromosomes. The exact location of a gene on a chromosome is its **locus.** Each chromosome has thousands of loci arranged in a definite manner, and the number and arrangement of genes on homologous chromosomes are identical. Genes that occupy homologous loci are **alleles,** or partner genes. Each individual, therefore, has 2 of each kind of gene, one on each chromosome of a pair of chromosomes.

Although genes usually remain stable from generation to generation, it is possible for them to undergo a change, or **mutation,** and thereby to transmit a new or altered trait to future generations. Mutation may occur spontaneously or may be induced by such environmental factors as radiation, medication, or viral infections. Both advanced maternal and paternal age favor mutation. In women, trisomy 21 is the classic example. In men over 30, fresh gene mutation accounts for sporadic cases of achondroplasia, hemophilia A, and Marfan's syndrome.

The human genome is estimated to contain 50,000–100,000 genes. Approximately 3400 genes are known. Combined information from family linkage studies, somatic cell hybridization, and gene dosage studies now permits human gene mapping, with 700 genes assigned to specific parts of specific chromosomes. Mapping has been of use in disease diagnosis, identification of heterozygotes, and prenatal diagnosis. Linkage studies can already reveal in utero mendelian disorders that are not biochemically identifiable. Another application is understanding gene interaction and regulation within the cell, for in human development it is important to understand the control mechanism that turns genes on and off.

McKusick VA: The morbid anatomy of the human genome. *Medicine* 1986;**65:**1.

## THE CHEMICAL BASIS OF HEREDITY (THE GENETIC CODE) (Fig 31–1)

Each chromosome contains only one DNA molecule, so that the typical human cell nucleus has 46 molecules of DNA. DNA has 2 functions. First, it is able to synthesize, or **replicate,** itself, thereby ensuring the integrity of hereditary transmission to future generations. Second, the sequential order of

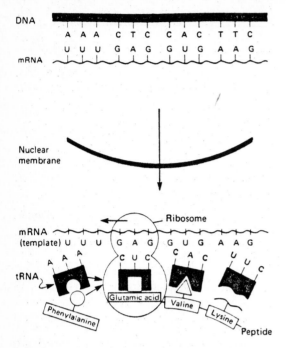

**Figure 31–1.** Diagrammatic representation of the way in which genetic information is translated into protein synthesis. (Reproduced, with permission, from Emery AEH: *Elements of Medical Genetics,* 6th ed. Churchill Livingstone, 1983.)

the bases (cytosine, guanine, adenine, thymine) of DNA acts as the **genetic code** that determines the development and metabolism of cells. DNA accomplishes this by directing the synthesis of its alter ego, messenger RNA (mRNA), which carries the genetic message out of the nucleus to the cytoplasm, where it becomes associated with the ribosomes that are the site of protein synthesis. Here the messenger RNA forms the template for sequencing particular amino acids. With the help of another RNA, transfer RNA (tRNA), the amino acids are incorporated into a polypeptide chain and then synthesized into specific proteins and enzymes.

## MODES OF INHERITANCE
## (Table 31–1)

### 1. MENDELIAN INHERITANCE

The essential definitions of modes of inheritance can be illustrated by studying the inheritance of a **single** characteristic carried by only **one** gene and not influenced by environmental factors.

Syndactyly (webbed fingers or toes) is a clinical example of this. Fig 31–2 illustrates a family tree with the abnormality. The gene for syndactyly is represented as **D** and the gene for normal interdigital spaces as **d.**

Each parent is represented by 2 genes, one of which came from the mother and the other from the father. Their genetic constitution has arbitrarily been designated Dd. The male parent (Dd) will produce sperms that are either D or d. The female parent will produce ova that are either D or d. The possible offspring are DD, Dd, or dd.

If we examine the parents and offspring for the presence of syndactyly, we find it in both parents (Dd and Dd) and 3 (DD, Dd, Dd) of the 4 offspring. Since these people have the same physical characteristic, ie, syndactyly, they are said to have the same **phenotype.** Their genetic composition, or **genotype,** is different, for it may be either Dd or DD. The genotype, therefore, may be the same as the phenotype, but it does not have to be. Since syndactyly is present if D is present, whether as one gene of a pair of genes (Dd) or as both genes (DD), it is a **dominant** trait. Normal digital spaces (d) are present only if d is on both genes (dd); thus, d is a **recessive** trait. If an individual's genetic constitution for interdigital spaces contains similar genes (DD, dd), the person is **homozygous** for that trait; if it contains dissimilar genes (Dd), the person is **heterozygous** for the trait.

Besides dominant and recessive inheritance, an intermediate, or **codominant, inheritance** may also occur. With codominance, both characteristics are expressed in the heterozygote. Hemoglobin S disease is an example of this. The S homozygote (SS) has sickle cell anemia; the S heterozygote (AS) has sickle cell trait, with both hemoglobin A and hemoglobin S, and the person without S (AA) has normal adult hemoglobin.

Inheritance is either **autosomal** or **X-linked (sex-linked)** depending on the chromosomal location of the gene. In investigating family trees for genetic disease, certain inheritance patterns with distinct features become evident. **Autosomal dominant inheritance** (Fig 31–2) has 3 criteria: (1) every affected person has an affected parent; (2) every affected person who marries a normal person has a 1:2 chance of having *each* offspring affected; and (3) every normal child of an affected person will have normal offspring. With **autosomal recessive inheritance,** the following characteristics are present: The vast majority of affected persons have parents who are normal in all outward appearances. In affected families, each child has a 1:4 chance of having a genetic defect. The offspring of an affected person and a normal person will be normal in most cases. If their offspring are affected, the "normal" parent is a heterozygote. When 2 affected persons marry, all their children will be affected. Lastly, the rarer the defect, the more likely it is that there is consanguinity in the family tree.

With **X-linked recessive inheritance,** there are 2 main characteristics: the defect is carried by females and exhibited by their sons, and affected males can pass the disease only through their daughters. Hemophilia A is an important clinical example of this.

**Table 31–1.** Some diseases with known modes of inheritance.*†

**Central nervous system**
Diffuse cerebral sclerosis (Pelizaeus-Merzbacher type): XD?, XR?
Diffuse cerebral sclerosis (Sholz type): XD?, XR?
Retinoblastoma: AD

**Digestive system**
Cystic fibrosis of the pancreas: AR
Hyperbilirubinemia
Congenital nonhemolytic jaundice with kernicterus (Crigler-Najjar): AR
Familial nonhemolytic jaundice (Gilbert's disease): AD
Chronic idiopathic jaundice (Dubin-Johnson): Probably AD
Chronic familial nonhemolytic jaundice (Rotor's syndrome): AD

**Genitourinary system**
Cystinosis: AR
Cystinuria: AR
Fanconi's syndrome (infantile and adult): AR
Nephrogenic diabetes insipidus: XR
Renal glycosuria: AD
Vitamin D-resistant rickets: XD

**Skin**
Albinism: AR
Anhidrotic ectodermal dysplasia: AR?
Xeroderma pigmentosum: AR

**Hematologic system**
Cell disorders
Congenital nonspherocytic hemolytic anemia (pyruvate kinase deficiency): AR
Sickle cell disease (homozygous hemoglobin S): AD
Sickle cell trait (heterozygous hemoglobin S): AD
Spherocytosis: AD
Thalassemia major (homozygous): AD
Thalassemia minor (heterozygous): AD
Plasma disorders
Congenital agammaglobulinemia: XR
Congenital afibrinogenemia: AR
Hemophilia A (factor VIII deficiency): XR
Hemophilia B (factor IX deficiency): XR
Hemophilia C (factor XI deficiency): AD
Deficiency of factor XII: AR
Deficiency of factor V: AR
Deficiency of factor VII: AR
Deficiency of factor X: AR
Von Willebrand's disease (deficiencies of factor VIII procoagulant [VIII:C], factor VIII-related antigen [VIIIR:Ag], and factor VIII-related ristocetin cofactor [VIIIR:WF or VIIIR:Rcf]: AD

**Musculoskeletal system**
Severe generalized familial muscular dystrophy (Duchenne's pseudohypertrophic muscular dystrophy): XR
Muscular dystrophy (facioscapulohumeral syndrome of Landouzy-Déjérine): AD
Progressive dystrophia ophthalmoplegica: AD
Myotonia atrophica: AD
Progressive muscular dystrophy (tardive type of Becker): XR
Charcot-Marie-Tooth peroneal muscular atrophy: AD, AR
Pseudohypoparathyroidism: XR
Periodic paralysis
Hyperkalemic: AD
Hypokalemic: AD
Normokalemic: AD

**Endocrine system**
Pituitary
Pituitary diabetes insipidus: AD
Thyroid
Familial cretinism with goiter—
Iodide trapping defect: AR
Iodide organification defect: AR?, AD?
Iodotyrosyl coupling defect: AR?
Deiodinase defect: AR
Abnormal serum iodoprotein: AR
Adrenal
Congenital virilizing adrenal hyperplasia: AR

**Metabolic disorders**
Carbohydrate:
Diabetes mellitus: AR
Galactosemia: AR
Glycogen storage disease (types I, II, III, IV, V, VI) (Von Gierke's disease): AR
Gargoylism (lipochondrodystrophy) (Hurler's disease): AR, XR
Hyperoxaluria: AR
Hereditary lactose intolerance: AR
Mucopolysaccharidoses—
Type I—Hurler's disease: AR
Type II—Hunter's disease: XR
Type III—Sanfilippo syndrome (heparitinuria): AR
Type IV—Morquio's disease: AR
Type V—Scheie's syndrome: AR
Type VI—Maroteaux-Lamy syndrome: AR
Fat:
The primary hyperlipidemias—
Type I—Familial hyperchylomicronemia (lipoprotein lipase deficiency): AR
Type II—Familial hyperbetalipoproteinemia (essential familial hypercholesterolemia): AD
Type III—hyperlipidemia (broad beta disease): AD
Familial combined hyperlipidemia (multiple lipoprotein type): AD
Familial hypertriglyceridemia: AD
Familial high-density lipoprotein disease (Tangier disease): AR
Gaucher's disease (cerebroside lipidosis): AR
Niemann-Pick disease (sphingomyelin lipidosis): AR
Tay-Sachs disease (infantile amaurotic idiocy): AR
Protein:
Amino acids—
Homocystinuria: AR
Phenylketonuria: AR
Porphyrias—
Congenital erythropoietic porphyria: AR
Erythropoietic porphyria: AR
Acute intermittent porphyria: AD
Porphyria cutanea tarda hereditaria: AD
Other—
Deficiency of pseudocholinesterase: AR
Deficiency of glucose-6-phosphate dehydrogenase: XD
Alkaptonuria: AR
Hyperuricemia: AD
Hereditary orotic aciduria: AR
Minerals:
Hepatolenticular degeneration (Wilson's disease): AR
Hemochromatosis: AD, AR

* AD = autosomal dominant; AR = autosomal recessive; XD = X-linked (sex-linked) dominant; XR = X-linked (sex-linked) recessive
† Reference: McKusick VA: *Mendelian Inheritance in Man: Catalogs of Autosomal Dominant, Autosomal Recessive and X-Linked Phenotypes.* Johns Hopkins Univ Press, 1986.

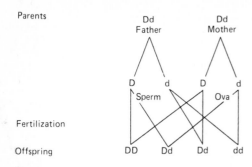

**Figure 31–2.** Mode of inheritance of syndactyly.

The gene for hemophilia A is carried on the X chromosome, and there is no homologous locus on the Y chromosome. Females, who have two X chromosomes, must have the gene for hemophilia present on both X chromosomes to have this recessive disease. Since the incidence of this gene in the population is low, the chance of 2 affected X chromosomes occurring together, although possible, is highly unlikely. Therefore, hemophilia is very rare in females. Because males have an XY chromosome composition, the hemophilia gene will be clinically expressed if it is present on the single X chromosome. Since the Y chromosome must come from the father, the affected X chromosome is from the mother, thereby giving the "mother-to-son" inheritance pattern. In the case of **X-linked dominant inheritance,** no fully dominant X-linked gene has been discovered in humans.

Genes do not always have an "all or none" action. A certain number of offspring may fail to show expression of a gene even though it may be a dominant gene or a homozygous recessive one. **Penetrance** is the statistical term that refers to the frequency with which a gene or genotype is morphologically manifest in the offspring. A comparable term, **expressivity,** refers to the degree of phenotypic expression of a trait (ie, forme fruste [incomplete expression] versus full expression). These variables make genetic analysis far more difficult.

Genetic disorders that are carried by a single gene have been most completely studied. They frequently have a characteristic somatic or biochemical defect that can be readily traced in many generations. Of the 3 distinct patterns of inheritance, there are 800 known dominant conditions, 550 known recessive conditions, and 100 known sex-linked conditions. On the whole, these genetic disorders of mendelian inheritance are rare. Perhaps 1% of all liveborn children will be affected with an autosomal disorder at some time in their lives. It is much more difficult to determine the mode of inheritance of the common diseases of possible genetic background (eg, arteriosclerosis), because the disease may be the result not only of genetic constitution but also of environmental factors (eg, diet).

## 2. POLYGENIC OR MULTIFACTORIAL INHERITANCE

There are a group of diseases with obvious genetic transmission but no chromosomal aberration and no clearcut mendelian inheritance pattern. They are characterized by familial clustering, varying frequencies in different racial or ethnic groups, and a greater frequency in monozygotic than in dizygotic twins. The inheritance pattern is said to be multifactorial or polygenic, and clinical disease is believed to be determined by the combined effect of environmental and genetic factors.

Recurrence risks are based on empiric data from the literature. Certain factors are known to increase the risk:

(1) A close relationship to the proband (patient). First-degree relatives have a higher rate of recurrence than second-degree relatives, etc.

(2) Occurrence in 2 or more members of a family.

(3) Severe disease in the proband.

(4) Disease in the proband of the rarely affected sex—eg, pyloric stenosis in a female.

(5) Disease with a strong genetic component—eg, gout.

When statistical data are not available for use in calculating the chances that future offspring will have the disease identified in the proband, a useful rough measure is that the maximum risk of occurrence of the disease in a first-degree relative is the square root of the incidence of the disease.

## CYTOGENETICS

Cytogenetics is the study of the chromosomal structure of cells. Because of the constancy of chromosomal number and morphology, classification of chromosomes is possible. The basic characteristics of chromosomes are (1) total length, (2) position of the centromere, (3) the length of the arms, (4) the presence or absence of satellites, and (5) the banding pattern (see below).

The 2 halves of the chromosome are called **chromatids.** A palely staining crossover point or primary constriction called the **centromere** (centrosome) divides the chromosome into 2 arm lengths. On some chromosomes there is a secondary constriction; the chromosomal material distal to this constriction is called a **satellite.**

In the Denver classification, chromosomes are arranged in 7 groups according to descending total length: group A (chromosomes 1–3); group B (chromosomes 4, 5); group C (chromosomes 6–12); group D (chromosomes 13–15); group E (chromosomes 16–18); group F (chromosomes 19, 20); and group G (chromosomes 21, 22). The X chromosome is in group C and the Y chromosome in group G. Staining techniques—quinacrine (Q), Giemsa (G), terminal (T), constitutive heterochromatin (C), and reverse (R)—disclose banded regions on each chromosome that are unique and allow absolute identification of the chromosome. These banding patterns vary with the stain and produce complementary rather than redundant information.

The chromosomal analysis is recorded by a uniform system of notation. First, there is the total chromosome count, followed by the sex chromosomes, and then any abnormalities thereafter. The autosomes are all designated by their numbers (1–22), and if the autosomes cannot be identified, the involved chromosome group is identified by its letter (A–G). A plus (+) or minus (−) sign indicates, respectively, a gain or loss of chromosomal material. The letter *p* represents the short arm of the chromosome, and the letter *q* represents the long arm. Other common symbols are *i* for isochromosome; *r* for ring chromosome; *s* for satellite; *ins* for insertion; *inv* for inversion; *mar* for marker; *del* for deletion; [:] for chromosomal break; [::] for chromosomal break and join; and *end* for endoreduplication. Translocations of material from one chromosome to another are identified by *t* followed by the numbers of the involved chromosomes in parentheses; the chromosome bands in which the breaks occur are identified in a second set of parentheses. ***Examples:*** The normal male is 46,XY; a girl with Down's syndrome is 47,XX,21+; a boy with cri du chat syndrome is 46,XY,5p–. A patient with chronic myelogenous leukemia is t(9;22)(q34;q11).

A modification of the Paris Conference nomenclature allows classification of the 850 bands now identified by prometaphase studies. The short arm (p) and the long arm (q) of each chromosome are divided into regions, bands, and subbands each of which is numbered from the centromere outward. A decimal point is placed between the band and subband designations. For example, 5p31.2 is chromosome 5, short arm, region 3, band 1, subband 2.

Harnden DG, Klinger HP (editors): An international system for human cytogenetic nomenclature (1985) ICSN 1985. *Birth Defects* 1985;**21**:1.

## Normal Methods of Cellular Division

Cells divide in one of 2 ways: by **mitosis** or by **meiosis.** In mitosis, a mother cell divides longitudinally to produce 2 daughter cells of exactly the same chromosomal number and composition as the mother cell. This type of cellular division is purely multiplicative (1 cell → 2 cells → 4 cells → 8 cells, etc). Meiosis occurs in the ovary or testis and involves 2 separate steps. The first step is **reduction-division,** in which the germ cell with a **diploid (2n)** number of chromosomes (46) produces 2 cells with a **haploid (n)** number of chromosomes (23). During this step, chromosomal material is exchanged between homologous chromosomes, thereby accounting for the random distribution of maternal and paternal genes. Crossovers do not normally occur between the X and Y chromosomes or between nonhomologous chromosomes. The second step is **equational division,** in which 4 daughter cells with a haploid number of chromosomes are formed by longitudinal division of the chromosomes produced in the first step of meiotic division. In the male, the 4 haploid cells are sperms. In the female, one of the 4 haploid cells is large and matures to eventually form an ovum; the other 3 haploid cells are small cells called **polar bodies,** and they undergo spontaneous degeneration.

## TYPES OF CHROMOSOMAL ABNORMALITIES

Chromosomal abnormalities can be those of number, structure, or a combination of both. They affect the autosomes as well as the sex chromosomes. Often they are associated with such factors as advanced parental age, radiation exposure, certain viral infections, and membership in a family with multiple cytogenetic defects. Once produced, these abnormalities are capable of perpetuating themselves.

These major structural changes may occur in a **balanced** or an **unbalanced** form. In the latter, there is a gain or loss of genetic material. In the former, there is no change in the amount of genetic material but only a rearrangement of it. It is possible, though not proved, that at the sites of breaks and new attachments of chromosome fragments there has been permanent structural or functional damage to a single gene.

### Abnormalities of Morphology

**A. Nondisjunction:** Nondisjunction is failure of a chromatid pair to separate in a dividing cell. If it occurs in either the first or second divisions of meiosis, this results in gametes with abnormal chromosomal patterns. If it occurs in mitosis, **mosaic** patterns occur, ie, one area of an organism will have one genetic pattern and another area of the same organism another genetic pattern.

In medical practice, patients with a mosaic genetic constitution present an incomplete and variable clinical picture with features of each of the genetic syndromes represented in the mosaic.

**B. Translocation:** (See Fig 31–3.) In simple translocation, there is an exchange of chromosomal material between 2 nonhomologous chromosomes.

**C. Deletion:** In deletion, there is a loss of chromosomal material owing to breakage of a chromatid during cell division.

**D. Duplication:** A chromosome segment is present more than once in a set of chromosomes. The repetition may occur in the same chromosome or in a nonhomologous chromosome.

**E. Occurrence of Isochromosomes:** An isochromosome is a chromosome in which the arms on either side of the centromere have the same genetic material in the same order, ie, the chromosome has at some time divided in such a way that it has a

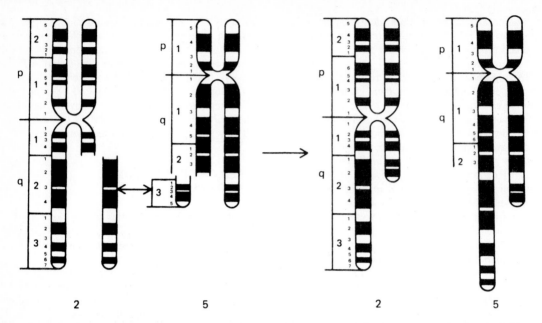

**Figure 31–3.** Reciprocal translocations. 46,XY,t(2;5)(q21;31). Breakage and union have occurred at bands 2q21 and 5q31 in the long arms of chromosomes 2 and 5, respectively. The segments distal to these bands have been exchanged between the 2 chromosomes. Note that the derivative chromosome with the lowest number (ie, No. 2) is designated first. (Reproduced, with permission, from Stanbury JE, Wyngaarden JB, Fredrickson DS [editors]: *The Metabolic Basis of Inherited Disease,* 4th ed. McGraw-Hill, 1978.)

double dose of the long arms and no short arms, or vice versa.

**F. Inversion:** Inversion occurs if, after fracture of a chromatid, the fragment reattaches itself to the same chromosome but in an upside down manner. The same genetic material is present but is distributed in a different order.

## Abnormalities of Chromosomal Number (Aneuploidy) (Table 31–2)

In aneuploidy, more or fewer than 46 chromosomes are present. A cell with more than 46 chromosomes is hyperdiploid, and one with fewer than 46 chromosomes is hypodiploid. If there is a balanced gain or loss of chromosomes or structural rearrangements, the cell is pseudodiploid. The following are all forms of aneuploidy:

**A. Monosomy:** (Chromosomal number is 45.) In monosomy, only one member of a pair of chromosomes is present. *Examples:* Stillborns, monosomy 21–22.

**B. Trisomy:** (Chromosomal number is 47.) Trisomy is caused by nondisjunction of a chromosome pair during the first meiotic division, with the result that 3 chromosomes are present instead of the usual 2. *Examples:* Trisomy 13; 18; 21.

**C. Polysomy:** (Chromosomal number is 48 or more.) Polysomy occurs when one chromosome is represented 4 or more times. *Example:* XXXXY.

**D. Complex Aneuploidy:** In complex aneu-

ploidy, 2 or more chromosomes have an abnormal variation in number; the structure of these chromosomes is normal. *Example:* Trisomy 21 and XXX in the same patient.

## METHODS OF STUDY OF CHROMOSOMAL ABNORMALITIES

Several laboratory tests are available for the study of patients with known or suspected chromosomal aberrations: (1) the study of cells for the presence of sex chromatin bodies in their nuclei; (2) chromosomal analysis; and (3) DNA analysis by gene-specific probes or linkage mapping. The first test is easily obtainable and relatively inexpensive and is used for screening. The chromosomal and DNA analyses are reliable but expensive tests performed by highly trained personnel, usually at medical centers.

### Sex Chromatin Analysis

**A. The X Chromosome:** The sex chromatin (Barr) body is a solid, well-defined planoconvex mass, approximately 1 $\mu$m in diameter, that is near or at the inner surface of the cell membrane in all tissues of the body. It is present during the interphase and is visible by light microscopy. It represents a single inactive condensed X chromosome. The number of Barr bodies in a cell is one less than the number of X chromosomes. Desquamated buccal, vaginal, and amniotic cells are usually studied. Females have an incidence of 40–60% and are chromatin-positive.

**Table 31–2.** Numerical abnormalities of sex chromosomes.*†

| Pheno-type | Sex Chromatin | Sex Chromosome | Chromosome Number | Incidence in Newborns | Clinical Picture |
|---|---|---|---|---|---|
| Female | Positive | XX | 46 | | Normal female. |
| Female | Few smaller than normal Barr bodies (7%) | Xx (partial deletion) | 46 | 0.05–0.15/1000 | Streak gonads. No secondary sex characteristics. Amenorrheic. |
| Female | Negative | XO | 45 | 0.1–0.3/1000 | Turner's syndrome. |
| Female | Positive for 2 Barr bodies | XXX | 47 | 0.7/1000 | Usually normal appearing female with mental retardation. Occasional menstrual distrubances and absence of secondary sex characteristics. |
| Female | Positive for 3 Barr bodies | XXXX | 48 | Rare | Normal female with mental retardation. |
| Female | Positive for 4 Barr bodies | XXXXX | 49 | Rare | Mental retardation with mongoloid facies and simian palmar crease. Skeletal defects similar to those of 49, XXXXY. |
| Her-maph-rodite | Positive | XX | 46 | Rare | Variable phenotype. Both testicular and ovarian tissue in gonads. |
| Male | Negative | XY | 46 | | Normal male. |
| Male | Positive for 1 Barr body | XXY | 47 | 1/1000 | Klinefelter's syndrome. |
| Male | Negative | XYY | 47 | 1/1000 | Undescended testes, ± mental retardation, irregularity of teeth. Tall (>6 feet). Radioulnar synostosis. |
| Male | Negative | XYYY | 48 | Rare | Mild psychomotor retardation, inguinal hernia, undescended testes, pulmonary stenosis, simian lines, dental dysplasia. |
| Male | Positive for 1 Barr body | XXYY | 48 | 1/25,000 | Klinefelter's syndrome. |
| Male | Positive for 2 Barr bodies | XXXY | 48 | Rare | Klinefelter's syndrome with more mental retardation and testicular atrophy. |
| Male | Positive for 3 Barr bodies | XXXXY | 49 | Rare | Mental retardation, hypoplastic external genitals, and skeletal defects. Facies suggestive of Down's syndrome. |

* Normal male and normal female included for comparison.
† Reference: Pitcher DC: Sex chromosome disorders. *CRC Crit Rev Clin Lab Sci* 1981;**13**:241.

Males do not possess the sex chromatin bodies and are therefore chromatin-negative.

**B. The Y Chromosome:** The Y chromosome can be detected in the interphase cells of all tissues of the body by its characteristic fluorescence with quinacrine mustard stain. The Y bodies have a 1:1 relationship with the Y chromosome. In the male, the Y body is seen in 25–50% of the interphase cells.

Recently, a DNA Y-specific probe has become available for identifying the Y chromosome.

### Chromosomal Analysis

Chromosome analyses are done by growing cells from biopsy in tissue culture; chemically inhibiting their mitoses; and then sorting, counting, and staining the chromosomes. Specimens are most often taken from the peripheral blood, bone marrow, skin, and testes. A statistically significant number of cells must be counted. Stains that reveal the banding patterns of chromosomes provide so much more useful information than other stains that they should be used if available. The results of these analyses appear in the literature as the **karyotype,** which is a drawing or photograph of a systematized array of chromosomes of a single cell.

The present indications for these highly technical procedures are as follows: (1) Patients with malformations consistent with autosomal trisomy or deletion syndromes. (2) Parents of patients with a trisomy syndrome if the mother is younger than 30 years of age or if there are other similarly affected siblings. (3) Parents of all children with Down's syndrome who are found to be of the translocation or mosaic type. (4) Patients with an abnormality on sex chromatin analysis. (5) Children who are grossly retarded physically or mentally, especially if there are associated anomalies. (6) All cases of intersex. (7) All females with evidence of Turner's syndrome, whether they are chromatin positive or chromatin negative. (8) All males with Klinefelter's syndrome, whether they are chromatin positive or chromatin negative. (9) Tall males (> 6 ft) with behavioral disorders. (10) Couples with multiple spontaneous abortions of unknown cause (see below). (11) Girls with primary amenorrhea and boys with delayed pubertal development. Up to 25% of patients with primary amenorrhea have a chromosomal abnormality. (12) Certain malignant and premalignant diseases (see pp 1044–1049). (13) Certain families and populations with chromosomal variants (polymorphism) that are valuable for linkage and genealogic studies. (14) Persons exposed to large amounts of radiation or those whose parents may have been exposed to chemical mutagens. The number, type, and duration of chromosomal abnormalities correlate well with the amount of radiation. (15) Infertile couples.

## DNA Analysis

Fetal DNA from the amniotic or trophoblastic cells is used for genetic diagnosis in certain circumstances: (1) when the primary genetic defect has been identified at the nucleotide level (eg, sickle cell disease); (2) when the gene for the disease has been cloned (eg, phenylketonuria, alpha and beta thalassemias); and (3) when a locus known to carry a disease is near a known polymorphism, thereby allowing diagnosis by linkage mapping. DNA can be polymorphic, ie, one or 2 normal but different nucleotide sequences can exist at a specific site. Because these variations are inherited and can act as markers, it is possible to examine DNA sequences to detect possible links between a polymorphic genetic marker and a locus known to cause disease. If these markers are detected near a locus known to cause a certain disease, then the potential for that disease is assumed to be present. The closer the marker to the locus known to cause disease, the more accurate the diagnosis. (For example, Duchenne's muscular dystrophy locus is loosely linked to a marker; cystic fibrosis and Huntington's disease are tightly linked to markers.)

If the patient does not have the known polymorphism, the method cannot be used.

## PRENATAL DIAGNOSIS

It is now possible to diagnose approximately 100 inborn errors of metabolism, more than 30 monogenic disorders, and an increasing number of structural defects in utero during the 12th–16th weeks of pregnancy by analysis of amniotic fluid and cells.

### Indications

The indications for prenatal diagnosis are as follows:

**(1) Advanced maternal age.** *Example:* Down's syndrome. The risk of Down's syndrome increases from 1:2000 live births at maternal age 20, to 1:300 at age 35, to 1:100 at age 40, and to 1:40 at age 45.

**(2) Carrier of X-linked disease.** *Examples:* Hemophilia A, Duchenne's muscular dystrophy. Male fetuses have a 50% chance of being affected and could be aborted if that is the parents' wish.

**(3) Known or possible carrier of a biochemical disease.** *Example:* Tay-Sachs disease. Enzymatic studies on cultured amniotic fluid cells identify over 80 inborn errors of metabolism. Before these complicated studies are undertaken, it should be established that both parents are heterozygotes.

**(4) Positive family history of a chromosomal defect.** This includes a documented chromosomal defect in a parent, a family history of a chromosomal defect, or a previous child or conceptus with a defined or undefined chromosomal defect. *Examples:* a parent who is a translocation carrier of Down's syndrome, an abortus with a proved trisomy.

**(5) Open neural tube defects.** *Examples:* Anencephaly, meningomyelocele. Maternal serum alphafetoprotein levels and sonography can be used to diagnose most open neural tube defects. If these tests are not definitive, alpha-fetoprotein levels in amniotic fluid can be measured as a nonspecific predictor.

### Methods

Ultrasound scanning is a safe noninvasive procedure that can diagnose gross skeletal malformations as well as bony malformations known to be associated with specific diseases (eg, Ellis-van Creveld disease).

Of the invasive procedures, amniocentesis and chorionic villus sampling are the most frequently used (see Table 31–3). The latter takes advantage of 2 facts: (1) trophoblastic cells of the chorionic villus have the same genetic constitution as the fetus; and (2) the trophoblastic cells are rapidly growing and dividing, allowing chromosomal analysis by direct technique in most instances. If chorionic villus sampling is successful, the mother is spared the prolonged waiting period for results as well as the physical and emotional trauma of a second-trimester abortion, if one is indicated.

Other prenatal diagnostic procedures—fetoscopy, fetography, and amniography—are more invasive and a definite risk to the mother and fetus. They are indicated only if the risk of abnormality is high and the information cannot be obtained by other means.

Of parents with indications for antenatal genetic diagnosis, 95% will be reassured that their baby does not have a genetic problem. Few of the conditions diagnosed are treatable; with many, however, appropriate management can be started on the first day of life.

Chervenak FA, Isaacson G, Mahoney MJ: Advances in the diagnosis of fetal defects. (Current Concepts.) *N Engl J Med* 1986;**315:**305.

**Table 31–3.** Comparison of the major invasive prenatal diagnostic methods.

| Method | Procedure | Laboratory Analysis | Waiting Time for Results | Advantages | Disadvantages |
|--------|-----------|---------------------|--------------------------|------------|---------------|
| Amniocentesis | At the 12th–16th weeks and by the transabdominal approach, 10–30 mL of amniotic fluid is removed for cytologic and biochemical analysis. Preceding ultrasound locates the placenta and identifies twinning and missed abortion. | 1. Amniotic fluid:<br>a. α-Fetaprotein<br>b. Limited biochemical analysis<br>c. Virus isolation studies<br>2. Amniotic cell culture: chromosomal analysis | 3–4 weeks | Twenty years of experience | Therapeutic abortion, if indicated, must be done in the second trimester. (RhoGam should be given to Rh-negative mothers to prevent sensitization.) Risks: approximately 1%<br>a. Fetal: puncture or abortion.<br>b. Maternal: infection or bleeding. |
| Chorionic villus sampling (CVS) | At the 8th–12th weeks, and with constant ultrasound guidance, the trophoblastic cells of the chorionic villa are obtained by transcervical endoscopic needle biopsy or aspiration. | 1. Direct cell analysis: chromosomal studies<br>2. Cell culture: limited biochemical analysis | 1–10 days | Three or 4 years of investigational experience | Therapeutic abortion, if indicated, can be done in the first trimester.<br>Risk: ~3%<br>a. Fetal: abortion<br>b. Maternal: bleeding and infection (uncommon). |

# CHROMOSOMAL DISORDERS

## Frequency

Chromosomal anomalies occur surprisingly often. In live newborns, the incidence of gross chromosomal defects is 0.5%; in live prematures, 2.5%; in stillbirths, 6.9%; and in spontaneous abortions, about 30%. The most frequent chromosomal defects are trisomy 18, triploidy, and 45,XO. With live births, trisomy of the sex chromosomes is most frequent. The XXX genotype occurs in 1:1000 female births and the XXY in 2:1000 male births. Down's syndrome (trisomy 21) is the most frequent autosomal anomaly. Its incidence is 1:2000 if the mother is age 25 and 1:100 if the mother is age 40 or over. Advanced paternal age accounts for one-fourth of cases. Trisomy 13 and 18 rates are 0.3:1000 and 0.2:1000 live births, respectively.

Chromosomal studies done on abortuses, stillbirths, and tissues of infants who die in the neonatal period can provide valuable information for explaining habitual abortions, monitoring a subsequent pregnancy, and furnishing genetic counseling.

## DISORDERS DUE TO ABNORMALITIES OF THE X & Y CHROMOSOMES

Most disorders of the sex chromosomes (Table 31–2) are compatible with life and do not display marked phenotypic abnormalities. They are primarily due to an excess number of sex chromosomes, but there are 2 important exceptions: Turner's syndrome (XO) and fragile X syndrome, a form of X-linked mental retardation. The latter was discovered in 1980 and, next to Down's syndrome, is the most common cause of mental retardation that can be specifically diagnosed. Its frequency is 1:2000 males. Before adolescence, the patient has moderate to severe nonspecific mental retardation, and after puberty, a significant portion of affected males have macro-orchidism, with testicular volumes 3–4 times normal size. A prominent jaw, large ears, and normal to enlarged head circumference may also be present. Neurologic problems include retardation of motor development, pronounced speech disability, hyperactivity, and concentration difficulties. Female carriers for fragile X syndrome may be normal, but a significant proportion have mental retardation of a less severe nature. Cytogenetically, the fragile site is at Xq27. Prenatal diagnosis is possible by chromosomal analysis of amniotic fluid cells.

Patients with sex chromosome abnormalities have diverse clinical features. The more frequent syndromes—XXY (Klinefelter's), XYY, and XO (Turner's)—do not have serious malformations associated with them. Longitudinal studies of patients with Klinefelter's syndrome reveal minor skeletal differences, a reduction in testicular volume, and, in one-third of cases, gynecomastia. Otherwise, there is a definite but small lowering of IQ (from the mean of 104 to 96), a slight but definite increase in abnormalities measured by behavioral and personality tests, and a definite increase in reading and more general learning disabilities. Unselected data on XYY males and XO females reveal a similar picture. In sex chromosomal syndromes prior to birth, additional or deficient genetic material is associated with growth retardation except where an extra Y chromosome is present. After birth, sex chromosomes behave differently. When there is additional X or (especially) Y material, individuals tend to be tall. In patients with only one X chromosome (Turner's syndrome), the average height is less than 1.5 m (5 ft); patients with multiple Y syndromes have an average height of over 1.8 m (6 ft). As the number of X and Y chromosomes increases, the disability increases. These include (singly or in combination) such problems as mental retardation, sterility, abnormal sex characteristics, and skeletal abnormalities.

At present, there are far more patients with multiple X syndromes than with multiple Y syndromes.

Ratcliffe SG, and Paul N (editors): Prospective studies on children with sex chromosome aneuploidy. *Birth Defects: Original Article Series* 1986;**22(3)**:1.

## AUTOSOMAL DISORDERS

Although autosomes far outnumber sex chromosomes, very few disorders were attributed to autosomal aberrations until staining techniques revealed a characteristic pattern for each autosome. Initially, patients with clinically identifiable syndromes—trisomy 13, 18, and 21—demonstrated severe growth defects and mental retardation in addition to multiple congenital defects and died early. The mean survival time for trisomy 13 is 130 days and for trisomy 21, 30 years. As more cases were found, it was apparent that the physical appearance became less characteristic with survival beyond the first few months. Now, with the use of banding techniques, hundreds of case reports are available describing partial deletions and partial trisomies for almost every chromosome. Identifiable cases include those with mental retardation and minor congenital anomalies as well as those with normal intelligence and minor defects, previously described as variations of normal. Patients now range in age from newborns to 50 years.

Correlation of autosomal defects and clinical findings is now possible and is facilitated by several International Registries of Chromosomal Variations in Man.

In addition, identification of carriers of balanced translocations allows genetic counseling and prenatal diagnosis to prevent recurrences.

The most prevalent autosomal disorder is Down's syndrome, or mongolism. Ninety-five percent of cases are due to trisomy 21, and the remaining 5% are due to translocations of D/21, 21/21, and 22/21 types. The trisomy 21 cases have an increasing frequency with advancing parental ages. Advanced maternal age accounts for 75% of cases and advanced paternal age for the remainder. The translocation cases account for the carrier state of Down's syndrome, for familial Down's syndrome, and for the occurrence of Down's syndrome in children of younger mothers. Physical examination cannot distinguish between Down's syndrome due to trisomy and that due to translocation.

There are a few identified relationships between chromosomal defects and psychiatric disorders. Family studies show that depressive disorders segregate with human leukocyte antigens (HLA), indicating that a gene contributing to depressive disorders must also be on chromosome 6. In 1987, studies of the Amish revealed that some cases of manic depression are caused by a dominant gene on the short arm of chromosome 11 (11p−).

Borgaonkar DS: *Chromosomal Variation in Man: A Catalogue of Chromosomal Variants and Anomalies,* 3rd ed. Liss, 1981.
Kolata G (editor): Manic depression gene tied to chromosome 11. *Science* 1987;**235**:1139.

## CANCER

Current chromosomal studies, now at a molecular level, support Boveri's 1914 hypothesis—ie, that cancer is caused by a change in genetic material at the cellular level.

**Oncogenes**—genes capable of causing malignant transformation in normal cells—have been discovered in experimental studies with the RNA tumor viruses. Currently, there are approximately 30 known oncogenes. They are named after the animal tumor virus from which they were identified—*myc* from avian myelocytomatosis virus, *abl* from Abelson murine leukemia virus, etc. Evidence from gene cloning and transfection studies reveals that these oncogenes are present in the human genome as well as throughout the animal kingdom. The oncogenes arose from preexisting normal cellular (c) genes (proto-oncogenes) that had been altered. Alterations can occur either in the structural or in the regulatory region of the proto-oncogene and are caused by viral or nonviral factors. In the structural area, mutations cause the synthesis of proteins of aberrant structure and function; in the regulatory area, there is an inappropriate amount of normal protein. For example, in chronic myelogenous leukemia, with its 9;22 translocation, the translocated *abl* proto-oncogene fuses to another unlinked gene and produces a hybrid protein that acts differently from the normal *abl* protein. In Burkitt's lymphoma, the normal regulation of the translocated *myc* proto-oncogene is lost, allowing production of an abnormal amount of a normal protein. The proteins encoded by oncogenes are now almost all known. Many of them are cellular growth factors; others have obscure functions. Many oncogenes are at the breakpoints of chromosomal translocations and deletions that are described with many types of cancer. It is still unclear how they are involved in the malignant transformation of the cell.

Studies of hereditary tumors reveal yet another factor in the causation of cancer—**anti-oncogenes,** ie, genes whose presence protects against cancer. For example, in cells of a retinoblastoma, there is a characteristic deletion on the long arm of chromosome 13 (13q14). Gene linkage studies reveal that in familial cases, this deletion occurs on one of the pair of chromosome 13. If, by somatic change, there is a similar deletion on the other chromosome 13, the cancer becomes expressed. The existing gene at chromosome 13q14 acts as an anti-oncogene, preventing the expression of the inherited chromosomal deletion.

## Predisposing Factors

Studies of cancer patients indicate that genetic factors play a role in only a small percentage of cases. With carcinoma of the stomach, breast, colon, prostate, and endometrium, a hereditary factor with a site-specific basis is operating, for relatives of patients with these types of cancer have a 3-fold higher risk of having the same type of cancer. Only rarely do the **mendelian laws of inheritance** apply. The classic examples are polyposis of the colon, Recklinghausen's neurofibromatosis, hereditary adenomatosis, basal cell nevus syndrome, and some cases of retinoblastoma. In general, the majority of cases of cancer are of unknown cause.

**Fragile sites** may also be important in the development of cancer. Fragile sites are chromosome gaps or breaks that occur when cultured cells are grown in media deficient in thymidine or folic acid. It appears that the fragile site has a unique DNA structure, and when its precursor substances are missing, the cell is prone to rearrangement. So far, 15 heritable fragile sites have been identified, 8 of which are located near chromosomal rearrangements known to be associated with leukemia and lymphoma. These fragile sites occur with a frequency of 0.2% and are inherited as simple mendelian codominant traits.

**Genetic instability** appears to contribute to the development of solid tumors. Bloom's syndrome, Fanconi's anemia, ataxia-telangiectasia, glutathione reductase deficiency, Kostmann's agranulocytosis, and pernicious anemia are autosomal recessive disorders that have a tendency toward chromosomal breakage and rearrangement in vitro. Furthermore, these disorders are associated with a fairly high incidence of neoplasia, chiefly leukemia and lymphoma. Studies of patients with ataxia-telangiectasia show that the anomalous clone is usually a structural rearrangement in 14. It is most often a translocation involving 14, 7, 6, and X. **Constitutional chromosomal anomalies** also contribute to the development of cancer. The risk of acute leukemia is increased 20-fold in patients with trisomy 21 (Down's syndrome). The leukemias in patients with Down's syndrome, unlike those in chromosomally normal children, are 3 times more likely to be acute nonlymphocytic leukemia (ANLL) rather than acute lymphocytic leukemia (ALL). Phenotypic females with an XY complement have a 25% greater risk of developing ovarian carcinoma. This is true whether or not mosaicism is present or the Y chromosome is intact or partially deleted. Tumors that develop in these patients are of different types, with gonadoblastoma occurring most frequently, sometimes as early as age 3. XXY males (Klinefelter's syndrome) have a 30-fold increase in the incidence of breast cancer as well as predisposition to acute nonlymphocytic leukemia. Patients with trisomy 21 or sex chromosome aneuploidy (XXX or XXY) have an increased incidence of retinoblastoma.

## The Leukemias

There is a remarkable specificity of chromosomal arrangements in patients with leukemia. When this cytogenetic information is combined with the FAB classification, it is possible to define subsets of patients in which response to therapy, clinical course, and prognosis are predictable (see Table 31–4).

The primary karyotypic change is the basis of one of the subclassifications of leukemia. It is felt to be related to the causation of the disease and thus may determine its nature. As secondary chromosomal changes occur, leukemia becomes more aggressive, often associated with drug resistance and reduced chance for a complete or long remission. Generally, the more complex and extensive the secondary changes, the worse the prognosis. Two situations are of particular importance in secondary leukemias. If there is a change in chromosome 5 (–5 or 5q–) and 7 (–7 or 7q–), the prognosis is very poor. These chromosomal changes occur after chemotherapy or other toxic exposure and are probably caused by them. On the other hand, Freireich reports that in 8 patients with secondary leukemias, those with an inv(16), t(15;17), or t(8q;21q) had a favorable response to chemotherapy and 87% achieved complete remission. Other cytogenetic findings have prognostic implications but to a lesser degree. If there are no chromosomal changes in bone marrow cells at the time of diagnosis, the survival time is longer than if any or all bone marrow cells have abnormal cytogenetics. The presence of double minute chromosomes or homogeneously staining regions on chromosomes indicates gene amplification and often the appearance of drug resistance.

Lastly, the least significant of all chromosomal changes is numerical alteration without morphologic abnormality. In acute lymphocytic leukemia, patients with the former finding have a better prognosis than those with the latter.

## Lymphomas & Other Hematologic Disorders

Far less cytogenetic information is available about lymphomas than about leukemia. In **Hodgkin's disease,** studies have been limited by the low yield of dividing cells and low number of clear-cut aneuploid clones, so that complete chromosomal analyses with banding are available for far fewer patients with Hodgkin's disease than for any other lymphoma. In Hodgkin's disease, the modal chromosomal number tends to be triploid or tetraploid. About one-third of the samples have a 14q+ chromosome. In **non-Hodgkin's lymphomas,** a new high-resolution technique of chromosome analysis has a 95% success rate. The modal number tends to be diploid. With the new International Formulation and Rappaport Classification of these lymphomas, there is a correlation be-

**Table 31–4.** Chromosomal changes in leukemias.

| | FAB Classification | Pathologic Classification | Chromosomal Subsets | Implicated Oncogene | Prognostic Factors and Survival |
|---|---|---|---|---|---|
| Acute nonlymphocytic leukemia (ANLL) | M1 | Acute myeloblastic leukemia without maturation (AML) | (1) t(q;22)(q34.1;q11.2), ie, Ph¹ chromosome | (1) c-*abl* | (1) Ph¹-positive patients have poor response to chemotherapy. Median survival: 9–10 months. |
| | | | (2) 5q/−5;7q−/−7;17<br>(3) del 3p and t with 3<br>(4) +21<br>(5) +8 | | (2) Poor prognosis.<br><br><br>(5) Median survival: 10 months. |
| | M2 | Acute myeloblastic leukemia with maturation (AML) | (1) t(8;21)(q22;q22) with Auer rods | (1) Hu-*ets*-2<br>c-*mos* | (1) Generally good prognosis (median survival 13 months), but worse if (1) loss of sex chromosome (X or Y) or (b) additional chromosome changes. Myeloblastoma reported in this subset. |
| | | | (2) t(q;22)(q34;q11), ie, Ph¹ chromosome | | (2) Poor prognosis. Occasional short-lived complete remissions. Short survival. |
| | | | (3) 5q/−5;7q−/−7<br>(4) del 3p and inv(3)<br>(5) +8 | | (3) Poor prognosis.<br><br>(5) Median survival; 10 months. |
| | | (6) } marrow basophilia<br>(7) } may be present | (6) t(6;q)(p22;q34)<br>(7) t(3;5)(q26;q22) | (6) c-*abl* | (6) Generally poor prognosis. |
| | | (8) Eosinophilia present | (8) inv(16) or 16q− | | (8) Relatively good prognosis. May have complete remission for 2 years or longer. |
| | M3 | Acute promyelocytic leukemia (APL) (hypergranular or microgranular) | (1) t(15;17)(q22;q11.2) | (1) c-*erb* A | (1) Generally poor prognosis (median survival 3 months). Additional chromosomal changes have poor prognosis. Increased incidence of disseminated intravascular coagulation (DIC). |
| | | | (2) i17 | | |
| | M4 | Acute myelomonocytic leukemia (AMMoL) | (1) Chromosome 11 involved<br>(2) t(q;22)(q34;q11), ie, Ph¹ chromosome<br>(3) 5q1−5;7q−/−7<br>(4) t(6;9)(p22;q34)<br>(5) +8 | | (2) Ph¹-positive patients have poor response to therapy.<br>(3) Poor prognosis.<br><br>(5) Median survival 10 months. |
| | | (6) } Eosinophilia<br>(7) } present<br>(8) } | (6) inv(16)(p13;q22)<br>(7) 16q−(q32)<br>(8) t(16;16)(p13;q22) | | (6) Relatively good prognosis.<br>(7) Relatively good prognosis.<br>(8) Good prognosis. Remission in 78% of patients (some remissions > 2 years). |
| | M5 | Acute monocytic leukemia (AMoL) | (1) Defects in 11q | | (1) Poor prognosis. |
| | | | (2) t(q;11) and del(11q)<br>(3) t(11;19)(q23;q12 or p12)<br>(4) +8 | (2) Hu-*ets*-2<br>(3) c-*Ha-ras*-1 | (2) Poor prognosis.<br>(3) Median survival 8 months.<br><br>(4) Median survival 10 months. |
| | M6 | Erythroleukemia | (1) Ph¹-positive | (1) c-*abl* | (1) Poor response to chemotherapy. |
| | | | (2) High chromosome count<br>(3) Major karyotypic changes<br>(4) −3 and t(3:?)<br>(5) dup 1<br>(6) +8 | | (6) Median survival 10 months. |
| | M7 | Acute megakaryoblastic leukemia | | | |

**Table 31–4 (cont'd).** Chromosomal changes in leukemias.

| | FAB Classi-fication | Pathologic Classification | Chromosomal Subsets | Implicated Oncogene | Prognostic Factors and Survival |
|---|---|---|---|---|---|
| **Acute lymphocytic** | L1 | **Common childhood variant; homogeneous population. Pathology:** Small blasts; nucleoli not evident; scanty cytoplasm, regularly shaped nucleus. | (1) 6q−<br>(2) t(1;19)(q23;q13)<br>(3) t(11;14)(q13;q32)<br>(4) High chromosome counts<br>(5) Ph¹-positive*<br>(6) Near heploid | (1) c-*myb*<br><br><br>(3) h-*ras*-1<br><br>(5) c-*abl* | (1) Good prognosis. Median survival > 36 months.<br>(2) Poor prognosis. Median survival 12 months.<br>(3) Poor prognosis.<br>(4) Good prognosis. Median survival 36 months.<br>(5) Very poor prognosis. Median survival 12 months.<br>(6) Median survival 8 months. |
| | | Common B or T cell | 9p− | | Poor prognosis. |
| | L2 | Common adult variant; heterogeneous population. **Pathology:** Large blasts, heterogeneous size; one or 2 large nucleoli; moderately abundant cytoplasm; irregularly shaped nucleus. | (1) t(q;22)(q34;q11)*<br>(2) t(4:11)(q21;q23)*<br>(3) bq−<br>(4) Other subsets:<br>　+21　11q−<br>　+8　t with 14q32<br>　i(17q) t with 11q<br>　7p−<br>(5) Near haploid | | (1) Very poor prognosis. Median survival 12 months.<br>(2) Very poor prognosis. Median survival 7 months.<br>(3) Intermediate to good prognosis.<br><br><br><br><br>(5) Median survival 12 months. |
| | | ? T cell | 9p− | | Poor prognosis. |
| | L3 | Burkitt cell type **Pathology:** Large blasts, homogeneous size; one or 2 prominent nucleoli; moderately abundant cytoplasm, often with cytoplasmic vacuolization; regularly shaped nucleus. | (1) t(8;14)(q24;q32)*<br>(2) t(2;8)<br>(3) t(8;22)(q24;q11 or 12)<br>(4) t(4;11)<br>(5) t(1;8;14)(q23;q24; q32) or t(3;8;14) (q14;) (q24;q32)<br>(6) 6q−<br>(7) 1q+ or +8/+8<br>(8) 14q+ | (1)<br><br><br><br>(4) c-*Ki-ras*-2 | (1) Very prognosis. Median survival 5 months.<br>(2) Poor prognosis. Median survival < 12 months.<br>(3) Poor prognosis. Median survival > 12 months.<br>(4) Poor prognosis. Median survival 8–10 months.<br><br><br>(8) Very poor prognosis. Median survival 6–9 months. |
| **Chronic myeloge-neous leukemia (CML)** | | | (1) t(q;22)(q34;q11) | (1) c-*abl*, c-*cis* | (1) Median survival 42 months. Patients with missing Y chromosome in marrow have longer survival. Blast phase with its poor response to therapy preceded by (i17q), extra Ph¹ chromosome, trisomy 8 and +19. Median survival 5 months. |
| | | | (2) Ph¹ chromosome variants (chromosome 22 always involved). | | (2) Same as (1), above. |
| | | | (3) Ph¹-negative. Frequent changes:<br>+8, −7, +21, −4, i(17q) | | (3) Poorer prognosis than Ph¹-positive CML. Median survival 12 months. |
| **Chronic lymphocytic leukemia (CLL)** | (1)<br>(2)<br>(3) | B cell<br>B cell and T cell<br>B cell and T cell | (1) Trisomy 12<br>(2) 14q+<br>(3) Translocation including 14 and 11. | (1) c-*ras* | (1) Median survival 14 months.<br>(2) Shortened survival time (42 months as compared to 60 months without 14q+). |
| **Prolymphocytic leukemia (PLL)** | | | (1) del(3)(p12)<br>(2) t(6;12)(q15;p13) | (1) c-*ras* | (2) Serious tendency toward vascular thrombosis. |
| **Acute hairy cell leukemia** | | | 6q−, +3, +12, +18, +14, +Y | | Any abnormal karyotype decreases survival time. |
| **Adult T cell leukemia** | | | (1) Trisomy 3; trisomy 7<br>(2) ? 14q11 | | (1) Complex chromosomal arrangements have poor prognosis. |

* Most frequent change.

tween the nonrandom chromosomal aberrations and the histologic type, but there are no data concerning the prognostic significance of the cytogenetic findings. By far the most information is available about **Burkitt's lymphoma,** a solid tumor of B cell origin. Ninety percent of patients with this disorder have a translocation between the long arm of chromosome 8 (8q–) and the long arm of chromosome 14 (14q+). The remainder have a t(8;2) or t(8;22). The translocated gene segment of chromosome 8, which contains the oncogene c-*myc*, is transposed directly into immunoglobulin loci on chromosomes 2, 14, and 22. The immunoglobulin loci now produce an abnormal amount of their encoded immunoglobulin—ie, chromosome 2 produces light-chain immunoglobulins with a kappa constant region, etc. These translocations occur in every Burkitt's lymphoma, whether it is of the African or non-African type, and whether it is Epstein-Barr virus (EBV)-positive or -negative. In **multiple myeloma,** about half of patients have abnormal cytogenetics. The clonal abnormalities found early in the disease are often present late in the disease.

There are limited cytogenetic studies of other hematologic disorders that have a recognized propensity for neoplastic transformation (Table 31–5). The limited studies do reveal that the chromosomal findings have therapeutic and prognostic significance.

## Solid Tumors
## (Table 31–6)

In solid tumors, there is far less cytogenetic information than there is for the leukemias, since it has been difficult to determine the primary karyotypic event.

Often, at the initial cytogenetic investigation of solid tumors, there are already multiple chromosomal changes. This is particularly true for the carcinomas, which have more complex karyotypes than the sarcomas. In addition, technical problems present difficulties in determining the primary karyotypic change. For example, solid tumors have a low mitotic index. They often have an infection that can either cause destruction of tumor cells or make cytogenetic analysis impossible. Until recently, cytogenetic analysis revealed chromosomes with a fuzzy appearance, making detailed analysis impossible.

Currently, the primary karyotypic event has been identified in 20 solid tumors. No clearly defined pattern emerges. In patients with transitional cell carcinoma of the urogenital tract, there is a uniform histologic appearance but several chromosomal subsets. These chromosomal alterations have no correlation with its clinical course, response to therapy, or prognosis. On the other hand, in synovial sarcoma, there is histologic variation but only one specific chromo-

**Table 31–5.** Chromosomal changes in myelodysplastic syndromes and other potentially malignant hematologic conditions.

| | Chromosomal Change | Prognostic Factors and Survival |
|---|---|---|
| Refractory anemia (RA) | (1) Any abnormal karyotype (89%)<br><br>(2) 5q– | (1) Risk of leukemia. About 7% of RA patients develop leukemia.<br>(2) Good prognostic factor. Slow development of illness.<br>Median survival: >60 months for both (1) and (2). |
| Refractory anemia with excess blasts (RAEB) | (1) Any abnormal karyotype (80%)<br><br><br>(2) 5q– | (1) High transformation to leukemia (ANLL). About 56% of RAEB patients develop leukemia.<br>(2) Good prognostic factor. Slow development of illness.<br>Median survival: 21 months for both (1) and (2). |
| Refractory anemia with excess blasts in transformation (RAEB-T) | | High incidence of transformation to ANLL (40% of patients). Median survival: 16 months. |
| Chronic myelomonocytic leukemia (CMMoL) | | 20% of patients develop ANLL. Median survival: 25 months. |
| Acquired idiopathic sideroblastic anemia (AISA) | Heterodiploidy. Disturbances in F chromosomes. | Median survival: >60 months. |
| Acute and chronic myelofibrosis | Nonspecific chromosomal abnormalities (40%). | 92% of patients with normal chromosomes respond to androgen therapy, whereas only 22% of patients with chromosomal abnormalities respond. |
| Polycythemia vera | (1) 20q– is the most consistent specific finding. Also +8, +9, 13q–.<br>(2) 5q–<br><br>(3) Appearance of subclones in patients with abnormal karyotype. | (1) No prognostic implications.<br><br>(2) Poor prognostic sign. Found in treated patients.<br>(3) Same as (2). |

**Table 31–6.** Specific (primary) chromosome changes in tumors.*

| Tumors | Chromosome Changes |
|---|---|
| **Benign** | |
| Meningioma | −22,22q− |
| Mixed tumors of salivary glands | t(3;8)(p21;q12), t(9;12)(p13−22;q13−15) |
| Lipoma | t(3;12)(q28;q14) |
| Colonic adenomas | 12q−,+8 |
| **Adenocarcinomas** | |
| Bladder | i(5p),+7,−9/9q−,11p− |
| Prostate | del(10)(q24) |
| Lung (SLCC) | del(3)(p14p23) |
| Colon | 12q−,+7,+8,+12,17(q11) |
| Kidney | del(3)(p21) |
| Uterus | 1q− |
| Ovary | 6q−,t(6;14)(q21;q24) |
| **Sarcomas** | |
| Liposarcoma (myxoid) | t(12;16)(q13;q11) |
| Synovial | t(X;18)(p11.2;q11.2) |
| Rhabdomyosarcoma (alveolar) | t(2;13)(q37;q14) |
| **Embryonal and other** | |
| Testicular (germ cell tumors) | i(12p) |
| Retinoblastoma | del(13)(q14)† |
| Wilms's tumor | del(11)(p13) |
| Neuroblastoma | del(1)(p32p36) |
| Malignant melanoma | del(6)(q11q27),i(6p),del(1) (p11p22),t(1;19)(q12;q13) |
| Ewing's sarcoma and peripheral neuroepithelioma | t(11;22) (q24;q12) |

* Reproduced, with permission, from Sandberg AA, Turc-Carel C: The cytogenetics of solid tumors: Relation to diagnosis, classification, and pathology. *Cancer* 1987;**59**:387.
† Associated with constitutional chromosome change.

somal translocation. Then there is the confusing problem of benign tumors having specific chromosomal changes—meningiomas, mixed salivary gland tumors, etc. However, cytogenetics has been of help in 2 situations: first, it can help identify the origin of tumors whose metastases have a confusing histologic picture; and second, it has helped identify the histogenesis of certain tumors, eg, Ewing's sarcoma.

Some investigators predict that—like leukemia and the lymphomas—solid tumors will have chromosomal subsets that will indicate causation, clinical course, response to therapy, and prognosis.

Bitter MA et al: Associations between morphology, karyotype, and clinical features in myeloid leukemias. *Hum Pathol* 1987;**18**:311.

Bloomfield CD: Chromosomal abnormalities identify high risk and low risk patients with ALL. *Blood* 1986;**67**:414.

Freireich EJ: Hematologic malignancies: Adult acute leukemia. *Hosp Pract* (June 15) 1986;**21**:91.

Jacobs RH et al: Prognostic implications of morphology and karyotype in primary myelodysplastic syndromes. *Blood* 1986;**67**:1765.

LeBeau MM, Rowley JD: Chromosomal abnormalities in leukemia and lymphoma: Clinical and biological significance. *Adv Hum Genet* 1986;**15**:1.

Mitelman F: *Catalog of Chromosomal Aberrations in Cancer,* 2nd ed. Vol 5 of *Progress and Topics in Cytogenetics.* Liss, 1985.

Sandberg AA: The chromosomes in human leukemia. *Semin Hematol* 1986;**23**:201.

Sandberg AA, Turc-Carel C: The cytogenetics of solid tumors. *Cancer* 1987;**59**:387.

## CHROMOSOMES & IONIZING RADIATION

The major problem of ionizing radiation is not the danger of lethal doses but of small doses that allow the cells to multiply after permanent alteration of their genetic material.

Detectable chromosomal changes occur after diagnostic and therapeutic x-ray as well as with beta and gamma radiation ($^{131}$I, $^{32}$P). These usually persist for a few hours to several weeks. In vitro studies reveal a direct relationship between the dose of ionizing radiation and the number of chromosomal abnormalities.

## VIRUSES, CHEMICALS, & CHROMOSOMES

For more than half a century, viruses and chemicals have been known to induce chromosomal aberrations in plants and animals. Only in the past decade have human chromosomal defects been proved to be caused by these agents. The measles, chickenpox, hepatitis, and rubella viruses may cause chromosomal aberrations in the leukocytes that may persist for several months after the clinical illness. Drugs such as ozone, analogous and intermediary metabolites of nucleic acids, and alkylating agents have deleterious effects on chromosomes. Studies of workers exposed to chemical solvents, insecticides, petroleum products, and anesthetic gases reveal an increased number of structural chromosomal abnormalities in their peripheral blood cells. Different carcinogens have different clonal abnormalities. Follow-up is being done to determine the incidence of fetal malformation and wastage as well as leukemia in these groups.

It is hoped that these new findings will add to our understanding of "spontaneous" chromosomal changes as well as chemical carcinogenesis.

## GENETIC COUNSELING

Genetic counseling is concerned with the scientific, psychologic, and social implications relating to the occurrence and risk of recurrence of a genetic disorder in a family.

The scientific basis for sound genetic counseling consists of (1) an accurate diagnosis, since closely related disorders—especially biochemical defects—may have very different prognoses and modes of inheritance; (2) a detailed family pedigree, showing affected and nonaffected members; and (3) knowledge about the natural history of the disease. A subcommittee of the American Society of Human Genetics lists 5 objectives of genetic counseling to help individuals or families:

[1] to comprehend the medical facts, including diagnosis, probable course of the disorder, and available management; [2] to appreciate both heredity's contribution to the disorder and the risk of recurrence in specific relatives; [3] to understand alternatives for dealing with the recurrence risk; [4] to choose and undertake an appropriate plan of action in view of risk, family goals, and ethical and religious standards; and [5] to adjust as well as possible to the disorder and/or to the risk of recurrence of the disorder.

The emotional impact of being informed that one is personally or closely affected by or involved in the transmission of some genetic disease may be overwhelming. After the interview during which the disorder and its recurrence risk have been discussed, follow-up communication at the physician's instance is desirable. One study reports that 21–75% of persons receiving genetic counseling did not understand or remember what they had been told. A following letter is a useful means of repeating and emphasizing important information and serves the family as documentary reference matter in the future. A phone call or home visit by personnel from the genetic clinic may disclose a need for further explanation or provide an opportunity to ask questions that have arisen since the interview.

To assist the clinician, the National Foundation has compiled an international directory of genetic services (see Bergsma reference, below).

Bergsma D (editor): *International Directory of Genetic Services,* 7th ed. Birth Defects Series. The National Foundation, New York, 1983.
Genetic Counseling: Report of the Subcommittee of the American Society of Human Genetics. *Am J Hum Genet* 1975;**27**:240.

# SELECTED HEREDITARY METABOLIC DISEASES

Garrod's original description in 1908 of 4 inborn errors of metabolism was regarded with interest, but these disorders were largely considered to be rare medical curiosities of little clinical importance. The several hundred hereditary metabolic disorders about which we now have at least some knowledge include common and uncommon, benign and serious diseases, metabolic disturbances involving almost every class of biochemical substance, and diseases of all organs and tissues of the body. Newly recognized metabolic disorders are being reported at a rapid rate, and this information has contributed greatly to the study of the molecular biology of humans and animals.

Information about metabolic abnormalities is not only important in furthering our understanding of hitherto obscure disease processes but also fundamental to a proper therapeutic approach to them. Old concepts of hereditary transmission of physical traits simply as dominant or recessive have had to be modified to explain the "asymptomatic carriers" of hereditary traits. Biochemical studies on relatives of patients with hereditary metabolic disorders may reveal deficiencies not clinically manifest. Recognition of the heterozygote carrier may be of extreme value from a eugenic point of view (in preventing potentially incompatible matings) and from the standpoint of the health of the individual (eg, in suggesting special dietary control, appropriate medication, and avoidance of drug idiosyncrasies).

Determination of the genetic basis of metabolic disorders is based on the family history and appropriate biochemical studies of the patient and available relatives. Biochemical studies may include the determination of essential blood constituents, abnormal protein molecules, specific enzymes, abnormal metabolites, electrolytes, renal transport mechanisms, and tolerance or restriction tests with food or chemicals.

Several of the hereditary metabolic disorders (eg, diabetes mellitus, hyperlipidemia, gout) as they relate to specific organ systems are discussed in other sections of this book.

## ABNORMALITY OF MOLECULAR STRUCTURE OF PROTEIN: METHEMOGLOBINEMIA

Congenital methemoglobinemia is a disease caused either by a deficiency of erythrocyte NADH dehydrogenase (required in converting methemoglobin to hemoglobin) or by the presence of one of 5 different abnormal hemoglobins, each designated as an M hemoglobin. The former is the more frequent form and is inherited as an autosomal recessive trait; the latter is autosomal dominant. Clinically, the disease is manifested by a persistent gray cyanosis not associated with cardiac or respiratory abnormality, and by easy fatigability, dyspnea, tachycardia, and dizziness with exertion. The venous blood is brown; the oxygen capacity of arterial blood is reduced, and excessive amounts of methemoglobin are present in the blood.

Oral administration of riboflavin, 120 mg/d, significantly decreases methemoglobin in the disease caused by enzyme deficiency. In addition, in some cases, continuous administration of methylene blue, 240 mg/d orally, will relieve the symptoms and cyanosis.

The prognosis for life is good. Pregnancies are not compromised. Heterozygotes can be identified by assays of enzyme activity. Toxic agents such as nitrites and aniline derivatives create a special hazard for NADH dehydrogenase-deficient patients. They cause a sudden increase in methemoglobin, which is tolerated poorly and may be fatal.

Mansour A: Methemoglobinemia. *Am J Med Sci* 1985;**289**:200.

## DISORDERS OF AMINO ACIDS

### Albinism

Albinism is a term that covers many clinical syndromes exhibiting hypomelanosis of the skin and eye due to inherited metabolic defects. Their incidence is 1:20,000. There are 3 forms of albinism: **ocular,** which is a sex-linked recessive trait as well as an autosomal recessive trait; **oculocutaneous,** which is autosomal dominant; and **cutaneous,** which is autosomal dominant. In the ocular form, the eye defect occurs alone. Clinical manifestations are photophobia, nystagmus, defective vision, and absence of binocular vision. The metabolic defect of ocular albinism is unknown. In the oculocutaneous form, defects in hair and skin pigmentation occur in addition to the ocular defects. The hypopigmented skin acquires folds and wrinkles easily when exposed to solar radiation. There is a high frequency of solar keratosis, basal cell carcinoma, and squamous cell carcinoma. Biochemically, patients with oculocutaneous albinism are divided into tyrosinase-positive and tyrosinase-negative, but the biochemical distinction does not separate the patients clinically. In both the ocular and oculocutaneous forms, there are abnormal optic pathways as well as rearrangements in the geniculocortical projections that account for the absence of binocular vision. The cutaneous form is a partial albinism or piebaldism that affects only the skin and hair. There is localized loss of melanocytes. Some patients have associated deafness.

There is no specific treatment. Sunlight should be avoided. Sunscreen preparations are useful. Dark glasses will help patients with photophobia.

### Alkaptonuria

Alkaptonuria is a rare autosomal recessive disease caused by a deficiency of the enzyme homogentisic oxidase. Since this enzyme is necessary in the intermediate metabolism of phenylalanine and tyrosine, its precursor, homogentisic acid, increases and is deposited in the connective tissues of the body to give them, grossly, a blue-black color and, microscopically, an ochre color (hence, ochronosis).

The cardinal features of alkaptonuria are pigmentation of the cartilage and other connective tissues, arthritis in later life, and signs of homogentisic acid in the urine. The blue-black pigmentation, not usually noticeable until age 20–30 years, is most apparent in the scleras of the eyes and pinnas of the ears. The arthritis may resemble rheumatoid arthritis clinically. The large joints of the body—mainly hips, knees, lumbosacral spine, and shoulders—may undergo acute inflammation followed by limitation of motion and ankylosis. In the urine, the homogentisic

acid causes a dark color (particularly when the urine is alkaline), and since it has reducing properties, it may give a false-positive result in Benedict's test for sugar.

Diagnosis rests on the identification of homogentisic acid in the urine by means of paper chromatography.

Since the disease has a prolonged, benign course, no attempts have been made to control phenylalanine and tyrosine in the diet. Degenerative arthritis is treated symptomatically. Vitamin C, a reducing agent, has been suggested as a means of decreasing pigment formation and deposition. There is no method for detection of the heterozygote.

### Phenylketonuria

Phenylketonuria (PKU) is one of the milestone diseases of medicine, for it was this disease in which the first biochemical cause of mental retardation was discovered and in which dietary treatment proved to be effective; prevention was thus made possible through early identification and treatment. It is an autosomal recessive disease whose incidence varies from 1:5000 in Irish persons and Scots to 1:300,000 in blacks, Ashkenazic Jews, and Finns. Clinically, the classic picture is represented by a blond, blue-eyed child with fair skin, eczema, and mental retardation. Seizures and behavioral problems are often present.

Since screening of newborns is widespread, the presenting problem is hyperphenylalaninemia in a healthy newborn infant. But hyperphenylalaninemia is no longer synonymous with phenylketonuria, for mass screening has revealed multiple causes of hyperphenylalaninemia. Thus far, 3 causes of hyperphenylalaninemia severe enough to require treatment have been defined. First, there is classic phenylketonuria due to phenylalanine hydroxylase deficiency. This form, accounting for 97% of cases, requires and responds to dietary treatment (to prevent mental retardation). The remaining 3% of cases are due to defects in 2 other enzymes that are involved not only in phenylalanine metabolism but also in biosynthesis of neurotransmitters such as dopamine, norepinephrine, and serotonin. Adequate therapy for this group requires $BH_4$, sepiapterin, levodopa, carbidopa, and 5-hydroxytryptophan in addition to the dietary regimen in order to prevent progressive neurologic degeneration.

Therapy consists of a restricted phenylalanine diet, with enough phenylalanine present to support adequate growth without causing mental impairment. The diet will not reverse or improve existing mental retardation, but if it is instituted before age 2 months, the child has a statistically significant chance of attaining normal intelligence. Blood phenylalanine levels are checked weekly to keep the blood level between 3 and 10 mg/dL. All agree that the diet should be maintained for 3–6 years, and some investigators feel it should be maintained for life. Recent studies suggest that there is a significant loss of intellectual function with discontinuation of the restricted diet in children with classic phenylketonuria before age 8. The severity of the IQ loss correlated with the duration of the unrestricted diet. Continuation of the diet also modified such symptoms as hyperkinesis, seizures, learning disorders, and eczema.

Genetics plays an important role in prevention. Once a patient is identified, the entire family and any subsequent offspring should be checked for phenylketonuria. If the mother has classic phenylketonuria, she can bear a normal infant, but there is an increase both in the rate of abortion and in the risk of bearing offspring with nonphenylketonuric mental retardation, microcephaly, and congenital heart disease. Limited studies suggest that the number of defective children born of mothers with phenylketonuria correlates directly with the maternal phenylalanine level. If the maternal blood phenylalanine is less than 480 μmol/L, the offspring are normal; if this level is 600–1200 μmol/L, there are some defective children; and when the level exceeds 1200 μmol/L, almost all offspring are defective. The current recommendation is to initiate therapy prior to conception.

The heterozygote can be identified and is free of any signs or symptoms of phenylketonuria. In 1985, prenatal diagnosis by a cloned phenylalanine gene probe became possible, permitting identification of 90% of families with previously affected children.

Holtzman NA et al: Effect of age at loss of dietary control on intellectual performance and behavior of children with phenylketonuria. *N Engl J Med* 1986;**314:**593.

Koch R et al: Maternal phenylketonuria. *J Inherited Metab Dis* 1986;**9(Suppl 2):**159.

## Homocystinuria

Homocystinuria, an autosomal disease with considerable genetic heterogeneity, is the second most common inborn error of amino acid metabolism. Its incidence is 1:200,000 live births. The vast majority of cases are due to a deficiency in the liver enzyme cystathionine synthase that causes an increase in the amount of methionine and other metabolites in blood and other body tissues. The cardinal signs and symptoms are due to defective collagen formation and occur in the eye, skeletal system, central nervous system, and cardiovascular system. Lens ectopia is typically present and may cause secondary glaucoma, myopia, retinal detachment, and cataract. The skeletal system consistently shows osteoporosis and genu valgum, and frequently there are chest, vertebral, and foot deformities. Mental retardation is present in half of cases. Major motor seizures are frequently present. The lethal complication is in the cardiovascular system, where multiple arterial and venous thromboses occur as a result of enhanced platelet stickiness. Occasionally, an abdominal aortic aneurysm may be present.

If ectopic lens is present, patients with homocystinuria may be wrongly diagnosed as having Marfan's syndrome. Diagnosis is suspected by a combination of clinical findings and excessive urinary homocysteine excretion, but definitive diagnosis requires the demonstration of reduced cystathionine synthase activity.

Treatment to achieve biochemical control should start as soon as the disease is diagnosed, for most clinical complications are irreversible. About half of patients respond to massive doses of pyridoxine. A daily dose of 500–1000 mg of pyridoxine, when effective, will cause a biochemical response in a few days; it should then be lowered until a minimum effective dose is found. A recent study of pyridoxine-resistant patients treated with betaine, 6 g/d, in addition to folate and pyridoxine showed biochemical improvement in all 10 patients and clinical improvement in 6. Studies in animals have shown that the vascular injury is induced by homocystine. A single dose of dipyridamole, 100 mg, combined with aspirin, 1 g, has also been reported to be effective in decreasing the incidence of thrombotic episodes.

Identification of heterozygotes is possible. Prenatal diagnosis is feasible but has not been reported.

Weilcken DE et al: Homocystinuria: The effects of betaine in the treatment of patients not responsive to pyridoxine. *N Engl J Med* 1983;**309:**448.

## DISORDERS OF CARBOHYDRATE METABOLISM

### Essential Fructosuria

Essential fructosuria is a rare metabolic disease (1:130,000) that is inherited as an autosomal recessive trait. It is an asymptomatic, harmless condition that is usually suspected by the finding of nonglucose-reducing sugar on routine urinalysis. Definitive diagnosis is made by means of paper chromatography of the urine.

### Hereditary Fructose Intolerance

Hereditary fructose intolerance is an autosomal recessive disease caused by the absence of the enzyme fructose-1-phosphate aldolase in the jejunum. As a result, fructose 1-phosphate accumulates in the liver and in the proximal tubules of the kidney. Hypoglycemia results not from hyperinsulinism but rather from failure of glucose release from the liver cells. Renal damage causes failure of acidification of the urine, as well as albuminuria and aminoaciduria. These derangements of liver and kidney function are reversible.

Clinically, the presenting symptoms are those of hypoglycemia and vomiting after the ingestion of fructose. In infants, the disease may progress to hepatosplenomegaly, failure to thrive, cachexia, and death. If the chronic state occurs, children and adults characteristically avoid sweets and fruits, and their teeth are in excellent condition. Studies reveal normal intelligence in spite of frequent hypoglycemic attacks.

Diagnosis is made by demonstrating marked and prolonged falls in the blood glucose and serum inorganic phosphorus levels during an intravenous fructose tolerance test.

Therapy consists entirely of avoiding fructose in fruits, vegetables, and sucrose-containing foods. Lack of recognition of the large amounts of fructose present in potatoes has resulted in some common failures in treatment. In hospitalized patients, intravenous fluids containing fructose must be avoided.

## Disorders of Galactose Metabolism

Galactosemia is a disturbance of galactose metabolism caused by an enzyme deficiency. The 3 enzymes involved are transferase, which accounts for 90% of cases; galactokinase, which accounts for 10% of cases; and in a newly described variant, epimerase.

In transferase deficiency, the toxicity syndrome is characterized by failure to thrive, vomiting, liver disease, cataracts, and mental retardation. Galactokinase deficiency, which is rarer, is mild and is mainly evidenced by cataracts. Epimerase deficiency involves only red cells, has no associated galactosemia, and is a benign disorder that is detected by screening procedures. The diagnosis is suggested by the detection of galactose in blood and urine and is confirmed by demonstration of enzyme deficiency in the peripheral red cells.

The disorder is treated by avoidance of galactose in foods. Nutramigen and soybean milks are effective substitutes for cow's milk. This diet is not harmful to the body, and it results in a striking regression of signs and symptoms: the cataracts get smaller, liver and renal abnormalities disappear, and growth resumes. Mental retardation, which is usually mild to moderate, is probably not altered.

Genetic studies play a highly significant role in these disorders. Since the heterozygotes can be identified by blood studies and the affected fetus identified by amniotic fluid or fetal blood analysis, a maternal diet free of galactose can be maintained during the pregnancy. In transferase deficiency, Donnell and others have reported 10 normal children and one with cataracts when this diet was used by mothers.

## Idiopathic Lactase Deficiency

Human infants have a high concentration of lactase at birth. This concentration falls rapidly in the first 4–5 years, and in many populations it reaches very low levels in adolescent and adult life. It is deficient in 3–19% of the adult white population, 70% of American blacks, 90% of American Indians, and virtually all Orientals.

Clinically, the characteristic history is that of a patient with a normal diet in infancy and childhood who begins to dislike or avoid milk in adolescence or adulthood. The symptoms range from bloating and flatulence to crampy abdominal pain and diarrhea. Repeated oral sugar tolerance tests are useful, but confirmation of the diagnosis requires demonstration of the enzyme deficiency by means of intestinal biopsy. Withdrawal of dietary lactose causes prompt disappearance of symptoms.

It is important to rule out secondary lactase deficiencies caused by intestinal disorders (eg, irritable colon, sprue, nonspecific intestinal injury, kwashiorkor), since these diseases are treatable.

## Glycogen Storage Diseases (GSD)

Glycogen storage diseases now constitute 12 separate entities, all of which are clinically and biochemically identifiable. Each has deficient activity of specific enzymes involved in the synthesis and degradation of glycogen, causing an accumulation of abnormal glycogen in any or all of the tissues of the liver, heart, skeletal muscle, kidney, and brain. The inheritance pattern is probably autosomal recessive (with the exception of type IXB, which is X-linked recessive).

Clinically, there is a wide range of symptoms and findings, varying from type IIA—which causes death in infancy—to type X—which, without therapy, is found in patients with hepatomegaly. In liver findings, the cardinal feature is hepatomegaly, which can be asymptomatic or associated with hypoglycemia and hyperlipidemia. Cardiac findings are those of a large, failing heart. If muscle involvement is present, there can be marked hypotonia or complaints of muscle pain and cramps on exercise. Kidney changes include bilateral enlargement, renal stones, and symptoms of hyperuricemia, as well as excess excretion of amino acids, phosphate, glucose, and galactose. Central nervous system involvement may include delayed motor and mental development, ataxia, hypotonia, spasticity, rigidity, and death.

Diagnosis, treatment, and prognosis depend on the exact definition of the biochemical defect by tissue evaluation. Many new (and as yet unproved) therapy procedures require precise diagnosis.

Prenatal diagnosis is indicated in types II and IVA, but in types I, II, VI, IX, and X, prenatal diagnosis is probably not indicated, because the conditions are compatible with normal life.

## DISORDERS OF LIPID METABOLISM

### Gaucher's Disease

Gaucher's disease is a lysosomal storage disease caused by a deficiency of the enzyme glucosylceramide β-glucosidase. Its substrate, glycocerebroside, accumulates in phagocytic cells throughout the body, primarily those of the liver, spleen, and bone marrow. The incidence ranges from 1 per 5000 to 1 per 10,000 among Jews of eastern European origin.

Clinically, it presents in 3 forms. The adult form, or type I, is characterized by splenomegaly, hepatomegaly, anemia, thrombocytopenia, and erosion of the cortices of long bones. Some adults may succumb as early as the third decade, but many are symptom-free until the seventh or eighth decade. Neurologic symptoms are rare. In type II, the infantile form, there is pronounced neurologic and little visceral involvement. Symptoms may occur by age 3 months, and death usually occurs by age 2. The third form, type III, or juvenile, has a wide variety of clinical signs and symptoms, including both neurologic and visceral involvement. These patients survive longer than do those with type II. Each clinical type is inherited as an autosomal recessive trait and "breeds true" (ie, is passed to the next generation without alteration).

Laboratory studies reveal an elevated serum acid phosphatase, but definitive diagnosis of this disorder requires the demonstration of a diminished leukocyte $\beta$-glucosidase level (7–15% of normal) or demonstration of Gaucher cells in the bone marrow by electron microscopy. MRI provides an excellent assessment of the degree of involvement in the bone, liver, and spleen in Gaucher's disease.

Treatment is supportive. Splenectomy is indicated only when hypersplenism occurs. Bone marrow transplantation performed in 3 patients resulted in normal enzyme content in the peripheral blood mononuclear cells and gradual disappearance to the abnormal lipid-containing histiocytes in the bone marrow but no enzymatic correction in the central nervous system. Prenatal diagnosis is possible for the 3 types of Gaucher's disease.

Rappaport JM, Barranger JA, Ginns EI: Bone marrow transplantation in Gaucher's disease. *Birth Defects: Original Article Series* 1986;**22**:107.

## Niemann-Pick Disease (Sphingomyelin Lipidosis)

Niemann-Pick disease is a rare autosomal recessive disorder characterized by the excessive storage of phospholipids, especially sphingomyelin, in the reticuloendothelial system. Manifestations occur early in infancy and consist primarily of hepatosplenomegaly and central nervous system involvement, with mental retardation and convulsions. Other symptoms and signs include diffuse pulmonary infiltration, cutaneous lesions, a cherry-red macular spot, gastrointestinal bleeding, lymph node enlargement, thrombocytopenia, anemia, and foam cells in hepatic or marrow biopsies. Definitive diagnosis is established by demonstrating sphingomyelinase deficiency in white blood cells and cultured skin fibroblasts.

Treatment is supportive. Death usually occurs during childhood. Prenatal diagnosis is possible.

## $G_{M2}$ Gangliosidoses (Tay-Sachs Disease)

Tay-Sachs disease is an autosomal recessive disease that is clinically apparent by age 5–6 months and invariably leads to death by age 3–4 years. The enzyme hexosaminidase A is absent, resulting in an accumulation of $G_{M2}$ ganglioside in the ganglion cells. The destruction of the ganglion cells is accompanied by glial proliferation and myelin degeneration. Clinically, psychomotor retardation, hypotonia, dementia, and blindness (associated with a cherry-red spot on the retina) occur. There are 2 rare variants, each with the same clinical and pathologic course but with different hexosaminidase defects.

The current application of genetic principles to this disease may well make it a model for genetic counseling for inborn errors of metabolism: the disease occurs primarily in Jews who have emigrated from northeastern Europe. With the advent of blood tests for hexosaminidase activity, discernment of the magnitude of the disease and identification of heterozygotes and affected fetuses are possible. In New York City, the carrier rate in the Jewish population is 1:30 and that in the non-Jewish population 1:300. With the help of synagogues, education and mass screening of this at-risk Jewish population have been undertaken, and genetic counseling has been given to the carriers. No specific therapy is available. Enzyme replacement is not available.

## DISORDERS OF PORPHYRIN METABOLISM

The porphyrins are cyclic compounds that are the precursors of heme and other important enzymes and pigments. Enzymatic defects in the heme synthetic pathways cause a group of disorders, the porphyrias, which may be either hereditary or acquired. These diseases have long been of interest because of their unusual range of clinical symptoms as well as the relative ease of identifying small amounts of porphyrin in the urine. Repeat studies indicate that the diverse clinical symptoms reflect the genetic heterogeneity of the disease.

The porphyrias are classified into 2 main categories, depending on whether the excessive porphyrin production takes place in the liver or in bone marrow. The classification is as follows:

> **Hepatic porphyrias**
> Acute intermittent porphyria
> Variegate porphyria
> Hereditary coproporphyria
> Porphyria cutanea tarda
> **Erythropoietic porphyrias**
> Congenital porphyria
> Erythropoietic protoporphyria

### Hepatic Porphyria

The hepatic porphyrias are a group of chemically and biochemically distinct diseases whose site of abnormal porphyrin metabolism is the liver.

**A. Acute Intermittent Porphyria:** This is an autosomal dominant disease with worldwide distribution. Its biochemical defect, a decrease in uroporphyrinogen-I synthase, seems to be generalized, for it has been reported in liver cells, erythrocytes, fibroblasts, and lymphocytes. The disease is clinically latent throughout adult life in about 90% of the people who inherit the gene defect. For the remaining 10%, the first symptoms occur at puberty or shortly thereafter. Characteristically, intermittent abdominal and neurologic manifestations occur with variable severity. The abdominal symptoms are often the presenting complaint. They may be mild, such as nausea and vomiting and colicky pain, but often they are severe enough to present as acute abdomen without fever or leukocytosis. There may be multiple surgical scars on the abdomen. Neurologic findings are just as variable, including paresthesia, hypesthesia, neuritic pain, wristdrop and footdrop, psychoses, convulsions, and quadriplegia. Significantly, there is no associated cutaneous sensitivity. Four exogenous factors may convert the latent disease to a manifest disease: drugs, steroids, starvation, and infection. The drugs include barbiturates, sulfonamides, and griseofulvin, and the steroids include estrogens. No doubt endogenous factors also play a role in precipitating an attack. Death due to respiratory paralysis may occur in 25% of patients with acute attacks.

Diagnosis is suspected by noting that freshly voided urine left standing in light and air turns dark. Definitive diagnosis is made by demonstrating increased porphobilinogens (PBG) and aminolevulinic acid (ALA) in the urine. A limited number of laboratories are able to demonstrate the enzymatic defect in erythrocytes.

**B. Variegate Porphyria:** This is an autosomal dominant disease first recognized in the Afrikaners of South Africa but now known in people in Sweden, the Netherlands, England, and the USA. Its biochemical defect is a deficiency of protoporphyrinogen oxidase. Clinical symptoms do not appear until the third decade. In addition to acute abdominal and neurologic manifestations such as those that occur in acute intermittent porphyria, cutaneous manifestations also appear, characterized by increased sensitivity of exposed skin to minor mechanical trauma and to light. Barbiturates and sulfonamides can induce the condition. Diagnosis rests on demonstration of continuous excretion of protoporphyrins and coproporphyrins in the feces.

**C. Hereditary Coproporphyria:** This autosomal dominant disease resembles variegate porphyria in its photosensitivity, abdominal and neurologic manifestations, and exacerbations. However, it is a much milder disease, and latent cases are frequent. The distinction is a biochemical one: in hereditary coproporphyria, there is a steady excretion of large amounts of coproporphyrin in the feces and, to a lesser extent, the urine. The enzymatic defect, a decrease in coproporphyrinogen oxidase, can be demonstrated in erythrocytes.

**D. Porphyria Cutanea Tarda:** Porphyria cutanea tarda, the most common form of porphyria, is an autosomal dominant disease caused by partial defi-

ciency of the enzyme uroporphyrinogen decarboxylase. Family studies indicate it can present as an overt, subclinical, or latent disorder. Although its distribution is worldwide, it is most common among the Bantu of Africa. It occurs more often in males, at middle age, with symptoms limited to the skin. Abdominal and neurologic manifestations do not occur. Photosensitivity is the major clinical finding, but hypertrichosis of the forehead and hyperpigmentation of the exposed skin are also prevalent. Estrogens, busulfan, barbiturates, phenytoin, and tolbutamide can induce the condition. For unknown reasons, all patients have evidence of liver dysfunction. This may be due to concomitant diseases (eg, alcoholic cirrhosis, tuberculosis, intestinal disease) as well as to overproduction of uroporphyrin, which in itself may be toxic to the liver. When the disease is of long duration, there is increased risk of hepatocellular carcinoma. Pathologically, there is hepatic parenchymal iron overload caused by increased saturation of iron-binding protein with iron. Biochemical evaluation indicates increased excretion of uroporphyrins with a variable amount of fecal porphyrins. A new method of measuring plasma porphyrins appears useful in diagnosis as well as in following the effectiveness of therapy.

A toxic form of this disease became apparent in 1956 when there was an explosive outbreak of porphyria in eastern Turkey. The chronic ingestion of hexachlorobenzene, a fungicidal agent used in wheat, inhibited hepatic uroporphyrinogen decarboxylase, thus causing the disease. No genetic factors were involved.

### Erythropoietic Porphyrias

**A. Congenital Porphyria:** Congenital erythropoietic porphyria is a very rare autosomal recessive disease with worldwide distribution. It is caused by an enzyme defect in the erythroid series of the bone marrow that results in an excess deposition of porphyrins in the tissues. Clinically, it presents as a well-defined syndrome in the newborn period or shortly thereafter. There is photosensitivity, erythrodontia (seen most readily with a Wood lamp), and fluctuating red urine that is usually associated with hemolytic anemia. The skin changes, occurring primarily on the hands and face, present as vesicles and bullae and progress to scarring and mutilation. The disease is slowly progressive, and death results from the hemolytic anemia or intercurrent infection. Splenectomy may be effective in decreasing hemolysis. Few patients survive beyond age 40. The clinical diagnosis is confirmed biochemically by demonstrating the porphyrinuria, especially of uroporphyrin I.

**B. Erythropoietic Protoporphyria:** Erythropoietic protoporphyria is an autosomal dominant disease with partial penetrance. Many latent forms exist, and these may be more common. The disease is mild, with clinical manifestations limited to the skin. It appears in childhood or early adolescence as a fluctuating solar urticaria or solar eczema. Intense painful itching, erythema, and edema occur and progress to chronic skin changes, particularly on the hands. Occasionally, there is mild hemolytic anemia. Liver disease due to porphyrin deposition occasionally occurs and may progress to cirrhosis. Cholelithiasis due to precipitated protoporphyrins may be present. Fluorescence microscopy confirms the diagnosis by demonstrating the excess protoporphyrin in the red cells.

## Treatment of Porphyrias

Preventive medicine is the most important feature in the long-term management of patients with porphyria. This includes a careful discussion of precipitating factors as well as information about prenatal diagnosis. Precipitating factors include infection, emotional stress, "crash" diets, and the use of drugs such as alcohol, estrogens, and barbiturates. Women who have acute attacks at the time of menstruation will be helped by contraceptives that prevent ovulation. A recent case report suggested that frequent attacks of porphyria related to the menstrual cycle can be prevented by administration of a long-acting agonist of luteinizing hormone-releasing hormone (LHRH). Patients with photosensitivity should avoid direct sunlight or should use dermatologic sunscreen preparations. The oral sun protective agent β-carotene (Solatene) in doses of 60–180 mg/d is effective.

Symptomatic treatment is important in the management of abdominal and neurologic manifestations. Mild abdominal symptoms can be controlled with the use of chlorpromazine or other phenothiazines; propoxyphene can be used in pain in the extremities; meperidine is effective in severe pain. Propranolol can stop persistent sinus tachycardia. Observation must be continuous, since progressive paralysis can cause respiratory failure, which in turn requires respiratory assistance. Physical therapy should be used to prevent secondary complications of neuropathy.

The acute attack of porphyria should be terminated as quickly as possible to prevent lasting neuronal damage. Hematin is the drug of first choice. At the dosage level of 3–4 mg/kg intravenously, there is a report of a dramatic recovery in 25 of 31 attacks in 20 patients, without any side effects. In 1978, there was a case report of the successful use of hematin prophylactically. Another method—high carbohydrate intake achieved with levulose, 400–500 mg/d intravenously—is also successful in treating acute attacks of porphyria. The clinical response is variable, and a rebound phenomenon with symptoms of a mild acute attack may occur 24–48 hours after infusion. Both hematin and high carbohydrate intake act by suppressing hepatic aminolevulinic synthase, thus reducing the overproduction of δ-aminolevulinic acid and porphobilinogen.

Recent isolated case reports indicate that large doses of propranolol also can be effective therapy for acute porphyria.

In cutaneous erythropoietic porphyria, hematin therapy, with its marked repressive effect on porphyrin synthesis, has produced remissions lasting several years. Splenectomy, which is helpful in the management of hemolytic anemia, may also reduce photosensitivity and porphyrin excretion.

In porphyria cutanea tarda, weekly venesections of 300–500 mL for 6 months usually result in clinical improvement that may last for months or years. It is postulated that the benefit may result either from (1) hemoglobin depletion, which may stimulate hemoglobin production by intermediate metabolites; or (2) depletion of iron stores. An alternative method of treatment consisting of chloroquine in small doses (100 mg twice weekly) results in clinical and biochemical remission in 6–12 months. At this dosage, there are usually no side effects. In some cases, plasmapheresis has been effective.

In erythropoietic protoporphyria, 3 patients who were treated with plasmapheresis and red cell exchange transfusion had prolonged clinical and biochemical remissions. Early recognition of liver disease in protoporphyria is important, for it may prove fatal. Cholestyramine, 4 g 3 times daily before meals, may reverse hepatic disease by binding protoporphyrin in the intestines and interrupting its enterohepatic circulation.

Abramowicz M (editor): Hemin infusions in acute intermittent porphyria. *Med Lett Drugs Ther* (April 13) 1984;**26**:42.

Anderson KE et al: Prevention of cyclical attacks of acute intermittent porphyria with a long acting agonist of luteinizing hormone-releasing hormone. *N Engl J Med* 1984;**311**:643.

Sekula SA, Tschen JA, Rosen T: The porphyrias. *Am Fam Physician* 1986;**33**:219.

Spiva DA et al: Erythropoietic protoporphyria: Therapeutic response to combined erythrocyte exchange and plasmapheresis. *Photodermatol* 1984;**1**:211.

# OTHER METABOLIC DISORDERS

## Cystic Fibrosis

Cystic fibrosis of the pancreas is one of the common inherited diseases among whites of European ancestry. This autosomal recessive disease has an incidence of 1:1500 white births and 1:17,000 black births in the USA. Its unknown defect involves all exocrine glands, causing high-protein, highly viscous secretions that readily obstruct the ducts of the body. These obstructions cause the major clinical manifestations of the disease.

Initially, cystic fibrosis was recognized only in infants and children, in whom it presented as meconium ileus in the newborn period or as chronic pulmonary and gastrointestinal disease in growth-retarded children. With the improvement of diagnostic tests, as well as with vigorous treatment, patients are now alive and functioning well in their mid 40s.

The major clinical signs and symptoms involve the gastrointestinal and pulmonary tracts. Pancreatic insufficiency with steatorrhea and azotorrhea is present in 95% of patients, but in adults, in contrast to children, it is rarely symptomatic. Twenty-five percent of adults have a meconium ileus equivalent (abnormal fecal accumulation) causing partial intestinal obstruction and intussusception. Generalized biliary cirrhosis, cholelithiasis (12%), and rectal prolapse may occur. These gastrointestinal complications contribute to the malnutrition and growth retardation in pediatric patients.

It is the disease in the pulmonary tract, however, that determines the life of the patient. It occurs in 97% of patients and is the major cause of morbidity and mortality. The tenacious secretions and their secondary infections cause sinusitis, chronic bronchitis, recurrent pneumonias, bronchiectasis, hyperaeration, and cor pulmonale. Nasal polyposis is a frequent finding (20–30%) but rarely requires therapy. Elsewhere, the sweat glands—with increased sodium and chloride secretion—can cause a depletion syndrome, especially in hot weather. The salt in the sweat may have a corrosive effect on metal and leather ornaments and clothing in direct contact with the skin. With respect to the reproductive tract, women can be fertile, whereas all affected men are sterile; atresia of the vas deferens and an abnormality in the exocrine glands cause sterility in the presence of spermatogenesis. Women who do not have pancreatic insufficiency tolerate pregnancy without undue hazard. Those with pancreatic insufficiency may have permanent deterioration of pulmonary function. Less common clinical manifestations are mono- or polyarticular arthropathy (8%) of the large joints and secondary amyloidoses (3 cases).

Diagnosis is readily and easily made in the presence of clinical symptoms by finding sodium and chloride concentrations greater than 60 meq/L in sweat induced by pilocarpine iontophoresis. The specimen should be 125–375 mg (average, 250 mg); a sweat sample of less than 40 mg is inadequate for accurate assay.

It is currently thought that the primary defect in cystic fibrosis is linked to the inability of chloride ions to cross the specialized epithelial cells of the exocrine glands, with the secondary effect that sodium ions fail to be resorbed. The clinical result and expression in the patient depend on the basic function of each organ involved. For example, in the skin there is increased sodium in the sweat. In other organs, the effects on basic function are still unclear.

Therapy should be vigorous and continuous, for recent studies have shown that adequately treated adult patients can have a successful intellectual, socioeconomic, and marital life. A high-calorie, low-fat diet with multivitamin supplementation is necessary, since absorption is incomplete. The adequate dose of pancreatic enzyme replacement (Cotazyme, Viokase) is determined by the clinical response of a good growth pattern, an improvement in stool consistency, and a decrease in the number of bowel movements. If the enzyme replacements are given with cimetidine, 20 mg/kg body weight/24 h, or sodium bicarbonate, 15 g/m$^2$/24 h, there is a significant decrease in fat and nitrogen excretion, presumably due to the prevention of acid-peptide destruction of the pancreatic enzymes in the stomach. A new form of pancrelipase supplement, enteric-coated microspheres in a gelatin capsule (Pancrease), passes intact through the stomach to the intestines, where it enhances fat absorption and allows a more normal diet. The daily average dose is about 5 tablets. The treatment of meconium ileus is, of course, surgical. The intussusception and fecal accumulation in adults require enemas of diatrizoate sodium (Gastrografin or Hypaque). Supplementary salt is needed, especially during hot weather, febrile episodes, and physical exertion; adults require over 4 g/d. For the respiratory tract, attention is directed to adequate drainage and prevention of infection. Adequate hydration, daily pulmonary percussion and drainage, bronchodilators, expectorants, and daily antibiotics are used in management. Patients with thick, tenacious sputum can use acetylcysteine (Mucomyst) for treatment, but this agent should not be used for prophylaxis. Many medical centers prescribe mist tents, but the efficacy of this method has not yet been proved. Recently, it has been noted that there is a need to avoid general anesthetics because subsequently there is degeneration of lung function. In managing the many complications of cystic fibrosis, a positive therapeutic environment should be provided in order to minimize the patient's anxiety and depression.

Prenatal diagnosis can be offered to affected families. For mothers with a known polymorphism near the cystic fibrosis locus on chromosome 7, prenatal diagnosis is by DNA analysis of chorionic villus samples. Otherwise, measurement of multiple enzymes—alkaline phosphatase (total and isoenzymes), aminopeptidase M, and γ-glutamyl transpeptidase—in the amniotic fluid at the 17th–19th weeks of pregnancy permits a 98% accurate diagnosis.

Boué JF: Prenatal diagnosis in 200 pregnancies with a 1–4 risk of cystic fibrosis. *Hum Genet* 1986;**74**:288.

Davis PB, di Sant'Agnese PA: Cystic fibrosis: Diagnosis and treatment: An update. *Chest* 1984;**85**:6.

Price JF: The need to avoid general anaesthesia in cystic fibrosis. *J R Soc Med* 1986;**79(Suppl 12)**:10.

Travis WD et al: Secondary (AA) amyloidosis in cystic fibrosis: A report of three cases. *Am J Clin Path* 1986;**85**:419.

## Primary Hyperoxaluria

Primary hyperoxaluria is an autosomal recessive disease characterized by continuous excessive synthesis of oxalic acid, leading to increased excretion of oxalates in the urine as well as to deposition of calcium oxalate in the tissues, especially the kidneys, synovia, and myocardium. Biochemically, there are 2 types, each with its own enzyme defect; clinically, they are indistinguishable.

The disease presents in childhood, usually before age 5 years. There is either asymptomatic gross hematuria or typical renal colic due to calcium oxalate stones. Rarely, there are symptoms of renal tubular acidosis. The clinical course is one of progressive renal insufficiency, leading to death by age 20 years.

Extrarenal manifestations are arthritis and cardiac disease. The disease can be simulated in animals and humans by pyridoxine deficiency.

Diagnosis depends on demonstration of excess renal oxalic acid excretion (normal, 60 mg of oxalic acid/1.73 m$^2$) in the absence of pyridoxine deficiency and ileal disease. The 2 types of the disease can be distinguished by measuring the amounts of glyoxylic, glycolic, and L-glyceric acid in the urine.

There is at present no specific treatment for hyperoxaluria. Pyridoxine, 2–200 mg daily, can markedly reduce oxalate excretion. The wide range of effective pyridoxine doses probably means that the patients who respond to low doses are either taking multivitamin tablets or are eating a diet rich in pyridoxine. Thiazide diuretics, eg, bendroflumethiazide, 2.5–5 mg daily, are helpful in stone prophylaxis, because they decrease the Ca:Mg ratio. All measures that reduce the risk of renal stones should be used, including forced fluids, a high-phosphate regimen, oral magnesium oxide, and allopurinol. Dietary restriction of oxalates has little effect on urinary oxalate excretion. Terminal renal failure is managed by chronic hemodialysis. In most cases, renal transplantation has not been successful, because oxalate crystals quickly accumulate in the transplanted kidney. There are rare cases of 3-year survivals. All siblings should be screened for hyperoxaluria, because early treatment of asymptomatic patients decreases the morbidity of the disease.

Yendt ER, Cohanim M: Response to a physiologic dose of pyridoxine in type 1 primary hyperoxaluria. *N Engl J Med* 1985;**312**:953.

## Marfan's Syndrome

Marfan's syndrome is a generalized disorder of the connective tissue, inherited as an autosomal dominant trait. In its classic form, it has a prevalence of 4–6 cases per 100,000 population, with no racial or ethnic predeliction. Its biochemical basis remains unknown. Clinically, it is manifested in the skeletal system, the eye, and the cardiovascular system, but in a given case there is such great variability in clinical expression that manifestations may not be present in all 3 systems.

The skeletal system characteristically shows extraordinarily long tubular bones, causing arachnodactyly and anomalous skeletal proportions. The patient is usually taller than might be expected on the basis of age and family background, but the excessive length of the arms and legs in relation to the trunk is even more indicative. Other skeletal anomalies include "tower skull," kyphoscoliosis, hyperextensibility of the joints, and genu recurvatum.

In the eye, 50–80% of the patients have lens dislocation that is bilateral, probably occurs in utero, and rarely progresses. Myopia and detached retinas are also described.

An elastin abnormality accounts for the weakness of the aortic media, leading to aortic regurgitation or aortic dilatation or dissection. Prolapse of the posterior mitral valve leaflet is present in 80% of cases. All patients are at risk for endocarditis.

Treatment is directed at the cardiovascular problems, for they account for 95% of the deaths. Echocardiography is the most sensitive means of detecting early aortic changes. Patients are examined yearly to follow the course of the slow but progressive aortic dilation. In adults, when the aortic diameter reaches 5.5 cm, the life-threatening complications of aortic rupture—dissection or aortic regurgitation—may occur. At this point, MRI is used to follow patients, for it allows more extensive visualization of the aorta. Prophylactic repair of the ascending aorta is now performed with a mortality rate of less than 10%. In addition, aortic valves have been successfully replaced. Medical management involves treatment with propranolol or reserpine to reduce the abruptness of ventricular ejection in the hope of protecting the aorta. With skeletal defects, treatment is primarily for scoliosis, which is the most deforming and disabling complication. Eyes are examined annually to diagnose refractive errors, prevent amblyopia, and detect early retinal detachment. The lens rarely requires removal.

Women with Marfan's syndrome have an increased rate of early spontaneous abortions. If patients have minimal cardiovascular disease, the risk of maternal death is low, but patients with preexisting aortic regurgitation, aortic root dilatation, or other severe cardiovascular disease have a significant risk of death from aortic dissection. Counseling regarding pregnancy risk requires evaluation of cardiovascular status, including echocardiographic determination of aortic root diameter.

In 1979, before cardiovascular surgery was available, the average survival age was 32 years. Survivors aged 82 years have also been reported.

Pyeritz RE: The Marfan syndrome. *Am Fam Physician* (June) 1986;**34**:83.
Pyeritz RE: Maternal and fetal complications of pregnancy in the Marfan's disease. *Am J Med* 1981;**71**:784.

## REFERENCES
### (For additional references, see Chapter 20.)

Fraser FC, Nora JJ: *Genetics of Man,* 2nd ed. Lea & Febiger, 1986.
Garrod AE: *Inborn Errors in Metabolism.* Oxford Univ Press, 1963.

Garver KL, Marchese SG: *Genetic Counseling for Clinicians.* Year Book, 1986.
Goodman RM, Gorlin RJ: *Atlas of the Face in Genetic Disorders,* 2nd ed. Mosby, 1977.

Harris H, Hirschhorn K (editors): *Advances in Human Genetics*. Plenum Press. [Annual.]

Kelley T: *Clinical Genetics and Genetic Counseling*. Year Book, 1986.

Porter IH, Hatcher NH (editors): *Prenatal Genetic Diagnosis and Treatment*. Academic Press, 1986.

*Prenatal Diagnosis*. [All issues; publication began in Jan 1981.]

Roman HL et al (editors): *Annual Review of Genetics*. Annual Reviews, Inc. [Annual.]

Smith DW: *Recognizable Patterns of Human Malformation*, 3rd ed. Saunders, 1982.

Stanbury JB et al (editors): *The Metabolic Basis of Inherited Disease*, 5th ed. McGraw-Hill, 1983.

Steinberg AG, Bearn AG: *Progress in Medical Genetics*. Grune & Stratton. [Annual.]

Thompson MW: *Genetics in Medicine*. Saunders, 1986.

Weatherall DJ: *The New Genetics and Clinical Practice*, 2nd ed. Oxford Univ Press, 1986.

# Malignant Disorders

*Sydney E. Salmon, MD*

The major features of this chapter are clinical aspects of cancer, including (1) unusual symptoms and syndromes that may be important in the diagnosis and management of cancer, (2) the diagnosis and treatment of emergency problems and complications of cancer, (3) the role of surgery and radiotherapy in primary cancer treatment, (4) cancer chemotherapy for advanced disease, and (5) adjuvant chemotherapy for micrometastases of primary cancers.

## THE PARANEOPLASTIC SYNDROMES

The clinical manifestations of cancer are usually due to pressure effects of local tumor growth; to infiltration or metastatic deposition of tumor cells in a variety of organs in the body; or to certain systemic symptoms. Except in the case of functioning tumors such as those of the endocrine glands, systemic symptoms of cancer usually are not specific, often consisting of weakness, anorexia, and weight loss. In the paraneoplastic syndromes, clinical findings may resemble those of primary endocrine, metabolic, hematologic, or neuromuscular disorders. At present, the mechanisms for such remote effects can be classed in 3 groups: (1) effects initiated by a tumor product (eg, carcinoid syndrome), (2) effects of destruction of normal tissues by tumor (eg, hypercalcemia with osteolytic skeletal metastases), and (3) effects due to unknown mechanisms (eg, osteoarthropathy with bronchogenic carcinoma). In paraneoplastic syndromes associated with ectopic hormone production, tumor tissue itself secretes the hormone that produces the syndrome. Ectopic hormones secreted by neoplasms are often "prohormones" of higher molecular weight than those secreted by the more differentiated normal endocrine cell. Autocrine growth factors secreted by neoplastic cells may also result in paraneoplastic syndromes.

The paraneoplastic syndromes are of considerable clinical importance for the following reasons:

(1) They sometimes accompany relatively limited neoplastic growth and may provide the clinician with an early clue to the presence of certain types of cancer. In some cases, early diagnosis may favorably affect the prognosis.

(2) The pathologic (metabolic or toxic) effects of the syndrome may constitute a more urgent hazard to the patient's life than the underlying cancer (eg, hypercalcemia, hyponatremia).

(3) Effective treatment of the tumor should be accompanied by resolution of the paraneoplastic syndrome, and, conversely, recurrence of the cancer may be heralded by return of the systemic symptoms. In some instances, rapid response to cytotoxic chemotherapy may briefly increase the severity of the paraneoplastic syndrome in association with tumor lysis (eg, hyponatremia with inappropriate antidiuretic hormone excretion). In some instances the identical symptom complex (eg, hypercalcemia) may be induced by entirely different mechanisms. Hypercalcemia may be due to secretions of parathyroid hormone, an osteoclast-activating factor, lymphotoxin, alpha tumor growth factor, prostaglandins, or other hormone secretion by the tumor or to direct invasion of the skeleton by metastases. In each situation, effective antitumor treatment usually results in return of serum calcium to normal, although supportive measures may also be of benefit.

Common paraneoplastic syndromes and endocrine secretions associated with functional cancers are summarized in Table 32–1.

List AF et al: The syndrome of inappropriate secretion of antidiuretic hormone (SIADH) in small cell lung cancer. *J Clin Oncol* 1986;**4**:1191.

## MANAGEMENT OF EMERGENCIES & COMPLICATIONS OF MALIGNANT DISEASE

Cancer is a chronic disease, but acute emergency complications may occur as a consequence of local accumulations of tumor (spinal cord compression, superior vena cava syndrome, malignant effusions, etc) or of more generalized systemic effects of cancer (hypercalcemia, opportunistic infections, disseminated intravascular coagulation, hyperuricemia, etc). Effective treatment of such complications is one of the most important aspects of management of the patient with advanced cancer.

**Table 32–1.** Paraneoplastic syndromes and certain endocrine secretions associated with cancer.

| Hormone Excess or Syndrome | Broncho-genic Carci-noma | Breast Carci-noma | Renal Carci-noma | Adrenal Carci-noma | Hepa-toma | Multiple Myeloma | Lym-phoma | Thy-moma | Prostatic Carci-noma | Pan-creatic Carci-noma | Chorio-carci-noma |
|---|---|---|---|---|---|---|---|---|---|---|---|
| Hypercalcemia | ++ | ++++ | ++ | ++ | + | ++++ | + | + | ++ | + | + |
| Cushing's syndrome | +++ | | + | +++ | | | | ++ | + | ++ | |
| Inappropriate ADH secretion | +++ | | | | | | + | | | + | |
| Hypoglycemia | | | | + | ++ | | + | | | | |
| Gonadotropins | + | | | | + | | | | | | ++++ |
| Thyrotropin | | | | | | | | | | | +++ |
| Polycythemia | | | +++ | + | ++ | | | | | | |
| Erythroid aplasia | | | | | | | | ++ | | | |
| Fever | | | +++ | | ++ | | +++ | ++ | | + | |
| Neuro-myopathy | ++ | + | | | | | | ++ | + | + | |
| Derma-tomyositis | ++ | + | | | | | | | | + | |
| Coagulopathy | + | ++ | | | + | + | | | +++ | +++ | |
| Thrombophle-bitis | | | + | | | | | | + | +++ | |
| Immunologic deficiency | | | | | | +++ | +++ | +++ | | | |

# SPINAL CORD COMPRESSION

Spinal cord compression by tumor mass is manifested by back pain, progressive weakness and sensory changes in the lower extremities, and blockage of contrast material as shown by myelography. It occurs as a complication of lymphoma or multiple myeloma, carcinomas of the lung, prostate, breast, and colon, and certain other neoplasms. Back pain at the level of the lesion occurs in over 80% of cases and may be aggravated by lying down, weight bearing, sneezing, or coughing; it usually precedes the development of neurologic symptoms or signs. Since involvement is usually epidural, a mixture of nerve root and spinal cord symptoms often develops.

The initial findings of impending cord compression may be quite subtle, and there should be a high index of suspicion when cancer patients develop back pain or weakness of the lower extremities. Prompt diagnosis and therapy are essential to prevent permanent spinal cord damage. Once paralysis develops, it is irreversible, whereas patients who are treated promptly may have complete return of function and may respond favorably to subsequent anticancer therapy.

While bone radiographs usually show evidence of vertebral metastases, they are not a substitute for myelography. However, magnetic resonance imaging (MRI) appears to offer an excellent noninvasive alternative to the myelogram and provides sagittal images of the entire spinal cord and vertebral canal. When the symptoms or neurologic examination are at all suggestive of a diagnosis of cord compression, an emergency CT myelogram or MRI scan should be performed. If a block is demonstrated on myelography, additional contrast is injected above the lesions, because of a tendency toward multiple lesions.

**Emergency treatment:** Radiation therapy to the involved area of the block and 2 adjacent vertebrae above and below represents the treatment of choice. The addition of chemotherapy is occasionally of use in treating lymphomas. Emergency surgery is indicated if there is doubt about the cause of the block or if the patient has failed previous radiation therapy.

Aside from this, decompression laminectomy is indicated only in patients with extremely rapid progression of signs and symptoms.

Rodicho LD et al: Early diagnosis of spinal epidural metastases. *Am J Med* 1981;**70**:1181.

# SUPERIOR VENA CAVA SYNDROME

Superior vena cava syndrome is a potentially fatal complication of bronchogenic carcinoma, lymphomas, and certain other neoplasms that metastasize to the mediastinum. It is characterized by brawny edema and flushing of the head and neck and dilated neck and arm veins, and it often develops gradually over 2–3 weeks. Partial syndromes may result from subclavian vein obstruction. The onset of symptoms is acute or subacute. Venous pressure in the upper extremities is increased, and bilateral brachial venography or sodium pertechnetate Tc 99m scanning demonstrates a block to the flow of contrast material into the right heart as well as large collateral veins. Although the underlying carcinoma is usually incurable when the condition develops, emergency therapy for this syndrome can provide effective palliation for prolonged periods of time (particularly in small-cell carcinoma). Treatment is sometimes indicated even when the diagnosis of cancer has not been confirmed histologically, since the syndrome is almost always due to cancer, and thoracotomy or mediastinoscopy may lead to death.

**Emergency treatment** consists of (1) intravenous administration of cyclophosphamide (1 g/m$^2$) through a central venous catheter or a lower extremity vein (to initiate tumor shrinkage); (2) intravenous injection of a potent parenteral diuretic (eg, ethacrynic acid) to relieve the edematous component of vena caval compression; and (3) mediastinal irradiation, starting within 24 hours, with a treatment plan designed to give a high daily dose but a short total course of therapy to rapidly shrink the local tumor even further. Intensive combined therapy will palliate the process in up to 90% of patients. In patients with a subacute presentation, radiation therapy alone usually suffices.

The ultimate prognosis depends on the nature of the primary neoplasm. Even in bronchochogenic carcinoma—other than small cell—occasional patients have slowly growing tumors that may not cause further symptoms for considerable periods of time.

Sculier JP, Feld R: Superior vena cava obstruction syndrome: Recommendations for management. *Cancer Treat Rev* 1985;**12**:209.

## MALIGNANT EFFUSIONS

The development of effusions in closed compartments such as the pleural, pericardial, and peritoneal spaces presents significant diagnostic and therapeutic problems in patients with advanced neoplasms. Most effusions due to cancer do not require emergency intervention, but they do if they accumulate rapidly or occur in the pericardial space. Direct involvement (thickening) of the serous surface with tumor appears to be the most frequent initiating factor in such cases. Benign processes such as congestive heart failure, pulmonary embolus, trauma, and infection (eg, tuberculosis) may be responsible, mimicking the effects of a neoplasm. Bloody effusions are usually due to cancer but occasionally are due to embolus with infarction or trauma. Chylous effusions may be associated with thoracic duct obstruction or may result from mediastinal lymph node enlargement in lymphoma. Cytologic or cell block examination of the fluid—or hook needle biopsy (eg, with the Cope pleural biopsy

needle)—should be used to prove that the effusion is truly neoplastic in origin before local therapy is used to prevent recurrence. Pericardial effusions should be tapped with continuous electrocardiographic monitoring or, alternatively, with the aid of ultrasonic localization. Pericardiocentesis is ideally carried out in a cardiac catheterization laboratory.

The management of effusions should be appropriate to the severity of involvement. Effusions due to lung, ovarian, and breast carcinoma often require more than simple drainage. Drainage of a large pleural effusion can be accomplished rapidly and with relative safety with a closed system using a disposable phlebotomy set connected to a vacuum phlebotomy bottle after the needle has been passed through the skin of the thorax. Thoracentesis performed in this fashion requires very little manipulation of the patient and prevents inadvertent pneumothorax associated with multiple changes of a stopcock connected to a syringe. Ultrasonography facilitates localization and removal of small or loculated effusions. For recurrent effusions, closed water-seal drainage with a chest tube for 3–4 days is an effective way to seal off the pleural space. Posttap radiographs are always indicated after thoracentesis to assess the results and rule out pneumothorax.

Recurrent effusions that do not respond to repeated taps or a chest tube may often be controlled by instillation of tetracycline, bleomycin, quinacrine, or mechlorethamine. The alkylating agent thiotepa and the antibiotic bleomycin appear to be preferable for suppression of malignant ascites, since they produce less local pain and discomfort in the peritoneum than do other agents.

The procedure is as follows: Most of the pleural, ascitic, or pericardial fluid is withdrawn. While a free flow of fluid is still present, tetracycline (200 mg), mechlorethamine (20–30 mg), thiotepa (30 mg), or bleomycin (60 mg) is instilled into the cavity. The solution should be freshly mixed at the time of injection. After the drug is injected and the needle withdrawn, the patient is placed in a variety of positions in order to distribute the drug throughout the cavity. On the following day, the remaining fluid is withdrawn from the body cavity. Inasmuch as at least half of the instilled drug is absorbed systemically from the cavity, use of alkylating agents is not advised for patients who already have significant pancytopenia or bone marrow depression due to chemotherapy. In such cases, bleomycin, quinacrine, or tetracycline is indicated, as these agents do not depress the bone marrow. Quinacrine is usually administered in a dose of 200 mg/d for 5 days, with daily drainage of residual fluid. Two or more daily doses of tetracycline are also frequently required.

Nausea and vomiting commonly follow the instillation of mechlorethamine but can often be controlled with prophylactic administration of an antiemetic agent prior to the procedure and at intervals afterward. Pleural pain and fever may occur after intracavitary administration of alkylating agents, tetracycline, or quinacrine but are more common with the latter compounds. Narcotic analgesics may be necessary. Bleomycin instillation may cause fever but generally is unassociated with significant toxicity. Recent tumor cloning studies have shown that when cytotoxic anticancer drugs are instilled locally and lead to resolution of malignant effusions, they are generally exerting a specific cytotoxic effect. Far higher local concentrations of these drugs are attained than when they are administered systemically. Such effusions can also act as "sanctuaries" in which viable tumor stem cells are protected from systemic chemotherapy. Once a pleural space or other potential space has been effectively sealed with such drug treatments, recurrent effusion is usually not a problem.

Hausheer FH, Yarboro JW: Diagnosis and treatment of malignant pleural effusion. *Semin Oncol* 1985;**12**:54.

## HYPERCALCEMIA

Hypercalcemia secondary to cancer is a fairly common medical emergency, particularly in breast carcinoma and multiple myeloma but also with a variety of other cancers. Bone metastasis is not an essential feature of the syndrome. Typical findings in addition to elevated serum calcium are anorexia, nausea and vomiting, constipation, polyuria, muscular weakness and hyporeflexia, confusion, psychosis, tremor, and lethargy; some patients are asymptomatic. Electrocardiography often shows a shortening of the QT interval. When the serum calcium rises above 12 mg/dL, sudden death due to cardiac arrhythmia or asystole may occur. The presence of hypercalcemia does not invariably indicate a dismal prognosis, especially in breast or prostate cancer.

In the absence of signs or symptoms of hypercalcemia, a laboratory report of elevated serum calcium should be repeated immediately to exclude the possibility of error.

Emergency treatment consists of (1) intravenous fluids, 3–4 L daily (starting with saline); (2) intravenous administration of a potent diuretic (such as furosemide) once saline infusion has been initiated and the volume status normalized; (3) prednisone, 60–80 mg/d orally for 4–5 days, followed by tapering; and (5) for severe hypercalcemia (> 15 mg/dL) or refractory cases, mithramycin (Mithracin), 25 µg/kg intravenously every other day for 2–4 doses. Although mithramycin therapy is often effective, the drug has significant toxicities, including potential hemorrhagic syndrome. Since only a limited number of doses are required, these complications are unlikely to occur. Mithramycin therapy should therefore be considered as part of the initial management of severe hypercalcemia and as an adjunctive agent in milder cases (see p 38). Most recently, there has been interest in use of the diphosphonates for the treatment of this complication.

Once the acute hypercalcemic episode has been treated, it is usually appropriate to begin systemic chemotherapy. In the case of breast cancer, hypercalcemia may appear as a "flare" after initiation of estrogen or antiestrogen therapy. Recent evidence suggests that when flares occurring after antiestrogen therapy are suppressed with analgesics and hypocalcemic agents, the patient will often achieve excellent remission with continued therapy. If chronic hypercalcemia persists—even if only to a moderate degree—the patient should be treated with small doses of prednisone alone or with calcitonin or oral sodium phosphate supplements (1–2 g/d) and encouraged to maintain a high fluid intake in the hope of preventing renal damage. When phosphate is used, if no alternative source of phosphate is available, disposable Fleet's Phospho-Soda enemas can be given orally. Intravenous sodium phosphate infusions are not advisable, since they are associated with extreme danger of metastatic calcification in addition to the hypernatremic effects. Chronic hypercalcemia that is refractory to the above measures can sometimes be managed with once-weekly mithramycin injection, 25 µg/kg intravenously. In most instances, when the cancer responds to chemotherapy, hypercalcemia subsides.

Insogna KL, Broadus AE: Hypercalcemia of malignancy. *Annu Rev Med* 1987;**38**:241.
Mundy GR et al: The hypercalcemia of cancer: Clinical implications and pathogenic mechanisms. *N Engl J Med* 1984;**310**:1718.

## HYPERURICEMIA & ACUTE URATE NEPHROPATHY

Increased blood levels of uric acid are often observed in patients with neoplasms who are receiving cancer chemotherapy. In this circumstance, hyperuricemia should be viewed as a preventable complication rather than as an acute emergency, inasmuch as uric acid formation can be inhibited with allopurinol. At present, hyperuricemia is most often a complication of treatment for hematologic neoplasms such as leukemia, lymphoma, and myeloma, but it may occur with any form of cancer that undergoes rapid destruction and release of nucleic acid constituents, and in some instances allopurinol will not have been given. Less commonly, certain rapidly proliferating neoplasms with a high nucleic acid turnover (eg, acute leukemia) may present with hyperuricemia even in the absence of prior chemotherapy. If the patient is also receiving a thiazide diuretic, the problem may be compounded by decreased urate excretion. Initial follow-up of patients receiving cancer chemotherapy should include measurements of serum uric acid and creatinine as well as complete blood counts. Rapid elevation of the serum uric acid concentration usually does not produce gouty arthritis in these patients but does present the danger of acute urate nephropathy. In this form of acute renal failure, uric acid crystallizes in the distal tubules, the collecting ducts, and the renal parenchyma. The danger of uric acid nephropathy is present when the serum urate concentration is above 15 mg/dL.

Prophylactic therapy consists of giving allopurinol, 100 mg orally 3 times daily, starting 1 day before initiation of chemotherapy. Allopurinol inhibits xanthine oxidase and prevents conversion of the highly soluble hypoxanthine and xanthine to the relatively insoluble uric acid. Patients who are to receive the purine antagonists mercaptopurine or azathioprine for cancer chemotherapy should be given only 25–35% of the calculated dose if they are also receiving allopurinol, inasmuch as the latter drug potentiates both the effects and toxicity of these drugs.

Emergency therapy for established severe hyperuricemia consists of (1) hydration with 2–4 L of fluid per day; (2) alkalinization of the urine with 6–8 g of sodium bicarbonate per day (to enhance urate solubility); (3) allopurinol, 200 mg 4 times daily orally; and (4) in severe cases, with serum urate levels above 25–30 mg/dL, emergency hemodialysis.

Since patients who suffer from this complication are often entering a stage of complete remission of the neoplasm, the prognosis is good if renal damage can be prevented.

## BACTERIAL SEPSIS IN CANCER PATIENTS

Many patients with disseminated neoplasms have increased susceptibility to infection. In some instances, this results from impaired host defense mechanisms (eg, acute leukemia, Hodgkin's disease, multiple myeloma, chronic lymphocytic leukemia); in others, it results from the myelosuppressive and immunosuppressive effects of cancer chemotherapy or a combination of these factors. In patients with acute leukemia and in those with granulocytopenia (< 600 granulocytes per microliter), infection is a medical emergency. Although fever alone does not prove the presence of infection, in these patients as well as in patients with multiple myeloma or chronic lymphocytic leukemia, it is highly suggestive. While infections in patients with myeloma or chronic leukemia are often due to sensitive organisms, patients with leukemia or pancytopenia are less fortunate, as resistant gram-negative organisms are more often responsible. Appropriate cultures (eg, blood, sputum, urine, cerebrospinal fluid) should always be obtained before starting therapy; however, one should not wait for results of these studies before initiating bactericidal antibiotic therapy. Gram-stained smears may show a predominant organism in sputum, urine, or cerebrospinal fluid.

### Emergency Treatment

In the absence of granulocytopenia and in nonleukemic patients, the combination of a third-generation cephalosporin with an aminoglycoside (tobramycin or gentamicin) has proved useful for patients with acute bacteremia. In the current era of intensive chemotherapy of acute leukemia, *Pseudomonas* bacteremia is the most frequent infection in granulocytopenic patients and may be fulminant and fatal within 72 hours. Initial treatment of febrile patients with acute leukemia and granulocytopenia should thus consist of 3 drugs: a cephalosporin, an aminoglycoside such as tobramycin, and an antipseudomonal beta-lactam antibiotic. Amphotericin B should be considered if the patient does not respond. If a causative organism is isolated, the combination is replaced with the best agent or agents; otherwise, the combination is continued until the infection has resolved.

Methods to reduce or eliminate granulocytopenia induced by cytotoxic drugs are currently being evaluated. These include the use of autologous bone marrow transplantation as well as evaluation of several new recombinant biologic products. The new biologicals, granulocyte colony-stimulating factor (GCSF) and granulocyte-macrophage colony-stimulating factor (GMCSF), directly stimulate human bone marrow progenitors to proliferate and cause leukocytosis. Several years of clinical investigation will be required to define the use of these exciting new agents.

Beutler SM et al: Preventing infection in neutropenic cancer patients. (Specialty conference.) *West J Med* 1983;**138**:690.

Higby DJ, Burnett D: Granulocyte transfusions: Current status. *Blood* 1980;**55**:2.

Kolata G: Research News: Clinical promise with new hormones. *Science* 1987;**236**:517.

## CARCINOID SYNDROME

Although tumors of argentaffin cells are rare and usually slow-growing, they synthesize and secrete a variety of vasoactive materials, including serotonin, histamine, catecholamines, prostaglandins, and vasoactive peptides. Carcinoid tumors usually arise from the ileum, stomach, or bronchi and tend to metastasize early; in most patients with small intestinal carcinoid tumors, development of the syndrome requires hepatic metastases.

The manifestations of carcinoid syndrome include facial flushing, edema of the head and neck (especially severe with bronchial carcinoid), abdominal cramps and diarrhea, asthmatic symptoms, cardiac lesions (pulmonary or tricuspid stenosis or insufficiency), telangiectases, and increased urinary 5-hydroxyindoleacetic acid (5-HIAA). Very severe acute symptoms occur in patients with bronchial carcinoids, beginning with disorientation and tremulousness followed by fever and flushing episodes that may last 3 or 4 days. Hypotension and pulmonary edema have also been observed. Even a small coin lesion in the lung may produce the entire syndrome, so that the lung tumor not be identified until after the diagnosis of carcinoid has been established biochemically. Qualitative tests for urinary 5-HIAA are positive in most instances and indicate that the patient is probably secreting 25–30 mg of 5-HIAA per day. False-negative results may occur in patients receiving phenothiazines, and false-positive results have been observed after ingestion of serotonin-rich foods such as bananas or walnuts or in patients taking cough syrups containing glycerol guaiacolate. Ideally, all drugs should be withheld for several days prior to the urine collection.

A provocative test for induction of the flush can be performed by injecting 5 μg of epinephrine (0.5 mL of 1:1000 solution diluted 100 times) intravenously. If the test is positive, the facial flush and some dyspnea usually appear within several minutes.

Emergency therapy for patients with bronchial carcinoids and prolonged flushing episodes consists of giving prednisone, 15–30 mg orally daily. The effect is dramatic, and treatment is usually continued for prolonged periods. However, the flushing itself may be due to kinins rather than serotonin, and corticosteroids may have no effect on kinin-mediated features of the syndrome. Abdominal cramps and diarrhea can usually be managed with diphenoxylate with atropine (Lomotil), alone or in combination with an antiserotonin agent such as methysergide maleate.

The $H_1$ histamine receptor antagonist cyproheptadine, the $H_2$ receptor blocker cimetidine, and phenothiazines may prove useful in prevention of flushing. Cyproheptadine is particularly useful because it is also a serotonin antagonist.

Patients with intestinal carcinoids may do well for 10–15 years with supportive therapy, and cancer chemotherapy may not be indicated. Because bronchial lesions cause more severe symptoms, chemotherapy with doxorubicin plus cyclophosphamide, streptozocin, or interferon alfa-2 should be considered if resection is not feasible or if metastases have occurred. Advanced-stage intestinal carcinoid patients may also benefit from such regimens.

Moertel CG: Treatment of the carcinoid tumor and the malignant carcinoid syndrome. *J Clin Oncol* 1983;**1**:727.

# PRIMARY CANCER TREATMENT: THE ROLE OF SURGERY & RADIATION THERAPY

Most human cancers present initially as localized tumor nodules and cause local symptoms. Depending on the type of cancer, initial therapy may be directed locally in the form either of surgery or radiation therapy. This is the treatment of choice for a variety of potentially curable cancers, including most gastrointestinal and genitourinary cancers, central nervous system tumors, and cancers arising from the breast, thyroid, or skin as well as most sarcomas.

In other circumstances, surgery may be used for palliation of noncurable cases or for reconstruction and rehabilitation.

Surgery initially often has both diagnostic and therapeutic effectiveness, since it provides access to tissue for diagnosis and permits pathologic staging of the extent of local and regional invasion as well as the first opportunity for removal of the primary neoplasm. While various imaging procedures are gaining increasing importance in evaluating the extent of cancer, it usually remains necessary for the surgeon to accurately identify those patients who can be potentially cured by local treatment alone.

For some specific sites, complete surgical removal of the tumor can be disfiguring, disabling, or unachievable. Under those circumstances, primary local treatment with ionizing radiation therapy may prove to be the treatment of choice. In other instances, surgery and radiation therapy are used in sequence.

Radiation therapy is usually delivered as brachytherapy or teletherapy. In brachytherapy, the radiation source is placed close to the tumor. This intracavitary approach is used for many gynecologic or oral neoplasms. In teletherapy, supervoltage radiotherapy is usually delivered with a linear accelerator, as this instrument permits more precise beam localization and avoids the complication of skin radiation toxicity. Various beam-modifying wedges, rotational techniques, and other specific approaches are used to increase the radiation dosage to the tumor bed while minimizing toxicity to adjacent normal tissues.

Well-oxygenated tumors are more radiosensitive than hypoxic tumors. Hypoxic tumors are often bulky, implying a potential synergistic role of debulking a neoplasm surgically prior to radiotherapy. Radiation therapy is normally delivered in a fractionated fashion, this method appears to have radiobiologic superiority by permitting time for recovery of normal host tissues (but not the tumor) from sublethal damage during the period of treatment. Various normal tissues (particularly the skin, mucosal surfaces, spinal cord, bone marrow, and lymphoid system) can exhibit early or late toxicity from radiation therapy and limit radiation dosage. Fractionated radiation doses are usually administered for 5 days per week until the desired total dose has been delivered, usually over the course of 4–6 weeks.

For most tumor types, there is a sigmoid curve of increasing rate of control of the local tumor with increasing radiation dose. Radiosensitive tumors usually exhibit radiosensitivity over the dose range of 3500–5000 cgy.

Radiation therapy can play a special role in curative treatment of tumors of the larynx (permitting cure without loss of the voice), carcinoma of the uterine cervix, and early-stage breast cancer and Hodgkin's disease.

Increasingly, the primary local therapy of cancer is integrated with systemic therapy, an approach that has proved to be superior for apparently localized tumor types with a high propensity for early metastatic spread and for which anticancer drugs are available.

This combined or adjuvant therapy approach will be discussed again later in this chapter.

# SYSTEMIC CANCER THERAPY

Use of cytotoxic drugs, hormones, antihormones, and biologicals has become a highly specialized and increasingly effective means of treating cancer and therapy is usually administered by a medical oncologist. Selection of specific drugs or protocols for various types of cancer has traditionally been based on results of prior clinical trials; however, many patients have drug-resistant tumors. Molecular mechanisms of drug resistance are now the subject of intense study. In many instances, specific drug resistance results from an amplification in the number of gene copies for an enzyme associated with drug resistance. A more general form of "multidrug resistance" to natural product anticancer drugs has also been described in association with expression of a 170-molecular-weight glycoprotein on the surface of tumor cells. This glycoprotein appears to be an energy-dependent transport pump that facilitates drug efflux from tumor cells. Strategies to overcome such multidrug resistance are now in development.

Cancer chemotherapy is usually curative in advanced stages of choriocarcinoma in women; in Burkitt's lymphoma and testicular tumors; and in some cases of acute leukemia, embryonal rhabdomyosarcoma, Hodgkin's disease, and diffuse histiocytic lymphoma. When combined with initial surgery and irradiation, chemotherapy also increases the cure rate in Wilms' tumor, and may provide long-term control of breast cancer and rectal cancer as well as bony osteogenic sarcomas. Combination chemotherapy provides significant palliation of symptoms along with prolongation of survival in many children with acute leukemia, Ewing's sarcoma, and retinoblastoma and in adults with Hodgkin's disease, non-Hodgkin lymphomas, mycosis fungoides, multiple myeloma, macroglobulinemia, carcinomas of the head and neck, thyroid, breast, esophagus, stomach, ovary, endometrium, and prostate, and small-cell carcinoma of the lung. Patients with carcinoma of the bladder or chronic leukemia also derive some relief of symptoms, although survival rates have not yet increased significantly. The results of currently available treatments are largely unsuccessful in squamous cancer of the lung as well as in metastatic melanoma and in adenocarcinomas of the colon, gallbladder, or pancreas.

While most anticancer drugs are used systemically, there are selected indications for local or regional administration (eg, intravesical therapy, intraperitoneal therapy, hepatic artery infusion).

A summary of the types of cancer responsive to chemotherapy and the current treatment of choice is offered in Table 32–2. In some instances (eg, Hodgkin's disease), optimal therapy may require a combination of therapeutic resources, eg, radiation therapy plus chemotherapy rather than chemotherapy alone. All patients with stage I or II Hodgkin's disease should receive radiation therapy. Table 32–3 outlines the currently used dosage schedules and the toxicities of the cancer chemotherapeutic agents. The dosage schedules given are for single-agent therapy. Combination therapy, as now used in advanced Hodgkin's disease, testicular tumors, and certain other neoplasms, requires reductions of the dosages shown—otherwise, the combined toxicity would be prohibitive. Such combination therapy should be attempted only by specialists in centers where adequate supportive services are available.

Hormonal therapy also plays an important role in cancer management. Hormonal therapy or ablation is important in palliation of breast and prostatic carcinoma, while added progestins are useful in suppression of endometrial carcinoma. Studies have shown that the 30% of women with metastatic breast cancer who show objective improvement with hormonal therapy have tumors that contain cytoplasmic estrogen and progesterone receptors. Patients whose tumors lack these receptor proteins are unresponsive to hormonal management but frequently respond to cytotoxic chemotherapy. Antiestrogens (eg, tamoxifen) and aromatase inhibitors (such as aminoglutethimide) that block peripheral conversion of adrenal androgens into estrogens have substantial additive effects to oophorectomy in women whose tumors are estrogen or progesterone receptor-positive. Thus, estrogen and progesterone receptor status should be assessed on all breast cancers at the time of mastectomy and on biopsy material (if available) from patients who manifest metastatic breast cancer. Antiestrogens such as tamoxifen have lower affinity for estrogen receptor protein than does endogenous estrogen. Therefore, the drug is of less value in the presence of functional ovaries. Although chemotherapy with drugs such as cyclophosphamide may depress ovarian function, oophorectomy is more effective and should be considered for premenopausal women who are to be treated with tamoxifen alone or in combination with cytotoxic agents. Androgen receptors remain difficult to measure in prostate cancer. In addition to estrogens, new hormonal approaches are also appearing in prostate cancer. These include the use of analogs of gonadotropin-releasing hormone and evaluation of aromatase inhibitors (eg, aminoglutethimide) and antiandrogens. Recombinant alfa-2 interferon has recently been approved by the FDA and have marked antitumor effects in hairy cell leukemia, moderate effects in lymphomas, chronic myelogenous leukemia, and the epidemic form of Kaposi's sarcoma (AIDS-associated), and lesser effects in multiple myeloma, metastatic melanoma, hypernephroma, and carcinoid syndrome. Their use together with other methods of treatment will probably increase significantly in the coming years.

**Table 32–2.** Cancers responsive to systemic agents.

| Diagnosis | Current Treatment of Choice | Other Valuable Agents |
|---|---|---|
| Acute lymphocytic leukemia | Induction: vincristine plus prednisone. Remission maintenance: mercaptopurine, methotrexate, and cyclophosphamide in various combinations. | Asparaginase, daunorubicin, VM-26,* carmustine, doxorubicin, cytarabine, allopurinol,† craniospinal radiotherapy. |
| Acute myelocytic and myelo-monocytic leukemia | Combination chemotherapy: thioguanine, cytarabine, and daunorubicin; or doxorubicin, vincristine, cytarabine, prednisone. | Methotrexate, mercaptopurine, allopurinol,† azacitidine,* AMSA, mitoxantrone.* |
| Chronic myelocytic leukemia | Busulfan. | Interferon, vincristine, mercaptopurine, hydroxyurea, melphalan, cytarabine, allopurinol.† |
| Chronic lymphocytic leukemia | Chlorambucil and prednisone (if indicated). | Vincristine, androgens,† allopurinol,† doxorubicin. |
| Hairy cell leukemia | Interferon. | Deoxycoformycin* (pentostatin). |
| Hodgkin's disease (stages III and IV) | Combination chemotherapy: mechlorethamine, vincristine, procarbazine, prednisone ("Mopp"). | Doxorubicin, bleomycin, vinblastine, dacarbazine ("ABVD"); lomustine, VM-26.* |
| Non-Hodgkin's lymphomas | Combination chemotherapy: cyclophosphamide, doxorubicin, vincristine, prednisone. | Bleomycin, lomustine, carmustine, VM-26,* AMSA, mitoxantrone,* interferon. |
| Multiple myeloma | Combination chemotherapy: melphalan, cyclophosphamide, doxorubicin, vincristine, carmustine. | Vindesine,* interferon, androgens.† |
| Macroglobulinemia | Chlorambucil. | Melphalan, interferon. |
| Polycythemia vera | Busulfan, chlorambucil, or cyclophosphamide; radiophosphorus P 32. | |
| Carcinoma of lung | Cyclophosphamide, doxorubicin, methotrexate, and lomustine (depends on cell type). | Cisplatin, quinacrine,† mitomycin, vincristine, etoposide, fluorouracil, vinblastine. |
| "Head and neck" carcinomas | Cisplatin and fluorouracil. | Hydroxyurea, doxorubicin, vinblastine, methotrexate, bleomycin. |
| Carcinoma of endometrium | Doxorubicin plus cyclophosphamide. | Progestins, fluorouracil, vinblastine, cisplatin. |
| Carcinoma of ovary | Cyclophosphamide and cisplatin. | Doxorubicin, melphalan, fluorouracil, vincristine, hexamethylmelamine,* bleomycin. |
| Carcinoma of cervix | Mitomycin, bleomycin, vincristine, and cisplatin. | Lomustine, cyclophosphamide, doxorubicin, methotrexate. |
| Breast carcinoma | (1) Combination of chemotherapy or tamoxifen (see text) if lymph nodes are positive at mastectomy. (2) Combination chemotherapy; hormonal manipulation for late recurrence (see text). | Cyclophosphamide, doxorubicin, vincristine, methotrexate, fluorouracil, mitomycin, vinblastine, mitoxantrone,* quinacrine,† prednisone,† megestrol, androgens, aminoglutethimide, and hydrocortisone. |
| Choriocarcinoma (trophoblastic neoplasms) | Methotrexate, alone or in combination with vincristine, dactinomycin, and cyclophosphamide. | Vinblastine, cisplatin, mercaptopurine, chlorambucil, doxorubicin. |
| Carcinoma of testis | Combination therapy: cisplatin, vinblastine, bleomycin or etoposide plus cisplatin. | Methotrexate, dactinomycin, mithramycin, doxorubicin, cyclophosphamide. |
| Carcinoma of prostate | Estrogens or leuprolide. | Doxorubicin plus cyclophosphamide, and cisplatin, estramustine, fluorouracil, progestins. |
| Wilms' tumor (children) | Vincristine plus dactinomycin after surgery and radiotherapy. | Methotrexate, cyclophosphamide, doxorubicin. |
| Neuroblastoma | Cyclophosphamide, cisplatin, doxorubicin, and vincristine. | Dactinomycin, daunorubicin, cisplatin. |
| Carcinoma of thyroid | Radioiodine ($^{131}$I), doxorubicin. | Bleomycin, fluorouracil, melphalan, cisplatin. |
| Carcinoma of adrenal | Mitotane. | Doxorubicin. |
| Carcinoma of stomach or pancreas | Fluorouracil plus doxorubicin and mitomycin. | Hydroxyurea, lomustine. |
| Carcinoma of colon | Fluorouracil. | Mitomycin, carmustine, cisplatin. |
| Carcinoid | Doxorubicin plus cyclophosphamide or interferon. | Dactinomycin, methysergide,† streptozocin. |
| Insulinoma | Streptozocin. | Doxorubicin, fluorouracil, mitomycin. |
| Osteogenic sarcoma | Doxorubicin, or methotrexate with citrovorum rescue initiated after surgery. | Cyclophosphamide, dacarbazine. |
| Miscellaneous sarcomas | Doxorubicin plus dacarbazine. | Methotrexate, dactinomycin, cyclophosphamide, vincristine, vinblastine. |
| Melanoma | Dacarbazine and dactinomycin. | Lomustine, cisplatin, mitomycin, vinblastine, interferon. |

*Note:* Interferon is now available as recombinant interferon alfa-a: Roferon (Roche, alfa 2A); Intron-A (Shering, alfa 2B).
* Investigational agent. Treatment available through qualified investigators and centers authorized by National Cancer Institute and Cooperative Oncology Groups.
† Supportive agent, not oncolytic.

**Table 32–3.** Single-agent dosage and toxicity of anticancer drugs.

| Chemotherapeutic Agent | Usual Adult Dosage | Acute Toxicity | Delayed Toxicity |
|---|---|---|---|
| **Alkylating agents** | | | |
| Mechlorethamine (nitrogen mustard, HN2, Mustargen) | 0.4 mg/kg IV in single or divided doses. | Nausea and vomiting | Moderate depression of blood count. Excessive doses produce severe bone marrow depression with leukopenia, thrombocytopenia, and bleeding. Alopecia and hemorrhagic cystitis occur with cyclophosphamide, while busulfan occasionally causes pigmentation and other unusual toxicities (see below). Acute leukemia may develop in 5–10% of patients receiving prolonged therapy with melphalan or chlorambucil. |
| Chlorambucil (Leukeran) | 0.1–0.2 mg/kg/d orally; 6–12 mg/d. | None | |
| Cyclophosphamide | 3.5–5 mg/kg/d orally for 10 days; 1 g/m² IV as single dose every 3–4 weeks. | Nausea and vomiting | |
| Melphalan (Alkeran) | 0.25 mg/kg/d orally for 4 days every 6 weeks. | None | |
| Thiotepa | 0.2 mg/kg IV for 5 days. | None | |
| Busulfan (Myleran) | 2–8 mg/d orally; 150–250 mg/course. | None | |
| Carmustine (BCNU, bischloroethylnitrosourea) | 200 mg/m² IV every 6 weeks. | Nausea and vomiting | Leukopenia and thrombocytopenia. Rarely hepatitis. Acute leukemia has been observed to occur in some patients receiving semustine. |
| Lomustine (CCNU) or semustine (methyl-CCNU) | 130 mg/m² orally very 6 weeks. | Nausea and vomiting | |
| Procarbazine (N-methyl-hydrazine, Matulane) | 50–300 mg/d orally. | Nausea and vomiting | Bone marrow depression, mental depression, monoamine oxidase inhibition. |
| Dacarbazine (dimethyl triazeno imidazole carboxamide, DTIC) | 250 mg/m²/d for 5 days every 3 weeks. | Anorexia, nausea, vomiting | Bone marrow depression. |
| Cisplatin (Platinol) | 50–100 mg/m² IV every 3 weeks. | Nausea and vomiting | Nephrotoxicity, mild otic and bone marrow toxicity, neurotoxicity. |
| **Structural analogs or antimetabolites** | | | |
| Methotrexate (amethopterin, MTX) | 2.5–5 mg/d orally; 15 mg intrathecally weekly or every other week for 4 doses. 20–25 mg IM twice weekly is well tolerated and may be preferable. | None | Oral and gastrointestinal tract ulceration, bone and marrow depression, leukopenia, thrombocytopenia. |
| Mercaptopurine (Purinethol, 6-MP) | 2.5 mg/kg/d orally. | None | Usually well tolerated. Larger dosages may cause bone marrow depression. |
| Thioguanine (6-TG) | 2 mg/kg/d orally. | None | Usually well tolerated. Larger dosages may cause bone marrow depression. |
| Fluorouracil (5-FU) | 15 mg/kg/d IV for 3–5 days, or 15 mg/kg weekly for at least 6 weeks. | None | Nausea, oral and gastrointestinal ulceration, bone marrow depression. |
| Cytarabine (Ara-C, Cytosar) | 100 mg/m²/d for 5–10 days given by continuous IV infusion, or in divided doses subcut or IV every 8 hours. | None | Nausea and vomiting, bone marrow depression, megaloblastosis, leukopenia, thrombocytopenia. |
| **Hormonal agents** | | | |
| Androgens | | | |
|   Testosterone propionate | 100 mg IM 3 times weekly. | None | Fluid retention, masculinization. There is a 10% incidence of cholestatic jaundice with fluoxymesterone. |
|   Fluoxymesterone (Halotestin) | 20–40 mg/d orally. | None | |
| Estrogens | | | |
|   Diethylstilbestrol | 1–5 mg 3 times a day orally. | Occasional nausea and vomiting | Fluid retention, feminization, uterine bleeding. |
|   Ethinyl estradiol (Estinyl) | 3 mg/d orally. | None | |
| Antiestrogen | | | |
|   Tamoxifen (Nolvadex) | 20 mg/d orally. | None | None |
| Progestins | | | |
|   Hydroxyprogesterone caproate (Delalutin) | 1 g IM twice weekly. | None | Occasional fluid retention. |
|   Medroxyprogesterone (Provera) | 100–200 mg/d orally; 200–600 mg orally twice weekly. | None | |
|   Megestrol acetate (Megace) | 40 mg 4 times a day orally. | none | |
| Adrenocorticosteroids | | | |
|   Prednisone | 20–100 mg/d orally or, when effective, 50–100 mg every other day orally as single dose. | None | Fluid retention, hypertension, diabetes, increased susceptibility to infection, "moon facies," osteoporosis. |

**Table 32–3 (cont'd).** Single-agent dosage and toxicity of anticancer drugs.

| Chemotherapeutic Agent | Usual Adult Dosage | Acute Toxicity | Delayed Toxicity |
|---|---|---|---|
| **Hormonal agents (cont'd)** Aromatase inhibitors Aminoglutethimide | 500 mg/d orally, along with hydrocortisone, 40 mg/d. | Initial drowsiness | Transient skin rash, which usually subsides with continued therapy. |
| Gonadotropin-releasing hormone inhibitors Leuprolide | 1 mg/d subcutaneously. | Usually none | Usually none. |
| **Biologic response modifiers** Interferon alfa-2 (recombinant) (Roferon, Intron-A) | 3–5 million IU subcutaneously daily or 3 times weekly. | Fever, chills, anorexia | Fatigue, weight loss, confusion. |
| **Natural products and miscellaneous agents** Vinblastine (Velban) | 0.1–0.2 mg/kg IV weekly. | Nausea and vomiting | Alopecia, loss of reflexes, bone marrow depression. |
| Vincristine (Oncovin) | 1.5 mg/m$^2$ IV (maximum: 2 mg weekly). | None | Areflexia, muscle weakness, peripheral neuritis, paralytic ileus, alopecia (below). |
| Dactinomycin (actinomycin D, Cosmegen) | 0.04 mg/kg IV weekly. | Nausea and vomiting | Stomatitis, gastrointestinal tract upset, alopecia, bone marrow depression. |
| Daunorubicin (daunomycin, rubidomycin) | 30–60 mg/m$^2$ daily IV for 3 days, or 30–60 mg/m$^2$ IV weekly. | Nausea, fever, red urine (not hematuria) | Cardiotoxicity, bone marrow depression, alopecia. |
| Doxorubicin (Adriamycin) | 60 mg/m$^2$ IV every 3 weeks to a maximum total dose of 550 mg/m$^2$. | Nausea, red urine (not hematuria) | Cardiotoxicity, alopecia, bone marrow depression, stomatitis. |
| Etoposide (Vepesid, VP-16) | 100 mg/m$^2$ IV daily for 5 days every 3 weeks. | Nausea and vomiting; occasionally, hypotension | Myelosuppression |
| Mithramycin (Mithracin) | 25–50 µg/kg IV every other day for up to 8 doses. | Nausea and vomiting | Thrombocytopenia, hepatotoxicity. |
| Mitomycin (Mutamycin) | 20 mg/m$^2$ every 6 weeks. | Nausea | Thrombocytopenia, leukopenia. |
| Bleomycin (Blenoxane) | Up to 15 mg/m$^2$ twice weekly to a total dose of 200 mg/m$^2$. | Allergic reactions, fever, hypotension | Fever, dermatitis, pulmonary fibrosis. |
| Hydroxyurea (Hydrea) | 300 mg/m$^2$ orally for 5 days. | Nausea and vomiting | Bone marrow depression. |
| Mitotane (o,p′-DDD, Lysodren) | 6–12 g/d orally. | Nausea and vomiting | Dermatitis, diarrhea, mental depression, muscle tremors. |
| **Supportive agents** Allopurinol (Zyloprim) | 300–800 mg/d orally for prevention or relief of hyperuricemia. | None | Usually none. Enhances effects and toxicity of mercaptopurine when used in combination. |
| Quinacrine (Atabrine) | 100–200 mg/d by intracavitary injection for 6 days. | Local pain and fever | None. |

## MECHANISMS OF ACTION OF CANCER CHEMOTHERAPEUTIC AGENTS

Although the emphasis in this chapter is on the empirical applications of cancer chemotherapy, the cytokinetics and mechanisms of drug action should be discussed briefly. At the clinical level of detectability of tumors, growth characteristics vary considerably between tumors of different histologic appearance or tissue of origin. The key cells in a cancer are the clonogenic **tumor stem cells,** which make up less than 1% of cancer cells but provide for population renewal and serve as the seeds of metastasis. Another useful concept is that of the "growth fraction"— the percentage of tumor cells that are proliferating at any given time. The leukemias, certain lymphomas, and genital tract tumors have relatively high growth fractions and are quite susceptible to treatment with drugs that have specific toxicity for proliferating cells. These drugs include cytarabine, mercaptopurine, thioguanine, methotrexate, fluorouracil, azacytidine,

vincristine, vinblastine, bleomycin, and certain steroid hormones. These drugs are therefore classed as **cell cycle specific (CCS)** agents, and their utility has proved to be greatest in tumors with high growth fractions such as those mentioned above. The sequential 4 phases of the cell cycle are G$_1$ (period of RNA and protein synthesis), S phase (period of DNA synthesis), G$_2$ (period of assembly of the mitotic spindle apparatus), and M (mitosis). Cytarabine is an excellent example of a drug with selective toxicity during just the S phase of the cell cycle, and its current use is virtually limited to the management of acute leukemia, in which it has had a major beneficial effect.

A second major group of drugs are classed as **cell cycle nonspecific (CCNS)** agents. Most of these drugs act by complexing with cellular DNA and are capable of doing this whether cells are proliferating or not. Examples are the alkylating agents (eg, mechlorethamine, cyclophosphamide, melphalan, carmustine), other chemical agents (cisplatin), and antibiotics such as dactinomycin, doxorubicin, and mitomycin. Such drugs are useful in the treatment of a variety of so-called "solid tumors," which generally have low growth fractions at the clinical phase of disease; but they are also quite useful in high growth fraction tumors. Tumor kinetics are far from static, however, and our strategy in cancer chemotherapy is now undergoing radical revision to exploit our expanding knowledge of cytokinetics, pharmacokinetics, selective cell line sensitivity, etc. Use of continuous infusion pumps and special routes of administration have also been important. The intraperitoneal route has been explored as a means of delivering high local concentrations of specific agents to the peritoneal space while minimizing systemic toxicity. Autologous bone marrow infusion has also been studied experimentally as a means of limiting bone marrow toxicity with high-dose therapy.

Drugs that have had the greatest value in humans are those that produce a fractional kill of at least 5–6 logs (100,000-fold to 1 million-fold reduction in tumor cell number) in animal tumor systems. Because patients with human tumors present with $10^{10}$–$10^{12}$ tumor cells, use of effective combination chemotherapy should be given serious consideration after a major reduction in the body burden of tumor is first accomplished with surgery or irradiation. A new strategy that has already been proved effective in Hodgkin's disease is the use of alternating non–cross-resistant combinations of drugs (eg, "MOPP-ABVD") for induction of remission. This approach has yet to be tested in other types of cancer. A theoretic scheme of strategies in cancer chemotherapy is shown in Fig 32–1. Mechanisms of action of biologicals such as the interferons remain unclear, but they appear to be suppressive agents and may act analogously to hormones, or in some instances (eg, with interleukin-2) in concert with the host's immune system.

## ADJUVANT CHEMOTHERAPY FOR MICROMETASTASES

One of the most important roles of cancer chemotherapy is undoubtedly as an "adjuvant" (to eradicate or suppress minimal residual disease) after "primary field" treatment with surgery or irradiation. Failures with primary field therapy are due principally to occult micrometastases of tumor stem cells outside the primary field. These distant micrometastases are usually present in patients with one or more positive lymph nodes at the time of surgery (eg, in breast cancer) and in patients with tumors having a known propensity for early hematogenous spread (eg, osteogenic sarcoma, Wilms' tumor). The risk of recurrent or metastatic disease in such patients can be extremely high (> 80%). Only systemic therapy can adequately attack micrometastases. Chemotherapeutic regimens that induce regression of advanced cancer may have curative potential (at the right dosage and schedule) when combined with surgery for high-risk "early" cancer.

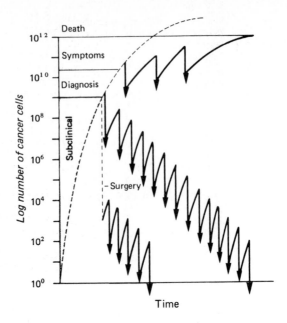

**Figure 32–1.** Relationship of tumor cell number to time of diagnosis, symptoms, treatment, and survival. Three alternative approaches to drug treatment are shown for comparison with the course of tumor growth when no treatment is given (dotted line). In the protocol diagrammed at top, treatment (indicated by the arrows) is given infrequently, and the result is manifested as prolongation of survival but with recurrence of symptoms between courses of treatment and eventual death of the patient. The combination chemotherapy treatment diagrammed in the middle section is begun earlier and is more intensive. Tumor cell kill exceeds regrowth; drug resistance does not develop; and "cure" results. In this example, treatment has been continued long after all clinical evidence of cancer has disappeared (1–3 years). This approach has been established as effective in the treatment of childhood acute leukemia, testicular cancers, and Hodgkin's disease. The recent introduction of the concept of "alternating non–cross-resistant" combination chemotherapy may further enhance this approach. In the treatment diagrammed near the bottom of the graph, early surgery has been employed to remove the primary tumor, and intensive adjuvant chemotherapy has been administered long enough (up to 1 year) to eradicate the remaining $10^3$ tumor stem cells that comprise the remaining occult micrometastases. This approach is now widely applied and appears effective in the treatment of breast cancer, rectal cancer, osteosarcoma, and Wilms' tumor.

Studies in experimental animals have shown that chemotherapy can eradicate small numbers of residual cancer cells after surgery. In other instances, micrometastases may be suppressed although not eradicated—such is the case when antiestrogen therapy is used in breast cancer.

The efficacy of adjuvant chemotherapy is also well established in pediatric neoplasms, eg, Wilms' tumor and rhabdomyosarcoma, where substantial improvement in survival has been obtained with adjuvant therapy. Recent studies have shown significant prolongation of survival in both pre- and postmenopausal women with stage II breast cancer who received adjuvant chemotherapy. In breast cancer, women with positive lymph nodes at breast cancer surgery have had prolonged disease-free survival from combination chemotherapy. Several useful combination chemotherapy regimens for adjuvant therapy for breast cancer are "CMF" (cyclophosphamide-methotrexate-fluorouracil), alone or with the addition of vincristine and prednisone (CMFVP), and "D/C" (doxorubicin-cyclophosphamide), alone or with the addition of fluorouracil. There is clear evidence of a dose-response effect of adjuvant cytotoxic chemotherapy, and low-dose protocols are generally ineffective. The antiestrogen tamoxifen has recently been shown to be a useful adjuvant in postmenopausal women and is most effective in treating cancers with positive hormone receptors. In osteogenic sarcoma, doxorubicin alone and in combination with other drugs has proved useful as an adjuvant. A recent report from the Gastrointestinal Tumor Study Group indicates that the 5-year relapse-free survival is improved in patients with rectal cancer when they receive postoperative radiotherapy and the combination of fluorouracil plus semustine.

Although it is still early to assess the overall results of these regimens, adjuvant chemotherapy should be considered as part of standard and indicated therapy in the patient groups discussed above. Thus, adjuvant chemotherapy should now be given serious consideration for patients who undergo primary surgical staging and therapy and are found to have a stage and histologic type of cancer known to be associated with a high risk of micrometastasis and for which effective chemotherapy is available. However, at present, adjuvant therapy remains investigational and unproved for a number of common tumors, including non–small-cell lung cancer, pancreatic cancer, and colon cancer. Adjuvant therapy is probably not indicated in early Hodgkin's disease or testicular carcinoma, since the cure rates with chemotherapy for these diseases when advanced and recurrent are high.

Eilber F et al: Adjuvant chemotherapy for osteosarcoma: Randomized prospective trial. *J Clin Oncol* 1987;5:21.

Salmon SE (editor): *Adjuvant Therapy of Cancer V*. Grune & Stratton, 1987.

## TOXICITY & DOSE MODIFICATION OF CHEMOTHERAPEUTIC AGENTS

A number of cancer chemotherapeutic agents have cytotoxic effects on rapidly proliferating normal cells in bone marrow, mucosa, and skin. Still other drugs such as the *Vinca* alkaloids produce neuropathy, and the hormones often have psychic effects. Acute and chronic toxicities of the various drugs are summarized in Table 32–3. Early recognition of significant toxicity is important to make certain that the ratio of benefit to toxic effects of treatment remains favorable. Appropriate dose modification usually minimizes these side effects, so that therapy can be continued with relative safety.

## Bone Marrow Toxicity

Depression of bone marrow is usually the most significant limiting toxicity in cancer chemotherapy. While autologous bone marrow transplantation can often reduce the myelosuppressive toxicity of high-dose chemotherapy, it is not yet clear that this will prove to be a generally useful strategy. Growth factors that stimulate myeloid proliferation (eg, granulocyte colony-stimulating factor (GCSF) and granulocyte-macrophage stimulating factor (GMCSF) are currently in clinical trial. These factors have the potential for markedly reducing the duration and severity of granulocytopenia after cytotoxic chemotherapy.

Commonly used short-acting drugs that affect bone marrow are the oral alkylating agents (eg, cyclophosphamide, melphalan, chlorambucil), procarbazine, mercaptopurine, methotrexate, vinblastine, fluorouracil, dactinomycin, and doxorubicin. In general, it is preferable to use alkylating agents in intensive "pulse" courses every 3–4 weeks rather than to administer in continuous daily schedules. This allows for complete hematologic (and immunologic) recovery between courses rather than leaving the patient continuously suppressed with a cytotoxic agent. This approach reduces side effects but does not reduce therapeutic efficacy. The standard dosage schedules that produce tumor responses with these agents often do induce some bone marrow depression. In such instances, if the drug is not discontinued or its dosage reduced, severe bone marrow aplasia may result in pancytopenia, bleeding, or infection. Simple guidelines to therapy can usually prevent severe marrow depression.

White blood counts (and differential counts), hematocrit or hemoglobin, and platelet counts should be obtained frequently. With long-term chemotherapy, counts should be obtained initially at weekly intervals; the frequency of counts may be reduced only after the patient's sensitivity to the drug can be well predicted (eg, 3–4 months) and cumulative toxicity excluded.

In patients with normal blood counts as well as normal liver and kidney function, drugs should usually be started at their full dosage and tapered if need be, rather than starting at a lower dose and escalating the dose to hematologic tolerance. When the dose is escalated, toxicity often cannot be adequately anticipated, especially if it is cumulative, and marrow depression is often more severe.

Drug dosage can usually be tapered on a fixed schedule as a function of the peripheral white blood count or platelet count (or both). In this fashion, smooth titration control of drug administration can usually be attained for oral alkylating agents or antimetabolites. A scheme for dose modifications is shown in Table 32–4. Alternatively, the interval between drug courses can be lengthened, thereby permitting more complete hematologic recovery.

Drugs with delayed hematologic toxicities do not always fit into such a simple scheme, and in general they should be administered by specialists familiar

**Table 32–4.** Scheme for dose modification of cancer chemotherapeutic agents.

| Granulocyte Count (/µL) | Platelet Count (/µL) | Suggested Drug Dosage (% of full dose) |
|---|---|---|
| > 3000 | > 100,000 | 100% |
| 2000–3000 | 75,000–100,000 | 50% |
| < 2000 | < 50,000 | 0% |

with the specific toxicities. Drugs requiring special precautions with respect to toxicity include doxorubicin, mitomycin, busulfan, cytarabine, bleomycin, mithramycin, carmustine, lomustine, semustine, and daunorubicin.

## Chemotherapy-Induced Nausea & Vomiting

A number of cytotoxic anticancer drugs induce nausea and vomiting as side effects. In general, these symptoms are thought to originate in the central nervous system rather than peripherally. Parenteral administration of single agents such as doxorubicin, etoposide, or cyclophosphamide frequently is associated with mild to moderate nausea and vomiting, whereas parenteral administration of nitrosoureas, dacarbazine, and particularly cisplatin usually causes severe symptoms, which can limit patient acceptance of chemotherapy. Combination chemotherapy with agents including those listed above can also cause severe symptoms. Recent advances in the study of antiemetics clearly reduce and often eliminate nausea and vomiting associated with drugs such as cisplatin. Cannabinoids (eg, tetrahydrocannabinol), are now commercially available (Marinol) as antiemetics for cancer patients receiving chemotherapy, but other agents are often preferable and cause fewer side effects. Metoclopramide (Reglan) is a particularly useful agent, especially when administered parenterally at a dosage of 1 mg/kg, both 30 minutes before and again 30 minutes after the administration of chemotherapy. Extrapyramidal signs may be induced with this drug but frequently can be suppressed with diphenydramine. Dexamethasone has antiemetic effects when administered at a dosage of 10 mg at similar intervals. Both of these agents are significantly more potent than conventional agents such as prochlorperazine, diphenhydramine, and thiethylperazine. Combinations of antiemetics (eg, metoclopramide along with dexamethasone and other agents) are often more effective than maximal doses of any one agent for blocking cisplatin-induced vomiting. Inclusion of diazepam in such combinations is often useful for its sedating effect. A patient receiving potent antiemetics along with chemotherapy on an outpatient basis must be escorted to and from the clinic, since the antiemetics often induce marked sedation and transient impairment of balance and reflexes.

Plezia PM et al: Immediate termination of intractable vomiting induced by cisplatin combination chemotherapy using an intensive five-drug antiemetic regimen. *Cancer Treat Rep* 1984;**68**:1493.

## Gastrointestinal & Skin Toxicity

Since antimetabolites such as methotrexate and fluorouracil act only on rapidly proliferating cells, they damage the cells of mucosal surfaces such as the gastrointestinal tract. Methotrexate has similar effects on the skin. These toxicities are at times more significant than those that have occurred in the bone marrow, and they should be looked for routinely when these agents are used.

Erythema of the buccal mucosa is an early sign of mucosal toxicity. If therapy is continued beyond this point, oral ulceration will develop. In general, it is wise to discontinue therapy at the time of appearance of early oral ulceration. This finding usually heralds the appearance of similar but potentially more serious ulceration at other sites lower in the gastrointestinal tract. Therapy can usually be reinstituted when the oral ulcer heals (1 week to 10 days). The dose of drug used may need to be modified downward at this point, with titration to an acceptable level of effect on the mucosa.

## Miscellaneous Drug-Specific Toxicities

The toxicities of individual drugs have been summarized in Table 32–3; however, several of these warrant additional mention, since they occur with frequently administered agents, and special measures are often indicated.

**A. Hemorrhagic Cystitis Induced by Cyclophosphamide:** Metabolic products of cyclophosphamide that retain cytotoxic activity are excreted into the urine. Some patients appear to metabolize more of the drug to these active excretory products; if their urine is concentrated, severe bladder damage may result. In general, it is wise to advise patients receiving cyclophosphamide to maintain a large fluid intake. Early symptoms include dysuria and frequency despite the absence of bacteriuria. Such symptoms develop in about 20% of patients who receive the drug. Should microscopic hematuria develop, it is advisable to stop the drug temporarily or switch to a different alkylating agent, to increase fluid intake, and to administer a urinary analgesic such as phenazopyridine. With severe cystitis, large segments of bladder mucosa may be shed and the patient may have prolonged gross hematuria. Such patients should be observed for signs of urinary obstruction and may require cystoscopy for removal of obstructing blood clots. Patients with tumors responsive to cyclophosphamide who develop severe cystitis should stop taking all drugs until the syndrome clears and should then be given different alkylating agents (eg, chlorambucil, melphalan, mechlorethamine) that lack this toxicity, as they are likely to be equally effective against the tumor.

**B. Vincristine-Induced Neuropathy:** Neuropathy is a toxic side effect that is peculiar to the *Vinca* alkaloid drugs, especially vincristine. The peripheral neuropathy can be sensory, motor, autonomic, or a combination of these effects. In its mildest form, it consists of paresthesias (''pins and needles'') of the fingers and toes. Occasional patients develop acute jaw or throat pain after vincristine therapy. This may be a form of trigeminal neuralgia. With continued vincristine therapy, the paresthesias extend to the proximal interphalangeal joints, hyporeflexia appears in the lower extremities, and significant weakness develops in the quadriceps muscle group. At this point, it is wise to discontinue vincristine therapy until the neuropathy has subsided. A useful means of judging whether peripheral motor neuropathy is significant enough to warrant stopping treatment is to have the patient attempt to do deep knee bends or get up out of a chair without using the arm muscles.

Constipation is the most common symptom of autonomic neuropathy associated with vincristine therapy. Patients receiving vincristine should be started on stool softeners and mild cathartics when therapy is begun; otherwise, severe impaction may result in association with an atonic bowel.

More serious autonomic involvement can lead to acute intestinal obstruction with signs indistinguishable from those of an acute abdomen. Bladder neuropathies are uncommon but may be severe.

These 2 complications are absolute contraindications to continued vincristine therapy.

**C. Methotrexate Toxicity and "Citrovorum Rescue":** In addition to standard uses of methotrexate for chemotherapy, this drug has some use in a very high dosage that would lead to fatal bone marrow toxicity if it were given without an antidote. The bone marrow toxicity of methotrexate can be prevented by early administration of citrovorum factor (folinic acid, leucovorin). If an overdose of methotrexate is administered accidentally, folinic acid therapy should be initiated as soon as possible, preferably within 1 hour. Intravenous infusion should be employed for large overdosages, inasmuch as it is generally advisable to give citrovorum factor repeatedly. Up to 75 mg should be given in the first 12 hours, followed by 12 mg intramuscularly every 4 hours for at least 6 doses.

Intentional high-dosage methotrexate therapy with citrovorum rescue should only be considered for osteosarcoma patients with good renal function.

Vigorous hydration and bicarbonate loading also appear to be important in preventing crystallization of high-dose methotrexate in the renal tubular epithelium. Daily monitoring of the serum creatinine is mandatory because methotrexate metabolism is slowed by renal insufficiency, and high-dosage methotrexate can itself cause renal injury. When high-dose methotrexate is used, folinic acid therapy should probably be started within 4 hours of the methotrexate dose and continued for 3 days (or longer if the creatinine level rises).

**D. Busulfan Toxicity:** The alkylating agent busulfan, frequently used for treatment of chronic myelogenous leukemia, has curious delayed toxicities including (1) increased skin pigmentation, (2) a wasting syndrome similar to that seen in adrenal insufficiency, and (3) progressive pulmonary fibrosis. Patients who develop either of the latter 2 problems should be switched to a different drug (eg, melphalan) when further therapy is needed. The pigmentary changes are innocuous and will usually regress slowly after treatment is discontinued; in this instance, change to a different compound is optional.

**E. Bleomycin Toxicity:** This antibiotic has found increasing application in cancer chemotherapy in view of activity in squamous cell carcinomas, Hodgkin's disease, non-Hodgkin's lymphomas, and testicular tumors. Bleomycin produces edema of the interphalangeal joints and hardening of the palmar and plantar skin as well as sometimes also inducing an anaphylactic or serum sickness-like reaction or a serious or fatal pulmonary fibrotic reaction (seen especially in elderly patients receiving a total dose of over 300 units). If nonproductive cough, dyspnea, and pulmonary infiltrates develop, discontinue the drug and institute antibiotic and high-dose corticosteroid therapy. Fever alone or with chills is an occasional complication of bleomycin treatment and is not an absolute contraindication to continued treatment. The fever may be avoided by prednisone administration at the time of injection. Moreover, fever alone is not predictive of pulmonary toxicity. About 1% of patients (especially those with lymphoma) may have a severe or even fatal hypotensive reaction after the initial dose of bleomycin. In order to identify such patients, it is wise to administer a test dose of 5 units of bleomycin first with adequate monitoring and emergency facilities available should they be needed. Patients exhibiting a hypotensive reaction should not receive further bleomycin therapy.

**F. Doxorubicin-Induced Myocarditis:** The anthracycline antibiotics doxorubicin and daunomycin both have delayed cardiac toxicity. The problem is greater with doxorubicin because it has a major role in the treatment of acute leukemia, sarcomas, breast cancer, lymphomas, and certain other solid tumors. Studies of left ventricular function and endomyocardial biopsies indicate that some changes in cardiac dynamics occur in most patients by the time they have received 300 mg/m$^2$. The *multiple-ga*ted (''MUGA'') radionuclide cardiac scan appears to be the most useful noninvasive test for assessing toxicity. Doxorubicin should not be used in elderly patients with significant intrinsic cardiac disease, and in general, patients should not receive a total dose in excess of 550 mg/m$^2$. Patients who have had prior chest or mediastinal radiotherapy may· develop doxorubicin heart disease at lower total doses. The appearance of a high resting pulse may herald the appearance of overt cardiac toxicity. Unfortunately, toxicity may be irreversible and frequently fatal at dosage levels above 550 mg/m$^2$. At lower doses (eg, 350 mg/m$^2$), the symptoms and signs of cardiac failure generally respond well to digitalis, diuretics, and cessation of doxorubicin therapy. Recent evidence suggests that cardiac toxicity can be correlated with high peak plasma levels obtained with intermittent high-dose bolus therapy (eg, every 3–4 weeks). Use of weekly injections or low-dose continuous infusion schedules appears to delay the occurrence of cardiac toxicity. Current laboratory studies suggest that cardiac toxicity may be due to a mechanism involving the formation of intracellular free radicals in cardiac muscle.

**G. Cisplatin Nephrotoxicity and Neurotoxicity:** Cisplatin is effective in testicular, bladder, and ovarian cancer as well as in several other types of tumor. Nausea and vomiting are common, but nephrotoxicity and neurotoxicity are more serious. Vigorous hydration plus mannitol diuresis may substantially reduce nephrotoxicity. The neurotoxicity of this drug is delayed and manifested as a peripheral neuropathy of mixed sensorimotor type and may be associated with painful paresthesias. The neuropathy may be secondary to hypomagnesemia, which can be induced by cisplatin. Therefore, the serum magnesium should be measured if neuropathy develops, and treatment with parenteral magnesium sulfate should be tried. These supportive measures do not appear to reduce the therapeutic effectiveness of cisplatin.

**H. Interferon Toxicities:** While alfa-2 interferon is generally well tolerated in the standard doses listed in Table 32–3, it has increasing toxicity with increasing doses and is more toxic in elderly patients. Tachyphylaxis often develops to the fever and chills. However, anorexia, fatigue, and weight loss can have cumulative effects and often represent dose-limiting toxicities and can be severe. In some patients, central nervous system symptoms develop and usually are manifested as confusion or heavy somnolence. Reduction in peripheral blood counts can develop, but this abnormality is usually not associated with significant bone marrow suppression. These interferon-induced side effects can sometimes be confused with the symptoms of progressive cancer. Fortunately, the side effects usually clear within 1 week after cessation of interferon therapy.

## EVALUATION OF TUMOR RESPONSE

Inasmuch as cancer chemotherapy can induce clinical improvement, significant toxicity, or both, it is extremely important to critically assess the beneficial effects of treatment in patients with advanced cancer to determine that the net effect is favorable. The most valuable signs to follow during therapy include the following:

**A. Tumor Size:** Significant shrinkage in tumor size can be demonstrated on physical examination, chest film or other x-ray, sonography, or radionuclide scanning procedure such as bone scanning (breast, lung, prostate cancer). CT scanning has assumed a significant role in evaluating tumor size and location for a wide variety of tumors and sites. Magnetic resonance imaging (MRI) appears to be the best noninvasive means of evaluating brain and spinal cord tumors and spinal cord compression, but CT scanning is also useful. Sonography has special utility in pelvic neoplasms.

**B. Marker Substances:** Significant decrease in the quantity of a tumor product or marker substance reflects a reduced amount of tumor in the body. Examples of such markers include paraproteins in the serum or urine in multiple myeloma and macroglobulinemia, chorionic gonadotropin in choriocarcinoma and testicular tumors, prostatic acid phosphatase in prostatic cancer, urinary steroids in adrenal carcinoma and paraneoplastic Cushing's syndrome, and 5-hydroxyindoleacetic acid in carcinoid syndrome. Tumor-secreted fetal antigens are becoming of increasing importance. These include alpha$_1$-fetoprotein in hepatoma, in teratoembryonal carcinoma, and in occasional cases of gastric carcinoma; ovarian tumor antigen (OC 125) in ovarian cancer; and carcinoembryonic antigen in carcinomas of the colon, lungs, and breast. Monoclonal antibodies are now used for measurement of a number of the tumor markers and offer the potential of delineating a number of additional markers for diagnostic purposes.

**C. Organ Function:** Return to normal function of organs that were previously impaired by tumor is a useful indicator of drug effectiveness. Examples of such improvement include the return to normal liver function (eg, increased serum albumin) in patients known to have liver metastases and improvement in neurologic findings in patients with cerebral metastases. Disappearance of the signs and symptoms of the paraneoplastic syndromes often falls in this general category and can be taken as an indication of tumor response.

**D. General Well-Being and Performance Status:** A valuable sign of clinical improvement is the general well-being of the patient. Although this finding is a combination of subjective and objective factors and may be partly a placebo effect, it nonetheless serves as a sign of clinical improvement in assessing some of the objective observations listed above. Factors included in the assessment of general well-being are improved appetite and weight gain and increased "performance status" (eg, ambulatory versus bedridden). Evaluation of factors such as activity status enables the physician to judge whether the net effect of chemotherapy is worthwhile palliation.

# REFERENCES

Baum M et al: Controlled trial of tamoxifen as single adjuvant agent in management of early breast cancer. *Lancet* 1985;**1**:836.

Bell DR et al: Detection of P-glycoprotein in ovarian cancer: A molecular marker associated with drug resistance. *J Clin Oncol* 1985;**3**:311.

Bonadonna G, Valagussa P: Current status of adjuvant chemotherapy for breast cancer. *Semin Oncol* 1987;**14**:8.

Brenner DE: Intraperitoneal chemotherapy: A review. *J Clin Oncol* 1986;**4**:1135.

Costanzi JJ et al: Phase II study of recombinant alpha$_2$ interferon in resistant multiple myeloma. *J Clin Oncol* 1985;**3**:654.

Curtis JE et al: High-dose cytosine arabinoside in the treatment of acute myelogenous leukemia: Contributions to outcome of clinical and laboratory attributes. *J Clin Oncol* 1987;**5**:532.

DeVita VT Jr: Progress in cancer management. *Cancer* 1983;**51**:2401.

DeVita VT Jr, Hellman S, Rosenberg SA (editors): *Principles and Practice of Oncology,* 2nd ed. Lippincott, 1985.

Durie BGM et al: Improved survival duration with combination chemotherapy induction: A Southwest Oncology Group Study. *J Clin Oncol* 1986;**4**:1227.

Fisher B et al: Influence of tumor estrogen and progesterone receptor levels on the response to tamoxifen and chemotherapy in primary breast cancer. *J Clin Oncol* 1983;**1**:227.

Fisher B et al: Ten year results from the National Surgical Adjuvant Breast and Bowel Project Clinical Trial evaluating the use of L-phenylalanine mustard in the management of primary breast cancer. *J Clin Oncol* 1986;**6**:929.

Golumb HM et al: Alpha-2 interferon therapy of hairy cell leukemia: A multicenter study. *J Clin Oncol* 1986;**4**:900.

Hainsworth JD et al: Successful treatment of resistant germ cell neoplasms with VP-16 and cisplatin: Results of a Southeastern Cancer Study Group Trial. *J Clin Oncol* 1985;**3**:666.

Hryniuck W: Average relative dose intensity and the impact on design of clinical trials. *Semin Oncol* 1987;**14**:65.

Ingle J et al: Randomized trial of diethylstilbestrol vs. tamoxifen in postmenopausal women with advanced cancer. *N Engl J Med* 1981;**304**:16.

Leichman L et al: Preoperative chemotherapy for carcinoma of the esophagus: A potentially curative approach. *J Clin Oncol* 1984;**2**:75.

Lenhard RE et al: Isotopic immunoglobulin: A new systemic therapy for advanced Hodgkin's disease. *J Clin Oncol* 1985;**3**:1296.

Link MP et al: The effect of adjuvant chemotherapy on relapse-free survival in osteosarcoma of the extremity. *N Engl J Med* 1986;*314*:1600.

Lippman ME (editor): *National Institutes of Health Consensus Development Conference on Adjuvant Chemotherapy and Endocrine Therapy of Breast Cancer.* NCI Monograph No. 1. National Cancer Institute, 1986.

Longo D et al: Twenty years of MOPP therapy for Hodgkin's disease. *J Clin Oncol* 1986;**4**:1295.

Osterlind K et al: Mortality and morbidity in long term surviving patients treated with chemotherapy with or without irradiation for small cell lung cancer. *J Clin Oncol* 1986;**4**:1044.

Perry MC: Toxicity of chemotherapy. *Semin Oncol* 1982;**9**:1. [Entire issue.]

Perry MC et al: Chemotherapy with or without radiation therapy in limited small cell carcinoma of the lung. *N Engl J Med* 1987;**316**:912.

Pritchard KI: Current status of adjuvant endocrine therapy for resectable breast cancer. *Semin Oncol* 1987;**14**:23.

Prosnitz LR, Kapp DS, Weissberg JB: Radiotherapy. *N Engl J Med* 1983;**309**:771.

Rosen ST et al: Radioimmunodetection and radioimmunotherapy of cutaneous T cell lymphomas using a [131]I-labeled monoclonal antibody. *J Clin Oncol* 1987;**5**:562.

Rosenberg SA: The low grade non-Hodgkin's lymphomas: Challenges and opportunities. *J Clin Oncol* 1985;**3**:299.

Rosenberg SA et al: A progress report on the treatment of 157 patients with advanced cancer using lymphokine-activated killer cells and interleukin-2 or high-dose interleukin-2 alone. *N Engl J Med* 1987;**316**:889.

Rosenberg SA et al: The treatment of soft tissue sarcomas of the extremities: Prospective randomized evaluations of (1) limb-sparing surgery plus radiation therapy compared with amputation and (2) the role of adjuvant chemotherapy. *Ann Surg* 1982;**196**:305.

Salmon SE: *Adjuvant Therapy of Cancer V.* Grune & Stratton, 1987.

Salmon SE, Sartorelli AC: Cancer chemotherapy. Chap 58 in: *Basic & Clinical Pharmacology,* 3rd ed. Katzung BG (editor). Appleton-Lange, 1987.

Salmon SE et al: Alternating combination chemotherapy improves survival in multiple myeloma. *J Clin Oncol* 1983;**1**:453.

Yeager AM et al: Autologous bone marrow transplantation in patients with acute nonlymphocytic leukemia, using ex vivo marrow treatment with 4-hydroperoxycyclophosphamide. *N Engl J Med* 1986;**315**:141.

# 33

# Immunologic Disorders

*Daniel P. Stites, MD, Samuel Strober, MD, & F. Carl Grumet, MD*

A wide variety of diseases in humans are associated with disorders of the immune response. Knowledge of immunoglobulin structure and function and of the cellular basis of immunity has resulted in a better understanding of these disorders. Diseases of immunity are usually caused by pathologic imbalances resulting from either excesses or deficiencies of immunocompetent cells or their products that disrupt normal homeostasis. This chapter provides a brief overview of basic and clinical immunology as an approach to the patient with immunologic disease.

## IMMUNOGLOBULINS & ANTIBODIES

### IMMUNOGLOBULIN STRUCTURE & FUNCTION

Immunoglobulins, which represent about 20% of plasma proteins, are specialized molecules that possess antibody activity. The basic unit of all immunoglobulins consists of 4 polypeptide chains linked by disulfide bonds. There are 2 identical heavy chains (molecular weight 55,000–70,000) and 2 identical light chains (molecular weight about 23,000). Both heavy and light chains have a C-terminal constant (C) region and an N-terminal variable (V) region. A hypervariable portion of the V regions of heavy and light chains together form the antibody combining site, which is responsible for the specific interaction with antigen.

Antibodies contain one of 5 classes of heavy chains ($\gamma$, $\alpha$, $\mu$, $\delta$, and $\epsilon$) and one of 2 types of light chains ($\kappa$ and $\lambda$). Either type of light chain can be associated with each of the heavy chain classes. Approximately 70% of human immunoglobulins have $\kappa$ light chains, and 30% have $\lambda$ light chains. About 10 million different antibody specificities are thought to exist in a given individual.

### Immunoglobulin Classes

**A. Immunoglobulin M (IgM):** IgM is made up of 5 identical basic immunoglobulin units. These units are connected to each other by disulfide bonds and a small polypeptide known as J chain. The molecular weight of IgM is about 900,000. The IgM molecule is found predominantly in the intravascular compartment and on the surface of B lymphocytes and does not normally cross the placenta. IgM antibody predominates early in immune responses; carbohydrate antigens such as blood group substances predominantly stimulate IgM.

**B. Immunoglobulin A (IgA):** IgA is present in the blood and relatively high concentration in saliva, colostrum, tears, and secretions of the bronchi and the gastrointestinal tract. Serum IgA is a single basic immunoglobulin unit, whereas secretory IgA is made up of 2 basic units connected to each other by J chain. A 70,000-molecular-weight molecule called secretory component is attached to the Fc portions. It is necessary to transport IgA into the lumens of exocrine glands, and it confers resistance to enzymatic destruction. Secretory IgA plays an important role in host defense mechanisms against viral and bacterial infections by blocking transport of microbes across mucosal surfaces.

**C. Immunoglobulin G (IgG):** IgG is a single basic immunoglobulin unit of MW 150,000 that comprises about 85% of total serum immunoglobulins. IgG is distributed in the extracellular fluid and is the only immunoglobulin that normally crosses the placenta. IgG binds complement via an Fc receptor present in the constant region of the $\gamma$ heavy chain. IgG binds to the surface of macrophages; this causes them to become killer cells.

**D. Immunoglobulin E (IgE):** IgE is present in serum in very low concentrations as a single immunoglobulin unit with $\epsilon$ heavy chains. Approximately 50% of patients with allergic diseases have increased serum IgE levels. IgE is a skin-sensitizing or reaginic antibody by virtue of attachment to mast cells. The specific interaction between antigen and IgE bound to the surface of mast cells results in the release of inflammatory products such as histamine, leukotriene, and chemotactic factors. These mediators can result in bronchospasm, vasodilation, smooth muscle contraction, and chemoattraction of many other inflammatory cells.

**E. Immunoglobulin D (IgD):** IgD is present in the serum in very low concentrations as a single basic immunoglobulin unit with $\delta$ heavy chains. IgD is found on the surface of most B lymphocytes in association with IgM, where it probably serves as a receptor for antigen.

Goodman JW: Immunoglobulins I: Structure and function. Chap 4, in: *Basic & Clinical Immunology*, 6th ed. Stites DP, Stobo JD, Wells JV (editors). Appleton-Lange, 1987.

Jeske DJ, Capra JD: Immunoglobulins: Structure and function. Chap 7, pp 131–165, in: *Fundamental Immunology.* Paul WE (editor). Raven Press, 1983.

## Immunoglobulin Genes

Genes that code for immunoglobulin light and heavy chain molecules undergo rearrangements in the DNA of B cells, which results in the synthesis and expression of immunoglobulin molecules. Clonal rearrangements of immunoglobulin genes in B cells have provided important evidence for an immunologic origin and typing of many leukemias and lymphomas.

Cleary ML et al: Immunoglobulin gene rearrangement as a diagnostic criterion of B cell lymphoma. *Proc Soc Natl Acad Sci USA* 1984;**81:**593.
Korsmeyer SJ, Waldmann TA: Immunoglobulins II: Gene organization and assembly. Chap 5 in: *Basic & Clinical Immunology,* 6th ed. Stites DP, Stobo JD, Wells JV (editors). Appleton-Lange, 1987.

## TEST FOR IMMUNOGLOBULINS

There are various ways of measuring antibody, including the following: (1) quantitative and qualitative determinations of serum immunoglobulins; (2) determination of isohemagglutinin and febrile agglutinin titers; (3) determination of antibody titers following immunization with tetanus toxoid, diphtheria toxoid, or pertussis vaccines; and (4) determination of the percentage of and absolute number of circulating B lymphocytes. The first method tests for the presence of serum immunoglobulins but not for the functional adequacy of the immunoglobulins. The second method tests for functional antibodies that are present in the serum of almost all individuals as a consequence of exposure to environmental antigens. The third method examines functional antibody activity in the serum after intentional immunization. The fourth method tests for the presence of the precursors of plasma cells that give rise to serum antibodies and is helpful in determining whether there has been a maturational arrest (see below).

The 2 most commonly used clinical tests of humoral immunity, which provide the first screening procedure for many diseases, are immunoelectrophoresis and quantitative immunoglobulin determinations.

### Immunoelectrophoresis

Immunoelectrophoresis is a screening device for semiquantitative estimates of the amounts of IgG, IgA, or IgM in the serum or other body fluids and for identifying abnormal immunoglobulin molecules such as myeloma (M) proteins. The absence of certain immunoglobulin classes or the presence of immunoglobulin molecules in abnormal concentrations may be apparent on immunoelectrophoresis.

Serum proteins added to gels are separated by their electrical charge and identified with appropriate antisera. The interaction between the class-specific antisera and the major serum immunoglobulin classes produces characteristic patterns in the gel. Abnormal immunoglobulins such as myeloma (M) proteins form a sharp arc that merges with the normal immunoglobulin arc of the same class. This method is useful in differentiating monoclonal from polyclonal increases in immunoglobulins and determining the immunoglobulin class of a paraprotein.

## Quantitative Immunoglobulin Determinations; Radial Diffusion & Nephelometry Techniques

Quantitative determinations of the serum IgG, IgA, and IgM levels can be carried out using the radial diffusion technique. Circular wells are cut in a gel plate impregnated with a specific antiserum directed against a single human immunoglobulin class. The radius or diameter of the circular precipitin ring is proportionate to the concentration of serum immunoglobulin. The precise immunoglobulin level is determined by comparing the diameter of the unknown serum to that of a standard containing known levels of immunoglobulins.

Determinations of the serum concentrations of IgM, IgG, and IgA can also be made accurately and rapidly by nephelometry. This method employs an instrument to measure the turbidity produced by the interaction of immunoglobulin and anti-immunoglobulin complexes. It is much more rapid than radial diffusion and is useful for measuring a wide spectrum of serum proteins. Quantitative immunoglobulin measurements do not differentiate between normal and abnormal immunoglobulin molecules, as does the immunoelectrophoresis procedure.

IgD levels have no recognized clinical use, and IgE levels must be measured with more sensitive techniques such as radioimmunoassay.

Stites DP, Rodgers RPC: Clinical laboratory methods for detection of antigens and antibodies. Chap 17 in: *Basic & Clinical Immunology,* 6th ed. Stites DP, Stobo JD, Wells, JV (editors). Appleton-Lange, 1987.

## DISEASES OF IMMUNOGLOBULIN OVERPRODUCTION (Gammopathies)

The gammopathies include those disease entities in which there is a disproportionate proliferation of a single clone of immunoglobulin-forming cells that produce a homogeneous heavy chain, light chain, or complete molecule. The amino acid sequence of the variable (V) regions is fixed, and only one type (κ or λ) of light chain is produced.

### Benign Monoclonal Gammopathy

The diagnosis is made upon finding a homogeneous (monoclonal) immunoglobulin (with either κ or λ chains but not both) in immunoelectrophoresis of the serum of an otherwise normal individual. The incidence of homogeneous immunoglobulins in the serum increases with age and may approach 3% in persons 70 years of age or older. A small percentage of apparently normal persons with a homogeneous serum immunoglobulin will go on to develop multiple myeloma. Parameters that suggest a favorable prognosis in "benign" monoclonal gammopathy include the following: (1) concentration of homogeneous immunoglobulin less than 2 g/dL, (2) no significant increase in the concentration of the homogeneous immunoglobulin from the time of diagnosis, (3) no decrease in the concentration of normal immunoglobulins, (4) absence of a homogeneous light chain in the urine, and (5) normal hematocrit and serum albumin concentration.

## Multiple Myeloma

This disease is characterized by the spread of neoplastic plasma cells throughout the bone marrow. Rarely, a single extraosseous plasmacytoma may be found. Anemia, hypercalcemia, increased susceptibility to infection, and bone pain are frequent. Certain diagnosis depends upon the presence of the following: (1) radiographic findings of osteolytic lesions or diffuse osteoporosis, (2) the presence of a homogeneous serum immunoglobulin (myeloma protein) or a single type of light chain in the urine (Bence Jones proteinuria), and (3) finding of an abnormal plasma cell infiltrate in the bone marrow biopsy (see Chapter 10).

## Waldenström's Macroglobulinemia

Waldenström's macroglobulinemia is characterized by a proliferation of abnormal lymphoid cells that have the features of both B cells and plasma cells. These cells secrete a homogeneous macroglobulin (IgM) that is easily detected and characterized by immunoelectrophoresis. Bence Jones proteinuria is present in 10% of cases. Clinical manifestations depend upon the physicochemical characteristics of the macroglobulin. Raynaud's phenomenon and peripheral vascular occlusions are associated with cold-insoluble proteins (cryoglobulins). Retinal hemorrhages, visual impairment, and transient neurologic deficits are common with high-viscosity serum. Bleeding diatheses and hemolytic anemia can occur when the macroglobulin complexes with coagulation factors or binds to the surface of red blood cells.

## Amyloidosis

Amyloidosis is manifested by impaired organ function from infiltration of the tissue with insoluble protein fibrils. Variations in composition of the fibrils can be largely correlated with the clinical syndromes (Table 33–1).

One chemical type of amyloid occurs (1) in a primary form, or (2) in company with plasmacytosis in bone marrow or lymphoid tissues. The protein fibrils in these entities are composed of immunoglobulin light chains or fragments of light chains, particularly the V region. This form of amyloid has been designated AL.

A nonimmunoglobulin protein (AA) is the major component of amyloid fibrils that form secondary to infection (osteomyelitis, tuberculosis), inflammation, rheumatoid arthritis, Hodgkin's disease, regional enteritis, renal cell carcinoma, leprosy, and intravenous drug abuse. The hereditary systemic amyloidosis associated with familial Mediterranean fever is composed of AA protein. The source of the protein is obscure, but it may be derived from the acute-phase reactant SAA (serum amyloid-associated).

Symptoms and signs of amyloid infiltration are related to malfunction of the organ involved, eg, nephrotic syndrome, chronic renal failure, cardiomyopa-

**Table 33–1.** Classification of amyloidosis.*

| | **Clinical Type** | **Common Sites of Deposition** | **Chemical Type of Fibril†** |
|---|---|---|---|
| **Familial** | Amyloid polyneuropathy (Portuguese, dominant inheritance) | Peripheral nerves<br>Viscera | $AF_p$<br>(prealbumin) |
| | Familial Mediterranean fever (recessive) | Liver, spleen, kidneys, adrenals | AA |
| **Generalized** | Primary | Tongue, heart, gut, skeletal and smooth muscles, nerves, skin, ligaments | AL |
| | Associated with plasma cell dyscrasia | Liver, spleen, kidneys, heart, adrenals | AL |
| | Secondary (infection, inflammation, etc) | Any site | AA |
| **Localized** | Lichen amyloidosis | Skin | AD |
| | Endocrine-related (eg, thyroid medullary carcinoma, diabetes mellitus, Addison's disease) | Endocrine organ (thyroid) | $AE$<br>($AE_t$) |
| **Senile** | | Heart<br>Brain | $AS_c$<br>$AS_b$ |

* Modified and reproduced, with permission, from Stites DP et al (editors): *Basic & Clinical Immunology,* 5th ed. Lange, 1984.
† AA = amyloid A, AD = amyloid dermatologic; AE = amyloid endocrine; AF = amyloid familial; AL = amyloid light chain; AS = amyloid senile.

thy, cardiac conduction defects, intestinal malabsorption, intestinal obstruction, carpal tunnel syndrome, macroglossia, peripheral neuropathy, end-organ insufficiency of endocrine glands, respiratory failure, obstruction to ventilation, and capillary damage with ecchymosis. Table 33–1 lists organs characteristically involved with each type of amyloid.

The diagnosis of amyloidosis is based on suspicion, family history, and preexisting long-standing infection or debilitating illness. Microscopic examination of biopsy (eg, gingival, renal, rectal) or surgical specimens is diagnostic. Fine-needle biopsy of subcutaneous abdominal fat is a simple and reliable method for diagnosing secondary systemic amyloidosis.

Treatment of localized amyloid "tumors" is by surgical excision. There is no effective treatment of systemic amyloidosis, and death usually occurs within 1–3 years. Treatment of the predisposing disease may cause a temporary remission or slow the progress of the disease, but it is unlikely that the established metabolic process is altered. Patients with plasma cell dyscrasia may occasionally respond to treatment with melphalan and prednisone. Colchicine may be of use in familial Mediterranean fever. Early and adequate treatment of pyogenic infections will probably prevent much secondary amyloidosis.

## Heavy Chain Disease
### (α, γ, μ)

These are rare disorders in which the abnormal serum and urine protein is a part of a homogeneous α, γ, or μ heavy chain. The clinical presentation is more typical of lymphoma than multiple myeloma, and there are no destructive bone lesions. Alpha chain disease is frequently associated with severe diarrhea and infiltration of the lamina propria of the small intestine with abnormal plasma cells μ chain disease is associated with chronic lymphocytic leukemia.

Glenner GG: Amyloid deposits and amyloidosis: The fibrilloses. (2 parts.) *N Engl J Med* 1980;**302:**1283, 1333.

Kyle RA, Bayrd ED: *The Monoclonal Gammopathies.* Thomas, 1976.

Kyle RA et al: Amyloidosis: Clinical and laboratory features in 229 cases. *Mayo Clin Proc* 1983;**58:**665.

# CELLULAR IMMUNITY

## CELL INVOLVED IN IMMUNITY

### Development of T & B Lymphocytes

Lymphocytes interact with antigens via specific receptors and thereby initiate immune responses of vertebrates. In birds, 2 lines of lymphocytes exist: one derived from the thymus and the other from the bursa of Fabricius. The thymus-derived cells are involved in cellular immune responses; the bursa-derived cells are involved in antibody responses. In mammals, T lymphocytes are analogous to the thymus-derived cells in birds and B lymphocytes are analogous to the bursa-derived cells.

Both T and B lymphocytes are derived from precursor or stem cells in the marrow. Precursors of T cells migrate to the thymus, where they develop some of the functional and cell surface characteristics of mature T cells. Thereafter, the cells migrate to the peripheral lymphoid tissues and enter the pool of long-lived lymphocytes that recirculate from the blood to the lymph. Further maturation of T cells occurs under the influence of a thymic hormones (eg, thymosin).

B cell maturation can be either antigen-independent or antigen-dependent. Antigen-independent maturation includes those stages of B cell development from precursor cells in the marrow through the virgin B cell (a cell that has not been exposed to antigen previously) found in the peripheral lymphoid tissues. The production and maturation of virgin B cells are ongoing processes even in adult animals. Antigen-dependent maturation occurs following the interaction of antigen with virgin B cells. Memory B cells and antibody-forming cells (plasma cells) are the final products of this developmental sequence. Many of the memory B cells are long-lived and recirculate from the blood to the lymph. Mature B cells in the periphery are found predominantly in primary follicles and germinal centers of the lymph nodes and spleen.

### Subpopulations of T Cells

T lymphocytes are heterogeneous with respect to their cell surface features (Table 33–2) and functional characteristics. At least 4 subpopulations of T cells are now recognized.

**A. Helper-Inducer T Cells:** These cells help to amplify the production of antibody-forming cells from B lymphocytes after interaction with antigen. Helper T cells also amplify the production of effector T cells for cell-mediated cytotoxicity.

**B. Cytotoxic or Killer T Cells:** These cells are generated after mature T cells interact with certain antigens such as those present on the surface of foreign cells. These cells are responsible for organ graft rejection and for cell-mediated killing of foreign cells in vitro.

**C. Suppressor T Cells:** These cells suppress the formation of antibody-forming cells from B lymphocytes. Suppressor T cells are regarded as regulatory cells that modulate humoral antibody formation. Alterations in these cells may play an important role in those disease entities in which there is an overproduction (systemic lupus erythematosus or autoimmune thyroiditis) or an underproduction (common variable agammaglobulinemia) of immunoglobulin. Cell-mediated immunity (ie, organ graft rejection) is also regulated by suppressor cells.

**D. Suppressor-Inducer T Cells:** These cells,

**Table 33–2.** Surface antigens detected by monoclonal antibodies on T and B cells.

| T Cell Antigens | | | B Cell Surface Antigens |
|---|---|---|---|
| Cluster of Differentiation* | Usual Designations | T Cell Subsets | |
| CD3 | Leu 4, OKT 3, T3 | All T cells | Ig heavy and light chains. |
| CD2 | Leu 5, OKT 11, T11 | All T cells with sheep red blood cell receptor | DR antigen. |
| CD4 | Leu 3, OKT 4, T4 | Helper-inducer T cells | B cell-specific antigens (B1, B2, Leu 12). |
| CD8 | Leu 2, OKT 8, T8 | Suppressor or cytotoxic T cells | Fc receptor. |

\* Proposed nomenclature for T cell antigens.

which have helper cell (not suppressor cell) surface antigens, amplify the development of suppressor T cells.

## Identification of T Cell Subpopulations With Monoclonal Antibodies

Monoclonal antibodies to T cell subpopulations are produced by immunizing mice or rats with human T cells and subsequently fusing the spleen cells of the animal with mouse myeloma cells to develop hybridoma cell lines. These hybridoma lines secrete monoclonal antibodies that identify cell surface antigens common to all human T cells (Table 33–2). Lymphocytes stained with fluorescein-labeled monoclonal antibodies are enumerated by microscopy or flow cystometry. About 75% of the peripheral blood lymphocytes of normal individuals are T cells; 50% are helper-inducer T cells, and 25% are suppressor or cytotoxic T cells.

Changes in the number or ratio of various T cell subsets occur in a wide variety of clinical conditions. For example, the ratio of helper to suppressor (H/S) cells in healthy individuals is about 1.6–2.2. In many acute viral infections, this ratio falls both as a result of decrease in helper/inducer cells and of increase in suppressor/cytotoxic cells. In AIDS and related HIV infections, H/S ratios are nearly always reduced—probably irreversibly—by the destructive effects of this lymphotropic virus. Among other clinical applications of the enumeration of these cells are the diagnosis of some immunodeficiencies, phenotyping of leukemias and lymphomas, and monitoring of immunologic changes following organ transplantation.

## T Cell Lymphokines

Many T cell functions can be mediated by lymphokines, which are humoral factors secreted by lymphoid cells. Most lymphokines are secreted when T cells are activated by antigens. Table 33–3 lists examples of lymphokines and their function which are released from antigen-stimulated lymphocytes.

Lymphokines are used in both diagnosis and experimental treatment of disease. The secretion of macrophage inhibitory factor (MIF) by peripheral blood lymphocytes in vitro has been used as a test of T

lymphocyte function. IL-2 is currently being tested as an anticancer treatment in selected patients.

## T Cell Antigen Receptors

T cells interact with several different types of cells during the regulation and mediation of immune responses. Examples of T cell interactions with other cells include presentation of antigens to T cells by macrophages, T cell-induced differentiation of B cells into antibody-secreting cells, and T cell killing of a variety of virus-infected cells. In all of these cell-cell interactions, T cells recognize foreign antigens on the surface of the non-T cell in association with other cell surface antigens that are coded for by the major histocompatibility gene complex of the non-T cell. T cells have cell surface receptors that recognize at least 2 different molecules; one recognition site binds to any single foreign antigen (viral, bacterial, etc) and the other binds to major histocompatibility antigens. An example of this "dual recognition" is observed in the killing of virus-infected target cells by cytolytic T cells. Cytolytic T cells taken from humans immunized to a given virus will kill virus-infected target cells if the target cells carry the same histocompatibility antigens as the immunized host.

These facts raise concerns about host defense against viral infection in bone marrow transplant recipients who do not share the MHC (HLA) antigens of the marrow donors. After marrow transplantation, donor T cells maturing in the host thymus are presumed to recognize foreign antigen in association with host-type histocompatibility antigens. However,

**Table 33–3.** Non–antigen-specific T cell lymphokines.

| Lymphokine | Function |
|---|---|
| T cell growth factor (TCGF, IL-2) | Promotes proliferation of T cells activated by antigens or mitogens |
| B cell growth factor (BCGF) | Promotes proliferation of B cells activated by antigens or mitogens |
| Macrophage inhibitory factor (MIF) | Inhibits motility of macrophages |
| Macrophage activating factor (MAF) | Promotes killing of bacteria and tumor cells by macrophages |
| Gamma interferon | Inhibits viral replication |

most antigen-presenting cells will bear donor-type histocompatibility antigens; this may lead to a severe immunodeficiency state, with a completely mismatched marrow transplant. Fortunately, at the present time, almost all transplant recipients share at least one HLA haplotype with the donor.

The structure of T cell antigen receptors and the genes that encode these glycoproteins have all recently been defined. The antigen recognition structure is a complex of 2 molecules, one containing variable alpha and beta chains and the other the monomorphic T3 (CD3) molecule. Genes encoding the beta chain have homology to immunoglobulin genes. Clonal rearrangement of T cell receptor genes proceeds during T cell development in a fashion similar to that of immunoglobulin genes in B cells. Recent studies have applied T cell receptor gene rearrangements to identify T cell leukemias, lymphomas, and mycosis fungoides, a rare malignant neoplasm of the skin.

Acuto O, Reinherz EL: The human T cell receptor. *N Engl J Med* 1985;**312**:1100.
deWeck AL: Lymphokines. *Springer Semin Immunopathol* 1984;**7**:271.
Stobo JD: T cells. Chap 7 in: *Basic & Clinical Immunology,* 6th ed. Stites DP, Stobo JD, Wells, JV (editors). Appleton-Lange, 1987.
Forman J: T cells: The MHC and function. *Immunol Rev* 1984;**81**:203.

## B Lymphocyte Subpopulations

Subpopulations of B cells that express different classes of surface markers are shown in Table 33–2. The majority of B cells express both IgM and IgD on the surface and are derived from pre-B cells found mainly in the bone marrow. Pre-B cells contain intracytoplasmic IgM but do not express surface immunoglobulin. Patients with congenital hypogammaglobulinemia frequently show a developmental arrest at the stage of the pre-B cell. The majority of patients with acquired hypogammaglobulinemia have a block of transition from the mature B cell to the plasma cell. Thus, most patients with this disease have normal numbers of circulating mature B cells.

B cells have been commonly identified by other surface markers in addition to immunoglobulins. These include the receptor for the Fc piece of immunoglobulins, B cell–specific antigens, and surface antigens coded for by the HLA-D genetic region in humans (Table 33–2). All mature B cells bear surface immunoglobulin that is the antigen-specific receptor. In contrast to the remarkable functional heterogeneity of T cells, B cells have only one major function, which is to develop into antibody-producing plasma cells.

## Other Cells Involved in Immune Responses

**A. Macrophages:** Macrophages are involved in the initial ingestion and processing of particulate antigens before interaction with lymphocytes. They play an important role in T and B lymphocyte cooperation in the induction of humoral antibody responses. In addition, they are effector cells for certain types of tumor immunity.

**B. NK (Natural Killer) Cells:** These lymphocytic cells, which are indirectly related to the T cell lineage, can kill a wide spectrum of target cells. They are recognized by the presence of specific surface antigens or Fc receptors. Many appear as large granular lymphocytes. Their role in host defense is probably the killing of virally infected cells and tumor cells in the absence of prior sensitization and without MHC restriction.

Leavitt D, Cooper MD: B cells. Chap 7 in: *Basic & Clinical Immunology,* 6th ed. Stites DP, Stobo JD, Wells, JV (editors). Appleton-Lange, 1987.
Schattner A, Duggan DB: Natural killer cells: Toward clinical application. *Am J Hematol* 1985;**18**:443.
Werb Z: Macrophages. Chap 7 in: *Basic & Clinical Immunology,* 6th ed. Stites DP, Stobo JD, Wells, JV (editors). Appleton-Lange, 1987.

## TESTS FOR CELLULAR IMMUNITY

### Techniques for Identification of Human B & T Cells

**A. B Cells:** Cell surface characteristics usually found on B but not T cells include the following: (1) easily detectable surface immunoglobulin, (2) specific antigens, (3) a receptor for the Fc portion of immunoglobulins that have been aggregated or complexed with antigen, and (4) DR antigens (Table 33–2).

Surface immunoglobulin is detected by direct fluorescence staining of live cell suspensions with fluorescein-conjugated heterologous antisera directed against human immunoglobulin. The receptor for aggregated immunoglobulin is identified by incubating lymphocytes in vitro with fluorescein-labeled IgG aggregates.

Specific B cell antigens and DR antigens are detected by immunofluorescence with monoclonal antibodies.

**B. T Cells:** T cell markers include specific surface antigens identified by monoclonal antibodies. Monoclonal antisera have been used in both immunofluorescence staining and in vitro cytotoxicity assays to identify T cell subsets (Table 33–2). T cells can also be detected in tissue sections or suspensions using enzyme-labeled antibodies that produce colors on incubation with particular substrates. Antibodies coupled to beads or colloidal gold can also be detected by microscopic examination when bound to lymphocytes. Approximately 75% of human peripheral blood lymphocytes are T cells and up to 25% are B cells.

**C. Flow Cytometry:** Flow cytometers are instruments that accurately measure the size, density, and at least 2 colors of immunofluorescent monoclonal antibodies on human lymphocytes. Ten thousand cells can be analyzed individually for the presence of all these parameters at once. This method greatly improves the accuracy, speed, and precision of phenotyping human T and B cells in the clinical laboratory.

## Procedures for Testing Cell-Mediated Immunity, or T Cell Function

**A. Skin Testing:** Cell-mediated immunity can be assessed qualitatively by evaluating skin reactivity following intradermal injection of a battery of antigens to which humans are frequently sensitized (ie, streptokinase, streptodornase, purified protein derivative, *Trichophyton, Dermatophyton,* or *Candida*). Anergy or lack of skin reactivity to all of these substances indicates a depression of cell-mediated immunity. Delayed hypersensitivity skin tests depend on complex interactions of T cells, macrophages, and other immunoreactants; thus, failure to respond cannot specifically identify a defect in a particular cell type.

**B. In Vitro Stimulation of Peripheral Blood Lymphocytes With Phytohemagglutinin or Allogeneic Lymphocytes (Mixed Lymphocyte Culture, MLC):** T lymphocytes are transformed to blast cells upon short-term incubation with phytohemagglutinin or allogeneic lymphocytes in vitro. Quantitative determinations of T cell activation can be made by following the cellular uptake of $^3$H-thymidine introduced into the culture medium. The in vitro uptake of $^3$H-thymidine by human peripheral blood lymphocytes serves as an indicator of T cell function and correlates well with the manifestations of cell-mediated immunity as measured by delayed hypersensitivity skin tests.

## APPLICATIONS OF T & B CELL TESTS

## Immunodeficiency Diseases

Thymic hypoplasia is associated with a marked decrease in the number of T cells in the peripheral blood. On the other hand, the absence of B cells in the blood is frequently found in X-linked agammaglobulinemia. Typing of blood T and B cells can aid in the diagnosis of these diseases in early childhood. Patients with acquired immunodeficiency syndrome (AIDS) have reduced numbers of T cells and reduced T helper and suppressor ratios.

## Lymphoproliferative Diseases

A marked increase in the number of peripheral blood lymphocytes that bear immunoglobulin of a single heavy chain class and light chain type represents a monoclonal proliferation of cells. Almost all patients with chronic lymphocytic leukemia and non-Hodgkin's lymphoma with blood involvement show this picture. On the other hand, lymphocytosis secondary to viral or bacterial infection is associated with a

normal percentage of B cells and the usual distribution of immunoglobulin classes on the cell surface.

Lymphocytic leukemias can be classified by phenotyping T and B cells, with implications for prognosis and, sometimes, treatment. Monitoring various T cell subsets is also useful in following patients with organ transplants.

Stites DP: Clinical laboratory methods for detection of cellular immune function. Chap 18 in: *Basic & Clinical Immunology,* 6th ed. Stites DP, Stobo JD, Wells, JV (editors). Appleton-Lange, 1987.

# IMMUNOLOGIC DEFICIENCY DISEASES

The primary immunologic deficiency diseases include congenital and acquired disorders of humoral immunity (B cell function) or cell-mediated immunity (T cell function). Most of these diseases are rare and—since they are genetically determined—occur almost exclusively in children. A classification of immunodeficiency disorders recommended by WHO is shown below:

Infantile X-linked agammaglobulinemia (see below)
Selective immunoglobulin deficiency (see below)
Transient hypogammaglobulinemia of infancy
X-linked immunodeficiency with hyper-IgM
Thymic hypoplasia (pharyngeal pouch syndrome, DiGeorge's syndrome) (see below)
Immunodeficiency with normal serum globulins or hyperimmunoglobulinemia
Immunodeficiency with ataxia-telangiectasia (see below)
Immunodeficiency with thrombocytopenia and eczema (Wiskott-Aldrich syndrome) (see below)
Immunodeficiency with thymoma
Immunodeficiency with generalized hematopoietic hypoplasia
Severe combined immunodeficiency (see below):
  (1) With dysostosis
  (2) With adenosine deaminase deficiency
Variable immunodeficiency (common, largely unclassified) (see below)
Acquired immunodeficiency syndrome (AIDS) (see below)

Ammann AJ: Immunodeficiency diseases. Chap 20 in: *Basic & Clinical Immunology,* 6th ed. Stites DP, Stobo JD, Wells JV (editors). Appleton-Lange, 1987.
Bergsma D et al (editors): *Immunodeficiency in Man and Animals.* (National Foundation–March of Dimes Original Article Series.) Sinauer Associates, 1975.
Cooper MD et al: Meeting report of the Second International Workshop on Primary Immunodeficiency Disease in Man. *Clin Immunol Immunopathol* 1974;**2**:416.

Stiehm ER, Fulginiti VA: *Immunologic Disorders in Infants and Children,* 2nd ed. Saunders, 1980.

## INFANTILE X-LINKED AGAMMAGLOBULINEMIA

This hereditary disorder results in a deficit in B cell function with essentially intact T cell function.

### Clinical Findings

The diagnosis is based on low IgG levels in serum, an X-linked pattern of heredity, intact cell-mediated immunity, and the absence of plasma cells in biopsy specimens of regional lymph nodes draining the site of recent antigenic stimulation, eg, DTP vaccine.

**A. Symptoms and Signs:** There are no symptoms during the first 5–6 months of life (probably due to presence of maternal antibody). Thereafter, the infant shows increased susceptibility to pyogenic infections (gram-positive organisms) and *Haemophilus influenzae,* resulting in recurrent furunculosis, pneumonia, and meningitis. There is normal susceptibility to viral exanthematous infections such as rubella, measles, and chickenpox. Other characteristic findings are chronic sinusitis, bronchiectasis, and arthritis of the large joints similar to rheumatoid arthritis.

**B. Laboratory Findings:** IgG levels in the serum are less than 200 mg/dL, serum IgA and IgM levels are less than 1% of normal, and isohemagglutinins are low or absent. The Schick test is positive, and antitoxin titers do not rise after vaccination with DTP vaccine. The peripheral lymphocyte count and delayed type hypersensitivity skin tests are normal. There are no B lymphocytes in the peripheral blood in most cases.

### Treatment

Recurrent bacterial infections can be prevented by the administration of gamma globulin for an indefinite period of time. The gamma globulin is usually administered intramuscularly at a dose of 0.2–0.4 mL/kg. Intravenous gamma globulin is also used at a dose of 100–400 mg/kg given over 2–4 hours. The need for repeated infusions can be determined by monitoring blood levels of IgG.

## THYMIC HYPOPLASIA (DiGeorge's Syndrome)

DiGeorge's syndrome is due to failure of embryogenesis of the third and fourth pharyngeal pouches. This results in aplasia of the parathyroid and thymus glands. The syndrome presents as a pure T cell functional deficiency with relatively intact B cell function.

### Clinical Findings

**A. Symptoms and Signs:** The major manifestations are neonatal tetany, hypertelorism, and increased susceptibility to viral, fungal, and bacterial infections. Infections are frequently lethal.

**B. Laboratory Findings:** Serum immunoglobulin levels are usually normal. Antibody responses may be low or normal, depending on the antigen used for immunization. Reactions to delayed hypersensitivity skin tests are absent, lymphocyte counts are low, and functional T cell assays are abnormal. Serum calcium is reduced, phosphorus is elevated, and parathyroid hormone is absent. Biopsy of lymph nodes shows normal germinal center formation but marked deficits in the thymus-dependent or paracortical areas.

### Treatment

Transplantation of fetal thymic tissue has been successful in reversing the deficits in cell-mediated immunity and raising the peripheral lymphocyte count to normal. The thymus-dependent areas of the lymph nodes of transplant recipients are also repopulated. Spontaneous remissions may occur.

## SEVERE COMBINED IMMUNODEFICIENCY

Both T and B cell function are markedly decreased in this entity, which is inherited in an autosomal recessive or X-linked pattern. A sporadic appearance in families also occurs. Dysostosis and adenosine deaminase deficiency occur in some cases.

### Clinical Findings

**A. Symptoms and Signs:** Increased susceptibility to infection is noted at 3–6 months of age. Death usually occurs within 2 years. In infancy, there is watery diarrhea, usually associated with *Salmonella* or enteropathic *Escherichia coli* infections. Pulmonary infections, usually with *Pseudomonas* and *Pneumocystis carinii,* are common, as is candidiasis in the mouth and diaper areas. Common viral exanthems such as chickenpox and measles are often lethal.

**B. Laboratory Findings:** Serum immunoglobulin levels are usually less than 1% of normal, and antibodies do not form in response to vaccinations such as DTP. The peripheral lymphocyte count is less than 2000/μL. Decreased delayed hypersensitivity is manifested by lack of skin reactivity to antigens. Lymph node biopsy shows no lymphocytes, plasma cells, or lymphoid follicles.

### Treatment

Passive administration of gamma globulin is temporarily effective. Bone marrow transplantation has been successful.

## IMMUNODEFICIENCY WITH THROMBOCYTOPENIA & ECZEMA (Wiskott-Aldrich Syndrome)

This disorder is characterized by eczema, thrombocytopenia, and recurrent bacterial and viral infections. Inheritance is X-linked, and affected individuals rarely survive more than 10 years. There appears to be a combined T and B cell functional deficit. IgM levels are low and isohemagglutinins absent, but IgG and IgA levels are normal. Cell-mediated immunity is impaired.

## IMMUNODEFICIENCY WITH ATAXIA-TELANGIECTASIA

Ataxia-telangiectasia begins in infancy with ataxia and choreoathetoid movements. Telangiectasia of the conjunctiva, face, arms, and eyelids is first noted 5–10 years later. Chronic sinusitis and respiratory infections follow, and death due to intercurrent pulmonary infection or lymphoreticular neoplasm occurs in the second or third decade. Approximately 80% of affected individuals lack serum and secretory IgA. In addition, there is a marked deficit in T cell function associated with a hypoplastic or dysplastic thymus gland. The disease is inherited in an autosomal recessive pattern.

## VARIABLE IMMUNODEFICIENCY

### Primary Acquired Hypogammaglobulinemia

Onset is in adulthood, with increased susceptibility to pyogenic infections; recurrent sinusitis and pneumonia progressing to bronchiectasis; spruelike syndrome with diarrhea, steatorrhea, malabsorption, and protein-losing enteropathy; and hepatosplenomegaly.

Arthritis of the type associated with congenital hypogammaglobulinemia and autoimmune diseases may occur. Serum IgG levels are usually less than 250 mg/dL; serum IgA and IgM levels are subnormal. Lymph node biopsy shows marked reduction in plasma cells. Noncaseating granulomas are frequently found in the spleen, liver, lungs, or skin.

Suppressor T cells inhibit B cells from producing antibody-forming cells in certain cases of adult-onset hypogammaglobulinemia. The absolute B cell count in the peripheral blood in these cases is normal. Although therapy at present is similar to that of congenital agammaglobulinemia, newer therapeutic goals may include elimination of suppressor T cells.

## SELECTIVE IMMUNOGLOBULIN DEFICIENCY

Absence of serum IgA with normal levels of IgG and IgM is found in a small percentage of normal individuals. Some cases of IgA deficiency may spontaneously remit. The associated deficiency of the IgG2 subclass is often associated with infections. Occasionally, a spruelike syndrome with steatorrhea has been associated with an isolated IgA deficit. Treatment

with commercial gamma globulin is ineffective, since IgA and IgM are not present in this preparation. Frequent infusions of plasma (containing IgA) are hazardous, since anti-IgA antibodies may develop, resulting in systemic anaphylaxis or serum sickness.

## ACQUIRED IMMUNODEFICIENCY SYNDROME (AIDS) (See also Chapter 21.)

AIDS is an example of a hitherto unrecognized form of immunodeficiency in which a chronic retroviral infection with HTLV-III/LAV/ARV (also called HIV—human immunodeficiency virus) in a susceptible host produces severe, life-threatening T cell defects. In addition to reduction of CD4 (T helper cells), there is an increase in CD8 (T suppressor cells), most of which have a cytotoxic phenotype.

B cell function is abnormal in that many infected individuals have marked hypergammaglobulinemia and fail to respond normally to antigens when immunized. Autoantibodies to T cells and circulating immune complexes are present. Clearly, only some infected individuals progress from health to ARC (AIDS-related complex) to AIDS, and usually over several years. The immunologic changes that occur in pre-AIDs are usually not as marked as in AIDS patients. The immunologic determinants of the clinical fate of persons infected with the AIDS virus are unknown.

Immunologic tests reveal a severe deficiency of T lymphocyte function and number, with little alteration in B lymphocyte numbers. Patients are frequently anergic. In vitro tests of peripheral blood T cell function such as proliferative responses to antigens and mitogens are markedly reduced or absent. The absolute lymphocyte count is severely decreased (frequently < 500 cells/μL), and the ratio of helper to suppressor/cytotoxic T cells is considerably lower than normal. The change in the latter ratio is due to a greater reduction in the absolute number of helper T cells in the peripheral blood as compared to suppressor/cytotoxic cells.

The causative virus is transmitted by sexual contact or intravenous routes, including blood transfusion. The disease is lethal in a high proportion of victims, especially those with Kaposi's sarcoma. Many studies with experimental antiviral therapy are in progress. No immunization is available.

Ammann AJ: Immunodeficiency diseases. Chap 20 in: *Basic & Clinical Immunology*, 6th ed. Stites DP, Stobo JD, Wells, JV (editors). Appleton-Lange, 1987.

Gallo RC: The AIDS virus. *Sci Am* 1987;**256**:46.

Levy JA: *AIDS: Pathogenesis and Treatment*. Marcel Dekker, 1987.

## SECONDARY IMMUNODEFICIENCY

Deficiencies in cell-mediated immunity, humoral immunity, or both have been associated with many diseases. Two examples of altered immunity secondary to underlying disease are discussed below.

## Immunodeficiency Associated With Sarcoidosis

The immunodeficiency associated with sarcoidosis is characterized by a partial deficit in T cell function with intact B cell function. Patients with sarcoidosis often are relatively nonreactive to intradermal injections of common antigens. However, complete lack of skin reactivity is infrequent. A positive reaction to purified protein derivative is usually noted during active infection with *Mycobacterium tuberculosis*. Serum immunoglobulin levels are normal or high, and specific antibody formation is generally intact.

## Immunodeficiency Associated With Hodgkin's Disease

A moderate to severe deficit in T cell function with intact B cell function is frequently found in Hodgkin's disease. Only 10–20% of patients with Hodgkin's disease show skin reactivity to common antigens, as compared to 70–90% of controls. Many patients show depressed responses to in vitro stimulation of peripheral blood lymphocytes with phytohemagglutinin. Serum immunoglobulins are normal, and specific antibody formation is intact except in agonal cases.

The clinical significance of depressed cell-mediated immunity in Hodgkin's disease is difficult to evaluate, since most patients are treated with potent immunosuppressive agents. Nevertheless, frequent infections with herpes zoster and *Cryptococcus* are probably related to immunodeficiency associated with the underlying disease.

Ammann AJ: Immunodeficiency diseases. Chap 22, in: *Basic & Clinical Immunology,* 6th ed. Stites DP, Stobo JD, Wells JV (editors). Appleton-Lange, 1987.

Rosen FS, Cooper MD, Wedgwood RJP: The primary immunodeficiencies. (2 parts.) *N Engl J Med* 1984;**311**:235, 300.

Stiehm ER, Fulginiti VA: *Immunologic Disorders of Infants and Children.* Saunders, 1980.

# AUTOIMMUNITY

Autoimmune diseases cannot be explained by a solitary cause or mechanism. Small amounts of autoantibodies are normally produced and may have physiologic roles in cellular interactions. The major theories regarding the development of autoimmune disease are (1) release of sequestered antigens, (2) the presence of abnormal clones, (3) shared antigens between the host and microorganisms, and (4) defects in helper or suppressor cell function and genetic susceptibility. In nearly all autoimmune diseases, multiple mechanisms of autoimmunity are operative and the exact causes are unknown.

## Cell-Mediated Autoimmunity

Certain autoimmune diseases are mediated by T cells that have become specifically immunized to autologous tissues. Cytotoxic or killer T cells generated by this aberrant immune response attack and injure specific organs in the absence of serum autoantibodies.

Diminished suppressor T cell activity results in disordered regulation of immune responses and may promote overactivity of other autoreactive mechanisms. The immune damage in nonorganic specific diseases such as systemic lupus erythematosus may be in part due to such a mechanism.

## Humoral Antibody-Mediated Autoimmunity

Several autoimmune diseases have been shown to be caused by humoral autoantibody in the absence of cell-mediated autoimmunity. The autoimmune hemolytic anemias, idiopathic thrombocytopenia, and Goodpasture's syndrome appear to be mediated solely by autoantibodies directed against autologous cell membrane constituents. In these diseases, antibody attaches to cell membranes, fixes complement, and thereby causes severe injury to the cell.

The existence of anti-receptor antibodies that compete with or mimic various physiologic agonists for cellular receptors is a specific autoimmune mechanism in several diseases. In Graves' disease, antibodies are present that compete with thyroid cells' TSH receptors and thereby stimulate thyroid hormone production. In rare instances of type I diabetes mellitus, anti-insulin receptor antibodies cause insulin resistance in peripheral target tissues. The anti-islet cell antibodies that are usually found in diabetes produce insulin deficiency by destroying islet cells in the pancreas.

In myasthenia gravis, antibodies to acetylcholine receptors of the myoneural junction block neuromuscular transmission and thereby produce muscle weakness.

## Immune Complex Disease

In this group of diseases (systemic lupus erythematosus, rheumatoid arthritis, some drug-induced hemolytic anemias and thrombocytopenias), autologous tissues are injured as "innocent bystanders." Autoantibodies are not directed against cellular components of the target organ but rather against autologous or heterologous antigens in the serum. The resultant antigen-antibody complexes bind nonspecifically to autologous membranes (eg, glomerular basement membrane) and fix complement. Fixation and subsequent activation of complement components produce a local inflammatory response that results in tissue injury.

Theofilopoulos AN: Autoimmunity. Chap 11 in: *Basic & Clinical Immunology,* 6th ed. Stites DP, Stobo JD, Wells, JV (editors). Appleton-Lange, 1987.

## AUTOIMMUNE DISEASES

The diagnosis and treatment of specific autoimmune diseases are described elsewhere in this book. Autoantibodies associated with certain autoimmune diseases are not usually implicated in the pathogenesis of tissue injury but are thought instead to be by-products of the injury (eg, autoimmune thyroiditis and antithyroglobulin antibody).

## TESTS FOR AUTOANTIBODIES ASSOCIATED WITH AUTOIMMUNE DISEASES

Assays for autoantibodies are similar to those used for detection of antibodies to heterologous antigens. Four commonly used methods are discussed below:

### Agglutination of Antigen-Coated Red Blood Cells

Red cells (human, sheep, etc) are incubated with tannic acid or other chemicals so that the cell surface becomes "sticky." The red cells are subsequently incubated with the specific antigen (eg, thyroglobulin), which is adsorbed to the cell surface. The antigen-coated cells are suspended in the unknown serum, and antibody is detected by red cell agglutination. Antigen-coated latex particles are substituted for red cells in the latex fixation test.

### Enzyme-Linked Immunoassays (ELISA)

Antibodies to various tissue antigens can be readily detected by ELISA tests. Extracted or purified antigens are fixed to a plastic microtiter well or beads. Patient's serum is added, and excess proteins are removed by washing and centrifugation. A second antibody coupled to an enzyme (eg, alkaline phosphatase) is added. The enzyme's substrate is then added, and color forms that is measured in a spectrophotometer. This test can also be adapted to antigen detection by placing the antibody on the plastic surface. ELISA assays have become widely applied in clinical laboratory testing.

### Immunofluorescence Microscopy

This technique is most frequently used for detection of antinuclear antibody. Frozen sections of mouse liver or other substrates are cut and placed on glass slides. Unknown serum is placed over the sections and washed away. A fluorescein-conjugated rabbit anti-human immunoglobulin is applied thereafter and washed. Antinuclear antibody specifically binds to the mouse cell nucleus, and the fluorescein conjugate binds to the human antibody. Fluorescence of the cell nucleus observed by fluorescence microscopy indicates a positive test.

### Complement Fixation

Specific antigen, unknown serum, and complement are incubated together. Sheep red blood cells coated with anti-sheep cell antibody are subsequently added to the reaction mixture for 30 minutes at 37 °C. Lysis of sheep cells indicates that complement is present (attaches to sheep cell surface). Lack of lysis indicates that complement has been consumed by the interaction of antibody in the unknown serum with the specific antigen. Lack of lysis is a positive test for the presence of specific antibody.

A list of autoimmune diseases and frequently associated autoantibodies is shown in Table 33–4. Many of the autoantibodies are not specific for a single disease entity (eg, antinuclear antibody, rheumatoid factor). Tests for the latter autoantibodies are best used as screening procedures in that a negative result makes the diagnosis of certain autoimmune diseases unlikely. For example, a negative antinuclear antibody test makes the diagnosis of systemic lupus erythematosus unlikely, since this antibody is detected in the serum of more than 95% of lupus patients.

**Table 33–4.** Some autoimmune diseases and their associated antibodies.

| Autoimmune Disease | Associated Autoantibodies |
| --- | --- |
| Autoimmune hemolytic anemia | Anti-blood group substance antibody |
| Autoimmune thyroiditis | Antithyroglobulin antibody |
| Chronic active hepatitis | Anti-smooth muscle, anticytoplasmic, antinuclear, anti-immunoglobulin (rheumatoid factor) antibody |
| Goodpasture's syndrome | Anti-basement membrane antibody |
| Idiopathic thrombocytopenic purpura | Antiplatelet antibody |
| Pemphigoid | Anti-basement membrane antibody |
| Pemphigus vulgaris | Anti-intercellular antibody |
| Pernicious anemia | Anti-parietal cell, anti-intrinsic factor antibody |
| Polymyositis | Antinuclear antibody |
| Primary biliary cirrhosis | Antimitochondrial antibody, antinuclear antibody |
| Rheumatoid arthritis | Anti-immunoglobulin (rheumatoid factor), antinuclear antibody |
| Scleroderma | Antinuclear antibody |
| Sjögren's syndrome | Anti-immunoglobulin, anti-salivary gland, antinuclear antibody |
| Systemic lupus erythematosus | Antinuclear, anti-DNA, anti-ENA (extractable nuclear antigen), anti-immunoglobulin, antilymphocyte, anti-red blood cell antibody |

# IMMUNOGENETICS & TRANSPLANTATION

## GENETIC CONTROL OF THE IMMUNE RESPONSE

The ability to mount a specific immune response is under the direct control of genes closely associated on the same chromosome with the structural genes for the major transplantation antigens. The major transplantation antigens are the cell surface glycoproteins (found on most cells of the body), which elicit the strongest transplantation rejection reaction when tissues are exchanged between 2 members of a particular species. In humans, this genetic region has been designated the **human leukocyte antigen (HLA)** complex because these antigens were first detected on peripheral blood lymphocytes. The complex includes antigens HLA-A, -B, -C, -DR, and others, each with many alleles.

The HLA region has been localized to chromosome 6, and the order of the different HLA loci is shown in Fig 33–1. Most (98%) of the time, the HLA complex is inherited intact as 2 haplotypes (one from each parent), and within any particular family, therefore, the number of different combinations found will be fairly small; eg, siblings have a 1:4 chance of being HLA-identical. In contrast, the number of antigen combinations among unrelated individuals is huge, resulting in probabilities of fewer than one in several thousand, depending upon the phenotype involved, of finding HLA-compatible individuals in a random donor pool. This is particularly important when compatible donors are needed for allosensitized patients requiring platelet transfusions or organ transplantation; family members have the highest likelihood of being compatible donors, whereas HLA compatibility between 2 unrelated individuals has a very low probability. HLA-A and -B typing is utilized for selection of compatible donors for platelet transfusions to allosensitized, thrombocytopenic recipients. Typing for these class I antigens as well as for HLA-D antigens is important in determining compatibility for organ transplantation. Typing for HLA markers is of value in studying associations between the HLA system and genetic control of disease susceptibility.

In the genetic region determining the structure of the mixed lymphocyte culture antigens and the major transplantation antigen complex, there are genes determining the ability to mount a specific immune response. These are called immune response, or **Ir,** genes. Although the exact mechanism of action of Ir genes is not yet known, it is clear that they affect the ability to recognize foreign antigens and to initiate the development of cellular and humoral immunity to these antigens. Genes with such a strong effect on specific immune responsiveness might be expected to have major effects on resistance or susceptibility to a wide variety of infectious, neoplastic, and autoimmune diseases.

Typing for HLA-D antigens has revealed extraordinarily strong associations between these genes and particular human diseases (see Table 33–5).

Schwartz BD: The human major histocompatibility HLA complex. Chap 6 in: *Basic & Clinical Immunology,* 6th ed. Stites DP, Stobo JD, Wells, JV (editors). Appleton-Lange, 1987.

## HLA TYPING

The standard method for detecting HLA-A, -B, and -C antigens is that of lymphocyte microcytotoxicity. Lymphocytes isolated from peripheral blood or lymph nodes are added to each well of a typing tray that has been preloaded with sera containing the appropriate cytotoxic alloantibody. After allowing for the alloantibodies to bind to target lymphocytes, complement is added. Those cells to which antibody has been specifically bound will have complement activated at the cell surface, resulting in cell death or lysis. By addition of a vital dye (eg, eosin, fluorescein diacetate, or trypan blue), viable and nonviable cells can be distinguished. It is thus possible to type for all of the known HLA-A, -B, and -C specificities. At present, the best sources of alloantisera are parous women, 10–30% of whom become sensitized during pregnancy to paternal antigens carried by the fetus. A few antibodies are also provided by individuals allosensitized by other causes, eg, transfusion or transplantation, and a few monoclonal antibodies are also used.

Typing for the class II antigens HLA-DR and -DQ is performed as described above, except that separated B lymphocytes are used as targets rather than unseparated peripheral blood lymphocytes. Antigens of the HLA-D and -DP series are detected by in vitro cellular reactivity. Lymphocytes of one individual will undergo DNA synthesis and proliferation upon encountering lymphocytes from another individual possessing foreign HLA-D antigens. Donor cells are irradiated or treated with mitomycin C to ablate their immune responsiveness. These "stimulator" cells are then mixed with peripheral blood lymphocytes of the recipient (responder) in this mixed leukocyte culture (MLR). A responder lacking the stimula-

```
          DQ   Bf
  —DP—DR—C2—B—C——A—
          D    C4
```

**Figure 33–1** Genetic map of the HLA region. The centromere is to the left. Bf, C2, and C4 are genes for components of the complement system.

**Table 33–5.** HLA and disease associations.

| Disease | Antigen | Frequency | | Relative Risk |
| --- | --- | --- | --- | --- |
| | | Patients (%) | Controls (%) | |
| Ankylosing spondylitis Caucasians | B27 | 79–100 | 4–13 | 87 |
| Japanese | B27 | 67–92 | 0–2 | 324 |
| Reiter's disease | B27 | 65–100 | 4–14 | 37 |
| *Salmonella* arthritis | B27 | 60–92 | 8–14 | 30 |
| Rheumatoid arthritis | DR4 | 70 | 28 | 6 |
| Psoriasis vulgaris | Cw6 | 87 | 33 | 13 |
| Graves' disease Caucasians | Dw3 | 50–54 | 4–26 | 4 |
| Japanese | Dw12 | 48 | 16 | 5 |
| Diabetes mellitus | DR3 heterozygotes | | | 3 |
| Diabetes mellitus | DR4 heterozygotes | | | 6 |
| Diabetes mellitus | DR3/DR4 heterozygotes | | | 33 |
| Acute lymphocytic leukemia | A2 | 83 | 44 | 6 |
| Systemic lupus erythematosus | DR4 | 73 | 33 | 5 |
| Narcolepsy | DR2 | 100 | 22 | > 400 |

tor's D antigen will respond by brisk DNA synthesis and proliferation that can readily be measured by DNA incorporation of tritiated thymidine. Responders possessing the D antigen of the donor will remain nonreactive.

HLA-DP antigens are identified by an extension of the MLR called primed lymphocyte typing. Following stimulation in a first MLR, the responder cells are restimulated in a secondary MLR by a different stimulator cell. If the 2 stimulator cells share a DP (or a D) antigen not possessed by the responder, the responder cells will demonstrate a brisk proliferative response.

Although technically demanding and requiring viable lymphoid cells and experienced laboratories, HLA typing is available at most large medical centers or blood banks.

Grumet FC: HLA serology—1983. Pages 207–220 in: *Advances in Immunobiology: Blood Cell Antigens and Bone Marrow Transplantation.* McCullough J, Sandler SG (editors). Liss, 1984.

Moen T: Primed lymphocyte typing (PLT): Application in typing for HLA-D locus determinants. Pages 71–82 in: *HLA Typing: Methodology and Clinical Aspects.* Vol 1. Ferrone S, Solheim BG (editors). CRC Press, 1982.

## CLINICAL TRANSPLANTATION

Organ transplants are commonly used in the treatment of many diseases. The main limitation to more widespread use of transplants is the scarcity of donor organs and the expense of these procedures. Failure to achieve completely successful grafts is primarily due to histoincompatibility and lack of totally safe and effective immunosuppressive regimens to halt rejection.

### Kidney Transplantation

End-stage renal disease is the indication for kidney transplantation. Kidneys from living related donors who are HLA-identical and also red blood cell ABO-matched have 90% survival at 1 year; less identical grafts have a somewhat lower survival rate. Transplants with matched cadaver kidney donors survive nearly as long, especially if the recipient does not contain antibodies to donor antigens. Donor screening is performed in all cases to avoid transmission of AIDS virus or other infectious agents. Pretreatment of recipients with blood transfusions from the donor appears to extend graft survival even longer. Graft rejection is manifested by diminishing renal function and is treated with immunosuppressive drugs (see below).

### Heart Transplantation

The indication for heart transplantation is end-stage cardiac disease clearly refractory to medical treatment. Donors and recipients are matched by excluding anti-HLA antibodies in the recipient, since there is rarely time for HLA typing. Rejection is diagnosed by endomyocardial biopsy and treated with immunosuppressants, particularly cyclosporine. Five-year survival is approximately 40% at selected centers.

### Lung Transplantation

Lung transplantation is currently combined with heart transplantation because of the poor results achieved with lung grafts alone. One-year survival may be as high as 70%.

## Liver Transplantation

Severe liver dysfunction without serious systemic complications of hepatic failure is the indication for liver transplantation. Children with developmental defects are typical recipients. Recipients are selected on the basis of ABO matching and organ size. HLA typing has not achieved practical results. One-year survival rates approach 70%.

## Pancreas & Islet Cell Transplants

The indications for these procedures—largely experimental at present—are pancreatic insufficiency and, in some cases, diabetes mellitus. Clinical results have been disappointing.

## Bone Marrow Transplantation

Leukemia, aplastic anemia, and congenital immunologic defects are currently the main indications for marrow transplants. HLA irradiation and immunosuppressive doses are used to prepare recipients. Graft-versus-host disease caused by attack of donor cells on histocompatible host cells may be fatal. This occurs more commonly in adults, which limits the use of bone marrow transplantation in this age group. Infections during the period of emerging immune competence can also present life-threatening problems.

The success rates of bone marrow transplantation are about 70% survival at 1 year in aplastic anemia, 40–75% survival at 1 year in various forms of leukemia, and extremely variable in immunologic deficiency diseases.

## Other Organs & Tissues

Transplantations of other organs—skin, cornea, bone, and heart valves—are now routine surgical procedures. Much further research remains to be done on transplantation of other organs—particularly neural tissue.

Garovoy MR et al: Clinical transplantation. Chap 23 in: *Basic & Clinical Immunology,* 6th ed. Stites DP, Stobo JD, Wells, JV (editors). Appleton-Lange, 1987.

## MECHANISM OF ACTION OF IMMUNOSUPPRESSIVE DRUGS

Therapies that suppress immune responses are used commonly to treat recipients of organ transplants and patients with autoimmune diseases or neoplasms. The most frequently used drugs and their modes of action are briefly summarized below.

**(1) Corticosteroids.** This group of drugs has potent anti-inflammatory and direct effects on immunocompetent cells. Corticosteroids inhibit cell-mediated immune responses more severely than antibody responses. T helper cells are preferentially reduced owing to redistribution. Neutrophils are increased owing to demargination and bone marrow release. Mono-

cytes and eosinophils are reduced. These cellular changes result in reduced inflammatory responses. Disruption of the interaction between T cells and macrophages appears to be an important mechanism, and corticosteroids have been shown to block the activation of T cells by interleukin-1 (IL-1) derived from macrophages. In addition, corticosteroids inhibit the expression of class II histocompatibility antigens on the macrophage surface, thereby interfering with presentation of antigen to T cells.

**(2) Cytotoxic drugs.** The most frequently used cytotoxic drugs are azathioprine and cyclophosphamide. Azathioprine is a derivative of mercaptopurine, an antagonist of purine synthesis. Azathioprine is a phase-specific drug that kills rapidly replicating cells. It inhibits proliferation of both T and B cells as well as macrophages. Cyclophosphamide is an alkylating agent that damages cells by cross-linking DNA. Although this cycle-specific drug is most effective in killing cells going through the mitotic cycle, it can also cause intermitotic cell injury and death. Cyclophosphamide can inhibit both cell-mediated and humoral immunity as well as inflammation. Azathioprine and cyclophosphamide are effective inhibitors of the production of serum antibodies.

**(3) Antimetabolites.** The most commonly used antimetabolite is methotrexate, an inhibitor of folic acid synthesis. Methotrexate inhibits rapidly proliferating cells in S phase and suppresses both cell-mediated and humoral immunity as well as inflammation.

**(4) Cyclosporine.** This cyclic polypeptide derived from a fungus has been used recently as an immunosuppressive drug in organ transplant recipients. Cyclosporine interferes with the secretion of interleukin-2 (IL-2) by T lymphocytes. Since IL-2 is necessary for T cell replication, this drug is a potent inhibitor of T cell proliferation and thereby inhibits T cell-mediated immune responses. Little effect has been shown on direct B cell immune responses or on inflammation. Its toxic effects are primarily on renal and hepatic function.

Seaman W: Immunomodulation. Chap 16 in: *Basic & Clinical Immunology,* 6th ed. Stites DP, Stobo JD, Wells, JV (editors). Appleton-Lange, 1987.

## ASSOCIATIONS BETWEEN HLA ANTIGENS & SPECIFIC DISEASES

In humans, very striking associations are observed between particular HLA antigens and specific diseases. These facts are important in relating HLA to diseases: HLA antigen frequencies vary substantially among different ethnic groups, and therefore control populations must be carefully selected. Appropriate statistical corrections must be made to compensate for the large number of antigens tested. Accurate clinical definition of disease is necessary to avoid diluting an HLA-disease association by mixing together diseases that are pathogenetically different but clinically similar. If the disease studied has a fatal outcome, then the proper disease phase must be selected to demonstrate associations. Some quantitative measure of strength of association is necessary to compare different HLA-disease relationships.

Table 33–5 is a partial list of HLA-disease associations. Studies have revealed that the strongest association is between HLA-B27 and ankylosing spondylitis, which holds in all ethnic groups but is more striking in Japanese people than in Caucasians studied. Other spondyloarthropathies (eg, Reiter's syndrome, arthritis following *Salmonella* or *Yersinia* infection) are also strongly associated with B27, suggesting that despite apparently different causes the pathogeneses of these diseases share some common factor related to the B27 marker. B27 is not specific for all arthritis; eg, rheumatoid arthritis associates not with that antigen but with DR4. Furthermore, disease associations are not restricted to B and DR; eg, psoriasis vulgaris is associated with a C locus antigen and acute lymphocytic leukemia with an A locus antigen. In diabetes mellitus, heterozygote individuals possess both the DR3 and the DR4 antigens and have a relative risk of 33, far greater than expected by simple addition

of risks for DR3 plus DR4. It also appears that a single mechanism may associate with different antigens in different ethnic groups. Among Caucasians studied in whom the Dw12 antigen is almost absent, Dw3 is associated with Graves' disease. Among Japanese people where Dw3 is almost completely lacking, Dw12 is associated with Graves' disease.

Sometimes combinations of antigens exhibit disease associations. This suggests either interaction among different genes affecting susceptibility or unusual linkage between the known HLA genes and some nearby gene actually responsible for the disease susceptibility.

There is promise of understanding HLA-disease relationships in the near future. At present, HLA and disease associations have clinical usefulness as a diagnostic aid (eg, B27 typing and ankylosing spondylitis) or in identifying individuals likely to have particularly good or bad (eg, hydralazine-induced lupus) responses to therapeutic regimens.

Grumet FC: HLA and disease. *Clin Immunol Rev* 1983;**2**:123.
Tiwari JL, Terasaki PI: *HLA and Disease Associations.* Springer, 1985.

---

## REFERENCES

Bellanti JA: *Immunology III,* 3rd ed. Saunders, 1985.
Fudenberg HH et al: *Basic Immunogenetics,* 3rd ed. Oxford Univ Press, 1984.
Hood LE et al: *Immunology,* 2nd ed. Benjamin/Cummings, 1984.

Paul WE, Fathman GG, Metzger H (editors): *Annu Rev Immunol* 1984–present. [Annual entire issue.]
Stites DP, Stobo JD, Wells JV (editors): *Basic & Clinical Immunology,* 6th ed. Appleton-Lange, 1987.

# Appendix

## CHEMICAL CONSTITUENTS OF BLOOD & BODY FLUIDS

### Validity of Numerical Values in Reporting Laboratory Results

The value reported from a clinical laboratory after determination of the concentration or amount of a substance in a specimen represents the best value obtainable with the method, reagents, instruments, and technical personnel involved in obtaining and processing the material.

**Accuracy** is the degree of agreement of the determination with the "true" value (eg, the known concentration in a control sample). **Precision** denotes the reproducibility of the analysis and is expressed in terms of variation among several determinations on the same sample. **Reliability** is a measure of the congruence of accuracy and precision.

Precision is not absolute but is subject to variation inherent in the complexity of the method, the stability of reagents, the accuracy of the primary standard, the sophistication of the equipment, and the skill of the technical personnel. Each laboratory should maintain data on precision (reproducibility) that can be expressed statistically in terms of the standard deviation from the mean value obtained by repeated analyses of the same sample. For example, the precision in determination of cholesterol in serum in a good laboratory may be the mean value ± 5 mg/dL. The 95% confidence limits are ± 2 SD, or ± 10 mg/

dL. Thus, any value reported is "accurate" within a range of 20 mg/dL. Thus, the reported value 200 mg/dL means that the true value lies between 190 and 210 mg/dL. For the determination of serum potassium with a variance of 1 SD of ± 0.1 mmol/L, values ± 0.2 mmol could be obtained on the same specimen. A report of 5.5 could represent at best the range 5.3–5.7 mmol/L. That is, the 2 results—5.3 and 5.7 mmol/L—might be obtained on analysis of the same sample and still be within the limits of precision of the test.

Physicians should obtain from the laboratory the values for the variation of a given determination as a basis for deciding whether one reported value represents a change from another on the same patient.

### Interpretation of Laboratory Tests

Normal values are those that fall within 2 standard deviations from the mean value for the normal population. This normal range encompasses 95% of the population. Many factors may affect values and influence the normal range; by the same token, various factors may produce values that are normal under the prevailing conditions but outside the 95% limits determined under other circumstances. These factors include **age; race; sex; environment; posture; diurnal** and **other cyclic variations; fasting** or **postprandial state, foods eaten; drugs;** and **level of exercise.**

Normal or reference values vary with the method employed, the laboratory, and conditions of collection and preservation of specimens. The normal values established by individual laboratories should be clearly expressed to ensure proper interpretation.

Interpretation of laboratory results must always be related to the condition of the patient. A low value may be the result of deficit or of dilution of the substance measured, eg, low serum sodium. Deviation from normal may be associated with a specific disease or with some drug consumed by the subject—eg, elevated serum uric acid levels may occur in patients with gout or may be due to treatment with chlorothiazides or with antineoplastic agents. (See Table 1.)

Values may be influenced by the method of collection of the specimen. Inaccurate collection of a 24-hour urine specimen, variations in concentration of the randomly collected urine specimen, hemolysis in a blood sample, addition of an inappropriate anticoagulant, and contaminated glassware or other apparatus are examples of causes of erroneous results.

**Table 1.** Some drugs affecting prothrombin time (Quick one-stage test) of patients receiving anticoagulant therapy with coumarin or phenindione derivatives.

| Prothrombin Time Increased By | Prothrombin Time Decreased By |
|---|---|
| Acetaminophen | Aminoglutethimide |
| Allopurinol | Antihistamines |
| p-Aminosalicyclic acid | Azathioprine |
| Amiodarone | Barbiturates |
| Androgens | Carbamazepine |
| Antibiotics (tetracyclines, | Contraceptives, oral |
| some cephalosporins [es- | Cyclophosphamide |
| pecially cefamandole, cefa- | Digitalis (in cardiac failure) |
| perazone, moxalactam], | Diuretics |
| erythromycin, chloram- | Ethchlorvynol |
| phenicol, metronidazole, | Glutethimide |
| sulfonamides) | Griseofulvin |
| Chloral hydrate | Mercaptopurine |
| Cholestyramine | Phenytoin |
| Cimetidine | Rifampin |
| Clofibrate | Vitamin K (in polyvitamin prep- |
| Disulfiram | arations and some diets) |
| Glucagon | Xanthines (eg, caffeine) |
| Heparin (Quick test increased; | |
| no effect on prothrombin- | |
| proconvertin [P and P] test) | |
| Hydroxyzine | |
| Indomethacin | |
| Mefenamic acid | |
| Methimazole | |
| Metronidazole | |
| Nalidixic acid | |
| Naproxen | |
| Oxyphenbutazone | |
| Phenylbutazone | |
| Phenyramidol | |
| Phenytoin | |
| Propylthiouracil | |
| Quinidine | |
| Quinine | |
| Salicylates (> g/d) | |
| Sulfinpyrazone | |
| Thyroid hormones | |
| Tricyclic antidepressants | |

*Note:* Whenever an unusual or abnormal result is obtained, all possible sources of error must be considered before responding with therapy based on the laboratory report. Laboratory medicine is a specialty, and experts in the field should be consulted whenever results are unusual or in doubt.

## Effect of Meals & Posture on Concentration of Substances in Blood

**A. Meals:** The usual normal values for blood tests have been determined by assay of "fasting" specimens collected after 8–12 hours of abstinence from food. With few exceptions, water is usually permitted as desired.

Few routine tests are altered from usual fasting values if blood is drawn 3–4 hours after breakfast. When blood is drawn 3–4 hours after lunch, values are more likely to vary from those of the true fasting state (ie, as much as +31% for AST [SGOT], −5% for lactate dehydrogenase, and lesser variations for

other substances). Valid measurement of triglyceride in serum or plasma requires abstinence from food for 10–14 hours.

**B. Posture:** Plasma volume measured in a person who has been supine for several hours is 12–15% greater than in a person who has been up and about or standing for an hour or so. It follows that measurements performed on blood obtained after the subject has been lying down for an hour or more will yield lower values than when blood has been obtained after the same subject has been upright. An intermediate change apparently occurs with sitting.

Values in the same subject change when position changes from supine to standing as follows: increase in total protein, albumin, calcium, potassium, phosphate, cholesterol, triglyceride, AST (SGOT), the phosphatases, total thyroxine, hematocrit, erythrocyte count, and hemoglobin. The greatest change occurs in concentration of total protein and enzymes (+11%) and calcium (+3 to +4%). In a series of studies, change from the upright to the supine position resulted in the following decreases: total protein, −0.5 g; albumin, −0.4 to −0.6 g; calcium, −0.4 mg; cholesterol, −10 to −25 mg; total thyroxine −0.8 to −1.8 μg; and hematocrit, −4 to −9%, reflecting hemodilution as interstitial fluid reenters the circulation.

A tourniquet applied for 1 minute instead of 3 minutes produced the following changes in reported values: total protein, +5%; iron, +6.7%; cholesterol, +5%; AST (SGOT), +9.3%; and bilirubin, +8.4%. Decreases were observed for potassium, −6%; and creatinine, −2.3%.

## Validity of Laboratory Tests*

The clinical value of a test is related to its specificity and sensitivity and the incidence of the disease in the population tested.

**Sensitivity** means percentage of positive results in patients with the disease. The test for phenylketonuria is highly sensitive: a positive result is obtained in all who have the disease (100% sensitivity). The carcinoembryonic antigen (CEA) test has low specificity: only 72% of those with carcinoma of the colon provide a positive result when the disease is extensive, and only 20% are positive with early disease. Lower sensitivity occurs in the early stages of many diseases—in contrast to the higher sensitivity in well-established disease.

**Specificity** means percentage of negative results among people who do not have the disease. The test for phenylketonuria is highly specific: 99.9% of normal individuals give a negative result. In contrast,

---

* This section is an abridged version of an article by Krieg AF, Gambino R, Galen RS: Why are clinical laboratory tests performed? When are they valid? *JAMA* 1975;**233:**76. Reprinted from the Journal of the American Medical Association. Copyright 1975. American Medical Association. See also Galen RS, Gambino SR: *Beyond Normality: The Predictive Value and Efficiency of Medical Diagnosis.* Wiley, 1975.

the CEA test for carcinoma of the colon has a variable specificity: about 3% of nonsmoking individuals give a false-positive result (97% specificity), whereas 20% of smokers give a false-positive result (80% specificity). The overlap of serum thyroxine levels between hyperthyroid patients and those taking oral contraceptives or those who are pregnant is an example of a change in specificity from that prevailing in a different set of individuals.

The **predictive value** of a positive test defines the percentage of positive results that are true positives. This is related fundamentally to the incidence of the disease. In a group of patients on a urology service, the incidence of renal disease is higher than in the general population, and the serum creatinine level will have a higher predictive value in that group than for the general population.

Formulas for definitions:

Before ordering a test, attempt to determine whether test sensitivity, specificity, and predictive value are adequate to provide useful information. To be useful, the result should influence diagnosis, prognosis, or therapy; lead to a better understanding of the disease process; and benefit the patient.

## SI Units (*Système International d'Unités*)

A "coherent" system of measurement has been developed by an international organization designated the General Conference of Weights and Measures. An adaptation has been tentatively recommended by the Commission on Quantities and Units of the Section on Clinical Chemistry, International Union of Pure and Applied Chemistry. SI units are in use in some European countries, and the conversion to SI will continue if the system proves to be helpful in understanding physiologic mechanisms.

Eight fundamental measurable properties of matter (with authorized abbreviations shown in parentheses) were selected for clinical use.

length: metre (m)
mass: kilogram (kg)
amount of substance: mole (mol)
time: second (s)
thermodynamic temperature: kelvin (K)
electric current: ampere (A)
luminous intensity: candela (cd)
catalytic activity: katal (kat)

Derived from these are the following measurable properties:

mass concentration: kilogram/litre (kg/L)
mass fraction: kilogram/kilogram (kg/kg)
volume fraction: litre/litre (L/L)
volume: cubic metre ($m^3$); for clinical use, the unit will be the litre (L)
substance concentration: mole/litre (mol/L)
molality: mole/kilogram (mol/kg)
mole fraction: mole/mole (mol/mol)
pressure: pascal (Pa) = newton/$m^2$

Decimal factors are as follows:

| Number | Name | Symbol |
|---|---|---|
| $10^{12}$ | tera | T |
| $10^9$ | giga | G |
| $10^6$ | mega | M |
| $10^3$ | kilo | k |
| $10^2$ | hecto | h |
| $10^1$ | deca | da |
| $10^{-1}$ | deci | d |
| $10^{-2}$ | centi | c |
| $10^{-3}$ | milli | m |
| $10^{-6}$ | micro | $\mu$ |
| $10^{-9}$ | nano | n |
| $10^{-12}$ | pico | p |
| $10^{-15}$ | femto | f |
| $10^{-18}$ | atto | a |

"Per"—eg, "per second"—is often written as the negative exponent. Per second thus becomes $\cdot s^{-1}$; per meter squared, $\cdot m^{-2}$; per kilogram, $\cdot kg^{-1}$. *Example:* cm/s = $cm \cdot s^{-1}$; g/$m^2$ = $g \cdot m^{-2}$; etc.

In anticipation that the SI system may be adopted in the USA in the next several years, values are reported here in the traditional units with equivalent SI units following in parentheses. SI conversion factors are presented in Tables 8 and 9 at the end of this section.

---

## COMMON CLINICAL VALUES IN TRADITIONAL & SI MEASUREMENTS*

---

### Albumin, Serum or Plasma:

See Proteins, Serum or Plasma.

### Aldolase, Serum:

Normal (varies with method): 3–8 units/mL (Sibley-Lehninger). Males, < 33 units; females, < 19 units (Warburg and Christian).

**A. Precautions:** Serum should be separated promptly. Avoid hemolysis. If there is to be any delay in the determination, the serum should be frozen.

**B. Physiologic Basis:** Aldolase, also known as zymohexase, splits fructose-1,6-diphosphate to yield dihydroxyacetone phosphate and glyceraldehyde 3-

---

* The values listed below and in the following section have been gleaned from many sources. Values will vary with method and individual laboratory.

phosphate. Because it is present in higher concentration in tissue cells than in serum, destruction of tissue results in elevation of serum concentration.

**C. Interpretation:** High levels in serum occur in myocardial infarction, muscular dystrophies, hemolytic anemia, metastatic prostatic carcinoma, leukemia, acute pancreatitis, and acute hepatitis. In obstructive jaundice or cirrhosis of the liver, serum aldolase is normal or only slightly elevated.

## Aminotransferases, Serum:

Normal (varies with method): AST (SGOT), 6–25 IU/L at 30 °C; SMA, 10–40 IU/L at 37 °C; SMAC, 0–41 IU/L at 37 °C. ALT (SGPT), 3–26 IU/L at 30 °C; SMAC, 0–45 IU/L at 37 °C.

**A. Precautions:** Avoid hemolysis. Remove serum from clot promptly.

**B. Physiologic Basis:** Aspartate aminotransferase (AST; SGOT), alanine aminotransferase (ALT; SGPT), and lactic dehydrogenase are intracellular enzymes involved in amino acid or carbohydrate metabolism: These enzymes are present in high concentrations in muscle, liver, and brain. Elevations of concentrations of these enzymes in the blood indicate necrosis or disease, especially of these tissues.

**C. Interpretation:**

**1. Elevated** after myocardial infarction (especially AST); acute infectious hepatitis (ALT usually elevated more than AST); cirrhosis of the liver (AST usually elevated more than ALT); and metastatic or primary liver neoplasm. Elevated in transudates associated with neoplastic involvement of serous cavities. AST is elevated in muscular dystrophy, dermatomyositis, and paroxysmal myoglobinuria.

**2. Decreased** with pyridoxine (vitamin $B_6$) deficiency (often as a result of repeated hemodialysis), renal insufficiency, and pregnancy.

**D. Drug Effects on Laboratory Results:** Elevated by a host of drugs, including anabolic steroids, androgens, clofibrate, erythromycin (especially estolate) and other antibiotics, isoniazid, methotrexate, methyldopa, phenothiazines, oral contraceptives, salicylates, acetaminophen, phenacetin, indomethacin, acetohexamide, allopurinol, dicumarol, carbamazepine, chlordiazepoxide, desipramine, imipramine, codeine, morphine, meperidine, tolazamide, propranolol, guanethidine, pyridoxine, and drugs that produce spasm of the sphincter of Oddi.

## Ammonia, Blood:

Normal (Conway): 10–110 $\mu$g/dL whole blood. (SI: 12–65 $\mu$mol/L.)

**A. Precautions:** Do not use anticoagulants containing ammonia. Heparin (ammonia-free) is the anticoagulant of choice. Plasma should be separated immediately in a refrigerated centrifuge and removed from the cells. Plasma may be stored briefly at 4 °C.

**B. Physiologic Basis:** Ammonia present in the blood is derived from 2 principal sources: (1) In the large intestine, putrefactive action of bacteria on nitrogenous materials releases significant quantities of ammonia. (2) In the process of protein metabolism, ammonia is liberated. Ammonia entering the portal vein or the systemic circulation is rapidly converted to urea in the liver. Liver insufficiency may result in an increase in blood ammonia concentration, especially if protein consumption is high or if there is bleeding into the bowel.

**C. Interpretation:** Blood ammonia is elevated in hepatic insufficiency or with liver bypass in the form of a portacaval shunt, particularly if protein intake is high or if there is bleeding into the bowel. Urea cycle metabolic defects may be seen in adults as well as children.

**D. Drug Effects on Laboratory Results:** Elevated by methicillin, ammonia cycle resins, chlorthalidone, and spironolactone. Decreased by monoamine oxidase inhibitors and oral antimicrobial agents.

## Amylase, Serum:

Normal (varies with method): 80–180 Somogyi units/dL serum. (One Somogyi unit equals amount of enzyme that will produce 1 mg of reducing sugar from starch at pH 7.2.) 0.8–3.2 IU/L.

**A. Precautions:** If storage for more than 1 hour is necessary, blood or serum must be refrigerated.

**B. Physiologic Basis:** Normally, small amounts of amylase (diastase), molecular weight about 50,000, originating in the pancreas and salivary glands, are present in the blood. Inflammatory disease of these glands or obstruction of their ducts results in regurgitation of large amounts of enzyme into the blood and increased excretion via the kidney.

**C. Interpretation:**

**1. Elevated** in acute pancreatitis, pseudocyst of the pancreas, obstruction of pancreatic ducts (carcinoma, stone, stricture, duct sphincter spasm after morphine), bowel infarction, and mumps. Occasionally elevated in renal insufficiency, in diabetic acidosis, in inflammation of the pancreas from a perforating peptic ulcer, and in small cell carcinoma of the lung. Rarely, combination of amylase with an immunoglobulin produces elevated serum amylase activity (macroamylasemia) because the large molecular complex (molecular weight at least 160,000) is not filtered by the glomerulus.

**2. Decreased** in acute and chronic hepatitis, in pancreatic insufficiency, and, occasionally, in toxemia of pregnancy.

**D. Drug Effects on Laboratory Results:** Elevated by morphine, codeine, meperidine, methacholine, sodium diatrizoate, and cyproheptadine. Perhaps elevated by pentazocine and thiazide diuretics. Pancreatitis may be induced by indomethacin, furosemide, chlorthalidone, ethacrynic acid, corticosteroids, histamine, salicylates, and tetracyclines. Decreased by barbiturate poisoning.

## Amylase, Urine:

Normal (varies with method): 40–250 Somogyi units/h.

**A. Precautions:** If the determination is delayed more than 1 hour after collecting the specimen, urine must be refrigerated.

**B. Physiologic Basis:** See Amylase, Serum. If renal function is adequate, amylase is rapidly excreted in the urine. A timed urine specimen (ie, 2, 6, or 24 hours) should be collected and the rate of excretion determined.

**C. Interpretation:** Elevation of the concentration of amylase in the urine occurs in the same situations in which serum amylase concentration is elevated. Urinary amylase concentration remains elevated for up to 7 days after serum amylase levels have returned to normal following an attack of pancreatitis. Thus, the determination of urinary amylase may be useful if the patient is seen late in the course of an attack of pancreatitis. An elevated serum amylase with normal or low urine amylase excretory rate may be seen in the presence of renal insufficiency or with macroamylasemia.

## Bicarbonate, Serum or Plasma:

Normal: 24–28 meq/L. (SI: 24–28 mmol/L.)

**A. Precautions:** Plasma or serum should be separated from blood cells and kept refrigerated in stoppered tubes.

**B. Physiologic Basis:** Bicarbonate-carbonic acid buffer is one of the most important buffer systems in maintaining normal pH of body fluids. Bicarbonate and pH determinations on arterial whole blood serve as a basis for assessing "acid-base balance."

**C. Interpretation:**

**1. Elevated in–**

**a. Metabolic alkalosis** (arterial blood pH increased) due to ingestion of large quantities of sodium bicarbonate, protracted vomiting of acid gastric juice, volume contraction, or accompanying potassium deficit.

**b. Respiratory acidosis** (arterial blood pH decreased) due to inadequate elimination of $CO_2$ (leading to elevated $P_{CO_2}$) because of chronic obstructive pulmonary disease, heart failure with pulmonary congestion or edema, or ventilatory failure due to any cause, including oversedation or narcotics.

**2. Decreased in–**

**a. Metabolic acidosis** (arterial blood pH decreased) due to diabetic ketoacidosis, lactic acidosis, starvation, persistent diarrhea, renal insufficiency, ingestion of excess acidifying salts or methanol, or salicylate intoxication.

**b. Respiratory alkalosis** (arterial blood pH increased) due to hyperventilation (decreased $P_{CO_2}$).

## Bilirubin, Serum:

Normal: Total, 1.1–1.2 mg/dL (SI: 3.5–19 μmol/L). Direct (glucuronide), 0.1–0.4 mg/dL. Indirect (unconjugated), 0.2–0.7 mg/dL. (SI: direct, up to 7 μmol/L; indirect, up to 12 μmol/L.)

**A. Precautions:** The fasting state is preferred to avoid turbidity of serum. For optimal stability of stored serum, samples should be frozen and stored in the dark.

**B. Physiologic Basis:** Destruction of hemoglobin yields bilirubin, which is conjugated in the liver to the diglucuronide and excreted in the bile. Bilirubin accumulates in the plasma when liver insufficiency exists, biliary obstruction is present, or the rate of hemolysis increases. Rarely, abnormalities of enzyme systems involved in bilirubin metabolism in the liver (eg, absence of glucuronyl transferase) result in abnormal bilirubin concentrations.

**C. Interpretation:**

1. Direct and indirect forms of serum bilirubin are elevated in acute or chronic hepatitis; biliary tract obstruction (cholangiolar, hepatic, or common ducts); toxic reactions to many drugs, chemicals, and toxins; and Dubin-Johnson and Rotor's syndromes.

2. Indirect serum bilirubin is elevated in hemolytic diseases or reactions and absence or deficiency of glucuronyl transferase, as in Gilbert's disease and Crigler-Najjar syndrome.

3. Direct and total bilirubin can be significantly elevated in normal and jaundiced subjects by fasting 24–48 hours (in some instances even 12 hours) or by prolonged caloric restriction.

**D. Drug Effects on Laboratory Results:** Elevated by acetaminophen, chlordiazepoxide, novobiocin, and acetohexamide. Many drugs produce either hepatocellular damage or cholestasis.

## Calcium, Serum:

Normal: Total, 8.5–10.3 mg/dL or 4.2–5.2 meq/L. Ionized, 4.2–5.2 mg/dL or 2.1–2.6 meq/L. (SI: total, 2.1–2.6 mmol/L; ionized, 1.05–1.3 mmol/L.)

**A. Precautions:** Glassware must be free of calcium. The patient should be fasting. Serum should be promptly separated from the clot.

**B. Physiologic Basis:** Endocrine, renal, gastrointestinal, and nutritional factors normally provide for precise regulation of calcium concentration in plasma and other body fluids. Since some calcium is bound to plasma protein, especially albumin, determination of the plasma albumin concentration is necessary before the clinical significance of abnormal serum calcium levels can be interpreted accurately.

**C. Interpretation:**

**1. Elevated** in hyperparathyroidism, secretion of parathyroidlike hormone by malignant tumors, vitamin D excess, milk-alkali syndrome, osteolytic disease such as multiple myeloma, invasion of bone by metastatic cancer, Paget's disease of bone, sarcoidosis, immobilization, and familial hypocalciuria. Occasionally elevated with hyperthyroidism and with ingestion of thiazide drugs.

**2. Decreased** in hypoparathyroidism, vitamin D deficiency (rickets, osteomalacia), renal insufficiency, hypoproteinemia, malabsorption, severe pancreatitis with pancreatic necrosis, and pseudohypoparathyroidism.

## Calcium, Urine
## (Daily Excretion):

Ordinarily there is a moderate continuous urinary calcium excretion of 50–150 mg/24 h, depending upon the intake. (SI: 1.2–3.7 mmol/24 h.)

**A. Procedure:** The patient should remain on a diet free of milk and cheese for 3 days prior to testing; for quantitative testing, a neutral ash diet containing about 150 mg calcium per day is given for 3 days. Quantitative calcium excretion studies may be made on a carefully timed 24-hour urine specimen.

**B. Interpretation:** On the quantitative diet, a normal person excretes 125± 50 mg (1.8–4.4 mmol) of calcium per 24 hours. In hyperparathyroidism, the urinary calcium excretion usually exceeds 200 mg/24 h (5 mmol/d). Urinary calcium excretion is almost always elevated when serum calcium is high.

## Chloride, Serum or
## Plasma:

Normal: 96–106 meq/L. (SI: 96–106 mmol/L.)

**A. Precautions:** Always use serum or plasma, not whole blood.

**B. Physiologic Basis:** Chloride is the principal inorganic anion of the extracellular fluid. It is important in maintenance of acid-base balance even though it exerts no buffer action. When chloride as HCl or $NH_4Cl$ is lost, alkalosis follows; when chloride is retained or ingested, acidosis follows. Chloride (with sodium) plays an important role in control of osmolarity of body fluids.

**C. Interpretation:**

**1. Elevated** in renal insufficiency (when Cl intake exceeds excretion), nephrosis (occasionally), renal tubular acidosis, hyperparathyroidism (occasionally), ureterosigmoid anastomosis (reabsorption from urine in gut), dehydration (water deficit), and overtreatment with saline solution.

**2. Decreased** in gastrointestinal disease with loss of gastric and intestinal fluids (vomiting, diarrhea, gastrointestinal suction), renal insufficiency (with salt deprivation), overtreatment with diuretics, chronic respiratory acidosis, diabetic acidosis, excessive sweating, adrenal insufficiency (NaCl loss), hyperadrenocorticism (chronic $K^+$ loss), and metabolic alkalosis ($NaHCO_3$ ingestion; $K^+$ deficit).

## Cholesterol, Serum or
## Plasma:

Normal: 150–265 mg/dL. (SI: 3.9–6.25 mmol/L.) See Table 2.

**A. Precautions:** The fasting state is preferred.

**B. Physiologic Basis:** Cholesterol concentrations are determined by metabolic functions, which are influenced by heredity, nutrition, endocrine function, and integrity of vital organs such as the liver and kidney. Cholesterol metabolism is intimately associated with lipid metabolism.

**C. Interpretation:**

**1. Elevated** in familial hypercholesterolemia

**Table 2.** Lipidemia: Ranges of population (USA) for serum concentrations of cholesterol (C), triglyceride (TG), low-density lipoprotein cholesterol (LDL-C), and high-density lipoprotein cholesterol (HDL-C).*

| Age | C (mg/dL) | TG (mg/dL) | LDL-C (mg/dL) Upper Limit | HDL-C (mg/dL) | |
|---|---|---|---|---|---|
| | | | | Male | Female |
| < 29 | 120–240 | 10–140 | 170 | 45 ± 12 | 55 ± 12 |
| 30–39 | 140–270 | 10–150 | 190 | | |
| 40–49 | 150–310 | 10–160 | 190 | | |
| > 49 | 160–330 | 10–190 | 210 | | |

* Reproduced, with permission, from Krupp MA et al: *Physician's Handbook*, 21st ed. Lange, 1985.

(xanthomatosis), hypothyroidism, poorly controlled diabetes mellitus, nephrotic syndrome, chronic hepatitis, bilary cirrhosis, obstructive jaundice, hypoproteinemia (idiopathic, with nephrosis or chronic hepatitis), and lipidemia (idiopathic, familial).

**2. Decreased** in acute hepatitis, alcoholic cirrhosis, and Gaucher's disease. Occasionally decreased in hyperthyroidism, acute infections, anemia, malnutrition, and apolipoprotein deficiency.

**D. Drug Effects on Laboratory Results:** Elevated by bromides, anabolic agents, trimethadione, and oral contraceptives. Decreased by cholestyramine resin, haloperidol, nicotinic acid, salicylates, thyroid hormone, estrogens, clofibrate, chlorpropamide, and neomycin.

## Creatine Kinase (CK) or
## Creatine Phosphokinase
## (CPK), Serum:

Normal (varies with method): 10–50 IU/L at 30 °C.

**A. Precautions:** The enzyme is unstable, and the red cell content inhibits enzyme activity. Serum must be removed from the clot promptly. If assay cannot be done soon after drawing blood, serum must be frozen.

**B. Physiologic Basis:** CPK splits creatine phosphate in the presence of ADP to yield creatine and ATP. Skeletal and heart muscle and brain are rich in the enzyme.

**C. Interpretation:**

**1. Elevated** in the presence of muscle damage such as with myocardial infarction, trauma to muscle, muscular dystrophies, polymyositis, severe muscular exertion, hypothyroidism, and cerebral infarction (necrosis). Following myocardial infarction, serum CK concentration increases rapidly (within 3–5 hours), and it remains elevated for a shorter time after the episode (2 or 3 days) than does AST or LDH.

**2. Not elevated** in pulmonary infarction or parenchymal liver disease.

**Table 3.** Creatine kinase isoenzymes.

| Isoenzyme | Normal Levels % of Total |
|---|---|
| (Fastest) Fraction 1, BB | 0 |
| Fraction 2, MB | 0–3 |
| (Slowest) Fraction 3, MM | 97–100 |

## Creatine Kinase Isoenzymes, Serum:

See Table 3.

**A. Precautions:** As for CK Normal (see above).

**B. Physiologic Basis:** CK consists of 3 proteins separable by electrophoresis. Skeletal muscle is characterized by isoenzyme MM, myocardium by isoenzyme MB, and brain by isoenzyme BB.

**C. Interpretation:** CK isoenzymes are increased in serum. CK-MM is elevated in injury to skeletal muscle, myocardial muscle, and brain; in muscle disease (eg, dystrophies, hypothyroidism, dermatomyositis, polymyositis); in rhabdomyolysis; and after severe exercise. CK-MB is elevated soon (within 2–4 hours) after myocardial infarction and for up to 72 hours afterward (high levels are prolonged with extension of infarct or new infarction); also elevated in extensive rhabdomyolysis or muscle injury, severe muscle disease, Reye's syndrome, or Rocky Mountain spotted fever. CK-BB is occasionally elevated in severe shock, in some carcinomas (especially small cell carcinoma or carcinoma of the ovary, breast, or prostate), or in biliary atresia.

## Creatinine, Serum or Plasma:

Normal: 0.7–1.5 mg/dL. (SI: 60–130 μmol/L.)

**A. Precautions:** None.

**B. Physiologic Basis:** Endogenous creatinine is excreted by filtration through the glomerulus and by tubular secretion at a rate about 20% greater than clearance of inulin. There are several methods for the determination of creatinine concentration. One of the most commonly used methods employs picrate (Jaffe reaction). Each method is susceptible to different interfering substances. The Jaffe reaction measures chromogens other than creatinine in the plasma. Because the chromogens are not passed into the urine, the measurement of creatinine in the urine is about 20% less than chromogen plus creatinine in plasma, providing, fortuitously, a compensation for the amount secreted. Thus, inulin and creatinine clearances for clinical purposes are comparable and creatinine clearance is an acceptable measure of glomerular filtration rate—except that with advancing renal failure, creatinine clearance exceeds inulin clearance owing to the secretion of creatinine by remaining renal tubules.

**C. Interpretation:** Creatinine is elevated in acute or chronic renal insufficiency, urinary tract obstruction, and impairment of renal function induced by some drugs. Materials other than creatinine may react to give falsely high results with the alkaline picrate method (Jaffe reaction): acetoacetate, acetone, β-hydroxybutyrate, α-ketoglutarate, pyruvate, glucose, bilirubin, hemoglobin, urea, and uric acid. Values below 0.7 mg/dL are of no known significance.

**D. Drug Effects on Laboratory Results:** Picrate method: Elevated by ascorbic acid, salicylates, barbiturates, sulfobromophthalein, methyldopa, trimethoprim, some penicillins, and many cephalosporins, all of which interfere with the determination by the alkaline picrate method.

## Glucose, Serum or Plasma:

Normal: Fasting "true" glucose, 65–110 mg/dL. (SI: 3.6–6.1 mmol/L.)

**A. Precautions:** If determination is delayed beyond 1 hour, sodium fluoride, about 3 mg/mL blood, should be added to the specimen. The filtrates may be refrigerated for up to 24 hours. Errors in interpretation may occur if the patient has eaten sugar or received glucose solution parenterally just prior to the collection of what is thought to be a "fasting" specimen.

**B. Physiologic Basis:** The glucose concentration in extracellular fluid is normally closely regulated, with the result that a source of energy is available to tissues, and no glucose is excreted in the urine. Hyperglycemia and hypoglycemia are nonspecific signs of abnormal glucose metabolism.

**C. Interpretation:**

**1. Elevated** in diabetes, hyperthyroidism, adrenocortical hyperactivity (cortical excess), hyperpituitarism, and hepatic disease (occasionally).

**2. Decreased** in hyperinsulinism, adrenal insufficiency, hypopituitarism, hepatic insufficiency (occasionally), functional hypoglycemia, and by hypoglycemic agents.

**D. Drug Effects on Laboratory Results:** Elevated by corticosteroids, chlorthalidone, thiazide diuretics, furosemide, ethacrynic acid, triamterene, indomethacin, oral contraceptives (estrogen-progestin combinations), isoniazid, nicotinic acid (large doses), phenothiazines, and paraldehyde. Decreased by acetaminophen, phenacetin, cyproheptadine, and propranolol.

## γ-Glutamyl Transpeptidase or Transferase, Serum:

Normal: Males, < 30 mU/mL at 30 °C. Females, < 25 mU/mL at 30 °C. Adolescents, < 50 mU/mL at 30 °C.

**A. Precautions:** Avoid hemolysis.

**B. Physiologic Basis:** γ-Glutamyl transferase (GGT) is an extremely sensitive indicator of liver disease. Levels are often elevated when transaminases and alkaline phosphatase are normal, and it is considered more specific than both for identifying liver impairment due to alcoholism.

The enzyme is present in liver, kidney, and pancreas and transfers C-terminal glutamic acid from a peptide to other peptides or L-amino acids. It is induced by alcohol.

**C. Interpretation:** Elevated in acute infectious or toxic hepatitis, chronic and subacute hepatitis, cirrhosis of the liver, intrahepatic or extrahepatic obstruction, primary or metastatic liver neoplasms, and liver damage due to alcoholism. It is elevated occasionally in congestive heart failure and rarely in postmyocardial infarction, pancreatitis, and pancreatic carcinoma.

### Iron, Serum:

Normal: 50–175 $\mu$g/dL. (SI: 9–31 $\mu$mol/L.)

**A. Precautions:** Syringes and needles must be iron-free. Hemolysis of blood must be avoided. The serum must be free of hemoglobin.

**B. Physiologic Basis:** Because of diurnal variation with highest values in the morning, fasting morning blood specimens are desirable. Iron concentration in the plasma is determined by several factors, including absorption from the intestine; storage in intestine, liver, spleen, and marrow; breakdown or loss of hemoglobin; and synthesis of new hemogloblin.

**C. Interpretation:**

**1. Elevated** in hemochromatosis, hemosiderosis (multiple transfusions, excess iron administration), hemolytic disease, pernicious anemia, and hypoplastic anemias. Often elevated in viral hepatitis. Spuriously elevated if patient has received parenteral iron during the 2–3 months prior to determination.

**2. Decreased** in iron deficiency; with infections, nephrosis, and chronic renal insufficiency; and during periods of active hematopoiesis.

### Iron-Binding Capacity, Serum:

Normal: Total, 250–410 $\mu$g/dL. (SI: 45–73 $\mu$mol/L.) Percent saturation, 20–55%.

**A. Precautions:** None.

**B. Physiologic Basis:** Iron is transported as a complex of the metal-binding globulin transferrin (siderophilin). Normally, this transport protein carries an amount of iron that represents about 30–40% of its capacity to combine with iron.

**C. Interpretation of Total Iron-Binding Capacity:**

**1. Elevated** in iron deficiency anemia, with use of oral contraceptives, in late pregnancy, and in infants. Occasionally elevated in hepatitis.

**2. Decreased** in association with decreased plasma proteins (nephrosis, starvation, cancer), chronic inflammation, and hemosiderosis (transfusions, thalassemia).

**D. Interpretation of Saturation of Transferrin:**

**1. Elevated** in iron excess (iron poisoning, hemolytic disease, thalassemia, hemochromatosis, pyridoxine deficiency, nephrosis, and, occasionally, hepatitis).

**2. Decreased** in iron deficiency, chronic infection, cancer, and late pregnancy.

### Lactate Dehydrogenase (LDH), Serum, Serous Fluids, Spinal Fluid, or Urine:

Normal (varies with method): Serum, 55–140 IU/L at 30 °C; SMA, 100–225 IU/L at 37 °C; SMAC, 60–200 IU/L at 37 °C. Serous fluids, lower than serum.

**A. Precautions:** Any degree of hemolysis must be avoided because the concentration of LDH within red blood cells is 100 times that in normal serum. Heparin and oxalate may inhibit enzyme activity. Remove serum from clot promptly.

**B. Physiologic Basis:** LDH catalyzes the interconversion of lactate and pyruvate in the presence of NADH or $NADH_2$. It is distributed generally in body cells and fluids.

**C. Interpretation:** Elevated in all conditions accompanied by tissue necrosis, particularly those involving acute injury of the heart, red cells, kidney, skeletal muscle, liver, lung, and skin. Commonly elevated with various carcinomas. Marked elevations accompany hemolytic anemias, the anemias of vitamin $B_{12}$ and folate deficiency, and polycythemia rubra vera. The course of rise in concentration over 3–4 days followed by a slow decline during the following 5–7 days may be helpful in confirming the presence of a myocardial infarction; however, pulmonary infarction, neoplastic disease, and megaloblastic anemia must be excluded. Although elevated during the acute phase of infectious hepatitis, enzyme activity is seldom increased in chronic liver disease.

**D. Drug Effects on Laboratory Results:** Decreased by clofibrate.

### Lactate Dehydrogenase (LDH) Isoenzymes, Serum:

Normal: See Table 4.

**A. Precautions:** As for LDH (see above).

**B. Physiologic Basis:** LDH consists of 5 separable proteins, each made of tetramers of 2 types, or subunits, H and M. The 5 isoenzymes can be distinguished by kinetics, electrophoresis, chromatography, and immunologic characteristics. By electrophoretic separation, the mobility of the isoenzymes corresponds to serum proteins $\alpha_1$, $\alpha_2$, $\beta$, $\gamma_1$, and $\gamma_2$. These are usually numbered 1 (fastest moving), 2, 3, 4, and 5 (slowest moving). Isoenzyme 1 is

**Table 4.** Lactate dehydrogenase isoenzymes.

|  | Isoenzyme | Percentage of Total (and Range) |
|---|---|---|
| (Fastest) | 1 ($\alpha_1$) | 28 (15–30) |
|  | 2 ($\alpha_2$) | 36 (22–50) |
|  | 3 ($\beta$) | 23 (15–30) |
|  | 4 ($\gamma_1$) | 6 (0–15) |
| (Slowest) | 5 ($\gamma_2$) | 6 (0–15) |

present in high concentrations in heart muscle (tetramer H H H H) and in erythrocytes and kidney cortex; isoenzyme 5, in skeletal muscle (tetramer M M M M) and liver.

**C. Interpretation:** In myocardial infarction, the α isoenzymes are elevated—particularly LDH 1—to yield a ratio of LDH 1:LDH 2 of greater than 1. Similar α isoenzyme elevations occur in renal cortex infarction and with hemolytic anemias.

LDH 5 and 4 are relatively increased in the presence of acute hepatitis, acute muscle injury, dermatomyositis, and muscular dystrophies.

**D. Drug Effects on Laboratory Results:** Decreased by clofibrate.

### Lipase, Serum:

Normal: 0.2–1.5 units.

**A. Precautions:** None. The specimen may be stored under refrigeration up to 24 hours prior to the determination.

**B. Physiologic Basis:** A low concentration of fat-splitting enzyme is present in circulating blood. In the presence of pancreatitis, pancreatic lipase is released into the circulation in higher concentrations, which persist, as a rule, for a longer period than does the elevated concentration of amylase.

**C. Interpretation:** Serum lipase is elevated in acute or exacerbated pancreatitis and in obstruction of pancreatic ducts by stone or neoplasm.

### Magnesium, Serum:

Normal: 1.8–3 mg/dL or 1.5–2.5 meq/L. (SI: 0.75–1.25 mmol/L.)

**A. Precautions:** None.

**B. Physiologic Basis:** Magnesium is primarily an intracellular electrolyte. In extracellular fluid, it affects neuromuscular irritability and response. Magnesium deficit may exist with little or no change in extracellular fluid concentrations. Low magnesium levels in plasma have been associated with tetany, weakness, disorientation, and somnolence.

**C. Interpretation:**

**1. Elevated** in renal insufficiency and in overtreatment with magnesium salts.

**2. Decreased** in chronic diarrhea, acute loss of enteric fluids, starvation, chronic alcoholism, chronic hepatitis, hepatic insufficiency, excessive renal loss (diuretics), and inadequate replacement with parenteral nutrition. May be decreased in and contribute to persistent hypocalcemia in patients with hypoparathyroidism (especially after surgery for hyperparathyroidism) and when large doses of vitamin D and calcium are being administered.

### Phosphatase, Acid, Serum:

Normal values vary with method: 0.1–0.63 Sigma units.

**A. Precautions:** Do not draw blood for assay for 24 hours after prostatic massage or instrumentation. For methods that measure enzyme activity, complete the determination promptly, since activity declines quickly; avoid hemolysis. For immunoassay methods, the enzyme is stable for 3–4 days when the serum is refrigerated or frozen.

**B. Physiologic Basis:** Phosphatases active at pH 4.9 are present in high concentration in the prostate gland, erythrocytes, platelets, reticuloendothelial cells, liver, spleen, and kidney. A variety of isoenzymes have been found in these tissues and serum and account for different activities operating against different substrates.

**C. Interpretation:** In the presence of carcinoma of the prostate, the prostatic fraction of acid phosphatase may be increased in the serum, particularly if the cancer has spread beyond the capsule of the gland or has metastasized. Palpation of the prostate will produce a transient increase. Total acid phosphatase may be increased in Gaucher's disease, malignant tumors involving bone, renal disease, hepatobiliary disease, diseases of the reticuloendothelial system, and thromboembolism. Fever may cause spurious elevations.

### Phosphatase, Alkaline, Serum:

Normal (varies with method): Bessey-Lowry, children, 2.8–6.7 units; Bessey-Lowry, adults, 0.8–2.3 units. Adults, King-Armstrong, 5–13 units: 24–71 IU/L at 30 °C; SMA, 30–85 IU/L at 37 °C; SMAC, 30–115 IU/L at 37 °C.

**A. Precautions:** Serum may be kept in the refrigerator for 24–48 hours, but values may increase slightly (10%). The specimen will deteriorate if it is not refrigerated. Do not use fluoride or oxalate.

**B. Physiologic Basis:** Alkaline phosphatase is present in high concentration in growing bone, in bile, and in the placenta. In serum, it consists of a mixture of isoenzymes not yet clearly defined. The isoenzymes may be separated by electrophoresis; liver alkaline phosphatase migrates faster than bone and placental alkaline phosphatase, which migrate together.

**C. Interpretation:**

**1. Elevated in–**

a. Children (normal growth of bone).

b. Osteoblastic bone disease—Hyperparathyroidism, rickets and osteomalacia, neoplastic bone disease (osteosarcoma, metastatic neoplasms), ossification as in myositis ossificans, Paget's disease (osteitis deformans), and Boeck's sarcoid.

c. Hepatic duct or cholangiolar obstruction due to stone, stricture, or neoplasm.

d. Hepatic disease resulting from drugs such as chlorpromazine and methyltestosterone.

e. Pregnancy.

**2. Decreased** in hypothyroidism and in growth retardation in children.

**D. Drug Effects on Laboratory Results:** Elevated by acetohexamide, tolazamide, tolbutamide, chlorpropamide, allopurinol, carbamazepine, cephaloridine, furosemide, methyldopa, phenothiazine, and oral contraceptives (estrogen-progestin combinations).

## Phosphorus, Inorganic, Serum:

Normal: Children, 4–7 mg/dL. (SI: 1.3–2.3 mmol/L.) Adults, 3–4.5 mg/dL. (SI: 1–1.5 mmol/L.)

**A. Precautions:** Glassware cleaned with phosphate cleansers must be thoroughly rinsed. The fasting state is necessary to avoid postprandial depression of phosphate associated with glucose transport and metabolism.

**B. Physiologic Basis:** The concentration of inorganic phosphate in circulating plasma is influenced by parathyroid gland function, action of vitamin D, intestinal absorption, renal function, bone metabolism, and nutrition.

**C. Interpretation:**

**1. Elevated** in renal insufficiency, hypoparathyroidism, and hypervitaminosis D.

**2. Decreased** in hyperparathyroidism, hypovitaminosis D (rickets, osteomalacia), malabsorption syndrome (steatorrhea), ingestion of antacids that bind phosphate in the gut, starvation or cachexia, chronic alcoholism (especially with liver disease), hyperalimentation with phosphate-poor solutions, carbohydrate administration (especially intravenously), renal tubular defects, use of thiazide diuretics, acid-base disturbances, and diabetic ketoacidosis (especially during recovery). Occasionally decreased during pregnancy and with hypothyroidism.

## Potassium, Serum or Plasma:

Normal: 3.5–5 meq/L. (SI: 3.5–5 mmol/L.)

**A. Precautions:** Avoid hemolysis, which releases erythrocyte potassium. Serum must be separated promptly from the clot, or plasma from the red cell mass, to prevent diffusion of potassium from erythrocytes. Platelets and leukocytes are rich in potassium; if these elements are present in large numbers (eg, in thrombocytosis or leukemia), the potassium released during coagulation will increase potassium concentration in serum. If these are sources of artifact, plasma from heparinized blood should be employed.

**B. Physiologic Basis:** Potassium concentration in plasma determines neuromuscular and muscular irritability. Elevated or decreased concentrations impair the capability of muscle tissue to contract.

**C. Interpretation:** (See Precautions, above.)

**1. Elevated** in renal insufficiency (especially in the presence of increased rate of protein or tissue breakdown); adrenal insufficiency (especially hypoaldosteronism); hyporeninemic hypoaldosteronism; use of spironolactone; too rapid administration of potassium salts, especially intravenously; and use of triamterene.

**2. Decreased in–**

a. Inadequate intake (starvation).

b. Inadequate absorption or unusual enteric losses—Vomiting, diarrhea, malabsorption syndrome, or use of sodium polystyrene sulfonate resin.

c. Unusual renal loss—Secondary to hyperadrenocorticism (especially hyperaldosteronism) and to adrenocorticosteroid therapy, metabolic alkalosis, use of diuretics such as chlorothiazide and its derivatives; renal tubular defects such as the de Toni-Fanconi syndrome and renal tubular acidosis; treatment with antibiotics that are excreted as anions (carbenicillin, ticarcillin); use of phenothiazines, amphotericin B, and drugs with high sodium content; and use of degraded tetracycline.

d. Abnormal redistribution between extracellular and intracellular fluids–Familial periodic paralysis or testosterone administration.

## Proteins, Serum or Plasma (Includes Fibrinogen):

Normal: See Interpretation, below.

**A. Precautions:** Serum or plasma must be free of hemolysis. Since fibrinogen is removed in the process of coagulation of the blood, fibrinogen determinations cannot be done on serum.

**B. Physiologic Basis:** Concentration of protein determines colloidal osmotic pressure of plasma. The concentration of protein in plasma is influenced by the nutritional state, hepatic function, renal function, occurrence of disease such as multiple myeloma, and metabolic errors. Variations in the fractions of plasma proteins may signify specific disease.

**C. Interpretation:**

**1. Total protein, serum–**Normal: 6–8 g/dL. (SI: 60–80 g/L.) See albumin and globulin fractions, below, and Table 5.

**2. Albumin, serum or plasma–**Normal: 3.5–5.5 g/dL. (SI: 33–55 g/L.)

**a. Elevated** in dehydration, shock, hemoconcentration, and administration of large quantities of concentrated albumin "solution" intravenously.

**b. Decreased** in malnutrition, malabsorption syndrome, acute or chronic glomerulonephritis, nephrosis, acute or chronic hepatic insufficiency, neoplastic diseases, and leukemia.

**3. Globulin, serum or plasma–**Normal: 2–3.6 g/dL. (SI: 20–36 g/L.) (See Tables 6 and 7.)

**a. Elevated** in hepatic disease, infectious hepatitis, cirrhosis of the liver, biliary cirrhosis, and hemochromatosis; disseminated lupus erythematosus; plasma cell myeloma; lymphoproliferative disease; sarcoidosis; and acute or chronic infectious diseases,

**Table 5.** Protein fractions as determined by electrophoresis.

| | Percentage of Total Protein |
|---|---|
| Albumin | 52–68 |
| $\alpha_1$ globulin | 2.4–4.4 |
| $\alpha_2$ globulin | 6.1–10.1 |
| $\beta$ globulin | 8.5–14.5 |
| $\gamma$ globulin | 10–21 |

**Table 6.** Gamma globulins by immunoelectrophoresis.

| | |
|---|---|
| IgA | 90–450 mg/dL |
| IgG | 700–1500 mg/dL |
| IgM | 40–250 mg/dL |
| IgD | 0.3–40 mg/dL |
| IgE | 0.006–0.16 mg/dL |

particularly endocarditis, tuberculosis, lymphogranuloma venereum, typhus, leishmaniasis, schistosomiasis, and malaria.

**b. Decreased** in malnutrition, congenital agammaglobulinemia, acquired hypogammaglobulinemia, and lymphatic leukemia.

**4. Fibrinogen, plasma**–Normal: 0.2–0.6 g/dL. (SI: 2–6 g/L.)

**a. Elevated** in glomerulonephritis, nephrosis (occasionally), and infectious diseases.

**b. Decreased** in disseminated intravascular coagulation (accidents of pregnancy such as placental ablation, amniotic fluid embolism, and violent labor; meningococcal meningitis; metastatic carcinoma of the prostate and occasionally of other organs; and leukemia), acute and chronic hepatic insufficiency, and congenital fibrinogenopenia.

**Sodium, Serum or Plasma:**

Normal: 136–145 meq/L. (SI: 136–145 mmol/L.)

**A. Precautions:** Clean glassware completely.

**B. Physiologic Basis:** Sodium constitutes about 140 of the 155 meq of cation in plasma. With its associated anions it provides the bulk of osmotically active solute in the plasma, thus affecting the distribution of body water significantly. A shift of sodium into cells or a loss of sodium from the body results in a decrease of extracellular fluid volume, affecting circulation, renal function, and nervous system function.

**C. Interpretation:**

**1. Elevated** in dehydration (water deficit), central nervous system trauma or disease, and hyperadre-

**Table 7.** Some constituents of globulins.

| Globulin | Representative Constituents |
|---|---|
| $\alpha_1$ | Thyroxine-binding globulin<br>Transcortin<br>Glycoprotein<br>Lipoprotein<br>Antitrypsin |
| $\alpha_2$ | Haptoglobin<br>Glycoprotein<br>Macroglobulin<br>Ceruloplasmin |
| $\beta$ | Transferrin<br>Lipoprotein<br>Glycoprotein |
| $\gamma$ | $\gamma$G $\gamma$D<br>$\gamma$M $\gamma$E<br>$\gamma$A |

nocorticism with hyperaldosteronism or corticosterone or corticosteroid excess.

**2. Decreased** in syndromes of elevated ADH, in water toxicity, in adrenal insufficiency; in renal insufficiency, especially with inadequate sodium intake; in renal tubular acidosis; as a physiologic response to trauma or burns (sodium shift into cells); in unusual losses via the gastrointestinal tract, as with acute or chronic diarrhea or with intestinal obstruction or fistula; and in sweating with inadequate sodium replacement. In patients with edema associated with cardiac or renal disease, serum sodium concentration is low even though total body sodium content is greater than normal; water retention (excess ADH) and abnormal distribution of sodium between intracellular and extracellular fluid contribute to this paradoxic situation. Hyperglycemia occasionally results in shift of intracellular water to the extracellular space, producing a dilutional hyponatremia. In the presence of hyperglycemia, serum sodium concentration will be reduced by 1.6 meq/L per 100 mg/dL glucose above 200 mg/dL. (Artifact: When measured by the flame photometer, serum or plasma sodium will be decreased in the presence of hyperlipidemia or hyperglobulinemia; in these disorders, the volume ordinarily occupied by water is taken up by other substances, and the serum or plasma will thus be "deficient" in water and electrolyte.)

**Thyroxine ($T_4$), Total ($TT_4$), Serum:**

Normal: Radioimmunoassay (RIA), 5–12 $\mu$g/dL (SI: 65–156 nmol/L); competitive binding protein (CPB) (Murphy-Pattee), 4–11 $\mu$g/dL (SI: 51–142 nmol/L).

**A. Precautions:** None.

**B. Physiologic Basis:** The total thyroxine level does not necessarily reflect the physiologic hormonal effect of thyroxine. Levels of thyroxine vary with the concentration of the carrier proteins (thyroxine-binding globulin and prealbumin), which are readily altered by physiologic conditions such as pregnancy and by a variety of diseases and drugs. Any interpretation of the significance of total $T_4$ depends upon knowing the concentration of carrier protein either from direct measurement or from the result of the erythrocyte or resin uptake of triiodothyronine ($T_3$) (see below). It is the concentration of free $T_4$ and of $T_3$ that determines hormonal activity.

**C. Interpretation:**

**1. Elevated** in hyperthyroidism, with elevation of thyroxine-binding proteins, and at times with active thyroiditis or acromegaly.

**2. Decreased** in hypothyroidism (primary or secondary), with decreased concentrations of thyroxine-binding proteins, and in chronic illness ("sick euthyroid").

**D. Drug Effects on Laboratory Results:** Increased by ingestion of excess thyroid hormone $T_4$. A variety of drugs alter concentration of thyroxine-binding proteins (see below), with parallel changes in total $T_4$ concentration. Decreased by ingestion of $T_3$, which inhibits thyrotropin secretion, with resultant decrease in $T_4$ secretion and concentration. $T_4$ synthesis may be decreased by aminosalicylic acid, corticosteroids, lithium, the thiouracils, methimazole, and sulfonamides. Total $T_4$ concentration may be reduced because of displacement from carrier protein-binding sites by aspirin, chlorpropamide, phenytoin, and tolbutamide. Cholestyramine may reduce $T_4$ concentration by interfering with its enterohepatic circulation.

## Thyroxine, Free, Serum:

Normal (equilibrium dialysis): 0.8–2.4 ng/dL. (SI: 10–30 pmol/L.) May be estimated from measurement of total thyroxine and resin $T_3$ uptake.

**A. Precautions:** None.

**B. Physiologic Basis:** The metabolic activity of $T_4$ is related to the concentration of free $T_4$. $T_4$ is largely converted to $T_3$ in peripheral tissue. ($T_3$ is also secreted by the thyroid gland.) Both $T_4$ and $T_3$ seem to be active hormones.

**C. Interpretation:**

**1. Elevated** in hyperthyroidism and at times with active thyroiditis.

**2. Decreased** in hypothyroidism, chronic illness.

**D. Drug Effects on Laboratory Results:** Elevated by ingestion of excess thyroid hormone $T_4$. Decreased by $T_3$, thiouracils, and methimazole.

## Thyroxine-Binding Globulin (TBG), Serum:

Normal as thyroxine, 12–28 $\mu$g $T_4$/dL. (SI: 150–360 $\mu$mol $T_4$/L.)

**A. Precautions:** None.

**B. Physiologic Basis:** TBG is the principal carrier protein for $T_4$ and $T_3$ in the plasma. Variations in concentration of TBG are accompanied by corresponding variations in concentration of $T_4$ with intrinsic adjustments that maintain the physiologically active free hormones at proper concentration for euthyroid function. The inherited abnormalities of TBG concentration appear to be X-linked.

**C. Interpretation:**

**1. Elevated** in pregnancy, in infectious hepatitis, and in hereditary increase in TBG concentration.

**2. Decreased** in major depleting illness with hypoproteinemia (globulin), nephrotic syndrome, cirrhosis of the liver, active acromegaly, estrogen deficiency, and hereditary TBG deficiency.

**D. Drug Effects on Laboratory Results:** TBG or binding capacity increased by pregnancy, estrogens and progestins (including oral contraceptives), chlormadinone, perphenazine, and clofibrate. Decreased by androgen, anabolic steroids, cortisol, prednisone, corticotropin, and oxymetholone.

## Triiodothyronine ($T_3$) Uptake, Serum; Resin ($RT_3U$) or Thyroxine-Binding Globulin Assessment (TBG Assessment):

Normal: $RT_3U$, as percentage of uptake of $^{125}$I-$T_3$ by resin, 25–36%; $RT_3U$ ratio (TBG assessment) expressed as ratio of binding of $^{125}$I-$T_3$ by resin in test serum/pooled normal serum, 0.85–1.15.

**A. Precautions:** None.

**B. Physiologic Basis:** When serum thyroxine-binding proteins are normal, more TBG binding sites will be occupied by $T_4$ in $T_4$ hyperthyroidism, and fewer binding sites will be occupied in hypothyroidism. $^{125}$I-labeled $T_3$ added to serum along with a secondary binder (resin, charcoal, talc, etc) is partitioned between TBG and the binder. The binder is separated from the serum, and the radioactivity of the binder is measured for the $RT_3U$ test. Since the resin takes up the non-TBG-bound radioactive $T_3$, its activity varies inversely with the numbers of available TBG sites, ie, $RT_3U$ is increased if TBG is more nearly saturated by $T_4$ and decreased if TBG is less well saturated by $T_4$.

**C. Interpretation:**

1. $RT_3U$ and $RT_3U$ ratio are increased when available sites are decreased, as in hyperthyroidism, acromegaly, nephrotic syndrome, severe hepatic cirrhosis, and hereditary TBG deficiency.

2. $RT_3U$ and $RT_3U$ ratio are decreased when available TBG sites are increased, as in hypothyroidism, pregnancy, the newborn, infectious hepatitis, and hereditary increase in TBG.

**D. Drug Effects on Laboratory Results:** $RT_3U$ and $RT_3U$ ratio are elevated by excess $T_4$, androgens, anabolic steroids, corticosteroids, corticotropin, anticoagulant therapy (heparin and warfarin), oxymetholone, phenytoin, and large doses of salicylate. $RT_3U$ and $RT_3U$ ratio are decreased by $T_3$ therapy; by estrogens and progestins, including oral contraceptives; and by thiouracils, perphenazine, and clofibrate.

## Thyroxine ($T_4$) Index: Calculation of "Corrected" $T_4$ From Values for Total $T_4$ ($TT_4$) and $RT_3U$ or $RT_3U$ Ratio:

Normal (varies with method):

$$\text{Free thyroxine index} = RT_3U \text{ (in \%)} \times TT_4 \text{ (in } \mu g/dL)$$

or

$$\text{Corrected } T_4 = RT_3U \text{ ratio} \times TT_4 \text{ (in } \mu g/dL)$$

**A. Precautions:** None

**B. Physiologic Basis:** This calculation yields a value for $TT_4$ corrected for altered TBG concentration. The concentration of free thyroxine ($FT_4$) per se depends on the equilibrium among $FT_4$, $T_4$ bound to TBG ($T_4TBG$), and unoccupied sites on TBG.

$$FT_4 + TBG \rightleftharpoons T_4 TBG$$

The index $FT_4I$ is more properly a value for $T_4$ "corrected" for variations in TBG.

**C. Interpretation:** $FT_4I$ is increased over $T_4$ in conditions in which $RT_3U$ ratio is increased (see Triiodothyronine Uptake).

$FT_4I$ is decreased below $T_4$ in conditions in which $RT_3U$ ratio is decreased.

**D. Drug Effects on Laboratory Results:** As for $RT_3U$ and $RT_3U$ ratio.

### Transaminases:
See Aminotransferases, above.

### Triglycerides, Serum:
Normal: < 165 mg/dL. (SI: < 1.65 g/L.) See also Table 2.

**A. Precautions:** Subject must be in a fasting state (preferably for at least 16 hours). The determination may be delayed if the serum is promptly separated from the clot and refrigerated.

**B. Physiologic Basis:** Dietary fat is hydrolyzed in the small intestine, absorbed and resynthesized by the mucosal cells, and secreted into lacteals in the form of chylomicrons. Triglycerides in the chylomicrons are cleared from the blood by tissue lipoprotein lipase (mainly adipose tissue), and the split products are absorbed and stored. Free fatty acids derived mainly from adipose tissue are precursors of the endogenous triglycerides produced by the liver. Transport of endogenous triglycerides is in association with $\beta$-lipoproteins, the very low density lipoproteins. (For further details, see Chapter 19.) In order to ensure measurement of endogenous triglycerides, blood must be drawn in the postabsorptive state.

**C. Interpretation:** Concentration of triglycerides, cholesterol, and lipoprotein fractions (very low density, low-density, and high-density) is interpreted collectively. Disturbances in normal relationships of these lipid moieties may be primary or secondary in origin.

**1. Elevated (hyperlipoproteinemia)–**

**a. Primary–**Type I hyperlipoproteinemia (exogenous hyperlipidemia), type IIb hyperbetalipoproteinemia, type III broad beta hyperlipoproteinemia, type IV hyperlipoproteinemia (endogenous hyperlipidemia), and type V hyperlipoproteinemia (mixed hyperlipidemia).

**b. Secondary–**Hypothyroidism, diabetes mellitus, nephrotic syndrome, chronic alcoholism with fatty liver, ingestion of contraceptive steroids, biliary obstruction, and stress.

**2. Decreased (hypolipoproteinemia)–**

**a. Primary–**Tangier disease ($\alpha$-lipoprotein deficiency), abetalipoproteinemia, and a few rare, poorly defined syndromes.

**b. Secondary–**Malnutrition, malabsorption, and, occasionally, with parenchymal liver disease.

### Urea Nitrogen & Urea, Blood, Plasma, or Serum:
Normal: Blood urea nitrogen, 8–25 mg/dL (SI: 2.9–8.9 mmol/L). Urea, 21–53 mg/dL (SI: 3.5–9 mmol/L).

**A. Precautions:** Do not use anticoagulants that contain ammonia (ammonium ion) if a urease method is used.

**B. Physiologic Basis:** Urea, an end product of protein metabolism, is excreted by the kidney. The urea concentration in the glomerular filtrate is the same as in the plasma. Tubular reabsorption of urea varies inversely with rate of urine flow. Thus, urea is a less useful measure of glomerular filtration than is creatinine, which is not reabsorbed. Blood urea nitrogen varies directly with protein intake and inversely with the rate of excretion of urea.

**C. Interpretation:**

**1. Elevated in–**

a. Renal insufficiency–Nephritis, acute and chronic; acute renal failure (tubular necrosis); and urinary tract obstruction.

b. Increased nitrogen metabolism associated with diminished renal blood flow or impaired renal function–Dehydration (from any cause), and upper gastrointestinal bleeding (combination of increased protein absorption from digestion of blood plus decreased renal blood flow).

c. Decreased renal blood flow–Shock, adrenal insufficiency, and, occasionally, congestive heart failure.

**2. Decreased** in hepatic failure, nephrosis not complicated by renal insufficiency, and cachexia.

**D. Drug Effects on Laboratory Results:** Elevated by many antibiotics that impair renal function, guanethidine, methyldopa, indomethacin, isoniazid, propranolol, and potent diuretics (decreased blood volume and renal blood flow).

### Uric Acid, Serum or Plasma:
Normal: Males, 3–9 mg/dL (SI: 180–530 $\mu$mol/L); females, 2.5–7.5 mg/dL (SI: 0.15–0.45 mmol/L).

**A. Precautions:** If plasma is used, lithium oxalate should be used as the anticoagulant; potassium oxalate may interfere with the determination.

**B. Physiologic Basis:** Uric acid, an end product of nucleoprotein metabolism, is excreted by the kidney. Gout, a genetically transmitted metabolic error, is characterized by an increased plasma or serum uric acid concentration, an increase in total body uric acid, and deposition of uric acid in tissues. An increase in uric acid concentration in plasma and serum may accompany increased nucleoprotein catabolism (blood dyscrasias, therapy with antileukemic drugs), use of thiazide diuretics, or decreased renal excretion.

**C. Interpretation:**

**1. Elevated** in gout, preeclampsia-eclampsia, leukemia, polycythemia, therapy with antileukemic drugs and a variety of other agents, renal insufficiency, glycogen storage disease (type I), Lesch-Nyhan syndrome (X-linked hypoxanthine-guanine phosphoribosyltransferase deficit), and Down's syndrome. The incidence of hyperuricemia is greater in Filipinos than in whites.

**2. Decreased** in acute hepatitis (occasionally), in treatment with allopurinol and probenecid and in inappropriate secretion of antidiuretic hormone.

**D. Drug Effects on Laboratory Results:** Elevated by salicylates (low doses), thiazide diuretics, ethacrynic acid, spironolactone, furosemide, triamterene, and ascorbic acid. Decreased by salicylates (large doses), methyldopa, clofibrate, sulfinpyrazone, and phenothiazines.

### Uric Acid, Urine:

Normal: 350–600 mg/24 h on a standard purine-free diet. (SI: 2–4 mmol/24 h.) Normal urinary uric acid/creatinine ratio for adults is 0.21–0.59; maximum of 0.75 for 24-hour urine while on purine-free diet.

**A. Precautions:** Diet should be free of high-purine foods prior to and during 24-hour urine collection. Strenuous activity may be associated with elevated purine excretion.

**B. Physiologic Basis:** Elevated serum uric acid may result from overproduction or diminished excretion.

**C. Interpretation:**

**1. Elevated** in renal excretion occurs in about 25–30% of cases of gout due to increased purine synthesis. Excess uric acid synthesis and excretion are associated with myeloproliferative disorders. Lesch-Nyhan syndrome (hypoxanthine-guanine phosphoribosyltransferase deficit) and some cases of glycogen storage disease are associated with uricosuria.

**2. Decreased** in renal insufficiency, in some cases of glycogen storage disease (type I), and in any metabolic defect producing either lactic acidemia or $\beta$-hydroxybutyric acidemia. Salicylates in doses of less than 2–3 g/d may inhibit renal secretion of uric acid.

Friedman RB et al: Effects of diseases on clinical laboratory tests. *Clin Chem* 1980;**26(Suppl 4)**:1D.

Hansten PD, Lybecker LA: Drug effects on laboratory tests. In: *Basic & Clinical Pharmacology*, 3rd ed. Katzung BG (editor). Appleton-Lange, 1987.

Lundberg GD, Iverson C, Radulescu G (editors): Now read this: The SI units are here. (Editorial.) *JAMA* 1986;**255**:2329.

Powsner EK: SI quantities and units for American medicine. *JAMA* 1984;**252**:1737.

Scully RE et al: Normal reference laboratory values: Case records of the Massachusetts General Hospital. *N Engl J Med* 1986; **314**:39.

Young DS: Implementation of SI units for clinical laboratory data. *Ann Intern Med* 1987;**106**:114.

# NORMAL LABORATORY VALUES

### (Blood [B], Plasma [P], Serum [S], Urine [U])

## HEMATOLOGY

**Bleeding time:** Ivy method, 1–7 minutes (60–420 seconds). Template method, 3–9 minutes (180–540 seconds).

**Cellular measurements of red cells:** Average diameter = 7.3 $\mu$m (5.5–8.8 $\mu$m).
Mean corpuscular volume (MCV): Men, 80–94 fL; women, 81–99 fL (by Coulter counter).
Mean corpuscular hemoglobin (MCH): 27–32 pg.
Mean corpuscular hemoglobin concentration (MCHC): 32–36 g/dL red blood cells (32–36%).
Color, saturation, and volume indices: 1 (0.9–1.1).

**Clot retraction:** Begins in 1–3 hours; complete in 6–24 hours. No clot lysis in 24 hours.

**Fibrinogen split products:** Negative > 1:4 dilution.

**Fragility of red cells:** Begins at 0.45–0.38% NaCl; complete at 0.36–0.3% NaCl.

**Hematocrit (PCV):** Men, 40–52%; women, 37–47%.

**Hemoglobin:** [B] Men, 14–18 g/dL (2.09–2.79 mmol/L as Hb tetramer); women, 12–16 g/dL (1.86–2.48 mmol/L). [S] 2–3 mg/dL.

**Partial thromboplastin time:** Activated, 25–37 seconds.

**Platelets:** 150,000–400,000/$\mu$L (0.15–0.4 × $10^{12}$/L).

**Prothrombin:** [P] Less than 2 seconds deviation from control.

**Red blood count (RBC):** Men, 4.5–6.2 million/$\mu$L (4.5–6.2 × $10^{12}$/L); women, 4–5.5 million/$\mu$L (4–5.5 × $10^{12}$/L).

**Reticulocytes:** 0.2–2% of red cells.

**Sedimentation rate:** Less than 20 mm/h (Westergren); 0–10 mm/h (Wintrobe).

**White blood count (WBC) and differential:** 5000–10,000/$\mu$L (5–10 × $10^{9}$/L).

| Myelocytes | 0 % |
| Juvenile neutrophils | 0 % |
| Band neutrophils | 0–5 % |
| Segmented neutrophils | 40–60% |
| Lymphocytes | 20–40% |
| Eosinophils | 1–3 % |
| Basophils | 0–1 % |
| Monocytes | 4–8 % |

Lymphocytes: Total, 1500–4000/$\mu$L

| B cell | 5–25% |
| T cell | 60–88% |
| Suppressor | 10–43% |
| Helper | 32–66% |
| H:S | >1 |

## BLOOD, PLASMA, OR SERUM CHEMICAL CONSTITUTENTS
### (Values vary with method used.)

**Acetone and acetoacetate:** [S] 0.3–2 mg/dL (3–20 mg/L).

**$\alpha$-Amino acid nitrogen:** [S, fasting] 3–5.5 mg/dL (2.2–3.9 mmol/L).

**Aminotransferases:**
Aspartate aminotransferase (AST; SGOT): [S] 6–25 IU/L at 30 °C; SMA, 10–40 IU/L at 37 °C; SMAC, 0–41 IU/L at 37 °C.
Alanine aminotransferase (ALT;SGPT) (varies with method used): [S] 3–26 IU/L at 30 °C; SMAC, 0–45 IU/L at 37 °C.

**Ammonia:** [B] 80–110 $\mu$g/dL (47–65 $\mu$mol/L) (diffusion method). Do not use anticoagulant containing ammonium oxalate.

**Amylase:** [S] 80–180 units/dL (Somogyi).

**$\alpha_1$-Antitrypsin:** [S] > 180 mg/dL.

**Ascorbic acid:** [P] 0.4–1.5 mg/dL (23–85 $\mu$mol/L).

**Base, total serum:** [S] 145–160 meq/L (145–160 mmol/L).

**Bicarbonate:** [S] 24–28 meq/L (24–28 mmol/L).

**Bilirubin:** [S] Total, 0.2–1.2 mg/dL (3.5–20.5 $\mu$mol/L). Direct (conjugated), 0.1–0.4 mg/dL (< 7 $\mu$mol/L). Indirect, 0.2–0.7 mg/dL (< 12 $\mu$mol/L).

**Calcium:** [S] 8.5–10.3 mg/dL (2.1–2.6 mmol/L). Values vary with albumin concentration.

**Calcium, ionized:** [S] 4.25–5.25 mg/dL; 2.1–2.6 meq/L (1.05–1.3 mmol/L).

**$\beta$-Carotene:** [S, fasting] 50–300 $\mu$g/dL (0.9–5.58 $\mu$mol/L).

**Ceruloplasmin:** [S] 25–43 mg/dL (1.7–2.9 $\mu$mol/L).

**Chloride:** [S or P] 96–106 meq/L (96–106 mmol/L).

**Cholesterol:** [S or P] 150–265 mg/dL (3.9–6.85 mmol/L). (See Lipid fractions.) Values vary with age.

**Cholesteryl esters:** [S] 65–75% of total cholesterol.

**$CO_2$ content:** [S or P] 24–29 meq/L (24–29 mmol/L).

**Complement:** [S] C3 ($\beta_{1C}$), 90–250 mg/dL. C4 ($\beta_{1E}$), 10–60 mg/dL. Total ($CH_{50}$), 75–160 mg/dL.

**Copper:** [S or P] 100–200 $\mu$g/dL (16–31 $\mu$mol/L).

**Cortisol:** [P] 8:00 AM, 5–25 $\mu$g/dL (138–690 nmol/L); 8:00 PM, < 10 $\mu$g/dL (275 nmol/L).

**Creatine kinase (CK):** [S] 10–50 IU/L at 30 °C.

**Creatine kinase isoenzymes:** See p 1097.

**Creatinine:** [S or P] 0.7–1.5 mg/dL (60–130 $\mu$mol/L).

**Cyanocobalamin:** [S] 200 pg/mL (148 pmol/L).

**Epinephrine:** [P] Supine, < 100 pg/mL (< 550 pmol/L).

**Ferritin:** [S] Adult women, 20–120 ng/mL; men, 30–300 ng/mL. Child to 15 years, 7–140 ng/mL.

**Folic acid:** [S] 2–20 ng/mL (4.5–45 nmol/L). [RBC] > 140 ng/mL (> 318 nmol/L).

**Glucose:** [S or P] 65–110 mg/dL (3.6–6.1 mmol/L).

**Glucose tolerance:** See p 752.

**Haptoglobin:** [S] 40–170 mg of hemoglobin-binding capacity.

**Hemoglobin A$_{1C}$:** [B] See p 753.

**Iron:** [S] 50–175 $\mu$g/dL (9–31 $\mu$mol/L).

**Iron-binding capacity:** [S] Total, 250–410 $\mu$g/dL (44.7–73.4 $\mu$mol/L). Percent saturation, 20–55%.

**Lactate:** [B, special handling] Venous, 4–16 mg/dL (0.44–1.8 mmol/L).

**Lactate dehydrogenase (LDH):** [S] 55–140 IU/L at 30 °C; SMA, 100–225 IU/L at 37 °C; SMAC, 60–200 IU/L at 37 °C.

**Lipase:** [S] < 150 units/L.

**Lipid fractions:** [S or P] Desirable levels: HDL cholesterol, > 40 mg/dL; LDL cholesterol, < 180 mg/dL; VLDL cholesterol, < 40 mg/dL. (To convert to mmol/L, multiply by 0.026.)

**Lipids, total:** [S] 450–1000 mg/dL (4.5–10 g/L).

**Magnesium:** [S or P] 1.8–3 mg/dL (0.75–1.25 mmol/L).

**Norepinephrine:** [P] Supine, < 500 pg/L (< 3 nmol/L).

**Osmolality:** [S] 280–296 mosm/kg water (280–296 mmol/kg water).

**Oxygen:**
   Capacity: [B] 16–24 vol%. Values vary with hemoglobin concentration.
   Arterial content: [B] 15–23 vol%. Values vary with hemoglobin concentration.
   Arterial % saturation: 94–100% of capacity.
   Arterial $P_{O2}$ ($P_{a_{O2}}$): 80–100 mm Hg (10.67–13.33 kPa) (sea level). Values vary with age.

**$P_{aCO2}$:** [B, arterial] 35–45 mm Hg (4.7–6 kPa).

**pH (reaction):** [B, arterial] 7.35–7.45 ($H^+$ 44.7–45.5 nmol/L).

**Phosphatase, acid:** [S] 1–5 units (King-Armstrong), 0.1–0.63 units (Bessey-Lowry). (See also p 1099.)

**Phosphatase, alkaline:** [S] Adults, 5–13 units (King-Armstrong). 0.8–2.3 (Bessey-Lowry); SMA, 30–85 IU/L at 37 °C; SMAC, 30–115 IU/L at 37 °C.

**Phospholipid:** [S] 145–200 mg/dL (1.45–2 g/L).

**Phosphorus, inorganic:** [S, fasting] 3–4.5 mg/dL (1–1.5 mmol/L).

**Potassium:** [S or P] 3.5–5 meq/L (3.5–5 mmol/L).

**Protein:**
   **Total:** [S] 6–8 g/dL (60–80 g/L).
   **Albumin:** [S] 3.5–5.5 g/dL (35–55 g/L).
   **Globulin:** [S] 2–3.6 g/dL (20–36 g/L).
   **Fibrinogen:** [P] 0.2–0.6 g/dL (2–6 g/L).
   **Separation by electrophoresis:** See Table 5.

**Prothrombin clotting time:** [P] By control.

**Pyruvate:** [B] 0.6–1 mg/dL (70–114 $\mu$mol/L).

**Serotonin:** [B] 5–20 $\mu$g/dL (0.3–1.15 $\mu$mol/L).

**Sodium:** [S or P] 136–145 meq/L (136–145 mmol/L).

**Specific gravity:** [B] 1.056 (varies with hemoglobin and protein concentration). [S] 1.0254–1.0288 (varies with protein concentration).

**Sulfate:** [S or P] As sulfur, 0.5–1.5 mg/dL (156–468 $\mu$mol/L).

**Transferrin:** [S] 200–400 mg/dL (23–45 $\mu$mol/L).

**Triglycerides:** [S] < 165 mg/dL (1.9 mmol/L). (See Lipid fractions.)

**Urea nitrogen:** [S or P] 8–25 mg/dL (2.9–8.9 mmol/L). Do not use anticoagulant containing ammonium oxalate.

**Uric acid:** [S or P] Men, 3–9 mg/dL (0.18–0.54 mmol/L); women, 2.5–7.5 mg/dL (0.15–0.45 mmol/L).

**Vitamin A:** [S] 15–60 $\mu$g/dL (0.53–2.1 $\mu$mol/L).

**Vitamin $B_{12}$:** [S] > 200 pg/mL (> 148 pmol/L).

**Vitamin D:** [S] Cholecalciferol ($D_3$): 25-Hydroxycholecalciferol, 8–55 ng/mL (19.4–137 nmol/L); 1,25-dihydroxycholecalciferol, 26–65 pg/mL (62–155 pmol/L); 24,25-dihydroxycholecalciferol, 1–5 ng/mL (2.4–12 nmol/L).

**Volume, blood (Evans blue dye method):** Adults, 2990–6980 mL. Women, 46.3–85.5 mL/kg; men, 66.2–97.7 mL/kg.

**Zinc:** [S] 50–150 $\mu$g/dL (7.65–22.95 $\mu$mol/L).

## HORMONES, SERUM OR PLASMA

**Pituitary:**
   Growth hormone (GH): [S] Adults, 1–10 ng/mL (46–465 pmol/L) (by RIA).
   Thyroid-stimulating hormone (TSH): [S] < 10 $\mu$U/mL.
   Follicle-stimulating hormone (FSH): [S] Prepubertal, 2–12 mIU/mL; adult men, 1–15 mIU/mL; adult women, 1–30 mIU/mL; castrate or postmenopausal, 30–200 mIU/mL (by RIA).
   Luteinizing hormone (LH): [S] Prepubertal, 2–12 mIU/mL; adult men, 1–15 mIU/mL; adult women, < 30 mIU/mL; castrate or postmenopausal, > 30 mIU/mL.
   Corticotropin (ACTH): [P] 8:00–10:00 AM, up to 100 pg/mL (22 pmol/L).

Prolactin: [S] 1–25 ng/mL (0.4–10 nmol/L).

Somatomedin C: [P] 0.4–2 U/mL.

Antidiuretic hormone (ADH; vasopressin): [P] Serum osmolality 285 mosm/kg, 0–2 pg/mL; > 290 mosm/kg, 2–12 + pg/mL.

**Adrenal:**

Aldosterone: [P] Supine, normal salt intake, 2–9 ng/dL (56–250 pmol/L); increased when upright.

Cortisol: [S] 8:00 AM, 5–20 μg/dL (14–55 μmol/L ); 8:00 PM, < 10 μg/dL (28 μmol/L).

Deoxycortisol: [S] After metyrapone, > 7 μg/dL (> 20 μmol/L).

Dopamine: [P] < 135 pg/mL.

Epinephrine: [P] < 0.1 ng/mL (< 0.55 nmol/L).

Norepinephrine: [P] < 0.5 μg/L (< 3 nmol/L).

See also Miscellaneous Normal Values.

**Thyroid:**

Thyroxine, free ($FT_4$): [S] 0.8–2.4 ng/dL (10–30 pmol/L).

Thyroxine, total ($TT_4$): [S] 5–12 μg/dL (65–156 nmol/L) (by RIA).

Thyroxine-binding globulin capacity: [S] 12–28 μg $T_4$/dL (150–360 nmol $T_4$/L).

Triiodothyronine ($T_3$): [S] 80–220 ng/dL (1.2–3.3 nmol/L).

Reverse triiodothyronine ($rT_3$): [S] 30–80 ng/dL (0.45–1.2 nmol/L).

Triiodothyronine uptake ($RT_3U$): [S] 25–36%; as TBG assessment ($RT_3U$ ratio), 0.85– 1.15.

Calcitonin: [S] < 100 pg/mL (< 100 ng/L).

**Parathyroid:** Parathyroid hormone levels vary with method and antibody. Correlate with serum calcium.

**Islets:**

Insulin: [S] 4–25 μU/mL (29–181 pmol/L).

C-peptide: [S] 0.9–4.2 ng/mL.

Glucagon; [S, fasting] 20–100 pg/mL (20–100 μg/L).

**Stomach:**

Gastrin: [S, special handling] Up to 100 pg/mL (47 pmol/L). Elevated, > 200 pg/mL.

Pepsinogen I: [S] 25–100 ng/mL.

**Kidney:**

Renin activity: [P, special handling] Normal sodium intake: Supine, 1–3 ng/mL/h; standing, 3–6 ng/mL/h. Sodium depleted: Supine, 2–6 ng/mL/h; standing, 3–20 ng/mL/h (1 ng/mL/h = 0.2778 ng/(L·s)).

**Gonad:**

Testosterone, free: [S] Men, 10–30 ng/dL; women, 0.3–2 ng/dL. (1 ng/dL = 0.035 nmol/L.)

Testosterone, total: [S] Prepubertal, < 100 ng/dL; adult men, 300–1000 ng/dL; adult

women, 20–80 ng/dL; luteal phase, up to 120 ng/dL.

Estradiol ($E_2$): [S, special handling] Men, 12–34 pg/mL; women, menstrual cycle 1–10 days, 24–68 pg/mL; 11–20 days, 50–300 pg/mL; 21–30 days, 73–149 pg/mL (by RIA). (1 pg/mL = 3.6 pmol/L.)

Progesterone: [S] Follicular phase, 0.2–1.5 mg/mL; luteal phase, 6–32 ng/mL; pregnancy, > 24 ng/mL; men, < 1 ng/mL. (1 ng/mL = 3.2 nmol/L.)

**Placenta:**

Estriol ($E_3$): [S] Men and nonpregnant women, < 0.2 μg/dL (< 7 nmol/L) (by RIA).

Chorionic gonadotropin: [S] Beta subunit: Men, < 9 mIU/mL; pregnant women after implantation, > 10 mIU/mL. (1 mIU/mL = 1 IU/L.)

## NORMAL CEREBROSPINAL FLUID VALUES

**Appearance:** Clear and colorless.

**Cells:** Adults, 0–5 mononuclears/μL; infants, 0–20 mononuclears/μL.

**Glucose:** 50–85 mg/dL (2.8–4.7 mmol/L). (Draw serum glucose at same time.)

**Pressure (reclining):** Newborns, 30–90 mm water; children, 50–100 mm water; adults, 70–200 mm water (avg = 125).

**Proteins:** Total, 20–45 mg/dL (0.2–0.45 g/L) in lumbar cerebrospinal fluid. IgG, 2–6 mg/dL (0.02–0.06 g/L).

**Specific gravity:** 1.003–1.008.

## RENAL FUNCTION TESTS

**_p_-Aminohippurate (PAH) clearance (RPF):** Men, 560–830 mL/min; women, 490–700 mL/min.

**Creatinine clearance, endogenous (GFR):** Approximates inulin clearance (see below).

**Filtration fraction (FF):** Men, 17–21%; women, 17–23%. (FF = GFR/RPF.)

**Inulin clearance (GFR):** Men, 110–150 mL/min; women, 105–132 mL/min (corrected to 1.73 $m^2$ surface area). (Divide by 60 = mL/s.)

**Maximal glucose reabsorptive capacity ($Tm_G$):** Men, 300–450 mg/min; women, 250–350 mg/min.

**Maximal PAH excretory capacity ($Tm_{PAH}$):** 80–90 mg/min.

**Osmolality:** On normal diet and fluid intake: Range 500–850 mosm/kg water. Achievable range, normal kidney: Dilution 40–80 mosm; concentration (dehydration) up to 1400 mosm/kg water (at least 3–4 times plasma osmolality).

**Specific gravity of urine:** 1.003–1.030.

## MISCELLANEOUS NORMAL VALUES

**Adrenal hormones and metabolites:**
  **Aldosterone:** [U] 2–26 $\mu$g/24 h (5.5–72 nmol). Values vary with sodium and potassium intake.
  **Catecholamines:** [U] Total, < 100 $\mu$g/24 h. Epinephrine, < 10 $\mu$g/24 h (< 55 nmol); norepinephrine, < 100 $\mu$g/24 h (< 590 nmol). Values vary with method used.
  **Cortisol, free:** [U] 20–100 $\mu$g/24 h (0.55–2.76 $\mu$mol).
  **11,17-Hydroxycorticoids:** [U] Men, 4–12 mg/24 h; women, 4–8 mg/24 h. Values vary with method used.
  **17-Ketosteroids:** [U] Under 8 years, 0–2 mg/24 h; adolescents, 2–20 mg/24 h. Men, 10–20 mg/24 h; women, 5–15 mg/24 h. Values vary with method used. (1 mg = 3.5 $\mu$mol.)
  **Metanephrine:** [U] < 1.3 mg/24 h (< 6.6 $\mu$mol) or < 2.2 $\mu$g/mg creatinine. Values vary with method used.
  **Vanillylmandelic acid (VMA):** [U] Up to 7 mg/24 h (< 35 $\mu$mol).

**Fecal fat:** Less than 30% dry weight.

**Lead:** [U] < 80 $\mu$g/24 h (< 0.4 $\mu$mol/d).

**Porphyrins:**
  Delta-aminolevulinic acid: [U] 1.5–7.5 mg/24 h (11–57 $\mu$mol).
  Coproporphyrin: [U] < 230 $\mu$g/24 h (< 350 nmol).
  Uroporphyrin: [U] < 50 $\mu$g/24 h (< 60 nmol).
  Porphobilinogen: [U] < 2 mg/24 h (< 8.8 $\mu$mol).

**Urobilinogen:** [U] 0–2.5 mg/24 h (< 4.2 $\mu$mol).

**Urobilinogen, fecal:** 40–280 mg/24 h (70–470 $\mu$mol).

# CARDIOPULMONARY RESUSCITATION (CPR)

## Basic Life Support

Time is a crucial factor in providing (1) emergency oxygenation and (2) circulation support. Prompt recognition of cardiac or respiratory arrest and rapid intervention are required. External support of respiration and circulation must be instituted just as soon as it can be established that the patient's unresponsiveness is due to apnea or apparent cardiac arrest. This necessitates rapid differentiation from other causes of sudden unconsciousness such as syncope, epilepsy, or choking on food. Delays of more than 3–4 minutes after the onset of respiratory or circulatory arrest decrease the chance of effective resuscitation and increase the possibility of permanent brain damage.

**A. Diagnose the Need for CPR:** Verify unconsciousness by gently shaking and calling to the victim. Call for help from the emergency medical service.

**Table 8.** SI Conversion table for values in clinical hematology.*†

| | B | blood |
| --- | --- | --- |
| | Erc(s) | erythrocyte(s) |
| | Sf | spinal fluid |

| Component | Present Unit | Conversion Factor | SI Unit Symbol | Significant Digits |
| --- | --- | --- | --- | --- |
| Erythrocyte count (B) | $10^6$/mm | 1 | $10^{12}$/L | X.X |
| Erythrocyte count (Sf) | mm$^{-3}$ | 1 | $10^6$/L | XX |
| Erythrocyte sedimentation rate [ESR] (BErc) | mm/h | 1 | mm/h | XX |
| Hematocrit (BErcs) vol. fraction | % | 0.01 | 1 | 0.XX |
| Hemoglobin (B) mass concentration | g/dL | 10 | g/L | XXX |
| Leukocyte count (B) | mm$^{-3}$ | 0.001 | $10^9$/L | XX.X |
|   Number fraction ["differential"] | % | 0.01 | 1 | 0.XX |
| Leukocyte count (Sf) | mm$^{-3}$ | 1 | $10^6$/L | XX |
| Mean corpuscular hemoglobin [MCH] (BErc) mass | pg | 1 | pg | XX |
| Mean corpuscular hemoglobin concentration [MCHC] (BErc) mass concentration | g/dL | 10 | g/L | XX0 |
| Mean corpuscular volume [MCV] (BErc) erythrocyte volume | $\mu$m$^3$ | 1 | fL | XXX |
| Platelet count (B) | $10^3$/mm$^3$ | 1 | $10^9$/L | XXX |
| Reticulocyte count (B)—adults | mm$^{-3}$ | 0.001 | $10^9$/L | XX |
|   Number fraction | % | 0.001 | 1 | 0.XXX |

* Data from Young DS: Implementation of SI units for clinical laboratory data. *Ann Intern Med* 1987;**106**:114.
† Current metric units × conversion factor = SI units.
SI units ÷ conversion factor = Current metric units.

**Table 9.** SI conversion factors for values in clinical chemistry.*†

| | | | |
|---|---|---|---|
| B | blood | Sf | spinal fluid |
| Erc(s) | erythrocyte(s) | U | urine |
| P | plasma | a | arterial |
| S | serum | v | venous |

| Component | Present Unit | Conversion Factor | SI Unit Symbol | Significant Digits |
|---|---|---|---|---|
| Acid phosphatase (S) | U/L | 16.67 | nkat/L | XX |
| Adrenocorticotropin [ACTH] (P) | pg/ml | 0.2202 | pmol/L | XX |
| Alanine aminotransferase [ALT] (S) | U/L | 0.01667 | μkat/L | X.XX |
| Albumin (S) | g/dL | 10.0 | g/L | XX |
| Adolase (S) | U/L | 16.67 | nkat/L | XX0 |
| Aldosterone (S) | ng/dL | 27.74 | pmol/L | XX0 |
| Aldosterone (U) | μg/24 h | 2.774 | nmol/d | XXX |
| Alkaline phosphatase (S) | U/L | 0.01667 | μkat/L | X.X |
| Amino acid nitrogen (P) | mg/dL | 0.7139 | mmol/L | X.X |
| Amino acid nitrogen (U) | mg/24 h | 0.07139 | mmol/d | X.X |
| δ-Aminolevulinate [as levulinic acid] (U) | mg/24 h | 7.626 | μmol/d | XX |
| Ammonia (vP) as ammonia [$NH_3$] | μg/dL | 0.5872 | μmol/L | XXX |
| Amylase (S) | U/L | 0.01667 | μkat/L | XXX |
| Androstenedione (S) | μg/L | 3.492 | nmol/L | XX.X |
| Angiotensin-converting enzyme (S) | nmol/mL/min | 16.67 | nkat/L | XX0 |
| $\alpha_1$-Antitrypsin (S) | mg/dL | 0.01 | g/L | X.X |
| Ascorbate (P) [as ascorbic acid] | mg/dL | 56.78 | μmol/L | X0 |
| Aspartate aminotransferase [AST] [SGOT] (S) | U/L | 0.01667 | ukat/L | 0.XX |
| Bicarbonate (B,P,S) | mEq/L | 1.00 | mmol/L | XX |
| Bilirubin, total (S) | mg/dL | 17.10 | μmol/L | XX |
| Bilirubin, conjugated (S) | mg/dL | 17.10 | μmol/L | XX |
| Calcitonin (S) | pg/mL | 1.00 | ng/L | XXX |
| Calcium (S) | mg/dL | 0.2495 | mmol/L | X.XX |
| Calcium ion (S) | mg/dL | 0.2495 | mmol/L | X.XX |
| Calcium (U), normal diet | mg/24 h | 0.02495 | mmol/d | X.X |
| β-Carotenes (S) | μg/dL | 0.01863 | μmol/L | X.X |
| Catecholamines, total (U) [as norepinephrine] | μg/24 h | 5.911 | nmol/d | XX0 |
| Ceruloplasmin (S) | mg/dL | 10.0 | mg/L | XX0 |
| Chloride (S) | mEq/L | 1.00 | mmol/L | XXX |
| Cholesterol (P) | mg/dL | 0.02586 | mmol/L | X.XX |
| Cholesterol esters (P) [as a fraction of total cholesterol] | % | 0.01 | 1 | 0.XX |
| Chorionic gonadotropin (P) [β-hCG] | mIU/mL | 1.00 | IU/L | XX |
| Complement, C3 (S) | mg/dL | 0.01 | g/L | X.X |
| Complement, C4 (S) | mg/dL | 0.01 | g/L | X.X |
| Copper (S) | μg/dL | 0.1574 | μmol/L | XX.X |
| Copper (U) | μg/24 h | 0.01574 | μmol/d | X.X |
| Coproporphyrins (U) | μg/24 h | 1.527 | nmol/d | XX0 |
| Cortisol (S) | μg/dL | 27.59 | nmol/L | XX0 |
| Cortisol, free (U) | μg/24 h | 2.759 | nmol/d | XX0 |
| Creatine (U) | mg/24 h | 7.625 | μmol/d | XX0 |
| Creatine kinase [CK] | U/L | 0.01667 | μkat/L | X.XX |
| Creatinine (S) | mg/dL | 88.40 | μmol/L | XX0 |
| Creatinine (U) | g/24 h | 8.840 | mmol/d | XX.X |
| Creatinine clearance (S,U) | mL/min | 0.01667 | mL/s | X.XX |

$$\text{Creatinine clearance corrected for body surface area} = \frac{\text{umol/L (urine creatinine)}}{\text{umol/L (serum creatinine)}} \times \text{mL/s} \times \frac{1.73}{A}$$

[where A is the body surface area in square meters ($m^2$)]

| Component | Present Unit | Conversion Factor | SI Unit Symbol | Significant Digits |
|---|---|---|---|---|
| Cyanocobalamin (S) [vitamin $B_{12}$] | pg/mL | 0.7378 | pmol/L | XX0 |
| Cystine (U) | mg/24 h | 4.161 | μmol/d | XX0 |
| Dehydroepiandrosterone (P,S) [DHEA] | μg/L | 3.467 | nmol/L | XX.X |
| Dehydroepiandrosterone sulphate [DHEA-S] (P,S) | ng/mL | 0.002714 | μmol/L | XX.X |
| 11-Deoxycortisol (S) | μg/dL | 28.86 | nmol/L | XX0 |
| Digoxin (P) | ng/mL | 1.281 | nmol/L | X.X |
| Disopyramide (P) | mg/L | 2.946 | μmol/L | XX |
| Electrophoresis, protein (S) | | | | |
| Albumin | % | 0.01 | 1 | 0.XX |
| $\alpha_1$-Globulin | % | 0.01 | 1 | 0.XX |
| $\alpha_2$-Globulin | % | 0.01 | 1 | 0.XX |
| β-Globulin | % | 0.01 | 1 | 0.XX |

**Table 9 (con't).** SI conversion factors for values in clinical chemistry.*†

| | | | |
|---|---|---|---|
| B | blood | Sf | spinal fluid |
| Erc(s) | erythrocyte(s) | U | urine |
| P | plasma | a | arterial |
| S | serum | v | venous |

| Component | Present Unit | Conversion Factor | SI Unit Symbol | Significant Digits |
|---|---|---|---|---|
| Electrophoresis, protein (S) (cont'd) | | | | |
| γ-Globulin | % | 0.01 | 1 | 0.XX |
| Albumin | g/dL | 10.0 | g/L | XX |
| α₁-Globulin | g/dL | 10.0 | g/L | XX |
| α₂-Globulin | g/dL | 10.0 | g/L | XX |
| β-Globulin | g/dL | 10.0 | g/L | XX |
| γ-Globulin | g/dL | 10.0 | g/L | XX |
| Epinephrine (P) | pg/mL | 5.458 | pmol/L | XX0 |
| Epinephrine (U) | μg/24 h | 5.458 | nmol/d | XX |
| Estradiol (S) | pg/mL | 3.671 | pmol/L | XXX |
| Estriol (U) | μg/24 h | 3.468 | nmol/d | XXX |
| Estrogens (S) [as estradiol] | pg/mL | 3.671 | pmol/L | XXX0 |
| Estrogens, placental (U) [as estriol] | mg/24 h | 3.468 | μmol/d | XXX |
| Estrone (P,S) | pg/mL | 3.699 | pmol/L | XXX |
| Estrone (U) | μg/24 h | 3.699 | nmol/d | XXX |
| Ethanol (P) | mg/dL | 0.2171 | mmol/L | XX |
| Fatty acids, nonesterified (P) | mg/dL | 10.00 | mg/L | XX0 |
| Ferritin (S) | ng/mL | 1.00 | μg/L | XX0 |
| α-Fetoprotein (S) | ng/mL | 1.00 | μg/L | XX |
| Fibrinogen (P) | mg/dL | 0.01 | g/L | X.X |
| Folate (S) | ng/mL | 2.266 | nmol/L | XX |
| Folate (Erc) | ng/mL | 2.266 | nmol/L | XX0 |
| Follicle-stimulating hormone [FSH] (P) | mIU/mL | 1.00 | IU/L | XX |
| Follicle-stimulating hormone [FSH] (U) | IU/24 h | 1.00 | IU/d | XXX |
| Fructose (P) | mg/dL | 0.05551 | mmol/L | X.XX |
| Galactose (P) [children] | mg/dL | 0.05551 | mmol/L | X.XX |
| Gases (aB) | | | | |
| P₀₂ | mm Hg (= Torr) | 0.1333 | kPa | XX.X |
| P_CO₂ | mm Hg (= Torr) | 0.1333 | kPa | X.X |
| Gastrin (S) | pg/mL | 1 | ng/L | XX0 |
| Globulins (S) [see immunoglobulins] | . . . | . . . | . . . | . . . |
| Glucagon (S) | pg/mL | 1 | ng/L | XX0 |
| Glucose (P) | mg/dL | 0.05551 | mmol/L | XX.X |
| Glucose (Sf) | mg/dL | 0.05551 | mmol/L | XX.X |
| γ-Glutamyltransferase [GGT] (S) | U/L | 0.01667 | μkat/L | X.XX |
| Growth hormone (P,S) | ng/mL | 1.00 | μg/L | XX.X |
| Haptoglobin (S) | mg/dL | 0.01 | g/L | X.XX |
| 5-Hydroxyindoleacetate (U) [as 5-hydroxyindole acetic acid; 5 HIAA] | mg/24 h | 5.230 | μmol/d | XXX |
| 17 Alpha-Hydroxyprogesterone (S,P) | μg/L | 3.026 | nmol/L | XX.X |
| Hydroxyproline (U) | mg/24 h/m² | 7.626 | μmol/(d·m²) | XX0 |
| Immunoglobulins (S) | | | | |
| IgG | mg/dL | 0.01 | g/L | XX.XX |
| IgA | mg/dL | 0.01 | g/L | XX.XX |
| IgM | mg/dL | 0.01 | g/L | XX.XX |
| IgD | mg/dL | 10 | mg/L | XX0 |
| IgE—0–3 years | IU/mL | 2.4 | μg/L | XX |
| 0–80 years | IU/mL | 2.4 | μg/L | XX |
| Insulin (P,S) | uU/mL | 7.175 | pmol/L | XXX |
| | mU/L | 7.175 | pmol/L | XXX |
| | μg/mL | 172.2 | pmol/L | XXX |
| Iron (S) | μg/dL | 0.1791 | μmol/L | XX |
| Iron-binding capacity (S) | μg/dL | 0.1791 | μmol/L | XX |
| Isoniazid (P) | mg/L | 7.291 | μmol/L | XX |
| Lactate (P) [as lactic acid] | meq/L | 1.00 | mmol/L | X.X |
| | mg/dL | 0.1110 | mmol/L | X.X |
| Lactate dehydrogenase (S) | U/L | 0.01667 | μkat/L | X.XX |
| Lactate dehydrogenase isoenzymes (S) | | | | |
| LD1 | % | 0.01 | 1 | 0.XX |
| LD2 | % | 0.01 | 1 | 0.XX |

**Table 9 (con't).** SI conversion factors for values in clinical chemistry.*†

| | | |
|---|---|---|
| B | blood | Sf | spinal fluid |
| Erc(s) | erythrocyte(s) | U | urine |
| P | plasma | a | arterial |
| S | serum | v | venous |

| Component | Present Unit | Conversion Factor | SI Unit Symbol | Significant Digits |
|---|---|---|---|---|
| Lactate dehydrogenase isoenzymes (S) (cont'd) | | | | |
| LD3 | % | 0.01 | 1 | 0.XX |
| LD4 | % | 0.01 | 1 | 0.XX |
| LD5 | % | 0.01 | 1 | 0.XX |
| Lead (B)—toxic | $\mu$g/dL | 0.04826 | $\mu$mol/L | X.XX |
| | mg/dL | 48.26 | $\mu$mol/L | X.XX |
| Lead (U)—toxic | $\mu$g/24 h | 0.004826 | $\mu$mol/d | X.XX |
| Lipase (S) | U/L | 0.01667 | $\mu$kat/L | X.XX |
| Lipids, total (P) | | | | |
| Lipoproteins (P) | mg/dL | 0.01 | g/L | X.X |
| Low-density [LDL]—as cholesterol | mg/dL | 0.02586 | mmol/L | X.XX |
| High-density [HDL]—as cholesterol | mg/dL | 0.02586 | mmol/L | X.XX |
| Lithium ion (S) | meq/L | 1.00 | mmol/L | X.XX |
| Luteinizing hormone (S) | mIU/mL | 1.00 | IU/L | XXX |
| Magnesium (S) | mg/dL | 0.4114 | mmol/L | X.XX |
| | meq/L | 0.500 | mmol/L | X.XX |
| Metanephrines (U) [as normetanephrine] | mg/24 h | 5.458 | $\mu$mol/d | XX.X |
| Nitrogen, total (U) | g/24 h | 71.38 | mmol/d | XX0 |
| Norepinephrine (P) | pg/mL | 0.005911 | nmol/L | X.XX |
| Norepinephrine (U) | $\mu$g/24 h | 5.911 | nmol/d | XX0 |
| Osmolality (P) | mosm/kg | 1.00 | mmol/kg | XXX |
| Osmolality (U) | mosm/kg | 1.00 | mmol/kg | XXX |
| Phosphate (S) [as phosphorus, inorganic] | mg/dL | 0.3229 | mmol/L | X.XX |
| Phosphate (U) [as phosphorus, inorganic] | g/24 h | 32.29 | mmol/d | XXX |
| Phospholipid phosphorus, total (P) | mg/dL | 0.3229 | mmol/L | X.XX |
| [human] placental lactogen (S) [hPL] | $\mu$g/mL | 46.30 | nmol/L | XX0 |
| Porphobilinogen (U) | mg/24 h | 4.420 | $\mu$mol/d | X.X |
| Porphyrins | | | | |
| Coproporphyrin (U) | $\mu$g/24 h | 1.527 | nmol/d | XXX |
| Protoprophyrin (Erc) | $\mu$g/dL | 0.0177 | $\mu$mol/L | X.XX |
| Uroporphyrin (U) | $\mu$g/24 h | 1.204 | nmol/d | XX |
| Uroporphyrinogen synthetase (Erc) | mmol/mL/h | 0.2778 | mmol/(L·s) | X.X |
| Potassium ion (S) | meq/L | 1.00 | mmol/L | X.X |
| Pregnanediol (U) | mg/24 h | 3.120 | $\mu$mol/d | XX.X |
| Pregnanetriol (U) | mg/24 h | 2.972 | $\mu$mol/d | XX.X |
| Progesterone (P) | ng/mL | 3.180 | nmol/L | XX |
| Prolactin (P) | ng/mL | 1.00 | $\mu$g/L | XX |
| Protein, total (S) | g/dL | 10.0 | g/L | XX |
| Protein, total (Sf) | mg/dL | 0.01 | g/L | X.XX |
| Protein, total (U) | mg/24 h | 0.001 | g/d | X.XX |
| Pyruvate (B) [as pyruvic acid] | mg/dL | 113.6 | $\mu$mol/L | XXX |
| Renin (P) | ng/mL/h | 0.2778 | ng/(L·s) | X.XX |
| Serotonin (B) [5-hydroxytryptamine] | $\mu$g/dL | 0.5675 | $\mu$mol/L | X.XX |
| Soidum ion (S) | meq/L | 1.00 | mmol/L | XXX |
| Sodium ion (U) | meq/24 h | 1.00 | mmol/d | XXX |
| Steroids | | | | |
| 17-Hydroxycorticosteroids (U) [as cortisol] | mg/24 h | 2.759 | $\mu$mol/d | XX |
| 17-Ketogenic steroids (U) [as dehydroepiandrosterone] | mg/24 h | 3.467 | $\mu$mol/d | XX |
| 17-Ketosteroids (U) [as dehydroepinandrosterone] | mg/24 h | 3.467 | $\mu$mol/d | XX |
| Ketosteroid fractions (U) | | | | |
| Androsterone | mg/24 h | 3.443 | $\mu$mol/d | XX |
| Dehydroepiandrosterone | mg/24 hr | 3.467 | $\mu$mol/d | XX |
| Etiocholanolone | mg/24 hr | 3.443 | $\mu$mol/d | XX |
| Testosterone (P) | ng/mL | 3.467 | nmol/L | XX.X |
| Theophylline (P) | mg/L | 5.550 | $\mu$mol/L | XX |
| Thyroid tests | | | | |
| Thyroid-stimulating hormone [TSH] (S) | $\mu$U/mL | 1.00 | mU/L | XX |
| Thyroxine [$T_4$] (S) | $\mu$g/dL | 12.87 | nmol/L | XXX |
| Thyroxine-binding globulin [TBG] (S) [as thyroxine] | $\mu$g/dL | 12.87 | nmol/L | XX0 |
| Thyroxine, free (S) | ng/dL | 12.87 | pmol/L | XX |
| Triiodothyronine [$T_3$] (S) | ng/dL | 0.01536 | nmol/L | X.X |
| $T_3$ uptake (S) | % | 0.01 | 1 | 0.XX |

**Table 9 (con't).** SI conversion factors for values in clinical chemistry.*†

| | | | |
|---|---|---|---|
| B | blood | Sf | spinal fluid |
| Erc(s) | erythrocyte(s) | U | urine |
| P | plasma | a | arterial |
| S | serum | v | venous |

| Component | Present Unit | Conversion Factor | SI Unit Symbol | Significant Digits |
|---|---|---|---|---|
| Transferrin (S) | mg/dL | 0.01 | g/L | X.XX |
| Triglycerides (P) [as triolein] | mg/dL | 0.01129 | mmol/L | X.XX |
| Urate (S) [as uric acid] | mg/dL | 59.48 | $\mu$mol/L | XX0 |
| Urate (U) [as uric acid] | g/24 h | 5.948 | mmol/d | XX |
| Urea nitrogen (S) | mg/dL | 0.3570 | mmol/L urea | X.X |
| Urea nitrogen (U) | g/24 h | 35.700 | mmol/d urea | XX0 |
| Urobilinogen (U) | mg/24 h | 1.693 | $\mu$mol/d | X.X |
| Vanillymandelic acid [VMA] (U) | mg/24 h | 5.046 | $\mu$mol/d | XX |
| Vitamin A [retinol] (P,S) | $\mu$g/dL | 0.03491 | $\mu$mol/L | X.XX |
| Vitamin B$_1$ [thiamine hydrochloride] (U) | $\mu$g/24 h | 0.002965 | $\mu$mol/d | X.XX |
| Vitamin B$_2$ [riboflavin] (S) | $\mu$g/dL | 26.57 | nmol/L | XXX |
| Vitamin B$_6$ [pyridoxal] (B) | ng/mL | 5.982 | nmol/L | XXX |
| Vitamin B$_{12}$ [cyanocobalamin] (P,S) | pg/mL | 0.7378 | pmol/L | XX0 |
| | ng/dL | 7.378 | pmol/L | |
| Vitamin C [see ascorbate] (B,P,S) | . . . | . . . | . . . | . . . |
| Vitamin D$_3$ | | | | |
| [cholecalciferol] (P) | $\mu$g/mL | 2.599 | nmol/L | XXX |
| 25-Hydroxycholecalciferol | ng/mL | 2.496 | nmol/L | XXX |
| 1$\alpha$,25-Dihydroxycholecalciferol | pg/mL | 2.385 | pmol/L | XXX |
| Vitamin E [$\alpha$-tocopherol] (P,S) | mg/dL | 23.22 | $\mu$mol/L | XX |
| D-Xylose (B) [25-g dose] | mg/dL | 0.06661 | mmol/L | X.X |
| D-Xylose excretion (U) [25-g dose] | % | 0.01 | 1 | 0.XX |
| Zinc (S) | $\mu$g/dL | 0.1530 | $\mu$mol/d | XX.X |
| Zinc (U) | $\mu$g/24 h | 0.01530 | $\mu$mol/d | XX.X |

* Data from Young DS: Implementation of SI units for clinical laboratory data. *Ann Intern Med* 1987;**106**:114.
† Current metric units × conversion factor = SI units.
SI units ÷ conversion factor = Current metric units.

Place the victim in the supine position on a flat, firm surface.

**B. Institute CPR in the *ABC* Sequence (Airway-Breathing-Circulation):**

**1. Airway–**

**a. Determine if breathing is absent–**Open the airway by positioning the neck anteriorly in extension. Determine if breathing is absent by obseгving the patient, listening for breathing, and holding a hand in front of the nose and mouth.

**b. If the patient is not breathing, take immediate steps to provide an airway–**In unconscious patients, the tongue becomes lax and may fall backward, blocking the victim's airway. Gently tip the victim's head backward as far as possible by lifting up the neck, near the base of the skull, with one hand and pressing down on the forehead with the other hand (Fig 1). Avoid hyperextending the victim's neck in accident cases when there is a possibility of neck fracture. In such an instance, keep mandible displaced forward by pulling strongly at the angle of the jaw (''chin lift'') or by lifting the angles of the mandible with both hands (''jaw thrust''). If mouth-to-mouth breathing is necessary and the rescuer decides to use the ''jaw thrust'' maneuver, the vic-

tim's nostrils should be closed by placing the check tightly against them.

**c. Clear the mouth and pharynx of foreign material** (eg, blood, vomitus) with the hooked index finger (''finger-sweep''), but avoid undue probing. Do not remove dentures but leave them in the mouth to obtain a better seal around the lips.

**2. Breathing–**

**a. If steps 1b and c fail to provide an airway, forcibly blow air through the mouth (keeping nose closed) or nose (keeping mouth closed) and quickly and fully inflate the lungs 4 times.** Exhaled air contains 16–18% oxygen. Watch for chest movement. If this fails to clear the airway immediately, foreign body airway obstruction is possible; roll the patient onto one side and deliver a sharp blow between the shoulder blades. If this measure also fails, use the Heimlich maneuver (see p 1117) and if required use an endotracheal (preferably orotracheal) tube. Perform a cricothyrotomy or tracheotomy if other measures fail.

**b. Feel the carotid or femoral artery for pulsations. If pulsations are present, give lung inflation by mouth-to-mouth breathing (keeping patient's nostrils closed), mouth-to-nose breathing**

**Table 10.** Therapeutic serum levels of some commonly used drugs.*†

| Drug | Therapeutic Range | | Toxic Level |
|------|------|------|------|
| | **Peak** | **Trough** | |
| **Antibiotics** | | | |
| Amikacin | 20–30 µg/mL | 1–8 µg/mL | >30 µg/mL |
| Kanamycin | 20–30 µg/mL | 1–8 µg/mL | >30 µg/mL |
| Gentamicin | 5–10 µg/mL | <2 µg/mL | >12 µg/mL |
| Tobramycin | 5–10 µg/mL | <2 µg/mL | >12 µg/mL |
| Netilmicin | 6–10 µg/mL | <2 µg/mL | >12 µg/mL |
| Chloramphenicol | 15–20 µg/mL | . . . | >25 µg/mL |

| Drug | Therapeutic Range | Toxic Level |
|------|------|------|
| **Antiarrhythmics** | | |
| Digoxin | 0.8–2 ng/mL | 2.5 ng/mL |
| Digitoxin | 10–22 ng/mL | 35 ng/mL |
| Lidocaine | 1.5–5 µg/mL | >7 µg/mL |
| Procainamide | 4–10 µg/mL | >16 µg/mL |
| Procainamide + n-acetylprocainamide | 10–30 µg/mL | >30 µg/mL |
| Quinidine | 2–5 µg/mL | >10 µg/mL |
| Disopyramide | 3–5 µg/mL | >7 µg/mL |
| **Antiepileptics** | | |
| Phenytoin | 10–20 µg/mL | >20 µg/mL |
| Phenobarbital | 15–40 µg/mL | >40 µg/mL |
| Primidone | 5–12 µg/mL | >15 µg/mL |
| Ethosuximide | 40–100 µg/mL | >150 µg/mL |
| Valproic acid | 50–100 µg/mL | >100 µg/mL |
| Carbamazepine | 8–12 µg/mL | >15 µg/mL |
| **Antidepressants** | | |
| Amitriptyline | 120–250 ng/mL | >500 ng/mL |
| Desipramine | 150–250 ng/mL | >500 ng/mL |
| Imipramine | 150–250 ng/mL | >500 ng/mL |
| Nortriptyline | 50–150 ng/mL | >500 ng/mL |
| Lithium | 0.6–1.4 meq/L | >2 meq/L |
| **Others** | | |
| Theophylline | 10–20 µg/mL | >20 µg/mL |
| Aspirin | 100–250 µg/mL | >300 µg/mL |
| Acetaminophen | . . . | >250 µg/mL |

\* See also Holford NHG: Clinical interpretation of drug concentrations. Chapter 67 in: *Basic & Clinical Pharmacology*, 3rd ed. Katzung BG (editor). Appleton & Lange, 1987.
† Plasma drug concentrations should be monitored when the drug has a narrow therapeutic range and the toxic level is near the upper range of the therapeutic range; when the therapeutic range is difficult to assess clinically; when the drug is given to achieve a therapeutic effect quickly and subsequent dosage must be modified; and when compliance with the prescribed dosage is in question.

**(keeping patient's mouth closed), or mouth-to-stoma breathing,** 12 times per minute—allowing about 2 seconds for inspiration and 3 seconds for expiration—until spontaneous respirations return. Observe rise and fall of the chest, avoiding excessive pressure that may cause gastric dilatation. Continue as long as the pulses remain palpable. Bag-mask techniques for lung inflation should be reserved for experts. If pulsations cease, follow directions as in 3, below.

**3. Circulation–If the carotid or femoral pulsations are absent, deliver a single, sharp, quick blow of the fist to the mid portion of the sternum (precordial thump)** *in case of witnessed cardiac arrest in the electrocardiographically monitored patient.* **If the response (return of pulsations) is not immediate, begin external cardiac compression** *without delay.* Alternate cardiac compression (closed heart massage) and pulmonary ventilation

(see above). Place the heel of one hand on the lower third of the sternum just above the level of the xiphoid. With the heel of the other hand on top of it and with fully extended arms, apply firm vertical pressure sufficient to force the sternum about 4–5 cm (1½–2 inches) downward (less in children) about once every second (60–80 per minute) (Fig 2). The compression should be smooth, and equal time should be allowed for compression and release. Avoid "quick jabs," which shorten the duration of compression. For children, use only one hand; for babies, use only 2 fingers of one hand, compressing 80–100 times per minute. After 15 sternal compressions, alternate with 2 quick, deep lung inflations. Repeat and continue this alternating procedure until it is possible to obtain additional assistance and more definitive care. If 2 operators are available, pause after every fifth compression while partner gives one mouth-to-mouth inflation. Check carotid pulse after 1 minute and every 5 minutes

**Table 11.** SI conversion table for therapeutic serum levels of some commonly used drugs.

| Drug | Present Unit | Conversion Factor | SI Unit Symbol | Significant Digits |
|---|---|---|---|---|
| **Antibiotics** | | | | |
| Amikacin | μg/mL | 0.0017 | umol/L | XX |
| Kanamycin | μg/mL | N/A | N/A | N/A |
| Gentamicin | μg/mL | N/A | N/A | N/A |
| Tobramycin | μg/mL | 0.00214 | umol/L | XX |
| Netilmicin | μg/mL | 0.0021 | umol/L | XX |
| Chloramphenicol | μg/mL | 0.00178 | umol/L | XX |
| **Antiarrhythmics** | | | | |
| Digoxin | ng/mL | 1.281 | nmol/L | X.X |
| Digitoxin | ng/mL | 1.31 | nmol/L | XX |
| Lidocaine | μg/mL | 4.267 | umol/L | X.X |
| Procainamide | μg/mL | 4.249 | umol/L | XX |
| N-Acetylprocainamide | μg/mL | 3.606 | umol/L | XX |
| Quinidine | μg/mL | 3.082 | umol/L | X.X |
| Disopyramide | μg/mL | 2.946 | umol/L | XX |
| **Antiepileptics** | | | | |
| Phenytoin | μg/mL | 3.964 | umol/L | XX |
| Phenobarbital | μg/mL | 43.06 | umol/L | XXX |
| Primidone | μg/mL | 4.582 | umol/L | XX |
| Ethosuximide | μg/mL | 7.084 | umol/L | XX0 |
| Valproic acid | μg/mL | 6.934 | umol/L | XX0 |
| Carbamazepine | μg/mL | 4.233 | umol/L | XX |
| **Antidepressants** | | | | |
| Amitriptyline | ng/mL | 3.605 | nmol/L | XX0 |
| Desipramine | ng/mL | 3.754 | nmol/L | XX0 |
| Imipramine | ng/mL | 3.566 | nmol/L | XX0 |
| Nortripytline | ng/mL | 3.797 | nmol/L | XX0 |
| Lithium | meq/L | 1 | mmol/L | X.X |
| **Others** | | | | |
| Theophylline | μg/mL | 5.550 | umol/L | XX |
| Aspirin | μg/mL | 0.0055 | mmol/L | X.XX |
| Acetaminophen | μg/mL | 6.616 | umol/L | XX0 |

thereafter. Resuscitation must be continuous during transportation to the hospital.

## Advanced Life Support (Fig 3)

Until spontaneous respiration and circulation are restored, there must be no interruption of artificial ventilation and cardiac massage while the attempt to (1) restart spontaneous circulation and (2) stabilize the cardiopulmonary circulation (steps A–D below) is being carried out. Three basic questions must be considered at this point: (1) What is the underlying cause, and is it treatable? (2) What is the nature of the cardiac arrest? If possible, determine the type of cardiac arrest by means of electrocardiography: (a) asystole, (b) shock or electromechanical dissociation (electrical activity without effective mechanical contraction), or (c) ventricular fibrillation. (3) What further measures will be necessary? Plan upon the assistance of a trained resuscitation team. Cardiac monitoring and assisted ventilation equipment, a DC defibrillator, emergency drugs, and adequate laboratory facilities are required.

**A. Provide for adequate prolonged oxygenation** *as soon as possible* by intubation, administration of 100% oxygen, and mechanically assisted ventilation. Promptly establish an intravenous line for long-term intravenous therapy and monitoring. Establish electrocardiographic monitoring immediately. Take the first of serial specimens for arterial blood gases, pH, and electrolytes.

**B. Epinephrine:** If a spontaneous effective heartbeat is not restored after 1–2 minutes of cardiac compression, give epinephrine (adrenaline), 5–10 mL of a 1:10,000 solution intravenously every 5 minutes as indicated. If an intravenous line has not been established, epinephrine can be administered via an endotracheal tube. Epinephrine may stimulate cardiac contractions and induce ventricular fibrillation that can then be treated by DC countershock (see below).

**C. Additional Circulatory Support:** If the victim has not had spontaneous pulsations with adequate ventilation for more than 5 minutes, administer 0.5–1 meq/kg of sodium bicarbonate intravenously. Ideally, additional bicarbonate therapy should be guided by blood gas determinations. Obviously, the therapy is directed at metabolic acidosis; however, excessive therapy will lead to alkalosis, which can depress myocardial function. In the absence of blood gas determinations, repeat one-half the original dose at 10-minute intervals.

Calcium is necessary for the normal inotropic action of the heart. However, previous protocols often led to grossly elevated calcium levels; this is especially

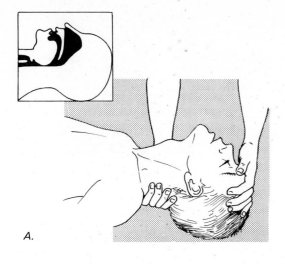

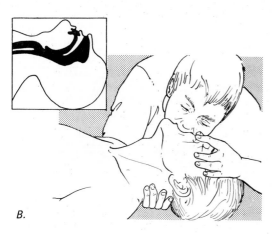

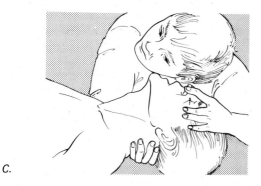

**Figure 1.** Proper performance of mouth-to-mouth resuscitation. **A:** Open airway by positioning neck anteriorly in extension. Inserts show airway obstructed when the neck is in resting flexed position and opening when neck is extended. **B:** Rescuer should close victim's nose with fingers, seal mouth around victim's mouth, and deliver breath by vigorous expiration. **C:** Victim is allowed to exhale passively by unsealing mouth and nose. Rescuer should listen and feel for expiratory air flow.

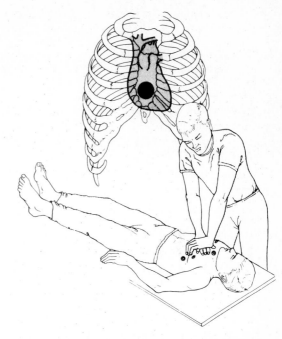

**Figure 2.** Technique of closed chest cardiac massage. Heavy circle in heart drawing shows area of application of force. Circles on supine figure show points of application of electrodes for defibrillation.

dangerous for patients receiving digitalis, as hypercalcemia can precipitate digitalis toxicity. In asystole or electromechanical dissociation, it is reasonable to administer intravenously 5 mL of a 10% calcium chloride solution. (*Caution:* This will precipitate in a line concurrently running sodium bicarbonate.) Though there is some controversy, it is probably not wise to repeat calcium administration unless there is prior reason to suspect hypocalcemia.

**D. Ventricular Arrhythmias:**

**1. Ventricular fibrillation–**If electrocardiography demonstrates ventricular fibrillation, maintain respiration and external cardiac massage until just before giving an external defibrillating shock. A DC countershock of 200–300 J is given across the heart, ie, with one electrode positioned to the right of the upper sternum and one paddle positioned just to the left of the left nipple in the anterior axillary line. Apply paddles *firmly,* as firm application will decrease impedance. If initial countershock fails, repeat the defibrillation with 300 J and again later at 360 J. If an attempt at defibrillation is successful but fibrillation subsequently recurs, do not increase the energy of defibrillation; instead, repeat the countershock at the previously successful energy level. This is recommended because repeated countershock decreases the resistance of the chest wall and because unnecessarily high energy may cause myocardial damage.

**2. Refractory ventricular fibrillation–**If cardiac function is still not restored, continue external

## CARDIORESPIRATORY ARREST

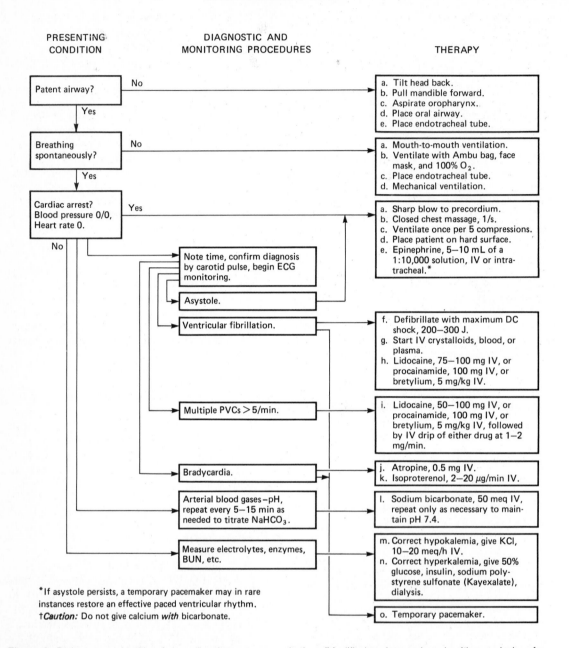

PRESENTING CONDITION     DIAGNOSTIC AND MONITORING PROCEDURES     THERAPY

*If asystole persists, a temporary pacemaker may in rare instances restore an effective paced ventricular rhythm.
†*Caution:* Do not give calcium *with* bicarbonate.

**Figure 3.** Patient care algorithm for cardiopulmonary resuscitation. (Modified and reproduced, with permission, from Shoemaker WC: A patient care algorithm for cardiac arrest. *Crit Care Med* [May-June] 1976;**4**:157.)

support of respiration and circulation and give bicarbonate and epinephrine as above. If cardiac action is reestablished but remains weak, give calcium chloride as above. If fibrillation persists or recurs, give **bretylium,** 350–500 mg intravenously as a bolus injection. If necessary, additional bretylium may be given as boluses of 700–1000 mg intravenously. If bretylium fails to suppress ventricular fibrillation, **lidocaine** may be tried as an initial 100-mg intravenous bolus injection; additional boluses of 50 mg may be given at 5- to 10-minute intervals, with the total dose not to exceed 225 mg. **Procainamide** may also be tried; this should be administered at a rate of 20 mg/min (100 mg every 5 minutes) to a total dose not exceeding 1 g. Procainamide is the most potent negative inotrope of these 3 antiarrhythmic drugs.

**3. Ventricular tachycardia**–For refractory or recurrent ventricular tachycardia, give a loading dose of lidocaine, 100 mg (or 1 mg/kg). If an infusion (2–4 mg/min) is not started promptly, a second loading dose of 0.5 mg/kg should be given in 5–10 minutes. If lidocaine is not successful, bretylium and procainamide can be tried as above. It may be necessary to use a pacemaker to override the abnormal rhythm.

**4. Severe sinus bradycardia**—In some instances of cardiac arrest with electrical sinus bradycardia (with a heart rate of < 60/min when associated with premature ventricular contractions or systolic blood pressure of < 90 mm Hg) or cardiac arrest with sinus bradycardia associated with a high degree of atrioventricular block, **atropine sulfate,** 0.4–0.6 mg intravenously, may be of value. Atropine is given intravenously in an initial dose of 0.5–1 mg; it may be repeated at 5-minute intervals to achieve the desired rate, with the total dose generally not exceeding 2 mg. **Isoproterenol** may be the treatment of choice for patients with profound bradycardia with complete heart block, and it may also be useful for treatment of profound bradycardia refractory to atropine. Give isoproterenol, 1 mg in 500 mL of 5% dextrose in water by intravenous infusion at a rate of 2–20 μg/min, and adjust the dose to increase the heart rate to approximately 60 beats/min. An electrical pacemaker may be necessary.

### Follow-Up Measures

When cardiac and pulmonary function have been reestablished and satisfactorily maintained, evaluation of central nervous system function deserves careful consideration. Decisions about the nature and duration of subsequent treatment must be individualized. Physicians must decide if they are ''prolonging life'' or simply ''prolonging dying.''

Support ventilation and circulation. Treat complications that might arise. Do not overlook the possibility of complications of external cardiac massage (eg, broken ribs, ruptured viscera).

Bass E: Cardiopulmonary arrest: Pathophysiology and neurological complications. *Ann Intern Med* 1985;**103:**920.

Ewy GA: Current status of cardiopulmonary resuscitation. *Mod Concepts Cardiovasc Dis* 1984;**53:**43.

Graver K: New trends in the management of cardiac arrest. *Am Fam Physician* (Feb) 1984;**29:**223.

Lo B et al; Do not resuscitate decisions: A prospective study at 3 teaching hospitals. *Arch Intern Med* 1985;**145:**1115.

Roth R et al: Out-of-hospital cardiac arrest: Factors associated with survival. *Ann Emerg Med* 1984;**13:**237.

Safar P: Cardiopulmonary-cerebral resuscitation. In: *Textbook of Critical Care.* Shoemaker WC et al (editors). Saunders, 1984.

Standards and guidelines for cardiopulmonary resuscitation (CPR) and emergency cardiac care (ECC). *JAMA* 1980;**244:**453. [Entire issue.]

# EMERGENCY TREATMENT OF FOOD CHOKING & OTHER CAUSES OF ACUTE AIRWAY OBSTRUCTION

Suspect life-threatening food choking in every case of respiratory distress or loss of consciousness that occurs while the patient is eating. A bolus of food (often poorly chewed meat) or other foreign object is usually lodged fairly high in the pharynx. Predisposing factors to acute airway obstruction include acute alcoholic intoxication, dentures, swallowing disorders due to any cause, and chronic obstructive pulmonary disease. In a hospital setting, elderly or debilitated patients who are sedated and have poor dentition are particularly prone to asphyxiation from large chunks of food.

The clinical picture of the choking patient may be mistaken for myocardial infarction, stroke, drug overdose, laryngospasm, or laryngeal edema.

If the unconscious patient is not breathing but can be ventilated, proceed with mouth-to-mouth or mouth-to-nose ventilation. If there is no pulse, institute CPR (see p 1108).

### Treatment (*Act quickly!*)

If airway obstruction is only partial, as evidenced by wheezing, forceful coughing, and adequate airway exchange, do *not* interfere with the patient's attempt to expel the foreign body. *If the patient is able to speak, even in a whisper, do not use the Heimlich procedure.*

*If there is progressive or complete airway obstruction* (ie, *the conscious patient is unable to speak, cough, or breathe* and often clutches the neck as a sign of choking distress) and it is not possible to ventilate the patient, perform the following in quick succession:

#### A. If Patient Is Sitting or Standing:

1. Deliver a rapid series of 4 hard, sharp blows with the heel of the hand to the interscapular portion of the patient's spine. If the back blows are ineffective, then

2. Apply 4 manual thrusts by the Heimlich procedure. Wrap arms around patient's waist. Make a fist with one hand and grasp the fist with the other. Place thumb side of fist against patient's abdomen just above the navel and below the rib cage (see Fig 4). Then press fist into the abdomen with a firm, quick upward thrust (not simply a squeeze or bear hug). When it is difficult to encircle the abdomen (eg, marked obesity, pregnancy), it may be necessary to utilize an alternative technique of forceful chest thrusts.

3. If the above maneuvers are unsuccessful, draw tongue away from the back of throat and try to remove the obstructing object with a forward sweep of the fingers.

4. If obstruction still persists, repeat the sequences until they are effective or the victim recovers.

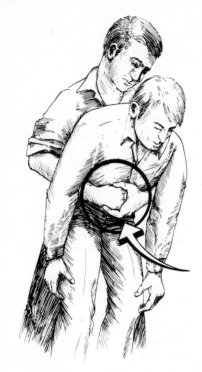

**Figure 4.** Heimlich procedure.

5. Those properly trained may use direct visualization with tongue blade and flashlight or laryngoscope for direct forceps extraction.

**B. With Patient Lying Down:** (When unconscious or when extremely heavy.)

1. Roll the patient onto one side and deliver a rapid series of 4 hard, sharp blows with the heel of the hand to the interscapular portion of the spine.

2. If the back blows are ineffective, quickly turn the patient to supine position (on back) and straddle his or her body. With one hand atop the other on the abdomen slightly above the navel, press the heel of the bottom hand into the abdomen with 4 quick upward thrusts, as above. Alternatively, the rescuer may position himself or herself exactly as for chest compressions (heel of hand on lower half of sternum) and exert 4 quick downward thrusts that will compress the chest cavity. If patient vomits, turn quickly on side and clear mouth to prevent aspiration.

3. Repeat the above sequences several times, if necessary.

4. Attempt direct visualization and forceps extraction if necessary.

If the above measures fail, it is necessary for trained operators to perform emergency circothyrotomy or tracheotomy.

Hoffman JR: Treatment of foreign body obstruction of the upper airway. *West J Med* 1982;**136**:11.

Standards and guidelines for cardiopulmonary resuscitation (CPR) and emergency cardiac care (ECC). *JAMA* 1980;**244**:453. [Entire issue.]

**Table 12.** Schedules of controlled drugs.*†

*Schedule I:* (All nonresearch use forbidden.)
 **Narcotics:** Heroin and many nonmarketed synthetic narcotics
 **Hallucinogens:**
  LSD
  MDA, STP, DMT, DET, mescaline, peyote, bufotenine, ibogaine, psilocybin, phencyclidine (PCP) (veterinary drug only)
 **Marihuana, tetrahydrocannabinols**
 **Methaqualone**

*Schedule II:* (No telephone prescriptions, no refills.)
 **Narcotics:**
  Opium
  Opium alkaloids and derived phenanthrene alkaloids: Morphine, codeine, hydromorphone (Dilaudid), oxymorphone (Numorphan), oxycodone (dihydrohydroxycodeinone, a component of Percodan, Percocet, Tylox)
  Designated synthetic drugs: Meperidine (Demerol), methadone, levorphanol (Levo-Dromoran), fentanyl (Sublimaze), alphaprodine (Nisentil), sufentanil (Sufenta)
 **Stimulants:**
  Coca leaves and cocaine
  Amphetamine (Benzedrine)
  Amphetamine complex (Biphetamine)
  Dextroamphetamine (Dexedrine)
  Methamphetamine (Desoxyn)
  Phenmetrazine (Preludin)
  Methylphenidate (Ritalin)
  Above in mixtures with other controlled or uncontrolled drugs
 **Depressants:**
  Amobarbital (Amytal)
  Pentobarbital (Nembutal)
  Secobarbital (Seconal)
  Mixtures of above (eg, Tuinal)

*Schedule III:* (Prescription must be written after 6 months or 5 refills.)
 **Narcotics:** The following opiates in combination with one or more active nonnarcotic ingredients, provided the amount does not exceed that shown:
  Codeine and dihydrocodeine: Not to exceed 1800 mg/dL or 90 mg/tablet or other dose unit
  Dihydrocodeinone (hydrocodone and in Hycodan): Not to exceed 300 mg/dL or 15 mg/tablet
  Opium: 500 mg/dL or 25 mg/5 mL or other dosage unit (paregoric)
 **Stimulants:**
  Benzphetamine (Didrex)
  Phendimetrazine (Plegine)
 **Depressants:**
  Schedule II barbiturates in mixtures with noncontrolled drugs or in suppository dose form
  Aprobarbital (Alurate)

**Depressants (cont'd):**
  Butabarbital (Butisol)
  Glutethimide (Doriden)
  Talbutal (Lotusate)
  Thiamylal (Surital)
  Thiopental (Pentothal)

*Schedule IV:* (Prescription must be rewritten after 6 months or 5 refills; differs from Schedule III in penalties for illegal possession.)
 **Narcotics:**
  Pentazocine (Talwin)
  Propoxyphene (Darvon)
 **Stimulants:**
  Diethylpropion (Tenuate)
  Mazindol (Sanorex)
  Phentermine (Ionamin)
  Fenfluramine (Pondimin)
  Pemoline (Cylert)
 **Depressants:**
  Benzodiazepines:
   Alprazolam (Xanax)
   Chlordiazepoxide (Librium)
   Clonazepam (Clonopin)
   Clorazepate (Tranxene)
   Diazepam (Valium)
   Flurazepam (Dalmane)
   Halazepam (Paxipam)
   Lorazepam (Ativan)
   Oxazepam (Serax)
   Prazepam (Centrax)
   Temazepam (Restoril)
   Triazolam (Halcion)
  Chloral hydrate
  Ethchlorvynol (Placidyl)
  Ethinamate (Valmid)
  Meprobamate (Equanil, Miltown, etc)
  Mephobarbital (Mebaral)
  Methohexital (Brevital)
  Methyprylon (Noludar)
  Paraldehyde
  Phenobarbital

*Schedule V:* (As any other [nonnarcotic] prescription drug; may also be dispensed without prescription unless additional state regulations apply.)
 **Narcotics:**
  Diphenoxylate (not more than 2.5 mg and not less than 0.025 mg of atropine per dosage unit, as in Lomotil)
  Loperamide (Imodium)
  The following drugs in combination with other active, nonnarcotic ingredients and provided the amount per 100 mL or 100 g does not exceed that shown:
  Codeine: 200 mg
  Dihydrocodeine: 100 mg

* Reproduced, with permission, from Katzung BG (editor): *Basic & Clinical Pharmacology,* 3rd ed. Appleton-Lange, 1987.
† Local or state laws may be at variance with federal schedule of controlled drugs.

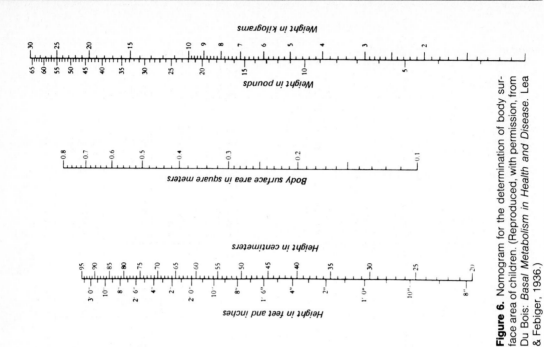

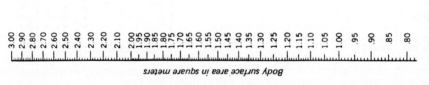

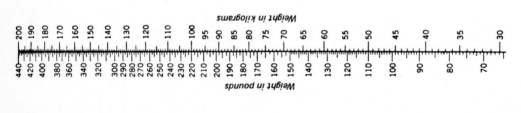

**Figure 6.** Nomogram for the determination of body surface area of children. (Reproduced, with permission, from Du Bois: *Basal Metabolism in Health and Disease.* Lea & Febiger, 1936.)

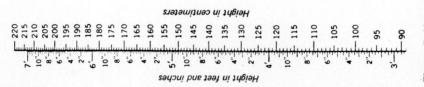

**Figure 5.** Nomogram for the determination of body surface area of children and adults. (Reproduced, with permission, from Boothby & Sandiford: *Boston MSJ* 1921;**185**:337. [Revised 1979.]

**Table 13.** Age-specific and age-adjusted death rates, United States, 1984. Both sexes, all races. Rates are per 100,000 population. Total deaths: male, 1,085,390; female, 961,490.*

| | All Ages | Age Under 1 Year | Age 1–14 | Age 15–24 | Age 25–34 | Age 35–44 | Age 45–54 | Age 55–64 | Age 65–74 | Age 75–84 | Age 85+ |
|---|---|---|---|---|---|---|---|---|---|---|---|
| | **All causes 886.7** | **All causes 1077.8** | **All causes 32.5** | **All causes 98.5** | **All causes 123.1** | **All causes 205.5** | **All causes 531.7** | **All causes 1289.6** | **All causes 2864.4** | **All causes 6416.5** | **All causes 14,890.1** |
| 1. | Heart disease 324.4 | Conditions from perinatal period 513.6 | Accidents 14.3 | Accidents 50.5 | Accidents 38.4 | Cancer 44.5 | Cancer 172.4 | Cancer 450.8 | Heart disease 1110.6 | Heart disease 2752.3 | Heart disease 7125.7 |
| 2. | Cancer 191.6 | Congenital anomalies 231.8 | Cancer 3.4 | Suicide 12.2 | Suicide 16.1 | Heart disease 37.1 | Heart disease 160.5 | Heart disease 444.7 | Cancer 830.0 | Cancer 1272.7 | Cerebrovasular disease 1796.6 |
| 3. | Cerebrovascular accidents 65.6 | Accidents 23.6 | Congenital anomalies 2.9 | Homicide 11.8 | Homicide 14.4 | Accidents 32.1 | Accidents 33.3 | Cerebrovascular disease 24.8 | Cerebrovascular disease 181.7 | Cerebrovascular disease 628.0 | Cancer 1559.1 |
| 4. | Accidents 40.1 | Heart disease 20.1 | Heart disease 1.3 | Cancer 5.5 | Cancer 12.6 | Suicide 14.3 | Cerebrovascular disease 24.8 | Chronic obstructive lung disease 46.6 | Chronic obstructive lung disease 147.3 | Chronic obstructive lung disease 265.9 | Pneumonia, influenza 853.0 |
| 5. | Chronic obstructive lung disease 29.8 | Septicemia 19.1 | Homicide 1.2 | Heart disease 2.5 | Heart disease 8.0 | Homicide 11.3 | Liver disease 22.6 | Accidents 37.3 | Diabetes mellitus 61.3 | Pneumonia, influenza 220.8 | Atherosclerosis 490.7 |
| 6. | Pneumonia, influenza 25.0 | Pneumonia, influenza 17.3 | Pneumonia, influenza 0.7 | Pneumonia, influenza 0.7 | Cerebrovascular disease 2.3 | Liver disease 10.3 | Suicide 16.9 | Liver disease 35.5 | Pneumonia, influenza 53.0 | Diabetes mellitus 124.2 | Chronic obstructive lung disease 336.9 |
| 7. | Diabetes mellitus 15.6 | Homicide 9.6 | Suicide 0.6 | Cerebrovascular disease 0.7 | Pneumonia, influenza 1.8 | Diabetes mellitus 4.1 | Diabetes mellitus 9.7 | Diabetes mellitus 26.8 | Accidents 50.8 | Accidents 109.7 | Accidents 270.4 |
| 8. | Suicide 12.3 | Kidney disease 6.3 | Conditions from perinatal period 0.4 | Chronic obstructive lung disease 0.4 | Diabetes mellitus 1.4 | Pneumonia, influenza 2.9 | Chronic obstructive lung disease 9.8 | Pneumonia, influenza 17.2 | Liver disease 38.0 | Athero-sclerosis 87.2 | Diabetes mellitus 212.8 |
| 9. | Chronic liver disease 11.3 | Cerebrovascular disease 3.3 | Septicemia 0.2 | Congenital anomalies 1.3 | Congenital anomalies 1.3 | Chronic obstructive lung disease 2.0 | Homicide 8.5 | Suicide 16.3 | Kidney disease 25.4 | Kidney disease 76.5 | Kidney disease 196.3 |
| 10. | Athero-sclerosis 10.4 | Cancer 2.5 | Cerebrovascular disease 0.2 | Diabetes mellitus 0.3 | Kidney disease 0.6 | Kidney disease 1.7 | Pneumonia, influenza 7.0 | Kidney disease 9.9 | Septicemia 19.9 | Septicemia 52.0 | Septicemia 129.8 |

* National Center for Health Statistics Monthly Vital Statistics Report (Sept 26) 1985;**33:**No. 13.

## CONVERSION TABLES

### Fahrenheit/Celsius Temperature Conversion
(°F = 9/5°C + 32; °C = 5/9 [°F − 32])

| °F | | °C | °F | | °C | °F | | °C |
|----|---|------|-----|---|------|-----|---|------|
| 90 | = | 32.2 | 97 | = | 36.1 | 104 | = | 40.0 |
| 91 | = | 32.8 | 98 | = | 36.7 | 105 | = | 40.6 |
| 92 | = | 33.3 | 99 | = | 37.2 | 106 | = | 41.1 |
| 93 | = | 33.9 | 100 | = | 37.8 | 107 | = | 41.7 |
| 94 | = | 34.4 | 101 | = | 38.3 | 108 | = | 42.2 |
| 95 | = | 35.0 | 102 | = | 38.9 | 109 | = | 42.8 |
| 96 | = | 35.6 | 103 | = | 39.4 | | | |

### Milliequivalent Conversion Factors

| meq/L of: | Divide mg/dL or vol% by: |
|-----------|--------------------------|
| Calcium | 2.0 |
| Chloride (from Cl) | 3.5 |
| (from NaCl) | 5.85 |
| $CO_2$ combining power | 2.222 |
| Magnesium | 1.2 |
| Phosphorus | 3.1 (mmol) |
| Potassium | 3.9 |
| Sodium | 2.3 |

### Approximate Length Equivalents

| Metric System | US System |
|---------------|-----------|
| 1 cm | 0.4 in |
| 1 m | 39.4 in |
| 1 km | 3281 ft (0.6 mi) |

### Metric System Prefixes (Small Measurement)

In accordance with the decision of several scientific societies to employ a universal system of metric nomenclature, the following prefixes have become standard in many medical texts and journals.

| k | kilo- | $10^3$ |
|---|-------|--------|
| c | centi- | $10^{-2}$ |
| m | milli- | $10^{-3}$ |
| μ | micro- | $10^{-6}$ |
| n | nano- (formerly millimicro, mμ) | $10^{-9}$ |
| p | pico- (formerly micromicro, μμ) | $10^{-12}$ |
| f | femto- | $10^{-15}$ |
| a | atto- | $10^{-18}$ |

### Household Equivalents (Approximate)

1 tsp = 6 mL
1 tbsp = 15 mL
1 oz (eg, medicine glass) = 30 mL
1 cup = 8 fluid oz = 240 mL
1 quart = 946 mL

### Apothecary Equivalents

| Metric | Approximate Apothecary Equivalents | Metric | Approximate Apothecary Equivalents | Metric | Approximate Apothecary Equivalents |
|--------|------------------------------------|--------|------------------------------------|--------|------------------------------------|
| 30 g | 1 oz | 0.12 g | 2 gr | 3 mg | 1/20 gr |
| 6 g | 90 gr | 0.1 g | 1½ gr | 2 mg | 1/30 gr |
| 5 g | 75 gr | 75 mg | 1¼ gr | 1.5 mg | 1/40 gr |
| 4 g | 60 gr | 60 mg | 1 gr | 1.2 mg | 1/50 gr |
| 3 g | 45 gr | 50 mg | 3/4 gr | 1 mg | 1/60 gr |
| 2 g | 30 gr | 40 mg | 2/3 gr | 0.8 mg | 1/80 gr |
| 1.5 g | 22 gr | 30 mg | 1/2 gr | 0.6 mg | 1/100 gr |
| 1 g | 15 gr | 25 mg | 3/8 gr | 0.5 mg | 1/120 gr |
| 0.75 g | 12 gr | 20 mg | 1/3 gr | 0.4 mg | 1/150 gr |
| 0.6 g | 10 gr | 15 mg | 1/4 gr | 0.3 mg | 1/200 gr |
| 0.5 g | 7½ gr | 12 mg | 1/5 gr | 0.25 mg | 1/250 gr |
| 0.4 g | 6 gr | 10 mg | 1/6 gr | 0.2 mg | 1/300 gr |
| 0.3 g | 5 gr | 8 mg | 1/8 gr | 0.15 mg | 1/400 gr |
| 0.25 g | 4 gr | 6 mg | 1/10 gr | 0.12 mg | 1/500 gr |
| 0.2 g | 3 gr | 5 mg | 1/12 gr | 0.1 mg | 1/600 gr |
| 0.15 g | 2½ gr | 4 mg | 1/15 gr | | |

## Pounds to Kilograms
(1 kg = 2.2 lb; 1 lb = 0.45 kg)

| lb | kg | lb | kg | lb | kg | lb | kg | lb | kg |
|----|----|----|----|----|----|----|----|----|----|
| 5 | 2.3 | 50 | 22.7 | 95 | 43.1 | 140 | 63.5 | 185 | 83.9 |
| 10 | 4.5 | 55 | 25.0 | 100 | 45.4 | 145 | 65.8 | 190 | 86.2 |
| 15 | 6.8 | 60 | 27.2 | 105 | 47.6 | 150 | 68.0 | 195 | 88.5 |
| 20 | 9.1 | 65 | 29.5 | 110 | 49.9 | 155 | 70.3 | 200 | 90.7 |
| 25 | 11.3 | 70 | 31.7 | 115 | 52.2 | 160 | 72.6 | 205 | 93.0 |
| 30 | 13.6 | 75 | 34.0 | 120 | 54.4 | 165 | 74.8 | 210 | 95.3 |
| 35 | 15.9 | 80 | 36.3 | 125 | 56.7 | 170 | 77.1 | 215 | 97.5 |
| 40 | 18.1 | 85 | 38.6 | 130 | 58.9 | 175 | 79.4 | 220 | 99.8 |
| 45 | 20.4 | 90 | 40.8 | 135 | 61.2 | 180 | 81.6 | | |

## Feet and Inches to Centimeters
(1 cm = 0.39 in; 1 in = 2.54 cm)

| ft | in | cm | ft | in | cm | ft | in | cm | ft | in | cm | ft | in | cm |
|----|----|----|----|----|----|----|----|----|----|----|----|----|----|----|
| 0 | 6 | 15.2 | 2 | 4 | 71.1 | 3 | 4 | 101.6 | 4 | 4 | 132.0 | 5 | 4 | 162.6 |
| 1 | 0 | 30.5 | 2 | 5 | 73.6 | 3 | 5 | 104.1 | 4 | 5 | 134.6 | 5 | 5 | 165.1 |
| 1 | 6 | 45.7 | 2 | 6 | 76.1 | 3 | 6 | 106.6 | 4 | 6 | 137.1 | 5 | 6 | 167.6 |
| 1 | 7 | 48.3 | 2 | 7 | 78.7 | 3 | 7 | 109.2 | 4 | 7 | 139.6 | 5 | 7 | 170.2 |
| 1 | 8 | 50.8 | 2 | 8 | 81.2 | 3 | 8 | 111.7 | 4 | 8 | 142.2 | 5 | 8 | 172.7 |
| 1 | 9 | 53.3 | 2 | 9 | 83.8 | 3 | 9 | 114.2 | 4 | 9 | 144.7 | 5 | 9 | 175.3 |
| 1 | 10 | 55.9 | 2 | 10 | 86.3 | 3 | 10 | 116.8 | 4 | 10 | 147.3 | 5 | 10 | 177.8 |
| 1 | 11 | 58.4 | 2 | 11 | 88.8 | 3 | 11 | 119.3 | 4 | 11 | 149.8 | 5 | 11 | 180.3 |
| 2 | 0 | 61.0 | 3 | 0 | 91.4 | 4 | 0 | 121.9 | 5 | 0 | 152.4 | 6 | 0 | 182.9 |
| 2 | 1 | 63.5 | 3 | 1 | 93.9 | 4 | 1 | 124.4 | 5 | 1 | 154.9 | 6 | 1 | 185.4 |
| 2 | 2 | 66.0 | 3 | 2 | 96.4 | 4 | 2 | 127.0 | 5 | 2 | 157.5 | 6 | 2 | 188.0 |
| 2 | 3 | 68.6 | 3 | 3 | 99.0 | 4 | 3 | 129.5 | 5 | 3 | 160.0 | 6 | 3 | 190.5 |

## Desirable Weights (Pounds)*
(See p 797.)

| | | Men (Ages 25–59) | | | | | Women (Ages 25–59) | | |
|------|--------|-------|--------|-------|------|--------|-------|--------|-------|
| **Height** Feet | Inches | **Small Frame** | **Medium Frame** | **Large Frame** | **Height†** Feet | Inches | **Small Frame** | **Medium Frame** | **Large Frame** |
| 5 | 2 | 128–134 | 131–141 | 138–150 | 4 | 10 | 102–111 | 109–121 | 118–131 |
| 5 | 3 | 130–136 | 133–143 | 140–153 | 4 | 11 | 103–113 | 111–123 | 120–134 |
| 5 | 4 | 132–138 | 135–145 | 142–156 | 5 | 0 | 104–115 | 113–126 | 122–137 |
| 5 | 5 | 134–140 | 137–148 | 144–160 | 5 | 1 | 106–118 | 115–129 | 125–140 |
| 5 | 6 | 136–142 | 139–151 | 146–164 | 5 | 2 | 108–121 | 118–132 | 128–143 |
| 5 | 7 | 138–145 | 142–154 | 149–168 | 5 | 3 | 111–124 | 121–135 | 131–147 |
| 5 | 8 | 140–148 | 145–157 | 152–172 | 5 | 4 | 114–127 | 124–138 | 134–151 |
| 5 | 9 | 142–151 | 148–160 | 155–176 | 5 | 5 | 117–130 | 127–141 | 137–155 |
| 5 | 10 | 144–154 | 151–163 | 158–180 | 6 | 6 | 120–133 | 130–144 | 140–159 |
| 5 | 11 | 146–157 | 154–166 | 161–184 | 5 | 7 | 123–136 | 133–147 | 143–163 |
| 6 | 0 | 149–160 | 157–170 | 164–188 | 5 | 8 | 126–139 | 136–150 | 146–167 |
| 6 | 1 | 152–164 | 160–174 | 168–192 | 5 | 9 | 129–142 | 139–153 | 149–170 |
| 6 | 2 | 155–168 | 164–178 | 172–197 | 5 | 10 | 132–145 | 142–156 | 152–173 |
| 6 | 3 | 158–172 | 167–182 | 176–202 | 5 | 11 | 135–148 | 145–159 | 155–176 |
| 6 | 4 | 162–176 | 171–187 | 181–207 | 6 | 0 | 138–151 | 148–162 | 158–179 |

* With indoor clothing weighing 5 pounds for men and 3 pounds for women.
† With shoes with 1-inch heels.
Source of basic data: *Build Study, 1979*. Society of Actuaries and Association of Life Insurance Medical Directors of America, 1980.

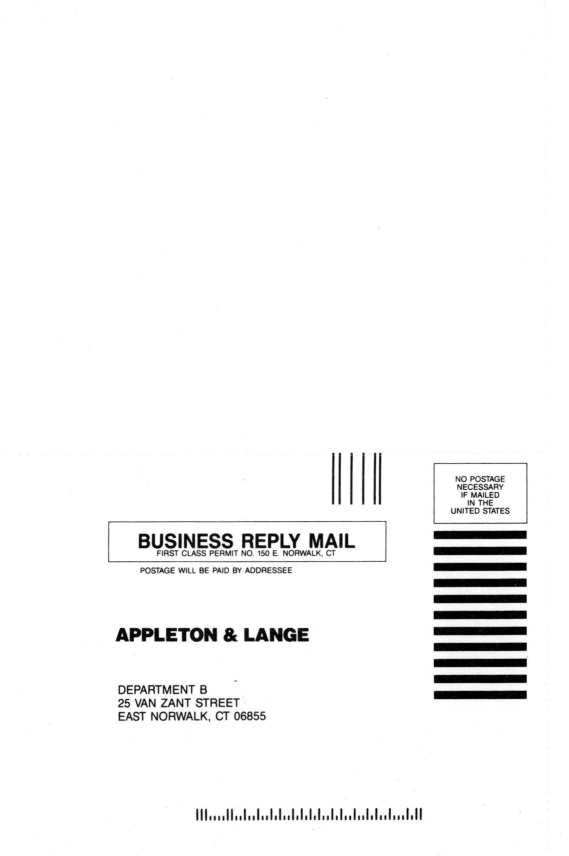